Blood Gases

	Arterial	Venous
Base excess	−3.0 to +3.0 mEq/L	−5.0 to +5.0 mEq/L
Bicarbonate (HCO_3)	18–25 mEq/L	18–25 mEq/L
pO_2	80–95 mm Hg	30–48 mm Hg
O_2 saturation	95–98%	60–85%
pCO_2	34–45 mm Hg	35–52 mm Hg
Total CO_2	23–30 mEq/L	24–31 mEq/L
pH	7.35–7.45	7.32–7.42

Hematology and Coagulation Tests

White blood cell (WBC) count	4.4–11.0 K/mm³
Hemoglobin	12.2–15.0 g/dL
Hematocrit	37.0–54.0%
Red blood cell (RBC) count	3.80–5.20 million/mm³
Mean corpuscular volume (MCV)	85.0–95.0 μm³
Mean corpuscular hemoglobin (MCH)	26.0–34.0 pg/cell
MCH concentration (MCHC)	32.6–36.0 g/dL
Red cell distribution width (RDW)	11.5–15.0%
Platelet count	150.0–420.0 K/mm³
Reticulocyte count	0.5–1.5% of RBCs

WBC differential
Neutrophils	38–70%
Lymphocytes	16–49%
Monocytes	2–9%
Eosinophils	0–5%
Basophils	0–2%

Sedimentation rate
Adult male	≤15 mm/hr
Adult female	≤20 mm/hr

Coagulation tests
Fibrinogen	200–400 mg/dL
Partial thromboplastin time (PTT)	60–85 seconds
Activated PTT	25–35 seconds
Prothrombin time (PT)	11–14 seconds

Note: The reference intervals shown are for adults and may vary according to technique or laboratory, or as new methods are introduced. Always consult the reference range for your own laboratory.

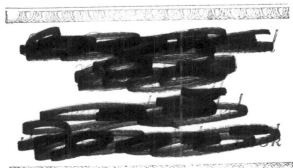

Family Medicine
Principles and Practice

Sixth Edition

Springer
New York
Berlin
Heidelberg
Hong Kong
London
Milan
Paris
Tokyo

Family Medicine
Principles and Practice

Sixth Edition

Robert B. Taylor, M.D.   Editor
Professor of Family Medicine
Oregon Health & Science University
    School of Medicine
Portland, Oregon

Associate Editors
Alan K. David, M.D.
Professor and Chairman
Department of Family and
    Community Medicine
Medical College of Wisconsin
Milwaukee, Wisconsin

Scott A. Fields, M.D.
Professor and Vice Chairman
Department of Family Medicine
Oregon Health & Science University
    School of Medicine
Portland, Oregon

D. Melessa Phillips, M.D.
Professor and Chairman
Department of Family Medicine
University of Mississippi School
    of Medicine
Jackson, Mississippi

Joseph E. Scherger, M.D., M.P.H.
Dean, College of Medicine
Florida State University College
    of Medicine
Tallahassee, Florida

With 160 Illustrations

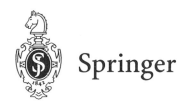 Springer

Robert B. Taylor, M.D.
Professor of Family Medicine
Department of Family Medicine
Oregon Health & Science University
   School of Medicine
Portland, OR 97201-3098, USA

Associate Editors

Alan K. David, M.D.
Professor and Chairman
Department of Family and
   Community Medicine
Medical College of Wisconsin
Milwaukee, WI 53226-0509, USA

D. Melessa Phillips, M.D.
Professor and Chairman
Department of Family Medicine
University of Mississippi School
   of Medicine
Jackson, MS 39216-4500, USA

Scott A. Fields, M.D.
Professor and Vice Chairman
Department of Family Medicine
Oregon Health & Science University
   School of Medicine
Portland, OR 97201-3098, USA

Joseph E. Scherger, M.D., M.P.H.
Dean, College of Medicine
Florida State University College
   of Medicine
Tallahassee, FL 32306-4300, USA

Library of Congress Cataloging-in-Publication Data
Family medicine : principles and practice / Robert B. Taylor, editor ; associate editors,
Alan K. David — [et al]. — 6th ed.
      p. ; cm.
   Includes bibliographical references and index.
   ISBN 0-387-95400-7
      1. Family medicine.   I. Taylor, Robert B.
      [DNLM: 1. Family Practice. WB 110 F197 2002]
   RC46 .F36 2002
   616—dc21   2001057671

ISBN 0-387-95400-7   Printed on acid-free paper.

Printed in the United States of America.

9 8 7 6 5 4 3 2 1   SPIN 10859867

www.springer-ny.com

Springer-Verlag   New York Berlin Heidelberg
A member of BertelsmannSpringer Science+Business Media GmbH

For this sixth edition and my last as editor, it seems fitting that I come full circle and repeat the dedication that I used in my book The Practical Art of Medicine, *published in 1972.*

Here it is:

When I began collecting information for this book, a colleague suggested that I write to his old preceptor—a small-town New England family physician who had served his patients and guided the destinies of medical students for decades. "He knows more practical medicine than any doctor I ever met. Once he spent an hour teaching me how to bandage a finger properly. Over and over we practiced, until I finally had it right."

My letter was never answered. The doctor had died the week before.

*"What a loss, that all his knowledge should die with him,"
I said.*

My friend smiled. "His knowledge didn't die with him."

I understood what he meant.

To this physician/teacher and the thousands like him—who over the years made the house calls, treated disease with ingenuity when medicine was lacking, offered comfort when medicine failed, and yet found time to pass their knowledge to the new generation of physicians—this sixth edition of Family Medicine: Principles and Practice *is dedicated.*

Preface

With the publication of this sixth edition, *Family Medicine: Principles and Practice* now spans four decades and two millennia. With each new edition, we attempt to address what is changing in family medicine and in health care, in general. Since the last edition, we have seen a maturing emphasis on evidence-based medicine and its progressive integration into the fabric of our discipline. There has been a burgeoning interest in complementary and alternative medicine. Advances in genetics are bringing what was once a basic science into the primary care office. There has been renewed enthusiasm for population-based medicine by family physicians and a new look at the ecology of health care.[1] The book has discussions of each of these important topics.

In addition, the sixth edition has new chapters on Family Issues in Health Care, Selected Problems of Aging, Home Care, and Medical Informatics, the Internet, and Telemedicine. Within other chapters, new topics have been added. These include: autistic spectrum disorder, HIV and AIDS in infants and children, Hantavirus infection, ischemic bowel syndromes, thrombotic thrombocytopenic purpura, hemolytic-uremic syndrome, the human genome, and helping patients with Medicare. Along with current traditional therapy, alternative/complementary medicine remedies are discussed in many chapters.

This edition, for the first time, has a list of Commonly Used Abbreviations, such as CBC, CT and HIV; see page xxxi. There are also tables of Laboratory Reference Values and commonly used ICD-9 codes printed inside the front and back covers.

With all these additions, what is the same in the sixth edition? First and foremost, the book continues to present the family practice approach to health care; as in previous editions, the lead authors of all chapters are family physicians. Also, the book's organization of chapters is the same format as that of the fourth and fifth editions, and thus readers will find the sixth edition's new information in a familiar "location." Finally, the book retains the clinical focus that has characterized all editions, telling the reader what the family physician needs to know in clinical practice, including family and community aspects of care.

The Associate Editors for this edition are: Alan K. David, M.D., Professor and Chairman of the Department of Family and Community Medicine, Medical College of Wisconsin; Scott A. Fields, M.D., Professor and Vice Chairman of the Department of Family Medicine of the Oregon Health & Science University (OHSU) School of Medicine; D. Melessa Phillips, M.D., Professor and Chairman of the Department of Family Medicine of the University of Mississippi School of Medicine; and Joseph E. Scherger, M.D., M.P.H., Dean of the College of Medicine of Florida State University. In preparing this sixth edition, I have been privileged to work with Coelleda O'Neil and Lily Cha at OHSU, and with Laurel Craven and Esther Gumpert, senior medical editors, at

Springer-Verlag-New York. I express heartfelt thanks to these individuals and to the book's 204 contributing authors.

The following is a personal note to all our readers:

This is the last edition for which I will serve as chief editor.

The book began with a 1975 lunch meeting in New York City with Springer-Verlag editor Charles F. (Chuck) Visokay, M.D. At that time I was in rural solo practice in New York's Hudson Valley, and had worked with Chuck on three previous medical books that I had written. Springer-Verlag New York Publishers decided to take a chance on the new specialty and a family physician who had never edited a multi-author volume. Chuck insisted that the book be clinical ("Otherwise nobody will buy it!"), and not solely "philosophical." We decided to integrate family practice concepts into all clinical chapters. Chuck's advice has proved to be sound, even though early editions have a number of chapters on the history of the specialty, the family life cycle, and the process of family medicine education.

The first two editions—published in 1978 and 1983—categorized clinical problems into definitive care, shared care, and supportive care problems, with inclusive lists of each that helped a number of family physicians define their bids for hospital privileges in newly formed clinical departments of family practice.

The support of the first four associate editors—John L. Buckingham, E.P. Donatelle, William E. Jacott, and Melville G. Rosen—helped a then-unknown family physician editor recruit authors for the first edition. Since then our other associate editors have been Thomas A. Johnson, Jr. and the four current associate editors listed previously. There has been remarkable continuity, which has helped a great deal in the book's evolution.

With each new edition, published every five years, the book has become more clinically oriented without losing the family medicine emphasis. The lists of disease categories were dropped in the third edition as no longer needed. With the fourth edition began the current format of relatively short, problem-focused chapters, a suggestion of associate editor Tom Johnson.

From the beginning, we have worked to compile a reference book that would be useful for physicians around the world. As a result, this book and its companion student textbook, *Fundamentals of Family Medicine*, have been translated into Spanish, Japanese, Chinese, Italian, and Russian. On my visits abroad, young physicians in Europe, Asia, Africa, and South America have exclaimed, "Dr. Taylor, I have read the big Family Medicine book." I hope that our efforts are helping to spread the message of family medicine around the world.

It has been a great honor and a privilege to serve as chief editor for six editions. I know that, in 1975, Chuck and I never envisioned the impact and longevity the book has enjoyed, thanks to the support of family physicians in both practice and academic settings.

Medical editor Charles F. Visokay died at his home April 27, 2002. I received the news while working on the manuscript for this sixth edition.

I will always be grateful to Chuck and to the Associate Editors and the hundreds of chapter authors represented in the six editions of the book. We always tried to make each edition the "best yet." Your work in writing and editing has helped define our discipline.

Although I step down as chief editor of this book, there will be a seventh edition 4 or 5 years from now. The next edition will have a new chief editor, whom I hope that you will support as you have helped and encouraged me over the past 28 years.

Robert B. Taylor, M.D.
Portland, Oregon, USA

Reference

1. Green LA, Yawn BP, Lanier D, Dovey SM. The ecology of medical care revisited. N Engl J Med 2001; 344:2021–5.

Clinical Practice Notice

Everyone involved with the preparation of this book has worked very hard to assure that information presented here is accurate and that it represents accepted clinical practices. These efforts include confirming that drug recommendations and dosages discussed in this text are in accordance with current practice at the time of publication. Nevertheless, therapeutic recommendations and dosage schedules change with reports of ongoing research, changes in government recommendations, reports of adverse drug reactions, and other new information.

A few recommendations and drug uses described herein have Food and Drug Administration (FDA) clearance for limited use in restricted settings. It is the responsibility of the clinician to determine the FDA status of any drug selection, drug dosage, or device recommended to patients.

The reader should check the package insert for each drug to determine any change in indications or dosage as well as for any precautions or warnings. This admonition is especially true when the drug considered is new or infrequently used by the clinician.

The use of the information in this book in a specific clinical setting or situation is the professional responsibility of the clinician. The authors, editors, or publisher are not responsible for errors, omissions, adverse effects, or any consequences arising from the use of information in this book, and make no warranty, expressed or implied, with respect to the completeness, timeliness, or accuracy of the book's contents.

Contents

Part I. The Principles of Family Medicine

Part II. The Practice of Family Medicine

A. The Person, Family, and Community
Preventive Care

Part III. Family Medicine Applications

Contributors

Allan V. Abbott, M.D., Professor of Family Medicine, Keck School of Medicine, University of Southern California, Los Angeles, CA

Cheryl A. Abboud, M.P.A., Administrator, Department of Pathology/Microbiology, University of Nebraska School of Medicine, Omaha, NE

Suraj A. Achar, M.D., Clinical Instructor of Family Medicine, University of California–San Diego School of Medicine, LaJolla, CA

Alan M. Adelman, M.D., M.S., Professor and Associate Chair, Department of Family and Community Medicine, Penn State University College of Medicine, Hershey, PA

John P. Allen, Ph.D., M.P.A., Chief, Treatment Research Branch, National Institute on Alcohol Abuse and Alcoholism, Rockville, MD

William A. Alto, M.D., M.P.H., Associate Professor of Family and Community Medicine, Dartmouth Medical School, Hanover, NH; Maine–Dartmouth Family Practice Residency, Fairfield, ME

Bruce Ambuel, Ph.D., Associate Professor of Family and Community Medicine, Medical College of Wisconsin, Milwaukee; Waukesha Family Practice Residency Program, Waukesha, WI

Kathryn M. Andolsek, M.D., M.P.H., Clinical Professor of Community and Family Medicine, Duke University School of Medicine, Durham, NC

David E. Anisman, M.D., Assistant Professor of Family Medicine, Uniformed Services University of the Health Sciences, Bethesda; Assistant Program Director, Family Practice Residency, Malcolm Grow Medical Center, Andrews Air Force Base, MD

Barbara S. Apgar, M.D., Clinical Professor of Family Medicine, University of Michigan Medical School, Ann Arbor, MI

José A. Arevalo, M.D., Associate Clinical Professor of Family and Community Medicine, University of California–Davis School of Medicine, Sacramento; Chief Medical Officer, Health Plan of the Redwoods, Santa Rosa, CA

Evan A. Ashkin, M.D., Clinical Assistant Professor of Family Medicine, The University of North Carolina School of Medicine, Chapel Hill, NC

John W. Bachman, M.D., Professor of Medicine, Mayo Medical School; Consultant, Department of Family Medicine, Mayo Clinic, Rochester, MN

Boyd L. Bailey, Jr., M.D., Associate Professor of Family Medicine, University of Alabama at Birmingham, School of Medicine; Director, University of Alabama–Selma Family Medicine Residency Program, Selma, AL

Robert A. Baldor, M.D., Associate Professor and Vice Chairman, Department of Family Medicine and Community Health, University of Massachusetts Medical School, Worcester, MA

Dennis J. Baumgardner, M.D., Professor of Family Medicine, University of Wisconsin Medical School, Madison; St. Luke's Family Practice Residency Program, Milwaukie, WI

Diane K. Beebe, M.D., Professor of Family Medicine, University of Mississippi School of Medicine, Jackson, MS

Kenneth M. Bielak, M.D., Associate Professor of Family Medicine, University of Tennessee-Knoxville School of Medicine, Knoxville, TN

Carol E. Blenning, M.D., Assistant Professor of Family Medicine, Oregon Health Science University School of Medicine, Portland, OR

Richard D. Blondell, M.D., Professor of Family and Community Medicine, University of Louisville School of Medicine, Louisville, KY

Patricia Ann Boken, M.D., Clinical Assistant Professor of Family Medicine, University of Pennsylvania School of Medicine, Philadelphia; Bryn Mawr Family Practice, Bryn Mawr, PA

Mark D. Bracker, M.D., Clinical Professor of Family and Preventive Medicine, University of California–San Diego School of Medicine, La Jolla, CA

Dan E. Brewer, M.D., Associate Professor of Family Medicine, University of Tennessee-Knoxville School of Medicine, Knoxville, TN

Steven P. Bromer, M.D., Assistant Clinical Professor of Family and Community Medicine, University of California–San Francisco School of Medicine, San Francisco, CA

Michael H. Bross, M.D., Medical Director, North Central County Health Center, Institute for Research and Education in Family Medicine, St. Louis, MO

Gregory L. Brotzman, M.D., Professor of Family and Community Medicine, Medical College of Wisconsin, Milwaukee, WI

Cora Collette Bruener, M.D., M.P.H., Department of Pediatrics, University of Washington Medical Center, Seattle, WA

Kenneth Brummel-Smith, M.D., Professor of Family Medicine, Oregon Health & Science University School of Medicine; Bain Chair, Providence Center on Aging, Providence Health System–Oregon, Portland, OR

Stephen A. Brunton, M.D., Director of Faculty Development, Stamford Hospital/Columbia University Family Practice Residency Program, Stamford, CT

Robert L. Buckley, M.D., Chairman and Executive Director of Medical Education, Resurrection Medical Center, Chicago, IL

Juan Carlos Buller, M.D., Staff Physician, San Diego Sports Medicine and Family Practice, San Diego, CA

Walter L. Calmbach, M.D., Associate Professor of Family and Community Medicine, Director of Sports Medicine Fellowship and South Texas Ambulatory Research Network (STARNET), University of Texas Health Science Center, San Antonio, TX

James F. Calvert, Jr., M.D., Associate Professor of Family Medicine, Oregon Health & Science University School of Medicine, Portland; Cascades East Family Practice Residency Program, Klamath Falls, OR

Bryan J. Campbell, M.D., Assistant Professor of Family and Preventive Medicine, University of Utah School of Medicine, Salt Lake City, UT

David C. Campbell, M.D., M.Ed., Clinical Professor of Community and Family Medicine, St. Louis University School of Medicine; The Institute for Research and Education in Family Medicine, St. Louis, MO

Douglas J. Campbell, M.D., Community Attending Physician, Good Samaritan Regional Family Practice Center, Yavapai Regional Medical Center, Prescott, AZ

Thomas L. Campbell, M.D., Professor, Department of Family Medicine and Department of Psychiatry, University of Rochester School of Medicine and Dentistry, Rochester, NY

G. Anne Cather, M.D., Associate Professor of Family Medicine, West Virginia University School of Medicine, Morgantown, WV

Frank S. Celestino, M.D., Associate Professor and Director of Geriatrics, Department of Family and Community Medicine, Wake Forest University School of Medicine, Winston-Salem, NC

Michael E. Clark, M.D., Assistant Professor of Family and Community Medicine, Dartmouth Medical School, Hanover, NH; Maine–Dartmouth Family Practice Residency Program, Augusta/Waterville, ME

Kathi D. Clement, M.D., Associate Professor of Family Medicine, University of Wyoming Family Practice Residency Program at Cheyenne, Cheyenne, WY

Richard D. Clover, M.D., Professor and Chairman, Department of Family and Community Medicine, University of Louisville School of Medicine, Louisville, KY

Kathy Cole-Kelly, M.S.W., M.S., Associate Professor of Family Medicine, Case Western Reserve University School of Medicine, Cleveland, OH

George C. Coleman, M.D., Associate Professor and Coordinator of Clinical Programs, Department of Family Practice, Virginia Commonwealth University School of Medicine, Medical College of Virginia Campus, Richmond, VA

Harry Colt, M.D., Assistant Professor of Family and Community Medicine, Dartmouth Medical School, Hanover, NH; Maine–Dartmouth Family Practice Residency Program, Fairfield, ME

Joyce A. Copeland, M.D., Clinical Assistant Professor of Family Medicine, Duke University School of Medicine, Durham, NC

Gerald M. Cross, M.D., Command Surgeon, United Sates Army FORSCOM, Atlanta, GA

Paul T. Cullen, M.D., Clinical Associate Professor of Family Medicine, University of Pittsburgh School of Medicine, Pittsburgh; Director, Washington Hospital Family Practice Residency Program, Washington, PA

R. Whit Curry, Jr., M.D., Professor and Chairman, Department of Community Health and Family Medicine, University of Florida College of Medicine, Gainesville, FL

William J. Curry, M.D., Assistant Professor of Family and Community Medicine, Pennsylvania State University School of Medicine, Hershey, PA

Peggy R. Cyr, M.D., Clinical Assistant Professor of Family Medicine, University of Vermont School of Medicine, Burlington, VT; Maine Medical Center Family Practice Residency, Portland, ME

Mel P. Daly, M.D., Family Physician, Greater Baltimore Medical Center, Baltimore, MD

James J. Deckert, M.D., Associate Clinical Professor of Family and Community Medicine, University of Missouri–Columbia, School of Medicine; Clinical Faculty, Mercy Family Medicine Residency Program and Geriatric Services, St. John's Mercy Medical Center, St. Louis, MO

Lanyard K. Dial, M.D., Associate Professor of Family Medicine, University of California-Los Angeles School of Medicine; Director, Family Practice Residency Program, Ventura County Medical Center, Ventura, CA

Lisa Grill Dodson, M.D., Assistant Professor of Family Medicine, Oregon Health & Science University School of Medicine, Portland, OR

Charles E. Driscoll, M.D., Clinical Professor of Family Medicine, University of Virginia School of Medicine, Charlottesville; Director, Family Practice Residency Program Centra Health, Lynchburg, VA

Jacquelyn S. Driscoll, R.N., Lynchburg, VA

Margaret V. Elizondo, M.D., Clinical Instructor of Family Medicine, University of California-San Diego School of Medicine, La Jolla; Grossmont Hospital, La Mesa, CA

Paul Evans, D.O., Associate Dean for Curricular Affairs and Associate Professor of Family Medicine, Oklahoma State University College of Osteopathic Medicine, Tulsa, OK

Enrique S. Fernandez, M.D., M.S.Ed., Family Physician, Miami, FL

Scott A. Fields, M.D., Professor of Family Medicine, Oregon Health & Science University School of Medicine, Portland, OR

Judith A. Fisher, M.D., Assistant Professor of Family Practice and Community Medicine, University of Pennsylvania School of Medicine, Philadelphia, PA

Cheryl A. Flynn, M.D., M.S., Assistant Professor of Family Medicine, Upstate Medical University, State University of New York, Syracuse, NY

John P. Fogarty, M.D., Professor and Chairman, Department of Family Medicine, University of Vermont College of Medicine, Burlington, VT

Josephine R. Fowler, M.D., Assistant Professor of Family Medicine, Boston University School of Medicine; Assistant Professor, Boston University School of Public Health, Boston MA

Stephen H. Fuller, PharmD., Associate Professor of Pharmacy Practice, Campbell University School of Pharmacy, Cary, NC

Valerie J. Gilchrist, M.D., Professor and Chair, Department of Family Medicine, Northeastern Ohio Universities College of Medicine, Rootstown; Associate Director, Aultman Family Practice Center, Aultman Hospital, Canton, OH

Dwenda K. Gjerdingen, M.D., Professor of Family Practice and Community Health, University of Minnesota School of Medicine, Minneapolis, MN

Rupert R. Goetz, M.D., Adjunct Associate Professor, Department of Psychiatry and Department of Family Medicine, Oregon Health & Science University School of Medicine, Portland, OR

Bruce W. Goldberg, M.D., Associate Professor of Family Medicine, Oregon Health & Science University School of Medicine, Portland, OR

Ronald H. Goldschmidt, M.D., Professor of Clinical Family and Community Medicine, University of California–San Francisco School of Medicine, San Francisco, CA

David B. Graham, M.D., Clinical Assistant Professor of Family Medicine, Oregon Health & Science University School of Medicine, Portland; Private Practice, Strawberry Wilderness Family Clinic, John Day, OR

Pepi Granat, M.D., Clinical Professor of Family Medicine and Community Health, University of Miami School of Medicine, Miami, FL

Joseph W. Gravel, Jr., M.D., Assistant Clinical Professor of Family Medicine and Community Health, Tufts University School of Medicine, Boston; Director, Tufts University Family Practice Residency Program, Malden, MA

Grant M. Greenberg, M.D., M.A., Clinical Instructor of Family Medicine, University of Michigan Medical School; East Ann Arbor Health Center, Ann Arbor, MI

James K. Gude, M.D., Clinical Professor of Family and Community Medicine, University of California–San Francisco School of Medicine, San Francisco, CA

Leonard J. Haas, Ph.D., Professor of Family and Preventive Medicine, University of Utah School of Medicine, Salt Lake City, UT

Richard I. Haddy, M.D., Professor of Family and Community Medicine, University of Louisville School of Medicine, Louisville, KY

Karen L. Hall, M.D., Associate Professor of Community Health and Family Medicine, University of Florida College of Medicine, Gainesville, FL

Michael B. Harper, M.D., Professor of Family Medicine, Louisiana State University Health Sciences Center, Shreveport, LA

Meg Hayes, M.D., Assistant Professor of Family Medicine, Oregon Health & Science University School of Medicine, Portland, OR

A. Kesh Hebbar, M.D., Assistant Professor of Family Medicine, Medical University of South Carolina, Charleston, SC

Darrell L. Henderson, M.S., Health Policy Analyst, American Academy of Family Physicians, Leawood, KS

Paula Cifuentes Henderson, M.D., Clinical Instructor of Family Medicine, University of California–Los Angeles School of Medicine, Los Angeles, CA

Michael Herbst, M.D., Associate Professor of Family Medicine, University of California–Los Angeles School of Medicine, Los Angeles; Faculty, Santa Monica–UCLA Family Practice Residency Program, Santa Monica, CA

Denise D. Hermann, M.D., Associate Clinical Professor of Medicine, Division of Cardiology, Department of Medicine, University of California–San Diego Medical Center, San Diego, CA

Kenneth A. Hirsch, M.D., Ph.D., Head, Inpatient Mental Health Services, Naval Medical Center, San Diego, CA

Joseph Hobbs, M.D., Professor of Family Medicine, Medical College of Georgia, Augusta, GA

Richard H. Hoffman, M.D., Assistant Clinical Professor of Family Practice, Virginia Commonwealth University School of Medicine, Medical College of Virginia Campus, Richmond; Associate Director, Chesterfield Family Practice Center, Columbia HCA Hospitals, Richmond, VA

William J. Hueston, M.D., Professor and Chairman, Department of Family Medicine, Medical University of South Carolina, Charleston, SC

Brian W. Jack M.D., Associate Professor and Vice Chair of Academic Affairs, Department of Family Medicine, Boston University School of Medicine, Boston, MA

David M. James, M.D., Associate Professor, Department of Family Medicine and Department of Emergency Medicine, State University of New York at Buffalo School of Biomedical Sciences, Buffalo, NY

Anthony F. Jerant, M.D., Assistant Professor of Family Medicine, University of California–Davis School of Medicine, Sacramento, CA

Thomas A. Johnson, Jr., M.D., Clinical Professor of Family and Community Medicine, University of Missouri–Columbia School of Medicine; Clinical Faculty, Mercy Family Medicine Residency Program, St. John's Mercy Medical Center, St. Louis, MO

Jeffrey G. Jones, M.D., M.P.H., Medical Director, St. Francis Traveler's Health Center, Indianapolis, IN

Sanford R. Kimmel, M.D., Professor of Clinical Family Medicine, Medical College of Ohio, Toledo, OH

John G. King, M.D., Associate Clinical Professor of Family Practice, Virginia Commonwealth University School of Medicine, Medical College of Virginia Campus, Richmond; Associate Director, Hanover Family Practice Center, VCU Health System Hospitals and Memorial Regional Medical Center, Mechanicsville, VA

George L. Kirkpatrick, M.D., Emergency Department Physician, Mobile Infirmary Medical Center, Mobile, AL

Michael S. Klinkman, M.D., M.S., Associate Professor of Family Medicine, University of Michigan School of Medicine, Ann Arbor, MI

Aubrey L. Knight, M.D., Associate Professor of Clinical Family Medicine, University of Virginia School of Medicine, Charlottesville; Director, Family Practice Education, Carilion Health System, Roanoke, VA

Bradley E. Kocian, M.D., Sports Medicine Fellow, University of Tennessee–Knoxville Medical Center, Knoxville, TN

Donald R. Koester, M.D., Associate Professor of Family Practice, University of Texas Southwestern Medical School, Dallas; McLennan County Family Practice Residency Program, Waco, TX

Lars C. Larsen, M.D., Professor of Family Medicine and Assistant Dean for Generalist Programs, The Brody School of Medicine at East Carolina University, Greenville, NC

Daniel T. Lee, M.D., Assistant Clinical Professor of Family Medicine, University of California-Los Angeles School of Medicine, Los Angeles; Faculty, Santa Monica-UCLA Medical Center Family Practice Residency Program, Santa Monica, CA

James E. Lessenger, M.D., Private Practice, Morinda Medical Group Inc., Porterville, CA

Richard B. Lewan, M.D., Associate Professor of Family and Community Medicine, Medical College of Wisconsin, Milwaukee; Director, Family Practice Residency Program, Waukesha Memorial Hospital, Waukesha, WI

Peter R. Lewis, M.D., Assistant Professor of Family and Community Medicine, Penn State University College of Medicine, Hershey, PA

Michael R. Lustig, M.D., Assistant Clinical Professor of Family Practice, Virginia Commonwealth University School of Medicine, Medical College of Virginia Campus, Richmond; Associate Director, Riverside Family Practice Center, Riverside Regional Medical Center, Newport News, VA

Patrick E. McBride, M.D., M.P.H., Professor of Medicine, University of Wisconsin Medical School, Madison, WI

Margaret E. McCahill, M.D., Clinical Professor, Department of Family and Preventive Medicine and Department of Psychiatry, University of California–San Diego School of Medicine, La Jolla, CA

Susan H. McDaniel, Ph.D., Professor , Department of Psychiatry (Psychology) and Department of Family Medicine, University of Rochester School of Medicine and Dentistry, Rochester, NY

Marc McKenna, M.D., Associate Professor of Community and Family Medicine, University of Pennsylvania School of Medicine, Philadelphia; Director, Chestnut Hill Hospital Family Practice Residency Program, Philadelphia, PA

Deborah S. McPherson, M.D., Assistant Director of Medical Education, American Academy of Family Physicians, Leawood, KS

James A. McSherry, M.B., Ch.B. (Deceased) Professor of Family Medicine and Psychiatry, The University of Western Ontario School of Medicine, London, Ontario, CN

Michael K. Magill, M.D., Professor and Chairman, Department of Family and Preventive Medicine, University of Utah School of Medicine, Salt Lake City, UT

Ronald L. Malm, D.O., Assistant Professor of Family Medicine, University of Wyoming Family Practice Residency Program at Cheyenne, Cheyenne, WY

Anthony D. Marcucci, M.D., Assistant Professor of Family Medicine, West Virginia School of Medicine, Morgantown, WV

David W. Marsland, M.D., Harris–Mayo Professor and Chair, Department of Family Practice, Virginia Commonwealth University School of Medicine, Medical College of Virginia Campus, Richmond, VA

Samuel C. Matheny, M.D., M.P.H., Claire Louise Caudill Professor and Chair, Department of Family Practice, University of Kentucky College of Medicine, Lexington, KY

Richard C. Mauer, M.D., Private Practice, Covenant Medical Center and Allen Memorial Hospital, Waterloo, IA

Todd J. May, D.O., Lieutenant Commander, Medical Corps, United States Naval Hospital, Camp Pendleton, CA

E.J. Mayeaux, Jr., M.D., Associate Professor of Family Medicine, Louisiana State University Health Sciences Center, Shreveport, LA

Alan L. Melnick, M.D., M.P.H., Assistant Professor of Family Medicine, Oregon Health and Science University School of Medicine, Portland; Health Officer, Clackamas County, OR

Susan Y. Melvin, D.O., Associate Clinical Professor of Family Medicine, University of California–Irvine College of Medicine, Irvine; Memorial Family Medicine Residency Program, Long Beach, CA

Donald B. Middleton, M.D., Professor, Department of Family Medicine and Clinical Epidemiology, University of Pittsburgh School of Medicine; Faculty, UPMC–St. Margaret Hospital Family Practice Residency Program, Pittsburgh, PA

Etan C. Milgrom, M.D., Associate Clinical Professor of Family Medicine, University of California–Los Angeles School of Medicine, Los Angeles, CA

Karl E. Miller, M.D., Associate Professor of Family Medicine, University of Tennessee–Chattanooga College of Medicine, Chattanooga, TN

Katherine E. Miller, M.D., Assistant Clinical Professor of Family Medicine and Community Health, Tufts University School of Medicine, Boston; Faculty, Tufts University Family Practice Residency Program, Malden, MA

William F. Miser, M.D., Associate Professor of Family Medicine, The Ohio State University College of Medicine and Public Health; Residency Director, The Ohio State University Family Practice Residency Program, Columbus, OH

Alicia D. Monroe, M.D., Associate Professor of Family Medicine, Brown Medical School, Providence; Memorial Hospital of Rhode Island, Pawtucket, RI

Laura Mosqueda, M.D., Associate Clinical Professor and Director of Geriatrics, Department of Family Medicine, University of California–Irvine College of Medicine, Irvine, CA

John B. Murphy, M.D., Professor of Family Medicine, Brown Medical School, Providence, RI

James E. Nahlik, M.D., Associate Clinical Professor of Community and Family Medicine, St. Louis University School of Medicine; Chief of Family Practice, Missouri Baptist Medical Center, St. Louis, MO

Laeth S. Nasir, M.B.B.S., Associate Professor of Family Medicine, University of Nebraska College of Medicine, Omaha, NE

Thomas S. Nesbitt, M.D., M.P.H., Associate Professor of Family Medicine and Assistant Dean for Regional Outreach, Telehealth and Continuing Medical Education; University of California–Davis School of Medicine, Sacramento, CA

Gary R. Newkirk, M.D., Clinical Professor of Family Medicine, University of Washington School of Medicine, Seattle; Program Director, Family Medicine Spokane Residency Training Program, Spokane, WA

Carole Nistler, M.D., Private Practice, Olmsted Community Hospital, Rochester, MN

William A. Norcross, M.D., Professor of Clinical Family Medicine, University of California-San Diego School of Medicine, La Jolla, CA

Mary Patricia Nowalk, Ph.D., R.D., Research Associate, Department of Family Medicine and Clinical Epidemiology, University of Pittsburgh School of Medicine, Pittsburgh, PA

Jim Nuovo, M.D., Associate Professor of Family and Community Medicine, University of California–Davis School of Medicine, Sacramento, CA

Michael L. O'Dell, M.D., Associate Professor of Family Medicine, University of Alabama–Huntsville School of Medicine, Huntsville, AL

Daniel K. Onion, M.D., M.P.H., Professor of Community and Family Medicine, Dartmouth Medical School, Hanover, New Hampshire; Maine–Dartmouth Medical Center, Augusta/Waterville, ME

David K. Ornstein, M.D., Assistant Professor of Surgery, Division of Urology, University of North Carolina School of Medicine, Chapel Hill, NC

Daniel J. Ostergaard, M.D., Vice President, International and Interprofessional Activities, American Academy of Family Physicians, Leawood, KS

Paul M. Paulman, M.D., Professor of Family Medicine, University of Nebraska College of Medicine, Omaha, NE

Dana W. Peterson, M.D., Private Practice, Presbyterian Hospital, Albuquerque, NM

Kent Petrie, M.D., Assistant Clinical Professor of Family Medicine, University of Colorado Health Sciences, Denver, CO

Doug Poplin, M.D., M.P.H., Medical Director, Saint Francis Occupational Health Center, Indianapolis, IN

Layne A. Prest, Ph.D., Associate Professor and Director of Behavioral Medicine, Department of Family Medicine, University of Nebraska School of Medicine, Omaha, NE

Mike Purdon, M.D., Clinical Instructor, University of Washington School of Medicine, Seattle, WA

Michael T. Railey, M.D., Assistant Professor of Community and Family Medicine, St. Louis University School of Medicine; Forest Park Hospital Family Medicine Residency Program, St. Louis, MO

Stephen Ratcliffe, M.D., M.S.P.H., Director, Family Practice Residency Program, Lancaster General Hospital, Lancaster, PA

James P. Richardson, M.D., M.P.H., Chief of Geriatric Medicine, Union Memorial Hospital, Baltimore, MD

Russell G. Robertson, M.D., Associate Professor of Family and Community Medicine, Medical College of Wisconsin, Milwaukee, WI

Jonathan E. Rodnick, M.D., Professor and Chairman, Department of Family and Community Medicine, University of California–San Francisco School of Medicine, San Francisco, CA

Glenn S. Rodriguez, M.D., Regional Medical Director of Quality Improvement and Health Services Integration, Providence Health System, Portland; Adjunct Associate Professor of Family Medicine, Oregon Health & Science University School of Medicine, Portland, OR

Joseph E. Ross, M.D., Assistant Clinical Professor of Family Medicine, University of Illinois-Rockford School of Medicine, Rockford, IL

George Saba, Ph.D., Associate Clinical Professor of Family and Community Medicine, University of California–San Francisco School of Medicine, San Francisco, CA

John Saultz, M.D., Professor and Chairman, Department of Family Medicine, Oregon Health & Science University School of Medicine, Portland, OR

Ted C. Schaffer, M.D., Clinical Assistant Professor, Department of Family Medicine and Clinical Epidemiology, University of Pittsburgh School of Medicine; Director, UPMC-St. Margaret Hospital Family Practice Residency Program, Pittsburgh, PA

Joseph E. Scherger, M.D., M.P.H., Dean, College of Medicine, Florida State University, Tallahassee, FL

Gordon T. Schmittling, M.S., M.S. Director of Research and Information Services, American Academy of Family Physicians, Leawood, KS

Jerome E. Schulz, M.D., Clinical Professor of Family Medicine, East Carolina University Brody School of Medicine; Pitt County Memorial Hospital, Greenville, NC

Thomas M. Schwartz, M.D., Clinical Assistant Professor of Family Medicine, Oregon Health and Science University School of Medicine; Faculty, Providence Milwaukie Family Practice Residency Program, Portland, OR

David Seaborn, Ph.D., Assistant Professor, Department of Psychiatry and Department of Family Medicine, University of Rochester School of Medicine and Dentistry, Rochester, NY

H. Russell Searight, Ph.D., Clinical Associate Professor of Community & Family Medicine, St. Louis University School of Medicine; Director of Behavioral Medicine, Forest Park Hospital Family Medicine Residency Program, St. Louis, MO

Patricia A. Sereno, M.D., M.P.H., Assistant Clinical Professor of Family Medicine and Community Health, Tufts University School of Medicine, Boston; Hallmark Family Health Center, Malden, MA

Allen F. Shaughnessy, Pharm.D., Clinical Associate Professor of Family Medicine, Medical College of Pennsylvania–Hahnemann School of Medicine, Philadelphia; Harrisburg Family Practice Residency Program, Harrisburg, PA

John P. Sheehan, M.D., Associate Clinical Professor of Medicine, Case Western Reserve University School of Medicine, Cleveland, OH

Ann K. Skelton, M.D., Clinical Associate Professor of Family Medicine, University of Vermont College of Medicine, Burlington, VT; Maine Medical Center Family Practice Residency, Portland, ME

David C. Slawson, M.D., B. Lewis Barnett, Jr. Professor of Family Medicine, University of Virginia School of Medicine, Charlottesville, VA

Charles Kent Smith, M.D., Dorothy Jones Weatherhead Professor of Family Medicine, Case Western Reserve University School of Medicine, Cleveland, OH

Gregory N. Smith, M.D., Clinical Assistant Professor, Department of Family Practice and Clinical Epidemiology, University of Pittsburgh School of Medicine; Director of Obstetrics Education and Clinical Training, UPMC–St. Margaret Hospital Family Practice Residency and Fellowship Program, Pittsburgh, PA

M. Rosa Solorio, M.D., M.P.H., Assistant Professor in Residence, Department of Family Medicine, University of California–Los Angeles School of Medicine, Los Angeles, CA

Jeannette E. South-Paul, M.D., Professor and Chair, Department of Family Medicine and Clinical Epidemiology, University of Pittsburgh School of Medicine, Pittsburgh, PA

David N. Spees, M.D., Clinical Instructor of Family Medicine, University of California–San Diego School of Medicine, La Jolla; Director, Travel Clinic, Sharp Rees–Stealy Medical Group, Inc., San Diego, CA

Michael R. Spieker, M.D., Director, Puget Sound Family Medicine Residency Program, Naval Hospital, Bremerton, WA

James H. Stein, M.D., Associate Professor of Medicine, University of Wisconsin Medical School, Madison, WI

Denise K.C. Sur, M.D., Associate Clinical Professor of Family Medicine, University of California–Los Angeles School of Medicine, Los Angeles; Faculty, Santa Monica–UCLA Medical Center Family Practice Residency Program, Santa Monica, CA

John E. Sutherland, M.D., Clinical Professor of Family Medicine, University of Iowa College of Medicine, Waterloo; Director, Northeast Iowa Family Practice Residency Program, Waterloo, IA

Angela W. Tang, M.D., Assistant Professor of Medicine, University of California–Los Angeles School of Medicine, Los Angeles; Department of Medical Education, Saint Mary Medical Center, Internal Medicine Residency, Long Beach, CA

Jeffrey L. Tanji, M.D., Associate Medical Director, Sports Medicine, University of California-Davis Medical Center, Sacramento, CA

Robert B. Taylor, M.D., Professor of Family Medicine, Oregon Health & Science University School of Medicine, Portland, OR

Marla J. Tobin, M.D., Family Physician, Warrensburg, MO

William L. Toffler, M.D., Professor of Family Medicine, Oregon Health & Science University School of Medicine, Portland, OR

Michael L. Tuggy, M.D., Clinical Assistant Professor of Family Medicine, University of Washington School of Medicine; Director, Swedish Family Medicine Residency Program, Seattle, WA

Marc Tunzi, M.D., Associate Clinical Professor of Family and Community Medicine, University of California–San Francisco School of Medicine, San Francisco; Director, Family Practice Residency Program, Natividad Medical Center, Salinas, CA

Margaret M. Ulchaker, M.S.N., R.N., C.D.E., NP-C., Clinical Instructor, Frances Payne Bolton School of Nursing, Case Western Reserve University, Cleveland, OH

Gail Underbakke, R.D., M.S., Nutrition Coordinator, Preventive Cardiology Program, University of Wisconsin Hospital and Clinics, Madison, WI

Richard P. Usatine, M.D., Associate Dean for Medical Education and Professor of Family Medicine, Florida State University College of Medicine, Tallahassee, FL

Daniel J. Van Durme, M.D., Associate Professor and Vice-Chairman, Department of Family Medicine, University of South Florida College of Medicine, Tampa, FL

E. Chris Vincent, M.D., Clinical Associate Professor of Family Medicine, University of Washington School of Medicine, Seattle, WA

Anne D. Walling, M.B., Ch.B., Professor of Family Medicine, University of Kansas School of Medicine, Wichita and Kansas City, KS

Eric Walsh, M.D., Associate Professor of Family Medicine, Oregon Health & Science University School of Medicine, Portland; Director, Oregon Health & Science University Family Practice Residency Program, Portland, OR

Gregg Warshaw, M.D., Professor of Family Medicine, University of Cincinnati College of Medicine, Cincinnati, OH

Howard N. Weinberg, M.D., Family Physician, Sentara Medical Group, Virginia Beach, VA

John M. Wilkinson, M.D., Assistant Professor of Family Medicine, Mayo Medical School; Consultant in Family Medicine, Mayo Clinic and Mayo Foundation, Rochester, MN

Mary Willard, M.D., Director, West Jersey–Memorial Family Practice Residency Program, Virtua Health, Voorhees, NJ

Christopher R. Wood, M.D., Assistant Professor, Family and Community Medicine, Medical College of Wisconsin, Milwaukee; Waukesha Family Practice Residency Program, Waukesha, WI

Wilma J. Wooten, M.D., M.P.H., Associate Clinical Professor of Family and Preventive Medicine, University of California–San Diego School of Medicine, La Jolla, CA

Lacey Wyatt-Henriques, M.D., M.P.H., Clinical Instructor of Family Medicine, University of California–Los Angeles School of Medicine, Los Angeles, CA

Allen S. Yang, M.D., Ph.D., Medical Oncology Fellow, MD Anderson Cancer Center, Houston, TX

Richard Kent Zimmerman, M.D., M.P.H., Associate Professor, Department of Family Medicine and Clinical Epidemiology, University of Pittsburgh School of Medicine, Pittsburgh, PA

Thomas J. Zuber, M.D., Associate Physician, Department of Family Medicine and Preventive Medicine, Emory University School of Medicine, Atlanta, GA

Robert G. Zylstra, Ed.D., L.C.S.W., Assistant Professor of Family Medicine, University of Tennessee–Chattanooga College of Medicine, Chattanooga, TN

Commonly Used Abbreviations

Abbreviation	Definition
ACE	Angiotensin-converting enzyme
ACTH	Adrenocorticotropic hormone
AIDS	Acquired immunodeficiency syndrome
ALT	Alanine aminotransferase (SGPT)
ANA	Antinuclear antibody
AST	Aspartate aminotransferase (SGOT)
bid	Twice a day
BP	Blood pressure
bpm	Beats per minute
BS	Blood sugar
BUN	Blood urea nitrogen
CBC	Complete blood count
CHF	Congestive heart failure
Cl$^-$	Chloride
CO$_2$	Carbon dioxide
COPD	Chronic obstructive pulmonary disease
CPR	Cardiopulmonary resuscitation
CSF	Cerebrospinal fluid
CT	Computed tomography
cu mm	cubic millimeter
CXR	Chest x-ray
d	Day, daily
dL	Deciliter
DM	Diabetes mellitus
ECG	Electrocardiogram
ESR	Erythrocyte sedimentation rate
FDA	United States Food and Drug Administration
FM	Family medicine
FP	Family physician
g	Gram
GI	Gastrointestinal
Hb	Hemoglobin
Hg	Mercury
HIV	Human immunodeficiency virus

Abbreviation	Definition
HMO	Health maintenance organization
hr	Hour
hs	Hour of sleep, at bedtime
HTN	Hypertension
IM	Intramuscular
INR	International normalized ratio
IU	International unit
IV	Intravenous
K^+	Potassium
kg	Kilogram
L	Liter
LD or LDH	Lactate dehydrogenase
mEq	Milliequivalent
μg	Microgram
mg	Milligram
min	Minute
mL	Milliliter
mm	Millimeter
mm^3	Cubic millimeter
MRI	Magnetic resonance imaging
Na^+	Sodium
NSAID	Nonsteroidal antiinflammatory drug
po	By mouth (*per os*)
PT	Prothrombin time
PTT	Partial thromboplastin time
q	Every
qd	Every day, daily
qid	Four times a day
qod	Every other day
RBC	Red blood cell
SC	Subcutaneous
sec	Second
SGOT	See AST
SGPT	See ALT
STD	Sexually transmitted disease
TB	Tuberculosis
tid	Three times a day
TSH	Thyroid stimulating hormone
U	Unit
UA	Urine analysis
WBC	White blood cell, white blood count
WHO	World Health Organization

Part I

The Principles of Family Medicine

1

Family Medicine: Now and Future Practice

Robert B. Taylor

In the beginning, the specialty of family practice had originated within the lifetimes of all its practitioners. Today family practice is in its fourth decade. Many of today's family physicians (FPs) were born following the pioneering efforts in the 1960s to begin the new specialty: family practice. Others were in grade school and high school while family physicians worked to attain credibility, hospital privileges, and curriculum time in medical schools. Some others have been on the sidelines, yet have benefitted from the specialty's success over the past 3-plus decades. Not all know the story of the family practice movement. For these reasons, I begin this book with an overview of the specialty's origin, evolution and current status.

One important function of reference books is to serve as historical records of milestones for a specialty and the thinking in a discipline during the time of each edition's life. Sometimes this record shows how much things have changed: In Osler's Modern Medicine, published in 1907, Dr. Osler (1849–1919) tells how to treat diabetes mellitus with opium and arsenic, although adding "the writer rarely resorts to them."[1] And sometimes a review of past writings reveals much that has not changed. Near the end of his career, Sir William Osler also wrote: "It is more important to know what patient has a disease, than what disease the patient has."[2] Osler added personal comments to many of his discussions, and since family medicine is arguably the most personal of all medical disciplines, this will be a "personal" chapter with some first-hand opinions, beliefs and anecdotes. What follows is a short history of the specialty, a discussion of current concepts important to the discipline, and some thoughts about future practice—based upon the author's 41 years of practice (three years in the US Public Health Service; 14 in rural general practice, then family practice; and 24 years in academic family medicine).

A Very Short History of the Specialty

Family practice in the United States of America evolved from general practice, which was the dominant force in health care until the early 20th century. Here is how it happened.

The Family Practice Approach

Medical care in the United States has been described as characterized by aggressive action, a mechanistic approach, problem orientation, and an emphasis on victory over disease.[3] This connotes that the good physician will record a comprehensive history, perform exhaustive testing, fix the defective organ, and cure the disease. Into this setting came family practice. In contrast to an aggressive assault on disease, family physicians championed *longitudinal health care*, which allowed both patient and physician to understand the nature of illness and to share decisions over time. A *relationship-based, biopsychosocial approach* integrated with the evolving new technology was advocated. The emphasis of family practice was on the *broad-based care of the person and family*, rather than a narrow focus on the disease problem. Finally, family physicians advocated *improving the quality of life*, particularly important when patients suffer chronic or terminal illness and victory over disease is not really possible. These principles, more often intuitively shared than explicitly articulated during the early years, guided subsequent historical events.

The Early Years

Family practice arose during the 1960s—the time of the Vietnam War, the civil rights movement, and social unrest in many areas of the world. These events coincided with a decline in access to broad-based health care in the United States, which occurred for a number of reasons: too few medical graduates to serve America's growing population, a trend toward specialization that began with World War II, and generalist training that was inadequate for an increasingly complex health care system. In response, the American public and far-sighted health care planners decried the fragmentation of American medicine and called for the creation of a physician who specialized in personal health care—the family physician.[4,5]

With the support of the American Academy of General Practice and U.S. general practitioners, in 1969 family practice became the 20th American medical specialty.

Four early decisions helped shape the future of the new specialty. A specialty certifying board—the American Board of Family Practice—was established in 1969; until 1979 a physician could qualify to sit for the certifying examination based on practice eligibility, but since then all candidates for specialty certification must be graduates of approved 3-year family practice residency programs. Three-year residency training programs were established, in contrast to the prior norm for general practitioners of a single year of internship perhaps supplemented by a 2-year general practice residency. Mandatory recertification was pioneered by the American Board of Family Practice, and all U.S. board-certified family physicians must take a recertification examination every 7 years; most other specialties have since followed this lead in various iterations. Finally, mandatory continuing medical education was required by the American Academy of Family Physicians and the American Board of Family Practice. The latter organization requires 300 hours of approved continuing medical education every 6 years as one component of the recertification process.

The new specialty began with 15 residency training programs, most converted from previous 2-year general practice training programs. Federal grant programs supported new departments of family medicine in medical school. And clinical departments of family practice were formed in community hospitals across America.

In 1986 the American Board of Family Practice adopted the current definition:

Family practice is the medical specialty which is concerned with the total health of the individual and the family. It is the specialty in breadth which integrates the biological, clinical, and behavioral sciences. The scope of family practice is not limited by age, sex, organ system, or disease entity. (Source: American Board of Family Practice, Lexington KY. Used with permission.)

From 1969 until today, the family practice movement continued to gain momentum, with solid gains in student interest, more residents in training, increased numbers of board-certified FPs in practice, and family physicians in leadership positions in clinical medicine and academia.

Family Practice in the United States

There are 797,000 physicians in the United States. Of this number, 69,000 are family physicians and 17,000 are general practitioners. Each year U.S. family physicians provide more office visits than the combined totals of physicians practicing general internal medicine and pediatrics.[6] Today there are 471 U.S. family practice residency training programs in community hospitals and academic medical centers. In the early years a few medical schools created departments of family medicine, often prompted by state legislative mandate or the prospect of federal grants; today almost all U.S. medical schools have departments of family medicine or other academic family medicine units.

In the beginning family practice entered the academic setting as both a new specialty and a social movement, aiming to refocus health care on the patient and family; this approach was not always well received. Today medical education and health care delivery are profoundly influenced by family medicine values, both through the impact of our presence throughout the health care system and through the power of our core mission of caring for the patient.

There are family medicine courses in almost all U.S. medical schools, teaching students family practice values and the family practice approach to health care. These courses—and the presence of family physicians in the academic medical centers—are demonstrating the importance of medical education in the office setting. Students who a generation ago would have never seen a multigenerational family of patients or cared for a patient with problems in multiple body systems are now learning to provide truly comprehensive health care, and are doing so in the offices of family physicians in the community.

In 1987 Pellegrino[7] commented: "The birth of Family Practice two decades ago, and its development as a genuine specialty within the bodies of both medical practice and academia is surely one of the most remarkable stories in contemporary medical history. The present success of family practice is a tribute to the intellectual foresight, astute social perceptions, and political acumen of a small group of dedicated general practitioners." Family conferences, shared decision making, home care, and community-based research are now respected components of 21st century health care. Family physicians are the only physicians who are distributed across America in the same geographic proportions as the American people. Also, during the 1990s family physicians were the only specialists whose incomes rose (38%) more than the general inflation rate for the decade (33%).[8] Today we see the continuation of this story as family physicians assume leadership in national medical organizations, hold important roles in determining health policy, and become deans of medical schools in the U.S. For further information about the history of family medicine, see Chapter 131, which provides a chronology of the evolution of family practice as a specialty in the U.S.

Family Practice Around the World

Family practice has a long history in Canada. In countries outside North America, family and general practice has evolved in various ways.[9] In Spain, for example, the Royal Decree of 1978 officially endorsed the specialty of family practice: "The family physician shall constitute the fundamental figure of the health system."[10] In England the general practitioner (GP) is the key provider in the National Health Service, and the countries of the European Economic Community (EEC) have agreed that postgraduate training in general practice should be a minimum of 2 full years, of which 6 months should be in an approved practice. There is a European Academy of Teachers of General Practice and a European Center for Research and Development in Primary Health Care.

Family practice residency programs exist in a number of Latin American countries, and an International Center for Family Medicine is located in Buenos Aires, Argentina. In Cuba the family physician is the chief provider in a comprehensive health plan for Cuban citizens. Family practice has played a role in the health care of Mexico since the 1970s.

In 14 Asian Pacific countries there is a core curriculum in family practice. Family practice is well established in South Korea, Malaysia, Singapore, Hong Kong, Taiwan, and the Philippines, as well as in Australia and New Zealand. Japan, Russia, India, and China now have family practice training programs. In the Ukraine, by government decree, pediatricians and internists are being retrained as family doctors to serve as the chief physicians in their new health care system. In 2001, the government of Vietnam declared a commitment to deploy trained family physicians in the 10,000 health centers serving the country's population of 67 million people.

There is family practice training in South Africa, Egypt, and Nigeria. An Arab Board of Family Practice oversees training in Saudi Arabia, Oman, Kuwait, and Jordan.

The nature of practice varies from country to country, and in some areas, such as the United States and Canada, family physicians often have an active role in hospital care. In other settings, such as in the United Kingdom and Latin America, family practice is chiefly office-based, often supplemented by home care.

The international group uniting family practice is the World Organization of National Colleges, Academies, and Academic Associations of General Practitioners/Family Physicians (WONCA), representing 53 member countries. WONCA held its 16th World Conference of Family Doctors in 2001 in Durban, South Africa, with the 17th World Conference scheduled for 2004 in Orlando, Florida, USA.

Philosophical Tenets and Their Impact on Medicine

The following values, concepts, and approach to health care are important to family physicians in the early 21st century and have influenced the global practice of medicine.

Enduring Values

Family physicians are bonded by shared beliefs. They value *continuing care* of the individual and family as beneficial to the patient–physician relationship and as an effective process of providing care. This continuity allows FPs to increase their knowledge of the patient at each office visit. *Comprehensive care* is an important tenet of family practice and involves full-service health care of both sexes and all ages "from conception to resurrection." Because FPs emphasize that the patient should receive appropriate care at the right place and at the right time, they place a high premium on *coordinated care*. This emphasis on coordinated care has made family physicians the ideal primary care clinicians in capitated care settings. Finally, a *family-centered approach* has been a cornerstone of family practice, with increasing recognition that our concept of family includes such diverse units as single-parent families, collective living groups, and same-sex couples. In my practice, a four-generation family of patients is not uncommon.

Relationship-based health care is the philosophical foundation of the specialty, and understanding personal accountability is the key to understanding family medicine. McWhinney[11] writes: "In general (family) practice, we form relationships with patients often before we know what illnesses the patient will have. The commitment, therefore, is to a person whatever may befall them." In my family practice I routinely ask about the patient's children, parents, job, dog, or cat; I tell my patients about my grandchildren. I become, in a sense, "a member of the family" (also see Chapter 4).

Family physicians have a community-based health care orientation. As individual practitioners, family physicians can profoundly influence the health of a community, and can also share their knowledge by serving on the boards of community agencies, such as a volunteer health clinic or adult day-care center. In addition, many FPs are leading efforts in population-based health care (see Chapter 6), extending from care of the illness of the individual to addressing community health problems such as smoking use or teen pregnancy.

Advances in Medical Thinking

Over the past three decades, family medicine has advanced medical thought in important ways, answering early skeptics who held that FPs had nothing to bring to the table of medical knowledge.[12] One of these is the use of *comprehensive clinical reasoning*, to include consideration of life events, the family's contribution to disease, and the impact of illness on the family (see Chapter 4). For example, as FPs we have all seen how juvenile diabetes can affect a family's dynamics in regard to relationships, family decision making, and the allocation of family resources. When the child with diabetes is sick, everything else in the household is of secondary importance and eventually relationships can be severely strained; early intervention by the family physician may avert family disruption (see Chapter 30).

Also, FPs have recognized *how problems of living can influence health*. Patients with stressful lives seldom present stress as a chief complaint. Instead they tell of fatigue, abdominal pain, and weight change—chief complaints that often represent a "ticket of admission" to health care. Recognition of the underlying cause of symptoms is important because, for example, a patient who has surgery that relieves chronic back pain may develop severe headaches if underlying life problems have not been identified and addressed.

A third area in which family medicine has advanced medical thinking is by teaching residents the *systems approach to health care*. In general systems theory there is a hierarchy of natural systems that includes molecules, cells, organs, body systems, person, family, community, nation, world, and so forth. To apply systems theory to medicine, if a person's pancreatic islet cells begin to make insufficient insulin, or if a farmer in Africa contracts AIDS, or if a community suffers an earthquake, all systems in the hierarchy are affected. Although family physicians have special expertise in "person" and "family," they need to consider the impact of disease on all systems, from small particles of matter to the biosphere.[13]

Family Medicine's Literature Heritage

Family medicine is developing a rich literature heritage. The papers describing our clinical research, practice methods, and advances in medical thought are being published in a growing number of publications. Although I will not attempt to list them all (in fear of offending by omission), there are currently at least six family practice journals worldwide, two major clinical reference books, four student textbooks, one textbook defining and examining the discipline, and at least four review books for board examinations.

These publications not only are important in presenting the family medicine approach to health care, but also allow the intergenerational transfer of values, methods, and thought—the "storytelling" of a specialty.

The Clinical Encounter as the Definable Unit of Family Practice

When future medical historians ask what was the major contribution of family medicine during its first half century, the answer might be the advances made in the traditional clinical encounter, adapting it to 21st century practice. The family physician's clinical encounter is analogous to the surgeon's surgical procedure, the gastroenterologist's endoscopy, or the radiologist's roentgenogram in that it is what we do. Its scope includes the FP's approach to undifferentiated problems, communication techniques, physician behavior, presentation of information to the patient and family, involvement of the patient and family in decisions, and ongoing care in the context of family and community. The office-based clinical encounter typically includes multiple problems, an average of 2.7 problems in one study.[14] By law it may be categorized as ranging from "minimal" to "high complexity." However long or short, the encounter is distinguished by a broad-based and longitudinal approach that is often not present in other specialties.

Over the past four decades, the family practice clinical encounter has become more streamlined, cost-effective, and (we hope) clinically relevant. The improvements have been achieved by the use of enhanced communication techniques, the use of "high-payoff questions," modern diagnostic and therapeutic instruments such as the fiberoptic nasopharyngoscope and the flexible sigmoidoscope, innovations in the style of documentation such as SOAP (subjective data, objective data, assessment, and plan) notes, advances in decision analysis, and the introduction of computer-based records.

In the new millennium, the clinical encounter is rapidly evolving to reflect the current advances in technology, with contact via the World Wide Web and telecommunications expanding our patient care capabilities, as described below.

Challenges to Family Practice

At this time the specialty faces several challenges. These include the increasing scope of primary care practice today, the growing tendency to consider health care a commodity rather than a professional service, and the current popularity of subspecialization among medical students.

The Increasing Complexity of Clinical Practice

Over the past few years, the scope of care provided by all primary care physicians has increased, chiefly because of capitation and the gatekeeper role.[15] In my solo family practice 20-some years ago, I saw 40 patients a day and yet I was usually on the way home by 5 P.M. Most of my patients had bronchitis, sprained ankles, earaches, lacerations, vaginitis, back pain, skin rashes, and so forth. Of course, like all FPs, I had some complex cases, such as my two female patients with systemic lupus erythematosus and the middle-aged man with amyotrophic lateral sclerosis, but those were the exceptions. This is no longer the case.

Today's office patient may have a half-dozen problems, and is more likely to be *sick* and to require more time than would be needed to treat an ear infection. Why the change? Today, most of my patients are capitated, chiefly with the Oregon Health Plan, and my care is most cost-effective when I see only those patients who really need office care. This means that many instances of back strain, flu, cystitis, vaginitis, and so forth receive advice through the nurse triage line, and only those who cannot be managed by telephone are given appointments. This also means that there are very few "easy" visits that allow me to catch up with my schedule. And even though a recent paper showed that the average duration of office visits increased by between 1 and 2 minutes from 1989 to 1998,[16] this small increase in my opinion is insufficient to account for the greater complexity of problems encountered in office practice.

Resisting the Commercialization of Medicine

Family physicians can take the lead in preventing medicine from being converted to a commodity.[17] Health care is not a hamburger or a toaster oven, although health maintenance organizations (HMOs) and the government often seem to act as though it were.

In 1969 one of family practice's initial roles was to combat the fragmentation of medicine.[4] At that time there was excessive specialization, and the patient with hypertension, joint pain, and a skin rash often needed to see three physicians. With the current presence of family practice, this is happily no longer the case. Today, the family physician's new role is to be the patient's advocate in a system that appears to treat health care as a commodity, often one to be rationed—using tight schedules, relative value units, incentive payments if the physician orders few tests and lower cost drugs, and severe financial penalties for minor coding errors. Even the term *provider* reinforces the "commodity" mentality.

What are family physicians to do? We *must* put the patient first, insist on affording the patient enough time so that we can do a good job, work to eliminate incentive payments that create ethical dilemmas for physicians, fight government efforts to criminalize administrative disagreements, and refuse to accept the insulting epithet *provider*.

Family Practice, Subspecialization, and Specialty Choice

Beginning in 1997, we saw a relative rise in the number of medical students entering subspecialty fields and a reciprocal decline in those selecting family practice and other primary care specialties as careers. Is this merely a sine wave that will correct in time? Perhaps. Progress is rarely a straight line, but occurs with peaks and valleys.

Family practice leaders are well aware of the trend, and are working to effect change through increased attention to student activities, efforts to close the income gap between primary care specialists and consulting specialists, and reduce the bureaucratic hassles inherent in managed care. In the meantime the current—and probably temporary—reduction in interest in FP careers may have a salutary effect; it will weed out the weak training programs in the system, and it will ensure that those joining our specialty at this time are the most firmly committed to the tenets of the specialty. In the end, the drop in FP trainee numbers may result in a stronger specialty in the future.

Current Trends and Future Practice

Tomorrow's health care will be shaped by current influences. In selecting what I believe to be the most significant influences on future practice, I chose from a long list that included the current focus on evidence-based health care (see Chapter 5), the medical and societal impact of HIV and AIDS (see Chapter 42), and the burgeoning interest in complementary and alternative medicine (see Chapter 128). The following are the four factors I believe most likely to influence family practice in the decade to come.

Information Technology and Human Relationships

Here we return to the evolving clinical encounter. The technologic influences on future practice include *medical technology* such as lasers, fiberoptics, and diagnostic ultrasound. It also includes *information technology* such as patient contact via e-mail or voicemail, information retrieval, computer-assisted charting, decision support systems, and the virtual house call.[18] Just as the automobile spelled the end of "horse and buggy" medicine, and the telephone allowed direct communication with the physician and the development of scheduled office practice, the Internet is profoundly changing the practice of medicine (also see Chapter 127).[19] Today, using asynchronous communication, I correspond with patients by e-mail about

their health problems. Sometimes the patient sends an e-mail at 2 A.M., knowing it will not be answered until the next day; this has saved a number of early morning telephone calls that were not emergencies. Sometimes the e-mail message is a prelude to an office visit. Occasionally I talk with patients by telephone as we simultaneously search the World Wide Web for clinical answers. The Internet is making the "digital house call" a reality. Face-to-face office visits are needed less often, and when they occur are longer in duration[16] and offer more value for time spent than in years past. With the Internet as part of comprehensive health care, FPs move one step further in actualizing their role as health advisor and consultant.

All the technology mentioned here is being used by FPs somewhere, and within a decade these functions will be the state of the art everywhere.

The Aging Population

The growing number of older people in the population is the reward for our success in battling infant diarrhea, accidental injuries, treatable infectious diseases, uncontrolled hypertension, and other causes of early death. According to the U.S. Bureau of the Census, there are currently 35 million people age 65 and older, and the number is projected to increase to more than 53 million by the year 2020. The fastest growing segment of our population is the group age 85 and older. Of course these are the people with multiple problems involving various organs and whose health care costs are the highest of any adult age group.

What is the likely impact on family practice? Family physicians need to prepare to serve an increasingly older patient panel, and must be positioned to compete with others who would claim greater expertise. We must insist upon a family practice approach, emphasizing continuity of care (there is no reason to change doctors when one turns 65), comprehensive care (the FP can care for a wider range of problems than any other physician), and family-oriented care (why fragment the care of the elderly and make it separate from the rest of the family?) (also see Chapters 23 to 26).

Globalization and Global Health Disparities

We see the effect of globalization in the economic marketplace: Price and wage differences between countries become a little narrower each year. Goods and jobs are increasingly moving freely across borders, as is information about lifestyle and economic opportunities.

The United States has yet to experience the full effect of globalization in health care. We in the United States spend billions of dollars annually for antianxiety medication while in other countries children die of infectious diseases for want of a vaccine or an inexpensive antibiotic. A woman in a developing country is 38 times more likely to die of pregnancy-related causes than a woman in the developed world. There are currently 35 million persons with AIDS worldwide, with an estimated 12 million AIDS orphans in Africa. These are, increasingly, problems shared by the global community and they represent both challenges and opportunities for all physicians.

U.S. Surgeon General David Satcher, M.D., Ph.D., a family physician, points out that 89% of the world's population lives in developing countries that bear 93% of the world's disease burden, but that account for only 11% of the world's health spending.[20] To phrase this another way, 89% of the world's health care resources are spent on 11% of the world's population. Dr. Satcher lists three "prescriptions" to improve health worldwide: supporting public health initiatives; enlisting allies such as computer specialists, economists, and patients; and challenging public health leaders to advocate for all health care consumers.

What about family practice and family physicians? Our roles may include controlling unnecessary health care expenditures in America and other developed countries, serving as physicians in developing countries, and advocating for sick persons whatever their nationality. We should also prepare to live and practice in a world where the differences in incomes, standard of living, and health care are much less than they are now.

Economic Policies and Health Care

Health policy is the "wild card." How national and state governments dictate eligibility for programs and the methods of making health care payments has a strong influence on how health care is provided. Witness what happens in those countries, such as Japan, in which the government controls health care payments, allows unrestricted access to any physician, and mandates relatively low fees. The result is many office visits for minor problems, long waits, very short visits, and frequent (and often medically unnecessary, at least by U.S. standards) follow-up visits for routine problems. The local saying is, "Three-hour wait, three-minute visit." It is, curiously, the opposite of the model that has resulted from capitated care in the U.S.—with increasingly complex problems seen in (slightly) longer office visits by primary care physicians.

In my home state of Oregon, we have seen how government can abruptly change health care. When it began, the Oregon Health Plan suddenly converted a large number of previously uninsured patients to being insured under the new state plan. This caused a major shift in where patients received care, as the newly insured patients sought to abandon the clinics that had struggled for years to provide their care and were courted by physicians in more "prestigious" settings. On the other hand, a state-mandated reduction in reimbursement can cause some physicians to withdraw from the plan, increasing the burden on those who remain.

On a national basis, a federal plan for universal access to health care will correct the disparity of 45 million Americans who lack insurance or other funding for health care. It will also profoundly affect how health care is delivered in America, depending on method of funding, how access is controlled, and how clinicians are paid. Let us hope that common sense and fairness prevail.

Caring for the World

Family medicine has been such a positive influence on health care worldwide that we would have had to invent it for the new millennium, if it did not already exist. Despite past pre-dictions to the contrary, family medicine has survived into the 21st century. A study reported in 2001 showed that each month a large portion of the U.S. population has health problems and almost 25% visit a physician's office.[21] Of those visits, more are to family physicians than to any other specialists (see Chapter 130). Approximately 11% of U.S. physicians are family physicians or general practitioners, and the number of FPs is growing.[6] Outside the U.S., there have been major successes in a number of other countries, as described earlier. Family medicine has done much more than survive; it has prospered and has had a powerful impact on health care delivery and medical education worldwide. It is a rapidly evolving discipline that brings a much-needed social conscience to medicine and, to some degree, is reinventing itself as it uses the new technology to expand its service role. The values of the specialty put people first—first before profit, first when there are ethical conflicts, and first before a single-minded emphasis on disease. In the 21st century, family physicians continue to care for the world. And all physicians should honor family practice's remarkable history of achievements and recognize its unlimited potential for future contributions to humankind.

Important Internet Sites

www.aafp.org   American Academy of Family Physicians
www.abfp.org   American Board of Family Practice
www.stfm.org   Society of Teachers of Family Medicine
www.globalfamilydoctor.com   World Organization of Family Doctors

References

1. Osler W. Osler's modern medicine, Vol. 1. Philadelphia: Lea Brothers, 1907;794–5.
2. Osler W. A way of life. Springfield, IL: CC Thomas, 1919.
3. Payer L. Medicine and culture. New York: Henry Holt, 1988.
4. Report of the Citizens' Commission on Graduate Education. The graduate education of physicians. Chicago: American Medical Association, 1966.
5. Report of the Ad Hoc Committee on Education for Family Practice of the Council on Medical Education. Meeting the challenge of family practice. Chicago: American Medical Association, 1966.
6. American Academy of Family Physicians: Facts about Family Practice: *www.aafp.org/facts/table01.html.*
7. Pellegrino ED. Family practice facing the 21st century; reflections of an outsider. In: Doherty WJ, Christianson CE, Sussman MB, eds. Family medicine: the maturing of a discipline. New York: Haworth Press, 1987.
8. Roberts R. The primary care mismatch. Family Practice News, May 15, 2001;31(10):9.
9. Haq C, Ventres W, Hunt V, et al. Where there is no family doctor: the development of family practice around the world. Acad Med 1995;70:370–80.
10. Gascon TG. *La medicina familiar e communitaria en Espana.* Rev Int Med Fam 1991;3:167–70.
11. McWhinney IR. Being a general practitioner: what it means. Eur J Gen Pract 2000;6:135–9.
12. Taylor RB. Family practice and the advancement of medical understanding. J Fam Pract 1999;48:53–7.

13. Taylor RB. Family: a systems approach. Am Fam Physician 1979;20(5):101–4.
14. Flocke SA, Frank SH, Wegner DA. Addressing multiple problems in the family practice office visit. J Fam Pract 2001;50: 211–6.
15. St. Peter RF, Reed MC, Kemper P, Blumenthal D. Changes in the scope of care provided by primary care physicians. N Engl J Med 1999;341:1980–5.
16. Mechanic D, McAlpine DD, Rosenthal M. Are patients' office visits with physicians getting shorter? N Engl J Med 2001;344: 198–204.
17. Pellegrino ED. The commodification of medical and health care: the moral consequences of a paradigm shift from a professional to a market ethic. J Med Philos 1999;24:243–66.
18. Ebell MH, Frame P. What can technology do to, and for, family medicine? Fam Med 2001;33:311–9.
19. Scherger JE. Primary care in 2001. Hippocrates 2001;14(3):26–32. Available at *www.hippocrates.com*.
20. Satcher D. Eliminating global health disparities. JAMA 2000; 284:2990–1.
21. Green LA, Yawn BP, Lanier D, Dovey SM. The ecology of medical care revisited. N Engl J Med 2001;344:2021–4.

2
Stages of Human Development

Kenneth Brummel-Smith and Laura Mosqueda

An understanding of the human developmental processes is a critical component of the family physician's role in continuing care. Patients often present to physicians with the superficial complaint of a medical concern when the true underlying problem relates to an adjustment to their own development or the response of the family to that adjustment. Whenever medical conditions develop in a family member, they are likely to have some impact on other members. Such conditions may have a more powerful effect when the illness occurs at the time of common stress points in the family life cycle, such as the birth of the first child or when an adolescent has been "acting up." Family physicians can be of great assistance in providing "anticipatory guidance," reassurance regarding the normality of such experiences, or assistance for those with a difficult adjustment. This chapter addresses the developmental characteristics during each stage of life and their impact on the care of the patient. Additionally, because the older population experiences a significant increase in medical problems, special attention is paid to the impact of illness on this stage of the developmental process.

Stages of Life

There is tremendous variability in human development, but certain similarities exist in most persons.[1] The notion that development ceases after adolescence is a myth. Each stage, from childhood to the end of life, is associated with specific developmental tasks (Table 2.1). Physical, psychological, and social development occur at different rates. Although the potential for maximal physical development is realized by age 30, psychological and social maturity are reached at later ages. Similarly, developmental tasks in each of these realms of our lives change as we age; the successful completion of these tasks prepares the person to move on in life, ready to meet the challenges of the next stage. Difficulty with the tasks can

increase the risk of psychosocial disruption and may even lead to medical problems. Hence, understanding the patient's presenting problem, within the context of the developmental process, will enable the family physician to provide comprehensive medical care. On the other hand, it may be that the concept of a linear progression of stages is a peculiarly Western one.[2] This point may be especially true when viewing the various components of the family life cycle and the development of the individual.

Childhood Stage

When dealing with a couple and the couple's first child, the family physician must be aware of the sometimes overwhelming learning experience that the parents are undergoing. Interpreting the infant's needs and dealing with the process of breast-feeding or baby foods are but two of many new experiences that must be mastered. Decisions regarding where the infant will sleep are sometimes troublesome. Some authors advocate training the child to be the master of his or her own sleep periods,[3] whereas others believe that having the child sleep with the parents can provide special benefits.[4] If there are other children in the family, the prospect of sibling rivalry must be addressed. When the parents take particular care to attend to the needs of the older children and involve them in the care of the new child, this adjustment usually goes smoothly.

As children reach 2 to 3 years, they begin to experiment with independent actions. This period provides trying times for parents but may also be viewed with wonder and amazement. For the parents, it is the beginning of a long stage of learning how best to set limits while promoting the child's independence. Many issues play out this theme; temper tantrums, negativity ("I'm not going to do it"), toilet training, thumb sucking, watching television, and masturbatory play are common concerns. For some children these issues are hardly prob-

Table 2.1. **Life Stages**

Infancy and childhood	Middle age
Adolescence	Retirement
Young adulthood	Old age

lematic, whereas for others their resolution may result in the family verging on total disruption. Children require consistent standards and cues, and they need to know what is expected of them; too much control or an expectation of meeting rigid expectations usually leads to stress with little likelihood of resolution. It is especially important that the parents are in basic agreement on the approach to the child. An understanding approach that fosters the child's independent decisions, within the limits of safety and the parents' personal needs, is likely to imbue the child with a sense of accomplishment and security. Above all, children need to be respected.

Parents have a huge impact on childhood development. Important determinants of that development include (1) the inherited temperamental qualities of the child, (2) parental practices and personality, (3) the quality of the child's school, (4) relationships with peers, and (5) the historical era in which the child is raised.[5] Discipline is often a difficult experience at this time. Interestingly, research has shown that verbal instructions are not effective at changing young children's problem behavior.[6] Explanations of future consequences related to a punishment procedure such as a time-out seem not to influence the behavior of toddlers and preschool-age children. Children at this stage of development have difficulty distinguishing causation from coincidence and fantasy from reality.[7] Fortunately, by age 6 children are usually developed enough to respond to reasoning and verbal instructions.

As they enter the late-childhood stage (ages 6 to 10) accidents become common. While most of these are minor, it should be recalled that death due to accidents is one of the most common causes of mortality in this age group. The family physician should proactively discuss accident prevention and safety awareness. Specific mention should be made about gun safety, as youngsters at this age explore their parent's rooms and may engage in play mimicking scenes they have seen on television.

The concept of gender socialization is important to consider. It appears that at an early age children begin to express gender-specific behaviors. Little girls may make their own dolls, and boys may fashion guns out of sticks. It is virtually impossible not to expose children to gender-identified material. Some parents may be upset that they have tried to raise their child in ways that discourage stereotyped behaviors, and yet the child still exhibits them. Still, a child should be given a wide range of opportunities for expression and exploration based on interest and aptitude rather than gender.

Role of the Family Physician

The family physician is often the counselor to young parents. Due to physical distance or unresolved family issues, parents may feel reluctant to discuss their parenting concerns with their own parents. The physician can explain the developmental processes that are operative, which may be especially helpful when parents are dealing with toddlers and preschool children. Reassuring the parent about the normality of such experiences and that they are doing a good job of parenting is often all that is needed. Eliciting from the parent their feelings and reactions to the child's behavior also helps to defuse the situation. As there are no "right" answers, encouraging parents to try alternative strategies is helpful. After all, doing more of what does not work, does not work. When recurrent behavioral problems are seen, the family system should be assessed for the presence of more serious discord, as the child's behavior may be a reflection of more substantial problems, such as impending divorce or abuse.

Adolescence Stage

The adolescent stage of human development is also a time of individuation and is perhaps the most turbulent (see Chapter 22). The body at puberty is going through tremendous change, a true metamorphosis. Rapid growth and hormonal changes affect the young person on a daily, often variable, basis. Perhaps it is a misnomer to term this period a "stage." So much change is occurring that it is more appropriately conceived of as an explosion! Psychosocially, the tasks of this stage are clear: begin separation from the family, develop a self-identity, develop a sexual identity, begin to depend on one's peers (rather than the family) for support, and start to formulate plans for a means of supporting ones self (Table 2.2). How these tasks are accomplished defines transition to a healthy adulthood.

The process of developing a self-identity is often one of the most stressful aspects of this stage for the adolescent's parents. It is interesting that exactly when adolescents are trying to be more independent from their parents, they become more dependent on their peers. In many cases, the adolescent chooses an adversarial path to this end. Whatever the parents believe, the opposite must be true! In reality, such dissension is usually a test, and if the groundwork of love and respect has been laid, deep inside the teen still looks to the parents for safety and guidance.

Sexual issues play a major role during this period. The majority of teens in the United States will have had intercourse by the time they graduate from high school. While sex is talked about more than in the past, there still is a great need for open, honest communication. Teens have a high pregnancy rate and frequently do not use barrier protection methods. Risk for human immunodeficiency virus (HIV) disease may also be increased due to teenagers' belief in their own indestructibility. Nonthreatening discussion of sexual issues by parents, sometimes aided by discussions with the family physician, is crucial to adolescents' acquisition of skills in coping with their newly developed sexuality.

Table 2.2 **Tasks of Adolescence**

Begin separation from the family
Develop a self-identity
Develop a sexual identity
Begin to depend on one's peers (rather than the family) for support
Start to formulate plans for a means of supporting oneself

By this age most gay and lesbian persons have become aware of their sexual orientation. It is also a time when open discussions about these discoveries can be extremely difficult. When all teenagers are dealing with trying to establish what is "normal," it is no surprise that in a society that generally discriminates against nonheterosexual orientations, these teens may experience special stresses. Although earlier work suggested that despite these stresses homosexual adolescents had an incidence of mental health problems that was no higher than that of the heterosexual population, recent research indicates that gay and lesbian adolescents are at high risk for depression and suicide.[8] Parents often have strong feelings and reactions to a child who is homosexual, and the family physician may play a critical role in helping the family find their way to acceptance and understanding.

As with younger children, teens need clear limits and standards. The difference is that they must also be involved and invested in the establishment of these limits. As the teenager moves through the continuum of change, increasing amounts of independent action should be not only allowed but also fostered. During this tumultuous time of change, the parents can assist the young person by proactively addressing issues like sex, drugs, and alcohol. Although young people may not respond with open discussion at that time, the message that there is safety in asking questions is established.

Role of the Family Physician

If approached sensitively, the family physician has the opportunity to truly serve the adolescent. Many issues at this stage may be perceived as "off limits" in the family. The physician, however, can address questions that teens may feel embarrassed to discuss with their parents, such as drug use, sex, or risk-taking.

Interviewing teenagers requires special skill, but the motivated physician can master this skill. The physician must address privacy issues. It is best to first discuss with the parents and child together your philosophy regarding confidentiality. If all interactions between the physician and the teen are to be privileged, it should be made clear and the commitment then maintained. The physician should advise teens that only in the rarest of circumstances (e.g., suicidal ideation) is anything divulged without their consent. Besides providing a great service, the elicitation of an adolescent's worries about sexual matters or feelings of depression can leave the physician feeling accomplished and satisfied, and it is well worth the effort.

Young Adulthood

For some time development was thought to cease with the adolescent years. It is now clear, however, that the later stages of life are filled with important developmental tasks. Erik Erikson[9] characterized young adulthood as being concerned with intimacy and the ability to form a meaningful and lasting relationship. Finding a partner, adjusting to the partner's lifestyle and expectations, and deciding on whether or when to have children are important aspects of this stage. It is also a time when the newly created family must adapt to the families of origin of each member (Table 2.3).

Young adults are usually quite concerned with mastery over their life. The full entry into adult life is often associated not only with marriage but also with establishing a career. The norm today is that both men and women must develop a method for meeting economic responsibilities, so most women work outside of the home. Women are often torn between desires to spend more time with children and their career demands. Decisions about child care are often troublesome to young families.

There is great variation during this period. For those who choose to marry, it is important to understand that a "perfect union" is not without discord. In fact, it appears that a strong affective bond requires more than just reciprocal gratification. It appears that discord and repair are necessary components of a lasting relationship. Successful repair turns despair into positive emotions.[10] A successful marriage has these characteristics: (1) power is shared by the partners, (2) there is a high level of mutual respect, (3) a level of self-disclosure that is satisfying to one another exists, (4) with greater self-disclosure there is increased opportunity to appreciate both similarities and differences, and (5) appreciation of similarities and differences leads to increased closeness and augmented individuation.

Though it is still perceived as being the norm by many people, the traditional "nuclear family" accounts for fewer than 25% of all families. Some individuals forsake marriage to pursue professional careers. Those who are gay or lesbian may only become fully aware of their orientation at this time. Single parents must struggle with significant financial concerns while trying to accomplish career development, and perhaps search for a mate. Persons who do follow a less traditional path must frequently cope with negative reactions of their families and the society and can use the support and understanding of a health care professional.

Financial concerns often affect families at this stage. Only 15% of American households are now supported solely by a male breadwinner, compared to 42% in 1960.[11] Some believe that a major threat to the family today is the broad-based cultural shift away from respect for activities that cannot be justified in terms of market dollar value.[12] Family functions are increasingly being "outsourced," as parents take on more roles outside of the home. This change affects both mothers and fathers as many more men are choosing to become stay-at-home dads.

Role of the Family Physician

Contacts with the physician during this stage are often made by women and are related to birth control, pregnancy, or well-child visits. Many opportunities are available for anticipatory guidance and counseling. The physician should assess the

---

Table 2.3. **Issues in Young Adulthood**

Forming meaningful and lasting relationships
Adjusting to the partner's lifestyle and expectations
Deciding on whether or when to have children
Adapting to the families of origin of each member
Career choices

stress level of the woman, and facilitate discussing her concerns about child rearing, her relationship with her partner, and her career. A frequent visit to the doctor by someone who is physically healthy is often an indicator of underlying psychosocial concerns.

Men in this age group see physicians much less often, making health-promotion–oriented interventions more sporadic and difficult. An ideal opportunity arises in the pregnant couple to encourage the father to attend prenatal or well-child visits.

Middle Age

Erikson[9] spoke of middle age as the time in life characterized by a conflict between generativity and stagnation. Generativity refers to the concern in establishing and guiding the next generation. It has been shown to be a strong predictor of subjective well-being, greater life satisfaction, and even greater work satisfaction.[13] This stage is often attended by consolidation of one's social and occupational roles. The uncertainty and testing of the young adult stage has passed. Many are firmly fixed in their careers, sometimes disproportionately so. Children are growing up and leaving home. For many, it is a time of relative economic stability and intellectual accomplishments. The question often arises concerning the appropriate goals in life. This is often termed the "mid-life crisis."

An important adaptation response to this stage is the development of new challenges to replace those already accomplished (Table 2.4). For some, this means changing jobs or duties within a job. Some take on added responsibilities or managerial roles. Others may increase their involvement in church and community affairs or exercise programs. Whatever the method, such endeavors are probably preferable to gaining all of one's sense of accomplishment through other people's activities, such as from one's spouse or children.

Much has been written about the "empty-nest" syndrome. Traditionally, this referred to a sense of loss and emptiness, especially in women, after the children left home. Research has been unable to document such a negative experience. Rather, it seems that the prime determinate of the parent's response to the children leaving is their own feelings of self-worth.

Daniel Levinson et al[14] described three overlapping stages in men's lives during this period: early (17–45 years), middle (40–65 years), and late (>60 years). The stages are separated by a transition period of 4 to 5 years. Within the stages there are specific patterns and developmental experiences. Levinson et al found remarkable similarities in the experiences of men from varied backgrounds and occupations. This type of research lends further evidence to the continual process of growth and development throughout the life span. Women during this stage have special transitions as well.[15] Traditionally, menopause was viewed as something fraught with problems: hot flashes, depression, and loss of femininity. Research has failed to bear out these ominous outcomes. Sexual activity may even increase when the couple is freed from the concerns of childbearing. Women may begin to fill the very useful role of a grandmother, assisting their children

Table 2.4. **Concerns in Middle Age**

Development of new challenges in career
Adjustment to children leaving home
Impact of age-related physical changes
Menopause
Divorce

in raising and teaching grandchildren. Some women embark on new careers or educational endeavors.

On the other hand, divorce at this stage of life can be particularly troublesome for women. Income falls precipitously, and if children are still home, the demands of parenting are usually carried out alone. Women tend to remarry less often than men (three quarters of divorced men and two thirds of divorced women remarry)[12] and may not have had a viable source of independent income before the divorce.

As one enters the forties and fifties, there is a growing awareness of the inevitable changes in one's body in response to aging. Aging becomes a physical reality, rather than just an intellectual concern. Weight gain is commonly seen and many report difficulty in reducing even with increased exercise. Illnesses, particularly in men, begin to rise in prevalence. Often there is a newfound desire to exercise to recover one's "lost youth."

In spite of all these potential changes, it may be surprising that life events have been shown to have very little influence on the levels of personality traits in individuals. However, in a longitudinal study of over 2000 subjects it does appear that the perception that one's family or social life were getting worse was associated with increased levels of anxiety, depression, and stress.[16]

Role of the Family Physician

One of the most important interventions by the family physician is to communicate the normality of these experiences. Some persons may be particularly upset that they are feeling unsatisfied with their lives at a time when they have accomplished so much. Health maintenance and disease screening interventions become more important. The patient needs to be taught that it is never too late to make positive changes in health status.

Retirement

Retirement, as a social phenomenon, is a relatively recent human experience. Much is still being learned about the positive and negative effects of retirement. In general, retirement that is freely chosen and well planned is strongly correlated with positive health outcomes (Table 2.5). Time for exercise, both physical and psychosocial, may increase. Many elders become involved in educational pursuits or advocacy programs. For some, the chance to travel is gratifying.

Opportunities for contact with grandchildren usually increase. While both child and grandparent usually appreciate increased contact, sometimes it can be stressful. Between 1980 and 1997, the number of children being raised by their grandparents rose by 33%.[12]

For most, retirement income is sufficient for their needs.[17] However, because of the shrinkage in real wages in the 1970s

Table 2.5. **Issues in Retirement**

Increased time with partner
Adjustment to change in life roles
Self-directed retirement usually a positive experience
Adjustment to change in income level
Increased risk of development of illness

and 1980s, Levy and Michel[18] noted that "the entire cohort of baby boomers will reach retirement (ages 55–64) with less than 50% of the net worth of their parents' cohort at a similar age: $143,000 versus $293,000."

Even when the retirement is planned, there are a number of developmental issues that the person must confront. Historically, men have viewed much of their self-worth in terms of their ability to produce on the job. This stage demands that the person reassess his sense of worth and come to some positive measures of worth outside of work. At present, over 45% of adult women are employed in jobs outside of the home.[19] Hence, these reactions may also be expected in women as this cohort ages. Retirement counselors are now available through the American Association of Retired Persons (AARP) or many large corporations to provide both economic and emotional planning to pre-retirees. They can assist with advance planning for retirement by offering advice on financial considerations or other activities.[20]

Retirement seems to take a negative toll when it is mandated based on age or comes unexpectedly. In these cases, it should be viewed as a risk factor for the development or exacerbation of health problems. Another risky situation is when the spouse's work outside of the home has enabled the couple to long avoid underlying problems. With retirement, much more time is spent by the couple together. They may find that for the first time in their lives together they have differences that need to be addressed directly.

Role of the Family Physician

The family physician can assist by broaching the subject of retirement with all patients. Education about the positive benefits of retirement can be provided. Encouragement of meeting with a retirement counselor may be useful. Scheduling an extra visit around the retirement for health maintenance purposes can also serve to emphasize healthy behaviors at this important transition period. Interviewing the spouse of the retiring partner is also advisable to assess how the spouse is adjusting. One should be particularly concerned when there is a sudden increase or a new onset of health problems. This may indicate a difficult adjustment situation.

Old Age

To some people, the concept that development occurs even in old age is an oxymoron. Much literature exists describing the tasks of this stage in primarily negative terms, such as "disengagement," "adjustment to losses," "and preparation for dying," and illness and significant changes in one's body and family are common during this stage. In contrast, little has been written until recently about the *positive* aspects of aging. In

fact, one's ability to adjust to the changes of life often determines whether the last years are viewed in a positive light.

Early studies in gerontology often characterized these years as with the term "disengagement".[21] More recent writers have rejected this notion in favor of recognizing that as we age we become more diverse, making such generalizations impossible. As a population, the older age group is more physiologically and socially diverse than perhaps any other age group. Such diversity is most likely due primarily to social factors and differential experiences of the meaning of old age. Income and education play a significant role in the maintenance of health through the later years. In this stage of life, approximately 7 years is added to healthy life expectancy when comparing the richest income group to the poorest.[22]

Persons in this stage usually take stock of their life. Most accomplishments in life have been made, although many of the world's greatest leaders have made their most significant contributions to society when they were well past their seventieth birthday. A positive adjustment to aging is found in those who can feel that, on balance, their life has been worthwhile and in those who willingly and consciously adapt to change. For some, a sense of legacy is felt through children and grandchildren. For others, it is measured in terms of accolades, writings, or other external measures. While in the earlier years people are often oriented toward happiness (a positive affective state), in the later years older people are more likely to be satisfied, a perception that one's personal goals have been achieved[17] (Table 2.6).

Regardless of income, the majority of older people perceive themselves as being in good health. This viewpoint is interesting considering that over 50% of those over age 75 are unable to perform at least one activity of daily living (e.g., bathing, dressing). This dichotomy probably can be explained by two perceptions: (1) that older people are remarkably adaptable and tend to view disability in a positive light, and (2) that some older people may be accepting of medically related changes that could potentially be reversed by better care. Older people are able to view changes in physical function with more equanimity than younger people faced with the same degree of impairment.[23] However, there is also a prevalent myth in our society that "old equals sick." Sickness is common, but it should not be considered normal.

A major theme in an older person's life may be that of loss: the loss of physical capabilities, functional reserves, income, and, perhaps most importantly, the loss of friends and family members. These losses can sometimes take a devastating toll on older persons (Table 2.7). It is not uncommon to have older patients go through a period in life when they experience the loss of a friend or family member to death on a monthly basis. It is a testament to the strength of older persons that this experience is so common yet so few become clinically depressed because of it.

On the other hand, older people do have a high incidence

Table 2.6. **Positive Reactions to Old Age**

Happiness—a positive affective state
Satisfaction—a perception that one's personal goals have been achieved

Table 2.7. **Losses in Old Age**

Physical capabilities	Changes in income
Functional reserves	Loss of friends and family members
Mild memory changes	

of depression and suicide. Older single white males have the highest rate of suicide of all age groups. Depression may affect as many as 30% of the population yet is often missed by primary care physicians.[24] Family physicians must develop skills in the detection and treatment of depressive disorders.

One area where there is a great deal of similarity among older persons is the almost universal fear of dependency. This fear far outweighs the fear of death in most geriatric patients. Many will make medical decisions based on the risk of becoming dependent or having to go to a nursing home. Some will decide to refuse treatment rather than burden their families with the high financial and emotional costs of long-term care (also see Chapters 23 and 24).

Role of the Family Physician

The older person uses the family physician for more than just medical care. People in this age group may be reticent to see a counselor but willing to discuss their innermost fears with their doctor. In most settings there are social workers available who are happy to assist the physician with initiation and coordination of referrals to social service agencies. Some physicians who have a high percentage of geriatric patients in their practice find that having a social worker in the office is invaluable. Unfortunately, many physicians spend too little time in the office with older persons.[25]

Death and Dying

Dying today is very different from dying in the early 1900s, when most of today's geriatric patients were born. At the turn of the century, most deaths occurred at home and the death rate in childhood was particularly high.[26] Most deaths currently affect people over the age of 65, and over 70% of Americans die in institutions, either hospitals or nursing homes.[27] Deaths in hospitals are often traumatic for surviving family members. The risk of an adverse health event may also be greater during times of bereavement, especially when the survivor is quite elderly.[28]

There is a strong presumption for prolonging life, almost at any cost, among many physicians. Older persons, and even some younger ones with terminal illness, may not share this value. Instead, the goals of relief of suffering, enhancement of function, and increasing the quality of life become predominant. But how should "quality of life" be defined? One person's perception of quality may be at odds with another's. Physicians are poor predictors of what older persons will consider to be low quality of life.[29] Older persons need open, honest appraisals from their physicians as to the interventions that may provide benefits and the limitations of medical care.

In the last 20 years, the hospice movement has helped people who are dying maintain a higher quality of life. Almost two thirds of hospice patients are over age 65.[30] By empha-

sizing patient-directed approaches to symptom control, even in those with no prospect for medical improvement, people can live more satisfying lives. The major objectives of care are pain control; prevention of constipation, depression, or other symptoms; involvement of families; and care at home or a home-like environment. Medicare has recognized the benefits of this approach by funding hospice care since 1982. The family physician will need to be skillful in assessing the presence of suffering and providing appropriate interventions. Unfortunately, recent research indicates that as many as 46% of patients die in pain that could have been better controlled[31] (also see Chapter 62).

Summary

Understanding the stages of life can help the family physician anticipate and explain common stresses experienced by patients. It is important to remember the great variability seen in individuals and the wide range of types of families that will be encountered in family practice. Because the burden of illness is increases with old age, particular attention should be paid to viewing the experience of aging from the patient's perspective. After all, becoming old is the one "condition" we all hope to acquire, especially when one considers the alternative.

References

1. Bridges, W. The seasons of our lives. Rolling Hills, CA: Wayfarer Press, 1977.
2. Seiden AM. Psychological issues affecting women throughout the life cycle. Psychiatr Clin North Am 1989;12:1–24.
3. Ferber R. Solve your child's sleep problems. St. Louis: Fireside, 1986.
4. Thevenin T. The family bed. Garden City Park, NY: Avery, 1987.
5. Kagan J. The role of parents in children's psychological development. Pediatrics 1999;104:164–7.
6. Blum NJ, Williams GE, Friman PC, Christophersen ER. Disciplining young children: the role of verbal instructions and reasoning. Pediatrics 1995;96:336–41.
7. Shonkoff JP. Pre-school. In: Levine MD, Carey WB, Crocker AC, eds. Developmental-behavioral pediatrics. Philadelphia: WB Saunders, 1991;39–47.
8. Bradford, J, Ryar, C. Rothblum, ED. National Lesbian Health Care Survey: implications for mental health care. J Consult Clin Psychol 1994;62:228–42.
9. Erikson EH. Childhood and society. New York: Norton, 1950.
10. Lewis JM. Repairing the bond in important relationships: a dynamic for personality maturation. Am J Psychiatry 2000;157: 1375–1378.
11. Rosen E. Men in transition. In: Carter B, McGoldrick M, eds. The expanded family life cycle: individual, family, and societal perspectives, 3rd ed. Boston: Allyn & Bacon, 1999;124–40.
12. Alessi G. The family and parenting in the 21st century. Adolesc Med: State of the Art Rev 2000;11:35–49.
13. Ackerman S, Zuroff DC, Moskowitz DS. Generativity in midlife and young adults: links to agency, communion, and subjective well-being. Int J Aging Hum Dev 2000;50:17–41.
14. Levinson D, Darrow CN, Klein EB, Levinson M, McKee B. The seasons of a man's life. New York, Alfred A. Knopf, 1978.
15. Sheehy G. Passages. New York: Bantam, 1984.

16 Costa PT, Herbst JH, McCrae RR. Personality at midlife: stability, intrinsic maturation, and response to life events. Assessment 2000;7:365–378.

17. Guillemard AM, Rein M. Comparative patterns of retirement: recent trends in developed societies. Annu Rev Sociol 1993; 19:459–503.

18. Levy F, Michel R. The economic future of American families: income and wealth trends. Washington, DC: The Urban Institute Press, 1991;101.

19. AFL-CIO. *www.aflcio.org/women/workers_rights.htm*, 2001.

20. Ekerdt DJ, Clark E. Selling retirement in financial planning advertisements. J Aging Studies 2001;15:55–68.

21. Cumming E, Henry W. Growing old: the process of disengagement. New York: Russell Sage Foundation, 1961.

22. Wilkens R, Adams O. Healthfulness of life: a unified view of mortality, institutionalization, and non-institutionalized disability research. Montreal: Institute for Research in Public Policy, 1978.

23. Whitbourne SK, Collins KJ. Identity processes and perceptions of physical functioning in adults: theoretical and clinical implications. Psychotherapy 1998;35(4):519–30.

24. Brakin RL, Schwer WA, Barkin SJ. Recognition and management of depression in primary care: a focus on the elderly. A pharmacotherapery overview of the selection process among the traditional and new antidepressants. Am J Ther 2000;7(3): 205–26.

25. Radecki SE, Kane RL, Solomon DH, Mendenhall RC, Beck JC. Do physicians spend less time with older patients? J Am Geriatr Soc 1988;36:713–8.

26. Gadow SA. A natural connection? Death and age. Generations 1987;11:15–18.

27. Lexis-Nexis. Statistical universe (2001), no. 129. Deaths by age and leading cause, 1997.

28. Rogers MP, Reich P. On the health consequences of bereavement. N Engl J Med 1988;319:510–2.

29. Uhlmann RF, Pearlman RA. Perceived quality of life and preferences for life-sustaining treatment in older adults. Arch Intern Med 1991;151:495–7.

30. Haupt BJ. An overview of home health and hospice care patients: 1996 national home and hospice care survey. Hyattsville, MD: Centers for Disease Control and Prevention/NCHS, 1998.

31. The SUPPORT principle investigators. A controlled trial to improve care for seriously ill hospitalized patients. JAMA 1995; 274:1591–98.

3

Cultural, Race, and Ethnicity Issues in Health Care

Enrique S. Fernandez, Jeannette E. South-Paul, and Samuel C. Matheny

The world is facing movements of peoples unparalleled in history. Even the heartland of the American continent, which has seen few new population groups since the European immigration of the 19th century, has felt the effects of this restive population shift during the late 1980s and 1990s. Physicians who themselves have had little experience outside their own cultural environment are now dealing with health and social issues of patients who approach their surroundings in profoundly different ways than they might themselves. Yet the differences have always been present.

Cultural groups exist in the United States in many forms, and each has the potential for its members to interpret their world in a different manner. In fact, the subtlety of the differences between peoples with common languages and outward appearances may cause even more misunderstandings and concerns than those with more obvious external dissimilarities.

Western Medicine in the Context of Race, Ethnicity, and Culture

The concepts of race, ethnicity, and culture frequently are addressed interchangeably. Racial distinctions are probably the ones most commonly made in clinical settings—often as part of a rote introductory clause in a patient history—and often have limited clinical utility, occasionally establishing misleading and potentially harmful patient stereotypes. An appreciation of how ethnic and cultural factors influence patient health and the clinical encounter is an important consideration when providing effective disease prevention, health promotion, and treatment interventions.

Race

Racial classifications are generally defined by physical characteristics (e.g., skin color, facial features, hair type) that are shared by a group of people. They form the basis for an assumption of a shared genetic heritage among groups of humans. A presumption of shared genetic traits by a group of people who bear superficial similarity might apply to inbred populations that are geographically isolated, but this distinction becomes less meaningful when one considers the intermingling of human populations over the centuries. When one considers that there is more genetic variation to be found within a given race than between two different races, ascribing genetic traits based on race designations alone adds little to the medical decision-making process.[1]

Ethnicity

The word *ethnic* is defined by the *American Heritage Dictionary* as, "of, or relating to, sizable groups of people sharing a common and distinctive racial, national, religious, linguistic, or cultural heritage." Derivations can also be linked with race. The word *ethnicity* is derived from the Greek terms *ethnos*, referring to the people of a nation or a tribe, and *ethnikos*, equating with "national" or "nationality."[2] Ethnicity thus refers to a group affiliation, which is normally expressed in terms of cultural characteristics. Although cultural characteristics are associated with ethnic groups, the members of such groups define and transmit cultural norms.

Culture

Culture can be described as the knowledge, skills, and attitudes learned and passed on from one generation to the next. Cultural identity is a dynamic, lifelong process that is constantly molded and refined by personal experience. Cultural identity thus incorporates a fluidity that defies conclusive statements about the characteristics of populations that share a common culture. Cultural norms can be modified by level of education, socioeconomic status, and the number of generations an individual is removed from the initial migration of his or her family from one society to another. Indeed, there are often more similarities to be found between two individuals of the same socioeconomic status who are from different cultures than between two individuals of the same culture who differ in socioeconomic status.[3] The degree of cultural identity determines the role that family plays for the individual, as well as communication patterns, affective styles, and personal values regarding level of control, individualism, collectivism, spirituality, and religious beliefs. Culture is also modified by age, sex, vocation, disability, and sexual orientation.

Health professionals often participate in a variety of cultures simultaneously: the culture of a family of origin, that of the family of a significant other, the profession entered, or even occasionally a culture dictated by other factors, such as sexual orientation. In turn, the patient presents with a variety of layers of the same cultural cake; recognizing these influences can be a complex, subtle, profound task. As physicians, it is useful to consider the origins of our medical model and how that model determines our approach to patients.

Western Medical Model

The Western medical model was developed in contemporary Western society as a powerful analytic tool to deal with illness. This model developed around the classical Greek myth of Pandora's box in which disease is an intrusion superimposed on humans from the outside. The concept defines the social system within which a defined professional group (i.e., physicians) takes responsibility for the care of persons with compromised function. The model determines the type of questions raised during the history-taking process. Emphasis on physical symptoms often predisposes the interviewer to neglect material of potentially great value (e.g., the social system of the patient). Indeed, cultural factors may create profound differences between patient and physician perceptions of health.

In our medical model, disease is defined as some form of abnormal structure or bodily function that leads to a specific pathology. In this context, disease is a condition most readily identified by the health professional, who attempts to place it in terms of the classification of disorders that has traditionally developed in Western medicine.

Illness, on the other hand, pertains more to the individual's feelings of a negative state of being or social function; it is the human experience of sickness. Illness then may be said to be the perception of the patient, whereas disease is the perception of the health provider. In many cases these two views of sickness coincide, but frequently there are major discrepancies between them. For example, a physician may detect an elevated blood pressure and communicate the diagnosis of hypertension to a patient, who feels perfectly well and has no symptoms but may feel ill only when beginning the antihypertensive medication. Conversely, a Mexican patient may decide that he or she is suffering from *susto*, or emotional fright. This description of a state of anxiety may fail to be identified by a physician but would be completely accepted and understood by anyone in this person's cultural group. Illness for the patient may have several distinct meanings. It may rep-

resent a threat to the individual, in that it may be perceived as possible punishment for a wrongdoing. Many cultures, including groups in the United States, have on occasion viewed various epidemics in this fashion, including human immunodeficiency virus (HIV) infection.

Illness may be also viewed as a loss, as with the loss of independence or the ability to communicate effectively, as would occur following a cerebrovascular accident or with other chronic, debilitating conditions. Conversely, illness may be viewed as a gain, in that there may be advantages to being ill that are more acceptable to society.

Clark[4] described, in her classic study of a Mexican-American community, a pregnant woman who had been struck by her husband. She sought the aid of a *curandera* to prevent a case of *susto* in her unborn child, as described above. This socially acceptable action allowed her to gain community sympathy against her husband for the physical abuse, which would otherwise have been denied her. The husband was convinced of the error of his ways, and the couple was reunited.[4]

Lastly, the illness may convey no particular significance to the individual patient and may be viewed as a normal part of life. Because biomedicine has been largely interested in the treatment of disease, little attention has been paid to interpreting the meaning of illness. Kleinman et al[5] noted that "because illness experience is an intimate part of social systems of meanings and rules for behavior, it is strongly influenced by culture." The lack of attention to illness, and therefore to culture, often results in noncompliance or dissatisfaction with health care delivery.

Population Demographic Shifts

Today minority populations—those who often do not subscribe to the Western biomedical model—are the fastest growing segments of the United States population, representing a substantial proportion of the work force for the 21st century.[6] Southeast Asians and Central Americans made up the largest numbers of immigrants in the late 1970s and 1980s. Census 2000 data revealed dramatic changes from what was initially projected from 1990 results. For the first time, non-Hispanic whites make up less than 70% of the overall population. African Americans and Hispanics each comprise 12% of the population, although Hispanics grew by 61% from numbers in 1990.[7] Asian Americans grew by more than 45% to make up 3.6% of the current population, while American-Indian representation remains low at 0.7%. Furthermore, the 2000 census allowed a change in options for self-identification. Subsequently, 6.8 million people identified themselves as multiracial.[8] Physicians of the 21st century will provide care to a population whose characteristics differ markedly from the population in the United States today. Over the next 30 years, the U.S. population will be larger by almost one third, it will be more diverse, and it will be older. The U.S. Census Bureau estimates that by the year 2050 only 52% of the American population will be white, 16% black, 22% Latino/Hispanic, and 10% Asian. These projected demographic trends will influence significantly the patterns of disease and the health care of the population.[9]

Morbidity and Mortality Variations

The health care system is a reflection of current American society. Lack of access to health care due to an inability to pay or lack of insurance, absence of translators when English is not the patient's language, differing health practices, psychosocial and environmental factors, and cultural differences are all major contributors to differences in health status among the various subgroups that comprise the American population.

Health Status of African Americans

A persistent gap exists in the United States between the health status of African Americans and that of white Americans. Infant mortality for African Americans continues to exceed that of whites and is merely a prelude to other negative health indicators through life: Being black is now considered a health hazard.[10] Even when income differences are factored in and financial access to prenatal care is ensured, African-American women use prenatal care later and less intensively.[11,12]

In 1990 the life expectancy at birth for African-American boys and girls was 64.5 and 73.6 years, respectively, whereas that for white boys and girls was 72.7 and 79.4 years, respectively. The infant mortality rate (per 1,000 births) in 1993 was 6.8 for whites compared with 16.5 for African Americans. There was a larger decline in mortality for African-American infants from 1992 to 1993 than for white infants, but the dramatic differences persist.[13]

Health Status of Hispanics

Hispanics are at increased risk for diabetes, hypertension, tuberculosis, HIV infection, alcoholism, cirrhosis, specific cancers, and violent deaths. Poverty and lack of health insurance are the greatest impediments to health care for Hispanics. One third to one fifth of various Hispanic populations (and one fifth of the African-American non-Hispanic population) are uninsured for medical expenses, compared with one tenth of the white non-Hispanic population.

Health Status of Native Americans

Native Americans suffer some of the worst health in the nation and the lowest social status even among minorities and underserved people. Access to health care for Native Americans is more difficult than for the rest of the U.S. population because of their geographic isolation in villages and communities that are large in area and have large reservations, poor transportation, lack of efficient communications systems, and lack of running water and sewage disposal. Travel may require long distances on dirt roads or by air. Native Americans are younger, less educated, less likely to be employed, and poorer than the general population. These factors, combined with high rates of sexually transmitted disease and drug use, favor the spread of HIV. Alcoholism exacts a terrible toll among many Native Americans. Tribal, cultural, educational, economic, and geographic diversity exist among Native Americans and affect their health care.[14]

Health Status of Asian-Pacific Americans

Important ethnic differences in risk factors indicate that Asian-Pacific American (APA) groups should be targeted for public health efforts concerned with obesity, hypertension, hypercholesterolemia, and smoking.[14] Conditions endemic in the country of origin and case rates for tuberculosis among APAs (44.5/100,000) are greater than for other minority groups: African Americans (29.1/100,000), Hispanics (20.6/100,000), and American Indians/Alaska Natives (14.6/100,000).[14]

Recognizing Cultural Differences

How we interpret and deal with illness is based on our explanations of illness—explanations that are specific to the social positions we occupy and the belief system we employ. These factors have been shown to modify how we perceive symptoms, what labels we attach to particular illnesses, and how we interpret these labels. How we communicate our health problems, the manner in which we present our symptoms, when and from whom we seek care, how long we remain in care, and our evaluation of that care are affected by cultural beliefs.[15]

Most health care providers have a collection of anecdotes about noncompliance by ethnically different patients. As these issues have been studied by medical sociologists and anthropologists, the focus of the problem has come to rest on the provider as much as on the patient. The "fallacy of the empty vessel" is a phrase coined by anthropologists to describe cross-cultural blindness. People tend to ignore parts of cultures (e.g. religion, health care traditions) that differ from their own. The anthropologist Hazel Weidman noted that orthodox health care providers often view Western health institutions as introducing something of significance into ethnic communities where nothing existed before. Thus the existing health traditions in such communities are ignored.

Borkan and Neher[16] developed a framework for use in family practice training programs, modeled after one developed by Bennett.[17] Bennett suggested a model with stages of individual development relative to cultural sensitivity. The Borkan and Neher model built on this model by recognizing the importance of ethnosensitivity to understanding the whole person and by advancing doctor–patient communication. They recognized that the individual trainee's relationship with other cultures may be more complex than implied by Bennett's model. The level of sensitivity exhibited by a trainee can vary according to the group encountered (e.g., sensitive and empathetic to Southeast Asians and culturally unaware with respect to Haitians).

Thus Borkan and Neher suggested a model of ethnosensitivity consisting of seven stages, with curricular strategies and goals to address each stage: (1) fear, (2) denial, (3) superiority, (4) minimization, (5) relativism, (6) empathy, and (7) integration. Fear is the most problematic stage because it may preclude any efforts to provide medical care. Denial can be addressed by attempting to heighten the awareness of trainees to cultural differences. Superiority is the stage where differences are recognized, but trainees tend to rank them according to their own value system. With minimization, cultural differences are viewed as unimportant against the background of basic human similarities. Ethnic and cultural differences are finally acknowledged in the relativism stage and are no longer seen as threatening. With empathy, the trainee can adopt the frame of reference of patients in order to experience events as they would. Integration is the most advanced level of physician awareness and allows the practitioner to become enmeshed in more than one culture.

Physicians and patients have their own cultural identities. Only by recognizing where one is on the cultural continuum can each encounter be placed in perspective. Knowing oneself and one's views and assumptions, therefore, is the first step in assessing and understanding others.

Individuals often submerge their identification with their past cultural traditions and adopt the traditions of their new country. Harwood[18] enumerated five major factors that may contribute to variation in an individual subscribing to the standards of a group of origin: (1) acculturation, (2) level of income, (3) occupation, (4) area of origin in the mother country, and (5) religion. The level of acculturation may be the most difficult to ascertain by a clinician; eight screening points are delineated for detecting those individuals who tend to be most acculturated into middle-class American standards:

1. Relatively high level of formal education
2. Greater generational removal from immigrant status
3. Low level of involvement within an ethnic or family social network
4. Experience with medical services that incorporates patient education and personal care
5. Previous experience with particular diseases in the immediate family
6. Immigration to this country at an early age
7. Urban, as opposed to rural, origin
8. Limited migration back and forth to the mother country

Harwood pointed out, however, that in times of stress, all individuals may revert to beliefs they do not consistently hold at other times.

Crucial Factors in the Cross-Cultural Clinical Encounter

It should be the goal of any clinical encounter that both the patient and the clinician are able to develop mutual understanding and feel comfortable in the relationship, and that quality health care is delivered in an efficient and timely manner beneficial to the patient. Several factors are necessary for successful physician–patient experience: an awareness of certain core cultural issues, an understanding of the meaning of illness to the patient, an ability for the physician to negotiate across this "cultural divide," and clarity of communication. Certain elements have been identified as essential for assessing the cultural attributes of a person, community, or group of people and have been termed the domains of culture.

Language

Word usage may not be the same in the cultures of the clinician and the patient, and care should be taken to use simple words that can be easily understood in communication. If a patient does not speak the language of the clinician or vice versa, it is especially important to attempt to alleviate areas of confusion. Up to one third of minority and immigrant households in the United States may be described as linguistically isolated. These are households where no one over the age of 14 speaks English. This poses significant challenges for the physician–patient encounter, especially when translators are not readily available.

A physician, newly arrived at his post on an Indian reservation in the southwestern United States, paid a courtesy call on the chair of the Tribal Council for the group with whom he was assigned. During the course of a half-hour of pleasant conversation, the chair told him that he hoped he would enjoy his stay and find the reservation pleasant. The physician answered by saying that he was sure that he would enjoy his tenure, but that his primary purpose here was to practice medicine and that his enjoyment of his setting was of secondary importance. Within a few hours, word had gotten out on the reservation that the physician had come to the reservation to "practice" (that is, experiment) on the tribe, a misunderstanding that nearly caused his transfer.

Time

Different cultures may hold different concepts of time, which can provide several areas of misunderstanding. For patients from certain cultures, being on time for an appointment may mean within a 15-minute window, within an hour, or within a half-day. The concept of future time may also vary. In some rural-based cultures, advising patients that they must undertake certain preventive measures to prevent illness at some future time may be difficult to fathom, as their consideration of time may exist only in the present or the next season.

Decision Makers

In some cultures, important decisions, including those involving medical care, may be a communal decision by the extended family or by a designated family leader instead of the spouse or other nuclear family members. In an attempt to expedite an important decision, physicians may alienate these designated decision makers or the patient. Conversely, when the family leader is the patient, other family members may be reticent to accept responsibility for decision making in the event of the incapacity of the family leader involved.

Illness Models

There may be significant differences of opinion between the clinician and the patient, and not just concerning the etiology of certain symptoms. The very recognition of certain conditions as "illness" by the patient and the physician may vary.

An African-American patient presented to a major city hospital emergency room, complaining of nervousness, "shakes," and weight loss over the past several months. He had been unable to sleep and expressed generalized anxiety. Upon more intensive questioning, it was determined by one of the nurses that he felt that one of his former female companions had placed a curse on him, known in the southern coastal region as "the root."

It was difficult in this case for the clinician to accept both the patient's explanation of the etiology of the symptoms and the very existence of the illness described.

Treatment and Effectiveness of Intercession

On occasion, the patient and clinician agree that significant illness is present, but the reasons for the illness and the appropriate treatment may differ significantly.

A woman who had recently moved to Los Angeles from central Mexico presented an 11-month-old child to a physician's office with signs of diarrhea and mild dehydration. The mother, through an interpreter, told the clinician that the child had *mollera caida*, literally "fallen fontanelle." Her method of treatment was to place salt on the fontanelle, turn the child upside down to fill out the sunken spots, and give the child *manzanilla* (chamomile) tea. The clinician, on the other hand, was concerned about the diarrheal etiology and wished to initiate oral rehydration.

Traditional Role of Healer

For better or worse, much of the outcome deriving from the encounter between the clinician and patient depends on the expectations and experiences of the patient in his or her cultural group. If the healer is expected to be omnipotent and make the diagnosis by observation only, questioning by the clinician may be taken as a sign of ignorance or incompetence. The healer may also have been an integral part of the community of the individual and be well respected and liked, or the converse may have been true. These attitudes may be transferred over to the clinician, who is unaware of the expectations bestowed by the patient.

Managing Cross-Cultural Differences

Cultural sensitivity training is implemented regularly in only a small number of medical schools. A 1991 study revealed that only 13% of schools offered cultural sensitivity courses to their students, with all but one being optional.[19] A national survey of family practice residencies in 1985 revealed that only 26% provided learning experiences in culturally sensitive health care.[20] However, a 1998 Association of American Medical Colleges' survey revealed that almost 70% of the 94 schools that responded taught courses in cultural competence. Fifteen percent plan to introduce it into the curriculum in the near future. Approximately one third (36%) of residencies offer some kind of formal teaching in this area.[21,22] The Liaison Committee on Medical Education also launched a new Diversity Standard in May 1999. It notes that students must understand and be able to deal with various belief systems, cultural biases, and other culturally determined factors that influence the manner in which different people experience illness and respond to advice and treatment. Furthermore, the Society of Teachers of Family Medicine (STFM) Task Force on Cross-Cultural Experiences published recommended curriculum guidelines to assist in training family physicians to provide culturally sensitive and competent health care.[23] The goal in such training is competence in recognizing bias, prejudice, and discrimination, using cultural resources, and overcoming cultural barriers to enhance primary care.

Cultural differences can easily lead to differences in the models by which a clinician or a patient might explain a presenting condition and the most effective course of management. Figure 3.1 suggests the ultimate goal in cross-cultural medicine: effective integration of patient and clinician knowledge to produce a shared model of care. When a clinician recognizes that a possibility exists for significant differences in the explanatory models of illness and the approach for management, it is necessary to supplement the traditional history to ascertain these issues and develop a plan for coming to some understanding with the patient.

LEARN Model

Berlin and Fowkes[24] developed an instrument useful to clinicians for negotiating the differences that may exist between

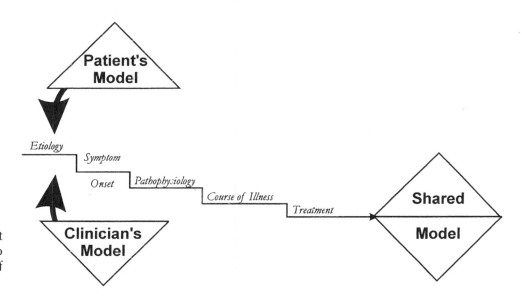

Fig. 3.1. Integration of patient and clinician knowledge to produce a shared model of care.

Listen with sympathy & understanding to
  the patient's perception of the problem

Explain your perceptions of the problem

Acknowledge and discuss differences &
  similarities

Recommend treatment

Negotiate treatment

Fig. 3.2. Managing cross-cultural differences: the LEARN model. (*Source:* Berlin and Fowkes,[24] with permission.)

patient and provider. The LEARN acronym is based on the following five steps (Fig. 3.2).

1. Listen. Ask the patient such questions as "What do you think is causing this problem?" "Why do you think it started in this way?" "What do you think this illness is doing to you?" "What do you fear the most about this illness?" "How severe is it?" "What do you think is going to happen to you?" "What kind of treatment do you think you should receive?" These questions give the clinician the framework to understand the patient's model of etiology of illness and the opportunity to demonstrate empathy and understanding.
2. Explain. With this step the clinician explains his or her interpretation of the medical condition. It may be nothing more than a supposition, but it is important that the clinician present an understanding based on Western medical tradition.
3. Acknowledge. It is important to acknowledge the patient's explanatory model and begin to develop areas where agreement can be met and conflicts between explanatory models can be resolved.
4. Recommend. In this stage, the clinician can recommend a plan for action that incorporates the patient's explanatory models of illness and those of the clinician.
5. Negotiate. Berlin and Fowkes consider this step the most important. It includes incorporating the patient's and clinician's understanding and plans. The final step may well be an amalgamation of the two belief systems that can be mutually tolerated.

In the case of the child with the *mollera caida*, the physician listened carefully to the mother's explanation of the cause of the sunken fontanelle. She then explained to the mother that in her view the cause of the sunken fontanelle was the diarrhea, but acknowledged the concern of the mother for restoring the fullness of the fontanelle. Because the mother was using boiled *manzanilla* tea, she negotiated with the mother to add sufficient nutrients to the tea to compose an oral rehydration solution and encouraged this part of the traditional treatment to continue.

Working with Translators

Special care is needed with interviews involving translators to ensure the accuracy and completeness of the information and the cooperation of the patient. Clinicians must view the translator as part of a team whose members collaborate to arrive at a competent plan for the patient:

1. Look at the patient when speaking. Always address the patient, not the interpreter, and speak in the first person directly to the patient, asking the interpreter to interpret in a direct fashion.
2. Use comforting body language, recognizing that it is instantaneously interpreted by the patient.
3. Whenever possible, explain to the interpreter in advance what you are trying to say and accomplish during the interview.
4. Assume that there will be misunderstandings, particularly when you are using nonprofessional interpreters.
5. Remain aware and test your patient's understanding. Some patients may understand your language even if they choose to use an interpreter; or, conversely, patients who speak fairly well in the language of the clinician may not have the same level of comprehension.
6. Keep the sentence structure simple, avoiding complex phrases.
7. If there are a significant number of patients in your practice who speak a particular language, it alleviates some misunderstanding if the clinician learns as much of the language as possible. This effort increases the trust of the patient and allows the clinician to more readily pick up errors by the interpreter.[25]
8. Be especially wary of the accuracy of interpretation from family members, particularly concerning the sexual or gynecologic history of female patients. In certain cultures it is taboo to discuss these topics with the patient, even when interpreting for the clinician. Also, in many cultures children are particularly problematic when acting as translators.

References

1. Cooper R, David R. The biological concept of race and its application to public health and epidemiology. J Health Polit Policy Law 1986;2:97–116.
2. Betancourt H, Lopez SR. The study of culture, ethnicity, and race in American psychology. Am Psychol 1993;48:629–37.
3. Greenbaum S. Race, ethnicity and culture. San Francisco: USF Center for Teaching Enhancement, 1992.
4. Clark M. Health in the Mexican American culture. Berkeley: University of California Press, 1959.
5. Kleinman A, Eisenberg L, Good B. Culture, illness, and care: clinical lessons from anthropologic and cross-cultural research. Ann Intern Med 1978;88:251–8.
6. Kehrer BH, Burroughs HC. More minorities in health. Menlo Park, CA: Kaiser Forums, 1994.
7. U.S. Bureau of the Census. Population change and distribution 1990 to 2000. Washington, DC: U.S. Census Brief, April 2001.
8. U.S. Bureau of the Census. Overview of race and hispanic origin, Washington, DC: U.S. Census Brief, March 2001.
9. Kehrer BH, Burroughs HC. More minorities in health. Menlo Park, CA: 1994.

10. Gates-Williams J, Jackson MN, Jenkins-Monroe V, Williams LR. The business of preventing African-American infant mortality [special issue]. West J Med 1992;157:350–6.
11. Murray JL, Bernfield M. The differential effect of prenatal care on the incidence of low birthweight among blacks and whites in a prepaid health plan. N Engl J Med 1988;319: 1385–91.
12. Kugler JP, Connell FA, Henley CE. Lack of difference in neonatal mortality between blacks and whites served by the same medical care system. J Fam Pract 1990;30(3):281–7.
13. Rosenberg HM, Ventura SJ, Maurer JD, Hauser RL, Freedman MA. Births and deaths. United States, 1995. Monthly Vital Statistics Rep 1996;45(3)S(2).
14. Lin-Fu JS. Asian and Pacific islander Americans: an overview of demographic characteristics and health issues. Asian Pac Islander J Health 1994;2:20–36.
15. Kleinman A, Eisenberg L, Good B. Culture, illness, and care: clinical lessons from anthropologic and cross-cultural research. Ann Intern Med 1978;88:251–8.
16. Borkan JM, Neher JO. A developmental model of ethnosensitivity in family practice training. Fam Med 1991;23:212–17.
17. Bennett MJ. A developmental approach to training for intercultural sensitivity. Int J Intercultural Rel 1986;10:179–96.
18. Harwooc A. Ethnicity and medical care. Boston: Harvard University Press, 1981.
19. Lum CK, Korenman SG. Cultural-sensitivity training in U.S. medical schools. Acad Med 1994;69:239–41.
20. McConarty PC, Farr F. Culture as content in family practice residencies. Presented at the Society of Teachers of Family Medicine 19th Annual Spring Conference, San Diego, May 1986.
21. Personal communication: teaching cultural competence: Danoff D, Asst VP for Medical Education, Washington, DC: AAMC.
22. Greene J. AM News 1999(25 Oct);8–9.
23. Like RC, Steiner P, Rubel AJ. Recommended core curriculum guidelines on culturally sensitive and competent health care. Fam Med 1996;27:291–7.
24. Berlin E, Fowkes WC Jr. A teaching framework for cross-cultural health care—application in family practice. West J Med 1983;934–8.
25. Freebairn J, Gwinup K. Cultural diversity and nursing practice. Irvine, CA: Concept Media, 1979.

4
Family Issues in Health Care

Thomas L. Campbell, Susan H. McDaniel, and Kathy Cole-Kelly

Caring for families is one of the defining characteristics of family practice. Families are the primary context within which most health problems and illnesses occur and have a powerful influence on health.[1] Most health beliefs and behaviors (e.g., smoking, diet, exercise) are developed and maintained within the family.[2] Marital and family relationships have as powerful an impact on health outcomes as biologic factors,[3] and family interventions have been shown to improve health outcomes for a variety of health problems.[4]

Family members, not health professionals, provide most of the health care for patients. Outside the hospital, health care professionals give advice and suggestions for the acute and chronic illness, but the actual care is usually provided by the patient (self-care) and family members. Chronic illness requires families to adapt and change roles to provide needed care. The aging of the population and increasing medical technology leads to a significant increase in the prevalence of chronic illness and disability and a rise in family caregiving.

Unfortunately, families are often neglected in health care. Our culture is individually oriented, valuing autonomy over connectedness. The impact of serious illness on other family members is often ignored. Family practice developed around the concept of caring for the entire family, yet many family physicians have received inadequate training in how to work with families. Some have even argued that it is not practical and takes too much time to work with families. The ability to work effectively and efficiently with families and to use them as a resource in patient care is an essential skill for all family physicians.

Despite rapid societal changes in the structure and function of families, the family remains the most important relational unit and provides individuals with their most basic needs for physical and emotional safety, health, and well-being.
The family can be defined as "any group of people related either biologically, emotionally, or legally."[5] This includes all forms of traditional and nontraditional families, such as un-

married couples, blended families, and gay and lesbian couples. The relevant family context may include family members who live a distance from the patient or all the residents of a community home for the developmentally delayed persons. In daily practice, family physicians are most often involved with family members who live in the same household.

Premises of a Family Systems Approach

There are three basic premises upon which a family systems approach is based. These premises are derived from systems theory, are supported by research, and help guide the clinical application of family systems.

1. A family systems approach is based on a biopsychosocial model of health care in which there is an interrelationship between biologic, psychological, and social processes. This approach places the patient and the illness in a larger framework involving multiple systems. The family-oriented physician must recognize and address the psychosocial factors as well as the biomedical factors in understanding patients and their illness. A systems approach emphasizes the interaction among the different levels of the larger systems and the importance of continuous and reciprocal feedback.
2. The family has an influence on physical and psychological health and well-being. This principle is well supported by research and has important implications for clinical practice. Clinicians must understand how the family can positively and negatively influence health and utilize the information to improve health care. There are several corollaries to this basic premise.
   a. The family is a primary source of many health beliefs and behaviors.

b. The family is an important source of stress and social support.

c. Physical symptoms may have an adaptive function within a family and be maintained by family patterns.

3. The family is the primary social context in which health care issues are addressed. Although the patient is the primary focus of medical care, the family is often the most important social context that must be understood and considered when delivering health care. It is not useful to think of the family as the "unit of care." Family physicians treat individuals within families, not families themselves. They must consider the family context and address family relationships when they influence health problems. This is important whether a physician cares for only one or every member of a family.

Doherty and Baird[6] have challenged the "illusion of the medical dyad" between the physician and patient and have described the relationship of the physician, patient, and family as a therapeutic triangle (Fig. 4.1). This triangle emphasizes that the family plays a role in all patient encounters regardless of whether family members are present and the need to be cognizant of both the patient–family relationship and the physician–family relationship.

Research on Families and Health

A large body of research has demonstrated the powerful influence that families have on health. There are many randomized controlled trials demonstrating the effectiveness of family interventions for medical disorders.[4] A recent Institute of Medicine report on families, health, and behavior reviewed the research on the influence of family relationships on the management and outcomes of chronic diseases.[7] Several general conclusions can be made from a review of this research:

1. Families have a powerful influence on health and illness. Numerous large epidemiologic studies have demonstrated that social support, particularly from the family, is health promoting. In an 1988 article in the journal *Science*, soci-

ologist James House et al[3] reviewed this research and concluded, "The evidence regarding social relationships and health increasingly approximates the evidence in the 1964 Surgeon General's report that established cigarette smoking as a cause or risk factor for mortality and morbidity from a range of disease. The age-adjusted relative risk ratios are stronger than the relative risks for all cause mortality reported for cigarette smoking."

Family support affects the outcome of most chronic medical illnesses. After suffering a myocardial infarction (MI), women with few or no family supports have two to three times the mortality rate compared to other women who are recovering from an MI.[8] Many stresses within the family, such as loss of a spouse and divorce, significantly impact morbidity and mortality.

2. Emotional support is the most important and influential type of family support. Social and family support can be divided into different types: instrumental, informational, and emotional. Instrumental support is the actual provision of services (e.g., driving the patient to the hospital) or caregiving (e.g., giving insulin injections) provided by family members. Informational support usually involves giving health-related information, such as advice on whether to seek medical care. Emotional support provides a listening ear, empathy, and the sense that one is cared about and loved. Although there is overlap among these categories, studies suggests that family emotional support has the most important influence on health outcomes and therefore cannot be replaced with social agencies or services that provide instrumental and informational support.

3. Marriage is the most influential family relationship on health. Even after controlling for other factors, marital status affects overall mortality, mortality from specific illnesses, especially cancer and heart disease, and morbidity. Married individuals are healthier than widowed, who are in turn healthier than either divorced or never-married individuals. Those who are married have healthier lifestyles and less disability, and they live longer. Bereavement or death of a spouse increases mortality, especially for men.[9] Separation and divorce is also associated with increased morbidity and mortality. Studies in psychoimmunology have shown that divorced and unhappily married men and women have poorer immune function than those in healthier marriages.[10]

4. Negative, critical, or hostile family relationships have a stronger influence on health than positive or supportive relationships. In terms of health, "being nasty" is worse than simply not being nice. Research in the mental health field with schizophrenia and depression first demonstrated that family criticism was strongly predictive of relapse and poor outcome.[11,12] Similar results have been found with smoking cessation,[13] weight management,[14] diabetes,[15] asthma, and migraine headaches. Physiologic studies have shown that conflict and criticism between family members can have negative influences on blood pressure,[16] diabetes control,[17] and immune function.

5. Family psychoeducation is an effective intervention for health problems. There is a wide range of types of family

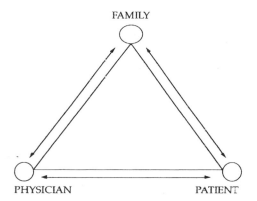

Fig. 4.1. Therapeutic triangle. (*Source:* Doherty and Baird.[6])

interventions that have been used for health problems, from simply providing family members with information about the disease to in-depth family therapy. The most consistently effective and studied family intervention seems to be family psychoeducation, in which family members are given training on how to manage and cope with the illness and provided with emotional and instrumental support.[18]

An excellent example of an effective, family psychoeducational intervention has been developed for family caregivers of Alzheimer disease (AD) patients.[19] In a randomized controlled trial, families attended individual and group instructional and problem-solving sessions where they learned how to manage many of the troublesome behaviors of patients with AD. They also participated in ongoing family support group and can access a crisis intervention service to help them with urgent problems. The caregivers who received this intervention were less depressed and physically healthier than those who did not, and AD patients were able to remain at home for almost a year longer than caregivers in the control group. The savings in nursing home costs were several times the cost of the interventions. This study should serve as a model for other family intervention programs.

This research establishes that families have a strong influence on overall health and on the outcome of specific illnesses. The impact is the greatest for illnesses in which there is a high burden on family caregivers. Effective family interventions range from complex, multifaceted programs (e.g., for AD patients) to educating family members about the illness (e.g., hypertension). To implement any of the interventions, family physicians must know how to work with families and use them as a resource in patient care.

Working with Families

Much of what has been written about working with families has focused on the family conference, the most formal and uncommon form of a family interview. It is useful to distinguish three approaches to working with families: the family-oriented approach with an individual patient, involving family members during a routine office visit, and the family conference or meeting (Table 4.1). In all of these contexts, medical care is enhanced by obtaining information about the family, assessing family relationships, and encouraging appropriate family involvement.

A Family-Oriented Approach with an Individual Patient

A family orientation has more to do with how one thinks about the patient than how many people are in the exam room. Since family physicians meet with individual patients more often than with family members, having a family-oriented approach to all patients is an important skill. This approach complements a patient-centered approach in which the physician explores the patient's experience of illness, an experience that occurs in a family or relational context. The patient's presenting complaint can be thought of as an entrance or window into understanding the patient in the context of the family. By exploring the patient's symptoms and illness, the physician can learn more about the patient's family, its relationship to the presenting complaint, and how the family can be used as resource in treatment. A key to being family oriented is choosing appropriate questions to learn about the psychosocial and family-related issues without the patient feeling that the physician is intruding or suggesting that the problem is "all in your head."

In a qualitative study of exemplar family physicians, Cole-Kelly and colleagues[20] examined the core components of a family-oriented approach with individual patients. These family physicians used both global family questions, such as "How's everyone doing at home?" as well as focused family-oriented questions, such as "How is your wife doing with that new treatment?" The exemplars frequently inquired about other family members and were able to keep a storehouse of family details in their minds that they frequently interspersed in the visits. The physician would commonly punctuate the end of the visit with a greeting to another family member: "Be sure to tell John I said hello."

A risk of being family-oriented with an individual patient is getting triangulated between family members—the one speaking to the physician and a family member being talked about. In Cole-Kelly et al's[20] study, the exemplar physicians were sen-

Table 4.1. **Working with Families**

	Family-oriented approach with individual patient	Involving family members in routine office visits	Family conference
Common medical situations	Acute medical problems Self-limiting problems	Well-child and prenatal care Diagnosis of a chronic illness Noncompliance Somatization	Hospitalization Terminal illness Institutionalization Serious family problem/conflict
Percent of time used by physician	60–75%	25–40%	2–5%
Length of visit	10–15 minutes	15–20 minutes	30–40 minutes
How scheduled	Routine care	May need to request family member attendance	Special scheduling and planning

Source: Adapted from McDaniel et al.[5]

sitive to the dangers of inappropriately colluding in a triangulated relationship with the patient and were very facile at avoiding those traps. The exemplars seemed to have an appreciation for the importance of understanding the concept of triangulation and to use it for their and the patient/family's advantage. The exemplars often explored family-oriented material during physical exams or while doing procedures, thus not using extra time for these areas of inquiry. Visits with a high family-oriented content occurred 19% of the time and family-oriented talk was low or absent in 52% of the visits. The visits that had the highest degree of family-oriented character were chronic illness visits and well-baby and child visits.

Asking some family-oriented questions can metaphorically bring the family into the exam room and provide a family context to the presenting problem.[21] Here are examples of family questions:

"Has anyone else in your family had this problem?" This question is often part of obtaining a genogram. It reveals not only whether there is a family history of the problem, but also how the family has responded to the problem in the past. The treatment used with one member of the family or in a previous generation may be a guide for the patient's approach to his/her illness or may describe how a patient does not want to proceed.

"What do your family members believe caused the problem or could treat the problem?" Family members often have explanatory models that strongly influence the patient's beliefs and behaviors regarding the health problem.[22] If the physician's treatment plan conflicts with what important family members believe or have recommended, it is unlikely the patient will comply.

"Who in your family is most concerned about the problem?" Sometimes another family member may be the one most concerned about the health problem and may be the actual person who really wants the patient to receive care. When the patient does seem concerned about the health problem or motivated to follow treatment recommendations, finding out who is most concerned may be helpful in creating an effective treatment plan.

"Along with your illness (or symptoms), have there been any other recent changes in your family?" This question is a useful way to screen for other additional stressors, health problems, and changes in the patient's family and how it is affecting the patient.

"How can your family be helpful to you in dealing with this problem?" Discovering how family members can be a resource to the patient should be a key element of all treatment planning.

These questions can be integrated into a routine 15-minute office visit with an individual patient and provide valuable family information relevant to the problem.

Genograms

Genograms or family trees are one key to a family-oriented interview with an individual patient. They are the simplest and most efficient method for understanding the family context of a patient encounter[23] (Fig. 4.2) and provide a psychosocial "snapshot" of the patient. Genograms provides crucial information about genetic risks and any family history of serious illnesses. With advances in genetic research, a detailed genogram should be an essential component of every patient's medical evaluation and database. Ideally a genogram should integrate genetic and psychosocial information.

The genogram can be started at an initial visit and added to during subsequent encounters. It may be quite simple and only include the current household and family history of serious diseases or provide more detailed information about family events and relationships. When possible, the genogram should include family members' names, ages, marital status, significant illnesses, and dates of traumatic events, such as deaths. Computerized genogram programs are available so that the genogram can be integrated into an electronic medical record.

Obtaining a genogram can be a particularly effective way to understand the family context and obtain psychosocial information from a somatically focused or somatizing patient. These patients often present with multiple somatic complaints and try to keep the focus of the encounter on their physical symptoms and distress. They are challenging patients, and it is often difficult to obtain family or psychosocial information from them. Since obtaining a family history is considered a routine part of a medical evaluation, it can often provide access to more relevant psychosocial illness. It provides a way to step back from the presenting complaints to obtain a broader view of patients and their symptoms in a manner that is acceptable to the patients. The genogram can also be used to screen for substance abuse and family violence.[23]

Involving Family Members in Routine Office Visits

Routine visits, in which one or more family members are present, are common and may be initiated by the patient, family members, or the clinician. These visits allow clinicians to obtain the family members' perspective on the problem or the treatment plan and answer the family members' questions. Family members accompany the patient to office visits in approximately one third of all visits, and these visits last just a few minutes longer than other visits. In some situations, they may be more efficient and cost-effective than a visit with an individual patient because a family member can provide important information about the health problem, or the visit may answer questions that might later arise. Family members may serve various roles for the patients, including helping to communicate patient concerns to the doctor, helping patients to remember clinician recommendations, expressing concerns regarding the patient, and assisting patients in making decisions. Physicians report that the accompanying family members improve their understanding of the patient's problem and the patient's understanding of the diagnosis and treatment.

There are many situations when a family physician may want to invite another family member to the next office visit. Partners and spouses are routinely invited to prenatal visits.

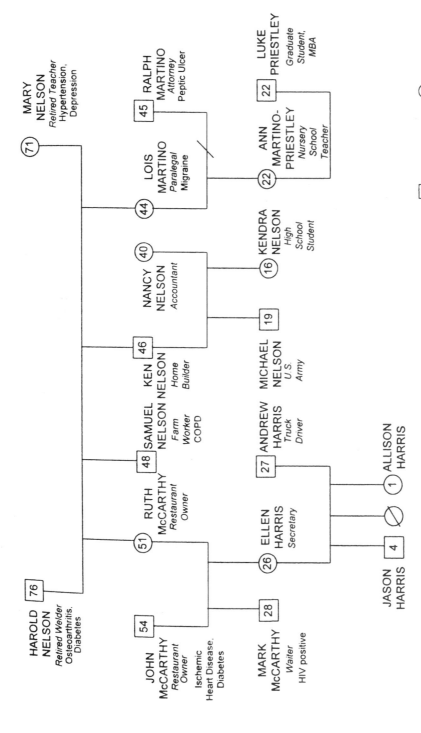

Nelson family genogram: family members, occupations, chronic health problems. Symbols used: ☐76, male, age 76; ○71, female, age 71; ○―○, marriage; ○―/―○, divorce; ⊘, deceased.

Fig. 4.2. Genogram.

Fathers and co-parents should be invited to well-child visits, especially when the child has a health or behavior problem. Whenever there is a diagnosis of a serious medical illness or concern about adherence to medical treatments, it is helpful to invite the patient's spouse or other important family members to come for the next visit. Elderly couples are usually highly dependent on each other. It can be particularly effective and efficient to see them together for their routine visits. Each can provide information on how the other one is doing and help with implementation of treatment recommendations. Consulting with family members during a routine visit is advised whenever the health problem is likely to have a significant impact on other family members or when family members can be a resource in the treatment plan.

Principles of Family Interviewing

The principles of interviewing an individual patient also apply to interviewing families, but there are additional complexities. One must engage and talk with at least one additional person, and there is opportunity for interaction between the patient and family members. In general, the physician must be more active and establish clear leadership in a family interview. This may be as simple as being certain that each participant's voice is heard ("Mrs. Jones, we haven't heard from you about your concerns about your husband's illness. Can you share those?") or may entail acting as a traffic cop with a large and vocal family ("Jim, I know that you have some ideas about your mother's care, but I'd like to let your sister finish talking before we hear from you.").

When interviewing families, establishing rapport and an initial relationship with each family member is particularly important. In a family systems approach, this is known as joining. An essential component of joining is making some positive contact with each person present so that each feels valued and connected enough to the physician to participate in the interview. Family members have often been excluded from health care discussions and decisions, even when they are present. They may not expect to be included in the interview or to be asked to participate in decision making. By making contact and shaking hands with each person, the physician is making clear that everyone is encouraged to participate in the interview.

There are several other important reasons for joining with family members at the beginning of the interview. The physician often has an established relationship with the patient, but may not have one with other family members, who may feel either left out or that their role is merely that of an observer. One common example of this occurs commonly during hospital rounds when there is a family member by the bedside. The usual approach is to either ask family members to leave during the interview or to ignore them. This is disrespectful of families and fails to use family members as a resource. It is recommended that the physician greet and shake hands with each family member and find out something about each person. At a minimum, this may be the family member's relationship with the patient and involvement in the patient's

health problems. It may also involve thanking them for their presence and help.

All the principles of good medical interviewing can be extended to family interviewing. It is helpful to encourage each family member to participate and to be as specific as possible when discussing problems. Individual and family strengths should be emphasized. Emotions that are present in any family member during the interview should be recognized and acknowledged: "Mr. Canapary, you look upset. Is there anything about your wife's health or her medical care that you are concerned about?" In addition, the physician must take an active role in blocking persistent interruptions and preventing one person from monopolizing the conversation.

Establishing a positive relationship with family members is particularly important and more challenging when there is conflict in the family. In these cases, a family member may assume that the physician has taken the side of the patient in the conflict. The physician must take extra steps to join with family members in conflict and establish one's neutrality. The goal in these situations is to develop an alliance with each family member and the patient without taking sides in the conflict. An exception to this goal is when family violence threatens and then safety must be the first priority.

In addition to establishing rapport and building a relationship through verbal communication, the physician can also make use of nonverbal strategies to enhance the relationship with the patient and family members. Just as it is important to be sure that the physician and an individual patient are in a comfortable sitting position and at eye level with one another, it is important also that other family members are sitting near enough that they can hear what's being said and be easily seen by the physician. This proximity will help the physician make eye contact with each person in the room.

Upon entering the room and seeing that one family member is sitting very far from the physician or isolated from other family members, the physician can gently motion the person to come closer to enhance the sense of everyone being included in the patient visit and being an important part of the encounter. Similarly, one family member might dominate both the verbal and nonverbal space in the encounter, making it difficult for the other family members to have as much involvement with the patient or physician. For these cases, the physician must "direct traffic," so all voices can be heard.

A physician who meets with multiple family members needs to learn how to avoid taking sides with one family member at the exclusion of another. It is very easy for the physician to unwittingly be pulled into unresolved conflicts between family members. In the case of an ill child, one parent may try to form a relationship with the physician that excludes the other parent. Or a wife can try to get the physician to side with her, hoping that the physician's alliance will bolster her position against her husband. To avoid getting caught in the middle of a triangle, the physician must listen to each member of the family but still remain neutral. Furthermore, the physician can assert that it won't be helpful to the family if the physician takes sides with one member against another. The physician can emphasize the importance of everyone

Table 4.2. **Dos and Don'ts of Family Interviewing**

Dos

Greet and shake hands with each family member.

Affirm the importance of each person's contribution.

Recognize and acknowledge any emotions expressed.

Encourage family members to be specific.

Maintain an empathic and noncritical stance with each person.

Emphasize individual and family strengths.

Block persistent interruptions.

Don'ts

Don't let any one person monopolize the conversation.

Don't allow family members to speak for each other.

Don't offer advice or interpretations early in a family interview.

Don't breach patient confidentiality.

Don't take sides in a family conflict, unless some one's safety is involved.

Source: Adapted from McDaniel et al.[5]

working together as the most beneficial way to enhance the health care of the patient (Table 4.2).

Family Conferences

A family conference is usually a specially arranged meeting requested by the physician, patient, or family to discuss the patient's health problem or a family problem in more depth than can be addressed during a routine office visit (see Table 4.1). All the principles of family interviewing discussed previously are used in a family conference. However, a family conference is usually longer than most office visits and involves more planning and structure.

Every family physician should have the skills to convene and conduct a family conference or meeting. In a randomized controlled trial, Karofsky and colleagues[24] examined the impact of an initial family conference for new pediatric patients and their families through a randomized controlled trial. The families that received the family conference had fewer subsequent visits for health problems or to the emergency room and more visits for health supervision (well-child visits). This study suggests that family conferences may be cost-effective by reducing health care utilization.

Meeting with entire families is most important when diagnosing and treating life-threatening illnesses. Family members are usually eager to obtain information from the physician and want to know how they can be helpful. Most physicians meet with a patient's family at the time of a hospitalization to explain a diagnosis and treatment plan. A family meeting at the time of hospital discharge should be routine. Usually family members must assume the responsibility for the care of the patient and need detailed information about the patient's condition and follow-up treatment. One study of couples coping with a myocardial infarction found that the best predictor of the wife's emotional well-being 6 months after her husband's heart attack was whether she had an opportunity to meet and talk with his physician prior to discharge.[25] Under managed care, hospital stays have shortened

dramatically, and patients are going home with significant health care needs that must be provided by family members or assisted by visiting nurses.

Family conferences should also be a routine part of palliative or end-of-life care, whether at home or in a hospice. Clarifying the patient's diagnosis and prognosis with the family can be very helpful for treatment planning. Family conferences are often essential to resolve conflicts about whether to move from curative to comfort care. Some family members may resist a patient's decision to stop chemotherapy or other medical treatments, often because they are not emotionally ready for the patient's death. If the decision can be discussed and emotional reactions shared in a family meeting, these problems or conflicts can be avoided. Finally, it is helpful to routinely meet with family members after a patient's death to answer questions, allow the sharing of grief, and assess how family members are coping. With large families or difficult problems, the physician may wish to ask a family therapist to help conduct the meeting.

Conducting a family conference requires skills in addition to those used when meeting with family members during a routine office visit. There are usually, but not always, more family members involved. A family assessment and some type of planned family intervention may be required. The reason for convening the family may involve difficult or conflictual issues, which require special skills to handle.

A detailed outline or blueprint for conducting a family conference has been described elsewhere.[5] Prior to meeting with the family, the physician should have a clear rational and initial plan for the conference. Here are the basic steps or phases of a family conference that can guide the physician.

Joining Phase

As discussed previously, it is particularly important to spend time to develop rapport with the family and get to know something about each family member at the beginning of the conference. This step is often neglected or given inadequate time by the inexperienced clinician. The family may want to discuss the problem or issue at the very outset, and the physician may lose the opportunity to join early and learn more about the family. The physician can stop the discussion of the problem and say, "I find it helpful to step back and learn a little bit more about each of you, before we discuss the problem." This joining phase, which may seem like social chat to the inexperienced, helps to create a sense of trust between the physician and family and an environment in which family members feel safe and supported. If the physician already knows the family well, this phase may be abbreviated but should not be eliminated.

Goal Setting

It is helpful to jointly establish goals for the conference with the family. This often begins with the physician's statement about why the family has been convened, for example, "to discuss your mother's illness and plans for further treatment." It is then useful to ask what the family wants to accomplish during the session. The family's goals may be quite different from the physician's, and they need to be respected and addressed. This is analogous to asking individual patients what they were hoping to achieve during a routine office visit.

Information Exchange

The physician may ask what the family knows about the patient's illness or problem. This is often more effective and informative than launching into a detailed description of the patient's problem without knowing the family's level of knowledge. It also allows the physician to directly address misunderstandings or misinformation and to identify whether family members have varying views of the problem. It is important to get the views of all the family members present, even if it's as simple as having a family member say he or she agrees with the others.

Obtaining further information about the family is usually very helpful in understanding the issues or problems that the family is dealing with. Gathering a more detailed genogram is an easy way to obtain this information, and families usually feel comfortable and often enjoy this process. It is crucial to identify family strengths and supports during the interview. These are the resources that the family members will use to cope with the problem or illness they are facing.

When conducting an interview with a large, conflictual, or enmeshed family, the physician usually needs to be more active than during interviews with individuals, directing the conversations between family members and managing arguments. Each family member should be encouraged to speak, and no one should be allowed to speak for someone else who is present. It is important not to let any one person monopolize the conversation, and to interrupt and solicit other family members' opinion on the topic.

Establishing a Plan

During this final phase, the physician should work with the family to develop a mutually agreed upon treatment plan and to clarify each person's role in carrying it out. The patient, physician, and family members should have input into the plan. For some families, this may require writing up a formal care plan that everyone can agree on.

Confidentiality

When working with family members, the family physician must maintain confidentiality with the patient. Prior to speaking with a family member, it is important that the physician is clear about what the patient feels can be shared and what, if anything, cannot be. A family member may bring up difficult or awkward concerns, but the physician may only disclose information the patient has approved (unless the patient is incompetent). In most cases, patients will agree that their care plan can be fully discussed with the family members. However, in family meetings involving adolescents or divorced parents, the rules for the meeting need to be clearly spelled out. The physician may remind families at the beginning: "John has agreed that I can talk with you about the options for his diabetes treatment. He, of course, will be the one who will make the final decisions, but we both think it will be helpful to have all of your thoughts about what

may be best." Such discussions value both the doctor–patient relationship as well as the patient–family relationships. The positive support of these relationships is only one of the positive outcomes of well-crafted family meetings.

Conclusion

The aging of the population, advances in medical research, and changes in our health care delivery system will continue to have dramatic impact on family issues in health care. There are increasing demands on families to provide care for aged and chronically ill patients, often without adequate services and insurance reimbursements. Family caregiving has led to an increasing burden on family members and poor physical and mental health for many caregivers. The role of the family in end-of-life decision making is only beginning to be addressed. Health care proxy laws allow patients to identify an individual, usually a close family member, to make medical decisions if the patient is unable to, but little research has been done on how patients make these choices, what they discuss with their designated health care agent, and whether family members follow the wishes of the patient. Because of the genetic revolution, we will soon have the ability to screen or test for hundreds of genetic disorders, but the impact of this technology on families is just beginning to be examined. Genetic counseling needs to address not only the genetic risks of the individual but also the implications for other family members. More family research is need in each of these areas.

One of the unique and distinguishing characteristics of family medicine is its emphasis on the family. No other medical specialty has a family focus or uses a family-oriented approach. Under our changing health care system, there is increasing recognition of the importance and cost-effectiveness of involving the family in all aspects of medical care. New models of care are being developed that emphasize teamwork, prevention, and collaboration with patients and their families. A family-oriented approach will become increasingly valued and effective model in the 21st century.

References

1. Campbell TL. The family's impact on health: a critical review and annotated bibliography. Fam Syst Med 1986;4(2,3):135–328.
2. Doherty WA, Campbell TL. Families and health. Beverly Hills, CA: Sage, 1988.
3. House JS, Landis KR, Umberson D. Social relationships and health. Science 1988;241(4865):540–5.
4. Campbell TL, Patterson JM. The effectiveness of family interventions in the treatment of physical illness. J Marital Fam Ther 1995;21(4):545–83.
5. McDaniel SH, Campbell TL, Seaburn DB. Family-oriented primary care: a manual for medical providers 2nd Edition. New York: Springer-Verlag, 2003.
6. Doherty WJ, Baird MA. Family therapy and family medicine: toward the primary care of families. New York: Guilford, 1983.
7. Weihs K, Fisher L, Baird MA. Families, health and behavior. Institute of Medicine report. Washington, DC: National Academy Press, 2001.

8. Berkman LF, Leo-Summers L, Horwitz RI. Emotional support and survival after myocardial infarction. A prospective, population-based study of the elderly. Ann Intern Med 1992;117(12): 1003–9.

9. Osterweis M, Solomon F, Green M. Bereavement: Reactions, consequences, and care. Washington DC: National Acadamy Press, 1984.

10. Kiecolt-Glaser JK, Fisher LD, Ogrocki P, Stout JC, Speicher CE, Glaser R. Marital quality, marital disruption, and immune function. Psychosom Med 1987;49(1):13–34.

11. Hooley JM, Orley J, Teasdale JD. Levels of expressed emotion and relapse in depressed patients. Br J Psychiatry 1986;148: 642–7.

12. Kanter J, Lamb HR, Loeper C. Expressed emotion in families: a critical review [Review]. Hosp Community Psychiatry 1987; 38(4):374–80.

13. Hooley JM, Richters JE. Expressed emotion: a developmental perspective. In: Cicchetti D, Toth SL, eds. Emotion, cognition, and representation. Rochester Symposium on Development Psychopathology. Rochester, NY: University of Rochester Press, 1995;133–66.

14. Fischmann-Havstad L, Marston AR. Weight loss maintenance as an aspect of family emotion and process. Br J Clin Psychol 1984;23(4):264–71.

15. Koenigsberg HW, Klausner E, Pelino D, Rosnick P. Expressed emotion and glucose control in insulin-dependent diabetes mellitus. Am J Psychiatry 1993;150(7):1114–5.

16. Ewart CK, Taylor CB, Kraemer HC, Agras WS. Reducing blood pressure reactivity during interpersonal conflict: effects of marital communication training. Behav Ther 1984;15(5):478–84.

17. Minuchin S, Baker L, Rosman BL, Liebman R, Milman L, Todd TC. A conceptual model of psychosomatic illness in children. Family organization and family therapy. Arch Gen Psychiatry 1975;32(8):1031–38.

18. McFarlane WR, Lukens E, Link B, Dushay R, Newmark M. Multi-family groups and psychoeducation in the treatment of schizophrenia. Arch Gen Psychiatry 1995;52(8):677–87.

19. Mittelman MS, Ferris SH, Shulman E, Steinberg G, Levin B. A family intervention to delay nursing home placement of patients with Alzheimer disease. A randomized controlled trial [see comments]. JAMA 1996;276(21):1725–31.

20. Cole-Kelly K, Yanoshik MK, Campbell J, Flynn SP. Integrating the family into routine patient care: a qualitative study. J Fam Pract 1998;47(6):440–5.

21. Cole-Kelly K, Seaburn D. Five areas of questioning to promote a family-oriented approach in primary care. Fam Syst Health 1999;17(3):348–54.

22. Wright LM, Bell JM, Rock BL. Smoking behavior and spouses: a case report. Fam Syst Med 1989;7(2):171–7.

23. McGoldrick M, Gerson R, Shellenberger S. Genograms: Assessment and intervention, 2nd ed. New York: W.W. Norton, 1999.

24. Karofsky PS, Rice RL, Hoornstra LL, Slater CJ, Kessinich CA, Goode JR. The effect of the initial family interview on a pediatric practice. Clin Pediatr 1991;30(5):290–4.

25. Fiske V, Coyne JC, Smith DA. Couples coping with myocardial infarction: an empirical reconsideration of the role of overprotectiveness. J Fam Psychol 1991;5(1):20–7.

26. McDaniel SH, Campbell TL, Hepworth J, Lorenz A. A manual of family-oriented primary care, 2nd edit. New York: Springer-Verlag. In Press.

5
Information Mastery: Practical Evidence-Based Family Medicine

Cheryl A. Flynn, Allen F. Shaughnessy, and David C. Slawson

Remember Marcus Welby? He symbolized the ideal family doctor—knowledgeable even about rare conditions, caring and compassionate, making multiple house calls with his little black bag, and devoting his complete attention and the best resources for the care of a single patient.

Fast forward to the new millennium, with health maintenance organizations (HMOs), schedules with 20 to 40 patients per day, and a huge information explosion, yet still having the responsibility of knowing the latest updates in medicine. As family doctors, we strive to maintain the characteristics embodied by that fictitious symbol—good history and physical examination skills, an understanding of the patient in the context of the family and community, and the ability to meld the two in diagnostic and therapeutic decision making. Yet with the exponential growth of information, and rapidly expanding medical technologies, it seems easy to blink an eye and miss some important new development. Lifelong learning skills and strategies to manage the jungle of medical information are the new survival tools for today's family doctors.

Enter evidence-based medicine (EBM), which is defined as "the conscientious, explicit, and judicious use of the current best evidence in making decisions about the care of an individual patient."[1] This practice encourages us to apply the highest quality information available at the time in the care of our patients. Critics argue that we have been using evidence all along; EBM is merely a new name for an old practice. But EBM is not simply the use of research in practice. Rather it is a systematic process to answer clinical questions with the best evidence. It requires lifelong learning skills not generally taught in medical school. A 1984 study found that physicians' knowledge of treating hypertension was inversely related to the year they graduated from medical school.[2] A later study demonstrated that those who attended a school where EBM was taught had no such knowledge decline.[3]

If EBM has been practiced all along, then why would an ophthalmologist from a well-respected institution advise jour-nal readers to use an eye patch to treat corneal abrasions despite knowing that there were seven randomized controlled trials showing no benefit and possible harm ("We've always done it this way")?[4,5] If our profession incorporates evidence into practice routinely, why were only two of 28 landmark trials implemented in practice in the 3 years following publication.[6] If you are a clinician who already is using the best evidence in practice, then we challenge you to train your colleagues and help train our future physicians, because clearly as a profession we do not routinely practice using the best evidence.

The newer definition of EBM is one that incorporates the best evidence, clinical experience, and patient perspective into medical management plans—a patient-centered evidence-based practice. This chapter outlines a new and more useful model of EBM, especially fitting for family physicians; offers practical strategies for using evidence in answering clinical questions; outlines a model for keeping up to date with the latest medical developments; and addresses some key concepts in the application of evidence in clinical practice.

Information Mastery

The traditional EBM model involves five steps to solve a clinical problem: developing answerable clinical questions, searching for and selecting the best evidence, evaluating the quality of that information, interpreting and applying it back at the patient level, and assessing one's practice. Although seemingly complete, this model has some limitations, especially for the busy family physician.

First is the lack of feasibility. It is estimated that the average physician generates about 15 clinical questions per day. Although some questions are simply "What is this drug?" or "What's the proper dose?" more than half are focused on identifying the best treatment or diagnosis strategies. Since it takes an average of 20 minutes to perform a Medline search, one would need several hours of uninterrupted time per week just to *find* the evidence for answering these questions. It is understandable, then, that the majority of the questions generated in practice remain unanswered. The unfortunate part is that half of the answers would have the potential to influence practice.[7]

A second, essential element of an evidence-based practice is the ability to keep up to date with the latest developments. To seek answers only to those questions we generate may leave us in the dark about new or previously unconsidered therapies. Worse still, it may result in medical gossip[8]—finding an answer to your question without the context of all the research of that area may result in the inappropriate application of the evidence.

Finally, the traditional EBM model presumes that the only source of medical information is the literature. Colleagues are the first source clinicians turn to for answers during practice.[9] The medical information system is expansive, and includes the World Wide Web beckoning from your personal computer, pharmaceutical representatives knocking at your door, and continuing medical education (CME) programs making broad-based medical recommendations. These sources are in addition to the estimated 6000 articles published each day in medical journals.[10] Family physicians need tools to help sort through this overwhelming quantity of medical information.

Information mastery (IM) was designed to be more user-friendly for busy clinicians. All sources of medical information are not equally useful, but depend on three factors:

$$Usefulness = \frac{Relevance \times Validity}{Work}$$

Here, *work* refers to any resources devoted to finding and using information. This conceptual model tells us that sources requiring little work are more useful. However, if an information source is either irrelevant or invalid, then regardless of the work, its usefulness will still be zero; all three factors must be balanced. The latter sections of this chapter offer practical tips and examples of ways to minimize work when answering clinical questions or attempting to stay current with medical information developments.

Determining Relevance: DOEs, POEs, and POEMs

One strategy to minimize work is to first assess relevance. Only if the source of information passes the relevance criteria do you need to follow through with a validity assessment. In medicine, we naturally create a hierarchy of relevance. It is uncommon that we'd apply data that were based solely on test tubes or animal models directly to our patients. Within clinical studies, there is also an additional hierarchy of data, that between disease-oriented and patient-oriented evidence. Disease-oriented evidence (DOE) refers to outcomes of pathophysiology, etiology, and pharmacology. Often these include test results and may also be called surrogate markers. We count them as important because we assume these interme-

diate outcomes are directly linked to the final outcomes. Consider guidelines that tell us to check for proteinuria in the diabetic patient. Why is the amount of protein in the urine important? Because it represents a marker for renal disease, we assume that less protein means that patients won't need dialysis or at least the need is delayed. Instead of assuming that an intervention that alters the quantity of proteinuria delays the need for dialysis or helps our diabetics live longer, why not study the final outcomes of morbidity and mortality? Insisting on evidence that is linked to final outcomes eliminates the assumption step and lets us know that what we are doing for our patients is more like to help than harm. These final outcomes are patient-oriented evidence (POEs) which are outcomes of mortality, quality of life, and disease prevention.

Why is this distinction so important? DOEs represent what ought to be based on our understanding of pathophysiology. What "ought to be," however, may not always turn out to be true. The medical literature is wrought with examples of medical decisions based on intermediate outcomes that were found not to withstand the longer term studies evaluating POEs: external fetal monitoring for low-risk pregnancies, calcium channel blockers for hypertension, antiarrhythmics for premature ventricular contractions after a myocardial infarction. These and other examples of POEs and DOEs are outlined in Table 5.1.

Two additional criteria must be considered when determining the relevance of medical information. First is the frequency with which the problem studied is encountered in your practice. Obviously, common problems are deserving of more attention. Second is deciding whether the information matters to you as a clinician. Would this evidence, if true, oblige you to change your current practice? If the perfect study were conducted demonstrating that penicillin treatment of strep pharyngitis prevented rheumatic heart disease, this should have little impact on our practices. However, a study demonstrating that estrogen replacement worsens urinary incontinence in postmenopausal women may offer motivation to not recommend this treatment to incontinent women. In this latter case, where our practice should be altered, the POE becomes a POEM, patient-oriented evidence that matters. The next step is validating the information to determine whether it should be applied.

Assessing the Validity of New Information

New research is believable only when it has been shown to be internally and externally valid. Internal validity is how well the evidence reflects the truth. To apply the results from a well-done study, the patient population needs to be similar enough to your patient or clinical population. This generalizability of the information to your own practice is external validity.

Determining validity is the hardest part of EBM for most people. Readers are often overwhelmed by statistical jargon and want to just accept that the editors have done that for them. Key validity considerations for different study types are outlined in Table 5.2. Readers can get a more detailed explanation from the

Table 5.1. **Examples of Disease-Oriented Evidence (DOEs) and Patient-Oriented Evidence that Matters (POEMs)**

DOEs	POEMs
DOEs that were supported by POEMs	
Pap smears detect premalignant cervical lesions.	Routine screening with pap smears decreases the rate of cervical cancer mortality.
Statins lower cholesterol.	In hyperlipidemic patients with cardiac disease, statins lower the risk of recurrent cardiac events and improve survival.
Beta-blockers and diuretics lower blood pressure in hypertensive patients.	Beta-blocker and diuretic treatment of hypertension decreases MI and stroke and increases survival.
DOEs that were contradicted by POEMs	
Antiarrhythmics eliminate PVCs seen on telemetry in patients post-MI.	Routine use of some antiarrhythmics increases mortality in post-MI patients.
External fetal monitoring (EFM) detects concerning fetal heart tracing patterns.	In uncomplicated pregnancy, use of EFM increases cesarean rates and no improvement in neonatal outcomes is noted.
Calcium channel blockers (CCBs) lower blood pressure in hypertensive patients.	CCBs have been shown to increase rates of stroke, MI, and mortality.[23]

MI = myocardial infarction; PVC = premature ventricular contraction.

"User's Guide" series (go to *http://www.cche.net/principles/content_all.asp*).[11] The IM worksheets offer a simplified version of validity assessment and can be obtained from the authors on request. One tip to lessen the work of evaluating study quality is to do this step as a group, for example in a resident journal club, or rotating responsibility among your clinical partners. Another option is to seek "prevalidated" sources, those where a known EBM/IM expert has done the quality evaluation for you.

The IM model tells us that focusing our attention on common, valid POEMs will maximize usefulness and help us offer the best care to our patients. When encountering any information source, first assess relevance (is it a common POEM that, if true, changes practice?), and, only if relevant, proceed to do the work of validating the evidence.

Practicing Information Mastery

The vast amount of medical information available to us can be a jungle of opportunities and traps. We choose to enter this jungle for one of four reasons: to refresh our memories of something forgotten (retracing), out of interest (sporting), to answer clinical questions (hunting), and to keep up to date (foraging). For medical problems with which we have less

clinical experience, our questions tend to be simplified: What are the causes of excessive vomiting in a 2-month-old? How does Crohn's disease usually present? These are background questions[12] and fall more into the first category of learning (or relearning). Sporting refers to seeking information that is uniquely interesting to us, our own research interests, or exploring the details about Aunt Agnes's zebra illness. Sporting, therefore, should be delegated to personal or academic time. Hunting and foraging have a direct impact on how we practice medicine and care for our patients every day and require the use of the best current information. This section offers practical suggestions for beginning your evidence-based practice: how to hunt, how to forage, and how to approach nonliterature sources of medical information. Remember, the usefulness equation is our model for all three: minimizing work, maximizing relevance, and maximizing validity.

Hunting

If a patient asks a question or one arises during patient care, we must find the answer. Right? Not necessarily. Doing so is the equivalent of reading every article encountered, and is likely not feasible. Thus the first consideration in hunting is deciding whether we actually need to hunt! This parallels the common criteria for relevance outlined above. A general rule

Table 5.2. **Key Validity Issues for Different Types of Articles**

Therapy	Diagnosis	Prognosis	Systematic reviews
Randomized controlled trial?	Cohort design?	Prospective following of an inception cohort?	Comprehensive search for studies?
Double blinding?	Consecutive enrollment of patients?	>80% follow-up?	A priori inclusion criteria defined?
Concealed allocation?	Appropriate reference standard applied to all patients?	Generalizability?	Validity assessment of included studies?
Explanation of follow-up and withdrawals?	Independent, blinded application of the new test?	Blind assessment of outcomes?	Test for homogeneity?
Intention to treat analysis?			Appropriateness of combining results?
Generalizability?			

to follow here is asking, "Will this answer apply to another patient before it becomes out of date?" If not, then it may not be worthwhile to hunt for the answer yourself. Suppose a patient with hairy cell leukemia asks your advice about the best treatment for her cancer. It's not likely that you as the family doctor will be prescribing that, nor is it likely that today's answer will be tomorrow's (or next year's) answer when you next encounter someone with this cancer. This question could be deferred to the patient's oncologist. Another patient whose psoriasis calms in the summer sun wonders if buying a light box for home use in the winter will help. Relative to other skin conditions, psoriasis is less common in primary care, but you will likely soon encounter other patients with this problem and proceeding to find an evidence-based answer is appropriate.

The next step is deciding when to hunt. Those newly in practice or those new to EBM will likely find it challenging to do evidence searches during busy office hours. Questions need not always be answered while patients are there; set a follow-up appointment and commit yourself to finding an answer before then. Keep a list of questions that arise during practice, prioritize them for relevance, and hunt for evidence-based answers whenever you can—during lunch or before returning patient phone calls, or when on call. Faculty might find some time during resident precepting. The bottom line here is to just do it; whatever steps you take toward answering clinical questions with evidence are steps toward an evidence-based practice. As your skills and information technology advance, finding answers "on the fly" will be easier. Programs that search multiple Internet sites simultaneously (TRIP, *http://www.tripdatabase.com*; SumSearch, *http://www.sumsearch.uthscsa.edu*), and newer evidence-based information tools (Medical Inforetriever, *http://www.medicalinforetriever.com*) are available on personal and handheld computers to bring evidence answers to the point of care.

Finally, knowing how and where to hunt is critical. Because a good answer begins with a good question, learning to ask well-constructed questions is the first step. Foreground questions are those specific questions about the best treatment or testing strategy; they arise more frequently as our medical experience increases and thus are best answered by using current evidence.[13] The four components of a good question form the PICO acronym:

*P*atient and problem information (age, race, severity of illness, setting, comorbid illnesses)
*I*ntervention proposed (which may represent medications, or advice, or screening tests)
*C*omparison group (no intervention, or standard of care)
*O*utcomes of interest (which should be POEMs).

This PICO format helps convert your clinical question into a search strategy that maximizes your chance of finding relevant information.

Developing reasonable searching techniques will also help minimize the work of hunting, although many busy clinicians will not have the time do to this on their own. A medical librarian (*http://www.crmef.org/curriculum*) can help train you to a sufficient level of skill for independent searching, addressing such things as Boolean search terms, truncation of keywords, and linking terms to medical subject headings. Established search strategies have been developed that help maximize the return of valid studies. For example, searching in PubMed offers the advantage of the clinical queries feature. Selecting the search purpose (therapy, diagnosis, prognosis, or etiology) links your clinical search terms with study design terms to improve the retrieval of more valid study types.

The last part of efficient hunting is knowing where to start. The medical information system can be envisioned as a pyramid (Fig. 5.1), with the most useful information, the most relevant and valid or predigested sources, at the top. Many of us were trained to look for evidence by searching Medline; however, this is the largest and least sorted database and therefore takes the most work to search. By starting at the top of

Drilling for the Best Information

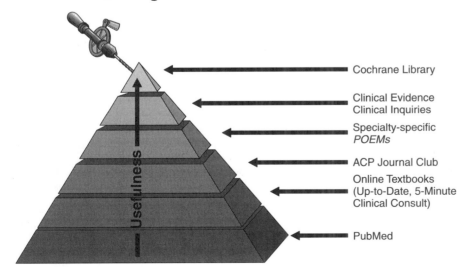

Cochrane Library

Clinical Evidence
Clinical Inquiries

Specialty-specific
POEMs

ACP Journal Club

Online Textbooks
(Up-to-Date, 5-Minute
Clinical Consult)

PubMed

Fig. 5.1. The medical information system depicted as a pyramid. The usefulness of the information increases as one climbs the pyramid.

Table 5.3. **Explanation of the Databases in the Information Pyramid (see Fig. 5.1).**

Database	Content/description	How to access
Cochrane Library	Database of SRs of therapeutics: high-quality MAs updated approximately every 2 years Database of abstracts of reviews of effectiveness DARE: validated summaries of published SRs/MAs Controlled Trials Registry	Cochrane SR abstracts available free online at *http://www.som.flinders.edu.au/fusa/cochrane/cochrane/revabstr/mainindex.htm* Full library available by subscription with quarterly updates
Clinical evidence	Text covering many clinical topics with full outline of evidence-supported treatments	In print; online version available from BMJ at *http://www.evidence.org*
Clinical inquiries	Database of evidence-based answers to a prioritized list of questions generated by FPs	2–4 are published each month in the JFP (available free online at *http://www.jfponline.com*) Soon will be housed in a searchable electronic database
JFP POEMs	Summaries of original research articles relevant to FPs with validity assessments	8 published each month in the JFP; search entire database of POEMs on the Web at *http://www.medicalinforetreiver.com*
ACP Journal Club	Critically appraised summaries of recent literature relevant to medical practice but not specifically for FPs	Available by subscription only
MD consult (5-minute consult)	Comprehensive collection of books, journals, news, and patient education sources	Available online for subscription fee (Accessed at *http://www.5mcc.com/*)
PubMed	National Library of Medicine's database with over 10 million citations Clinical queries feature links your search with built-in filters to better find validly designed studies for therapy, diagnosis, etiology, and prognosis	Accessed free at *http://www.ncbi.nlm.nih.gov.entrez/*

ACP = American College of Physicians; BMJ = *British Medical Journal*; EBM = evidence-based medicine; FP = family practitioner; JFP = *Journal of Family Practice*; MA = meta-analysis; SR = systematic review.

the pyramid of sources and drilling down only as far as necessary to find a relevant and valid answer to the question, much time can be saved. The pyramid also shows us which databases are the most relevant and valid. Table 5.3 contains further information on each of these databases, as well as tools to search through the various databases.

It will likely take time and practice for the average clinician to develop efficient hunting skills. However, even asking questions and considering the quality of the evidence one finds are simple first steps in the continuum toward a more evidence-based practice.

Foraging

Doctors cite journal reading as one key method for keeping up to date; many of us have a bedside stack. In reality, though, we do a poor job of reading journals (or else there would be no stack!). Nor do we succeed at incorporating that information into practice. Instead of reading the stack, consider scanning the stack for relevant evidence. Read only the abstract conclusion and ask yourself the relevance question: Is this a common POEM that will change my practice? Read on to validate only those articles that pass the relevance criteria. In this way IM limits what we need to read, but also increases the responsibility of carefully assessing the information deemed relevant.

Even better strategies can be developed to forage the medical literature with less work and more likelihood of retrieving relevant and valid information. Four basic principles apply to a practical foraging strategy: (1) regularly casting a broad net, (2) being aware of the best sources of information, (3) using relevance criteria to screen information for usefulness, and (4) developing a retrieval system.

Since family physicians see a broad range of patients and problems, we especially have a need to be far-reaching in our attention to the medical literature. Scanning the most respected journals and all of our own specialty journals still leaves us at risk for missing a potentially relevant article. For example, a well-done trial was published in *Neurology* in 1998 demonstrating effective migraine prophylaxis from high-dose riboflavin.[13] Most family physicians do not read *Neurology* regularly and would have missed this potentially useful information. Since less than 4% of original research represents POEMs,[14] a lot of sieving is required to identify the few nuggets of gold. Even the journals with the highest POEM:DOE ratios—*JAMA, Lancet, British Medical Journal, Annals of Internal Medicine, Journal of Family Practice (JFP)*—have at most one or two articles per issue pertinent for family doctors.[14]

By perusing "POEM bulletin boards," we can let others do this filtering work for us. *JFP POEMs* is a site that can reduce the work of foraging. Editors scan more than 90 journals monthly, using the IM criteria to select articles of relevance specifically to family doctors. Eight of 25 to 30 relevant articles are selected each month and the summaries of the critical appraisal and key population and outcome information are published in the *JFP*. These reviews can be found and searched online at *www.medicalinforetriever.com*. The remaining studies are critically appraised and summarized in both the *Evidence-Based Practice* newsletter and the daily e-mail electronic newsletter (*InfoPointer*).

Other abstracting services do similar work. The American College of Physicians Journal Club (ACPJC) publishes validated summaries of original research. Although they cite relevance to medical practice as selection criteria, ACPJC does not target primary care specifically, nor does it use the IM relevance criteria.[15] Other services (Tips from Other Journals, Journal Watch) highlight potentially relevant research without a formal validity assessment. These may best be used by scanning the summaries and applying the relevance criteria to identify truly relevant information for your practice. Unfortunately, needing to personally perform a validity assessment greatly increases the work involved in applying the information into practice. Thus, secondary sources offering both relevant and valid information are preferred.

Newer electronic services are emerging that further lessen the work. Medical InfoPointer (*www.medicalinforetriever. com*) is an abstracting service that carefully evaluates research for relevance and validity and delivers a short synopsis with a "bottom line" recommendation of one article each day via e-mail. Bandolier on the Web (*bandolier@pru.ox.ac.uk*) is a British evidence-based medicine resource that will e-mail its monthly table of contents to interested readers.

Regardless of the strategies employed, the final and essential step of foraging is to create a retrieval system. The traditional version of this was cutting the article out from the journal and filing it your cabinet in some reasonable ordering system. Today's clinician needs to "file" the key information (population and intervention details, outcomes assessment and magnitude of results, and the original citation) in an electronic system on handheld or personal computer to make it available quickly during patient care. Web-based software (e.g., Avant go) makes it possible to download Web pages to store in your electronic folders. Many of the foraging sites above also have searching capabilities—so if you remember that the riboflavin article for migraine prophylaxis was in *JFP* POEMs, you can quickly search that database to retrieve the answer in a matter of seconds. The paper version of foraging is still a great first step toward better information mastery. But ultimately, technology phobia or not, you'll likely need to develop some simple computer skills in searching and filing or you'll be left behind.

Other Medical Information Sources

As a general rule, when evaluating the usefulness of any source of information consider the work, the relevance, and the validity of the information. A sampling of information sources are highlighted below using the usefulness equation as the guide.

Medical Literature that Is Not Original Research

Summary reviews are those that paint a broad landscape of a clinical topic; they likely include the classic presentation, epidemiology, and diagnostic and therapeutic suggestions. We may be enticed by these reviews; they seem to be a low-work option, one stop shopping. Yet because the authors usually do not specify their methods for finding or evaluating the evidence, we are often not sure of the relevance and quality of information upon which recommendations are based. In fact, the quality of these reviews varies inversely with the level of expertise of the author,[16] suggesting that authors may begin with their conclusions and report only the data that support their recommendations, while ignoring contradictory reports! When reading summary reviews, if you stumble across advice that is contrary to your current practice, check whether the recommendation is based on a POEM, and if so (or if you can't tell), consider finding the original study yourself to evaluate the true usefulness. This added work makes this type of article less useful in the long run. Summary reviews may best be reserved for retracing, or when we have background rather than foreground questions.

Similar issues exist for clinical practice guidelines (CPGs). The intent of CPGs is to provide recommendations supported by available information that help clinicians make medical decisions. However, the quality of these seemingly low-work sources can vary greatly, from purely consensus-based opinion to a summary and synthesis of only quality evidence. Characteristics of quality CPGs include a brief summary statement for each recommendation, a long reference section pointing to original research, a methods section explaining how evidence was obtained and evaluated, and a detailed discussion of the evidence. Identifying an evidence table, a balance sheet, or some indication of the strength of the supporting evidence increases the likelihood of the CPG being evidence-linked. The relevance varies between and within CPGs; scanning for recommendations that are POEM-based can help identify those that are more relevant. Specific criteria for evaluating the validity of CPGs have been developed.[17]

Continuing Medical Education (CME)

Doctors cite attendance at CME programs as the second most common strategy to keep up to date. Yet the passive, lecture-based CME rarely improves knowledge and almost never changes behavior. Since most CME talks are similar in structure to the summary type reviews, we may be falsely lulled into thinking we're learning a lot when in fact we're not. Interactive educational processes and those that incorporate an audit/feedback system are more likely to influence us. But to truly make CME useful requires your attention and participation as a member of the audience. Keep your ears open for any recommendation by the speaker that would change your current practice. Ask follow-up questions about the evidence on which the speaker based her suggestions. Was it POEM data? What was the quality of the data? Are the references available? Implement only those that are valid POEMs.

Experts

In the context of medical information, an expert is anyone of whom we ask a clinical question. Most often we turn to "content experts," those with more expertise in the topic of inquiry. Yet the answers they give can often be quite subjective, based more on experience than valid data.[18,19] Clinical scientists are those with expertise in evaluating information for validity but may not necessarily be content experts. The best experts are YODAs (your own data analyzers),[20] who have and share the evidence basis for their recommendations, balancing it with their clinical experience. Our suggestion is to seek out the YO-DAs in your own community. When referring patients or asking questions of your consultants, include specific requests for the source of their recommendations. It may be solely experience based, but knowing this will help you keep your eyes and ears open for valid POEMs in the future.

Pharmaceutical Representatives

Pharmaceutical representatives (PRs) are seemingly the source of medical information that requires the least amount of effort—they come to *you* often bringing lunch! Frequently the information they supply is not relevant (DOE based) or the methodology of the studies isn't sound. This serves to remind us that work must be balanced with relevance and validity to define usefulness. Ask for their sources to assess the usefulness of their information.

Even more helpful may be to ask PRs explicitly for the information needed to decide if their suggested therapy is better than what you currently prescribe. The STEPS mnemonic is a helpful way to remember these key questions. *S*afety refers to the long-term absence of harmful drug effects, whereas *t*olerability is the significance of more short-term side effects. Since we cannot judge whether a patient's headache is more significant than his stomach upset, the best measure of tolerability is pooled dropout rates from placebo-controlled trials. This information tells us who had side effects of any kind severe enough to warrant discontinuing the medication. *E*ffectiveness is not only whether the medication works—for POEM outcomes—but how well it works. We need to consider the clinical significance of the data presented (see application section). *P*rice refers to the cost not only of the medication but also of any associated monitoring required. *S*implicity is the ease of the medication regimen from the patient's perspective, and may influence compliance.

Application of Evidence

Clinical Significance

An important consideration in the application of evidence to individual patients is the clinical significance of the effect. It is not sufficient to ask whether one treatment is better than another; we need also to ask *how much* better. For example, one of the currently available antivirals is proven to shorten the duration of symptoms in adults with influenza (i.e., the statistical difference). But the amount of benefit is approximately a half day less of symptoms (i.e., the clinical difference). In the course of a 7-day illness, this may not seem worth the expense or risk of intestinal side effects to most patients. Yet to a busy stockbroker, taking the drug to possibly be able to return to work 4 hours sooner may be worthwhile.

Clinical experience and patient perspective are the basis for deciding the clinical significance of such a finding.

The number needed to treat (NNT) is another measure of clinical significance. Calculated as the inverse of the rate difference, NNT tells us how many patients need to be treated for one to receive benefit. Consider two patients with elevated cholesterol: first is a 63-year-old male smoker with hypertension, total cholesterol of 250, and a high-density lipoprotein (HDL) of 35; the other is a 37-year-old woman with a total cholesterol of 328 and an HDL of 40. The statins have been shown to lessen the risk of a cardiac event by approximately 30%.[21] Intuitively we'd encourage the man to take lipid-lowering medication more so than the woman, because his cardiac risk is greater. NNT allows us to quantify the benefit for each. Using incidence data from the Framingham study[22] to calculate baseline risk, the man's 10-year risk of a cardiac event decreases from 30.4% to 20% and the woman's from 3.2% to 2.2% if treated with a statin. This yields NNTs of 9.6 and 100, respectively. Thus, the same medication yields a very different level of clinical benefit for each patient and should influence who receives treatment.

Clinical Jazz

If EBM were solely medical decision making based on evidence, it would become what critics call cookbook medicine, and could be done by computers. Either that, or we'd be paralyzed, unable to care for patients at all because there just aren't valid POEM data for much of what we do. Yet if we practiced only experience-based medicine, we may still be bloodletting our preeclamptic patients because some of them got better. Lest we consider this an unrealistic example, how many of us are victims of the latest bad experience bias? Objective evidence of this bias is seen in obstetricians whose cesarean section rates increase following an adverse event.[23] Clinical experience is important, but as the sole evidence source it is fraught with biases that would never be acceptable if presented in a research article: small sample sizes, lack of blinding or randomization, lack of standardized outcome measurements, and nonrandom loss to follow-up.

EBM is not really in competition with clinical experience. The newer definition of EBM integrates the use of evidence, balanced with clinical judgment and the patient's preferences. In the IM model, this is clinical jazz. And like fine jazz music, it requires structure—the evidence of valid POEMs—along with improvisation—our clinical experience. Following this structure can actually be liberating. Basing our decisions on well-done outcomes-based research helps us avoid being ping-ponged between conflicting recommendations and may increase our confidence with medical decision making. The simplicity of the structure allows us ample room for improvisation. We use our judgment every time we make a decision in the absence of ideal evidence: POEMs with study flaws, or valid DOEs, or no existing evidence addressing our clinical questions. A key component of EBM in these situations is the awareness that our decisions are based on this lesser-than-ideal level of evidence and keeping our eyes open to replace that information when better quality data are available.[24]

Conditions with multiple valid POEMs, such as hypertension, provide opportunities to improvise as well. We rely on our clinical experience to apply most research data, since the patients we see in our offices are rarely as healthy, nor is our follow-up as rigorous, as those in randomized controlled trials.

Finally, our artistry and communication skills are needed to negotiate with patients whose preferences differ from the evidence. One patient may refuse colon cancer screening, despite high-quality relevant data in support of flexible sigmoidoscopy; a mother may demand a computer tomography (CT) scan to evaluate her child, who has an acute headache but a normal exam and evidence demonstrating no need for a CT scan. A restricted view of EBM would suggest we only perform those services with evidence to support them; patient-centered medicine may seem like bowing to the patient's wishes regardless of the evidence. Clinical jazz is harmonizing the evidence, our experience, and our patients' views together to come to a reasonable decision. This is a true evidence-based medical practice!

References

1. Sackett DL, Rosenberg WMC, Gray JAM, Haynes RB, Richardson WS. Evidence based medicine: what it is and what it isn't. BMJ 1995;312:71–2.
2. Evans DE, Haynes RB, Gilbert JR, et al. Educational package on hypertension for primary care physicians. Can Med Assoc J 1984;130:719–22.
3. Shin JH, Haynes RB, Johnston ME. Effect of problem-based, self-directed undergraduate education on life-long learning. Can Med Assoc J 1993;148:969–76.
4. Slawson DC, Shaughnessy AF. Treatment of corneal abrasions. JAMA 1996;275(11):837.
5. Flynn CA, D'Amico F, Smith G. Should we patch corneal abrasions? J Fam Pract 1998;47:264–70.
6. Fineburg HV. Clinical evaluation: how does it influence medical practice? Bull Cancer 1987;74:333–46.
7. Ely JW, Oheroff JA, Ebell MH, et al. Analysis of questions asked by family doctors regarding patient care. BMJ 1999;319: 358–61.
8. Slawson DC, Shaughnessy AF, Bennett JH. Becoming a medical information master: feeling good about not knowing everything. J Fam Pract 1994;38:505–13.
9. Connelly DP, Rich EC, Curley SP, Kelly JT. Knowledge resource preferences of family physicians. J Fam Pract 1990;30: 353–9.
10. Arndt KA. Information excess in medicine. Overview, relevance to dermatology, and strategies for coping. Arch Dermatol 1992;128:1249–56.
11. Oxman AD, Sacket DL, Guyatt GH. Users' guides to the medical literature. I. How to get started. JAMA 1993;270:2093–5.
12. Asking answerable clinical questions. In: Sackett DL, Straus SE, Richardson WS, Rosenberg W, Haynes RB, eds. Evidence-based medicine: How to practice and teach EBM, 2nd ed. Edinburgh: Churchill Livingstone, 2000;13–27.
13. Schoenen J, Jacquy J, Lenaerts M. Effectiveness of high-dose riboflavin in migraine prophylaxis: a randomized controlled trial. Neurology 1998;50:466–70.
14. Ebell MH, Barry HC, Slawson DC, Shaughnessy AF. Finding POEMs in the medical literature. J Fam Pract 1999;48:350–5.
15. Slawson DC, Shaughnessy AF. Becoming an information master. Using "medical poetry" to remove the inequities in health care delivery. J Fam Pract 2001;50:51–6.
16. Oxman AD, Guyatt GH. The science of reviewing research. Ann NY Acad Sci 1993;703:125–33.
17. Hayward RSA, Wilson MC, Tunis SR, Bass ER, Guyatt G. Users' guides to the medical literature. VIII. How to use clinical practice guidelines. A. Are the recommendations valid? JAMA 1995;274:570–4.
18. Slawson DC, Shaughnessy AF. Obtaining useful information from expert-based sources. BMJ 1997;314:947–9.
19. Chalmers TC. Informed consent, clinical research and the practice of medicine. Trans Am Clin Climatol Assoc 1982;94:204–12.
20. Shaughnessy AF, Slawson DC, Bennett JH. Becoming an information master: a guidebook to the medical information jungle. J Fam Pract 1994;39:489–99.
21. LaRosa JC, He J, Vupputuri S. Effect of statins on risk of coronary disease: a meta-analysis of randomized controlled trials. JAMA 1999;282:2340–6.
22. Anderson KM, Odell PM, Wilson PW, Kannel WB. Cardiovascular disease risk profiles. Am Heart J 1990;121:293–8.
23. Turretine MA, Ramirez MM. Adverse perinatal events and subsequent cesarean rates. Obstet Gynecol 1999;94:185–9.

6
Population-Based Health Care

Bruce W. Goldberg

The past two decades have witnessed extensive changes within our health care system. An abundance of new diagnostic technologies and therapeutic advances have emerged. Concomitantly, doubts about the efficacy of some technologies, concerns about escalating health care costs, the increasing numbers of individuals without health insurance or access to care, and growing consumer and corporate interest have led to changes in the organization and delivery of health care services. Today's health care system attempts to link effectiveness to the improvement of public health outcomes, and seeks to reduce costs. Consumers and policy makers are looking for the right mix of efficacious, cost-effective technology delivered in a highly personal and consumer friendly setting.

Family physicians are assuredly qualified to bring forth many of the improvements that policy makers, consumers, and professionals are seeking. Family practice has proved that it can deliver exceptional primary care to individuals and families. The specialty has been built upon the commitment to quality, personal attention, and interpersonal relationships that all patients seek. It has proven that it can deliver cost-effective care while at the same time improving quality. As first-contact providers of primary health care, family physicians are in a position to support efforts to improve access to care. However, to function effectively within a health care system that links effectiveness to the improvement of public health outcomes will require an additional set of skills. Family physicians will need to expand beyond the traditional one-to-one physician–patient model and acquire the knowledge and skills for population-based clinical practice.[1,2]

The term *population-based medicine* or *population-based health care* has emerged over the past 10 years and has been defined in a number of ways.[1,3–5] It represents a transformation of medicine from that solely focused on the individual patient to also include a focus on broader populations or denominators. These two distinct approaches are not mutually exclusive but rather complementary. As physicians seek to improve the health of individuals they must also consider a greater population and look to improve the outcome of their interventions at the level of both the individual and the population.

A number of forces have led to the development and growing application of population-based health care. The growth of managed care, with its attention to discrete panels of patients, capitated payments, and incentives based on population health indices, has been a powerful influence. However, perhaps more significant has been the increased emphasis on both clinical and cost effectiveness, concerns about appropriate resource allocation, and greater attention to public health outcomes. In addition, the development of computer-based information technology now provides tools that greatly enhance and make more accessible the practice of population-based health care.

Population-based medicine is now recognized as an important component of both medical practice and medical education. The Association of American Medical Colleges affirmed that physicians need to be committed to using systematic approaches for promoting and maintaining the health of both individuals and the populations of which those individuals are members.[3] They identified population-based medicine as one of the contemporary issues in medicine that will require changes in the design and content of educational programs to be more in concert with this developing trend.

Throughout this chapter, the term *population-based health care* is used to denote an expanded set of physician obligations and an approach to medical care that places the individual patient within the context of the larger community and places the physician responsible for optimizing the health of both individual patients and the population from which the patient comes. This chapter reviews the rationale for family physicians' involvement in population-based health care and the skills necessary to be successful at it.

Toward a New Model

Medical practice changed dramatically during the 20th century. At the start of the 20th century most physicians were community-based general practitioners. Medical care was primarily provided in the doctor's office or the patient's home, and the role of technology and the hospital were limited. In 1910 Abraham Flexner[6] called for a transformation of medical education into the academic, teaching hospital model currently used by all medical schools in the United States.

By 1960 most physicians were specialists and an increasing amount of care was provided in the hospital (see Chapters 1 and 130). Concomitant with this move toward specialists, large numbers of new and technologically advanced diagnostic tests and therapeutic agents rapidly became available. Physicians not only had new treatments but also, for the first time, the technology to prevent diseases such as polio, smallpox, and tetanus. The beliefs that disease could be conquered by technology and that health was the absence of disease became dominant societal paradigms.

Despite all the medical advances, it soon became clear that our health care system was in disarray. Medical care was too costly for the indigent, and there was both a shortage and maldistribution of physicians. The Medicare and Medicaid programs were enacted, and the 1964 Health Professional Assistance Amendments eventually led to a dramatic increase in the number of health providers trained in the United States.[7] The prevailing beliefs about medical care began to change from a disease-oriented approach toward a more ecologic model. In 1961 White and his colleagues[8] wrote:

It is now time for health professions, and particularly for faculty members with clinical interests, to join their colleagues from the other disciplines, and to accord medical-care research and teaching the same priority they have accorded research in the fundamental mechanisms of pathologic processes. Investigation and teaching directed at improved understanding of the ecology of medical care and ways of favorably modifying it eventually should reduce the time lag between developments in the laboratory and delivery to the consumers of new knowledge accruing from the vast sums of money that the latter are currently paying for disease-oriented research.

The ecologic model of medical care views health as a naturally occurring state that is affected by an assortment of interrelated factors: (1) environment—physical and social; (2) access to health care services—preventive, curative, and rehabilitative; (3) heredity; and (4) personal lifestyle.[9,10] Through this ecologic model, medicine is recognized as a social institution that can improve health by both curing disease and improving the way we organize and deliver health care. This ecologic philosophy and a series of changes in our health care system have prompted an appeal for physicians to adopt a more population-based perspective.[1,11]

A Transforming Health Care System

The current transformation of our health care system has been driven by problems in three domains: cost, quality, and access. The cost of providing medical care has risen at a dramatic rate and an ever-increasing portion of our gross domestic product is being devoted to health. As a result we have seen a variety of complex changes in the organization, financing, and delivery of health care. Since the mid-1980s there has been a marked alteration in community-based medical practices. Free-standing individual and small group practices are vanishing across the United States as a dramatic horizontal and vertical consolidation within the health delivery system is taking place.[1] Care is now increasingly organized and delivered by large health care systems, not individual practices or hospitals.

Simultaneously, there has been a move away from fee-for-service reimbursement toward capitation. Under such arrangements, physicians and health care systems are paid not for the individual services they render, but rather for providing care for an identified population. There has been much debate about the ethics of capitation and its ability to provide the appropriate incentives. Whether it will continue as a system for provider reimbursement remains to be seen.[12] However, it appears that it will continue as the means by which health plans are paid.

Concerns about the quality of health care being delivered and the cost of paying for inappropriate or ineffective services have led to increased importance being placed on practice guidelines, treatment algorithms, outcomes measurements, and evidence-based medicine. Practice guidelines and treatment algorithms help individual physicians provide appropriate care while at the same time assisting with resource allocation. When based on rigorous review of the available literature, rather than individual experience, guidelines and algorithms assist physicians in the development of population-based clinical skills.[13]

Efforts to evaluate the appropriateness and effectiveness of care are moving away from "process measures" and toward a more outcomes-oriented approach. Measuring the quality of care often focuses on the activities carried out by providers when treating patients (process measures). For example, in individuals with asthma, assessing quality of care through process measures might include determining if spirometry is performed, inhaled corticosteroids are appropriately prescribed, vital signs are monitored, or appropriate follow-up care is arranged. On the other hand, an outcomes-oriented approach might assess quality by determining the number of emergency room visits or hospital admissions for asthmatics within a year. Process measures tend to be readily available and indeed are necessary if providers are to evaluate and improve their delivery systems, although research has not clearly demonstrated a correlation between commonly used process measures and the desirable outcomes that result from receiving medical care. As such, many experts now believe that directly measuring the outcomes or the results of care is the best way to evaluate quality.[14]

Issues surrounding access to health care have compelled medicine to consider a more population-based perspective. The large number of Americans without health insurance or with inadequate health insurance has prompted examination of unmet needs and health risks across the entire population. From both economic and ethical perspectives, there is renewed emphasis on bringing the uninsured into the health care system and ensuring that access is available to all citizens. Access has been recognized as an important issue among insured populations as well. Managed care plans are now being appraised based on their ability to provide access for an entire population. The percentage of members with visits to primary care providers and the existence of access standards for various services have become important measures of health plan performance[15] (see Chapter 130).

Family Practice: A Population-Based Specialty

In many ways, family practice has always been a population-based specialty. It emerged during the late 1960s from growing discontent with the biomedical philosophy and a health care system that was dominated by specialist physicians who confronted individuals from the standpoint of an organ system. Family practice moved away from the biomedical philosophy and embraced a more ecologic or biopsychosocial model. Fundamental to family practice was a holistic view of the individual, a belief in health promotion and disease prevention, and care of the patient in the context of family and community. The concept of caring for patients in the context of family and community attests to the specialty's value of maintaining a population-based perspective.

As an academic discipline, family medicine has provided leadership for an expanded view of health and advanced medical knowledge in a variety of areas. On an individual patient level, family medicine has recognized the importance of the interaction between patient and physician and its effects on patient outcomes and satisfaction. Similarly, family practice has increased our understanding of family dynamics and how to treat individuals in the context of their families. At the population level, family medicine has been a leader in advancing the concepts and practice of community-oriented primary care (COPC).

Essentials for Population-Based Health Care

To solve clinical problems at the individual level, physicians utilize an array of tools and a characteristic approach to the patient encounter learned and practiced through many years of clinical training. Likewise, the practice of population-based medicine requires a distinct set of tools and a characteristic approach to problem solving. Described below are the essential requirements for the practice of population-based health care.

Defined Population

Fundamental to population-based practice is an identifiable population. Often referred to as the "denominator," in the context of population-based practice the population is that group of individuals to whom health care is delivered and the level at which its effectiveness and outcomes are measured. Although superficially it often appears simplistic, defining or enumerating the denominator population is a pivotal and intricate task.

As initially conceived, COPC described the denominator population as a geographic community for which the physician was responsible.[16,17] Such a definition has not easily been adopted within the United States. In the U.S., family physicians have commonly viewed their active patients as their denominator population. Such a restricted interpretation excludes many patients who might consider themselves part of a physician's practice but who themselves had not made an office visit during the past few years. When considered from the perspective of population-based preventive services, such a definition excludes many patients in need of screening procedures or immunizations but who had not recently been in the office. Similarly, such an interpretation might exclude intervening with individuals at high risk for developing a particular disease. As such, it is important for family physicians to consider not only whom they see in the office but also whom they do not see. Within a managed care setting, this task can be greatly simplified as family physicians receive lists of members assigned to them.

The definition of a population clearly changes depending on one's vantage point. Managed care organizations would certainly define their membership as their population and so they direct efforts at improving health across a variety of practices. Alternatively, individual practitioners or even health systems might enumerate, or actually list, all individuals in their patient population who have or who are at risk for a particular problem or condition.

Epidemiology

Successfully addressing problems from a population perspective requires that physicians have knowledge and understanding of the basic epidemiologic and demographic characteristics of their population. Additionally, they must understand the natural history of conditions and disease processes within their particular community. This is often difficult for primary care physicians whose primary locus of education has been the hospital or tertiary care setting. In such settings physicians are taught to care for problems from the perspective of the most infrequent, uncommon, and most complicated cases, and then are expected to extrapolate to patterns that prevail in the community.

Physicians should also have some basic knowledge and skill in epidemiology and access to individuals with advanced expertise in the field. Consider, for example, a common medical problem such as hypertension. Assessing the effectiveness of pharmacologic treatment for the hypertensive patient requires one to measure an individual's blood pressure. Assessing the effectiveness of a population-based intervention to decrease the incidence of hypertension in a community requires using fundamental epidemiologic techniques. Physicians therefore require basic knowledge about data collection, existing data sets, data analysis, sample sizes, statistical techniques, and extrapolating information from secondary data sets. The skills necessary to perform modest, practice-based epidemiologic investigations and to integrate them into the process of clinical care has been termed "primary care epidemiology."[18]

Informatics

To successfully practice population-based health care requires efficient management of large amounts of information (see

Chapter 127). The increasing availability and growth of information and database technology within medical practice has greatly enhanced the analysis of population-based data. It is, therefore, imperative that physicians maintain basic proficiency with emerging data management technology.

Computerized databases containing basic demographic information about a physician's practice can rapidly provide information to assist in enumerating the population. Computerized reminder systems to increase the provision of preventive services and improve certain clinical conditions are already being widely used.[19,20] The addition of computerized clinical information including diagnoses, medication lists, and laboratory, physical examination, and diagnostic testing data provides a powerful mechanism for improving outcomes. For example, using a clinical information database, it is now possible for a practice to readily identify individuals at high risk for certain conditions and to identify practice patterns or treatment modalities that are more likely to result in favorable outcomes.

Teamwork

Unlike the family physician of the 1960s who was likely to practice alone, today's family physicians practice as part of groups and complex organizations. The ability to function effectively as part of a health care team and not simply as the sole provider of care is therefore important for the effective practice of population-based health care. Although population-based health care can be practiced in relative isolation, it is far more effective when harnessing the skills and expertise of a variety of health professionals.[21] Population-based health care moves beyond the model of a physician seeing a patient and making a clinical intervention. Rather, it entails a more comprehensive approach that, depending on the problem being addressed, may necessitate the skills of a variety of health professionals. The effective use of subspecialists, nurses, public health professionals, health educators, and community resources is essential. To be successful in working with such multidisciplinary groups requires excellent leadership and communication skills.

Evidence-Based Medicine

Evidence-based medicine is a process and philosophy that integrates the best external evidence with individual clinical expertise and patient choice[22] (see Chapter 5). It is a four-step process that includes formulation of a question, searching the literature, appraising the validity of information, and applying it. The application of information includes the ability to consolidate it with clinical judgment in medical practice. As such, this process and philosophy differ greatly from the expert-based approach that has often been at the foundation of clinical medicine.

Evidence-based medicine has often been discussed in reference to the decisions that clinicians make when caring for individuals. The data upon which to base clinical decisions primarily come from population-based studies. Yet these studies often neglect patient individuality and clinician judgment. In this regard, the feasibility of applying evidence-based medicine to the hundreds of decisions that primary care physicians need to make everyday has been questioned. However, when approaching clinical problems from a population-based perspective, it is a much more practical and effective tool.

Appraising the literature and applying it to populations are the most complex and daunting of the four-step evidence-based medicine process. Applying the best available evidence to bring about improvement in a population's health is the essence of population-based health care and perhaps its greatest challenge. Methods for appraising the validity of evidence in the literature have matured over the past few years but the field is still evolving and challenges exist.[23] Perhaps in greatest need of development are the mechanisms by which evidence and recommendations can be put into practice. For example, the U.S. Preventive Services task force has done an outstanding job in appraising the literature and making recommendations regarding the performance of clinical preventive services.[24] However, real challenges remain in the application of this information and in translating the synthesis and distillation of knowledge into practice. While few doubt the benefit of screening for hypertension in the general population or for breast cancer in women over 50, the real challenge is in the widespread adoption of such screening practices by physicians, patients, policy makers, and communities. To do this requires teamwork and skills beyond those of the individual physician.

Social and Ethical Considerations

Intrinsic to population-based care and medical practice are a number of social and ethical considerations that include, but are not limited to, equity, access, advocacy, and the allocation and distribution of resources. Analogously, some fear that population-based medicine may undermine the physician–patient relationship and the role of physicians in advocacy for their individual patient.[25] However, caring for populations and individuals need not be antithetical, but rather complementary. This is consistent with the ethos of family practice that considers care in the context of community.

Consider access to health care. For the individual patient, the physician needs to assure access to their services. Are there sufficient appointment slots? Is there an easy means to contact the physician for information and advice? Extending that beyond the individual physician, one must also consider access to specialty care, ancillary services, and hospital care. However, population-based health care takes such considerations and expands them to the level of the population. Rather than just considering the issue of access for an individual patient, the physician is now compelled to look at the needs of the entire population.

One Model for Population-Based Health Care

A number of approaches to population-based health care have been described.[4,21,26] All advocate a systematic approach to denominator and problem identification, intervention, and evaluation. Their structures are similar and, interestingly, resemble those used by continuous quality improvement programs. COPC is one approach to population-based health care that can help family physicians balance their obligations to the individual patient with that of society at large. In view of family medicine's rich history of participation in the development and application of COPC, it has been chosen for illustration below.

COPC Philosophy

Community-oriented primary care was proposed decades ago as a practical way to integrate the principles of community medicine and public health into the delivery of primary care health care. Despite compelling appeals for its widespread use, its successful application in the United States has been limited.[27] As our health care system moves toward greater recognition of the importance of population-based health care, COPC is again emerging as an excellent model for the practice of population-based health care.[9]

Community-oriented primary care is a systematic strategy to address the health care of the community and individuals in an integrated fashion.[16,28] An example is adult-onset diabetes. On the individual level, the family physician is concerned with maintaining the patient's glycemic control and preventing complications that can result from the disease. It involves a skilled clinical assessment that requires a medical history and physical examination, laboratory testing, pharmacologic management, and patient education regarding diet and exercise. Care at the community or population level would also concern itself with glycemic control and preventing complications, but accomplishing this goal among an entire population necessitates a different approach. It might require identifying individuals with poor glucose control, determining the reasons for poor control, and developing an intervention or program to improve their health. Likewise it might mean setting up a system to ensure that all diabetics have a yearly retinal examination or to determine the frequency at which certain complications occur in a particular denominator population.

At the population level the physician might want to address other questions: What is the contribution of diabetes to the morbidity and mortality of the population? Are diagnostic and treatment resources being used efficiently? What are the population's knowledge and attitudes toward diabetes, obesity, and exercise? How many diabetics are being treated, and how many are adequately controlled? Finally, in the COPC model, one would ideally look to prevent diabetes from occurring among high-risk individuals rather than solely seeking to improve their treatment.

COPC Process

The COPC paradigm can easily be utilized within a primary care practice. Such a practice must be comprehensive and able to provide the array of services necessary to meet the needs of the population it serves. Care must be accessible and continuous over time. Furthermore, the primary care provider must act as the coordinator of care when multiple individuals are involved in delivering services and information.

The COPC process provides a methodology for identifying and addressing the major health problems of a population. It applies the principles of management to the planning and implementation of health care. The COPC process requires four elements.

1. Defining and characterizing the community or denominator population
2. Identifying health and health care problems
3. Intervention or modification of practice patterns
4. Monitoring the impact of the intervention

These four elements are organized into a cycle (Fig. 6.1) through which decisions are continually influenced by feedback of population-based information.[29]

Defining or enumerating the characteristics of the denominator population is the initial step in the COPC cycle. As discussed previously, it is important for family physicians to take an expansive view of their population and consider those individuals who do not regularly seek care in the office. Ideally, physicians should be able to list all individuals in their population and describe their sociodemographic characteristics, cultural beliefs, and health-related behaviors.

Once a population is defined, the family physician can identify and prioritize its significant health problems and major health risks. Subsequently, intervention strategies can be planned to address them. Ideally, this goal is best accomplished with the substantive involvement of individuals from the denominator population. It is perhaps the inclusion of the community that distinguishes COPC from population-based health care.[30]

With a program in place, emphasis shifts to surveillance. The purpose of surveillance is to collect information that assesses the impact of the intervention. Surveillance may utilize primary data collection, such as information collected in

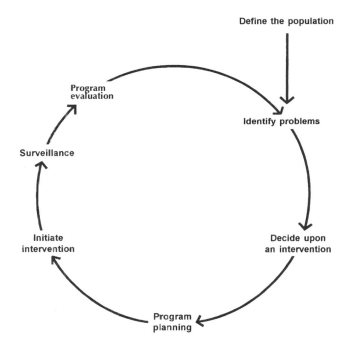

Fig. 6.1. The community-oriented primary care cycle.

population surveys, or it may rely on secondary data collected from clinical encounters or other available data sets. Regardless of the methods used, it is important that the appropriate surveillance techniques and evaluation methods have been developed prior to beginning an intervention. Once an intervention is completed, it may be impossible to collect important information retrospectively.

The final step in the COPC cycle is program evaluation. Both process and outcome evaluations should be performed. Process evaluations can help identify problems in the design and implementation of an intervention. Outcomes-based evaluations assist in determining the extent to which an intervention had its desired effect. Like interventions, evaluations should concentrate on the denominator population; assessing only the numerator population can convey erroneous information.[31] Finally, evaluations should focus on both the positive and the negative impacts of a program.

Summary

Changes in the way health care is organized, delivered, and financed has brought about the need for physicians to expand their practice beyond the level of the individual patient to also provide care for populations. To solve clinical problems at the individual level, physicians utilize an array of tools and a characteristic approach to the patient encounter learned and practiced through many years of clinical training. Basic epidemiology, teamwork, informatics, evidence-based medicine, and a systematic process provide physicians with the necessary tools and an approach to solving problems on the population level.

References

1. Greenlick MR. Educating physicians for population-based clinical practice. JAMA 1992;267:1645–8.
2. Geyman JP, Bliss E. What does family practice need to do next? A cross-generational view. Fam Med 2001;33:259–67.
3. Association of American Medical Colleges. Contemporary issues in medicine—medical informatics and population health: report II of the medical school objectives project. Acad Med 1999;74:130–41.
4. Weiss K. A look at population-based medical care. Dis Mon 1998;44:353–69.
5. Ferguson JH. Curative and population medicine: bridging the great divide. Neuroepidemiology 1999;18:111–9.
6. Flexner A. Medical education in the United States and Canada. Bulletin 4. New York: Carnegie Foundation for the Advancement of Teaching, 1910.
7. Zervanos NJ. A century of medical educational reform: family practice, a specialty whose time has come. Fam Med 1996;28: 144–6.
8. White KL, Williams TF, Greenberg BG. The ecology of medical care. N Engl J Med 1961;265:885–92.
9. Wright RA. Community-oriented primary care, the cornerstone of health care reform. JAMA 1993;269:2544–7.
10. Freymann JG. The public's health care paradigm is shifting: medicine must swing with it. J Gen Intern Med 1989;4:313–9.
11. O'Connor PJ. Community-oriented primary care in a brave new world. Arch Fam Med 1994;3:493–4.
12. Bodenheimer TS. Capitation's uncertain future. J Gen Intern Med 2001;16:281–2.
13. Bero L, Rennie D. The Cochrane collaboration: preparing, maintaining, and disseminating systematic reviews of the effects of health care. JAMA 1995;274:1935–8.
14. Siu AL, McGlynn EA. Choosing quality of care measures based on the expected impact of improved care on health. Health Serv Res 1992;27:619–50.
15. HEDIS 2001, vol. 1. Washington, DC: National Committee for Quality Assurance, 2000.
16. Kark SL. The practice of community oriented primary health care. London: Appleton-Century-Crofts, 1981.
17. Kark SL, Kark E. An alternative strategy in community health care: community-oriented primary health care. Isr J Med Sci 1983;19:707–13.
18. Mullan F, Nutting PA. Primary care epidemiology: new uses of old tools. Fam Med 1986;18:221–5.
19. Ebell MH, Frame P. What can technology do to, and for, family medicine. Fam Med 2001;33:311–9.
20. Dickey LL, Gemson DH, Carney P. Office system interventions supporting primary care-based health behavior change counseling. Am J Prev Med 1999;17:299–308.
21. Taplin S, Galvin MS, Payne T, Coole D, Wagner E. Putting population-based care into practice: real option or rhetoric? J Am Board Fam Pract 1998;11:116–26.
22. Sackett DL, Rosenberg WM, Gray JA, Haynes RB, Richardson WS. Evidence based medicine: what it is and what it isn't. BMJ 1996;312:71–2.
23. Mulrow CD, Cook D, eds. Systematic reviews: synthesis of best evidence for health care decisions. Philadelphia: American College of Physicians, 1998.
24. Harris RP, Helfand M, Woolf SH, et al. Current methods of the U.S. Preventive Services Task Force: a review of the process. Am J Prev Med 2001;20(3S):21–35.
25. Feldman DS, Novack DH, Gracely E. Effects of managed care on physician-patient relationships, quality of care, and the ethical practice of medicine: a physician survey. Arch Intern Med 1998;158:1626–32.
26. Rivo ML. It's time to start practicing population-based health care. Fam Pract Manag 1998;5:37–46.
27. Longlett SK, Kruse JE, Wesley RM. Community-oriented primary care: critical assessment and implications for resident education. J Am Board Fam Pract 2001;14:141–7.
28. Tollman S. Community oriented primary care: origins, evolution, applications. Soc Sci Med 1991;32:633–42.
29. Abramson JH. Community-oriented primary care—strategy, approaches, and practice: a review. Public Health Rev 1988;16: 35–98.
30. Henley E, Williams RL. Is population-based medicine the same as community-oriented primary care? Fam Med 1999;31:501–2.
31. Nutting PA, Barrick JE, Logue SC. The impact of a maternal and child health program on the quality of prenatal care: an analysis by risk group. J Community Health 1979;4:267–79.

Part II

The Practice of Family Medicine

7

Clinical Prevention

Anthony F. Jerant

Background

Definition and Focus

Clinical prevention involves the maintenance and promotion of health and the reduction of risk factors that result in injury and disease. The elements of clinical prevention include screening tests, counseling interventions, and immunizations, as well as chemoprophylaxis, the use of drugs or biologics taken by asymptomatic persons to reduce the risk of developing a disease. This chapter provides the tools for family physicians to meet the formidable challenge of providing clinical prevention services in an evidence-based manner. While mass screening is an important public health tool, the material in this chapter mostly concerns the individualized screening that is offered during single physician–patient encounters. Detailed information regarding lifestyle counseling can be found in Chapter 8. Consistent with the approach of the U.S. Preventive Services Task Force (USPSTF), the focus of this chapter is primary and secondary prevention. *Primary prevention* is the reduction of risk factors for diseases before they occur, whereas *secondary prevention* is the identification and treatment of diseases or conditions at an early stage. Both primary and secondary prevention concern asymptomatic individuals. *Tertiary prevention*, which reduces the future negative health effects of diseases or conditions that have already become symptomatic, is discussed in many other chapters in this book.

The Ongoing Need for Clinical Preventive Services

Tremendous successes in clinical prevention have been realized in the last 50 years. For example, mortality due to coronary heart disease has declined by approximately 50%, and more than half of this decline can be attributed to preventive interventions such as reducing cigarette smoking and detecting and treating hyperlipidemia. The greater than 90% reductions in morbidity and mortality due to measles, mumps, rubella, smallpox, pertussis, tetanus, and *Haemophilus influenzae* type b resulting from mass vaccination programs are an even greater prevention success story.[1]) Nevertheless, the most common underlying causes of death in the United States reflect an ongoing need to improve and expand the delivery of clinical preventive services (Table 7.1).[2]

The leading health indicators in *Healthy People 2010*, a blueprint for public health resulting from collaboration between hundreds of state and federal agencies and organizations, were clearly developed with this list in mind (Table 7.2).[3] Because the average life expectancy in America lags behind that of nearly 20 other nations, one of the main goals of *Healthy People 2010* is to increase life expectancy and years of healthy life. There are 467 specific objectives within 28 focus areas derived from population data, many pertinent to clinical prevention (Table 7.2). The full report is available on the World Wide Web (WWW) at *http://www.health. gov/healthypeople*. *Healthy People 2010* provides a critical link between public health and clinical practice. Approaching every patient with the focus areas in mind will help in detecting the most prevalent contributors to early morbidity and mortality. For example, in the focus area for cancer, one objective is to increase the proportion of adults who receive colorectal cancer screening from 35% to a target of 50%. A 55-year-old patient who has not undergone screening might be informed that while it can reduce the risk of death due to colorectal cancer, only one in three eligible Americans receives such screening. Subsequently, the patient's genetic and environmental history, health habits, and preferences can be used to develop a personalized colorectal cancer prevention plan.

Table 7.1. **Actual Causes of Death in the United States in 1990**

Cause of death	Estimated number of deaths	Percent of total deaths
Tobacco use	400,000	19
Diet / activity patterns	300,000	14
Alcohol	100,000	5
Microbial agents	90,000	4
Toxic agents	60,000	3
Firearms	35,000	2
Sexual behavior	30,000	1
Motor vehicles	25,000	1
Illicit use of drugs	20,000	<1
Total	1,060,000	50

Source: McGinnis and Foege,[2] with permission.

Evidence-Based Clinical Prevention

Principles of Screening

Seven principles should be considered in evaluating a potential screening intervention:

1. The disease or condition in question must lead to substantial morbidity or mortality. Several conditions consistently account for the greatest disease burden in our society. This burden can be quantified using the disability-adjusted life year (DALY), the sum of the years of life lost due to premature mortality and the years of life lost due to disability in a population (Table 7.3).[4] Screening patients for these conditions and underlying risk factors should be given the highest priority.

2. The screening test employed to detect the condition should be accurate. An ideal screening test has both a high sensitivity (low false-negative rate) and high specificity (low false-positive rate). In practice, screening tests seldom meet this ideal. For example, the CAGE acronym screening tool for alcohol abuse and dependence (see Chapter 59) has fair specificity (76–96%) but relatively low sensitivity (74–78%) at the most commonly used definition of abnormal (two or more affirmative responses). Lowering the abnormal cutoff to one or more affirmative responses would increase the number of problem drinkers detected (sensitivity 86–90%) but would also lead to more false positives (specificity 52–93%).[5] The trade-off between sensitivity and specificity is a characteristic of all screening tests.

3. The disease or condition should have a high incidence and/or prevalence. Screening is effective for some conditions only when individuals reach a certain age, are of a certain gender, or possess certain risk factors that place them at increased risk for developing the conditions. Stated another way, as the prevalence of a disease or condition increases, the positive predictive value (PPV) of a test increases, regardless of its sensitivity and specificity:

$$PPV = \frac{(Sensitivity \times Prevalence)}{[(Sensitivity \times Prevalence)] + [(1 - Specificity) \times (1 - Prevalence)]}.$$

Another way to estimate the overall "yield for effort" of a screening intervention is the number needed to screen (NNS),[6] which is analogous to the concept of number needed to treat (NNT) in clinical therapeutics. NNS is calculated by taking the reciprocal of the absolute risk reduction (ARR) conferred by screening:

$$NNS = 1/ARR$$
$$= 1/[(No.\ of\ outcome\ events/No.\ of\ screened\ patients) - (No.\ of\ outcome\ events\ /\ No.\ of\ controls)]$$

For example, the NNS to prevent one death due to tuberculosis (TB) in programs involving intravenous drug abusers ranges from 103 to 4650, while in studies involving individuals with no identifiable risk factors for TB, the NNS to prevent one death due to TB ranges from 132,690 to 606,797.[7] These figures provide clinically tangible estimates of the yield of TB screening and reinforce the concept that the PPV of a screening test increases as the incidence of the condition in question increases in the screened population.

4. The disease or condition should have an asymptomatic period during which it can be detected. Diseases with long asymptomatic periods, such as cervical cancer, are easier to target with screening than diseases with a short preclinical duration, such as leukemia. However, for conditions with a long preclinical duration, *lead-time bias* can make it appear that a group of screened patients survives longer than a

Table 7.2. **Healthy People 2010 Leading Health Indicators and Focus Areas Pertinent to the Clinical Prevention Encounter**

Leading indicators	Focus areas
Access to health care	Arthritis, osteoporosis, and chronic back conditions
Environmental quality	
Immunization	Cancer
Injury and violence	Chronic kidney disease
Mental health	Diabetes
Overweight and obesity	Disability and secondary conditions
Physical activity	Family planning
Responsible sexual behavior	Heart disease and stroke
Substance abuse	Human immunodeficiency virus
Tobacco use	Immunization and infectious disease
	Injury and violence prevention
	Maternal, infant, and child health
	Nutrition and overweight
	Oral health
	Physical activity and fitness
	Respiratory diseases
	Sexually transmitted diseases
	Substance abuse
	Tobacco abuse
	Vision and hearing

Source: Healthy People 2010,[3] with permission.

Table 7.3. **Estimated Top 10 Leading Causes of Disability-Adjusted Life Years (DALYs) in the United States, 1996**

	Men			Women		
Rank	Cause	DALYs	% of total DALYs	Cause	DALYs	% of total DALYs
	All conditions	18,314,401	100	All conditions	15,886,327	100
1	Ischemic heart disease	1,969,256	10.75	Ischemic heart disease	1,181,298	7.45
2	Road traffic collisions	933,953	5.10	Unipolar major depression	1,073,911	6.77
3	Lung/bronchus cancers	812,675	4.44	Cerebrovascular disease	836,345	5.27
4	HIV/AIDS	773,640	4.22	Lung/bronchus cancers	549,963	3.47
5	Alcohol abuse/ dependence	736,572	4.02	Osteoarthritis	521,443	3.24
6	Cerebrovascular disease	673,877	3.68	Breast cancer	514,729	3.21
7	Homicide and violence	567,322	3.10	COPD	510,084	3.19
8	COPD	545,350	2.98	Dementia/CNS degenerative disorder	506,858	3.16
9	Self-inflicted	541,640	2.96	Diabetes mellitus	500,932	2.90
10	Unipolar major depression	477,040	2.60	Road traffic collisions	459,489	2.61

CNS = central nervous system; COPD = chronic obstructive pulmonary disease.

Source: Michaud et al.[4] copyright 2001, American Medical Association, with permission.

group that is not screened. In reality the screened patients may simply be finding out they have the disease earlier, during its asymptomatic phase. To avoid attributing benefit to a screening program that suffers from lead-time bias, screening decisions should be based on comparisons of actual mortality rates, rather than on measures that are affected by the time elapsed since diagnosis, such as 5-year survival rates. A second problem related to preclinical disease duration is called *length-time bias.* Less aggressive cases have a longer asymptomatic period and are more likely to be detected by screening than more aggressive cases. Thus, a screening program may appear to improve survival when it is actually only detecting more indolent cases that have a better prognosis. Prostate cancer screening has been criticized for many reasons, including strong concerns about lead-time and length-time bias.

5. The disease or condition should have a widely available and acceptable treatment known to improve outcomes. Many conditions that are otherwise worthy candidates for screening are not currently amenable to treatments that change their natural history. For example, dementia accounts for a substantial number of DALYs (Table 7.3) but fails to meet this criterion.

6. The screening procedure should entail reasonable health risks and financial cost. Screening cost estimates should include not only the cost of an initial screening test but also costs related to repeat office visits, specialty referrals, additional testing, false positives, and complications. Formal cost-effectiveness analyses of preventive interventions account for all of these factors. The end point of such analyses is often the ratio of dollar cost per quality-adjusted life year (QALY), the product of the number of years of life and the quality of those years as measured from 0 (indifference between life and death) to 1 (full health) on a questionnaire. Thus, a screening test that provides an average of 12 more years of life with a quality rating or *utility* of 0.4 is said to provide 4.8 QALYs. Although there is no universal agreement on what dollar cost/QALY ratio

cut-point defines a cost-effective screening program, Table 7.4 provides a comparative listing of ratios for some widely accepted preventive practices.[8] Cost-effectiveness must be considered from the societal perspective, but clinicians can greatly influence the costs of screening programs by taking an evidence-based approach.

7. The screening procedure should be acceptable to the patient and society. The yield of a screening program is decreased if many candidates are unwilling to undergo testing. For example, colorectal cancer screening via flexible sigmoidoscopy is supported by research evidence, but the rate of patient adherence to a physician's recommendation for flexible sigmoidoscopy is only 35%, partially due to test discomfort and inconvenience.

Family physicians can effectively individualize the following general clinical prevention guidelines by considering

Table 7.4. **Median, Minimum, and Maximum Estimated Cost-Utility Ratios for Various Preventive Interventions**

Preventive service	Median $/QALY	Minimum $/QALY	Maximum $/QALY
Immunizations and vaccinations	1500	Cost-saving	140,000
Screening tests			
Cardiovascular disease	3300	950	130,000
Neoplasms	18,500	Cost-saving	140,000
Other diseases	11,500	Cost-saving	450,000
Counseling			
HIV risk behaviors	1200	Cost-saving	2400
Cardiovascular risk factors	74,000	Cost-saving	8,900,000

QALY = quality-adjusted life year.

Source: Reprinted by permission of Elsevier Science from Stone et al.[8]

Table 7.5. **Interventions Considered and Recommended for Prevention, Birth to 10 Years; Leading Causes of Death: Perinatal Conditions, Congenital Anomalies, Sudden Infant Death Syndrome (SIDS), Injuries**

Interventions for the general population

SCREENING
Height and weight
Blood pressure
Vision screen (age 3–4 years)
Hemoglobinopathy screen (birth)[a]
Phenylalanine level (birth)[b]
T_4 and/or TSH (birth)[c]

COUNSELING
Injury prevention
Child safety car seats (age <5 years)
Lap shoulder belts (age ≥5 years)
Bicycle helmet; avoid bicycling near traffic
Smoke detector, flame retardant sleepwear
Hot water heater temperature <120–130°F
Window/stair guards, pool fence
Safe storage of drugs, toxic substances, firearms, and matches
Syrup of ipecac, poison control phone number
CPR training for parents/caregivers

Diet and exercise
Breast-feeding, iron-enriched formula, and foods (infants and toddlers)
Limit fat and cholesterol; maintain caloric balance; emphasize grains, fruits, and vegetables
Regular physical activity
Substance use
Effects of passive smoking*
Antitobacco message*
Dental health
Regular visits to dental care provider*
Floss, brush with fluoride toothpaste daily*
Advice about baby bottle tooth decay*
IMMUNIZATIONS
See Tables 7.6 and 7.7
CHEMOPROPHYLAXIS
Ocular prophylaxis (birth)

Interventions for high-risk populations (see detailed high-risk definitions in footnotes)

POPULATION	POTENTIAL INTERVENTIONS
Preterm or low birth weight	Hemoglobin/hematocrit (high risk 1 [HR1])
Infants of mothers at risk for HIV	HIV testing (HR2)
Low income; immigrants	Hemoglobin/hematocrit (HR1); purified protein derivative (PPD (HR3)
TB contacts	PPD (HR3)
Native American/Alaska Native	Hemoglobin/hematocrit (HR1); PPD (HR3); hepatitis A vaccine (HR4); pneumococcal vaccine (HR5)
Travelers to developing countries	Hepatitis A vaccine (HR4)
Residents of long-term care facilities	PPD (HR3); hepatitis A vaccine (HR4); influenza vaccine (HR6)
Certain chronic medical conditions	PPD (HR3); pneumococcal vaccine (HR5); influenza vaccine (HR6)
Increased individual or community lead exposure	Blood lead level (HR7)
Inadequate water fluoridation	Daily fluoride supplement (HR8)
Family history of skin cancer; nevi, fair skin, eyes, hair	Avoid excess/midday sun, use protective clothing* (HR9)

[a]Whether screening should be universal or targeted to high-risk groups will depend on the proportion of high-risk individuals in the screening area, and other considerations.

[b]If done during first 24 hours of life, repeat by age 2 weeks.

[c]Optimally between day 2 and 6, but in all cases before newborn nursery discharge.

*The ability of clinician counseling to influence this behavior is unproved.

HR1—Infants age 6–12 months who are living in poverty; black, Native American, or Alaska Native; immigrants from developing countries; preterm and low birth weight infants; infants whose principal dietary intake is unfortified cow's milk.

HR2—Infants born to high-risk mothers whose HIV status is unknown. Women at high risk include past or present injection drug use; persons who exchange sex for money or drugs, and their sex partners; injection drug–using, bisexual, or HIV-positive sex partners currently or in past; persons seeking treatment for sexually transmitted diseases (STDs); blood transfusion during 1978–1985.

HR3—Persons infected with HIV, close contacts of persons with known or suspected TB, persons with medical risk factors associated with TB, immigrants from countries with high TB prevalence, medically underserved low-income populations (including homeless), residents of long-term care facilities.

HR4—Persons >2 years old living in or traveling to areas where the disease is endemic and where periodic outbreaks occur (e.g., countries with high or intermediate endemicity; certain Alaska Native, Pacific Island, Native American, and religious communities). Consider for institutionalized children aged ≥2 years. Clinicians should also consider local epidemiology.

HR5—Immunocompetent persons >2 years old with certain medical conditions, including chronic cardiac or pulmonary disease, diabetes mellitus, and anatomic asplenia. Immunocompetent persons ≥2 years old living in high-risk environments or social settings (e.g., certain Native-American and Alaska-Native populations).

Table 7.5. (Continued)

HR6—Annual vaccination of children ≥6 months old who are residents of chronic care facilities or who have chronic cardiopulmonary disorders, metabolic diseases (including diabetes mellitus), hemoglobinopathies, immunosuppression, or renal dysfunction.

HR7—Children about age 12 months who (1) live in communities in which the prevalence of lead levels requiring individual intervention, including residential lead hazard control or chelation, is high or undefined; (2) live in or frequently visit a home built before 1950 with dilapidated paint or with recent or ongoing renovation or remodeling; (3) have close contact with a person who has an elevated lead level; (4) live near lead industry or heavy traffic; (5) live with someone whose job or hobby involves lead exposure; (6) use lead-based pottery; or (7) take traditional ethnic remedies that contain lead.

HR8—Children living in areas with inadequate water fluoridation (see Table 7.8)

HR9—Persons with a family history of skin cancer, a large number of moles, atypical moles, poor tanning ability, or light skin, hair, and eye color.

T_4 = thyroxine; TSH = thyroid-stimulating hormone.

Source: U.S. Preventive Services Task Force,[9] with permission.

each of these seven screening principles and the way they apply to their specific practice settings and patient populations.

Clinical Preventive Services Guidelines

The 1996 recommendations of the USPSTF, found in the *Guide to Clinical Preventive Services*, 2nd edition,[9] were chosen as the primary resource for this section for several reasons. First, the recommendations are generated using an explicit evidence-based approach, and the items listed in the age-specific recommendation tables are those for which the USPSTF concluded that there is either good or fair evidence to support the recommendation. Second, in contrast to the recommendations of organizations such as the American Cancer Society (ACS) and medical professional groups, the recommendations are not directly tied to public awareness efforts and professional or political agendas. Finally, the USPSTF makes recommendations throughout the life cycle and is thus highly relevant to family physicians. A revised third edition of the guide is scheduled to appear in 2002, and new recommendations and updates are being posted on the WWW as they are released; go to *www.ahrq.gov/clinic/uspstfix.htm*.

General Recommendations for All Age Groups

In general, new patients should undergo a comprehensive history and physical examination, have a health risk appraisal completed, and be educated regarding age-specific preventive services. Previous health records should be obtained to avoid duplication of services, and additional services may be added routinely based on the individual's risk profile. Because the evidence base is continually growing and changing, family physicians must frequently update their clinical prevention protocols as new evidence becomes available.

Birth to Ten Years (Table 7.5)

Period Immediately Following Birth

Screening for congenital conditions is the first priority in prevention for newborns. All 50 states require testing for phenylketonuria and congenital hypothyroidism, but states vary regarding other mandated tests. In addition to mandated screening tests, infants born to mothers at risk for human immunodeficiency virus (HIV) infection but whose infection status is unknown should be considered for HIV testing. From the time of birth and throughout childhood, it is important to be aware of family psychosocial and socioeconomic factors such as poverty and parental substance abuse that place children at increased risk for multiple adverse health outcomes and developmental problems. For example, parents who smoke tobacco must be counseled regarding the risks to infants of passive smoke exposure, including higher rates of otitis media and lower respiratory tract infections. Counseling of smoking mothers has been shown to reduce their children's exposure to environmental tobacco smoke, regardless of the mothers' eventual cessation status.[10]

Passive tobacco smoke exposure is also associated with an increased risk for sudden infant death syndrome (SIDS),[11] a leading cause of death in this age group. The USPSTF has not produced a recommendation regarding optimal infant sleep position, but substantial evidence suggests that SIDS is associated with the prone sleep position. Further, although no definite causal link has been established, populations in which physician counseling and media efforts has led to increased use of the supine sleeping position have observed decreased rates of SIDS, resulting in an American Academy of Pediatrics (AAP) recommendation that physicians counsel all parents to place infants to sleep on their backs on a firm surface.[12] A dialogue regarding breast-feeding should ideally be begun during the early prenatal period. Nevertheless, because it is associated with lower rates of otitis media and infectious diarrhea,[13] physicians should encourage all mothers to breast-feed at the time of birth. This protective effect follows a dose-response relationship so that infants who are not exclusively breast-fed still benefit. Newborns should ideally receive their first hepatitis B vaccination, using a thimerosal-free formulation, prior to discharge from the hospital.

Infancy to Age Two

Ensuring that appropriate growth is being maintained is an important preventive task in this group. Very low birth weight

Table 7.6. **Recommended Childhood Immunization Schedule United States, 2002**

	range of recommended ages			catch-up vaccination				preadolescent assessment			
Age Vaccine	Birth	1 mo	2 mo	4 mo	6 mo	12 mo	15 mo	18 mo	24 mo	4–6 yr	11–12 yr	13–18 yr
Hepatitis B[1]	Hep B #1	only if mother HBsAg(−)									Hep B series	
		Hep B #2			Hep B #3							
Diphtheria, Tetanus, Pertussis[2]		DTaP	DTaP	DTaP			DTaP		DTaP		Td	
Haemophilus influenzae Type b[3]		Hib	Hib	Hib		Hib						
Inactivated Polio[4]		IPV	IPV		IPV				IPV			
Measles, Mumps, Rubella[5]						MMR#1				MMR#2	MMR#2	
Varicella[6]						Varicella			Varicella			
Pneumococcal[7]		PCV	PCV	PCV	PCV				PCV	PPV		

Vaccines below this line are for selected populations - - - - - -

Hepatitis A[8]									Hepatitis A series		
Influenza[8]					Influenza (yearly)							

This schedule indicates the recommended ages for routine administration of currently licensed childhood vaccines, as of December 1, 2001, for children through age 18 years. Any does not given at the recommended age should be given at any subsequent visit when indicated and feasible. ▨ Indicates age groups that warrant special effort to administer those vaccines not previously given. Additional vaccines may be licensed and recommended during the year. Licensed combination vaccines may be used whenever any components of the combination are indicated and the vaccine's other components are not contraindicated. Providers should consult the manufacturers' package inserts for detailed recommendations.

1. Hepatitis B vaccine (Hep B). All infants should receive the first dose of hepatitis B vaccine soon after birth and before hospital discharge; the first dose may also be given by age 2 months if the infant's mother is HBsAg-negative. Only monovalent hepatitis B vaccine can be used for the birth dose. Monovalent or combination vaccine containing Hep B may be used to complete the series; four doses of vaccine may be administered if combination vaccine is used. The second dose should be given at least 4 weeks after the first dose, except for Hib-containing vaccine which cannot be administered before age 6 weeks. The third dose should be given at least 16 weeks after the first dose and at least 8 weeks after the second dose. The last dose in the vaccination series (third or fourth dose) should not be administered before age 6 months.

Infants born to HBsAg-positive mothers should receive hepatitis B vaccine and 0.5 mL hepatitis B immune globulin (HBIG) within 12 hours of birth at separate sites. The second dose is recommended at age 1–2 months and the vaccination series should be completed (third or fourth dose) at age 6 months.

Infants born to mothers whose HBsAg status is unknown should receive the first dose of the hepatitis B vaccine series within 12 hours of birth. Maternal blood should be drawn at the time of delivery to determine the mother's HBsAg status; if the HBsAg test is positive, the infant should receive HBIG as soon as possible (no later than age 1 week).

2. Diphtheria and tetanus toxoids and acellular pertussis vaccine (DTaP). The fourth dose of DTaP may be administered as early as age 12 months, provided 6 months have elapsed since the third dose and the child is unlikely to return at age 15–18 months. **Tetanus and diphtheria toxoids (Td)** is recommended at age 11–12 years if at least 5 years have elapsed since the last dose of tetanus and diphtheria toxoid-containing vaccine. Subsequent routine Td boosters are recommended every 10 years.

3. Haemophilus influenzae type b (Hib) conjugate vaccine. Three Hib conjugate vaccines are licensed for infant use. If PRP-OMP (PedvaxHIB® or ComVax® [Merck]) is administered at ages 2 and 4 months, a dose at age 6 months is not required. DTaP/Hib combination products should not be used for primary immunization in infants at ages 2, 4 or 6 months, but can be used as boosters following any Hib vaccine.

4. Inactivated polio vaccine (IPV). An all-IPV schedule is recommended for routine childhood polio vaccination in the United States. All children should receive four doses of IPV at ages 2 months, 4 months, 6–18 months, and 4–6 years.

5. Measles, mumps, and rubella vaccine (MMR). The second dose of MMR is recommended routinely at age 4–6 years but may be administered during any visit, provided at least 4 weeks have elapsed since the first dose and that both doses are administered beginning at or after age 12 months. Those who have not previously received the second dose should complete the schedule by the 11–12 year old visit.

6. Varicella vaccine. Varicella vaccine is recommended at any visit at or after age 12 months for susceptible children, i.e. those who lack a reliable history of chickenpox. Susceptible persons aged ≥13 years should receive two doses, given at least 4 weeks apart.

7. Pneumococcal vaccine. The heptavalent **pneumococcal conjugate vaccine (PCV)** is recommended for all children age 2–23 months. It is also recommended for certain children age 24–59 months. **Pneumococcal polysaccharide vaccine (PPV)** is recommended in addition to PCV for certain high-risk groups. See MMWR 2000;49(RR-9);1–35.

8. Hepatitis A vaccine. Hepatitis A vaccine is recommended for use in selected states and regions, and for certain high-risk groups; consult your local public health authority. See MMWR 1999;48(RR-12);1–37.

9. Influenza vaccine. Influenza vaccine is recommended annually for children age ≥6 months with certain risk factors (including but not limited to asthma, cardiac disease, sickle cell disease, HIV, diabetes; see MMWR 2001;50(RR-4):1–44), and can be administered to all others wishing to obtain immunity. Children aged ≤12 years should receive vaccine in a dosage appropriate for their age (0.25 mL if age 6–35 months or 0.5 mL if aged ≥3 years). Children aged ≤8 years who are receiving influenza vaccine for the first time should receive two doses separated by at least 4 weeks.

For additional information about vaccines, vaccine supply, and contraindications for immunization, please visit the National Immunization Program Website at www.cdc.gov/nip or call the National Immunization Hotline at 800-232-2522 (English) or 800-232-0233 (Spanish).

Approved by the Advisory Committee on Immunization Practices (www.cdc.gov/nip/acip), the American Academy of Pediatrics (www.aap.org), and the American Academy of Family Physicians (www.aafp.org).

children, an increasing population, often have postnatal growth rates that lag behind those of term infants. Special growth curves, produced by several formula manufacturers, should be utilized until "catch up" growth is achieved, usually at about 3 years of age. Injury prevention counseling should also be emphasized. Injuries account for two of every five deaths in children aged 1 through 4, four times the number of deaths due to birth defects, the second leading cause of death in this age group. Clinicians must also remain alert to the various presentations of family violence, which may include injuries initially attributed to accidents. While the debate regarding lead screening in childhood continues, the USPSTF and Centers for Disease Control and Prevention (CDC) currently recommend a selective approach. Children should be screened if they live in areas with risk for lead exposure, belong to groups that may be at risk (such as the poor), or are found to be at risk based on a "yes" answer to any of the following three questions: (1) Does the child live in or regularly visit a house that was built before 1950? (2) Does the child live in or regularly visit a house that was built before 1978 with recent (within the last 6 months) or ongoing renovations or remodeling? (3) Does the child have a sibling or playmate who has or did have lead poisoning? Physicians must also be aware of local policies, since some states mandate screening.

Table 7.6 provides the most recent universal childhood immunization schedule.[14] Recent changes include the addition of pneumococcal conjugate vaccination and, in certain areas, hepatitis A vaccination. Unfortunately, many children receive immunizations late or not at all, placing them at risk for infectious diseases and increasing the chance of community infectious disease outbreaks in vaccinated individuals.[15] Physician failure to review immunization status at each visit and unnecessary practice policies against vaccination in certain circumstances, such as in the presence of acute minor illness with low-grade fever, are important causes of missed opportunities to vaccinate.[16] Evidence-based vaccination protocols, provider education, and immunization flow sheets may help to reduce missed opportunities. A "catch-up" schedule should be employed for children who have fallen behind to rapidly return them to full coverage (Table 7.7).[17] The Immunization Action Coalition produces excellent resources for both physicians and parents on the WWW: *http://www.immunize.org/*.

To help prevent dental caries, children who live in communities with low levels of fluoride in the water should be prescribed fluoride supplements beginning at 6 months of age. Other dental preventive efforts include counseling parents to put children to bed without a bottle and recommending periodic dentist visits beginning at around age 3.

Table 7.7. **Minimal Age for Initial Childhood Vaccinations and Minimal Interval Between Vaccine Doses by Type of Vaccine***

Vaccine type	Minimal age for dose 1	Minimal interval between doses 1 and 2	Minimal interval between doses 2 and 3	Minimal interval between doses 3 and 4
Hepatitis B	Birth	1 month	2 months	*a*
DtaP (DT)*b*	6 weeks	4 weeks	4 weeks	6 months
Combined DTwP-Hib*c*	6 weeks	1 month	1 month	6 months
Hib (primary series)				
HbOC	6 weeks	1 month	1 month	*c*
PRP-T	6 weeks	1 month	1 month	*c*
PRP-OMP	6 weeks	1 month	*c*	
Inactivated poliovirus	6 weeks	4 weeks	4 weeks*d*	*e*
Pneumococcal conjugate	6 weeks	1 month	1 month	*c*
MMR	12 months*f*	1 month		
Varicella	12 months	4 weeks		

DtaP (DT diphtheria and tetanus toxoids and acellular pertussis vaccine (diphtheria and tetanus toxoids vaccine); DTwP-Hib = diphtheria and tetanus toxoids and whole-cell pertussis vaccine–*Haemophilus influenzae* type b conjugate vaccine; HbOC = oligosaccharides conjugated to diphtheria CRM197 toxin protein; PRP-T = polyrigosylribitol phosphate polysaccharide conjugated to tetanus toxoid; PRP-OMP = polyribosylribitol phosphate polysaccharide conjugated to a meningococcal outer membrane protein; MMR = measles-mumps-rubella.

*The minimal acceptable ages and intervals may not correspond with the optimal recommended ages and intervals for vaccination. For current recommended routine schedules, see Table 7.6.

*a*The final dose of hepatitis B vaccine is recommended at least 4 months after the first dose and no earlier than 6 months of age.

*b*The total number of doses of diphtheria and tetanus toxoids should not exceed six each before the seventh birthday.

*c*The booster doses of Hib and pneumococcal vaccines that are recommended following the primary vaccination series should be administered no earlier than 12 months of age and at least 2 months after the previous dose.

*d*For unvaccinated adults at increased risk of exposure to poliovirus with less than 3 months but more than 2 months available before protection is needed, three doses of inactivated poliovirus (IPV) should be administered at least 1 month apart.

*e*If the third dose is given after the third birthday, the fourth (booster) dose is not needed.

*f*Although the age for measles vaccination may be as young as 6 months in outbreak areas where cases are occurring in children younger than 1 year, children initially vaccinated before the first birthday should be revaccinated at 12 to 15 months of age and an additional dose of vaccine should be administered at the time of school entry or according to local policy. Doses of MMR or other measles-containing vaccines should be separated by at least one month.

Adapted from Epidemiology and Prevention of Vaccine-Preventable Diseases, 6th ed,[17] with permission.

Table 7.8. **Interventions Considered and Recommended for Prevention, Age 11 to 24 Years; Leading Causes of Death: Injuries, Homicide, Suicide, Malignancies, Heart Disease**

Interventions for the general population

SCREENING
Height and weight
Blood pressure[a]
Papanicolaou (Pap) test (women)[b]
Chlamydia screen[c]
Rubella serology or vaccination history (females >12 years old)
Assess for problem drinking

COUNSELING
Injury prevention
Lap/shoulder belts
Bicycle/motorcycle/all-terrain vehicle (ATV) helmets*
Smoke detector*
Safe storage/removal of firearms*
Substance use
Avoid tobacco use
Avoid underage drinking and illicit drug use*
Avoid alcohol/drug use while driving, swimming, boating, etc.*

Sexual behavior
Sexually transmitted disease (STD) prevention; abstinence*; avoid high-risk behavior*; condoms/female barrier with spermicide*
Diet and exercise
Limit fat and cholesterol; maintain caloric; balance; emphasize grains, fruits, and vegetables
Adequate calcium intake (females)
Regular physical activity*
Dental health
Regular visits to dental care provider*
Floss; brush with fluoride toothpaste daily*

IMMUNIZATIONS
See Tables 7.6 and 7.7
Rubella (females >12 years old)[d]

CHEMOPROPHYLAXIS
Multivitamin with folic acid (females planning/capable of pregnancy)

Interventions for high-risk populations (see detailed high-risk definitions in footnotes)

POPULATION	POTENTIAL INTERVENTIONS
High-risk sexual behavior	RPR/VDRL (HR1); screen for gonorrhea (female) (HR2), HIV (HR3), chlamydia (female) (HR4); hepatitis A vaccine (HR5)
Injection or street drug use	RPR/VDRL (HR1); HIV screen (HR3), hepatitis A vaccine (HR5); PPD (HR6); advice to reduce infection risk (HR7)
TB contacts; immigrants, low income	PPD (HR6)
Native Americans, Alaska Natives	Hepatitis A vaccine (HR5); PPD (HR6); pneumococcal vaccine (HR8)
Travelers to developing countries	Hepatitis A vaccine (HR5)
Certain chronic medical conditions	PPD (HR6); pneumococcal vaccine (HR8); influenza vaccine (HR9)
Settings where adolescents and young adults congregate	Second MMR (HR10)
Susceptible to varicella, measles, mumps	Varicella vaccine (HR11); MMR (HR12)
Blood transfusion between 1975 and 1985	HIV screen (HR3)
Institutionalized persons; health care/lab workers	Hepatitis A vaccine (HR5); PPD (HR6); influenza vaccine
Family history of skin cancer; nevi, fair skin, eyes, hair	Avoid excess/midday sun; use protective clothing* (HR13)
Prior pregnancy with neural tube defect	Folic acid 4.0 mg (HR14)
Inadequate water fluoridation	Daily fluoride supplement (HR15)

[a]Periodic blood pressure (BP) for persons aged ≥21 years.

[b]If sexually active at present or in the past: q ≤ 3 years. If sexual history is unreliable, begin Pap tests at age 18 years.

[c]If sexually active.

[d]Serologic testing, documented vaccination history, and routine vaccination against rubella (preferably with MMR) are equally acceptable alternatives.

*The ability of clinician counseling to influence this behavior is unproven.

HR1—Persons who exchange sex for money or drugs, and their sex partners; persons with other STDs (including HIV); and sexual contacts of persons with active syphilis. Clinicians should also consider local epidemiology.

HR2—Women who have two or more sex partners in the last year; a sex partner with multiple sexual contacts; exchanged sex for money or drugs; or a history of repeated episodes of gonorrhea. Clinicians should also consider local epidemiology.

HR3—Men who had sex with men after 1975; past or present injection drug use; persons who exchange sex for money or drugs, and their sex partners; injection drug-using, bisexual, or HIV-positive sex partner currently or in the past; blood transfusion during 1978–1985; persons seeking treatment for STDs. Clinicians should also consider local epidemiology.

HR4—Sexually active females with multiple risk factors including history of prior STD; new or multiple sex partners; age under 25; nonuse or inconsistent use of barrier contraceptives; cervical ectopy. Clinicians should also consider local epidemiology.

HR5—Persons living in, traveling to, or working in areas where the disease is endemic and where periodic outbreaks occur (e.g., countries with high or intermediate endemicity; certain Alaska-Native, Pacific Island, Native-American, and religious communi-

Table 7.8. (Continued)

ties); men who have sex with men; injection or street drug users. Vaccine may be considered for institutionalized persons and workers in these institutions, military personnel, and day care, hospital, and laboratory workers. Clinicians should also consider local epidemiology.

HR6—HIV positive, close contacts of persons with known or suspected TB, health care workers, persons with medical risk factors associated with TB, immigrants from countries with high TB prevalence, medically underserved low-income populations (including homeless), alcoholics, injection drug users, and residents of long-term facilities

HR7—Persons who continue to inject drugs.

HR8—Immunocompetent persons with certain medical conditions, including chronic cardiac or pulmonary disease, diabetes mellitus, and anatomic asplenia. Immunocompetent persons who live in high-risk environments or social settings (e.g., certain Native-American and Alaska-Native populations).

HR9—Annual vaccination of residents of chronic care facilities; persons with chronic cardiopulmonary disorders, metabolic diseases (including diabetes mellitus), hemoglobinopathies, immunosuppression, or renal dysfunction; and health care providers for high-risk patients.

HR10—Adolescents and young adults in settings where such individuals congregate (e.g., high schools and colleges), if they have not previously received a second dose.

HR11—Healthy persons aged ≥13 years without a history of chickenpox or previous immunization. Consider serologic testing for presumed susceptible persons aged ≥13 years.

HR12—Persons born after 1956 who lack evidence of immunity to measles or mumps (e.g., documented receipt of live vaccine on or after the first birthday, laboratory evidence of immunity, or a history of physician-diagnosed measles or mumps).

HR13—Persons with a family or personal history of skin cancer, a large number of moles, atypical moles, poor tanning ability, or light skin, hair, and eye color.

HR14—Women with previous pregnancy affected by neural tube defect who are planning pregnancy.

HR15—Persons aged <17 years living in areas with inadequate water fluoridation (see Table 7.8).

Source: U.S. Preventive Services Task Force,[9] with permission.

Two to Ten Years

Early detection of cardiovascular disease risk factors should be a major focus of screening beginning in early childhood. The body mass index (BMI) is a practical indicator of the appropriateness of weight for height in children age 2 and older and can be plotted on recently updated growth curves. Although a low BMI can indicate poor nutrition or an underlying medical disorder, elevated BMI in childhood is a more common problem that is reaching epidemic proportions in the U.S. For children 6 and older, a BMI from the 85th to the 95th percentile indicates overweight, whereas a BMI above the 95th percentile indicates obesity. Childhood obesity is associated with a host of immediate and long-term health risks, including increased rates of obesity and early mortality in adulthood.[18] Early identification should be followed by frequent monitoring and parental counseling regarding appropriate diet and nutrition (also see Chapter 53). Physicians should also screen children for a sedentary lifestyle, a major contributor to childhood obesity, and provide counseling regarding physical activity. All children should receive periodic blood pressure measurement throughout this period, and those with measurements that persistently exceed the 95th percentile values in tables based on gender, age, and height should receive further evaluation. Such tables are available on the WWW: *http://www.nhlbi.nih.gov/health/prof/ heart/hbp/hbp_ped.htm.*[19] The USPSTF and other organizations recommend cholesterol measurement only in children at high risk for adult coronary artery disease. Risk factors include a family history of premature cardiovascular disease or family members with cholesterol levels greater than 240 mg/dL.

Injury prevention counseling should be continued throughout this period. Thirty-three percent of injuries in this age group are due to violence, and 67% are due to unintentional injuries. Simple measures that reduce injury-related mortality in children, such as the use of helmets when bicycling, should be emphasized. Firearm safety should also be reviewed. Safe sun precautions should be periodically reviewed for children at increased risk for skin cancer, including those with a family history, a large number of moles, atypical moles, poor tanning ability, or light skin, hair, and eye color. The immunization series outlined in Table 7.6 should be continued as appropriate throughout childhood, so that all children will have received the full complement of vaccinations by the age of 12. Because purified protein derivative (PPD) testing of all children is exceedingly expensive and results in many false-positive tests, the USPSTF and CDC recommend a selective approach to screening based on the risk of exposure to TB. Exposure risk factors include birth or prior residence in a region where TB is highly prevalent, such as Southeast Asia, and close exposure to persons known or suspected to have TB.[20] (also see Chapter 84).

Eleven to Twenty-Four Years (Table 7.8)

This period includes adolescence, a developmental period that poses unique clinical prevention challenges (also see Chapter 22). Although comprehensive guidelines for preventive care in this age group have been proposed, evidence to support many of the items included is lacking. It is especially unclear whether physician counseling is capable of changing adolescent health behaviors and impacting on key adverse health outcomes. An important principle of prevention for this age group is opportunistic delivery of services. Since adolescents seldom visit a physician specifically for preventive care, every clinic visit by

Table 7.9. **Interventions Considered and Recommended for Prevention, Age 25 to 64 Years; Leading Causes of Death: Malignancy, Heart Disease, Injuries, HIV, Suicide, and Homicide**

SCREENING
- Blood pressure
- Height and weight
- Total blood cholesterol (men beginning age 35, women beginning age 45)
- Papanicolaou (Pap) test (women)[a]
- Fecal occult blood test[b] and/or sigmoidoscopy (≥50 years)
- Mammogram ± clinical breast exam (women 50–69 years)[c]
- Assess for problem drinking
- Rubella serology or vaccination history (women of childbearing age)[d]

COUNSELING
- Substance use
  - Tobacco cessation
  - Avoid alcohol/drug use while driving, swimming, boating, etc.*
- Diet and exercise
  - Limit fat and cholesterol; maintain caloric balance; emphasize grains, fruits, and vegetables
  - Adequate calcium intake (women)
  - Regular physical activity*

Injury prevention
- Lap/shoulder belts
- Motorcycle/bicycle/ATV helmets*
- Smoke detector*
- Safe storage/removal of firearms*

Sexual behavior
- STD prevention; avoid high-risk behavior*; condoms/female barrier with spermicide
- Unintended pregnancy: contraception

Dental health
- Regular visits to dental care provider*
- Floss, brush with fluoride toothpaste daily*

IMMUNIZATIONS
- Tetanus-diphtheria (Td) boosters
- Rubella (women of childbearing age)[d]

CHEMOPROPHYLAXIS
- Multivitamin or folic acid (women planning or capable of pregnancy)
- Discuss hormone prophylaxis (peri- and postmenopausal women)

Interventions for high-risk populations (see detailed high-risk definitions in footnotes)

POPULATION	POTENTIAL INTERVENTIONS
High-risk sexual behavior	RPR/VDRL (HR1); screen for gonorrhea (female) (HR2), HIV (HR3), chlamydia (female) (HR4); hepatitis B vaccine (HR5); hepatitis A vaccine (HR6)
Injection or street drug use	RPR/VDRL (HR1); HIV (HR3); hepatitis B vaccine (HR5); hepatitis A vaccine (HR6); PPD (HR7); advice to reduce infection risk (HR8)
Low income; TB contacts; immigrants; alcoholics	PPD (HR7)
Native Americans/Alaska Natives	Hepatitis A vaccine (HR6); PPD (HR7); pneumococcal vaccine (HR9)
Travelers to developing countries	Hepatitis B vaccine (HR5); hepatitis A vaccine (HR6)
Certain chronic medical conditions	PPD (HR7); pneumococcal vaccine (HR9); influenza vaccine (HR10)
Blood product recipients	HIV screen (HR3); hepatitis B vaccine (HR5)
Susceptible to measles, mumps, rubella	MMR (HR11); varicella vaccine (HR12)
Institutionalized persons	Hepatitis A vaccine (HR6); PPD (HR7); pneumococcal vaccine (HR9); influenza vaccine (HR10)
Health care/lab workers	Hepatitis B vaccine (HR5); hepatitis A vaccine (HR6); PPD (HR7);
Family history of skin cancer; fair skin, eyes, hair	Avoid excess/midday sun; use protective clothing* (HR13)
Previous pregnancy with neural tube defect	Folic acid 4.0 mg (HR14)

[a]Women who are or have been sexually active and who have a cervix: q ≤ 3 years.

[b]Annually.

[c]Mammogram q 1–2 years, or mammogram q 1–2 years with annual clinical breast examination.

[d]Serologic testing, documented vaccination history, and routine vaccination (preferably with MMR) are equally acceptable.

*The ability of clinician counseling to influence this behavior is unproven.

HR1—Persons who exchange sex for money or drugs, and their sex partners; persons with other STDs (including HIV); and sexual contacts of persons with active syphilis. Clinicians should also consider local epidemiology.

HR2—Women who exchange sex for money or drugs, or who have had repeated episodes of gonorrhea. Clinicians should also consider local epidemiology.

HR3—Men who had sex with men after 1975; past or present injection drug use; persons who exchange sex for money or drugs, and their sex partners; injection drug-using, bisexual, or HIV-positive sex partner currently or in the past; blood transfusion during 1978–1985; persons seeking treatment for STDs. Clinicians should also consider local epidemiology.

HR4—Sexually active females with multiple risk factors including: history of prior STD; new or multiple sex partners; age under 25; nonuse or inconsistent use of barrier contraceptives; cervical ectopy. Clinicians should also consider local epidemiology.

Table 7.9. (Continued)

HR5—Blood product recipients (including hemodialysis patients), persons with frequent occupational exposure to blood or blood products, men who have sex with men, injection drug users and their sex partners, persons with multiple recent sex partners, persons with other STDs (including HIV), travelers to countries with endemic hepatitis B.

HR6—Persons living in, traveling to, or working in areas where the disease is endemic and where periodic outbreaks occur (e.g., countries with high or intermediate endemicity; certain Alaska-Native, Pacific Island, Native-American, and religious communities); men who have sex with men; injection or street drug users. Vaccine may be considered for institutionalized persons and workers in these institutions, military personnel, and day care, hospital, and laboratory workers. Clinicians should also consider local epidemiology.

HR7—HIV positive, close contacts of persons with known or suspected TB, health care workers, persons with medical risk factors associated with TB, immigrants from countries with high TB prevalence, medically underserved low-income populations (including homeless), alcoholics, injection drug users, and residents of long-term facilities.

HR8—Persons who continue to inject drugs.

HR9—Immunocompetent persons with certain medical conditions, including chronic cardiac or pulmonary disease, diabetes mellitus, and anatomic asplenia. Immunocompetent persons who live in high-risk environments or social settings (e.g., certain Native-American and Alaska-Native populations).

HR10—Annual vaccination of residents of chronic care facilities; persons with chronic cardiopulmonary disorders, metabolic diseases (including diabetes mellitus), hemoglobinopathies, immunosuppression, or renal dysfunction; and health care providers for high-risk patients.

HR11—Persons born after 1956 who lack evidence of immunity to measles or mumps (e.g., documented receipt of live vaccine on or after the first birthday, laboratory evidence of immunity, or a history of physician-diagnosed measles or mumps).

HR12—Healthy adults without a history of chickenpox or previous immunization. Consider serologic testing for presumed susceptible adults.

HR13—Persons with a family or personal history of skin cancer, a large number of moles, atypical moles, poor tanning ability, or light skin, hair, and eye color.

HR14—Women with previous pregnancy affected by neural tube defect who are planning pregnancy.

Source: U.S. Preventive Services Task Force,[9] with permission.

an adolescent should be viewed as an opportunity to provide prevention. Unfortunately, very low rates of clinical preventive services delivery have recently been observed for the typical adolescent visit.[21] Although adolescents may initially be hesitant to discuss health risk behaviors, they appear to become more willing to do so with repeated physician efforts.[22] Appointment invitation letters can increase the number of visits made by adolescents specifically to receive preventive services.[23]

Between 50% and 75% of all deaths in this age group are due to unintentional injuries, suicides, and homicides. Providing brief counseling regarding proven injury prevention measures is prudent. Important recommendations regarding motor vehicle injury reduction might include not driving at night for the first year after a driver's license is obtained, not riding in a car with an intoxicated individual, and always using a three-point seat restraint.[24] Cardiovascular risk reduction measures such as recommending tobacco avoidance and regular exercise and screening for obesity should be continued. For sexually active teens, contraception and sexually transmitted disease (STD) avoidance counseling are critical. The third USPSTF has released an advance statement regarding chlamydia, the most common STD in the United States, recommending screening all women who are sexually active and aged 25 or younger; have more than one sexual partner; have had an STD in the past; and do not use condoms consistently and correctly, regardless of age. Periodic screening for other STDs in sexually active teens and young adults should also be considered.

Because most alcohol problems begin in early adulthood, the USPSTF recommends screening for problem drinking for all adolescents and young adults using either "careful history-taking" or a standardized questionnaire such as the CAGE. Although finding insufficient evidence to recommend for or against routine screening for other drug abuse, given the increasing prevalence of amphetamine and other illicit drug use in many areas, physicians should have a low threshold for questioning young people about drug use (also see Chapter 60).

In addition to ensuring that a tetanus booster is administered at about 10 years after the last childhood tetanus vaccination, physicians should inform college students about the increased risk of meningococcal infection in crowded dormitory settings and provide them with information regarding meningococcal vaccination.[25]

Twenty-Five to Sixty-Four Years (Table 7.9)
Women's Health Issues

Although preconception counseling is important for all young women, an opportunistic approach must be taken since few specifically request such care (see Chapter 10). Women planning pregnancy or at risk for unintended pregnancy should be advised to take folic acid, 0.4 to 0.8 mg/day, beginning at least 1 month prior to conception and continuing throughout the first trimester of pregnancy to reduce the risk of neural tube defects. This dose can be obtained by taking a prenatal vitamin daily. Physician advise about folic acid has been shown to dramatically increase patient compliance with this recommendation.[26] Screening for cervical cancer using the Papanicolaou (Pap) smear is recommended every 1 to 3 years for all women who have been sexually active and who have a cervix. Although the most cost-effective interval for repeat testing is controversial, the most important things physicians can do to reduce the incidence of cervical cancer are to ensure that as many women as possible receive at least some screening and to ensure that abnormal results are followed up appropriately. Of women who develop invasive cervical cancer, 50% have never had a Pap smear, 10% have not had a Pap smear within 5 years of diagnosis, and 10% have not received appropriate follow-up of a prior precancerous result.[27]

Breast cancer screening should be offered as women enter middle age, but the optimal time of initiation remains an emotionally charged, controversial issue (see Chapter 107). The USPSTF recommends screening with mammography alone or mammography plus clinical breast examination (CBE) for all women of ages 50 to 69. The task force found insufficient evidence to recommend for or against mammography or CBE for women of ages 40 to 49 or 70 and older, and for teaching patient breast self-examination at any age. In 1997, a National Institutes of Health (NIH) consensus panel initially issued a statement agreeing with the USPSTF position. Shortly after, following a storm of rebuttals by academicians, politicians, and professional interest and advocacy groups, the panel reversed its statement, recommending initiation of periodic mammography and CBE for all women beginning at age 40, as is advocated by the ACS. Unfortunately, these conflicting recommendations and the complexity of the medical literature in this area have greatly confused patients and physicians. It is clear that the potential mortality benefit from breast cancer screening in women of ages 40 to 49 is much smaller than that obtained by screening women of ages 50 to 75, and that beginning screening at an earlier age results in a higher lifetime incidence of false-positive tests.[28] For now, physicians must review the evidence, form their own conclusions, and then use an "informed consent" approach in negotiating a plan with patients. The National Cancer Institute's Breast Cancer Risk Assessment Tool may help in developing individualized recommendations: *http://bcra.nci.nih.gov/brc/*.

Physicians should also provide counseling to reduce the risk of osteoporosis by encouraging women to remain physically active, consume 1000 to 1500 mg of calcium daily, and avoid tobacco use. Bone density measurement may be indicated in women with significant risk factors for osteoporosis such as Caucasian ancestry, petite body frame, low body weight, tobacco use, excessive alcohol and caffeine intake, and prolonged corticosteroid use (see Chapter 122). During the perimenopause, discussion regarding hormone replacement therapy (HRT) should be initiated. Although long-term HRT reduces the risk of osteoporosis and associated fractures, its use is associated with a slight increase in the incidence of breast cancer, and its potential benefit in the primary and secondary prevention of cardiovascular disease remains unproved. Thus, an "informed consent" approach to counseling is advised, with careful weighing of patient preferences and risk factors for osteoporosis, heart disease, and breast cancer.

Men's Health Issues

Prostate cancer is the second leading cause of death for men over age 55, and African-American men have a slightly higher incidence of prostate cancer than other men. While acknowledging its clinical importance, the USPSTF found a lack of evidence to recommend for or against screening for prostate cancer with digital rectal examination (DRE), serum prostate-specific antigen (PSA), or other tests. Evidence that early diagnosis of prostate cancer improves long-term survival is lacking, and there are potential costs and psychological burdens related to the expected high number of false-positive screening tests is large[29] (see Chapter 98). Refinements in PSA testing are promising but have not yet been properly evaluated. Despite these concerns, the ACS recommends annual DRE for all men starting at age 40, annual PSA testing beginning at age 40 for African-American men and those with a history of prostate cancer, and annual PSA testing beginning at age 50 for all others. The lack of a clear evidence base for prostate cancer screening and the conflicting recommendations of various organizations have created confusion among physicians and patients alike. As with breast cancer screening in women under age 50, an "informed consent" approach to counseling and educating patients should be utilized. Because prostate neoplasms usually grow slowly, men with a life expectancy of less than 10 years should generally not be screened.

Issues of Importance to Both Men and Women

In addition to its importance as a major cardiovascular disease risk factor, tobacco use has been linked to increased risk for cervical, bladder, lung, and other cancers. Strong counseling regarding smoking cessation, adequate physical activity, and a prudent diet are part of general cancer prevention efforts (see Chapter 8). The USPSTF found insufficient evidence to recommend for or against routine screening for skin cancer by primary care providers or counseling patients to perform periodic skin self-examinations. However, because one in six Americans will develop skin cancer during their lifetime and the incidence of malignant melanoma has increased rapidly during the past decade, physicians should briefly assess skin cancer risk in all individuals (see Chapter 117). Those at increased risk should be advised to avoidance of sun exposure, particularly between 10 A.M. and 3 P.M., and to use protective clothing such as shirts and hats when outdoors. The USPSTF found insufficient evidence to recommend for or against advising sunscreen use. For patients at increased risk for malignant melanoma, such as those with familial atypical mole and melanoma syndrome, referral to a skin cancer specialist for evaluation and surveillance should be considered.

Screening for colorectal cancer should be offered to all average-risk men and women beginning at age 50 (see Chapter 92). The USPSTF recommends annual fecal occult blood testing (FOBT), periodic flexible sigmoidoscopy (FS), or both, stating that there is insufficient evidence to make more specific recommendations. Colonoscopy can detect proximal adenomas and neoplasms, but it is more expensive than FS, is associated with a higher risk of complications such as perforation, and has not been shown to be superior in reducing colorectal cancer mortality. Modeling studies suggest that annual FOBT combined with FS every 5 years, beginning at age 50, is the most cost-effective approach to screening and may reduce colorectal cancer mortality by 50% to 80%.[30] As for cervical cancer screening, the major focus in colorectal cancer detection should be to ensure that as many eligible people as possible receive at least some type of screening. Less than half of eligible patients have undergone FOBT or FS within the preceding 5 years.[31] Medicare provides reimbursement for screening FOBT and FS and, beginning in July 2001, will also reimburse for screening colonoscopy once every 10 years. Even a single colonoscopy at 55 years of age may reduce colorectal cancer mortality by 30% to 50%.[30] Patients who are reluctant to undergo colorectal cancer screening may be willing to have "once in a lifetime" screening. More aggressive screening should be considered for those at increased risk for colorectal cancer, such as those with a family history of colorectal cancer or adenomatous polyps.[32]

Outside of cancer screening measures, cardiovascular disease prevention should be the major focus of preventive efforts in this age group, including periodic blood pressure screening. The third USPSTF has issued an advanced recommendation to periodically test total cholesterol levels in all men of ages 35 and older and all women of ages 45 and older (see Chapter 119). This extends the recommendations of the second USPSTF, which supported routine cholesterol screening only through age 65. High-density lipoprotein (HDL) and low-density lipoprotein (LDL) screening is recommended for individuals at high risk for cardiovascular disease. The American College of Physicians (ACP) recommends periodic total cholesterol screening in men of ages 35 to 65 and women of ages 45 to 65, with follow-up HDL testing for individuals with elevated levels.[33] Treatment decisions in the ACP recommendations are based on the ratio of total to HDL cholesterol, based on research indicating that higher ratios confer increased risk for cardiovascular disease. By contrast, the National Cholesterol Education Program's (NCEP) Adult Treatment Panel III recommends that a routine fasting lipoprotein profile (total, HDL, and LDL cholesterol and triglyceride levels) be obtained every 5 years in all adults of ages 20 or older.[34] As for the cancer screening controversies outlined above, physicians must weigh the evidence supporting each recommendation and collaborate with patients to determine the appropriate course of action.

Tobacco cessation counseling should be provided when applicable, and information on a low-fat diet that is rich in fresh fruits and vegetables and on regular physical activity should be conveyed. The incidence of obesity is increasing at an alarming rate in the United States, conferring increased risk for major cardiovascular risk factors such as hypertension and elevated cholesterol. Periodic weight and height assessment and BMI surveillance should be provided, with further evaluation and intervention offered to those individuals who are overweight (BMI 25.0–29.9) or obese (BMI ≥30.0). Although the USPSTF found insufficient evidence to recommend for or against screening for diabetes mellitus in asymptomatic adults, given its association with obesity and its role as a cardiovascular risk fac-

tor, physicians should have a low threshold for obtaining screening fasting serum glucose levels (see Chapter 120). Diabetes screening should also be considered for those with a family history of diabetes and those from high-risk ethnic groups, including Hispanics and Native Americans. Physicians often have difficulty determining the overall level of cardiovascular disease risk for individuals of varying age and either gender in the face of multiple risk factors. Coronary disease risk prediction score sheets which account for multiple variables, may be useful in this regard.[35] The score sheets are also available on the WWW: *http://www.nhlbi.nih.gov/about/framingham/riskabs.thm*. Derived from the predominantly white, middle-class Framingham Heart Study population. they may be less accurate when applied to other types of individuals.

The USPSTF found insufficient evidence to recommend for or against routine aspirin prophylaxis for the primary prevention of myocardial infarction or stroke. Because it is associated with a small increase in the risk of hemorrhagic stroke,[36] aspirin chemoprophylaxis should be employed mostly for those patients with risk factors for cardiovascular disease. Moderate alcohol consumption may reduce the risk of cardiovascular disease, but routine physician endorsement of moderate alcohol use for patients who are not already drinking is not recommended given the high prevalence of problem drinking in the U.S. Indeed, the USPSTF recommends screening for problem drinking in all adults and questioning regarding other drug abuse in those considered at increased risk.

Age 65 and Older (Table 7.10)

This group includes both the "young old" (ages 65 to 79) as well as the "oldest old" (ages 80 and beyond), which is now the fastest growing segment of the U.S. population (also see Chapters 23 and 24). However, there is tremendous physiologic variability in the elderly that makes recommendations for prevention based on age alone risky. In both chronologic and physiologic terms, aging impacts on some of the criteria for preventive interventions outlined earlier in this chapter. For example, prostate cancer screening is not indicated for many individuals in this group given the long interval between detection via screening and the earliest time of expected impact on mortality. In addition, older adults may wish to focus primarily on quality of life during their remaining days. Screening interventions that are associated with inconvenience and discomfort may not be desired, regardless of their potential to reduce mortality. Finally, there is a limited evidence base to support many preventive interventions in this age. Physicians must discuss these gaps in evidence, the risks and benefits of screening, and the quality of life goals of older adults before embarking on screening interventions.

The USPSTF recommends annual influenza vaccination as well as a single immunization against *Streptococcus pneumoniae* for all adults of ages 65 and older. Periodic vision and hearing screening are also suggested because the incidence of both functional vision and hearing problems increases dramatically with aging, rising from about 10% at age 65 to approximately 40% by age 90. Injuries, particularly falls, remain an important source of morbidity and mortality in this

Table 7.10. **Interventions Considered and Recommended for Prevention, Age 65 and Older; Leading Causes of Death: Heart Disease, Malignancies (Lung, Colorectal, Breast), Cerebrovascular Disease, Chronic Obstructive Pulmonary Disease, Pneumonia, and Influenza**

SCREENING
Blood pressure
Height and weight
Total blood cholesterol
Fecal occult blood test[a] and/or sigmoidoscopy
Mammogram ± clinical breast exam[b] (women ≤69 years)
Papanicolaou (Pap) test (women)[c]
Vision screening
Assess for hearing impairment
Assess for problem drinking
COUNSELING
Substance use
Tobacco cessation
Avoid alcohol/drug use while driving, swimming, boating, etc*
Limit fat and cholesterol; maintain caloric balance; emphasize grains, fruits, vegetables
Adequate calcium intake (women)
Regular physical activity*

Injury prevention
Lap/shoulder belts
Motorcycle and bicycle helmets*
Fall prevention*
Safe storage/removal of firearms*
Smoke detector*
Set hot water heater to <120–130°F
CPR training for household members
Dental health
Regular visits to dental care provider*
Floss, brush with fluoride toothpaste daily*
Sexual behavior
STD prevention; avoid high-risk sexual behavior*; use condoms*
IMMUNIZATIONS
Pneumococcal vaccine
Influenza (a)
Tetanus-diphtheria (Td) boosters
CHEMOPROPHYLAXIS
Discuss hormone prophylaxis (peri- and postmenopausal women)

Interventions for high-risk populations (see detailed high-risk definitions in footnotes)

POPULATION	POTENTIAL INTERVENTIONS
Institutionalized persons	PPD (HR1); hepatitis A vaccine (HR2); amantadine/rimantadine (HR4)
Chronic medical conditions; TB contacts; low income; immigrants; alcoholics	PPD (HR1)
Persons ≥75 years, or ≥70 years with risk factors for falls	Fall prevention intervention (HR5)
Family history of skin cancer; nevi, fair skin, eyes hair	Avoid excess/midday sun; use protective clothing* (HR6)
Native Americans/Alaska Natives	PPD (HR1); hepatitis A vaccine (HR2)
Travelers to developing countries	Hepatitis A vaccine (HR2); hepatitis B vaccine (HR7)
Blood product recipients	HIV screen (HR3); hepatitis B vaccine (HR7)
High-risk sexual behavior	Hepatitis A vaccine (HR2); HIV screen (HR3); hepatitis B vaccine (HR7); RPR/VDRL (HR8); advice to reduce risk of infection (HR9)
Injection or street drug use	PPD (HR1); hepatitis A vaccine (HR2); HIV screen (HR3); hepatitis B vaccine (HR7); RPR/VDRL (HR8); advice to reduce risk of infection
Health care/lab workers	PPR (HR1); hepatitis A vaccine (HR2); amantadine/rimantadine (HR4); hepatitis B vaccine (HR7)
Persons susceptible to varicella	Varicella vaccine (HR10)

[a]Annually.

[b]Mammogram q 1–2 years, or mammogram q 1–2 years with annual clinical breast exam.

[c]All women who are or have been sexually active and who have a cervix. Consider discontinuation of testing after age 65 years if previous regular screening with consistently normal results.

*The ability of clinician counseling to influence this behavior is unproven.

HR1—HIV positive, close contacts of persons with known or suspected TB, health care workers, persons with medical risk factors associated with TB, immigrants from countries with high TB prevalence, medically underserved low-income populations (including homeless), alcoholics, injection drug users, and residents of long-term facilities.

HR2—Persons living in, traveling to, or working in areas where the disease is endemic and where periodic outbreaks occur (e.g., countries with high or intermediate endemicity; certain Alaska-Native, Pacific Island, Native-American, and religious communities); men who have sex with men; injection or street drug users. Vaccine may be considered for institutionalized persons and workers in these institutions, military personnel, and day care, hospital, and laboratory workers. Clinicians should also consider local epidemiology.

HR3—Men who had sex with men after 1975; past or present injection drug use; persons who exchange sex for money or drugs, and their sex partners; injection drug-using, bisexual, or HIV-positive sex partner currently or in the past; blood transfusion during 1978–1985; persons seeking treatment for STDs. Clinicians should also consider local epidemiology.

HR4—Consider for persons who have not received influenza vaccine or are vaccinated late; when the vaccine may be ineffective due to major antigenic changes in the virus; for unvaccinated persons who provide home care for high-risk persons; to sup-

Table 7.10. (Continued)

plement protection provided by vaccine in persons who are expected to have a poor antibody response; and for high-risk persons in whom the vaccine is contraindicated.

HR5—Persons aged 75 years and older; or aged 70–74 with one or more additional risk factors, including use of certain psychoactive and cardiac medications (e.g., benzodiazepines, antihypertensives); use of ≥4 prescription medications; impaired cognition, strength, balance, or gait. Intensive individualized home-based multifactorial fall prevention intervention is recommended in settings where adequate resources are available to deliver such services.

HR6—Persons with a family or personal history of skin cancer, a large number of moles, atypical moles, poor tanning ability, or light skin, hair, and eye color.

HR7—Blood product recipients (including hemodialysis patients), persons with frequent occupational exposure to blood or blood products, men who have sex with men, injection drug users and their sex partners, persons with multiple recent sex partners, persons with other STDs (including HIV), travelers to countries with endemic hepatitis B.

HR8—Persons who exchange sex for money or drugs, and their sex partners, persons with other STDs (including HIV); and sexual contacts of persons with active syphilis. Clinicians should also consider local epidemiology.

HR9—Persons who continue to inject drugs.

HR10—Healthy adults without a history of chickenpox or previous immunization. Consider serologic testing for presumed susceptible adults.

Source: U.S. Preventive Services Task Force,[9] with permission.

group but are more likely to occur while performing simple daily tasks such as walking to the bathroom at night. Fall prevention measures including regular exercise, environmental hazard reduction, and avoiding sedating medications should be discussed with all older individuals. Those who are frail, have had prior falls, or are at ongoing high risk for falls may benefit from a multifactorial intervention that includes home assessment and a hip-protective undergarment.[37] End of life planning is also an important preventive care topic for older patients. The value of medical advance directives in improving primary care physicians' and lay surrogates' accuracy in predicting a patient's wishes for care is unclear. However, advance directive discussions and documentation may improve the prediction of patients' wishes by hospital-based physicians and may improve patients' sense of well-being and satisfaction with care.[38] Finally, many elders live in poverty, and many reside in assisted living and skilled nursing facilities. These older adults are often frail and may face substantial socioeconomic disadvantages. Screening these individuals for nutritional adequacy, social isolation, depression, and the ability to perform basic and instrumental activities of daily living should be considered.

The Process of Delivering Preventive Care

The Move Toward Accountability in Preventive Services Delivery

Physicians are now being held accountable for offering and delivering evidence-based preventive services. Quality of care models such as the Health Plan Employer Data and Information Set (HEDIS) seek to provide health care purchasers and consumers with a standard against which individual plans can be compared and evaluated. The HEDIS 2001 measures are heavily weighted toward clinical prevention, including items such as breast cancer screening rates, childhood immunization status, and rates of advising smokers to quit. Health plans

and clinicians that fail to meet quality thresholds for these indicators are at risk for declining patient enrollment as consumers transfer their care to "higher performers." Nevertheless, delivering individualized, evidence-based clinical preventive services remains a formidable challenge. This section provides a list of issues hindering the delivery of optimal clinical preventive services and provides potential solutions suggested by the research literature.

Organizational Issues and Potential Solutions

Issue 1: Time Constraints of the Clinical Encounter

There is a finite amount of time that can be spent with each patient, and in this time the physicians must address a range of concerns in addition to providing clinical preventive services. In the landmark Direct Observation of Primary Care (DOPC) study, one third of 4401 patient encounters included discussion of at least one preventive service, but only 3% of the all encounter time was allotted to preventive services.[39] Time pressures will increase with the aging of the population, as more patients present with multiple chronic diseases, conditions, and functional limitations.

Potential Solutions. Physicians must employ the incremental approach to clinical prevention that is endorsed by the USPSTF. The most urgent priorities for prevention can be addressed first, leaving others for future encounters. Standard "scripts" or minipresentations concerning common preventive topics may increase efficiency.

Issue 2: Limited Dissemination of New Findings and Evidence-Based Prevention Guidelines

The dissemination of evidence-based prevention guidelines in textbooks and journals has limited impact. Such resources, while valuable, rapidly become out of date and may not be readily available at the point of patient care.

Potential Solutions. Evidence-based summary resources that present up-to-date information in a rapid-use format include Patient-oriented evidence that matters (POEMs), *http://www.jfponline.com*; clinical evidence, *http://www.clinicalevidenceonline.com/*; the Cochrane Library, *http://www.updateusa.com/clibhome/clib.htm*; and the ACP Journal Club, *http://www.acponline.org/journals/acpjc/jcmenu.htm*. The Internet is already an established tool for the delivery of recommendations at the point of care. In the near future, palm-top computers will allow even better point of care access to recommendations.

Issue 3: Competing and Conflicting Recommendations

Many organizations publish recommendations advocating clinical preventive services that are not evidence-based. Clinicians may become confused by conflicting guidelines and are often faced with patients requesting interventions that are promoted by these organizations but not supported by rigorous evidence.

Potential Solutions. The USPSTF recommendations should be utilized whenever possible, and patients should be informed about the levels of evidence for specific interventions. Prevention plans that account for local practice characteristics and patient risk factors, preferences, and beliefs can then be negotiated.

Issue 4: Lack of Office Systems Organized to Provide Effective Preventive Services

Office systems used by practices with successful prevention efforts include designated roles for staff at all levels, paper and computer-based health risk appraisal tools, reminder systems, patient education materials, and record systems, and a quality monitoring and improvement process.

Potential Solutions. The best-known set of materials aimed at improving clinical prevention is Put Prevention into Practice (PPIP). The PPIP kit is paper-based and includes flow sheets, patient-held prevention records, a clinician handbook, prevention prescription pads, medical record reminder stickers, patient reminder postcards, and posters for waiting and examination rooms. Implementing the PPIP office system has been shown to modestly increase the rates of delivery of multiple USPSTF-recommended preventive services. However, dissemination of PPIP has been slow and limited, the absolute increase in rates of delivery for specific services is small, and the positive effects related to its implementation diminish beyond 1 year of follow-up.[40] Both paper and computer-based reminder systems, including those linked to comprehensive electronic medical records, have been shown to improve rates of preventive services delivery, and the impact appears greatest when the reminder is provided to the physician at the time of a patient visit.[41] As for PPIP, the number of practices utilizing such resources is small and their absolute impact has been limited.

The smaller than anticipated impact of these tools has led to the recognition that the problem of low preventive service delivery rates is a complex, systems issue. The DOPC study suggests there are two major differences between practices delivering limited preventive services and those providing higher levels of these services: (1) the degree of pro-activity in dealing with competing practice demands, and (2) physician philosophy.[42] Practices with the greatest need to improve preventive care may be the least likely to implement programs like PPIP due to overwhelming competing demands, such as a practice that is heavily weighted toward acute medical care or physicians with a low "prevention orientation." Developing and testing approaches to dealing with competing demands in primary care and changing physician behavior should be given the highest priority. In the meantime, adapting generic materials to individual practice circumstances and enlisting nonphysician clinic staff in prevention efforts are useful first steps. For example, modification of PPIP flow sheets to meet local needs may result in better acceptance of the materials and higher rates of flow sheet completion,[43] and simple mailed or telephone call reminders provided by nonphysician staff can increase childhood immunization "up to date" rates.[44] In the future, remote home-based health risk appraisals, conducted using the Internet and other distance communications technologies, are likely to become routine.

Issue 5: Poor Reimbursement for Preventive Services

In 1988 less than 5% of health care expenditures in the United States was allocated to prevention, and only one third of those expenditures were allocated to clinical prevention.[45] Tobacco cessation counseling and hearing, vision, and blood pressure screening are all endorsed by the USPSTF for older adults, yet none are covered by Medicare. Paradoxically, many states mandate coverage for screening services not recommended by the USPSTF.

Potential Solutions. Physicians must remain advocates for a preventive health care agenda, making sure local congressional representatives and health plans are aware of shortfalls and misplaced priorities.

Physician and Patient Issues and Potential Solutions

Issue 1: Failure to Adopt and Maintain a Prevention Orientation

Despite the proven benefits of many clinical preventive efforts, some physicians have a practice style that de-emphasizes prevention. In the DOPC study, physicians with a higher volume practice had lower up-to-date rates of preventive screening and counseling services and immunizations.[46] Female physicians have consistently been shown to offer more clinical preventive services than male physicians, and the effect is not limited to gender-specific interventions.[47] In addition, some patients do not embrace the concept of clinical prevention.

Potential Solutions. All physicians, and particularly males and those working in high-volume settings, should carefully examine their practice style to ensure it is prevention-centered. Physicians must open a dialogue with patients who do not have a prevention orientation by providing individually tailored information and collaborating to determine the areas in which the patient is most ready to accept preventive interventions.

Issue 2: Holding on to Non–Evidence-Based Beliefs and Practices

Given the time constraints of the modern clinical encounter, it is critical to discard disproved and questionable preventive practices. Focusing on such services reduces the amount of time and money that can be devoted to providing evidence-based services and compounds many of the issues listed above. For example, the "complete physical" appointment accounts for as much as one third of physicians' time spent seeing patients in some practices, yet many elements of this venerable activity have no proven value.

Potential Solutions. Physicians must let go of non–evidence-based prevention ideas as part of the solution to the competing demands issue. Since many patients never make checkup visits, preventive services are best delivered over time, during acute illness and other visits. Making the shift away from the "complete physical" model will require patient education, since people have come to expect certain low-yield maneuvers and interventions. A caring, "high-touch" manner can be conveyed to patients without resorting to the misleading reassurance of a normal heart and lung examination. Patients who request non–evidence-based interventions should be congratulated for their interest in prevention and their health. The dialogue should focus on the reasons for the patient's concern about the health issue in question. The evidence to support the intervention should be summarized and placed in the context of the individual. Finally, a prevention plan is negotiated. Although some patients may still insist on non–evidence-based interventions, most will be satisfied with this approach.

Issue 3: Failure to Account for Varying Patient Health-Belief Models

The United States is increasingly multicultural, and culture and ethnicity impact on every aspect of preventive care, from genetics to health behavior. Some traditional cultural health belief models do not include the Western construct of the concept of prevention.

Potential Solutions. Physicians should learn about the ethnic groups, cultures, and socioeconomic strata represented in their patient population. A rapid overview can be obtained using the U.S. Census Bureau's WWW site at *http://www.census.gov*, which includes color maps and tables detailing the ethnic distribution of local neighborhoods, language spoken at home, and aggregate family incomes. Becoming involved in community cultural and ethnic activities is an important next step. Perhaps the most important skill in providing multicultural care is to approach each patient without relying on cultural stereotypes. Differing degrees of acculturation and interindividual variability in beliefs make such generalizations dangerous.

Issue 4: Poor Preventive Communication Skills

Just as physicians must learn key physical examination and history-taking skills to diagnose acute medical illnesses, they must also acquire and maintain the communication skills needed to provide optimal clinical prevention. These skills include the ability to (1) translate research and statistics into lay terms, (2) determine patient readiness to modify a health risk behavior, and (3) negotiate a clinical prevention plan.

Potential Solutions. Health systems increasingly offer communication skills training to physicians, recognizing that deficiencies result in poorer health care outcomes and higher costs. Although the best method of conveying health risk information to patients remains unclear, helping patients to understand how a health problem develops (its antecedents) and to recognize what could happen to them as a result (its consequences) may be more successful than simply providing numerical risk information.[48] In determining a patient's readiness to change a risk behavior, the transtheoretical model provides a useful framework (Table 7.11).[49] The model illustrates that changes in behavior occur gradually, through a predictable series of steps. Individuals seldom skip steps, so that the physician's role is to assist them in moving to the next stage of change rather than to push them toward behavior change in one giant leap. The model also acknowledges that most individuals undergo behavior relapses after successful change. Knowledge of the model may remove the sense of fatalism many physicians feel when trying to help patients change their behaviors and reinforce the importance of providing the right input at the right stage. For example, repeatedly pressuring a smoker at the precontemplation stage to pick a quit smoking date may create an adversarial relationship, reinforcing the negative behavior and making it less likely the individual will consider cessation. Instead, acknowledging the lack of readiness to quit, spending a few moments to explore the reasons for smoking, and providing education about the harmful health effects of smoking may encourage patient contemplation, setting the stage for eventual cessation.

Table 7.11. **Ladder of Behavioral Change**

Model stage	Patient manifestations
Precontemplation health	Not thinking about change; may be resigned to behavior; feeling of no control; denial of problem; may believe consequences are not serious
↓ ↑ Contemplation	Weighing benefits and costs of the current behavior and the proposed change
↓ ↑ Preparation	Experimenting with small changes in behavior
↓ ↑ Action	Taking a definitive action to change
↓ ↑ Maintenance	Maintaining the new behavior over time
↓ ↑ Relapse	Experiencing normal part of the process of change; often feel demoralized, may interpret small "slips" as irrevocable slide back to prior behavior

Source: Prochaska et al,[49] with permission.

Issue 5: Failure to Recognize and Acknowledge the Harms of Screening

Clinical prevention saves many lives but also has potential harms, such as complications of diagnostic procedures and patient anxiety. Physicians generally underemphasize the harms of screening in a well-intentioned effort to help as many people as possible. For example, although FOBT has been shown to reduce the relative risk of colorectal cancer death by 33%, the absolute reduction in all-cause mortality associated with testing is only 0.3% and the false-positive rate is high. Many screened individuals must undergo potentially morbid procedures such as colonoscopy to realize the small absolute reduction in mortality. In addition, some physicians continue to offer worthless services due to misguided medicolegal concerns. Patients have also been conditioned by the health care system and the media to believe all preventive care is more beneficial than harmful. These beliefs and practices place patients at an unjustifiably increased risk of harm.

Potential Solutions. When possible, decisions regarding whether to offer a preventive service should be based on absolute reductions in all-cause mortality rather than relative reductions in disease-specific outcomes. Harm counseling must be provided when screening also has the potential for adverse consequences. The informed consent model, developed for clinical research, should be applied. For interventions with proven benefit and minimal or no adverse consequences, such as counseling regarding infant car seat use, informed consent is not necessary.

References

1. Ten great public health achievements: United States, 1900–99. MMWR 1999;48:241–64.
2. McGinnis JM, Foege WH. Actual causes of death in the United States. JAMA 1993;270:2207–12.
3. U.S. Department of Health and Human Services. Healthy people 2010 2nd ed.: With understanding and improving health and objectives for improving health. 2 vols. Washington, DC: U.S. Government Printing Office, November 2000.
4. Michaud CM, Murray CJL, Bloom BR. Burden of disease: implications for future research. JAMA 2001;285:535–9.
5. Schorling JB, Buchsbaum DG. Screening for alcohol and drug abuse. Med Clin North Am 1997;81:845–65.
6. Rembold CM. Number needed to screen: development of a statistic for disease screening. BMJ 1998;317:307–12.
7. Rose DN. Benefits of screening for latent *Mycobacterium tuberculosis* infection. Arch Intern Med 2000;160:1513–21.
8. Stone PW, Teutsch S, Chapman RH, Bell C, Goldie SJ, Neumann PJ. Cost-utility analyses of clinical preventive services: published ratios, 1976–97. Am J Prev Med 2000;19:15–23.
9. U.S. Preventive Services Task Force. Guide to clinical preventive services, 2nd ed. Baltimore: Lippincott Williams & Wilkins, 1996.
10. Hovell MF, Zakarian JM, Matt GE, Hofstetter CR, Bernert JT, Pirkle J. Effect of counseling mothers on their children's exposure to environmental tobacco smoke: a randomized controlled trial. BMJ 2000;321:337–42.
11. Cook DG, Strachan DP. Health effects of passive smoking—10: summary of effects of parental smoking on the respiratory health of children and implications for research. Thorax 1999;54: 357–66.
12. Willinger M, Hoffman HJ, Wu K, et al. Factors associated with the transition to nonprone sleep positions of infants in the United States. JAMA 1998;280:329–35.
13. Scariati PD, Grummer-Strawn LM, Fein SB. A longitudinal analysis of infant morbidity and the extent of breast feeding in the United States. Pediatrics 1997;99:E5.
14. Zimmerman RK. The 2001 recommended childhood immunization schedule. Am Fam Physician 2000;63:151–4.
15. Feikin DR, Lezotte DC, Hamman RF, Salmon DA, Chen RT, Hoffman RE. Individual and community risks of measles and pertussis associated with personal exemptions to immunizations. JAMA 2000;284:3145–50.
16. Santoli JM, Szilagyi PG, Rodewald LE. Barriers to immunization and missed opportunities. Pediatr Ann 1998;27:366–74.
17. Epidemiology and prevention of vaccine-preventable diseases, 6th ed. Atlanta: Centers for Disease Control and Prevention, 2000.
18. Schonfeld-Warden N, Warden CH. Pediatric obesity: an overview of etiology and treatment. Pediatr Clin North Am 1997; 44:339–61.
19. National High Blood Pressure Education Program. Update on the task force report (1987) on high blood pressure in children and adolescents: a working group report from the National High Blood Pressure Education Program. Bethesda, MD: National Heart, Lung, and Blood Institute, 1996.
20. American Thoracic Society/Centers for Disease Control and Prevention. Targeted tuberculin testing and treatment of latent tuberculosis infection. Am J Respir Crit Care Med 2000;161 (part 2):S221–47.
21. Merenstein D, Green L, Fryer GE, Dovey S. Shortchanging adolescents: room for improvement in preventive care by physicians. Fam Med 2001;33:120–3.
22. Steiner BD, Gest KL. Do adolescents want to hear preventive counseling messages in outpatient settings? J Fam Pract 1996; 43:375–81.
23. Knishkowy B, Palti H, Schein M, Yaphe J, Edman R, Baras M. Adolescent preventive health visits: a comparison of two invitation protocols. J Am Board Fam Pract 2000;13:11–16.
24. Grossman D. Adolescent injury prevention and clinicians: time for instant messaging. West J Med 2000;172:151–2.
25. Meningococcal disease and college students: recommendations of the Advisory Committee on Immunization Practices (ACIP). MMWR 2000;49:11–20.
26. Patuszak A, Bhatia D, Okotore B, Koren G. Preconception counseling and women's compliance with folic acid supplementation. Can Fam Physician 1999;45:2053–7.
27. Cervical cancer. National Institutes of Health consensus statement. Bethesda, MD: National Institutes of Health, 1996.
28. Ernster VL. Mammography screening for women aged 40–49: a guidelines saga and a clarion call for informed decision making. Am J Public Health 1997;87:1103–6.
29. Coley CM, Barry MJ, Fleming C, Fahs MC, Mulley AG. Early detection of prostate cancer. Part II: estimating the risks, benefits, and costs. American College of Physicians. Ann Intern Med 1997;126:468–79.
30. Frazier AL, Colditz GA, Fuchs CS, Kuntz KM. Cost-effectiveness of screening for colorectal cancer in the general population. JAMA 2000;284:1954–61.
31. Screening for colorectal cancer—United States, 1997. MMWR 1999;48:116–21.
32. American Gastroenterological Association. Colorectal cancer screening: clinical guidelines and rationale. Gastroenterology 1997;112:594–42.
33. American College of Physicians. Guidelines for using serum cholesterol, high-density lipoprotein cholesterol, and triglyceride levels as screening tests for preventing coronary heart disease in adults. Part 1. Ann Intern Med 1996;124:515–7.

34. Expert Panel on Detection, Evaluation, and Treatment of High Blood Cholesterol in Adults. Executive summary of the Third Report of the National Cholesterol Education Program (NCEP) Expert Panel on Detection, Evaluation, and Treatment of High Blood Cholesterol in Adults (Adult Treatment Panel III). JAMA 2001;285:2486–97.

35. Wilson PWF, D'Agostino RB, Levy D, Belanger AM, Silbershatz H, Kannel WB. Prediction of coronary heart disease using risk factor categories. Circulation 1998;97:1837–47.

36. He J, Whelton PK, Vu B, Klag MJ. Aspirin and risk of hemorrhagic stroke: a meta-analysis of randomized controlled trials. JAMA 1998;280:1930–5.

37. Kanus P, Parkkari J, Niemi S, et al. Prevention of hip fracture in elderly people with use of a hip protector. N Engl J Med 2000;343:1506–13.

38. Ditto PH, Danks JH, Smucker WD, et al. Advance directives as acts of communication: a randomized controlled trial. Arch Intern Med 2001;161:421–30.

39. Stange KC, Zyzanski SJ, Jaen CR, et al. Illuminating the "black box": a description of 4454 patient visits to 138 family physicians. J Fam Pract 1998;46:377–89.

40. Melnikow J, Kohatsu ND, Chan BKS. Put prevention into practice: a controlled evaluation. Am J Public Health 2000;90:1622–5.

41. Jerant AF, Hill DB. Does the use of electronic medical records improve surrogate patient outcomes in outpatient settings? J Fam Pract 2000;49:349–57.

42. Stange KC. One size doesn't fit all: multimethod research yields new insights into interventions to increase prevention in family practice. J Fam Pract 1996;43:358–60.

43. Moser SE, Goering TL. Implementing preventive care flow sheets. Fam Pract Manag 2001;8:51–3.

44. Udovic SL, Lieu TA. Evidence on office-based interventions to improve childhood immunization delivery. Pediatr Ann 1998;27:355–61.

45. Estimated national spending on prevention: United States, 1988. MMWR 1988;41:529–31.

46. Zyzanski SJ, Stange KC, Langa D, Flocke SA. Trade-offs in high-volume primary care practice. J Fam Pract 1998;46:397–402.

47. Kreuter MW, Strecher VJ, Harris R, Kobrin SC, Skinner CS. Are patients of women physicians screened more aggressively? A prospective study of physician gender and screening. J Gen Intern Med 1995;10:119–25.

48. Rothman AJ, Kiviniemi MT. Treating people with information: an analysis and review of approaches to communicating health risk information. J Natl Cancer Inst Monogr 1999;25:44–51.

49. Prochaska JO, DiClemente CC, Norcross JC. In search of how people change: applications to addictive behaviors. Am Psychol 1992;47:1102–14.

8
Health Promotion

Richard Kent Zimmerman and Mary Patricia Nowalk

Lifestyle Factors and Risk of Disease

Reduction in risk for a variety of chronic diseases can be achieved through the adoption and maintenance of healthy lifestyles. Smoking, low levels of physical activity, excess body weight, and other conditions related to high-fat, calorically dense diets contribute to development or worsening of many forms of cancer, coronary heart disease (CHD), diabetes, osteoarthritis, gallbladder disease, sleep apnea, and hypertension (Fig. 8.1). An estimated 700,000 deaths (33%) in the United States in 1990 were attributable to tobacco use, dietary factors, and activity patterns.[1] Health promotion practices by primary care physicians in the form of assessment, assistance with lifestyle change, and encouragement in general, are low cost in comparison to the benefit to patients.

Tobacco Use

Prevalence of Smoking in the United States

It is estimated that 48 million adult Americans (25%) currently smoke.[2] Approximately 3,000 young people become regular smokers each day, and the number of frequent smokers among high school students has increased to 16%.[3] Demographic characteristics of persons more likely to smoke are male gender, socioeconomic status below poverty level, education level less than 13 years, and Native-American and Alaskan-Native ethnicity.[4]

Impact of Tobacco on Health

Smoking has long been recognized as the single largest cause of preventable death in the United States, causing more than 430,000 deaths annually.[5] Smoking contributes to morbidity and mortality both directly and indirectly. Byproducts of tobacco are among the most potent of human carcinogens and are linked to 30% of all cancer deaths annually, especially neoplasms of the lung, mouth and throat, pancreas, kidney, bladder, and uterine cervix.[1] Smoking is responsible for 180,000 deaths due to cardiovascular disease and is related to respiratory illness such as bronchitis and emphysema, gastrointestinal disorders, and cerebrovascular disease. Smoking during pregnancy accounts for about one fifth of low birth weight neonates and about one twentieth of perinatal deaths.

Environmental tobacco smoke (ETS) contains over 4,000 chemical compounds, many of which are toxic and/or known carcinogens. ETS causes an estimated 3,000 deaths from lung cancer and 35,000 to 40,000 deaths from heart disease and a variety of respiratory problems among nonsmokers. Among children, ETS increases the risk of lower respiratory tract infections, resulting in 7,500 to 15,000 hospitalizations, exacerbation of asthma, and increased ear infections.[2]

In the United States alone, the financial burden of medical treatment for smoking-related diseases, lost productivity and earnings, and premature death total nearly $100 billion.[3] In 1990 cigarette smoking resulted in 5 million estimated years of potential life lost prior to life expectancy.[6]

Smoking Cessation

The health benefits of smoking cessation are immediate and profound. Within a half hour of quitting, blood pressure returns to precigarette levels. After only 1 day, the risk of heart attack decreases. Lung function improves by as much as 30% within 3 months.[7] Smoking cessation reduces all-cause mortality as well as the risk of cancer, myocardial infarction, stroke, chronic obstructive pulmonary disease mortality, peripheral artery disease, and low birth weight.[8] Although the risk of CHD death is reduced by 50% in 1 year, a 50% re-

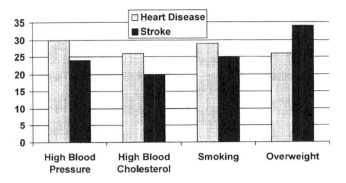

Fig. 8.1. Prevalence of modifiable risk factors for heart disease and stroke.

Table 8.1. **The 5 A's for Brief Intervention**

Ask about tobacco use.	Identify and document tobacco use status for every patient routinely (e.g., at every visit)
Advise to quit.	In a clear, strong and personalized manner, urge every tobacco user to quit
Assess willingness to make a quit attempt.	Is the tobacco user willing to make a quit attempt at this time?
Assist in quit attempt.	For the patient willing to make a quit attempt, use counseling and pharmacotherapy to help him or her quit
Arrange followup.	Schedule follow-up contact, preferably within the first week after the quit date

Source: Modified from Fiore, et al.[5]

duction in the risk of cancer requires approximately 10 years. Compared to women who smoke throughout pregnancy, those who stop by the 30th week of gestation have infants with higher birth weights and lower perinatal mortality.

Although many adults express interest in quitting, it is not easily achieved. Nicotine is the addictive drug in tobacco; however, other factors contribute to tobacco dependence. They include habit cued by daily activities, pleasure, and self-medication to reduce negative affect and withdrawal symptoms.[9] Furthermore, nicotine produces euphoria similar to that from other addictive psychomotor stimulants and has addictive pharmacologic and behavioral properties that are similar to heroin and cocaine. Symptoms of nicotine withdrawal include depression, irritability, restlessness, headache, fatigue, increased appetite. Both the smoking habit and its associated activities, as well as nicotine withdrawal symptoms, make smoking cessation physically and psychologically difficult. Recidivism is high. Therefore, tobacco dependence is increasingly viewed as a chronic disease that requires ongoing assessment and intervention.

Interventions to Assist Patients in Tobacco Use Cessation

The U.S. Public Health Service has recently issued clinical practice guidelines for treating tobacco use and dependence.[5] This comprehensive document challenges health care providers to treat tobacco dependence as a chronic disease and to recognize that effective treatments are available, and recommends health system changes that promote assessment and treatment and reimburse providers for their efforts. The guidelines recommend using the five A's: Ask about tobacco use, Advise to quit, Assess willingness to quit, Assist in quit attempt, and Arrange follow-up (Table 8.1). An algorithm is available to guide the process (Fig. 8.2). The primary interventions to reduce tobacco use are counseling, support, and pharmacotherapy.

All patients who are willing to attempt to quit should be provided with counseling. There is a strong dose-response relationship between the amount of counseling time provided

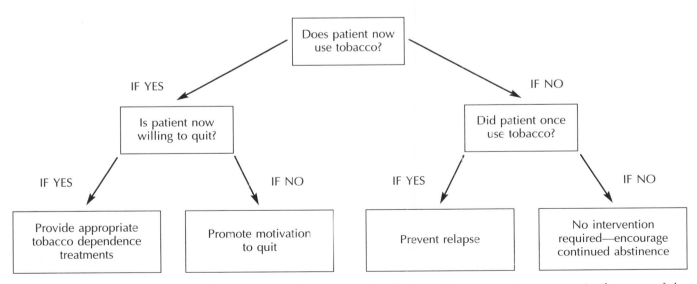

Fig. 8.2. Algorithm for treating tobacco use. Relapse prevention interventions are not necessary in the case of the adult who has not used tobacco for many years. (Modified from Fiore et al.[5])

Table 8.2. **Estimated Abstinence Rates for Pharmacotherapies for Smoking Cessation**

Pharmacology	Estimated abstinence rate (%)	Placebo (%)
Bupropion SR*	30.5	17
Nicotine gum (2 mg)	24	17
Nicotine inhaler	23	10
Nicotine nasal spray	30.5	14
Nicotine patch	18	10
Two nicotine therapies	28.6	—

Source: Modified from Fiore, et al.[5]
*Bupropion sustained release formula.

and successful quitting.[5] Some of the topics that can be discussed are setting a plan for quitting, problem-solving skills, relapse prevention, obtaining social support, the availability of pharmacotherapy, and scheduling follow-up visits with the clinician to assist with cessation efforts. Telephone support, initiated either by the provider or by the patient, has also been recommended as part of a multicomponent smoking cessation program.[10]

It is now recommended that all patients without contraindications be offered pharmacotherapy such as bupropion or nicotine replacement therapy (Table 8.2). Clonidine and nortriptyline are second-line medications and may be considered if the aforementioned first-line medications are not effective. Information to guide choice of pharmacotherapy is given in Table 8.3.

A meta-analysis estimated the abstinence rate for bupropion SR at 30.5% compared to 17% for placebo (Table 8.2). Possible adverse effects include seizures, bronchospasm, and atrioventricular (AV) block. The dose is 150 mg orally for 3 days and then 150 mg twice a day for 7 to 12 weeks. In one study, the abstinence rates at 12 months were 15.6% in the placebo group, 16% in the nicotine-patch group, 30% in the bupropion group, and 35.5% in the group given both bupropion and the nicotine patch.[11]

Cessation rates at one year for counseling (4–9%) double for nicotine patches (9–25%).[5] Similar rates are noted for nicotine gum (Table 8.2).[12] Nicotine patches may cause skin irritation, dizziness, tachycardia, headache, nausea, vomiting. Nicotine gum can cause throat irritation, mouth ulcers, hiccups, nausea, and tachycardia. Side effects of nicotine nasal sprays are nasal and throat irritation, which generally subside after 1 to 2 weeks. Inhalers also cause coughing and throat irritation.

Weight gain is often a concern of smokers, yet research has shown that weight gain during quitting averages 10 pounds, with women gaining more weight than men. Because the health risks of smoking are more immediate and dangerous than the risks of modest weight gain, potential weight gain should not prevent attempts at smoking cessation. Many of the behavioral techniques used to quit smoking can later be modified and used to shape dietary behavior for weight loss.

Table 8.3. **Prescribing Pharmacotherapy for Smoking Cessation**

Question	Comment
What factors should a clinician consider when choosing among the five first-line pharmacotherapies?	Because of the lack of sufficient data to rank-order these five medications, choice of a specific first-line pharmacotherapy must be guided by factors such as clinician familiarity with the medications, contraindications for selected patients, patient preference, previous patient experience with a specific pharmacotherapy (positive or negative), and patient characteristics (e.g., history of depression concerns about weight gain).
Are pharmacotherapeutic treatments appropriate for lighter smokers (e.g., 10–15 cigarettes/day)?	If pharmacotherapy is used with light smokers, clinicians should consider reducing the dose of first-line nicotine pharmacotherapies. No adjustments are necessary when using bupropion SR.
Which pharmacotherapies should be considered with patients particularly concerned about weight gain?	Bupropion SR and nicotine replacement therapies, in particular nicotine gum, have been shown to delay, but not prevent, weight gain.
Are there pharmacotherapies that should be especially considered in patients with a history of depression?	Bupropion SR and nortriptyline appear to be effective with this population.
Should nicotine replacement therapies be avoided in patients with a history of cardiovascular disease?	No. The nicotine patch in particular is safe and has been shown not to cause adverse cardiovascular effects.
May tobacco dependence pharmacotherapies be used long-term (e.g., 6 months or more)?	Yes. This approach may be helpful with smokers who report persistent withdrawal symptoms during the course of pharmacotherapy or who desire long-term therapy. A minority of individuals who successfully quit smoking use ad libitum medications (gum, nasal spray, inhaler) long-term. The use of these medications long-term does not present a known health risk. Additionally, the FDA has approved the use of bupropion SR for a long-term maintenance indication.
May pharmacotherapies ever be combined?	Yes. There is evidence that combining the nicotine patch with either nicotine gum or nicotine nasal spray increases long-term abstinence rates over those produced by a single form of pharmacotherapy. Bupropion SR combined with nicotine therapy increases abstinence rates.

Source: Modified from Fiore, et al.[5]

Smokers who are unwilling to quit should be advised of the risks of continued smoking and the personal benefits of quitting. It is recommended that these issues be addressed at every visit,[5] when feasible.

It is also important to prevent initiation of tobacco use. Most adults report that they started smoking as teenagers.[2] Antitobacco messages should be given to children and young adults to reduce the chances that a person will begin smoking. A meta-analysis of behavioral impact of antitobacco messages showed that the best results occur from programs with a social reinforcement orientation.[13] Using role playing and extended practice, such programs develop abilities to recognize social pressure, develop skills to resist it, and identify immediate social (bad breath) and physical (decreased athletic ability) consequences of tobacco use.

Tobacco dependence treatment during routine physician visits has been shown to be cost-effective and in fact has been called the "gold standard" for preventive medicine.[5] The average cost per smoker of effective smoking cessation treatment is estimated to be $165.61.[3] One early meta-analysis found that 5.8% more smokers remained abstinent in the intervention groups (counseling, literature, nicotine replacement therapy, or a combination) than the control groups after 1 year of follow-up.[14] Although this effect may seem modest, the impact (effect size) when applied to the entire United States is large.

Resources

Several organizations have resources available for patients and clinicians, including the American Academy of Family Physicians (1-800-274-2237; *www.aafp.org*), the National Cancer Institute (1-800-4CANCER; *www.nci.nih.gov*), the American Lung Association (212-315-8700; *www.lungusa.org*), the American Cancer Society (1-800-ACS-2345; *www.cancer.org*), and the U.S. Public Health Service (*www.surgeongeneral.gov*), which recently released a clinical practice guideline on treating tobacco use and dependence.

Sedentary Lifestyle and Exercise

Impact on Health

A sedentary lifestyle increases the risk of mortality from all causes. A prospective cohort study revealed increases in all-cause mortality from 18.6 per 10,000 for the most fit men to 64 per 10,000 for the least-fit men.[15] A similar increase was seen in women; the corresponding values were 8.5 and 39.5 per 10,000, respectively. Other data show that the relative risk (RR) of death from coronary heart disease is double (RR 1.9; 95% confidence interval 1.6–2.2) for sedentary versus active occupations.[16] Overall, exercise can add up to 2 years of life and eliminate one third of the excess deaths due to coronary heart disease.

Other benefits of exercise include better mental health, lower risk of hip fracture, and lower risk of adult-onset diabetes mellitus (DM). In one cohort study, each 500-kcal increase in energy expended on leisure-time physical activity resulted in a 6% reduction in risk of developing DM.[17] Despite the evidence about the benefits of exercise, more than half of the adults in the United States do not engage in regular physical activity.

Effects of Starting Exercise

Persons who start exercising at a moderate level (≥4.5 metabolic equivalents) have a 23% lower risk of death than those who do not exercise (95% confidence interval 4–42%).[18] Furthermore, men who change their status from unfit to fit experience a 44% reduction in mortality.[19] Each minute increase in maximal treadmill time results in a 7.9% decrease in mortality.[19]

Exercise improves cardiovascular fitness, lipoprotein profiles, insulin sensitivity, pulmonary physiology, and bone mass (Table 8.4). The most important change is improved myocardial oxygen balance, which occurs by improved blood supply to the heart, reduced heart rate, reduced blood pressure, and improved stroke volume. Improved fibrinolysis, decreased platelet aggregation, lower sensitivity to catecholamine, and decreased insulin resistance also contribute to the decrease in mortality and morbidity from coronary heart disease.

Moderate exercise has mental health benefits as well. In anxious sedentary adults, it increases aerobic fitness, decreases tension and anxiety, decreases depression, decreases confusion, and increases perceived coping ability.[20] Moderate exercise has also been shown to reduce tension and anxiety in the general population[21] (see Chapters 31 and 32).

Concerns about starting an exercise program include injury rates and potential impact on arthritis. In a study of elderly persons who were starting an exercise program, injury rates were 9% for strength training, 5% for walking, and 57% for jogging, although there was one person who discontinued exercising due to injury.[22] Running has not been shown to accelerate the development of radiographic or clinical osteoarthritis of the knees.[23] Thus, beginning an exercise program with more strenuous activities such as jogging may lead to an increased rate of injuries, especially in the elderly, but does not predispose to arthritis.

Cost-effectiveness data reveal that the cost for each quality-adjusted life year gained from physical activity is $11,313, which is similar to that from other interventions to prevent coronary heart disease.[24]

Counseling to Increase Exercise

In one study, brief physician advice to patients about exercise resulted in increased duration but not frequency of exercise.[25] Another study found that risk factor education and counseling in the primary care office increased regular exercise.[26] Although exercise has been shown to increase longevity and physician advice may be effective, many physicians do not routinely incorporate the exercise counseling into their practices.

Experts from the American College of Sports Medicine (ACSM) and the Centers for Disease Control and Prevention

Table 8.4. **Physiologic Effects of Exercise**

System affected	Effect
Cardiovascular	Improved balance between myocardial oxygen demand and supply by reduced heart rate, reduced blood pressure, increased blood supply to the myocardium, and improved stroke volume Increased size of heart muscle, contractility, and chamber size Probably reduced risk for lethal ventricular arrhythmias due to lower ischemia, high fibrillation threshold, and lessened adrenergic response to stress Lower systolic blood pressure by 3–11 mm Hg, lower diastolic blood pressure by 3–8 mm Hg, depending on initial blood pressure Increased blood volume
Lipids and blood	Increased high-density lipoprotein (HDL) (5–15% increase), perhaps decreased low-density lipoprotein (LDL), decreased total cholesterol/HDL ratio Decreased platelet adhesiveness Enhanced fibrinolysis
Obesity and insulin	Increased insulin sensitivity and decreased resistance Decreased obesity, particularly central obesity
Pulmonary	Increased functional capacity and decreased nonfunctional residual volume Increased diffusion
Bone and muscle	Increased bone mass; probably slows decline in bone density with age for women Greater muscle mass

Source: Adapted in part from the work of Douglas McKeag, M.D., with permission.

(CDC) concluded that every adult should exercise for 30 minutes on most days of the week at a moderate intensity level of 3 to 6 metabolic equivalents (Met).[27] Examples of activities at various Met levels are given in Table 8.5. The ACSM and CDC noted that because enjoyment of an activity is related to participation, moderate-intensity activities are more likely to be continued than high-intensity ones. Consequently, they recommended "30 minutes or more of moderate-intensity physical activity on most, preferably all, days of the week." They noted that the health benefits of physical activity accrue in proportion to the total amount of activity performed, measured as calories or minutes of activity. Furthermore, the daily 30 minutes of exercise can be accrued over shorter intervals, as three 10-minute bouts of exercise result in a significant increase in maximal oxygen uptake, although

the increase was not as high as for 30 minutes of continuous exercise.[28]

One study of nonvigorous energy expenditure (<6 Met) did not find decreased mortality in men even if a large amount of time and energy is spent in the nonvigorous activities.[29] Other data suggest a linear dose-response relation between activity and health (except for the most vigorous levels or more than 3000 kcal per week).[8] Hence sedentary persons should increase their activity to a moderate level, and modestly active persons should increase their activity to 6 to 7 Met or higher.

Stress Testing Prior to Exercise

Persons with cardiac risk factors such as hypercholesterolemia, hypertension, diabetes mellitus, tobacco use, or a family history of heart disease may need an exercise stress test prior to beginning an exercise program. Persons of age 40 years or younger with two or more cardiac risk factors and persons of ages 41 years or older with one or more cardiac risk factors generally should have an exercise stress test prior to beginning an exercise program.

Exercise Prescription

The exercise prescription should identify activity, frequency, duration, intensity, and program elements. These aspects of the exercise prescription should be individualized to the patient; activity, frequency, and duration have been discussed previously. Intensity is based on a set percentage of the maximal predicted heart rate (MPHR), which can be determined by the formula $220 - \text{age}$ (Table 8.6). Sedentary persons may start by achieving 60% of MPHR and gradually progress to higher percentages; 90% is the maximum recommended. Program elements should include warm-up for 5 minutes with stretching exercises, the activity itself, and a 2- to 3-minute cool-down period.

Table 8.5. **Examples of Activities to Achieve Various Levels of Metabolic Equivalents**

Metabolic equivalents	Examples
2–3	Bowling, strolling, golf (power cart)
4–5	Walking 3.5 mph, cycling 8.0 mph, golf (carrying clubs), light carpentry, raking leaves, table tennis (ping-pong), dancing (e.g., foxtrot), calisthenics, doubles tennis, painting
6–7	Walking 5 mph, cycling 11 mph, singles tennis, splitting wood, snow shoveling, hand lawn mowing, square dancing, water-skiing, light downhill skiing, ice skating, roller skating, swimming
8–9	Jogging 6 mph, cycling 13 mph, vigorous basketball, social squash or handball
10–11	Running 7 mph, racquetball
≥12	Running 8–10 mph, vigorous competitive sports (e.g., competitive handball or squash)

Table 8.6. **Heart Rates According to Age**

Age (Years)	Heart rate (bpm)		
	60% of maximum	90% of maximum	Maximum
20	120	180	200
30	114	171	190
40	108	162	180
50	102	153	170
60	96	144	160
70	90	135	150

The formula for maximum predicted heart rate is 220 − age and may not be accurate if rate-altering medications such as β-blockers are being taken.

Nutrition

Good nutrition is essential throughout the life span to ensure proper growth and development, maintenance of health, recovery from acute illness, and prevention of chronic disease. In the United States, undernutrition resulting from inadequate food intake exists only in certain high-risk population groups. However, overnutrition and nutrient imbalances contributing to overweight, obesity, and a variety of chronic diseases are widespread among Americans. Unlike smoking or alcohol use, eating is a daily behavior that cannot be completely eliminated. Moreover, eating behavior is entwined with religious, cultural, and regional traditions that are not easily abandoned. Despite recommendations for healthful eating, taste and cost have been found to best predict food choices,[30] and individuals will preferentially choose foods with which they are more familiar.[31] This section addresses principles of good nutrition for maintenance of health and prevention of chronic diseases for the general population.

Caloric Needs

Caloric needs are determined by basal metabolic rate (BMR) and level of physical activity. BMR is highest during periods of growth and development, is proportional to the percentage lean body mass, and generally decreases with age. BMR accounts for approximately 80% of total caloric needs in sedentary persons and 60% for very active individuals. Table 8.7 shows recommended caloric intake for adults. Maintaining caloric intake near these levels will help adults prevent weight gain. A caloric excess of only 100 kcal/day will result in a 10-lb weight gain in 1 year. Therefore, it is essential to make routine adjustments in caloric intake or expenditure to maintain one's weight. To lose weight, it is necessary to reduce caloric intake below levels needed to maintain weight or to increase caloric needs through physical activity. In addition to increasing caloric expenditure, physical activity also helps to increase BMR among sedentary individuals and to offset the decrease in BMR that accompanies caloric restriction.

Dietary Fat

Dietary source of calories is just as important for prevention of chronic disease as is total intake of calories. High fat intake, especially saturated fat has been linked to CHD, colon cancer, and breast cancer. Reduction of total fat and saturated fat intakes has been shown to reduce blood cholesterol levels, and lower total and saturated fat intakes are associated with decreased risk of hyperlipidemia and CHD. Although total fat and saturated fat intakes have declined over the past 30 years, they are still above recommended levels, at 33% and 11%, respectively.[32] Current guidelines recommend a maximum 30% of calories from all types of fat, with <10% saturated fat, 60% or more from carbohydrates, and 10% from protein. In a 2,000-kcal diet, the total fat intake should be <65 g, saturated fat <20 g, carbohydrate 300 g, and protein 50 g. Recent guidelines issued by the National Heart, Lung, and Blood Institute (NHLBI) recommend saturated fat intake of <7% of calories and cholesterol intake <200 mg/day for individuals at high risk of CHD.[33]

Fat is the most calorically dense macronutrient providing 9 kcal/g, compared with about 4 kcal/g for both carbohydrates and protein. Nutrition fact labels on most foods provide consumers with the information needed to determine whether or how much of a given food is an appropriate choice.

The Food Guide Pyramid

A simple way to ensure that individuals eat a balanced diet is to base food choices on the Food Guide Pyramid (Fig. 8.3). The pyramid recommends 6 to 11 servings from the bread, cereal, rice, and pasta group, 3 to 5 servings from the vegetable group, 2 to 4 servings from both the milk, yogurt, and cheese group and the meat, poultry, fish, dry beans, eggs, and nuts group. Individuals with lower caloric needs should eat the smaller number of servings and those with higher caloric needs should eat the larger number of recommended servings. Within each food group there is a wide variety of foods available and selection of foods from all groups is encouraged.

Studies have shown inverse relationships between physical activity levels and intake of nutrients associated with chronic disease, i.e., fat, saturated fat, and cholesterol. More active individuals consumed more fiber, vitamins, calcium, and less total fat and saturated fat than sedentary individuals.[34,35]

Table 8.7. **Recommended Daily Calorie Intake by Gender, Age, and Activity Level**

Age (years)	Calorie intake		
	Low activity	Moderate activity	High activity
Men			
19–24	2300	3000	3700
25–50	2300	3000	3800
51+	2000	2600	3200
Women			
19–24	1800	2200	2600
25–50	1800	2200	2600
51+	1700	2000	2400

Source: Adapted from data from the National Research Council. Recommended dietary allowances, 10th ed. Washington, DC: National Academy Press. 1989:29, 330; compiled by the National Food Processors Association.

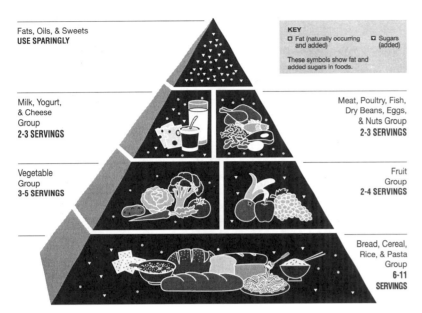

Fig. 8.3. Food Guide Pyramid.

The recently revised Dietary Guidelines for Americans[36] address the interactions among diet, body weight, and physical activity by encouraging all Americans to make sensible food choices, be physically active on a daily basis, and achieve a healthy body weight. The Food Guide Pyramid is the daily food choice guide incorporated into the dietary guidelines.

Weight Control and Weight Maintenance

Recent guidelines on the treatment of overweight and obesity[37] have highlighted the need for comprehensive evaluation and treatment of a health condition that has reached epidemic proportions. There are an estimated 97 million Americans who are overweight or obese. Both conditions lead to increased risk of diabetes, hypertension, CHD, stroke, gallbladder disease, osteoarthritis, dyslipidemia, sleep apnea, and cancer of the colon, breast, prostate, and endometrium. All-cause mortality also increases with increasing body weight.[37]

Overweight is defined as body mass index (BMI) = 25–29.9 kg/m^2; obese is BMI >30 kg/m^2. To determine BMI using pounds and inches, BMI = [weight (lbs.) $\times$ 703] ÷ [height (in.) $\times$ height (in.)]. Alternatively, waist circumference can be used as a measurement of weight related risk. For men, waist circumference >40 inches (102 cm) and for women, waist circumference >35 inches (88 cm) are considered to be high risk. Among those who are overweight, goals for weight loss should be to (1) reduce body weight; (2) maintain a lower body weight over the long term; and (3) at a minimum, prevent further weight gain.

The role of the health care provider is to assess level of overweight and other risk factors, assess patient's readiness to attempt weight loss, assist patient in setting realistic goals, provide patient with behavioral techniques for achieving goals, and provide support and follow-up. An appropriate weight loss goal for most patients is 1 to 2 lbs/week, or a caloric deficit of 3500 to 7000 calories. Intake and increases in activity should reflect such a difference from baseline levels. Specific techniques to facilitate weight loss include self-monitoring; realistic goal setting; making small changes; substituting lower calorie foods; increasing nutrient-dense, low-calorie foods; and increasing physical activity. Techniques used may vary from person to person. For patients with severe obesity or moderate obesity with comorbidities, pharmacotherapy or surgery may be considered.

Other Important Nutrients

Several other nutrients warrant special mention because of their association with a number of chronic diseases. These include calcium, fiber, vitamins, and other minerals. Calcium intake over the lifetime, but especially before age 30, is associated with peak bone mineral density and ultimately to the risk of osteoporosis. The greater the bone mineral density, the less susceptible bone is to breakage due to bone resorption that occurs with aging, but especially following menopause. Calcium intake of 1300 mg for adolescents and 1000 mg for adults,[38] while not difficult to achieve, requires thoughtful food selection. Dairy products are the primary source of calcium; however, replacement of liquid milk by other beverages such as carbonated drinks, sport drinks, and coffee contributes to low average calcium intakes. Calcium fortification of such foods as orange juice, breakfast cereals, and other grain products should help to reverse this trend. Patients should be encouraged to choose calcium-fortified products if they do not regularly consume dairy products.

Fiber, though not a nutrient per se, is an essential part of a healthful diet, as it provides bulk, aids digestion and elimination, and may lower low-density lipoprotein levels. Dietary fiber, the nondigestible portion of plant foods, is found in whole grains, vegetables, and fruits that are consumed in a state as close to natural and as unrefined as possible. High-fiber diets are generally lower in total and saturated fat, and are associated with lower risk of CHD and several forms of cancer including colon cancer (also see Chapters 76 and 92).

Daily needs for vitamins and minerals can generally be met with consumption of a varied, balanced diet as delineated in the Food Guide Pyramid. For individuals whose intake is limited by choice or amount of foods, a multivitamin/mineral supplement is recommended. Most adolescent girls and premenopausal women should take an iron supplement, as it is difficult to meet the recommended daily intake (15 mg) from foods alone. Women intending to conceive should be aware of recommendations to increase folate consumption before conception; pregnant women should consume 600 μg folate per day. Many grain foods are also fortified with folate, along with other B vitamins. Several vitamins (fat soluble) and minerals (such as selenium) are dangerous in large amounts. Toxic levels of these nutrients can be attributed to use of high-dose, single-nutrient supplements.

Herbals and Other Supplements

Dietary supplements, herbals, botanicals, enzymes, and metabolites are part of a growing multibillion dollar business. Some of the reasons people are turning to such products are prevention or treatment of chronic disease, supplementation of poor diet, weight loss, and distrust or cost of approved pharmaceuticals. Yet most dietary supplements are not regulated by the Food and Drug Administration (FDA). The responsibility for identity, purity, quality, strength, and composition of dietary supplements is left to the manufacturer.[39] It is important to assess patients' use of dietary supplements, as many supplements interact with medications or may influence diagnostic test results. Furthermore, some patients may delay treatment for certain conditions because they are using dietary supplements.

Resources

There are many resources available for clinician and patient reference regarding nutrition and weight loss issues, including the American Dietetic Association (800/366–1655), National City for Nutrition and Dietetics Information Line (*www.eatright.org*), Food and Nutrition Board of the Institute of Medicine (*www4.nas.edu/IOM/IOMhome.nsf*), Food and Nutrition Information Center (*www.nalusda.gov/fnic*), and the Food and Drug Administration (*www.fda.gov*). The Practical Guide for the Identification, Evaluation, and Treatment of Overweight and Obesity in Adults can be obtained from NHLBI at *www.nhlbi.nih.gov*.

References

1. McGinnis JM, Foege WH. Actual causes of death in the United States. JAMA 1993;270(18):2207–12.
2. American Cancer Society. Cancer facts and figures 1998: tobacco use. Available at *www.cancer.org/statistics/cff98/tobacco.html*.
3. U.S. Department of Health and Human Services. Treating tobacco use and dependence: a systems approach. Washington, DC: DHHS, November 2000.
4. Centers for Disease Control and Prevention. Cigarette smoking among adults—United States, 1995. MMWR 1997;46(51):1217–20.
5. Fiore MC, Bailey WC, Cohen SJ, et al. Treating tobacco use and dependence: clinical practice guideline. Rockville, MD: U.S. Department of Health and Human Services, Public Health Service, June 2000.
6. Centers for Disease Control and Prevention. Cigarette smoking-attributable mortality and years of potential life loss—United States, 1990. MMWR 1993;42:645–9.
7. The American Cancer Society. Quitting smoking. Available at *www2.cancer.org/cid/676.00/index.htm*.
8. U.S. Preventive Services Task Force: Guide to clinical preventive services, 2nd ed. Baltimore: Williams & Wilkins, 1996.
9. Fiore MC, Jorenby DE, Baker TB, Kenford SL. Tobacco dependence and the nicotine patch: clinical guidelines for effective use. JAMA 1992;268:2687–94.
10. Task Force on Community Preventive Services. Recommendations regarding intervention to reduce tobacco use and exposure to environmental tobacco smoke. Am J Prev Med 2001;20(2S):10–15.
11. Jorenby DE, Leischow SJ, Nides MA, et al. A controlled trial of sustained-release bupropion, a nicotine patch, or both for smoking cessation. N Engl J Med 1999;340(9):685–91.
12. Silagy C, Mant D, Fowler G, Lodge M. Meta-analysis on efficacy of nicotine replacement therapies in smoking cessation. Lancet 1994;343:139–42.
13. Bruvold WH. A meta-analysis of adolescent smoking prevention programs. Am J Public Health 1993;83:872–80.
14. Kottke TE, Battista RN, DeFriese GH, Brekke ML. Attributes of successful smoking cessation interventions in medical practice: a meta-analysis of 39 controlled trials. JAMA 1988;259:2882–9
15. Blair SN, Kohl HW, Paffenbarger RS, Clark DG, Cooper KH, Gibbons LW. Physical fitness and all-cause mortality: a prospective study of healthy men and women. JAMA 1989;262:2395–401.
16. Berlin JA, Colditz GA. A meta-analysis of physical activity in the prevention of coronary heart disease. Am J Epidemiol 1990;132:612–28.
17. Helmrich SP, Ragland DR, Leung RW, Paffenbarger RS. Physical activity and reduced occurrences of non-insulin-dependent diabetes mellitus. N Engl J Med 1991;325:147–52.
18. Paffenbarger RS, Hyde RT, Wing AL, Lee I, Jung DL, Kampert JB. The association of changes in physical activity level and other lifestyle characteristics with mortality among men. N Engl J Med 1993;328:538–45.
19. Blair SN, Kohl HW, Barlow CE, Paffenbarger RS, Gibbons LW, Macera CA. Changes in physical fitness and all-cause mortality: a prospective study of healthy and unhealthy men. JAMA 1995;273:1093–8.
20. Steptoe A, Edwards S, Moses J, Mathews A. The effect of exercise training on mood and perceived coping ability in anxious adults from the general population. J Psychosom Res 1989;33:537–47.
21. Moses J, Steptow A, Mathews A, Edwards S. The effects of exercise training on mental well-being in the normal population: a controlled trial. J Psychosom Res 1989;33:47–61.
22. Pollock ML, Carroll JF. Injuries and adherence to walk/job and resistance training programs in the elderly. Med Sci Sports Exerc 1991;23:1194–200.
23. Lane NE, Michel B, Bjorkengren A, et al. The risk of osteoarthritis with running and age: a 5-year longitudinal study. J Rheumatol 1993;20:461–8.
24. Centers for Disease Control and Prevention. Public health focus: physical activity and the prevention of coronary heart disease. MMWR 1993;42:669–72.
25. Lewis B, Lynch W. The effect of physician advice on exercise behavior. Prev Med 1993;22:110–21.
26. Logsdon DN, Lazaro CM, Meier RV. The feasibility of behavioral risk reduction in primary medical care. Am J Prev Med 1989;5:249–56.
27. Pate RR, Pratt M, Blair SN, et al. Physical activity and public health: a recommendation from the Centers for Disease Control

and Prevention and the American College of Sports Medicine. JAMA 1995;273:402–7.

28. DeBusk RF, Stenestrand U, Sheehan M, Haskell WL. Training effects of long versus short bouts of exercise in healthy subjects. Am J Cardiol 1990;65:1010–3.

29. Lee I, Hsieh C, Paffenbarger RS. Exercise intensity and longevity in men: the Harvard alumni health study. JAMA 1995; 273:1179–84.

30. Glanz K, Basil M, Maibach E, Goldberg J, Snyder D. Why Americans eat what they do: taste, nutrition, cost, convenience, and weight control concerns as influences on food consumption. J Am Diet Assoc 1998;98(10):1118–26.

31. Nowalk MP, Wing RR, Koeske R. The effect of tasting food samples on the use of recipes distributed in nutrition counseling. J Am Diet Assoc 1986;86(12):1715–6.

32. Kennedy ET, Bowman SA, Powell R. Dietary-fat intake in the US population. J Am Coll Nutr 1999;18(3):207–12.

33. National Institutes of Health, National Heart, Lung, and Blood Institute. ATP III guidelines at-a-glance quick desk reference. NIH publication no. 01-3305. Bethesda, MD: NIH, May 2001.

34. Gillman MW, Pinto BM, Tennstedt S, Glanz K, Marcus B,

Friedman RH. Relationships of physical activity with dietary behaviors among adults. Prev Med 2001;32:295–301.

35. Eaton CB, McPhillips JB, Gans KM, Garber CE. Cross-sectional relationship between diet and physical activity in two southeastern New England communities. Am J Prev Med 1995;11(4): 238–44.

36. U.S. Department of Agriculture, U.S. Department of Health and Human Services. Nutrition and your health: dietary guidelines for Americans, 5th ed. Home and Garden bulletin no. 232. Washington, DC: Department of Agriculture, 2000.

37. National Institutes of Health, National Heart, Lung, and Blood Institute, North American Association for the Study of Obesity. The practical guide: identification, evaluation, and treatment of overweight and obesity in adults. NIH publication no. 00-4084. Bethesda, MD: NIH, October 2000.

38. National Academy of Sciences. 1997–1998 dietary reference intakes (DRI): 1989 recommended daily allowances (RDA). Washington, DC: National Academy Press, 1998.

39. U.S. Food and Drug Administration, Center for Food Safety and Applied Nutrition. Overview of dietary supplements. January 3, 2001. Available at *www.cfsan.fda.gov/~dms/ds-oview.html*.

9

Health Care of the International Traveler

David N. Spees

Health care of the international traveler starts with pretravel education and prevention and ends with posttravel evaluation for exposures to diseases not normally encountered in the country of origin.

Travel History

The goals of the pretravel visit are (1) education of the traveler, (2) assessment of the risk of exposure to preventable diseases, and (3) provision of preventive and prophylactic care. The travel history is the most important component for assessing risk. Critical elements include the type and purpose of the trip, departure date, itinerary, duration and degree of risk, climate and altitude, mode of travel, and place of sleep. This additional information complements the standard medical history and evaluation. Figure 9.1 is a sample history form.

Trip Risk Assessment

The risk of encountering health problems during travel correlates directly with the type of trip. Exposure increases in about the following order of trip type: Cruises are the least hazardous, as passengers spend the nights aboard, limiting exposure to indigenous diseases and arthropods. Pleasure and adventure seekers require special attention depending on their definition of "pleasure" or "adventure"; some are only sightseers, whereas others are seeking sexual encounters. Business trips can be lonely and prolonged. This isolation from family and familiar mores can result in behaviors or pleasures not normally risked. The most hazardous common trip for travelers is a safari, typically to East Africa. Most safaris are physically comfortable, but exposure to insect-borne disease, local water, and native food is frequent. Of higher risk are visits to family and friends or others living on the local economy of developing countries, such as teachers, students, and missionaries. These visitors often travel with children, feel pressure to conform to local customs, do not want to offend local hosts and relatives with their Western differences, are in close contact with indigenous people, and have high exposure to insect-borne disease. Many immigrants return to their native countries having lost their previous partial immunities (e.g., against malaria and diarrhea) and underestimate their risk and that of their children. Travelers at the highest risk are trekkers, campers, bikers, and rafters. Although they are usually better prepared by more pretravel self-education and are more aware of their risks, they are also more adventuresome, more medically compromising, and often financially unwilling to purchase expensive medications and vaccines.

Medical History

Certain factors in the medical history have special significance to travel medicine. The medical history form in Figure 9.1 highlights these key factors. The existence of any of these conditions or allergies may preclude trips of certain types and may be contraindications to vaccines and medications, such as antimalarial drugs, specifically prescribed for travelers. Implications of a positive reply are covered in the sections Prevention and Preexisting Diseases, below.

Prevention

The purpose of the patient's pretravel visit is to obtain preventive services. Elements of prevention should include education, immunizations, prophylaxis for malaria and high altitude illness, and medication for traveler's diarrhea.

Pretravel Education

Education is central to the travel visit. Its role is risk reduction and preparedness for possible problems or aggravation

Patient name _____ Age _____

Today's date _____   Departure date _____

Type of trip:

_____ Cruise   _____ Studying

_____ Pleasure/adventure   _____ Teaching

_____ Business   _____ Missions

_____ Safari   _____ Trekking

_____ Family/friends   _____ Rafting

Itinerary:

City/province/country   No. of days

_____

_____

_____

_____

Will you be:

_____ Staying exclusively on a cruise ship?

_____ Staying in a hotel?

_____ Staying in a home?

_____ Climbing above 8,000 ft/2500m?

_____ Camping?

_____ Entering a jungle?

Medical history:

Do you have any of the following?

_____ Asthma   _____ Kidney/bladder trouble

_____ Heart trouble   _____ High blood pressure

_____ Ulcers/prior   _____ Diabetes
      stomach surgery   _____ Psoriasis

_____ Arthritis   _____ Weak immunity

_____ Bronchitis/
      emphysema

List other medical problems: Current medications:

1.   1.

2.   2.

3.   3.

Allergies:

_____ None known

_____ Neomycin/streptomycin/polymyxin B

_____ Eggs

_____ Other medication allergies—please list

Have you ever had red measles? _____ Or after 1956
had the red measles vaccine? _____

Pregnant?

_____ Yes/maybe   _____ Impossible

_____ No, type of contraception

Fig. 9.1. Medical history form.

of existing problems. A checklist of those education items (Fig. 9.2) can be used as a prompt for the patient visit.

Water and Food Safety

The maxim is, "Cook it, boil it, peel it, or forget it." Boiling clean water for 3 minutes at any altitude is sufficient. A 1-minute boil will pasteurize water for most situations. Bottled water is generally safe, if the sealed cap is removed only in the tourist's presence. Chlorine and iodine tablets are available in camping stores and sufficiently kill organisms for the immunocompetent; iodine is more efficacious. Water filters are not recommended because of insufficient testing or inadequate filtering of viruses. Avoid all tap water and ice cubes, even if mixed in alcoholic beverages. Milk is often unpasteurized, as are dairy products. All meats and vegetables should be thoroughly cooked and served steaming hot. Avoid all cold buffets, chilled desserts, and salads. Peeling the intact skins of fruits before eating is safe.

Insect Avoidance

The traveler cannot contract certain diseases, fortunately, unless bitten by the vector. Bites of the mosquito, tick, tsetse fly, sandfly, or flea are avoided by applying a repellant containing 20% to 50% diethyltoluamide (DEET) (Sawyer, Repel, Cutter, others) on all exposed skin surfaces. Prolonged or excessive applications of high concentrations can be toxic to young children. Long-sleeve shirts and long pants are essential wear in malarious or dengue areas. Spraying or soaking clothes, mosquito nets, and tents with permethrin (Duranon, Sawyer, others) significantly reduces the number of bites and incidence of malaria.

First-Aid Kit

Inclusion of an antipyretic/analgesic, a topical antibiotic, an insect repellent with 20% to 50% DEET, a sunscreen with an ultraviolet A (UVA) and B (UVB) with sun protection factor (SPF) of 15 or more, an antihistamine, and possibly ipecac

Most travelers	Individualized advice
___ Vaccines required/ needed	___ Malaria prophylaxis
___ Vaccine side effects	___ Poisoning/-quine toxicity
___ Food and water safety	___ High altitude sickness
___ Insect/sun avoidance	___ Freshwater exposure/ schistosomiasis
___ Traveler's diarrhea	___ Overseas pharmacies/ over the counter drugs
___ First aid kit/ medications	___ STDs/HIV
___ General/transport safety	___ Rabies/animals

Fig. 9.2. Educational items reviewed.

and an antifungal gynecologic cream are advisable. It is also the logical place to put any medical records and abnormal electrocardiograms (ECGs).

General Safety Advice

A seatbelt is always used in a taxi, or one should sit in the back seat; it is advisable to be assertive with unsafe drivers. Display of any valuables and money should be avoided. Travelers should never travel with anything they cannot afford to have stolen. In a closed space with a gas heater, a window should be cracked open. The lower stories in hotels are safest, and the nearest operative fire exit should be identified. Antimalarial, chlorine, and iodine tablets in proximity to bored traveling children are a hazardous combination, perhaps warranting ipecac in the cabin bag.

Jet Lag

The best method to entrain circadian rhythms is unknown, although certain measures are helpful. Before travel, adjusting to the new time zone by 1 hour per 24-hour period is helpful. At the destination, taking 5 mg of melatonin at bedtime for the first few days shortens the duration. In the mornings at the destination, bright light is helpful, as is a high-protein breakfast with a caffeinated beverage. Alcohol should be avoided and liberal hydration employed. A prescription hypnotic such as zolpidem (Ambien) also promotes sleep at night.

Motion Sickness

Effective agents for prophylaxis of motion sickness in adults include transdermal scopolamine (Transderm SCOP) applied 8 hours before motion or dimenhydrinate (Dramamine) 50 to 100 mg taken 1 hour before motion and then every 4 to 6 hours. Either may impair performance or produce unacceptable anticholinergic side effects, particularly in the elderly.

Local Practitioners and Pharmacies

Developing-world pharmacies frequently allow the purchase of most medications over the counter. However, wishing to be certain of "curing the problem" and pleasing the patient, local practitioners and pharmacists often overprescribe. For example, traveler's diarrhea might be treated for bacterial causes with chloramphenicol in addition to one or more antiparasitic drugs. The U.S. embassy can provide names of reputable practitioners and hospitals.

Freshwater and Schistosomiasis

All freshwater must be assumed to be fecally contaminated. After any accidental tropical or semitropical freshwater exposure, one should towel off quickly to minimize the risk of schistosomiasis and other waterborne diseases.

Sexually Transmitted Diseases

The anonymity of travel combined with open prostitution places many travelers at risk of sexually transmitted diseases (STDs), including human immunodeficiency virus (HIV) infection. Some individuals travel explicitly for sexual encounters. Openly addressing this possibility with travelers can promote defensive behaviors and encourage safe sex.

Commonsense Advice

(1) Hand-carry all medications in original containers. (2) The first-aid kit should include a copy of any abnormal or unusual ECG, radiologic report, and recent hospital discharge summary. (3) The traveler should verify insurance policy coverage and consider the purchase of medical evacuation insurance. (4) Nasal/sinus congestion should be treated early and aggressively before flying. (5) An injection is never accepted without personally observing the unbroken seals of the sterile needle, syringe, and medication.

Immunizations

Travel vaccines fall into two categories: required and recommended. Unless otherwise stated, most vaccines can be administered simultaneously. A notable exception to coincident administration is immune serum globulin with measles vaccine.

Required Immunizations

The only World Health Organization (WHO) regulated vaccine currently required by countries is yellow fever vaccine. These countries are listed in Health Information for International Travel (HIIT) with updates in Summary of HIIT (Table 9.1). Both cholera and meningococcal vaccines have been required in the past. Until a better cholera vaccine is available, cholera vaccine is unlikely to become officially required even in epidemic conditions. Meningococcal vaccine has been required by Saudi Arabia 10 days before the annual hajji to Mecca.

Only an approved yellow fever vaccination center can administer this vaccine. Some public health departments allow individual practitioners to be a designated center. It is a fastidious live viral vaccine that requires careful handling and use within 1 hour of reconstitution. Serious reactions are uncommon in those less than 65 years old.

Recommended Immunizations

Physicians are familiar with the routine vaccines: tetanus/diphtheria, influenza, and pneumococcal vaccines. The most frequently recommended additional prophylactic agents are immune serum globulin or hepatitis A vaccine, a polio booster, a measles booster, and typhoid vaccines. Special situations might require meningococcal, hepatitis B, Japanese encephalitis, or rabies vaccines. Most authorities are uncertain as to what duration of travel justifies the risk of prophylactic vaccination.

Table 9.1. **Resources for International Travel**

Centers for Disease Control and Prevention (CDC). Health Information for International Travel and Summary of Health Information for International Travel: *http://www.cdc.gov/* (choose Travelers' Health). International Travelers' Hotline: 1-877-394-8747

International Society of Travel Medicine: *http://www.istm.org*

Travel and Tropical Medicine Manual, 3rd edition, Elaine Jong and Russell McMullen, editors. Philadelphia: WB Saunders, 2001

Table 9.2. **Vaccines for International Travel**

Vaccine	Age	Booster interval	Booster dose and route	Primary series	Comments
Hepatitis A (Harvix/Vaqta)	>18 years	Once at 6–18 months	IM in deltoid	1 dose	Trip <5 months; add immune serum globulin (ISG) if departing in <2–4 weeks
	1–18 years		IM in deltoid	1 dose	Not Food and Drug Administration (FDA) approved in 1–2 year olds
Immune serum globulin (ISG)	All	3 months	0.02 mL/kg	None	Trip <3 months; Not with measles, mumps, rubella (MMR)
Typhoid Oral Ty21a	6 years	q5y	1 cap qod at bedtime × 4	4 caps	Not with antibiotics, mefloquine, or Malarone
Injectable Typhim Vi	≥2 years	q2y	0.5 mL IM	One dose	Few side effects
Tetanus/diphtheria	≥7 years	5–10 years	0.5 mL SC	Three doses	
Polio (eIPV)	≥18 years	Once in adults	See insert/SC	3 doses	Not if streptomycin or neomycin anaphylaxis
Measles/Measles, mumps, rubella (MMR)	Born after 1956	Age dependent	0.5 mL SC	One dose, two doses in lifetime	Not with ISG
Meningococcus (ACYW-135)	≥3 months	q3y	See insert/SC	One dose	Less effective in <4 year olds; booster in 2 years
Hepatitis B	All	none	Age dependent	IM deltoid, three doses	Consider accelerated schedules; see text
Influenza	Usual	1 year	Usual/SC	1 dose	Give in spring for Southern Hemisphere
Yellow fever	≥9 months	10 years	0.5 ml SC	One dose	Call Centers for Disease Control (CDC) if needed for <9-month-old
Japanese encephalitis	≥1-year-old	≥3 years	1.0 mL SC	Three doses	Observe for 30 min after each dose
Rabies	All at risk	≥2 years or check titer	1.0 ml IM deltoid or 0.1 ml ID	Three doses	ID route contraindicated with antimalarials

DPaT, *Haemophilus influenzae* type b (HIB), varicella and pneumococcus vaccines per usual schedules.
Oral cholera and tick-borne encephalitis vaccines are not available in the United States.
Pregnancy or immunocompromise may contraindicate vaccination.

On occasion, elderly patients or persons reared in the developing world and who later immigrated to the United States are found who either never received a primary vaccination series, or their immunization status is unknown. These patients should complete the primary series before traveling. If they are starting their journey before adequate completion of the primary series, they should be informed of the possible inadequacy of their vaccine status. The primary series should be completed on return or continued overseas if safely available.

Recommended vaccines are discussed below in order of approximate frequency of administration to travelers. See Table 9.2 for dosage and frequency.

Hepatitis A or Immune Serum Globulin. Hepatitis A vaccine or the prophylactic agent immune serum globulin (ISG) before each trip is recommended for every traveler to the developing world unless there is evidence of immunity. The vaccine is preferable in most situations. If departure is shorter than the 2 to 4 weeks it takes for adequate efficacy of the vac-

cine, ISG and the vaccine may be administered together with little effect on subsequent protection by the vaccine. A booster dose of hepatitis A vaccine 6 to 18 months later will probably give lifetime immunity.

Tetanus/Diphtheria. A tetanus/diphtheria booster dose is given every 10 years. Consider a booster after a 5-year interval in high-risk situations. Those situations include trips with likelihood of a cut or puncture wound where sterile needles or properly stored vaccine may be unavailable.

Typhoid. Typhoid vaccination is recommended when the risk of exposure during the protective duration of the vaccine totals more than 5 to 6 weeks. Ty21a, a four-dose oral vaccine, replaces injectable vaccine for routine use in travelers age 6 years and older. The efficacy (>60%) of Ty21a is equal to that of injectable vaccine. Its protection lasts 5 years, and side effects are unusual and mild. Ty21a capsules contain live, attenuated bacteria and should be kept refrigerated and taken on an empty stomach with a cool or tepid beverage. The capsules are taken every other day and separated by several days from antibiotics, mefloquine, and Malarone. Injectable typhoid vaccine, Typhim Vi, is useful for those 2 to 6 years old; it has few side effects and needs only one dose as a primary series, but lasts only 2 years.

Poliomyelitis. Injectable enhanced polio vaccine (eIPV) is a safe, effective booster. It is given as a one-time adult booster if traveling to an endemic area. If the patient's primary series is incomplete or unknown and there is not enough time to complete the primary series before travel, a single booster dose of either injectable or oral (OPV) vaccine is recommended. It is not needed for the polio-free Western Hemisphere and some countries of the Western Pacific.

Measles/Rubella. For patients born after 1956, a second booster of measles vaccine is suggested. It is given at least 2 weeks before ISG or its efficacy cannot be ensured. In female travelers, combine it with rubella unless immunity to rubella is known. Pregnancy is contraindicated during the next 3 months. Frequently, the traveler is departing before the 2-week interval needed between ISG and measles vaccine. Use of ISG takes priority, with or without hepatitis A vaccine.

Meningococcus. Meningococcal meningitis is periodically epidemic in parts of Nepal and in a band across sub-Saharan Africa stretching from Mali to Ethiopia and Uganda. It will probably continue to be required by Saudi Arabia for pilgrims on hajji to Mecca. The quadrivalent A,C,Y,W-135 vaccine should be administered at least 10 days before arrival; it has few side effects.

Hepatitis B. Seroconversion is common for those residing in the developing world.[1] Therefore, hepatitis B is recommended for (1) travelers staying 6 months or longer, (2) pleasure seekers who might be sexually exposed, and (3) medical personnel. The primary series takes 6 months to complete, but a schedule with Engerix-B given at 0, 1, and 2 months produces excellent seroprotection,[2] with an additional booster suggested at 12 months if exposure continues. A more accelerated schedule of the same vaccine given on days 0, 7, and 21 or 28 has also resulted in good immunogenicity at 12 months[3] (see Chapter 90).

Influenza. Influenza may spread throughout an airliner.[4] Therefore, influenza vaccine use is encouraged during the usual influenza season in the Northern Hemisphere and during the spring and early summer for travelers to the Southern Hemisphere (see Chapter 39).

Rabies. Many countries are highly endemic for rabies. Travelers are not at high risk, but the expensive vaccine and rabies immune globulin are not available in most countries. Long-term travelers, children, cyclists, and pet adopters should consider preexposure vaccination.

Cholera. The injectable cholera vaccine is no longer produced. The rare risk of this disease to travelers makes this vaccine rarely indicated, even during epidemics. Oral vaccines are more promising and available in other countries.

Japanese Encephalitis. A mosquito-borne arboviral infection, Japanese encephalitis is the leading cause of viral encephalitis in Asia. The Japanese encephalitis vaccine is indicated for travelers spending more than 30 days in the rural areas of countries on the Pacific Rim from India to China and east to the Philippines and Japan. The greatest risk is during the rainy season, April to October, and is minimal in urban areas. The three-dose primary series is administered over 14 or, preferably, 30 days and must be finished 10 days before travel begins. HIIT has a table of risk by country.

Malaria Prophylaxis

The need for an antimalarial prescription is a common reason for travel consultation. The most important advice is the mosquito avoidance measures described earlier. The second important component is prescribing the best antimalarial prophylaxis. Areas of the world with chloroquine-sensitive malaria, though shrinking, are still found in Mexico, Central America, and the Middle East. For simplicity, one could assume that all malarious areas are chloroquine-resistant. None of the prophylactic and mosquito avoidance measures are 100% effective.

Mefloquine (Lariam)

Probably the most prescribed antimalarial, mefloquine, is effective in both chloroquine-resistant and chloroquine-sensitive areas. It is taken once weekly starting 1 to 2 weeks before arrival in the malarious area, taken once weekly during possible exposure, and continued for 4 weeks after the last possible exposure. Most side effects, which are usually transient and occur during the first two doses, consist of dizziness, strange dreams, and insomnia. It has been reported to cause serious neuropsychiatric adverse effects in 1/10,600 users.[5] These effects are seizures, anxiety, depression, or psychotic episodes. Therefore, it should not be used in travelers with epilepsy or serious psychiatric illness. It is relatively contraindicated in those with cardiac conduction abnormalities and the first trimester of pregnancy. Resistance is rare.

Atovaquone/Proguanil (Malarone)

Atovaquone/proguanil (Malarone) is the newest antimalarial and available in adult and pediatric doses. It is very effective prophylaxis for chloroquine-resistant malaria and can be use in children weighing more than 11 kg. Ingested with food or a milky drink, one starts 2 days before exposure, continues daily during exposure and daily for only 7 days after last possible exposure. Its cost is prohibitive for exposures longer than about 7 days. However, side effects are infrequent and the same as a placebo.

Doxycycline

Effective against chloroquine-resistant malaria in lieu of mefloquine, possible phototoxic side effects limit the general use of doxycycline in tropical areas. Start 1 day before possible malaria exposure, continuing daily during exposure and for 4 weeks after the last possible exposure. Its use requires meticulous application of a sunscreen (SPF >15) with UVA-blocking properties; women should carry an antimonilial vaginal cream. Doxycycline is contraindicated in children under 8 years old.

Chloroquine Phosphate (Aralen)

Chloroquine phosphate is useful in chloroquine-sensitive malarious areas. The dosage is one 500 mg tablet (Aralen) in adults and 5.0 mg/kg of the base weekly in children, starting 1 week before possible exposure, weekly during exposure, and for 4 weeks after the last possible exposure. Side effects of chloroquine, which are infrequent, consist of dizziness or gastrointestinal upset, and the drug can precipitate a flare of psoriasis. For children, mixing it in jam lessens its bitter taste. It is toxic in overdose and should be stored in a childproof container.

Primaquine Phosphate

Useful for postexposure elimination of the hepatic forms of *Plasmodium vivax* and *Plasmodium ovale*, there is little indication for primaquine in the returning short-term traveler. However, even without symptoms, it should be considered if the exposure period is longer than 6 months. Before administration, a normal glucose-6-phosphate dehydrogenase (G6PD) level should be confirmed.

Traveler's Diarrhea

The incidence of traveler's diarrhea (TD) ranges from 4% to more than 50%; it is the most preventable and easily treatable disease of travelers. For perspective, 4% of European travelers to the United States acquire TD,[6] and the attack rate for the developing world ranges from 20% to 56%.[7] A National Institute of Health (NIH) consensus conference defined TD as a syndrome characterized by a twofold or greater increase in the frequency of unformed bowel movements. Commonly associated symptoms include abdominal cramps, nausea, bloating, urgency, fever, and malaise. Episodes of TD usually begin abruptly, occur during travel or soon after returning home, and are generally self-limited. TD typically results in four or five loose or watery stools per day. The median duration of diarrhea is 3 to 4 days. Ten percent of the cases persist longer than 1 week, approximately 2% longer than 1 month, and less than 1% longer than 3 months.[8] Rapid treatment can shorten the duration to a matter of hours, an important factor for expensive tourist and short business trips. Bacterial etiologies account for 37% to 72+% of cases. The most common bacteria, in approximate order of frequency, are enterotoxigenic *Escherichia coli*, *Shigella*, *Campylobacter jejuni*, *Salmonella*, and *Vibrio* spp. The most common viral etiologies (responsible for up to 36% of cases of TD) are rotavirus and Norwalk viruses.[7] Parasites, primarily *Giardia lamblia* and *Entamoeba histolytica*, cause up to 9% of cases. Frequently more than one pathogen is found during a diarrheal illness, and 20% to 50% of cases of TD remain unexplained.[8]

Prophylaxis

Generally, antibiotic prophylaxis is avoided. The first line of prevention is food and water safety and vaccination; these points were covered earlier in the chapter (see Prevention). Prophylaxis is justified in special circumstances where the risk of TD must be minimized and requires a short duration of antibiotic exposure. These situations might include an international sporting event, a honeymoon, or an intense, high-level business meeting. Agents with prophylactic efficacy include bismuth subsalicylate (Pepto-Bismol) 2 tablets qid; norfloxacin (Noroxin) 400 mg qd; ciprofloxacin (Cipro) 500 mg qd; ofloxacin (Floxin) 300 mg qd; and perhaps, doxycycline (Vibramycin) 100 mg qd.

Treatment

Rapid treatment of adults can reduce the duration of TD to 1 day or less. The fluoroquinolones provide the broadest coverage against the bacterial etiologies of TD. Their cost limits widespread use in developing countries, resulting in infrequent resistance to this class of antibiotics. If there is no fever or bloody diarrhea, start with two loperamide (Imodium) capsules after the first loose stool and continue at the usual doses of loperamide. If the diarrhea continues after the third loose stool, give two tablets of either ciprofloxacin 500 mg or norfloxacin 400 mg. Most TD stops at this point, but if it still continues give one tablet of the fluoroquinolone bid for 3 days. Rifaximin, a luminal antibiotic dosed at 400 mg tid for three doses appears promising and available in Europe. Distant second-line alternatives are bismuth subsalicylate 30 mL every half-hour for eight doses or doxycycline 100 mg two bid for 3 days. Antidiarrheal agents are not recommended for children. Azithromycin (Zithromax) at usual doses has some efficacy. Oral rehydration solution (ORS) is the best treatment for young children. ORS packets promoted by WHO are available in most developing-world pharmacies or clinics. Mixed in 1 L of safe water, they are safe and effective. Introduce safe foods of the same consistency as the diarrheal stools.

High-Altitude Illness

The axiom is "climb high, but sleep low." The incidence of high-altitude illness increases with ascent above 2500 m (8200 feet). The prevalence is 9% at 2850 meters (9350 feet) and 34% at 3650 meters (12,000 feet).[9] Common to the syndromes of acute mountain sickness (AMS), high-altitude pulmonary edema (HAPE), and high-altitude cerebral edema (HACE) are rapid ascent and tissue hypoxia. The latter results from the lower partial pressure of oxygen at high altitudes. AMS ranges from a mild illness (headache being the most common symptom, followed by nausea or lassitude) to a severe illness (vomiting, dyspnea at rest, ataxia, mental impairment, or cyanosis). HAPE can develop after several days, usually during sleep, with symptoms of extreme dyspnea, cough, rales, mild fever, and cyanosis. HACE can develop after several days of mild AMS, presenting with progressively severe lassitude, decreasing alertness, psychosis, focal neurologic signs, and eventual coma. Predisposing factors to these syndromes are poorly understood but include more exertion and prior residence at less than 3000 feet.

The best prophylaxis is slow ascent, less than about 300 m (1000 feet) per day. For rapid ascents above 3000 m (9800 feet) lasting more than 12 hours, consider prophylaxis with 125 to 250 mg acetazolamide (Diamox) bid, starting 24 hours before ascent and continuing during the first 2 to 4 days at high altitude. Over-the-counter analgesics are adequate for the headache. Acetazolamide can be reserved to treat mild cases of AMS. Although dexamethasone (Decadron) 4 mg q6h can be used for prophylaxis, it is usually reserved for treatment of severe AMS, HAPE, or HACE. Once dexamethasone is started, high-flow oxygen and descent should begin emergently.

Preexisting Diseases

Several diseases noted by the history form require elucidation. Generally, travelers should treat aggravation of a preexisting disease early and aggressively. Travelers must be prepared for the disease exacerbations they can manage.

Bronchitis/Emphysema

Patients with chronic obstructive pulmonary disease (COPD) may require arterial blood gas determinations before travel (see Chapter 83). Aircraft maintain cabin pressure equivalent to 2438 m (8000 feet) or less. This altitude results in a fall of partial pressure of arterial oxygen (PaO_2) to approximately 60 mm Hg in healthy individuals. Though prediction of hypoxemia in the COPD patient is difficult, patients with a preflight PaO_2 of less than 70 mm Hg or oxygen saturation of less than 93% should receive supplemental oxygen from the airline during the flight.[10] Individuals with preflight hypercapnia or vital capacity of less than 50% should travel by land or obtain specialty consultation.

Asthma

Because of the frequency of upper respiratory infections and pollution in the developing world, the traveler should expect to experience an exacerbation of asthma (see Chapter 83). Travelers should follow their peak flow readings and must know how to self-medicate with antibiotics and corticosteroids to the limit of their ability.

Heart Disease

Airline travel should be restricted for 4 to 8 weeks after myocardial infarction and supplemental oxygen considered for the following 4 months (see Chapter 76). A general rule is that the cardiac patient should be able to walk 100 yards and climb 12 steps,[11] although an exercise treadmill test will give a more precise functional capacity.

Ulcers/Prior Stomach Surgery

Prohibit airline travel for 10 to 14 days after abdominal surgery[12] (see Chapter 87). The minimum time after laparoscopy using CO_2 inflation is unknown, but airline travel should be safe after 48 hours. As hypochlorhydria and H_2-blockers diminish the stomach's natural barrier to traveler's diarrhea and cholera, consider prophylaxis or aggressive treatment and liberalize indications for vaccination.

Physical Handicap/Arthritis

Special provisions for handicap needs should be made in advance with the airline. Information on travel for the handicapped can be obtained from most organizations for seniors or for the specific handicap. Arthritides should be well controlled with the expectation of some aggravation (see Chapters 112,113).

Posttravel Evaluation

Well Traveler

Most returning short-term travelers do not need evaluation. Arbitrarily, those who have had an exposure of 6 months in the developing world should have a complete blood count to check for anemia and eosinophils and one to three fecal examinations for ova and parasites. A history of other possible exposures guides additional testing.

Symptomatic Traveler

For the symptomatic traveler the history should focus on symptoms or illnesses during the travel. It should consider sexual and freshwater exposures, prophylactic compliance, and the exact travel itinerary to determine possible exposures. This risk assessment guides the evaluation. Whatever the symptoms, if malaria exposure was possible, start with examination of thick and thin blood smears. If the illness continues or the index of suspicion is high, the malaria smears should be repeated as frequently as every 6 hours. A technologist experienced in reading malaria smears is preferable, as the parasitic load may be light in nonimmune travelers but the patient very ill. Urinalysis, a fresh fecal specimen for culture, and three specimens for ova and parasites often reveal most of the common problems. Otherwise, evaluation of a febrile illness can proceed in an orderly, routine fashion. Tests to consider early in the evaluation would be those for liver function, malaria antibodies, hepatitis serologies, schistosomiasis serology, HIV screen, and rickettsial serologies. A rapid plasma reagin test for syphilis and an intermediate-strength purified protein derivative skin test screen for the great imitators.

Summary

Staying healthy abroad is not always easy, but pretravel education with proper prophylaxis and vaccination can prevent the most common maladies. The world is shrinking, and it has never been easier for patients to savor its differences, its mystery, and its excitement. The family physician can take the lead in preventing the resurgence of the old scourges such as malaria and diphtheria and in limiting the spread of emerging diseases.

References

1. Steffen R. Hepatitis A and hepatitis B: risks compared with other vaccine preventable diseases and immunization recommendations. Vaccine 1993;11:518–20.
2. Marsano L, Greenberg R, Zetterman R, et al. Comparison of a rapid hepatitis B immunization schedule to the standard schedule for adults. Am J Gastroenterol 1996;91(1):111–5.
3. Bock HL, Löscher T, Scheiermann N, et al. Accelerated schedule for hepatitis B immunization. J Travel Med 1995;2:213–17.
4. Klontz KC, Hynes NA, Gunn RA, et al. An outbreak of influenza A/Taiwan1/86(H1NI) infections at a naval base and its association with airplane travel. Am J Epidemiol 1989;129:341–8.
5. Schlagenhauf P. Mefloquine for malaria chemoprophylaxis 1992–1998: a review. J Travel Med 1999;6:122–133.
6. Steffen R. Epidemiologic studies of traveler's diarrhea, severe gastrointestinal infections, and cholera. Rev Infect Dis 1986; 8(suppl 2):S122–30.
7. Castelli F, Carosi G. Epidemiology of traveler's diarrhea. Chemotherapy 1995;41(suppl 1):20–32.
8. Travelers' diarrhea: National Institutes of Health consensus development conference statement. JAMA 1985;253:2700–4.
9. Maggiorini M, Buhler B, Walter M, et al. Prevalence of acute mountain sickness in the Swiss Alps. BMJ 1990;301(6756): 853–5.
10. Cottrell JJ. Altitude exposures during aircraft flight. Chest 1988; 92:81–4.
11. Kusumi RK. Medical aspects of air travel. Am Fam Physician 1981;23:125–9.
12. AMA Commission on Emergency Medical Services. Medical aspects of transportation aboard commercial aircraft. JAMA 1982;247:1007–11.

10
Preconception Care

Josephine R. Fowler and Brian W. Jack

Family physicians have practiced risk reduction in preparation for pregnancy for many years as part of such activities as premarital counseling, family planning, and genetic counseling. In recent years there is a growing realization that poor obstetric outcomes may be prevented by more comprehensively assessing and modifying medical, psychosocial, and behavioral risk before pregnancy. This concept, called preconception care, can help couples make decisions regarding the timing of conception and can improve their readiness for pregnancy.[1]

The goals of preconception care are (1) to ensure that a woman and her partner are healthy and practicing healthy lifestyles before pregnancy, (2) to ensure that couples have the opportunity to address risky behaviors that might result in poor pregnancy outcomes, and (3) to reduce the likelihood of unwanted pregnancies. Many of the medical conditions, personal behaviors, and psychosocial risks associated with negative pregnancy outcomes can be identified and modified before conception. Many health care options are limited by the time a woman becomes pregnant. A comprehensive preconception care program can benefit women desiring pregnancy by reducing risks, promoting healthy lifestyles, and increasing readiness for pregnancy.

Development of the concept of preconception care was identified as a priority in the 1990s.[1–3] The U.S. Public Health Service underscored the importance of preconception care by including among the health promotion and disease prevention objectives for the year 2000 a recommendation to increase to at least 60% the proportion of primary care providers who offer age-appropriate preconception care and counseling.[4] This chapter describes the role of the family physician in providing preconception care and discusses components of the preconception visit.

Role of the Family Physician

All family physicians care for young men and women and should be aware of preconception needs.[5,6] Family physicians should include consideration of the potential for pregnancy as a part of the usual health care for men and women of reproductive age and should assess and discuss the implications of a woman's present health status on a possible pregnancy. Attention to the health of prospective parents before they conceive is a natural extension of family practice, as it requires that family physicians extend their prevention and health promotion skills to couples of reproductive age. Family physicians are already aware of many of the concerns that are the source of the preconception visit. All family physicians can practice preconception care, regardless of whether or not they provide prenatal, labor, and delivery services.[7] Preconception care can be most effectively provided as part of ongoing primary care. Family physicians can include preconception care as part of such standard clinical encounters as routine health maintenance; school, work, or premarital examinations; family planning visits; negative pregnancy tests; and well-child care for another member of the family. At such visits family physicians should address smoking, diet and nutrition, the importance of early entry to prenatal care, and effective family planning, and clarify choices about lifestyle, education, and occupation that might affect the decision to become pregnant. Family physicians should begin education early with young men about responsible fatherhood and sexuality. Men should be engaged in preparing for fatherhood, and the evaluation of risks should be encouraged to support efforts by their partners to lower reproductive risk.

Content of Preconception Care

Preconception care includes the provision of health education individualized to a woman's or couple's needs (health promotion), a thorough and systematic identification of risks (risk assessment), and the initiation of actions to address those risks (interventions).

Health Promotion

Health promotion that applies to all women of childbearing age is an important component of preconception care and consists of counseling and education to support healthful behavior about pregnancy and parenting (see Chapter 8). In family practice, education about pregnancy, birth, and parenting occurs throughout the parenting years. The preconception visit is an opportunity for more intensive involvement. Table 10.1 lists the content of the health promotion component of preconception care.

An objective of preconception care is to assess a woman's readiness for pregnancy. Unwanted and unintended pregnancy is a major problem in the United States. Unintended pregnancy is associated with delays in the initiation of prenatal care and behaviors that increase the risk for adverse birth outcomes.[8] Because interventions to prevent unwanted pregnancy must occur before conception, preconception health promotion supports the idea that women can choose whether to become pregnant and includes counseling about pregnancy planning, spacing, and contraception. These visits offer opportunities for reproductive education about such topics as sexuality, information sources on pregnancy and parenting, pregnancy planning, and readiness for pregnancy, including the option of delaying or not having children. For many women, the recognition that they can take control and direct the course of their own lives, rather than being at the mercy of external forces, is a necessary component of adopting control of their reproductive potential.

Table 10.1. **Content of Preconception Care: Health Promotion by Education and Counseling**

Education about pregnancy, birth, and parenting

Discuss good dietary habits and optimal weight

Exercise programs

Identify adverse health behaviors including tobacco, alcohol, and illicit drugs

Identify environmental exposures

Review current medications including risks and benefits

Discuss safe sexual practices

Review family planning options including birth spacing

Discuss prevention of unwanted pregnancy including imparting knowledge, influencing attitudes, and enhancing life options

Emphasize the importance of early prenatal care

Counseling about the availability of social, financial, and vocational assistance programs

Make arrangements for ongoing primary care

Through health promotion activities, the family physician can provide counseling about the availability of social programs, including vocational training, that might be considered an alternative to pregnancy. The interventions available include imparting knowledge, influencing attitudes, providing access to contraceptives, and enhancing life options. Family planning, education, and social services needed to provide these interventions should be considered part of preconception care. If a woman and her partner opt to delay pregnancy, the preconception visit offers the family physician an opportunity to discuss methods of contraception. Careful, consistent use of contraception and conscientiously planning pregnancy can improve fetal outcome, reduce the number of abortions, have an impact on child abuse and neglect, and reduce health care costs. Counseling to promote and support healthful behavior should foster the idea that women can choose healthy behaviors. The preconception visit offers an opportunity to discuss many health options, including exercise programs, dietary habits, and optimal weight. Health promotion should include helping women with smoking cessation, discussing risks associated with alcohol and drug use, and identifying resources for assistance with substance abuse and risky behaviors. Counseling about avoiding teratogenic medications or choosing alternative regimens is also important before pregnancy. The preconception visit offers an opportunity to provide information on avoidance of occupational hazards and exposure to environmental toxins. Working mothers can be counseled about workplace hazards, legal rights of pregnant workers, and child-care options. Counseling about safe sexual practices and ways to prevent sexually transmitted diseases (STDs) including human immunodeficiency virus (HIV) is important before pregnancy.

Preconception care should stress the value of early enrollment for prenatal care. Knowledge about publicly funded prenatal programs, eligibility requirements, and application processes may help low-income women plan for risk reduction visits before and during pregnancy. This information may encourage women to enroll early for prenatal care once they are pregnant. Women should be encouraged to maintain an accurate menstruation calendar along with a record of the discontinuation of oral contraceptives and of any nonmenstrual bleeding. It might allow more accurate dating of conception, which can better identify those women who are truly postdates and require intervention, and can reduce the number of women erroneously considered postmature.

Risk Assessment

Another aim of preconception care is to identify risks in women's medical, reproductive, family, and psychosocial history, nutritional and behavioral risks, and maternal exposures. Comprehensive risk assessment allows the family physician and the woman to identify her alterable risks for poor pregnancy outcome before conception occurs. Preconception risk assessment includes the history, physical examination, and laboratory testing. Table 10.2 lists the content of the risk assessment component of preconception care.

Figure 10.1 shows the preconception risk factors as a percentage of the total risk factors identified at the time of a neg-

Table 10.2. **Content of Preconception Care: Risk Assessment**

History (examples of important conditions, behaviors, or exposures are listed after each category)

Reproductive history: menstrual, sexual, contraceptive, obstetric, breastfeeding

Infectious disease history: human immunodeficiency virus, hepatitis B, hepatitis C, toxoplasmosis, rubella, varicella, and bacterial vaginosis

Exposure to teratogens: occupational exposures (heavy metals, organic solvents), medications (gold, lithium, isotretinoin, folic acid antagonists, valproic acid, and warfarin)

Medical history: cardiovascular disease, diabetes mellitus, seizure disorder, thyroid disease, immune thrombocytopenia, and pulmonary embolism

Family and genetic history: Tay-Sachs disease, β-thalassemia, α-thalassemia, sickle cell anemia, cystic fibrosis, advanced maternal age, family history of genetic disease, previously affected pregnancy

Nutrition: food habits, attitudes, use of vitamins and minerals, food allergies, availability of food, bulimia, anorexia, pica, phenylketonuria

Psychosocial risks: lack of adequate financial resources, inadequate housing, inadequate medical insurance, communication difficulties, barriers to medical care, inadequate pregnancy readiness, lack of personal support, deficient coping skills, living in an abusive situation, psychiatric conditions, extremes of work or exercise

High-risk behaviors: smoking, alcohol, and substance abuse

Physical examination: general physical examination including blood pressure and pulse, height, weight, pelvic and breast examinations

Laboratory testing

Offered to all women: urine dipstick for protein and glucose, hemoglobin or hematocrit determination, hepatitis B and HIV testing, Papanicolaou smear

Offered to high-risk women: screening for gonorrhea, syphilis, *Chlamydia* bacterial vaginosis, hemoglobinopathies, Tay-Sachs disease, abnormal parental karyotype; purified protein derivative (PPD); toxoplasmosis, herpes simplex, and cytomegalovirus titers; toxicology testing for illicit drugs

ative pregnancy test in one study.[9] The figure demonstrates the importance of a comprehensive preconception risk assessment. Using this comprehensive approach, preconception risk was identified in more than 90% of women. In another study, when only four risks were analyzed (smoking, alcohol use, being underweight, and delayed initiation of prenatal care), 59% of mothers with planned pregnancies and 66% of those with unplanned pregnancies had an indication for preconception counseling.[10]

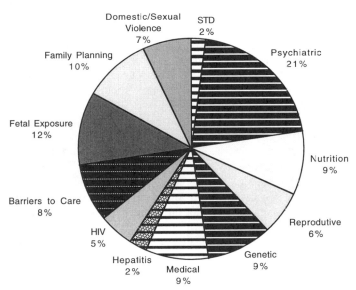

Fig. 10.1. Preconception risk factors as percent of total risks at the time of a negative pregnancy test. (From Jack et al,[9] with permission.)

Reproductive History

Preconception assessment includes a discussion of a woman's menstrual, sexual, contraceptive, and obstetric history. A history of past pregnancy outcomes should include the number and length of previous pregnancies and the presence of complications, such as fetal death, prematurity or postdatism, intrauterine growth retardation, macrosomia, hemorrhage, surgical delivery, gestational diabetes mellitus, or pregnancy-induced hypertension. Breastfeeding and contraceptive history provide information useful for prospective counseling.

Infectious Disease History

Human Immunodeficiency Virus

All family physicians should provide preconception screening, diagnosis, education, and counseling about HIV for women of childbearing age. Perinatal transmission of HIV has become a major cause of illness and death. Eighty-five percent of women with HIV infection are of childbearing age and there are about 7,000 births per year to HIV-infected women in the United States. In the absence of treatment, the risk of perinatal transmission is 15% to 40% and varies with maternal factors such as p24 antigenemia, $CD8^+$ and $CD4^+$ lymphocyte counts, and placental membrane inflammation. Sixty-five to seventy percent of vertical transmission occurs at labor and delivery. Risk factors associated with increased vertical transmission include breastfeeding, use of fetal scalp electrodes, prolonged rupture of membranes, and high viral load and CD4 counts.[11] An important turning point occurred in 1994 when the AIDS Clinical Trial Group demonstrated that zidovudine administered to a group of HIV-infected women during pregnancy and labor and to their newborns reduced the risk of perinatal HIV infection by two thirds, from 25.5% to 8.3%.[12] Limitations of the study are that these women had mild disease, had not received previous treatment, and long-term effects were not known. Recent recommendations favor multidrug regimen for HIV-infected women[11] (see Chapter 42).

All women should be offered HIV counseling and testing before pregnancy. Women who test negative for HIV should be counseled about safe sexual practices. Those women testing positive must be informed of the risks of vertical transmission to the infant and the associated morbidity and mortality. These women should be offered contraception. Those choosing pregnancy must be counseled about the availability of treatment to prevent vertical transmission and the importance of early prenatal care.

Hepatitis

Each year in the United States more than 300,000 persons, primarily young adults, become infected with hepatitis B virus (HBV) and 6% to 10% of adolescent and adult patients develop a chronic carrier state (see Chapter 90). An estimated 16,500 births occur to HBV-infected women each year in the United States. Without the availability of HBV vaccine, approximately 4300 newborns annually would acquire HBV infection from their mothers.[13] HBV infection acquired during infancy progresses to chronic disease (chronic active or persistent infection) in more than 95% of cases. These infections lead to early death during adulthood due to cirrhosis or hepatoma in 25% to 50% of cases.[14] Women at ongoing risk for HBV (sexual contacts of HBV-infected persons, users of IV drugs, prostitutes, institutionalized women, and Southeast Asians[15]) can be tested for evidence of previous or ongoing HBV infection, and if susceptible, these women should be vaccinated before they become pregnant.[16]

Hepatitis C virus (HCV) infection increases the risk of developing cirrhosis and hepatocellular carcinoma. Women with HCV infection should be counseled that the most likely route of transmission is through infected blood or blood products, and that risk of perinatal transmission to the newborn if they become pregnant is currently estimated to be about 3% to 4%.

Toxoplasmosis

About one third of adult women in the United States have antibodies to toxoplasmosis (see Chapter 44); the remainder may be at risk for a primary maternal infection during pregnancy that can result in congenital infection. Prospective studies performed in the United States have established an incidence of congenital toxoplasmosis of 1.1 per 1000 live births. Of children born to mothers who had toxoplasmosis during pregnancy, approximately 8% are severely affected at birth. The rest are affected with mild disease or subclinical infection but are at risk for late sequelae such as chorioretinitis, mental retardation, and sensorineural hearing loss. Severe fetal effects are more likely if infection is acquired during the first or second trimester.[17]

Preconception testing for immunity to *Toxoplasma gondii* by measuring its immunoglobulin G (IgG) antibody titer provides physicians with information of use for counseling women, especially those at high risk for acquiring toxoplasmosis. Women already immune can be reassured that they cannot become infected during pregnancy. Women who are susceptible should be counseled before pregnancy about properly cooking meat and avoiding close contact with cats and cat litter or soil that may contain cat feces. Raw meat and the feces of newly infected cats are the only sources for the *Toxoplasma* protozoa at a time during its life cycle when it can infect humans.[18,19]

Because the acute infection in the adult is usually subclinical, preconception testing can help the physician identify whether an acute infection during pregnancy is due to *T. gondii*. The frequency of subclinical infection limits the value of routine toxoplasmosis testing. Some evidence indicates that treatment during pregnancy of women who seroconvert may lessen neonatal problems. Antibody testing during pregnancy that demonstrates *Toxoplasma* infection in a woman who had negative titers before pregnancy indicates that infection has occurred. In the absence of such preconception information, interpretation of titers obtained during pregnancy may be difficult. Thus preconception testing might lead to a prompt diagnosis and timely treatment decisions.[19]

Rubella

Rubella infection during pregnancy, particularly during the first 16 weeks, can result in spontaneous abortion, stillbirth, or a baby with the congenital rubella syndrome (see Chapter 18). The incidence of rubella has declined by more than 99% since 1969, the year the rubella vaccine was licensed.[20] However, serologic surveys of various populations found 10% to 20% of women of childbearing age lack serologic evidence of immunity to rubella. Preconception screening and vaccination prior to pregnancy can prevent congenital rubella syndrome. A history of rubella during childhood is frequently inaccurate. Even with such a history, women who have not been tested previously, who have not received two doses of the measles/mumps/rubella (MMR) vaccine, and by history are not pregnant should receive the vaccine without any testing. Since the virus is a live virus, there is a theoretical risk of intrauterine infection in women who begin pregnancies within 3 months. Should conceptions occur soon after vaccination, women can be reassured that their fetuses are not at appreciable risk. Several large series have identified no case of vaccination-related congenital defect.[21]

Varicella

The availability of varicella vaccine, the rare occurrence of a congenital varicella syndrome, and the severity of neonatal disease in infants of women contracting varicella late during pregnancy suggest a benefit for preconception immunization of those women who do not have a history of chickenpox[22] (see Chapter 18). Women of childbearing age without a history of chickenpox can receive a two-dose varicella vaccine. Because the vaccine contains live virus, it should not be given to pregnant women, and women who have been vaccinated should be advised to avoid becoming pregnant for 1 month.[23]

Bacterial Vaginosis

Bacterial vaginosis (see Chapter 102) has been associated with delivery of low birth weight infants,[24] and treatment of women with bacterial vaginosis during pregnancy reduces the risk of premature delivery[25] (see Chapter 14). There might be benefits to identifying and treating women with bacterial vaginosis before conception. However, as with asymptomatic bacteriuria, the frequency of recurrence might limit the value of preconception detection.

Exposure to Teratogens

Routine assessment of hobbies, habits, and home and employment environments might identify exposures associated with adverse reproductive consequences and that can be minimized during the preconception period. The effects on human pregnancy of most of the chemicals in occupational use are unknown, but several, such as heavy metals and organic solvents, have been implicated in a variety of reproductive disorders. It is prudent to educate women for whom pregnancy is a possibility about such hazards and to provide them with the facts available about the teratogenic potential of any chemical or environmental agent to which they are exposed.[26]

Medications

The family physician should ask about the use of prescription and nonprescription drugs and provide information on the safest choices; how to avoid drugs associated with fetal risk is discussed as well. Early prenatal care entry should be stressed for those women who require careful monitoring of medications during pregnancy. Routine preconception modification of therapeutic regimens, including elimination of known teratogenic drugs such as gold, lithium, isotretinoin, folic acid antagonists, anticonvulsants, and warfarin, can reduce anomalies. For example, isotretinoin (Accutane), a treatment for severe, recalcitrant cystic acne, is highly teratogenic, causing craniofacial defects, malformations of the cardiovascular and central nervous systems, and defects of the thymus. Among fetuses who survive until 20 weeks' gestation the malformation rate is 23%. An estimated 4000 women ages 15 to 44 per year have an approved indication for this drug, but 65,000 women of reproductive age receive a prescription.[27]

Preconception counseling of women for whom drugs are essential might lead to postponement or avoidance of pregnancy. In some cases, alternative drugs can be prescribed or the dosages reduced. For example, women requiring anticoagulation should be encouraged to switch to heparin before conception.

Medical History

Preconception care includes the detection and optimal control of specific medical conditions. Advances in the effectiveness of medical treatment and the increased rate of pregnancy by women in their late thirties have led to an increase in the frequency of women with chronic diseases deciding to conceive. For women with preexisting chronic medical conditions, preconception care should include assessment of the likelihood of pregnancy affecting the mother's health and of the medical condition affecting the pregnancy. For women with certain conditions, it might include advice regarding the timing or avoidance of pregnancy.

Cardiovascular Disease

Cardiovascular diseases including hypertension (see Chapters 75 and 76) are the most common chronic conditions among women of childbearing age. Some women with cardiovascular disease would benefit from evaluation and treatment before pregnancy. Some have conditions of great importance to pregnancy, such as rheumatic heart disease or congenital cardiac defects. Evaluation of the presence and severity of disease for such conditions can be helpful when counseling women regarding the potential impact of pregnancy on their health. For some women, corrective surgery is indicated prior to conception.[28] Women who are found to have a congenital cardiac defect might benefit from genetic counseling.

Diabetes Mellitus

Improved control of maternal glucose and antepartum fetal surveillance has led to a significant reduction in the perinatal mortality rate seen during pregnancies complicated by insulin-dependent diabetes mellitus (IDDM) (see Chapter 120). Today the leading causes of perinatal mortality during pregnancies complicated by IDDM are major congenital malformations. Whereas the risk of major malformations in the general population is 2% to 3%, these malformations are observed in approximately 10% of pregnancies complicated by IDDM. Although virtually any organ system can be affected, the most characteristic abnormalities include sacral agenesis, complex cardiac defects, spina bifida, and anencephaly. These malformations occur during the critical period of fetal organogenesis, approximately 5 to 8 weeks after the last menstrual period.[29]

The increased rate of congenital malformations in infants born to mothers with IDDM is significantly reduced when these women maintain excellent blood glucose control during organogenesis. At least six clinical studies have demonstrated that women who optimize glucose control prior to conception reduce their risk of having a fetus with major malformations to that of the nondiabetic population.[30] Women with near-normal glycosylated hemoglobin levels are at the lowest risk of delivering an infant with a congenital malformation, and women with the highest levels have nearly a 25% risk of a major malformation in their offspring. Prevention of these congenital malformations through preconception care saves an estimated $1720 per delivery.[31]

Seizures

Preconception care is especially applicable to women with seizure disorders (see Chapter 64), as they are at high risk because of their disease and the medications required for seizure control. The risk of major malformations, minor anomalies, and dysmorphic features is two- to threefold higher in infants of mothers with epilepsy who receive treatment with antiepileptic drugs compared with the risk for infants of mothers without epilepsy.

Women with idiopathic epilepsy who are seizure-free for 2 years or more and have a normal electroencephalogram should be offered a trial period free of the antiepileptic medication before attempting pregnancy. Adequate time should be allowed to assess these results because hypoxic seizure early in pregnancy can have severe consequences.

Medications such as valproic acid have been associated with neural tube defects and others such as phenytoin and phenobarbital are associated with malformations. If anticonvulsant medications are required during pregnancy and if the woman plans to become pregnant, the least toxic medication should be initiated before pregnancy and the medication adjusted frequently to keep serum levels in the lowest effective range.[32,33]

Treated Medical Disease

Women with a history of successfully treated medical disease nonetheless can be at serious jeopardy during pregnancy. For example, women whose thyroid glands have been ablated for Graves' disease might have circulating thyroid-stimulating antibodies that can induce thyrotoxicosis in their fetuses.[34] Women with hypothyroidism should be optimally treated before pregnancy.[35]

Women with a history of immune thrombocytopenia might convey a risk of hemorrhage to their fetus. Women with a history of pulmonary embolism should be counseled regarding the risk of recurrence during pregnancy and the need for early prenatal enrollment and careful medical and obstetric monitoring throughout pregnancy if they choose to conceive.[28]

For some women, careful monitoring of the waxing and waning nature of their disease may allow the physician to counsel the woman regarding optimal timing of pregnancy. For example, women with systemic lupus erythematosus can be monitored for the presence of lupus anticoagulant or anticardiolipin antibodies associated with a high risk of midtrimester loss. These women might benefit by timing their pregnancies to occur when their disease is in remission, including the absence of antibodies, or following suppressive therapy.[36,37]

Family and Genetic History

The ideal time for genetic investigation and counseling is before a couple attempts to conceive. The identification of genetic risk can be accomplished by a careful genetic history (see Chapter 16). Patients with a specific indication such as advanced maternal age, a family history of genetic disease, or a previously affected pregnancy should be offered preconception genetic counseling. Carrier screening to determine if the parents are heterozygous for certain genetic conditions and therefore at increased risk for conceiving offspring with these disorders is of special significance because it allows relevant counseling before the first affected pregnancy. Common disorders for which genetic screening is recommended include Tay-Sachs disease for people of Eastern European or French Canadian ancestry; β-thalassemia for those of Mediterranean, Southwest Asian, Indian Pakistani, or African ancestry; α-thalassemia for people of Southeast Asian ancestry; sickle cell anemia for people of African descent[38]; and cystic fibrosis for those with a family history of the disease.[39] The family history also might reveal other risks for genetic diseases, such as fragile X disease or Down syndrome.

If either member of a couple is affected by genetic disease or has an affected relative, the couple should be referred for genetic counseling and possible genetic testing. Genetic counseling explains the risk and, if necessary, arranges for diagnostic tests such as chorionic villous sampling or amniocentesis early in pregnancy. Such determinations could influence a couple's decision to conceive or adopt and could alter the clinical management of the pregnancy and newborn.

Preconception screening not only provides a couple more time to consider their options and make plans, but also adds to the number of options available. For couples identified to be at risk during pregnancy, confirmatory testing only provides the option of induced abortion. When testing is done before conception, additional options include not bearing children, artificial insemination, in vitro fertilization, surrogate pregnancy, and adoption.

Prevention of Neural Tube Defects

The preconception visit should include nutritional counseling to ensure that the diets of all women who might bear children contain an adequate amount of folic acid. It has been well demonstrated that a large portion of spina bifida and anencephaly can be prevented by using dietary folic acid supplementation when it is taken before conception and continued through the first trimester of pregnancy. In 1991 a large randomized trial of women who had had a previous child with a neural tube defect (NTD) conclusively demonstrated that 4-mg doses of folic acid before and during early pregnancy resulted in a 71% reduction of recurrence of NTDs.[40] This study did not address the possible benefit of lower doses of folic acid, although other studies have suggested that lower doses might result in comparable reductions.

Additionally, there appear to be excellent prospects for substantially reducing, through use of folic acid, the number of NTDs among U.S. women who have not had a prior NTD-affected pregnancy.[41] The U.S. Public Health Service now recommends that all women of childbearing age who are capable of becoming pregnant should consume 0.4 mg of folic acid per day for the purpose of reducing their risk of having a pregnancy affected with spina bifida or other NTD. Because the effects of higher intakes are not well known but include complicating the diagnosis of vitamin B_{12} deficiency, care should be taken to keep the total folate consumption at less than 1 mg per day.[42]

Implementing these recommendations might provide the opportunity for primary prevention of as many as 60% of these serious birth defects.[43] A woman's risk of having a child with a NTD was found to be associated with early pregnancy red blood cell folate levels in a continuous dose-response relationship. This finding suggests that it might be possible to identify and supplement women with low folic acid levels and thereby prevent NTDs.[44]

Nutrition

A woman's nutritional status at conception can have profound effects on reproductive outcome. At the preconception visit a complete dietary history includes a history of food habits, attitudes, use of vitamins and mineral supplements, food allergies, knowledge about proper nutrition, and the availability of food (see Chapter 8). Lactose intol-

erance should be identified and the adequacy of dietary calcium assessed. The family physician also should assess the
woman for conditions such as bulimia, anorexia, pica, or
hypervitaminosis. Once identified, nutritional counseling
and in some cases treatment of an underlying emotional
condition should be initiated. Women who are at nutritional
risk should be provided an individualized dietary intervention, possibly with the aid of a nutritionist. Low-income
families and women with special nutritional needs should
be assisted to obtain additional food from such sources as
the Aid to Families with Dependent Children (AFDC) food
stamp program and the WIC (Women, Infants, and Children) program as soon as possible. In some instances, the
use of food pantries, soup kitchens, and similar facilities
may need to be recommended.

Preconception assessment of nutrition status should identify women who are underweight or overweight. Women who
are underweight and subsequently gain little weight during
pregnancy are at high risk of fetal and neonatal morbidity and
mortality.[45] At the other extreme, marked obesity is associated with gestational diabetes, NTDs, hypertension, macro-
somic infants, and resultant prolonged labor and shoulder dystocia.[46] Thus management plans for both underweight and
overweight are best developed before pregnancy.

Calcium

The current calcium intake recommendation for pregnant
women and adolescent females is 1200 to 1500 mg per day,
but the reported median intake is 600 to 700 mg per day,
which is insufficient to ensure optimal gestational blood pressure regulation.[47] There is now adequate evidence to recommend that every woman of reproductive age should be advised to consume the current recommended level of calcium.[48]

Vitamin A

The recommended dietary allowance for women is 2700 IU
of vitamin A per day. Currently, about 1% to 2% of women
average more than 10,000 IU of vitamin A from supplements.
Evidence in humans suggests that more than 10,000 IU of vitamin A per day is teratogenic, resulting in cranial/neural crest
defects.[49] Women in the reproductive age group are advised
to avoid consuming vitamin A at these levels and should consume liver products only in moderation, as they contain large
amounts of vitamin A. Women with a history of a previous
pregnancy resulting in a fetus with an NTD should be advised
not to attempt to achieve high doses of folic acid (i.e., 4 mg)
by taking multivitamins because of the possibility of ingesting harmful levels of vitamin A.

Phenylketonuria

Infants born to women with classic phenylketonuria (PKU)
and a maternal blood phenylalanine level of more than 20
mg/dL are likely to have microcephaly and mental retardation and are at increased risk of congenital heart disease and
intrauterine growth retardation. Dietary restrictions that result in lowered levels of maternal phenylalanine during the
earliest weeks of gestation appear to reduce the risk of fetal
malformation.[50,51]

Psychosocial Factors

Preconception risk assessment provides an opportunity to
identify risks related to personal, social, and psychological
characteristics (see Chapters 2, 3, and 4). Risks of a personal
nature include lack of adequate financial resources such as
low income, inadequate housing or medical insurance, or
communication difficulties. Real or perceived barriers to family planning or early prenatal care enrollment can be detected.
Psychological risks that can be identified by a sensitive interviewer include inadequate pregnancy readiness, lack of
personal support, deficient coping skills, high stress and anxiety, and psychiatric conditions. Extremes of physical work,
exercise, and other activity should be assessed.

Victims of domestic violence should be identified precon-
ceptionally, as they are likely to be abused during pregnancy
(see Chapter 28). Up to 25% of obstetric patients are physically abused while pregnant. Such assaults can result in placental separation; antepartum hemorrhage; fetal fractures;
rupture of the uterus, liver, or spleen; and preterm labor. Information about available community, social and legal resources, and a plan for dealing with the abusive partner should
be made available to abused women.[52]

Implementing a comprehensive preconception care program for many women includes addressing barriers to access
to medical care. After these barriers are identified, advice,
counseling, education, and developing a personal relationship
with a family physician before pregnancy might successfully
address some of these impediments.

Good social support around the time of childbirth is important to the mental and physical health of the new mother.[53]
Preconception evaluation should include an assessment of social support and family function. The family physician can
assess social supports available to help identify potential problems such as domestic violence, parenting difficulties, and
other stresses that may affect pregnancy or child rearing.

High-Risk Behaviors

Queries regarding a patient's social and lifestyle history
should seek to identify behaviors that might compromise reproductive outcome.

Smoking

Smoking (see Chapter 8) contributes to many obstetric problems, such as preterm delivery, intrauterine growth retardation,
abruptio placentae, placenta previa, and spontaneous abortion.
Each year tobacco-related products are responsible for an estimated 32,000 to 61,000 infants born with low birth weight (representing 11% to 21% of low birth weight births) and 14,000
to 26,000 infants who require admission to a neonatal intensive care unit. Tobacco use is also responsible for an estimated
1900 to 4300 infant deaths resulting from perinatal disorders
and 1200 to 2200 deaths from sudden infant death syndrome.[54]
Nevertheless, 25% to 30% of pregnant women in the United
States smoke, and many women still smoking are unaware of
the risks.[55,56] Given the benefits of smoking cessation, all
women who smoke should be offered advice and counseling
about methods designed to help them stop. For some women

the benefits to their future infants provide additional motivation necessary for successful smoking cessation. Because many women require multiple attempts prior to success, preconception intervention is particularly worthwhile.

Alcohol Intake

Alcohol intake (see Chapter 59) early in pregnancy can have devastating consequences for the fetus. Fetal alcohol syndrome outranks Down syndrome and spina bifida in prevalence and is the leading known cause of mental retardation.[57] Alcohol is a teratogen. Alcohol causes fetal wastage, growth retardation, organ anomalies, neurosensory problems, and mental retardation. Only 55% of women questioned in a 1985 study had heard of the fetal alcohol syndrome and fewer than 25% knew it includes congenital defects.[56] A safe level of alcohol consumption during pregnancy has not been established. The adverse effects of alcohol might begin early in pregnancy, before a woman realizes she is pregnant. An estimated 11% of women who drink 1 to 2 oz of absolute alcohol a day during the first trimester have babies with features consistent with the prenatal effects of alcohol.[58] All women of childbearing age should be given accurate information about the consequences of alcohol consumption during pregnancy, the likelihood that effects begin early during the first trimester, and that no safe level of consumption has been established. Those women who currently have an alcohol-related problem should be identified and educated as to the risks of alcohol consumption, and efforts should be initiated to assist them in stopping.

Substance Abuse

Use of cocaine, heroin, and other substances (see Chapter 60) during pregnancy may lead to spontaneous abortion, premature delivery, abruptio placentae, fetal growth retardation, congenital anomalies, and fetal or neonatal death.[59,60] An estimated 10% to 15% of women use cocaine, heroin, methadone, amphetamines, PCP, or marijuana during pregnancy.[61] A careful history to identify use of illegal substances should be obtained as part of the preconception risk assessment. Occasional recreational use might not be considered by the woman to be a problem, nor might she be aware of the dangers of such occasional use during early pregnancy. Use of cocaine during the first trimester, possibly before the woman is aware that she is pregnant, is associated with abruption and with congenital defects even if the woman does not continue to use it later during the pregnancy.[62]

The preconception interview provides an opportunity for women to be educated about the risks and for occasional drug users to be encouraged to abstain, especially if they are not actively preventing pregnancy. Those women identified as users of cocaine or other illicit substances should be encouraged to maintain effective birth control until their substance abuse has been properly treated.

Physical Examination and Laboratory Testing

Preconception care should include all aspects of regular age-appropriate preventive care for women, including physical examination and laboratory testing. Important elements of the physical examination include blood pressure and pulse, height, weight, and pelvic and breast examinations.

Laboratory tests offered to all women at a preconception evaluation include rubella titer, urine dipstick for protein and glucose, hemoglobin or hematocrit determination to detect iron deficiency anemia, hepatitis B surface antigen, HIV testing, and toxicology screening for illicit drugs. A Papanicolaou smear can be prepared, so if cervical dysplasia is detected, it can be treated before conception, which is safer than during pregnancy.

Women in high-risk groups can be offered other laboratory testing including tests for gonorrhea, syphilis, and *Chlamydia*, and bacterial vaginosis screening so infection can be treated before conception. Laboratory assessment can also include titers for toxoplasmosis and screening for hemoglobinopathies, Tay-Sachs disease, and abnormal parental karyotype for selected women. A purified protein derivative (PPD) test should be done in areas where tuberculosis is prevalent, so if treatment is necessary it can precede pregnancy. The Expert Panel on the Content of Prenatal Care noted that preconception testing of women for herpes simplex and cytomegalovirus could prove beneficial for some women.[63]

Interventions

Interventions to reduce risks are a critical component of preconception care. With the knowledge gained from preconception risk assessment, medical and psychosocial interventions can take place. Preconception identification of women with risks provides the opportunity for appropriate treatment, pregnancy planning, early entry into prenatal care, or recommendations to avoid pregnancy.

Table 10.3 lists the content of the intervention component of preconception care. Some preconception risks are easily identified and effective interventions available (e.g., rubella vaccination). Other risks, such as smoking, are certainly worthy of identification, although initial attempts at treatment are not always effective. Some conditions, particularly psychosocial risks, are not easily treated but might benefit from evaluation or counseling by the family physician or by involvement of appropriate community services.

A complete program of preconception care includes comprehensive follow-up by the family physician. For preconception care to be most effective, intervention services must be available and coordinated at the community level. Coordination of medical and community services such as visiting nurses, social workers, mental health counselors, and nutritionists, among others, is needed to provide continuous, comprehensive coordinated care of women at medical and psychosocial risk.

Preconception care is most effective when the woman and her partner are properly motivated. Many social and cultural influences, including attitudes and values projected at home and through the schools, churches, peer groups, and public media, contribute to decisions by men and women during their teenage and early adult years regarding sexuality and childbearing. The receptiveness of couples to preconception care

Table 10.3. **Content of Preconception Care: Interventions**

Treatment with 0.4 mg of folic acid per day; women with a prior neural tube defect (NTD)-affected pregnancy should take an additional 4.0 mg of folic acid for 1 month before pregnancy

Treatment of medical disease; women with diabetes mellitus should enter a program for intensive control of their blood glucose

Modification of chronic disease medications to decrease maternal or fetal risk during pregnancy

Vaccination for rubella, hepatitis B, and varicella

Counseling, education, and testing in regard to HIV, hepatitis B, bacterial vaginosis, and other infections

Nutrition counseling or referral; all women of reproductive age should consume 1200 to 1500 mg of calcium per day

Substance abuse counseling or referral to treatment programs

Home visitation to treat psychosocial risks

Referral to social service agencies for services and support

Initiation of treatment or referral for psychiatric conditions

Provision of contraception and family planning services

Provision of safe shelters

Financial assistance and planning including medical assistance

Vocational training

Provide information of local community resources

---

is heightened at certain times, such as during a family planning visit when a woman is considering stopping her method of birth control, at the time of a negative pregnancy test, or at a premarital visit.

Successful preconception care identifies women at highest risk so resources can be directed to those most in need. Unfortunately, women at social risk, who are at increased risk of poor pregnancy outcome, often encounter barriers to obtaining health services, including preconception counseling and care. Thus women most likely to benefit from preconception care include those least likely to have access to it. Optimally, to reach women most in need, family physicians must make preconception care available in settings that offer special opportunities to reach high-risk women, such as community health centers, sexually transmitted disease clinics, substance abuse treatment centers, women's shelters, halfway houses, and detention centers.

References

1. U.S. Public Health Service Expert Panel on the Content of Prenatal Care. Caring for our future: the content of prenatal care. Washington, DC: U.S. Department of Health and Human Services, 1989.
2. Jack B, Culpepper L. Preconception care: risk reduction and health promotion in preparation for pregnancy. JAMA 1990; 264:1147–9.
3. Jack B, Culpepper L. Preconception care. In: Merkatz IR, Thompson JE, Mullen PD, Goldenberg RL, eds. New perspectives on prenatal care. New York: Elsevier, 1990;69–88.
4. Healthy people 2000: midcourse review and 1995 revisions. Washington, DC: U.S. Department of Health and Human Services, Public Health Service 2000.
5. Jack BW, Culpepper L. Preconception care. J Fam Pract 1991; 32:306–15.
6. Gjerdingen DK, Fontaine P. Preconception health care: a critical task for family physicians. J Am Board Fam Pract 1991;4: 237–50.
7. Jack B. Preconception care (or how all family physicians "do" OB). Am Fam Physician 1995;51:1807–8.
8. Miller CA. Wanting children. Am J Public Health 1992;82: 341–3.
9. Jack BW, Campanile C, McQuade W, Kogan MD. The negative pregnancy test: an opportunity for preconception care. Arch Fam Med 1995;4:340–5.
10. Adams MM, Bruce FC, Shulman HB, Kendrick JS, Brogan DJ. Pregnancy planning and preconception counseling. Obstet Gynecol 1993;82:955–9.
11. HIV Infection in Pregnancy. ACOG Educational Bulletin. January 1997:232.
12. Connor EM, Sperling RS, Gelbert R, et al. Reduction of maternal-infant transmission of human immunodeficiency virus type 1 with zidovudine treatment: Pediatric AIDS Clinical Trials Group Protocol 076 Study Group. N Engl J Med 1994;331: 1173–80.
13. Centers for Disease Control Immunization Practices Advisory Committee. Prevention of perinatal transmission of hepatitis B virus: prenatal screening of all pregnant women for hepatitis B surface antigen. MMWR 1988;37:341–6.
14. Stevens CE, Toy PT, Tong MJ, et al. Perinatal hepatitis B virus transmission in the United States: prevention by passive-active immunization. JAMA 1985;253:1740–5.
15. Centers for Disease Control. Changing patterns of groups at high risk for hepatitis B in the United States. MMWR 1988;37: 429–32.
16. Margolis HS, Coleman PJ, Brown RE, et al. Prevention of hepatitis B virus transmission by immunization: an economic analysis of current recommendations. JAMA 1995;274:120–8.
17. Wilson CB, Remington JS. What can be done to prevent congenital toxoplasmosis? Am J Obstet Gynecol 1980;138:357–63.
18. Krick JA, Remington JS. Toxoplasmosis in the adult—an overview. N Engl J Med 1978;298:550–3.
19. Fuccillo DA, Madden DL, Tzan NR, et al. Difficulties associated with serological diagnosis of *Toxoplasma gondii* infections. Diagn Clin Imunol 1987;5:8–13.
20. Centers for Disease Control. Rubella and congenital rubella syndrome—United States, 1985–1988. MMWR 1989;38:172–88.
21. Centers for Disease Control. Rubella vaccination during pregnancy—United States, 1971–1988. MMWR 1989;38:289–93.
22. Paryani SG, Avrin AM. Intrauterine infections with varicella-zoster virus after maternal varicella. N Engl J Med 1986;34: 1542.
23. American Academy of Pediatrics Committee on Infectious Diseases. Recommendations for the use of live attenuated varicella vaccine. Pediatrics 1995;95:761–6.
24. Hillier SL, Nugent RP, Eschenbach DA, et al. Association between bacterial vaginosis and preterm delivery of a low birthweight infant. N Engl J Med 1995;333:1737–42.
25. Hauth JC, Goldenberg RL, Andrews WW, et al. Reduced incidence of preterm delivery with metronidazole and erythromycin in women with bacterial vaginosis. N Engl J Med 1995;333: 1732–6.
26. Culpepper L, Thompson JE. Work during pregnancy. In: Merkatz IR, Thompson JE. Mullen PD, Goldenberg R, eds. New perspectives on prenatal care. New York: Elsevier, 1990;211–34.
27. Teratology Society. Recommendations for isotretinoin use in women of childbearing potential. Teratology 1991;44:1–6.

28. Barrett JM, Van Hooydonk JE, Boehm FH. Pregnancy-related rupture of arterial aneurysms. Obstet Gynecol Surv 1982;37:557–66.

29. Steel JM, Johnston FD. Prepregnancy management of the diabetic. In: Chamberlain G, Lumley J, eds. Prepregnancy care: a manual for practice. Chichester: Wiley, 1986;165–82.

30. Kitzmiller JL, Gavin LA, Gin GD, et al. Preconception care of diabetes: glycemic control prevents congenital anomalies. JAMA 1991;2645:731–6.

31. Elixhauser A, Weschler JM, Kitzmiller JL. Cost-benefit analysis of preconception care for women with established diabetes mellitus. Diabetes Care 1993;16:1146–57.

32. Taysi K. Preconceptional counseling. Obstet Gynecol Clin North Am 1988;15:167–78.

33. Delgado-Escueta AV, Janz D. Consensus guideline: preconception counseling, management, and care of the pregnant women with epilepsy. Neurology 1992;42:149–60.

34. Momotani N, Noh J, Oyanagi H, Ishikawa N, Ito K. Antithyroid drug therapy of Graves' disease during pregnancy: optimal regimen for fetal thyroid status. N Engl J Med 1986;315:24–8.

35. Man EB, Brown JF, Surunaian SA. Maternal hypothyroxinemia: psychoneurological deficits of progeny. Ann Clin Lab Sci 1991;21:227–39.

36. Lockshin MD, Druzin ML, Goei S, et al. Antibody to cardiolipin as a predictor of fetal distress or death in pregnant patients with systemic lupus erythematosus. N Engl J Med 1985;313:152–6.

37. Lubbe WF, Butler WS, Palmer SJ, Liggins GC. Fetal survival after prednisone suppression of maternal lupus-anticoagulant. Lancet 1983;1:1361–3.

38. Antenatal diagnosis of genetic disorders. Technical bulletin no. 108. Washington, DC: American College of Obstetricians and Gynecologists, 1987.

39. Lemna WK, Feldman GL, Kerem B-S, et al. Mutation analysis for heterozygote detection and the prenatal diagnosis of cystic fibrosis. N Engl J Med 1990;322:291–6.

40. MRC Vitamin Study Research Group. Prevention of neural tube defects: results of the Medical Research Council Vitamin Study. Lancet 1991;338:131–7.

41. Czeizel AE, Dudas I. Prevention of the first occurrence of neural-tube defects by periconceptional vitamin supplementation. N Engl J Med 1992;327:1832–5.

42. Recommendations for the use of folic acid to reduce the number of cases of spina bifida and other neural tube defects. MMWR 1992;41:1–8.

43. Werler MM, Shapiro S, Mitchell AA. Periconceptional folic acid exposure and risk of occurrent neural tube defects. JAMA 1993;269:1257–61.

44. Daly LE, Peadar NK, Molloy A, Weir DG, Scott JM. Folate levels and neural tube defects: implications for prevention. JAMA 1995;274:1698–702.

45. Naeye RL. Weight gain and the outcomes of pregnancy. Am J Obstet Gynecol 1979;135:3–9.

46. Johnson SR, Kolberg BH, Varner MWS, Railsback LD. Maternal obesity and pregnancy. Surg Gynecol Obstet 1987;164:431–7.

47. Bucher HC, Guyatt G, Cook RJ, et al. Effect of calcium supplementation on pregnancy induced hypertension and pre-eclampsia: a meta-analysis of randomized controlled trials. JAMA 1996;275:1113–7.

48. McCarron DA, Hatton D. Dietary calcium and lower blood pressure: we can all benefit [editorial]. JAMA 1996;275:1128–9.

49. Rothman KJ, Moore LL, Singer MR, et al. Teratogenicity of high vitamin A intake. N Engl J Med 1995;333:1369–73.

50. Drogari E, Smith I, Beasley M, Lloyd JK. Timing of strict diet in relation to fetal damage in maternal phenylketonuria. Lancet 1987;2:927–30.

51. Platt LD, Koch R, Azen C, et al. Maternal phenylketonuria collaborative study, obstetric aspects and outcome: the first 6 years. Am J Obstet Gynecol 1992;166:1150–62.

52. Gazamarian JA, Lazoricks S, Spitz AM, et al. Prevalence of violence against pregnant women. JAMA 1996;275:1915–20.

53. Thompson JE. Maternal stress, anxiety, and social support during pregnancy: possible direction for prenatal intervention. In: Merkatz IR, Thompson JE, Mullen PD, Goldenberg R, eds. New perspectives on prenatal care. New York: Elsevier, 1990;319–35.

54. DiFranza JR, Lew RA. Effect of maternal cigarette smoking on pregnancy complications and sudden infant death syndrome. J Fam Pract 1995;40:385–94.

55. Williamson DF, Serdula MK, Kendrick JS, Binkin MJ. Comparing the prevalence of smoking in pregnant and nonpregnant women, 1985 to 1986. JAMA 1989;261:70–4.

56. Fox SH, Brown C, Koontz AM, Kessel SS. Perceptions of risks of smoking and heavy drinking during pregnancy: 1985 NHIS findings. Public Health Rep 1987;102:73–9.

57. Waren KR, Bast RJ. Alcohol-related birth defects: an update. Public Health Rep 1988;103:638–42.

58. Hanson JW, Streissguth AP, Smith DW. The effects of moderate alcohol consumption during pregnancy on fetal growth and morphogenesis. J Pediatr 1978;92:457–60.

59. Hadeed AJ, Siegel SR. Maternal cocaine use during pregnancy: effect on the newborn infant. Pediatrics 1989;84:205–10.

60. MacGregor SN, Keith LG, Chasnoff IJ, et al. Cocaine use during pregnancy: adverse perinatal outcome. Am J Obstet Gynecol 1987;157:686–90.

61. National Association for Perinatal Addiction Research and Education. Innocent addicts: high rate of prenatal drug abuse found. ADAMHA News. Rockville, MD: National Institute on Drug Abuse, October 1988.

62. Chasnoff IJ. Cocaine: effects on pregnancy and the neonate. In: Drugs, alcohol, pregnancy and parenting. Dordrecht: Kluwer, 1988;97–103.

63. Whitley RJ, Goldenberg RL. Infectious disease in the prenatal period and recommendations for screening. In: Merkatz IR, Thompson JE, Mullen PD, Goldenberg RL, eds. New perspective on prenatal care. New York: Elsevier, 1990;363–406.

11
Normal Pregnancy, Labor, and Delivery

Margaret V. Elizondo and Joseph E. Scherger

Pregnancy and birth are normal physiologic processes for most women. The cesarean delivery rate of nearly 25%, which has persisted in the United States for many years now, is a reflection of the degree of medical intervention in the birth process. Unfortunately, modern medicine has been guilty of using a disease model for the management of pregnancy and birth, resulting in higher than expected rates of complications. At least 90% of women should have a normal birth outcome without medical intervention.[1]

The disease model for pregnancy and birth took hold during the 1920s led by a Chicago obstetrician, Joseph DeLee, who questioned what is normal and pioneered efforts to improve medically on the "cruelty of nature."[2] During this period, childbirth in America went from the home to the hospital, and the legacy of hospital interventions in the birth process began. Much good has come from modern hospital obstetric care, with maternal mortality having decreased to low levels; moreover, infant mortality has steadily declined for populations having access to perinatal care. Modern prenatal care also developed during the first half of the 20th century; and with a focus on good nutrition and screening for problems during pregnancy, it has improved birth outcome.[3]

A renewed respect for normal childbirth came about as a reaction to hospital interventions, led by Dick-Read[4] during the 1930s and 1940s, Lamaze during the 1950s,[5] Kitzinger[6] during the 1960s, and eventually a social movement in America during the 1970s with the widespread development of childbirth education. Odent's[1] *Birth Reborn* represents a culmination of the effort to rediscover normal pregnancy and birth.

Technologic obstetrics, with its steady focus on improving the uncertainty of nature and sparing women the pain of childbirth, continues to march onward. Prenatal care has become preoccupied with serial ultrasound evaluations and screening for α-fetoprotein (AFP) abnormalities, gestational diabetes, genetic disorders, and every potentially infectious agent. Continuous electronic fetal monitoring, developed during the early 1970s, quickly became the standard of care in most American hospitals, despite little evidence of benefit and cumulative evidence that it causes unnecessary cesarean interventions.[7,8] Epidural anesthesia has become so commonplace in some hospitals that labor units are quiet and nurses have little experience helping women through natural labor.

Approximately 30% of U.S. family physicians provide maternity care. The current lack of access to prenatal care for many women in both rural and urban areas is a compelling reason for more family physicians to deliver these services. Knowledgeable about scientific medicine, yet with a humanistic approach to pregnancy and birth similar to that of midwives, the family physician is well suited to provide a balance between nature and technology and may be a guiding force to appropriate maternity care.[9]

This chapter focuses on normal pregnancy and delivery from a perspective of family-centered care. Family-centered maternity care has been defined by the International Childbirth Association as care that focuses on how the birth of a child affects the entire family. A woman who gives birth forms new relationships with those close to her, and all family members take on new responsibilities to each other, the baby, and the community. Family-centered maternity care is an attitude rather than a specific program. It respects the woman's individuality and need for autonomy and requires that a woman be guided, not directed, and that she be allowed to make her own decisions in accordance with her goals.[10] The family physician, as physician for the woman, the father, and the children, is well suited to provide family-centered maternity care. This chapter reviews the principles and practice of normal pregnancy, labor, and delivery.[11]

Prenatal Care

Current prenatal care begins before conception. This important early phase of preventing complications is referred to as preconception care and is detailed in Chapter 10. Prenatal care after conception should begin as early as possible, as health screening and intervention early during pregnancy may improve birth outcome. For example, taking folic acid in doses present in multivitamins during the first 6 weeks of pregnancy provides a three- to fourfold reduction in the chance of neural tube defects in the offspring.[12] Early screening and intervention is useful for control of diabetes, genetic testing, changing teratogenic drugs such as phenytoin (Dilantin), treating infections, and lifestyle modifications of such factors as smoking, alcohol use, recreational drugs, and maternal nutrition.

The traditional approach to prenatal care, developed early during the 20th century, has been modified by an expert panel convened by the U.S. Public Health Service.[13] Rather than a single comprehensive initial visit followed by monthly visits until the third trimester, this panel recommended more intensive intervention early in pregnancy if risk factors exist that can be modified. For example, women who smoke, have poor nutrition, or have a high-risk home environment may benefit from frequent visits and a multidisciplinary team approach early in pregnancy. Women at low risk may require fewer visits than are scheduled with the traditional protocol.

Health Promotion

All those who care for childbearing women should approach pregnancy as an opportunity to promote the health and well-being of the family (see Chapter 8). Counseling to reinforce healthful behaviors and education about pregnancy, childbirth, and parenting are crucial parts of perinatal care—not "extras."

Table 11.1 is an outline of topics to be covered in the education of all pregnant women and their support persons.[14] Experienced parents require only an abbreviated program, focusing on selected areas of interest to them. Preparation for natural childbirth (birth without regional or systemic analgesic drugs) and for vaginal birth after a previous cesarean section can reduce maternal anxiety and the rates of operative delivery and associated complications.[15] Childbirth preparation classes, often run by hospitals, clinics, or private childbirth educators, fulfill this function well. The benefits of breast-feeding for baby and mother should be discussed with women and their family members prior to or early during pregnancy and then modeled at delivery. The effectiveness of education on preventing low birth weight has not been proved.[3] However, information about smoking, alcohol and drug use, prevention of sexually transmitted infection, and mobilizing family supports and social services in the community are likely to be beneficial.

Motivation to adopt more healthy behaviors is probably stronger during pregnancy than at most other times, though a woman may curb behavior such as smoking during pregnancy only to resume it after delivery. All family members involved should be educated on the benefits of a non-smoking household, including decreased incidence of sudden infant death syndrome (SIDS) and respiratory illnesses.[16]

Abstention from alcohol and recreational drugs is also important. Alcohol exposure during gestation is a more common cause of mental retardation than Down syndrome.[17] The prevalence of cocaine use during pregnancy is reported at 17%

Table 11.1. **Sample Topics for Birth and Parenting Classes**

Early pregnancy
Nutrition; optimum weight gain; iron, calcium, vitamin supplements
Exercise and sex during pregnancy
Common symptoms and remedies: fatigue, nausea/vomiting,
    backache, round ligament pain, syncope, constipation
Danger signs: bleeding, contractions, dysuria, vaginitis weight loss
Psychology of pregnancy: body image, libido; need for security; education for self-help; changing family roles; acceptance of pregnancy
Fevers, hot tubs, saunas
Environmental and occupational hazards and how to mitigate them; stress management
Exposure to infectious agents (e.g., toxoplasmosis, rubella, HIV, varicella)
Avoidance of tobacco, alcohol, x-rays, other drugs
Resources available for pregnant and parenting families

Late pregnancy
Common symptoms and remedies: heartburn, backache "loose joints," hemorrhoids, edema, insomnia
Nutrition/fetal growth
Avoidance of tobacco and other drugs
Potentially serious symptoms: edema, bleeding, headache meconium-stained fluid, decreased fetal movements
Exercise (e.g., Kegel's, pelvic tilt), sex, travel (avoid prolonged sitting because of risk of deep vein thrombosis)
Occupational adjustments (avoid excessive exertion, prolonged standing, stress) and postpartum plans
Breast-feeding
Signs of labor
Stages of labor
Techniques for pain control (and practice relaxation, visualization)
Cesarean section, vaginal birth after cesarean, other potential interventions
Birth plan; importance of labor companion and early parent–infant contact
Positions for labor and birth
Seat belt use; infant car seats
Circumcision
Sibling preparation

Postpartum/parenting
Care of the perineum, Kegel's exercises
Practical support for breast-feeding
Reasons to contact provider (e.g., maternal hemorrhage, fever, increased pain; infant jaundice, respiratory distress)
Postpartum exercises
Nutrition, especially calcium and iron
Rest and sleep
Return to work
Sex, contraception
Sibling adjustment
Infant immunizations and preventive care schedule
Infant growth and development: normal expectations and parenting issues at each age

in some populations but often is not admitted to the physician.[18] With a paucity of research on substance use by women and few treatment programs accepting pregnant women, this area is a challenge to professionals caring for them (see Chapter 60).

Women will often ask for advice on working during pregnancy. The physician should review the effects of physical exertion and prolonged standing during pregnancy, occupational and environmental hazards (e.g., heat, heavy metals, anesthetic gases, x-rays, and possibly cathode ray tubes). Daycare and health care workers need to be apprised of the risks of certain infectious disease exposures in pregnancy.[19] Physicians should also be prepared to counsel on the legal rights of pregnant workers, child care, and breast-feeding issues. In general, women may continue moderate activities, but should strive to keep their heart rate <140 and their temperature within 1 to 2 degrees of normal.[20] Attention should be given to appropriate hydration, and women at risk for preterm labor may need to curtail some activities as pregnancy progresses.

Nutrition and weight should be closely monitored during prenatal care (see Chapter 8). Physicians must be knowledgeable about nutritional requirements and offer practical suggestions for management of nausea and vomiting, gastroesophageal reflux, constipation, backache, and hemorrhoids. Anticipatory guidance about body image changes, risks of obesity, and ways of modifying the diet within various constraints (e.g., vegetarianism, lactose intolerance) are also important considerations. Optimal weight gain during pregnancy varies depending on the prepregnancy weight. An underweight woman may benefit from gaining 40 pounds, whereas an obese woman might do well gaining 10 to 15 pounds. The normal weight gain of 25 to 35 pounds is often exceeded without harm to the fetus. Nutritional advice to pregnant women should focus on a high-quality, high-protein diet with a steady, gradual weight gain profiled to the woman's size and eating habits. Pregnant women should be instructed to avoid the presence of cat feces and eating raw meat (toxoplasmosis). Caffeine intake should be limited.

Prenatal Screening

The purpose of prenatal screening is to identify problems that could affect the outcome of pregnancy and for which effective interventions are available. The number of conditions for which screening is available seems limitless. Therefore, the choice of items should be based on a rational assessment of the current literature, legislation, medicolegal climate, cost-effectiveness, and treatment effectiveness. Each screening test should be evaluated to ensure that the benefits of the test and the planned intervention outweigh the risks and complications. Prenatal screening should be discussed with each patient at the first prenatal visit.

Traditional medical teaching focuses on screening for medical conditions using blood tests, ultrasonography, amniocentesis, and physical examination. A comprehensive approach would also include screening through questioning about family and social dysfunction, such as single parent status, a history of domestic abuse, substance abuse, economic hardship, and work-related stresses. The relation between psychosocial stress and outcome of pregnancy is now well established.[21,22] Physicians should be knowledgeable about public social service programs available to support pregnant patients and their families.

Table 11.2 outlines the screening tests offered to most patients. Genetic history determines which patients are offered special testing such as hemoglobin electrophoresis (e.g., African Americans, who are at higher risk for sickle cell disease, or those of Asian or Mediterranean background, who are at higher risk for thalassemia). Testing for Tay-Sachs disease and cystic fibrosis carrier states is becoming more common, and some authorities recommend screening more than just those with a family history of these disorders.[23,24] All women who will be 35 years of age or older by their due date should be offered amniocentesis and/or chorionic villus sampling (CVS) for chromosomal analysis. CVS has the advantage of testing earlier in gestation (generally 10 to 14 weeks) and providing results rapidly (a few days). It is only available through experienced perinatologists, though, and may be associated with a slightly higher complication rate than amniocentesis. Amniocentesis has the advantage of measuring amniotic fluid AFP level as well as analyzing chromosomes, so that neural tube defects (NTDs) can be more readily detected.[23] Amniocentesis is generally performed at 14 to 20 weeks and results return in about 10 days. Other women with personal or family history of genetic problems, including Down syndrome (trisomy 21), should have the opportunity to meet with a genetics counselor, if possible, and review options for prenatal testing.

The expanded AFP screen (triple marker) uses blood levels of AFP, human chorionic gonadotropin (hCG), and unconjugated estriol (uE$_3$) to screen for NTDs, Down syndrome,

Table 11.2. **Common Screening Tests in Pregnancy**

Initial
  Blood type/Rh factor/antibody screen (indirect Coombs' test)
  Complete blood count (CBC)
  Rubella immunoglobulin G (IgG)
  Rapid plasma reagin (RPR)
  Hepatitis B surface antigen
  Urinalysis and culture
  Papanicolaou smear
  Gonorrhea culture (GC)/chlamydia
  Consider screening for bacterial vaginosis
  Offer human immunodeficiency virus (HIV) testing
  Hemoglobin electrophoresis, if indicated
  Consider Tay-Sachs and cystic fibrosis genetic testing
  Purified protein derivative (PPD), if indicated
10–20 weeks
  Offer triple marker [expanded α-fetoprotein (AFP) screening]
    at 15–20 weeks (16–18 ideally)
  Consider chorionic villus sampling (CVS) or amniocentesis,
    if indicated
  Offer ultrasonography for fetal age and anatomy (generally
    17–20 weeks)
24–28 weeks
  Screen for gestational diabetes (1-hour 50-g glucose load)
  Repeat CBC
  Repeat antibody screen (ABS) if Rh negative (Give RhoGAM
    at 28 weeks)
32–36 weeks
  Group B streptococcal screening (35–37 weeks)
  Repeat CBC, if indicated
  Repeat GC/chlamydia/RPR, if indicated

and trisomy 18; 85% of NTDs are detected by an increase in AFP level, but this result can also indicate multiple gestation, abdominal wall defects, congenital nephrotic syndrome, maternal hemorrhage, fetal demise, inaccurate dating, and even normal pregnancy. A low level of AFP may also be found with fetal demise, inaccurate dating, and normal pregnancy, or may be associated with molar gestation or Down syndrome. Down syndrome is also associated with increased hCG levels and decreased uE_3 levels; 60% of Down syndrome cases are detected using these three markers. Trisomy 18 is associated with low levels of all three markers.[25] If the initial triple marker screening is abnormal, it may be necessary to repeat the test or to order a diagnostic ultrasound scan to confirm gestational age and evaluate for fetal abnormalities (see Chapter 16). Amniocentesis may be indicated to measure amniotic fluid AFP and for chromosome evaluation. Because expanded AFP screening is widely available and is considered standard by some, the test should be discussed with all patients, with a mutual agreement of patient and practitioner regarding its use. The screening is done between 15 and 20 weeks' gestation, optimally at 16 to 18 weeks.

Routine ultrasonography currently falls into a gray area. In the United States, a National Institutes of Health (NIH) consensus conference recognized 27 indications for prenatal ultrasonography that result in examinations in most pregnancies.[26] The American College of Obstetricians and Gynecologists recommended adherence to these guidelines.[27] In most of Western Europe, ultrasonography is done routinely at 16 to 18 weeks. The benefits and cost-effectiveness of universal screening are still controversial and are the subject of ongoing study.[28,29]

Screening for gestational diabetes mellitus (GDM) is generally recommended for all pregnant patients at 24 to 28 weeks' gestation. A 50-g glucose solution is given and plasma glucose measured 1 hour later. An abnormal value of 140 or more is further evaluated with a 3-hour 100-g glucose tolerance test, following measurement of fasting plasma glucose. Two or more abnormal values on this test confirm the diagnosis of GDM. One abnormal value may warrant retesting in 4 to 6 weeks.

The Expert Committee on the Diagnosis and Classification of Diabetes Mellitus allows a small subset of women to forgo routine screening: those who are under 25 years of age, of normal weight, with *no* family history of diabetes, and *not* of Hispanic, Native-American, Asian, or African-American background, are at very low risk for GDM.[30] Women with the above risk factors, however, and others including prior GDM or glucosuria, may benefit from earlier screening, in addition to routine screening at 24 to 28 weeks (see Chapter 120).

Bacterial vaginosis has been associated with preterm birth. Metronidazole (Flagyl) (500 mg po bid × 7 days) and clindamycin (300 mg po bid × 7 days) have been shown to decrease preterm birth rates in women with bacterial vaginosis.[31] It is unclear if asymptomatic women should be screened routinely. Group B streptococcal (GBS) infection can be devastating to newborns. The Centers for Disease Control and Prevention (CDC) reports that 10% to 30% of women carry this bacteria in the genital region, though fewer than 1% of infants are actually infected.[32] Despite this low rate of infection, given the mortality rate of up to 20%, screening for GBS in pregnant women is becoming standard. The outer vagina, perineum, and rectum are cultured at 35 to 37 weeks, with positive carriers treated with intravenous antibiotics intrapartum (penicillin 5 million units intravenously followed by 2.5 million units every 4 hours or clindamycin 900 mg intravenously every 8 hours until delivery). The CDC also endorses another strategy to prevent GBS disease, based on risk factors rather than universal screening. In this case, mothers are treated with intrapartum antibiotics only if they have risk factors such as previous infant with invasive GBS disease, GBS bacteriuria in this pregnancy, delivery at <37 weeks' gestation, ruptured membranes >18 hours, or intrapartum temperature of 100.4°F or greater.

Risk Assessment

The outcome of screening is identification of patients at risk for complications during pregnancy. Conventional risk assessment divides patients into low-, medium-, and high-risk categories. Because most family physicians are trained to care for low- and medium-risk patients, and to refer or share the care of high-risk patients with perinatal specialists, proper risk assessment is crucial. Table 11.3 indicates risk factors recognized by the American Board of Family Practice, the American College of Obstetricians and Gynecologists, and the American Academy of Pediatrics.[3,33] Family physicians in some areas and with appropriate training provide obstetric care for high-risk patients, but the classification of risk status remains important for guiding clinical care. The prenatal record should conveniently assist in the evaluation and indication of risk status.

High-risk categories should not be absolute contraindications to care by family physicians. For example, family physicians may be the best qualified to handle high-risk social situations and substance abuse. Because of broad medical training, family physicians may have more experience than some obstetricians in an area dealing with medical problems, such as thyroid or pulmonary disease. Consultation does not preclude shared care. Some high-risk problems may resolve during the pregnancy, and the birth may be a low-risk event.

Prenatal Visits

The schedule of prenatal visits has traditionally been every 4 weeks through the 28th week of pregnancy, every 2 weeks until the 36th week of pregnancy, and then weekly until delivery. A U.S. Public Health Service report suggested that low-risk patients require fewer visits, whereas patients with risk factors may need modified or intensive care.[13] For example, risk factors identified early in pregnancy, such as smoking, alcohol or drug use, family dysfunction, or lack of social support, should be aggressively managed with frequent visits early during pregnancy. Subsequent risk factors, such as elevated blood pressure or preterm labor, require more frequent visits beginning as soon as the condition develops.

The initial prenatal visit consists of a detailed history, phys-

Table 11.3. **Obstetric Risk Criteria**

Category I: higher risk factors	Category II: medium risk factors
Initial prenatal factors	*Initial prenatal factors*
Age ≥40 or ≤16	Ages 35–39, 16–17
Multiple gestation	Drug dependence/alcohol abuse
Preexisting or insulin-dependent diabetes	High-risk family—lack of family/social support
Chronic hypertension	Uterine or cervical malformation or incompetence
Renal failure	Contracted pelvis
Heart disease, class II or greater	Previous cesarean section
Hyperthyroidism	Multiple spontaneous abortions (>3)
Rh isoimmunization	Grand multiparity (>8)
Chronic active hepatitis	History of gestational diabetes
Convulsive disorder	Previous fetal or neonatal demise
Isoimmune thrombocytopenia	Hypothyroidism
Severe asthma	Heart disease, class I
HIV infection	Severe anemia (unresponsive to iron)
Significant hemoglobinopathy (e.g. sickle cell disease)	Pelvic mass or neoplasia
Subsequent prenatal and intrapartum factors	Prior deep vein thrombosis/pulmonary embolism
Vaginal bleeding, second or third trimester	Prior preterm delivery
Pregnancy-induced hypertension (or toxemia),	Pyelonephritis
moderate or severe	Threatened preterm labor
Fetal malformation, by α-fetoprotein (AFP) screening,	Preterm rupture of membranes
ultrasonography, or amniocentesis	*Subsequent prenatal and intrapartum factors*
Abnormal presentation: breech, face, brow, transverse	Gestational diabetes, diet-controlled
Intrauterine growth retardation	Pregnancy-induced hypertension (toxemia), mild
Polyhydramnios/oligohydramnios	Pregnancy at >41 weeks, obtain appropriate
Pregnancy >42 weeks or <35 weeks	fetal/placental tests
Abnormal fetal/placental tests	Active genital herpes
Persistent severe variable or late decelerations	Positive high or low AFP screen
Macrosomia	Estimated fetal weight >10 pounds (4.5 kg) or
Cord prolapse	<5.5 pounds (2.5 kg)
Mid-forceps delivery	Abnormal nonstress test
	Arrest of normal labor curve
	Persistent moderate variable decelerations or poor
	baseline variability
	Ruptured membranes beyond 24 hours
	Second stage beyond 2 hours
	Induction of labor

ical examination, and laboratory assessment. A complete physical examination is performed as early as possible. The pelvic assessment, which includes a bimanual examination, is helpful for dating the pregnancy and evaluating the pelvic structure. Screening laboratory investigations are undertaken as stated above. Accurate dating of the pregnancy is critically important for prenatal care, including the proper performance and interpretation of screening tests, and avoidance of unnecessary testing due to a misdiagnosis of prematurity or postdates. If dating is not clear from the initial visit, an ultrasound scan should be performed promptly to establish an accurate due date. Ultrasound dating is less accurate the further pregnancy progresses. Clinical dating is based on number of weeks since the start of the last menstrual period (LMP), assuming the usual 4-week cycle, with the due date (estimated date of confinement, EDC) being 40 weeks after the start of the LMP. Uterine size grows in a predictable manner in normal pregnancies, with fundal height (measured from the symphysis pubis to the top of the uterus, in centimeters) roughly equal to estimated gestational age (EGA) between 20 and 36 weeks. Prior to an EGA of 20 weeks, the uterus, on bimanual exam, is roughly lemon size at 6 weeks, orange size at 8 weeks,

grapefruit size at 10 weeks, and cantaloupe size at 12 weeks, filling the pelvis at that point.[34]

First-trimester prenatal care (up to 14 weeks) includes a determination of the patient's well-being during pregnancy, a review of family and lifestyle issues, and a reevaluation of the risk status. The clinical assessment includes measuring maternal weight gain, blood pressure, uterine growth, detecting fetal heart tones by Doppler ultrasonography, and counseling patients toward a healthy pregnancy. Common problems in the first trimester include nausea, vomiting, and gastroesophageal reflux. Patients should be counseled to eat frequent small meals and may use antacids such as calcium carbonate (e.g., Tums) or magnesium hydroxide (e.g., Maalox/Mylanta). Prenatal vitamins may help some patients, but be intolerable to others. Severe nausea and vomiting, associated with significant weight loss, ketonuria and/or electrolyte abnormalities, should be investigated with laboratory testing to rule out medical conditions associated with nausea and vomiting, and ultrasonography to rule out twin or molar gestation.[23] These cases may require intravenous hydration and antiemetics, with informed consent regarding teratogen issues with medication use.

Vaginal bleeding should be investigated carefully to rule out infection, threatened abortion, or placental abnormality, though patients may often report self-limited bleeding after sexual intercourse or vaginal exam. Rh-negative patients need to receive RhoGAM intramuscularly after episodes of vaginal bleeding, and after procedures such as amniocentesis.

Second-trimester prenatal care (14 to 28 weeks) includes confirmation of the estimated date of delivery by quickening (perception of fetal movements) at 18 to 20 weeks or earlier, uterine size at the umbilicus at 20 weeks, and fetal heart tones being heard using a fetoscope at 20 weeks. The fetus may be evaluated by ultrasonography if fetal age or size is in doubt. Health education during the second trimester includes planning for labor and delivery through childbirth education classes, initial discussion of infant feeding including encouragement of breast-feeding, and planning for parenting by recommending reading and/or classes. Mothers should be instructed to report symptoms that would indicate a pregnancy risk, such as vaginal bleeding, significant edema (especially of the face or fingers), continuous headache, blurring of vision, abdominal pain, persistent vomiting, chills, fever, dysuria, leakage of amniotic fluid, or change in frequency or intensity of fetal movements.

More frequent visits are generally made during the third trimester to evaluate for elevated blood pressure or other signs of preeclampsia, such as sudden excessive weight gain or edema, or significant proteinuria. Labor signs are taught to the patient with careful attention to the possibility of preterm labor. Fetal presentation is determined by Leopold's maneuvers, or by digital vaginal exam and/or ultrasonography when in question. Labor and delivery preferences of the mother and father should be clarified, and a completed prenatal record, including documentation of the parent's birth request, should be given to the patient or sent to the hospital. Predelivery lactation consultation should be considered in patients with nipple abnormalities that might preclude normal breast-feeding.

Other pregnancy complaints such as varicosities, hemorrhoids, and backaches are common in the latter part of pregnancy. Patients should avoid prolonged standing at this point in pregnancy, and may find relief with maternity support hose. Constipation, which aggravates hemorrhoids, can be alleviated with proper hydration and fiber laxatives. Back pains late in pregnancy should always be evaluated with the specter of preterm labor in mind. Tylenol is considered safe to use in recommended doses at any gestational age.

Fetal Assessment

Methods have been developed to assess the well-being of the fetus during pregnancy, including fetal movement records ("kick counts"), the nonstress test (NST), nipple stimulation or oxytocin contraction stress test (CST), and ultrasonography for amniotic fluid evaluation. These methods are used according to accepted protocols when risk factors are present that may jeopardize the fetus. They are routinely applied when pregnancy continues past 41 weeks, or earlier for certain conditions, such as diabetes, hypertension, decreased fetal movement, polyhydramnios/oligohydramnios, intrauterine growth retardation (IUGR), Rh sensitization, or previous unexplained stillbirth. Some authorities recommend that women monitor fetal movements regularly during the third trimester of pregnancy. Family physicians should understand these methods and be aware of their relative usefulness, including their sensitivity, specificity, and predictive values.[35]

Duration of Pregnancy

The normal duration of human pregnancy has considerable variation. The bell-shaped curve of human pregnancy is illustrated in Figure 11.1. The median is just past 280 days, or 40 weeks, from the last menstrual period. Two standard deviations from the mean would be 37 to 43 weeks. About 10% of pregnancies reach 42 weeks, confirming the normalcy of postdates pregnancy for many women. However, as pregnancies extend beyond 42 weeks, conditions such as oligohydramnios, passage of meconium into the amniotic fluid, macrosomia, and dysmaturity with potential IUGR, increase in frequency and can cause significant risk for the fetus.[23]

Labor and Delivery

Labor

Labor in the first stage is defined as progressive dilation of the cervix with uterine contractions. The early (latent) phase of labor occurs up to 4 cm dilation and is variable in duration. Progress during this phase is often slow because of the time needed for effacement of the cervix.

The active phase of labor is more rapid and predictable, yet there is still considerable individual variation. With frequent, regular contractions, the average is 1.2 cm dilation per hour in primigravidas and 1.5 cm per hour in multigravidas, but flexibility is important. Friedman[36] attempted to describe labor, not to define parameters women must follow. Arrest of labor is present where there has been no cervical dilation for 2 hours during this active phase.

When the pregnant patient presents in labor, her prenatal record must be carefully reviewed and risk assessment done. Decisions regarding need for antibiotics (e.g., positive group B streptococcus screening or prolonged rupture of membranes) should be made early. Current or recent active genital herpes is an indication for cesarean delivery to avoid neonatal herpes infection.

Support and observation are the hallmarks of managing normal labor. Women in labor should be given as much freedom of movement as possible. During the first stage of labor the blood pressure and the frequency and duration of contractions are measured every 15 to 30 minutes. The fetal heart rate should be monitored during and immediately after a contraction every 30 minutes during the first stage by whatever method is most convenient (electronically, Doppler ultrasonography, or fetoscopic auscultation). Intermittent fetal heart rate monitoring is preferable to continuous monitoring in normal or low-risk patients, as continuous monitoring interferes with freedom of movement and has a high false-positive rate.[7,8] Continuous electronic fetal monitoring in low-

Fig. 11.1. Distribution of duration of pregnancy, in days from last menstrual period to birth, among 383,484 singleton, noncesarean births with certain menstrual dates in Sweden, 1976–1980. Vertical lines are drawn at 259, 280, and 294 completed days. The line has been drawn between day-to-day percentage values, without any smoothing of the curve ("raw data"). (From Bergsjo et al,[43] with permission.)

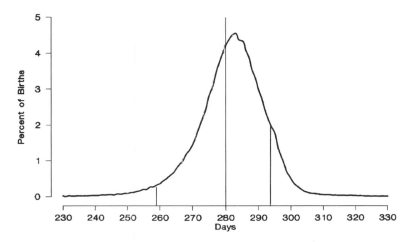

risk patients has resulted in three times the diagnosis of fetal distress and twice the frequency of cesarean sections without improving birth outcome.[37]

Women succeed best during the second stage of labor (expulsion of the fetus) when they are allowed and encouraged to use their instincts about pushing. Prolonged breath-holding and Valsalva maneuvers should be avoided, as they may result in decreased oxygenation of the placenta and fetal hypoxia. Women push more effectively and are in less pain when upright: sitting, squatting, kneeling, or standing.[38] Fatigued or hypotensive women may push while lying on their side. The dorsal lithotomy position should be avoided to prevent inferior vena cava compression, with resultant maternal hypotension and fetal distress. The fetal heart rate should be monitored every 15 minutes during the second stage in low-risk patients.[39]

Support During Labor

Continuous emotional support of the woman during labor enhances the birth process. It may be provided by a labor support team consisting of the nurse, the delivering physician or midwife, the father, and any other person close to the mother. A "doula" is a lay person trained to provide continuous support to the woman in labor and may be provided by the hospital to ensure that all women in labor receive optimal emotional support for labor and birth. Support during labor may reduce the need for intrapartum medication and technologic intervention.[40]

Intrapartum Analgesia and Anesthesia

Because all medications given during labor have side effects for both the mother and fetus, none is given routinely. Pain during labor may be managed by nonpharmacologic methods primarily, such as support from labor attendants, change of position, rest, physical contact, ambulation, and a warm shower or bath. Labor and birth without medication may be preferable for the woman and her partner. Some women benefit from pain medication during labor. A short-acting narcotic given parenterally during the first stage of labor may help the woman cope, and it may even facilitate dilation of the cervix.

Lumbar epidural anesthesia has become increasingly common and provides effective pain relief. It has a place in the management of dystocia and is of benefit for cesarean section. Its use during labor should be carefully considered, not elective. Studies in Europe and North America have shown that elective use of epidural anesthesia during labor increases the need for oxytocin augmentation and may increase the cesarean rate.[36,41] Documented effects of epidural anesthesia on labor include decreased uterine activity, prolongation of the first stage of labor, relaxation of the pelvic diaphragm predisposing to minor malpresentation, decreased maternal urge and ability to push, prolonged second stage of labor, and increased use of instrumental vaginal delivery.[42]

Despite these effects, epidural anesthesia has become almost routine in many hospitals, including hospitals with residency programs, and is requested by many women. If women and their birth attendants hope to avoid epidural anesthesia, prenatal education, support during labor, and management of the birthing environment must receive high priority.

Delivery

Normal delivery of the infant should occur in whatever position is comfortable for the woman, and the physician should be as flexible as possible with birth positions. The infant's head should remain flexed during delivery to lessen the diameter presenting to the perineum. An episiotomy is avoided unless the infant is large or delivery must occur quickly. Sometimes delivery of the head can be more controlled by gently pushing between contractions. After the head is delivered the physician should not rush to deliver the shoulders. The physician should assess for shoulder dystocia (Is the infant's head tightly retracted to the perineum?), check for a nuchal cord and reduce or clamp and cut it if necessary, suction the mouth and nose, and allow spontaneous delivery of the shoulders. The anterior and posterior shoulders should be delivered during a contraction with limited traction. Patience and gentleness result in fewer perineal lacerations.

The delivered infant is assessed immediately for color, tone, and respiratory effort. If no resuscitation efforts are necessary, the infant is placed against the mother for bonding,

warming, and drying. Clamping and cutting the cord and assigning of Apgar scores may follow these initial steps.

Delivery of the placenta (third stage of labor) should not
be attempted until separation has occurred from the uterus (up
to 30 minutes). Placental separation is likely when there is a
sudden gush of blood, the uterus becomes globular or firm
and rises in the abdomen, and the cord protrudes farther out
of the vagina. Gentle traction on the cord and suprapubic pressure to avoid uterine inversion spontaneously delivers the placenta. The placenta is examined for completeness, number of
vessels, and abnormalities. The mother is examined for cervical, vaginal, or perineal lacerations. Most first-degree lacerations (skin or mucosal tears) do not require suturing. Conditions that require action immediately postpartum include
hepatitis immunization of infants from mothers with positive
hepatitis B surface antigen, rubella vaccine for susceptible
women, and RhoGam for Rh-negative women.

Summary

The family physician can be skillful in the management of
normal pregnancy, labor, and delivery. Inclusion of this joy-
ous part of the family life cycle into the physician's practice
has numerous benefits for diversifying the practice and bonding the family with the physician. The family physician may
play an important role in advocating the proper support and
management of normal pregnancy, labor, and delivery in an
environment filled with extensive technology.

Acknowledgment

Some of the material in this chapter has been published in
a paper by members of the Working Group on Teaching Family-Centered Perinatal Care of the Society of Teachers of Family Medicine (with permission).[11]

References

1. Odent M. Birth reborn. New York: Pantheon, 1984.
2. Wertz RW, Wertz DC. Lying-in: a history of childbirth in America. New Haven: Yale University Press, 1989.
3. American Academy of Pediatrics and the American College of
   Obstetricians and Gynecologists. Guidelines for perinatal care,
   4th ed. Elk Grove Village, IL: American Academy of Pediatrics,
   1997.
4. Dick-Read G. Childbirth without fear, 2nd ed. New York:
   Harper & Row, 1959.
5. Karmel M. Thank you, Dr. Lamaze. Philadelphia: Lippincott,
   1959.
6. Kitzinger S. The experience of childbirth. New York: Pelican,
   1967.
7. Freeman R. Intrapartum fetal monitoring—a disappointing
   story. N Engl J Med 1990;322:624–6.
8. Banta HD, Thacker SB. The case for reassessment of health care
   technology. JAMA 1990;264:235–40.
9. Larimore WL, Reynolds JL. Family practice maternity care in
   America: ruminations on reproducing an endangered species—
   family physicians who deliver babies. J Am Board Fam Pract
   1994;7:478–88.
10. International Childbirth Education Association. Definition of fam-
    ily-centered maternity care. Int J Childbirth Educ 1987;2(1):4.
11. Scherger JE, Levitt C, Acheson LS, et al. Teaching family cen-
    tered perinatal care in family medicine. Parts 1 and 2. Fam Med
    1992;24:288–98, 368–74.
12. Willett WC. Folic acid and neural tube defect: can't we come
    to closure? Am J Public Health 1992;82:666–8.
13. Expert panel on the content of prenatal care: the content of pre-
    natal care. Washington, DC: US Public Health Service, 1989.
14. Nichols FH, Humenick SS. Childbirth education: practice, re-
    search and theory. Philadelphia: WB Saunders, 1988.
15. Scott JR, Rose NB. Effect of psychoprophylaxis (Lamaze prepa-
    ration) on labor and delivery in primiparas. N Engl J Med
    1976;294:1205–7.
16. Blair PS, Fleming PJ, Bensley D, et al. Smoking and sudden in-
    fant death syndrome: results from 1993–5 case-control study for
    confidential inquiry into stillbirths and deaths in infancy. BMJ
    1996;313:195–198.
17. U.S. Preventive Services Task Force. Guide to clinical preven-
    tive services. Baltimore: Williams & Wilkins, 1989;289–95.
18. Volpe JJ. Effect of cocaine use on the fetus. N Engl J Med
    1992;327:399–404.
19. Crump WJ. The pregnant day-care worker: What are the infec-
    tious risks? Fam Pract Recert 2000;22(11):21–28.
20. Copeland JA, Andolsek KM. Exercise in pregnancy. In: An-
    dolsek KM, ed. Obstetric care: standards of prenatal, intra-
    partum, and post-partum management. Philadelphia: Lea &
    Febiger; 1990;113–16.
21. Gjerdingen DK, Froberg DG, Fontaine P. The effects of social
    support on women's health during pregnancy, labor and deliv-
    ery, and the postpartum period. Fam Med 1991;23:370–5.
22. Williamson HA, LeFevre M, Hector M. Association between
    life stress and serious perinatal complications. J Fam Pract
    1989;29:489–96.
23. Gabbe SG, Niebyl JR, Simpson JL, eds. Obstetrics: normal and
    problem pregnancies, 3rd ed. New York: Churchill Livingstone,
    1996.
24. National Institutes of Health Consensus Development Confer-
    ence. Genetic testing for cystic fibrosis. Arch Intern Med
    1999;159:1529–39.
25. American College of Obstetricians and Gynecologists. Mater-
    nal serum screening. ACOG educational bulletin no. 228. Wash-
    ington, DC: ACOG, 1996.
26. U.S. Department of Health and Human Services, Public Health
    Service, National Institutes of Health. Diagnostic ultrasound im-
    aging in pregnancy. NIH publication no. 84-667. Washington,
    DC: Government Printing Office, 1984.
27. American College of Obstetricians and Gynecologists. Ultra-
    sonography in pregnancy. ACOG technical bulletin no. 187.
    Washington, DC: ACOG, 1993.
28. Bucher H, Schmidt JG. Does routine ultrasound scanning im-
    prove outcome in pregnancy? Meta-analysis of various outcome
    measures. BMJ 1993;307:13–17.
29. Ewigman BG, Crane JP, Frigoletto FD, et al. Effect of prenatal
    ultrasound screening on perinatal outcome. N Engl J Med
    1993;329:821–7.
30. The Expert Committee on the Diagnosis and Classification of
    Diabetes Mellitus. Report of the Expert Committee on the Di-
    agnosis and Classification of Diabetes Mellitus. Diabetes Care
    1997;20:1183–1197.
31. McGregor JA, French JI, Parker R, et al. Prevention of prema-
    ture birth by screening and treatment for common genital in-
    fections: results of a prospective controlled evaluation. Am J
    Obstet Gynecol 1995;173(1):157–167.
32. Centers for Disease Control and Prevention. Prevention of peri-
    natal group B streptococcal disease: a public health perspective.
    MMWR 1996;45(RR-7):1–24.

33. American Board of Family Practice. Normal pregnancy: reference guide 17. Lexington, KY: American Board of Family Practice, 1983.

34. Fox GN. Teaching first trimester uterine sizing. J Fam Pract 1985;21:400–1.

35. American College of Obstetricians and Gynecologists. Antepartum fetal surveillance. ACOG practice bulletin no. 9. Washington, DC: ACOG, 1999.

36. Friedman EA. Disordered labor: objective evaluation and management. J Fam Pract 1975;2:167–72.

37. Neilson JP. Electronic fetal heart rate monitoring during labor: information from randomized trials. Birth 1994;21(2):101–4.

38. Olsen R, Olsen C, Cox NS. Maternal birthing positions and perineal injury. J Fam Pract 1990;30:553–7.

39. American College of Obstetricians and Gynecologists. Fetal heart rate patterns: monitoring, interpretation, and management. ACOG technical bulletin no. 207. Washington, DC: ACOG 1995.

40. Kennell J, Klaus M, McGrath S, et al. Continuous emotional support during labor in a U.S. hospital. JAMA 1991;265: 2197–201.

41. Ramin SM, Grambling DR, Lucas MJ, et al. Randomized trial of epidural versus intravenous analgesia during labor. Obstet Gynecol 1995;86:783–9.

42. Johnson S, Rosenfeld JA. The effect of epidural anesthesia on the length of labor. J Fam Pract 1995;40:244–7.

43. Bergsjo P, Denman DW III, Hoffman HY, et al. Duration of human singleton pregnancy. Acta Obstet Gynecol Scand 1990;69: 197–207.

12
Medical Problems During Pregnancy

José A. Arevalo and Thomas S. Nesbitt

All primary care physicians should have an understanding of the interaction of various medical conditions with pregnancy. Whereas only some family physicians provide primary obstetric care, nearly all care for women during their childbearing years. Medical conditions that coexist with pregnancy may profoundly affect the course of pregnancy, and pregnancy may have a significant effect on the course of particular medical conditions. In addition, many medical conditions decrease the patient's chances of having a successful pregnancy if they are not diagnosed and addressed during the preconception period. For example, failure to adequately control a patient with insulin-dependent diabetes mellitus prior to conception may have disastrous consequences during the first few weeks of pregnancy, often before the patient seeks prenatal care. This chapter addresses conditions that may exist in pregnant patients.

Infections

Urinary Tract Infections

Urinary tract infection (UTI) constitutes the most common important infectious complication of pregnancy (also see Chapter 95). Bacteria continue to be responsible for the predominance of UTI in pregnancy; viruses and fungi are rarely the cause. These infections usually occur as one of three distinct clinical presentations or a combination: (1) asymptomatic bacteriuria, (2) acute cystitis, or (3) pyelonephritis. Controversy still exists regarding the role of pregnancy as a risk factor for infection of the urinary tract. Intestinal/perineal flora can gain entry to the urinary system by ascending the urethra into the lower urinary tract. Retrograde movement of the organisms, particularly if vesicoureteric reflux is present, can lead to infection of the upper urinary tract. Proposed risk factors for UTIs include relative immunosuppression of pregnancy, lower socioeconomic class, diabetes mellitus, and sickle cell disease.[1]

Asymptomatic Bacteriuria

Historically, asymptomatic bacteriuria (ASB) is defined as 100,000 colonies or more per milliliter of *one* organism from a midstream urine culture or 1,000 to 10,000 colonies per milliliter of *one* organism on a catheterized specimen in a woman without traditional symptoms of a lower UTI, such as dysuria, urinary frequency, and urgency or suprapubic pain.[2] The prevalence of ASB during pregnancy is about 2% to 10% in pregnant women, similar to that in the nonpregnant state. The most common organisms identified in ASB, accounting for 85% to 90% of all organisms isolated, are *Escherichia coli, Klebsiella, Enterobacter, Streptococcus, Staphylococcus, Proteus, Pseudomonas,* and *Citrobacter.* Although pregnancy does not increase the prevalence of ASB, it does increase the risk of progression from asymptomatic to symptomatic disease. The significance of ASB during pregnancy is that, if untreated, 20% to 30% of affected women develop acute pyelonephritis during the third trimester. Screening and treatment of ASB have been shown to reduce the rate to 3%.[3,4] Routine urine culture at 12 to 16 weeks as a screening test is recommended. Use of leukocyte esterase or nitrite testing in pregnant women may be cost-effective if the prevalence of ASB is low.[4]

Cystitis

Acute cystitis during pregnancy is characterized by significant bacteriuria associated with the presence of symptoms of lower UTI and the absence of signs of systemic infection. Occurring primarily during the second trimester of pregnancy, cystitis is usually associated with negative initial screening urine cultures.[5] Studies have shown that treatment of ASB results in a dramatic decline in the number of cases of subsequent pyelonephritis, but the incidence of acute cystitis does not appear to change.[5] The diagnosis of cystitis is similar during pregnancy and the nonpregnant state and is typified by symptoms of urinary frequency, urgency, dysuria, and suprapubic discomfort, and a urine culture with 100,000 colonies or more per milliliter. Symptomatic lower UTI may be difficult to identify during pregnancy because these symptoms are also found frequently in pregnant women with sterile urine. Thus the diagnosis is based primarily on finding a positive urinalysis or urine culture in a pregnant woman with typical symptoms. Fever, nausea, vomiting, flank pain, and chills are usually absent in women with uncomplicated cystitis. The physical examination is normal except for suprapubic tenderness. In most cases an adequate, clean-catch midstream urine sample is cloudy and malodorous, and it tests positive to nitrite. Microscopic examination of the urine usually discloses white (WBCs) and red blood cells (RBCs), bacteria, and a positive nitrite test.

Management of Lower UTIs

Although ampicillin/amoxicillin is still widely used to treat uncomplicated UTI, recent reports of increasing resistance call for consideration of a 5- to 7-day course of a first-generation cephalosporin, a short-acting sulfa drug, or nitrofurantoin (cure rates between 50% and 90%). Single-dose antimicrobial therapy, such as 2 g of cephalexin, may be just as effective, but recently some experts have recommended at least 3 days of therapy.[6] Urine cultures should be prepared 1 to 2 weeks after initial therapy and then monthly for the remainder of the pregnancy. If this therapy fails to eradicate the infection, the patient should be retreated with high-dose antimicrobial therapy (according to the sensitivity of the organism) for at least 3 weeks.

Pyelonephritis

Acute pyelonephritis, occurring primarily during the latter half of pregnancy complicates about 1% to 2% of all gestations.[7,8] With routine screening and treatment of ASB the expected 20% to 30% rate of subsequent pyelonephritis can be reduced to about 3% to 6%.[3,8] Acute pyelonephritis is principally a clinical diagnosis, typically presenting with fever, chills, flank pain, nausea, vomiting, and malaise. Microscopic evaluation of the urine should demonstrate pyuria and occasionally bacteriuria. It is unlikely that in an adequately collected specimen the urine would fail to demonstrate pyuria. The urine culture can be negative in true pyelonephritis if the laboratory reports more than 100,000 colonies, the affected urethra is obstructed, or the infection is anaerobic.

Because of the possibility of preterm labor and/or septic complications, pregnant women presenting with pyelonephritis should be hospitalized for intravenous antimicrobial therapy and close monitoring. Recently, hospital stays of less than 24 hours and home therapy have been advocated for selected lower risk patients. Because of the potential risk of preterm labor and fetal distress, the initial evaluation should initially include a short course of external fetal monitoring. Frequent assessment of vital signs and urine output with careful evaluation of fluid status is crucial in seeking signs of septic shock. Increasing resistance to ampicillin by Enterobacteriaceae call for initial therapy with a second- or third-generation cephalosporin or an aminoglycoside such as gentamicin.[9] Because one fourth of pyelonephritis patients initially present with a rise in their serum creatinine as a consequence of dehydra-

tion, caution must be used when treating with an aminoglycoside to prevent nephrotoxicity. Creatinine assays are done before and after aminoglycoside treatment if there is evidence of impaired renal function or suspicion that therapy with the aminoglycoside must continue after the third day. The aminoglycoside can be discontinued once the culture results demonstrate sensitivity to a less toxic antibiotic.

Eighty-five percent of patients with pyelonephritis are afebrile and asymptomatic by 48 hours and 95% by 72 hours.[9] Once the patient is afebrile for 24 hours, oral antibiotics can be substituted to complete a full 14-day course. If the fever continues beyond 48 hours, the possibility of urinary obstruction or renal anomalies exists and further studies are indicated. Many experts recommend nitrofurantoin suppressive therapy for the remainder of the pregnancy.[7]

Listeriosis

Listeriosis during pregnancy is caused by *Listeria monocytogenes*, a gram-positive rod shown to cause stillbirths, amnionitis, spontaneous abortions, neonatal infections, and maternal bacteremia. Most maternal infections are detected during the third trimester but may be missed because of the nonspecific flu-like symptoms. This infection is primarily food-borne, and approximately half of all reported cases of human listeriosis are pregnancy related. *Listeria* infections are usually detected by culturing the organism from blood, cerebrospinal fluid, or amniotic fluid.

Early maternal antibiotic therapy has been shown to reduce the high mortality and morbidity in infected neonates. Ampicillin, with addition of an aminoglycoside, is the treatment of choice. Alternative regimens include trimethoprim/sulfamethoxazole or erythromycin. Prevention in the form of counseling pregnant women to avoid eating unpasteurized milk products, raw eggs, or partially cooked meats is recommended.[10]

Viral Hepatitis

Hepatitis A

Hepatitis A is caused by a single-stranded RNA virus of the family Picornaviridae (see Chapter 90). Transmitted primarily via the fecal-oral route, this infection has a worldwide distribution and is usually acquired from contaminated food or via sexual contact. The incubation period varies from 10 to 50 days. The symptoms of malaise, anorexia, nausea with occasional vomiting, and fatigue may mimic normal pregnancy. Pregnant women with hepatitis A virus (HAV) may develop icterus, jaundice, and right upper quadrant abdominal tenderness. Antibody to anti-HAV immunoglobulin M (IgM) is positive during the icteric phase and persists 4 to 6 months. The HAV does not cross the placental membranes, and so intrauterine infection does not occur; however, cases of miscarriage or premature labor have been associated with acute hepatitis A infection.

Treatment is primarily supportive, as fulminant hepatic injury and death are uncommon. Hospitalization is rarely necessary unless the patient has severe nausea and vomiting and is in danger of dehydration. A single intramuscular immune gamma globulin dose of 0.02 mL/kg is recommended as pre- and postexposure prophylaxis in individuals who are household, close personal, and sexual contacts of persons with documented hepatitis A. A hepatitis A vaccine (Havrix; SmithKline-Beecham Biologicals, Philadelphia) is a killed, formalin-inactivated vaccine prepared from whole virus grown in human diploid cells and is recommended as prophylaxis.[11] No data regarding the safety of this vaccine have been reported for pregnant women.

Hepatitis B

More than 400 million people worldwide are infected chronically with the hepatitis B virus (HBV) and the World Health Organization estimates that HBV is responsible for over one million deaths annually. HBV, a DNA hepadnavirus, is known to result in chronic active hepatitis, chronic persistent hepatitis, cirrhosis, and hepatocellular carcinoma. Multiple lines of evidence indicate that perinatal infection is responsible for a significant share of these infections through vertical transmission in certain high-risk populations.[12] In the United States about 40% of infants born to mothers who are hepatitis B surface antigen (HBsAg) positive become infected. Up to 10% of adults infected with HBV become persistently infected and are at risk for the same chronic complications. Treatment of acute infection with HBV is supportive, observing for, and promptly treating, dehydration.

Although the prevalence of this virus is significantly lower in the United States than in other parts of the world (e.g., Asia and Africa), compelling evidence demands that physicians who care for pregnant women screen for HBV to identify infants who would benefit from vaccination. Screening is accomplished by testing serum for HBsAg. The specificity and sensitivity rates are considered to be sufficiently high to justify prophylactic immunization of the newborn when the maternal test is positive. This is accomplished by vaccinating the newborn at birth with hepatitis B immune globulin (HBIg) and hepatitis B vaccine (HBVac). Follow-up vaccinations with HBVac only are recommended at 1 and 6 months, with routine testing for HBsAg and hepatitis B core antibody (anti-HBC) 12 to 18 months after birth. Several vaccine formulations using recombinant DNA technology are currently available in the United States.

Transplacental infection of the fetus is rare. Women with positive HBsAg tests should be evaluated for the presence of chronic liver disease by a thorough history and physical examination with evaluation of aminotransferase and γ-glutamyltransferase (GGT) levels. Consideration for maternal treatment using antiviral therapy to prevent serious chronic sequelae is indicated. Close intimate contacts should be offered evaluation, and those with negative HBsAg and anti-HBC should be offered routine vaccination with HBVac.[13]

Hepatitis C

Hepatitis C, like hepatitis B, is transmitted through body fluids and has the major risk factors of multiple blood product transfusions, intravenous drug use, and multiple sexual partners. At one time approximately 20% to 40% of acute viral hepatitis in the United States was classified as non-A, non-B because serologic markers for HAV and HBV were absent.[14] It is now generally accepted that most non-A, non-B hepatitis is due to the hepatitis C virus (HCV). This RNA-containing virus is related to the pestiviruses. Serologic testing can identify antibodies to HCV, although the antibody remains an unreliable predictor because of the delay in seroconversion after exposure. Approximately 50% of those infected with this virus develop biochemical evidence of chronic liver disease and one quarter will progress to cirrhosis.

Interferon-α and ribavirin combination therapy appear to confer a more acceptable sustained virologic response than treatment with interferon alone; however, inadequate experience in pregnancy precludes definitive recommendations for widespread use. Vertical transmission occurs in 4% to 50% and may be enhanced in the presence of human immunodeficiency virus (HIV).[15] Neonatal risk is highest when acute HCV infection occurs in the mother during the third trimester of pregnancy. Acute infection during the first or second trimester does not pose a significant risk to the fetus.

Hepatitis D

Delta hepatitis is due to a defective RNA virus (HDV) that has been demonstrated to co-infect individuals with active HBV infection. Infection with this agent occurs only when HBsAg is present. Transmission of HDV is similar to that of HBV except for rare reports of neonatal transmission. Most individuals affected are intravenous drug abusers or their sexual contacts. Superinfection with HDV results in an 80% likelihood of chronic hepatitis in those with previous hepatitis B. At present no specific therapy is available for HDV once infection occurs. Therefore, the key factor for preventing transmission of HDV lies in the prevention of HBV infection.[16]

Varicella

Varicella zoster virus is classified in the herpes virus group. Varicella infection in the form of chickenpox is one of the most communicable diseases in our society, with up to 90% of young adults demonstrating immunity for varicella zoster[17] (also see Chapters 18 and 116). Although not completely understood, it is believed that transmission of this disease is through respiratory droplets and direct contact. The classic eruption of chickenpox, which usually begins on the head and neck and progresses to the trunk, is usually not confused with other infections.

Varicella zoster infections during pregnancy appear to be most significant during the first 20 weeks and in the third trimester. Infection early in pregnancy may result in congenital varicella-zoster syndrome, which manifests as skin lesions, limb deformities, and central nervous system (CNS) or ocular anomalies. The risk of this syndrome appears to be about 2% for infants in women who have varicella infections in the first 20 weeks.[18]

The other significant period of risks is in the late third trimester, specifically if the mother develops the disease 5 days before to 2 days after delivery. The risks of transmitting chickenpox during this period is 10% to 20%, and, if untreated, the case fatality rate is 30%.[19] Varicella late in pregnancy warrants attempts to delay delivery until 5 to 7 days after the onset of illness. If this is not possible, the neonate should be given varicella-zoster immune globulin immediately after birth and should be isolated from the mother until lesions that might contact the baby have crusted.[19]

Nonimmune pregnant women with a significant exposure should receive zoster varicella immune globulin (ZVIG), which is 60% to 80% effective in preventing infection if given in the first 96 hours after exposure.[19] Nonimmune women seen in the preconception period should be immunized and avoid pregnancy for 3 months.

Tuberculosis

Screening and Active Disease

Tuberculosis (TB) in humans is caused by an acid-fast bacillus of the species *Mycobacterium tuberculosis* or *Mycobacterium bovis* (see Chapter 84). About 1% of all women of childbearing age are tuberculin-positive, with much higher rates among particular groups such as Native Americans, immigrants from Asia or Central America, and homeless women. According to the Centers for Disease Control and Prevention, the number of reported cases of new tuberculosis cases in the United States has been on a downward trend since the TB epidemic peaked in 1992, declining by 7% from 1999 to 2000.[20] Once identified, active disease in a pregnant women is usually easily treated; nonetheless, the most significant risk of untreated infection is to the newborn. Newborn infection can result in serious consequences such as tuberculous meningitis.[21] Recent reports of increasing rates of HIV infection along with increasing rates of multidrug-resistant tuberculosis have prompted public health experts to urge more comprehensive screening.

Infection with tuberculosis in the United States occurs primarily though the inhalation of microdroplets by a susceptible host. The lower two thirds of the lungs are the site of most early lesions. Most healthy individuals overcome the infection and show no evidence that infection has occurred other than a positive tuberculin skin test. The tuberculosis bacillus has the unique ability to lie dormant for decades only to reactivate when the immune system begins to falter. If immunosuppression occurs because of age, poor nutrition, other chronic illness, or drugs, the infection can advance, leading to progressive disease. Active disease during pregnancy may be masked by nonspecific symptoms. Pregnant women most commonly present with apical upper lobe disease most likely due to reactivation of a previously acquired infection. Although pregnancy was at one time considered a risk factor for reactivation, evidence does not support this hypothesis, and most experts maintain that other underlying factors play a more pivotal role in the development of active disease.

All high-risk pregnant women should be screened for tuberculosis using the 5 tuberculin unit (TU) Mantoux intradermal test (purified protein derivative; PPD). Tuberculin skin testing has been found to be safe during pregnancy. Physicians should question each woman to ensure she has not had a previous positive test. Multipuncture tests (e.g., Mono-Vacc or Tine) have been shown to produce a high false-negative rate in adults, thereby limiting their usefulness as a screening study. Interpretation of the tuberculin skin test has been revised to identify three distinct risk groups[22] (see Chapter 84). A positive PPD test requires exclusion of active disease through a complete history and physical examination and with a posteroanterior chest radiograph (the lateral view adds lit-

tle to the evaluation) using abdominal shielding. If the chest radiograph is suggestive of active disease or symptoms are present, sputum smears and cultures should be obtained. Numerous foreign-born persons have been vaccinated in their native country with the bacille Calmette-Guérin (BCG) vaccine, an attenuated form of *M. bovis*. Although false-positive reactions may occur as a result of BCG, many experts recommend that a prior history of BCG not be considered as the primary factor in interpreting a positive PPD.[23]

Persons with a positive PPD test should undergo a thorough physical examination looking for physical signs of TB. Those lacking evidence of active infection should receive isonicotinic acid hydrazide (INH) (isoniazid) prophylaxis for a 9-month course if they meet the criteria defined in recent guidelines. Briefly, these criteria recommend INH prophylaxis in persons under 35 years of age who are from high-prevalence countries; medically underserved, low-income, high-prevalence populations; or long-term care facilities. Treatment of latent infections using INH is also recommended in persons of any age with HIV infection or who are at risk of HIV infection or other medical conditions that increase the risk of TB, or those with a close contact with patients who have been newly diagnosed with TB or have recently been identified as new skin test converters. Screening for HIV infection may also be indicated for recent converters. Patients with possible exposure to drug-resistant TB should be treated according to current recommendations for multidrug preventive therapy. Directly observed therapy—observation of the patient by a health care worker as the medication is taken—may be indicated in patients who are unlikely to be compliant.

Therapy

If active pulmonary tuberculosis is identified, treatment consists of a 9-month course of isoniazid (300 mg/day) and rifampin (10 mg/kg/day) with the addition of pyridoxine at 25 mg/day. If regional variation predicts a high rate of multidrug resistance, ethambutol (15–25 mg/kg/day) is added with the imperative that cultures be prepared prior to initiating therapy. Streptomycin, pyrazinamide, and ethionamide should not be used during pregnancy because of the risk of fetal toxicity.

Preventive Therapy

Women of ages 35 years or younger and who are identified as PPD positive with a negative chest radiograph should be offered preventive therapy *after delivery* of isoniazid 300 mg/day for a minimum of 6 months. Careful monitoring for hepatotoxicity is indicated for the first 3 months, particularly in Latino patients.[22]

Parasitic Infections

See Chapter 44.

Toxoplasmosis During Pregnancy

Toxoplasmosis, increasingly being recognized as an important infection during pregnancy,[24] is caused by *Toxoplasma gondii*, a protozoan parasite. The disease is usually asymptomatic in pregnant women. Humans most commonly become infected with this organism through (1) cat feces, which contaminates soil or is found in cat boxes; (2) ingesting undercooked meat or raw milk; or (3) vertical transmission from mother to fetus. Infection of the fetus can occur only in women who acquire infection during pregnancy. Previously infected women have immunity, which protects the fetus from becoming infected. Overall, approximately 40% of nonimmune pregnant women who are infected with *Toxoplasma* transmit the infection to the fetus. The rate of transmission is higher if the woman is infected during the third trimester.

The major complications of congenital toxoplasmosis are microencephaly, mental retardation, cerebral calcification, and meningoencephalitis with resultant hydrocephalus. Impaired vision or even blindness can also occur. In addition, these infants may have thrombocytopenia, skin rash, jaundice, or hepatosplenomegaly.[24] Immunocompetent women who acquire *Toxoplasma* infection during pregnancy often present with minimal clinical findings, requiring the clinician to be alert to signs and symptoms in women at risk. In some women, however, a mononucleosis or flu-like syndrome occurs. Symptoms may include malaise, lymphadenopathy, rash, hepatosplenomegaly, and the appearance of atypical lymphocytes on the peripheral smear.[24]

Laboratory diagnosis involves measuring antibodies to the organism in the maternal serum. A positive result should be confirmed by a reference laboratory. Once the diagnosis of maternal infection has been established, an attempt should be made to document placental passage. Ultrasound and fetal blood sampling have been used, and more recently a specific gene of the organism in amniotic fluid has been used with polymerase chain reaction (PCR) testing.[25,26] Treatment of patients with fetal infection has been recommended to include pyrimethamine and either sulfadiazine or sulfadoxine.[26,27] Pyrimethamine is generally contraindicated during the first trimester of pregnancy due to potential teratogenic effects.[26,28] Folinic acid (calcium leucovorin) should be given along with pyrimethamine and sulfadiazine to reduce marrow toxicity. Neonatal treatment is also recommended. For acutely infected women without documented fetal involvement, spiramycin has been recommended.[26]

The key to managing toxoplasmosis during pregnancy is prevention.[24] First, the major source of *Toxoplasma* is cats, and therefore pregnant women with cats should be carefully counseled on preventive measures. If the cat does come into the home, the litter box should be emptied daily, and the pregnant woman should avoid any contact with the cat box or cat feces. If this is unavoidable, precautions should be taken to avoid any contact with the cat feces or used litter, such as wearing gloves and carefully discarding the litter. Second, because raw meat is a possible source, meat in the pregnant woman's home should always be stored at the proper temperatures and cooked thoroughly.

Hematologic Disorders

Iron Deficiency Anemia

Anemia, defined as a hemoglobin concentration of less than 11.0 g/dL in the first and third trimesters and less than 10.5 g/dL in the second trimester, is considered one of the most frequent maternal complications during pregnancy, with iron deficiency the most common cause (see Chapter 125). It is estimated that a single normal pregnancy costs the mother 1000 mg of iron.[29] Moreover, obligatory menstrual blood loss during the childbearing years results in relatively limited iron stores in most women. During pregnancy, maternal plasma volume expansion and fetoplacental demand for iron serves to lower the packed cell volume (PCV) even in the healthy iron-sufficient woman. Iron intestinal absorption increases from about 1 mg/day in the nonpregnant state to about 3 mg/day during the third trimester. For many women, dietary iron stores are not sufficient to replenish the obligatory maternal iron loss, and so supplemental iron is necessary. The symptoms of iron deficiency anemia (IDA) mimic the complaints brought on by the pregnancy itself with fatigue, malaise, irritability, pallor, headache, paresthesias, and pica. The fetus rarely endures significant morbidity due to maternal IDA, as iron is preferentially transferred to the fetoplacental unit even with severe maternal IDA. However, reports of intrauterine growth retardation and stillbirths have been reported with severe IDA of less than 6.5 g/dL.[30]

If possible, all pregnant women with screening hemoglobin levels less than 10.5 g/dL should have a thorough review of their blood smear. For women with moderate anemia (hemoglobin ≥9.0 and ≤10.5) in whom other reasons for anemia have been excluded, a presumptive diagnosis of iron deficiency and a diagnostic trial of iron supplementation (200–300 mg of elemental iron/day) is warranted. Usually an elevated reticulocyte count (5–8%) and an increase of at least 1 g/dL in the hemoglobin concentration are then seen by the third week. If compliance is assured and reticulocytosis fails to appear, serum iron, total iron-binding capacity (TIBC), and serum ferritin should be measured and hemoglobin electrophoresis undertaken.

Thalassemia

The thalassemias (see Chapter 126) are a group of hematologic disorders typified by a defect in the synthesis of one (or more) of the four polypeptides that make up the hemoglobin molecule, resulting in a decrease in the production of hemoglobin. People from the Mediterranean and Southeast Asia are disproportionate affected, although this disorder is found worldwide. Homozygous expression, usually identified during childhood, has a poor prognosis and consequently is rarely found in pregnant women. Heterozygous thalassemias (thalassemia intermedia and thalassemia minor) are relatively common in certain populations and can be diagnosed during routine screening of pregnant women. Most patients with heterozygous thalassemia demonstrate no specific clinical findings except for a mild microcytic anemia with hypochromia and microcytosis [mean cell volume (MCV) 65–75 fentoliter (fl)]. Heterozygous β-thalassemia may demonstrate an elevated level of hemoglobin A_2 on electrophoresis. The diagnosis in pregnant women is usually suspected when the patient fails to respond to an iron challenge and has normal serum iron levels, TIBC, ferritin, and hemoglobin electrophoresis. The importance of identifying this condition lies in providing genetic counseling and in withholding iron therapy to prevent iron overload.

Clotting Disorders

See Chapter 81.

Thrombophlebitis and Thromboembolic Disorders

Pregnancy increases the risk for thrombosis because of increasing lower extremity venous distention through mechanical obstruction of venous drainage by the enlarging uterus and hormonal effects on the venous system. In addition, levels of all of the procoagulants increase in the plasma except for factor XI and XIII. Other risk factors for thrombosis—obesity, dehydration, edema, and lower extremity varicosities—may also be present during pregnancy. Moreover, the risk for deep venous thrombosis (DVT) and pulmonary embolism (PE) increases significantly in the postpartum state if other comorbidities are present such as cesarean section, infection, obesity, prolonged bed rest, and malignancy.[31]

Deep Venous Thrombosis

Deep venous thrombosis has been reported to occur in 0.1% to 3.0% of all deliveries and is 3 to 16 times more common after delivery by cesarean section.[31] The diagnosis of DVT is complicated by the poor sensitivity of the classic lower extremity signs and symptoms of pain, tenderness, edema, erythema, a palpable cord, and a positive Homan sign (pain in the posterior calf with dorsiflexion of the affected foot) usually in the postpartum period. Because of the strong association between DVT and subsequent PE, confirmatory tests must be used before initiating therapy. Thrombosis diagnosed by clinical means alone is confirmed in fewer than half of the cases.[32] Most pregnancy-associated venous thromboses originate in the distal venous system but can extend into the iliac or femoral veins where the potential for embolization is higher. During pregnancy, the use of noninvasive diagnostic testing is limited because radioactive iodine employed for fibrinogen scanning is contraindicated and single impedance plethysmography has a comparably low sensitivity. Although venography has been called the "gold standard," many experts cite concern about the high rate of ionizing radiation, the technical difficulties, and the possibility that the procedure itself may predispose to thrombosis as reasons not to use venography routinely to diagnose DVT. Duplex ultrasound scanning and color Doppler ultrasonography with compression[33] have higher diagnostic sensitivity for proximal lower extremity thrombosis especially during the first and second trimesters but are inferior for identifying DVT of the calf veins. Both these tests are subjective and highly dependent on the skill of the examiner. Magnetic resonance imaging (MRI) has proved useful for diagnosing DVT in pregnant women.[34]

Pulmonary Embolism

Pulmonary embolization (see Chapter 81) during pregnancy continues to be a major cause of maternal mortality in the United States. Typically, the patient is in the puerperium but may be postpartum by several weeks. Tachypnea, dyspnea, and pleuritic chest pain in a pregnant woman should immediately alert the physicians to the possibility of PE, especially in patients at high risk. Hypoxemia is usually present with an arterial Po_2 less than 85 mm Hg and accompanying hypocarbia and respiratory alkalosis. Unless the embolus is massive, the electrocardiogram (ECG) and chest radiographs are typically nonspecific.

Ventilation-perfusion lung scanning is considered to be highly sensitive for PEs during pregnancy, especially in women without prior lung disease. Findings consistent with lobar or segmental profusion defects with adequate ventilation and no corresponding defects on chest radiography are highly correlated with PE on pulmonary angiography.[31] Pulmonary arteriography is usually reserved for cases in which the V/Q scan is indeterminate and the suspicion of PE is high. Recently the use of the helical computed tomographic angiography has been considered equivalent to pulmonary angiography, although this resource is not universally available.[35] Treatment of venous thromboembolic (VTE) disease consists of anticoagulation with unfractionated heparin, bed rest, and analgesics. Use of subcutaneous low molecular weight heparin (LMWH) has been shown to be equally effective in the treatment of VTE and has the added advantage of a much lower incidence of heparin-induced thrombocytopenia than heparin and a lower incidence of osteoporosis.[36] Many experts now recommend the use of unfractionated or LMWH during pregnancy followed by warfarin therapy after delivery.[37] Oral anticoagulants are not favored as treatment for DVT/PE by most experts because of the increased risk of fetal embryopathy.[38]

Thrombocytopenia

Significantly decreased platelet counts during pregnancy may be caused by a number of conditions (see Chapter 126), the most common of which are preeclampsia [including the HELLP syndrome (hemolytic anemia, liver dysfunction, coagulation changes)], systemic lupus erythematosus (SLE), drug-induced thrombocytopenia, gestational thrombocytopenia, and immune thrombocytopenic purpura. Thrombotic thrombocytopenic purpura (TTP) in pregnant women has been reported fewer than 100 times and is beyond the scope of this chapter. TTP in general is discussed elsewhere in the text, as are SLE and preeclampsia. Gestational thrombocytopenia is of unknown etiology but may be due to an acceleration of platelet destruction process associated with pregnancy.[39] The platelet count in gestational thrombocytopenia usually ranges from 50,000/ mm^3 to 150,000/ mm^3. These patients usually require no therapy.[39]

Immune thrombocytopenic purpura (ITP) is more common in women and generally has its onset during the first three decades of life. The frequency of this condition during pregnancy is about 0.1% to 0.2%. The disorder is caused by maternal immunoglobulin G (IgG) antiplatelet glycoprotein specific antibodies.[39] These antibodies cross the placenta and can result in decreased fetal platelet counts. The mechanism of platelet sequestration and destruction is discussed elsewhere in this text under the general discussion of ITP. Differentiating ITP from gestational thrombocytopenia can be difficult if the low platelet count is first discovered in pregnancy, and therefore the clinician should use the services of an experienced laboratory for the evaluation. Because some of the other causes of thrombocytopenia can be far more serious, it is critical that other potential causes of thrombocytopenia be ruled out.

The major concern in this condition is hemorrhage. Spontaneous bleeding is uncommon with platelet counts above 20,000/mm^3; however, close monitoring of all pregnant women with ITP is warrented.[40] Treatment for this condition includes glucocorticoids, intravenous immunoglobulin (IVIg), and, in severe cases, splenectomy. Some have recommended treating only if platelet counts drop below 20,000/mm^3 in the prenatal period but attempting to keep platelet counts above 50,000/mm^3 after 36 weeks.[41] During the prenatal period, platelet transfusions have limited benefit because of subsequent rapid destruction of the transfused platelets and should be reserved for acute hemorrhage or at the time of procedures.

Labor and delivery raises the most significant concerns, particularly for the fetus. Studies have shown a poor correlation between maternal and fetal platelet counts in ITP.[40] Recent work suggests that the risk to the fetus in ITP is less than previous thought and that a conservative approach may be warrented.[40] Horn et al[40] suggested the following approach in labor and delivery: have platelets available for maternal counts below 50,000/ mm^3, avoid epidural anesthesia for counts below 80,000/mm^3, avoid scalp electrode or scalp sampling, avoid traumatic delivery such as vacuum-assisted delivery, and promptly repair perineal lacerations.[40]

Endocrine Disorders

Diabetes

Few other areas in perinatal medicine have realized such dramatic improvement than diabetes in pregnancy. Maternal and neonatal adverse outcomes have been dramatically reduced primarily as a consequence of intensive medical management. Diabetes mellitus can be classified as primary (no contributing cause) or secondary when hyperglycemia is a consequence of other medical conditions (see Chapter 120). The most common forms of primary diabetes are type 1, formerly known as insulin-dependent diabetes mellitus (IDDM); type 2, formerly known as non–insulin-dependent (NIDDM); and gestational (type 2-G) diabetes. Type 1 typically presents in the second or third decades and is an autoimmune disorder that is characterized by insulin deficiency and a tendency toward ketonemia if exogenous insulin is not administered. In contrast, type 2 typically is diagnosed after age 40 in obese individuals who have early hyperinsulinemia and relative insulin resistance and who are resistant to ketosis in the absence of exogenous insulin. Gestational diabetes is defined as having its onset or initial recognition during pregnancy. The diagnosis of diabetes during pregnancy is dependent on the presence of relative hyperglycemia and whether the hyperglycemia predates the onset of the pregnancy.

Women with pregestational, type 1 or type 2 diabetes have

been shown to suffer significantly elevated rates of adverse maternal and neonatal outcomes such as preeclampsia, congenital anomalies, prematurity, neonatal metabolic derangements, macrosomia, respiratory distress syndrome, asphyxia, and stillbirths if they are not adequately monitored and managed. Normalization of blood glucose levels before and during the early weeks of pregnancy has been shown to reduce the risks of congenital anomalies and miscarriages.

Approximately 90% of diabetes in pregnancy can be classified as gestational diabetes. Methodologic issues and imprecise definitions confound the exact contribution to adverse outcomes from uncontrolled gestational diabetes. A consensus has arisen regarding the importance of screening women at high risk for gestational diabetes, as fetal macrosomia, neonatal hypoglycemia, hyperbilirubinemia, and hypocalcemia may be higher in infants born to women with gestational diabetes.[42]

During pregnancy, insulin antagonistic hormone levels increase (e.g., human placental lactogen, prolactin, cortisol, and progesterone), creating a relative insulin resistance. The results of these changes are seen during the latter half of pregnancy, with reduced fasting blood glucose levels and exaggerated postprandial glucose and insulin levels compared to the nonpregnant state. The National Diabetes Data Group has recommended that all pregnant women be screened for glucose intolerance utilizing a 50-g oral glucose challenge at 24 to 28 weeks regardless of the timing of the last meal. The American College of Obstetrics and Gynecology (ACOG) recommended the same screening tests but limited its use to women age 30 or older. A venous plasma value of 140 mg/dL (7.8 mmol/L) or more 1 hour later should be followed by a standard 3-hour glucose tolerance test. The Fourth International Workshop-Conference on Gestational Diabetes recommended the Carpenter and Coustan modification of the original O'Sullivan and Mahan criteria in 1998. The diagnosis is secure if at least two of the readings exceed these values: fasting, ≥95 mg/dL; 1 hour, ≥180 mg/dL; 2 hours, ≥155 mg/dL; and 3 hours, ≥140 mg/dL.[43]

Once the diagnosis is made, maternal education and dietary consults are critical. Recommended weight gain is 11 to 16 kg (24–35 lb) with a diet consisting of 30 kcal/kg body weight, not to exceed 2500 kcal/day. Careful monitoring of the plasma or capillary glucose is recommended, keeping the fasting level less than 105 mg/dL and the 1-hour level less than 140 mg/dL. Fetal ultrasonography is recommended during the third trimester to evaluate fetal growth, amniotic fluid volume, and malformations. If the glucose levels remain satisfactory, antepartum fetal testing or early delivery is not indicated. If the glucose levels exceed those outlined, the patient is referred to a perinatologist for follow-up. It is the practice of most family practice centers to refer all type 2-G patients who require insulin therapy.

Thyroid Disorders

Diseases involving thyroid function are frequent in women, affecting more than 1 in 500 pregnancies.[44] The hormonal changes that occur during the normal pregnant state significantly increase thyroid-binding globulin by stimulating hepatic biosynthesis. Regulatory mechanisms in most patients keep free thyroid hormone at euthyroid levels. It is therefore important when assessing thyroid function in the pregnant woman to measure free thyroid hormone as well as thyroid-stimulating hormone (TSH) using a sensitive bioassay. Thyroid diseases are covered elsewhere in this text (see Chapter 121). This section focuses on common thyroid diseases in relation to pregnancy.

Hyperthyroidism

Hyperthyroidism represents most of the newly diagnosed thyroid disease that occurs during pregnancy. The most common cause of this condition is Graves' disease. Hyperthyroidism during pregnancy must be treated because of the risks of stillbirth, premature birth, and low birth weight.[44] It should also be noted that women with hyperemesis may have underlying transient hyperthyroidism.[44] Thyroid-stimulating immunoglobulin crosses the placenta, resulting in stimulation of the fetal thyroid gland. Antithyroid medications such as propylthiouracil (PTU) and methimazole also cross the placenta, affecting fetal thyroid function. Optimal management for the hyperthyroid pregnant patient achieves high normal free thyroid hormone levels using as little medication as possible. PTU is the drug of choice as it has low rates of placental transfer and because methimazole has a questionable association with congenital malformations of the scalp.[45] Frequent monitoring of the pregnant patient on PTU is necessary to minimize the amount of drug required to keep the patient in the euthyroid state. Surgical treatment has little place in the treatment of the pregnant hyperthyroid patient.

Hypothyroidism

Untreated hypothyroidism during pregnancy is unusual, as it is associated with a high rate of infertility. Nonetheless, when pregnancy does occur in the hypothyroid patient, rates of abortion, fetal growth retardation, preeclampsia, abruption, stillbirths, and congenital malformations are increased.[44] With proper treatment the incidence of these adverse outcomes is reduced to near-normal levels.[46] Women on thyroid medication who wish to attempt pregnancy should be evaluated to document the hypothyroid state. If results cast doubt on a definite diagnosis of hypothyroidism, discontinuation of medication for 1 month while the patient uses contraception may be appropriate. At the end of this time a TSH assay is performed. If the diagnosis is confirmed, the patient is given an appropriate dose of L-thyroxine (T_4) titrated by following the serum TSH level; titration may take as long as 2 months. Pregnant patients presenting on thyroid medication should continue medication because of the risk of the hypothyroid state in the untreated state. In these patients the adequacy of therapy should be assessed by determining the free T_4 and TSH levels. Patients in whom the diagnosis of hypothyroidism is made during pregnancy should be treated with doses of 0.05 to 0.10 mg L-thyroxine and free T_4 and TSH levels determined at approximately 4 weeks. The dose is then adjusted, keeping the patient in the euthyroid state. L-Thyroxine does not pass the placental barrier and therefore should not directly affect thyroid hormone regulation in the fetus.

Respiratory Disorders

Gestational changes in the physiology of the respiratory system may lead to alterations in symptoms, which may affect underlying respiratory tract diseases. The primary alterations in pulmonary function are hyperventilation secondary to increasing progesterone levels during pregnancy. This increased minute ventilation leads to a decrease in PCO_2 to 27 to 32 mm Hg with a compensatory increase in the renal excretion of bicarbonate and, in some women, to a sensation of dyspnea. Other pulmonary function parameters change little except for a moderate decrease in the functional residual volume.[47]

Rhinitis

Nasal congestion develops frequently during pregnancy, as the nasal pharynx becomes edematous and hyperemic, often leading to increased mucus secretion. Allergic rhinitis (see Chapter 39) is common in patients of childbearing age and may be difficult to distinguish from physiologic changes. Occasionally, allergic rhinitis during pregnancy is complicated by nasal polyposis, which most often regresses after delivery. Rhinitis caused by viruses such as rhinovirus, or "the common cold," occurs in most adults at least once or twice a year. Pregnant women are likely to also experience this condition. It can be differentiated from the above conditions, as viral rhinitis is more often associated with a low-grade fever, myalgias, headache, and often a nonproductive cough.

The physiologic mucosal edema and congestion that often accompany pregnancy is not treated, if possible. In addition, treatment of allergic rhinitis during the first trimester is discouraged. Use of sympathomimetic drugs, specifically phenylpropanolamine and pseudoephedrine, during the first trimester has been associated with congenital malformations. These drugs may also cause constriction of the uterine vessels and reduced uterine blood flow at any time during pregnancy. Antihistamines should also be avoided during the first trimester. Diphenhydramine has been associated with malformations in at least one large study.[48] Chlorpheniramine appears to be safer but probably should also be avoided during the first trimester.[48] Newer antihistamines, such as fexofenadine and loratadine, should be avoided as there are inadequate studies documenting the safety of their use during pregnancy, although animal studies suggest that cetirizine may be safe.[48] The limited study regarding other complications has led to the recommendation that this drug be used only when the benefit clearly outweighs the risk to the fetus. The use of intranasal beclomethasone has not been associated with significant congenital anomalies.[48] Treatment of viral upper respiratory infections is mainly supportive, with fluids, bed rest, and acetaminophen to lower the temperature. It is generally believed that the use of acetaminophen as an antipyretic at all stages of pregnancy is beneficial in avoiding the potential teratogenic effects associated with significant fever.

Lower Respiratory Infections

Bronchitis and pneumonia during pregnancy occur as in the general population and commonly in smokers. In pregnant patients the two most common organisms responsible for pneumonia are *Mycoplasma pneumoniae* and *Streptococcus pneu-*

moniae. Pneumonia during pregnancy may be associated with significant complications, such as bacterial empyema and respiratory failure, which may be partly due to the decreased tidal volume secondary to the enlarging uterus later in the pregnancy. The clinician should not hesitate to confirm the diagnosis of pneumonia during pregnancy with a chest radiograph. It should also be kept in mind that pulmonary embolism can mimic pneumonia in pregnant women. Confirmed pneumonia in a pregnant patient requires hospitalization for observation and antibiotic therapy. Ambulatory therapy may be considered in selected cases as long as frequent and close follow-up is assured. In all instances antibiotic therapy should be guided by culture results and/or local epidemiologic microbiologic considerations including resistance patterns.

Asthma

Asthma (see Chapter 83) complicates fewer than 1% of all pregnancies, and several studies have shown that well-controlled asthma does not appreciably affect the outcome of pregnancy. Education on avoidance of exacerbating influences, the importance of medication adherence, and the proper use of peak flow meters is essential to help minimize the severity of acute attacks. Routine medications such as β_2-agonist, mast cell inhibitors, inhaled corticosteroids, and theophylline are considered safe in pregnancy. Leukotriene inhibitors are controller medications that have not been adequately studied in pregnancy and should be reserved for the exceptional case. Fortunately, asthmatic episodes during pregnancy usually occur in women with a history of asthma who can provide a comparison of the severity of attacks. Women who present with acute dyspnea or respiratory distress should be immediately evaluated. Those with a history of hospitalization for asthma, and particularly a history of incubation, require close observation and immediate therapy. Physical examination should concentrate on the vital signs, looking for the presence of fever (temperature >38.0°C), tachycardia [>120 beats per minute (bpm)], tachypnea (respiration rate >30), and pulsus paradoxus of 12 mm or more. The severity of the bronchospasm should be evaluated with spirometry or peak flowmeters. For acute asthma, the Po_2 is usually decreased; thus careful evaluation of the Pco_2 and pH is indicated. If the pH is elevated and the Pco_2 is below normal for pregnancy, the attack is considered mild. A decreased Po_2 with a normal Pco_2 (for pregnancy) and a normal pH is a moderate attack. A Pco_2 above 38 with pH ≤ 7.35 are ominous signs, indicating the need for management in an intensive care unit. Therapy is centered around rehydration and administration of a β_2-agonist, theophylline, and corticosteroids. Expectorants are not effective, and those with iodine are contraindicated during pregnancy because of concern over fetal goiter.[49]

Cardiovascular Disease: Chronic Hypertension

The definitions and classifications of hypertensive disease (see Chapter 75) during pregnancy have been confusing. Two expert groups have come together to define hypertensive conditions of pregnancy in the hope of establishing a standard nomenclature.[50] This group has recommended clarifying four conditions that involve hypertension during pregnancy. The first is *preeclampsia/eclampsia,* previously referred to as toxemia. This condition is described elsewhere in the book. A second condition, *transient hypertension of pregnancy,* is less well understood; it involves transient hypertension without proteinuria and edema. This condition resolves after pregnancy but may return with subsequent pregnancies. These patients appear to be at greater risk for chronic hypertension later in life.[50] *Chronic hypertension,* the topic of this section, involves hypertension prior to pregnancy or sometimes diagnosed early in pregnancy but not induced by the pregnant state. The fourth hypertensive condition during pregnancy is a combination of *chronic hypertension* and *superimposed preeclampsia* (see Chapter 13). Chronic hypertension in women of childbearing age mainly consists of essential hypertension. Chronic hypertension, which affects approximately 1% to 3% of pregnancies,[51] constitutes a risk to pregnancy with an increased associated risk of placental abruption, acute renal failure, intrauterine growth retardation, and prematurity.[51] Superimposed preeclampsia occurs in as many as 5% to 50% of patients with chronic hypertension and may partially explain the increased risks of other complications.[51]

In patients without an established diagnosis of chronic hypertension but who are found to be hypertensive during pregnancy, it is sometimes difficult to determine whether the hypertension was caused by pregnancy or was preexisting hypertension discovered during pregnancy. Determining the etiology of hypertension is particularly a problem when women without previous blood pressure measurements are not seen until the second trimester. Chronic hypertension is less likely to be associated with proteinuria or nondependent edema. Also, a uric acid level of less than 5 mg/dL is more likely found with chronic hypertension, as an elevated uric acid level is a sensitive marker of preeclampsia. Blood urea nitrogen (BUN) and creatinine levels are rarely helpful for differentiating the two. In cases of hypertension with elevated liver function and decreased platelets, preeclampsia with the HELLP syndrome is strongly suspected.

Treatment of chronic hypertension during pregnancy is controversial. Expert panel recommendations include treatment of pregnant women with diastolic blood pressures higher than 105 mm Hg, and systolic pressure at or above 160 mm Hg, treating lower pressures only if there are other significant risk factors, such as renal disease or end-organ damage.[52] Previous authors have reported no benefit of treating pregnant women with diastolic blood pressures below 110 mm Hg. Most experts continue to recommend methyldopa as the drug of choice because of its long history of safety during pregnancy.[47] Work evaluating beta-blockers in pregnant women has shown these agents to be efficacious for treatment of hypertension. However, atenolol and metoprolol have been associated with intrauterine growth retardation when treatment was started before midpregnancy.[53] Labetolol has shown promise and is generally believed to be safe during pregnancy. Angiotensin-converting enzyme inhibitors are contraindicated, as they have been associated with fetal death.[48]

Gastrointestinal Disorders

See Chapter 87.

Reflux Esophagitis

Heartburn, or gastroesophageal reflux disease (GERD), is characterized by a burning, epigastric or retrosternal discomfort usually affecting women during late pregnancy. The differential diagnosis includes angina, achalasia, esophagitis, and esophageal stricture (also see Chapter 87). This common disorder results from reflux of gastric secretions resulting from mechanical effects of the enlarging uterus and the effects of progesterone in decreasing lower esophageal sphincter tone. Reflux is aggravated by increased intraabdominal pressure, heavy meals, and the recumbent position.

Treatment is focused on avoiding aggravating factors, eating frequent light meals, and elevating the head of the bed. Magnesium and aluminum antacids taken 1 to 3 hours after meals and at bedtime are helpful and safe so long as maternal renal function is normal. Histamine-2 receptor antagonists (H$_2$RA) may provide relief in carefully selected resistant cases where peptic ulcer disease has been excluded. Caution should be exercised when using proton pump inhibitors in pregnancy because of limited data establishing their safety and efficacy.

Peptic Ulcer Disease

Pregnancy does not appear to influence the incidence of peptic ulcer disease (PUD).[54] The typical pain of PUD is described as gnawing or burning that usually appears about 30 minutes after meals in patients with gastric ulcer and 90 minutes to 3 hours after meals in those with duodenal ulcer. The pain characteristically is localized to the mid-epigastrium. Physical examination is unremarkable except for nonspecific abdominal tenderness, and unless there is active bleeding, laboratory tests are normal. Active bleeding may produce an iron deficiency anemia that is difficult to differentiate from anemia of poor nutrition.

Pregnant women with typical peptic symptoms should be initially treated with antacids and H$_2$RA. If symptoms persist despite these medications, consideration should be given to screening and treatment for *Helicobacter pylori* infection. The diagnosis of *H. pylori* can be made using a urea breath test, stool antigen tests, serology, or through biopsy techniques. Triple therapy regimes consisting of proton pump inhibitors (PPIs) and antibiotics have been shown to provide symptomatic relief as well as reduce ulcer recurrences and complications, although as noted above PPIs have not been studied extensively in pregnancy. Esophagogastroduodenoscopy (EGD) is reserved for persistent cases since radiographic studies are not routinely recommended in pregnancy.

Skin Disorders

Virtually any skin condition (see Chapter 115) that can occur in the nonpregnant state can occur during pregnancy, and some are exacerbated by pregnancy. Some skin changes carry no significance but raise concern among patients. Because of the increase in melanocyte-stimulating hormone, there is increased pigmentation in all dark areas of the skin, such as melanocytic nevi. The clinician must be aware that this is a normal occurrence while maintaining a critical eye for lesions that may have undergone malignant transformation. Some conditions are unique to pregnancy, and they form the focus of this discussion.

Pruritus Gravidarum

Pruritus gravidarum is a common condition, the frequency of which is increased during late pregnancy. It is characterized by generalized pruritus, and its etiology may be multifactorial. A form of pruritus in pregnancy is associated with bile salt accumulation leading to jaundice, thought to be secondary to hormonal interference with bile salt excretion. There are no specific lesions associated with these conditions.

An antipruritic lotion or oatmeal baths may help relieve the mild itching. Antihistamines such as chlorpheniramine may be used after midpregnancy in more severe cases, but these agents provide minimal relief with significant bile salt accumulation. In these cases, it may be necessary to use cholestyramine to bind bile salts, along with vitamin K supplementation.

Prurigo Gestationalis

Prurigo gestationalis affects 0.5% to 2.0% of pregnancies and occurs during the later weeks of the second trimester.[55] Lesions of this condition are 1- to 2-mm excoriated papules that occur on the extensor surfaces. They are intensely pruritic. Topical and oral antipruritics are usually sufficient treatment. If antihistamines are used, as noted above, the safety is greater after midpregnancy and if limited to those drugs with a safety track record such as chlorpheniramine.

Pruritic Urticarial Papules and Plaques

Pruritic urticarial papules and plaques (PUPPs) typically occur late in pregnancy in primigravida patients.[55] Lesions nearly always begin on the abdomen and in some cases spread symmetrically to involve other parts of the body, sparing the face. The lesions commonly begin in striae as red papules frequently surrounded by a thin, pale halo. As the condition progresses, the lesions may become confluent and form urticarial plaques or even target lesions. Despite the urticarial appearance, the lesions are not transient. The condition resolves spontaneously during the perinatal period and rarely lasts beyond the first postpartum week.[56] No significant maternal or fetal complications have been reported.[55] Symptomatic treatment for the itching is all that is required and includes low-potency topical steroids, antihistamines, cool compresses, and oatmeal baths.

Herpes Gestationalis

Herpes gestationalis, a rare, blistering disease of pregnancy, is believed by some to be a variant of bullous pemphigoid. Because of its potentially significant consequence to mother and fetus, it should be managed in conjunction with a dermatologist or perinatologist.

Impetigo Herpetiformis

Impetigo herpetiformis may be triggered by pregnancy. This condition was previously thought probably to be a form of pustular psoriasis.[56] Its onset is usually in the third trimester. The manifestations of this disease include superficial pustular lesions on an erythematous base beginning in the intertriginous areas and spreading to the thighs. There also may be mucous membrane involvement. This condition requires consultation because of its potential to progress to a more severe state associated with maternal and fetal mortality and morbidity.

Neurologic Disorders

Seizure Disorders

See Chapter 64.

Seizure disorders are the most frequent major neurologic event in pregnancy.[57] Multiple studies have addressed the effect of pregnancy on the frequency of seizures.[58] The results have been remarkably inconsistent. It appears, however, that approximately 50% to 60% of patients experience no significant change in the frequency of seizures; 30% to 45% of pregnant patients have been reported to have an increase in seizure activity[57,58] and the remaining patients have a decrease.

Although spontaneous abortions and prematurity are not increased in the epileptic patient, there is a slight increase in the rate of stillbirths.[57] This increase may be partially explained by noncompliant patients who experience status epilepticus with prolonged apnea hypoxia and acidosis. The incidence of preeclampsia is not higher among epileptic women, but it is important to differentiate eclamptic from noneclamptic seizures during the third trimester or postpartum in the epileptic patient.

One major effect of seizure disorders on pregnancy stems from the effects of anticonvulsive medication. Much controversy remains regarding anticonvulsive medication during pregnancy. Trimethadione is contraindicated during pregnancy because of the high risk of adverse effects on the fetus.[57] Phenytoin carries a relative risk of carcinogenesis, teratogenesis, and coagulopathy.[57] Valproic acid has been associated with a 1% to 2% incidence of spina bifida. Carbamazepine, although initially thought to be relatively safe for pregnancy, has been associated with craniofacial and neural tube defects.[59] Phenobarbital is associated with possible teratogenesis, neonatal depression, and coagulopathy.[57] Deficiency of vitamin K–dependent clotting factors have been particularly associated with phenytoin, primidone, and barbiturates, and folic deficiency with all anticonvulsants. This has led to the recommendation of folic acid supplementation to all mothers on anticonvulsant drugs, strict adherence to maternal serum α-fetoprotein (MSAFP) testing at 16 to 18 weeks, and comprehensive ultrasound examination at 18 to 22 weeks, as well as the standard intramuscular injection vitamin K for

the neonate.[57] Unfortunately, newer anticonvulsants have not been demonstrated to be any safer during pregnancy than those discussed above.

In summary, epileptic women contemplating pregnancy should be informed that the risk of complications is clearly greater than in nonepileptic patients, although approximately 90% of epileptic women can expect to have a normal pregnancy. These patients should be counseled prior to conception regarding vitamin replacement and anticonvulsant medication. Because no medication is completely safe, each patient should be advised of its risks. Ideally, seizure medications should be adjusted during the preconception period. The choice of seizure medication during pregnancy should be made in consultation with a neurologist or specialist in maternofetal medicine.

Migraine

Migraine headaches, with onset usually during the teenage and young adult years, have long been known to occur more commonly in women than in men (see Chapter 63). Pregnancy has a variable effect on the frequency and severity of migraine symptoms, although most women experience improvement.[60] Fluctuations in the pattern of migraine during pregnancy are believed to be related to changes in the estrogen level. Nonetheless, the presentation and clinical findings during pregnancy are similar to those of the nonpregnant state.

Treatment of migraine consists of rest, removal from noxious stimuli, occasional acetaminophen use, and if necessary antiemetics. The "triptans" (sumatriptan, zolmitriptan, naratriptan), ergotamine alkaloids, and isometheptene mucate (Midrin) should be avoided during pregnancy. Nonsteroidal antiinflammatory drugs (NSAIDs) such as ibuprofen can be used intermittently until the 34th week of pregnancy; however, prolonged use, particularly late in pregnancy has been associated with premature closure of the ductus arteriosus. Narcotics use should be judiciously reserved for the recalcitrant, severe cases along with consideration of prophylaxis using propranolol.

Bell's Palsy

Unilateral inflammation and edema of the seventh cranial nerve as it exits from the stylomastoid foramen results in acute peripheral facial paralysis, or Bell's palsy (see Chapter 67). This neuropathy occurs more frequently during pregnancy, and the cause remains elusive. More than 70% of patients recover completely without therapy. Although once used routinely, corticosteroid therapy for Bell's palsy has been questioned. Symptomatic treatment consists of reassurance, an eye bandage at night, and artificial tears during the day. The benefit of surgical decompression has not been established.

Carpal Tunnel Syndrome

Compression of the median nerve as it enters the palm of the hand can lead to carpal tunnel syndrome (see Chapter 67). As many as 25% of pregnant women complain of numbness, tingling, and burning of the palmar and dorsal surfaces of the first three fingers and the latter aspect of the fourth finger. The syndrome can also involve the entire hand. Physical examination may demonstrate a positive Phalen sign: reproduction of the patient's symptoms with maximal flexion of the wrist for about 1 minute. The Tinel sign when tapping over the course of the median nerve elicits a report of pins and needles over the median nerve distribution. Symptoms often affect both hands.

If no motor weakness or atrophy is present, resting the hands by the use of volar splinting at night may be helpful. Diuretic use is contraindicated during pregnancy, and NSAIDs provide little symptomatic relief. Injection of the carpal tunnel with a long-acting corticosteroid and lidocaine has been shown to offer some relief. Surgical decompression is reserved for recalcitrant cases usually after delivery.

References

1. Naeye RL. Causes of the excessive rates of perinatal mortality and prematurity in pregnancies complicated by maternal urinary-tract infection. N Engl J Med 1979;300:819–28.
2. Harris RE. The significance of bacteriuria during pregnancy. Obstet Gynecol 1979;53:71–3.
3. Kass EH. The role of asymptomatic bacteriuria in the pathogenesis of pyelonephritis. In: Quinn EL, Kass EH, eds. Biology of pyelonephritis. Boston: Little, Brown, 1960;399–412.
4. Whalley PJ. Bacteriuria of pregnancy. Am J Obstet Gynecol 1967;97:723–38.
5. Harris RE, Gilstrap LC. Cystitis during pregnancy: a distinct clinical entity. Obstet Gynecol 1981;57:578–80.
6. Dujff P. Maternal and perinatal infections. In: Gabbe SG, Niebyl JR, Simpson JL, eds. Obstetrics normal and complicated pregnancies. New York: Churchhill Livingstone, 2001.
7. Duff P. Pyelonephritis in pregnancy. Clin Obstet Gynecol 1984;27:17–31.
8. Kass EH. Pyelonephritis and bacteriuria: a major problem in preventive medicine. Ann Intern Med 1962;56:46–53.
9. Fan YA, Pastorek JG, Miller JM, Mulvey J. Acute pyelonephritis in pregnancy. Am J Perinatol 1987;4:324–6.
10. Smith JL. Foodborne infections during pregnancy. J Food Prot 1999;62:818–29.
11. Westblom TU, Gudipati S, DeRousse C, Midkiff BR, Belshe RB. Safety and immunogenicity of an inactivated hepatitis A vaccine: effect of dose and vaccination schedule. J Infect Dis 1994;169:996–1001.
12. Nishioka K. Predominant mode of transmission of hepatitis B virus: perinatal transmission in Asia. In: Vyas GN, Dienstag JL, Hoofnagle JH, eds. Viral hepatitis and liver disease. Orlando, FL: Grune & Stratton, 1984;424–32.
13. Arevalo JA. Hepatitis B in pregnancy. West J Med 1989;150: 668–74.
14. Advisory Committee on Immunization Practices. Protection against viral hepatitis. MMWR 1990;39(suppl 2):1–26.
15. Paccagnini S, Principi N, Massironi E, et al. Perinatal transmission and manifestation of hepatitis C virus infection in a high risk population. Pediatr Infect Dis J 1995;4:195–9.
16. Hoofnagle JH. Type D (delta) hepatitis. JAMA 1989;261: 1321–5.
17. Fox GN, Strangavity JW. Varicella-zoster virus infections in pregnancy. Am Fam Physician 1989;39:89–98.
18. Yankowitz J, Pastorek JG. Viral diseases. In: James DK, Steer PJ, Weiner CP, Gonik B, eds. High risk pregnancy: management options, 2nd rev. ed. London: Saunders, 2000:531–4.
19. Duff P. Infections in pregnancy. In: Ling FW, Duff P, eds. Obstetrics and gynecology: principles for practice, 1st ed. New York: McGraw-Hill. 2000;125–7.
20. Centers for Disease Control. U.S TB cases decline seven percent in 2000, reaching an all-time low. Press release 12 Jun 2001. *http://www.cdc.gov/nchstp/tb/pubs/pressrelease/061201.htm.*
21. Vo QT, Stettler W, Crowley K. Pulmonary tuberculosis in pregnancy. Prim Care Update Obstet Gynecol 2000;7:233–49.
22. Centers for Disease Control. Screening for tuberculosis and tuberculosis infection in high-risk populations: recommendations of the Advisory Committee for the Elimination of Tuberculosis. MMWR 1990;38:1–12.
23. American Thoracic Society. Diagnostic standards and classification of tuberculosis. Am Rev Respir Dis 1990;142:725–35.
24. Bakht FR, Gentry LO. Toxoplasmosis in pregnancy: an emerging concern for family physicians. Am J Fam Pract 1992;45:1683–90.
25. Hohlfeld P, Daffos F, Costa JM, et al. Prenatal diagnosis of toxoplasmosis with a polymerase-chain reaction test on amniotic fluid. N Engl J Med 1994;331:695
26. Gagne SS. Toxoplasmosis. Primary care update. Obstet Gynecol 2001;3:122–6.
27. Daffos F, Forestier F, Capella-Pavilosky M, et al. Prenatal management of 746 pregnancies at risk for congenital toxoplasmosis. N Engl J Med 1988;318:271–5.
28. Duff P. Infections in pregnancy. In: Ling FW, Duff P, eds. Obstetrics and gynecology: principles for practice, 1st ed. New York: McGraw-Hill, 2000;123–5.
29. Danforth D. Other complications and disorders due to pregnancy. In: Danforth D. ed. Obstetrics and gynecology, 4th ed. Philadelphia: Harper & Row, 1982;482.
30. McFee JG. Iron metabolism and iron deficiency during pregnancy. Clin Obstet Gynecol 1979;22:799–812.
31. Rutherford SE, Phelan JP. Deep venous thrombosis and pulmonary emboli in pregnancy. Crit Care Obstet 1991;18:345–70.
32. Laros RK, Alger LS. Thromboembolism and pregnancy. Clin Obstet Gynecol 1979;22:871–88.
33. Polak JF, Wilkinson DL. Ultrasonographic diagnosis of symptomatic deep venous thrombosis in pregnancy. Am J Obstet Gynecol 1991;165:625–9.
34. Spritizer CE, Evans AC, Kay HH. Magnetic resonance imaging of deep venous thrombosis in pregnant women with lower extremity edema. Obstet Gynecol 1995;85:603–7.
35. Garg K, Welsh CH, Feyerabend AJ, et al. Pulmonary embolism: diagnosis with spiral CT and ventilation-perfusion scanning—correlation with pulmonary angiographic results or clinical outcome. Radiology 1998;208:201–8.
36. Monreal M, Lafoz E, Olive A, del Rio L, Vedia C. Comparison of subcutaneous unfractionated heparin with a low molecular weight heparin (Fragmin) in patients with venous thromboembolism and contraindications to coumarin. Thromb Haemost 1994;71:7–11.
37. Sellman JS, Holman RI. Thromboembolism during pregnancy. Risks, challenges, and recommendations. Postgrad Med 2000; 109:71–84.
38. Ginsberg JS, Hirsh J, Turner DC, et al. Risks to the fetus of anticoagulant therapy during pregnancy. Thromb Haemost 1989; 61:189–96.
39. Samuels P. Hematologic disorders. In: Ling FW, Duff P, eds. Obstetrics and gynecology: principles for practice, 1st ed. New York: McGraw-Hill, 2000;123–5.
40. Horn EH, Davies J, Keane L. Other hematologic conditions. In: James DK, Steer PJ, Weiner CP, Gonik B, eds. High risk pregnancy management options, 2nd rev. ed. London: Saunders, 2000;487–9.
41. Letsky EH, Greaves M. Guidelines on investigation and management of thrombocytopenia in pregnancy and neonatal alloimmune thrombocytopenia. Br J Haematol 1996;95:21–6.

42. Landon MB. Diabetes mellitus and other endocrine diseases. In: Ling FW, Duff P, eds. Obstetrics and gynecology: principles for practice, 1st ed. New York: McGraw-Hill, 2000;231–6.

43. Sacks DA, Abu-Fadil S, Greenspoon JS, Fotheringham N. Do the current standards for glucose tolerance testing represent a valid conversion of O'Sullivan's original criteria? Am J Obstet Gynecol 1989;161:638–41.

44. Landon MB. Diabetes mellitus and other endocrine diseases. In: Ling FW, Duff P, eds. Obstetrics and gynecology: principles for practice, 1st ed. New York: McGraw-Hill, 2000;231–6.

45. McCarroll AM. The placental transfer of propylthiouracil, methimazole and carbamazepine. Arch Dis Child 1976;51:532–6.

46. Montoro M. Successful outcomes of pregnancy in women with hypothyroidism. Ann Intern Med 1981;94:31–5.

47. Collop NA, Harman EM. Pulmonary problems in pregnancy. Comp Ther 1990;16:17–23.

48. Briggs GG, Freeman RK, Yaffe SJ. Drugs in pregnancy and lactation, 5rd ed. Baltimore: Williams & Wilkins, 1998.

49. Huff RW. Asthma in pregnancy: medical problems in pregnancy. Med Clin North Am 1989;73:653–60.

50. Cunningham FG, Lindheimer MD. Hypertension in pregnancy. N Engl J Med 1992;326:927–31.

51. Siba BM. Diagnosis and management of chronic hypertension in pregnancy. Obstet Gynecol 1991;78:451–61.

52. Egerman RS. Hypertensive disorders during pregnancy In: Ling FW, Duff P, eds. Obstetrics and gynecology: principles for practice, 1st ed. New York: McGraw-Hill, 2000;245–7.

53. Butters L, Kennedy S, Rubin PC. Atenolol in essential hypertension during pregnancy. BMJ 1990;301:587–9.

54. Michaletz-Onody PA. Peptic ulcer disease in pregnancy. Gastroenterol Clin North Am 1992;21:817–26.

55. Gordon MC, Landon MB Dermatologic disorders. In: Gabbe SG, Niebyl JR, Simpson JL, eds. Obstetrics: normal and problem pregnancies, 3rd rev. ed. New York: Churchill Livingstone, 1996;1283–7.

56. Kennedy CTC, Kyle P. Skin disease. In: James DK, Steer PJ, Weiner CP, Gonik B, eds. High risk pregnancy: management options, 2nd rev. ed. London: Saunders, 2000;919–23.

57. Samuels P. Neurologic disorders. In: Ling FW, Duff P, eds. Obstetrics and gynecology: principles for practice, 1st ed. New York: McGraw-Hill, 2000;191–9.

58. Patterson RM. Seizure disorders in pregnancy. Med Clin North Am 1989;73:661–6.

59. Jones KL, Lacros RV, Johnson KA, Adams J. Pattern of malformations in children of women treated with carbamazepine. N Engl J Med 1989;320:1661–6.

60. Carhuapona JR, Tomlinson MW, Levine SR. Neurological diseases. In: James DK, Steer PJ, Weiner CP, Gonik B, eds. High risk pregnancy: management options, 2nd rev. ed. London: Saunders, 2000;803–8.

13
Obstetric Complications During Pregnancy

Carol E. Blenning

This chapter focuses on the following four complications of pregnancy: spontaneous abortion, ectopic pregnancy, preterm labor, and hypertension associated with pregnancy. Their definition, epidemiology, etiology, pathophysiology, diagnosis, prevention, and management are discussed.

Spontaneous Abortion

Spontaneous abortion (SAB) is the involuntary loss of pregnancy prior to 20 weeks' gestation. Recurrent spontaneous abortion (RSA) is defined as three or more consecutive SABs.

Epidemiology

SAB is fairly common, occurring in about 20% of known pregnancies. First-trimester vaginal bleeding occurs in 30% of pregnancies, and about half of these go on to spontaneously abort early (first trimester). Most (80%) of SABs occur early, in the first trimester.[1] But due to lack of patient recognition and/or failure to access health care services, preclinical (undiagnosed) cases push the rate of SAB toward 50% of pregnancies.

Etiology

Etiologies vary widely but most, especially first trimester, are secondary to a major genetic anomaly, e.g., trisomy, triploidy, and monosomy. In clinical practice, the etiologies of early losses are not usually discovered. Other etiologies can be divided into internal and external environmental factors.

Internal factors include uterine anomalies [such as from maternal diethylstilbestrol (DES) exposure], leiomyomata, incompetent cervix, uncontrolled insulin-dependent diabetes mellitus, progesterone deficiency due to luteal phase defect, and immunologic factors, which can be autoimmune or alloimmune.[1] The less common alloimmune reaction occurs when there is maternal rejection of the paternal component of the fetus as a foreign body. More commonly, maternal antibodies interfere with the pregnancy. Antiphospholipid antibodies (APLAs) include lupus anticoagulant and anticardiolipin antibodies. Of women with RSA and systemic lupus erythematosus (SLE), 80% are APLA positive, but whether this is associative or causative is still unclear.[2]

External environmental factors include substances, toxins, infections, and trauma. Ten cigarettes smoked per day increases the risk of SAB, daily alcohol consumption can triple the risk, and four cups of coffee per day has also been proven to raise the risk. Medications such as warfarin, anticonvulsants, and chemotherapeutic agents are associated with SAB, and 5 rads of irradiation at implantation is the minimum lethal dose. Occupational exposure to arsenic, lead, formaldehyde, benzene, or ethylene oxide is also a risk factor. Maternal infections add risk, as does increasing maternal or paternal age.[2]

With RSA there is a usual chance of a subsequent successful pregnancy (70–90%). Early losses, usually aneuploid, are generally nonrecurring, whereas late losses are often euploid and involve a maternal abnormality, but are much less common overall (consider positive APLA or cervical incompetence).[2]

Diagnosis

Clinically, women often present with vaginal bleeding (VB) and/or cramping. A history should include date of the last menstrual period (LMP) and menstrual history; birth control method used, if any; possible date of conception; and obstetric and gynecologic histories. Establishment of gestational age (GA) is very important. Physical examination should include vital signs; abdominal, speculum, and bimanual exams (the bimanual examiner should be accurate within 2 weeks GA); checking the cervix for dilation (a normal undilated cervix will not admit ring forceps); and listening for fetal heart tones, which are generally heard by external Doptone in the 9- to 12-week window. Progesterone levels can be helpful. A value of less than 5 indicates a nonviable pregnancy, greater than 25 supports the likelihood of viability of 99%, and values in between need to be followed and supported by other data.[1]

To aid in diagnosis, serial ultrasound examinations are preferred, if available, to quantitative β-human chorionic gonadotropin (β-hCG) levels. Ultrasound diagnosis can consist of loss of cardiac motion or development of yolk sac without fetal pole in weekly, serial exams. Expected landmarks, given GA by LMP, are as follows:

Number of weeks	Landmark	β-hCG level
<5	Possible gestational sac	<1500
6–7	Gestational sac 5 to 8 mm with yolk sac	1500
7	5- to 10-mm embryo in 25-mm gestational sac	>20,000
8	Cardiac motion seen when embryo is 20 mm	

Early presenters should be reevaluated when the gestational sac is expected to be 25 mm in size, calculated by an expected rate of growth of 1.1 mm per day. Cardiac motion without VB carries a risk of SAB of 4.2%, while the presence of VB raises the risk to 12.7%. When the gestational sac is >25 mm without an embryo or the gestational sac is distorted, an abnormal pregnancy outcome is almost assured.[1] β-hCG values aid in diagnosis when GA is <6 weeks, no gestational sac is seen, or when ultrasound is not available. Levels that fail to rise 66% in 48 hours indicate a pregnancy that is not progressing normally.[1]

Differential diagnoses to consider with vaginal bleeding include normal pregnancy, ectopic pregnancy, trophoblastic disease, and nonobstetric problems such as cervical polyps, friable cervix, and cervical cancer. With pain, possible diagnoses include ectopic pregnancy, pelvic inflammatory disease, ovarian cyst, and appendicitis. Fever and anorexia combined with abdominal pain or tenderness point toward an infectious etiology. During pregnancy the appendix is often pushed toward the abdominal right upper quadrant and can present more like a gallbladder or large bowel process.[3]

Prevention

Though expectant management is often recommended to the patient with threatened abortion in the form of bed rest, there is still no proof that this is effective.[4] For women with RSA, workup is indicated and should include parental karyotyping with chromosomal banding, and immunologic studies. Women positive for APLA have better outcomes on heparin (10,000 units sc q12 h) vs. aspirin (80 mg daily) or prednisone (40 mg daily).[2] For RSA, administration of hCG has not yet been proven advantageous, nor have various immunologic treatments, including paternal cell immunization, third-party donor leukocytes, trophoblast membranes, and intravenous immunoglobulin.[5,6] It is recommended to avoid administration of the influenza vaccine during the first trimester, though the correlation to SAB is unclear.[7]

Management

Nonsurgical management of SAB is a more available option with the use of high-resolution vaginal ultrasound, which allows for a better and earlier estimate of the volume of products of conception retained. One study showed that the use of misoprostol safely and effectively reduced the need for surgical management in the form of dilation and curettage. Misoprostol taken by mouth 400 mg every 4 hours, maximum dose 1200 mg, resulted in complete expulsion of products of conception in about half of the patients when evaluated by repeat ultrasound at 24 hours. These patients also had fewer complications than those who received surgical management. The remaining patients went on to dilation and curettage, though they had more bleeding and required more analgesia. The gastrointestinal side effects of misoprostol are usually manageable and did not prove to have clinical relevance.[8]

Surgical management by vacuum aspiration has been compared to sharp curettage and is not only faster, but also associated with less bleeding and pain. Complications are rare (uterine perforation) and appear to be comparable between the two methods.[9] Rh immune globulin, minidose, should be administered in the Rh-negative woman.[2] Management of the patient with SAB should always include attention to her emotional state. Up to 10% of women experience an acute stress disorder following SAB, and up to 1% demonstrate posttraumatic stress disorder 4 weeks later. They recover much better with support and debriefing. Some avail themselves of professional counseling and all should be offered this option.[10]

Ectopic Pregnancy

Ectopic pregnancy is a fertilized ovum that implants outside the intrauterine cavity. More than 95% of ectopic pregnancies occur in the fallopian tubes, 2.5% are in the cornua, and the rest implant in or on the ovaries, cervix, or abdominal cavity. Rupture and hemorrhage occur when the site cannot accommodate the placental attachment or growing embryo.[11]

Epidemiology

The incidence of ectopic pregnancy is 19.7 per 1000 pregnancies in North America. With rupture it causes 10% to 15% of maternal deaths and is the leading cause of first-trimester maternal mortality. The incidence has more than quadrupled in the past three decades, especially among women over 35 years of age and in nonwhite ethnic groups. Increases in risk factors account for this more than does improvement in early diagnosis. Case fatality (3.8 per 10,000 cases) is only 10% of what it was three decades ago, owing to improved diagnosis, but risk of death is still disproportionately greater among black women and other nonwhite minorities.[11]

Etiology

Almost all ectopic pregnancies are accounted for by interference with fallopian tube function, either anatomic (such as scarring and blockage) or functional (decreased mobility of the tube). Anatomic factors include tubal damage from pelvic inflammatory disease, previous ectopic pregnancy, and prior tubal or pelvic surgery. There is a 15% to 20% risk of recurrent ectopic following one salpingostomy and a 32% risk following two. Functional factors include endometriosis; use of hormones to promote ovulation and fertility; infertility itself (associated with abnormal tubal function); DES exposure *in utero*, which causes not only anomalies but also tubal dysfunction; and cigarette smoking, which is dose related and may cause impairment of tubal ciliary action. Other associative factors include multiple sexual partners, early age at first intercourse, and douching. These factors play an indirect role by increasing the risk of sexually transmitted disease (STD) and/or ascending pelvic infection. Intrauterine devices (IUDs), on the other hand, do not increase risk for ectopic pregnancy.[11] One meta-analysis ranked risks into three categories: strong, moderate, and slight. Strong risks were previous ectopic, tubal surgery and DES exposure. Moderate risks included history of infection (gonorrhea, chlamydia, or pelvic inflammatory disease), greater than one sexual partner, and smoking (either past or present). Slight risks were prior abdominal or pelvic surgery, douching, and intercourse before 18 years of age.[12]

Diagnosis

The most common presentation of ectopic pregnancy is a patient with abdominal pain and spotting, 6 to 8 weeks after her last menstrual period. The three most common signs and symptoms are abdominal pain, abdominal tenderness, and vaginal bleeding, though any number of the following also occur: adnexal tenderness, pain radiating to the shoulder, cervical motion tenderness, normal to slightly enlarged uterus, palpable adnexal mass, syncope, hypovolemic shock, and history of infertility, IUD use, or previous ectopic pregnancy.[13] Leaking or rupture should be suspected in the patient with hypotension or abdominal tenderness with guarding and rebound. Identification of risk factors and a high level of suspicion are important as 40% to 50% of ectopic pregnancies are misdiagnosed at the first emergency department visit.[11] Important laboratory studies include urine hCG and serum β-hCG. Serum progesterone greater than or equal to 25 ng/mL is 97.5% sensitive in ruling out ectopic pregnancy, but the combination of hCG and ultrasound provides an even greater sensitivity. Creatine kinase and fetal fibronectin levels do not have adequate enough sensitivities to be reliable in the diagnosis of ectopic pregnancy.[11]

The accuracy of ultrasound can be described by its discriminatory zone, which is the serum β-hCG level above which the gestational sac should be seen. For abdominal ultrasound the discriminatory zone is greater than 6500 mU/mL and for vaginal ultrasound it is greater than 1500. A culdocentesis results in recovery of nonclotting bloody fluid in the case of ectopic pregnancy, whereas yellow- or straw-colored fluid suggests rupture of ovarian cyst. This procedure is rarely necessary now with the availability of ultrasound. If the patient is hemodynamically unstable or has multiple signs and symptoms of ectopic pregnancy, she should go straight to laparoscopy. In the stable patient too early for clear evidence

of ectopic, serial β-hCG determinations can be followed. They double approximately every 48 hours in the normal pregnancy. When β-hCG does not increase 66% in 48 hours, the pregnancy is not progressing normally. When an apparent intrauterine pregnancy is failing and tissue is passed, these products of conception should be checked for chorionic villi. If chorionic villi are not present or if the serum β-hCG level has not fallen at least 15% in 12 hours following loss of products, ectopic pregnancy should be suspected.[11]

When ultrasound is not readily available, patients can be clinically triaged. For hemodynamically stable first-trimester patients with abdominal pain or vaginal bleeding, high-risk cases are those with peritoneal signs or definite cervical motion tenderness (95% specificity). Of those remaining (not high risk), intermediate-risk cases have no fetal heart tones, no tissue at the os, no midline pelvic cramping, and the presence of pain or tenderness, including cervical motion and uterine or adnexal tenderness (96–100% sensitive). All remaining cases are considered low risk and carry less than 1% chance of ectopic pregnancy.[14]

Management

Ectopic pregnancy can be managed either medically or surgically. Expectant management can be effective, as 68% to 77% of ectopics resolve without intervention. But because those cases that resolve spontaneously are not readily predictable, expectant (and close) follow-up is only advised if the β-hCG is low and falling, and if pregnancy size measures less than 3.5 cm on ultrasound.[11]

Methotrexate, at a dose of 50 mg per square meter of body surface area given intramuscularly, is now the mainstay of medical management and is most successful when the β-hCG level is less than 15,000 mU/mL (93% successful), whether or not there is free peritoneal fluid seen on ultrasound.[15] Its mechanism of action targets rapidly dividing cells, such as those found in trophoblastic tissue. Side effects of nausea, vomiting, diarrhea, and urinary frequency are usually mild, however, due to the low dose needed for treatment. Patients rarely experience changes in buccal mucosa, bone marrow, and skin. Absolute requirements for use of methotrexate include hemodynamic stability, ultrasound findings consistent with ectopic pregnancy, reliable follow-up, and no contraindications to use of methotrexate (immunodeficiency, blood dyscrasias alcoholism, chronic liver disease).[11] Relative requirements include pregnancy less than 3.5 cm size without rupture, lack of cardiac motion, and β-hCG less than 5,000 mU/mL. Serial β-hCGs determinations must be followed and, though a single dose is 71% effective, if they are not falling, a second dose of methotrexate (84–94% effective) versus laparoscopy can be considered. Ninety percent of patients diagnosed early with ectopic pregnancy are treatable with methotrexate.[16] Each resolved, unruptured ectopic pregnancy saves $3000 when treated medically, with similar efficacy and complication rates compared to surgical management.[17]

Laparotomy is used when the patient is not hemodynamically stable or if laparoscopy is not possible. For pregnancy in the ampulla a linear salpingostomy is performed with healing by secondary intention. A fimbria pregnancy can be "milked" out. For pregnancy located in the isthmus, that segment is excised and later microscopically reanastomosed. Salpingectomy is indicated when there is uncontrolled bleeding, extensive tubal damage, a recurrent ectopic pregnancy in the same tube, or if sterilization is desired. Complications to surgical management include recurrence (5–20%) and incomplete removal of trophoblastic tissue (single-dose methotrexate can be given in the high risk patient).

β-hCG levels must be followed to a level of less than 5 mU/mL in all cases, regardless of management. The rare instance of heterotopic pregnancy (one per 2600 pregnancies in the United States and Europe but 3% risk with fertility treatments) is challenging to diagnose. Half are identified after rupture of the ectopic pregnancy, and surgical treatment is required if the remaining intrauterine pregnancy is desired.[11]

Preterm Labor

Preterm labor (PTL) is labor occurring between 20 and 37 completed weeks of gestation. Labor is defined as four uterine contractions (UCs) within 20 minutes or eight UCs within 60 minutes, combined with at least one of the following criteria: premature rupture of membranes (PROM), cervical dilation beyond 2 cm, effacement greater than 50%, or documented change of the cervix. Preterm premature rupture of membranes (PPROM) is when ROM occurs more than 1 hour before onset of labor (premature) and before 37 weeks GA (preterm).[18]

Epidemiology

PTL affects 1 in 10 U.S. births and causes 75% of the neonatal deaths that are not attributable to congenital malformations. Despite improved survival and decreased morbidity with advances in perinatology and neonatology, the rate of PTL has not changed, and may even be increasing. In 25% of preterm births (PTBs) the labor was induced due to either maternal or fetal indicators. Thirty percent of PTBs are associated with premature rupture of membranes. PTBs are preventable in less than half of the women presenting in labor prior to 37 weeks' gestation. Thus, it is important to identify PTL early or, when possible, before it occurs, by identification of risk factors.[18]

Etiology

Preconception risk factors include smoking, substance use, poor nutrition, STDs, and stressful working conditions. It is valuable to address these factors, to extend family planning services, and to treat hypertension, diabetes, and other preexisting medical conditions, especially in women who are medically underserved, in both urban and rural settings.

Clinical factors associated with PTL range from general maternal factors to uterine and fetal factors. Women with no prenatal care, those of color or in lower income groups, those under 18 or over 40 years of age, those who are underweight, and, as mentioned above, users of tobacco or other substances

are at increased risk. A history of PTL followed by PTB (subsequent pregnancy PTL risk ranges from 17–37%), or second-trimester miscarriage also raises risk. Uterine factors include greater uterine volume, trauma, infection, uterine anomalies such as bi- and unicornuate uterus and fibroids (especially submucosal and subplacental fibroids), retained IUD, and abnormal implantation of the placenta. Infections more likely to result in PTB are gonorrhea, chlamydia, syphilis, trichomonas, bacterial vaginosis, group B streptococcus, chorioamnionitis, asymptomatic bacteriuria, and acute pyelonephritis. Trauma and DES exposure can cause painless cervical dilation or incompetence, and can require cerclage. Fetal factors that play a role in PTL include intrauterine fetal demise (IUFD), intrauterine growth retardation (IUGR), and congenital anomalies.

Several markers have been thought to be of value in identifying the woman at risk for PTL. These include cytokine, estradiol-17, β, estriol, and progesterone. But fetal fibronectin (FFN) is the most promising, especially when used for its negative predictive value. A negative FFN gives a woman a 3 in 1000 chance of having a PTB within the following week. The positive predictive value gives risk of PTB as high as 83% in the presence of symptoms. FFN is discussed further in the next subsection.[18]

Diagnosis

The best diagnosis is early diagnosis, which means a patient must be educated to recognize the signs and symptoms of PTL. Patients need to know what to do in case of cramping, pelvic pressure, UCs greater than four per hour, increased vaginal discharge, backache, and low back pain.[18] Routine cervical examination as an attempt to improve early identification is not useful in the patient without risk factors, possibly useful if there is increased risk, and not a known cause of PTL.[19]

The routine use of transvaginal ultrasound is not recommended in diagnosing PTL, even with risk factors. But it does offer a more standardized measure of cervical length up to 4 cm. A normal third-trimester cervix measures 3.5 to 4.8 cm; 1.5 cm correlates with 50% effacement and 1.0 cm with 75%. These values are more useful in primiparous women, whereas dilation of the internal os is a better measure for the multiparous. A shorter cervix is associated with increased relative risk, especially in women with risk factors.[19]

FFN is an adhesive substance that lies between the embryonic and inner uterine surfaces. Its presence in cervical and vaginal fluids is unusual after 20 weeks' gestation (less than 10% of women) and rare after 24 weeks, when it can represent a detachment of fetal membranes from decidua. UCs in the presence of a positive FFN triples the risk of PTB. The FFN test is 10 times better at predicting PTB when compared with other factors and signs. At 14 days its negative predictive value is 99%, and a positive test is a better predictor at 7 days than dilatation or UC frequency. Positive predictive value decreases with increasing gestational age, however. It may help predict chorioamnionitis and infection, especially when combined with UC monitoring. The FFN test is expensive to run (though the test equipment is not) and not valid if the cervix has been examined within 24 to 48 hours. Thus, many practitioners will collect the specimen before doing the digital exam, and then discard the tube if the test is not indicated.[19]

Because PTB is associated with increased UCs more than 24 hours prior to delivery, home monitoring of uterine activity is thought to be of diagnostic use. There is evidence that it reduces PTBs in singleton pregnancies at increased risk for PTL, but only one study has demonstrated this in twin gestations. Home monitoring with daily nurse contact applied to the general population did not result in earlier diagnosis, or decreased PTBs or neonatal morbidity. The United States Preventive Services Task Force finds insufficient evidence to recommend for or against the use of home uterine activity monitoring as a screening tool. It is supported in cases with a history of PTB.[19]

Prevention

Treating PTL and PTB costs over $3 billion per year.[19] Unfortunately, prevention of PTL is fairly limited. In general, treatment of infections is important. Urinary tract infections (including pyelonephritis) respond to antibiotics with good outcomes, though in pregnancy there is no optimal medication.[20] The evidence concerning treatment of bacterial vaginosis (BV) is conflicting. One review showed that recurrence of PTB is reduced when women with a history of PTB are screened and treated early in pregnancy (although it is unclear if this is also associated with neonatal well-being).[21] Other evidence found that treating women who were asymptomatic but positive for BV at 16 to 24 weeks' gestation showed no difference in any measure used, including PTB rates at 37, 35, and 32 weeks, premature rupture of membranes, hospitalization for PTL, use of tocolytic therapy, vaginal infection, use of neonatal intensive care unit (NICU), or neonatal death. Even women at increased risk did not experience improved rates of PTB.[22] Also, there is not enough evidence to show that women with threatened PTL who receive magnesium maintenance have a lower incidence of PTB.[23]

Management

The approach to the patient who is suspected of having PTL should include a thorough history and physical examination. Important elements of the history include evaluation of the dating accuracy and identification of risk factors. Examinations include a clean-catch urinalysis, sterile speculum exam (consider obtaining FFN specimen first), microscopy (wet mount and potassium hydroxide slides, smear to check for ferning), and collection of gonorrhea, chlamydia, and group B streptococcus (GBS) tests. Digital exam for cervical dilation should be avoided in the presence of PPROM. Assessment of fetal heart tones and evaluation for UCs must be done. UCs every 15 minutes or less require treatment. Uterine irritability should respond to a bolus of 500 cc of intravenous fluids (lactated Ringer's or normal saline). If UCs persist following the bolus when the rate is reduced to 100 cc/hour, then terbutaline can be administered subcutaneously (0.25 mg). Ultrasound can help determine gestational age, fetal presentation, placental position, presence of anomalies, and amount of amniotic fluid. Amniocentesis is useful in assessing fetal lung maturity and in evaluating for chorioamnionitis. Amniotic fluid should be sent for Gram stain, glucose, lecithin/sphingomyelin (L/S) ratio, and culture and sensitivity.[18]

Treatment of PTL generally includes the use of parenteral tocolytics, steroids, and antibiotics. Each medication has its indications, contraindications, and complications, and patients must be clearly apprised to allow for the most informed consent.[18]

The parenteral tocolytics most commonly used are magnesium sulfate, β-mimetics (ritodrine and terbutaline), indomethacin, and calcium channel blockers (nifedipine). A newer oxytocin receptor inhibitor, antocin, is not widely used yet. Indications for tocolytic use are regular UCs and cervical change, though tocolysis is much less effective if the cervix is beyond 3-cm dilation. Contraindications to tocolysis include a nonreassuring fetal heart rate tracing, eclampsia, severe preeclampsia, a singleton IUFD, chorioamnionitis, fetal maturity, and maternal hemodynamic instability. Table 13.1 lists the specific tocolytic contraindications.[18]

Magnesium sulfate ($MgSO_4$) is an effective tocolytic with a low side-effect profile. It is known to act centrally, reducing risk of seizures by blocking neuromuscular transmission. It may also work as a calcium antagonist to reduce UCs. The loading dose is 4 to 6 g given IV over 15 to 30 minutes, followed by a drip of 1 to 4 g/hour to maintain a serum magnesium level of 4 to 6 mEq. The drip should be maintained until there are no UCs for a 12- to 24-hour period. Then terbutaline 2.5 to 5 mg po is usually given 30 minutes before discontinuing the $MgSO_4$ drip, and then every 2 to 4 hours, though oral terbutaline used following the acute phase of PTL is not proven effective. Maternal side effects and complications due to $MgSO_4$ include nausea, vomiting, headache, pulmonary edema, and, at toxic levels, hypotension, respiratory depression, muscle paralysis, tetany, and cardiac arrest. Fetal effects can include decreased muscle tone and lethargy. Calcium gluconate is an effective antidote.[18,19]

Of the β-mimetics ritodrine and terbutaline, only the former (IV use) is Federal Drug Administration (FDA)-labeled

---

Table 13.1. **Contraindications to Tocolysis in Preterm Labor**

Specific tocolytic agents
  β-mimetic agents
    Maternal cardiac rhythm disturbance or other cardiac disease
    Poorly controlled diabetes, thyrotoxicosis, or hypertension
  Indomethacin
    Asthma
    Coronary artery disease
    Gastrointestinal bleeding (active or past history)
    Oligohydramnios
    Renal failure
    Suspected fetal cardiac or renal anomaly
  Magnesium sulfate
    Hypocalcemia
    Myasthenia gravis
    Renal failure
  Nifedipine
    Maternal liver disease

for treatment of PTL. Despite that, terbutaline is commonly used and is also available in oral form. These medications stimulate β_2-receptors, causing relaxation of uterine and lung smooth muscle, with little action at the cardiac β_1-receptors (increased inotropy). Ritodrine is given 0.05 to 0.1 mg/minute IV, increasing every 15 minutes to as much as 0.35 mg/minute. Monitoring is important with IV use because of the risk of hypotension and tachycardia. Terbutaline is often given subcutaneously, 0.25 mg every 1 to 6 hours. Though maintenance oral terbutaline has not proven to be any more effective than simple observance following successful tocolysis of acute PTL, it is used in adjusted doses to minimize UCs and hold maternal heart rate between 90 and 105, and is discontinued between 35 and 37 weeks' gestation. Cardiac ischemia is possible, so any chest pain or arrhythmia should result in discontinuing the drug and doing an electrocardiogram. To prevent the complication of pulmonary edema, a low-sodium diet and fluid restriction of 2.5 to 3 L IV/day is instituted, respiratory rate and lung exam are checked frequently, and input, output, and weight are monitored. Hypotension, hypokalemia, hyperglycemia, and ketoacidosis are also potential complications. Blood glucose should be checked every 12 hours for nondiabetics and every 2 hours for diabetics. A baseline glucose is also useful.[18,19]

Second-line tocolytics include indomethacin and calcium channel blockers. Indomethacin inhibits prostaglandins and the production of cytokines that trigger labor. It is indicated for pregnancies less than 32 weeks' gestation, but use is limited to 48 hours due to potential fetal side effects of oligohydramnios and transient loss of patency of the ductus arteriosus. It can be given rectally, 100 mg every 1 to 2 hours as needed, or 25 mg orally every 4 to 6 hours. Potential complications include hepatitis, renal failure, and gastrointestinal bleeding.

Calcium channel blockers inhibit smooth muscle contractions, causing uterine relaxation. Nifedipine is given by mouth in a 30-mg loading dose, followed by 20 mg every 4 to 8 hours for the first 24 hours, then 10 mg every 8 hours as maintenance until 35 to 37 weeks' gestation. Its efficacy is similar to that of ritodrine. It can cause transient hypotension.[18]

Steroids are now an essential part of the management of PTL. This class of medication is the only treatment shown to improve fetal survival in PTL cases presenting between 24 and 34 weeks' gestation. In neonates, the use of corticosteroids reduces the incidence of intraventricular hemorrhage and respiratory distress syndrome, and also reduces mortality, even when administered less than 24 hours before birth,

though the most efficacy is appreciated starting at 24 hours after dosing and lasting for 7 days. There are also better outcomes for PTL at 30 to 32 weeks' gestation with PPROM and no chorioamnionitis. Betamethasone can be given (12 mg IM every 24 hours for two doses) or dexamethasone (6 mg IM every 12 hours for four doses). Readministration at 7 days is of questionable benefit except in cases with 24 to 34 weeks GA and risk of PTB within 7 days.[24] No long-term maternal or neonatal adverse effects have been reported, though steroids given with tocolytics increase the risk of maternal pulmonary edema, especially in the setting of maternal infection, fluid overload, or multiple gestation. Benefits of therapy are less pronounced when membranes are ruptured as opposed to intact. Use of steroids does not affect the diagnosis of infection, and risk of subsequent infection is minimal.[18,19] There is also a significant reduction in the incidence of necrotizing enterocolitis (10–80%). The National Institutes of Health (NIH) has published recommendations, but a more active dissemination of the information is needed to improve use of this beneficial tool.[25,26] Table 13.2 summarizes the benefits and risks.[27] Untreated, suspected intrauterine infection is an important contraindication.

Antibiotics are important in the management of PTL in treating STDs, urinary tract infections, respiratory and vaginal infections, and in the patient positive for GBS or at risk for this infection. With PPROM, antibiotics can lengthen the pregnancy and reduce the incidence of clinical chorioamnionitis, despite only questionable benefit to the infant. Overall reduction (maternal and neonatal) in infectious morbidity is demonstrated, but improved neonatal morbidity and mortality in the short and long term are unproven.[28] Antibiotics indicated for PPROM are as follows: 2 g ampicillin IV q6h plus 250 mg erythromycin IV q6h for 48 hours, followed by 250 mg amoxicillin po q8h plus 333 mg erythromycin base po q8h for 5 days, or 2 g ampicillin IV q6h for 24 hours and then 500 mg ampicillin po q6h until discharge or delivery.[19]

Without the condition of PPROM, antibiotics are not proven effective. PPROM cases between 24 and 32 weeks' gestation do respond to antibiotics with reductions in neonatal death, respiratory distress syndrome (RDS), sepsis, intraventricular hemorrhage, and necrotizing enterocolitis. One review found that even when membranes are intact, in the setting of PTL, antibiotics help prolong the pregnancy and reduce risk of maternal infection and neonatal necrotizing enterocolitis without, however, showing any significant reduction in RDS or neonatal sepsis and even having an association

Table 13.2. **Benefits and Risks of Prenatal Corticosteroid Administration in Preterm Labor**

	Maternal risks	Neonatal risks	Neonatal benefits
Short term	Pulmonary edema (with tocolytics) Infection (with PPROM) Compromised diabetic control Compromised screening for gestational diabetes	Infection (rare) Adrenal suppression	Lower mortality Less respiratory distress syndrome Less intraventricular hemorrhage Less need for oxygen and ventilatory support Lower neonatal costs, shorter NICU stays
Long term	None serious	Unknown	Less long-term neurodevelopmental disability Increased survival

NICU = neonatal intensive care unit; PPROM = preterm premature rupture of membranes.

with increased perinatal mortality.[29] Because GBS has an association of preterm labor and increased morbidity and mortality in neonates, prophylaxis is recommended for rupture of membranes greater than 18 hours, GBS-positive culture, GBS bacteriuria, or history of prior GBS-infected neonate. Broader spectrum coverage is indicated for intrapartum temperature equal to or greater than 38.0°C (100.4°F). For PPROM not in labor, GBS culture should be checked, and either prophylaxis given until culture is negative or prophylaxis begun when culture turns positive. If the 35- to 37-week GA GBS screening culture is negative, prophylaxis is not indicated. For GBS prophylaxis, penicillin G 5 million units IV is given, then 2.5 million units IV q4h until delivery or, for penicillin-allergic patients, clindamycin 900 mg IV q8h until delivery. One conclusion safely made is that antibiotics should be used judiciously and with clear indications in the patient with PTL.[18,19]

Other miscellaneous agents and therapies have been investigated in the treatment of PTL. Thyrotropin-releasing hormone (TRH) was thought to be effective, when used with steroids, in improving fetal lung development in a very preterm gestation. But, in fact, an increased risk was found: infants required ventilatory support more frequently, had lower 5-minute Apgar scores, and poor 12-month outcomes.[30]

Amnioinfusion has not been proven effective in treatment of PPROM. Though there was a decrease in the number of severe fetal heart rate decelerations per hour in the first stage of labor, there has been no established improvement of outcomes in cesarean section rates, Apgar scores, or neonatal death rates.[31]

Vitamin K usage in very preterm neonates is controversial. Trials of poorer quality suggest it improves coagulability and thus reduces rates of intraventricular hemorrhage, whereas trials of better quality do not.[32]

Phenobarbital helps diminish fluctuations in blood pressure and blood flow in the brain and, by this mechanism, was thought to prevent ischemic injury in the very preterm birth. But further studies of better quality do not demonstrate the benefits seen in earlier studies. There are no differences seen in neurodevelopmental abnormalities at 18 to 36 months of age, and maternal sedation is a common side effect.[33]

Finally, professional psychosocial support is important in the event of preterm birth. Also, there are social disadvantages associated with low birth weight. Social workers, midwives, nurses, and trained lay persons who provide emotional support, tangible assistance, information, and advice help improve psychosocial outcomes in these families, even in the absence of improved medical outcomes.[34]

Hypertension Associated with Pregnancy

Definition

Hypertension (HTN) in pregnancy is divided into three categories: pregnancy-induced hypertension (PIH), pregnancy-aggravated hypertension (PAH), and coincidental hypertension. HTN in pregnancy is defined by systolic blood pressure (SBP) >140 mm Hg or diastolic blood pressure (DBP) >90 mm Hg. Also, a relative rise in either measurement can be significant. For women with a rise in SBP of 30 and/or a rise in DBP of 15, 30% to 55% go on to develop PIH. For women with increases of less than 30 and 15 mm Hg, only 15% develop PIH (also see Chapter 75).

By definition, PIH occurs only during the latter half of pregnancy and resolves within 24 hours after delivery. It includes a spectrum of clinical scenarios, ranging from HTN alone and transient HTN, to mild and severe forms of preeclampsia, to eclampsia, when at least one convulsion occurs in association with preeclampsia syndrome. Preeclampsia is PIH with proteinuria and/or pathologic edema, and persistence of hand and face edema after arising. Mild preeclampsia includes mild elevation of DBP (less than 100 mm Hg), trace to 1+ proteinuria (<100 mg on spot test or <300 mg/day), mild elevation of liver function tests (LFTs), and otherwise no symptoms. The severe form involves DBP ≥110 mm Hg, 2+ proteinuria or greater than 4 g per 24 hours, markedly increased LFTs, and any of the following: headache, visual changes, upper abdominal pain, decreased urine output, elevations of creatine and bilirubin, thrombocytopenia, and, especially with PAH, IUGR and pulmonary edema. Mild preeclampsia can progress rapidly to its severe form. The grand mal convulsions of eclampsia do not usually occur more than 48 hours following delivery, though they can occur as late as 10 days postpartum. Ten percent of eclamptic convulsions occur before the onset of overt proteinuria.

PAH is underlying HTN worsened by pregnancy and can have superimposed preeclampsia/eclampsia, especially after 24 weeks GA.

Coincidental HTN (>140/90 mm Hg) occurs before pregnancy or before 20 weeks GA (except in the case of gestational trophoblastic disease, which causes early HTN) and persists long after the pregnancy is over.[35]

Epidemiology

Preeclampsia affects 5% to 7% of pregnancies, especially nulliparous women (70% of women with preeclampsia are nulliparous) and those over 40. Multiparous women at risk are those with multiple gestation or hydrops. African-American and Latina women are at increased risk, compared to Caucasians. Controlling for race, lower socioeconomic status also increases risk, as does a family history of preeclampsia, lack of prenatal care, diabetes, and chronic hypertension.[35] Superimposed HELLP (hemolysis, elevated liver enzymes, low platelets) syndrome affects 4% to 12% of cases of preeclampsia-eclampsia, or 0.2 to 0.6% of all pregnancies.[36] In developed countries, eclampsia occurs once in every 2000 deliveries. This figure is 20 times greater in developing countries. Worldwide, eclampsia causes more than 50,000 maternal deaths annually.[37] Access to prenatal care is the key to prevention of eclampsia.

Etiology

The morbidity and mortality associated with preeclampsia/eclampsia is caused, at the cellular level, by severe vasospasm, which causes microangiopathic hemolysis, microvascular damage, and platelet activation. The liver undergoes periportal hemorrhage and fibrin deposition. A defect in nitric oxide metabolism may contribute to the development of preeclampsia and HELLP. Maternal mortality due to complications of HELLP is 2%, whereas the perinatal mortality reaches 33%; 4% to 38% of cases involve disseminated intravascular coagulation (DIC) and 2% experience rupture of a hepatic hematoma, which is often fatal.[38]

Diagnosis

Symptoms of preeclampsia include headache, visual disturbance, abdominal pain, swelling, malaise, and nausea/vomiting (50%). Severe headache is often a precursor to eclamptic convulsion. Visual changes and epigastric and right upper quadrant abdominal pain are also ominous. Physical exam findings include elevated blood pressure (see definition, above), inappropriate weight gain (60%), right upper quadrant abdominal tenderness, edema (see definition, above) and hyperreflexia. Laboratory studies that suggest preeclampsia include proteinuria (1+ or higher), thrombocytopenia (<100,000 platelets/mm³), abnormal LFTs [aspartate aminotransferase (AST) and alanine aminotransferase (ALT) can range from 200 to 700 U/L, lactate dehydrogenase (LDH) >600 U/L, elevated bilirubin], coagulopathy, and elevated uric acid (>5 mg/dL). Of note is that there is no correlation between elevated blood pressure, abnormal LFTs, and abnormal liver biopsy.[38]

Prevention

Preventing preeclampsia is somewhat uncertain. There appears to be no impact from the amount of salt intake.[39] Calcium supplementation helps women at high risk of gestational hypertension and women of communities with low calcium intake, though the beneficial dose is unknown.[40] Studies have shown that 1.5 to 2 gm of calcium per day lowered blood pressure and may have lowered rates of PTB, cesarean section, IUGR, and perinatal mortality. But even though it may have reduced preeclampsia, it was not shown to lower the rate of eclampsia, and poor outcomes were found because of this. But the risk and cost is low, so treating even low-risk women may be worth it in terms of risks and benefits.[41]

Antiplatelet agents (low-dose aspirin) have shown small to moderate benefits in preventing preeclampsia (15% reduction). The difficulty is determining which patients to treat, when to begin treatment, and the proper dose. An 8% drop in PTB and 14% decrease in neonatal mortality have been demonstrated, despite no reduction in the rate of small for gestational age (SGA) babies.[42]

Management

Ambulatory management is reasonable if PIH is mild and blood pressure is less than 140/90. Bed rest is recommended, the patient should be seen at least twice weekly to monitor for signs and symptoms of preeclampsia, and fetal growth should be assessed. Hospital management is indicated for SBP ≥140 mm Hg sustained, DBP ≥90 mm Hg sustained, or evidence of severe preeclampsia. These patients need a complete history and physical; daily weights; admission test for proteinuria, and at least every 2 days thereafter; blood pressure checks every 4 hours; laboratory studies to include creatinine, uric acid, LFTs, hematocrit, and platelets; and measurements of fetal growth and amniotic fluid. The ultimate treatment of PIH is delivery, but management decisions depend on the severity of PIH, gestational age, and condition of the cervix. Management can include expectant observation (and the use of medications), labor induction, or immediate delivery.[35]

Medical management offers few options. Magnesium sulfate (MgSO₄) is superior to diazepam and phenytoin in the management of eclampsia. Though maternal death rates are similar, MgSO₄ is associated with fewer recurrences of convulsion. The number needed to treat (NNT) for magnesium sulfate is only eight patients when measuring recurrence of seizure, compared to the other two drugs.[37] One review of MgSO₄ vs. diazepam also showed fewer Apgar scores less than seven at 5 minutes and fewer neonates who stayed longer than 7 days in NICU in cases treated with MgSO₄.[43] MgSO₄ vs. phenytoin revealed a lower maternal risk of pneumonia, ventilation, and ICU admission. There were fewer neonatal deaths, admissions to NICU, and fewer stays in NICU longer than 7 days.[44] MgSO₄ vs. a lytic cocktail demonstrated less respiratory depression when treating eclampsia.[45]

For treatment of preeclampsia, MgSO₄ is a better anticonvulsant. It reduces the rate of eclampsia significantly, compared to placebo and phenytoin, though MgSO₄-treated cases resulted in cesarean more often.[46] Colloid as a plasma volume expander has not proven effective, however, in preeclampsia treatment.[47]

Antihypertensive agents exhibit little difference in treating hypertension, except that diazoxide causes hypotension, and ketanserin is not as effective as hydralazine.[48] Treating mild to moderate hypertension (140–169/90–109) reduces the risk of developing severe hypertension by 50%. But there is no significant difference seen in preeclampsia, neonatal mortality, PTB, and SGA. No antihypertensive stands out, except that methyldopa may be associated with increased risk of neonatal mortality.[49] In general, beta-blockers lower the risks of developing severe hypertension and of requiring a second antihypertensive. They may be associated with an increase in SGA infants, but effects on PTB and perinatal mortality are uncertain. No significant differences were noted between beta-blockers and methyldopa, hydralazine, and nicardipine.[50]

According to American College of Obstetrics and Gynecology (ACOG) Guidelines, PIH is a pregnancy-related condition that stands as an indication for antepartum fetal surveillance.[51]

The management of HELLP is delivery. Steroids postpartum help to raise platelet levels, and lower ALT and blood pressure. Strategies not effective include plasmapheresis, antithrombotics, and immunosuppression. Laboratory abnormalities peak 1 to 2 days postpartum and return to normal 3 to 11 days postpartum. HELLP carries a 3.4% risk of recurrence.[38]

Following delivery, magnesium should be continued for 24

hours. Intravenous hydralazine can be used to keep DBP under 110. Patients should be seen 2 weeks postpartum and, if still hypertensive at that time, should start antihypertensive therapy, generally with either diuretic or beta-blocker therapy. These women with persistent elevation of blood pressure now have chronic hypertension and should receive appropriate patient education.[35]

References

1. Wolkomir MS, ed. ALSO (Advanced Life Support in Obstetrics) course syllabus, 3rd ed. Kansas City: AAFP, 1996;5–18.
2. Abortion. In: Cunningham FG, MacDonald PC, Gant NF, Leveno KJ, Gilstrap LC, eds. Williams' obstetrics, 19th ed. East Norwalk, CT: Appleton and Lange, 1993;665–78.
3. Walling AD. Acute appendicitis in pregnancy. Am Fam Physician 2000;62:232.
4. Threatened abortions. Dialog 2000;8:item 5.
5. Scott JR, Pattison N. Human chorionic gonadotropin for recurrent miscarriage (Cochrane Review). In: The Cochrane Library, issue 2. Oxford: Update Software, 2001.
6. Scott JR. Immunotherapy for recurrent miscarriage (Cochrane Review). In: The Cochrane Library, issue 2. Oxford: Update Software, 2001.
7. Preboth M. ACIP issues recommendations for the 2000–2001 influenza season. Am Fam Physician 2000;62:233–6.
8. Miller K. Nonsurgical management of spontaneous abortion. Am Fam Physician 2000;61:194–7.
9. Forna F, Gulmezoglu AM. Surgical procedures to evacuate incomplete abortion (Cochrane Review). In: The Cochrane Library, issue 2. Oxford: Update Software, 2001.
10. Bowles SV, James LC, Solursh DS, et al. Acute and post-traumatic stress disorder after spontaneous abortion. Am Fam Physician 2000;61:1689–96.
11. Tenore JL. Ectopic pregnancy. Am Fam Physician 2000;61:1080–8.
12. Ankum WM, et al. Risk factors for ectopic pregnancy: a meta-analysis. Fertil Steril 1996;65:1093–9. Available at *www.jr2.ox.ac.uk/bandolier/booth/hliving/Ectopreg.html*.
13. Sadovsky R. Diagnosing and managing ectopic pregnancy. Am Fam Physician 2001;63:761–2.
14. Sadovsky R. Prediction model to estimate risk for ectopic pregnancy. Am Fam Physician 2000;61:2504–6.
15. Kirchner JT. Methotrexate in the treatment of ectopic pregnancy. Am Fam Physician 2000;61:2228–31.
16. Methotrexate treatment of bleeding. Dialog ed-Fasolino E 2000;8:item 10.
17. Walling AD. Single dose methotrexate therapy for ectopic pregnancy. Am Fam Physician 2000;62:427–31.
18. Von Der Pool BA. Preterm labor: diagnosis and treatment. Am Fam Physician 1998;57:2457–64.
19. Weismiller DG. Preterm labor. Am Fam Physician 1999;59:593–602.
20. Vazquez JC, Villar J. Treatments for symptomatic urinary tract infections during pregnancy (Cochrane Review). In: The Cochrane Library, issue 2. Oxford: Update Software, 2001.
21. Brocklehurst P, Hannah M, McDonald H. Interventions for treating bacterial vaginosis in pregnancy (Cochrane Review). In: The Cochrane Library, issue 2. Oxford: Update Software, 2001.
22. Kirchner JT. The role of bacterial vaginosis in preterm labor. Am Fam Physician 2000;62:652–5.
23. Crowther CA, Moore V. Magnesium for preventing preterm birth after threatened preterm labour (Cochrane Review). In: The Cochrane Library, issue 2. Oxford: Update Software, 2001.
24. Preboth M. NIH statement on antenatal corticosteroids. Am Fam Physician 2001;63:794–7.
25. GRiP—steroids in preterm delivery, March 1994; band 2–2. Available at *www.jr2.ox.ac.uk/bandolier/band2/b2–2.html*.
26. Leviton LC. Methods to encourage the use of antenatal corticosteroid therapy for fetal maturation. A randomized controlled trial. JAMA 1999;281:46–52. Available at *www.jr2.ox.ac.uk/bandolier/band79/b79-2.html*.
27. Anyaegbunam WI, Adetova AB. Use of antenatal corticosteroids for fetal maturation in preterm infants. Am Fam Physician 1997;56:1093–6.
28. Kenyon S, Boulvain M. Antibiotics for preterm premature rupture of membranes (Cochrane Review). In: The Cochrane Library, issue 2. Oxford: Update Software, 2001.
29. King J, Flenady V. Antibiotics for preterm labour with intact membranes (Cochrane Review). In: The Cochrane Library, issue 2. Oxford: Update Software, 2001.
30. Crowther CA, Alfirevic Z, Haslam RR. Prenatal thyrotropin-releasing hormone for preterm birth (Cochrane Review). In: The Cochrane Library, issue 2. Oxford: Update Software, 2001.
31. Hofmeyr GJ. Amnioinfusion for preterm rupture of membranes (Cochrane Review). In: The Cochrane Library, issue 2. Oxford: Update Software, 2001.
32. Crowther CA, Henderson-Smart DJ. Vitamin K prior to preterm birth for preventing neonatal periventricular haemorrhage (Cochrane Review). In: The Cochrane Library, issue 2. Oxford: Update Software, 2001.
33. Crowther CA, Henderson-Smart DJ. Phenobarbital prior to preterm birth for preventing neonatal periventricular haemorrhage (Cochrane Review). In: The Cochrane Library, issue 2. Oxford: Update Software, 2001.
34. Hodnett ED. Support during pregnancy for women at increased risk of low birthweight babies (Cochrane Review). In: The Cochrane Library, issue 2. Oxford: Update Software, 2001.
35. Hypertensive disorders in pregnancy. In: Cunningham FG, MacDonald PC, Gant NF, Leveno KJ, Gilstrap LC, eds. Williams' obstetrics, 19th ed. East Norwalk, CT: Appleton and Lange, 1993;764–9,783–90.
36. O'Hara Padden M. HELLP syndrome: recognition and perinatal management. Am Fam Physician 1999;60:829–36.
37. Duley L. Which anticonvulsant for women with eclampsia? Evidence from the Collaborative Eclampsia Trial. Lancet 1995; 345:1455–63. Available at *www.jr2.ox.ac.uk/bandolier/band17/b17-5.html*.
38. Hunt CM, Sharara AI. Liver disease in pregnancy. Am Fam Physician 1999;59:829–36.
39. Duley L, Henderson-Smart D. Reduced salt intake compared to normal dietary salt, or high intake, in pregnancy (Cochrane Review). In: The Cochrane Library, issue 2. Oxford: Update Software, 2001.
40. Atallah AN, Hofmeyr GJ, Duley L. Calcium supplementation during pregnancy for preventing hypertensive disorders and related problems (Cochrane Review). In: The Cochrane Library, issue 2. Oxford: Update Software, 2001.
41. Bucher HC, et al. Calcium supplementation and hypertension of pregnancy. Am Fam Physician 1996;54:1061–2.
42. Knight M, Duley L, Henderson-Smart DJ, King JF. Antiplatelet agents for preventing and treating pre-eclampsia (Cochrane Review). In: The Cochrane Library, issue 2. Oxford: Update Software, 2001.
43. Duley L, Henderson-Smart D. Magnesium sulphate versus diazepam for eclampsia (Cochrane Review). In: The Cochrane Library, issue 2. Oxford: Update Software, 2001.
44. Duley L, Henderson-Smart D. Magnesium sulphate versus phenytoin for eclampsia (Cochrane Review). In: The Cochrane Library, issue 2. Oxford: Update Software, 2001.
45. Duley L, Gulmezoglu AM. Magnesium sulphate versus lytic cocktail for eclampsia (Cochrane Review). In: The Cochrane Library, issue 2. Oxford: Update Software, 2001.

46. Duley L, Gulmezoglu AM, Henderson-Smart DJ. Anticonvulsants for women with pre-eclampsia (Cochrane Review). In: The Cochrane Library, issue 2. Oxford: Update Software, 2001.

47. Duley L, Williams J, Henderson-Smart DJ. Plasma volume expansion for treatment of women with pre-eclampsia (Cochrane Review). In: The Cochrane Library, issue 2. Oxford: Update Software, 2001.

48. Duley L, Henderson-Smart DJ. Drugs for rapid treatment of very high blood pressure during pregnancy (Cochrane Review). In: The Cochrane Library, issue 2. Oxford: Update Software, 2001.

49. Abalos E, Duley L, Steyn DW, Henderson-Smart DJ. Antihypertensive drug therapy for mild to moderate hypertension during pregnancy (Cochrane Review). In: The Cochrane Library, issue 2. Oxford: Update Software, 2001.

50. Magee LA, Duley L. Oral beta-blockers for mild to moderate hypertension during pregnancy (Cochrane Review). In: The Cochrane Library, issue 2. Oxford: Update Software, 2001.

51. Preboth M. ACOG guidelines on antepartum fetal surveillance. Am Fam Physician 2000;62:1184–8.

14
Problems During Labor and Delivery

Stephen Ratcliffe and Kent Petrie

This chapter provides an overview of common problems faced by the family physician during labor and delivery. The anticipation, early recognition, and prevention of problems are emphasized as well as management strategies. Except when otherwise specified, level-one evidence as represented by a randomized controlled trial (RCT), systematic reviews, or meta-analyses of RCTs will be used to support the recommendations.

Dystocia or difficult labor accounts for more than 50% of cesarean sections (CSs) performed on nulliparous women. After a slow decline of the CS rate in the United States during the 1990s, there was a 4% increase in the rate from 22.0% in 1999 to 22.9% in 2000.[1] The American College of Obstetrics and Gynecology's (ACOG) vaginal birth after previous cesarean section (VBAC) policy of October 1998 states that the ability to perform a CS during an attempted VBAC should be immediately available.[2] The CS rate has begun to increase during this decade because of this more restrictive approach to VABCs.[1] It is important that family physicians utilize a systematic, evidence-based approach to achieve the safest, lowest primary CS rate for their nulliparous patients.

Active Management of Labor

To recognize and treat dystocia, the practitioner should have an understanding of the concepts of the active management of labor (AML) model, which was developed at the National Maternity Hospital in Dublin, Ireland. This model has been used to keep CS rates at the 6% to 8% level over the past 30 years.[3] The AML model is *only* for the nulliparous patient and employs the following components:

- Childbirth education stresses how a diagnosis of labor is made, and that once this diagnosis is made the labor will not last more than 12 hours and women will receive continuous support in labor.

- A diagnosis of labor is made when there are regular, painful contractions and there is complete cervical effacement, rupture of membranes, or a bloody show.

- Upon admission, patients undergo an amniotomy, do not receive continuous fetal heart rate monitoring, receive continuous labor support from their midwife, and are encouraged to ambulate.

- Within 2 hours of labor diagnosis, patients receive oxytocin augmentation if they are not following a labor curve or partogram that documents a 1 cm per hour cervical dilation. The Irish model uses the high-dose oxytocin regimen that starts at 6 mU/minute dose with dosing increments of 6 mU every 20 minutes until a maximum dose of 40 mU/minute is reached.

- During stage two, oxytocin is initiated if failure to descend is noted. Pushing is delayed until the head is on the vaginal floor (approximately +2 station).

- All nulliparous labors are reviewed on a weekly basis to monitor adherence to the AML protocol.

Dystocia

Diagnosis

A diagnosis of dystocia is made for the *nulliparous* woman when, during the active phase of labor, there is a failure to make progressive cervical dilation and fetal head descent according to agreed-upon criteria. When the progress of labor is slower than that described by Friedman,[4] a cervical dilation rate of less than 1 cm per hour during the active phase of labor, this is known as a *protraction* disorder. When there has been no progress over a 2-hour period during the active phase, this is known as an *arrest of labor*. Protraction and arrest disorders may occur in either stage one or two of labor.

Factors Associated with Dystocia in Nulliparous Patients[5]

There is evidence based on cohort studies that if a nulliparous woman is admitted to the labor ward (less than 3-cm dilation) or if she receives regional anesthesia prior to 5-cm dilation, she is at increased risk of having dystocia and cesarean intervention.[5] Once in active labor, women are at an increased risk of dystocia and cesarean intervention if they do not receive continuous emotional support or if they receive continuous electronic fetal heart rate (FHR) monitoring. The use of regional (epidural) anesthesia is associated with a prolongation of stage one and two labor and an increase in operative vaginal deliveries but is not associated with an increased overall rate of cesarean section.

O'Driscoll et al[3] estimate that inadequate uterine contractions account for 85% of dystocia. In the Irish experience, true cephalopelvic disproportion (CPD) occurs in only one of every 250 nulliparous deliveries. In the United States, the diagnosis of CPD as the reason for dystocia is made 10 times more often. Amniotomy performed after 3-cm dilation, a routine component of AML, decreases the incidence of dystocia but is not, as a single intervention, associated with a decrease in cesarean intervention.[6] Ambulation in labor, as a single intervention, has no direct effect on the incidence of dystocia and CS intervention.[7]

Fetal factors associated with an increased risk of dystocia and cesarean intervention include fetal macrosomia, malpresentation, malposition (persistent occiput posterior), and fetal anomalies such as hydrocephalus.

The management of stage two in the United States appears to be markedly different from that used in the AML model. An RCT that replicated the AML model in the U.S. has had similar CS rates during stage one compared to the Irish outcomes, but had an eightfold increase in CS rates during stage two.[8]

Recognition and Management[5]

Clinicians should differentiate latent from active-phase labor in nulliparous patients. The diagnosis of dystocia occurs in the active phase when protracted or arrested labor occurs. Recognition of these labor disorders may be aided with the use of labor curves. Malpositions such as occiput posterior may be treated with a change in labor positions. Selected use of amniotomy can be used when the fetal head is engaged. Use of oxytocin augmentation is the mainstay of treatment for dystocia. Some clinicians use an intrauterine pressure catheter (IUPC) to document adequate strength of uterine contractions. Rouse et al[9] demonstrated in a prospective cohort study that delaying cesarean intervention for arrest of labor from 2 to 4 hours resulted in a marked decrease in CS rates (26% to 8%). This level-two evidence should be replicated in RCTs before a recommendation is made to manage arrest of labor in this fashion.

Dystocia that occurs in stage two can be treated by initiating an oxytocin infusion, doing a manual rotation of a persistent occiput posterior position, changing maternal pushing positions, allowing the fetal head to "rest and descend" to a +2 to +3 position prior to pushing, and selectively using vaginally assisted deliveries when the fetal station is +2 or lower.

Chorioamnionitis[10]

Chorioamnionitis is an infection of the amniotic membrane and space. It is commonly associated with preterm labor in that up to 13% of women who labor prematurely have positive amniotic fluid cultures. The incidence of this condition in the term pregnancy is between 0.5% and 2%. The major risk factors for chorioamnionitis include multiple vaginal exams (eight exams compared to zero to two exams, odds ratio = 5.1) and labor lasting more than 12 hours compared to <3 hours (odds ratio = 4.1).

Pathophysiology

Chorioamnionitis usually is polymicrobial in nature including aerobic and anaerobic bacteria from the intestinal tract. Other infectious agents such *Mycoplasma hominis, Ureaplasma urealyticum*, and *Chlamydia* have also been implicated. Chorioamnionitis increases the risk of postpartum endometritis and may result in significant maternal and neonatal morbidity and mortality.

Diagnosis

The classic signs and symptoms of chorioamnionitis include maternal fever; uterine tenderness; fetal tachycardia; foul-smelling lochia; and maternal chills, fever, and rigor. These signs and symptoms may be absent in the woman having preterm labor. Lieberman et al[11] have demonstrated that women who have epidural anesthesia have an increased risk of low-grade intrapartum temperatures that are often mistaken for chorioamnionitis. A leukocytosis with a left shift is a sensitive marker of infection but may miss some infections.

Management

The treatment of preterm premature rupture of the membranes (PPROM) with antibiotics is associated with a prolongation in time from rupture of membranes to delivery, a decrease in the incidence of neonatal sepsis, respiratory distress syndrome, and prolonged mechanical ventilation.[12] The treatment of PPROM with antibiotics is not associated with an improvement in neonatal mortality. There is recent evidence that the use of amoxicillin/sulbactam should be avoided because of an increased incidence of neonatal necrotizing enterocolitis.[13] Antibiotics commonly used to treat PPROM include ampicillin and erythromycin.

Broad-spectrum antibiotics such as ampicillin, 2 g every 6 hours, and gentamicin, 120 to 140 mg loading dose followed by 1 to 1.5 mg/kg intravenously every 8 hours, are used to treat chorioamnionitis in the term pregnancy. This coverage is usually sufficient despite the presence of anaerobic bacteria in up to 50% of infections. Clindamycin, 500 to 750 mg every 6 hours, can be added if anaerobic coverage is used. There is preliminary evidence that the addition of clindamycin may be useful to lower the incidence of postpartum endometritis if the patient with chorioamnionitis needs to undergo cesarean intervention.[14]

Prevention

Locksmith et al,[15] in a large cohort analysis, demonstrated that the treatment of group B streptococcus (GBS) carriers with intrapartum antibiotics compared to treatment of women with GBS risk factors resulted in a decrease in the incidence of chorioamnionitis (relative risk 0.7, confidence interval 0.6–0.8). In this study, the screening of 23 women for GBS at 35 to 37 weeks' gestation resulted in four women receiving antibiotics in labor and preventing one case of chorioamnionitis.

Shoulder Dystocia

Although shoulder dystocia is an uncommon obstetric emergency (occurring in 0.15% to 0.60% of all deliveries), all practitioners should be prepared to manage this potentially devastating delivery complication. Shoulder dystocia is defined as impaction of the anterior shoulder against the symphysis pubis after the fetal head has delivered. The incidence increases with fetal weight, but prediction of macrosomia is of limited assistance for avoiding shoulder dystocia, as more that 50% of cases occur with fetuses weighing less than 4000 g.[16] Antepartum risk factors include maternal diabetes, maternal obesity and excessive weight gain, narrow anteroposterior (AP) diameter on clinical pelvimetry, and a history of previous shoulder dystocia. This complication frequently occurs in low-risk patients.[17]

Diagnosis

The physician should also be aware of intrapartum risk factors. A prolonged active phase of the first stage of labor, a prolonged second stage, head bobbing during the second stage, and the need for assisted delivery by vacuum or forceps may be clues to potential shoulder dystocia. If upon delivery the fetal head immediately retracts onto the perineum and the anterior shoulder does not deliver with modest downward traction, shoulder dystocia is diagnosed.

Management

Response to this obstetric emergency must be expeditious and deliberate. It is helpful to prepare in advance and develop and practice an institutional protocol. The protocol should include notification of extra personnel, recording the timing and sequence of maneuvers used to resolve the dystocia, and preparation for newborn resuscitation. Carlan et al[18] developed a logical order of maneuvers (the HELPER-R mnemonic, Table 14.1), which has been widely taught and has proved useful for emergency management of shoulder dystocia. Permanent injury to the fetus is rare but can occur even in the well-managed case. The newborn should be carefully examined for brachial plexus injuries and fractures of the clavicle and humerus. Thorough documentation and communication with the patient and her support person are important.

Intrapartum Fetal Surveillance

The fetus is generally well adapted to extract oxygen from the maternal circulation during normal labor and delivery. Complications may subject the fetus to decreased oxygenation, however, leading to potential damage to organ systems and even fetal death. Oxygen delivery is dependent on uterine blood flow and can be affected by uterine hyperstimulation, maternal position, and conduction anesthesia. Complications such as preeclampsia, abruptio placentae, placenta previa, and chorioamnionitis can further alter blood flow and oxygen exchange within the placenta. The umbilical cord is vulnerable to prolapsed or compression during labor, further disrupting oxygen delivery to the fetus. Any of these complications can be more serious in premature or growth-retarded fetuses, which are more susceptible to the effects of hypoxia and acidosis. It is the goal of intrapartum fetal surveillance techniques to detect fetal hypoxia and

---

Table 14.1. **HELPER-R: A Stepwise Approach to Shoulder Dystocia Management**

Help: Call for assistance for delivery, anesthesia, and newborn resuscitation

Episiotomy: Although shoulder dystocia is not a soft tissue obstruction, episiotomy may facilitate access to the baby's shoulders and posterior arm if internal rotation maneuvers are necessary

Legs: Flexion and abduction of the maternal hips (McRoberts maneuver) is highly effective for relieving dystocia

Pressure: Assistant applies external suprapubic pressure with a closed fist while downwards traction is applied to the fetal head; avoid fundal pressure, which further drives the anterior shoulder into the pubic symphysis

Enter vagina: Rotating the shoulder to an oblique position with relation to the maternal pelvis may relieve obstruction; it may be accomplished by two finger pressure over the posterior aspect of the anterior shoulder (Rubin maneuver) or pressure over the anterior aspect of the posterior shoulder (Woods screw maneuver)

Roll: At any point the physician may elect to place the patient on all-fours; this position facilitates spontaneous rotation, improves maternal expulsive forces, and allows easy access to the posterior arm if necessary[35]

Remove the posterior arm: pass a hand into the vagina under the posterior shoulder and follow the arm to the elbow; flex the forearm and sweep the arm over the chest to deliver the posterior arm and shoulder first, allowing the anterior shoulder to slide under the symphysis

Source: Modified with permission from Carlan et al,[18] American Family Physician. Copyright © American Academy of Family Physician. All Rights Reserved.

acidosis or their combination (asphyxia) to allow timely intervention.[19]

Surveillance Methods

Fetal Heart Rate Monitoring

The fetal central nervous system (CNS) is susceptible to hypoxia. Because the fetal heart rate (FHR) is under CNS control thorough sympathetic and parasympathetic reflexes, FHR pattern changes can indicate decreased CNS oxygenation or reflex responses. Normally the baseline FHR can range from 120 to 160 beats per minute (bpm). Tachycardia (>160 bpm) or bradycardia (<120 bpm) can indicate CNS hypoxia. A more important baseline pattern, however, is the variability of the FHR, which represents the difference in rate from beat to beat. Normal FHR variability (>6 bpm) implies that the CNS is adequately oxygenated at the time of observation. Periodic FHR changes fall into well-defined patterns. Accelerations of FHR with contractions or fetal movements are normal findings in well-oxygenated fetuses. Variable decelerations (abrupt in onset and cessation and variable in duration, depth, and shape) are caused by umbilical cord compression and may indicate fetal compromise if severe or persistent. Early decelerations (mirroring the contraction) are due to a vagal reflex response to head pressure and are usually benign. Late decelerations (smooth decelerations with onset and nadir delayed 10 to 30 seconds after the onset and apex of the contraction) are secondary to transient fetal hypoxia in response to decreased placental perfusion during contractions.

These FHR patterns can be evaluated by auscultation (DeLee stethoscope or Doppler sonography) or by electronic monitoring (external or internal). With the advent of liberal use of continuous electronic FHR monitoring (EFM) during the 1970s, there was great hope that intrapartum asphyxia could be virtually eliminated. Large retrospective studies using historical controls were encouraging. It was simply assumed that continuous EFM would be more effective than intermittent auscultation in detecting the compromised fetus. Numerous RCTs, however, have not confirmed the original hope for the improved newborn outcomes. RCTs of continuous EFM compared to intermittent auscultation have shown no decrease in perinatal morbidity and mortality, no improvement in Apgar scores, no improvement in immediate neurologic outcomes, and no reduction in cerebral palsy. The incidence of neonatal seizures is decreased when continuous EFM is used with fetal scalp sampling versus intermittent monitoring, but only in pregnancies complicated by postdates, prolonged rupture of membranes, or use of oxytocin.[20] The use of continuous EFM is associated with an increased frequency of the diagnosis of fetal distress and increased rates of instrumental delivery and cesarean section.

These studies prompted ACOG to recommend intermittent auscultation as a reasonable alternative to EFM, monitoring the FHR for 1 minute after contractions every 30 minutes during the first stage of labor and every 15 minutes during the second stage in low-risk patients. High-risk patients may be monitored every 15 minutes during the first stage and every 5 minutes during the second stage.[19] Many institutions still advocate the use of an EFM admission test strip for 20 minutes on admission to labor and delivery or prior to being sent home after a labor check.[21]

The current classification scheme for FHR patterns divides patterns into two categories: reassuring and nonreassuring (Table 14.2). Fetal distress—progressive hypoxia and acidosis—is fortunately rare, the diagnosis of which cannot be made by the FHR tracing alone. The use of this term should be abandoned. It is far more clinically relevant to describe FHR patterns and their severity and outline management plans accordingly.[22]

Fetal Scalp pH Monitoring

Fetal scalp sampling to determine the presence of fetal acidosis has been shown to lower the false-positive rate of continuous EFM, thereby lowering the rate of both forceps and cesarean deliveries.[20] A fetal scalp pH of 7.25 or above is reassuring; an intermediate result of 7.20 to 7.24 should be repeated; pH less than 7.20 warrants expeditious delivery. As a clinical alternative to scalp pH testing, numerous studies have demonstrated a correlation between spontaneous or inducible FHR accelerations with nonacidotic fetuses. Accelerations may be induced by scalp stimulation[23] or vibroacoustic stimulation with an artificial larynx.[24]

Fetal Pulse Oximetry

Hardware and software are currently available to monitor continuous fetal pulse oximetry via a small prove placed on the fetal cheek or temple. In 2000, the Food and Drug Administration (FDA) approved the first commercial monitor. Though less invasive than scalp pH, sensor placement is difficult, with frequent hair, caput, and meconium interference. Membranes must be ruptured for placement. In a recent RCT, fetal pulse oximetry did not demonstrate a decrease in overall cesarean section rates in the presence of nonreassuring FHR tracings.[25] This technology must be demonstrated to be efficacious in multiple randomized controlled clinical trials before widespread use for fetal surveillance is recommended.

Management of Nonreassuring Fetal Surveillance: General Measures

When the physician encounters nonreassuring FHR patterns, general measures to improve fetal oxygenation and placental perfusion should be instituted. Maternal oxygen may be administered by mask. Uterine blood flow can be improved by moving the laboring patient to a lateral recumbent or knee-chest position. Oxytocin infusion can be discontinued to re-

Table 14.2. **Reassuring and Nonreassuring Fetal Heart Rate (FHR) Patterns[36]**

Reassuring pattern	Nonreassuring pattern
Baseline	
Normal rate	Bradycardia or tachycardia
Normal variability	Poor or absent variability
Periodic changes	
Accelerations	Early decelerations
	Late decelerations
	Variable decelerations
	Prolonged decelerations

duce the stress of uterine contractions. Maternal hypotension may resolve with intravenous fluids to restore intravascular volume or by administering ephedrine (2.5–10.0 mg IV) to restore vascular tone reduced by epidural block.

Tocolytic Administration

Uterine activity often contributes to nonreassuring FHR patterns or low scalp pH. Tocolytic treatment decreases or abolishes uterine activity, removing the ischemic effect of uterine contractions and improving the metabolic condition of the fetus prior to delivery. Tocolytics may be particularly important to buy time when unavoidable delays in effecting operative delivery are encountered. Randomized controlled trials have shown terbutaline (0.25 mg SC or 0.125–0.25 mg IV) to be more effective than magnesium sulfate (2–4 g IV over 20 minutes), with transient maternal tachycardia the only side effect.[26]

Amnioinfusion

Oligohydramnios may result in cord compression and compromise of fetal oxygenation, and it may be associated with nonreassuring FHR patterns, fetal acidosis, and fetal demise.

When recognized through recurrent variable decelerations or low amniotic fluid volume seen on ultrasonography or in association with thick meconium, oligohydramnios can be treated by amnioinfusion, infusing warmed saline through an intrauterine pressure catheter. A continuous infusion technique is effective, infusing a loading dose of 250 to 500 mL at 10 to 15 mL/min followed by a maintenance dose of 1 to 3 mL/min. RCTs of saline amnioinfusion have demonstrated reduced rates of cesarean delivery for fetal distress, improved Apgar scores, and improved neonatal outcomes in the setting of meconium-stained fluid.[27]

Delivery

If fetal surveillance again returns to reassuring patterns (resolution of abnormal FHR patterns, improved scalp pH) after the use of the general treatment measures, tocolytic administration, and/or amnioinfusion, labor may be allowed to continue under close observation while preparations are made for possible operative delivery. Clinical judgment must be applied in each case to determine the safest mode of delivery (vaginal or cesarean). A useful algorithm for surveillance of the laboring patient is shown in Figure 14.1.

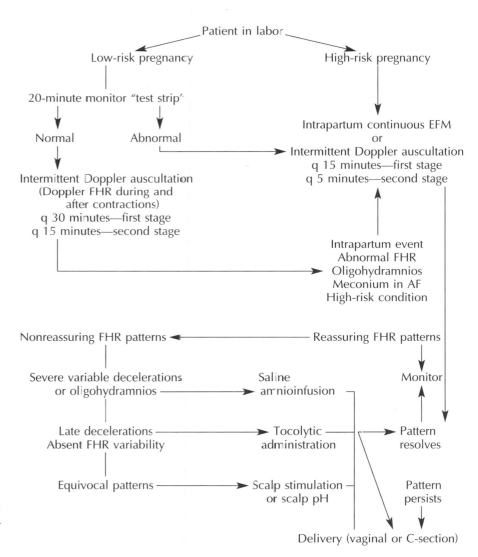

Fig. 14.1. Labor monitoring. EFM = electronic FHR monitoring; FHR = fetal heart rate, AF = amnionic fluid.

Bleeding Complications During Labor

The three most dangerous bleeding complications during labor are vasa previa, placental abruption and placenta previa. A heavy bloody show may be the only sign that alerts the physician to one of these obstetric emergencies.[28]

Vasa Previa

Bleeding from vasa previa is a rare but life-threatening fetal hemorrhage from the rupture of fetal vessels in a velamentous insertion of the cord (cord vessels run in fetal membranes and insert into the edge of the placenta, sometimes crossing the cervix).

Diagnosis

Rapid diagnosis is crucial because fetal mortality is greater than 50%. In most cases, fetal distress is evident on electronic fetal heart rate monitoring. If the FHR is reassuring, a modified Apt test can be performed on the vaginal pool blood to test for the presence of fetal hemoglobin.

Treatment

Treatment of vasa previa with evidence of fetal distress is immediate cesarean section with neonatal resuscitation available.

Placental Abruption

Placental abruption occurs when there is premature separation of the placenta prior to birth. It is thought to occur because of disease of the decidua and uterine blood vessels.[29] This theory is supported by the strong association between hypertension (both preexisting and pregnancy-induced) and placental abruption. Among women experiencing a placental abruption, about half have hypertension. Other associated risk factors for placental abruption include abdominal trauma, grand multiparity, uterine anomalies, nutritional (folate) deficiencies, short umbilical cord, cigarette smoking, cocaine use, a history of abruption, and advanced maternal age.

Abruptions are classified into one of three types: grade I, not accompanied by fetal distress (40%); grade II, presenting with moderate bleeding and often fetal distress (45%); and grade III, accompanied by severe bleeding that may lead to consumptive coagulopathy and often fetal death (15%).[30]

Diagnosis

Third-trimester bleeding occurs in 80% of placental abruptions and pain in about 50%. Uterine irritability is common with grade I abruptions, and with increasing severity (grades II and III) contractions may become tetanic. Port wine–stained amniotic fluid may be seen in cases where the hemorrhage dissects through the amniotic membranes with occult abruption. Ultrasonography often does not detect a clot underneath the placenta, and a normal scan should not delay treatment. Abruption remains a clinical diagnosis. There is much overlap of clinical signs and symptoms for the three grades of placental abruption, and a high index of suspicion is important.

Treatment

The maternal and fetal status must be carefully and continually assessed. Patients are often hemodynamically unstable and intravenous access (peripheral and central) is critical to correct hypotension. Blood products should be immediately available. With mild (grade I) abruption without fetal distress, half of the patients safely deliver vaginally. When a nonreassuring FHR tracing is present, an emergency cesarean is usually necessary, keeping in mind that disseminated intravascular coagulation (DIC) is uncommon in the presence of a viable fetus. This operative approach results in a lower perinatal mortality rate. In the presence of DIC, expeditious delivery of fetus and placenta should be accompanied by use of blood products and fresh frozen plasma. Cryoprecipitate is used sparingly because of its potential to carry blood-borne infections. Heparin has not been found to be of use for this form of DIC.

Placenta Previa

Placenta previa occurs when the mature placenta covers or is proximate to the internal cervical os. It is seen in 0.4% to 0.6% of all births. It is more common in multiparas and has a recurrence rate of 4% to 8%. There is a significant relation between placenta previa and a history of cesarean section, dilation and curettage, spontaneous abortion, and evacuation of retained products of conception.[31] This point supports the theory that a major reason for a blastocyst implantation situated low in the uterine segment is previous endometrial or myometrial disruption. Other predisposing factors associated with placenta previa include increased maternal age, multiple pregnancy, and abnormal fetal lie during the third trimester. There are three categories of placenta previa:

1. Total previa: the internal os is completely covered by the placenta.
2. Partial previa: the placenta covers only a portion of the internal os.
3. Marginal previa: the placenta is proximate to the os but is not covering it.

During the early second trimester, a placenta previa can be visualized via ultrasonography 5% to 8% of the time. If partial or marginal, it tends to resolve in 95% of cases with upward migration of the placenta and 10-fold lengthening of the lower uterine segment. Placenta previa is associated with increased perinatal morbidity and mortality, particularly when a woman presents with active bleeding secondary to a placenta previa during the second trimester.

Diagnosis

The diagnosis is usually established using ultrasonography, often when the woman is still asymptomatic. Ultrasound error rates in placental localization are 3% to 7%. Possible explanations for this error rate include placental migration, overdistention of the urinary bladder, low-lying myometrial contractions, uterine fibroids, and extraembryonic blood clots. More extensive use of the transvaginal ultrasound probe decreases this false-positive rate. The classic clinical presentation of a placenta previa is profuse, bright red, painless vaginal bleeding.

Treatment

Once diagnosed, management of this disorder is usually conservative: bed rest until 37 to 38 weeks' gestation so long as there is not enough bleeding to pose a threat to the mother and fetus. Women with a placenta previa are delivered by 36 weeks' gestation 50% of the time. The usual mode of delivery is cesarean section. Marginal and partial previa can sometimes be managed expectantly for a vaginal delivery if preparations are made for an immediate cesarean. The availability of blood products for transfusion is essential for safe management of this condition.

Postpartum Hemorrhage[32,33]

Every practitioner must know how to recognize and promptly manage a postpartum hemorrhage (PPH). The classic definition of a PPH occurs when there is maternal blood loss that exceeds 500 cc in the first 24 hours after birth. The incidence of this is approximately 5%. A severe PPH occurs when this loss exceeds 1000 cc and occurs in 1% to 2% of deliveries. PPH accounts for 25% of all causes of maternal mortality and in developed countries results in maternal mortality in 1 in 1000 deliveries. PPH also results in maternal morbidity such as anemia, increased need for transfusion, adverse effects on breastfeeding, and sequelae of hemorrhagic shock including acute tubular necrosis and pituitary infarct (Sheehan's syndrome). Antenatal risk factors for PPH, include preeclampsia, nulliparity, multiple gestation, previous PPH and previous C-section. Intrapartum risk factors include prolonged third stage, arrest of fetal descent, vaginal/perineal lacerations, use of episiotomy, assisted delivery, and augmented labor.[32]

Etiology

Approximately 70% of PPH is caused by uterine atony; 20% is due to cervical, vaginal, and perineal lacerations; and 10% is due to placental factors such as retained placental and abnormal uterine attachment (placenta accreta, encreta, and percreta). Underlying maternal coagulopathies play an important causative role in only 1% of PPHs.

Recognition/Management

Family physicians must maintain a low threshold to recognize and manage a PPH. They should be alerted to this possibility when managing many of the above antenatal and intrapartum conditions. Although uterine atony needs to remain the primary suspect when excessive maternal bleeding is noted, the delay in diagnosing a significant laceration may result in additional quantity of bleeding that could have been prevented. As soon as the clinician has noted excessive maternal bleeding, the ABCs of an emergency should be initiated. Extra help should be summoned. Oxygen may be administered. One or two large-bore intravenous lines should be started and a vigorous fluid resuscitation with normal saline or lactated Ringer's begun. The clinician should begin these maneuvers automatically while beginning a vigorous bimanual uterine massage. A concurrent search for a vaginal or perineal laceration should be done. If these maneuvers do not arrest the PPH, the following medications can be used to help treat uterine atony: oxytocin, 20 units (IM or IV); methylergonovine (Methergine), 0.2 mg (IM) and 15-methyl prostaglandin $F_{2\alpha}$ (Hemabate) 0.25 mg IM or intramyometrially. The reader is referred to an obstetrics text or the Advanced Life Support in Obstetrics (ALSO) manual for a more complete discussion of treatment strategies.[33]

Prevention

There is high-quality, category A evidence that the active management of stage three reduces the incidence of PPH. This consists of giving oxytocin (20 U in 1000 cc of lactated Ringer's solution at 200 cc/hour) at the time of the delivery of the anterior shoulder followed by early umbilical cord clamping and applying controlled cord traction. The active management of stage three compared to expectant management is associated with a reduction in moderate PPH (>500 cc blood loss; number needed to prevent one moderate PPH is 10) and severe PPH (>1000 cc blood loss; number needed to treat to prevent one severe PPH is 65).[34]

References

1. National Center for Health Statistics, Centers for Disease Control. Births: preliminary data for 2000, vol 29(5), (PHS, 2001) 1120.
2. ACOG Practice Bulletin. Vaginal birth after previous cesarean delivery. Number 2, October 1998. Clinical management guidelines for obstetrician-gynecologists. American College of Obstetricians and Gynecologists. Int J Gynaecol Obstet 1999; 64:201–8.
3. O'Driscoll K, Foley M, MacDonald D. Active management of labor as an alternative to cesarean section for dystocia. Obstet Gynecol 1984;63:485–90.
4. Friedman EA. Labor: Clinical evaluation and management, 2nd ed. New York: Appleton, Century, Crofts, 1978.
5. Cline M. Management of labor abnormalities. In: Ratcliffe S, Baxley E, Byrd J, Sakornbut E, eds. Family practice obstetrics. Philadelphia: Hanley and Belfus, 2001;415–22.
6. Fraser W, Marcoux S, Moutquin M, et al. Effect of early amniotomy on the risk of dystocia in the nulliparous women. N Engl J Med 1993;328:1145–9.
7. Bloom S, McIntire D, Kelly M, et al. Lack of effect of walking on the labor and delivery. N Engl J Med 1998;339:76–9.
8. Frigoletta F, Leiberman E, Long J, et al. A clinical trial of active management of labor. N Engl J Med 1994;333:745–50.
9. Rouse DJ, Owen J, Hauth JC. Active-phase labor arrest: oxytocin augmentation for at least 4 hours. Obstet Gynecol 1999; 93:323–8.
10. Ratcliffe S. Chorioamnionitis. In: Ratcliffe S, Baxley E, Bryd J, Sakornbut E, eds. Family practice obstetrics, 2nd ed. Philadelphia: Hanley and Belfus, 2001;448–53.
11. Lieberman E, Lang J, Frigoletta F, et al. Epidural analgesia, intrapartum fever, and neonatal sepsis evaluation. Pediatrics 1997;99:415–9.
12. Kenyon S, Boulvain M. Antibiotics for preterm premature rup-

ture of membranes (Cochrane Review). In: The Cochrane Library, issue 1. Oxford: Update Software, 2001.

13. Kenyon S, Taylor D, Tarnou-Mordi W. Broad spectrum antibiotics for spontaneous preterm labour: the ORACLE II randomized trial. Lancet 2001;357:989–94.

14. Turnquest M, How H, Cook C, et al. Chorioamnionitis: is continuation of antibiotic therapy necessary after cesarean section? Am J Obstet Gynecol 1998;179:1261–6.

15. Locksmith G, Clark P, Duff P. Maternal and neonatal infection rates with three different protocols for prevention of group B streptococcal disease. Am J Obstet Gynecol 1999;180:416–22.

16. Morrison JC, Sanders JR, Magann EF, et al. The diagnosis and management of dystocia of the shoulder. Surg Gynecol Obstet 1992;175:515–22.

17. Naef RW, Martin JN. Emergent management of shoulder dystocia. Obstet Gynecol Clin North Am 1995;22:247–59.

18. Carlan SJ, Angel JL, Knuppel RA. Shoulder dystocia. Am Fam Physician 1991;43:1307–11.

19. American College of Obstetricians and Gynecologists. Fetal heart rate patterns. Monitoring, interpretation, and management. ACOG technical bulletin no. 207, July 1995.

20. Thacker SB, Stroup DF. Continuous electronic fetal heart monitoring during labor (Cochrane Review). In: The Cochrane Library, issue 1. Oxford: Update Software, 2001.

21. Ingemarsson A. Admission test: a screening test for fetal distress in labor. Obstet Gynecol 1986;68:800–6.

22. Sweha A, Hacker TW, Nuovo J. Interpretation of the electronic fetal heart rate during labor. Am Fam Physician 1999;59:2487–500.

23. Clark SL, Gimouksy ML, Miller FC. The scalp stimulation test: a clinical alternative to fetal scalp blood testing. Am J Obstet Gynecol 1984;224:148–52.

24. Smith CV, Nguyen HN, Phelan JP. Intrapartum assessment of fetal wellbeing: a comparison of fetal acoustic stimulation with acid-base determinations. Am J Obstet Gynecol 1986;155:726–32.

25. Garite TJ, Dildy GA, McNamara YH, et al. A multicenter controlled trial of fetal pulse oximetry in the intrapartum management of non-reassuring fetal heart rate patterns. Am J Obstet Gynecol 2000;183:1049–58.

26. Kulier R, Hofmeyr GJ. Tocolysis for suspected intrapartum fetal distress (Cochrane Review). In: The Cochrane Library, issue 1. Oxford: Update Software, 2001.

27. Hofmeyer GJ. Amnioinfusion prophylactically versus therapeutically for Intrapartum oligohydramnios (Cochrane Review). In: The Cochrane Library, issue 1. Oxford: Update Software, 2001.

28. Byrd J. Intrapartum bleeding. In: Ratcliffe SD, Baxley EG, Byrd JE, Sakornbut EL, eds. Family practice obstetrics, 2nd ed. Philadelphia: Hanley and Belfus, 2001;453–7.

29. Lowe TW, Cunningham FG. Placenta abruption. Clin Obstet Gynecol 1990;33:406–13.

30. Ananth CV, Berkowitz GS, Savitz DA, et al. Placenta abruption and adverse perinatal outcomes. JAMA 1999;282:1646–51.

31. Miller DA, Chollet JA, Goodwin TM. Clinical risk factors for placenta previa–placenta accreta. Am J Obstet Gynecol 1997;177:210–4.

32. Combs C, Murphy E, Laros F. Factors associated with postpartum hemorrhage with vaginal birth. Obstet Gynecol 1991;77:69–74.

33. Anderson J, Etches D, Smith D. Postpartum hemorrhage: third stage emergency. Advanced life support in obstetrics manual, 4th ed. Kansas City: American Academy of Family Physicians 2001.

34. McDonald S, Elbourne D, Prendiville WJ. Active versus expectant management in the third stage of labour (Cochrane Review). In: The Cochrane Library, issue 1. Oxford: Update Software, 2001.

35. Meenan AL, Gaskin IM, Hunt P, et al. A new (old) maneuver for the management of shoulder dystocia. J Fam Pract 1991;32:625–9.

36. Parer JT. Handbook of fetal heart rate monitoring. Philadelphia: WB Saunders, 1997.

15
Postpartum Care

Dwenda K. Gjerdingen

The months following childbirth are characterized by physical, mental, and social changes that affect mothers and other family members. These changes may result from the childbirth event, the stresses and demands of caring for an infant, increased exposure to infectious illnesses, and the family's adaptation to a new member. To support individuals through this transition, it is important that health care providers give effective routine care, recognize and manage early and delayed postpartum problems as they occur, and provide education to families that optimizes their health during this time.

Early Postpartum Period

Routine Care

The early postpartum period is generally characterized by minor to moderate discomforts often related to changes in the breasts and genital organs or to episiotomy or cesarean section wounds (Table 15.1).[1–14] Serious complications may arise, however, and to recognize such problems early all new mothers should be carefully observed within the first few hours after delivery by monitoring their temperature, blood pressure, pulse, uterine fundus, and vaginal flow. Unless contraindicated, oxytocic agents are used routinely during the immediate postpartum period to reduce the risk of postpartum hemorrhage.

Several measures may help to alleviate early postpartum discomfort. Nonsteroidal antiinflammatory drugs (e.g., ibuprofen) or narcotics ease pain due to uterine cramps or surgical wounds. Perineal pain often responds to such local measures as ice packs, witch hazel, tub baths, or topical anesthesia. Painful hemorrhoids are also relieved by these measures, as well as by stool softeners, topical steroids, dietary fiber, fluids, and increased activity. Severe hemorrhoids that do not improve over time may require surgical excision.

For women who choose to breast-feed, instruction is offered regarding feeding techniques and breast care, which includes gently cleansing and drying the areola and nipple after each feeding. Subsequent engorgement may be treated by warm compresses prior to nursing and a frequent feeding schedule. Focal areas of engorgement, thought to be secondary to plugged ducts, often respond to massaging the affected area while nursing. Sore, cracked nipples are managed by careful cleansing and air-drying after feeding, using moisturizing creams, and scheduling shorter, more frequent periods of nursing. Factors that may help to promote breast-feeding in the early postpartum period include breast-feeding on demand, rooming in during the postpartum hospital stay, and avoiding formula, pacifiers, and test-weighing after breast-feeding.[13] Beyond the early postpartum period, the duration of breast-feeding appears to be greater for mothers who do not return to full-time work.[14] Women who choose not to breast-feed may suffer breast engorgement and pain for the first few weeks after delivery. These symptoms can be somewhat relieved by local applications of cold, fluid restriction, and a supportive brassiere, but drugs are not routinely recommended to prevent lactation. Although modest bone loss during lactation has been observed, no long-term adverse bony effects have been noted for breast-feeding mothers, regardless of calcium intake.[15]

Prescription of drugs to nursing mothers requires careful consideration of their effect on the newborn. Drugs contraindicated during breast-feeding include tetracycline, chloramphenicol, antineoplastic agents, iodine-containing substances, ergot alkaloids (bromocriptine, ergotamine), gold, combination oral contraceptives (because they may decrease milk supply), cyclophosphamide, cyclosporine, doxorubicin, lithium, methotrexate, phenindione, drugs of abuse, and radiopharmaceuticals. Other drugs that should be used with caution include sulfonamides, metronidazole, salicylates, antihistamines, psychotropic agents, phenobarbital, ethanol,

Table 15.1. **Early Postpartum Problems**

Problem	Frequency
Discomfort from sutures	Most women with surgical wounds
Back pain	>67%[1]
The "blues"	50–80%[2]
Breast engorgement and pain	41% of breast-feeding women[3]
Nipple soreness	38% of breast-feeding women[3]
Bacteriuria	25–34% after cesarean section[4]
Endometritis	2.6% after cesarean section; 0.17% after vaginal delivery[5]
Postcesarean wound infection	4%[5]
Carpal tunnel syndrome	3%[6]
Urinary retention	2–18%[7]
Postpartum hemorrhage	1.5–20%[8]
Urinary tract infection	1–7% of cesarean sections[9]
Preeclampsia/eclampsia	5%[10]
Episiotomy infection	0.5–0.6%[11]
Thromboembolism	0.007%[12]
Anemia	a
Hemorrhoids	a
Constipation	a

"Early postpartum" here refers to the period within a few days after delivery.
[a]Exact frequencies during the early postpartum period are not readily available.

nicotine, and large amounts of caffeine. Women who desire contraception while nursing can choose between barrier and progesterone-only hormonal contraceptives (e.g., progestin minipill or medroxyprogesterone injection).

Postpartum urinary retention—seen most commonly among women who have had a cesarean section, epidural anesthesia, or their first vaginal delivery—has been defined as the absence of spontaneous micturition within 6 hours of delivery or, in patients who have been catheterized, within 6 hours after the catheter has been removed.[7] When urinary retention is diagnosed, treatment may begin with conservative measures, such as administering oral analgesics, ambulating, or taking a warm bath. If these measures are unsuccessful, the patient should be intermittently catheterized every few hours until she is able to void. Indwelling catheters are avoided because of the associated risk of urinary tract infections. Urinary incontinence is also a problem for some women after they deliver, especially if the delivery was associated with perineal trauma.

Women with D-negative blood who have not been sensitized to the D antigen, and who have delivered D-positive infants, should receive RhD (Rhesus factor) immune globulin 300 μg IM within 72 hours of delivery to prevent hemolytic disease in future pregnancies. Many hospitals have routine protocols for screening mothers' and infants' blood and for administering immune globulin when indicated so that this important procedure is not overlooked.

Women who have had cesarean sections require additional postoperative observation and care. They are at increased risk for several problems, including endometritis, parametritis, peritonitis, superficial wound infection, urinary tract infec-

tions, sepsis, pneumonia, paralytic ileus, hemorrhage, pulmonary embolus, and deep venous thrombosis. Measures commonly used to prevent thromboembolic and hemorrhagic complications include early ambulation and postoperative use of oxytocic agents. Women undergoing cesarean section who are at risk for endomyometritis (i.e., those who have been in labor or have had ruptured membranes for at least 6 hours) may benefit from single-dose prophylactic antibiotics, such as ampicillin/sulbactam, cefazolin, or cefotetan, administered IV after the cord has been clamped.[16]

Problems such as postpartum hemorrhage and infection are major causes of morbidity and mortality, regardless of whether the delivery was by cesarean section or done vaginally. These complications, therefore, demand immediate recognition and attention.

Postpartum Hemorrhage

Conventionally, postpartum hemorrhage has been defined as a blood loss of more than 500 mL following the birth of a baby.[8] Because estimates of postpartum blood loss vary considerably, there is a wide range in the reported prevalence of postpartum hemorrhage, from 1.5% to 20.0%.[8]

Hemorrhage may occur in the form of a sudden massive gush or a steady flow, either of which can produce severe hypovolemia. Vital signs may not change until large volumes of blood have been lost. Hence it is important to initiate intravenous fluid therapy early during the course of bleeding, and blood replacement with packed red blood cells and fresh frozen plasma should be considered if the hemorrhage continues.

Critical to the management of postpartum hemorrhage is early determination of the source of bleeding. Uterine atony, the most common cause of postpartum hemorrhage, should be suspected with the clinical finding of a large, boggy uterus. It is usually effectively managed with uterine massage and drugs that promote uterine contraction, such as oxytocin (Pitocin), 10 to 40 units IV in 1000 mL lactated Ringer's solution, or 10 units IM; methylergonovine maleate (Methergine), 0.2 mg IM q2–4h, and prostaglandin $F_{2\alpha}$ ($PGF_{2\alpha}$; Hemabate), 0.25 mg IM q15–60 min. Less commonly, postpartum hemorrhage may result from vaginal or cervical lacerations or a ruptured or inverted uterus. Therefore, when bleeding continues without known cause, the uterus, cervix, and vagina should be carefully examined. Rarely, bleeding may result from a coagulopathy, which when suspected should be confirmed by laboratory tests such as the prothrombin time, partial thromboplastin time, platelet count, fibrinogen level, fibrin split products assay, and clot retraction test.

When postpartum hemorrhage fails to respond to conservative measures or minor surgical repair, transcatheter embolization of the internal iliac artery may be attempted. This procedure is believed by many to be superior to arterial ligation or hysterectomy because of its higher success and lower complication rates, avoidance of surgical risks, fertility preservation, and shorter hospitalizations.[17,18] If bleeding continues unabated, internal iliac artery ligation or abdominal hysterectomy should be considered.

Occasionally, abnormal bleeding occurs after the first postpartum day. Late postpartum hemorrhage may be due to abnormal involution of the placental site, endometritis, or retained placental fragments, the latter of which can be detected by ultrasonography. Initial treatment consists of intravenous fluids and pharmacologic therapy with oxytocin, methylergonovine, or prostaglandins, plus antibiotics. Curettage is not used routinely because of its tendency to disrupt the placental site and provoke further bleeding; rather, it is used only if retained placental fragments are identified or if the bleeding does not respond to more conservative therapy. Patients who have had any degree of hemorrhage resulting in anemia are placed on oral iron therapy after their condition has stabilized.

Recognizing the life-threatening complications that sometimes result from massive postpartum hemorrhage—adult respiratory distress syndrome, disseminated intravascular coagulation, empty-sella syndrome, and eventual death—it is imperative that postpartum hemorrhage be quickly recognized and efficiently managed.

Postpartum Fever/Infection

Any patient with a fever over 100.4°F during the first 24 hours postpartum should be completely evaluated to rule out such potentially life-threatening causes as early streptococcal infection, transfusion reaction, or thyroid crisis. Other sources of fever that may present within the first 2 to 3 days after delivery include atelectasis, urinary tract infection, and pneumonia. Infections of the breasts, surgical wounds, and gynecologic organs and tissues are usually seen after the third postpartum day. Women who have had cesarean sections are at greatest risk for endometrial, surgical wound, urinary tract, and respiratory infections. The diagnosis and treatment of the more common postpartum genitourinary infections are shown in Table 15.2. (also see Chapter 95).

Subsequent Postpartum Health

After their discharge from the hospital, new mothers often continue to deal with a variety of physical and mental concerns. Problems that arise from childbirth, along with others that result from the demands of caring for an infant, may persist for some time. Symptoms that occur at increased frequency during the first few weeks after delivery include breast and vaginal/perineal discomfort, constipation and hemorrhoids, decreased appetite, hot flashes and sweating, acne, dizziness, hand numbness, emotional tension, fatigue, and depression.[21-23] Several of these problems (breast and vaginal symptoms, constipation and hemorrhoids, fatigue, dizziness, and depression) may continue for several months, and are often joined by other later-appearing problems, such as respiratory infections, hair loss, and thyroiditis.[21,24] The evaluation and management of several delayed postpartum problems are shown in Table 15.3.[25-28]

Return to Work

Most women who have babies now return to, or enter, the work force after childbirth, and the postpartum well-being of these women is linked to several work-related variables. There is early evidence that the mother's mental health is related to longer maternity leaves and shorter postleave working hours.[29] In addition, a woman's return to work is often accompanied by her infant's placement in day care, which exposes the infant, mother, and other family members to a variety of infectious diseases. Finally, many women decrease or discontinue breast-feeding with their return to work, a change that may result in breast symptoms for the mother and diminished immunologic protection for the baby.

Mothers might preserve their sense of well-being during this time by arranging for adequate time off work after delivery and limiting work hours initially. Parents should be encouraged to discuss maternity/parental leave arrangements openly with their employers during pregnancy, and this discussion should include such issues as job guarantees, anticipated duration of leave, salary and health insurance coverage during leave, number of work hours, opportunity to breast-feed during the workday, child care benefits, and ability to care for a sick infant.

Fathers' and Siblings' Postpartum Well-Being

Although most of the literature on postpartum disorders focuses on symptoms experienced by mothers, fathers and other family members may also wrestle with "postpartum" disturbances. For example, fathers may experience such problems as fatigue, irritability, headaches, depression, difficulty concentrating, insomnia, nervousness, restlessness, insufficient sleep, sexual problems, worries about the future, and coping with visitors.[30,31] Siblings may show behavioral changes in response to the addition of a new baby to the family (see Chapter 19). Commonly seen "negative" reactions are confrontations with the mother or infant and anxiety behaviors.[32] It is likely that these behaviors are at least partially a result of the loss of attention and sense of displacement that these children feel when the infant arrives; therefore, efforts should be made to provide regular, positive interactions between parents and the other children. Recognizing that fathers and siblings may experience their own set of postdelivery problems, it is important that they not be forgotten at this time. These individuals could be monitored either directly (e.g., by having them present at the postpartum visit) or indirectly, by asking the mother about the well-being of other family members. Concerns thus identified could be addressed by follow-up visits.

Marital Well-Being

For many couples the birth of a child, particularly the first child, is followed by feelings of marital dissatisfaction. For some couples this dissatisfaction is severe enough to constitute a crisis, whereas for others only slight difficulties are noted. On average, the decline in marital satisfaction persists until the child reaches school age, after which time it improves.[33] Specific marital changes observed during the post-

Table 15.2. **Diagnosis and Treatment of Postpartum Infections**

Type of infection	Clinical presentation	Diagnostic studies	Treatment
Endometritis	Fever, plus one or more of the following: uterine tenderness, foul smelling lochia, and leukocytosis of >12,000 after exclusion of other sources of infection, which develop within the first 5 days after delivery[5]	White blood count (WBC) or complete blood count (CBC), blood cultures, endometrial cultures; isolates: aerobic streptococci, anaerobic gram-positive cocci, aerobic and anaerobic gram-negative bacilli[7]	Clindamycin + gentamicin; if no improvement within 48 hours, add ampicillin or vancomycin (if penicillin allergic), continue until afebrile for 48 hours and clinically improved, then discontinue;[19] may also use later generation extended cephalosporins[11]; intravenous therapy alone is adequate and need not be followed by oral therapy[11]
Cesarean or episiotomy wound infection	Symptoms of infection: inflammation, discharge, wound dehiscence, sometimes fever	WBC or CBC and wound cultures; most common isolate is penicillin-resistant *Staphylococcus aureus*; other possible organisms: *S. epidermidis*, enterococci, group A or B streptococci, *Escherichia coli, Klebsiella* sp., *Clostridium perfringens*[4]	Early infections, occurring within 24–48 hours, are often caused by β-hemolytic streptococci and respond to parenteral penicillin; later infections are opened, drained, and treated with broad-spectrum antibiotics; infections with *C. perfringens* require surgical debridement and broad-spectrum antibiotics (e.g., clindamycin + ampicillin + gentamicin)
Urinary tract infection	Dysuria, urinary frequency, hematuria, fever	Urinalysis and urine culture; severe infections: also CBC and blood cultures; isolates: *E. coli*, enterococci, *Proteus* species, *Klebsiella, S. epidermidis, Pseudomonas, Enterobacter*, group B streptococci, *S. aureus*[4]	Antibiotics: amoxicillin, trimethoprim/sulfamethoxazole, cephalexin or cefazolin, or nitrofurantoin
Mastitis	Fever, chills, tachycardia, malaise, breast erythema (whole or part)	Culture milk of affected breast, US may help identify an abscess	Warm compresses, rest, frequent nursing, antibiotics (dicloxacillin, first-generation cephalosporin, erythromycin, or vancomycin); for abscess: drain, discontinue nursing, give antibiotics
Septic pelvic thrombo-phlebitis	High fever, tachycardia, acute abdominal pain radiating to the flank, groin, or upper abdomen; abdominal examination may be normal, or a woody vessel may be palpated in the vagina or parametria	WBC, blood cultures, abdominopelvic CT or MRI	Intravenous antibiotics, using a protocol similar to that described for endometritis; heparin does not give additional benefit[20]
Necrotizing fasciitis	Sudden onset of severe pain, hypotension, tachypnea, tachycardia, hypo- or hyperthermia; incision site: red, gray, or black discoloration; ulcers, bullae, crepitus, sensory changes, discharge, edema	Frozen sections showing necrosis, PMN infiltration, fibrinous thrombi, angiitis, microorganisms, absence of muscular involvement	Affected tissue aggressively debrided; broad-spectrum antibiotics for aerobes and anaerobes[11]

US = ultrasonography; CT = computed tomography; MRI = magnetic resonance imaging; PMN = polymorphonuclear neutrophils.

Table 15.3. **Delayed Postpartum Problems**

Problem	Clinical manifestation/evaluation	Treatment
Anemia	Fatigue, decreased hemoglobin	If iron deficiency anemia, treat with oral iron (ferrous sulfate 325 mg, 1–2 tablets daily)
Carpal tunnel syndrome	Symptoms, including hand numbness, tingling or pain, usually occur during pregnancy; a few women first notice symptoms days to weeks after delivery, and these symptoms persist for an average of 6.5 months[25]; examination may show positive Tinel and Phalen signs and abnormal nerve condition	Most cases resolve with conservative measures, such as avoidance of provocative activities and use of diuretics, nonsteroidal antiinflammatory drugs, steroid injections, and night splints; surgery may be necessary if the patient has thenar atrophy or incapacitating symptoms of long duration
Constipation	Seen in nearly 20% of women at 1 month postpartum and may persist for months[21]	Dietary fiber and fluid, exercise, stool softeners
Depression	Occurs in 10–20% of postpartum women[26]; characterized by depressed mood, markedly diminished interest or pleasure in most activities, significant change in appetite or weight, insomnia or hypersomnia, psychomotor agitation or retardation, fatigue, feelings of worthlessness or inappropriate guilt, difficulty concentrating, and recurrent thoughts of death or suicide; organic causes of depression (e.g., anemia, thyroid disease, or medication side effects) should be investigated	Mild symptoms: observe and support; moderate to severe symptoms: antidepressant- and/or psychotherapy; when antidepressants are elected for non-breast-feeding women, selective serotonin reuptake inhibitors (SSRIs) are recommended as first-line agents; for breast-feeding women, the risks and benefits of antidepressant therapy should be weighed as the effects of antidepressant on the nursing infant are largely unknown[27]; some experts believe that amitriptyline, nortriptyline, desipramine, clomipramine, and sertraline are drugs of choice for breast-feeding women, as they have not been found in quantifiable amounts in nurslings, and no adverse infant events have been reported[23]
Fatigue	Observe for associated symptoms of pallor fever, mood disturbances, and exertional dyspnea to rule out anemia, infection, thyroid disorder, psychological disorders, cardiomyopathy	Treat associated disorders; allow adequate rest; obtain help with child care and household tasks
Hair loss	Peaks at 6 months postpartum, when it is noticed by approximately 20% of mothers[21]	Changes are usually self-limited; if they persist, thyroid evaluation is considered
Perineal discomfort	Discomfort resulting from an episiotomy, genital lacerations, or vaginal atrophy may persist weeks or months after delivery; prolonged pain is more common with mediolateral than midline episiotomy; dyspareunia related to vaginal atrophy, caused by decreased levels of estrogen, may be prolonged by breast-feeding	Discomfort caused by vaginal atrophy: estrogen creams. For nursing mothers: lubricating jellies (e.g., K-Y Jelly, Replens, Astroglide)
Thyroiditis	Postpartum thyroiditis presents in approximately 5% of women; hyperthyroid phase—at 1–3 months postpartum: associated with fatigue, palpitations, a small painless goiter, and low TSH; hypothyroid phase—between 3 and 6 months postpartum: associated with symptoms of depression, cognitive impairment, goiter, high TSH, and elevated microsomal antibodies[24]	Symptomatic hyperthyroidism: beta-blockers; hypothyroidism: levothyroxine (Levothroid, Synthroid); attempt withdrawal of levothyroxine at about 12 to 18 months postpartum; women who have had postpartum thyroiditis should be observed long-term, as some eventually develop permanent hypothyroidism
Urinary stress incontinence	Primary symptom is urinary incontinence, occurring with activities that increase intraabdominal pressure, such as coughing or sneezing	Kegel exercises, observation, and hysterectomy with bladder repair if symptoms persist and interfere with daily function

TSH = thyroid-stimulating hormone.

partum period include increases in marital conflict, fewer positive interchanges between partners, less frequent leisure activities, and movement to a more traditional division of household labor.[34]

Couples also experience changes in sexual activity after childbirth. They resume intercourse at an average of 7 weeks postpartum; however, there are wide variations, with 19% of women resuming intercourse within the first month, and 19% not until 4 months postpartum or later.[35] An important cause of postpartum decline in sexual activity is women's perineal discomfort related to episiotomies, perineal or vaginal tears, vaginal atrophy, or insufficient lubrication; this discomfort continues for an average of 3 months (range of 1 to greater than 12 months).[36] Other causes of reduced sexual activity include vaginal bleeding or discharge, fear of injury, a decreased sense of attractiveness, breast-feeding, and other child-care responsibilities. Together, these factors may result in distraction, time constraints, and fatigue. Unlike mothers, fathers do not tend to lose interest in sexual activity after childbirth, but their sexual activity declines in response to their partner's lack of interest,[37] which may in turn provoke further marital discord.

Important to the mother's (and likely the father's) postpartum well-being and marital happiness are the emotional support and practical help provided by the partner, friends, and relatives. To foster parents' mutual support, it may be useful to discuss specific techniques of support that partners can use with one another, such as planned parental (maternity, paternity) leave, scheduling time together, providing individual free time for one another, and sharing household and child-care responsibilities.

The postpartum period is a time of dynamic change for all family members, and this change is often accompanied by physical, emotional, and marital difficulties. The impact of these problems can be moderated by preparing the couple for postpartum changes during prenatal visits, by monitoring for problems during the immediate postpartum period and subsequent months, and by effectively managing problems that arise.

References

1. Ostgaard HC, Andersson GB. Postpartum low-back pain. Spine 1992;17:53–5.
2. Hopkins J, Marcus M, Campbell SB. Postpartum depression: a critical review. Psychol Bull 1984;95:498–515.
3. Graef P, McGhee K, Rozycki J, et al. Postpartum concerns of breastfeeding mothers. Nurse Midwif 1988;33(2):62–6.
4. Leigh DA, Emmanuel FXS, Sedgwick J, Dean R. Post-operative urinary tract infection and wound infection in women undergoing caesarean section: a comparison of two study periods in 1985 and 1987. J Hosp Infect 1990;15:107–16.
5. Chaim W, Bashiri A, Bar-David J, Shoham-Vardi I, Mazor M. Prevalence and clinical significance of postpartum endometritis and wound infection. Infect Dis Obstet Gynecol 2000;8:77–82.
6. Gould JS, Wissinger HA. Carpal tunnel syndrome in pregnancy. South Med J 1978;71:144–5.
7. Saultz JW, Toffler WL, Shackles JY. Postpartum urinary retention. J Am Board Fam Pract 1991;4:341–4.
8. Gilbert L, Porter W, Brown VA. Postpartum hemorrhage—a continuing problem. Br J Obstet Gynaecol 1987;94:67–71.
9. Miller JM. Maternal and neonatal morbidity and mortality in cesarean section. Obstet Gynecol Clin North Am 1988;15:629–38.
10. Cunningham FG, MacDonald PC, Gant NF, et al. Williams' obstetrics, 20th ed. Stamford, CT: Appleton & Lange, 1997.
11. Calhoun BC, Brost B. Emergency management of sudden puerperal fever. Obstet Gynecol Clin North Am 1995;22:357–67.
12. Paraskevaides EC. Deep venous thrombosis in pregnancy and the puerperium. Aust NZ J Obstet Gynaecol 1989;29:220–4.
13. Centouri S, Burmaz T, Ronfani L, et al. Nipple care, sore nipples, and breastfeeding: a randomized trial. J Hum Lact 1999;15:127–132.
14. Fein SB, Roe B. The effect of work status on initiation and duration of breast-feeding. Am J Public Health 1998;88:1042–6.
15. Eisman J. Relevance of pregnancy and lactation to osteoporosis? Lancet 1998;352:504–5.
16. Noyes N, Berkeley AS, Freedman K, Ledger W. Incidence of postpartum endomyometritis following single-dose antibiotic prophylaxis with either ampicillin/sulbactam, cefazolin, or cefotetan in high-risk cesarean section patients. Infect Dis Obstet Gynecol 1998;6:220–3.
17. Hansch E, Chitkara U, McAlpine J, El-Sayed Y, Dake MD, Razavi MK. Pelvic arterial embolization for control of obstetric hemorrhage: a five-year experience. Am J Obstet Gynecol 1999;180:1454–60.
18. Vedantham S, Goodwin SC, McLucas B, Mohr G. Uterine artery embolization: an underused method of controlling pelvic hemorrhage. Am J Obstet Gynecol 1997;176:938–48.
19. Brumfield CG, Hauth JC, Andrews WW. Puerperal infection after cesarean delivery: evaluation of a standardized protocol. Am J Obstet Gynecol 2000;182:1147–51.
20. Brown CE, Stettler RW, Twickler D, Cunningham FG. Puerperal septic pelvic thrombophlebitis: incidence and response to heparin therapy. Am J Obstet Gynecol 1999;181:143–8.
21. Gjerdingen DK, Froberg DG, Chaloner KM, McGovern PM. Changes in women's physical health during the first postpartum year. Arch Fam Med 1993;2:277–83.
22. Gruis M. Beyond maternity: postpartum concerns of mothers. Am J Matern Child Nurs 1977;2:182–8.
23. Harrison MJ, Hicks SA. Postpartum concerns of mothers and their sources of help. Can J Public Health 1983;74:325–8.
24. Lucas A, Pizarro E, Granada ML, Salinas I, Foz M, Sanmarti A. Postpartum thyroiditis: epidemiology and clinical evolution in a nonselected population. Thyroid 2000;10:71–7.
25. Wand JS. The natural history of carpal tunnel syndrome in lactation. J R Soc Med 1989;82:349–50.
26. Steiner M. Perinatal mood disorders: position paper. Psychopharmacol Bull 1998;34:301–6.
27. Briggs GG, Freeman RK, Yafee SJ. Drugs in pregnancy and lactation, 5th ed. Baltimore: Williams & Wilkins, 1998.
28. Wisner KL, Perel JM, Findling RL. Antidepressant treatment during breast-feeding. Am J Psychiatry 1996;153:1132–7.
29. Gjerdingen DK, Chaloner KM. The relationship of women's postpartum mental health to employment, childbirth, and social support. J Fam Pract 1994;38:465–72.
30. Clinton JF. Physical and emotional responses of expectant fathers throughout pregnancy and the early postpartum period. Int J Nurs Stud 1987;24:59–68.
31. Chalmers B, Meyer D. What men say about pregnancy, birth and parenthood. J Psychosom Obstet Gynecol 1996;17:47–52.
32. Stewart RB, Mobley LA, Van Tuyl SS, Salvador MA. The firstborn's adjustment to the birth of a sibling: a longitudinal assessment. Child Dev 1987;58:341–55.
33. Bigner JJ. Parent–child relations: an introduction to parenting, 5th ed. Columbus, OH: Merrill (Prentice Hall), 1998.
34. Belsky J, Pensky E. Marital change across the transition to parenthood. Marriage Fam Rev 1988;12:133–56.
35. Byrd JE, Hyde JS, DeLamater JD, Plant A. Sexuality during pregnancy and the year postpartum. J Fam Pract 1998;47:305–8.
36. Abraham S, Child A, Ferry J, Vizzasrd J, Mira M. Recovery after childbirth: a preliminary prospective study. Med J Aust 1990;152:9–12.
37. Gielen AC, O'Campo PJ, Faden RR. Interpersonal conflict and physical violence during the childbearing years. Soc Sci Med 1994;39:781–7.

16
Genetic Disorders

John W. Bachman

In family medicine, knowledge of genetics is useful in evaluating the risk a patient may have for a genetic disorder and to counsel patients about possible risks associated with any future childbearing. Today's family physician assumes many roles in managing genetic issues (Table 16.1). The explosion in science centering on genetics requires all primary care physicians to be aware of the pragmatic advances in this field.

The Basic Science of Genetics

There are 50,000 to 100,000 genes located in the 46 chromosomes of the human cell. Each gene is composed of one copy originating from the paternal side and the other from the maternal side. Genes are composed of DNA, and the ultimate products of most genes are proteins. The coding for a gene is its genotype. The physical result in the organism is its phenotype. It may not necessarily mean that the organism with the gene is expressed by its phenotype (recessive gene).

Most changes in the DNA of genes do not result in a disease; these are called polymorphisms. A change in the DNA of a gene that results in an abnormal protein that functions poorly or not at all is called a mutation. The same mutation in a gene does not necessarily produce the same physical findings in affected persons. This difference is called gene expression. Alleles are alternative forms of a gene at a specific location on a chromosome. A single allele for each locus is inherited from each parent. Damage to DNA is corrected by DNA repair genes. Mutations of repair genes lead to an increased risk for cancer.

Types of Testing

Indirect Analysis–Linkage Analysis

This type of testing is used when the location of a gene is not known or it is too difficult to test for directly. It is used primarily in families and requires that one affected person be tested to determine whether the gene is located near some genetic material that can be measured, such as another gene or a segment of DNA. If a marker is found, it can be used in other family members to assess whether they might have the gene. (You find the gene by knowing the company it keeps.) A geneticist might order this testing in a patient if there is a clustering of a disease in the family.

Direct Mutation Analysis

This type of genetic analysis involves looking for the specific mutation on the gene by one of several techniques. Common ones include Southern blot analysis, multiplex polymerase chain reaction, and direct sequencing of the gene. It does not rely on testing other members of the family. A family physician or geneticist ordering this type of testing is looking for a specific mutation on a gene, usually because of observing a patient's phenotype. A limitation of this technique is that a disease may be caused by multiple mutations. An example is cystic fibrosis, which is the result of the loss of phenylalanine at position 508 in about 70% of cases. The other 30% of cases are caused by hundreds of other mutations on the gene. Therefore, it is unrealistic to check for all of them when screening an individual. Another issue is that sometimes more than two genes are involved and account for the same phenotype.

Molecular Cytogenetic Analysis

Chromosome rearrangements can be detected by fluorescence in situ hybridization (FISH). The technique involves preparing a fluorescent probe that identifies either the abnormal region (a visible color appears on examination) or a normal region (no color appears). The technique is quick but often requires follow-up studies.

Table 16.1. **The Roles of Family Physicians in Genetic Medicine**

Identify individuals who are at increased risk for genetic disorders or who have a disorder

Use common prenatal genetic screening methods and effectively use genetic testing to care for individuals

Recognize the characteristics of common genetic disorders

Provide ongoing care for individuals with genetic disorders by monitoring health and coordinating referrals

Provide informed options about genetic issues to patients and their families

Be aware of genetic services for patients with various genetic disorders for appropriate referral

Types of Genetic Disorders

The types of genetic disorders that the patients of family physicians may have can be classified as follows:

1. Chromosome disorders: These disorders are caused by the loss, gain, or abnormal arrangement of one or more chromosomes. Their frequency in the population is about 0.2%.
2. Mendelian disorders: These disorders are single-gene defects caused by a mutant allele at a single genetic locus. The transmission pattern is divided further into autosomal dominant, autosomal recessive, X-linked dominant, and X-linked recessive. Their frequency is about 0.35%.
3. Multifactorial disorders: These disorders involve interactions between genes and environmental factors. The nature of these interactions is poorly understood. It includes cancers, diabetes, and most other diseases that develop during a patient's life. The risks of transmission can be estimated empirically, and their estimated frequency in the population is about 5%.
4. Somatic genetic disorders: Mutations arise in somatic cells and are not inherited. They often give rise to malignancies. Although the mutation is not inherited, it often requires a genetic predisposition.
5. Mitochondrial disorders: These disorders arise from mutations in the genetic material in mitochondria. Mitochondrial DNA is transmitted through only the maternal line.

Each of these groups of disorders, except mitochondrial disorders, is discussed below.

Chromosome Abnormalities

Down Syndrome

The most frequent chromosome disorder (1 in 800 births in the United States) is the one associated with Down syndrome. Down syndrome is caused primarily by nondisjunction during development of the egg, with failure of a chromosome 21 pair to segregate during meiosis. The event is random. Another cause (3–4% of cases) is a robertsonian translocation, in which chromosome 21 attaches to another chromosome.

Although the amount of genetic material is normal, the number of chromosomes is 45 instead of 46. The offspring of a parent with a robertsonian translocation have a 25% chance of having a Down syndrome karyotype. Karyotyping is required for all newborn children with Down syndrome to rule out robertsonian translocation. Another cause of Down syndrome (1–2% of cases) is nondisjunction after conception that leads to a mosaic pattern of inheritance, in which some cells are trisomy 21 and others are normal. A normal karyotype initially in a child with classic Down syndrome is possibly explained by mosaicism and requires chromosome analysis of other tissue. Down syndrome can be diagnosed during the prenatal period (see Chapter 11). The definitive tests are amniocentesis and chorionic villus sampling. Indications for either procedure are as follows[1]:

1. Robertsonian translocation and previous birth of a child with Down syndrome: For women younger than 30 years, the risk for recurrent Down syndrome is about 1%. For those older than 30, the risk is the same as that for other women of their age. The risk for recurrence in a patient with a robertsonian translocation is high.
2. Increasing maternal age: The risks for Down syndrome and other chromosome disorders according to maternal age are listed in Table 16.2. Prenatal diagnosis should be offered to women older than 35 years, who in fact comprise the largest group referred for genetic testing prenatally. About 25% of all Down syndrome births can be detected when age is used as a criterion.
3. Low serum levels of maternal α-fetoprotein: When testing for neural tube defects, another subset of pregnant women can be identified as being at risk for having a child with Down syndrome. Because the liver of a fetus with Down syndrome is immature, α-fetoprotein levels are lower than normal. Another 20% of fetuses with Down syndrome can be identified with this test (amniocentesis rate of 5% of a pregnant population being tested). The test also can be used to adjust patients older than age 35 years into a lower risk group.
4. Triple test: The risk for Down syndrome can be ascertained by measuring the serum levels of α-fetoprotein, estrogen, and human chorionic gonadotropin (hCG). The serum hCG level is higher and that of unconjugated estriols is lower in a pregnant woman whose fetus has Down syndrome. Detection rates of 60%, with an amniocentesis rate of 5% of a pregnant population being tested, have been reported.

All biochemical tests used for screening can produce false-positive results. It is important to confirm gestational age with ultrasonography before proceeding with amniocentesis to evaluate abnormal serum findings. Generally, routine screening exclusively with multiple biochemical markers is not recommended. None of the screening studies can guarantee that a child does *not* have Down syndrome. The definitive diagnostic study is amniocentesis or chorionic villus sampling. The advantage of chorionic villus sampling is earlier detection of Down syndrome so an abortion can be performed earlier during the pregnancy. The disadvantage is that the sampling is not useful for detecting neural tube defects.

Table 16.2. **Chromosome Abnormalities in Liveborn Infants, by Maternal Age**[a]

Maternal age (years)	Risk for Down syndrome	Total risk for chromosome abnormalities[b]
20	1/1667	1/526
21	1/1667	1/526
22	1/1429	1/500
23	1/1429	1/500
24	1/1250	1/476
25	1/1250	1/476
26	1/1176	1/476
27	1/1110	1/455
28	1/1053	1/435
29	1/1000	1/417
30	1/952	1/385
31	1/952	1/385
32	1/769	1/322
33	1/602	1/286
34	1/485	1/238
35	1/378	1/192
36	1/289	1/156
37	1/224	1/127
38	1/173	1/102
39	1/136	1/83
40	1/106	1/66
41	1/82	1/53
42	1/63	1/42
43	1/49	1/33
44	1/38	1/26
45	1/30	1/21
46	1/23	1/16
47	1/18	1/13
48	1/14	1/10
49	1/11	1/8

[a]Because sample size for some intervals is relatively small, 95% confidence limits are sometimes relatively large. Nonetheless, these figures are suitable for genetic counseling.

[b]47,XXX excluded for ages 20 to 32 years (data not available).

Source: Simpson,[16] by permission of Bailliere Tindall.

When counseling patients, a family physician should discuss the cost of the studies, the risks, and the concerns of the parents. During a discussion about children with Down syndrome, important points that should be made include the 33% chance of cardiac abnormalities, the presence of other congenital conditions, intellectual development to the level of the third to ninth grade, and the ability of most children to leave home and live independently as adults. Although it once was thought that only women who would have an abortion should undergo testing for Down syndrome, it is acceptable to use the tests to identify a high-risk pregnancy that may require care at a tertiary medical center.

At birth, a child with Down syndrome is identified on the basis of the following physical examination findings: hypotonia, craniofacial features of brachycephaly, oblique palpebral fissures, epicanthal folds, broad nasal bridge, protruding tongue, and low-set ears. The child may have Brushfield spots; short, broad fingers; a single flexion crease in the hand (the so-called simian crease, which is present in 30% of children with

Down syndrome and about 5% of normal children); and a wide space between the first two toes. About a third of the children have recognizable congenital heart disease, and the risk of duodenal atresia and tracheoesophageal fistula is increased. It is important to recognize congenital heart disease during the newborn period, and echocardiography is mandatory. Irreversible pulmonary hypertension with no recognizable signs can develop by 2 months. Ophthalmologic examination for cataracts, hearing tests, thyroid tests, and a complete blood cell count for leukemoid reaction should be performed.

An effective method has been described for informing parents that their child has Down syndrome. The basic principle is to tell both parents as soon as possible, with the baby present, in a quiet, private room. The child is referred to by name, and the information is provided by a credible person who can provide a balanced point of view. This person then gives the parents his or her telephone number should they have additional questions, and the family is given time to absorb the information. Other suggestions include providing information about the National Down Syndrome Society (1-800-221-4602) and having other parents of children with Down syndrome visit the new parents.

During the first 5 years of life, it is important to check for hypothyroidism annually, evaluate vision and hearing at 6-month to 1-year intervals, and provide special education (see Chapter 17). Growth charts are available online.[2] All children with Down syndrome should stay with the family, and most can be mainstreamed into kindergarten. It is important to use standard measures for Down syndrome to monitor growth and development. A child with Down syndrome often has a problem with verbal learning in school and does much better with visual learning. Resources for enhancing education are available from the National Association for Down Syndrome. A comprehensive resource for health supervision is available.[3] Before children with Down syndrome participate in sports, instability of the atlantodens must be assessed on cervical radiographs. Children who require intubation also may need evaluation. How frequent these radiographs should be obtained is debatable. No child has become paralyzed in the Special Olympics, and 90% of children in whom paralysis developed because of instability showed symptoms during the preceding month.

Most people with Down syndrome are able to leave home, work, and form relationships. Counseling them about contraceptive measures is appropriate. Alzheimer disease occurs in 25% of adults with Down syndrome.

Turner Syndrome

Turner syndrome has an incidence of about 1 in 2000 births.[4] The syndrome involves errors in one of the X chromosomes, such as the absence of one X chromosome (60% of cases), a structural abnormality of an X chromosome (20% of cases), or mosaicism involving the X chromosome of at least one cell line (20% of cases). Cases now are often discovered with prenatal amniocentesis and ultrasonography.

Heart Lesions

Many Turner syndrome patients have left-sided heart lesions, such as postductal coarctation (up to 20%) and bicuspid aortic valves (up to 50%), with or without stenosis. With time, distention of the ascending aorta may develop, leading to damage, possible dilation, dissection, and premature atherosclerosis. Echocardiography is recommended during infancy and the second decade of life. Bicuspid valves are an indication for prophylactic treatment for subacute bacterial endocarditis.

Bone Abnormalities

Osteoporosis is common with Turner syndrome, and calcium supplementation is important. Medical therapy may be indicated depending on bone density. Other skeletal characteristics include micrognathia, short metacarpals, genu valgum, scoliosis, and a square, stocky appearance.

Puberty

Oocytes degenerate by the time of birth in most cases of Turner syndrome. Between the ages of 12 and 15, puberty is induced with estrogens, and after 12 months progesterone is added to the regimen. Pregnancy has occurred in spontaneously menstruating patients. These patients usually have a mosaic pattern. In medical centers that specialize in in vitro fertilization, pregnancy rates of 50% to 60% have been reported with the use of both sister and anonymous donors.

Stature

Failure of growth occurs in virtually all patients with Turner syndrome. Often intrauterine growth failure is mild, height increases normally until age 3, growth velocity is progressive until age 14, and the adolescent growth phase is long. The short stature responds to treatment with growth hormone. It should begin when the stature is less than the fifth percentile (usually at age 2–5 years). Estrogen treatment may commence in adolescence.

Other Common Problems

Glucose intolerance, hearing loss over time, hypothyroidism (up to 50% by the time of adulthood), and congenital urinary tract abnormalities are more common among patients with Turner syndrome (35–70%) than in the general population. Fetal lymphedema may cause webbing of the neck, a low posterior hairline, and auricular malrotation.

Studies to consider for patients with Turner syndrome include chromosome karyotyping, thyroid function tests (annually), a baseline evaluation of the kidneys, and echocardiography.

Klinefelter Syndrome

Klinefelter syndrome is characterized by a 47,XXY karyotype.[3,4] It has an incidence of 1.7 in 1000 male infants. The disorder usually is diagnosed at puberty or during an infertility evaluation. In adolescents, its characteristics include gynecomastia (40%), small testicles (<2.5 cm long), tall stature, and an arm span that is greater than the person's height. Klinefelter syndrome is the most common cause of hypogonadism in males; testosterone levels are about half the normal value. The follicle-stimulating hormone and lactate dehydrogenase levels are increased. Treatment includes testosterone and occasionally mastectomy for gynecomastia.

Other Chromosome Abnormalities

Trisomy 18 is the second most common trisomy (1 in 8000 births).[3,4] Fewer than 10% of affected infants survive to age 1 year. Trisomy 13, the third most common trisomy, has an incidence of 1 in 20,000 births. Fifty percent of affected children die during the first month, and fewer than 5% survive beyond age 3. Cri du chat syndrome is due to a deletion involving chromosome 5. The incidence is 1 in 20,000 births. The clinical features include severe mental retardation, hypotonia, and a kitten-like cry. Life expectancy is the same as that for other patients with similar IQs.

Mendelian Disorders

Genogram

Knowledge of the family history is a powerful weapon for preventing premature death.[5] The first step in detecting a mendelian disorder involves constructing a genogram of the family history. Although genograms are used by fewer than 20% of family physicians, they are useful for showing patterns of genetic inheritance. One study indicated that three fourths of patients referred for genetic counseling had another significant family disorder that could affect pregnancy. Reports have demonstrated that 90% of doctors are able to interpret data from a genogram written by other colleagues. To save time, a medical assistant can initially question a patient about the family history of genetic disorders before a physician obtains a complete medical history. The information collected includes the following:

1. Demographic data: the names of relatives and their birth dates, ages, sexes, spontaneous abortions, places of residence, and dates of death.
2. Medical disorders: a listing of the diseases experienced by family members
3. Social factors: relationships and the nature of these relationships
4. Other data: previous family crises

When a genogram is constructed, squares are used to represent male members and circles to represent female members. Three generations should be represented, and each generation is on a horizontal row. A first-degree relative is a parent, sibling, or child. A second-degree relative is an aunt, uncle, nephew, niece, grandparent, or grandchild.

Dominant Disorders

With classic dominant inheritance, the affected person has a parent with the disorder. The parent usually mates with someone who does not have the genetic disorder, and the offspring have a 50% chance of having the disorder. Typically, predisposition for the disorder is carried on one chromosome, and expression of the disorder is modified by the chromosome makeup of the other parent. The dominant condition usually does not alter the ability to reproduce but tends to alter materials that provide structure to a body. Examples of dominant disorders include Marfan syndrome, Huntington disease, neurofibromatosis, achondroplasia, and familial hypercholesterolemia. About 6% of cases of breast cancer are inherited dominantly. For construction of a genogram, an excellent screening question for dominant disorders is, "Has anyone in your family had a serious disorder during adolescence or middle age?" Diseases that seem to be present in each generation tend to be dominant.

Recessive Disorders

With classic recessive-disorder inheritance, both mates have a gene for the disorder. The offspring have a 25% chance of having a normal gene pattern, a 50% chance of being a carrier, and a 25% chance of having the disorder. Carriers tend to have a reproductive advantage in certain environments; for example, sickle cell trait carriers are more resistant to falciparum malaria than noncarriers. The disorders tend to involve enzymes, and siblings who have the disorder tend to have the same severity because there is no modifying gene as in a dominant disorder. If untreated, recessive disorders tend to cause death at an early age.

Screening questions that are useful for revealing recessive disorders include "Has anyone in your family had stillbirths?" and "Has anyone in your family had children who died or were seriously ill during early childhood?" An important consideration when screening for recessive disorders[6] is to inquire about the nationality of the patient. Certain nationalities are associated with recessive disorders. For example, in patients of Caribbean, Latin American, Mediterranean, or African descent, hemoglobin testing should be performed to screen for sickle cell anemia or thalassemia disorders (see Chapter 126). Patients of Ashkenazi Jewish origin should be screened for Tay-Sachs disease and possibly Gaucher disease (1 in 450 births). There are exceptions to this tendency. For example, hemochromatosis is a very common recessive disorder and is often frequently missed because the symptoms occur late in life.

In addition to the medical history, laboratory screening tests performed in the newborn detect recessive disorders. States require that many of these tests be performed. Examples are phenylketonuria, galactosemia, congenital adrenal hyperplasia, and hemoglobinopathy tests. The ideal time for conducting these laboratory studies is 72 hours after birth, although with early hospital dismissal of newborns, this timing is difficult. The American Academy of Pediatrics recommends that screening tests be performed in all infants before dismissal from the hospital. If the infant is dismissed less than 24 hours after birth, the screening tests should be repeated before the infant is 2 weeks old. Many medical clinics recommend rescreening if dismissal occurs at 48 hours. The diagnoses of phenylketonuria and hypothyroidism may be missed if the infant is not retested after early dismissal. In some states, other newborn screening tests are performed to detect galactosemia (incidence of 1 in 50,000 births; it involves a defect in the enzyme for converting glucose to galactose), hemoglobinopathies, and congenital adrenal hyperplasia. Follow-up data for children with abnormal screening results have been published.[7]

Newborns who become progressively more ill usually are thought to have a septic condition. An inborn error of metabolism should be considered in a newborn who vomits and becomes progressively comatose. Also, it is important to remember that a mother who has phenylketonuria should be placed on a rigorous phenylalanine-free diet when pregnant to ensure that her condition does not cause mental retardation in the fetus. Ideally, this diet is started during the preconception period.

Cystic Fibrosis

A recessive disorder currently discussed widely is cystic fibrosis.[8,9] Nearly 30,000 people in the United States have this disorder. It is carried by about 1 in 25 Caucasians in the U.S., and these carriers often do not have a family history of cystic fibrosis. The clinical characteristics of cystic fibrosis include pancreatic insufficiency (85% of patients), pulmonary disease characterized by recurrent infections and bronchiectasis, and failure to grow. In more than 60% of patients, the diagnosis is made during the first year of life. Interestingly, the diagnosis is made in 5% of patients after age 15 years. Most authorities believe that early diagnosis prevents pulmonary damage in early life, but, currently, routine screening of infants is not recommended.[10] The diagnosis is based on the concentration of chloride in sweat being greater than 60 mEq/L and clinical suspicion of the disease. Improvements in antibiotics, physiotherapy, and nutrition have increased the average age of survival from 4 years in 1960 to 30 years in 1995. Current advances in treatment include agents that break down mucus and trials for gene therapy. The mucus produced in a patient with cystic fibrosis provides an excellent medium for *Pseudomonas* and other bacteria that damage lungs. Cross-infection has led to cystic fibrosis organizations' discouraging camps for patients and developing guidelines for limiting this problem. The gene associated with cystic fibrosis was identified in 1989 on chromosome 7 and encodes the protein cystic fibrosis transmembrane conductance regulator, which is a chloride channel in cells. The failure of this channel to work properly causes excess chloride in sweat and changes in fluid balance, which in turn cause thickened mucus in the lungs. The most common defect in cystic fibrosis cells is the absence of phenylalanine in the protein (deletion). Testing is recommended for patients with a family history of cystic fibrosis and their partners. There are more than 150 mutations of the cystic fibrosis gene, and testing can detect 85% of the carriers.

Multifactorial Disorders

Neural Tube Defects

Neural tube defects (NTDs) are the disorders most commonly screened for prenatally.

Physiology

α-Fetoprotein is synthesized in the yolk sac, gastrointestinal tract, and liver. The protein enters the amniotic fluid through urination, secretions, and transudation from blood vessels, and small amounts leak into the maternal serum.

Incidence

The incidence of NTDs is 1 to 2 in 1000 births. A family history of NTDs and diabetes in the mother increase the risk significantly. If the mother's diet is supplemented with folic acid before conception, the incidence of NTDs decreases. These defects are associated with high mortality, high morbidity, and long-term developmental disability.

Screening

Of every 1000 pregnant females who are tested at 16 to 18 weeks' gestation in the U.S., about 25 to 50 have increased levels of maternal serum α-fetoprotein (msAFP) and 40 to 50 have low levels.[9,10] The mothers with high levels of msAFP can undergo ultrasonography to determine gestational age or the presence of a multiple gestation or significant abnormality. An alternative is to repeat the test within 1 to 2 weeks for mothers with abnormally high or low levels of the protein. If the repeat studies confirm the previous abnormal results, ultrasonography is performed. After screening with ultrasonography, about 17 of the patients with increased levels of msAFP and 20 to 30 of those with low levels have no findings that explain the abnormal values. Amniocentesis should be performed in these patients. Of the 17 patients with high levels, one or two have a fetus with a significant NTD, whereas 1 in 65 of those with a low msAFP have a fetus with a chromosome abnormality (1 in 90 chance of Down syndrome). For a pregnant female with an abnormally high msAFP level and a fetus with no NTD, the risk of stillbirth, low birth weight, neonatal death, and congenital anomalies is increased. Excellent summaries are available.[11]

Other Disorders

The overall risk for recurrent cleft lip, with or without cleft palate, is 4% if a sibling or parent has the abnormality and 10% if it is present in two previous siblings. Lip pits or depressions on the lower lip of a newborn may be the manifestation of an autosomal-dominant trait; the recurrence rate for a sibling is 50%.

Generally, the incidence of multifactorial disorders is less than 5%. The incidence of recurrence is 2% to 5% for cardiac anomalies, 1% to 2% for tracheoesophageal fistula, 1% to 2% for diaphragmatic hernia, 6% to 10% for hypospadias, and 4% to 8% for hip dislocation.

General Considerations in Counseling Patients

In North America about 8% of pregnancies meet the criteria for performing amniocentesis or chorionic villus sampling. The following are basic points for prenatal testing:

1. All patients have the right to receive information about the genetic risk associated with a pregnancy. It allows parents to make an informed choice about having a child with an abnormality.
2. All patients have the right to refuse testing. What a patient decides to do about any given risk factor is entirely up to the patient. Genetic testing is voluntary, except for what a

state requires (e.g., neonatal screening for phenylketonuria, hypothyroidism, and other inborn errors of metabolism).
3. Referral to a geneticist is useful for difficult cases or patients with complex or unusual genetic disorders.
4. Genetic screening is not expected to detect all genetic disorders in a given population.

Cancer and Genetics

Certain families have an increased risk for specific cancers.[12] Many of these families have an identifiable gene associated with the disorder. Possession of the gene does not automatically mean that cancer will develop in the patient. Most genes can be altered by environmental factors and by other genes. In some families a defective gene is inherited, such as for retinoblastoma. With time there is a somatic mutation of the other normal copy of the gene. With colorectal carcinoma there is a multistep process in which a cell mutates and forms a family of abnormal cells, one of which mutates to form another cell line. Over time, these accumulated multiple mutations form a cell line that is cancer. Consequently, a risk can be predicted on the basis of the history of the gene being found in other families. One of the most important concepts to remember is that if an abnormal cancer gene is found in a patient who is not a member of a family with a history of cancer, there is minimal evidence for determining risk for the patient for that cancer. Most single-gene disorders that predispose to cancer are rare. Colon cancer and breast cancer, described below, are exceptions to this rule.

Colon Cancer (Also See Chapter 92)

Inherited colon cancer represents 5% to 10% of colon cancer cases and about 30% of adult genetic referrals. It is reassuring to family members that no matter how extensive the family history of colon cancer, the risk for development of colon cancer never exceeds 50% in a family member.

Familial Adenomatous Polyposis (Gardner Syndrome)

Familial adenomatous polyposis has an incidence of 1 in 10,000 and makes up less than 1% of colon cancers. It is caused by having an autosomal-dominant gene located on chromosome 5 (APC gene). Predictive testing of first-degree relatives is appropriate, and those who have the gene need colon studies starting at age 12 years. Once several polyps are found, colon resection is recommended. Regular surveillance afterward is needed to assess potential cancers in the upper intestinal tract.

Hereditary Nonpolyposis Colon Cancer

Most observers believe that hereditary nonpolyposis colon cancer accounts for 2% of colon cancers and is the result of a defect on hMSH2 found on chromosome 2 or four other genes. They are autosomal dominant. All genes in this group are mismatch repair genes. The genes function in repairing abnormal DNA. Consequently, for a tumor to appear it must be altered and the genes for repair absent. This is called the "two-hit hypothesis." Colonoscopy is the preferred method of screening at intervals of 18 months to 3 years depending on the family history. Suggested surveillance guidelines can be found in the literature.[13]

Breast Cancer (Also see Chapter 107)

Among all women with breast cancer, 20% to 30% have at least one relative with breast cancer. Among these cases, 5% to 10% are caused by mutations in *BRCA1* and *BRCA2* genes. Inherited breast cancer has the clinical features of younger age at onset (less than 45), bilaterality, and cancer at other sites. The genes are tumor-suppressor genes (they repair damaged DNA), and the loss of both alleles is required for the initiation of tumors. Testing is reasonable in patients with the following:

1. One first-degree relative age 30 years or less with breast cancer or a male relative with breast cancer.
2. Two first-degree relatives with breast cancer, one of whom is younger than 50 years or both are younger than 60 years, or one has bilateral breast cancer or both have ovarian cancer.
3. One first-degree relative with breast cancer and one first-degree relative with ovarian cancer.
4. One first-degree relative and one second-degree relative with breast cancer if the sum of their ages at onset is less than 110 or one has bilateral disease.
5. Two second-degree relatives with breast cancer if the sum of their ages is 60 or less.
6. *BRCA1* gene: The first identified gene for breast cancer is located on chromosome 17, and more than 600 mutations have been detected. A woman carrying a mutation is estimated to have a 56% to 87% lifetime risk of having breast cancer and a 15% to 45% chance of having a lifetime risk of ovarian cancer.
7. *BRCA2* gene: The second gene for breast cancer was detected in 1995 and has more than 150 mutations. The lifetime risks for development of breast cancer (37–87%) and ovarian cancer (10–20%) are somewhat less than the risks associated with the *BRCA1* gene.

Human Genome

On June 26, 2000, the Human Genome Project and Celera Genomics jointly announced that the human genome had been sequenced. The development of genetic information brought on by the sequencing of the human genome is accelerating. How useful is knowledge about sequencing of the human genome to clinicians? It certainly bodes well for a single mendelian gene. However, most common diseases rely on several genes. The situation has been described well by Holtzman and Marteau[14]:

It would be revolutionary if we could determine the genotypes of the majority of people who will get common diseases. The complexity of the genetics of common diseases casts doubt on whether accurate prediction will ever be possible. Alleles at many different gene loci will increase the risk of certain diseases only when they are inherited with alleles at other loci, and only in the presence of specific environmental or behavioral factors. Moreover, many combinations of predisposing alleles, environmental factors, and behavior could all lead to the same pathogenic effect.

The basic science of the human genome is not yet being applied in the family physician's office, but its use will follow predictable patterns. The first stage is identification of a gene that causes an illness. The second stage is development of methods to do genetic testing in a physician's practice. With the ability to identify the gene come the issues of carrier testing, presymptomatic genetic screening, and odds of the gene being fully expressed. Currently, gene therapy for altered DNA is restricted to protocols.

Current research efforts revolve around single nucleotide polymorphisms (SNPs, or "snips"). These are fragments of DNA that vary by a single DNA alteration. There are thousands of these fragments, and they make up less than 0.1% of a human's DNA. They determine the essential differences between individuals. The first application of SNPs is in drug use. For example, Glaxo developed a medication called alosetron hydrochloride (Lotronex) for irritable bowel syndrome. It was withdrawn from the market because 43 people had side effects. By analyzing DNA from patients who had side effects, it is hoped that the DNA difference that led to the side effect could be determined. Testing patients for this difference before the drug is used might lead to safe use. The use of SNPs to determine which patients are susceptible to medication reactions will probably be the first application that family physicians will use widely. Testing most likely will be done with a biochip made up of DNA strands; when a patient's DNA is compared with the chip, differences will be highlighted, pointing to significant problems with prescribing medication or eventually subtyping diseases such as diabetes and autoimmune diseases.

Finally, it is important to consider that genetic sequencing of pathogens will yield promising treatments. *Mycobacterium tuberculosis* and *Treponema pallidum* are examples of organisms whose genomes are now known.

Web Sites of Value

A reasonable way of keeping up with innovations is to use the Internet. The following sites are useful:

The Human Genome Projects Information: *http://www.ornl.gov/hg-nis.*
A useful site that includes maps, genes, and diseases is the GENATLAS query: *http://bisance.citi2.fr/GENATLAS/menu_an.htm.*
PubMed has extensive resources for genetics[15]: *http://www.ncbi.nlm.nih.gov/Genbank/index.html.* At this time the site is more useful to basic science. It has *Molecular Biology of the Cell,* a textbook, online.
Montana State publishes a series of education topics quarterly. It is located at *http://www.mostgene.org/gd/gdlist.htm.*
George Washington University produces lectures of high quality in its Frontiers in Clinical Genetics: *http://www.frontiersingenetics.com/main.htm.*

OMIM—Online Mendelian Inheritance in Man: *http://www.ncbi.nlm.nih.gov/Omim*. The site tends to be comprehensive but focuses on basic sciences.

A society-based site for education, National Coalition of Health Professional Education in Genetics: *http://www.nchpeg.org*.

GeneClinics: *http://www.geneclinics.org*. An excellent all-around site for information that is current and well supported for clinicians.

GeneTests: *http://www.genetests.org/*. This site has materials and directories for genetic testing.

The genetics and rare conditions site of the University of Kansas has information for patients, *http://www.kumc.edu/gec/geneinfo.html*, and providers, *http://www.kumc.edu/gec/prof/geneelsi.html*.

Acknowledgment

Portions of this chapter were previously published in Bachman JW. Medical genetics. In: Breslow L, ed. Encyclopedia of public health. New York: Macmillan Publishers 2001, with permission of the publisher.

References

1. Layman LC. Essential genetics for the obstetrician/gynecologist. Obstet Gynecol Clin North Am 2000;27:555–66.
2. Richards G. Growth charts for children with Down syndrome. Available at *www.growthcharts.com/index.htm*.
3. Cunniff C, Frias JL, Kaye C, et al. Health supervision for children with Down syndrome. Pediatrics 2001;107:442–9.
4. Saenger P. Turner's syndrome. N Engl J Med 1996;335:1749–54.
5. Jolly W, Froom J, Rosen MG. The genogram. J Fam Pract 1980;10:251–5.
6. Buist NR, Tuerck JM. The practitioner's role in newborn screening. Pediatr Clin North Am 1992;39:199–211.
7. Pass KA, Lane PA, Fernhoff PM, et al. US newborn screening system guidelines II: follow-up of children, diagnosis, management, and evaluation. Statement of the Council of Regional Networks for Genetic Services (CORN). J Pediatr 2000;137(suppl):S1–46.
8. Robinson P. Cystic fibrosis. Thorax 2001;56:237–41.
9. Welsh MJ, Smith AE. Cystic fibrosis. Sci Am 1995;273:52–9.
10. Genetic testing for cystic fibrosis. NIH Consensus Statement 1997;15:1–37.
11. Congenital disorders. Screening for neural tube defects—including folic acid/folate prophylaxis. In: Guide to clinical preventive services, 2nd ed. 2001. Available at *www.cpmcnet.columbia.edu/texts/gcps/gcps0052.html*.
12. Weitzel JN. Genetic counseling for familial cancer risk. Hosp Pract 1996;31:57–69.
13. Cole TR, Sleightholme HV. ABC of colorectal cancer. The role of clinical genetics in management. Br Med J 2000;321:943–6.
14. Holtzman NA, Marteau TM. Will genetics revolutionize medicine? N Engl J Med 2000;343:141–4.
15. McEntyre J, Lipman D. PubMed: bridging the information gap. Can Med Assoc J 2001;164:1317–9.
16. Simpson JL. Screening for fetal and genetic abnormalities. Baillieres Clin Obstet Gynaecol 1991;5:675–96.

17

Problems of the Newborn and Infant

Richard B. Lewan, Christopher R. Wood, and Bruce Ambuel

Family-centered care offers diverse opportunities for reducing risk and improving the health of newborns and infants. Premarital, preconception, and prenatal visits allow assessment for genetic disorders, ensure healthy lifestyle changes (e.g., nutrition), provide preconception vitamins, manage chronic diseases such as diabetes, and intervene when prenatal disorders such as toxemia threaten. Optimal care requires preparation for emergencies (e.g., neonatal resuscitation, sepsis), management of common problems, timely referral for complicated conditions, and prevention through early identification of feeding, growth and developmental problems, and family violence. Full family involvement prepares each member for new roles, recruits participation in healthy habits, and maintains cohesiveness when problems arise.

Newborn Care

Newborn Resuscitation

Skillful resuscitation can prevent lifelong complications of common neonatal emergencies. Proper preparation for the distressed newborn begins with a search for risk factors with each delivery. Participation in a resuscitation course or hospital-based practice sessions promotes teamwork and leadership. Then team members can develop and maintain skills using an organized plan of assessment and intervention. Figure 17.1 outlines an intervention protocol for a term newborn based on meconium, respiratory effort, heart rate, and color. This figure can be posted with a list of tested equipment in a visible location in the resuscitation area. Ready access must be provided to the equipment and medications listed. When time permits, all equipment is laid out and tested. Prior to obtaining intravenous access, epinephrine and naloxone can be given by endotracheal tube followed by 1 to 2 mL of saline. Basic resuscitation skills for a depressed newborn include (1) controlling the thermal environment with proper use of a ra-

diant warmer and rapid, thorough drying; (2) positioning, suctioning, and gentle tactile stimulation; (3) catheter suctioning of meconium from the airway on the perineum followed by gentle bulb syringe suctioning after delivery and adding prompt tracheal suctioning of any meconium through an endotracheal tube if the newborn is not vigorous (e.g., if depressed respirations, tone or heart rate below 100 beats per minute; repeat until clear unless the heart rate is low); (4) providing immediate bag and mask ventilation for newborns with apnea, gasping, or poor respiratory effort; and (5) administration of naloxone or IV normal saline if indicated. Effective positioning and skillful assisted ventilation revive most distressed neonates. Short delays greatly prolong recovery time and increase the risk of complications.

Advanced skills for patients without immediate consultation include (1) endotracheal tube placement with ventilation for patients not responding or requiring more prolonged bag and mask ventilation; (2) chest compressions at 120 per minute for a sustained heart rate of less than 60 beats per minute (cycles of three compressions followed by one breath); (3) central circulation access through the umbilical venous catheter because peripheral intravenous access is often unsuccessful; and (4) chest puncture at the fourth intercostal space in the anterior axillary line with a 21-gauge angiocatheter or butterfly for tension pneumothorax.[1]

Stabilization for Transfer to the Nursery or Transport to Intensive Care

Postresuscitation priorities include assessment for emergent anomalies, maintenance of basic needs, effective communication with and support of the family, and deciding on the level of care required. Pulse oximetry and a cardiorespiratory monitor are used to monitor ongoing success. Oxygen saturations should be kept at 88% to 92% for preterm newborns and 92% to 94% for term newborns. Baseline tests for un-

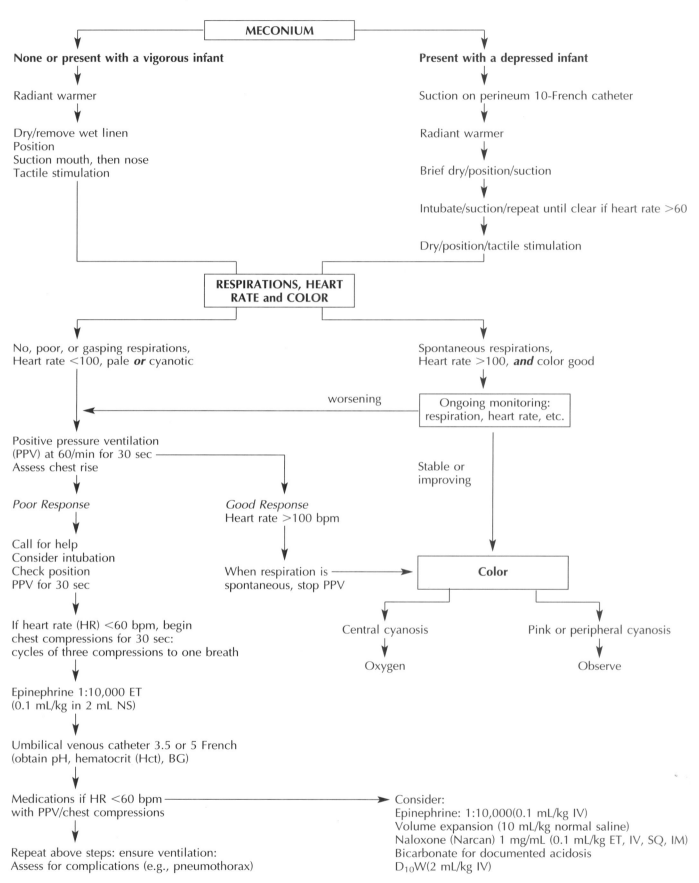

Fig. 17.1. An intervention protocol for a term newborn. NS = normal saline; BG = blood glucose; ET = endotracheal.

stable newborns include a chest radiograph, complete blood count (CBC), glucose, and blood gases (arterial if possible, otherwise capillary). A sepsis workup and other laboratory tests may then be considered. Ventilatory support is needed for persistent respiratory distress, apnea, or deteriorating blood gases (especially Pco_2 >60 with acidosis). Feedings should then be avoided and a nasogastric tube placed. Intravenous fluids are started with 10% dextrose in water ($D_{10}W$) at 65 to 80 mL/kg/day for the first 24 hours. Timely transport of unstable or high-risk neonates for tertiary care enhances outcome (e.g., early surfactant therapy for hyaline membrane disease).

Giving Bad News to Parents After Delivery

Family physicians will confront situations where they need to discuss bad news with parents regarding their newborn. These situations can range from a stillbirth, to a neonatal death, to a multisystem serious anomaly, or to isolated problems such as cleft palate. Studies have surveyed patients and family members to determine how they believe physicians should give bad news.[2] These studies have covered a wide range of patient and family experiences including cancer, birth defects, traumatic injury and death, etc. Four common themes emerge from this work indicating that patients want (1) a clear, direct statement of the news; (2) time to talk together in private; (3) openness to emotion; and (4) ongoing involvement in decision making.[2] In addition, when physicians are discussing bad news with parents regarding a newborn, parents prefer that the physician talk to both parents together and early. Parents also prefer that the physician, when possible, discuss the news with the baby present and being held by a parent or the physician.[3,4]

Common Problems in the Nursery

Low Birth Weight Newborns

Every hospital should provide a standard graph that allows plotting of weight to gestational age (by dates and examination) to identify newborns who are premature (<37 weeks), small for gestational age (SGA) (weight <10th percentile), or both. Once classified, problems unique to each can be prevented or anticipated. For example, prematurity is associated with hyaline membrane disease, apnea, jaundice, and intracranial hemorrhage. Asymmetric SGA newborns (small trunk relative to head size, caused by uteroplacental insufficiency) are at risk for asphyxia, meconium aspiration, hypoglycemia, hypothermia, and polycythemia. Symmetric SGA [small head and body, caused by genetic or TORCH (toxoplasmosis, other agents, rubella, cytomegalovirus, herpes simplex) syndromes] adds risk for congenital malformations and poor subsequent catch-up growth. All may be at risk for sepsis.

Those newborns cared for in a level I nursery are ready for discharge when they are (1) medically stable, (2) tolerating feedings well with consistent weight gain, (3) able to maintain stable body temperature in an open crib for 24 hours, and (4) free of apneic or bradycardic spells requiring intervention for a number of days (or home monitoring is established), and when their caregivers are educated and able to cope with the infant at home, and discharge planning is complete.

Postterm Newborns

After 42 weeks' gestation, some newborns are large and at risk for birth trauma and asphyxia. Others are postmature with absent lanugo and vernix, long nails, thin and scaly skin, abundant scalp hair, increased alertness, and low birth weight (SGA due to placental insufficiency with the risks described above). Early feedings are indicated.

Neonatal Sepsis

Sepsis is often accompanied by nonspecific signs and symptoms, making early detection difficult; 2/1000 neonates have bacterial sepsis. Risk increases with preterm labor, premature rupture of membranes, or intrapartum fever. Group B streptococcus (GBS) and *Escherichia coli* are responsible for 70% of the bacterial infections, and *Listeria monocytogenes,* enterococcus, staphylococcus, and other gram-negative bacteria (e.g., *Haemophilus influenzae*) are responsible for most of the rest. Early manifestations include temperature instability, lethargy, and poor feeding. Only about 50% have a temperature higher than 37.8°C (100°F) axillary. Prompt evaluation and careful observation every few hours can clarify when a thorough workup is needed. Hepatosplenomegaly, jaundice, petechiae, seizures, stiff neck, and bulging fontanel occur late and denote a poor prognosis.

Group B streptococcal infection is associated with 20% mortality and often presents at or just after birth with rapid deterioration, unexplained apnea, tachypnea, respiratory distress, or shock. Late-onset disease (mean 24 days) usually presents as meningitis. Intrapartum chemoprophylaxis based on the 1996 Centers for Disease Control and Prevention (CDC)[5] recommendation reduces morbidity and mortality of neonatal GBS infections.

Diagnosis

Helpful studies include CBC, chest radiography, and cultures of blood, cerebrospinal fluid (CSF), and urine. Catheterization or suprapubic aspiration are preferable for culture. The CSF may contain up to 32 white blood cells (WBC)/mm^3 during the first few days, so a Gram stain and protein and glucose levels in the CSF should be checked. Surface cultures are no longer recommended.

Treatment

Antibiotics should be initiated quickly with a combination of ampicillin (200 mg/kg/day IV or IM divided tid for infants during the first week of life, tid thereafter) plus gentamicin (2.5 mg/kg per dose bid for the first week, tid thereafter). Dosages are reduced for low birth weight infants or if meningitis is excluded. Because viruses and noninfectious disorders can produce sepsis-like illness, antibiotics can be stopped at 48 hours with sterile cultures unless the suspicion for infection continues to be high. Treatment is then continued intravenously at least 7 days while monitoring gentamicin levels.

If the latter assay is not available, cefotaxime can be used instead of gentamicin. Methicillin (or vancomycin if resistance is possible) should replace ampicillin when starting antibiotics after 3 days of life. Bacteremia is treated for 7 to 10 days or 5 to 7 days after a clinical response is noted. Meningitis requires at least 14 days of therapy depending on the response and causative organism.[6]

Respiratory Distress

Tachypnea, grunting, nasal flaring, retractions, cyanosis, apnea, or stridor should be evaluated with a chest radiograph, blood gases, glucose, and hematocrit. Early-onset causes include hyaline membrane disease (HMD), meconium aspiration, transient tachypnea of the newborn (TTN), or "wet lung," and less commonly in utero acquired pneumonia or congenital defects compromising the respiratory tract. At several hours after birth sepsis, metabolic abnormalities, cardiac failure, and intraventricular hemorrhage become more likely.

Hyaline membrane disease affects preterm newborns who manifest "stiff" lungs, hypercarbia, hypoxia, and a "groundglass" (reticulonodular) radiograph with air bronchograms. Signs are usually present within minutes after birth and progressively worsen after. Rapid stabilization and early surfactant therapy improves outcome. Meconium aspiration usually occurs after 34 weeks, causing airway obstruction and edema often within hours of birth. Radiography reveals hyperinflation and possibly pneumothorax. After resuscitation, aggressive support with ventilation and oxygen should maintain the PO_2 above 80 mm Hg. Sepsis workup and antibiotic coverage are indicated for HMD and meconium aspiration because the risk of pneumonia is increased.

Transient tachypnea of the newborn presents just after birth in term or preterm newborns and improves significantly within 24 hours. Tachypnea, little hypoxia or hypercarbia, and radiographic findings of perihilar streaking (not reticulonodular) and fluid in the fissures are common. Oxygen requirements gradually decrease after the first few hours. If the course is atypical or there is a risk of sepsis, neonatal pneumonia and other causes must be considered.

Apnea

A respiratory pause of 20 seconds (shorter if cyanosis or bradycardia occurs) strongly suggests pathology in the term infant. Apnea of prematurity should not occur before 1 day or after 7 days of life. The evaluation begins with a history about the event including respiratory effort, color, tone, relation to feeding, and unusual movement. Vital signs (for thermal disorders), a careful cardiorespiratory and neurologic examination, CBC, and calcium, magnesium, and electrolyte levels are assessed. Based on the suspicion, an electrocardiogram (ECG), echocardiogram, arterial blood gases, electroencephalogram (EEG), head computed tomography (CT) scan, or reflux studies may be needed. Management of the underlying problem and resolution of apnea associated with desaturations or bradycardia for several days allow discharge. Pnuemography does not predict the risk of sudden infant death syndrome. Evidence to support the use of home monitoring is lacking. It is not indicated in asymptomatic preterm patients.

Cyanosis

Blue hands and feet are sometimes normal or may be due to slowed circulation. Trunk and mucous membrane involvement (i.e., central cyanosis) after the first 20 minutes of life requires rapid evaluation. If hypothermia, hypoglycemia, narcotic respiratory depression, hypotension, and choanal atresia are not found, causes may include pulmonary, cardiac, neurologic and metabolic disorders as well as polycythemia, sepsis, and acidosis. Intermittent cyanosis with alternating "spells" of apnea and periods of normal breathing suggests a neurologic disorder. Involvement in the upper or lower part of the body or continuous cyanosis without respiratory signs strongly suggests a cardiac cause, especially if a PO_2 of 100 mm Hg is not achieved when the infant is placed in 100% oxygen for 20 minutes. Hypoxia should be reversed with oxygenation and assisted ventilation in preparation for rapid referral.

Hypotension and Shock

After quick assessment including repeated vital signs and obtaining essential laboratory tests (i.e., CBC, coagulation studies, glucose, electrolytes and pH, calcium, cultures, and if indicated the Kleihauer-Betke test), volume expansion with normal saline (10 mL/kg over 30 minutes) should be undertaken promptly for suspected hypovolemia, sepsis, or neurogenic causes. Once stabilized, the history and physical examination can direct further study. Any suggestion of sepsis requires a workup and antibiotic coverage. If cardiogenic causes are likely, inotropic agents may be indicated and should be considered when volume expansion is ineffective.

Cardiac Murmurs (Also See Chapter 78)

Soft, benign murmurs are common during the first 24 hours of life, but early loud murmurs suggest valvular stenosis or regurgitation. Murmurs of cardiac shunts may be heard at 72 hours but more often at 2 to 3 weeks. Loud murmurs, abnormal heart sounds, or findings suggesting cardiac disease (i.e., cyanosis, poor color or feeding, tachycardia, bradycardia, abnormal blood pressure, respiratory distress, or hepatomegaly) necessitate a prompt ECG, chest radiograph, and, if pathology is suspected, cardiology consultation. All neonates require careful auscultation at the 2-week visit.

Jaundice

Jaundice is noted in at least 50% of Caucasian newborns, with 6% having total serum bilirubin (TSB) levels higher than 12.9 mg/dL. Higher levels are noted in Asian and American Indian newborns. Kernicterus leading to death or severe neurologic handicap is preventable if bilirubin levels do not exceed 25 to 30 mg/dL (lower in sick premature neonates). Two important errors are likely sources of the rising incidence of kernicterus now seen even in healthy term newborns. First, delayed recognition due to early discharge occurs if the newborn is not reassessed by day 3 of life. Second, delayed evaluation for and treatment of hemolysis, makes it more likely that exchange transfusion will be needed.

Diagnosis

Icterus, best detected by blanching blood from the skin, is first noted in the face and progresses to the feet as TSB levels rise. While recent studies suggest unreliability of the clinical exam in estimating TSB, if icterus does not reach the umbilicus in low-risk newborns, the TSB is unlikely to be more than 12 mg/dL.[7] Transcutaneous bilirubinometry estimates TSB but is inaccurate with rapid progression, after phototherapy, or with dark skin. TSB levels must be measured for severe or rapid-onset jaundice. Inaccuracy of ±1 mg/dL should be considered when following TSB trends.

Physiologic jaundice is common with a typical pattern of unconjugated hyperbilirubinemia, reaching an average peak of 6 mg/dL by day 3 and resolution within 1 week in term infants and within 2 weeks in preterm infants. A search for pathologic jaundice is needed with (1) icterus during the first 24 hours (assess quickly for hemolysis), (2) TSB rising more than 5 mg/dL per day, (3) TSB exceeding 15 mg/dL in term infants and 10 mg/dL in preterm infants, (4) icterus lasting longer than 10 days in term infants and 21 days in preterm infants, and (5) a direct bilirubin level exceeding 1.5 mg/dL. Review the maternal, perinatal, and family history for risk factors, reexamine, determine the infant's blood type and Rh, and perform a direct Coombs' test (on cord blood saved from the delivery, if possible). If these tests are normal, an exaggerated physiologic jaundice pattern is likely. If hemolysis is found without ABO incompatibility, hematocrit, blood smear, and red blood cell defect tests [e.g., glucose-6-phosphate dehydrogenase (G6PD)] may be indicated. A sepsis evaluation is unnecessary if the only clinical finding is unconjugated hyperbilirubinemia. The direct bilirubin level should be checked if jaundice persists or cholestasis is suspected (light stool, dark urine, jaundice with a green tinge).

Treatment

Despite the trend of high TSB levels before treatment, earlier treatment is needed for those at risk of kernicterus (i.e., hemolysis, asphyxia, and prematurity). Jaundice during the first 24 hours of life requires prompt evaluation and consideration for exchange transfusion if hemolysis is found.

TSB ranges are recommended for starting phototherapy in healthy term newborns as follows: TSB of 12 to 15 mg/dL at 24 to 48 hours, 15 to 18 mg/dL at 48 to 72 hours, and 17 to 20 mg/dL at more than 72 hours.[8] Increasing or high TSB levels (i.e., 20 mg/dL at 24 to 48 hours, 25 mg/dL at more than 48 hours) require intensive (double or special lights) phototherapy. If very high TSB levels do not decline 1 to 2 mg/dL within 6 hours or higher levels are encountered (i.e., 25 mg/dL at 25 to 48 hours and 30 mg/dL at any time), exchange transfusion should be added. Phototherapy precautions include increasing fluids by 15 mg/kg/day, patching eyes, and monitoring for temperature instability. A transient rash, green stools, lethargy, irritability, and abdominal distention may occur. Phototherapy can be stopped when the TSB falls by 5 mg/dL or below 14 mg/dL.[7] A rebound rise

is uncommon. Home phototherapy (using a fiberoptic blanket) with uncomplicated jaundice and a reliable family allows breast-feeding and bonding to proceed with minimal interruption. If jaundice persists or bronze discoloration is noted, fractionate the bilirubin (i.e., direct) to search for cholestasis.

Breast-feeding is associated with elevated bilirubin levels beginning on the third day. More frequent feeding (i.e., 10 times in 24 hours without supplements unless milk production is low) reduces TSB levels. Breast-milk jaundice is a delayed, sometimes alarming, common form of jaundice. It begins after the third day, peaks by the end of the second week, and gradually resolves over 1 to 4 months. If the evaluation previously described reveals no pathologic cause, parental preference should strongly influence whether to breast-feed frequently (formula supplement if low output), begin phototherapy, or interrupt breast-feeding. Interruption of breast-feeding for 48 hours, while confirming the diagnosis with an abrupt decline in TSB, increases the risk of breast-feeding failure significantly and is usually unnecessary.

Hypoglycemia

Newborn blood glucose levels should be higher than 40 mg/dL. Hypoglycemia can occur without risk factors or symptoms. The most common symptoms are "jitteriness," hypothermia, poor feeding, apnea, apathy, abnormal cry, hypotonia, and seizures. A capillary glucose strip from a warmed heel allows screening of high-risk or symptomatic infants. Any value less than 45 mg/dL must be confirmed by venipuncture. Hypoglycemic injury is prevented by keeping newborns warm and initial monitoring every 30 minutes with early caloric support if high risk. Oral feeding can be attempted for levels more than 25 mg/dL. If symptomatic, a bolus of $D_{10}W$ (2 mL/kg) over 2 to 3 minutes is followed by an infusion of 8 mg/kg/min. The glucose strip is rechecked at 15 minutes and then hourly until three consecutive normal values occur.

Metabolic Disorders

Unexplained poor feeding, vomiting, lethargy, convulsion, or coma in a previously healthy newborn suggests an inborn error of metabolism even during the first few hours of life. After excluding hypoglycemia and hypocalcemia, plasma ammonia, bicarbonate, and pH should be checked. Early consultation and treatment avoids severe metabolic and neurologic disturbances.

Anemia

A central venous hematocrit less than 45% in newborns delivered after 34 weeks is often caused by blood loss and less often by hemolysis or congenital anemias. Careful review of the history, physical examination, red blood cell (RBC) indices, and peripheral smear can guide further evaluation. Coombs' test, reticulocyte count, and Kleihauer-Betke stain of maternal blood to look for fetomaternal transfusion may be needed. If the newborn is without compromise and has a hematocrit over 20%, observation is indicated. Shock requires repeated 5 mL/kg infusions over 5 minutes of crossmatched or O-negative blood until symptoms are alleviated. Severe hemolysis may require exchange transfusion.

Polycythemia

A hematocrit of more than 65% venous or 70% capillary may cause plethora, subsequent jaundice, and hyperviscosity. If the infant is symptomatic (lethargy, apnea, irritability, seizures, feeding difficulties, respiratory distress, cyanosis, hypoglycemia) and after confirming the hematocrit elevation, a partial exchange transfusion should be given to lower the hematocrit to 50%.

Birth Injuries

Head injuries include soft tissue swelling and bruising of the scalp resulting from vertex delivery (caput succedaneum), slow subperiosteal hemorrhage limited to the surface of one cranial bone that does not cross the midline or bruise (cephalohematoma), and skull fracture that requires treatment only if severely depressed. Clavicle fracture, the most common fracture, manifests as limited arm movement and crepitus over the injury. Immobilization of the affected arm and shoulder may be considered. This fracture often is undetected initially and may be found during the first outpatient visit.

Erb's palsy (neuritis of C5-C6 roots due to delivery trauma) causes arm adduction and internal rotation, elbow extension and pronation, and wrist flexion ("waiter's tip" posture). Five to nine percent have diaphragm paralysis. Early improvement or hand grasp suggests a favorable prognosis. Recovery is complete within 3 to 6 months. If no shoulder, arm, or clavicle fractures exist, the infant's sleeve can be pinned in a functional position for 1 week followed by gentle passive exercises.

Human Immunodeficiency Virus Infection in Neonates and Infants

Approximately 7000 women with HIV give birth annually in the United States. Without intervention, 1750 newly infected infants would be born every year. If currently recommended prevention practices are implemented, this number should decrease to somewhere between and 70 to 522 infants. Some have suggested that the best way to decrease this number even further is to prevent HIV transmission to fathers and mothers. The AIDS Clinical Trial Group (ACTG) protocol 076 demonstrated that if previously untreated HIV-positive pregnant women with CD4 counts >200/mm^3 are treated with zidovudine [ZDV or azido-thymidine (AZT)], the risk of vertical HIV transmission drops from 25.5% to 8.3%. Multidrug regimens along with scheduled cesarean section and avoidance of breast-feeding has been suggested to decrease the rate of transmission to 1%. However, research is still needed to assess the overall effect of multidrug regimens in pregnancy. Women should be offered counseling with an HIV expert because of the complex and varied treatment regimens, and considerations for their own health. Protocol 076 recommended that pregnant women should be started on oral ZDV (100 mg five times daily) as early as 14 weeks gestation. It is continued through delivery (loading dose

of 2 mg/kg over 1 hour and then continuous infusion of 1 mg/kg/hour), and given to the newborn during the first 6 weeks of life (2 mg/kg every 6 hours, beginning 8 to 12 hours after birth).[9] All pregnant women should be screened for HIV and those positive started on ZDV.[10]

In utero infection causes 30% to 50% of the cases of vertical transmission. These infants typically have a more virulent infection with laboratory evidence of infection at birth.[11] Most of the other cases of vertical transmission occur intrapartum through exposure to infected cervical and vaginal secretions. The rate of such transmission is almost doubled when delivery follows rupture of membranes of more than 4 hours duration. A large meta-analysis of cohort studies found that scheduled cesarean section prior to labor decreased the incidence of transmission by 50%.[12,13] All factors relating to the health of the mother, the infant, and the providers must be considered when making this decision. The use of the intrapartum and neonatal portions of protocol 076 significantly decreases transmission, even in those women who have not received antepartum ZDV or cesarean section.[14] Urging HIV positive mothers to use formula instead of breast milk can further decrease the chance of vertical transmission.[15]

Newborns of HIV-positive mothers who did not receive either antepartum or intrapartum ZDV should be started on the neonatal arm of the ACTG protocol 076 within 24 hours of birth. If a woman at high risk for acquiring HIV delivers with an unknown HIV status, the CDC recommends that both the mother and infant should be screened for HIV.[10] Infants whose mothers received multidrug therapies should be monitored more closely in the antepartum period.

Infant Diagnosis

It is imperative that infants infected with HIV be quickly identified to ensure early use of antiretroviral therapies and to prevent opportunistic infections. In the majority of infected infants, physical examination at birth is normal, making early identification more difficult. Presenting symptoms are often subtle and include failure to thrive, lymphadenopathy and hepatosplenomegaly, chronic or recurrent diarrhea, interstitial pneumonia, and persistent oral thrush. The diagnosis depends on laboratory testing. Any infant exhibiting any of the above symptoms who is born to a mother at high risk for HIV, or who exhibits any other signs of immunocompromise, should be tested. Certainly all infants born to HIV-positive mothers should also be tested. The initial screen should be the DNA polymerase chain reaction (PCR) test. If this is negative, it should be repeated at 2 weeks, 1 to 2 months, and 3 to 6 months. If at any point the PCR is positive, it should be confirmed by HIV culture as soon as possible. Treatment can be started while the culture is pending.[15,16]

Treatment of Infants

Due to the rapidly changing and complex nature of HIV treatment recommendations, management of the HIV-infected infant should be done by or in conjunction with a consultant. A detailed discussion of management will thus not be offered; however, a few general concepts should be kept in mind. Prevention of *Pneumocystis carinii* pneumonia (PCP) is one of

Table 17.1. **Approaches to Common Neonatal Anomalies**

Abnormality	Causes	Evaluation/treatment
Head		
Macrocephaly (head size >97%)	May be normal; hydrocephalus; genetic and metabolic disorders	Check for neurologic impairment; consider ultrasonography, head computed tomogram (CT)
Microcephaly (head size <3%)	Cerebral dysgenesis; prenatal insults; other syndromes; familial	Head CT or magnetic resonance imaging, maternal phenylalanine level
Large fontanels	Skeletal disorders; chromosomal anomalies; hypothyroidism; high intracranial pressure	Check for neurologic impairments
Small fontanels	Hyperthyroidism; microcephaly; craniosynostosis	Check for neurologic impairments
Craniotabes (softening of cranial bones giving a "ping-pong ball" sensation)	Prematurity; if local, benign bone demineralization; if generalized, syphilis or osteogenesis imperfecta	Should recalcify and harden over 3 months If persists, Venereal Disease Research Laboratory (VDRL); check for blue sclera and fractures
Eyes		
Abnormal red reflex ("white pupil")	50% of patients have cataracts	Ophthalmologic evaluation
Nasolacrimal duct obstruction (6% of newborns; overflow tearing or mucopurulent drainage; erythema)	Incomplete canalization of duct with residual membrane near nasal cavity; 96% resolve spontaneously by 1 year	Nasolacrimal massage tid; topical antibiotics for mucopurulent drainage; surgery at 9–12 months, earlier if severe
Ears		
Any significant ear anomaly and preauricular pits/fistulas		Check for hearing impairment and possible renal abnormalities
Mouth/palate		
Long philtrum, thin upper lip, small jaw, large tongue		Check for genetic abnormalities
Epstein's pearls (2–3 mm white papules on the gums or palate)	Keratogenous cysts	Spontaneous resolution in weeks; reassurance
Short lingual frenulum ("tongue-tie")	Normal	Clip if feeding impaired; tip of tongue notches when extruded or cannot touch upper gums
Cleft lip or palate	Isolated variant; some genetic anomalies	Feeding assessment; lip repair usually at 3 months, palate by 1 year; revision of repair at 4–5 years; speech therapy
Neck		
Fistulas, sinuses, or cysts midline or anterior to the sterno-cleidomastoid (SCM); may retract with swallow	Branchial cleft anomalies; thyroglossal duct cysts	Nonemergent surgical referral
Neck		
Cystic hygroma (soft mass of variable size in the neck or axilla)	Dilated lymphatic spaces (failure of drainage into jugular vein)	Semiurgent surgical referral as lesion can expand rapidly
Congenital torticollis (tilting of the infant's head due to SCM spasm)	Usually an isolated muscular defect from traumatic delivery; appears at 2 weeks	Early physical therapy usually successful in 2–3 months; ortho referral if persists
Skin		
Umbilical cord granuloma	Vascular, red/pink granulation tissue after cord separation	Apply silver nitrate 1–3 times protecting surrounding skin; excise if persists
Café-au-lait spots (flat, light brown macules usually <2 cm)	Consider neurofibromatosis if more than four spots larger than 5 mm	No treatment
Hemangiomas (often raised, red, vascular nodules, deeper lesions appear blue; usually <4 cm; onset during first 3–4 weeks, increases over 6–12 months)	Multiple lesions suggest possible dissemination involving internal organs	Most involute and disappear by 7–9 years of age; observe without treatment unless involving vital structures, ulceration or infection; evaluate further if multiple.
Mongolian spots (gray-blue plaques, up to several centimeters, often lumbosacral, may appear elsewhere)	Hyperpigmentation, seen in up to 70% of nonwhite infants	Benign; most fade over first year; document location since sometimes confused with abuse during infancy

(Table continues on next page)

Table 17.1. **Approaches to Common Neonatal Anomalies (*Continued*)**

Abnormality	Causes	Evaluation/treatment
Nevi (variably sized light to dark congenital; brown macules; some others appear later during infancy)	Congenital giant (>20 cm) may undergo malignant degeneration	No treatment needed, although some advise removal of congenital nevi at puberty; refer giant nevi for evaluation
Petechiae (normal only on head or upper body after vaginal births)	Infection or hematologic problem if abnormal	If abnormal, check CBC and look for signs of TORCH syndrome
Port-wine stains (permanent vascular macules)	Possible associated ocular or central nervous system (CNS) abnormalities	Cosmetic problem only, unless other abnormalities found
Subcutaneous fat necrosis (hard, purplish, defined areas on cheeks, back, buttocks, arms, or thighs, appearing during the first week)	Necrosis of fat from trauma or asphyxia	Spontaneous resolution over several weeks; rare complication of fluctuance or ulceration
Abdomen/gastrointestinal		
Mass	Genitourinary (GU) in 50% (either kidney or bladder)urinary	Emergent ultrasound (US) of urinary tract
Single umbilical artery	31% have other congenital defects	Careful clinical exam for other defects
Delayed passage of meconium (99% of healthy term neonates pass meconium within 24 hours)	Small bowel obstruction with bilious vomiting (atresias, malrotations, meconium ileus) or large bowel obstruction (Hirschsprung's, anorectal atresias, meconium plug syndrome)	Anal inspection and rectal exam; if distended, abdominal x-ray and consider contrast enema, anorectal manometry and rectal biopsy; vomiting or distention requires rapid surgical evaluation
Intestinal atresia (bilious vomiting with variable degrees of distention)	If duodenal, resorption of lumen occurred. If jejunoileal, mesenteric vascular injury	Nasogastric (NG) tube, lab, chest and supine/upright abdominal x-ray; contrast enema; surgery
Meconium ileus (distended at birth, x-ray with distended loops and bubbly picture of air/stool in right lower quadrant; absent air/fluid levels)	Abnormal meconium trapping resulting in small bowel obstruction; usually caused by cystic fibrosis	Supine/upright abdominal x-ray; treat with hyperosmolar gastrograffin enema (successful in two thirds), otherwise surgery; check sweat chloride test
Meconium plug syndrome (most common distal obstruction)	Inspissated colorectal meconium; diffuse gaseous distention of intestinal loops on x-ray; no air fluid levels)	Abdominal x-ray; contrast enema is diagnostic and often therapeutic; search for other causes if symptoms continue
Genitourinary tract		
Ambiguous genitalia (if gonads are palpable, likely to be male)	Virilization of genetic female (esp. congenital 21-hydroxylase deficiency) or undermasculinized male	Obtain karyotype and 17α-hydroxy-progesterone quickly; withhold diagnosis of sex until karyotype complete
Hypospadias (urethral opening proximal to tip of glans; may be associated chordee: abnormal penile curvature)	Isolated defect unless other GU anomalies present; 10–15% have first-degree relative with hypospadias	Avoid circumcision; repair 6–12 months of age by experienced surgeon; check for cryptorchidism and hernia; siblings at increased risk
Cryptorchidism (failure of testicular descent; 20% bilateral; long-term complications of infertility and cancer if left untreated)	May be normal: seen in 30 % of preterm, 4% of term; if bilateral, consider ambiguous genitalia; if hypospadias and bilateral, consider urologic or endocrine problems	Observe for descent by 6 months; if not, treatment by 1 year of age; if bilateral, obtain karyotype; if also hypospadias, do full urologic and endocrine evaluation
Hydrocele (scrotal swelling that transilluminates but does not reduce during the exam)	Persistence of processus vaginalis distally without communication to the abdominal cavity	If no hernia, most spontaneously resolve in 3–12 months; prompt surgical referral if hernia or increasing size; persistence beyond 1 year makes hernia likely
Inguinal hernia (inguinal bulge that extends toward or into the scrotum; larger with crying or straining)	Processus vaginalis persists and communicates with abdominal cavity	If reducible, prompt referral for surgery to avoid incarceration; if irreducible, emergent referral
Musculoskeletal		
Syndactyly (fusion of two or more digits)	Sporadic or autosomal dominant with varying expressivity	Depending on site, surgery between 6 and 18 months of age

(Table continues on next page)

Table 17.1. **Approaches to Common Neonatal Anomalies** *(Continued)*

Abnormality	Causes	Evaluation/treatment
Polydactyly (more than five digits)	Sporadic or autosomal dominant (e.g., 5th finger in blacks)	If no cartilage/bone, remove early, otherwise surgery at 6–18 months
Metatarsus adductus (forefoot supinated and adducted; may be flexible or rigid; ankle range of motion must be normal)	Hereditary "tendency," but often due to uterine crowding; 10% association with hip dysplasia requires careful exam	If flexible and overcorrects into abduction, no treatment; if corrects only to neutral, use corrective shoe for 4–6 weeks and reassess; if rigid, needs early casting
Talipes equinovarus (clubfoot; variably rigid foot, calf atrophy, hypoplasia of tibia, fibula, and foot bones)	Multifactorial with autosomal dominant component; 3% risk in sibs and 20% to 30% for offspring of affected parent	Anteroposterior (AP) and stress dorsiflexion lateral x-ray; early serial casting; if persists, surgery by 6–12 months (90% success rate)
Nervous system		
Spina bifida occulta (spinal defect with cutaneous signs: patch of abnormal hair, dimple, lipoma, hemangioma)	Nonfusion of posterior arches of spine; may be tethering of cord or sinus to spinal space with risk of infection; clinical exam for other defects	Examine for neurologic deficits; US to document defect if cutaneous signs; nonemergent referral to neurosurgeon if dermal sinus or tethering suspected; prompt referral if deficits present

the most important goals of HIV management. All infants between 6 weeks and 1 year of age either born to HIV-positive mothers or proved to be HIV infected should receive prophylaxis with 150 mg of trimethoprim and 750 mg of sulfamethoxazole/m²/day divided twice daily and given 3 days weekly. However, if later HIV infection can be reasonably excluded, PCP prophylaxis can be discontinued. Close attention should be paid to nutritional status. Development should be monitored closely so that physical or occupational therapy can be started in a timely manner if needed. Children should be monitored for signs and symptoms of neoplastic disease, as the effect of retroviral therapies on young children is yet unknown.[15,17] See Chapter 42 for additional information on management of the HIV-infected child.

Approaches to Common Neonatal Anomalies

Table 17.1 provides a brief overview of common anomalies encountered by those caring for newborns.

Guidelines for Early Hospital Discharge of the Newborn

Resurgence of kernicterus demonstrates the risk of early discharge in a changing health care environment. Careful assessment of medical risk and stability, completed education of parents on proper care and warning signs, and secured early medical follow-up are essential components of care prior to discharge between 6 and 24 hours. Examples of eligibility criteria are adequate prenatal care, uncomplicated and low-risk pregnancy and delivery, 5-minute Apgar score over 6, weight over 2500 g, gestational age more than 37 weeks, normal vital signs, stable medical condition including jaundice, completed physician examination, normal glucose, at least two successful feedings, voiding of urine, appropriate parent–newborn interaction, proper car seat, plans for completion of metabolic screening by 7 days of life, and ability of the parents to follow verbalized instructions. A home visit at 2 to 3 days of life by a physician or trained nurse improves infant assessment, early identification of problems, and ongoing educational efforts.

Infant Care

Well-Child Care and Normal Development

Well-infant visits, with an emphasis on answering parents' questions and providing anticipatory guidance, are critical during this period of rapid transitions. They facilitate the accommodation of the family to its newest member while building a relationship of trust with the physician. Cultural and socioeconomic issues, familial expectations and stresses, and an assessment of the infant's physical environment should be addressed, preferably starting prenatally. To allow early treatment of disabilities, each visit should include a systematic age-appropriate physical exam and assessment of fine and gross motor development, sensory function, language expression and comprehension, and social behavior. These visits also provide an opportunity to administer immunizations and obtain screening tests as discussed in Chapter 7. Performing this variety of tasks is simplified by the use of standardized forms.

Nutrition, Feeding, and Associated Problems

Future mothers typically decide by the second trimester of their pregnancy what nutrition, breast milk or formula, they will provide their newborns. Thus, whenever possible, discussion about the advantages and disadvantages of these two forms of nutrition should occur early in pregnancy.

Breast Milk

It is generally recognized that breast milk is the preferred form of sustenance for newborns and young infants due to its better digestibility and enhancement of infant immunity. Breastfeeding allows the infant to share the mother's immunity to the pathogens present in the community at any given time. It also results in significant reductions in the incidence of gastrointestinal infections and otitis media as well as perhaps other respiratory infections. Although two of the principal immunologic factors have their highest concentrations in the colostrum the immunologic protection increases with the duration of breast-feeding and is greatest for serious and persistent infections.[18,19] Considering costs of formula, visits to doctors offices, and hospital admissions, some suggest that it is much less expensive to breast-feed.[20]

Infection and Chemicals. Breast milk, unfortunately, can transmit pathogens from the mother to the infant. Thus in developed countries the presence of maternal HIV, septicemia, active tuberculosis, and typhoid fever is an absolute contraindication to breast-feeding while the presence of hepatitis B and cytomegalovirus are relative contraindications.

When seeking to explain any unexpected change in the behavior of a breast-fed infant, it is always important to examine the diet and drug history of the mother. Nicotine can cause infant irritability and reduces both the amount of milk produced and the letdown. Alcohol should be avoided for 1 to 2 hours prior to breast-feeding for each drink consumed. Marijuana is excreted for several hours after even occasional use and cocaine is excreted for 24 to 36 hours.[18]

Vitamin Supplementation. Vitamin D supplementation (400 IU) is needed in those mothers receiving little sunlight, and possibly those whose skin is darkly pigmented. Because the fluoride content of breast milk is low, the totally breast-fed baby may be supplemented with 0.25 mg of fluoride daily starting after 6 months of life. A full-term totally breast-fed infant should receive supplemental iron (2 mg/kg up to 15 mg/day) after 4 months of age and a preterm infant from birth.[18]

Supporting Breast-Feeding. Physician support is often critical to a mother's successfully breast-feeding. Prenatal visits provide an ideal opportunity for early encouragement. In addition to infant benefits, maternal health benefits should be discussed such as emotional impacts and reduced incidence of breast and ovarian cancer. Cultural and personal factors must be factored into decision making so that the patient is not pressured into a decision that may later result in failure and emotional disappointment.

After delivery, reassure mothers that it is rare not to be able to provide adequate milk for their infants and that infants often require 3 to 4 days to nurse effectively. Advise mothers that breast-fed infants often feed every 2 to 4 hours and that developing a feeding routine is often a compromise between the infant's spontaneous pattern and the mother's schedule. When problems arise the assistance of a lactation specialist can often be invaluable.

Formula

The vast majority of infants will thrive on cow's milk–based formula. Thus for those mothers who cannot breast-feed long-term, a good compromise may be to encourage breast-feeding for the initial few weeks after birth, and then to primarily use formula and breast-feed only a couple of times daily. In most cases such part-time breast-feeding can be accomplished as long as a nipple with a small hole is used so that the formula feeding more closely reproduces breast-feeding.

Differences between the brands of formula are generally insignificant. True infant intolerance to cow's milk–based formulas is unusual, and soy protein formulas are of value only if lactase intolerance is strongly suspected, such as after a prolonged episode of diarrhea. Even then a trial of cow's milk formula should be attempted again every 2 to 4 weeks since the intolerance is usually transient.

Because formulas do not contain fluoride, suggest the use of powdered forms mixed with fluoridated water. Low-iron formulas offer no advantages over regular iron fortification because constipation from iron is quite rare.

Advancing Infant Diet

Infants should remain on either breast milk or formula until 12 months of age because the introduction of whole cow's milk before this age increases the risk of occult gastrointestinal bleeding and iron deficiency anemia. At 12 months of age, a child should generally be placed on whole or 2% milk to provide the extra calories available from the milk fat, then gradually switched to skim milk by 2 or 3 years of age in those eating well (30% of calories from fat).

Introducing nonmilk foods into the diet prior to age 4 to 6 months neither benefits the infant nor increases the likelihood of the infant sleeping through the night. On the other hand, as infants approach 12 months of age, introducing such foods can avoid making the diet too protein-dense, especially if there is a focus on whole cereals, green vegetables, legumes, and fruits. This accustoms children at a young age to nutritionally balanced high-fiber diets.

Some generally accepted guidelines for introducing nonmilk foods are the following: separate the introduction of new foods by at least 3 days to more easily determine the cause of any food intolerance; start with easily digested foods such as cereals, especially rice, and yellow vegetables; postpone such potential allergens as citric fruits, wheat, and eggs until 9 to 12 months of age; and minimize the risk of airway obstruction by avoiding spongy foods (e.g., hot dogs and grapes) and foods with kernels (e.g., corn and nuts). Once a normal child is eating a balanced diet there is no need for supplemental vitamins and iron. Fluoride, though, should be supplemented if the supply in the water system is less than 0.6 ppm.

Obesity

The significance of being overweight as an infant is unclear. Three quarters of such infants become normal-weight adults and most obese adults are not obese as infants. However, when there is a genetic predisposition to obesity, especially if associated with a strong family history of cardiovascular disease, hypercholesterolemia, and diabetes, it is reasonable to encourage primary prevention. This can include breast-feeding and delaying introduction of solids as well as avoiding overfeeding by not using the bottle as a pacifier and using a small spoon to feed solids. However, restriction of fat prior to the age of 2 years can result in a failure to consume adequate calories and other nutrients.[21]

Colic

The syndrome of colic is defined by paroxysms of irritability, fussing, or crying with the infant seeming to be in

Table 17.2. **Approaches to Common Problems of the Infant**

HEENT (head, ears, eyes, nose, and throat)

Thrush (pearly white pseudomembranes on the oral mucosa). Causes: transmission from vaginal mucosa during delivery; contaminated fomites (nipples—both breast and bottle, toys, teething rings). Rx: clean fomites (boil bottle nipples, toys); oral nystatin, 200,000–500,000 U q4–6h until clear ×48 hours.

Nasolacrimal duct obstruction (see Table 17.1). Symptoms usually delayed until days to weeks after birth. Rx: nasolacrimal massage tid and cleansing of eyelids with warm water; topical antibiotics (sulfacetamide or gentamicin drops) for secondary conjunctivitis.

Strabismus (misalignment of eyes). Screen with corneal light reflex and cover test. Rx: ophthalmology referral for persistent deviation > several weeks or any deviation >4 months of age.

Hearing loss. Screening either mandatory after delivery or for those at risk: family history; congenital infection; craniofacial abnormalities; birth weight <1500 g; hyperbilirubinemia requiring exchange transfusion; severe depression at birth; bacterial meningitis. Screening: otoacoustic emissions testing or auditory brainstem response. Treatment by 6 months can greatly improve future language development.

Teething (painful gums secondary to eruption of teeth with irritability, drooling). Fever and other systemic effects not caused by teething. Rx: chewing on soft cloth, teething ring, dry toast hastens eruption; topical and systemic analgesia.

Skin problems

Circumcision. Elective procedure performed only on healthy, stable newborns using preferably a penile block. Contraindicated if any genital abnormalities. Advantages: decreased incidence of phimosis and urinary tract infection. Risks (small): hemorrhage; sepsis; amputation; urethral injury; removal of excessive foreskin with painful scarring. Risk of general anesthesia is added since it is often used after the neonatal period.

Diaper dermatitis (erythematous, scaly eruptions that may advance to papulovesicular lesions or erosions; may be patchy or confluent; genitocrural folds often spared). Due to reaction to overhydration of skin, friction, and/or prolonged contact with urine, feces, chemicals such as in diapers, and soaps. Rx: frequent changing of diapers; exposure to air; bland, protective topical ointment (petrolatum, zinc oxide) after each diaper change; advanced cases may require 1% hydrocortisone ointment.

Candidal superinfection (pronounced erythema with sharp margins, satellite lesions, involvement of genitocrural folds). Rx: topical antifungal; treat associated thrush.

Milia (superficial 1–2 mm inclusion cysts). Common on face and gingiva. Requires no Rx.

Miliaria (clear or erythematous papulovesicles in response to heat or overdressing; especially in flexural areas). Resolves with cooling.

Seborrheic dermatitis (most commonly greasy yellow scaling of scalp or dry white scaling of inguinal regions; may be more extensive). Rx: generally clears spontaneously; may require 1% hydrocortisone cream; mild antiseborrheic shampoos for scalp lesions; mineral oil with gentle brushing after 10 minutes for thick scalp crusts.

Atopic dermatitis (intensely pruritic, dry, scaly, erythematous patches). Acute lesions may weep. Typically involves face, neck hands, abdomen, and extensor surfaces of extremities. Genetic propensity with frequent subsequent development of allergic rhinitis and asthma. Consider evaluation for food and other allergens. Rx: mainstay is avoidance of irritants (temperature and humidity extremes, foods, chemicals) and drying of the skin (frequent bathing, soaps) with frequent application of lubricants (apply to damp skin after bathing); severe disease usually requires topical steroids; acute lesions may require 1:20 Burrow's solution and antihistamines (diphenhydramine, hydroxyzine).

Heart murmur

Innocent or functional (typically diminished with decreased cardiac output, i.e., standing).

Newborn murmur. Onset within first few days of life that resolves by 2–3 weeks of age. Typically soft, short, vibratory, grade I–II/VI early systolic murmur located at lower left sternal border that subsides with mild abdominal pressure.

Still's murmur. Most common murmur of early childhood. May start in infancy. Typically loudest midway between apex and left sternal border. Musical or vibratory, grade I–III early systolic murmur.

Pulmonary outflow ejection murmur. May be heard throughout childhood. Typically soft, short, systolic ejection murmur, grade I–II and localized to upper left sternal border.

Hemic murmur. Heard with increased cardiac output (fever, anemia, stress). Typically grade I–II high-pitched systolic ejection murmur heard best in aortic/pulmonic areas.

Pathologic or organic murmurs. Any diastolic murmur. Consider when a systolic murmur has one or more of the following: grade III or louder, persistent through much of systole, presence of a thrill, abnormality of second heart sound, or a gallop. Other ominous signs: congestive heart failure, cyanosis, tachycardia. Evaluation: chest x-ray (CXR), electrocardiogram (ECG), and if persistent or any distress then cardiology consult.

Gastrointestinal

Constipation (intestinal dysfunction in which the bowels are difficult or painful to evacuate). Associated failure to thrive, vomiting, moderate to tense abdominal distention, or blood without anal fissures requires ruling out organic disease (Hirschsprung's, celiac disease, hypothyroidism, structural defects, lead toxicity). Common causes are anal fissures, undernutrition, dehydration, excessive milk intake, and lack of bulk. Less common with breast-feeding. Rarely caused by iron-fortified cereals. Rx: in early infancy increase amount of fluid or add sugars (Maltsupex); later add juices (prune, apple) and other fruits, cereals, and vegetables; may add further artificial fiber (Citrocel); severe disease may require brief use of milk of magnesia (1–2 tsp), docusate sodium, and glycerin suppositories and when persistent requires ruling out of organic disease.

(Table continues on next page)

Table 17.2.

Gastroesophageal reflux. Vomiting noted in 95% by 6 weeks old, resolving in 60% by age 2. Associated growth delay in 60%, aspiration pneumonia in 30% of affected infants, esophagitis and hemoccult positive stool, chronic cough, wheezing. Consider cow's-milk allergy. Dx: mild cases confirmed by history and therapeutic trial. If more severe, esophageal pH probe and barium fluoroscopic esophagography. Endoscopy if esophagitis is suspected. Rx: position prone for neonates; elevate head of bed for older infants. Thickened feedings with cereal; acid suppression if esophagitis. If more severe, consider metoclopramide (side effects are common); surgery if medical therapy fails.

Pyloric stenosis (nonbilious vomiting immediately after feeding becoming progressively more projectile). 4:1 male:female preponderance. Onset 1 week to 5 months after birth (typically 3 weeks). May be intermittent. Dx: palpation of pyloric mass (typically 2 cm in length, olive shaped) that may be easier to palpate after vomiting; ultrasound preferred method to confirm difficult cases (90% sensitivity). Rx: surgery after rehydration.

Anemia

Improved nutrition has reduced incidence but infants remain at significant risk. Additional risk factors: low socioeconomic status, consumption of cow's milk prior to age 6 months, use of formula not iron fortified, low birth weight, prematurity. Effects: fatigue, apathy, impairment of growth, and decreased resistance to infection. Causes: iron deficiency most common (usually sufficient birth stores to prevent occurrence prior to age 4 months), sickle cell disease, thalassemia, lead toxicity. Screening: hemoglobin (Hgb) or hematocrit (Hct) between ages 6 and 9 months (some recommend only for infants with risk factors). Rx: if microcytic give trial of iron (elemental iron, Feosol, 3–6 mg/kg/day); if not microcytic or unresponsive to iron consider other causes (family history, environment).

Sleep disturbances (when the infant's sleeping pattern disrupts the parent's sleep).

Seventy percent of infants can sleep through the night by age 3 months. Most 6-month-olds no longer require nighttime feeding. Screening: a sudden change in sleeping pattern should prompt a search for new stresses, physical (infection, esophageal reflux, etc.) or emotional (new surroundings or household members, etc.). Rx: establish realistic parental expectations (consider the natural sleeping patterns of the infant); allow the infant awakening at night to learn how to fall asleep by himself (keep bedtime rituals simple and put the infant in his bed awake; do not respond to infant's first cry; keep interactions during the night short and simple; provide a security object for older infants); slowly change undesirable sleeping patterns (move bedtime hour up and awaken infant earlier in the morning; decrease daytime napping).

---

pain and difficult to console without apparent cause. Episodes typically last for a total of more than 3 hours a day but rarely occur daily. They most often occur in the afternoon or evening and between the ages of 2 weeks and 4 months. Because half of all infants can present with this picture, the other factor that seems to define these babies is that one or both parents have difficulty dealing with this facet of the infant's behavior. Parental behavior, however, does not seem to be a cause of the colic, only a response. Before infants are given the diagnosis of colic, they should have a thorough physical exam to identify an acute processes such as infection or intussusception, especially if the onset is sudden.

Treatment of Colic

A principal focus is on reassuring parents that the process is a common, self-limited one and providing them with some basic measures to try. These include providing motion as in a mechanical swing, rocker, or papoose, or exposure to a steady hum such as in a car or a vacuum cleaner; snug bundling; warmth such as a warm water bottle on the stomach; and burping well and frequently during and after feeding. Often the physician's most important roles are providing support over time and legitimizing the parents' sense of frustration, and even anger, with the situation. The physician should also encourage parents to help each other with caring for the infant, and whenever possible to enlist the help of others so that they have an opportunity to take a break. When all else fails, parents may need permission to periodically shut the door and let the infant "cry it out."[22]

Infants with more prolonged, severe bouts of crying, especially if intermittent throughout the day, may have at least a partial organic cause. If such a child seems to pass a lot of gas with relief, some physicians prescribe simethicone (Mylicon), although studies have not revealed benefit. Constipation should be treated as it would in other infants (Table 17.2). Frequent vomiting, especially if accompanied by poor feeding and failure to thrive, suggests gastroesophageal reflux. If a trial of antacids is not effective, further workup is indicated. With signs of allergy (eczema, asthma) or a strong family history of allergies, milk allergy should be considered. Finally, although anticholinergic agents have been advocated in the past, their efficacy probably has more to do with their sedating effect than any specific effect on the gastrointestinal muscles. Because they have a potential for severe side effects, their use is discouraged.

Failure to Thrive

Failure to thrive (FTT) is a failure to grow at an appropriate rate, with weight crossing two major channels on the recently updated National Center for Health Statistics (NCHS) growth curve or falling below the 5th percentile for age and sex after correcting for parents' stature, prematurity, growth retardation at birth, and race.[23,24] Because of a high prevalence of FTT in urban and rural areas (5–10%) and significant morbidity (developmental delay, permanent cognitive deficits, behavioral disorders, short stature, chronic physical problems, and medical illness), it is advisable to begin following any child whose weight declines across one NCHS channel or if a parent suspects a growth problem.[25]

Diagnosis

Although the consequences of malnutrition sometimes obscure the original causes, a thorough history and physical examination detect most organic, behavioral, family, and environmental problems that contribute to FTT. This initial assessment should include (1) prior records including growth charts and prenatal history (prematurity, growth retardation); (2) nutrition (diet, behavior); (3) development (cognitive, motor, behavioral, emotional); (4) social context (parental knowledge, family dysfunction, drug abuse, social support, isolation); and (5) environment (poverty, shelter, toxic exposures to lead or pesticides). Diagnostic studies can follow in a stepwise manner, with step 2 studies chosen based on history, physical exam, and severity.[26]

Step 1: CBC, fasting chemistry panel, electrolytes, urinalysis, lead level

Step 2: thyroid, stool (culture, ova and parasites, fat), sweat chloride, tuberculosis, HIV, skeletal survey, renal studies

Treatment

Hospitalization is indicated when there is (1) severe malnutrition; (2) suspected abuse or neglect; (3) a need to observe parent–child interaction or a documented problem with interaction; (4) family dysfunction (e.g., barriers to follow-up, disorganization, depression, chemical dependence, violence); (5) need for further diagnostic workup; or (6) failure of outpatient treatment. Outpatient treatment may be appropriate when FTT is moderate (infant's weight is more than 60% the average weight for age *and* more than 85% average for height). Weekly follow-up may be lengthened after sustained weight gain. Collaborative, interdisciplinary treatment involves the parents, physician, social worker, nutritionist, and psychologist. It implements one or more of the following strategies: (1) treating organic factors first; (2) implementing a written nutritional plan for meals and snacks with caloric intake 1.5 to 2.0 times normal; (3) beginning a vitamin supplement; (4) supporting parents with mealtime observation and coaching; (5) treating specific family problems that interfere with the family's ability to care for the infant (misunderstanding, depression, drug abuse); (5) enlisting social support (family, friends, church); (6) mobilizing community and economic resources for the family; (7) establishing continuity of care and access to the treatment team; and (8) promoting parental competence.

Fever

In children under 3 years of age, if a source for the fever cannot be found, or if otitis media is found, 3% to 11% have occult bacteremia. The risk is even higher in infants under the age of 3 months who have an 8.6 % risk of having a serious bacterial infection.[27,28] Timely evaluation prevents treatment delays. Clinicians must counsel parents carefully and avoid unnecessary testing because the sepsis evaluation creates marked parental anxiety (e.g., 30% believing their infant is dying). In an attempt to provide a framework for evaluation of these children, a set of guidelines was published in *Pedi-*

atrics in 1993 that presents a reasonable outline of how to approach this vexing problem.[27] The basic elements of the guidelines, with some variations proposed by others are as follows[28-30]:

Toxic-Appearing Infants

Children with signs of sepsis (e.g., lethargy, poor perfusion, hypoventilation, hyperventilation, cyanosis) should be hospitalized for a full septic workup with blood urine and spinal fluid cultures. If no source is initially found, a chest x-ray is indicated for infants with high fever and leukocytosis. They should then be placed on antibiotics pending culture results. In those younger than 1 to 2 months of age, antibiotic choices should follow the recommendations made earlier in this chapter for neonates. Older children are most frequently treated with either cefotaxime, 50 mg/kg, IV, q8h, or ceftriaxone, 100 mg/kg, IV, q24h.

Low-Risk Infants

The clinical criteria defining this group are the following: previously healthy, nontoxic appearance, no focal bacterial infection (except otitis media), and ability to be closely monitored by caregivers. Laboratory criteria are WBC count of 5,000 to 15,000/mm^3 (<1500 bands/mm^3); normal urinalysis [<5 WBCs/high power field (hpf)]; and when diarrhea present, <5 WBCs/hpf in stool. Most would recommend obtaining the urine sample by catheterization.

Younger Than 29 Days Old

The guidelines recommend admitting all such infants with rectal temperatures >38°C (100.4°F) for the septic workup described earlier in this chapter for neonates, without or without antibiotic coverage, pending culture results. Recent research confirms serious bacterial infection can be missed in nontoxic, febrile infants who meet the above low-risk laboratory criteria.[30] However, some still would recommend performing all or part of the same workup as an outpatient because the probability of a serious bacterial infection is only 0.2% among infants meeting the criteria defining low risk.[28] Automatic admission of all febrile infants has significant cost implications, and risk of iatrogenic complications.[31] If treated as an outpatient, all infants must be reevaluated within 24 hours. If blood cultures were performed and were positive, these infants should be admitted for sepsis evaluation and parenteral antibiotics. If a urine culture was obtained and was positive, and there is a persistent fever, the infant should be admitted for septic evaluation and parenteral antibiotics; however, outpatient treatment with oral antibiotics can be used if the patient is afebrile and well.

Infants 29 to 90 Days Old (Rectal Temperatures >38°C)

These infants can be managed as outpatients. Some recommend culturing both urine and blood, others only one of these, and some add a lumbar puncture and analysis. If there is any suspicion of bacteremia, most would recommend getting at least a blood culture and giving a dose of parenteral antibiotics, most often IM ceftriaxone, 50 mg/kg (maximum of 1 g). These infants should be reevaluated within 24 hours, and positive cultures should be treated as for outpatients <28 days old; however, blood cultures positive for *Streptococcus pneumoniae,* known to be sensitive to penicillin, can be treated with oral penicillin or amoxicillin. Otherwise treatment should be based on clinical appearance at the time of reevaluation.

Infants 3 to 36 Months Old

There is no need to screen for occult bacteremia in infants with temperatures <39°C (102.2°F). However, those infants with persistent fever for more than 2 to 3 days, worsening clinical appearance, or temperatures ≥39°C without an apparent source of the fever, other than otitis media, constitute a higher risk group. They should be evaluated with a WBC count. If the count is ≥15,000/mm^3, a blood culture is indicated, as well as injection of a parenteral antibiotic (most commonly IM ceftriaxone, 50 mg/kg up to a maximum of 1 g), while the culture is pending. In addition, a urine sample by catheter should be cultured from all boys <6 months of age or girls <2 years of age who are treated with antibiotics. This higher risk group should be reevaluated and treated as described above for outpatient infants 28 to 90 days old.

Sudden Infant Death Syndrome

Sudden infant death syndrome (SIDS) is the leading cause of death in infants past the neonatal period, peaking at age 2 months. Characterized by being unexpected and without apparent cause, despite thorough postmortem examination, it represents a collection of etiologies all involving an abnormality of cardiorespiratory regulation. This divergence of etiologies has so far frustrated attempts to develop reliable screening and prevention methods. Many have recommended using electronic home monitoring of apnea and bradycardia for those infants judged to be at high risk, including siblings of SIDS casualties, infants who had apparent life-threatening episodes, and those with the other risk factors cited below. However, such monitors have generally had little effect on reducing the incidence of SIDS in part because of frequent poor parent compliance with their use. When employed, they can be discontinued if there are no episodes of true apnea for 16 consecutive weeks. The use of event recorders with the monitors has made identifying apneic episodes more objective and seems to allow shorter periods of monitoring.

At this time the greatest impact on reducing the incidence of SIDS involves targeting those risk factors known to be associated with a two- to threefold increase in the risk of SIDS. These include maternal smoking or drug use, poor prenatal care, complications of delivery and prematurity, shared sleep surface, soft sleeping surface, bedding that can cover the face, and prone (stomach) sleeping position. Infants who have no medical contraindications should be placed for sleep in the supine (back) or side position. There are no controlled studies demonstrating efficacy, but retrospective studies have showed a strong correlation between sleeping position and SIDS.[32–34]

Other Common Problems of the Infant

Table 17.2 provides short summaries of other frequent problems of infancy and their management.

Family and Community Issues

Child Care

More than 50% of infants under 1 year of age have parents who work outside the home. The physician can encourage parents to use paid and unpaid leave to maximize time with their child during the first year of life and to select child care carefully. A quality child-care setting supports normal infant development, but many settings fail to protect health and safety or provide adequate developmental stimulation. Children in day care are 2 to 18 times more likely to contract certain infectious disease including enteric pathogens, respiratory pathogens, and herpesvirus infections.[26] Parents can find quality programs in both private homes and child care centers; nonprofit centers generally provide higher quality care than for-profit centers.[35] Parents can compare several programs by making scheduled and unscheduled visits to observe the emotional atmosphere and sanitation. The optimal adult/child ratio before 1 year of age is 1:3 and should not exceed 1:4. The day-care provider should have and carefully follow written policies to minimize the spread of infectious disease. Staff should (1) be trained in child development; (2) be paid sufficiently to minimize turnover; (3) enjoy their interactions with children, respond positively to children's accomplishments, and attend quickly when a child is upset; and (4) wash their hands after diapering and before food preparation, use disposable tissue for wiping runny noses, and routinely wash changing tables. After enrollment, encourage parents to continue occasional unscheduled visits and to investigate sudden changes in their child's behavior such as withdrawal, anxiety, or agitation.

Families and Infants: Risks and Resources

Normal infant development is promoted by fostering a family's strengths and resources but is threatened by individual, family, and environmental risk factors (see Chapter 4). Infant risk factors include chronic illness, physical handicap, low birth weight, growth failure, and developmental delay. Family factors include physical or sexual abuse, family violence, neglect, parental depression, chemical dependence, and chronic illness. Environmental factors include poverty and environmental toxins such as lead. Table 17.3 outlines systematic approach for identifying some common resources and risks for early family development. When possible, screening for such risk factors should start prenatally. Early intervention programs promote healthy development and prevent developmental delay even when infants and families face serious medical, psychosocial, and environmental obstacles. Effective early intervention has five elements:

1. *Crisis intervention.* Take quick action to treat immediate threats to safety (e.g., family violence, physical or sexual abuse, severe neglect).
2. *Family-centered care.* Collaborate with parents and avoid labeling a child or parent. Describe the challenge the family faces and the strengths and resources they have to assist them. Teach parents about the unique needs and abil-

Table 17.3. **Assessing Resources and Risks for Early Family Development**

Concept	Interview questions
Social support	Do you have at least one friend or relative you can turn to for support and advice?
	Do you work, attend school, or participate in a religious community?
Housing	Do you have any concerns about housing?
Child care	Do you have any concerns about child care?
Transportation	Do you have any concerns about transportation?
Finances	Will you have any problems paying for food and clothing? Vitamins and medications? Health care?
Safety	During the past year, has anyone you know:
	Made you afraid for your safety?
	Pushed, kicked, slapped, hit, or otherwise hurt you?
	Forced sexual or physical contact?
	Tried to control your activities, your friends, or other parts of your life?
	Do you have any guns in your house?
	Do you have any concerns about safety or violence in your neighborhood?
	Do you use a seat belt when you ride in a car?
	Do you use an infant or car seat for each infant and toddler in your family?
	Do your children always use a seat belt?
Personal health	In general, how healthy do you consider yourself? (Excellent, good, fair, or poor)
STD and HIV Risk	Have you ever had herpes, gonorrhea, chlamydia, trichomonas, genital warts, or a pelvic infection?
	Have you had two or more sexual partners in the past year?
Emotions	During the last 30 days, how much of the time have you felt downhearted and blue? (Very little, sometimes, often, most of the time)
Alcohol and drugs	Have your parents had any problems with alcohol or drugs?
	Does your partner have any problems with alcohol or drugs?
	Have you had any problems in the past with alcohol or drugs?
	During the past 30 days, on how many days did you have at least one drink of alcohol?
	During the past 30 days, on how many days did you have five or more drinks of alcohol in a row, that is, within a couple of hours?
Tobacco	Does anyone in your home smoke tobacco?
	Do you currently smoke or use tobacco?

HIV = human immunodeficiency virus; STD = sexually transmitted disease.

ities of their infant. Be optimistic and adapt your interventions to the family's culture.

3. *Social support.* Help families identify supportive family, friends, church, or mutual-help groups.
4. *Community resources.* Help parents mobilize community resources to treat specific needs of the infant and family (e.g., specialized day care, parenting classes).
5. *Ecologic model of intervention.* Assess the individual infant, family, and physical environment and customize your intervention to use the family's specific strengths. Continue to coordinate the involvement of multiple professionals and ensure that the overall plan remains suitable for the family. Serve as an advocate and catalyst to ensure the treatment team addresses unanswered questions.

Chaotic families disrupted by family violence, sexual abuse, or chemical dependence may be difficult to work with, as these same problems tend to disrupt the doctor–patient relationship. It is important that family-centered care be respectful, culturally sensitive, and nonstigmatizing. The physician can take a leadership role by helping the team and family focus on the developmental potential of the infant and family.

Partner Violence (Also See Chapter 28)

One in five pregnant women experience partner violence (domestic violence) during their pregnancy, with higher rates among adolescent girls.[36] Partner violence has a well-documented negative impact on both maternal and infant health. Pregnant women who are being abused are more likely to delay seeking prenatal care, and experience higher rates of depression, anxiety, suicide attempts, alcohol or other drug abuse, and tobacco smoking. Abused women are more likely to experience pregnancy that is unwanted. Intentional injury, often the result of domestic violence, is one of the leading causes of death among pregnant women. Although the health impact of partner violence on infants needs additional study, current research shows that infants born to abused women are more likely to have low birth weight and experience premature birth. Family physicians can play a valuable role by implementing standard screening for partner violence among all pregnant patients. The most effective strategy involves screening at multiple times during the pregnancy, using written questions as well as patient interview, and using questions with demonstrated reliability and validity.

Infants of Substance-Abusing Mothers

Drug abuse during pregnancy significantly increases the risk for low birth weight, growth retardation, microcephaly, and other anomalies. Fetal alcohol syndrome includes the well-described triad of growth retardation before or after birth, nervous system abnormalities, and midfacial hypoplasia. Cardiac and renal systems may also be affected. Infants are typically irritable, have difficulty feeding, and show disorganized sleep patterns. The full syndrome occurs with heavy drinking throughout pregnancy but lower levels of exposure also affect development. The specific effects of prenatal exposure to cocaine and other drugs of abuse are less well described. Exposure to one substance is often confounded by abuse of other drugs and social and environmental factors (e.g., diet and prenatal care) that correlate with chemical dependence and are known to affect infant outcome.[37]

Parents should be encouraged to seek treatment for chemical dependence at any point during pregnancy or after birth. When maternal drug abuse is suspected, infants should be evaluated and treated for acute withdrawal symptoms and then referred for developmental assessment and early intervention.

Adolescent Parents

Adolescent parents are often perceived as high risk, when in fact adolescent girls who have access to appropriate resources, including pre- and postnatal care, give birth to healthy infants and raise children who are well adjusted. True risk factors are poverty, lack of access to health care, family violence, and substance abuse. Adolescents who grow up in a family with violence, sexual abuse, or chemical dependence initiate sexual intercourse at an earlier age than the general population and experience a higher rate of pregnancy.

When working with adolescent parents, (1) expect a positive outcome while offering respect and dignity; (2) encourage family support, if appropriate, including support of the father and his family; (3) encourage use of community resources (child care, parenting classes, education, early intervention programs); (4) initiate family planning early during the pregnancy; and (5) encourage continued education and delay of the birth of another child (delay by as little as 6 months and completion of high school improves long-term social and economic outcome).

Public Policy

Federal law PL99-457 encourages states to develop programs that identify and provide services to children at risk from birth to age 3 years. By statute these early intervention programs are to be individualized, family-centered, and involve the primary care physician. Implementation varies from state to state, making it important for physicians to familiarize themselves with local programs and resources.

References

1. Zaichkin J, Kattwinkel J, eds. International guidelines for neonatal resuscitation: an excerpt from the guidelines 2000 for cardiopulmonary resuscitation and emergency cardiovascular care: international consensus on science. Pediatrics 2000;106(3):1–16.
2. Ambuel B, Mazzone M. Breaking bad news and discussing death. Prim Care 2001;28(2):249–67.
3. Krahn GL, Hallum A, Kime C. Are there good ways to give 'bad news'? Pediatrics 1993;91(3):579–82.
4. Sharp MC, Strauss RP, Lorch SC. Communicating medical bad news: parents' experiences and preferences. J Pediatr 1992;121: 539–46.
5. Centers for Disease Control and Prevention. Prevention of perinatal group B streptococcal disease: a public health perspective. MMWR 1996;45(RR-7):1–24.
6. Klein JO. Bacterial sepsis and meningitis. In: Remington JS, Klein JO, eds. Infectious diseases of the fetus and newborn, 6th ed. Philadelphia: WB Saunders, 2001.
7. Moyer VA, Ahn C, Sneed S. Accuracy of clinical judgment in neonatal jaundice. Arch Pediatr Adolesc Med 2000;154:391–4.
8. Dennery PA, Seidman DS, Stevenson DK. Neonatal hyperbilirubinemia. N Engl J Med 2001;344(8):581–90.
9. Centers for Disease Control and Prevention. Zidovudine for the prevention of HIV transmission from mother to infant. MMWR 1994;43:285–8.
10. Centers for Disease Control and Prevention. U.S. Public Health Service recommendations for human immunodeficiency virus counseling and voluntary testing for pregnant women. MMWR 1995;44(RR-7):3–11.
11. Davis SF, Byers RH, Lindegren ML, et al. Prevalence and incidence of vertically acquired HIV infecton in the United States. JAMA 1995;247:952.
12. Landesman SH, Kalish LA, Burns DN, et al. Obstetrical factors and the transmission of human immunodeficiency virus type 1 from mother to child. N Engl J Med 1996;334:1617–23.
13. The International Perinatal HIV group. The mode of delivery and the risk of vertical transmission of human immunodeficiency virus type 1—a meta-analysis of 15 prospective cohort studies. N Engl J Med 1999;340(13):977–87.
14. Centers for Disease Control and Prevention. Public Health Service task force recommendations for the use of antiretroviral drugs in pregnant women infected with HIV-1 for maternal health and reducing perinatal HIV-1 transmission in the United states. MMWR 1998;47(RR-2):16–17.
15. Chadwick EG, Yogev R. Pediatric AIDS. Pediatr Clin North Am 1995;42:969–92.
16. Luzuriaga K, Sullivan JL. DNA polymerase chain reaction for the diagnosis of vertical HIV infection. JAMA1996;275:1360–1.
17. Mofenson, Lynne M. Care and counseling of HIV-infected pregnant women to reduce perinatal HIV transmission. UpToDate (http://www.uptodate.com), May 2, 2000.
18. Lawrence PR. Breast milk: best source of nutrition for term and preterm infants. Pediatr Clin North Am 1994;41:925–42.
19. Dewey KG, Heinig MJ, Nommsen-Rivers LA. Differences in morbidity between breast-fed and formula-fed infants. J Pediatr 1995;126:696–702.
20. Montgomery AM. Breastfeeding and postpartum maternal care. Prim Care 2000;27(1):237–50.
21. Hardy SC, Kleinman RE. Fat and cholesterol in the diet of infants and young children: implications for growth, development, and long-term health. J Pediatr 1994;125:S69–75.
22. Treem WR. Infant colic: a pediatric gastroenterologist's perspective. Pediatr Clin North Am 1994;41:1121–38.
23. Drotar D. Failure to thrive (growth deficiency). In: Roberts MC, ed. Handbook of pediatric psychology. New York: Guilford, 1995;516–36.
24. Leung AKC, Robson WLM, Fagan JE. Assessment of the child with failure to thrive. Am Fam Physician 1993;48:1432–8.
25. Ambuel JP, Harris B. Failure to thrive: a study of failure to grow in height or weight. Ohio State Med J 1963;59:997–1001.
26. Behrman RE, Kliegman RM, Jenson HB. Nelson textbook of pediatrics, 16th ed. St. Louis: WB Saunders, 2000.
27. Baraff LJ, Bass JW, Fleisher GR, et al. Practice guideline for the management of infants and children 0 to 36 months of age with fever without source. Pediatrics 1993;92:1–12.
28. Grubb NS, Lyle S, Brodie JH, et al. Management of infants and children 0 to 36 months of age with fever without a source. J Am Board Fam Pract 1995;8:114–9.

29. Young PC. The management of febrile infants by primary-care pediatricians in Utah: comparison with published practice guidelines. Pediatrics 1995;95:623–7.

30. Baker D. Evaluation and management of infants with fever. Pediatr Clin North Am 1999;46(6):1061–72.

31. Slater M, Krug S. Evaluation of the infant with fever without source: an evidence based approach. Emerg Med Clin North Am 1999;17(1):97–126, viii–ix.

32. Freed GE, Steinshneider A, Glassman M, Winn K. Sudden infant death syndrome prevention and an understanding of selected clinical issues. Pediatr Clin North Am 1994;41:967–89.

33. AAP Task Force on Infant Positioning and SIDS. Positioning and SIDS. Pediatrics 1992;89(6Pt1):1120–6.

34. Kemp JS, Unger B, Wilkins D, et al. Unsafe sleep practices and an analysis of bed-sharing among infants dying suddenly and unexpectedly: results of a four-year population based, death-scene investigation study of SIDS and related deaths. Pediatrics 2000;106(3):E41.

35. Phillips DA, Howes C, Whitebook M. The social policy context of child care: effects on quality. Am J Community Psychol 1992;20(1):25–52.

36. Hamberger LK, Ambuel B. Spousal abuse in pregnancy. Prim Care Clin North Am. 2001; 3:203–24.

37. Singer L, Farkos K, Kliegman R. Childhood medical and behavioral consequences of maternal cocaine use. J Pediatr Psychol 1992;17:389–406.

18
Communicable Diseases of Children

Dennis J. Baumgardner

The communicable diseases of childhood are a source of significant disruption for the family and a particular challenge to the family physician. Although most of these illnesses are self-limited and without significant sequelae, the socioeconomic impact due to time lost from school (and work), costs of medical visits and remedies, and parental anxiety are enormous. Distressed parents must be treated with sensitivity, patience, and respect for their judgment, as they have often agonized for hours prior to calling the physician. They are usually greatly reassured when given a specific diagnosis and an explanation of the natural history of even the most minor syndrome. It is essential to differentiate serious from benign disorders promptly (e.g., acute epiglottitis versus spasmodic croup), recognize serious complications of common illnesses (e.g., varicella encephalitis), and recognize febrile viral syndromes (e.g., herpangina), thereby avoiding antibiotic misuse. To this end, differential diagnosis is the primary emphasis of this chapter.

Common Cold

An infant or child with "a cold," as described by the parent or caretaker, may have one of several viral-like respiratory syndromes.[1,2] A "bad cold" may represent simply that, or it may be a specific, sometimes serious, disorder such as bronchiolitis. A common cold is defined as an acute viral disease consisting of nasal stuffiness, sneezing, coryza, throat irritation, and minimal to no fever. Routine laboratory studies are unnecessary, and the required treatment is minimal. If signs and symptoms deviate from these criteria, the history, physical examination, and appropriate laboratory studies often define one of several other more specific respiratory syndromes, as summarized in Table 18.1, which also outlines management of the common cold and these particular respiratory syndromes.

Key points are that (1) a significant pharyngitis is not present with most colds; (2) most colds are 3- to 7-day illnesses (except for lingering cough and coryza for up to 2 weeks); and (3) abrupt worsening of symptoms or development of high fever mandates prompt reevaluation. Tonsillopharyngitis (hemolytic streptococci, Epstein-Barr virus, adenovirus, *Corynebacterium*) usually manifests as a sore throat, fever, erythema of the tonsils and pharynx with swelling and edema, often headache, and cervical adenitis. In addition to entities listed in Table 18.1, colds must also be differentiated from allergic rhinitis, asthma, nasal or respiratory tree foreign bodies, adenoiditis, otitis media, sinusitis, diphtheria, influenza, bronchitis, respiratory mycoplasmal and chlamydial infections, measles prodrome, and pneumonia.[2] Specific viral diagnosis (culture or rapid diagnostic testing) is generally unnecessary for the common cold but may be useful to confirm specific syndromes such as pharyngoconjunctival fever or when used for the first few cases of an outbreak of similar illnesses, especially to confirm agents such as influenza A or B or the respiratory syncytial virus.

Croup

Croup is a spectrum of viral respiratory syndromes characterized by varying degrees of inspiratory stridor, cough, and hoarseness due to laryngeal-region obstruction. These syndromes include laryngitis (older children and adults) and nonrecurrent and spasmodic croup (diseases of young children caused predominantly by parainfluenza 1 viruses). Prompt diagnosis and assessment of the severity of croup-like illnesses are essential. Table 18.1 lists salient features of croup syndromes and the often-similar life-threatening illnesses acute epiglottitis and bacterial tracheitis (a superinfection).[1–10] In addition, laryngeal diphtheria must always be considered in conjunction with croup; it is differentiated by immunization history, relatively slow progression of the disease, greater degree of hoarseness, and pharyngeal signs of diphtheria.[2,6,7]

Respiratory Syncytial Virus

The respiratory syncytial virus (RSV) is the major cause of bronchiolitis and pneumonia in young children, with outbreaks occurring, with regularity, yearly during the winter and early spring. An abrupt increase in bronchiolitis and pediatric pneumonia in a community suggests RSV infection, which may be confirmed by performing viral cultures or rapid diagnostic tests in initial cases. Naturally acquired immunity to RSV is incomplete, and repeated infections are common, although the primary encounter generally results in the most severe illness. Bronchiolitis must be differentiated from asthma, an often-difficult task. Asthma is favored by the following factors: age over 1 year, atopic family history, repeated attacks, sudden onset without prodrome, and a prompt response to β-agonists (see Chapter 83).[9,10]

The common respiratory viruses vary in pathogenesis, with signs and symptoms of rhinovirus, coronavirus, and respiratory syncytial virus infections resulting largely from the host response. Influenza and adenoviruses can lyse infected cells and cause inflammation by direct tissue damage. RSV, influenza, parainfluenza, rhinovirus, adenovirus, and others can exacerbate asthma. Current investigations are exploring the ability of childhood RSV and adenovirus infection to cause asthma or chronic obstructive lung disease later in life, perhaps in concert with cigarette smoke and host genetic factors.[11,12]

Acute Parotid or Cervical Swelling

Parotid gland enlargement results in visible swelling distributed fairly evenly above and below the angle of the jaw; the swelling of acute cervical adenitis remains below the jaw. Elevated serum amylase may differentiate parotitis from cervical adenitis, abscess, or other mass but is not specific for mumps. Exudation of pus is seen with suppurative parotitis, which may be caused by *Staphylococcus, Streptococcus, Haemophilus influenzae,* or other bacteria. Other causes of acute parotitis include viruses—influenza, parainfluenza, Coxsackie, enterocytopathogenic human orphan virus (ECHO), Epstein-Barr, cytomegalovirus (CMV), herpes, human immunodeficiency virus (HIV), lymphocytic choriomeningitis—and certain drugs.[2,13] Juvenile recurrent parotitis is a childhood disease of unknown etiology typified by recurrent attacks of acute unilateral or bilateral parotid swelling with pain, fever, malaise, and sometimes purulent exudate.[13]

Acute unilateral cervical adenitis[2,14] in children is usually caused by β-hemolytic streptococci or *Staphylococcus aureus,* and it generally is a result of spread from local infections of the head, neck, or teeth. Usual findings are a large, tender, unilateral cervical mass, with or without overlying erythema, fever, and leukocytosis. The diagnosis may be made on clinical grounds, but needle aspiration of the inflamed node for Gram and acid-fast stains and cultures is often useful. A skin test for tuberculosis should be considered. Complications may include node suppuration or bacteremia.

Initial empiric antibiotic therapy is oral dicloxacillin, cephalexin, or amoxicillin/clavulanic acid (Augmentin). Incision and drainage should generally be performed for fluctuant or pointing nodes. Close follow-up is mandatory. Causes of bilateral acute cervical adenitis are infectious mononucleosis, tularemia, and diphtheria. Subacute disease may be caused by nonspecific viral pharyngitis, β-hemolytic streptococci, cat-scratch fever, mycobacteria, and fungi.[2,14]

Mumps

Mumps virus infects only humans and causes a systemic illness, which may serve as a prototype for other systemic viral illnesses. It is spread primarily by respiratory droplets. The usual incubation period is 16 to 18 days (range 12–25 days). The period of communicability ranges from 7 days before swelling to 9 days after. The disease is most common during late winter and spring in North America, where a few thousand cases still occur each year. Mumps is predominantly a disease of school-age children.[1,15,16]

Clinical Presentations and Diagnosis

Approximately 30% of infections are subclinical. The classic symptoms are bilateral or unilateral parotid gland swelling (present for up to 10 days) and fever up to 40°C (104°F) lasting 1 to 6 days. Parotitis may be preceded by several days of nonspecific symptoms including malaise, fever, headache, myalgias, anorexia, and, rarely, a rash. Other salivary glands may be swollen as well. The clinical diagnosis is made after observation of typical signs and symptoms in patients with outbreak-associated disease or known mumps exposure; however, diagnostic testing for measles should be done for 2 or more days of parotitis without other obvious cause. Mumps virus may be isolated from throat washings, urine, cerebrospinal fluid (CSF), and other bodily fluids. A variety of serologic tests are available.[1,15,16]

Serious sequelae may occur without observable parotitis. Meningeal signs are present in about 10% of cases, but meningoencephalitis is rare.[1] Most encephalitides are characterized by fever, vomiting, meningismus, headaches, and sometimes seizures, and the CSF shows lymphocytosis.[17] Most patients experience full recovery, but persistent sequelae include paralysis, seizures, cranial nerve palsies, and hydrocephalus.[15] Other mumps-related neurologic sequelae may occur. Hearing should be tested following mumps, as loss may occur even in the absence of encephalitis.

Mumps orchitis[18] is rarely seen in prepubertal boys but occurs in up to 35% of adolescents. It is generally unilateral and follows parotitis (if present) by 4 to 8 days (up to 6 weeks); the average duration is 7 to 10 days. Symptoms and signs include gradual testicular pain and swelling and often fever. Epididymitis or reactive hydrocele may occur. Impaired fertility occurs in 13% of cases, but complete sterility is infrequent.

A self-limited monoarticular or migratory polyarthritis may occur 1 to 3 weeks after parotitis (if present). Fever is often present along with variable elevations of the erythrocyte sedimentation rate (ESR).[19,20] Other rare complications of mumps include miscarriage, thyroiditis, nephritis, pancreatitis, myocarditis, mastitis, ataxia and other systemic manifestations.[1,15]

Management and Prevention

Treatment of viral parotitis, including mumps, is supportive and may include analgesics/antipyretics, fluids, and rest. Bed

Table 18.1. **Selected Respiratory Tract Syndromes in Children**[1,2]

Syndrome	Usual etiologic agents	Typical clinical presentation
Common cold[2,3]	Viral agents: rhino-, corona-, para-influenza, respiratory syncytial (RSV); adeno-, influenza; occasional: entero-, Coxsackie-, reo-; *Mycoplasma pneumoniae*	*Children:* Throat irritation, nasal stuffiness; then sneezing, clear rhinorrhea; followed in 1–3 days by more purulent rhinorrhea, nasal obstruction, subjective sore throat. May have malaise, myalgias, chilly feelings, headache, anorexia, mild fever, cough. *Nasopharyngitis:* Same as above plus objective evidence of pharyngitis. *Infants:* Coryza, often nasal congestion, irritability, restlessness. More often febrile than children. May have feeding/sleep disturbance, vomiting, diarrhea.
Pharyngoconjunctival fever[5]	Adenoviruses	Abrupt onset of fever, pharyngitis, conjunctivitis (less common if unassociated with swimming); often headache, anorexia, cervical adenopathy, adenoid hypertrophy, eye discomfort, flushed face. May have malaise, myalgias, gastrointestinal symptoms, migratory palpebral erythema. May persist 2 weeks.
Herpangina	Coxsackie A and B, and echoviruses ? Herpes simplex virus	Sudden onset of fever up to 41.1°C (106°F) followed by 1–14 small papular to vesicular to ulcerative lesions on erythematous base on anterior tonsillar pillars, soft palate, uvula, tonsils, posterior buccal mucosa. May have anorexia, drooling, sore throat, coryza, headache, abdominal/back pain, vomiting, diarrhea.
Pertussis (whooping cough)	Toxicogenic strains of *Bordetella pertussis* (whooping cough syndrome can be caused by *B. parapertussis, B. bronchiseptica, C. trachomatis, C. pneumoniae, M. pneumoniae,* adenoviruses)	Catarrhal stage: mild upper respiratory symptoms with cough; can progress to paroxysmal state: severe bursts of cough with inspiratory whoop followed by emesis. Mild or no fever. Whoop may be absent in older children or <6 months old. Apnea common in those <6 months old. Duration of uncomplicated cases: 6–10 weeks.
Laryngotracheitis (nonrecurrent croup)[6,7]	Parainfluenza virus types 1–3; influenza virus, adenovirus, RSV, measles; *Mycoplasma pneumoniae*	Most common ages 3 months to 3 years; male: female, 1.5:1; prodrome (2–5 days) of mild fever, rhinorrhea, malaise, sore throat, cough; then onset of barking seal-like (croupy) cough, gradually increasing inspiratory stridor, fever up to 40.6°C (105°F), hoarseness, mildly inflamed pharynx. Wheezing if laryngotracheobronchitis. Duration: 2–7 days.
Spasmodic croup[6]	Same as nonrecurrent croup	Same ages as nonrecurrent croup; male/female 6:1. Minimal to no prodrome. Sudden nocturnal onset of croupy cough, history dyspnea and inspiratory stridor. No fever. Often family or history of prior attacks and/or allergy/asthma history. Duration: 2–4 hours/episode.

Diagnosis	Management	Complications	Prevention
Clinical. Viral cultures or diagnostic tests not routinely warranted. Rule out tonsillo-pharyngitis (see text).	Increased fluids, saltwater nose drops/sprays and/or increased humidification; dextromethorphan or codeine cough suppressant at bedtime in children if cough disturbs sleep. Warm saltwater gargles and/or judicious use of antiseptic/anesthetic throat sprays/lozenges if nasopharyngitis. Consider ibuprofen or acetaminophen if significant fever or aches, although acetaminophen and aspirin may increase rhinovirus symptoms and prolong viral shedding.[4] Efficacy of echinacea and other herbals is unproved. Studies on zinc lozenges are mixed. New antivirals being studied.[3]	Secondary infections: otitis media, acute sinusitis, bacterial adenoiditis, pharyngitis, pneumonia; rarely: meningitis, encephalitis if young infant/immunocompromised (adenovirus).	Good hand-washing. Isolation of patients impractical. Crowd/contact avoidance if susceptible to complications.
Clinical. For specific diagnosis: conjunctival/pharyngeal viral culture; rapid antigen tests; paired serology.	Same as nasopharyngitis. *Avoid* steroid-containing ophthalmic preparations.	Superficial keratitis; secondary infections: sinusitis, otitis media, bacterial conjunctivitis.	Adequate pool chlorination. Exclude ill persons from pools ≥2 weeks after recovery. Good hand-washing.
Clinical. For specific etiology: viral culture of lesions, throat or rectum.	Fluids, supportive care. Useful local treatment of oral lesions: mixture of equal parts of viscous lidocaine 2% (Xylocaine), diphenhydramine (Benadryl) elixir, aluminum/magnesium hydroxide (antacid); four drops to lesions prior to feeding up to five times/day (dispense 6 mL if infant).	Rarely: myocarditis, meningitis, encephalitis.	General preventative measures not necessary. Avoid unnecessary exposure to known cases. Good hand-washing and hygiene.
Nasopharyngeal culture on special media (notify Lab in advance). Many false-negative cultures. Serology problematic. New tests being researched.	Supportive care. Hospitalize infants and those with severe disease. Erythromycin 40–50 mg/kg/day PO in four divided doses (maximum 2 g/day) for 14 days may ameliorate disease if started in catarrhal stage; thereafter limits spread to others. (Trimethoprim/sulfa, newer macrolides unproved alternative.)	Severe disease in infants. Pneumonia, seizures, encephalopathy. Case-fatality rate 0.5% in <6-month-olds in U.S.	Respiratory isolation: for 5 days after initiation of erythromycin (3 weeks after onset of paroxysms if untreated). Prophylaxis: same 14 day antibiotic regimen as for treatment for household, day care, and other close contacts of all ages. Immunization: universal, usually given as DPT vaccine.[1]
Clinical. Correct diagnosis essential. Funneling of tracheal lumen (steeple sign) on frontal x-ray most consistent finding, but nonspecific, and often not present.	Humidified air (oxygen if needed based on oximetry). Severe: dexamethasone 0.6 mg/kg IM; nebulized epinephrine (racemic epinephrine 2.25% or L-epinephrine 1:1000) 0.25 or 0.5 mL in 2–3 mL normal saline (anticipate rebound stridor); hospitalize unless improvement sustained for 2–3 hours, reliable follow-up. Moderate: dexamethasone 0.15–0.6 mg/kg PO (most cost-effective choice) or IM or one or more doses of nebulized budesonide 2 mg; consider epinephrine. Mild: close parental observation; consider nebulized budesonide.	Severe airway obstruction requiring intubation (uncommon), rare: respiratory failure, pulmonary edema, pneumothorax/mediastinum. Laryngotracheopneumonitis. Bacterial tracheitis.	No specific recommendations.
Clinical. Correct diagnosis essential.	Avoid overtreatment! Humidification. Mild sedative at bedtime to prevent further attacks if certain of diagnosis. May need to be treated as above if cannot promptly differentiate from nonrecurrent croup.	Nonspecific, similar to common cold.	No specific recommendations.

(Table continues on next page)

Table 18.1. **Selected Respiratory Tract Syndromes in Children**[1,2] (*Continued*)

Syndrome	Usual etiologic agents	Typical clinical presentation
Acute epiglottitis[7]	*Haemophilus influenzae* type b; rarely: staphylococci, streptococci, others	Typically 3–8 years old (less often <1 year, or adult). Prodrome uncommon. Abrupt onset and rapid progression of fever, marked apprehension, variable degrees of respiratory distress. No cough. May have sore throat, dysphagia, drooling, delirium, stridor, choking sensation. Looks toxic, has cherry-red epiglottis, is in a sitting forward position with protruding chin/tongue; leukocytosis with left shift. (If <2 years, may appear like croup at first.)
Bacterial tracheitis[7,8]	*Staphylococcus aureus, Moraxella catarrhalis,* streptococci, *H. influenzae,* others	Combined symptoms of croup and epiglottis. Slow or rapid clinical progression following croup-like onset; high fever, toxicity, stridor, bandemia.
Bronchiolitis[9,10]	RSV (up to 75%), adenovirus, Para-influenza- and influenza viruses, rhinovirus, mumps, *Mycoplasma pneumoniae*	Age ≤2 years (especially ≤6 months) prodrome of coryza, fever to 40°C (104°F), gradually deepening cough (may be paroxysmal and induce emesis, no whoop); then dyspnea, tachypnea, prolonged expiration, chest wall retractions, wheezing and/or rales/rhonchi (apnea possible in young infants). Chest x-ray: hyperinflation, multiple interstitial infiltrates.

rest and medications have not been shown to prevent mumps orchitis, but rest, scrotal elevation, ice packs, and antiinflammatory medications may ease scrotal symptoms.[18]

Mumps patients should have respiratory isolation and be excluded from school or day care until all manifestations have cleared. This period lasts 9 days after the onset of parotid swelling.[1] Mumps immune globulin is of no value. Mumps vaccine[1,15] does not prevent infection following known exposure but may be given in this setting to protect against subsequent exposures. Live mumps vaccine is usually given in a two-step regimen with measles and rubella vaccines (MMR). Outbreaks may occur despite high vaccination rates.[16]

Kawasaki Disease

Kawasaki disease (mucocutaneous lymph node syndrome) is an acute vasculitis that primarily affects infants and young children.[21–24] It must be included in the differential diagnosis of fever, cervical adenitis, acute exanthems, and other mucocutaneous diseases. The etiology is unknown, but is likely infectious, perhaps involving bacterial superantigens. There are no known socioeconomic or climatic risk factors and no

evidence of person-to-person spread. Most cases occur in children younger than 5 years; it is rare under 6 months, and the male/female ratio is 1.4:1.0. It is worldwide and most prevalent in persons of Oriental descent.

Clinical Presentation and Diagnosis

Kawasaki disease is diagnosed on the basis of 5 days or more of fever *and* at least four of the following principal clinical features: (1) changes in peripheral extremities (acute: erythema and edema of hands/feet; convalescent: membranous desquamation of fingertips); (2) polymorphous exanthem; (3) bilateral, painless, nonexudative conjunctival injection; (4) changes in lips and oral cavity, such as erythema and cracking of lips, strawberry tongue, diffuse injection of oral and pharyngeal mucosa; and (5) acute, nonpurulent cervical lymphadenopathy (≥1.5 cm in diameter), usually unilateral.[20,21] Patients with features of Kawasaki disease who do not fulfill the criteria should be considered to have it if coronary artery disease is detected by echocardiography or coronary angiography. Young children particularly may have atypical disease (not fulfilling all criteria). A high index of suspicion must be used to avoid delayed

Diagnosis	Management	Complications	Prevention
Clinical features plus either enlarged epiglottis (thumb sign) on slightly extended lateral neck x-ray, or experienced, controlled view of epiglottis with intubation standby. Epiglottic and blood cultures for retrospective confirmation. Direct antigen test for *H. influenzae* of blood and urine may be helpful.	Advanced planning/rapid diagnosis. Intensive care. Endotracheal/nasotracheal intubation. Ceftriaxone (Rocephin) or cefotaxime (Claforan) intravenously if *H. influenza*; appropriate empiric antibiotics if other agents suspected. (Racemic epinephrine, corticosteroids *not* indicated.)	Abrupt airway obstruction with risk of death. Extra-epiglottic metastatic infection rare, despite bacteremia.	*H. influenzae* type b vaccine (has reduced incidence). Rifampin prophylaxis for *all* nonpregnant household contacts (if *H. influenzae*) with at least one contact. Day-care: give if ≥two invasive cases over 60-day period. Dosage 20 mg/kg (maximum 600 mg) daily by mouth ×4 days.[1]
Direct laryngoscopy and bronchoscopy. Usually normal epiglottis but subglottic narrowing, purulent tracheal secretions. Positive tracheal cultures.	Rapid bronchoscopy/diagnosis. Intensive care. Endotracheal intubation or tracheostomy frequently required. Antibiotics (empirical choice vancomycin/ceftriaxone).	Respiratory arrest, sepsis, tracheal damage. Toxic shock syndrome if staph (rare)	For *H. influenzae* type b, see above.
Clinical and epidemiologic grounds (see text). Viral culture and/or rapid antigen tests for RSV.	Supportive care, hydration, oxygen, respiratory monitoring. Individualize treatment. Minimal to no benefit from bronchodilating agents; epinephrine aerosols may be more beneficial than albuterol. Corticosteroids of no clear benefit.	Apnea/respiratory failure most likely first 48–72 hours after onset of dyspnea. Bronchospasm. Respiratory abnormalities later in life still being investigated. Association of RSV with otitis media, SIDS, CNS disorders, myocarditis, heart block.	Contact isolation for young children/infants. Large droplet precautions, cohort nursing, careful hand-washing and eye/nose goggles in the hospital. Breast-feeding seems to lower incidence. Avoid second-hand smoke. RSV immunoglobulin for prophylaxis of high-risk populations.[1]

diagnosis. A typical case[21,22] usually begins with fever up to 40°C (104°) for 4 to 5 days to 4 weeks, the onset of which is followed shortly by bilateral conjunctival injection. A fairly generalized morbilliform or urticaria-like rash appears within 5 days of illness, characterized by perineal area desquamation and erythema of the lips, pharynx, tongue, and hands and feet (with induration). Finger and toe desquamation usually begins 10 to 20 days after onset of fever. Clinical reexacerbations may occur, and skin peeling may recur for several years.

Other noncardiac signs and symptoms that may be present, by system, include the following[21,22]: (1) gastrointestinal: vomiting, diarrhea, abdominal pain, gallbladder hydrops, ileus, mild jaundice, or transaminase level elevation; (2) blood: elevated ESR, positive C-reactive protein, leukocytosis with left shift, mild anemia, thrombocytosis (after 2–3 weeks); (3) urinary: sterile pyuria, proteinuria; (4) skin: transverse furrows of fingernails during convalescence, peripheral gangrene; (5) respiratory: cough, rhinorrhea, pulmonary infiltrate; (6) musculoskeletal: arthralgias, arthritis; (7) neurologic: aseptic meningitis, irritability, facial palsy; (8) sensory: hearing loss, tympanitis, uveitis.

Cardiovascular Complications

Early in the disease, signs of myocarditis become apparent in 25% of patients and include tachycardia, gallop rhythm, electrocardiogram (ECG) changes, pericardial effusion, and mitral or aortic valve insufficiency. Heart failure or shock can occur. The major feature affecting the otherwise excellent prognosis for Kawasaki disease is coronary artery involvement. Coronary dilatation may be noted as early as 6 days to 4 weeks after the onset of fever. Frank coronary artery aneurysms may occur and can be identified by skilled echocardiography in most cases. Fortunately, most aneurysms resolve within 1 to 2 years.[21–23]

Management

Goals of management are control of the acute inflammatory process and prevention of coronary artery involvement (which may include empiric treatment of possible cases). Aspirin (80–100 mg/kg/day in four divided doses) is initiated once the diagnosis is tentatively made. A single infusion of intravenous gamma globulin (2 g/kg) is given, and a repeat dose should be considered if fever is persistent. After resolution of fever and other inflammatory signs, aspirin is continued at a single daily dose of 3 to 5 mg/kg/day for its antiplatelet effect. It may be discontinued at 6 to 8 weeks if no coronary involvement is present. Aspirin is continued at 3 to 5 mg/kg/day indefinitely if coronary involvement is present. Dipyridamole (Persantine) is used if the patient is aspirin intolerant, and added to aspirin in selected cases of coronary involvement.[21,22]

An echocardiogram is obtained as soon as the diagnosis of Kawasaki disease is suspected and repeated at 2 to 3 weeks and at 6 to 8 weeks if initially negative. All patients with significant coronary artery disease are followed initially and subsequently in conjunction with a cardiovascular team experienced in the treatment of Kawasaki disease complications. Guidelines for comprehensive follow-up are based on risk level.[23] The overall prognosis is good. Those with large aneurysms or coronary artery obstruction are the most at risk.

Viral Exanthems

Many viruses produce exanthems in children. Like mumps (discussed above), many of these systemic illnesses are subclinical or occasionally produce significant and varied sequelae. The major entities and their management are summarized in Table 18.2.[24–32] The diagnosis is largely clinical, but some overlap does occur (e.g., mild forms of measles resembling other exanthems and roseola-like illnesses caused by enteroviruses and other agents). Laboratory tests that may be helpful include (1) serology for measles and rubella; (2) rubella culture; (3) immunoglobulin M (IgM) titers for parvovirus B19; (4) Tzanck smear, direct immunofluorescence, serology, or culture for varicella-zoster, herpes, and other viruses.[1,25]

Other childhood viral exanthems,[25] with and without fever,

Table 18.2. **Major Exanthem Producing Viral Diseases in Childhood[24,25]**

Disease	Agent	Epidemiology: incubation period	Transmission	Period of contagion	Rash: description	Distribution of rash
Measles (rubeola)[26]	Measles virus (paramyxovirus)	8–12 days until symptoms; avg. 14 days until rash	Direct contact with infectious droplets; airborne spread	3–5 days before rash to 4 days after	Purplish-red, maculopapular, blotchy	Generalized after distal spread from hairline, will include palms/soles
Rubella (German measles)	Rubella virus (togavirus)	14–23 days	Direct or droplet nasopharyngeal secretion contact	7 days before rash to 14 days after (up to 1 year if congenital)	Diffuse, discrete, reddish-pink, macular	Starts on face, spreads distally to trunk and extremities
Roseola (exanthem subitum)[28,29]	Human herpesvirus 6B and 7	5–15 days (mean of 9–10 days) for human herpes virus 6B	Horizontally by saliva; 95% of cases are 6 months–3 years old	Unknown (probably maximal during febrile phase)	Rose-pink macules and papules	Starts on trunk, spreads to head and extremities

include the maculopapular, petechial, purpuric, or vesicular exanthems of enterovirus and adenovirus infections. Hand-foot-mouth disease (usually Coxsackie virus), presents as macules and vesicles of the hands and feet following a prodrome, in association with oral vesicles and ulcers. A papular purpuric gloves and socks syndrome is caused by parvovirus B19, Coxsackie, and other viruses, and a variety of skin manifestations are associated with parvovirus B19.[24,30,31] A unilateral laterothoracic (eczematous or scarlatiniform) exanthem has been described and is presumably of viral origin.[24] A variety of infections produce symmetric, flat-topped erythematous papules of the face, buttocks, and extremities (Gianotti-Crosti syndrome) in young children. Similarly, a number of viruses, particularly rubella and parvovirus, may cause the STAR complex (*s*ore throat, elevated *t*emperature, *a*rthritis, and pruritic urticarial *r*ash).[33] Zoster, characterized by vesicles and bullae on an erythematous base in dermatomal distribution, may occur in children of all ages following acquisition of the varicella-zoster virus (see Chapter 116). Viral exanthems must be differentiated from bacterial (e.g., scarlet fever), rickettsial, and parasitic infections; the rash of mononucleosis, particularly following amoxicillin, drug and toxin-mediated eruptions; and other dermatologic disorders (see Chapters 38, 115, 116).

Viral Gastroenteritis

Viral gastroenteritis is the most common identifiable cause of acute childhood diarrhea in the United States, with rotavirus the most frequent agent in young children. Annual rotavirus epidemics begin in Mexico during late fall and progress systemat-

Duration of rash	Clinical presentation: fever	Other symptoms	Course	Management	Complications	Congenital infection	Prevention
4–7 days	Moderate to high, 5 days or more	Conjunctivitis, coryza, cough, Koplik's spots (white spots on red oral mucosa opposite first/second molars).	Fever, cough, conjunctivitis starts first; rash appears on days 3–7; mild, modified course seen if partial passive immunity; atypical if older vaccine used; severe, may lack rash if immunocompromised.[27]	Supportive. Vitamin A if 6 months to 2 years old hospitalized with complications, or if >6 months with risk factors or malnutrition.[1]	Otitis media, croup, bronchopneumonia, diarrhea, encephalitis, subacute sclerosing panencephalitis, hearing loss, thrombocytopenic purpura, others.	Preterm labor, miscarriage, low birth weight.	Live attenuated measles vaccine usually given as MMR. Recommendations for special situations available.[1] For exposed susceptibles: measles vaccine; consider immune globulin (IG) 0.25 ml/kg/M for normal hosts (within 6 days), 0.5 mL/kg if immunocompromised.[1]
3–4 days	Mild	Headache, malaise, coryza; post-auricular sub-occipital, posterior cervical adenopathy; polyarthralgia (arthritis).	Starts with adenopathy and malaise; fever and rash begin on day 3.	Supportive.	Encephalitis, thrombocytopenia.	Risk of fetal infection and congenital rubella syndrome (fetal death, prematurity, congenital defects).	Live rubella vaccine usually given as MMR.
Hours to days	High, continuous up to 40.6°C (105.1 °F)	Coryza, diarrhea, red pharyngeal papules, otitis media, cough, lymphadenopathy; WBC count normal or low.	Abrupt fever and irritability for 3–7 days; rash starts with resolution of fever (rash may be absent)	Supportive, control of fever consider ganciclovir if severe and immunocompromised	Seizures, encephalitis, thrombocytopenia; virus may persist, then reactivate; in immunosuppressed may cause fever, hepatitis, pneumonia, bone marrow suppression.	Rare intrauterine or perinatal transmission postulated; no anomalies reported.	None.

Table 18.2. **Major Exanthem Producing Viral Diseases in Childhood**[24,25] *(Continued)*

Disease	Agent	Epidemiology: incubation period	Transmission	Period of contagion	Rash: description	Distribution of rash
Erythema infectiosum (fifth disease)[30,31]	Parvovirus B-19	4–21 days	Presumed respiratory secretions and blood; school/day care outbreaks occur (attack rates up to 50% in households)	Before rash appears (≥7 days after illness if aplastic crisis)	Intense erythema of cheeks (perhaps ears) with circumoral sparing ("slapped cheeks") often followed in 1 day by symmetric, reticulated red maculopapular rash	Body rash starts on extremities (not palm/ soles), spreading centrally or caudally (may be atypical/ rubelliform)
Chickenpox	Varicella-zoster virus (a herpes-virus)	10–22 days	Direct contact with lesions or airborne droplets	1–2 days before rash to 5 days after (and for duration of vesicles)	Scattered erythematous macules that vesiculate, rupture and crust (often all types of lesions seen at presentation).	Progressive, diffuse, includes scalp

ically across the continent, reaching the Northeast by spring. Nosocomial and day-care outbreaks are common. Although rotavirus infections occur most often in children 6 months to 2 years of age, all ages are affected, including one third of parents of affected children (see Chapter 94). The virus lyses enterocytes of the upper jejunal villi, which frequently induces a secondary lactose intolerance of up to 3 weeks' duration. As with most viral causes of gastroenteritis, the resulting diarrhea is usually watery and nonbloody, and fever, if present, is mild. Three days of vomiting usually precedes or accompanies 3 to 10 days of diarrhea, which may result in considerable dehydration. Fever and abdominal pain may also occur.[1,34–36]

Norwalk virus causes community and common source outbreaks in school-age and older children and adults. Symptoms last 12 to 60 hours with nausea (predominant symptom), vomiting, and diarrhea followed in up to half of the children by fever, chills, headache, myalgias, and malaise. Adenovirus type 40 and 41 infections peak in children younger than 2 years of age and cause a 5- to 12-day rotavirus-like illness in which diarrhea predominates.[1,35]

Astrovirus and caliciviruses other than Norwalk virus occasionally cause a milder rotavirus-like illness. Respiratory symptoms often occur in conjunction with gastroenteritis viruses, but it is usually coincidental.[35]

Duration of rash	Clinical presentation: fever	Other symptoms	Course	Management	Complications	Congenital infection	Prevention
Cheeks: 1–4 days Body rash: fluctuation with environmental changes for weeks	Mild or none	Arthralgias/arthritis, may be prolonged[33]; may have mild respiratory symptoms without rash; may be asymptomatic or atypical.	Rash and other symptoms jointly may follow by 7–10 days prodrome of fever, headache, malaise, myalgias, sore throat, coryza.	Supportive. Consider IV immunoglobulins if hematologic complications or chronic infection in immunodeficient patients.	Encephalitis, hepatitis, others. Chronic anemia in immunodeficient patients; aplastic crisis if chronic hemolytic anemia (often fever, malaise, myalgias without rash).	Fetal hydrops and death: risk if proven maternal infection (<20 weeks' gestation) <10%; risk from prenatal exposure 1–3%. Anomalies not associated.	Good hygiene and hand washing. Routine occupational exclusion of pregnant women not recommended (avoid aplastic cases).
Several days (may be chronic in AIDS)	Mild or none	Moderate to intense pruritus, mucous membrane lesions, arthritis, thrombocytopenia, hepatitis	May have mild constitutional prodrome. Rash, fever, other symptoms appear concurrently.	Supportive. Avoid salicylates and corticosteroids. Symptomatic relief for pruritus (antihistamines, calamine, colloidal oatmeal baths). IV acyclovir if immunocompromised. Oral acyclovir 20 mg/kg (max. 800 mg) four times daily for 5 days reduces fever, lesions, constitutional symptoms if started within 24 hours of rash,[32] but may be best reserved for ≥12 years or high risk.[1] Local treatment for oral lesions as for herpangina (Table 1).	Otitis media, Reye syndrome, meningitis, encephalitis, glomerulonephritis, cerebellar ataxia, transverse myelitis, pneumonia, bacterial superinfection, including predisposition to life-threatening invasive group A β-hemolytic streptococcal infections.	Maternal infection <20–28 weeks' gestation may yield congenital anomalies. Maternal infection within 5 days of delivery may yield severe neonatal disease.	Varicella vaccine at 12–18 months old; catch-up immunization by 12 years if no history of chickenpox. Varicella-zoster immune globulin (VZIG) for all susceptible exposed persons at risk for progressive disease— follow guidelines[1]; postexposure vaccine if susceptible but not high risk.

Diagnosis

When infants and children are seen in the office with mild symptoms and historical and physical findings consistent with one of the above viral syndromes, no special diagnostic tests are indicated. Certain historical factors (e.g., travel, exposure, or drugs) suggest other nonviral etiologies. Bloody diarrhea suggests invasive enteric bacteria, progressive *Escherichia coli* 0157:H7, pseudomembranous colitis (*Entamoeba*), or even Crohn's disease in an adolescent. Stool cultures should be reserved for patients with historical evidence of bacterial infection, high fever, blood or mucus in the stool, fecal leukocytes, or immune deficiency. Ova and parasite examinations, including *Cryptosporid-*

ium and *Cyclospora*, are done if historical evidence or prolonged diarrhea is present. Rapid tests are available for *Giardia* and *Cryptosporidium*. Rapid viral diagnosis by commercial antigen detection kits is available for rotavirus and adenovirus. Paired serology and emerging antigen detection tests may be used for other viruses as well. Viral tests are probably most useful for confirming the etiology early during outbreaks, for severe cases, and for suspected disease at unusual ages or seasons.[1,35,36]

Aside from diagnostic clues, the physical examination focuses on estimation of the hydration and hemodynamic state (mucous membrane moisture, tears, skin turgor, capillary refill time) and fontanel, orthostatic, or mental status changes. Significantly dehydrated children (10% or greater body-weight loss), especially infants, should be hospitalized for aggressive intravenous therapy, along with those with severe illness or electrolyte abnormalities.[34,36]

Management

Children without vomiting or dehydration may simply continue an age-appropriate diet emphasizing complex carbohydrates, lean meats, fruits, vegetables, and yogurt. Additionally, oral rehydration solution 10 mL/kg may be given for each diarrheal stool. Outpatient management of viral diarrhea with dehydration includes oral rehydration solution, 50 mL/kg for mild dehydration (3–5% body-weight loss), or 100 mL/kg for moderate (6–9% body weight loss), *plus* replacement of estimated ongoing fluid losses, given over four hours. Hydration and illness status is then reassessed.

Vomiting is not a contraindication to oral rehydration (use small, frequent administration). Breast-feeding infants may be managed by continuing breast-feeding, and supplementing with oral rehydration solution. Age-appropriate diet as described above should be resumed once dehydration is corrected and emesis resolves. Some experts choose lactose-free formula for the first 2 to 3 weeks, whereas others advocate this practice only if there is evidence of secondary lactose intolerance such as exacerbation of diarrhea with reintroduction of lactose containing foods, particularly if acid range stool pH and stool-reducing substances of 0.5% or greater are documented.

Rehydration with clear liquids such as soft drinks, commercial sports drinks, gelatin water, and apple juice is not recommended due to the inappropriately high carbohydrate content and osmolality. Caffeine, plain water, tea, and excessive use of soups (high-sodium content) must be avoided.

There is no evidence that one oral rehydration solution is superior to another. All commercial preparations appear to be effective and safe, provided the child is hemodynamically stable. Specific antidiarrheal and antiemetic medications are generally not indicated.[34,36]

Most agents of viral gastroenteritis are spread by the fecal-oral (and possibly respiratory) route. Contaminated water, food, and fomites may be important. Prevention involves good hygiene, sound advice for travel (care in the use of water or food), boiling of shellfish, and meticulous handwashing. A rotavirus vaccine was withdrawn due to an association with intussusception.

Pinworms

Humans are the only natural host of the pinworm *Enterobius vermicularis,* a 1-cm, white, thread-like helminth responsible for millions of infections in the United States. It is most common in school-age children, regardless of socioeconomic status, and is most prevalent among family members, in institutions, and in areas of crowding. Oral ingestion of eggs begins a 15- to 43-day life cycle that involves temporary attachment of larvae in the duodenum, habitation and copulation of adult worms in the cecum and adjacent gut, and migration of gravid females out of the anus at night to deposit thousands of eggs in the perianal and perineal regions. Although larvae may

reenter through the anus, reinfection of the patient and infection of others generally occurs via the fecal-oral route, most commonly under the fingernails of the patient. Linens and furry animals may act as fomites.[37,38]

Clinical Presentation and Diagnosis

A large proportion of patients are asymptomatic, and the classic symptoms of perianal itching, restless sleep, and irritability may be no more common among infected than uninfected children. Occasionally, the parasite migrates to cause vulvo-vaginitis-urethritis (most common), salpingitis, prostatitis, and bowel, liver, and other organ system disease. Anorexia, weight loss, and personality changes (due to the misconceived stigmata associated with having pinworms) are sometimes seen. Unless peritoneal invasion occurs, eosinophilia is not present.

Parents may observe worms on an infected child by nocturnal flashlight examination of the anal verge, but the parasites may be confused with white thread. The cellophane tape test detects 50% of infections on the first examination and 99% if five examinations are done. A clear piece of cellophane tape is placed against the areas of the perianal region early in the morning, then placed face down on a clean glass slide and brought to the physician's office for microscopic examination.[37,38]

Management

Because pinworm infection spreads within families and may be asymptomatic, initial treatment of all family members is best. The medication kills only adult worms, so retreatment of symptomatic individuals 2 weeks after the initial therapy may improve cure rates. Mebendazole 100 mg (Vermox chewable tablets) in a single dose for adults and children is generally effective. Albendazole in a single oral dose of 400 mg is an alternative. Both agents are not recommended in pregnancy. Preventive measures such as frequent hand and fingernail washing, avoidance of digit sucking, and decontamination of clothing, sleeping quarters, and toilet seats may decrease reinfection, but may not justify the associated increased psychological trauma and stigmata associated with pinworms.[37,38]

References

1. American Academy of Pediatrics. Report of the Committee on Infectious Diseases, 25th ed. Elk Grove Village, IL: American Academy of Pediatrics, 2000.
2. Upper airway infections. In: Feigin RD, Cherry JD, eds. Textbook of pediatric infectious diseases, 4th ed. Philadelphia: WB Saunders, 1998;128–241.
3. Turner RB, Schaffner W. Will anything work for the common cold? Patient care 2000;34(22):15–24.
4. Graham NMH, Burrell CJ, Douglas RM, Debelle P, Davies L. Adverse effects of aspirin, acetaminophen, and ibuprofen on immune function, viral shedding, and clinical status in rhinovirus-infected volunteers. J Infect Dis 1990;162:1277–82.
5. Giladi N, Herman J. Pharyngoconjunctival fever. Arch Dis Child 1984;59:1182–3.

6. Klassen TB. Croup—a current perspective. Pediatr Clin North Am 1999;46:1167–78.

7. Rosekrans JA. Viral croup: current diagnosis and treatment. Mayo Clin Proc 1998;73:1102–7.

8. Bernstein T, Brilli R, Jacobs B. Is bacterial tracheitis changing? A 14-month experience in a pediatric intensive care unit. Clin Infect Dis 1998;27:458–62.

9. Hall CB, McCarthy CA. Respiratory syncytial virus. In: Mandell GL, Bennett JE, Dolin R, eds. Principles and practice of infectious diseases, 5th ed. Philadelphia: Churchill Livingstone, 2000:1782–801.

10. Horst PS. Bronchiolitis. Am Fam Physician 1994;49:1449–53.

11. Busse WW. The role of the common cold in asthma. J Clin Pharmacol 1999;39:241–5.

12. Hogg JC. Childhood viral infection and the pathogenesis of asthma and chronic obstructive lung disease. Am J Respir Crit Care Med 1999;160:526–8.

13. Whitelaw CC, Kallis JM. Pediatric facial swelling. Acad Emerg Med 1998;5:146–202.

14. Berman S, Schmitt BD. Acute cervical adenitis. In: Hay WW Jr, Groothuis JR, Hayward AR, Levin MJ, eds. Current pediatric diagnosis and treatment. 12th ed. Norwalk, CT: Appleton & Lange, 1995;485–7.

15. Wharton M, Cochi SL, Williams WW. Measles, mumps and rubella vaccines. Infect Dis Clin North Am 1990;4:47–73.

16. Caplan CE. Mumps in the era of vaccines. Can Med Assoc J 1999;160:865–6.

17. McDonald JC, Moore DL, Quennec P. Clinical and epidemiologic features of mumps meningoencephalitis and possible vaccine-related disease. Pediatr Infect Dis J 1989;8:751–5.

18. Manson AL. Mumps orchitis. Urology 1990;36:355–8.

19. Gordon SC, Lauter CB. Mumps arthritis: a review of the literature. Rev Infect Dis 1984;6:338–44.

20. Cheek JE, Baron R, Atlas H, Wilson DL, Crider RD Jr. Mumps outbreak in a highly vaccinated school population. Arch Pediatr Adolesc Med 1995;149:774–8.

21. Gersony WM. Diagnosis and management of Kawasaki disease. JAMA 1991;265:2699–703.

22. Applegate BL. Kawasaki syndrome. Postgrad Med 1995;97(2):121–6.

23. Dajani AS, Taubert KA, Takahashi M, et al. Guidelines for long-term management of patients with Kawasaki disease. Circulation 1994;89:916–22.

24. Resnick SD. New aspects of exanthematous diseases of childhood. Dermatol Clin 1997;15:257–66.

25. Frieden IJ, Resnick SD. Childhood exanthems. Pediatr Clin North Am 1991;38:859–87.

26. Arguedas AG, Deveikis AA, Marks MI. Measles. Am J Infect Control 1991;19:290–8.

27. Kaplan LJ, Daum RS, Smaron M, McCarthy CA. Severe measles in immunocompromised patients. JAMA 1992;267:1237–41.

28. Hall CB, Long CE, Schnabel KC, et al. Human herpesvirus-6 infections in children. N Engl J Med 1994;331:432–8.

29. Leach CT. Human herpes virus-6 and -7 infections in children: agents of roseola and other syndromes. Curr Opin Pediatr 2000;12:269–74.

30. Cherry JD. Parvovirus infections in children and adults. Adv Pediatr 1999;46:245–69.

31. Magro CM, Dawood MR, Crowson AN. The cutaneous manifestations of human parvovirus B19 infection. Hum Pathol 2000;31:488–97.

32. Dunkle LM, Arvin AM, Whitley RJ, et al. A controlled trial of acyclovir for chickenpox in normal children. N Engl J Med 1991;325:1539–44.

33. Jundt JW, Creager AH. STAR complexes: febrile illness associated with sore throat, arthritis, and rash. South Med J 1993;86:521–8.

34. Burkhart DM. Management of acute gastroenteritis in children. Am Fam Physician 1999;60:2555–63.

35. Lieberman JM. Rotavirus and other viral causes of gastroenteritis. Pediatr Ann 1994;23:529–35.

36. Murphy MS. Guidelines for managing acute gastroenteritis based on a systematic review of published research. Arch Dis Child 1998;79:279–84.

37. Mahmoud AAF. Intestinal nematodes (roundworms). In: Mandell GL, Bennett JE, Dolin R, eds. Principles and practice of infectious diseases, 5th ed. New York: Churchill Livingstone, 2000:2939–40.

38. Russell LJ. The pinworm, *Enterobius vermicularis*. Prim Care 1991;18:13–24.

19
Behavioral Problems of Children

James E. Nahlik and H. Russell Searight

Family physicians deal with a wide range of behavioral problems. The methods used to treat children are variable and require flexibility on the part of the family physician. This requirement is not surprising to the experienced physician, who is able to comfort a 3-year-old who sits on the mother's lap as well as to chat about "cool" topics with the preteen. The methods to change behaviors, though, are derived from the principles of behavioral modification. In this chapter we examine several common behavioral problems of children. The diagnoses are defined according to the *Diagnostic and Statistical Manual of Mental Disorders*, 4th edition (DSM-IV)[1] whenever possible. The physician must learn how to recognize when psychopathology is present and how to foster more adaptive behavior in family and school contexts.

Behavior Modification

A practical way to initiate modification of children's behavior is to "catch them being good," which puts into practice the power of positive reinforcement. This principle is effective for all age groups and for many behaviors. A common example is at the dinner table when the 3-year-old is reluctant to start his dinner. His mother or father may then compliment him when he simply takes a sip of milk. The child usually thrives on this sort of attention and usually seeks more compliments by starting to eat. Parents are sometime skeptical about this approach and ask why they would interrupt the child, for example, who is happily playing with a puzzle. The mother is afraid that he will stop this good behavior if interrupted. But praising the good behavior builds children's self-esteem, and helps them to persist in the quiet time. An example for older children is to admire the results of a routine household chore they have undertaken. Intermittent positive reinforcement, also a useful tool, originally was demonstrated in mice when they were rewarded with food when they

pressed a bar. If they were rewarded intermittently, instead of every time they pressed the bar, they were much more diligent in the desired task. We do not need to teach parents to be intermittent, as they are physically unable to praise children each time they "catch them being good." Positive reinforcement can be taken a step further when necessary by making agreements, or contracts, for rewards other than words of praise. A favorite snack has been used commonly, but it can lead to obesity if overdone. Other positive rewards depend on the child's needs and age.

Punishment, or negative reinforcement, is periodically required. The classic description is training horses to walk by holding a carrot on a stick in front of their nose. The carrot, of course, is an example of positive reinforcement. If the horses do not respond, the trainer resorts to punishment: "Hit them with the stick." This may or may not work for horses, but in practice we advocate punishments that are nonviolent. There is a long tradition of slapping or spanking in our society, but the current repercussions of child abuse and spouse abuse must prompt concern about the appropriateness of such punishment today. Physical punishment models aggression, and it offers no alternatives to the child.[2]

One option is the "time-out" concept.[2] This form of punishment is effective for children over 2 years of age and up to 12 years. There is an assigned "time-out chair" or other location such as a corner or the staircase. Children are removed from their undesirable behavior and told to stay at the "time-out" location. A timer is then set to the number of minutes equivalent to their age (e.g., a 5-year-old is expected to sit for 5 minutes). While in "time-out" they are not allowed to ask questions or play but are reminded to think about their behavior. When the time expires, they can be greeted by a hug, ending the incident. Older children may require other negative reinforcements such as doing an extra chore, being grounded, or sustaining other losses of privilege. On occasion the parent must ignore the child's inappropriate behavior. Ultimately children must be able to gain self-control for them to function in society.

Attention-Deficit/Hyperactivity Disorder

Children with attention-deficit/hyperactivity disorder (AD/HD) can be frustrating to the parents and the family physician. Children with this disorder are affected in all areas of their interaction with the world, and diagnosis, treatment, and management are time-consuming and labor-intensive. The criteria for diagnosis contained in the DSM-IV are clinically useful for establishing the diagnosis (Table 19.1).

The family physician must utilize these criteria and if the diagnosis is established select the best treatment(s). This disorder is reported to occur in 3% to 5% of school-age children according to the DSM-IV.[1] However, recent studies suggest that the prevalence rate may approach 8%. AD/HD is described as a single disorder with subtypes, and the DSM-IV identifies some children who were missed by earlier classifications. Children who are not hyperactive but who cannot sustain attention (more often girls) can now be classified as AD/HD—predominantly inattentive type (DSM classification number 314.00). The classic "fidgety Phil," who is hyperactive and impulsive, can be diagnosed as AD/HD—predominantly hyperactive-impulsive type (314.01). The additional criteria of the DSM-IV help rule out children whose problems do not ap-

pear before age 7, those who have trouble at home but not in school (or vice versa), and those whose symptoms occur because of another psychological process. These children are apt to have other diagnoses that can affect their school performance such as learning disabilities, conduct disorder, anxiety, and depression[3] (see Chapters 31 and 32). The physician must also determine if there is a medical condition affecting the child's behavior. The most common complicating factors are hearing or vision impairment unrecognized by the parent. Less likely medical conditions that can present as hyperactivity are hyperthyroidism, lead toxicity, allergies, and seizure disorders.

Diagnosis

These children present by several routes, including referral by the schoolteacher. The schools rely on the physician to make the diagnosis and to recommend a treatment plan. Teachers and parents should be asked to provide information on the child's behavioral history, which can be done with a questionnaire, such as the Conners,[4] or by careful interview in the office. The history should include a family history, prenatal facts, and a medical history of the child. The physical examination of the child includes hearing and vision screening tests and observation of developmental markers. Growth parameters and blood pressure are important for diagnosis and for baseline when initiating medications. Signs of chronic illnesses such as anemia or allergies may explain some problematic behaviors. Children with AD/HD—predominantly hy-

---

Table 19.1. Diagnostic and Statistical Manual of Mental Disorders (DSM) Criteria for Attention-Deficit/Hyperactivity Disorder

A. At least six of the following symptoms of inattention or hyperactivity-impulsivity must be evident:
  Inattention
    Lack of attention to details or careless mistakes in schoolwork, work, or other activities
    Difficulty sustaining attention in tasks or play activities
    Impression of not listening when spoken to directly
    Failure to follow through on instructions or finish schoolwork or duties
    Difficulty organizing tasks and activities
    Avoidance or dislike of tasks that require sustained mental effort (e.g., schoolwork or homework)
    Tendency to lose things necessary for tasks or activities (e.g., toys, school assignments, pencils, books, or tools)
    Distractions by extraneous stimuli
    Forgetfulness in daily activities
  Hyperactivity
    Fidgeting with hands or feet or squirming in seat
    Not remaining seated when expected
    Running about or climbing excessively (or subjective feelings of restlessness in older persons)
    Difficulty engaging in leisure activities quietly
    Often "on the go" or "driven by a motor"
    Excessive talking
  Impulsivity
    Tendency to blurt out answers before questions have been completed
    Difficulty awaiting turn
    Tendency to interrupt or intrude on others (e.g., butting into conversations or games)
The additional criteria defined in the DSM-IV are as follows:
B. Some hyperative-impulsive or inattentive symptoms that caused impairment were present before age 7 years.
C. Some impairment from the symptoms is present in two or more settings [at school (or work) and at home].
D. There must be clear evidence of clinically significant impairment in social, academic, or occupational functioning.
E. The symptoms do not occur exclusively during the course of a pervasive developmental disorder, schizophrenia, or
    other psychotic disorder and are not better accounted for by another mental disorder (e.g., mood disorder, anxiety
    disorder, dissociative disorder, or a personality disorder).

Source: Reprinted with permission from the Diagnostic and Statistical Manual of Mental Disorders, Fourth Edition, Text Revision. Copyright 2000 American Psychiatic Association.

peractive-impulsive type—may show multiple contusions or abrasions from their haphazard activities, and a few clip the tags out of their shirts as they cannot tolerate extraneous stimulation.[5] The neurologic examination must rule out motor disturbances, tics, and sensory impairment. Blood tests are not routinely indicated. Occasionally the history and physical examination dictate evaluating the blood count, thyroid-stimulating hormone (TSH), or lead level. Ultimately the diagnosis is secured by fulfilling the diagnostic criteria through documentation of six DSM-IV behaviors (Table 19.1).

Treatment

Once the diagnosis of AD/HD is secure, treatment usually begins in several areas. The parent or teacher is often expecting pills, but the physician also should emphasize skills.[6] Instruction about developing behavioral skills is crucial to help the parent and student understand that medication may be used for only a short period (months) to help the student become diligent in gaining organizational skills and an increasing ability to focus. For instance, students can be taught list-making to allow them to concentrate on one task at a time.[6] Behavior modification, psychotherapy, family therapy, and support groups are indicated for many AD/HD children and their families. Treatment with medication is often initiated at the first office visit or later if the behavior modifications take first priority.[7]

The psychostimulant medications are beneficial in 70% to 80% of patients with AD/HD.[8] Stimulants are remarkably safe, have few side effects, and have not been shown to result in persisting adverse effects. The mechanism of action is postulated to be increased arousal in the areas of the brain that control impulses and attention. Stimulants block the reuptake of dopamine and norepinephrine into the presynaptic neurons. The increased availability of dopamine and norepinephrine normalizes the patients' behavior while it is in the circulation. Parents often ask, "Why stimulate the hyperactive child?" The answer is that these medications stimulate the part of the brain specifically involved with attention. AD/HD patients who are prescribed methylphenidate show increases in the striatal perfusion in the frontal lobes. The left frontal lobe is postulated to be the site for impulse control.[9] The stimulant medication used most often is methylphenidate (Ritalin), which has a duration of action of 3 to 5 hours. The methylphenidate dose is usually initiated at 5 mg twice each day, before breakfast and before lunch. The child's behavior is closely monitored, and if problems continue, the dose is increased slowly up to a maximum daily dose of 0.6 mg/kg. Many children require a dose of 10 or 20 mg twice each day, and sometimes three times each day. The second dose is usually given after lunch, but it can be problematic for teachers and administrators or cause a stigma to the student. The sustained-release form of methylphenidate may be helpful for children who need higher doses but have difficulty taking medication at school. This long-acting formulation has the same bioavailability as the regular tablet, with slower absorption. A once-a-day preparation of methylphenidate encapsulated in an oral osmotic (OROS) release delivery system was approved in 2000. In controlled trials this OROS

methylphenidate (Concerta) acted similarly to thrice daily immediate-release methylphenidate.[10]

Dextroamphetamine (Dexedrine) has been shown to be as effective as methylphenidate for decreasing overactivity, impulsivity, and inattention in children with AD/HD. Some children unresponsive to methylphenidate have responded to dextroamphetamine and vice versa. Dextroamphetamine may be preferable in patients with a history of tics, depression, or anxiety. It costs less, is started at a dose of 5 mg, and is titrated similarly to methylphenidate. The spansule form of dextroamphetamine (Dexedrine spansules) is uniquely suited to small children who are unable to swallow tablets. This capsule may be opened and sprinkled onto food that is to be eaten immediately.[7] It is indicated for children as young as 3 years. Adderall, a recemic mixture of d- and l-amphetamine has been demonstrated to be equally effective as methylphenidate.[11] Adderall's behavioral effects may last up to 6 hours. Dosing ranges from 5 to 20 mg once or twice per day. Other stimulants such as methamphetamine and pemoline are useful in selected cases (Table 19.2). The most common adverse effects of the stimulants are insomnia and anorexia. Slowed growth has been reported in addition to abdominal pain, headache, dizziness, and irritability. These side effects usually lessen with continued medicine, and they all resolve when the medication is discontinued. Pemoline can cause hepatotoxicity, so liver function tests should be done prior to and periodically during therapy.

Several nonstimulant medications are being used successfully for AD/HD. Clonidine, guanabenz, desipramine, and other antidepressants can be considered for the patient who is unresponsive to the stimulants. Occasionally patients with comorbid disorders such as anxiety respond to treatment with medications for the other disorder. Older treatments for attention problems, such as diets low in sugar or preservatives, have not withstood controlled trials.

Children with AD/HD can be energetic and accomplished in many areas. They can be guided to devote their extra energies to productive tasks such as scouting, sports, school assignments, and self-improvement. When these skills are successfully implemented, children experience higher self-esteem, with a reduced need for medication or other forms of therapy. Some children require long-term use of the stimulants, even through high school and college.

Learning Disabilities

At least 3% to 5% of school-age children are learning-disabled.[1] The definition of a learning disability varies, as educators, psychologists, neurologists, pediatricians, and language pathologists frequently employ distinct diagnostic criteria. A frequent standard is a significant difference between the measured intelligence quotient (IQ) and a standardized academic test. According to the DSM-IV, academic test scores in a given skill should be 1 to 2 standard deviations (SD) below the measured IQ.[1]

Learning disabilities (315.2) tend to occur in one or more of several key areas, including reading, spelling, numerical

Table 19.2. **Pharmacotherapy for Attention-Deficit/Hyperactivity Disorder in Children**

Medication	Initial dose	Maximum dose	Side effects of class
Stimulants			
Methylphenidate (Ritalin)	5 mg bid	60 mg/day	Tachycardia
Methylphenidate oral osmotic (OROS) delivery system (Concerta)	18 mg qd	54 mg/day	Hypertension Insomnia Anorexia
Dextroamphetamine (Dexedrine)	2.5 mg bid	40 mg/day	Headache Irritability
Pemoline (Cylert)	18.75 mg qd	75 mg/day	Precipitation of tics
Tricyclic antidepressants (given at bedtime)			
Imipramine (Tofranil)	25–50 mg/day	5 mg/kg/day	Sedation
Desipramine (Norpramin)	25–50 mg/day	5 mg/kg/day	Dry mouth
Amitriptyline (Elavil)	25–50 mg/day	5 mg/kg/day	Urinary retention Constipation Blurred vision Hypertension Arrhythmias
Central-acting antihypertensive			
Clonidine (Catapres)	0.05 mg/day	0.008 mg/kg/day	Hypotension Dry mouth Dizziness Constipation Headache Drowsiness

Source: Searight et al,[3] with permission.

calculation, or written expression. A child may exhibit evidence of a learning disability in more than one academic skill area, although the child's global level of intellectual functioning is assumed to be at least average. Additionally, the family physician should be sure to establish that the child's hearing and vision are not impaired before a learning disability is seriously considered. Environmental health factors, such as elevated lead levels, should also be ruled out. It is assumed that the learning-disabled child has had adequate exposure to formal education; thus the diagnosis is often not assigned until at least the second grade.

The causes of learning disabilities have not been precisely established, but these conditions are probably caused by multiple factors. Fennell[12] suggested four etiologic types: (1) established neurologic histories (e.g., seizure disorders); (2) neurologic "soft signs" or pronounced developmental delays; (3) learning disabilities without positive neurologic signs; and (4) learning disabilities secondary to a psychiatric disorder such as depression. From an educational perspective, children with learning problems secondary to emotional issues or environmental deprivation are excluded from the learning-disabled category.

Although learning disabilities are diagnosed in terms of academic skills, they are usually attributable to a more fundamental deficit in receptive or expressive language, decoding written or orally presented material, or visuospatial skills. Dyslexia, termed specific reading disability in DSM-IV, is the most common learning disability. Reading is a complex activity involving visual perceptual, linguistic, and sequencing skills. Currently, dyslexia's core deficit is believed to be a failure to understand that written and verbal content can be broken down into basic phonetic units. A related deficit in mapping sounds onto specific letters is also present.[13] Developmentally, early indicators of possible dyslexia include delayed language development and difficulty with identifying and naming letters of the alphabet, with verbal recall, and with generating words beginning with the same letter (e.g., ball, black, baby).[12]

The family physician can play a valuable role in assisting the child who has a suspected learning disability, and thus assisting the parents. The family doctor may be the first professional contacted when a child is performing poorly in school. A learning disability should always be considered when evaluating children with academic problems, particularly elementary school children. Although the learning-disabled child may have a long history of consistently poor school performance, the higher functioning child may not be detected until later in elementary school, such as in the fourth or fifth grade. At later grade levels, there is greater emphasis placed on independent work skills, such as reading on one's own or writing essays in which children must organize their writing without external aids such as a structured workbook. The physician should also consider other childhood disorders such as AD/HD. When disruptive behavior is present in addition to poor academic performance, the primary problem may be conduct or oppositional defiant disorder, either alone or in conjunction with a learning disability. A relatively sudden drop in academic performance should alert the physician to an emotional problem such as depression, family stress, or substance abuse. To formally document a learning disability, children need to undergo testing with the Wechsler Intelligence Scale for Children–III (WISC-III) or the Wechsler Preschool and Primary

Scale of Intelligence–Revised (WPPSI-R) as well as educational tests such as the Woodcock-Johnson. These tests can be administered and interpreted by a clinical or school psychologist. Public Law 94-142 guarantees all children with special needs an appropriate education in the least restrictive environment. Family physicians can be instrumental in educating parents and encouraging them to seek diagnostic and educational services for their child.

Conduct Disorders

Conduct disorders are some of the most common behavioral problems of children. Up to 50% of patients under 18 receiving outpatient psychiatric care have a conduct disorder diagnosis (312.8). The defining feature is a persistent behavior pattern involving violation of others' rights and the failure to abide by socially accepted rules.[1] Conduct-disordered children and adolescents usually exhibit at least one of the following symptom clusters: (1) aggression toward people or animals (or both); (2) property destruction (i.e., vandalism); (3) lying ("conning" others or theft); (4) serious violations of rules such as multiple school truancies or running away from home overnight.

The prevalence of conduct disorders in the United States appears to be increasing, particularly in inner city areas. For boys under age 18, prevalence rates range from 6% to 16% with a 2% to 9% range among girls.[1] DSM-IV describes two conduct disorder subtypes: childhood onset, which appears before age 10, and the adolescent type, characterized by no significant behavioral difficulties until age 10 or older. The adolescent-onset type is usually less severe and has a better prognosis.[12] Like most

psychiatric syndromes, conduct disorder is diagnosed primarily through the history (Table 19.3). It is important for the physician to obtain information about the patient from all possible vantage points. There is considerable evidence that children and adolescents underreport problem behaviors. Additionally, "conning" others is a common symptom of conduct disorder, and this deliberate deception may extend to the medical interview.

The family physician should seriously entertain a conduct disorder diagnosis when evaluating young adolescents and preadolescents who are using drugs, alcohol, or cigarettes or who are engaging in sex. Conduct-disordered children often have little empathy or concern for others' feelings and have few or no significant emotional attachments. There are indications that children with earlier-onset conduct problems are more psychologically disturbed[13] and engage in more serious destructive behavior, such as cruelty to animals and arson. Adolescent-onset conduct disorder increasingly occurs in the context of gang activity. This variation generally reflects assimilation to gang subculture and is associated with less psychological disturbance.[14–16] The physician should have a "behavioral threshold" to distinguish lower level noncompliance and misbehavior from more severe psychiatric disturbance. A childhood history of conduct disorder is found among most adults with antisocial personality disorder. Of all conduct disorder symptoms, aggression is the most consistent over time.[17] In addition to age of onset, severity is related to the frequency and variety of antisocial behaviors and its presence in various settings (e.g., home, school, community).

Conduct disorder is often found among children with two other disruptive behavior patterns: AD/HD and oppositional

Table 19.3. **DSM-IV Criteria for Conduct Disorder**

A. A repetitive and persistent pattern of behavior in which the basic rights of others or major age-appropriate norms or rules are violated, as manifested by the presence of three or more of the following criteria during the past 12 months, with at least one criterion present during the past 6 months.
   Aggression to people or animals
      1. Often bullies, threatens, or intimidates others
      2. Often initiates physical fights
      3. Has used a weapon that can cause physical harm to others (e.g., bat, brick, knife, gun)
      4. Has been physically cruel to people
      5. Has been physically cruel to animals
      6. Has stolen while confronting a victim (e.g., mugging, purse snatching, extortion, armed robbery)
      7. Has forced someone into sexual activity
   Destruction of property
      8. Has deliberately engaged in fire setting with the intention of causing serious damage
      9. Has deliberately destroyed others' property (other than by fire setting)
   Deceitfulness or theft
      10. Has broken into someone else's house, building, or car
      11. Often lies to obtain goods or favors or to avoid obligations (i.e., "cons" others)
      12. Has stolen items of nontrivial value without confronting a victim (e.g., shoplifting but without breaking and entering; forgery)
   Serious violations of rules
      13. Often stays out at night despite parental prohibitions, beginning before age 13 years
      14. Has run away from home overnight at least twice while living in parental or parental surrogate home (or once without returning for a lengthy period)
      15. Is often truant from school, beginning before age 13 years
B. The disturbance in behavior causes clinically significant impairment in social, academic, or occupational functioning.
C. If the individual is age 18 years or older, criteria are not met for antisocial personality disorder.

Source: Reprinted with permission from the Diagnostic and Statistical Manual of Mental Disorders, Fourth Edition, Text Revision. Copyright 2000 American Psychiatic Association.

defiant disorder.[18] Oppositional defiant disorder (313.81) is characterized by frequent argumentative and negativistic verbalizations, temper tantrums, and refusal to comply with adult requests. Oppositional defiant children, like those with conduct disorder, often are reared in families with inconsistent discipline, although the parents are more likely to be depressed than overtly antisocial. Conduct disorder is distinguished from AD/HD and oppositional defiant disorder by an emphasis on aggressive, illegal, and overtly destructive acts. Both hereditary and environmental factors are implicated in the etiology of conduct disorder. Support for genetic involvement comes from twin studies in which adoptees were separated at birth (see Chapter 16). The offspring had higher rates of delinquency when one of the biologic parents had antisocial personality disorder. The family environments of conduct-disordered children are often chaotic, with supervision and discipline either nonexistent or sporadic.[14,19] Fathers are often absent or exhibit antisocial behavior.[14] Direct observation of these families has shown little parental warmth, few positive verbalizations toward their children, and failure to monitor children's activities.[19]

Because of these parental issues, conduct disorder has a guarded prognosis. Successful behavioral intervention for these children includes the following: (1) targeting two or three behaviors on which to focus for a several-week period; (2) consistently rewarding desired behaviors: with young children, rewards are often tangible (e.g., cookies), and for older children "points" redeemable for privileges are employed; (3) implementing mild punishments such as "time-out" or removal of privileges (access to television); and (4) monitoring and supervising children (with adolescents, knowledge of their whereabouts is particularly important). All of these principles must be implemented consistently. It is also important for parents to engage in positive exchanges with their children to break the cycle of coercion and behavioral escalation.[19] Similar strategies are used for oppositional defiant children with particular emphasis on rewarding appropriate communication.

Anxiety Disorders

Although anxiety disorders affect both children and adults, there are several syndromes unique to pediatric patients, including separation anxiety and overanxious disorders. These disorders share some features, including chronic worry, social avoidance, and excessive desire for proximity to the primary caregiver.

Separation anxiety is a normal developmental process that begins midway through the first year, peaks at around 15 months, and then gradually declines through the third year. By contrast, separation anxiety disorder (309.21) is characterized by unrealistic, persistent worry about harm befalling a parent or caregiver or fears of death or an accident that could render the caregiver inaccessible. These children also may refuse to sleep in their own beds or attend school. DSM-IV estimates that about 4% of children and adolescents have separation anxiety disorder.[1] Families of these children are often close-knit. The physician encountering separation anxiety should encour-

age the parents to provide a balance between support and age-appropriate independence. For example, children who refuse to sleep in their own bed should not be taken into the parents' bed but should be permitted to sleep with a night-light and favorite toy or music in their room. In extreme cases they could be allowed to sleep on a carpet near the parents' bed as a transitional step toward sleeping alone. Similarly, school refusal should not be accepted, and the child is sent to preschool as scheduled. Carrying a "transitional object," such as a family photograph, might be effective in reducing anxiety.

Overanxious disorder (313.0) is a label often applied to generalized anxiety when it occurs in elementary school children and young adolescents.[1] These children experience excessive anticipatory anxiety around situations where they are evaluated. Their response includes considerable self-consciousness, excessive rumination about future events, and functional somatic complaints including headaches and stomachaches.[14] They are highly self-critical and frequently request adult reassurance. Outwardly, these children appear restless or tense because of their inability to relax.

A closely related condition is social anxiety disorder, with an average onset at age 12. Unrealistic fears of social embarrassment, particularly in front of unfamiliar people, characterize this condition.[1] As a result of multiple episodes of panic-like anxiety, the child begins to avoid a broad range of interpersonal situations. There is growing evidence that selective serotonin reuptake inhibitors are helpful for pediatric separation, generalized, and social anxiety disorders.[20] Behavioral interventions include relaxation training and structured social interaction.

The physician can recommend that the parents provide the child with increased opportunities for peer interaction, which should be done in a gradual manner with initial activities conducted with one peer present for several hours before moving to small social groups. Parents can also be encouraged to help the child by role-playing social exchanges. For children who require formal psychological treatment, a referral to social skills or peer activity therapy group is most helpful.

Phobias (300.20) are common in both children and adults. The overall lifetime prevalence for specific phobias is about 10%. Pediatric phobias are distinct from common childhood fears of the dark, strangers, and animals. The degree of fear is disproportionate, and the phobic situation is avoided or tolerated with great discomfort. For a child to be diagnosed as phobic, the distress or avoidance should result in impaired social, academic, or family functioning. Preoccupation and anticipatory anxiety about the phobic object or situation is also common. The treatment of choice is relaxation training (deep breathing with the possible addition of systematic tensing and relaxation of muscle groups) coupled with graded exposure to the phobic stimulus.[21]

Obsessive-Compulsive Disorder

Obsessive-compulsive disorder (OCD) (300.3) in children and adolescents appears to be underdiagnosed. Until recently the disorder was not recognized in children. However, retrospective studies of adults with OCD indicated that about 40% of these patients reported onset during childhood and adolescence.[22] The average age of onset appears to be about 13 years.[23] Whereas adult-onset OCD occurs about equally across genders, childhood onset appears to be more common in boys.[23] The prevalence in children and adolescents appears to be about 1%.[24]

Obsessive-compulsive disorder is characterized by repetitive intrusive anxiety-provoking thoughts (obsessions) and ritualistic actions (compulsions). The repetitive behaviors have no function except to temporarily reduce anxiety. Common obsessions involve fears of contamination by dirt or germs, aggressive acts toward self or others, and orderliness and scrupulosity. Common compulsions include washing, checking (e.g., locks, ovens), counting, or straightening objects. Childhood OCD may differ from this adult picture by including compulsions without corresponding obsessions and odd behaviors such as finger-licking.[22] Tics are common, and there appears to be a linkage between childhood OCD and Tourette's syndrome.[22]

Multimodal treatment including medication, behavioral therapy, and family intervention is most helpful with OCD children. Both clomipramine[22] and sertraline[25] used successfully with adults also appear to benefit OCD children. When the selective serotonin reuptake inhibitors (SSRIs) are prescribed, doses higher than the usual starting dose are often required. Behavioral treatment, emphasizing gradual exposure to anxiety-provoking situations, has also been successful.[14] Parents are often overinvolved with OCD children and may contribute to their social isolation. Thus family therapy that focuses on increased community activities and promotes greater independence in the child is likely to have an additive effect with pharmacotherapy and behavioral exposure.

Other Treatable Behavioral Problems

This section covers several common abnormal behaviors of children. Tics, thumb sucking, and nail biting are never life threatening, but parents often ask what can be done with the child who exhibits these behaviors. Physicians often appropriately suggest that it be ignored, although some treatment may be considered. Habit reversal is a comprehensive behavior therapy treatment approach that includes multiple treatment components.[26] It involves defining the abnormal behavior, requiring the subject to recognize when the behavior occurs, and then recommending a competing response component, such as making a fist or grasping an object.

Tic Disorder

Tics are brief, rapid, repetitive, stereotypic movements or utterances that involve contractions of groups of muscles in one or more parts of the body. This section covers the most common transient tic disorder of childhood (307.21) and does not address the more serious Tourette's syndrome. The transient tic disorder differs from Tourette syndrome in that it is pres-

ent for at least 4 weeks but no longer than 12 months. Transient tic disorders occur at some time in about 25% of children. Some parents are upset or aggravated by these nervous habits, but the tics often fade if ignored. When treatment is required, the principles of behavior modification are important. Relaxation training, self-monitoring, and habit reversal have all been studied for transient tic disorder, with varying success. When these children were treated with self-monitoring plus the competing response (described above), the subjects were successful in reducing the tics by about 80%.[26] This behavior modification program requires some time from both the patient and the provider but is preferred to the use of medications.

Thumb Sucking

Sucking of the thumb is a relatively common activity among young children, with an incidence of 30% to 40% among preschoolers and 10% to 20% in children over age 6.[26] Thumb sucking may have a psychological benefit in toddlers. This substitute form of nurturing allows them to consolidate emotions and handle their stresses. The habit can adversely affect a child's dental health, however, and has been associated with an anterior open bite, malocclusion, narrowing of the dental arches, mucosal trauma, and deformity of the thumb. These children are also prone to infections such as yeast or impetigo around the mouth and paronychia of the thumb. Thumb sucking (307.9) may also have an impact on social acceptance of children, who are viewed as less intelligent or less happy. One way to avoid thumb-sucking problems is by early use of an orthodontic pacifier, as the "binky" is more easy to remove from the child's environment. Despite all of the possible problems, treatment of thumb sucking is generally ineffective until the child is at least 4 years old, or even older if the child has experienced a traumatic loss. When treatment is required, a form of habit reversal was found to be successful in 47% of subjects at a 3-month follow-up.[26]

Nail Biting

Nail biting (307.9) occurs in up to 45% of teenagers and lesser numbers of children under age 12. It is often harmless but may cause paronychia, nail loss, and even dental problems. An unattractive habit, nail biting has been well studied with a variety of treatments. Elimination of nail biting was accomplished in 15% of children treated with bitter-tasting substances, 40% of those treated with habit reversal, and 57% of those with competing responses.[26] The competing-response patients were taught to make a fist or grasp an object for 3 minutes when the biting urge was recognized. They were also instructed to groom the nails and cuticles on a regular basis. The bitter-tasting substances are easy to administer and inexpensive but are not usually effective for reducing the behavior. Success can best be accomplished when the nail biters themselves have decided to cease the habit and are thus motivated to keep their hands busy in other ways.

One study evaluated pharmacologic treatment of nail biting. Leonard et al[27] evaluated 25 adult subjects in a 10-week double-blind crossover trial of clomipramine hydrochloride and desipramine hydrochloride. The clomipramine was significantly better than the desipramine for eliminating nail biting. These researchers also noted significant difficulty in recruiting subjects to participate in and complete the study.

Temper Tantrums

Temper tantrums (312.1) are a notoriously common problem in children aged 2 to 6 years. The "terrible twos" should more positively be described as the "testing twos" because it gives way to the autonomy of the 3-year-old. These stages of behavioral development are important for the child and the parent to weather. The parents must learn that temper tantrums are not deliberate misbehavior but the way their child tests their limits. The children must be given rules and discipline, but the parents must avoid emotionally demeaning actions and harsh physical discipline. Child-rearing practices are rarely formally taught. To change the child's behavior, parents often rely on techniques based on their own upbringing. The family physician's office often permits direct observation of inappropriate discipline, and then the physician can explain behavior modification in terms appropriate to the parent. The most important practice for the parents to understand is consistency. They must set and maintain limits for the child and set clear consequences for any misbehavior.[2]

Temper tantrums are usually a response of children not getting their way during a specific encounter. The tantrums can be worse if the child is sleepy or ill. Temper tantrums are most upsetting to parents when they occur in public places, which is when parents should be the most consistent. The parents may choose to ignore the child until the tantrum is over. Young children can be embraced firmly to prevent them from harming themselves. Using the "time-out" corner for 1 minute for each year of age can be effective. Children then know that they must get themselves cooled down before the timer is up, or they may gain another "time-out" period. When the tantrum is over, children can be counseled on what went wrong, what they should do differently in the future, and how to regain self-control.

Stuttering

Stuttering (307.0) is a speech articulation disorder characterized by repetition and unusual prolongations of sounds, syllables, or words (e.g., "m-m-m-my dog-g-g is bl-bl-bl-black"). There may also be hesitations or pauses disrupting the normal speech flow and rhythm.[1,28]

Stuttering is distinguished from normal developmental language dysfluency by the repetition pattern. In stuttering, word segments are repeated and sounds are prolonged. In contrast, normal language development includes repetition of whole words and phrases. Stuttering's prevalence is about 1% among prepubescent children and drops to about 0.8% among adolescents.[1] The disorder is more common among boys by a factor of about 3:1.[14] Stutterers are more likely to have family members with the same condition. For many children, the onset of stuttering occurs at about age 2 to 3 years when expressive language is developing.[14] A significant proportion of these children do not begin stuttering until they start school.[14]

Poor coordination of airflow with impaired articulation and resonance combine to impair timing of sounds comprising speech.[28] The apparent increase in stuttering with school attendance suggests that external stress may be contributory.[14] Additional support for the role of stress is that stuttering is more pronounced during public speaking, while talking on the phone,[1] or when interacting with authority figures. Stuttering may disappear when singing or reading aloud. Up to 70% of young children stop stuttering on their own.[1] Young children's stuttering will benefit from parental strategies including face-to-face eye contact with the child during all verbal exchanges, not finishing the child's utterances, and using questions that the child can answer with just a few words.

A dilemma for the primary care physician is whether to refer the stuttering child for speech therapy. Relaxation training including deep breathing to reduce muscle tension in the throat and chest has been employed as one component of successful treatment. Effective stuttering therapies also include attention to language skills. Strategies include gradually increasing the complexity of verbalization and mental preparation of conversational content. In addition to addressing the peer rejection that stuttering children often experience, early intervention may also help to improve language skills.

Sleep Disturbance

Sleep problems (307.40) in children are common and frustrating to parents (see Chapter 56). The sleepless child often disrupts the entire family and affects the adult members at work. Their crying and begging can usually overwhelm new and even experienced parents. The parents get free advice from their neighbors and relatives that may exacerbate the problem. It is important to know what normal sleep is at different ages and to know strategies for intervention. The normal hours required for sleep decrease as the child grows older. The average newborn sleeps 15 to 16 hours every day. At 1 year it is about 13 to 14 hours including the daytime nap of 1 to 2 hours.[29] At 3 years of age the child sleeps about 12 hours, then at 5 years requires about 11 hours of sleep and no daytime nap. There is wide variation in these average sleep requirements, and most children vary from night to night. The serum levels of growth hormone are highest during sleep, so when children are in a "growth spurt" they may sleep more. Most children can go to bed at an appropriate time, fall asleep within minutes, and stay asleep until a reasonable hour in the morning. Sometimes problems occur if the living arrangements do not allow a good routine or suitable surroundings to allow healthy sleep.

Development of Good Sleep Patterns

Bedtime rituals or routines are the most important elements of successful sleep. Such routines vary with age but should not vary significantly from night to night. For example, at 4 months of age the baby usually has the diapers changed and sleep garments in place. They may be fed and rocked and then placed in the crib when still awake, thereby conditioning them to settle themselves to sleep. This step is important so when they naturally wake up during the night they can settle themselves back to sleep. Toddlers require a different ritual when preparing for bed, because bedtime means separation. One parent must schedule the time to assist them with a routine each night, such as washing and brushing teeth, changing clothes, and reading a bedtime story. Ideally, this special time together occurs regularly at an agreed time. But children quickly learn to stretch the limits, and so the rules must be enforced. Infants and toddlers may use a transitional object such as a stuffed animal or a security blanket. This object gives them a feeling of control over their world because it does not leave and is there when they awaken. School-age children may use a posted list of the bedtime routine, but they still appreciate some time with the parent before going to sleep. Discussion of their school day or the parent's workday can be comforting and provide closure.

Colic (789.0) is probably the most common cause of significant sleep disturbance during the first year of life. Frequently, colicky infants are overly sensitive to the surroundings or stimulation. Chaos in their environment is unpleasant, and they respond by crying. Adequate time spent crying can alleviate this exhibition of tension. Children may be permitted to cry for 15 to 30 minutes, if the parents are in agreement. They then usually fall asleep; if still awake, their basic needs should be rechecked. If the diaper is dry and no fever or source of pain is found, they should be comforted and laid in bed. Other illnesses certainly can disrupt sleep, and appropriate treatment of febrile illness is important.

There is much truth to the expression about babies getting days and nights confused. The proper explanation is sleep-phase shifts. There can be an early sleep-phase syndrome or a late sleep-phase syndrome. An example of early sleep phase is the baby who goes to bed nicely at 6 P.M. but then wakes up at 4:00 or 5:00 A.M. The parents may become distraught because the child wakes up so early, which interrupts some of their important sleep time. All that has happened is that the baby has started his circadian rhythm to sleep early and wakes up the appropriate 10 to 11 hours later. This problem is corrected by gradually, over 10 to 15 days, keeping children awake later. This change helps them to sleep later. The late sleep-phase syndrome is more common in older children and in disrupted families when the children stay up late and then are difficult to arouse in the morning. The remedy is to set a time for awakening and then gradually adjust the bedtime earlier to reach the needed amount of time in bed. One efficient time to solve this problem is during the month of October, when, in most states, the clocks are set back for the end of daylight savings time. At this window of opportunity, simply do not change the clocks in the children's room, and so they are then going to bed (and getting up) an hour earlier.

Sleep walking (307.46) and sleep talking are common, but usually harmless sleep problems that bother parents. They are both forms of partial wakings that occur during non–rapid-eye-movement (non-REM) sleep. It usually occurs within 1 to 4 hours of falling to sleep, at the end of the first or second sleep cycle. When the awakenings are intense and frightening, they are called "sleep terrors." This problem is more common among adolescents and preadolescents. These children may wake up briefly, but they have only a vague memory of something having happened. Frequently psychological stress has occurred but not necessarily a major emotional problem. The treatment of most partial awakenings is to ignore them unless children leave their bed and get into dangerous situations. If they do, they can be awakened or protected from falling until they are awake. If there is emotional stress, the cause may need to be addressed.

Nightmares and bad dreams are common and occur only during REM sleep, when all dreams occur. During REM sleep the body cannot move, so only the memories of the dreams are harmful. When children wake up from a nightmare, they are truly frightened and need full reassurance and support. These episodes are most common in children ages 3 to 6 but can occur at any age. They may represent deep-seated issues for the children to discuss, but mostly the dream explains itself.

Family Bed

In most Western cultures, allowing children to sleep in the parents' bed is not permissible, with rare exceptions such as illness or significant loss. But it is a common and accepted practice in many developing countries, and in those families it is culturally normative. Studies have shown that people sleep best when alone in bed, as the movements and arousals of another person stimulate awakenings.[29] It is important for children to sleep alone in order to separate from the parent without high anxiety and to promote eventual independence. Sleeping in their parents' bed can make children feel confused and anxious, as it blurs the boundaries that they had understood. Sometimes insecure adults are the ones comforted by the toddler, and they are in need of counseling. From time to time the scenario can be avoided by gently returning the children to their own bed as often as needed. When absolutely necessary, a pillow and blanket can be placed on a carpet in the parents' room.

Summary

Behavioral problems in children are common and can usually be alleviated by intervention in the office. The principles of behavior modification have been practiced and refined over the years for practical usage today. To institute these practices the family physician sometimes must schedule extra time with the family or assign a staff member for specific tasks. The families of such patients have considerable trust in the family doctor, and with this trust, knowledge, and experience, the patients often improve and appreciate the interventions as they get older.

References

1. American Psychiatric Association. Diagnostic and statistical manual of mental disorders, 4th ed. Washington, DC: APA, 1994.

2. Novak LL. Childhood behavior problems. Am Fam Physician 1996;53:257–62.
3. Searight HR, Nahlik JE, Campbell DC. Attention-deficit/hyperactivity disorder: assessment, diagnosis, and management. J Fam Pract 1995;40:270–9.
4. Conners CK. Rating scales for use in drug studies with children. Psychopharmacol Bull 1973; special issue: psychopharmacology in children: 60.
5. Nahlik JE. New thoughts on attention-deficit/hyperactivity disorder. Hosp Pract 1995;30:70–2.
6. Jones C. Attention deficit disorder strategies for school age children. San Antonio, TX: Communication Skill Builders (Harcourt Brace, Psychological Corp.), 1994.
7. Nahlik JE, Searight HR. Diagnosis and treatment of attention-deficit/hyperactivity disorder. Primary Care Rep 1996;2(8): 65–74.
8. Safer DJ. Major treatment considerations for attention-deficit hyperactivity disorder. Curr Probl Pediatr 1995;25:137–43.
9. Sieg KG, Gaffney GR, Preston DF, Hellings JA. SPECT brain imaging abnormalities in attention deficit hyperactivity disorder. Clin Nucl Med 1995;20(1):55–60.
10. Wilens TE, Spencer TJ. The stimulants revisited. Child Adolesc Psychiatr Clin North Am 2000;9(3):573–603.
11. Pelham WE, Gangy EM, Chronic AM, et al. A comparison of morning-only and morning/late afternoon Adderall to morning-only, twice-daily, and three times-daily methylphenidate in children with attention-deficit/hyperactivity disorder. Pediatrics 1999;10(suppl):36–41.
12. Fennell EB. The role of neuropsychological assessment in learning disabilities. J Child Neurol 1995;10(suppl):36–41.
13. Shaywitz SE. Dyslexia. N Engl J Med 1998;338:307–12.
14. Schwartz S, Johnson JH. Psychopathology of childhood: a clinical experimental approach. New York: Pergamon, 1985.
15. Loeber R. Antisocial behavior: more enduring than changeable? J Am Acad Child Adolesc Psychiatry 1991;30:393–7.
16. Zuckerman M. Beyond the sensation seeking motive. Hillsdale, NJ: Erlbaum, 1979.
17. Farrington DP. Childhood aggression and adult violence: early precursors and later life outcomes. In: Pepler J, Rubin KH, eds. The development and treatment of childhood aggression. Hillsdale, NJ: Erlbaum, 1991:169–78.
18. Barkley R. Attention deficit hyperactivity disorder: a handbook for diagnosis and treatment. New York: Guilford, 1990.
19. Webster-Stratton C. Annotation: strategies for helping families with conduct disordered children. J Child Psychol Psychiatry 1991;32:1047–62.
20. The Research Unit on Pediatric Psychopharmacology Anxiety Study Group. Fluvoxamine for the treatment of anxiety disorders in children and adolescents. N Engl J Med 2001;17: 1279–85.
21. Kratchowill TR, Morris RJ. The practice of child therapy, 2nd ed. New York: Pergamon, 1991.
22. Rapoport JL, Leonare HL, Swedo SE, Leane MC. Obsessive-compulsive disorder in children and adolescents: issues in management. J Clin Psychiatry 1993;54(suppl):27–9.
23. Hanna GL. Demographic and clinical features of obsessive-compulsive disorder in children and adolescents. J Am Acad Child Adolesc Psychiatry 1995;34:19–27.
24. Rapoport JL, Ismond DR. DSM-IV training guide for diagnosis of childhood disorders. New York: Brunner/Mazel, 1996.
25. March JS, Biederman J, Wolkow R, et al. Sertraline in children and adolescents with obsessive-compulsive disorder: A multicenter randomized controlled trial. JAMA 1998;280:1752–6.
26. Peterson AL, Campise RL, Azrin NH. Behavioral and pharmacological treatments for tic and habit disorders: a review. Dev Behav Pediatr 1994;15:430–41.
27. Leonard HL, Lenane MC, Swedo SE, Rettew DC, Rapoport JL. A double-blind comparison of clomipramine and desipramine treatment of severe onychophagia (nail biting). Arch Gen Psychiatry 1991;48:821–7.
28. Lawrence M, Barclay DM. Stuttering: a brief review. Am Fam Physician 1998;57:2175–8.
29. Ferber R. Solve your child's sleep problems, 1st Fireside ed. New York: Simon & Schuster, 1986.

20
Musculoskeletal Problems of Children

Mark D. Bracker, Suraj A. Achar, Todd J. May,
Juan Carlos Buller, and Wilma J. Wooten

Torsional and Other Variations of the Lower Extremity

Gait Abnormalities

Rotational problems resulting in gait abnormalities are the most common orthopedic conditions in the pediatric age group. Parents are frequently concerned that their child will grow up deformed or be unable to play sports as they observe in-toeing or out-toeing and seek medical attention. Recent studies, however, have shown athletes with internal tibial torsion are faster than age-matched controls.[1] Most rotational abnormalities resolve spontaneously as musculature develops, and knowing this fact is reassuring to parents. Rarely, conditions remain fixed and require surgical correction at an older age. Torsional deformities may be due to problems in the foot (metatarsus adductus), tibia (torsion), or femur and hip (femoral anteversion). Angular abnormalities (bowlegs, knock-knees) generally resolve spontaneously as well. Certain terminology has been recommended as well as specific testing used to evaluate gait (Fig. 20.1).

Terminology

Definitions of the terms used in this chapter are as follows:

Angle of gait (foot progression angle): Angle of the intersection between the foot axis and the line progression. It is the result of static and dynamic influences from the foot to the hip. This angle remains relatively stable at 8 to 12 degrees of out-toeing through growth. There is a wide range of normal values varying from 3 degrees in-toeing to 20 degrees out-toeing; in one study of 130 children, 4.5% had an in-toeing gait.[2] Abnormalities anywhere along this kinetic chain (including hip, leg, and foot) can change the angle of gait.

Femoral antetorsion: Anteversion beyond the normal range [2 standard deviations (SD)].

Femoral anteversion: Angular difference between the forward inclination of the femoral neck and the transcondylar femoral axis (Fig. 20.2).

Foot axis: Imaginary line bisecting the long axis of the foot from the mid-heel through the middle to the metatarsal heads.

Internal and external femoral rotation: The child lies prone with the knees flexed to 90 degrees, the pelvis is stabilized, and the angle of gravity-assisted internal (medial rotation) and external rotation (lateral rotation) of each leg is measured.

Thigh–foot angle: Measures tibial torsion. The child lies prone and flexes the knees to 90 degrees; the angle is then placed in neutral position. Looking down at the sole of the foot, an imaginary line through the long axis of the foot is measured against the long axis of the femur. The angle between these two axes is the thigh–foot angle.

Evaluation and Interpretation

The medical history is obtained first and includes the type of deformity, apparent time of onset, amount of progression, family history, and previous treatment. A complete musculoskeletal and neurologic examination is performed, and finally a torsional (rotational) profile is generated to determine the severity and level of deformity (Fig. 20.3).

Foot Progression Angle. It is important to watch the child walk as naturally as possible. When being observed, children may initially try to control the amount of in-toeing to please the parent or physician. Keep in mind also that the amount of in-toeing becomes worse when a child is fatigued. In-toeing is expressed as a negative value (12–10 degrees) and out-toeing as a positive value. The normal value range for the foot progression angle is wide, and severe deformity above the foot may exist with a normal angle.

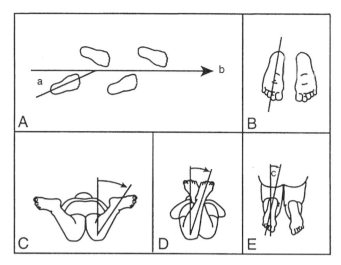

Fig. 20.1. Tests for torsional deformities (see text for full discussion). (A) Foot progression angle (a) is formed by the foot axis (B) and the line of progression (b). (B) Foot axis. (C) Measurement of internal femoral rotation. (D) Measurement of external femoral rotation. (E) Thigh-foot angle (c) is formed by the longitudinal axis of the femur and the foot axis. (From Lillegard and Kruse,[50] with permission.)

Hip Rotation. With the child in the prone position, the knees are flexed to 90 degrees with the pelvis level. The thigh is then rotated medially (internal rotation of the hip) by gravity alone. Lateral rotation is measured with the child in the same position by allowing the legs to cross. The diagnosis of medial femoral torsional deformity/femoral anteversion is made if medial rotation is more than 70 degrees. Total joint laxity must be taken into consideration by concurrent reduction in lateral rotation. Restriction of lateral rotation during early infancy is thought to be due to intrauterine position.

Tibial Rotation. Tibial rotation, the most difficult measurement to make accurately, requires assessment of the thigh–foot angle (TFA). The TFA increases from early childhood to mid-childhood. Internal tibial rotation is expressed as a negative angle. A negative value up to 20 degrees is considered normal during infancy. Medial tibial torsion exists if the TFA is more than 20 degrees. During early childhood the tibia rotates laterally.

Foot. The sole of the foot is observed to determine its shape; the lateral border is normally straight. Metatarsus adductus is the characteristic appearance of a "bean-shaped foot" with a wide space between the first and second toes, prominence at the base of the fifth metatarsal bone, and convexity at the lateral side of the foot. Metatarsus adductus is often present in conjunction with tibial torsion.

Clinical Patterns and Management

In-toeing (Metatarsus Adductus). The terms *metatarsus adductus* (MA) and *metatarsus varus* are used interchangeably.

MA occurs when the forefoot bones are deviated medially at the tarsal–metatarsal junction, causing the foot to appear to curve inward at the midfoot (bean-shaped foot). It is probably caused by a combination of intrauterine position and genetic predisposition and can be either flexible or rigid. Studies dispute the belief that hip dysplasia is higher among patients with metatarsus varus than in the general population.[3] On physical examination the foot is convex laterally and concave medially. The lateral border of the base of the fifth metatarsal may appear prominent. With the heel held in neutral position and pressure directed laterally at the first metatarsal head, a flexible deformity corrects to neutral but does not overcorrect as do normal feet. One helpful test is to stroke the lateral border of the foot, noting if the infant reflexly corrects the deformity. Treatment for flexible MA involves having the parents passively correct the range of deformity (as described above) with each diaper change. Due to the high rate of spontaneous resolution and the history of natural resolution, no treatment has been shown to be superior. These treatments vary from observation to casting to bracing night or day, or both, to orthopedic shoes. Children with rigid MA require cast correction and are best treated before 6 months of age and worked up for other neuromuscular disorders. If begun during the first month of life, correction can often be obtained within 6 to 8 weeks of casting by a knowledgeable orthopedist. After age 8 months, cast correction is almost impossible due to foot stiffness and active kicking by robust toddlers.

The reasons for treating these feet remain controversial, and specific treatment indications vary among orthopedic surgeons. It is currently believed that residual MA is not linked to adult degenerative arthritis.[1] Surgical correction is rarely indicated. When needed, Heyman-Herndon soft tissue releases are advised for children under age 4 years, and multi-

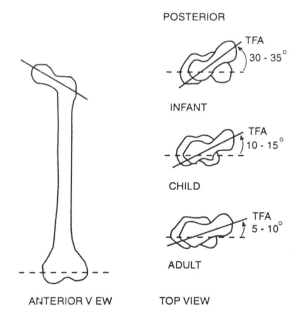

Fig. 20.2. Transcondylar femoral axis (TFA) as it would be measured radiographically in degrees of rotation.

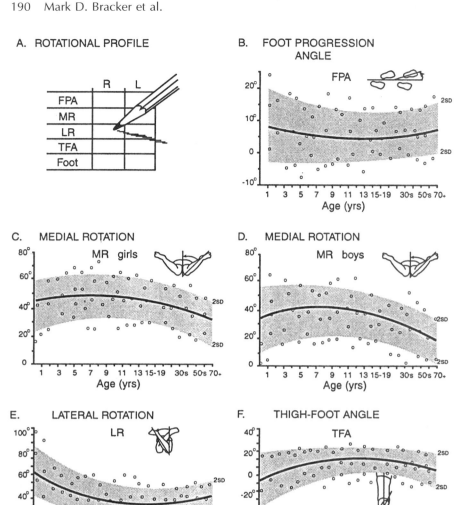

A. ROTATIONAL PROFILE

B. FOOT PROGRESSION ANGLE

C. MEDIAL ROTATION

D. MEDIAL ROTATION

E. LATERAL ROTATION

F. THIGH-FOOT ANGLE

Fig. 20.3. (A) Torsional profile. (B–F) Range of normal values by age group and sex. (From Engel and Staheli,[2] with permission.)

ple metatarsal osteotomies are recommended for older children.[4] In severe cases requiring surgical correction, associated heel valgus is common and must be addressed or the child will be further disabled because correction of the forefoot alone removes the stable tripod of the foot.

Tibial Torsion. In-toeing can also be due to excessive internal tibial torsion (medial tibial version). It can be clinically estimated using the TFA described previously. Normally the tibia is externally rotated 5 degrees at birth and 15 degrees at skeletal maturity. Correction is almost always spontaneous. Bracing, splints, twister cables, and shoe modifications have not been shown to be effective and are not recommended, as most of these deformities correct spontaneously by 3 to 4 years of age.[5] Developmental correction may be delayed if the child sleeps prone with the legs internally rotated or sits with the knees flexed and feet internally rotated. Although there is no proved benefit of altering the child's sitting position, parents may be instructed to encourage the child to avoid these positions. Derotational osteotomy is reserved for severe deformity, including significant functional and cosmetic disability, internal rotation of more than 85 degrees, external rotation of less than 10 degrees, radiographic anteversion of

more than 45 degrees, or external tibial rotation of less than 35 degrees. The child must be at least 7 to 8 years old.[6]

Femoral Anteversion. The angle between the femoral neck axis and the transcondylar axis of the distal femur is called femoral version (Fig. 20.2). Femoral anteversion (FA) decreases from an average of 40 degrees at birth to about 15 degrees at skeletal maturity. Children commonly sit on their knees with their feet out to the sides in the classic W position. With femoral anteversion the in-toeing is worse at the end of the day when compensating muscles fatigue. FA presents by age 3 to 4 years and resolves slowly over the next 5 years and is more common in girls than boys.

Infants normally have limited medial rotation due to a tight hip capsule, and external rotation to 90 degrees is common. External rotation decreases to around 55 degrees by age 3 and slowly decreases thereafter. Internal rotation increases from 35 degrees at birth to 60 degrees by age 6, at which time it is slightly greater than external rotation. From birth to 2 years of age the total range should be 120 degrees, decreasing to 95 to 110 degrees thereafter.

Treatment for an in-toeing gait due to excessive femoral anteversion, termed medial femoral torsion, is almost always simple observation, as 85% resolve with spontaneous derotation of the proximal femur during normal growth. Bony derotation occurs up to age 8 and in some cases into adolescence. Surgery is rarely indicated; it is reserved for severe, uncompensated medial femoral torsion causing significant functional and cosmetic problems during late childhood. In rare severe cases, a proximal femoral derotation osteotomy can be done safely at age 9 or 10.

Angular Abnormalities of the Knee

Newborns generally have a genu varus of approximately 15 degrees due physiologically to intrauterine positioning. Parents frequently note bowed legs as their child starts to stand. Children with superimposed internal tibial torsion actually look more bowed than they are. Children progress from genu varus in the newborn until 24 months and then start to develop genu valgus to about 15 degrees by age 4 years. Then by 6 to 7 years of age, this valgus begins to correct to 5 to 6 degrees, where it essentially remains to adulthood. Pathologic genu valgum or varus should be evaluated for metabolic disorders, inflammatory disease, tumors, osteochondrodysplasia, posttraumatic conditions, congenital abnormalities, osteogenesis imperfecta, or Blount's disease as possible causes.

Bowlegs

Excessive genu varus deformities with a tibial-femoral angle of more than 20 degrees should be investigated if they have not started correcting by 2 years of age. Growth charts should be carefully reviewed along with developmental and family history. Evaluation should include physical exam, gait observation, knee ligament laxity assessment, rotational evaluation, and foot position. Appropriate laboratory and standing radiographic studies should be ordered. The posteroanterior (PA) standing radiographs must be taken with the child's feet together or a shoulder width apart and neutral rotation with the patella pointing directly forward. The physis should be carefully examined. A tibiofemoral angle of more than 20 degrees in toddlers indicates severe physiologic bowing, or Blount's disease. Severe physiologic bowing is characterized radiographically as follows.

1. Medial metaphyseal beaking of the proximal fibula and distal femur
2. Medial cortical thickening
3. Varus angulation of more than 20 degrees based on the metaphyseal-diaphyseal angle
4. No pathologic changes in the proximal tibial epiphysis

After other etiologies have been ruled out and severe physiologic bowing is diagnosed, spontaneous correction can be expected by 7 to 8 years of age. If significant deformity persists past age 8, corrective tibial osteotomy is necessary in certain cases.

Blount's Disease

Osteochondrosis deformans tibiae, or Blount's disease, is due to defective formation of the posterior medial border of the proximal tibial epiphysis and may be difficult to distinguish from severe physiologic bowing. Blount's disease is more common in blacks than whites and is associated with obesity

and early walking. Radiographic findings after 18 to 24 months are angulation under the posterior medial proximal epiphysis, metaphyseal irregularity, beaking of the proximal tibia, and wedging of the proximal epiphysis. Another radiographic sign that has been found useful to diagnose Blount's disease is the metaphyseal-diaphyseal (MD) angle. The angle is derived from drawing a line along the lateral tibial cortex on a standard PA radiograph, and then drawing a line perpendicular to the tibial cortex line and one through the epiphysis. If the angle between the epiphysis and tibial cortex perpendicular line is greater than 11 degrees, Blount's disease is diagnosed.[7] Most of these children require corrective bracing or surgery and should be referred as soon as identified.

Knock-Knees

Genu valgus (knock-knees) can be apparent, physiologic, or pathologic. Apparent valgus may be due to large thighs, joint laxity, or poor muscle tone. Most cases are idiopathic or physiologic. Pathologic causes include juvenile rheumatoid arthritis, rickets, trauma, endocrine disturbance, and infection. Most children have a slight genu valgus that generally resolves by 6 years of age; it can become excessive later during childhood or early adolescence when the normal valgus fails to resolve. Genu valgus may represent an acceleration of normal angulation caused by abnormal forces across the knee. Standing PA radiographs with the feet pointing straight ahead may be obtained to document the tibiofemoral angle and to rule out underlying disease. Young children with this problem tend toward spontaneous resolution. With older children, knock-knees is less likely to correct completely.

Surgical correction of severe knock-knees deformity causing significant functional or cosmetic problems should be performed 1 year before the end of physeal growth in the femur (girls, 10–11 years old; boys, 12–13 years old). A staple encircles the femoral physis, which continues to grow laterally but not medially.[8]

Problems of the Feet

Toe Walking

The tiptoe gait characteristic of beginning toddlers should give way to an adult-like pattern by 2 years of age. Neuromuscular conditions such as cerebral palsy or spinal cord lesions such as spina bifida, tethered cord, and diastematomyelia can produce foot deformity, which can be appropriately evaluated diagnostically or referral made if toe walking persists beyond age 2.

Clubfoot

Talipes equinovarus (clubfoot), which occurs in approximately 1/1000 births,[9] is characterized by talar plantar flexion, hindfoot varus, forefoot adduction, and soft tissue contractures, resulting in a cavus foot deformity (Fig. 20.4).[10] It is thought to be secondary to intrauterine position in a genetically predisposed fetus but is also associated with congenital hip dislocation, myelomeningocele, and arthrogryposis. The major deformity of clubfoot is in the subtalar complex, with shortening and medial deviation of the talus with displacement of the navicular medially.[11] Radiographs confirm the severity of deformity,

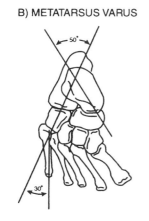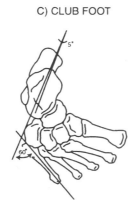

A) NORMAL   B) METATARSUS VARUS   C) CLUB FOOT

Fig. 20.4. Bone alignment. (A) Normal foot. (B) Metatarsus adductus (varus). (C) Clubfoot, demonstrating Kite's angle. Note Kite's angle is increased in metatarsus varus and decreased in club foot.

allow comparisons over time, and are essential for judging the type of surgical correction needed.

Treatment by an experienced orthopedic surgeon is an acquired skill that is becoming a lost art. Proper intervention involves reduction of the displaced navicular on the head of the talus and mobilization of tight capsules and tendons through manipulation followed by placement in a series of carefully molded corrective casts. The need for extensive surgery is reduced if casting is early and effective with 30% to 50% correction obtained.[12] Operative intervention is indicated if complete correction cannot be obtained or maintained. Recognition and treatment of clubfoot deformity should be initiated in the newborn nursery; therefore, recognition and referral of this entity are imperative. Parents should be reassured it is normal for the affected foot and calf to be smaller throughout the child's life.

Cavus Foot

Pes cavus, or cavus foot, is a fixed equinus and pronation deformity of the forefoot in relation to the hindfoot, usually resulting from an underlying neuromuscular condition: spinal dysraphism (spina bifida, lipoma, tethered cord, diastematomyelia), Charcot-Marie-Tooth disease, Friedreich's ataxia, or cord tumor. Occasionally, cases are familial or idiopathic. When unilateral, a spinal disorder is almost always the cause. All cavus feet demonstrate excessive plantar flexion of the first ray with pronation of the forefoot in relation to the hindfoot. The workup includes family and neurologic history and exam, weight-bearing radiographs of the feet, and strong consideration of a referral to the orthopedist. Corrective shoes and inserts are not effective for treating cavus feet. Surgical management, best undertaken after age 4 or 5 years, is directed toward medial and plantar release (plantar fascia, short flexors, adductor hallucis) followed by weekly cast changes to gain full correction.[13]

Flatfoot

Flexible Flatfoot

All children have flatfeet at birth. Some of these feet remain flat and asymptomatic and are a normal physiologic variant. The normal foot may appear flat until the child is 3 to 5 years old. Reasons include ligament laxity, flexibility of cartilage, neuromuscular development, and the presence of subcutaneous fat that occupies space in the arch. The support ligaments gradually tighten to form the longitudinal arch, increasing definition with normal growth. As a result, the true flexible flatfoot is difficult to diagnose clinically before the child is 2 years old.

The cause is primarily laxity of the ligaments that normally support the bones forming the arch. The laxity is frequently familial and is sometimes associated with Down, Marfan, and Ehlers-Danlos syndromes, all of which include excessive ligament laxity. Testing is done by having the child dorsiflex the great toe or stand on tiptoe (looking for the formation of an arch). Observed from the rear, the patient may have calcaneal valgus when bearing weight, shifting to varus position when standing tiptoe (a reflection of subtalar flexibility).[14]

Radiographic evaluation aids in confirming the diagnosis, localizing the malaligned joints, and ruling out other possibilities in the differential diagnosis. Anteroposterior and lateral radiographs are obtained with the patient standing so the feet are in the weight-bearing position.

No treatment is necessary for the asymptomatic foot, as there is gradual improvement with growth and development; the greatest improvement is seen by age 4. Recent studies have shown no greater incidence of painful adult feet in children with flexible flat feet.[12] The use of arch supports in asymptomatic children with flexible flatfoot has not been shown to make a difference in terms of altering the radiographic or clinical outcome.[14] For the occasional child who does develop a symptomatic flexible flatfoot, correction with an orthosis may be indicated. Medial longitudinal arch supports are helpful, and a medial heel wedge is added if calcaneal valgus is present.

Rigid Flatfoot

A rigid flatfoot is flat both sitting and standing; it may be due to underlying conditions such as infection, old trauma, congenital vertical talus, or tarsal coalition. Rigid pes planus with normal (nonspastic) peroneals is usually caused by an old infection of the tarsus, rheumatoid arthritis, or injury resulting in ankylosis and deformity that persists after the symptoms of the original pathology have subsided.[15] Rigid pes planus with associated spasm of the peroneus muscles, termed peroneal spastic flatfoot, is most often secondary to tarsal coalition or less commonly tarsal joint arthritis, tuberculosis, or old trauma. The decreased range of motion is due primarily to ankylosis, and the peroneal spasm is probably secondary to stress from the rigid tarsus. This stress results in painful strains, which initiate reflux muscle spasms of the peroneals.[15] Deformity of the foot secondary to cerebral palsy is common. Typically, the spastic flatfoot occurs in an ambulatory diplegic individual. In this case contracture of the Achilles tendon is the primary problem. Tarsal coalitions may be identified on plain radiographs but are often cartilaginous and best identified with a computed tomography (CT) scan. Orthopedic surgeons must exercise care regarding patient selection for surgery. All foot surgery is characterized by several weeks to months of disability during the postoperative period. The adolescent patient is not immune to reflux sympathetic dystrophy. Therefore, a specific diagnosis is mandatory, and patient expectations of postsurgical results should be discussed preoperatively. The patient with diffuse foot pain is a poor surgical candidate.

Elbow–Radial Head Subluxation

Epidemiology

Subluxation of the head of the radius, also known as "pulled elbow" or "nursemaid's elbow," is subluxation of the annular ligament into the radiohumeral joint. Commonly seen in preschool children 2 to 4 years old, the peak incidence occurs between 1 and 3 years of age. Injury after 5 years of age is rare and is most likely due to abnormal anatomic physiology. Salter and Zaltz[16] found that the annular ligament in children older than 5 years of age is thicker and more firmly attached to the periosteum at the radial neck. Boys are more frequently injured than girls, and the injury is diagnosed more often on the left side than the right side.

Traction may occur when lifting a child by one arm at the wrist or hand or swinging a child by both arms. Although this trauma may be slight, subluxation occurs owing to this longitudinal traction while the elbow is extended and the forearm pronated, resulting in a transverse tear of the annular ligament at its distal attachment to the radial neck. When the forearm is pronated, the radial head has its narrowest diameter in the anteroposterior plane. The radial head protrudes through the tear and migrates distally with proximal recession of the annular ligament into the radiocapitellar joint. Once traction is released, the annular ligament is trapped between the radial head and the capitellum, and full reduction of the radial head is blocked.

Diagnosis

The injured child presents by refusing to use the affected limb but may not complain of pain. Often the shoulder is suspected to be the culprit. At presentation, the arm is held at the side with elbow partially flexed and the forearm pronated. Clinical findings include tenderness to palpation over the radial head and decreased range of motion at the elbow. Radiographs may show soft tissue swelling but are usually negative. Al-

though the elbow is a commonly injured joint in children, interpretation of the radiograph may be difficult owing to joint anatomy. Because the radial epiphysis is not ossified, subluxation is diagnosed on clinical grounds.

Treatment

Reduction of the radial head is possible if the proximal edge of the annular ligament does not extend beyond the widest part of the radial head. Reduction of the annular ligaments is achieved by supination of the forearm, flexion of the elbow, and simultaneous pressure over the radial head. This maneuver is also achieved when manipulating the elbow to obtain an anteroposterior roentgenogram. An audible click may be heard with reduction associated with significant relief. Often the arm can be used immediately after reduction. Immobility is not necessary. The prognosis is excellent after successful reduction, with only a 5% recurrence rate.[16] On the rare occasion when closed reduction is unsuccessful, surgical referral is warranted. After an open reduction, immobilization of the elbow is recommended in a plaster splint at 90 degrees of flexion with the forearm in neutral position. Mobilization can be started within 1 week.

Classification

The traumatic cause of radial head subluxation, as noted above, is axial traction. In rare cases nontraumatic causes have been identified. Idiopathic subluxation may be due to congenital conditions. In the three cases reported by Southmayd and Ehrlich,[17] the radial head was observed to be enlarged and deformed. Patients presented with no history of trauma but experienced pain and limitation of the range of motion at the elbow. The cause of this condition remains unknown. Other nontraumatic causes of radial head subluxation have been associated with Apert syndrome. In such cases subluxation occurs early, even at birth, and may be the consequence of developmental deformity of abnormal cartilage tissue.

Problems of the Hip and Lower Extremity

Transient Synovitis of the Hip

Transient synovitis of the hip (TSH), a self-limited unilateral disease of unknown etiology, is the most common disorder causing a limp in children. TSH is most common between the ages of 2 and 10 years (average 6 years) and occurs more frequently in boys. The condition often parallels or follows a viral upper respiratory infection and has been considered by some to represent a viral or perhaps "viral-immune response" disorder affecting the hip.[18] The few biopsies reported for this benign, transitory disease have revealed only nonspecific inflammatory congestion and hypertrophy of the synovial membrane

Children with TSH present with an ill-defined limp, hip or knee pain, and possibly a low-grade fever. The hip is often held flexed, abducted, and externally rotated to provide for

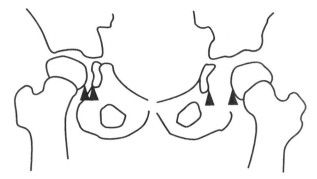

Fig. 20.5. Teardrop distance is the interval between the ossified part of the femoral head or neck and the acetabulum (arrowheads). The teardrop distance is a useful criterion for early diagnosis of Legg-Calvé-Perthes disease and is also a good indicator of the presence of excess joint fluid caused by sepsis. In 96% of normal subjects the teardrop distance in both hips is the same or differs by only 1 mm or less.

maximum joint volume. A complete blood count may show mild leukocytosis without a left shift. The erythrocyte sedimentation rate (ESR) may be elevated, exceeding 20 mm/hour in nearly one third of patients.[19] Radiographs may show capsular swelling characterized by increased distance between the medial acetabulum and the ossified part of the femoral head (Fig. 20.5). Ultrasound examination has been used increasingly as a diagnostic tool to detect hip disorders because of its high sensitivity for demonstrating effusion in the hip joint.

It may be difficult to differentiate TSH from early septic arthritis; and if clinical suspicion is high, the hip should be aspirated. Initial treatment is bed rest, usually at home, but occasionally hospitalization is required to perform studies needed to rule out sepsis and thus allay parental and physician concern.

Symptoms may last up to 7 to 10 days but rarely more than 2 weeks. Failure to resolve with rest should lead to a more extensive workup to exclude juvenile rheumatoid arthritis, sacroiliac joint infection, osteomyelitis of the ileum, and osteoid osteoma, each of which may mimic TSH. A few patients with TSH (1–3%) go on to develop Legg-Calvé-Perthes disease within a year.[20] Therefore, patients with TSH should have their hips examined once or twice during the year following acute presentation. Radiographs are unnecessary if hip motion is full.

Septic Hip

A septic hip is considered a medical emergency, as surgical drainage of pus soon after onset of symptoms prevents destruction of the femoral head and neck. Accumulating fluid and pus containing destructive enzymes rapidly elevate the intraarticular pressure and permanently injure vessels and articular cartilage. Microorganisms usually enter the hip joint by bacteremia, the result of distant infection (skin or subcutaneous abscess, otitis media, pharyngitis, pneumonia, or umbilical infection). In neonates nosocomial infection may occur via catheters or venipuncture.

In neonates and infants, the early stages of septic hip may be mistaken for cellulitis, venous thrombosis, superficial abscess, and sciatic nerve palsy. Unilateral swelling of the thigh or leg may indicate a ruptured septic hip with extravasation of pus into the thigh fascial planes. Older children usually present as apprehensive, toxic, and experiencing constant hip pain. Typical septic arthritis of the hip in infants and children can be recognized without difficulty. The child is febrile with the thigh in a position of flexion, abduction, and external rotation. The pain is worse with any hip movement. A site of infection and portal of entry into the bloodstream such as skin abscess, otitis media, or pneumonia is usually present.

Laboratory testing may show an elevated complete blood count (CBC), ESR, and C-reactive protein. C-reactive protein rises within 6 to 8 hours, while the ESR may not rise for 24 to 48 hours. There is considerable overlap between TSH and septic arthritis. No combination of physical exam or laboratory findings is 100% sensitive or specific in diagnosing septic arthritis of the hip.[19] Aspirating pus from the hip joint remains critical for diagnosis and early decompression. Blood cultures and cultures from other sites are obtained before initiating antibiotics (see Chapter 43). *Staphylococcus* and gram-negative organisms are commonly found in newborns. In children 1 to 18 months of age, *Haemophilus influenzae* is a frequent cause of septic hip. *Salmonella* can infect a hip in patients with sickle cell disease. Intravenous antibiotics should be started following needle aspiration and culture, but antibiotics alone cannot cure septic hip. Treatment must include surgical decompression.

Slipped Capital Femoral Epiphysis

Slipped capital femoral epiphysis (SCFE) is the most common serious disorder of the hip in adolescents. The peak age incidence is 11 years for girls and 14 years for boys; the incidence in the general population is approximately 2 per 100,000 with a male to female ratio of 2.5:1.0.[21] SCFE is characterized by sudden or gradual medial displacement of the femoral neck from the capital femoral epiphysis. The epiphysis remains in the acetabulum, resulting in a retroversion deformity of the femoral neck. The goals of treatment for a patient with a SCFE are to stabilize the slip and prevent further displacement while avoiding the complications of avascular necrosis, chondrolysis, and early osteoarthritis.

The etiology is multifactorial and ill-defined. Classification of SCFE has been traditionally based on duration of symptoms. Slips have been divided into acute (symptoms <3 weeks), acute-on-chronic (symptoms of mild pain for >3 weeks with a recent sudden exacerbation), and chronic (symptoms >3 weeks).[22] Newer classification schemes attempt to address the question of stability because unstable slips have a poorer prognosis.[23,24]

With an acute slip, mild symptoms are present for a short time before the displacement occurs; minimal trauma may then cause an acute separation, with pain so severe the child cannot bear weight on the affected side. Patients with the chronic form have hip pain localized to the groin, buttock, or

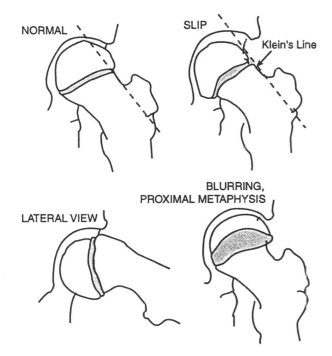

Fig. 20.6. Left slipped capital femoral epiphysis. A line drawn along the superior aspect of the femoral neck (Klein's line) barely intersects with the femoral head compared to the normal right side, a sign of slipping of the left femoral head.

lateral hip. Occasionally, the child has only knee pain. There is a decrease in abduction, flexion, and internal rotation, and as the hip is gently flexed it may roll into external rotation.

The clinical diagnosis of SCFE requires radiographic confirmation of femoral head displacement. Radiographic assessment must include both hips in anteroposterior (AP) and lateral views. Both hips are included because bilateral disease occurs in one third of cases.[25] The earliest changes may be subtle, only showing widening or irregularity of the epiphyseal plate (Fig. 20.6). Since initial displacement occurs posteriorly, the true lateral or "frog" lateral views are most sensitive to detect early SCFE. On the AP view the Klein's line drawn along the superior femoral neck should intersect 20% of the lateral femoral head (Fig. 20.6). When the diagnosis is suspected from the clinical findings, but plain radiographs are not conclusive, magnetic resonance imaging (MRI) is the best study to demonstrate the subtle widening and irregularity of the physis and even early slippage of the femoral head.[26]

Surgery is the only reliable treatment for SCFE. Results are best if it is performed soon after diagnosis because outcomes depend on early stabilization. Any attempt to reduce a chronic slip produces avascular necrosis.

In children who have unilateral disease at diagnosis, nearly 20% may go on to develop bilateral disease. Most often sequential slips will occur within 18 months, although reports have documented cases that occur up to 5 years after initial diagnosis.[25] Frequent follow-up examination is recommended until definite radiographic evidence of physeal closure is noted.

Developmental Dysplasia of the Hip

The term *developmental dysplasia of the hip* (DDH) describes a spectrum of disorders: frank dislocation, partial dislocation (subluxation), instability, and acetabular dysplasia. Because many of these findings are not present at birth, the term *developmental dysplasia* has replaced the older term *congenital hip dislocation*. The reported incidence of all forms of DDH is 2 to 6/1000 and is influenced by genetic and environmental factors. The etiology of DDH is multifactorial. The female to male ratio is 5:1. Hormonal factors play a role in joint laxity. Mechanical factors increasing the risk of DDH include oligohydramnios, primigravida, and breech presentation. Intrauterine positioning may explain the 3:1 predominance of left hip involvement. One in five children with DDH has a positive family history.[27,28]

In the newborn, Barlow and Ortolani tests (Fig. 20.7) are the most reliable tests for diagnosis and should be part of every well-baby examination (see Chapter 17). The infant is examined relaxed and supine, with one of the examiner's hands stabilizing the pelvis. The other hand holds the hip to be examined with the thumb in the groin and the index or long finger over the greater trochanter. The hip is flexed to 90 degrees and adducted past the midline while a gentle outward force is made by the thumb. The hip may be felt to dislocate during adduction (positive Barlow sign). The hip is then abducted and gently lifted. Relocation of the dislocated femoral head may be felt (a pop is not heard), which is a positive Ortolani's reduction test. A positive test is felt as a "clunk." The high-pitched click that is often heard is normal and unrelated to DDH.

In the child over 2 to 3 months of age, muscle tightness may mask dislocation or reduction. Clinical signs are more subtle as the child approaches walking age, but the following abnormalities should always be sought during well-child examinations: an asymmetric hip abduction, one knee lower than the other (positive Galeazzi's sign), and asymmetric thigh

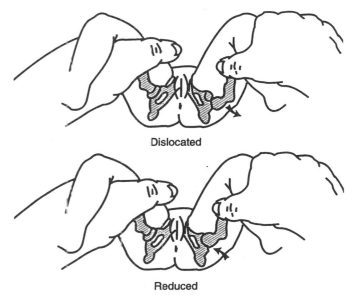

Fig. 20.7. Barlow and Ortolani tests.

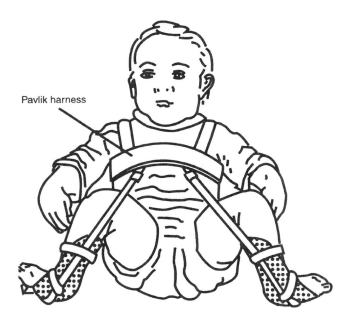

Fig. 20.8. Pavlik harness on a newborn. The hips are fully flexed, then fall out passively into abduction.

creases. Unfortunately, these clinical examinations do not identify all neonates with DDH, in part because some cases are missed on initial examination and other children develop instability later. Standard radiographs are difficult to interpret until the femoral head begins to ossify at 3 to 6 months of age. During dynamic ultrasonography a modified Barlow maneuver is used for the hip evaluation, increasing the accuracy of diagnosing hip instability after 6 weeks of age.[29,30]

Neonatal hip instability or dislocation can be treated with a Pavlik-type harness (Fig. 20.8) with 85% to 90% success in infants up to 6 to 8 months of age.[31,32] This harness holds the infant's hips in a flexed and abducted position, directing the femoral head into the developing acetabulum. Pavlik harness use requires close ultrasound or radiographic monitoring and frequent clinical follow-up. Most hips stabilize after 2 to 3 months. Dislocated hips diagnosed at 6 to 18 months of age often require closed or open surgical reduction under anesthesia, followed by spica cast immobilization.

Legg-Calvé-Perthes Disease

Legg-Calvé-Perthes disease (LCPD) is avascular necrosis of the femoral head in otherwise clinically normal children. LCPD typically presents between 4 and 8 years of age, with the boy/girl ratio approximately 5:1. Bilateral involvement occurs in approximately 10%.[20] Interesting parallels exist between LCPD and "constitutional delay of growth." Children with LCPD are often small for age, and thin, with bone age that is delayed by 1 to 2 years. Recent studies have proposed a link with familial thrombotic disorders, such as the factor V Leiden mutation.[33] Age at onset is an important indicator of outcome; children under 6 years of age often do well without specific treatment, whereas children over 9 years have a worse prognosis.[20]

Catterall[34] has classified LCPD according to radiographic

findings of the percent of the femoral head that is avascular (Fig. 20.9). The ultimate Catterall classification may not be determined for 6 to 9 months after the initial onset.[35] The history and physical findings can vary markedly depending on the stage of the disease process. During the early stages, the history is most often that of a limp or increasing groin, thigh, or knee pain. The physical findings at this time are similar to those of a child with an "irritable hip"; the initial synovitis may cause a decrease in range of motion on internal and external rotation, and there may be muscle atrophy of the thigh or calf consistent with an antalgic gait. With later, more severe stages of LCPD, there may be contractures of the adductor and hip flexor musculature in addition to restricted internal and external rotation.

Techniques for diagnosing LCPD and determining its prognosis include radiography, technetium scanning, MRI, arthrography, and CT scans. They are all equally useful, and each has advantages and disadvantages. Laboratory evaluation is normal.

LCPD is a self-healing disorder and there is no evidence that any treatment speeds the return of blood flow to the femoral head.[20] The main treatment objectives are to relieve muscle spasm, regain range of motion, and contain the femoral epiphysis within the acetabulum to minimize deformation of the femoral head. Orthopedic consultation is recommended. Nonsurgical treatment includes the use of a spica cast, removable orthosis, and braces. Surgical options for more severe disease include soft tissue procedures to release the adductors and bony procedures to mechanically realign the hip.[36] Long-term outcomes are good for most children, although approximately 10% to 15% develop deteriorating symptoms and degenerative arthritis that may require hip arthroplasty.[37] Most patients with LCPD can participate in sports.

Apophyseal Injuries
Apophysitis of the Hip

Apophyseal injury involving the anterosuperior and anteroinferior iliac spines, iliac crest, and ischial tuberosity typically occurs in active adolescents. Major abdominal and hip muscles either insert or originate at these sites of bone growth. The condition is most common in distance runners and dancers and is associated with muscle–tendon imbalance and rapid growth (see Chapter 52). Adolescents present with vague, dull pain related to activity located near the hip. Should a single traumatic episode exceed the strength of the physis, an avulsion fracture through the growth plate occurs. Radiographs may be useful for evaluating acute trauma and ruling out other hip pathology. Treatment includes rest from the offending activity followed by a program of stretching and progressive strengthening of the abdominal and hip muscles (Table 20.1). Depending on their size and displacement, acute fractures may be treated with rest or open-reduction internal fixation.

Sinding-Larsen-Johansson Syndrome

Sinding-Larsen-Johansson syndrome is an apophyseal injury to the inferior pole of the patella. The condition is thought

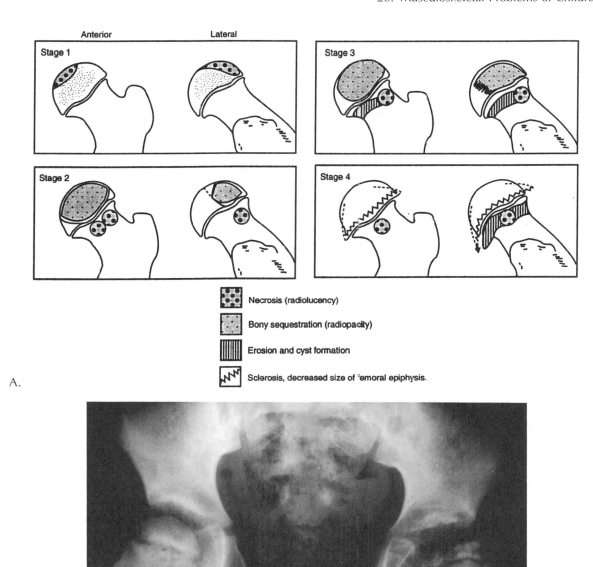

A.

B.

Fig. 20.9. (A) Catterall classified Legg-Calvé-Perthes disease into four stages. Stage 1: Necrosis is present at the anterior aspect of the femoral head as noted by the dotted areas. Lysis is present, but there is no bony sequestration. Stage 2: Bony sequestration is present as noted by the central areas of radiopacity. A medial and lateral column of normal bone protects the central area from collapse. Stage 3: Extensive bony sequestration diminishes support and increases the chance of residual deformity. Metaphyseal cyst formation is noted by the line-slashed areas. Stage 4: Total involvement produces significant residual deformity shown by the jagged areas that indicate sclerosis and decreased size of the femoral head. (From Gerberg and Micheli,[45] with permission.) (B) Legg-Calvé-Perthes disease. Radiograph shows severe changes of the entire left femoral head due to avascular necrosis. (From Lillegard and Kruse,[50] with permission.)

Table 20.1. **Apophyseal Injuries**

Injury	Age (years)	Site	Presentation	Differential diagnosis	Treatment
Sever's disease	8–13	Posterior calcaneus	Heel pain with activity	Achilles tendinitis, stress fracture	Heel cups, RICE, decrease activity, NSAIDs
Osgood-Schlatter disease	Boys: 10–15 Girls: 8–13	Tibial tuberosity	Anterior knee pain	PFD, OCD, stress fracture	RICE, activity modification, NSAIDs
Sindig-Larsen-Johannson syndrome	10–13	Inferior pole of patella	Anterior knee pain	PFD, OCD, stress fracture	RICE, activity modification NSAIDs
Apophysitis of the hip	9–13	ASIS, AIIS, iliac crest, ischial tuberosity	Dull ache around the hip	Muscle strain, stress fracture	RICE, stretching program, NSAIDs

Source: Peck,[58] with permission.
NSAIDs = nonsteroidal antiinflammatory drugs; PFD = patellofemoral dysfunction; OCD = osteochondritis dissecans; RICE = rest, ice, compression, and elevation; ASIS = anterosuperior iliac spine; AIIS = anteroinferior iliac spine.

to result from multiple episodes of traction-induced micro-trauma at an immature, inferior patellar pole, with resultant calcification and ossification at this junction. It is commonly seen in active preteen boys (10–12 years old), who complain of pain over the inferior pole of the patella or at the proximal quadriceps patellar junction that is worsened by running or stair climbing. Point tenderness is noted at the patella–quadriceps or patella–patellar tendon junctions. The remainder of the knee examination is usually normal. Radiographs may be normal or show varying amounts and shapes of calcification or ossification at the patellar junction.

It is important to advise the patient and family that it is a self-limited condition that improves with rest and attainment of skeletal maturity. Activity modification, use of a knee sleeve, ice, massage, and antiinflammatory medication are usually helpful for reducing discomfort.

Osgood-Schlatter Disease

Osgood-Schlatter disease, the most common apophyseal disorder, was independently described in 1903.[38] The condition is found most commonly in boys age 10 to 15 years and in

girls 2 years earlier; it is often bilateral (20–30% of cases). On examination, exquisite tenderness may be noted over the anterior tibial tubercle, with prominence and swelling at that location. Pain worsens during running, jumping, and ascending or descending stairs. Resisted extension of the knee at 90 degrees of flexion causes pain. Radiographs are obtained to exclude the possibility of osteomyelitis and arterial-venous malformations. A discrete separate ossicle is noted at the tibial tubercle in as many as 50% of reported cases.

The patient and family must understand that 12 to 18 months may be required to allow spontaneous resolution by physiologic epiphysiodesis. Treatment with ice, antiinflammatory medication, and an appropriately contoured knee pad relieves symptoms. The level of sporting activity is balanced with tolerance and severity of symptoms. If symptoms progress to disability with activities of daily living, a brief course (7–10 days) of knee immobilization usually resolves the discomfort. Steroid injections into the tibial tubercle should never be done. Rare, persistent cases that fail to respond to a lengthy trial of conservative therapy may resolve with surgical removal of the bony ossicle overlying the tibial tubercle.

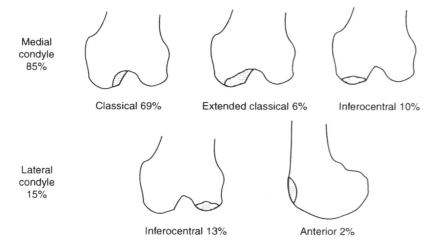

Medial condyle 85%

Classical 69%   Extended classical 6%   Inferocentral 10%

Lateral condyle 15%

Inferocentral 13%   Anterior 2%

Fig. 20.10. Distribution of osteochondritis dissecans by body location.

Sever's Disease

In 1912 Sever[39] described a benign inflammatory condition to the calcaneal apophysis in active adolescents. The sports most commonly associated with Sever's disease are soccer and running. The disease presents with unilateral or bilateral (60%) posterior heel pain in the 8- to 13-year-old athlete. It is associated with accelerated growth, tight heel cords, and other biomechanical abnormalities. Patients present with tenderness at the insertion of the Achilles tendon on the calcaneus. Radiographs may show partial fragmentation and increased density of the os calcis, thereby ruling out other rare causes of heel pain, such as unicameral bone cyst or a stress fracture. Activity modification, stretching of the gastrocnemius–soleus complex, ankle inverters and everters, and heel cups have all proved helpful. Children may return to sports without limitation 2 to 4 weeks after symptoms resolve.

Osteochondritis Dissecans

Osteochondritis dissecans (OCD) is characterized by separation of a fragment of bone with overlying articular cartilage from the surrounding normal bone. OCD most commonly affects the medial aspect of the lateral femoral condyle, but is also seen in the talar dome and humeral capitellum (Fig 20.10). OCD can occur in all large joints. The incidence is estimated to be 15 to 30 cases per 100,000 persons. OCD may be more common than is currently known because asymptomatic lesions are discovered only incidentally. Risk factors include repetitive microtrauma as seen in throwing sports or gymnastics. OCD has a familial predisposition. Contralateral joint involvement is noted in 20% to 30% of patients with OCD of the knee.

Without proper management the disease may progress through four stages: stage 1, thickening of the articular cartilage (stable); stage 2, fragment in situ and beginning of demarcation of the articular cartilage (stable); stage 3, partial detachment (unstable); and stage 4, complete detachment of the fragment and formation of a loose body (unstable).[40] OCD may be viewed as a stress fracture of the involved subchondral bone and requires differentiation from epiphyseal dysplasia, ossification defects, and acute osteochondral fracture. Symptoms include vague joint pain, catching, restricted range of motion, and pain with activity or range of motion. Plain radiographs reveal most lesions. Radioisotope scanning may be used if onset is acute and x-rays are negative. MRI is the gold standard for staging once the diagnosis is made.

Conservative treatment, including avoidance of stressful or painful activities and restricted weight bearing for periods ranging from 2 to 6 months may be successful in selected patients. Predictors of good clinical outcomes with conservative management include open joint physis, and small lesions that are stable on MRI.[41] Not all lesions heal spontaneously, and surgery may be required to stimulate new bone growth. Most orthopedic surgeons prefer arthroscopic drilling of the lesion from inside the joint.

Problems of the Spine

Spondylolysis and Spondylolisthesis

Spondylolysis is an acquired condition in which there is a bony defect on one or both sides of the pars interarticularis (Fig. 20.11), usually at the L5-S1 level. The incidence of spondylolysis is about 5% in preadolescent North American children and rises to 12% in gymnasts and divers.[42] The defect is not apparent at birth but develops usually between 5 and 10 years of age.[43] Thus vigorous athletic activity in children may produce repetitive stress on the developing pars.

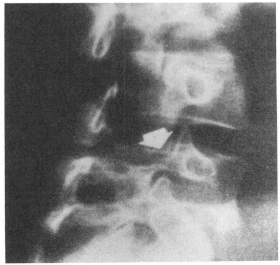

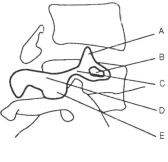

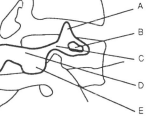

Fig. B

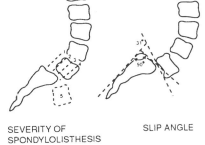

SEVERITY OF
SPONDYLOLISTHESIS

SLIP ANGLE

Fig. C

A

Fig. 20.11. Spondylolysis, and spondylolisthesis (right). (A) Radiographic representation of an abnormal elongation (greyhound sign) of the pars interarticularis, or the "neck" of a scotty dog (arrow). Other defects, such as sclerosis or lysis in the pars, are best visualized in this "neck." (From Lillegard and Kruse,[50] with permission.) (B) "Scotty dog." A = superior articular process (ear); B = pedicle (eye); C = pars interarticularis (neck); D = lamina (body); E = inferior articular process (front leg). (C) Severity of spondylolisthesis and slip angle.

When bilateral pars defects are present at a single vertebral level, translation (slip) of the vertebral body may occur in adjacent vertebrae, which is termed spondylolisthesis. Four distinct types of spondylolisthesis have been described: dysplastic, isthmic, degenerative, and traumatic. Most cases in children and adolescents are of the dysplastic or isthmic type, whereas degenerative changes of the facet joints may result in spondylolisthesis in older adults without spondylolysis of the pars interarticularis.

Spondylolysis and spondylolisthesis may be asymptomatic or may present with low back pain occasionally radiating to the buttocks. Physical examination may show lumbosacral tenderness and accentuation of pain by hyperextension of the spine with one leg raised off the ground and flexed 90 degrees at the hip and knee (one-leg hyperextension test). Patients with significant spondylolisthesis have a classic appearance of a short torso and flat buttocks, often standing with their knees held in modest extension. Neurologic status, including bladder function, must be assessed, although neurologic deficit is unusual and is seen in about 35% of those with more than 50% slippage of the vertebrae.[43]

Radiographs should include anteroposterior, lateral, and oblique views of the lumbar spine. The pars defect is best seen on the oblique film (Fig. 20.11) and is unilateral in about 20% of patients. The pars defect appears as a band or break in the "Scotty dog's neck" (pars interarticularis) of L5. Sclerosis of the opposite pars may be present. A standing spot lateral view of L5-S1 allows accurate assessment of a possible slip. Scoliosis is commonly associated with spondylolisthesis. Bone scans show increased activity on one or both sides in symptomatic spondylolysis but are not routinely required.

If asymptomatic, no treatment is required, and there is no need to limit contact sports. For a mildly symptomatic patient, temporary reduction of activity is all that is needed. If symptoms are alleviated, progressive activity is permitted. Symptoms that are sudden in onset, traumatically induced, or do not resolve with rest do heal—much as any fracture would heal—after 10 to 12 weeks of immobilization in a plastic body jacket or a Boston-type spinal orthosis. In general, once symptoms resolve, the child can resume normal activities, although advice regarding return to rigorous spine-bending athletic events (gymnastics, diving, downed lineman in football) is controversial (see Chapter 52).

With spondylolisthesis, if slippage is less than 30% and symptoms are minimal, treatment is conservative. With persistent pain unresponsive to treatment or slippage more than 30% to 50%, spinal fusion is recommended. Such fusion is generally at the L5-S1 level and includes L4 if slippage is more than 50%.[44]

Idiopathic Scoliosis

Idiopathic scoliosis is defined as lateral deviation of the spine of more than 10 degrees (measured by the Cobb method),[45] with structural change and without congenital anomalies of the vertebrae. It is inherited in an autosomal-dominant manner with variable penetrance or a multifactorial condition. It

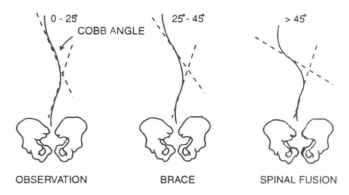

Fig. 20.12. Measuring the Cobb angle and treatment of idiopathic scoliosis.

occurs in approximately 2% of the population. Normally, only about one fifth to one sixth of this group require treatment.[46]

Scoliosis is a painless condition usually identified by shoulder, scapular, or pelvic asymmetry during school screening or routine physical examination. Forward bending (Adam's) testing is done with the child standing straight and bending forward with palms together and knees straight. Truncal asymmetry, most commonly right rib prominence, may be seen. Any limb length irregularity should be noted and corrected by placing blocks under the short leg and leveling the pelvis prior to examination. Neurologic examination is normal. Initial radiologic evaluation consists of standing PA and lateral spine films on a long cassette to include the pelvis. The curve is measured using the Cobb method[45] (Fig. 20.12). If a structural curve of 10 to 20 degrees is identified, orthopedic referral is recommended. Painful scoliosis or an atypical curve pattern (apex left thoracic) is indicative of possible underlying neurologic problems, such as syringomyelia or spinal cord lesion, and is probably not idiopathic scoliosis.

The risk of curve progression is higher in young children, in those with large curves or double curves, and in girls. Bracing is usually initiated for curves of more than 20 degrees with documented progression and growth remaining or for curves initially 30 degrees or more. Curves of more than 45 to 50 degrees are usually not amenable to bracing, so surgery is recommended, as the risk of continued progression after skeletal maturity is high in this group.[46]

Scheuermann's Disease

Scheuermann's disease (juvenile kyphosis) is defined as an abnormal increase in thoracic kyphosis (normal 20–40 degrees) during puberty with at least 5 degrees of anterior wedging of at least three or more adjacent vertebrae. It is to be distinguished from postural round back, which is more flexible and lacks radiographic changes in the vertebrae.[47] The etiology is unclear, but a familial incidence is noted in 30% to 48% of cases. It occurs in about 1% of the population and is more common in boys.

Clinically, it is possible to distinguish two forms of juvenile kyphosis. Thoracic Scheuermann's disease has an apex of the curve at T7–9, and thoracolumbar Scheuermann's disease has an apex at T11-12. Cosmetic deformity is often the chief complaint. Pain is usually aching and occurs more commonly with the thoracolumbar form.

Radiographs should include standing posteroanterior and lateral scoliosis films. Hyperextension lateral films help to determine the flexibility of the curve. Radiographs show irregularity of the vertebral endplates, anterior wedging of 5 degrees or more of three or more adjacent vertebrae, Schmorl's nodes, and increased kyphosis measured between T4 and T12 by the Cobb method.

Kyphosis may worsen during the growing period. Curves of 40 to 60 degrees may be treated by a trial of hyperextension exercises if the curve is supple and demonstrates active correction. Curves of 60 to 75 degrees are treated with a Milwaukee brace or underarm orthosis with a breastplate. Bracing is begun if the vertebral end plates are not fused to the vertebral body, with full-time wearing for 6 to 12 months and then part-time (about 16 hours/day) for 6 months or until the end plate fuses. Bracing is less effective for curves of more than 65 to 75 degrees or after skeletal maturity. Surgery may be indicated for cosmesis, progressive deformity despite bracing, or intractable pain. No long-term cardiopulmonary problems have been identified.[48,49]

References

1. Karoll LA. Rotational deformities in the lower extremities. Curr Opin Pediatr 1997;9:77–90.
2. Engel FM, Staheli LT. The natural history of torsional and other factors influencing gait in early childhood. Clin Orthop 1974; 99:12–17.
3. Wells L. Common lower extremity problems in children, primary care. Clin Office Pract 1996;23(2):299–303.
4. Brink DS, Levitsky DR. Cuneiform and cuboid wedge osteotomies for correction of residual metatarsus adductus: a surgical review. J Foot Ankle Surg 1995;34:371–8.
5. Fabray G, MacEwen GD, Shands AR Jr. Torsion of the femur: a follow-up study in normal and abnormal conditions. J Bone Joint Surg 1973;55A:1726–38.
6. Kling TF, Hensinger RN. Angular and torsional deformities of the lower limbs in children. Clin Orthop 1983;176:136–47.
7. Bruce RW Jr. Torsional and angular deformities. Pediatr Clin North Am 1996;43(4):867–81.
8. Mielke CH, Stevens PM. Hemiepiphyseal stapling for knee deformities in children younger than 10 years: a preliminary report. J Pediatr Orthop 1996;16:423–9.
9. Cummings RJ, Lovell WW. Operative treatment of congenital idiopathic club foot. J Bone Joint Surg 1988;70A:1108–12.
10. Ponseti IV. Congenital clubfoot, the results of treatment. J Bone Joint Surg 1963;45A:261–9.
11. Cowell H. Talocalcaneal coalition and new causes of peroneal spastic flatfoot. Clin Orthop 1972;85:16–22.
12. Hoffinger SA. Evaluation and management of pediatric foot deformities. Pediatr Clin North Am 1996;43:1091–111.
13. Paulos L, Samuelson KM. Pes cavovarus: review of a surgical approach using selective soft tissue procedures. J Bone Joint Surg 1980;62A:942–53.
14. Wenger DR, Mauldin D, Speck G, Morgan D, Lieber R. Corrective shoes and inserts as treatment for flexible flatfoot in infants and children. J Bone Joint Surg 1989;71A:800–10.
15. Steward M. Miscellaneous afflictions of the foot. In: Campbell's operative orthopedics. St. Louis: Mosby, 1980;1703.
16. Salter RB, Zaltz C. Anatomic investigation of the mechanism of injury and pathologic anatomy of "pulled elbow" in young children. Clin Orthop 1971;77:134.
17. Southmayd W, Ehrlich MB. Idiopathic subluxation of the radial head. Clin Orthop 1976;121:271.
18. Hardinge K. The etiology of transient synovitis of the hip in childhood. J Bone Joint Surg 1970;52B:100–7.
19. Del Beccaro M, Champoux A, Bockers T, Mendelman P. Septic arthritis versus transient synovitis of the hip: The value of screening laboratory tests. Ann Emerg Med 1992;21(12): 1418–22.
20. Roy DR. Current concepts in Legg-Calve-Perthes Disease. Pediatr Ann 1999;28(12):748–52.
21. Busch M, Morrisy R. Slipped capital femoral epiphysis. Orthop Clin North Am 1987;18:637–47.
22. Fahey JJ, O'Brien ET. Acute slipped capital femoral epiphysis: review of the literature and report of ten cases. J Bone Joint Surg 1965;47A:1105–27.
23. Kallio PE, Paterson DC, Foster BK, Lequene GW. Classification in slipped capital femoral epiphysis. Clin Orthop 1993; 294:196–203.
24. Loder RT, Richards BS, Shapiro PS, Reznick LR, Aronsson DD. Acute slipped capital femoral epiphysis: the importance of physical stability. J Bone Joint Surg 1993;75A:1134–40.
25. Loder RT, Aronson DD, Greenfield ML. The epidemiology of bilateral slipped capital femoral epiphysis. J Bone Joint Surg 1993;75A:1141–7.
26. Umas H, Liebling M, Moy L, Harmamati N, Macy N, Pritzker H. Slipped capital femoral epiphysis: a physeal lesion diagnosed by MRI, with radiographic and CT correlation. Skel Radiol 1998;27:139–44.
27. Committee on Quality Improvement and Subcommittee on Developmental Dysplasia of the Hip. American Academy of Pediatrics: clinical practice guideline: early detection of developmental dysplasia of the hip. Pediatrics 2000;105(4): 896–905.
28. Gerscovich EO. Radiologists' guide to the imaging in the diagnosis and treatment of developmental dysplasia of the hip. Skel Radiol 1997;26:386–97.
29. Rosendahl K, Markestad T, Lie RT. Ultrasound in the early diagnosis of congenital dislocation of the hip: the significance of hip stability versus acetabular morphology. Pediatr Radiol 1992;22:430–3.
30. Graf R. Hip semiography: how reliable? Sector scanning versus linear scanning? Dynamic versus static examination? Clin Orthop 1992;281:18–21.
31. Weinstein SL. Congenital hip dislocation: long-range problems, residual signs and symptoms after successful treatment. Clin Orthop 1992;281:69–74.
32. Harris IE, Dickens R, Menelaus MB. Use of the Pavlic harness for hip displacements: when to abandon treatment. Clin Orthop 1992;281:29–33.
33. Gruppo R, Glueck CJ, Wall E, Roy D, Wang P. Legg-Perthes disease in three siblings, two heterozygous and one homozygous for the factor V Leiden mutation. J Pediatr 1998;132(5):885–8.
34. Catterall A. The natural history of Perthes' disease. J Bone Joint Surg 1971;53B:37–53.
35. Gershuni DH. Preliminary evaluation and prognosis in Legg-Calvé-Perthes disease. Clin Orthop 1980;150:16–22.
36. Herring JA. The treatment of Legg-Calve-Perthes disease. J Bone Joint Surg 1994;76A(3):448–57.
37. McAndrew MP. Weinstein SL. A long-term follow-up of Legg-Calve-Perthes disease. J Bone Joint Surg 1984;66A(6):860–9.
38. Osgood RB. Lesions of the tibial tubercle occurring during adolescence. Boston Med J 1903;148:114–17.
39. Sever JW. Apophysitis of the os calcis. NY Med J 1912;95: 1025–9.

40. Obedian RS, Grelsamer RP. Osteochondritis dissecans of the distal femur and patella. Clin Sports Med 1997;16:157–74.

41. De Smet AA. Omer AI, Graf BK. Untreated osteochondritis dissecans of the femoral condyles: prediction of patient outcome using radiographic and MR findings. Skel Radiol 1997;26:463–7.

42. Wiltse LL, Newman PH, Macnab I. Classification of spondylolysis and spondylolisthesis. Clin Orthop 1976;117:23–9.

43. Hensinger RN. Spondylolysis and spondylolisthesis in children and adolescents. J Bone Joint Surg 1989;71A:1098–107.

44. Boxall D, Bradford DS, Winter RB, Moe JH. Management of severe spondylolisthesis in children and adolescents. J Bone Joint Surg 1979;61:479–95.

45. Sorensen KH. Scheuermann's juvenile kyphosis. Copenhagen: Munksgaard, 1964.

46. Hensinger RN, Greene TL, Hunter LY. Back pain and vertebral changes simulating Scheuermann's kyphosis. Spine 1982;6:341–2.

47. Bradford DS. Juvenile kyphosis. In: Bradford DS, Lonstein JE, Moe JH, et al, eds. Moe's textbook of scoliosis and other spinal deformities, 2nd ed. Philadelphia: WB Saunders, 1987;347–68.

48. Cobb J. Outline for study of scoliosis. AAOS Instruct Course Lect 1948;5:261–275, Ann Arbor: J. W. Edwards.

49. Moe JH, Byrd JA III. Idiopathic scoliosis. In: Bradford DS, Lonstein JH, Moe JH, et al, eds. Moe's textbook of scoliosis and other spinal deformities, 2nd ed. Philadelphia: WB Saunders, 1987;191–232.

50. Lillegard W, Kruse R. In Taylor RB, eds. Family medicine: principles and practice, 4th ed. New York: Springer-Verlag, 1993.

21
Selected Problems of Infancy and Childhood

Sanford R. Kimmel

The interactional model of human development recognizes that each child has a genetic potential that is shaped through life experiences.[1] Central nervous system (CNS) attributes are inherited, but a warm, nurturing, loving environment is necessary for individuals to reach their maximum fulfillment. The family physician should follow the neurodevelopment of the child from infancy into adulthood and identify significant deviations from the norm. Table 21.1 lists biologic and psychosocial factors in the etiology of abnormal development.

Developing Child and an Approach to Abnormal Development

Developmental Surveillance and Screening

At preventive health care visits, the family physician should assess the child's developmental skills (see Chapter 7). Assessment can be accomplished through directly questioning the parent and examining the child on a number of age-appropriate parameters (surveillance) or using a formal developmental assessment tool (e.g., Denver II Developmental Screening Test, Early Language Milestone Scale). Surveillance presupposes a familiarity with developmental milestones and an ability to distinguish significant delay from normal variation. Standardized screening tests are generally more time-consuming but can be administered by nonphysicians after specific training to ensure reliability.

Language Delays in the Infant and Toddler

During the first 3 years of life, children learn basic language rules and a significant basic vocabulary (Table 21.2). They also develop the motor skills needed to express these words verbally. Language delays may result from sensory organ deficits (hearing), CNS dysfunction, environmental deprivation, or a combination of these factors. Consequently, a hearing assessment is the first step in the workup of the language-delayed child. As the physician subsequently investigates other potential causes of the delay, a speech-language pathologist can quantify the delay and provide therapy.

Motor Delays in the Infant

The infant develops gross motor skills in a continuum that progresses from head to toe. The newborn has no significant control over large muscle groups. During the first 2 months of life babies attain neck muscle control such that they can hold their head up when placed in a prone position. By 4 months of age they have control over the shoulder girdles such that they can lift the chest off a flat surface when placed prone. The average 6-month-old can sit without support, having developed control over the hip girdle. Between 9 and 12 months of age there is a progression from pulling to stand, to cruising (walking while holding onto a fixed object), and then to walking without support. Significant delays in this progression may be due to sensory organ deficit (e.g., blindness), CNS dysfunction (e.g., static encephalopathy), peripheral nervous system pathology (e.g., lower motor neuron disease), or muscular disease. The history and neuromuscular examination help differentiate among these causes.

Early Intervention

Handicaps identified early in life allow a systematic approach that attempts to address all of the needs of the child and tries to minimize the stress created by the handicap on the family. This approach is called early intervention. By federal mandate, early intervention teams are set up by school systems. The teams generally consist of nurses, social workers, physical therapists, occupational therapists, speech and language pathologists, and educators. Close collaboration between the

Table 21.1. **Factors Contributing to Abnormal Development**

Biologic factors
  Genetic
    Identifiable structural anomalies of the chromosomes
      (e.g., trisomy 21, fragile X syndrome)
    Abnormalities at the level of the gene not identified by
      standard cytogenetics
  Prenatal
    Infection
    Trauma
    Toxicity
    Malformations of unknown intrauterine cause
    Metabolic
  Perinatal
    Birth injury including asphyxia
  Neonatal
    Infection
    Central nervous system injury as a result of prematurity
      and its treatment
  Postneonatal
    Trauma
    Infection
    Toxic (e.g., lead)
    Metabolic
    Neoplastic
Psychosocial factors
  Environmental deprivation
    Child neglect
    Loss of a loved one
    Inappropriate parenting
  Child abuse
    Physical
    Psychological

team and physician is mandatory to maximize the outcome of the developmentally delayed child. The family physician must know how to refer children to the local early intervention program and should communicate openly with team members.

Developmental Problems in the Preschool and School-Age Child

Neurodevelopmental competence occurs along a continuum ranging from superior skills in all areas (gifted children) to seriously delayed skills in most areas (mental retardation). Children with generally average to above-average neurodevelopmental skills (normal intelligence) are said to have a

Table 21.2. **Key Language Milestones During the First 5 Years of Life**

Age	Skill
Newborn	Alert; cries, throaty sounds
2 Months	Coos
4 Months	Laughs, squeals
6 Months	Monosyllabic repetition (babbling)
12 Months	First word
18 Months	Five- to six-word vocabulary; puts two words together
2 Years	Many words; follows two-step directions
3 Years	Uses appropriate grammatic structure (subject-verb-object)

learning disability when they have one or more significant weaknesses that preclude educational achievement at a level predicted by their overall intelligence. When children are suspected of having superior abilities or when they are not achieving well educationally, formal psychometric testing (intelligence testing and academic achievement testing) is done. Although it is common to label children as gifted or learning disabled, it is more important that the family physician help children maximize their achievement. The physician should assist the parents in serving as the child's advocate to ensure that appropriate placement and curricular changes are made in the school system. When significant neurodevelopmental handicaps are identified, the family physician must see to it that the child has an appropriate medical assessment to determine the cause of the delays.

Mental Retardation

The diagnosis of mental retardation is based on a measured intelligence quotient (IQ) that is at least 2 standard deviations below the median. Testing should be culturally, linguistically, and behaviorally appropriate. Using the Wechsler Intelligence Scale for Children, mental retardation may be categorized as mild with an IQ of 50 to 70, moderate with an IQ of 35 to 49, severe with an IQ of 20 to 34, and profound with an IQ below 20.[2] No more than 5% of cognitively disabled individuals have severe or profound mental retardation.[2]

Mental retardation may be caused by multiple factors including structural malformations of the brain, metabolic abnormalities, or acquired deficits such as CNS infection. For example, Down syndrome occurs in 1 in 1000 births (see Chapter 16) and fragile X syndrome has an incidence similar to that of Down syndrome in males.[2] Children living with economic, physical, and emotional hardship are often more vulnerable to biologic insults because of inadequate nutrition and access to appropriate care.[3]

Because there are many factors causing mental retardation, one specific cause is often not pinpointed in an individual child. Management of the child with mental retardation must consequently be individualized. In addition, how children utilize their specific strengths and weaknesses in adapting to the environment is more important than labeling the degree of the disability. The family physician should identify the strengths, abilities, and resources of the child and the family and collaborate with resources in the community in order to maximize care.

Autistic Spectrum Disorder

Prevalence and Etiology of Autistic Spectrum Disorder

Autistic spectrum disorder (ASD) represents a continuum of pervasive developmental disorders (PDDs) ranging from classic autism to Asperger's syndrome. Approximately 70% of autistic children in a United Kingdom study were mentally retarded, whereas 100% of the children with Asperger's syndrome had normal intelligence.[4] Most children were classified as having PDD not otherwise specified (PDD-NOS), and most of these children had intelligence in the normal range.[4] The prevalence of autism is generally believed to be 1 in 1000 children and that of ASD 1 in 500 children.[5] The U.K. study suggested a higher prevalence of greater than 6 per 1000 for all PDDs.[4] The ratio of affected boys to girls is approximately 4:1.[5,6]

Genetic factors are strongly implicated in the etiology of ASD as evidenced by high rates in monozygotic twins (60–90%); however, the recurrence rate for isolated ASD is from 3% to 7%.[5] ASD is also seen in tuberous sclerosis, fragile X syndrome, metabolic disorders such as untreated phenylketonuria, and congenital infections such as rubella.[6] Concern that ASD might be caused by the measles-mumps-rubella (MMR) vaccine has been rejected at the population level by a 2001 Institute of Medicine (IOM) report.[7] However, the IOM report noted that it did not "exclude the possibility that MMR vaccine could contribute to ASD in a small number of children."[7]

Characteristics of Children with Autistic Spectrum Disorder

Children with ASD have language deficits ranging from never developing verbal language to coherent speech with subtle differences in usage.[6] They also have more difficulty with receptive language than solely mentally retarded children who usually understand language better than they can speak it.[6] Children with ASD have deficits in social interactions, displaying poor eye contact, preferring to play alone, or lacking in empathy. They do not look back and forth between an item of interest and a caregiver (joint attention), unlike the typical older infant.[6] However, most autistic children are capable of developing an attachment with a loved family member.[5]

Parents usually become concerned about their child's development at age 18 months but may not seek help for an additional 6 months.[5] Poor eye contact, repetitive or stereotypic behaviors, and inability to elicit a social smile, understand simple commands, or engage in pretend play at the appropriate developmental ages suggest that the child should be evaluated for ASD or other developmental disorders.[5] Children with language delays should always have an audiologic and speech and language evaluation. Chromosome analysis should be performed if dysmorphic features are present. An electroencephalogram is indicated if symptomatic or subclinical seizures are suspected because 20% to 30% of children with ASD have seizures developing during early childhood or adolescence.[5]

Management of the Autistic Child

Parents should understand that children with ASD vary widely in their abnormal behaviors, intelligence, and prognosis. Broad goals are to improve the communication, social, adaptive, behavioral, and academic skills of the child with ASD while decreasing maladaptive and repetitive behaviors.[5] The best means of accomplishing this must be individualized according to the strengths of the child, family, and community.

Infants and toddlers should be enrolled in early intervention programs. The Young Autism Project at UCLA has demonstrated that an intensive system (40 hours/week) of breaking tasks into small increments with reinforcement resulted in higher IQ scores and better expressive speech for some children.[5,6] Higher functioning children should be mainstreamed in the public school system, assisted by teaching aides and tutors to provide increased attention, speech therapy, or other necessary help. The Treatment and Education of Autistic and Communication-Handicapped Children Curriculum (TEACCH) promotes the use of structured learning situations.[5] Appropriately trained parents have implemented TEACCH-based programs at home.

Psychopharmacologic medications may be used as adjunctive treatment to prevent self-injurious or aggressive behavior and treat associated conditions such as depression and attention-deficit/hyperactivity disorder (AD/HD).[5] Currently used drugs include risperidone, selective serotonin reuptake inhibitors (SSRIs), and clonidine hydrochloride. Physicians prescribing these medications should be very knowledgeable about their use because they may cause a variety of adverse effects. For example, in some children with ASD, traditional stimulant use may increase aggressiveness and stereotypical behavior.[5] There is no single pharmacologic, nutritional, or behavioral intervention that cures children with ASD. It is thus understandable that some parents may turn to unproven alternative treatments. Parents desiring further information may contact the Autism Society of America at *http://www.autism-society.org*.

Environmental Influences

All phases of a child's development may be affected by environmental influences. The fetus may be exposed in utero to toxic substances from maternal smoking, alcohol, illicit drugs, or inadvertent exposure to harmful chemicals or elements such as lead. Children are at particular risk from environmental toxins because of their greater metabolic rate and hand-to-mouth activity. Rapid cellular growth and differentiation and retention of toxins in bone and adipose tissue also enhance toxicity.[8]

Lead Intoxication as a Model of Environmental Influences

Sources of Lead

Lead is ubiquitous in the environment. Lead-based paint was available until the mid-1970s and is present in an estimated 57 million occupied housing units built prior to 1980.[9] In deteriorated housing, contaminated dust and soil as well as flaking paint chips ingested by the child (pica) are a major source of lead. Remodeling an older home also places the inhabitants at risk for lead intoxication if the house is not properly deleaded.

Drinking water is another source of lead if lead-containing pipes or fixtures or lead-soldered joints are present in the plumbing system. Children may absorb more than 50% of the lead they drink in water, which is more completely absorbed than lead found in food.[9] If the plumbing cannot be replaced, cold water should be run for several minutes prior to using and should not be boiled. Hot water from the tap should not be used for drinking, as hot or acidic liquids leach lead from pipes and lead-containing vessels.

Family members whose occupations (e.g., radiator repair) or hobbies expose them to high levels of lead may subsequently expose children by wearing work garments or bringing scrap material home. Some ethnic groups use folk remedies containing lead, such as the use of azarcon or greta for digestive disorders in Hispanic populations.[10] The use of unleaded gasoline has resulted in lower airborne levels of lead, but localized exposure may occur during sandblasting, demolition, or incineration of solid waste.

Symptoms of Lead Poisoning

Infants, young children, and the fetuses of pregnant women are at greatest risk for the adverse effects of lead. Poor nutrition may compound these effects. Diminished IQ, hearing, birth weight, and subsequent growth may be seen with lead levels as low as 10 μg/dL. Nerve conduction velocity slows at 20 μg/dL, but peripheral neuropathy and frank anemia may not become apparent until the lead level reaches 70 μg/dL. Encephalopathy, colic, and nephropathy may not appear until a level of 80 to 100 μg/dL is reached.[9] Prolonged lead exposure has also been linked with an increased risk for antisocial and delinquent behavior.[11]

Screening for Lead Poisoning

A 1999 National Health and Nutrition Survey of 19 states found that 7.6% of children younger than 6 years old had blood lead levels (BLLs) of 10 μg/dL or higher.[12] Low-income children living in older housing were 30 times more likely to have a BLL greater than 10 μg/dL than middle-income children in newer housing.[12] Because young children enrolled in Medicaid are three times more likely than non-Medicaid children to have an elevated BLL, federal regulations require they have a blood lead test at ages 12 and 24 months.[13] Children ages 36 to 72 months enrolled in Medicaid who have not previously been screened should also have a blood lead test. Screening should be considered in children with developmental delays and pica, children who have emigrated from countries where lead poisoning is common, and victims of abuse or neglect. Children with unexplained neurologic symptoms, recurrent abdominal pain, hearing loss, anemia, developmental delay, autism, or other behavior disorder may also warrant testing for lead toxicity.[9]

Venous blood lead levels are preferred for screening. Capillary (fingerstick) samples are acceptable only if properly collected.[14] Children who regularly reside in houses built before 1960, have siblings with a history of lead poisoning, or live with adults whose jobs or hobbies involve exposure to lead are considered at high risk. They should have their initial screening done at 6 months of age, and children at low risk should begin at 12 months of age. Guidelines for screening and intervention are described in Table 21.3. Iron deficiency enhances lead absorption and often coexists with lead toxic-

---

Table 21.3. **Childhood Lead Screening and Intervention**

Lead level venous blood (μg/dL)	Intervention
<10	No action necessary, retest age 24 months
10–14	Obtain a confirmatory venous blood lead level (BLL) within 1 month; if still within this range, provide education to decrease blood lead exposure; repeat BLL within 3 months
15–19	Obtain a confirmatory venous BLL within 1 month; if still within this range, take a careful environmental history; provide education to decrease blood lead exposure and decrease lead absorption; repeat BLL test within 2 months
20–44	Obtain a confirmatory venous BLL within 1 week; if still within this range, conduct a complete medical history (including an environmental evaluation and nutritional assessment) and physical examination; provide education to decrease blood lead exposure and to decrease lead absorption; either refer the patient to the local health department or provide case management that should include a detailed environmental investigation with lead hazard reduction and appropriate referrals for support services; if the BLL is >25 μg/dL, consider chelation (not currently recommended for BLLs <45 μg/dL), after consultation with clinicians experienced in lead toxicity treatment
45–69	Obtain a confirmatory venous BLL within 2 days; if still within this range, conduct a complete medical history (including an environmental evaluation and nutritional assessment) and a physical examination; provide education to decrease blood lead exposure and to decrease lead absorption; either refer the patient to the local health department or provide case management that should include a detailed environmental investigation with lead hazard reduction and appropriate referrals for support services; begin chelation therapy in consultation with clinicians experienced in lead toxicity therapy; complete lead abatement of child's home prior to return
≥70	Hospitalize the patient and begin medical treatment immediately in consultation with clinicians experienced in lead toxicity therapy; obtain a confirmatory BLL immediately; the rest of the management should be as noted for management of children with BLLs between 45 and 69 μg/dL

Source: Adapted from American Academy of Pediatrics Committee on Environmental Health,[14] with permission.

ity. Serum iron studies are indicated whenever elevated lead levels of 15 μg/dL or higher are present.[9]

Management of Lead Poisoning

Reducing exposure to lead is the cornerstone of managing the child with lead intoxication. The source(s) of lead in the environment should be investigated and the child removed from the environment if necessary. Vacuuming lead-contaminated dust may aerosolize lead particles and should not be performed. All lead-based paint should be removed or made permanently inaccessible.[9] Scraping, sanding, and especially the use of heat guns or torches increase the environmental exposure to lead.[15] Complete lead abatement should be carried out only by a certified contractor.

Chelation therapy for children with an initial blood lead level of 25 to 44 μg/dL is controversial because it has not been proved to prevent or reverse neurotoxicity.[16] Some children with lead levels in this range may benefit from (oral) chelation therapy if blood lead levels persist despite intensive environmental abatement. Children with blood lead levels of 45 μg/dL or higher require referral to a team skilled in chelation therapy. Children with blood lead levels of 70 μg/dL or more or with symptoms of lead poisoning constitute a medical emergency requiring hospitalization and treatment with CaNa$_2$ ethylenediaminetetraacetic acid (EDTA) and dimercaprol (BAL).[16]

Although approved only for treating individuals with blood lead levels over 45 μg/dL, succimer (Chemet) appears to be an effective oral chelating agent with high selectivity for lead. It is less likely to chelate essential metals such as iron or zinc and to precipitate encephalopathy than CaNa$_2$EDTA.[16] The child should be monitored for gastrointestinal symptoms, rashes or other allergic reactions, reversible neutropenia, and increases in liver transaminases while succimer therapy is being administered.[16]

Following chelation therapy, children should not be discharged from the hospital until they can go to a lead-free environment. Blood lead levels should be rechecked 7 to 21 days after treatment and the children seen weekly or every other week for 4 to 8 weeks and then monthly for 6 to 12 months.[9]

Childhood Injury Prevention

In the United States injuries cause more deaths among children ages 1 to 19 years than all diseases combined. Recent data indicate that annually more than 16,000 children die[17] and almost 11 million are treated in emergency departments for nonfatal injuries.[18] Many injuries are preventable and result from the interaction of an agent, host, and environment. Preventive strategies include (1) education to modify people's behavior to avoid or eliminate the hazard; (2) legislation to require behavior or conditions that promote safety; and (3) passive means of protection through product or environmental design[19] (see Chapter 7).

Motor Vehicle Injuries

Injuries to motor vehicle occupants are the major cause of death in children 0 to 19 years old.[20] Rear-facing safety seats should be used for infants weighing 20 lb (9 kg) or less, and forward-facing seats should be used for toddlers weighing 40 lb (18 kg) or less. Children 4 years old and heavier than 40 lb should use a booster seat with a lap belt until they weigh 80 lb and are 9 years old. The adult seatbelt and shoulder harness is then used. Infant seats should be anchored to the rear seat in vehicles with passenger-side airbags, as these devices deploy with explosive force. Children 12 years of age and younger should also sit in the rear seat, as airbags may be dangerous to them. However, airbags may be lifesaving for adolescent motorists who have a higher motor vehicle fatality rate and are less likely to use active restraints than younger children. The use of alcohol also plays a major role in adolescent crash fatalities.

Homicide and Suicide

Violent behavior precipitated by alcohol may lead to homicide and is now the second leading cause of injury death among children and first among infants younger than 1 year old.[21] Most homicide deaths occur among boys and almost half among African Americans. At least 75% of male homicides are inflicted with firearms.[17] Although the causes of violence are multifactorial, heavy exposure to television violence increases the likelihood of aggressive and antisocial behavior, especially among boys.[22]

Boys also account for over 80% of suicides, which is the third leading cause of injury death among children.[17] Whites and nonblack minority boys have higher suicide rates. Over 60% of suicides among children ages 1 to 19 years were caused by firearms, about 30% by suffocation, e.g., hanging, and approximately 6% by poisoning.[17] The presence of a gun in the house increases the risk for suicide 10-fold.[20] Media broadcasts of suicides may prompt imitative behavior by susceptible teenagers.[22]

Drowning

Drowning is the fourth leading cause of injury death and the second leading cause of unintentional injury death in children[17] (also see Chapter 50). Fencing pools with a lockable enclosure that is at least 4 feet high and providing proper supervision can prevent pool drownings among young children. Avoiding alcohol use could potentially prevent the 40% of adolescent drownings in which alcohol is a contributing factor.[20]

Fires and Burns

Fires and burns are the third major cause of unintentional injury death among children (see Chapter 50).[17] It is estimated that more than 70% of the deaths due to house fires could be prevented by functioning smoke alarms.[20] Lowering the temperature of the hot-water heater to 49°C (120°F) greatly decreases the risk of scald burns.[23]

Pedestrian Injuries

Pedestrian injuries are an important but declining cause of injury-related deaths of children under age 15 years.[20] Rerouting and slowing traffic in addition to well-demarcated walkways and crossing aids may improve pedestrian safety. Children under age 6 years should not cross streets alone.[23]

Bicycle Injuries

Bicycle-related injuries are responsible for more than 500,000 emergency department visits and more than 300 childhood deaths annually in the United States.[20] Head injuries are the most common cause of death and disability from these injuries. Bicycle helmets have been shown to decrease the risk of serious head injury by 85% and brain injury by 88%.[24]

Safety Counseling

The family physician should counsel parents about injury prevention during routine anticipatory guidance (Table 21.4). The Injury Prevention Program (TIPP) is a safety education package available through the American Academy of Pediatrics at *www.AAP.org*. It consists of age-appropriate information sheets. Injury prevention material may also be obtained from the National SAFE KIDS Campaign, which is cosponsored by the American Academy of Family Physicians.[23]

Enuresis

Enuresis is the involuntary voiding of urine beyond the developmental age of anticipated control, usually 5 years for girls and 6 years for boys. Primary enuresis occurs in children who have never been dry for extended periods, and secondary enuresis is the onset of wetting after a continuous dry period of more than 6 months.[25] Nocturnal (nighttime) enuresis is usually primary, while diurnal (daytime) enuresis often indicates voiding dysfunction or significant underlying pathology.[26]

Nocturnal enuresis is more common among boys than girls and occurs in approximately 15% of 5-year-old children. Spontaneous resolution occurs at a rate of 15% per year, leaving only 1% to 2% of adolescents enuretic. Enuresis occurs in more than 40% and 70% of children when one and both parents, respectively, have a history of enuresis.[25]

Evaluation

Although most children have uncomplicated primary nocturnal enuresis, a careful history and physical examination, including neurologic assessment, should be performed to detect potential organic or psychological causes (Table 21.5). A urinalysis and urine culture should always be done to check for urinary tract infection, diabetes mellitus, or underlying kidney disease. A dilute urine specific gravity measurement in a first morning-voided specimen suggests diabetes insipidus or other disorder affecting renal concentrating ability. Abnormal findings from the history and physical examination or urinalysis suggest the need for further imaging studies such as renal ultrasonography or intravenous pyelography and voiding cystourethrography (see Chapter 95). Urologic referral may also be indicated.[25]

Table 21.4. **Age-Appropriate Safety Counseling**

Age	Child's abilities	Related safety risks and counseling
Newborn	Immobile	Smoke detectors, parental smoking Set hot water temperature to 120°F Infant car seat, parents "buckle up" Infant sleep on back to prevent sudden infant death syndrome (SIDS)
Infant	Rolls over Reaches for objects Puts objects in mouth Sits unsupported Crawls Pulls to stand, cruises Seeks hidden objects	Falls from high surfaces Burns from hot liquids, cigarettes Choking and aspiration Toddler car seat, bicycle-mounted seats Safety gates, infant walker hazards Burns from stove, harmful objects in reach Drawer and cabinet locks
Toddler/preschooler	Walks, runs, climbs Gets into or onto anything Moves toward autonomy Inquisitive and persistent Uses tricycles and playground equipment	Supervise crossing street, in or near water Safe enclosed play area Use car seats despite resistance No guns or store guns locked and unloaded Bicycle helmet, resilient surfaces
School-age child	Increasing independence Rides bicycle Overestimates abilities Shows increasing ability to follow rules, and assume responsibility Unsupervised play	Traffic hazards, and "rules of the road" Bicycle helmets, bicycle safety Water safety, swimming lessons Seat belt use, pedestrian safety
Adolescent	Risk-taking behavior and substance abuse Response to peer pressure	Automobile safety, drinking and driving; bicycle and/or motorcycle helmet Violence prevention counseling

Source: Adapted from Glotzer and Weitzman,[23] with permission.

Table 21.5. **Organic and Secondary Causes of Childhood Enuresis**

Symptom or sign	Clinical disorder
Psychological stress (e.g., new sibling or home, separation or death of parent)	Secondary enuresis
Urinary urgency, frequency, or dysuria	Urinary tract infection, hypercalciuria, drugs (e.g., methylxanthines)
Urinary urgency, daytime dribbling Sitting on foot to compress perineum—girls Crossing legs, grabbing penis—boys	Primary voiding disorder (e.g., pediatric unstable bladder and detrusor sphincter dyssynergia)
Polydipsia, polyuria, weight loss	Diabetes mellitus, diabetes insipidus, renal concentrating defects
Weak urinary stream, daytime/nighttime wetting	Obstructive uropathy (e.g., posterior urethral valves)
Constipation, soiling, fecal impaction	Detrusor sphincter dyssynergia, neurogenic bladder
Distended bladder, sensation incomplete emptying	Obstructive uropathy, neurogenic bladder
Abnormal reflexes, gait, perineal sensation, lumbosacral abnormalities, lax anal sphincter	Neurogenic bladder (e.g. spina bifida)
Continuous urinary dribbling	Ectopic ureter
Vaginitis, trauma to external genitalia	Sexual abuse, foreign body

Source: Adapted from Warady et al,[26] with permission.

Treatment

Nocturnal enuresis usually resolves spontaneously, so reassurance and education of the child and parents are important. Parents in the United States may view bed-wetting as a significant problem, and some deal with it by punishment.[27] The children must not be blamed but should be encouraged to participate in the treatment of their condition. Placing stars on a calendar for dry nights followed by a small reward for consecutive dry nights provides positive reinforcement. The child should void before going to bed, but frequent awakening at night to prevent wetting is seldom helpful. A child who has a small bladder capacity may benefit by increasing the time between daytime voiding and practicing stream interruption during voiding. Normal bladder capacity (in ounces) approximately equals age (in years) +2 up to 11 years of age. Measuring the child's urine volume once a week assesses progress.[25]

"Enuresis alarms" have a cure rate of about 70% when used in motivated children over 7 years of age with a supportive family. They cause the child to wake up and suppress the micturition reflex and ultimately inhibit the reflex with the child asleep. Those that utilize sensors in the underwear with a small battery-operated audio or tactile alarm attached to the child's pajamas are safer than the traditional mattress pad and bell. The alarm should be continued until the child has been dry for 4 weeks. Relapses may be retreated with an equally good success rate.[25]

Pharmacologic therapy is more popular, as it may offer a more rapid response; however, it has more side effects and is more expensive. Oxybutynin chloride (Ditropan) is useful for children with daytime frequency or urgency that is associated with uninhibited bladder contractions that is not secondary to an organic cause. The starting dose is 5 mg for children who are least 6 years old and may be increased up to two or three times per day. Anticholinergic side effects include dry mouth, blurred vision, and drowsiness.[28] For nocturnal enuresis, the tricyclic antidepressant imipramine hydrochloride (Tofranil) suppresses uninhibited bladder contractions, increases bladder outlet resistance, and has a strong inhibitory action on bladder smooth muscle.[29] An initial dose of 10 mg 1 to 2 hours before bedtime can be given to children age 6 years or older. The dose can be gradually increased to obtain a satisfactory response. The maximum dose is 50 to 75 mg for older children and adolescents.[25] Higher doses do not increase efficacy but do increase the risk of side effects, including an increase in pulse rate, blood pressure, nervousness, sleep disturbances, parkinsonian effects, or postural hypotension.[29] Overdose can result in cardiac arrhythmias, seizures, coma, and death. Enuretic relapses are frequent with discontinuation of the drug and may be avoided by gradually tapering the dosage.

Desmopressin (DDAVP) is a synthetic analogue of antidiuretic hormone (ADH) that increases renal water resorption and urine concentration while decreasing urinary volume. Some enuretic patients with normal bladder capacity do not demonstrate the nocturnal increase in ADH found in nonenuretic children.[30] An initial dose of one spray in each nostril (20 μg total) at bedtime may be increased by one spray (10 μg) per week to a maximum of two sprays in each nostril. Rapid short-term improvement occurs in 70% of children with nocturnal enuresis.[31] In one Swedish study, 31% of patients aged 6 to 12 years old became dry and 24% had at least a 90% reduction in wet nights after one year.[31] Its rapid onset of action makes it especially useful for short-term situations such as staying overnight at friends' homes or at camp.[29] Desmopressin tablets require 20-fold higher doses then the nasal spray and have decreased absorption when taken with meals. A response rate of about 80% has been reported with 400 μg orally.[31] The drug is expensive, and relapses may occur once the drug is stopped. Side effects of DDAVP include transient headache, nausea, abdominal pain, and nasal congestion. Water intoxication with hyponatremia is rare but can occur if large amounts of water are ingested prior to taking the desmopressin.[31]

Encopresis

Encopresis is the regular, voluntary, or involuntary passage of feces into inappropriate places (e.g., underwear) by a child who is developmentally 4 years of age or older.[32] Primary encopresis occurs when the child has not been continent of stool for at least 1 year. Secondary encopresis is present when fecal incontinence occurs after the child has been continent for at least 1 year.[32] Encopresis is four to five times more common among boys, and secondary encopresis accounts for 50% to 60% of cases.[32] Organic causes of soiling, such as inflammatory bowel disease, hypothyroidism, hypercalcemia, and aganglionic megacolon, should be excluded.[33]

Functional fecal retention may occur owing to fear of defecating in a strange place, prior pain due to a rectal fissure, oppositional behavior, or occasionally fear of the toilet.[34] The child's effort to withhold stools may be accompanied by grunting and becoming red-faced, which may be interpreted as "trying." Increased rectal volume and pressure may cause loss of the urge to defecate and result in soiling during play or relaxation.[35] Seepage around hard, impacted stools may produce "paradoxical diarrhea."[36] Frequent or continued soiling may ostracize the child from his peers and family and lead to emotional maladjustment.[36] Successful treatment of the soiling often leads to improvement in the child's behavior.[32]

Management

The parents and the child should be educated about the causes of encopresis and that full evacuation of the colon is necessary for resumption of normal function.[32] The child should sit on the toilet for 5 to 10 minutes two or three times a day, usually after meals to take advantage of the gastrocolic reflex. Successful bowel movements should be noted by stars or stickers placed on a calendar and a reward given when reasonable targets are achieved.[35]

Mild retention and constipation can be treated by adding fiber to the diet and softening the stool. An oral laxative such as senna or bisacodyl is occasionally necessary.[35] More severe cases require a complete colorectal cleanout. Mineral oil may be used in children over 1 year of age not at risk for pulmonary aspiration. An initial dose of 15 to 30 mL per year of age per day up to a maximum of 240 mL/day may be given for 3 or 4 days.[33] Maintenance mineral oil therapy (maximum 60–90 mL/day) is required to keep the stools soft and regular for a period of 6 to 12 months. It can be taken cold, mixed with orange juice, or in emulsified form (Kondremul, Milkinol). Phosphate enemas can cause hyponatremia and should be avoided.[33]

References

1. Thomas A, Chess S. Dynamics of psychological development. New York: Brunner-Mazel, 1980.
2. Crocker AC, Nelson RP. Mental retardation. In Levine MD, Carey WB, Crocker AC, eds. Developmental-behavioral pediatrics, 3rd ed. Philadelphia: WB Saunders, 1999;551–9.
3. Shonkoff JP. Mental retardation. In: Behrman RE, Kliegman RM, Jenson HB, eds. Nelson textbook of pediatrics, 16th ed. Philadelphia: WB Saunders, 2000;125–9.
4. Chakrabarti S, Fombonne E. Pervasive developmental disorders in preschool children. JAMA 2001;285:3093–99.
5. Committee on Children with Disabilities, American Academy of Pediatrics. Technical report: the pediatrician's role in the di-

agnosis and management of autistic spectrum disorder in children. Pediatrics 2001;107:e85. *www.pediatrics.org/cgi/content/full/107/5/e85.*
6. Teplin SW. Autism and related disorders. In: Levine MD, Carey WB, Crocker AC, eds. Developmental-behavioral pediatrics, 3rd ed. Philadelphia: WB Saunders, 1999;589–605.
7. Institute of Medicine Immunization Safety Review Committee, Stratton K, Gable, A, Shetty P, McCormick M, eds. Immunization safety review: measles-mumps-rubella vaccine and autism. Washington, DC: National Academy Press, 2001;1–11.
8. Mayer JL, Balk SJ. A tip-toe through the toxins. Contemp Pediatr 1988;5:22–40.
9. Centers for Disease Control. Preventing lead poisoning in young children: a statement by the Centers for Disease Control. Atlanta: US Department of Health and Human Services, 1991;1–105.
10. Centers for Disease Control. Lead poisoning associated with use of traditional ethnic remedies—California, 1991–1992. MMWR 1993;42:521–4.
11. Needleman HL, Riess JA, Tobin MJ, Biesecker GE, Greenhouse JB. Bone lead levels and delinquent behavior. JAMA 1996;275:363–9.
12. Centers for Disease Control and Prevention. Blood lead levels in young children—United States and selected states, 1996–1999. MMWR 2000;49:1133–7.
13. Advisory Committee on Childhood Lead Poisoning Prevention. Recommendations for blood lead screening of young children enrolled in Medicaid: targeting a group at high risk. MMWR 2000;49(RR14):1–13.
14. American Academy of Pediatrics Committee on Environmental Health. Screening for elevated blood lead levels. Pediatrics 1998;101:1072–8.
15. Amitai Y, Brown MJ, Graef JW, Cosgrove E. Residential deleading: effects on the blood lead levels for lead-poisoned children. Pediatrics 1991;88:893–7.
16. Committee on Drugs, American Academy of Pediatrics. Treatment guidelines for lead exposure in children. Pediatrics 1995;96:155–60.
17. National Center for Injury Prevention and Control. *http://webapp.cdc.gov/cgi-bin/brok.* May 15, 2001.
18. Centers for Disease Control and Prevention. National estimates of nonfatal injuries treated in hospital emergency departments—United States, 2000. MMWR 2001;50:340–6.
19. Greensher J. Recent advances in injury prevention. Pediatr Rev 1988;10:171–7.
20. Rivara FP, Grossman DC. Prevention of traumatic deaths to children in the United States: how far have we come and where do we need to go? Pediatrics 1996;97:791–7.
21. Brenner RA, Overpeck MD, Trumble AC, DerSimonian R, Berendes H. Deaths attributable to injuries in infants, United States, 1983–1991. Pediatrics 1999;103:968–74.
22. Strasburger VC. Children, adolescents, and television. Pediatr Rev 1992;13:144–51.
23. Glotzer D, Weitzman M. Childhood injuries: issues for the family physician. Am Fam Physician 1991;44:1705–16.
24. Thompson RS, Rivara FP, Thompson DC. A case-control study of the effectiveness of bicycle safety helmets. N Engl J Med 1989;320:1361–7.
25. Rushton HG. Nocturnal enuresis: epidemiology, evaluation, and currently available treatment options. J Pediatr 1989;114:691–6.
26. Warady BA, Alon U, Hellerstein S. Primary nocturnal enuresis: current concepts about an old problem. Pediatr Ann 1991;20:246–55.
27. Moffatt MEK. Nocturnal enuresis: psychologic implications of treatment and nontreatment. J Pediatr 1989;114:697–704.
28. Kimmel SR. Evaluation and management of childhood enuresis. Fam Pract Recert 2000;22:59–66.

29. Himsl KK, Hurwitz RS. Pediatric urinary incontinence. Urol Clin North Am 1991;18:283–93.
30. Nørgaard JP, Rettig S, Djurhuus JC. Nocturnal enuresis: an approach to treatment based on pathogenesis. J Pediatr 1989;114: 705–10.
31. Läckgren G, Hjälmås K, van Gool J, et al. Nocturnal enuresis: a suggestion for a European treatment strategy. Acta Paediatr 1999;88:679–90.
32. Howe AC, Walker CE. Behavioral management of toilet training, enuresis, and encopresis. Pediatr Clin North Am 1992;39:413–32.
33. Seth R, Heyman MB. Management of constipation and encopresis in infants and children. Gastroenterol Clin North Am 1994;23:621–36.
34. Di Lorenzo C. Constipation. In: Hyman PE, Di Lorenzo C, eds. Pediatric gastrointestinal motility disorders. New York: Academy Professional Information Services, 1994;129–43.
35. Nolan T, Oberklaid F. New concepts in the management of encopresis. Pediatr Rev 1993;14:447–51.
36. Christophersen ER. Toileting problems in children. Pediatr Ann 1991;20:240–4.

22
Health Care of the Adolescent

M. Rosa Solorio and Lacey Wyatt-Henriques

The majority of adolescent medical visits are made to family physicians: 37% of the 60 million annual visits in the United States.[1] Adolescents generally view physicians as credible and valued sources of health-related information.[2] Over 70% of adolescents are seen by a physician annually, on average making three visits per year. They are routinely seen for acute problems such as upper respiratory infections or routine prenatal care for older adolescents.

The American Medical Association Department of Adolescent Health, with the assistance of a scientific advisory board, developed and published Guidelines for Adolescent Preventive Services (GAPS). The GAPS report is the first comprehensive set of recommendations for adolescent preventive strategies.[3] It comprises 24 recommendations in four general areas: (1) health care delivery, (2) health guidance, (3) screening, and (4) immunizations. Physician-based interventions are strongly recommended in all categories.

In the United States, approximately three fourths of all deaths among persons aged 10 to 24 years result from only four causes: motor-vehicle crashes, other unintentional injuries, homicide, and suicide. Substantial morbidity and social problems among persons also result from unintended pregnancies and sexually transmitted diseases (STDs), including human immunodeficiency virus (HIV) infection. Associations have been found between alcohol/substance use and more risk-taking in adolescents, such as being more likely to have unprotected intercourse, being involved with violence, and motor vehicle accidents (MVAs).

Notable ethnic differences on risky behaviors are that white adolescents are more likely to smoke cigarettes, drink alcohol, and attempt suicide in the younger years than blacks or Hispanics; black youths are more likely to have had sexual intercourse compared to whites and Hispanics; both black and Hispanic youths are more likely to engage in violence compared to whites.[4] The effect of race/ethnicity, income, and family structure on adolescent risk factors has been studied, and findings suggest that these factors provide only limited understanding of adolescent risk behaviors.[4]

Approach to the Adolescent and Family/Confidentiality

The physician's role is to provide factual health information and practical advice to the adolescent patient. The CAGE questionnaire can be used to screen for high-risk behaviors (see Chapter 59).[5] Quality health care begins with the establishment of trust, respect, and confidentiality between the physician and the adolescent. Parents and adolescents need to be aware of the adolescent's right to privacy, but that if an adolescent is believed to be in danger, the parents will be notified. It is important to address parental concerns in the clinic and meeting with the parents first may be a good idea. After hearing the parents' concerns the physician can then meet with the adolescent alone so he or she feels free to discuss personal concerns. Because the confidentiality law varies from state to state, it is important for physicians to familiarize themselves with the law in their state. The conditional confidentiality that a physician may offer an adolescent is a dependent on the health care legal rights of the adolescent in that particular state. Laws usually focus on contraception, pregnancy care, abortion, STD treatment, HIV testing, drug abuse treatment, mental health treatment, and the legal emancipation of minors. The physician needs to quickly identify adolescents at risk to appropriately target interventions.

Growth and Somatic Changes

Physical growth and sexual maturation are major physiologic changes of adolescence. Assessing pubertal development is an important skill for family physicians. Tanner's classic staging

Table 22.1. **Tanner Stages of Development: Girls**

Stage/Mean age	Breast	Pubic hair	Other physical changes
1	Flat, prepubertal	No true pubic hair	Preadolescent
2/10.8 Years	Small raised breast bud	Sparse growth, downy hair at sides of labia	Growth spurt begins
3/11.8 Years	General enlargement and raising of breast and areola	Pigmentation, coarsening, and curling with increased amount	Growth decelerates; 25% of girls experience menarche
4/13.2 Years	Areola and papilla form; contour separate from that of breasts	Adult pubic hair, limited in area	About 65% of girls experience menarche
5/14.6 Years	Adult breast, areola; resume same contour as breast tissue	Adult hair, classic female escutcheon	About 10% of girls experience menarche

Source: Adapted from Tanner,[6] with permission.

of physical development is shown in Tables 22.1 and 22.2 (6) and Figures 22.1 and 22.2. Although both boys and girls reach completion of puberty at about the same age, girls begin the transition from preadolescence Tanner stage 1 to stage 2 about 1 year earlier than boys. The duration of puberty for girls is about 4 years, beginning at a mean age of 10.8 years. The overall duration of puberty in boys is about 3 years, beginning at a mean age of 11.8 years. Growth spurts usually occur at an earlier stage of development in girls, accounting for the height discrepancy between boys and girls during early adolescence.

At the onset of puberty there is an increase in gonadotropin-releasing hormone (GnRH), follicle-stimulating hormone (FSH), luteinizing hormone (LH), and the sex hormones. In girls the gonadotropins lead to ovarian development and the production of estrogen and then to secondary sexual characteristics. The main growth spurt in girls occurs between ages 11 and 13, with the growth of the spinal column accounting for most of this growth.[6] Increased estrogen levels lead to epiphyseal closure and cessation of growth during late adolescence. Women's final stature tends to be smaller than men's owing to the earlier onset of sexual maturation and epiphyseal closure. The weight increase in girls is mostly due to added adipose tissue. Axillary hair growth and sweat gland enlargement occurs about 2 years after the onset of puberty and is androgen dependent. The onset of menarche is usually after breast and pubic hair have been completed and after the height spurt (Tanner stage 4).

In boys, LH leads to an increase in testicular size and development of the testicular Leydig cells, which produce testosterone, and then secondary sex characteristics. FSH stimulates development of the seminiferous tubules of the testes, leading to spermatogenesis and fertility during mid- to late adolescence. In boys, enlargement of the testes is the first sign of sexual maturation (Tanner stage 2).[6] The penis also begins to increase in size, and both the testes and the penis reach an adult size over a 2- to 4-year period. Pubic hair appears during Tanner stage 2 and spreads onto the medial thighs by Tanner stage 5. Facial hair usually appears on the upper lip after Tanner stage 3.

Temporary breast tenderness and thelarche (breast bud development) is a common and temporary condition that occurs in 40% of boys and can persist approximately 1.5 years. Thelarche is most likely caused by estrogen stimulation, but there is no evidence of hormonal difference between those with and without this condition. Thelarche is more often bilateral than unilateral and occurs in thin as well as obese boys. All boys should be offered reassurance about this benign, self-limited problem.

The growth spurt in boys occurs between Tanner stages 3 and 4. During Tanner stage 3 boys go through spermarche (first ejaculation), at a mean age of 13. Adult fertility is associated with Tanner stage 4. Axillary hair growth and sweat gland enlargement usually occur 2 years after the onset of puberty.

Table 22.2. **Tanner Stages of Development: Boys**

Stage/Mean age	Genitals	Pubic hair	Other physical changes
1	Testes: volume 1.5 cc; phallus: child-like	None	Preadolescent
2/11.8 Years	Testes: 1.6–6.0 cc; scrotum: reddened thinner; phallus: no change	Sparse growth of downy hair at base of penis	Percent of body fat increases from 4.3% to 11.2%.
3/12.8 Years	Testes: 6–12 cc; scrotum: greater enlargement; phallus: increased length	Pigmentation, coarsening, and curling with increased amount	Growth spurt begins in 25%
4/13.9 Years	Testes: 12–20 cc; scrotum: further enlargement and darkening; phallus: increased length and circumference	Adult pubic hair with spread to lateral aspect thighs	Growth spurt begins in most
5/14.8 Years	Testes: 20 cc; scrotum and phallus: adult	Adult pubic hair	Apex strength

Source: Adapted from Tanner,[6] with permission.

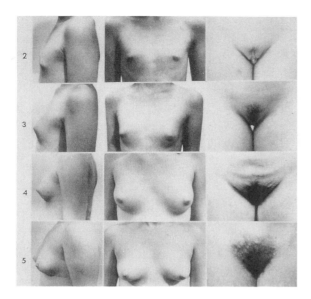

Fig. 22.1. Tanner stages 2 to 5 (A–D) of development: girls. (With permission from James Farrow, M.D., Department of Adolescent Medicine, University of Washington.)

Concerns About Growth and Development

Concerns about growth and sexual development often bring the teenager to the attention of the physician. Common complaints in girls include problems with delay of onset of menarche. If the girl is age 13 to 14 and has signs of pubertal development such as breast buds (Tanner stage 2), she can be reassured that menarche will occur within 2 to 5 years. It is normal for menses to be irregular for the first 2 years because of anovulatory cycles. Girls may also be concerned about being too tall. If a girl is at Tanner stage 4 and menstruating, she has completed most of her growth. Because estrogen leads to closure of epiphyseal growth plates there are rarely more than 2.5 inches of growth in height after menarche.

Boys are more likely to present with concerns of short stature. Short stature may lead to teasing at school and may affect a boy's self-esteem. Constitutional delay in pubertal development is the most common cause of short stature among adolescent boys, and a sequential growth record showing linear growth is seen. The family history may reveal a pattern of delayed growth and sexual maturation, although no specific inheritance pattern has been identified.

Precocious puberty in girls is defined as the onset of breast or pubic hair development before the age of 8 years and in boys as testicular enlargement before the age of 9.5 years. Pubertal delay in girls is defined as no breast development by age 13 or if more than 5 years has elapsed between the beginning of breast development and menarche, and in boys as the absence of testicular enlargement by age 13.5 or if more than 5 years has elapsed from the beginning to completion of pubertal development.[7]

For both genders, organic diseases of the hypothalamic-pituitary-gonadal axis and other major systemic illnesses must be ruled out as a specific cause of delay in growth or sexual maturation. Most patients who have organic disease, such as growth hormone deficiency or hypothyroidism, do not follow a given percentile on the growth chart but begin to deviate from their prior growth patterns, plateauing at the time the disorder manifests clinically. With constitutional delays, it is at the time of the pubertal growth spurt that patients appear to be falling behind. In the case of short stature, a general workup includes a complete history, physical examination, review of linear growth over time, radiography of the hand or wrist to determine skeletal age, and possibly laboratory evaluations for inflammatory disorders of the bowel, renal failure, anemia, and thyroid and growth hormone deficiency. The adolescent who has less than a 4-year discrepancy between chronologic age and skeletal age as measured by radiography is unlikely to have growth hormone deficiency.

Psychological Developmental Tasks

There is a tendency to focus on the physiologic problems of adolescents, but an understanding of the psychological changes and tasks of adolescence is as important as understanding the physical changes (Table 22.3). In general, fail-

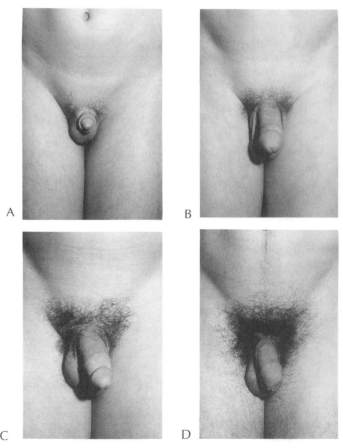

Fig. 22.2. Tanner stages 2 to 5 (A–D) of development: boys.

Table 22.3. **Psychosocial Tasks During Adolescence**

Establishment of autonomy	Psychosocial-psychosexual development	Future orientation
Early (11–14 years): shift from family to peer group	Acceptance of physical change	Concrete cognition
Middle (14–17 years): development of identity and asserting independence	Establishment of peer relations	
Late (>17 years): emotional and economic independence	Evolution of personal values; development of responsible behavior	Vocational and life style choices

Source: Adapted from Kellerman J, Katz ER. The adolescent with cancer: theoretical, clinical and research issues. J Pediatr Psychol 1977;2:127–31, with permission.

ure to complete one of these tasks may lead to delay in subsequent psychological maturation.

Connectedness with one caring adult, a positive body image, and an absence of concern about abuse or domestic violence have been shown to be psychologically protective factors for adolescents regardless of race, class, or gender.[8] There are family and cultural variations in developmental themes, and it is important to consider and ask about them with each adolescent. Studies focusing on self-image and adjustment of adolescents into age-appropriate roles have provided empiric support for the hypothesis that adolescence is for the most part a relatively stable period of development and that most adolescents are well adjusted.

Health Maintenance for Adolescents

A useful technique for interviewing adolescents begins with directed nonthreatening questioning—"What school do you go to? What grade are you in? How do you feel about school?"—followed by increasingly open-ended questions. Spending time with adolescents alone and giving them adequate time to respond to questions is also important. The use of questionnaires that adolescents can complete before the interview may save time and lead to more complete answers. A useful mnemonic, SAFE TEENS, may be used to remember important areas to discuss with adolescents at the time of their visit (Table 22.4).[9] As with all interviews the physician should consider the adolescent's concerns before proceeding with his or her own agenda.

As many as 20% of adolescents are inadequately immunized. Important immunizations in this age group include a tetanus and diphtheria (Td) booster between ages 11 and 12. Rubella screening by the history, prior immunizations, or antibody levels should be documented in all girls. Mumps-measles-rubella (MMR) immunization should be repeated if the patient has not had a booster since infancy. Hepatitis B

Table 22.4. **Mnemonic for Preventive Care of the Adolescent**

S	Sexuality
A	Accidents
F	Firearms/homicides
E	Emotions/suicides
T	Toxins (tobacco, alcohol, drugs)
E	Environment (school, home, friends)
E	Exercise
N	Nutrition
S	Shots/immunizations

Source: Schubiner AH. Preventive health screening in adolescent patients. Prim Care 1989;16:211–30.

immunization is recommended for all adolescents not previously immunized. Tuberculin skin testing [purified protein derivative (PPD)] and immunizations such as influenza should be provided to adolescents in high-risk categories (also see Chapter 7).

As in children, it is wise to monitor growth with a linear growth and weight chart, documenting the Tanner stage at each visit to keep track of pubertal development. At each visit, take a few minutes to discuss developmental milestones and provide anticipatory guidance (Table 22.5).

Physical Examination

For girls the first pelvic examination should be done after the onset of sexual activity or as symptoms dictate to obtain a Papanicolaou (Pap) smear and cultures as appropriate. In the absence of symptoms, a pelvic examination is not needed prior to sexual activity. It is important to make this examination as positive an experience as possible to demonstrate respect for the patient and to encourage compliance with future needed examinations: have a medical assistant present during the examination, explain the reasons for the examination, pay special attention to draping, perform the exam in an unhurried manner, and use a pediatric speculum. For boys, explain the parts of the genital region that will be examined and the reasons for doing so. If an erection occurs during the examination, it is important to comment on it as a normal event to decrease adolescent concern. Teaching points during the general examination include normal anatomy and teaching females about breast self-examination and boys (if more than Tanner stage 4) about testicular self-examination.

Adolescence and Nutrition

The growth rate during adolescence is second only to that during infancy, so an adequate diet is important (Table 22.6). Whether adolescents are active or sedentary, they should eat a variety of foods from the basic food groups. Unfortunately, many adolescents eat unbalanced diets in which fat and sugar furnish a large percentage of their total calories. A daily diet composed of 50% to 60% carbohydrates, 15% to 25% fat, and 15% to 20% protein meets the needs of any active teenager. Nutritional supplements are usually unnecessary if the adolescent follows a balanced diet. Exercise does not increase de-

Table 22.5. **Adolescent Health Care Maintenance**

Age	Developmental milestones	Anticipatory guidance	
Early Age 10–14 F 10–13 M 12–14	Peer relationships Increased body awareness Can begin abstract thinking	Patient: Parents:	Confidentiality School Family relations Sexual development Puberty/reproduction Safety: vehicles/seatbelts/helmets Confidentiality Limit setting (fair rules) Review adolescent development
Middle Age 13–16 F 13–16 M 14–17	Independence/dependence issues Peer group influence Abstract thinking Sexual awareness	Patient: Parents:	Scheduling appointments alone School performance Family relationships Sexual activity—partner selection/condoms Contraception/STDs/HIV Self-breast examination/self-testicular examination Safety: vehicles, seatbelts, helmets, firearms Substance use/abuse Peer relationships (best friend)/gang membership Increased independence Mood swings Risk awareness Parental involvement in school
Late Age 16–18	Body image/gender role secured Planning for future Close friendships	Patient: Parents:	Sexuality Peer relations Future plans Safety: vehicular/firearms Substance use/abuse Accept sexuality Support individuation

Source: Adapted from Shore WB, Braveman PA, Mellin L. Health maintenance for adolescents. In: Taylor, ed. Family medicine, 4th ed. New York: Springer, 1993.

mands for nutrients much beyond the normal increases of the growing body, although high levels of physical activity may increase caloric needs 1000 to 3000 kcal/day. Calcium may be recommended (up to 1500 mg/day) for female athletes with inadequate intake or a significant family history of osteoporosis.

It is important to ask adolescents about dieting practices irregardless of their weight, as research suggests that higher body mass index is not associated with the initiation of dieting, as some underweight and even very underweight girls begin to diet. Discuss proper fluid intake with adolescents. Many drink excessive carbonated or caffeinated drinks, which leads to further fluid loss instead of replenishing fluids. Thirst is not always a good indicator of fluid needs. Emphasize fluid intake with athletes, as they may underestimate the amount of fluid lost during exercise.

Obesity

The National Longitudinal Study of Adolescent Health Survey using the smoothed version of the National Health and Nutrition Examination Survey (NHANES I) 85th percentile cutoff for obesity indicates that 26.5% of the adolescent population (ages 12–19) is obese. Ethnic differences exist and the rates are highest for blacks (30.9%), followed by Hispanics (30.4%) whites (24.2%), and Asians (20.6%). All groups showed more obesity among males than among females, except for blacks (27.4% for males and 34.4% for females). Hispanic and Asians adolescents born in the U.S. are more than twice as likely to be obese as are first-generation immigrants in similar ethnic groups. From 1965 to 1996, a shift occurred in the adolescent diet—increases in higher-fat foods and in the consumption of soft drinks.[10] These trends may compromise the health of the future U.S. population because obesity is associated with chronic health conditions such as cardiovascular disease, diabetes, and cancer.

Characterization as being overweight leads to stigmatization, and undue attention to body size may increase the incidence of eating disorders among children and adolescents.[11] It is important to focus on the preventable aspects of obesity, monitor adolescent weight, and make recommendations early in the course of weight increases. The best advice to adolescents and their parents is to increase exercise and decrease fatty food intake (also see Chapter 53).

Eating Disorders

Eating disorders such as anorexia nervosa and bulimia nervosa are complex illnesses and are the third most common chronic illness in adolescent females (after obesity and asthma) with a prevalence of up to 5%.[12] Over the past decade

Table 22.6a. Dietary Reference Intakes (DRIs): Recommended Intakes for Individuals (Food and Nutrition Board, Institute of Medicine, National Academies): Vitamins

Life stage group	Vitamin A (μg/d)[a]	Vitamin C (mg/d)	Vitamin D (μg/d)[b,c]	Vitamin E (mg/d)[d]	Vitamin K (μg/d)	Thiamin (mg/d)	Riboflavin (mg/d)	Niacin (mg/d)[e]	Vitamin B_6 (mg/d)	Folate (μg/d)[f]	Vitamin B_{12} (μg/d)
Males											
9–13 y	**600**	**45**	5*	**11**	60*	**0.9**	**0.9**	**12**	**1.0**	**300**	**1.8**
14–18 y	**900**	**75**	5*	**15**	75*	**1.2**	**1.3**	**16**	**1.3**	**400**	**2.4**
19–30 y	**900**	**90**	5*	**15**	120*	**1.2**	**1.3**	**16**	**1.3**	**400**	**2.4**
Females											
9–13 y	**600**	**45**	5*	**11**	60*	**0.9**	**0.9**	**12**	**1.0**	**300**	**1.8**
14–18 y	**700**	**65**	5*	**15**	75*	**1.0**	**1.0**	**14**	**1.2**	**400**[g]	**2.4**
19–30 y	**700**	**75**	5*	**15**	90*	**1.1**	**1.1**	**14**	**1.3**	**400**[g]	**2.4**
Pregnancy											
≤18 y	**750**	**80**	5*	**15**	75*	**1.4**	**1.4**	**18**	**1.9**	**600**[h]	**2.6**
19–30 y	**770**	**85**	5*	**15**	90*	**1.4**	**1.4**	**18**	**1.9**	**600**[h]	**2.6**
Lactation											
≤18 y	**1200**	**115**	5*	**19**	75*	**1.4**	**1.6**	**17**	**2.0**	**500**	**2.8**
19–30 y	**1300**	**120**	5*	**19**	90*	**1.4**	**1.6**	**17**	**2.0**	**500**	**2.8**

Note: This table (taken from the DRI reports, see *www.nap.edu*) presents recommended dietary allowances (RDAs) in **bold type** and adequate intakes (AIs) in ordinary type followed by an asterisk (*). RDAs and AIs may both be used as goals for individual intake. RDAs are set to meet the needs of almost all (97% to 98%) individuals in a group. For healthy breast-fed infants, the AI is the mean intake. The AI for other life stage and gender groups is believed to cover needs of all individuals in the group, but lack of data or uncertainty in the data prevent being able to specify with confidence the percentage of individuals covered by this intake.

[a]As retinol activity equivalents (RAEs). 1 RAE = 1 μg retinol, **12** μg β-carotene, 24 μg α-carotene, or 24 μg β-cryptoxanthin. The RAE for dietary provitamin A carotenoids is twofold greater than retinol equivalents (RE), whereas the RAE for preformed vitamin A is the same as RE.

[b]Cholecalciferol. 1 μg cholecalciferol = 40 IU vitamin D.

[c]In the absence of adequate exposure to sunlight.

[d]As α-tocopherol. α-Tocopherol includes *RRR*-α-tocopherol, the only form of α-tocopherol that occurs naturally in foods, and the *2R*-stereoisomeric forms of α-tocopherol (*RRR*, *RSR*, *RRS*, and *RSS*-α-tocopherol) that occur in fortified foods and supplements. It does not include the *2S*-stereoisomeric forms of α-tocopherol (*SRR*, *SSR*, *SRS*, and *SSS*-α-tocopherol), also found in fortified foods and supplements.

[e]As niacin equivalents (NE). 1 mg of niacin = 60 mg of tryptophan; 0–6 months = preformed niacin (not NE).

[f]As dietary folate equivalents (DFE). 1 DFE = 1 μg food folate = 0.6 μg of folic acid from fortified food or as a supplement consumed with food = 0.5 μg of a supplement taken on an empty stomach.

[g]In view of evidence linking folate intake with neural tube defects in the fetus, it is recommended that all women capable of becoming pregnant consume 400 μg from supplements or fortified foods in addition to intake of food folate from a varied diet.

[h]It is assumed that women will continue consuming 400 μg from supplements or fortified food until their pregnancy is confirmed and they enter prenatal care, which ordinarily occurs after the end of the periconceptional period—the critical time for formation of the neural tube.

Source: Adapted from National Academy of Sciences. Recommended Daily Allowances 2001. Washington, DC: National Academy Press, 2001.

Table 22.6b. **Dietary Reference Intakes (DRIs): Recommended Intakes for Individuals, Elements**

Life stage group	Calcium (mg/d)	Copper (μg/d)	Fluoride (mg/d)	Iodine (μg/d)	Iron (mg/d)	Magnesium (mg/d)	Phosphorus (mg/d)	Selenium (μg/d)	Zinc (mg/d)
Males									
9–13 y	1300*	**700**	2*	**120**	**8**	**240**	**1250**	**40**	**8**
14–18 y	1300*	**890**	3*	**150**	**11**	**410**	**1250**	**55**	**11**
19–30 y	1000*	**900**	4*	**150**	**8**	**400**	**700**	**55**	**11**
Females									
9–13 y	1300*	**700**	2*	**120**	**8**	**240**	**1250**	**40**	**8**
14–18 y	1300*	**890**	3*	**150**	**15**	**360**	**1250**	**55**	**9**
19–30 y	1000*	**900**	3*	**150**	**18**	310	**700**	**55**	**8**
Pregnancy									
≤18 y	1300*	**1000**	3*	**220**	**27**	**400**	**1250**	**60**	**13**
19–30 y	1000*	**1000**	3*	**220**	**27**	**350**	**700**	**60**	**11**
Lactation									
≤18 y	1300*	**1300**	3*	**290**	**10**	**360**	**1250**	**70**	**14**
19–30 y	1000*	**1300**	3*	**290**	**9**	**310**	**700**	**70**	**12**

Note: This table presents recommended Dietary Allowances (RDAs) in **bold type** and adequate intakes (AIs) in ordinary type followed by an asterisk (*). RDAs and AIs may both be used as goals for individual intake. RDAs are set to meet the needs of almost all (97% to 98%) individuals in a group. For healthy breast-fed infants, the AI is the mean intake. The AI for other life stage and gender groups is believed to cover needs of all individuals in the group, but lack of data or uncertainty in the data prevent being able to specify with confidence the percentage of individuals covered by this intake.

Sources: Dietary Reference Intakes for Calcium, Phosphorus, Magnesium, Vitamin D, and Fluoride (1997); Dietary Reference Intakes for Thiamin, Riboflavin, Niacin, Vitamin B_6, Folate, Vitamin B_{12}, Pantothenic Acid, Biotin, and Choline (1998); Dietary Reference Intakes for Vitamin C, Vitamin E, Selenium, and Carotenoids (2000); and Dietary Reference Intakes for Vitamin A, Vitamin K, Arsenic, Boron, Chromium, Copper, Iodine, Iron, Manganese, Molybdenum, Nickel, Silicon, Vanadium, and Zinc (2001). These reports may be accessed via *www.nap.edu.*

Adapted from National Academy of Sciences. Recommended Daily Allowances 2001. Washington, DC: National Academy Press, 2001.

many authors have noted that anorexia nervosa and bulimia nervosa are detectable in all social classes and that higher socioeconomic status is not a major factor in the prevalence of these conditions. With anorexia nervosa food intake is severely limited, and with bulimia nervosa binge-eating episodes are followed by attempts to minimize the effects of overeating by vomiting, cathartics, exercise, or fasting.

The application of formal diagnostic criteria such as those in the *Diagnostic and Statistical Manual of Mental Disorders,* 4th edition (DSM-IV) has limited application to the adolescents with eating disorders. The wide variability in the rate, timing, and magnitude of both height and weight gain during normal puberty, the absence of menstrual periods during early puberty along with the unpredictability of menses soon after menarche, and the normal lack of psychological awareness regarding abstract concepts (e.g., self-concept, motivation to lose weight or affective states) limits the application.[13] All adolescents with an eating disorder should be evaluated for comorbid psychiatric illness. More research is needed to learn about the aspects of eating disorders that are particularly relevant to adolescents.

The only way to diagnose this condition is by the physician taking a detailed history on nutrition and dieting in the adolescent. Unfortunately, biologic features such as pubertal delay, growth retardation, or the impairment of bone mineral acquisition may occur at subclinical levels of eating disorders in adolescents. The diagnosis of an eating disorder should be considered not only in an adolescent who meets established diagnostic criteria but in any adolescent patient who engages in potentially unhealthy weight control practices or demonstrates obsessive thinking about food, weight, shape, or exercise.[13] Consider an eating disorder in any teenager who fails to attain or maintain a healthy weight, height, body composition, or stage of sexual maturation for gender and age.[13] Eating disorders may lead to irreversible effects on the physical and emotional growth and development of adolescents. In some cases these disorders are fatal. Therefore, the threshold for intervention in adolescents should be lower than that in adults. Most physical complications in adolescents with an eating disorder improve with nutritional rehabilitation and recovery from the eating disorder. Some of the medical complications that are potentially reversible are growth retardation if the disorder occurs before closure of the epiphyses, pubertal delay or arrest, and impaired acquisition of peak bone mass during the second decade of life (this would increase the risk of osteoporosis during adulthood).

Adolescents with eating disorders require evaluation and treatment focused on biomedical and psychosocial features of these complex, chronic health conditions. Assessment and ongoing management should be interdisciplinary and is best accomplished by a team consisting of medical, nursing, nutritional, and mental health disciplines. Family therapy is frequently an important part of treatment[13] (also see Chapter 35).

Hospitalization of an adolescent with an eating disorder is required in the presence of significant malnutrition; physiologic or physical evidence of medical compromise (e.g., vital sign instability, dehydration, or electrolyte disturbances) even in the absence of significant weight loss; arrested growth and development; failure of outpatient treatment; acute food refusal; uncontrollable bingeing, vomiting, or purging; family dysfunction that prevents effective treatment; and acute medical or psychiatric emergencies.[13]

Depression

Depression is a common problem that affects adolescents yet it remains significantly underdiagnosed. One screening tool that may be used for depression is the Beck Depression Inventory for Primary Care.[14] One general population study found that 27% of high school students were moderately depressed and 5% severely depressed. Depression is more common in females. Strong predictors of depression in adolescents are depression in one or both parents, low parental support, and loss of a parent through death or separation. The multitude of sociodemographic, biologic, and personal factors contributing to the development of depression are not well understood.

Adolescents with depression may present with somatic symptoms such as headaches and gastrointestinal complaints, which may include food intolerance, abdominal pain, and nausea. The primary care physician can treat depression in adolescents through counseling if trained in this area or through a counseling referral to an adolescent psychologist or psychiatrist, depending on the severity of the depression and the level of functioning of the adolescent. In cases of major depression, especially if there is active suicidal ideation, hospitalization is required and evaluation by a psychiatrist is needed.

Bipolar affective disorder (BPD), originally thought to be rare in childhood, is now diagnosed even in the prepubertal age group.[15] There appears to be a genetic predisposition to this disorder, but environmental factors are also considered important. Early recognition may lead to early treatment and reduce both short- and long-term morbidity and mortality.[15] Referral to an adolescent psychiatrist is recommended (also see Chapter 32).

Affective disorders have been associated with substance use and heavy drinking in adolescents, and therefore physicians need to screen youths with these conditions for substance use. In addition, screening youths for a history of emotional, physical, and sexual abuse as well as family violence is considered important as some of the behaviors exhibited by these youth may represent posttraumatic stress disorder (PTSD), which may be confused with psychotic features of BPD and schizophrenia.

Suicide

Suicide affects young people from all races and socioeconomic groups. Although suicide rates peaked in the 1990s and have continued to decline since, it continues to be the third-leading cause of death among adolescents. Many experts believe that numerous "accidental" deaths are actually suicides. Boys tend to have more fatal outcomes than girls when attempting suicide because of their use of more lethal methods, namely firearms and hanging. Adolescent girls most often attempt suicide by ingesting pills.

Conditions that have been associated with suicide include depression, BPD, conduct disorder, psychosis, alcohol and drug use, family history of suicide, being gay or bisexual, and a history of physical or sexual abuse. Studies indicate that gay and bisexual adolescents have a two to three times higher incidence of attempted suicide. Episodic despondence can occur in any adolescent, including a high achiever, leading to self-destructive behavior. A sense of hopelessness also correlates with suicidal intention and may occur without symptoms of depression.

Family physicians should not hesitate to question adolescents in general about suicidal thoughts. Asking an adolescent such questions does not precipitate the behavior. Most adolescents are relieved that someone cares enough to ask if they have been considering suicide and someone has heard their cry for help. Never dismiss suicidal thoughts as unimportant.

To assess an adolescent with suicidal thoughts, determine the sequence of events that preceded the threat, identify current problems and conflicts, and assess the degree of suicidal intent. Prior to allowing the young person to leave the clinical setting, the physician should assess the individual's coping resources and access to support systems, and the attitudes of the individual and the family toward intervention and follow-up.[16] An adolescent who has active suicidal plans or has attempted suicide requires hospitalization and consultation with mental health professionals. A brief hospital stay allows complete medical and psychological evaluation and prompt initiation of therapy (also see Chapter 33).

Tobacco Use

Tobacco use is a major health hazard for adolescents It is at this stage that addiction may begin and continue into adulthood. It is estimated that tobacco use kills more Americans each year than alcohol, cocaine, crack, heroin, homicide, suicide, car accidents, firearms, and acquired immunodeficiency syndrome (AIDS) combined. Despite laws that prohibit minors from purchasing tobacco, 80% of current smokers began smoking before age 18. Current statistics show that 12.8% of middle school and 34.8% of high school students smoke tobacco. Physicians need to screen all patients during routine visits on tobacco use.

The National Cancer Institute and the American Academy of Pediatrics issued a paper on clinical interventions to prevent tobacco use by children and adolescents.[17] Physicians' offices have been identified as effective sites for smoking cessation intervention. It is estimated in adult studies that approximately 10% of patients quit following physicians' recommendations. This rate could be higher with ongoing participation by the physician in a smoking cessation intervention. Just as important is the physician's active role in community-wide efforts to curb tobacco smoking. Organizations that have smoking cessation programs include the American Cancer Society, the American Health Foundation, the

Table 22.7. **Potential Physical Findings: Drug-Specific**

Site	Alcohol	Marijuana	Cocaine	LSD, mushrooms, peyote	Inhalants	Heroin, narcotics
Eyes	Periorbital edema; bloodshot; conjunctivitis; scleral icterus	Red/bloodshot; photophobia; conjunctivitis; nystagmus; diplopia; reduced accommodation	Pupils dilated; mydriasis	Nystagmus; perceptual illusions; flashbacks	Reddened	Constricted pupils, lacrimation
Nose	Rhinorrhea	—	If snorting: septum erythematous possibly perforated; epistaxis	—	Erythematous nasal passage	Rhinorrhea, sniffing, sneezing
Mouth	Odor of alcohol; poor dental hygiene	Dry green-gray coated tongue; poor dental hygiene	If smoking: brown-coated tongue; cheilosis; brown deposits on teeth	—	—	Poor dental hygiene
Chest	Tachycardia/bradycardia; decreased respirations; high blood pressure	Gynecomastia; upper respiratory infections	Rapid respirations; murmur; tachycardia; complaint of chest pain; arrhythmia; high blood pressure	—	—	Decreased pulse, respiration, and blood pressure
Abdomen	Palpable enlarged liver; epigastric tenderness; nausea/vomiting; distended abdomen	—	—	—	—	Hepatomegaly; severe cramping; nausea/vomiting
Genitourinary	Hemorrhoids resulting from diarrhea or constipation; blood in stool	Decreased sperm count	—	—	—	Constipation; in withdrawal: diarrhea
Skin	Jaundiced; easily bruised; petechiae; telangiectasia; reduced turgor; palms erythematous	—	Dry or diaphoretic; if smoking: small burns on fingers, hands, abdomen	Warm	—	Ashen, dry excoriated; in withdrawal: goose-bumps
General	Slurred speech; ataxic gait; malnutrition	Weight gain; lethargy; adolescent cigarette smoker	Hyperreflexia; weight loss; emaciated; in withdrawal: anergic, irritable, depressed	Hyperreflexia	Neurologic sequelae; headache	In withdrawal: joint and muscle ache, hyporeflexia

Source: Acee A, Smith D. The crash after crack. Am J Nursing 1987;87:614–7. Robin H, Michaelson J. Drug abuse—recognition and diagnosis. Chicago: Yearbook Publishers, 1988.

American Heart Association, the American Lung Association, and the March of Dimes Birth Defects Foundation.

The key to helping adolescents is prevention and early intervention. Encouraging parents and older siblings to serve as nonsmoking role models is important. Future research needs to determine which models are most effective for pre-vention and for smoking cessation in adolescent patients. Elimination of tobacco use requires a comprehensive strategy that includes health professional interventions, policy changes, advertising restrictions, comprehensive school-based programs, community activities, and advocacy approaches (see Chapter 8).

Other Substance Abuse

Drug abuse affects adolescents in all cultural and socioeconomic groups. Drug use may represent simple adolescent experimentation or significant abuse that interferes with the adolescent's development and daily life. Oral or inhaled drugs are most common, and intravenous drug use is uncommon during this age group. There is an association between psychiatric comorbidities and substance use. Therefore, careful assessment of the drug use pattern as well as associated psychiatric comorbidities is essential. Drugs in frequent use include alcohol, marijuana, and cocaine. New drugs such as Ecstasy, a hallucinogenic drug, and Ice, a metamphetamine, are popular with some adolescents.

A study of the prevalence of drug usage in white suburban adolescents and African-American urban adolescents who received care through private physicians' offices found that the rates of drug use were higher for the white suburban youths.[18] Stereotypes of drug abuse occurring only in minorities, the poor, and the uneducated interfere with the recognition of this problem in many adolescents.

The drug-abusing adolescent differs from the adult-using population in the length of time it takes to reach what substance abuse experts call a crisis point. The crisis point is the moment at which something happens in an addict's life that causes the addict or someone in power to decide that something is wrong and that some form of intervention is required.[19] The teen may be failing in school, may be truant, may be moody, or may be unmanageable in many areas. The average adult alcoholic may take up to 15 years to reach a crisis, but the average adolescent takes approximately 2 years to arrive at this same point. Thus adults who have been drinking excessively for 6 months have a less serious problem than a teen who has been drinking in the same manner and for the same length of time.

Diagnosing an adolescent with chemical dependence is not difficult once the physician has learned how to obtain a drug history. Adolescents may present with trouble in three main areas: family, school, or legal problems. The physician should assess the patient for drug-related symptoms[19] such as slurred speech or hyperactivity (Table 22.7). Urine testing alone should not be used to establish drug dependence, and adolescents should never be tested without their knowledge and consent. False positives as well as false negatives can occur. For example, an adolescent who is prescribed cough medicine may test positive for codeine. Different drugs remain in the system for different lengths of time. An adolescent who last smoked marijuana several weeks before the examination may test positive at the time of urine testing (Table 22.8).

Reasons for drug use are multifactorial and include family substance use, poor relationships with parents, child abuse and neglect, perceived peer drug use, failure in school, low self-esteem, early antisocial behavior, and psychopathology, particularly depression. In general, physicians should address the issue of drug abuse in routine clinical interactions and should make appropriate referrals to facilities for further assessment and treatment. As a primary care provider for an adolescent, the physician's role should be advocating for the

Table 22.8. **Detection Limits of Commonly Abused Drugs[a]**

Drug	Limits of sensitivity (μg/mL)	Approximate duration of detectability (days)
Cannabinoids (marijuana)	20 ng/mL	3–5[b]
Phencyclidine (PCP)	0.5	8
Cocaine metabolites		2–3
Codeine	0.5	2
Methadone	0.5	3
Amphetamine	0.5	2

[a]Factors of dose, frequency, route of administration, and the person's health have dramatic effects on these values.

[b]In rare circumstances, these substances may be present for weeks in heavy users.

Source: Adapted from McCunney RJ. Drug testing: technical complications of a complex social issue. Am J Ind Med 1989; 15:589–600.

patient and helping parents understand the problem. Parents are sometimes willing to recognize problems in their child's life but are unwilling to see problems in their own lives. If a family is functioning poorly, the entire family may benefit from counseling. Continued substance abuse recovery for the adolescent in the family with impaired dynamics is almost impossible.

The wide array of therapeutic approaches to substance abuse suggests there is not one best way to control or solve this problem. Therapeutic interventions include inpatient treatment, ambulatory treatment, group and individual counseling, and self-help groups. It is difficult to assess the rates of success for the various programs, as there is no standard methodology for reporting and follow-up.

In terms of prevention, adolescents report that newspapers and television are their most common source of information. Therefore, using mass media to educate adolescents about substance use may be effective. Some school-based prevention programs have been shown to be effective in decreasing illicit drugs.

Adolescent Sexual Health

National statistics indicate that half of high school students report having had sexual intercourse, and of these only half use condoms regularly. Adolescents are sexually active and need and want advice from physicians on how to be decrease the risks of STDs/HIV. Some studies indicate that adolescents would prefer that their physicians discuss with them STD/HIV risks instead of their parents or their teachers. Parents, of course, have a most influential role on adolescent sexual behavior. Since families are the most proximal and fundamental social system influencing child development, they provide many of the factors that protect adolescents from engaging in sexual risk behaviors. However, this only occurs if there is open and effective communication about sexuality where the adolescent can learn about familial sexual norms and where norms are safe ones.[20] If adolescents don't receive sexual information from their families, they turn to their peers for information. Physicians, therefore, have an important role to play in sexual education if adolescents have not yet received appropriate information from their parents or peers. Assessing the type of sexual information that an adolescent has and correcting misconceptions is important.

A complete discussion on the contraceptive methods available is indicated for the sexually active adolescent. For most sexually active adolescents, pregnancy is unintended. Physicians can reduce unintended pregnancies by making all adolescents aware of the existence of emergency contraception (ECP) or the "morning-after pill." ECPs reduce the risk of pregnancy by 75% if taken within 72 hours of unprotected intercourse. Vomiting and nausea are common side effects from ECPs and can compromise their efficacy, and therefore routine pretreatment with an antiemetic is recommended (see Chapter 101).

Important items for the physician to include in a discussion of sexuality with adolescents include sexual behavior, number of male partners, number of female partners, condom use, contraception use, and screening for sexual abuse. It is important to assess sexual behavior and not sexual orientation, as some youth who are homosexual may not describe themselves as such despite their behavior. If a youth is found to be at risk for STD/HIV, laboratory screening is indicated after obtaining informed consent. State laws vary on the age that an adolescent may provide consent for HIV testing. Primary care physicians tend to deliver STD/HIV preventive services to adolescents at rates far below those recommended by current guidelines.[21] This is now taking on special significance because the Centers for Disease Control and Prevention (CDC) estimates that 50% of new HIV infections are estimated to occur among people under the age age 25, typically through sexual transmission. Nationally, the HIV epidemic has shifted from white homosexual males to African Americans and Hispanics, women, and adolescents. The adolescents most at risk are homosexual and bisexual males, females who have sex with bisexuals (usually the fact that the male is bisexual is unknown to the female), and homeless youths who trade sex for money.

It is now becoming imperative that we identify youths at risk for HIV and that we offer them timely HIV testing before they transmit the infection to others. Most youths do not become aware of their serostatus for about 10 years, resulting in substantial opportunity for infecting others.[22] It is estimated that only 16% of youths living with HIV are aware that they carry the infection, which is much lower than the estimate for adults (67%).[23] When youths know they are infected, 70% report changing their sexual behavior, and 50% of those using intravenous drugs stop their use.[24] Thus, there are substantial benefits to society from early diagnosis of this infection. Alcohol and other oral drugs play a significant role in placing youths at risk for STD/HIV, as they have a disinhibiting effect on sexual restraint. Adolescents who use substances may be less likely to practice safe sex.

Sexual abuse as well as dating violence is unfortunately common in adolescents. If physicians don't ask, the adolescent is not likely to be forthcoming with such sensitive information. If an adolescent has been sexually abused, physi-

cians are required by law to report the incident to proper authorities.

Legal and Ethical Considerations

Several major legal issues routinely confront physicians: Whose consent is required for treating an adolescent? What information is confidential, and under what circumstances may it be disclosed? What are the possible sources of payment for an adolescent's care? The controlling legal principles are a matter of state law, and ensuring that adolescents have access to necessary health care requires the resolution of many complex legal and ethical issues dealing with confidentiality. Research suggests that many adolescents, particularly those age 14 or older, are as competent as adults to give informed consent for medical treatment. In addition to the basic requirement of consent for any medical care, the law requires physicians to obtain informed consent for treatment. Failure to obtain consent as required by law includes potential liability for the tort of battery (defined as the unauthorized touching of another person), negligence, or malpractice. Legal provisions that enable minors to give their consent for care and that protect the confidentiality of that care are considered critical elements for access to care in this age group.[25]

References

1. Igra V, Millstein S. Current status and approaches to improving preventive services for adolescents. JAMA 1993;269:1408–13.
2. Millstein SG. A view of health from the adolescent's perspective. In: Millstein SG, Peterson AC, Nightingale EO, eds. Promoting the health of adolescents: new directions for the twenty-first century. New York: Oxford University Press, 1993;97–118.
3. Elster AB, Kuznets NJ. AMA guidelines for adolescent preventive services (GAPS): recommendations and rationale. Baltimore: Williams & Wilkins, 1994.
4. Blum RW, Beuhring T, Shew ML, Bearinger LH, Sieving RE, Resnick MD. The effects of race/ethnicity, income, and family structure on adolescent risk behaviors. Am J Public Health 2000;90(12):1879–84.
5. Ehrman, WG, Matson SC. Approach to assessing adolescents on serious or sensitive issues. Pediatr Clin North Am 1998; 45(1):189–204.
6. Tanner JM. Growth at adolescence. London: Blackwell, 1962; 1–39, 156–75.
7. Root AW. Endocrinology. II. Aberrations of sexual maturation. J Pediatr 1973;83:187–200.
8. Resnick MD, Blum RW, Harris L. Risk and protective factors in adolescent health compromising behaviors. Presented at the Society of Adolescent Medicine Annual Meeting, March 1992.
9. Schubiner HH. Preventive health screening in adolescent patients. Prim Care 1989;16:211–30.
10. Cavadini C, Siega-Riz, Popkin BM. US adolescent food intake trends from 1965 to 1996. West J Med 2000;173(6):378–83.
11. Maloney MJ, McGuire J, Daniels SR, Specker B. Dieting behavior and eating attitudes in children. Pediatrics 1989;84:482–9.
12. Fisher M, Golden N, Katzman DK. Eating disorders in adolescents: a background paper. J Adolesc Health 1995;16:420–37.
13. Kreipe RE, Golden NH, Katzman DK, Fisher M. Eating disorders in adolescents: a position paper for the Society of Adolescent Medicine. J Adolesc Health 1995;16:476–80.
14. Winter LB, Steer RA, Jones-Hicks L, Beck AT. Screening for

major depression disorders in adolescent medical outpatients with the Beck Depression Inventory for Primary Care. J Adolesc Health 1999;24(6):389–94.

15. Robb AS. Bipolar disorder in children and adolescents. Curr Opin Pediatr 1999;11(4):317–22.

16. Gispert M, Wheeler K, Marsh L, et al. Suicidal adolescents: factors in evaluation. Adolescence 1985;20:753–62.

17. Epps RP, Manley MW. Clinical interventions to prevent tobacco use by children and adolescents. In: Glynn TJ, Manley MW, eds. How to help your patients stop smoking. Appendix G. NIH publ. no. 92-3064. Washington, DC: US Department of Health and Human Services, Public Health Service, National Institutes of Health, 1992;61–7.

18. Farrow JA, Schwartz RH. Adolescent drug and alcohol usage: a comparison of urban and suburban pediatric practices. J Natl Med Assoc 1992;84:409–13.

19. Myers DP, Andersen AR. Adolescent addiction: assessment and identification. J Pediatr Health Care 1991;5(2):86–93.

20. Perrino T, Gonzalez-Soldevilla A, Pantin H, Szapocznik J. The role of families in adolescent HIV prevention: a review. Clin Child Fam Psychol Rev 2000;3:81–96.

21. Schuster MA, Bell RM, Petersen LP, Kanouse DE. Communication between adolescents and physicians about sexual behavior and risk prevention. Arch Pediatr Adolesc Med 1996;150(9): 906–13.

22. Centers for Disease Control and Prevention. 1998 Guidelines for treatment of sexually transmitted diseases. MMWR 1998; 47(RR-1):1–118.

23. Centers for Disease Control and Prevention. Statistical projections/trends May 13, 1999; available at *http://www.cdc.gov/nchstp/hiv_aids/hivinfo/vfax/260210.ht.*

24. Rotheram-Borus MJ, Murphy DA, Swendeman D, et al. Substance use and its relationship to depression, anxiety, and isolation among youth living with HIV. Int J Behav Med 2000;6: 293–311.

25. English A. Treating adolescents: legal and ethical considerations. Adolesc Med 1990;74:109–12.

23
Selected Problems of Aging

Lanyard K. Dial

The population of our nation is slowly and irreversibly growing older. We have moved from the youth-oriented society that has been the status quo since the establishment of our country to a population now dominated by older adults. In fact, the fastest growing segment of all age groups is that segment of people over the age of 85. This dramatic shift is altering, and will continue to alter, the health care system of our country. Seniors disproportionately use all aspects of health services. Practicing family physicians will find that their daily visits will include more and more patients who are elderly. This chapter provides information on issues that are common to this population and covers topics of both a clinical and a social/functional nature. These choices reflect the breadth of medical needs in older individuals.

Selected Clinical Issues

Frailty

The aging of our patient population has forced us to face the fact that many patients will develop functional losses and frailty. Frailty is not a pure medical diagnosis nor a classic clinical syndrome; it is more an overall statement of the condition of an individual. It is best thought of as a decline in a person's function to a level that requires assistance with all instrumental activities of daily living (IADLs) and one or more activities of daily living (ADLs)[1,2] (Table 23.1). Without interventions, frail individuals progress to lose further physical and social function causing institutionalization and death. Frailty is not just a medical condition or in the realm of just the physician, but can be perceived by all who know the individual and have watched the development of this state. Clear definitions or objective parameters for frailty are still lacking. Typically a "frail" individual shows some or many of the features listed in Table 23.2.

Without a clear scale or lab measurement, the best approach for the physician is to recognize that frailty exists, that it is virtually inevitable unless one has a rapid demise, and that the most reliable understanding comes from a comprehensive functional assessment. The patient's initial presentation for medical care is typically either acute, such as a fall, a fracture, or an abrupt change in mental function, or a chronic decline commonly known as "failure to thrive." In either case, the underlying considerations for the physician are similar, and a systematic approach is needed to identify and prevent this condition or to determine its cause and treatment options.

Frailty and functional loss results from the interaction of three major processes (Fig. 23.1):

The effects of the natural aging process on organ and tissue functions
The damage resulting from disuse and abuse
The derangements caused by both acute and chronic diseases

Natural Aging Progressing to Frailty

As we age, our organs and tissues become less resilient, and less able to rebound from insults. Fortunately, many of our organs are paired or are designed with a significant reserve; for example, we can live in a nonfrail state with the function of only one eye or on only 20% of either liver or kidney function. But at some point even natural aging can lead to enough dysfunction that the individual becomes frail. Figure 23.2 depicts the downsloping line of function with age. Without major illnesses, the age at which one starts on the loss of function downslope and the slope of the loss is different for each individual. A professional athlete who is no longer competitive at the age of 30 may complain of loss of reflex or musculoskeletal function. A heavy laborer may notice a decline in ability to perform certain job tasks in the 3rd or 4th decade. Most Americans begin to sense a loss of function in their 4th or 5th decade as they notice less endurance or strength, joint stiffness or muscle aches, or loss of the resilience that they

Table 23.1. **Definitions of ADLs and IADLs**

Activities of daily living (ADLs)	Instrumental activities of daily living (IADLs)
Ability to perform basic self-care tasks: *Dressing*—ability to dress oneself appropriately *Eating*—ability to self-feed *Ambulating*—ability to manuever in one's environment *Toileting*—ability to use toilet facilities *Hygiene*—ability to clean oneself, including hair and teeth	Ability to use instruments and interact with the environment to perform tasks necessary for independent function: *Shopping*—ability to obtain necessary tems for care (food, clothing, hygiene needs) *Housekeeping*—ability to keep environment clean *Accounting*—ability to manage money and simple finances *Food preparation*—ability to prepare foods for eating *Transportation*—abiltity to use modes of transportation to get necessary items

had as a youth. The vast majority of people don't begin to seek medical care for age-related functional decline until their 6th or 7th decade of life. However, frailty from normal aging alone seems most commonly to begin somewhere in the 8th decade, although there are who reach their 9th decade and 10th decades in nonfrail states.

Disuse and Abuse Causing Frailty

One of the clearly recognized principles of frailty in aging is that the natural state of healthy aging is altered by both abuse and disuse. Many individuals do not age well as a result of some form of abuse to their organs and tissues. Common abuses include over exposure to the ultraviolet (UV) rays of the sun, or indulgences in alcohol, tobacco, or drugs. Loss of function and frailty occurs at an earlier age in such people. Abuse can also be the result of repetitive trauma or the forces of obesity on our musculoskeletal system. A key focus of the field of preventative geriatrics is how to avoid functional loss and frailty from disuse. Inactivity causes progressive loss of both physical and psychological function. The benefits to an elder's gait, strength, and physical function by participation in regular nonstrenuous exercise such as Tai Chi are well documented.[3,4] Even elders who have severe physical limitations can have both physical and psychological benefit from simple exercises.

Diseases that Can Cause Frailty

Perhaps the largest area of impact is the recognition and treatment of diseases that lead to frailty. Chronic illnesses can hasten the rate of decline in natural function and the onset of any acute illness can move an individual from a well-functioning elder into a frail state. Illnesses that can cause frailty span

physical, social, and psychological boundaries. Table 23.3 lists some of the most common conditions that lead to loss of function in the elderly.

Treating the Frail Elder

Reversing or stabilizing the functional level of a frail elder depends on recognizing the condition and determining the major etiologic factors. Poor appetite and the resultant weight loss can be reversed with some behavioral changes and the judicious use of medications (Table 23.4).

In situations where the progressive loss cannot be halted or reversed, the appropriate management is to transition into a palliative care approach. The life expectancy of frail individual varies, but it is important to recognize that many frail elders will live for a number of years at a functional level in which they are dependent on a caregiver for support in their basic activities. Understanding the patients' functional losses and pairing their needs with an appropriate level of services is the key.

Spontaneous Leg Movement Disorders

Older adults are more prone to develop a variety of idiopathic disorders of movement of the lower extremity. Taken together, these can be grouped as spontaneous leg movement disorders. They include restless leg syndrome, periodic limb movement disorder, and nocturnal leg cramps.[5]

Restless Leg Syndrome

Restless leg syndrome (RLS) is a poorly understood neurologic disorder that causes patients to experience unpleasant sensations in their legs usually while at rest. Most patients describe

Table 23.2. **Common Clinical Findings in "Frail" Elder**

Dependence in all IADLs
Dependence in one or more ADLs
Anorexia
Weight loss
Loss of muscle bulk
Weakness
Decreased ambulation
Increased instability—more falls
Dementia and episodic delirium
Decreased social interactions
Urinary and fecal incontinence
Pressure sores

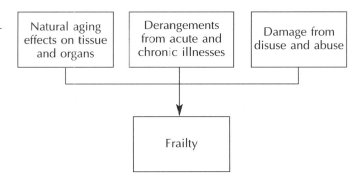

Fig. 23.1. Three processes that contribute to frailty.

Development of a Frail State

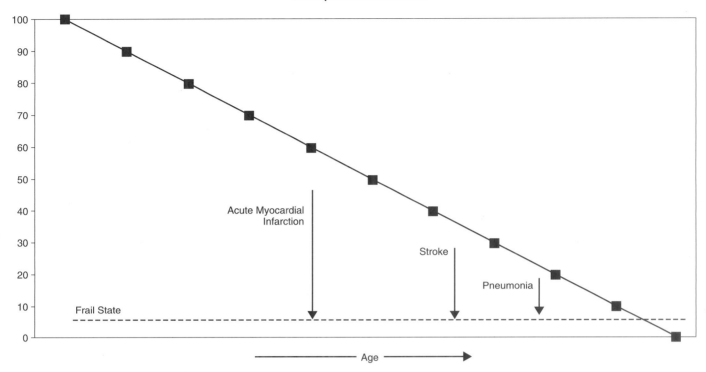

Fig. 23.2. A gradual decline of functional level with normal aging leads to a frail state. Patients move rapidly into a frail state with the onset of an acute illness. Vertical axis represents percent of full function.

a pulling, drawing, crawling type of discomfort of their calves. It has also been reported to occur in the thighs and feet. These sensations occur during times when the legs are at rest, most commonly at nighttime while lying in bed. RLS is a benign condition, usually causing insomnia and its attendant consequences (such as daytime fatigue, reduced concentration, and dysthymia). RLS affects between 10% and 20% of seniors. Younger patients can be affected, and in them there is a more common familial pattern. Patients with underlying neuropathies are more prone to RLS. Some cases have been reported due to mineral deficient states such as vitamin B_{12}, folate, magnesium, or most commonly iron.[6] The other association is with an elevated blood urea nitrogen seen in uremic states.

The diagnosis of RLS is based on history. Patients can present with a complaint of leg symptoms typical for RLS, or of insomnia, in which case the discovery of the unpleasant leg sensations occurs with questioning.

The current standard requires a yes answer to all of the following four questions[7,8]:

Do you experience unpleasant sensations like pulling, drawing, or crawling in your legs?
Do these sensations occur predominantly at rest?
Are these symptoms worse in the evening or nighttime?
Do these sensations cause you to have an urge to move, and does moving improve them?

There are no physical findings to support the history, and so the diagnosis is purely subjective. Some sophisticated sleep centers can electronically monitor leg movements and central nervous system (CNS) activity during rest to confirm the diagnosis if necessary. Patients should be evaluated for neuropathies, mineral deficiencies, and uremia. In addition, patients with RLS have a higher incidence of depression and anxiety disorders and these should be looked for and treated appropriately.

The treatment of RLS begins with increased daily muscle stretches and exercise. Medications should be reserved for those with excessive sleep disturbances. The current recommended therapy is with dopamine and its agonists. This comes from research that has given rise to a theory that RLS may result from a decline in CNS dopamine activity. Table 23.5 lists the most common dopaminergic agents used in the treatment of RLS. Therapy can usually reduce or eliminate symptoms in 80% to 90% of patients. Also used are analgesics such as acetaminophen, nonsteroidal antiinflammatory medication or opioids. The use of sedatives such as benzodiazepines, although historically a common choice, should be avoided in the elderly because of their excessive sedation and associated complications.[7–10]

Periodic Limb Movement Disorder

Periodic limb movement disorder (PLMD) is a related condition to RLS.[5] About 80% of patients with RLS experience PLMD. PLMD is defined as involuntary repetitive contractions of muscles of the leg occurring every 20 seconds to 1 minute during sleep. It has also been called "nocturnal myoclonus." PLMD increases with age such that it occurs in up to 80% of

Table 23.3. **Common Conditions Leading to Loss of Function and Frailty**

Chronic medical illnesses	Endocrine diseases
	Diabetes
	Hypothyroidism
	Organ failure
	Liver
	Renal
	Heart
	Chronic lung disease
	Cancer
	Degenerative neurologic diseases
	Alzheimer's disease
	Parkinson's disease
	Sensory diseases
	Deafness
	Blindness
	Arthritis
Acute medical illnesses	Infections
	Acute blood loss
	Medication reactions
	Acute vascular event
	Coronary
	Cerebral
	Pulmonary embolus
	Hospitalizations and surgeries
Psychological illnesses	Depression
	Psychosis
	Grief
Social conditions	Isolation
	Poverty
	Abuse
	Loss of caregiver

Table 23.4. **Treatment for Elders with Poor Appetite and Weight Loss**

Nonpharmacologic methods to increase nutrition	Frequent small meals high in protein and fat
	Supplements as meal replacements or nighttime snacks combined with exercise program
	Increase socialization around meals
Medications to boost appetite	Megestrol acetate
	Dronabinol
	Steroids
	Antidepressants (methylphenidate, mirtazipine)
	?Growth hormone

patients over the age of 65. Patients with PLMD may present with insomnia if the movements cause recurrent awakening, or they may be brought in by complaints from their bed partner. The evaluation and treatment parallels that of RLS.

Nocturnal Leg Cramps

Nocturnal leg cramps (NLCs) are painful muscles spasms of the muscles in the leg, usually the calf, that last for a few seconds to a few minutes. Most people experience them periodically, but for some they are a nightly bother. They are benign, but they can cause significant discomfort and disturb an individual's resting pattern. They are associated with inade-

quate fluid intake or dehydration from diuretic use or water loss. Medical conditions associated with increased NLC include calcium and phosphorus imbalances, uremia, hypothyroidism, and Addison's disease. Crampy pain of the calf at rest, usually during the night, does not indicate vascular disease.

Preventing NLCs begins with increasing fluid balance and performing nightly stretching exercises of the calf muscles. If the patient experiences cramps, then the legs should be extended at the knee and the foot dorsiflexed, pulling the toes toward the head.

Quinine use for nocturnal leg cramps should be avoided. In 1995 the Food and Drug Administration (FDA) decided quinine was not effective for nocturnal leg cramps, may be unsafe, and ordered its removal from the over-the-counter market.[9–11] It is still available by prescription but it can cause significant side effects including nausea, vomiting, diarrhea, hearing loss, tinnitus, vasodilatation, flushing, diaphoresis, and hypotension. Serious life-threatening cardiac rhythm disturbances can occur in some patients with high doses.[11] The use of tonic water at bedtime has been suggested as it contains small amounts of quinine and will increase fluid balance.

Constipation

Constipation is an extremely common occurrence throughout life, and the elderly experience this problem with increased frequency. In some, constipation is simply a nuisance, but it can signify serious underlying disease and it can create serious problems. Constipation alone can create abdominal pain,

Table 23.5. **Dopaminergic Medications Used to Treat Restless Leg Syndrome**

Generic medication	Trade name	Dosing	Mechanism of action	Side effects
L-dopa + carbidopa	Sinemet Sinemet CR	100–500 mg of L-dopa at bedtime	Direct dopamine supplementation	Nausea, dyskinesia, hypotension
Bromocriptine	Parlodel	1.25–10 mg at bedtime	Dopamine agonist	Nausea, dyskinesia
Pergolide	Permax	0.05–2 mg at bedtime	Dopamine agonist	Nausea, dyskinesia, nasal congestion
Pramipexole	Mirapex	0.125–1 mg at bedtime	Dopamine agonist	Nausea, dyskinesia
Ropinirole	Requip	0.25–2 mg at bedtime	Dopamine agonist	Nausea, dyskinesia

colonic/rectal overdistention colonic obstruction, rectal prolapse sigmoid volvulus, or urinary/fecal incontinence.

An exact definition of constipation is difficult and probably unnecessary except for research purposes. For many patients, the presenting symptoms include painful bowel movements, the need to strain to have bowel movements, hard stools, infrequent stools, the feeling of incomplete evacuation, or the need to use some type of laxative/enema or digitalization to have a bowel movement.

Risk Factors

The self-reported prevalence of constipation increases with age and occurs more commonly in females than males. Less exercise, sedentary lifestyle, diseases that create immobility and the use of a variety of medications are the most significant risk factors in the elderly.[12] Many underlying diseases and many medications are associated with an increase in the frequency of the complaint of constipation (Tables 23.6 and 23.7). Despite folklore, there have been a number of studies that show that low dietary fiber consumption and fluid intake are not independent risk factors for developing constipation.

Evaluation

The initial assessment must involve a complete history and physical exam to determine potential underlying causes. A recent change in bowel habits, if not clearly associated with a new disease or medication, requires a prompt evaluation for underlying colonic disease. A thoughtful look at the patient's medication list will frequently find potential inciting agents. A blood sample should be obtained to check for thyroid function, electrolytes, and underlying anemia. Elderly patients with new symptoms of constipation, associated weight loss, or anemia should undergo a colonoscopy as the procedure of choice (also see Chapter 92). Colon transit evaluation or manometric evaluation are available, but rarely necessary.

Management of Constipation

For most healthy elders, providing good bowel habit suggestions such as increasing physical activity and drinking plenty of liquids will be adequate. In addition, specific foodstuffs can be recommended such as fresh or dried fruits, vegetables, and foods high in soluble fibers such as grains, bran, nuts, and beans. A "colon cocktail" is a commonly used food mixture to maintain stool softness and consistency. The mixture is equal quantities of prune juice, applesauce, and psyllium, and is usually made as one cup of each. This mixture is kept refrigerated, and the patient takes 1 to 2 tablespoons each day.[13]

Table 23.6. **Diseases Associated with Chronic Constipation in the Elderly**

Neuropsychiatric disorders	Nonneuropsychiatric disorders
Multiple sclerosis	Hypothyroidism
Parkinson's disease	Diabetes mellitus
Spinal cord injury	Hypercalcemia
Autonomic neuropathies	Hypokalemia
Depression	Systemic sclerosis
Stroke	Obstructing colonic lesions
	Dehydration

Table 23.7. **Medications Associated with Constipation**

Anticholinergics
Anticonvulsants
Antihypertensives
Antiparkinsonsian drugs
Opiates
5-HT$_3$-antagonists
Nonsteroidal antiinflammatories
Chronic laxative abuse
Tricyclic antidepressants
Calcium channel blockers
Aluminum antacids
Bismuth
Calcium
Iron
Diuretics
Barium

When medications are considered, be cognizant that laxatives are available in a variety of forms, including bulk agents, lubricants, osmotically active agents, and stimulants (Table 23.8). The choice of which agent for which patient depends on the patient's underlying colon status. Lubricants are poor choices overall in that they have serious risks (lipoid aspiration) and distasteful side effects (anal seepage).[14] Most ambulatory and healthy patients who fail to respond to changes in habits and foodstuffs can be given bulk agents as their first line of drug therapy. These agents cause a increase in stool volume, a decrease in colon transit time, and an improvement in stooling consistency. Osmotically active agents are the best second choice in these patients and frequently the most effective. All of these agents are nonabsorbed, mild agents whose main side effects are increased bloating and gas.

When these agents fail, then stimulant agents become the necessary drugs of choice. Stimulants alter colonic motility and can alter fluid and electrolyte transport into the stool. They should be restricted in their use to two to three times a week to prevent overstimulation and atony of the bowel. The last resort for severe constipation is the addition of rectal suppositories and/or enemas to stimulate colon evacuation.

In demented patients, postsurgical patients, and patients on chronic narcotics, the choice of laxatives changes. These patients do very poorly on bulking agents creating a larger volume of impacted stool.[14] The most successful therapy is a combination of osmotic and stimulant medications with the use of suppositories or enemas periodically to induce evacuation. Such combinations, started early and used consistently, can prevent most constipation complaints in such elders.

Social/Functional Issues

Community-Based Assistive Services and Living Arrangements

Most seniors reach a point at which they require assistance with their daily needs. The options at this point are dependent on many variables including the seniors' specific needs, their resources in terms of family and friends, their financial circum-

Table 23.8. **Drug Therapy for Constipation**

Drug groups and specific medications	Common doses	Comments
Bulk agents		Effective at 12–72 hours; inexpensive; side effects include gas, bloating
Methycellulose (Citrucil)	1–4 tbsp/day	
Psyllium (Metamucil, Konsyl)	1 tbsp qd–tid	
Barley malt extract (Maltsupex)	12–32 g bid	
Calcium polycarbophil (FiberCon)	1 tablet qd–qid	
Lubricants		Effective within 8 hours; distasteful to some; mild efficacy
Mineral oil	1–2 tbsp bid	
Osmotics		Effective at 4 to 8 hours; nonabsorbable; treats moderate to severe constipation
Lactulose (Cephulac)	2–4 tbsp, repeat q4h prn	
Sorbitol (70%)	2–4 tbsp, repeat q4h prn	
Polyethylene glycol	8–25 g per day	
Ricinoleic acid (castor oil)	1–2 tsps, repeat q4h prn	
Stimulants		Most effective; can induce GI cramping, 6–12 hours
Senna (Senokot)	1–2 tabs qd	
Bisacodyl (Dulcolax)	5-mg tabs or 10-mg suppositories	
Enemas		Last resort in healthy patients; used frequently in combinations with stimulants in patients who are demented, hospitalized, or on chronic narcotics; effective within 15–30 minutes
Tap water		
Sodium phosphate/biphosphate (Fleet)	4.5 oz enema once	

stances, and the available assistive services and living arrangements. The goal for the physician is to assist the patient in finding the appropriate services and living arrangements.

Assistive Services

Informal support for seniors comes from family and friends. Formal support services are part of every community. There are a variety of formal assistive services designed to support seniors who are living in noninstitutionalized settings.[3,4,13] Support services come from both governmental organizations and private organizations. Information and referral services are available to find the type of services that people need. Table 23.9 provides a description of the most common services available.

Table 23.9. **Formal Community-Based Support Services for Seniors**

Community-based services	Description
Senior centers	Central location for group activities for seniors such as games, crafts, health fairs, etc.; usually has a congregate meal program
Adult day care	Provides daytime supervised activities for seniors in a group setting; some can accommodate patients with dementia
Day hospitals	Similar to adult day care, provides daytime supervised activities for seniors in a group setting plus medical services (usually rehabilitation services or nursing services for parenteral medication)
Nutrition programs	Provides meals to seniors; can be at congregate sites such as day care or senior centers; can be home delivered program such as meals-on-wheels
Housekeeping services	Provides simple housekeeping services such as house cleaning, washing, shopping, or food preparation
Home repair services	Provides necessary home repair services such as installation of safety equipment (bath railing, locks), repair of steps or simple plumbing or electrical needs
Security services	Provides for easy contact to emergency services; commonly a necklace or button that contacts a local emergency room.
Telephone contact services	Provides for a daily telephone call to ensure that the individual is in no need
Transportation services	Provides transportation for seniors into the community; sometimes limited to appointments for health care needs
Case management	Provides a coordinator of care for a senior who can assist in financial and social service needs
Respite care	Provides for short-term care for a senior so that a live-in caregiver can have a break (respite) from care

Alternative Living Arrangements

Many seniors find themselves in need of living arrangements other than the single family home/apartment because of failing health. There are a variety of options depending on the level of services needed.

Independent Living Facilities. Independent living facilities (ILFs) are for the senior who needs minimal services but prefers to have them centralized. Such housing usually is an apartment or a bungalow that is associated with a facility that provides services in a centralized location. Usually ILFs provide for a congregate meal service, exercise facility, group activities, and a group transportation system. Most of these facilities provide for an easy transition to the assisted living mode.

Board and Care Facilities. The board and care facilities are also called group homes or residential care facilities. These are living arrangements in which a number of unrelated seniors live together providing for a reduced cost of services and more supervision of care. The residents can have their own room, or share a room, and have access to a cooperative living room, dining room, and kitchen. There is nonprofessional staff support at these facilities that does the housecleaning, meal preparation, and can assist residents in the taking of medication. These facilities are frequently licensed by the state and have surveys that monitor their care.

Assisted Living Facilities. An assisted living facility offers an independent living arrangement with support from licensed professional staff. Commonly people share living rooms, dining rooms, and recreational facilities, but live in their own apartment-like room. The intent of this type of living arrangements is to provide for aging in place, in which seniors can have increasing help from staff as they age while staying in their same place.

Continuing-Care Retirement Communities (CCRCs). CCRCs are all-inclusive facilities that provide the levels of care necessary for the aging individual. They require substantial financial resources that are paid as a lump sum up front and a fixed monthly expense, or a variable monthly expense depending on the level of services needed. Most provide for independent living, assisted living, and more dependent supervised living up to and including a skilled nursing facility.

How to Help Seniors Understand Medicare

Medicare Structure

Medicare is the federal government program of health coverage available to seniors, permanently disabled adults, and those on end-stage renal dialysis. It was enacted into law in 1965 and it is currently the nation's largest source of payment for medical care, insuring almost 40 million beneficiaries. Its fundamental structure is two different insurance plans, part A and part B, which receive revenues from different sources and pay for different types of services (Table 23.10).[15,16] In addition to the part A or B plans, Medicare dollars can flow into existing health maintenance organizations (HMOs), preferred provider organizations (PPOs), and other structured health plans that then can offer to provide beneficiaries with expanded services (particularly a limited formulary medication benefit). These programs are called "Medicare+Choice" plans.

Medicare Finances[15–17]

Some 89% of all Medicare revenue comes from people less than 65 years old through taxes and interest on the trust fund, and only 11% comes from the elderly covering monthly premiums, deductibles, and copayments. Total Medicare annual expenditures exceed $215 billion. Approximately 85% of patients with Medicare have some form of supplemental insurance to help pay for deductible costs, copayments, and uncovered expenses (especially prescription drug costs). Fifteen percent of patients have Medicaid supplemental insurance, 35% have an employer-sponsored plan, 25% have purchased a private supplemental plan (so-called Medigap policies), and 10% have supplemental plans through a variety of public (state and federal) programs.

Table 23.10. **Medicare Fundamentals**

	Part A	Part B
Financing	From Social Security Tax into Medicare Hospital Insurance Trust Fund Supplemental Trust Fund	25% from enrollees @ premium $45/mo; 75% general tax revenue; all into Medicare Supplemental Trust Fund
Coverage	Hospital care Home health care Hospice care Skilled nursing homes	Physician visits Emergency room care Lab and x-rays PT and OT services Mental health services Durable medical equipment
Reimbursement	Payments through Medicare intermediaries to hospitals, hospices, skilled nursing homes, and home health based on per episode, per diagnosis, or per day; deductible for hospitalization, $759	Payment through carriers; patient is responsible for $100 annual deductible and 20% copayment for most services

OT = occupational therapy; PT = physical therapy.

Table 23.11. **Medicare-Covered Services**

Type of services	Specific covered areas
Physician services	Medical care by any practitioner provided in an office, hospital, outpatient facility, nursing home hospice, or at home; includes all physician services—primary care and specialty care, surgery, pathology, radiology
Health maintenance screening procedures	*Breast cancer*—annual mammography *Cervical cancer*—Pap and pelvic exam—q 2 years; annually for high risk *Colon cancer*—annual fecal occult blood and flexible sigmoidoscopy or colonoscopy every 4 years; high-risk patients—flex sig, or colonoscopy covered as screening exam every 2 years *Prostate cancer*—Digital rectal exam and PSA annually *Glaucoma screening*—annual for high-risk individuals *Bone mineral density*—DEXA scanning *Immunizations*—hepatitis B, influenza, pneumococcal, tetanus (postinjury)
Mental health services	Outpatient therapy by a physician or a psychologist or care provided in a comprehensive rehabilitation program
Hospital care	Semiprivate room, specialty units, laboratory, x-ray, medications, supplies, blood (first three units paid by patient), meals, nursing care (not private duty) Care must be ordered by a physician and stay approved by a peer-review organization
Hospital outpatient services	Diagnostic lab and x-ray tests as outpatient (including those with independent laboratories), medical supplies, emergency room visits, ambulatory surgery, ambulance transportation
Outpatient medications	Non-HMO benefits limited—coverage for Immunosuppressants after organ transplantation Erythopoietin for patients with end-stage renal disease on dialysis Oral anticancer agents Clotting factors for patients with hemophilia
Physical and occupational therapy	Covered whether provided by hospital or independent provider
Nutritional therapy	Coverage for medical nutritional therapy for diabetics or patients with renal disease
Home health care	Intermittent services (up to 21 days) provided by home skilled nursing, home-health aides, physical therapists, occupational therapists, speech therapists
Durable medical equipment	Covered equipment assistive devices, beds, oxygen equipment; prosthetic devices (except dental)

Covered Services

Medicare is an extensive insurance plan with coverage extending from hospital to home and from physicians to therapists. Its coverage is complex and subject to a variety of deductibles and copayments. Table 23.11 lists covered services, including those passed in the fall of 2000 due to be enacted during the 2002 year.[18,19]

There are important areas of health care needs not covered by Medicare. Prescription drug coverage is the most hotly debated at the time of this writing.[20] In addition, Medicare does not cover any dental care, hearing or vision services, podiatric foot care, or any type of custodial nursing or home care.

Assessing Driving Competency

Competency assessment for driving is a complex undertaking because of the many variables involved, but the need cannot be ignored. Older adults drivers have the highest fatality rate per crash and per mile driven of all age groups.[21] Combine this with the fact that the number of elderly drivers is increasing and we are faced with a clear mandate to assess an

Table 23.12. **Potential or Mild Functional Losses Associated with Increased Driving Risks**

Cognitive loss	Visual-spatial losses more important than memory in early disease Slowed central processing of information ("slowed reaction time")
Motor loss	Loss of grip strength and wrist function Limitations in rotation of neck Limitation in upper and lower extremity motion/strength
Sensory loss	Visual loss—visual fields, central acuity, night vision, and increased glare Hearing loss—especially bilateral hearing loss Patients with combined visual and hearing loss at highest risk
Loss of consciousness	Any seizure disorder Medical diseases (cerebrovascular, cardiac arrythmias, diabetes, medication use, alcohol use) that have caused loss of consciousness within last year

elder's competency to drive. The licensing and testing requirements vary from state to state across our country but it is the expectation that physicians can identify potentially impaired drivers and initiate referral.

Driving is a cornerstone issue for many seniors as it provides access to shopping, food, and socialization. It is a quality of life issue that can affect one's sense of well-being and self-worth. Identifying the at-risk senior is the challenge. Age or any specific medical illness or use of any specific medication alone is a poor predictor of driving ability. An easy-to-identify at-risk individual is one who has had a recent accident or moving violation. Another group of at-risk elders are those with extensive functional losses.[22,23] The difficulty for physicians is in judging the significance of potential losses or mild losses of function. Table 23.12 lists the most commonly cited causes of potential or mild functional losses correlated with driving impairment.

Once the physician has determined that the individual elder is at risk, then a discussion should be undertaken with the patient and their family about restricting driving. In many states, the Department of Motor Vehicles has a driving competency assessment program that puts seniors through written and performance tests to determine continued licensure. In states where this is unavailable, it is the role of the family physician to suggest driving restrictions. This is best approached by emphasizing the risk to the elderly driver. Another important factor is to assist the patient and family with contacts to available services to fill in for the loss of driving independence.

References

1. Rockwood K, Stolee P, McDowell I. Factors associated with institutionalization of older people in Canada: testing a multifactorial definition of frailty. J Am Geriatr Soc 1996;44: 578–82.
2. Balducci L, Stanta G. Cancer in the elderly: cancer in the frail patient, a coming epidemic. In: Hematology/oncology clinics of North America. Philadelphia: WB Saunders, 2000;235–50.
3. Kane RL, Ouslander JG, Abrass IB. Essentials of clinical geriatrics, 4th ed. New York: McGraw-Hill, 1999.
4. Cassel CK, Cohen HJ, Larson EB, et al. Geriatric medicine, 3rd ed. New York: Springer-Verlag, 1997.
5. Mahowald MW, Schenck CH. Sleep disorders: parasomnias including the restless legs syndrome. In: Clinics in chest medicine. Philadelphia: WB Saunders, 1998;183–202.
6. Rothdach AJ, Trenkwalder C, Haberstock J, Keil U, Berger K. Prevalence and risk factors of RLS in an elderly population: The MEMO study. Neurology 2000;54:1064–8.
7. Chokroverty S, Jankovic J. Restless legs syndrome: a disease in search of identity. Neurology 1999;52:907–10.
8. Werra R. Restless legs syndrome. Am Fam Physician 2001;63: 1048–52.
9. Leg disorders (restless legs syndrome, intermittent claudication, and nocturnal leg cramps): patient education handout, 2000. Available at *www.mdconsult.com*.
10. Cobbs EL, Duthie EH, Murphy JB, ed. Geriatric review syllabus: a core curriculum in geriatric medicine, 4th ed. Dubuque, IA: Kendall/Hunt Publishing Co. for the American Geriatric Society, 1999.
11. Nordt SP, Clark RF. Acute blindness after severe quinine poisoning. Am J Emerg Med 1998;16:214–5.
12. Talley NJ, Fleming KC, Evans JM, et al. Constipation in an elderly community: a study of prevalence and potential risk factors. Am J Gastroenterol 1996;91:19–25.
13. Dial LK. Conditions of aging: the Academy collection. Baltimore: Williams & Wilkins, 1999.
14. Wald A. Constipation. In: Medical clinics of North America. Philadelphia: WB Saunders, 2000;1231–46.
15. Iglehart JK. The American health care system: Medicare. N Engl J Med 1999;340:327–32.
16. What every medical resident needs to know about the Medicare program: medical education and training, 5th ed. Washington, DC: Health Care Financing Administration, 1999.
17. Pawlson LG. Financing, coverage, and costs of health care for older persons. In: Cobbs EL, Duthie EH, Murphy JB, eds. Geriatric review syllabus: a core curriculum in geriatric medicine, 4th ed. Dubuque, IA: Kendall/Hunt Publishing Co. for the American Geriatric Society, 1999;42–9.
18. Moon M. Health policy 2001:Medicare. N Engl J Med 2001; 344:928–31.
19. Directors Newsletter. Am Acad Fam Physicians 2001(March 29);2–3.
20. Inglehart JK, Health policy 2001: Medicare and prescription drugs. N Engl J Med 2001;344:1010–4.
21. Sims RV, Owsley C, Allman RM, Ball K, Smoot TM. A preliminary assessment of the medical and functional factors associated with vehicle crashes by older adults. J Am Geriat Soc 1998;46:556–61.
22. Retchin SM, ed. Medical considerations in the older driver. In: Clinics in geriatric medicine, vol 9. Philadelphia: WB Saunders, 1993;92.
23. Gallo JJ, Rebok GW, Lesikar SE. The driving habits of adults aged 60 years and older. J Am Geriatr Soc 1999;47:335–41.

24
Common Problems of the Elderly

James P. Richardson and Aubrey L. Knight

Older patients are a challenging but satisfying part of most family physicians' practices. Optimal care of geriatric patients occurs when the precepts of continuity of care, the team approach to the management of illness, the importance of the family, and the biopsychosocial model are followed. Because of the prevalence of chronic disease in the elderly, cure may be elusive, but appropriate care always improves the quality of the older adult's life. Some common problems of the elderly are reviewed in this chapter. More complete discussions may be found in textbooks of geriatric medicine.[1,2]

Urinary Incontinence

Urinary incontinence (UI) is defined as an involuntary loss of urine sufficient to be a problem. UI is a common clinical entity, affecting 15% to 30% of community-dwelling older adults. The prevalence is twice as high in women as in men. Institutionalized, hospitalized, and homebound elders have higher prevalence rates. It translates into a huge cost burden in both economic and human terms. UI is more common in the elderly population, but there are other identifiable risk factors, including pregnancy, urinary tract infection, medications, dementia, immobility, diabetes mellitus, estrogen deficiency, pelvic muscle weakness, and smoking.

Types of Urinary Incontinence

Most cases of UI can be divided into one of five causes: (1) involuntary loss of urine with a strong urinary urgency (urge incontinence); (2) urethral sphincter pressure insufficient to hold urine (stress incontinence); (3) too high urethral resistance or insufficient bladder contractions (overflow incontinence); (4) chronic impairment of physical or cognitive function (functional incontinence); and (5) a combination of features of more than one type (mixed incontinence) (Table 24.1).

Urge incontinence, also referred to as detrusor instability, occurs when the involuntary bladder contractions overcome the normal resistance of the urethra. This type of incontinence is likely the most common cause of problematic incontinence, affecting up to 70% of persons with incontinence. The three basic mechanisms of action for this type of incontinence are loss of brain inhibition, as might occur with a stroke or in parkinsonism; involuntary detrusor contractions, as might occur with a urinary tract infection; and loss of the normal voiding reflexes. It is characterized by a strong desire to void followed by a loss of urine, often on the way to the bathroom.

Stress incontinence, also referred to as sphincter insufficiency, is most frequently encountered in postmenopausal women and is the result of reduced intraurethral pressure. The loss of urine occurs when there is an associated increase in intraabdominal pressure, such as during coughing, sneezing, or laughing.

Overflow incontinence is the result of the bladder not emptying properly. It can be secondary to an atonic or hypotonic detrusor or an obstruction of the bladder outlet from an enlarged prostate, urethral stricture, or stone. Detrusor hypoactivity can result from diabetes mellitus, lower spinal cord injury, or drugs. Overflow incontinence is characterized by a variety of symptoms that may be confused with symptoms more frequently associated with urge or stress incontinence. The urinary stream is often weak, and there is the sensation of incomplete emptying of the bladder.

Functional incontinence occurs in persons who, despite normal urinary tract functioning, are incontinent. It results from physical, psychiatric, or cognitive dysfunction or environmental limitations. This type of incontinence is frequently seen in the hospital setting when restraints or bed rails are utilized.

Mixed incontinence is common in older persons and usually is associated with features of stress and urge incontinence.

Table 24.1. **Treatment of Urinary Incontinence**

Type	Signs and symptoms	Treatment
Urge (detrusor instability)	Inability to get to toilet Large volume loss Normal postvoid residual (PVR)	Treat underlying condition Prompted voiding Bladder training Anticholinergic agents
Stress (sphincter insufficiency)	Urine loss with increased intraabdominal pressure Small volume loss Normal PVR	Pelvic muscle exercises Estrogen α-Adrenergic agents Surgical correction
Overflow (outlet obstruction or hypoactive bladder)	Constant urine loss Abdominal pain/distention High PVR	Treat underlying condition α-Adrenergic blockers Intermittent catheterization Surgical correction
Functional	Inability or unwillingness to be continent Large or small volume loss Normal PVR	Treat underlying condition Remove hindrances

Evaluation

The evaluation of UI has as its goal confirmation of the diagnosis, identification of any reversible causes, and identification of factors that require further diagnostic or therapeutic interventions. History focuses on the neurologic and urologic systems. Additionally, complete review of the medications, both prescribed and over the counter, is necessary. This phase should be accompanied by detailed exploration of the UI symptoms, including duration, frequency, timing, precipitants, and amount of urine lost. Associated symptoms such as nocturia, dysuria, hesitancy, urgency, hematuria, straining, and frequency should be noted. Finally, it is important to inquire about such conditions as diabetes mellitus, neurologic diseases, or urologic problems. At the conclusion of the initial visit, if the patient cannot characterize the incontinence, a bladder record should be kept for several days.[3]

The physical examination focuses on abdominal, neurologic, and genitourinary tract examinations. Specifically, during the abdominal examination the bladder is palpated. The physician assesses both cognitive function and nerve roots S2–3 during the neurologic examination. In men, the physician examines the genitalia to detect abnormalities of the foreskin, glans penis, and perineal skin and does a rectal examination, testing for perineal sensation, sphincter tone, fecal impaction, and prostatic enlargement. In women, a pelvic examination is done to assess perineal skin condition, pelvic prolapse, pelvic mass, and muscle tone. Finally, one can perform the cough stress test to observe urine loss with a full bladder.

Additional tests performed to evaluate all patients with UI include urinalysis and assessment of postvoid residual (PVR). A PVR of more than 100 mL is strongly suggestive of incomplete emptying of the bladder. The patient should be observed for leakage of urine while straining with a full bladder. Urine flow can be calculated simply by dividing the amount voided by the time it takes to void. A rate slower than 10 to 15 mL/sec is considered abnormal. Selected patients have a urine culture or blood testing that might include blood urea nitrogen (BUN), creatinine, glucose, calcium, electrolytes, and urine cytology. Further testing, including intravenous pyelography, ultrasonography, and computed tomography (CT), or referral to a specialist should be pursued when indicated by the history, physical examination, and simple testing.

Management

The first step in management is to identify and treat any reversible factors, remembering that there may be more than one cause. Seemingly small improvements may make a big difference to patients, and in many patients cure is possible. The type of UI dictates further treatment. Management can be behavioral, surgical, or pharmacologic. Many of the medications used to treat UI can, if used in the wrong circumstance, worsen the symptoms. Dosages listed below are average; both starting and maintenance doses must be individualized.

Nonpharmacologic Therapy

Clinical guidelines from the Agency for Health Care Policy and Research (AHCPR)[3] recommend behavioral therapy in the form of bladder training, prompted voiding, or pelvic muscle exercises for most forms of UI. Bladder training is most effective in the setting of urge incontinence but also may be helpful for other forms of UI. It involves behavioral education through the use of urge inhibition and scheduled voiding; it requires a cognitively intact individual. Prompted voiding, the nonpharmacologic treatment of choice in the cognitively impaired incontinent individual, involves scheduled voiding and requires prompting by the caregiver. Pelvic muscle exercises (Kegel's exercises), a regimen of planned, active exercises of the pelvic muscles to increase periurethral muscle strength, are particularly helpful in women with stress incontinence (see Chapter 104).

Other nonpharmacologic means of managing stress UI include biofeedback with or without electrical stimulation, collagen injection into the periurethral area, and vaginal pessaries. Nonpharmacologic treatments for overflow incontinence include intermittent catheterization, indwelling urethral or suprapubic catheters, external collection systems, and protective undergarments. Chronic indwelling catheters should not be viewed as a viable treatment option except when all else has failed or when there is accompanying local skin breakdown.

Pharmacologic Agents

Postmenopausal women with stress incontinence should use topical or oral estrogen in postmenopausal doses unless contraindicated. For those with an intact uterus, a progestin is added. α-Adrenergic agents such as pseudoephedrine (Sudafed, 15–30 mg PO tid) are also helpful in the setting of stress incontinence.

Anticholinergic agents such as oxybutinin (Ditropan, 2.5–5.0 mg PO tid or qid), tolterodine (Detrol, 1.0–2.0 mg PO bid), propantheline (Pro-Banthine, 7.5–30.0 mg PO tid), dicyclomide (Bentyl, 10–20 mg PO tid), and imipramine (Tofranil) or desipramine (Norpramin) (both at 25–100 mg PO a day) are often effective for urge incontinence. Anticholinergic medications should be used with caution, especially in the elderly, because of their side effects (confusion, constipation, and dizziness—see below).

In patients with overflow incontinence, bethanechol (Urecholine, 10–50 mg PO tid) can help facilitate bladder emptying. Men with prostatic hypertrophy and overflow incontinence can likely benefit from the α-adrenergic blockers prazosin (Minipress), terazosin (Hytrin), or doxazosin (Cardura) (all titrated up to 1–5 mg PO per day), or tamsulosin (Flomax), at either 0.4 or 0.8 mg PO per day (see Chapter 98).

Surgical Treatment

Surgical therapy is indicated in certain circumstances. Stress incontinence with urethrocele has an 80% to 95% 1-year success rate with suspension of the bladder neck.[3] Obstructive overflow incontinence with prostatic enlargement is often best treated with prostate surgery. Patients with urge incontinence and detrusor instability refractory to medical therapy often benefit from augmentation cystoplasty.

Falls

Falls are common, alarming, and worrisome to patients, their families, and their physicians. Most falls by the elderly do not result in serious consequences, but some cause hip fractures, other injuries, and rarely death. Unintentional injury is the sixth leading cause of death among the elderly, and most of these deaths are the result of falls.[4] Frequent falls may lead to consideration of a change in living arrangements or a severe limitation in socialization. Studies have clarified both the evaluation and management of patients who fall.[5–10]

The cause of a fall that results from loss of consciousness, a stroke or seizure, or an accidental or intentional blow to the body usually is easily discerned and managed. In most cases, however, the cause of a fall is not readily apparent. Falls may be classified as extrinsic (caused by slips or trips), intrinsic (caused by poor gait or balance, impaired sensation or proprioception, or cognitive impairment), nonbipedal (e.g., a fall out of bed), or nonclassifiable. Risk factors for falls from prospective studies include older age, white race, cognitive impairment, medication use, chronic diseases such as arthritis and Parkinson disease, foot problems, dizziness, and impaired muscle strength, gait, and balance.[5] Acute illnesses such as pneumonia, sepsis, and myocardial infarction also may present with a fall.

Most falls occur in the patient's home, and the home environment is usually a factor in these falls. Many falls occur on stairs, with injuries more likely to occur while descending rather than climbing stairs. Other hazards are electrical cords, uneven surfaces such as throw rugs or carpeting, or objects left on the floor. Poor lighting may contribute to these hazards.

Medication use is a potentially easily modifiable risk factor for falls. Long-acting benzodiazepines, barbiturates, antidepressants [including selective serotonin reuptake inhibitors (SSRIs)], and neuroleptics are associated with an increased risk of falls. Diuretics and other antihypertensive medicines also may increase the risk of falls by producing postural hypotension (see below and Chapter 75).

Numerous trials have been completed that examine methods of fall reduction and injuries due to falls. Low-level exercise appears to reduce the frequency of falls but may not reduce the number of falls resulting in medical treatment[6] or fractures.[7] The multisite FICSIT (Frailty and Injuries: Cooperative Studies of Intervention Techniques) trial has demonstrated a modest decline in frequency of falls for the groups that underwent a variety of exercise interventions.[8] One FICSIT site used a multidisciplinary program to identify and reduce risk factors for falls. The intervention group underwent environmental hazard assessment, review of medications, treatment of postural hypotension, and physical therapy to improve strength and treat any balance or gait impairments. The rate of falls during the following year was reduced by 31%. In another FICSIT study, this time of tai chi, a low-intensity exercise derived from Chinese martial arts, falls were cut by almost half.[9] Known risk factors can be used to target the elderly for interventions, but because some elderly without risk factors experience falls as well, probably all elderly should be questioned periodically about falls. At this time, effective strategies for the practicing physician include (1) a home assessment to eliminate environmental hazards, such as throw rugs, unlit stairs, or poorly arranged furniture (by the physician during a housecall or a home care agency); (2) review of all medications, with elimination of problematic drugs when possible; (3) office evaluation of gait and balance (by the physician with a screening instrument[10] or by a physical therapist); (4) detection and treatment of postural hypotension or other chronic diseases that may cause weakness with standing (e.g., congestive heart failure, chronic obstructive pulmonary disease); (5) detection and treatment of sensory losses, including poor vision and proprioception (e.g., vitamin B_{12} deficiency); and (6) physical, medical, or surgical therapy for arthritis or other musculoskeletal disorders, especially when the feet are involved (see Chapters 111 and 112).

Postural Hypotension

Postural or orthostatic hypotension is defined as a drop in systolic blood pressure of at least 20 mm Hg 1 minute after a patient changes from a supine to a standing position. Syncope or near-syncope may be presenting symptoms, but elderly persons with postural hypotension may complain of nonspecific symptoms such as weakness, fatigue, or difficulty concentrating.

The most common causes of postural hypotension in older people are deconditioning, usually due to a long hospitalization requiring prolonged bed rest and loss of compensating autonomic reflexes, and medications, especially diuretics, tricyclic antidepressants, neuroleptics, antihypertensives, and dopaminergic drugs [e.g., levodopa (Sinemet)]. Treatment is the same for these patients. Deconditioned patients should be encouraged to gradually increase their activity, under the supervision of a physical therapist if necessary. Salt intake can be liberalized for most patients without heart failure. Raising the head of the bed on blocks 4 to 6 inches high also helps improve postural hypotension by stimulating autonomic reflexes and fluid retention. Offending drugs should be eliminated whenever possible. Patients with hypertension can be switched from a diuretic to a calcium channel blocker, angiotensin-converting enzyme inhibitor, or a beta-blocker, as these classes of antihypertensives have a low incidence of postural hypotension when used alone. Until the postural hypotension improves, patients should be reminded to change positions slowly to give compensating mechanisms some time to work. Patients also can be instructed to tighten their calf muscles while standing, thereby decreasing the pooling of blood in the legs.

Patients with rarer causes of postural hypotension (e.g., Shy-Drager syndrome) may need to be evaluated and treated by a neurologist experienced in these conditions. In severe cases, salt tablets and fludrocortisone (Florinef) may be necessary.

Polypharmacy

Elderly patients consume a disproportionate number of drugs; consequently, they suffer a disproportionate number of adverse drug reactions. Inappropriate overprescribing, or polypharmacy, has been defined as taking too many drugs, using drugs for too long a time, or using drugs at too high a dose. The recent Institute of Medicine report has drawn attention to the number of adverse events that occur in hospitals, many of which are due to adverse drugs reactions.[11] Careful attention to appropriate prescribing can avoid many of these problems.

Risk Factors

Several risk factors for polypharmacy have been identified. Older adults with chronic medical problems often consult several physicians. Vague complaints may tempt physicians to prescribe, or patients or their families may pressure physicians to prescribe. Both hospitalization and nursing home placement usually result in more medications being prescribed. Medication is often added to a patient's regimen to treat the side effects of another drug. Physiologic changes of aging, including decreased body water and increased proportion of fat, can change the volume of distribution of some drugs and other pharmocokinetic characteristics and make the older person more prone to adverse drug effects.

Problematic Drug Classes

Neuroleptics, long-acting benzodiazepines, and tricyclic antidepressants have been associated with hip fractures resulting from falls[12] (see above and Chapters 31 and 32). Antihypertensive agents can also lead to falls. Benzodiazepines, especially those with long half-lives, are associated with cognitive impairment. Anticholinergic drugs, such as those given for urinary incontinence or irritable bowel syndrome, also may worsen cognition or may even lead to delirium (see below). Cardiovascular drugs and nonsteroidal antiinflammatory drugs (NSAIDs) have high rates of adverse effects. Drug–drug interactions are less frequent causes of adverse effects, but the potential for these problems increases as the number of drugs taken increases.

Principles of Prescribing

Simple changes in a patient's drug regimen can result in substantial improvements in a patient's condition. The following principles, modified from those first espoused by Vestal,[13] are helpful when prescribing for older adults.

1. Evaluate the need for drug therapy. Drug therapy is not always necessary or helpful.
2. Make a diagnosis before prescribing. The potential for adverse reactions is reduced when a specific drug is given for a specific, confirmed diagnosis.
3. A careful drug history is essential. Patients do not always immediately recall drugs prescribed by other physicians.
4. Know the pharmacology of the drugs you prescribe, especially with respect to the influence of the changes of aging. Patient reactions are more predictable when the prescriber uses few drugs in each drug class.
5. Start with small doses and titrate slowly to the desired response. Establish reasonable goals, stopping titration when the goals are achieved or side effects develop.
6. Keep the regimen simple to encourage compliance. Once- or twice-a-day dosing is ideal. Careful instruction should be given to both the patient and a relative or friend, if possible.
7. Review all medications regularly and discontinue those that are ineffective or no longer indicated. Ask the patient to throw all the drugs in their medicine cabinet into a paper bag and bring them to the office for review twice a year.
8. Remember that drugs cause illness. A new symptom may not be the result of a chronic or new medical condition. Always eliminate drug causes first.

Pain Management

Pain, acute or chronic, is one of the most common complaints of older individuals. Evaluating and treating pain syndromes in the elderly can be difficult. Many elderly patients are stoic. Cognitive impairment, especially in residents of nursing homes, may cause physicians to question the reliability of complaints of pain. Painful syndromes such as acute myocardial infarction and intraabdominal emergencies often present atypically or even silently in the elderly population. As a result, elderly patients are at risk for both over- and undertreatment of pain syndromes. Other consequences of improperly treated pain include depression, malnutrition, polypharmacy, cognitive dysfunction, and immobility. Acute pain is defined by its distinct onset and duration of less than 6 weeks; chronic pain lasts longer. Guidelines to the management of pain have been published.[14–16]

WHO Analgesic Ladder

Drug therapy is the cornerstone of treatment of acute and chronic pain due to cancer. The World Health Organization (WHO) analgesic ladder organizes drug therapy into three steps: (1) nonopioid drugs, (2) low-dose opioids, and (3) higher-dose opioids.[16] Treatment is begun with nonopioids, and opioid drugs are added as necessary. It is important to realize that when opioid–acetaminophen combinations are used [e.g., acetaminophen with codeine (Tylenol no. 3), oxycodone with acetaminophen (Percocet)], patients should receive no more than 4000 mg of acetaminophen per day. Adjuvant therapy, such as tricyclic antidepressants, caffeine, or anticonvulsants, may be added at any step.

Acute Pain

In the older patient with acute pain, physicians should determine the etiology of the pain while simultaneously making the patient comfortable. Rest, ice, compression, and elevation comprise the mainstay of treatment for acute injuries. In the elderly population, however, the period of rest should not exceed 48 to 72 hours, and early mobilization is encouraged. Physicians should start with the safest analgesics, such as acetaminophen, and add or substitute stronger analgesics as necessary. With respect to drug therapy, special considerations apply to the elderly. Older persons are more sensitive to the analgesic properties of opioids and to their side effects, such as sedation and respiratory depression. In addition, constipation and central nervous system (CNS) effects (e.g., delirium and depression) are more common in elderly patients treated with narcotics. NSAIDs should be used with care because of their gastrointestinal, renal, and hepatic effects, especially in the frail elderly. Some physicians believe that older patients have higher pain thresholds, but there is no experimental evidence to support this belief.[14]

Chronic Cancer Pain[15,16]

As in the case of patients with acute pain, the WHO analgesic ladder is followed for those with chronic pain, beginning with nonopioids such as acetaminophen and NSAIDs, adding opioids as necessary. NSAIDs may be particularly effective in cancer patients with bony metastases. Tricyclic antidepressants and the anticonvulsants carbamazepine (Tegretol) and valproic acid (Depakote) are usually helpful for neuropathic pain, although side effects (orthostatic hypotension, constipation, dry mouth) may limit the use of tricyclics.

Several principles help the physician provide optimal relief of cancer pain. Wide variation exists in the response of elderly patients to analgesics. Titration must be done carefully, with frequent follow-up to ensure that the drug is effective. Patients who have pain most of the day should receive their drugs regularly, not as needed. Side effects are treated aggressively. For example, sedation due to opioids can be particularly bothersome but can be treated by adding a stimulant such as caffeine or dextroamphetamine (Dexedrine). Long-acting morphine (MS Contin), oxycodone (OxyContin), and fentanyl patches (Duragesic) are helpful for patients with severe cancer pain, but care must be taken when calculating equianalgesic doses.[14] Other patients may require patient-controlled analgesia (PCA), continuous epidural morphine, or local radiation therapy. Lastly, nonpharmacologic adjunctive therapies including exercise, transcutaneous nerve stimulation, acupuncture, chiropractic manipulation, or prayer may aid in the treatment of pain (see Chapter 61).

Nutrition

There are few data regarding the nutritional requirements in the aged population. Similarly, the effect of nutrition on the aging process in humans is unclear. Poor nutritional status, however, does contribute to the morbidity of chronic illnesses and worsens the prognosis when an older person becomes ill. Protein–calorie malnutrition is the most common nutritional abnormality in the elderly. In one study, hospitalized elders had a 44% prevalence of protein–calorie malnutrition as defined by height/weight and serum albumin.[17] Conversely, up to 25% to 30% of older persons are overweight, defined as a body mass index (BMI) >28. Obesity increases the likelihood of developing coronary artery disease, diabetes mellitus, hypertension, and sleep apnea.

Many factors increase the risk for malnutrition in the elderly. A decrease in the acuity of taste and smell with aging lessens the enjoyment of eating. Poor dentition or poorly fitting dentures may lead to chewing difficulties. Swallowing disorders are more common in older persons, and gastrointestinal motility declines with age. Other risk factors for malnutrition include depression, poverty, social isolation, certain medications, and dementia. Such conditions as pressure ulcers, chronic infections, malabsorption, sepsis, malignancy, and alcoholism can increase the metabolic demands and result in malnutrition.

Nutritional Assessment

The key to the evaluation of malnutrition in the elderly is a high index of suspicion (see Chapter 8). Patients are asked about symptoms such as nausea, vomiting, anorexia, swallowing difficulties, and abdominal pain. They are also asked about any new medications, diagnoses, or social issues. A careful weight history is obtained and the weight loss expressed as a percentage of the patient's usual weight. Weight loss of more than 10% of the patient's usual weight usually represents severe malnutrition.

Physical signs of malnutrition may be difficult to recognize in the elderly. Anthropometric measures such as weight, height, BMI, and skinfold thickness can be helpful for the initial assessment. The total lymphocyte count, hemoglobin, serum albumin, and cholesterol levels are important screening tests. Transferrin and prealbumin levels are more sensitive measures of short-term undernutrition, but are more expensive. The farther the results are below normal values, the greater is the degree of malnutrition present. The Nutrition Screening Initiative (NSI) focused on the need for primary care physicians to consider the nutritional aspects of medical care.[18] The NSI developed a screening tool useful for evaluating risk for malnutrition.

Treatment

Treatment of malnutrition begins while efforts are made to identify the sources of nutrient losses and conditions that increase the metabolic needs. Additionally, nutritional support begins early in those individuals who are at increased risk for malnutrition. In the nonstressed elderly, approximately 22 to 25 kcal/kg body weight is required. This support increases to 30 kcal/kg in the severely stressed elderly.

Oral supplementation with food is optimal. The goal is to optimize the types of food and consistency of the diet to improve the nutritional status of the individual. The addition of liquid supplemental feedings can also improve nutritional status. When there is refusal or an inability to swallow, enteral tube feeding with a small-bore nasogastric tube or gastrostomy/jejunostomy tube is required. The decision on which of these methods to use depends on patient preference, suspected length of time the feedings will be necessary, and patient tolerance to each method. Feeding can occur in a continuous fashion or with intermittent bolus feeds. Each of these methods of feeding carries a risk of aspiration. Diarrhea is a frequent complication in the tube-fed patient.

When poor nutrition is related to depression, treatment of the depression is imperative. Buproprion (Wellbutrin) is an antidepressant that is less likely to adversely affect appetite compared to the SSRIs. Mirtazapine (Remeron) is another antidepressant that has the favorable side effect of improved appetite and weight gain in severely depressed older adults. Megestrol acetate (Megace) is a progesterone preparation that is widely studied as an appetite stimulant in cancer and acquired immunodeficiency syndrome (AIDS) patients and may be useful for older populations.

Total parenteral nutrition (TPN) is indicated in the elderly patient when there is an inability to use the gut to meet nutrient needs. Complications are more likely to occur in the elderly population, but it should not preclude the use of TPN in the appropriate clinical setting in an elderly patient. As with younger individuals, the use of TPN necessitates careful monitoring of the electrolyte and glucose levels as well as renal function.

Health Promotion and Disease Prevention

Elderly patients are living longer and longer. Average life expectancy for a 65-year-old man is at least 15 years more, and women live even longer. Thus it is important that physicians consider health promotion activities for their elderly patients,

just as they do for children and younger adults.[19,20] Among the interventions that are probably helpful in the elderly are (1) immunizations for influenza, pneumococcal disease, and tetanus-diphtheria; (2) counseling for injury prevention (car safety belts, smoke detectors, hot water heater temperature (<120°F) and for smoking cessation; (3) cervical cancer screening for women who have not been previously screened; (4) guaiac stool testing, sigmoidoscopy, or colonoscopy to detect colorectal cancer; and (5) hormone replacement therapy and calcium supplementation for women at risk of osteoporosis. Currently, no evidence exists to support the use of prostate-specific antigen screening in men older than 69 years or mammography screening for breast cancer in women older than 69 years, although physicians may choose to screen some older individuals for these conditions (see Chapter 7).[20] The United States Preventive Services Task Force now recommends cholesterol screening for healthy elderly who will live long enough to realize the benefits of therapy.

Evaluating and Managing Nursing Home Patients

Every physician who takes care of older patients has some interaction with a nursing home. For some family physicians, this interaction may be limited to referring their office patients for admission when they can no longer remain in the community. Increasingly, however, family physicians will be asked to assume larger roles in nursing homes. Only about 5% of the elderly reside in nursing homes, but the lifetime chance of an older person being admitted to a nursing home is about 40%.[21]

Evaluating Elderly Patients for Nursing Home Placement

Most nursing home residents are admitted to a long-term-care facility from the hospital. Not uncommonly physicians are asked to certify that an elderly person living in the community needs nursing home care. Usually these patients and their families present at a time of crisis. Patients may have been found wandering in the neighborhood, or they may have suffered recurrent falls and are thought to be unsafe in their home. Loss of function, usually as a result of cognitive impairment, is the common denominator.[22]

Careful assessment is important because a less restrictive environment may be a better solution and because patients and families often are not aware of these possibilities. Physicians should evaluate these patients thoroughly, focusing on their functional abilities, such as activities of daily living (ADLs, such as bathing, eating, dressing) and instrumental activities of daily living (IADLs, such as using the phone or buying groceries). A mental status examination is important, as patients may appear relatively intact on casual questioning but be severely impaired (see Chapter 25). Patients and family members should be questioned closely regarding the possibility of major depression, which has a high incidence among severely medically ill elderly and nursing home residents. Medicines are reviewed to see if any can be eliminated, especially those that may impair function (see above). The social history explores personal and financial resources that could support other care options, and advance directives are reviewed. For patients found to require the services of a nursing home, a complete assessment provides an opportunity to stabilize chronic illnesses or to complete any evaluations that might be necessary prior to admission.

Integrating Nursing Home Practice into the Office Practice

Family physicians can provide continuity of care for their elderly patients who are admitted to nursing homes by continuing to follow them after their admission. To avoid disrupting an office practice, however, it is wise for the physician to limit privileges to just a few facilities. Ideally, these nursing homes are near the physician's office, home, or hospital, so visits can be incorporated into the usual workday. Another benefit of limiting privileges to a few homes is that the physician becomes more familiar with the nursing staff and capabilities of those facilities.[22]

After building up a sizable census, it is practical to set aside a half-day every 1 or 2 weeks to make rounds. Routine nursing home rounds gives the physician a chance to consult with the resident's usual nurses and observe patients during therapy or other activities. Fewer phone calls from the nursing staff usually result as well. To minimize disruptions in the office, some physicians ask nursing homes to call at previously agreed-on times for routine problems.

Physicians with an interest in the organization and administration of nursing homes may wish to work as a medical director. Most medical directors approve policies and procedures, act as liaisons with the medical staff, supervise employee health issues, address quality improvement, and help keep the facility abreast of new regulations or medical treatments. New medical directors can find resources to help them through the American Medical Directors Association (10480 Little Patuxent Parkway, Suite 760, Columbia, MD 21044; phone 1-800-876-AMDA).

Pressure Sores

Pressure sores are defined as changes in the skin and underlying tissue that result from pressure over bony prominences. If not attended to, these forces cause ulceration. The best treatment for pressure sores is prevention, but even under the best conditions it is not always possible.

Epidemiology

The incidence of pressure sores is greatest among the elderly population, especially during long hospital or nursing home confinements.[23–25] Additionally, patients with spinal cord injuries or cerebrovascular disease are at risk for the development of pressure sores. Factors that may contribute to the likelihood of developing pressure sores include nutritional deficiencies, volume depletion, increased or decreased body weight, anemia, fecal incontinence, renal failure, diabetes, malignancy, sedation, major surgery, numerous metabolic disorders, cigarette smoking, and being bed- or chair-bound. Finally, the aging skin itself, because of reduced epidermal thickness and elasticity, increases the risk for pressure changes.

Etiology

There are four primary mechanisms in the development of pressure sores: pressure, shearing forces, friction, and moisture.[26] More than 90% of pressure sores occur over the bony prominences of the lower part of the body. The amount of time and pressure necessary to cause tissue damage depends on the number of risk factors present. The second etiologic factor, shearing forces, are caused by the sliding of adjacent surfaces. This sliding results in compression of capillary flow in the subcutaneous layer. An example of shearing forces is elevation of the head of the bed, which causes the body to slide down producing a shear in the sacral and coccygeal region. Friction is the force created when two surfaces move across each other, such as would occur when maneuvering a patient on the bed. The impact of friction damages the epidermis, which is already vulnerable in the elderly. This damage accelerates the onset of ulceration. Finally, moisture increases the risk of pressure ulceration. A high correlation exists between urinary or fecal incontinence and ulceration. Because of the increased risk of skin infection, the presence of a sacral pressure sore is an indication for a chronic indwelling urethral catheter in the incontinent patient.

Clinical Evaluation

The best method for evaluating a pressure sore is to classify the sore by its severity. There are several classification schemes for pressure sores. The National Pressure Ulcer Advisory Panel has proposed a staging system[27] that divides pressure sores into four grades, depending on the depth of tissue involvement.

Grade I pressure sore (Fig. 24.1A): Acute inflammatory response in all layers of the skin. The clinical presentation of a grade I pressure sore is a well-defined area of nonblanchable erythema of the intact skin.

Grade II pressure sore (Fig. 24.1B): Presents as a break in the epidermis and dermis, with surrounding erythema, induration, or both. It is caused by an extension of the inflammatory response leading to a fibroblastic response.

Grade III pressure sore (Fig. 24.1C): Inflammatory response characterized by an irregular full-thickness ulcer extending into the subcutaneous tissue but not through underlying fascia. There is often a draining, foul-smelling, necrotic base.

Grade IV pressure sore (Fig. 24.1D): Penetrates the deep fascia, eliminating the last barrier to extensive spread. Clinically, it resembles a grade III sore except that bone, joint, or muscle can be identified.

The complications of pressure sores are associated with significant morbidity and mortality. Most of the complications occur with grade III and IV sores and include cellulitis, os-

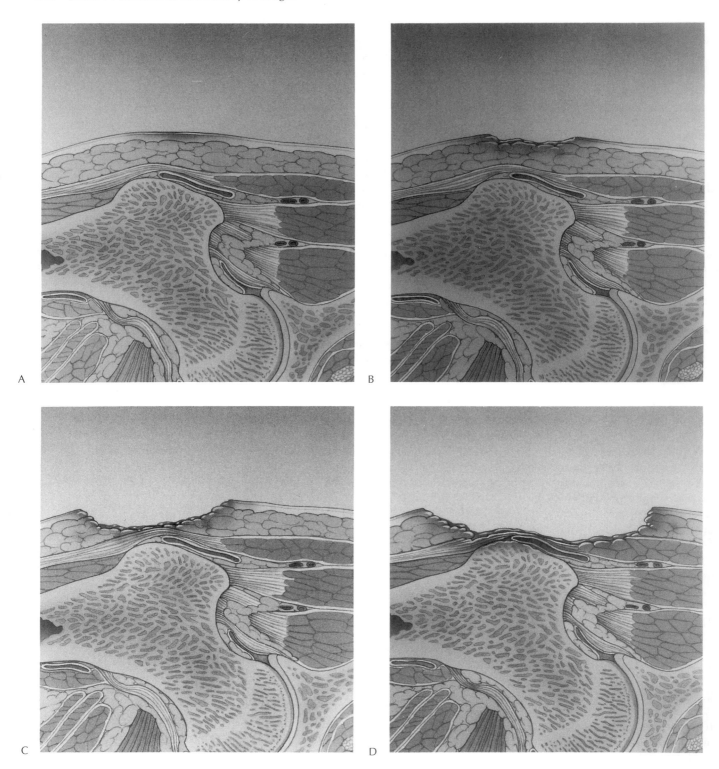

Fig. 24.1. National Pressure Ulcer Advisory Panel staging system. (A) Grade I pressure sore, characterized by inflammatory reaction of the epidermis and dermis. It presents clinically as nonblanchable erythema over an area of pressure. (B) Grade II pressure sore, characterized by epidermal and dermal skin breakdown with surrounding erythema. (C) Grade III pressure sore, characterized by an ulcer extending into the subcutaneous tissue, frequently with necrosis. (D) Grade IV pressure sore, characterized by extension of the ulcer beyond the fascial layer and thus involving muscle, bone, or other structures. (From National Pressure Ulcer Advisory Panel,[27] with permission.)

teomyelitis, septic joints, pyarthrosis, and tetanus. Tetanus may complicate pressure sores, and for this reason immunoprophylaxis against tetanus is recommended in patients with pressure sores.[28]

Prevention

Because of the great morbidity and mortality associated with pressure sores and the financial burden incurred by treating this problem, their prevention is the primary goal of physicians and health care facilities taking care of patients at risk. Identifying persons at risk is the first step in employing intensive preventive measures.

Persons at risk should undergo frequent assessment and be placed in an environment that enhances soft tissue viability, which can be achieved through the use of proper positioning techniques and support surfaces. At the time of positioning, the patient's skin is examined for areas of redness that indicate early pressure changes. When repositioning, the patient is lifted, not dragged, from a bed or wheelchair to avoid friction and subsequent damage to the epidermis. Elevating the head of the bed to more than 30 degrees is avoided to minimize the shearing forces.

Special pads, beds, and mechanical devices are available and prevent pressure sores by altering the pressure over bony prominences. Devices such as gel pads, foam cushions, wheelchair cushions, and sheepskin pads are practical for preventing pressure sores at specific anatomic sites. No single device has yet been developed that is effective in preventing all pressure sores. Static flotation mattresses, low air loss mattresses, alternating air pressure mattresses, and air-fluidized beds help to prevent and treat pressure sores. These beds tend to relieve pressure by using air or buoyancy to keep the patient's weight evenly distributed. Such devices, however, cannot be relied on as a substitute for basic nursing care.

Preventive care of pressure sores also involves improvement of medical conditions that predispose the individual to the development of pressure changes. In particular, nutritional deficiencies, incontinence, and immobility should be minimized. Nutritional status is assessed on admission to the hospital or nursing home: Once a pressure sore has developed, nutritional status usually is already severely compromised and is difficult to correct.

Management

The first step in the management of pressure sores is assessing the extent of the sore and patients' overall status, including their nutritional state. Regardless of the grade of the sore, adherence to the principles of prevention outlined above remain important.

Wound Cleansing and Debridement

The primary goal of therapy for pressure sores is to create an environment that promotes healthy granulation tissue. Wounds are cleansed as atraumatically as possible with normal saline-soaked gauze, wound irrigation, and whirlpool baths. Most antiseptics, such as hydrogen peroxide and povidone-iodine, are cytotoxic and should be avoided.

Necrotic tissue prevents healing and creates favorable conditions for bacterial contamination. The ideal method for debriding pressure sores is sharp dissection of the necrotic tissue. Enzymatic debridement using such agents as fibrinolysin, collagenase, and dextranomer should be used only during intervals between surgical debridement to help dissolve thin necrotic layers that are less accessible to excision.[29] The inability of these agents to penetrate eschar or to remove large amounts of tissue limits their usefulness. There is no proof that topical antibiotics are superior to careful cleansing and wet-to-dry dressings. In addition, topical antibiotics may sensitize the tissue, promote the appearance of resistant organisms, and have systemic toxicity.[26]

Dressings

Once the wound is clean with granulation tissue visible, the use of dressings that promote healing is advisable. The cardinal rule is to keep the ulcer moist and the surrounding skin dry.[30] Additional factors when selecting dressings include exudate control and caregiver time requirements. Dressing options include saline-soaked gauze and occlusive dressings. The appeal of the occlusive dressings is that they can usually remain on the pressure sore for several days, whereas gauze dressings should be changed several times daily. This convenience is particularly useful for outpatient management of pressure sores. These dressings should be avoided in the presence of clinical infection.

Managing Complications

The two most frequently encountered complications are nonhealing and infection. For clean wounds that fail to heal, reassessment of the patient's overall status and a 2-week trial of a broad-spectrum topical antibiotic are recommended.[30] In patients who are operative candidates, surgical repair of the nonhealing wound may be considered. When these wounds are complicated by bacteremia, soft tissue infection, or osteomyelitis, appropriate systemic antibiotics are employed.

Delirium

Delirium is a syndrome of acutely altered mental status. Delirium is frequent in older persons, especially those with dementia, typically occurring in ill inpatients and nursing home residents. Delirium may the only presenting symptom of many acute illnesses as well, including sepsis syndrome and other infections, myocardial infarction, surgical emergencies, adverse drug reactions, volume depletion, and electrolyte disturbances. Failure to recognize and appropriately treat delirium contributes to worse outcomes in these patients, regardless of etiology.

Delirium is diagnosed in the setting of a fluctuating level of consciousness, accompanied by inattentiveness and poor recent memory. Unlike dementia patients (if not delirious), these patients present acutely and do not have a normal level of consciousness. Typically, speech is incoherent or disorganized. The level of consciousness may vary from hyperalert to comatose.

Evaluation and Management

As noted above, possible etiologies are numerous, and usually there is more than one cause. Treatment requires continual assessment and reassessment of causes, beginning first with a careful examination of the nervous system. Laboratory testing should include a complete blood count (CBC), chemistry panel, and liver function tests. Additional tests that may be helpful include thyroid function tests, a B_{12} level, and drug levels. Correcting electrolyte abnormalities, treating infections, and eliminating sedatives (especially benzodiazepines) and anticholinergic drugs (e.g., tricyclic antidepressants, antihistamines, drugs for urge incontinence, etc.) are the most productive strategies. Helpful environmental alterations include clear communication to delirious patients (with repeated reorientation), having a calming family member present, ensuring adequate lighting, reducing noise, and allowing uninterrupted sleep.[31] Neuroleptics are the drugs of choice, whether patients are agitated or lethargic. Low-dose oral haloperidol (Haldol) is usually sufficient in older adults. Patients may be given 0.5 to 1 mg orally or parenterally. This dose may be repeated until the patient is sedated as long as hypotension does not occur (blood pressure should be checked at least every half-hour). Benzodiazepines may worsen behavior because of disinhibition effects, but are useful for delirium that results from alcohol withdrawal or seizures.

References

1. Hazzard WR, Bierman EL, Blass JP, Ettinger WH, Halter JB, Ouslander JG, eds. Principles of geriatric medicine, 4th ed. New York: McGraw-Hill, 1999.
2. Adelman AM, Daly MP, eds. 20 common problems in geriatrics. New York: McGraw-Hill, 2001.
3. US Department of Health and Human Services. Clinical practice guideline: urinary incontinence in adults. AHCPR publ. no. 92-0038. Rockville, MD: DHHS, 1992;38–65.
4. Koogler CE, Wolf SL. Falls. In: Hazzard WR, Bierman EL, Blass JP, Ettinger WH, Halter JB, Ouslander JG, eds. Principles of geriatric medicine, 4th ed. New York: McGraw-Hill, 1999; 1535–46.
5. King MB, Tinetti ME. Falls in community-dwelling older persons. J Am Geriatr Soc 1995;43:1146–54.
6. Hornbrook MC, Stevens VJ, Wingfield DJ, et al. Preventing falls among community-dwelling older persons: results from a randomized trial. Gerontologist 1994;34:16–23.
7. Vetter NJ, Lewis PA, Ford D. Can health visitors prevent fractures in elderly people? BMJ 1992;304:888–90.
8. Province MA, Hadley EC, Hornbrook MC, et al. The effects of exercise on falls in elderly patients: a pre-planned meta-analysis of the FICSIT trials. JAMA 1995;273:1341–7.
9. Wolf SL, Barnhart HX, Kutner NG, et al. Reducing frailty and falls in older persons: an investigation of Tai Chi and computerized balance training. J Am Geriatr Soc 1996;44:489–97.
10. Shumway-Cook A, Brauer S, Woollacott M. Predicting the probability of falls in community-dwelling older adults using the Timed Up and Go Test. Phys Ther 2000;80:896–903.
11. Kohn LT, Corrigan JM, Donaldson MS, eds. To err is human: building a safer health system. Washington, DC: National Academy Press, 2000.
12. Ray WA, Griffin MR, Schaffner W, et al. Psychotropic drug use and the risk of hip fracture. N Engl J Med 1987;316:363–9.
13. Vestal R. Clinical Pharmacology. In: Hazzard WR, Andres R, Bierman EL, Blass JP, eds. Principles of geriatric medicine and gerontology, 2nd ed. New York: McGraw-Hill, 1990;201–11.
14. Acute Pain Management Guideline Panel. Acute pain management: operative or medical procedures and trauma; clinical practice guideline. AHCPR publ. no. 92-0032. Rockville, MD: Agency for Health Care Policy and Research, Public Health Service, US Department of Health and Human Services, 1992.
15. American Geriatrics Society Panel on Chronic Pain in Older Persons. The management of chronic pain in older persons. J Am Geriatr Soc 1998;46:635–51.
16. World Health Organization. Cancer pain and palliative care: report of a WHO expert committee. World Health Organization Technical Report Series 804. Geneva: WHO, 1990;1–75.
17. Wilson WG, Vaswani S, Liu D, et al. Prevalence and causes of undernutrition in medical outpatients. Am J Med 1998;104:56–63.
18. White JV, Dwyer JT, Posner BM, Ham RJ, Lipschitz DA, Wellman NS. Nutrition Screening Initiative; development and implementation of the public awareness checklist and screening tools. J Am Diet Assoc 1992;92:163–7.
19. Richardson JP. Health maintenance for the elderly. In: Taylor RB, ed. The manual of family practice, 2nd ed. Philadelphia: Lippincott, Williams & Wilkins, 2002;28–32.
20. United States Preventive Services Task Force. Guide to clinical preventive services, 2nd ed. Baltimore: Williams & Wilkins, 1996.
21. Kemper P, Murtaugh CM. Lifetime use of nursing home care. N Engl J Med 1991;324:595–600.
22. Richardson JP. Outpatient evaluation for nursing home admission. In: Yoshikawa TT, Cobbs EL, Brummel-Smith K, eds. Ambulatory geriatric care, 2nd ed. St. Louis: Mosby-Year Book, 1998;113–7.
23. Brandeis GH, Morris JN, Nash DJ, Lipsitz LA. The epidemiology and natural history of pressure ulcers in elderly nursing home residents. JAMA 1990;264:2905–9.
24. Reuler JB, Cooney TG. The pressure sore: pathophysiology and principles of management. Ann Intern Med 1981;94:661–6.
25. Guralnik JM, Harris TB, White LR, Cornoni-Huntley JC. Occurrence and predictors of pressure sores in the National Health and Nutrition Examination Survey follow-up. J Am Geriatr Soc 1989;36:807–12.
26. Knight AL. Medical management of pressure sores. J Fam Pract 1988;27:95–100.
27. National Pressure Ulcer Advisory Panel. Pressure ulcers prevalence, cost and risk assessment: consensus development conference statement. Decubitus 1989;2(2):24–8.
28. Richardson JP, Knight AL. The prevention of tetanus in the elderly. Arch Intern Med 1991;151:1712–17.
29. Seiler WO, Stahelin HB. Decubitus ulcers: treatment through five therapeutic principles. Geriatrics 1985;40:30–44.
30. Pressure Ulcer Guideline Panel. Pressure ulcer treatment. Am Fam Physician 1995;51:1207–22.
31. Meagher DJ. Delirium: optimising management. BMJ 2001;322:144–9.

25
Alzheimer's Disease and Related Dementias

Gregg Warshaw

Cognitive impairment is common in the older adult and often represents an underlying, undetected clinical condition. When accompanied by other medical or social problems, cognitive impairment can precipitate stressful problems for and require decisions from families, caregivers, and clinicians. A thorough history is critical for successful diagnosis and treatment. Initially, the history should include a careful review, with both patient and family, of the chronologic course of the changes in mental status. The pace of the progression and the duration of the symptoms are particularly important. A patient with a history of deteriorating cognitive function over months or years presents a different diagnostic and treatment problem from one who presents with a mental status change over days or weeks (delirium). This chapter reviews the assessment of dementia and the current understanding of the etiology of Alzheimer's disease (AD) and proposes management strategies for patients with dementias and their families.

Dementia

Reversible Dementia

The first task for the clinician is to determine if the long-term deterioration represents a reversible or arrestable process of cognitive impairment. Caution is required in diagnosing the impairment as an irreversible dementia. There is a long list of potentially reversible conditions that can present as chronic deterioration of cognitive function, the most common of which are the memory impairments associated with medications or depressive illness. The other reversible causes of chronic confusion are rare in patients over age 70, probably accounting for fewer than 5% of all cases. Table 25.1 lists potential reversible or arrestable etiologies of dementia.

A thorough patient history and physical examination are invaluable for determining the possible cause of the chronic confusion. A home assessment is frequently beneficial for evaluating an individual because the patient usually demonstrates optimal mental functioning in a familiar environment. The most important historical information is the duration of symptoms. Family members or neighbors can help document the length and progressive course of the illness. It is important to determine if there has been a dramatic clinical course; a steady, slow, subtle change; or a wide fluctuation of changes of mental status. Sudden onset is not consistent with AD.

It is useful to have an objective test for mental status, such as a simple, easily repeatable mental status questionnaire to document the progression.[1] Figure 25.1 is an example of a commonly used short screening examination for cognitive impairment. This questionnaire is not diagnostic but represents an objective, brief assessment tool. Well-educated, intelligent adults can score near normal on a screening test and still have a progressive dementia. A measure of functional capacity should also be obtained from family or friends. When office cognitive testing and family observations are discordant, more formal neuropsychological testing may be required.

Focal neurologic findings, seizures, and gait disturbance are features that are rare early in the course of AD. Although the clinical course of AD may consist of good and bad days, the general trend should be slow deterioration. Periods of steady improvement are not consistent with the diagnosis. A common variant presentation of AD includes impairment of language, perception, and other cognitive functions prior to clearly documented loss of short-term memory. Detailed criteria for the clinical diagnosis of AD are established.[2]

Laboratory Evaluation

Depending on the circumstances and clinical information, some of the procedures listed in Table 25.2 should be performed. These tests are selected to exclude the possible causes of confusion listed in Table 25.1.[3] Computed tomography (CT) of the brain is appropriate in the presence of a history

Table 25.1. **Potentially Reversible or Arrestable Etiologies of Dementia**

Metabolic, toxic, or systemic factors
  Pernicious anemia
  Dehydration
  Hypercalcemia
  Hyperlipidemia
  Hypoxemia/anoxia/pulmonary embolism
  Hyperthyroid, hypothyroid
  Cushing syndrome
Intracranial infections
  Cryptococcal meningitis
  Neurosyphilis/syphilitic gumma
  Whipple's disease
  AIDS/toxoplasmosis
Other intracranial disease
  Subdural hematoma
  Neoplasm
  Normal-pressure hydrocephalus
Depression ("pseudodementia")
Seizures (see Chapter 64)
Drug-induced
  Alcohol, psychotropic agents
  Neuroleptics, antidepressants
  Anxiolytics/sedatives/hypnotics
  Amantadine, levodopa
  Bromocriptine, antihistamines
  Hypoglycemic agents, anticonvulsants
  Analgesics, cimetidine
  Carbon monoxide, antimicrobials
  Organophosphates
  Heavy metals (lead, mercury, thallium, manganese)
Immunologic factors
  Granulomatous angiitis
  Limbic encephalitis
Miscellaneous factors
  Sensory deprivation/intensive care unit psychosis
  Fecal impaction

estimated 5% of adults 65 years of age and older suffer severe, chronic, irreversible cognitive impairment. Another 5% exhibit moderate degrees of impairment. Cognitive impairment is age-correlated as well; the estimated prevalence in 80-year-olds increases to 22%.[6] The incidence of AD is approximately 14 times higher among persons older than 85 years than among those 65 to 69 years of age.[7] Although half of persons in long-term care facilities display cognitive impairment, most impaired adults are at home and are unknown to or uninvestigated by clinicians.

Impaired memory, especially recent memory, typically indicates initially the clinical syndrome of chronic dementia. Other changes are impaired judgment, loss of insight, flat-

suggestive of a mass, focal neurologic signs, or dementia of brief duration. Magnetic resonance imaging (MRI) is more sensitive than CT for detecting small infarcts, mass lesions, and subcortical structures; however, a noncontrast CT is adequate for the assessment of most dementia patients. Although some clinicians recommend that an MRI be obtained if vascular dementia is suspected, white-matter changes revealed by T2-weighted MRI images generally are not related to dementia and can be overinterpreted.[4] Attempts to identify a reliable diagnostic test for AD continue. Positron emission tomography (PET), single photon emission computed tomography (SPECT), and MRI spectroscopy scans have identified areas in brains of AD patients that show reduced metabolic activity.[5] The availability and costs of these procedures, however, limit their use in routine diagnostic work.

Progressive Dementia

In most chronic cognitively impaired older adults, the observed deterioration is not secondary to a reversible disease or to drug reactions. The underlying cause of chronic, progressive deterioration of cognitive functioning is an irreversible change in the structure and function of the brain. An

	Maximum score
Orientation	
What is the (year) (season) (date) (day) (month)?	5
Where are we (state) (county) (town) (hospital) (floor)?	5
Registration	
Name three objects (1 second to say each). Then ask the patient all three after you have said them. Give one point for each correct answer.	3
Attention and calculation	
Begin with 100 and count backward by 7 (stop after five answers). Alternatively, spell "world" backward.	5
Recall	
Ask for three objects repeated above.	3
Language	
Show a pencil and a watch, and ask the patient to name them.	2
Repeat the following: "No ifs, ands, or buts."	1
A three-stage command: "Take a paper in your right hand, fold it in half, and put it on the floor."	3
Read and obey the following: (show written item). *Close your eyes..*	1
Write a sentence.	1
Copy a design (intersecting polygons).	1
Total score possible	30

Fig. 25.1. Folstein Mini-Mental State Examination. Of a possible score of 30, patients with moderate to advanced dementia generally score below 20; those with early dementia, depression, or both have a score in the range 20 to 25. Normal older adults score in the range 28 to 30. (From Folstein et al,[1] with permission.)

Table 25.2. **Laboratory Assessment of Chronic Confusion**

1. Complete blood count
2. Biochemical screening
3. Serum vitamin B_{12} level
4. Serum electrolytes
5. Thyroid function tests
6. Urinalysis
7. Drug levels
8. Arterial blood gases
9. Serologic tests for syphilis
10. Human immunodeficiency (HIV) antibodies
11. Chest films
12. Skull films
13. Electroencephalogram (EEG)
14. Lumbar puncture (spinal fluid analysis)
15. Head CT or MRI scan

Depending on the circumstances and clinical information, some or all of the procedures should be performed. (Items 1–5 are obtained in most instances.)

tening of affect, and eventually change in personality. As the illness progresses these changes are commonly followed by trouble swallowing, walking, controlling bladder and bowel functions, and maintaining mobility. AD, the most frequent cause of dementia in this age group, probably accounts for at least 50% of the progressive dementias in the elderly. Estimates suggest that it is the fourth or fifth leading cause of death in the United States. The next most common causes of dementia are vascular disease, alcohol-related dementia, and dementia with Lewy bodies (DLBs). Recent research has determined that DLBs may be the underlying pathology in up to 20% of cases of presumed AD. Whether DLB is a variant of Alzheimer's Disease or a separate process remains unclear. The recommended diagnostic criteria for DLB include the observation of at least one of the following: fluctuation in cognitive skills, recurring, detailed visual hallucinations, or Parkinson's symptoms (especially muscle rigidity and loss of spontaneous movement).[8] Other causes of permanent damage to the brain in this age group are relatively rare. Progressive dementias occur in association with Parkinson's disease in about 15% of cases. Other rare causes of chronic dementias include acquired immunodeficiency syndrome (AIDS: apathy and depression are early symptoms), and Pick's disease (frontal lobe and speech disturbances predominate) (see Chapters 41 and 66).

Alzheimer's Disease

Causes

Although pathologists have recognized changes in brain cell anatomy characteristic of AD, the cause of this disease remains unknown. The pathologic changes in the brains of AD patients are distinctive of the illness, including neurofibrillary tangles and neuritic plaques; analysis of these lesions is central to current research. The recent development of a model in mice for the amyloid pathology of AD has led to considerable new research.[9] Amyloid is the chief component of the neuritic plaques. An approach to immunizing mice to prevent

the development of the amyloid brain pathology has been promising, however, the importance of the amyloid plaques to the development of the clinical symptoms of AD is not yet clear. Many other hypotheses about the cause of the disease have been tested. The fact that there is an accumulation of aluminum—30 times the normal amount—in the brains of AD patients examined at autopsy initially suggested aluminum toxicity as a cause, but a causal relation has not been established; accumulation of aluminum may be a secondary phenomenon. Some rare chronic brain diseases have been shown to be viral in etiology, but no virus has been isolated from AD patients. Disturbance in the immune system has been suggested, but as with the aluminum hypothesis further work is needed to identify the relation between such abnormalities and the disease. Finally, there is some evidence that increased educational and occupational attainment may reduce the risk of developing AD.[10]

Alzheimer's disease has a genetic component; the risk for an individual in a family with AD increases by a factor of three or four.[11,12] The importance of the genetic risk in AD is complicated by the fact that the diagnosis is not always certain, and that many individuals within families may not live to an old enough age to manifest symptoms. The two basic types of AD are familial (FAD) and sporadic AD. FAD accounts for fewer than 10% of all AD cases. It is associated with gene mutations on chromosomes 1, 14, and 21. Most FAD cases are characterized by earlier onset (many before age 60). The apolipoprotein E (apoE) gene on chromosome 19 has been linked to sporadic, late-onset AD.[13] ApoE is a substance that helps transport cholesterol in the blood. The *apoE* gene has three alleles: *apoE2*, *apoE3*, and *apoE4*. Having one copy (30% of U.S. population) or two copies (2% of U.S. population) of the *apoE4* allele may increase a person's risk to develop AD. At age 70 about 50% of those with *apoE4/4* have developed AD, compared to 28% with *apoE3/4* and 6% with *apoE2/4* and *apoA3/3*. *apoE2* in particular appears to be protective for AD. Individuals with mild cognitive impairment that progresses to AD are more likely to carry the *apoE4* allele.[14] Using PET scans, it has been demonstrated that cognitively normal middle-aged adults who are homozygous for the *apoE4* allele have reduced glucose metabolism in the same regions of the brain as do patients with probable AD.[15] In summary, the *apoE4* allele is neither necessary nor sufficient for the development of AD, and some with it live into the ninth decade with no signs of dementia. At this time it is not recommended that *apoE* status be used in routine clinical practice for diagnosis or for predictive testing.[16]

Drug Treatment

The role of neurotransmitters is an active area of current AD research. The focus is on acetylcholine metabolism. There is consistent evidence that enzymes related to the cholinergic system are reduced in brains of patients with AD. Current research of the cholinergic hypothesis includes testing the correlation between cholinergic dysfunction and cognitive impairment and study of whether the enhancement of cholinergic function decreases the severity of the cognitive deficit. Numerous acetylcholine precursors, cholinesterase inhibitors, and cholinergic agonists are being tested in human clinical trials.[17]

Specific treatment of the memory loss associated with AD is currently limited to acetylcholine agonists: tacrine (Cognex), donepezil (Aricept), and rivastigmine (Exelon). All three medications have a similar magnitude of cognitive effect. One third of patients who reach a therapeutic level obtain some benefit from acetylcholine agonists. Expected treatment responses may include improvement in short-term memory or functional capabilities, or a slowing of clinical decline. Dramatic responses are rare. These medications have been most effective in patients with mild to moderate symptoms.

With tacrine initial dosing is 10 mg po qid. At 6-week intervals, if the medication is tolerated, the dose can be increased by 40 mg/day, not to exceed a total dose of 160 mg/day. The most serious adverse event associated with tacrine is hepatotoxicity associated with elevations in alanine aminotransferase (ALT). ALT levels should be measured every other week for at least the first 16 weeks of tacrine therapy. Elevations above three times normal require dose reduction or withdrawal of the medication. Other side effects include nausea, diarrhea, dizziness, headache, myalgia, and ataxia. Theophylline doses may need to be reduced if coadministered with tacrine.

Donepezil is not associated with hepatotoxicity and can be taken once a day. Initial dosing is 5 mg/day, and the dose can be raised to 10 mg/day if side effects are tolerated (including nausea, diarrhea, dizziness, headache, myalgia, and ataxia).

Rivastigmine is also not associated with hepatotoxicity. It is prescribed on a twice-a-day schedule. The occurrence of nausea, vomiting, or loss of appetite may be more frequent than with donepezil, and a low starting dose of the medication is recommended (1.5 mg bid for 2 weeks, with subsequent increases of 3 mg/day, at 2- to 4-week intervals, as tolerated, up to a maximum dose of 6 mg bid).

Ginkgo biloba is a widely utilized, natural compound that may have some benefit in the treatment of AD. It has been studied extensively, with positive outcomes, but many of the clinical trials have been criticized for weak study design. A recent well-designed, 24-week trial with 214 subjects demonstrated no benefit. The recommended dose of ginkgo is 120 to 160 mg/day of the pure extract. Ginkgo can inhibit platelet aggregation, and increases in bleeding time can be seen, especially in association with other anticoagulants or antiplatelet therapy.

Interventions designed to slow or stop the neurodegenerative basis for AD have been tested with the objective of delaying the onset or slowing the progression of the disease. Trials of estrogen therapy in middle age and older women have been disappointing. High doses (1,000 IU bid) of vitamin E may have some impact on the rate of progression of AD. It is not yet known if lower doses (400 IU bid) would have a similar effect. Also, regular use of nonsteroidal antiinflammatory medications has been associated with a lower incidence of AD.

Management

Common management problems physicians face when caring for AD patients include demanding behavior, wandering at night, accusatory challenges, incontinence, delirium, and depression. AD is similar to other chronic illnesses (e.g., arthritis, heart disease) in that good medical management can slow functional decline and limit unnecessary complications. To be effective, the family physician should be available, interested, and willing to talk with the family. Patients should see their doctor every 4 to 6 months. Even if all is going well, it is important for the doctor to be aware of the patient's current mental and physical condition. The mental status of AD can be further impaired by many other disorders, such as heart disease or infections. Recognition and aggressive treatment of a coexisting illness can result in a noticeable improvement in the patient's mental condition.

Many older people are taking several prescription medications, and even if the medications are being prescribed appropriately and being taken correctly, any medication poses a threat to the AD patient. A regular and careful review of the patient's medications is one of the most important aspects of good management. Sedative drugs, antihypertensive medications, and cardiac medications are just a few examples of drugs that can further impair the brain and worsen the functional mental status of patients.

It is important that AD patients have optimal hearing and vision. Decreased sensory input secondary to poor vision or deafness may aggravate existing confusion and result in paranoia, delusions, or hallucinations. Careful hearing and vision evaluations should be part of the routine medical care of these patients.

Adjusting the Environment

Simple care in adjusting a demented person's environment can avoid unnecessary accidents and limit confusion. In general, the patient should be allowed as much freedom as possible, but structure in the daily schedule and familiar positioning of objects in the environment is important. Meal routines, medication routines, and exercise should all occur at regular times. Bedtime should be set at the same time each evening. Clutter and furniture that has sharp corners or is unstable are to be avoided. The environment must be checked for any possible poisons or potential hazards for the patient. AD patients have difficulty evaluating the environment and in new situations are prone to accidental falls. Hospitals and nursing homes report that falls are most common during the first several weeks of a patient's stay. It is also possible that medications or coexisting illnesses (e.g., Parkinson's disease or an unsuspected anemia) can be the cause of falling; therefore, any AD patient who suddenly develops instability or falling should undergo thorough medical evaluation.

Depression and Dementia

Depression is a common accompaniment of dementia, particularly during the early stages.[18] It may be necessary to initiate treatment with antidepressant medications in patients with mild or moderate dementia who appear depressed (see Chapter 32). Sometimes the patient's mood elevates and cognition improves. Nortriptyline (Pamelor) 10 to 25 mg/day, and serotonin reuptake inhibitors [e.g., sertraline (Zoloft) 25 to 50 mg/day; citalopram (Celexa) 10 to 20 mg/day] are good choices. Depressed patients are also more likely to use alcohol or tranquilizers, which has a catastrophic effect on their mental functioning. Rather than being depressed, some demented patients, particularly late in the disease, are simply apathetic and listless. It can be helpful to encourage activities by trying to reinvolve the patient at a comfortable level in some activities. Occasionally, the patient becomes upset or agitated even with a small amount of stimulation.

Wandering

Wandering is a frequent, serious problem that warrants careful consideration. Patients should be evaluated for pain or other discomfort. When confused patients are taken to new places, they may feel lost or believe they are not where they are supposed to be. Patients with AD who are hospitalized require frequent general reassurance about where they are, which sometimes increases their comfort and ease of management. When wandering appears to be aimless, it is sometimes helpful to plan daily exercise for the patient to see if it can reduce wandering during other parts of the day. Physical restraints are a last resort and are used only in consultation with the patient's family. Reclining geriatric chairs are preferred rather than tying arms and bodies into chairs. Many people with AD are restless at night, and this "sundowning" can be challenging. A sedating tranquilizer is just as likely to aggravate the problem as to help.

If medication is prescribed for wandering or nighttime agitation, it should be used only after all nondrug interventions have been tried and a medical evaluation is completed to eliminate potential coexisting medical problems. If paranoid or violent behavior is a predominant symptom, an antipsychotic medication can be used [e.g., haloperidol 0.5 to 3.0 mg/day, or risperidone (Risperdal) 0.25 to 2 mg/day]. For agitation without psychotic features, an antianxiety agent can be prescribed (e.g., lorazepam 0.5 to 4.0 mg/day or buspirone 10 to 30 mg/day). Some anticonvulsants have also been helpful for the management of aggression associated with AD [carbamazepine (Tegretol) 50 to 100 mg bid, valproate (Depakote) 125 to 250 mg bid]. All psychotropic medications prescribed to AD patients have the potential to affect cognitive function adversely or worsen agitation. Careful evaluation of the target symptom response and side effects is essential.

Catastrophic Reactions

Anger, overreacting, or catastrophic reactions are common in dementing patients. These reactions frequently occur at the time of family gatherings or in health care facilities. People with dementia often become excessively upset and may experience rapidly changing moods. Strange situations, confusion, groups, or noise may precipitate reactions wherein the patients may weep, blush, or become agitated, angry, or stubborn. They may strike out at those trying to help them. It is important to accept these behaviors as symptoms of dementing illness. Efforts to orient the patient to the environment and simplify tasks help avoid these reactions.

Incontinence

Urinary incontinence is a common problem in the later stages of AD, and when it develops a medical evaluation is indicated

(see Chapter 24). Potentially treatable causes may be found (e.g., infections or an enlarged prostate gland). If the incontinence is the result of the AD, it usually represents an inability of the brain to inhibit bladder contractions (urge incontinence or detrusor instability). It results in the bladder emptying without the patient being able to choose when and where it should occur. Supervised toileting programs that encourage voiding prior to the patient developing the urge to urinate can frequently lead to considerable improvement. Adjunct therapy includes the use of bladder relaxant medication [e.g., oxybutynin 5 to 15 mg/day or tolterodine (Detrol) 1 to 2 mg po bid]. It is important to emphasize that fluid restriction is not an acceptable treatment for urinary incontinence. Patients with AD are at risk for dehydration (they may forget to drink enough liquids), which can lead to worsening of their mental condition.

Fecal or stool incontinence is less common than urinary incontinence but does occur in the later stages of AD. Once again a medical evaluation is essential. Reversible causes for this problem include stool impactions (constipation leading to incontinence), laxative misuse, poor dietary habits, bowel infections, or other bowel disease. If a reversible condition is not found, it usually means that the brain damage resulting from the dementia has led to the problem. Bowel training programs can help to regulate stooling and can be supervised by family, caregivers, or visiting nurses.

Alzheimer's Disease Special Care Units

In an attempt to develop improved environments for AD victims, many health facilities have developed special outpatient and inpatient programs for these patients.[19] Adult day-care programs for individuals with dementia are sponsored by community health agencies, hospitals, and nursing homes. The goals of these programs are to allow patients to function in safe environments and participate in activities that are stimulating but not frustrating. Music, interacting with pets, and gardening are examples of frequently successful activities. An important achievement of day-care programs has been to relieve stress on home caregivers. This respite has enabled family caregivers to keep their relatives at home further into the course of the illness.

Inevitably in many cases AD patients eventually require rest home or nursing home care. Some assisted living and nursing home facilities have developed special units especially designed for the demented patient. These units encourage activity and exercise. The environment is free of hazards and disturbing stimulation. As with day-care programs, appropriate activities are encouraged. The use of physical restraints or sedatives is discouraged.

Families of Individuals with Alzheimer's Disease

The family physician caring for a patient with AD can provide crucial support to the family and caregivers. Families of AD patients have frequent questions and need advice and information. The issues on the minds of relatives change as the disease progresses. Table 25.3 reviews the common family issues that occur during the early, middle, and late stages of AD.

Table 25.3. **The Family and Alzheimer's Disease: Framework for Professional Providers**

Early stage
  Family issues
    Denial
    Cure seeking
    Cover-ups
    Asking the patient to try harder
    Fear
  Areas to assess
    Premorbid personalities and relationships
    Previous and concurrent caregiving responsibilities
    Informal supports: family and community
  Interventions
    Conduct a medical evaluation, provide primary care
      and information
    Discuss: coping with ambiguities, embarrassing
      situations; how, when, and what to tell whom;
      coping with role changes, modifying expectations;
      enhancing support system; legal/financial precautions
Middle stage
  Family issues
    Protection versus allowing risks
    Role fatigue or overload
    Behavior, mood, and sleep disorders management
    Isolation
    Preliminary grief
  Areas to assess
    Caregiver health status, tolerance for stress
    Family conflicts regarding care
    Cultural/religious proscriptions
    Community resources (e.g., respite, day care)
  Interventions
    Prescribe respite and ways to conserve energy
    Discuss: coping with crushed expectations;
      helplessness, anger, guilt; replacing lost
      confidante; accepting help: review old promises,
      how much, when, from whom?
Late stage
  Family issues
    Terminal care
    Guilt
    Limbo status
  Areas to assess
    Family attitudes toward terminal care, nursing homes
    Losses and gains with institutional care
  Interventions
    Encourage locating and evaluating long-term care
      facilities
    Discuss: coping with feelings and decisions regard-
      ing terminal care; planning for surviving family;
      coping with separation, new freedom; meeting
      altruistic needs

Source: Modified from Gwyther LP. Care of Alzheimer's pa-
tients: a manual for nursing home staff. American Health Care
Association, Washington, DC, and the Alzheimer's Disease and
Related Disorders Association, Chicago, 1985, with permission.

Conclusion

Cognitive impairment in the older person requires precise diagnosis. The previous assumption that senility during old age
is inevitable is not supported by evidence and should be rejected. Progressive cognitive impairment does occur in a sig-

nificant minority of the elderly, and a thorough evaluation occasionally uncovers a treatable cause of cognitive impairment.
In cases of AD or multiinfarct dementia, multidisciplinary approaches to treatment of the patient and family can significantly ease the burden conferred by these tragic illnesses.

Resources for Relatives and Caregivers

Selected Books on Caring for the Alzheimer's Patient

Cohen D, Eisdorfer C. The loss of self. New York: W.W.
  Norton and Company, 2001.
Mace NL, Rabins PV. The 36 hour day. New York: Warner
  Books, 2001.
Powell LS, Courtice K. Alzheimer's disease: a guide for fam-
  ilies. Cambridge, MA: Perseus Publishing, 1992.

Organizations

Additional information is available from local chapters of the
Alzheimer's Association and from the Alzheimer's Associa-
tion National Office or the National Institute on Aging's
Alzheimer's Disease Education and Referral Center (ADEAR):

Alzheimer's Association
  919 North Michigan Avenue, Suite 1000
  Chicago, Illinois 60611-1676
  1-800-272-3900
  www.alz.org
Alzheimer's Disease Education and Referral Center
  P.O. Box 8250
  Silver Spring, Maryland 20907-8250
  1-800-438-4380
  www.alzheimers.org

References

1. Folstein MF, Folstein SE, McHugh PR. "Mini mental state": a
   practical method for grading the cognitive state of patients for
   the clinician. J Psychiatr Res 1975;12:189–98.
2. McKhann G, Drachman D, Folstein M, et al. Clinical diagnosis
   of Alzheimer's disease: report of the NINCDS-ADRDA work
   group. Neurology 1984;34:939–44.
3. NIH Consensus Conference. Differential diagnosis of dementing disease. JAMA 1987;2580:3411–6.
4. Small GW, Rabins PV, Barry PP, et al. Diagnosis and treatment
   of Alzheimer Disease and related disorders. JAMA 1997;278:
   1363–71.
5. Budinger TF. Future research in Alzheimer's disease using imaging techniques. Neurobiol Aging 1994;15(suppl):s41–8.
6. National Institute on Aging. Progress report on Alzheimer's disease, 1999. Bethesda, MD: National Institutes of Health, 1999.
7. Hebert LE, Scherr PA, Beckett LA, et al. Age-specific incidence
   of Alzheimer's disease in a community population. JAMA 1995;
   273:1354–9.
8. McKeith LG, Galasko D, Kosaka K, et al. Consensus guidelines

for the clinical and pathologic diagnosis of dementia with Lewy bodies (DLB): report of the consortium on DLB international workshop. Neurology 1996;47:1113–24.

9. Schenk D, Barbour R, Dunn W, et al. Immunization with amyloid-beta attenuates Alzheimer-disease-like pathology in the PDAPP mouse. Nature 1999;400:173–7.

10. Stern Y, Gurland B, Tatemichi TK, et al. Influence of education and occupation on the incidence of Alzheimer's disease. JAMA 1994;271:1004–10.

11. Breitner JCS. Clinical genetics and genetic counseling in Alzheimer's disease. Ann Intern Med 1991;115:601–6.

12. Breitner JCS, Silverman JM, Mohs RC, Davis KL. Familial aggregation of Alzheimer's disease. Neurology 1988;38:207.

13. Saunders AM, Strittmatter WJ, Schmechel D, et al. Association of apolipoprotein E allele epsilon 4 with late-onset familial and sporadic Alzheimer's disease. Neurology 1993;43:1467–72.

14. Peterson RC, Smith G, Ivnik RJ, et al. Apolipoprotein E status as a predictor of the development of Alzheimer's disease in memory-impaired individuals. JAMA 1995;273:1274–8.

15. Reiman EM, Caselli RJ, Yun LS, et al. Preclinical evidence of Alzheimer's disease in persons homozygous for the epsilon 4 allele for apolipoprotein E. N Engl J Med 1996;334:752–8.

16. Statement on use of apolipoprotein E testing for Alzheimer Disease. American College of Medical Genetics/American Society of Human Genetics Working Group on ApoE and Alzheimer's disease. JAMA 1995;274:1627–9.

17. Mayeux R, Sano M. Treatment of Alzheimer's Disease. N Engl J Med 1999;341:1670–9.

18. Lazarus LW, Newton N, Cohler B, et al. Frequency and presentation of depressive symptoms in patients with primary degenerative dementia. Am J Psychiatry 1987;144:41–5.

19. Holmes D, Ory M, Teresi J. Special dementia care: research, policy, and practice issues. Alzheimer Dis Assoc Disord 1994; 8(suppl 1):13–55.

26
Elder Abuse

Karl E. Miller and Robert G. Zylstra

There are many similarities between elder abuse and child abuse. One could argue, however, that at-risk seniors are frequently more difficult to identify than at-risk children due to social isolation, and problematic to treat given their assumed legal competence. For many abused and neglected older individuals, a visit to their family physician may be the only point of contact with a professional capable of both identifying their concerns and coordinating needed interventions.

Estimates regarding the incidence of elder abuse vary, due in large part to differing research objectives and reporting guidelines. Perhaps the best recent investigation is the 1998 National Elder Abuse Incidence Study, published by the U.S. Administration on Aging (AOA).[1] The AOA estimated that in 1996 approximately 450,000 noninstitutionalized elderly persons aged 60 and over were victims of abuse and/or neglect, or about 1% to 2% of the total population. Including self-neglect as a reporting category increases this figure an additional 20%. Even more disturbing, however, is the finding that of this number approximately 80% went unreported to adult protective service (APS) agencies. Failure to identify elder abuse and take appropriate action can have tragic results, as the risk of death among elderly individuals who experience abuse is three times greater than that of the general population.[2] Therefore, it is imperative for family physicians to develop the skills necessary to identify elderly patients at risk for abuse and create an effective management strategy. In addition, family physicians need to be able to develop strategies to assist patients and their caregivers prevent abuse even before it takes place.

This chapter covers the current definitions of abuse, risk factors for abuse associated with both the elderly and their caregivers, and barriers that elderly patients and their physicians face when dealing with abuse issues. It also reviews how to assess suspected elderly abuse victims, reporting guidelines, and treatment and prevention strategies.

Abuse Categories

Commonly used definitions related to elder abuse and neglect are as follows (1):

Physical abuse: Willful infliction of physical pain or injury. Examples include hitting, slapping, shaking, striking with objects, and use of physical or chemical restraints.

Sexual abuse: Nonconsensual sexual contact, including rape, unwanted touching, sexual advances, or innuendoes.

Psychological abuse: Conduct resulting in mental or emotional anguish. This includes threats to institutionalize or withhold medication, nutrition, or hydration.

Financial or material exploitation: Misappropriating an older person's assets for someone else's benefit. Examples include theft and blackmail as well as coercion to change wills or other legal documents counter to the victim's best interest.

Neglect: Failure to provide the goods or services necessary for maintaining health and avoiding harm or illness. Neglect may be active, as seen with intentional refusal to provide for basic needs associated with activities of daily living such as hygiene assistance, medications, food, and physical assistance when needed for personal safety. Neglect may also be passive and unintentional, the result of caregiver ignorance or inability to provide for the patient's basic needs.

Self-neglect is frequently omitted or reported separately in statistical summaries. Described in one study as "a pattern of intentionally neglecting prescribed self-care activities despite available resources and knowledge,"[3] self-neglect is difficult to define due to conflicting individual and ethnic perspectives. Concerns regarding mental competence frequently complicate intervention, as do ethical issues related to patient autonomy.

Risk Factors

There are a number of characteristics common to many victims of abuse and neglect. These include the following: female, age greater than 75, poor health, low income, isolation, alcohol abuse, and history of mental illness or domestic violence.[4,5] One important characteristic is the development of dementia. This disease frequently has a subtle onset that can go unrecognized for several years. Identifying those elderly individuals with early-onset dementia is an important component of any comprehensive geriatric assessment (see Chapters 24 and 25). Cognitive impairments greatly limit individuals' ability to care for themselves, while impaired decision-making capabilities limit the autonomy and subsequent ability of depressed individuals to protect themselves from abusive and/or neglectful situations. While cause-and-effect relationships are difficult to establish, there does appear to be a significant comorbid association between psychiatric illness and elder abuse.[6]

Similarly, there are warning signs associated with those who are at risk of abusing or neglecting others. These include the following: male, financial dependence on the victim, history of substance abuse, history of prior violent acts, and current or prior history of psychiatric disorders.[7] Another important characteristic to recognize is caregiver burnout. Elderly patients who depend on others for care can generate significant amounts of stress for caregivers. While caregivers may be able to cope with day-to-day demands, they may decompensate when a crisis develops or simply exhaust themselves over time. It is vital that family physicians identify caregiver stress and coordinate the support services necessary to relieve these stressors.

Identification Barriers

Patient-Related

One obstacle to recognizing elder abuse is that a substantial number of elderly individuals are socially isolated.[1] A significant number live alone, and many are dependent on caregivers or other individuals for transportation. Physical limitations can further contribute to isolation by making it more difficult for the elderly to travel.

Other patient-related barriers to recognition of abuse include fear of retribution. Older individuals may be reluctant to discuss problems with health care providers due to concern that it will only make matters worse or result in nursing home placement.[8] Cognitive impairments may prevent some individuals from recognizing the abusive nature of their situation, while others may rationalize that the treatment they receive is "normal" or acceptable given their circumstances.

Physician-Related

Physician barriers reducing the likelihood of identifying elder abuse are primarily knowledge-based. The strongest factor in predicting physician recognition of elder abuse is an under-standing of the associated risk factors listed above.[9] Physicians also underestimate the prevalence of elder abuse, do not know how to assess for abuse, and fail to develop a systematic plan for how to respond to identified abuse.[9] Denials regarding the presence of abuse, reluctance to intervene, and fear of reprisal further hamper appropriate identification.

Assessment

Appropriate assessment of elderly patients where abuse is suspected includes a careful history and a targeted physical examination. Whenever possible, the initial portion of the history should be taken with both the patient and caregiver present. This allows for the physician to observe their relationship, with particular attention given to anxiety on the part of the patient or an overbearing attitude on the part of the caregiver.

Following the interview with both the patient and caregiver, the patient must be interviewed privately.[5] Information should be obtained regarding current health status, living arrangements, financial status, emotional stressors, and social support. A history of alcohol and drug abuse, for the patient as well as for other members of the household, should also be included,[10] as should a sexual history regarding any unwanted advances or physical contact.[5]

Any individual suspected of being abused should have a comprehensive physical examination, which is best performed with the patient completely undressed. General signs in an elderly individual suggesting abuse include appearance of poor physical care and signs of psychosocial distress. Particular attention should be given to the patient's general appearance, skin integrity, neurologic status, and musculoskeletal and genitourinary systems.[10] A complete skin examination should include evaluation for bruising on flexor surfaces, bruises of different ages, and burns. Assessment of neurologic status should take into consideration cognitive function, which is critical to the successful performance of activities of daily living. Assessment of ambulatory skills, an important component in establishing if reported injuries occurred secondary to falls or represent signs of abuse, should also be considered as part of the neurologic evaluation. Musculoskeletal examination should consider possible signs of injury that cannot be explained by the patient's history, whereas genitourinary examination includes findings suggestive of sexual abuse.

When elder abuse is suspected it is important to carefully document all findings. In addition to a written note, documentation should also include a diagram of all injuries noted during the examination. If possible, dated Polaroid photographs should be taken of each injury. X-rays of any injured area should be performed and if there is any suspicion that the elderly patient may have suffered a head injury, a computed tomography brain scan should be done. If clinical findings suggest malnutrition or dehydration, laboratory testing (e.g., complete blood count, blood urea nitrogen, creatinine, total protein and albumin levels) should be requested to document findings consistent with either of these conditions.

As alluded to earlier, an important component of assessing for elder abuse includes observing caregiver and patient interactions. Defensiveness and/or irritability on the part of caregivers may be a sign of burnout.[11] Prompt identification and intervention may be instrumental in preventing the occurrence of abuse or reducing the likelihood of continuing abuse.

Management

Whenever feasible, discuss concerns related to suspected abuse or neglect directly with the patient. To the extent that patients are competent to understand the process, include them in the treatment plan and enlist their active support and participation. Involve professionals from other disciplines to assist in the evaluation. Hospital social workers and case managers offer additional skills and are generally knowledgeable regarding available community services. Even after referring the patient to an outside agency, remain involved. Continued contact with a trusted family physician can significantly enhance the intervention process.

Prevention

Prevention of elder abuse starts by identifying those at risk. Family physicians who have developed long-term relationships with patients and their families have a distinct advantage in assessing and addressing patient as well as caregiver risk factors. Home health care professionals or other home-based service providers can further extend this advantage by observing both the elderly patient and the caregivers in the home environment. Combining office and home-based assessment can provide primary care physicians an excellent opportunity to determine the appropriate level of care needed.

Community Services

The best adjunct to care provided by a family physician is coordination with community agencies staffed with interdisciplinary teams trained to deal with abuse and neglect situations from a social as well as medical perspective. A number of communities are looking to volunteer providers as well in an effort to expand the scope of available services.[12]

Reporting Guidelines

Less than half of primary care physicians diagnosed elder abuse in the past year,[13] and even fewer reported a case to the authorities.[14] One dilemma related to reporting is a perceived conflict regarding doctor–patient confidentiality. Unlike child abuse, where legal statutes clearly protect the rights of minors, elder abuse happens to adults who most often are presumed to be legally competent and autonomous decision makers. While physicians are expected to respect patient au-

tonomy, they must also balance this right with the potential risk for injury that may occur if the suspected abuse is not reported.

While all states require health care providers to report suspected elder mistreatment,[15] specific legal requirements vary from state to state. Reports made in good faith are immune from civil liability. Failure to report can be considered negligence and is punishable by fines, imprisonment, or loss of license.

Strategies found to be helpful when reporting suspected elder abuse include identifying and collaborating with a single agency such as adult protective services, having an accessible directory of alternative community resources, and providing an educational package for the patient and family members that includes a description of the warning signs of caregiver stress and available community support services.[9] Physicians also need to be familiar with guidelines for detection and management of suspected abuse cases and standard protocols for documenting suspected abuse.[5] By following these guidelines physicians can improve their care of elder abuse victims while at the same time reduce the potential for conflict with family members or the legal system.

Conclusion

Proper care of elderly individuals at risk for abuse can and should be provided by family physicians. Adequate understanding of the associated warning signs and a working relationship with supportive community services, combined with a meaningful doctor–patient relationship, can have a significant impact on the emotional as well as physical well-being of older patients.

References

1. Administration on Aging. The National Elder Abuse Incidence Study: final report, September 1998. Available at *www.aoa. dhhs.gov/abuse/report/*.
2. Lachs MS, Williams CS, O'Brien S, Pillemer KA, Charlson ME. The mortality of elder mistreatment. JAMA 1998;280:428–32.
3. Reed PG, Leonard VE. The analysis of the concept of self-neglect. ANS Adv Nurs Sci 1989;12:39–53.
4. Lachs MS, Williams C, O'Brien S, Hurst L, Horwitz R. Risk factors for reported elder abuse and neglect: a nine-year observational cohort study. Gerontologist 1997;37:469–74.
5. Swagerty DL, Takahashi PY, Evans JM. Elder mistreatment. Am Fam Physician 1999;59:2804–8.
6. Dyer CB, Pavlik VN, Murphy KP, Hyman DJ. The high prevalence of depression and dementia in elder abuse and neglect. J Am Geriatr Soc 2000;48:205–8.
7. Dolan VF. Risk factors for elder abuse. J Insur Med 1999; 31:13–20.
8. Kruger RM, Moon CH. Can you spot the signs of elder mistreatment? Postgrad Med 1999;106:169–73,177–8.
9. Krueger P, Patterson C. Detecting and managing elder abuse: challenges in primary care. The Research Subcommittee of the Elder Abuse and Self-Neglect Task Force of Hamilton-Wentworth. Can Med Assoc J 1997;157:1095–100.

10. Marshall CE, Benton D, Brazier JM. Elder abuse. Using clinical tools to identify clues of mistreatment. Geriatrics 2000;55: 42–4,47–50,53.
11. Mendonca JD, Velamoor VR, Sauve D. Key features of maltreatment of the infirm elderly in home settings. Can J Psychiatry 1996;41:107–13.
12. Hiatt SW, Jones AA. Volunteer services for vulnerable families and at-risk elderly. Child Abuse Negl 2000;24:141–8.
13. McCreadie C, Bennett G, Gilthorpe MS, Houghton G, Tinker A. Elder abuse: do general practitioners know or care? J R Soc Med 2000;93:67–71.
14. Rosenblatt DE, Cho KH, Durance PW. Reporting mistreatment of older adults: the role of physicians. J Am Geriatr Soc 1996; 44:65–70.
15. Subcommittee on Health and Long-Term Care of the Select Committee on Aging, House of Representatives. Elder abuse: a decade of shame and inaction. Washington, DC: US Government Printing Office, 1992.

27
Child Abuse and Neglect

Susan Y. Melvin

Child maltreatment has persisted throughout history, from the practice of infanticide during the first century to the intergenerational abuse seen today. In 1962 the battered child syndrome was defined in the medical literature.[1] In 1974 the Child Abuse Prevention and Treatment Act (CAPTA) was passed requiring mandatory reporting of abuse in every state by designated personnel, including physicians, educators, social workers, and law enforcement officials. Since then, as victims themselves became parents, the long-term effects of child abuse and neglect have become evident. Chemical dependence, eating disorders, affective disorders, dysfunctional relationships, violence, and posttraumatic stress disorder have been identified more frequently in adults who were abused as children.[2]

Although child abuse crosses all socioeconomic and cultural backgrounds, some children are at greater risk. Younger parents are at greater risk than older to abuse their children. Single-parent families and families in poverty are at greater risk. Other risk factors include drug and alcohol abuse, depression and psychiatric disorders, poor social support, and social isolation.

Domestic violence and its impact on maltreatment often begins in utero (see Chapter 28). Frequently violence starts or escalates during pregnancy and has a significant impact on fetal morbidity and mortality, including miscarriage and low birth weight.[3] Additionally, studies show that children in homes where domestic violence exists are not spared. Ninety percent of children are aware of the violence directed at their mother, and 70% of children in battered women's shelters are themselves victims of physical abuse.[4]

Chemically abusing parents are more frequently perpetrators of sexual and physical abuse and neglect.[5] Others who are at increased risk for maltreatment include children in dysfunctional homes, where the family's roles and boundaries are poorly defined; children living without a natural parent; children with low self-esteem; and children with physical, mental, or behavioral problems.[6] The possible combination of factors is extensive. A history of abuse leaves a child at risk for abuse to recur.

It is rare for a child to voluntarily disclose a history of abuse to a physician, although it can happen. It is more likely that the child tells a trusted friend, teacher, or relative. If a child discloses a history of abuse, it is not the physician's responsibility to validate the statements, only to report to the appropriate agency, which then investigates. The physician should be supportive and express belief in the child's statements. Some behavioral indicators (Table 27.1)[7,8] may cue a physician to pursue the history. These indicators are not specific for child maltreatment, however, but represent a child's response to any kind of significant stress. Those stresses may include attending a new school, recent divorce of parents, or abuse.

The history provides the most important information for identifying child abuse and neglect. If a caregiver is unable to give a reasonable explanation for a child's injuries or the physical findings and history are not compatible, child abuse probably exists. Contradictions in the history or delays in seeking treatment for an injury may indicate abuse.

The physicians' role is to support and protect the child. Historical information should be obtained privately as appropriate for the age of the child. Questions should be open-ended and not leading, and vocabulary should be appropriate for the child's developmental level. Any information disclosed must be received without expression of disbelief or shock and then recorded and reported appropriately.

Neglect

Neglect is the most common form of maltreatment, representing 50% of reported cases of child abuse.[9] Even at this level, neglect is seriously underreported.[5] Neglect, defined as

Table 27.1. **Behavioral Indicators Associated with Neglect and Abuse of Children and Adolescents**

Clinging
Irritability
Regression: bowel/bladder, withdrawal, thumb sucking
Night terrors, sleep walking, afraid to sleep alone
Eating disorders or difficulties
Change in school performance: distracted, hyperactive
Acting out among peers: antisocial, aggressive behavior
Restricted social life
Suicide, depression, anxiety, phobic disorders
Decreased self-esteem
Overt abnormal sexual activity for age: coercive fellatio,
    insertion of objects into the vagina or rectum,
    simulated intercourse
Delinquency, running away
Substance abuse
Prostitution
Psychosomatic complaints, especially gastrointestinal or
    genitourinary

the failure of a parent or guardian to provide for the child's basic needs, manifests as lacking adequate food, clothing, shelter, medical care, education, safety, and nurturing. Identifying neglect is understandably difficult and must take into account the socioeconomic, educational, and functional levels of the parents. However, if children are to be protected, as the law states, it is mandatory that physicians report neglect. Neglect may be less dramatic than physical abuse but is equally damaging and represents more deaths.

The physical signs of neglect include malnutrition, poor hygiene, and inadequate clothing for the environment. Inadequate growth in a child may be due to poor caloric intake. Failure to thrive is associated with neglect in over 50% of case. Children who fall off the growth curve may need to be hospitalized for investigation and evaluation of organic causes. Behavioral signs relate to lack of supervision, poor school attendance, and exploitation, such as when a child is asked to beg or steal. Repeated ingestion of toxic substances demonstrates a lack of supervision. A child with excessive home responsibilities, such as caring for siblings or doing housework, and role reversal, in which the child becomes responsible for the parent, are examples of neglect. Medical neglect may be more easily identified and includes lack of appropriate medical care for acute or chronic conditions, lack of immunizations, poor dental care, and failure to thrive. Religion-motivated neglect can be identified when it limits medical intervention and should be reported by law.

Emotional Abuse

Family dynamics that undermine the development of healthy self-esteem in children can be classified as emotionally abusive. Frequently emotional abuse accompanies physical abuse and neglect but can occur in isolation. Terrorizing or abandoning a child are obvious forms of emotional abuse. However, more subtle forms such as lack of love or nurturing can be more difficult to identify. Expectations that are not com-

patible with growth and development, excessive responsibility, denigrating comments, and an attitude conveying that the child's presence is a burden are common examples of emotional abuse. Because this type of abuse is difficult to define, referral to a mental health professional may be appropriate. Signs may include excessive seriousness, lack of spontaneity, withdrawal, lack of confidence, aggression, and acting out.

Physical Abuse

Although it is not the most common form of child maltreatment, physical abuse is more easily identified. Recognizing injury patterns is essential, requiring the physician to review the history and seriously consider the developmental capacity of the child as it relates to an injury.

Dermatologic Manifestations

The most important part of the evaluation for physical abuse is examining the skin. A thorough examination requires that the child be undressed, gowned, and completely examined. Injury in locations usually concealed from public view often represents intentional injury.

Bruising

The skin mirrors the objects used to inflict injury. Common objects include belts, buckles, looped cords (electric), sticks, whips, fly swatters, coat hangers, spatulas, spoons, brushes, combs, teeth, and hands. Identifying injuries in different stages of healing supports the suspicion of ongoing intentional injury. Intentional injury should be considered when bruising occurs on padded areas such as buttocks, genitalia or portions of the face. Accidental bruising is more common over bony areas such as the forehead or the anterior tibial surfaces. Bruising caused by bleeding disorders may be mistaken for physical abuse. When bruising is the major manifestation, hematologic evaluation is required, including a complete blood count, prothrombin time, partial thromboplastin time, and bleeding time.

Burns

Burns are present in 12% of all physical abuse cases.[10] Nonaccidental burns can be inflicted by hot liquids or heated objects (see Chapter 50). The difficulty of diagnosing intentional burns is that children, once toddling, may pull or spill a hot liquid on themselves. However, the child must be developmentally capable of performing the task described in the parent's or guardian's history: For example, a nonambulatory child would have difficulty pulling something off the stove. The caregiver's history, considerations of the child's developmental abilities, and the pattern of the burn are necessary to determine the origin of the injury.

Discrepancies in any area are indicative of nonaccidental trauma. Intentional scald burns occur when a hot liquid is thrown at a child or when a child is immersed in hot water. The degree of injury depends on the temperature of the liquid and the duration of exposure. Common sites of injury with accidental splash burns include the head, face, chest, and abdomen, sites that would be affected if the child pulled hot liquid off a stove or table. Neither inflicted nor accidental splash burns are uniform in depth.

Immersion burns are uniform in depth and often are symmetric because the child is forcibly held in the water. Immersion burns often represent a form of punishment by parents with poor coping skills. For example, a parent may become frustrated during toilet training and immerse the child's buttocks in hot water as a form of punishment. Physical findings would show symmetric burns of the buttocks and legs, usually sparing the flexor creases of hips, knees, and ankles as the child tried to withdraw from the pain. Another form involves immersing the hands as a disciplinary act, which manifests as a glove-like, symmetric burn. Accidental immersion burns can occur, especially in homes where hot water thermostats are set above 120°F,[11] but these burns are not symmetric because the child's natural response is to struggle to get out of the water, and additional splash burns are evident. Children who are physically disabled and dependent on a caregiver to lift them in and out of the bathtub are at greatest risk for accidental immersion burns.

Mechanical burns occur when skin comes in contact with a hot object, accidentally or intentionally. The burns take the shape of the heated object and may be easily recognized. Burns on the feet, hands, or mouth may be accidental, resulting from curiosity or exploration. However, burns on the dorsum of the hands, the back, head, or buttocks are unlikely to be accidental. Although the diameter of a cigarette is 0.7 cm, when it is held against a child's skin it classically results in a 1.0-cm round lesion. Typical sites for cigarette burns are the dorsum of the hands, back, and buttocks, but such burns can occur anywhere.

Rope burns look like abrasions, are usually seen around the wrist or ankle, and sometimes are seen at the angle of the mouth if a child has been gagged. Rope burns usually are not an isolated finding and require further evaluation, especially for signs of sexual abuse.

Bites

Bite marks are easily recognized, symmetric, crescent-shaped bruises, sometimes with petechial hemorrhage; occasionally there is a break in the skin (see Chapter 47). Human bites are easily differentiated from animal bites. Animal bites result in puncture wounds and are narrower in diameter. Human bites tend to crush and tear. It is common for siblings to bite each other. However, if the diameter of the bite between the canine teeth is more than 3 cm, it usually represents an adult bite. Human bites are associated with a high rate of infection and may cause cellulitis.

Ocular Injuries

All children who have suspected nonaccidental injuries should undergo careful ophthalmologic evaluation (see Chapter 70). Trauma not otherwise visible may be evident in the retinal examination. Retinal hemorrhages are often associated with head trauma, including that seen with the shaken baby syndrome.[12]

Eye injuries result from common accidental as well as nonaccidental trauma. Common eye injuries associated with abuse include hyphema, dislocated lens, retinal detachment, rupture of the globe, blow-out orbital fractures, and retinal and conjunctival hemorrhages.[13]

Central Nervous System Injuries

Most deaths caused by physical abuse of children are secondary to intracranial injury.[14] Unfortunately, infants can have a fatal head injury without external evidence of trauma, as in the shaken baby syndrome. This syndrome is most common in infants under 6 months of age. The baby presents with lethargy, vomiting, and seizures. They may present with a more severe picture: unresponsive, comatose, or in respiratory arrest. They may have a bulging fontanel and enlarging head. In the absence of findings related to viral illness, reflux, or colic, there must be a high index of suspicion for nonaccidental trauma. These acceleration–deceleration injuries result in a high rate of mortality and an even higher rate of morbidity with lifelong disability.[12] Accidental trauma rarely causes intracranial injuries in infants unless it occurs in a motor vehicle accident or similar major trauma.[15]

Skull Fracture

A skull fracture due to minor trauma is rare. A parent or guardian who describes minor trauma as the cause of a skull fracture should be reported for abuse and further investigated. Skull fractures that suggest abuse include depressed, nonparietal fractures with complex configurations, multiple calvarial fractures, bilateral fractures that cross the suture lines, and fractures associated with intracranial injuries. Accidental fractures typically are simple, single, linear, and parietal; they are rarely associated with intracranial injury unless they result from major trauma.[16]

Intracranial Injuries

The most common cause of subdural hematoma in children is abuse, and most of these children present with a tense fontanel and seizures. In children under 2 years of age the subdural hematomas frequently are bilateral.[16] Other intracranial injuries include cerebral edema, infarction, atrophy, and subarachnoid hemorrhage.

Diagnostic Imaging

Plain radiographs of the skull are the most sensitive means for identifying fractures. However, computed tomography (CT) is most helpful for distinguishing the extent of intracranial injuries. Magnetic resonance imaging (MRI) may be helpful for diagnosing small subdural hematomas.

Skeletal Injury

Fifty percent of fractures in infants younger than 1 year of age have been found to be nonaccidental. It is difficult for a small child to exert enough force to fracture a bone. In contrast, accidental fractures occur more commonly in school-age children. Fractures in infants may cause crying, swelling, or bruising, and the child may favor the arm or leg.

Metaphyseal fractures of the long bones are considered diagnostic of abuse.[17] The forces required to produce these injuries rarely occur with an accidental fall. Pulling or twisting, using the arm or leg as a handle for shaking, or a direct blow causes the injury. The most common fractures are termed "corner" and "bucket-handle" lesions. A corner fracture is a small chip fracture that is pulled away from the peripheral margin of the metaphysis, such as might happen with a sudden jerk of an extremity. A bucket-handle fracture is a larger crescent-shaped bone fragment that pulls away and tips into an oblique plane. Subperiosteal hemorrhage and periosteal new bone formation are associated with these fractures. Metaphyseal fractures commonly involve the tibia, distal femur, and proximal humerus (see Chapters 110 and 111). Diaphyseal fractures are common with abuse but are less specific for it. Shaft fractures are more common in the older infant and require direct impact or a torsional force that results in a spiral fracture.[17] The younger the child, the more likely the fracture is nonaccidental.

Accidental rib fractures are rare outside of major trauma. The most common site of rib fractures with nonaccidental trauma is near the costovertebral junction.[17] The fractures are usually multiple and are often difficult to identify radiographically before callus formation (10–14 days after injury), especially as the ribs are rarely displaced. In children under 2 years of age, rib fractures usually are caused by manual compression and in older children by direct blows. Studies suggest that fractures of the first rib in children are frequently related to abuse, with possible mechanisms including impact force, compressive force, and shaking or acute axial load (slamming), which can cause an indirect fracture.[18] In the absence of major trauma or underlying bone disease, rib fractures should be considered specific evidence for physical abuse.

Other skeletal injuries from abuse include vertebral fractures, which may occur with sudden hyperflexion, hyperextension injuries. Uncommon fractures involve the shoulder, sternum, and scapula.

A complete skeletal survey is indicated for all children younger than 2 years of age when physical abuse or neglect is suspected. The survey should include the entire axial and appendicular skeleton. A "baby-gram" or single radiograph is not adequate. Skeletal surveys are rarely indicated after 5 years of age. Instead, request appropriate specific imaging.

Nontraumatic causes of fracture are uncommon to rare. They include osteogenesis imperfecta, osteomyelitis, syphilis, scurvy, rickets, and neoplasia.

Visceral Trauma

Abdominal injuries are second only to head trauma for causing death of abused children. Victims tend to be infants, and often bruises or other marks are not visible. Injuries often involve multiple organs, including rupture of the liver or spleen, transection of the pancreas, or bowel obstruction secondary to hematoma. The history is often vague or misleading, and frequently there is a significant delay in seeking medical attention.

Other Forms of Physical Abuse

Less common forms of physical abuse include passive inhalation of free-base cocaine, intentional drowning or suffocation, gunshot wounds, and poisoning. Munchausen syndrome by proxy is recognized more now than in the past. It is defined as an illness in the child that has been inflicted by a parent or guardian for the adult's secondary gain. The child may undergo repeated evaluations, hospitalizations, and procedures. When the child is separated from the parent the symptoms resolve.[19]

Sexual Abuse

Child sexual abuse has been defined as the exploitation of children for the sexual gratification or profit of an adult or a person in a position of power, such as an older child or adolescent.[20] Sexual abuse may include fondling, oral copulation, mutual masturbation, sodomy, complete and vulvar coitus, and child pornography and prostitution. To intervene on the child's behalf, the clinician must recognize the behavioral[7,8] (Table 27.1), medical[7] (Table 27.2), and physical[8] (Table 27.3) signs of sexual abuse. Estimates of prevalence indicate that one of three girls and one of every five boys before the age of 18 have been sexually molested.[21]

It is common to have normal physical findings on exam even in cases where there is a known perpetrator. But the history is most critical to intervention. The interview should be nonthreatening. Questions should be open-ended. Spontaneous disclosures made by the child should be well docu-

Table 27.2. **Medical Signs and Symptoms Indicating Sexual Abuse of Children and Adolescents**

Unexplained genital irritation, injury, or scarring
Bruising, scratches, or bites not consistent with history
Difficulty walking or sitting
Sperm on clothing
Grasp marks
Blood stains on underwear
Pain in genital or anal area, or both
Enuresis, encopresis, or both
Penile swelling, discharge, or both
Recurrent atypical abdominal pain
Unexplained recurrent urinary tract infections
Proctitis
Any sexually transmitted disease
Pregnancy in a pubescent girl

Table 27.3. **Physical Findings Associated with Child Sexual Abuse**

Reflex relaxation of pelvic or pubococcygeal muscles when child is touched lateral to the introitus
Reflex relaxation of anal sphincter with lateral retraction of the buttocks (anal wink)
Hymenal diameter ≥1 cm in a prepubescent girl
Genital scarring
Presence of vaginal discharge or odor
Pigmentary changes (labial or perianal skin), pallor, or erythema
Loss of gag reflex
Extreme compliance (child is emotionally distant during examination)

mented verbatim. Documentation should be timed and dated. If the alleged abuse was greater than 72 hours prior to presentation, consider reporting and deferring exam to a child sexual abuse exam center if available.

Physical Examination

Patience is required when performing a genital examination on a child who may have been a victim of abuse. A child should not be forced to undergo a genital examination, but parents and a supportive environment assist in getting the required task accomplished. If the abuse is thought to be recent (within 72 hours) a forensic evaluation is necessary, including cultures from the throat, vagina, and rectum. Efforts should be made to collect hair and semen samples as well. Speculum examinations are not necessary; cultures are taken from the vagina with a cotton swab. Visual inspection and documentation of any bruising, skin tears, and abrasions should be recorded. Most states provide rape kits that assist the collection procedure. If available, a forensic physician should be present at the initial examination so the process does not have to be repeated. Genital exams should document a description of the labia, clitoris, urethra, hymen, vestibule, posterior fourchette, and anus. Clear color photographs may be helpful for documentation, but a standard diagram of the perineum with findings is adequate.

When a child is touched lateral to the introitus and reflex relaxation of the pelvic muscles occurs, sexual abuse should be suspected. Children who have been chronically sodomized may have a similar reflex relaxation of the anal sphincter with lateral retraction of the buttocks. Loss of gag reflex may indicate chronic oral copulation. Genital scarring, changes in pigment, and discharge may indicate abuse.

Commonly with child sexual abuse there are no physical findings. Anatomic hymenal variations are normal, and clinical experience on the part of the examiner is essential if the diagnosis of an abnormal hymen secondary to abuse is to be diagnosed. However, child abuse is suspected if a prepubescent girl has a hymenal diameter of more that 1 cm.[6] Hymenal lacerations most commonly occur with digital or penile penetration and are evident in the posterior hymenal segment. Straddle injuries may result in laceration of the anterior hymenal segment.[22]

Sexually Transmitted Disease

A child who has any sexually transmitted disease should be evaluated for abuse (see Chapter 41). Chlamydia and gonorrheal infections outside the newborn period are fairly specific for sexual abuse, but either can be acquired at birth as the infant passes through the birth canal.[23] Condyloma acuminata may also be acquired during the birth process. Because of a 20-month incubation period, the mode of transmission may be difficult to identify. Yet sexual transmission of this virus in children has been clearly established. Genital herpes in a prepubescent child should elicit concerns about abuse, although cases of self-inoculation have been noted.

Herpes simplex may also be acquired during the birth process, and syphilis and human immunodeficiency virus (HIV) can be acquired in the birth canal and go unnoticed for years. These diseases may also represent sexual abuse, however, and so require further evaluation. Children with non-neonatal cases of trichomoniasis have a high probability of sexual abuse. Bacterial vaginosis does not appear to be naturally occurring in prepubertal girls and may be considered an indicator of sexual abuse.[23]

Reporting

The physician's legal responsibility is to report suspected child abuse or neglect to the appropriate agency and provide protection for the child until the appropriate authority assumes that role. It is not the physician's responsibility to investigate or validate the situation. The reporting agency usually is the local law enforcement agency or the state's child protective services. Physicians cannot be held civilly or criminally responsible for reporting suspected abuse unless an intentionally false report is made.

Treatment and Prevention

Abused children need to be assured that they are physically all right, that the situation was not their fault, that they are not alone, and that it has happened to others. Physicians must use caution when making promises to children. The situation may get worse before it gets better, especially if the child requires more examinations, is removed from the home, or ends up in a lengthy court battle.

Referral to trained professionals in the area of child abuse is advisable as soon as the abuse is identified, even before the physical examination if possible. The psychological intervention is essential for alleviating the lifelong sequelae of abuse.

Child abuse is a disease of the "family," and the family physician is in a unique position not only to recognize abuse but also to identify those at high risk who are in situations where intervention can occur. Preventive therapy may include referral to a psychologist for family therapy and clarification of new roles, boundaries, expectations, methods of communication, and discipline. It also includes recognizing children with low self-esteem and those who are socially isolated, and then making a referral before the child becomes a victim. Family physicians taking care of couples who deal with conflict by violence have a responsibility to the children of those relationships, as studies show children in homes of domestic violence are also victims. Any child with a history of abuse is at risk for being a victim again and should be in treatment. Parents or guardians with a history of abuse or with poor coping and parenting skills may be helped by psychotherapy and parenting classes. Many opportunities exist for intervention by physicians.

Other forms of prevention include educating parents to communicate with their children about the possibilities of abuse and to teach children the differences between "good" and "bad" touching. Parents should also be encouraged to develop a "no-secrets rule" in the household to ensure the flow of communication. Physicians should also encourage parents to teach their children the correct anatomic terminology for genitalia and bodily functions, which assists children in their communication.

References

1. Kempe CH. The battered child syndrome. JAMA 1962;181: 1742.
2. Egami Y, Ford DE, Greenfield SF, et al. Psychiatric profile and sociodemographic characteristics of adults who report physically abusing or neglecting children. Am J Psychiatry 1996;153: 921–7.
3. Jones RF. Domestic violence: let our voices be heard. Obstet Gynecol 1993;81:1–4.
4. Groves BM, Zuckerman B, Marahs S, et al. Silent victims: children who witness violence. JAMA 1993;269:262–4.
5. Jaudes PK, Ekwo E, Van Voorhis J, et al. Association of drug abuse and child abuse. Child Abuse Negl 1995;19:1065–75.
6. Finkelhor D, Hoteling G, Lewis IA, et al. Sexual abuse in a national survey of adult men and women: prevalence, characteristics and risk factors. Child Abuse Negl 1990;14:19–28.
7. Gale J, Thompson RJ, Moran T, et al. Sexual abuse in young children: its clinical presentation and characteristic patterns. Child Abuse Negl 1988;12:163–70.
8. Krug RD. Recognition of sexual abuse in children. Pediatr Rev 1986;8:25–30.
9. Dubowitz H, Giardino A, Gustavson E. Child neglect: guidance for pediatricians. Pediatr Rev 2000;21:4.
10. Showers J, Garrison KM. Burn abuse: a four year study. J Trauma 1988;28:1581–3.
11. Yeoh C, Nixon JW, Dickson W, et al. Patterns of scald injuries. Arch Dis Child 1994;71:156–8.
12. American Academy of Pediatrics. Shaken baby syndrome: inflicted cerebral trauma, statement of the committee on child abuse and neglect. Pediatrics 1993;92:872–5.
13. Munger CE, Peiffer RL, Bouldin TW, et al. Ocular and associated neuropathologic observations in suspected whiplash shaken infant syndrome: a retrospective study of 12 cases. Am J Forensic Med Pathol 1993;14:193–200.
14. American Academy of Pediatrics, Section on Radiology. Diagnostic imaging of child abuse. Pediatrics 2000;106:6.
15. Goldstein B, Kelly MM, Bruton D, et al. Inflicted versus accidental head injury in critically injured children. Crit Care Med 1993;21:1328–32.
16. Zimmerman RA, Bilaniuk LT. Pediatric head trauma. Neuroimaging Clin North Am 1994;4:349–66.
17. Merten DF, Carpenter BL. Radiologic imaging of inflicted injury in the child abuse syndrome. Pediatr Clin North Am 1990; 37:815–37.
18. Strouse PJ, Owings CL. Fractures of the first rib in child abuse. Radiology 1995;197:763–5.
19. Boros SJ, Ophoven JP, Anderson R. Munchausen syndrome by proxy: a profile for medical child abuse. Aust Fam Physician 1995;24:768–73.
20. Paradise JE. The medical evaluation of the sexually abused child. Pediatr Clin North Am 1990;37:839–62.
21. Sgroi S. Handbook of clinical intervention in child sexual abuse. Lexington, MA: Lexington Books, 1985.
22. Adams JA, Harper K, Knudson S, et al. Examination findings in legally confirmed child sexual abuse: it's normal to be normal. Pediatrics 1994;94:310–6.
23. Argent AC, Lachman PI, Hanslo D, et al. Sexually transmitted diseases in children and evidence of sexual abuse. Child Abuse Negl 1995;19:1303–10.

28
Domestic Violence

Valerie J. Gilchrist

Although domestic violence may refer to all aspects of family violence, this chapter focuses on intimate partner violence (IPV). Over 95% of such abuse involves a man abusing his female partner. Although several studies have shown an almost equal number of episodes of violence perpetrated by men and by women, others show that women use violence for self-defense and escape while men use violence for control, punishment, or attention.[1] Regardless of motivation the result is both injury and fear in the female partner.[2,3]

An intimate partner's physical, emotional, or sexual abuse effects up to 50% of women in the United States at some time in their lives.[3-5] While the lifetime prevalence varies by definition of abuse, population studied, and methodology, this figure may be an underestimation because high-risk populations such as those hospitalized, homeless, institutionalized, or incarcerated are excluded. Thirty percent of female homicides in 1996 were committed by partners or expartners.[6] Battery is the single greatest cause of injury to women.[3,6]

Background

Cycle of Violence

IPV is cyclic.[7] After an abusive episode there is the *honeymoon phase*, during which the abuser is apologetic, often courting the victim with gifts and attention, promising that he will never hurt her again. This phase invariably shifts into the *tension-building phase*, during which the woman lives in an atmosphere of extreme tension and fear as her partner threatens and isolates her. The tension-building phase ultimately culminates in the *violent phase* of battery and abuse. With repetition the cycle increases in frequency and severity.

The goal of the abuse is power and control by the perpetrator. Figure 28.1 depicts tactics employed by batterers. On-

going ego-battering erodes the victim's self-image. She is systematically stripped of the resources that would allow her to leave: her self-respect, pride, career, money, friends, and family. She often sees no options except trying to make do in her situation and hoping that somehow she can prevent further violence.[8-10]

Abused Women

Women who are divorced or separated, younger, and of a lower socioeconomic status (SES) report higher prevalence rates of abuse, but there is no characteristic premorbid personality profile of the abused woman.[9] Women who have been previously traumatized will have more severe symptoms with IPV.[11]

Abusing Men

Batterers do not lose control but rather take control. Common characteristics include dependency on and jealously of their partners, a belief in traditional gender roles, a high need for control, difficulty with trust, and a refusal to accept responsibility for their violent behaviors.[12] Abusing men are not a homogeneous population. Men who batter only within their families are the least violent, and rarely have criminal records or exhibit psychopathology. Men who exhibit passive-aggressive, dependent, or borderline personality characteristics are more violent, and those who are antisocial engage in both partner and extrafamilial violence.[13,14] Ninety percent of men who batter have no criminal record.[8] The use of alcohol or drugs by the abuser is associated with increased violence.[15,16]

Abuse in Homosexual Relationships

Abuse in gay and lesbian relationships is similar in form, prevalence, and precipitants to heterosexual relationships.

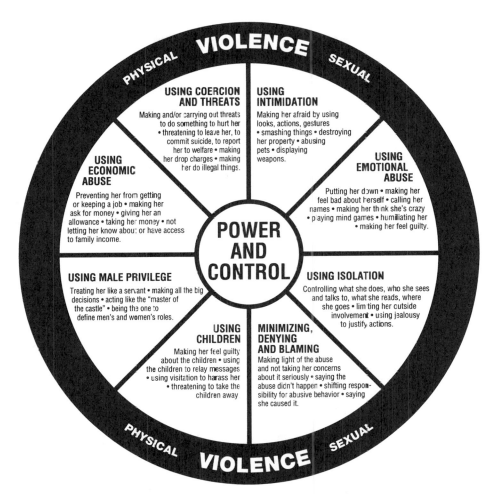

Fig. 28.1. Power and control wheel illustrates many components of domestic violence, all of which are ultimately enforced by the threat or actuality of physical and sexual violence. (From the Domestic Abuse Intervention Project, Minnesota Program Development, 202 E. Superior, Duluth MN 55802, with permission.)

However, there may be pressures within the gay community not to reveal violence, there are fewer social resources, and IPV is less commonly recognized by clinicians. Batterers may use homophobic control threatening to "out" their partner. If the batterer is human immunodeficiency virus (HIV) positive, he may use this as an infective threat or a guilt-inducing control strategy. If the partner is HIV positive, the batterer may threaten to reveal this or to deny care or medication. Also, without expected gender stereotypes the batterer may use the illusion of mutual battery to maintain control.[17]

Special Populations

Up to 50% of adolescents report dating violence, and IPV for pregnant adolescents is especially high.[5,18] Many adolescent victims of IPV have also been subjected to abuse in their family of origin.[18]

Older women also experience IPV, often for many years. They are frequently financially dependent on their partner. Children may provide resources or apply pressure to keep the relationship intact. Abuse may intensify with the stress of caregiving.[19]

Immigrant women who are victims of IPV often have few resources. They may not speak English well, may fear the police and authority, especially if they are undocumented, and may live in a setting that sanctions abuse or view abuse as a "private" matter.[5]

Clinical Presentation

Battered women present with repeated, increasingly severe physical injuries, self-abuse, and psychosocial problems including depression, drug or alcohol abuse, and suicide attempts.[3,5] The battering injuries are often inconsistent with the explanation provided, bilateral, and only in areas covered by clothing. There may be contusions, lacerations, abrasions, pain without obvious tissue injury, evidence of injuries at different times, and evidence of rape. A partner, if present, may be controlling, overly solicitous, and reluctant to leave.

Twenty-five percent of battered women report receiving medical care, and 10% require hospital treatment; however, most abused women present for routine, not emergency, medical care, and most injuries do not require hospitalization.[3,10]

Abused women are more likely to define their health as poor, and they have more hospitalizations, surgical procedures, pelvic pain, sexually transmitted diseases, functional gastrointestinal problems, chronic headaches, and chronic pain problems in general.[3,4,10] Poor health is just as significantly associated with psychological IPV as physical assault.[4] Abused women and their children use more health care services.[5,20] Fear of abuse has limited partner notification of HIV status.[10] IPV precipitates unemployment, homelessness, and poverty for women.[4,14]

Surveys in family practice settings revealed current abuse in 10% to 50% of women, with a lifetime prevalence of up to 40%. The diagnosis of depression was the strongest indicator of domestic violence.[5,20]

As many as 50% of women who visit emergency departments are battered, and studies in these settings reveal a lifetime prevalence of 11% to 54% depending on the definition of abuse and the method used. Victims present equally with trauma and nontraumatic complaints and more often in the evening or night.[21]

Up to one in five women are battered during pregnancy and this may become more frequent in the postpartum period.[5,20] Pregnancy may incite the initial episodes of abuse but most often there is preceding abuse.[22] Abused women have more unintended pregnancies, are twice as likely to delay seeking prenatal care, twice as likely to miscarry, and four times as likely to have a low birth weight infant, and these infants are 40% more likely to die during the first year of life.[20]

One third to one half of women presenting to mental health centers have been battered.[3,10] The diagnosis of borderline personality disorder and substance abuse are particularly common.[5,11,14,20] IPV was found in 55% of a sample of depressed women.[23] Domestic violence is a cause of posttraumatic stress disorder (PTSD). The severity of both PTSD and depression correlate directly with the intensity of the abuse.[5,20] One in 10 victims of abuse will attempt suicide[3] (also see Chapters 32 and 33).

After battery, victims have demonstrated a ninefold increased risk for drug abuse, and the use of alcohol increased 16-fold.[10,11] There is concurrent use of alcohol and drugs during 25% to 80% of the battering episodes, and this is a marker for more severe injury.[16] The presence of substance abuse should initiate questions about violence.

Children

Forty-seven percent of children entering domestic violence shelters have been abused, and in 45% to 60% of child abuse cases there is concurrent domestic violence.[20] Children are inevitably aware of the violence and suffer from the consequences of the violence. These include direct injury while trying to intervene, decreased nuturance and social support because of maternal depression, and family dislocations with potential social and economic disadvantage.[20,24] Children's symptoms include internalizing symptoms (somatic complaints, disturbed sleep, withdrawal, anxiety, depression), externalizing behaviors (aggression, cruelty to animals, defiance

of authority, destructiveness), and defects in social competence (school achievement, peer relations, self-confidence, and participation in sports and other extracurricular activities).[20,24] Children's symptoms increase with the severity, frequency, content, and resolution of parental conflict and if there is concurrent child abuse.[24,25] These children are predisposed to later enactment of abuse against, or victimization by, an intimate partner.[14]

Diagnosis

Battered women may lack money for medical care or transportation to medical facilities, or they may be prevented by their abuser from seeking medical care. Victims may withhold information from clinicians because they feel ashamed, humiliated, or that the injuries are not serious or are deserved. Victims also may lie about the source of injuries in an effort to protect the partner or children or because of fears of retribution for any disclosure or police involvement. Many women disclose abuse only after numerous inquiries.[5,26]

The single most important step medical professionals can take is to *ask every woman, confidentially,* if she is being or has been abused. Domestic violence cuts across all ages and socioeconomic, racial, ethnic, religious, and professional groups, although social and ethnic backgrounds may influence both the victim's and the perpetrator's perception of domestic violence. Domestic violence occurs at a frequency comparable to breast cancer and is more common than other conditions for which screening is routine. Questioning communicates to the patient that the problem is not trivial, shameful, or irrelevant. It opens the area to further conversation and may begin the process of the abused woman's leaving the relationship.[9]

It is important for physicians to remain nonjudgmental and relaxed because abused women are extremely sensitive to nonverbal cues. While general questions about a relationship with a partner may be a good way to open conversation ("How are things going at home? How do you resolve differences?"), explicit direct questioning is most effective.[5,6] Ask about nonviolent but psychologically abusive acts ("Are you insulted, threatened?"), and about the use of force such as grabbing or restraining, pushing, or throwing objects (be specific about the type of objects thrown). Ask about forced sex, clubbing, beating, choking, and the use of weapons. Ask about her fear: "Do you feel safe in your current relationship?" She may also fear a partner from whom she has separated but who is threatening or stalking her. Negative responses to lower levels of violence do not preclude positive responses to more severe violence.

Physician Barriers

Domestic violence is a complex social problem that requires physicians to step beyond the biomedical paradigm and confront their own personal feelings and social beliefs.[27–29] In unselected patients, physicians identified only 1.5% to 8.5% of victims.[5] Clinicians consistently underestimate the prevalence of IPV among their patients.[28] Physician education and chart reminders have been successful in increasing the identification of IPV.[30,31]

Physicians feel they have not been trained to deal with domestic violence and there is little they can do.[27,28] Physicians working with IPV recognize that it is not a problem that they can "fix" but one that requires time, as well as working with both the patient and community agencies. These physicians recognize cues, frame questions to reduce discomfort and validate concerns, and focus on establishing trust and emotional safety for women.[26]

Physicians rarely discover the abusers in their practice because they appear normal. If incidents are discovered, abusers commonly accuse their partners of exaggeration, do not define their actions as violent, or dismiss the incident as an exception. Physicians must not rationalize, minimize, or excuse the abuser's violence. Family therapy is not appropriate in a setting of violence.[3]

Management

The quality of medical care a battered woman receives often determines if she will follow through with referrals to legal, social service, and health care agencies.[9] It is critical for the physician to breach the battered woman's isolation and to validate her view of reality by telling her that spouse abuse is a crime, that she does not deserve abuse, that things can improve, and that her feelings of defeat are a result of the abuse.[9,11]

Physicians may inadvertently retraumatize the woman by blaming her, or insisting she leave, not realizing women are at the greatest risk of being brutally beaten or killed when they leave their abuser.[3,10,15,27,32] Physicians may diagnose anxiety, depression, or substance abuse without realizing these are a result of ongoing abuse. This labels the victim, delays appropriate intervention, and, if psychoactive drugs are prescribed, increases the risk of suicide.[20,27,29]

Physicians must not only diagnose domestic violence but also establish its severity and the woman's risk. Immediate

Table 28.1. Features Associated with Increasing Risk of Intimate Partner Violence

Increasing frequency of violence
Increasing severity of injuries
The presence of weapons
Substance abuse
Unemployment
Threats and overt forced sexual acts
Threats of suicide or homicide
Surveillance
Abuse of children, pets, other family members, or the destruction of treasured objects
Increasing isolation
Extreme jealousy and accusations of infidelity
Failure of multiple support systems
A decrease or elimination of remorse expressed by the batterer

Table 28.2. The Components of an Abused Woman's Safe Plan

Places to which she could flee—one primary and two backups
    Telephone numbers
    Transportation
Cash
Bag packed for her and children
Documents (or copies)
    Driver's license
    Birth certificates
    Social security card
    Welfare card
    Health and other insurance policies
    Bank statements
    Protection orders/restraining orders
    Immigration papers
An extra set of keys to home and car
Evidence of abuse such as names and addresses of witnesses, pictures of injuries, and medical reports
Something meaningful for each child (blanket, toy, book), but if the children are old enough, she should talk to them about safety—how to call for help and where to go to keep themselves safe

danger must be assessed. The best way to ascertain the woman's risk is to ask: "Are you safe tonight? Can you go home now? Are your children safe? Where is your batterer now?" If she says she is in immediate danger, the physician should believe her and begin to explore safer options. Continued support, validation, risk assessment, documentation, and practical advice comprise the "treatment" of domestic violence. At each visit immediate danger must be assessed, features associated with increasing risk reviewed (Table 28.1), a safe plan established or reviewed (Table 28.2), and documentation provided. Scheduled follow-up visits provide the patient opportunities to acknowledge the validity of her experiences, the difficulties in her situation, and the chance to reassess her options. By facilitating rather than directing change, physicians can focus on the process of empowerment rather than on the outcome of leaving.[27] Physician behaviors that have been found particularly helpful or unhelpful by battered women are summarized in Table 28.3.[33,34]

Documentation

The physician's documentation provides the history and evidence of abuse. The abused woman needs to know that her records are confidential unless she decides to use them. Notes should be nonjudgmental and precise, and should document the chronology. The chief complaint and a description of abusive events should use the patient's own words. Include a complete description of any injuries with body diagrams, specifying the type, number, size, location, and age of any injuries, and the explanation offered. Photographs should be taken before medical treatment, if possible, and should include a reference object (such as a ruler) to convey relative size, and the face of the woman in at least one. All photographs should be dated and kept with the consent form.[35] The physician's record should

Table 28.3. **The Desirability of Common Physician Behaviors Identified by Abused Women**

Desirable behaviors
  Performing a careful, sensitive medical examination
  Asking for concerns or questions
  Listening
  Expressing emotional support
  Providing reassurance that the beating was not the
    woman's fault
  Being compassionate and respectful
  Noticing body language
  Stating that abuse is wrong under any circumstances
  Asking or offering to call the police
Undesirable behaviors
  Not scheduling a follow-up visit
  Insisting that the woman get away from her abuser
  Calling the police without the woman's permission
  Treating physical injuries without asking how they occurred
  Recommending couple counseling
  Going along with the patient's explanation of the injury,
    even if inconsistent with injuries
  Acting as if the abuse was not serious because the physical
    injuries were not serious
  Acting as if he/she did not care that an assault had
    occurred
  Telling the woman things could be worse

also include the results of diagnostic procedures, referrals, and recommended follow-up, and should record any contact with the abuser. The badge number of the investigating officer, if the police are notified, should be noted.[36]

The Process of Leaving

Separation from an abusive partner is an ongoing process.[14,32,37,38] Abusers respond predictably when their partner leaves, first trying to locate her, and apologizing and promising to change, but if the woman does not return, then they become threatening, embarrassing her in public or harassing her. Women are five times more likely to be murdered by their partner during the separation than before the separation or after divorce. Seventy-five percent of calls to the police and 73% of emergency room visits occur after separation.[5,32]

Most women eventually leave or change an abusive relationship, but it may involve returning repeatedly and may take years.[14,32] In one longitudinal study, after $2^1/_2$ years three fourths of the battered women were no longer in violent relationships; 43% had left, and in 32% the violence ended.[14] Women report going through stages of *reclaiming their self* as they separate from their abusive partners.[38] Initially they are shocked, fearful, and ashamed, and want to deny the abuse. After recurrent abuse, they problem solve, trying to change their behaviors or the circumstances to avoid or minimize abuse and hoping for improvement. Isolation, power imbalance, and alternating abusive and kind behaviors predispose victims to the formation of strong emotional attachments to their abusers and explain why battered women struggle to separate themselves emotionally from their abusers and often return after leaving.[9,11] Eventually, abused women realize that no matter what they do the abuse is unavoidable and they need to separate both

emotionally and physically. The ability of a woman to separate depends on her resources, both material (job, housing, social supports, legal services, and child support) and psychological (self-esteem, resisting self-blame).[32,37] Subsequent violence by her partner, especially threats against the children and inadequate legal protection, are often cited by women as a reason to return to an abusive relationship. Eventual recovery from an abusive relationship is characterized by establishing a safe and separate living situation, grieving the loss, and later developing a new sense of oneself and one's abuse history.[20,32,37,38]

Legal Issues

Battered women may take civil actions, which include filing a protective order or seeking an injunction or restraining order. They may also choose to file criminal charges, including prosecution for assault and battery, aggravated assault or battery, harassment, intimidation, or attempted murder. However, the legal response to domestic violence is less than optimal. The woman is likely to know whether the batterer will adhere to court orders.[3,36] Physicians should refer batterers to an appropriate state-certified batterer treatment program, but also need to realize that the enrolment of the batterer in a program, or even a restraining order, in no way guarantees a woman's safety.[12,39]

Most states require reporting of criminal assaults; however, some states now have mandatory reporting of domestic violence. These laws have not increased reporting, and without the necessary support services this has put victims at risk and fearful of confiding in their physicians, and physicians become conflicted about their obligations to report versus their concern for their patient's safety.[36,40] The Joint Commission on Accreditation of Health Care Organizations require policies for the identification and assessment of abuse victims and the education of providers.[36]

Prevention

Primary prevention of domestic violence will be achieved only by challenging the roles of violence and patriarchy in society. This includes educating parents and teens about nonviolent problem-solving strategies and questioning gender stereotypes both in individual patient interactions and through school- or community-based programs.[8,10,18,41,42] *Secondary prevention* includes the interruption and elimination of intergenerational abuse of all kinds, challenging popular media images of gendered violence, and treating the cofactors of alcohol and substance abuse.[18,42] *Tertiary prevention* can be achieved by identifying victims and their abusers and helping each one. When available, battered women's shelters are effective, although few of the women in need can access them. Court-ordered programs for male batterers have had some success in the reduction of battery. Education, referral, outreach, and brief intervention programs by clinicians or volunteers have been shown to increase women's adoption of safe behaviors and to decrease abuse.[43,44] Comprehensive community-based programs for the identification and treatment of both victims and perpetrators are the most effective.[11,18]

Family and Community Issues

Treatment of domestic violence requires working in partnership with community agencies not only for individual patients but also as an advocate for increased and coordinated services, public education, and research.[41,45] It is hoped that the recent passage of the federal Violence Against Women Act of 2000 will increase services for families. Many communities and states operate toll-free 24-hour domestic violence hotlines. Excellent Web-based resources are available, but victims need to be warned about Internet tracking by abusers and cyber stalking.[46] Some recommended sites for victims and professionals include the following: Family Violence Prevention Fund, *http://www.fvpf.org*; Crisis Support Network, *http://crisis-support.org*; Violence Against Women Office of Department of Justice, *http://www.ojp.usdoj.gov/vamo*; Minnesota Center Against Violence and Abuse, an electronic clearing house, *http://www.mincava.umn.edu*; Centers for Disease Control and Prevention's National Center for Injury Prevention and Control and Family and Intimate Violence Prevention Program, *http://www.cdc.gov/ncipc/dvp/fivpt/fivpt.htm*; and the National Coalition Against Domestic Violence, *http://www.ncadv.org/*. The National Domestic Violence Hot Line is 1-800-799-SAFE.

Families that engage in one form of family violence are likely to engage in others.[8] Family physicians are in a unique position to interrupt the cycle of violence and to effect positive change in the lives of both the victims and the abusers, as well as the children affected by domestic violence.

References

1. Hamberger LK, Lohr J, Bonge D, Tolin D. An empirical classification of motivations for domestic violence. Violence Against Women 1997;3(4):401–23.
2. Cascardi M, Langhinrichsen VD. Marital aggression: impact, injury, and health correlates for husbands and wives. Arch Intern Med 1992;152:1178–84.
3. American Medical Association. Diagnostic and treatment guidelines on domestic violence. Chicago: AMA, 1992.
4. Coker AL, Smith PH, Bethea L, King MR, McKeown RE. Physical health consequences of physical and psychological intimate partner violence. Arch Fam Med 2000;9:451–7.
5. Nauman P, Langford D, Torres S, Campbell J, Glass N. Women battering in primary care practice. Fam Pract 1999;16(4):343–52.
6. Sisley A, Jacobs LM, Poole G, Campbell S, Esposito T. Violence in America: a public health crisis B domestic violence. J Trauma Injury Infect Crit Care 1999;46(6):1105–13.
7. Walker LE. The battered woman syndrome. New York: Springer, 1984.
8. Gelles RJ, Cornell CP. Intimate violence in families, 2nd ed. Newbury, CA: Sage, 1990.
9. Burge SK. Violence against women as a health care issue. Fam Med 1989;21:368–73.
10. Stark E, Flitcraft A. Women at risk: domestic violence and women's health. Thousand Oaks, CA: Sage, 1996.
11. Herman JL. Trauma and recovery. New York: Basic Books, 1992.
12. Cardin AD. Wife abuse and the wife abuser: review and recommendations. Counseling Psychol 1994;22(4):539–82.
13. Holtzworth-Munroe A. A typology of men who are violent toward their female partners: making sense of the heterogeneity in husband violence. Curr Direct Psychol Sci 2000;9(4):140–3.
14. Johnson M, Ferraro K. Research on domestic violence in the 1990s: making distinctions. J Marriage Fam 2000;62:948–63.
15. Kyriacou DN, Anglin D, Taliaferro E, et al. Risk factors for injury to women from domestic violence. N Engl J Med 1999; 341(25):1892–8.
16. Brookoff D, O'Brien KK, Cook CS, Thompson TD, Williams C. Characteristics of participants in domestic violence: assessment at the scene of domestic assault. JAMA 1997;277(17):1369–73.
17. West CM. Leaving a second closed: outing partner violence in same-sex couples. In: Jasinski JL, Williams LJ, eds. Partner violence: a comprehensive review of 20 years of research. Thousand Oaks, CA: Sage 1998;163–83.
18. Stringham P. Domestic violence. Prim Care 1999;26(2):373–84.
19. Phillips LR. Domestic violence and aging women. Geriatr Nurs 2000;21(4):188–93.
20. Campbell J, Lewandowski L. Mental and physical health effects of intimate partner violence on women and children. Psychiatr Clin North Am 1997:20(2):353–74.
21. Olson L, Anctil C, Fullerton L, et al. Increasing emergency physician recognition of domestic violence. Ann Emerg Med 1996;27(6):741–6.
22. Martin SL, Mackie L, Kupper LL, Buescher PA, Moracco KE. Physical abuse of women before, during and after pregnancy. JAMA 2001;285(12):1581–4.
23. Scholle SH, Rost KM, Golding JM. Physical abuse among depressed women. J Gen Intern Med 1998;13:607–13.
24. Anderson SA, Cramer-Benjamin DB. The impact of couple violence on parenting and children: an overview and clinical implications. Am J Fam Ther 1999;27:1–19.
25. Dubowitz H, Black MM, Kerr MA, et al. Type and timing of mothers' victimization: effects on mothers and children. Pediatrics 2001;107(4):728–35.
26. Gerbert B, Caspers N, Bronstone A, Moe J, Abercrombie P. A qualitative analysis of how physicians with expertise in domestic violence approach the identification of victims. Ann Intern Med 1999;131:578–84.
27. Warshaw C. Domestic violence: changing theory, changing practice. J Am Med Wom Assoc 1996;51(3):87–91.
28. Snugg NK, Thompson RS, Thompson DC, Maiuro R, Rivara FP. Domestic violence and primary care: attitudes, practices and beliefs. Arch Fam Med 1999;8:301–6.
29. Gremillion DH, Kanof EP. Overcoming barriers to physician involvement in identifying and referring victims of domestic violence. Ann Emerg Med 1996;27(6):769–73.
30. Wiist WH, McFarlane J. The effectiveness of an abuse assessment protocol in public health prenatal clinics. Am J Public Health 1999;89:1217–21.
31. Thompson RS, Rivara FP, Thompson DC, et al. Identification and management of domestic violence: a randomized trial. Am J Prev Med 2000;19(4):253–63.
32. Landenburger KM. The dynamics of leaving and recovering from an abusive relationship. J Obstet Gynecol Neonatal Nurs 1998;27(6):700–6.
33. Hamberger LK, Ambuel B, Marbella A, Donze J. Physician interaction with battered women: the women's perspective. Arch Fam Med 1998;7:575–82.
34. Rodriguez MA, Szkupinski Quiroga S, Bauer HM. Breaking the silence: battered women's perspectives on medical care. Arch Fam Med 1996;5(3):153–8.
35. Bryant W, Panico S. Physician's legal responsibilities to victims of domestic violence. NC Med J 1994;55(9):418–21.
36. Hyman A. Domestic violence: legal issues for health care practitioners and institutions. J Am Med Wom Assoc 1996;51(3):101–5.
37. Rothery M, Tutty L, Weaver G. Tough choices: women, abu-

sive partners and the ecology of decision-making. Can J Community Mental Health 1999;18(1):5–18.

38. Merritt-Gray M, Wuest J. Counteracting abuse and breaking free: the process of leaving revealed through women's voices. Health Care Wom Int 1995;16:399–412.

39. Capshew T, McNeece CA. Empirical studies of civil protection orders in intimate violence: a review of the literature. Crisis Intervent 2000;6(2):151–67.

40. Mills L. Mandatory arrest and prosecution policies for domestic violence: a critical literature review and the case for more research to test victim empowerment approaches. Criminal Justice Behav 1998;25(3):306–18.

41. Candib LM. Primary violence prevention: taking a deeper look. J Fam Pract 2000;49(10):904–6.

42. Foshee VA, Bauman KE, Arriaga XB, et al. An evaluation of safe dates, an adolescent dating violence prevention program. Am J Public Health 1998;88(1):45–50.

43. McFarlane J, Parker B, Soeken K, Silva C, Reel R. Safety behaviors of abused women after an intervention during pregnancy. J Obstet Gynecol Neonatal Nurs 1998;27:64–9.

44. Sullivan CM, Bybee DI. Reducing violence using community-based advocacy for women with abusive partners. J Consult Clin Psychol 1999;67:43–53.

45. Chalk R, King P. Assessing family violence interventions. Am J Prevent Med 1998;14(4):289–92.

46. Finn J. Domestic violence organizations on the Web: a new arena for domestic violence services. Violence Against Women 2000;6(1):80–102.

29
Sexual Assault

Diane K. Beebe

Sexual assault is a violent crime. The term is used interchangeably with rape and is defined as any forced attempt or completed act of vaginal, anal, or oral penetration by a part of the accused's body or foreign object without the victim's consent. Force may be physical or psychological coercion.[1] Lack of consent may include being under age 18 years or having impaired mental functioning owing to drugs, alcohol, sleep, or unconsciousness.

Occurrence

One of 6 women, more than 17 million, and one of 33 men, nearly 3 million, in the United States age 18 and older report having been victims of a completed or attempted sexual assault. There is a lifetime prevalence of rape of nearly 18% for women and 3% for men,[2] although some studies place it as high as 39% for women.[3] Of the women victims, more than half were younger than age 18 when they experienced their first attempted or completed rape.[2]

These statistics underestimate the true number of sexual assaults occurring annually in the United States. Many such crimes on the homeless, on those living in group facilities, and on those unavailable for surveying go unaccounted. As reported by victims, less than one third of incidents are reported to law enforcement.[4] Women assaulted by a partner are significantly less likely to report the assault. Victims are reluctant to report it because they fear embarrassment, the assailant, or other people finding out, and they feel a sense of responsibility for the assault.[3] The most common reason for not reporting was that it was considered a personal matter. Victims who do report cite the fear of a repeat assault by the offender.[4,5] Because the rates of arrest and conviction for sexual assault are low, victims may feel a sense of futility. Rates of arrest vary, depending on state laws mandating reporting or arrest.

In nearly three out of four incidents, the offender was known to the victim, with approximately 60% of these assaults occurring at the home of the victim, a friend, a relative, or a neighbor. Sexual assaults by strangers are more likely to occur on the street or in commercial property. Two thirds of sexual assaults occur between 6 P.M. and midnight.[4]

Impact

Apart from the tremendous personal burden for victims and their families, the economic burden of sexual assault includes health care costs, lost income from work, and legal or court-related activities.[5] Women victims of sexual assault have an increased number of physician and emergency room visits for up to 3 years following the assault.[6]

Female Victims

The annual rate of sexual assault in the United States is 8.7 rapes per 1000 women age 18 and older.[2] Over 90% of female rapes involve a single assailant.[5] In the U.S., the highest rates of sexual assault occur in the below 35 age group; however, 2% to 3% of all sexual assaults occur in postmenopausal women. As the only age group predominantly assaulted by strangers, older women are particularly vulnerable due to decreased physical strength, stamina, and mobility. Many elderly women live alone and have caregivers, often strangers, in their homes.[6]

Male Victims

The victimization rate for males in the U.S. is 1.2 rapes per 1000 men age 18 and older, accounting for over 111,000 rapes annually.[2] Male sexual assault does not occur only in institutions. Assault by strangers and multiple assailants are more common among men. Men are more likely to sustain serious injuries, with a higher rate of anal assault than for women. Men are less likely to report the crime and more likely to seek treatment for nongenital injuries.[6,7] Expected to be in control, to be able to defend themselves, and to be the sexual aggressor, men fear the shame, societal disbelief, and potential judgment of being homosexual. Male sexual assault suggests nothing regarding the sexual orientation of the victim or the perpetrator. Most perpetrators identify themselves as heterosexual.[8]

Intimate Partner Violence

Nearly 64,000 women a year, 56 per 100,000, are victims of sexual assault by their intimate partner.[1] An intimate partner is a current or former spouse, an opposite- or same-sex cohabiting partner, a boyfriend or girlfriend, or a date. Approximately 6% of all sexual assaults are by a current spouse.[5] Women often feel socially pressured to have sexual relations with their husbands, regardless of their feelings about the situation or the type of sexual activity. Sex may be used as a bargaining tool against anger, extramarital affairs, or limitations of money and other resources. Marital sexual assault is more frequent in marriages characterized by other forms of violence or involving alcoholic husbands. Laws against spousal sexual assault now exist in most states. The effects on victims of marital sexual assault may be more severe than victims of stranger sexual assault. Long-term effects include distrust of men, an increased phobia of intimacy, and sexual dysfunction.[9]

Date Rape

One of the most important risk factors for date and acquaintance rape is prior victimization or past sexual abuse. Reported rates of date rape in the college population range from 13% to 27% of women, with approximately 50% reporting some type of unwanted sexual contact.[10] Victims and perpetrators often view the occurrence of date sexual assault differently, with perpetrators seeing no harm done. Risk factors for date rape in women include views that condone sexual aggression, younger current age and age at first date, previous sexual activity, greater age difference between the man and the woman, and alcohol use by either the victim or the perpetrator. Concern over substance-related rape is increasing with the using of "date-rape drugs" such as flunitrazepam (Rohypnol), a potent sedative.[10,11] Lacking color, taste, or odor, the drug is often unintentionally ingested, and effects appear in less than 30 minutes. Impaired memory and judgment, loss of inhibition, confusion, and eventual unconsciousness make the victim vulnerable to attack.[12] Dating violence is not limited to younger women. Studies have shown that, similar to younger women, over 65% of women over 40 years reported unwanted affection and physical contact on dates.[13]

Family Physician's Role

Most victims of sexual assault are more likely to seek help from their primary care physician than from mental health professionals, sexual assault crisis centers, or victim assistance programs.[14] The function of the physician is not to determine if a sexual assault has occurred. Rape is a legal, not a medical, term, and the commitment of a crime is determined by the courts. The physician's responsibilities involve treatment of physical injuries, history documentation, careful physical examination, evidence collection, prevention of sexually transmitted disease and pregnancy, psychological support, and arrangements for follow-up counseling.[6] Physicians should be involved in training personnel, developing hospital protocols, and addressing the medical, psychological, safety, and legal needs of victims.[15] A community plan should utilize the cooperative efforts of law enforcement agencies, local governments, courts, hospitals, and other relevant organizations to provide total care for victims.

Care of the Victim

Only one third of women who sustain injuries seek medical care,[2] with women assaulted by a stranger more likely to seek treatment.[3] The patient should be examined in a private, quiet area in the emergency room or clinic. The patient's verbal and signed consent for examination, for evidence collection, and for release of information to law enforcement must be obtained. Explanation of each step is important to allow the patient as much control as possible over the situation.[6] If available, a specially trained rape crisis counselor should be called to remain with the victim. A friend or relative should bring the victim a change of clothes and may remain with the victim throughout the examination if desired.

History

Questioning should be nonjudgmental so that the victim's feelings of self-blame for the assault are not heightened. The written record should carefully record the patient's account of the incident. The pertinent history is outlined in Table 29.1.[6]

Physical Examination

Nearly a third of female rape victims sustain injuries, and the risk of injury increases if the assailant is a current or former intimate partner.[2] The sooner evidence is collected after an assault, the better, preferably within 72 hours.[16] The patient should disrobe carefully over a clean cloth or paper sheet so that any debris or hair present on the clothes may be recov-

Table 29.1. **Pertinent History**

General medical history: allergies, medications, immunizations, illnesses
Sexual history: date of last consensual intercourse, contraceptive use, last menstrual period, past genitourinary infections
Assault history: number and sex of assailants, relationship of perpetrator to victim, types of sexual assault including ejaculation, physical violence including use of weapons, foreign objects or restraints, use of drugs or alcohol, specifics (date, time, location) of assault
Postassault activities: change of clothing, douching, bathing, urination, defecation, mouth rinsing

ered. Only the victim should handle the clothes to avoid contamination. The clothes are placed in paper, not plastic, bags, as plastic may enhance bacterial growth on blood or body fluid stains. In female victims the most common sites of extragenital trauma are the mouth, throat, wrists, arms, breasts, and thighs.[17] A careful description of the findings is essential. Drawings and diagrams of injuries, noting the location, size, and color of wounds, burns, lacerations, or abrasions are helpful. The use of a Wood's lamp is routine to examine the perineal and inner thigh area, though not all seminal stains are detectable with a Wood's lamp.[16] Any fluorescent areas are swabbed with cotton swabs for collection. Vaginal swabs should be obtained even if there are no visible pooled secretions. Pubic hair should be combed over a sheet of paper to catch any material that can identify the assailant; plucked or cut pubic and head hairs can be used to identify which hairs belong to the victim. Scrapings from under fingernails are collected if the victim reports a struggle.[16]

The vaginal examination is performed gently with a small speculum lubricated only with water. Lubricants may be spermicidal and interfere with wet mounts. The hymen, vaginal walls, cervix, and rectum are examined for lacerations or abrasions. Examination with a colposcope is superior to gross visualization alone in detecting genital trauma. Toluene blue may also increase detection of perineal lacerations.[7] Bimanual pelvic examination is performed to assess any masses or tenderness. In male victims, testicles are examined for evidence of trauma.

Collection of Evidence

Evidence should be collected regardless of the initial decision of the victim about pursuing criminal prosecution of the alleged assailant. Evidence not collected cannot be retrieved should the victim later decide to file charges. A "chain of evidence" must ensure that each step of evidence collection is documented by the person collecting and handling the specimens. All collected specimens should be air-dried, sealed, dated, and transported by a police officer to a local crime laboratory. Results of collected tests are not returned to the physician; therefore, duplicate samples pertinent to proper medical treatment should be collected at the time of the examination.[18]

Secretions are collected with cotton swabs from the vagina, rectum, and oral cavity. Forensic analysis can detect the presence of spermatozoa and seminal plasma components. Motile sperm may be recovered from the vagina for several hours following ejaculation. Nonmotile sperm may be detected for 24 hours in the vagina and rectum, but may be recovered from cervical mucus for several days.[19] Douching, urination, and administration of oral contraceptives, which change the cervicovaginal environment, decrease the likelihood of sperm recovery after an assault.[20] Less than 50% of sexual assault cases will have seminal evidence recovered; however, crime lab analysis will commonly find evidence of semen that is not noted in the emergency room. Sperm has been found in 45% of cases where sperm was not noted in the emergency department.[7] The mouth is swabbed for detection of sperm and acid phosphatase even if the victim has eaten, drunk, brushed

the teeth, or gargled. Spermatozoa may be recovered from the oral cavity, although salivary enzymes usually destroy seminal fluid within hours.[19] The absence of sperm does not preclude sexual assault.[21] Fifty percent of assailants experience impotence or ejaculatory dysfunction.[22] An absence of sperm may also be due to vasectomy or azoospermia of the assailant.[21] In these cases, penile epithelial cells still exfoliate into the vagina and may be detected with enhanced techniques for identification of nonsperm male cells in cervicovaginal smears.[20] All swabs are sent to a forensic laboratory for determination of the enzyme acid phosphatase and the plasma glycoprotein p30. Both are present in high concentrations in prostatic secretions and are best detected within 48 hours after coitus.[19]

Genetic typing of semen, blood, and vaginal fluid can help identify an assailant. These fluids contain high levels of four genetic markers: ABO blood group antigens, phosphoglucomutase, peptidase A, and deoxyribonucleic acid (DNA). Since 80% of the population secretes blood group antigens into other body fluids, the victim's secretor status must be determined by blood and saliva analysis. Peptidase A and phosphoglucomutase are present in semen regardless of secretor status.[16,19]

Sexually Transmitted Disease Prevention

The risk of acquiring a sexually transmitted disease (STD) from a sexual assault is estimated at 5% to 10%. The risk of human immunodeficiency virus (HIV) transmission in a single sexual assault is estimated at less than 0.1% and may be related to factors such as the type of penetration, number of assailants, and viral load of the assailant.[6] There are no formal recommendations for HIV prophylaxis. The risks, side effects, cost, and need for close monitoring and follow-up testing should be discussed with each victim.[6,23] Positive cultures and studies from specimens obtained up to 24 hours after the assault may represent preexisting disease. Diseases with long incubation periods may not be detected if follow-up is incomplete. Table 29.2 outlines recommended examinations and treatment for STDs[6,24] (also see Chapter 41).

Pregnancy

The risk of pregnancy from a single rape is estimated to be up to 5% in fertile victims.[6] Preexisting pregnancy can be determined by serum human chorionic gonadotropin β-subunit assay. Physicians are obligated to offer treatment for the prevention of pregnancy and document patient counseling (Table 29.2). Pregnancy prophylaxis must be administered within 72 hours of the assault. The teratogenicity and 1% failure rate of postcoital medications should be explained.[18] If the patient does not desire immediate treatment, a serum pregnancy test may be repeated in a week.

Emotional Reactions and Psychological Sequelae

Sexual assault victims may display a variety of emotions immediately following an attack. The *expressed style*, with visible agitation, anxiety, and crying, is often exhibited. However, many victims present with the quiet, calm, seemingly

Table 29.2. **Sexually Transmitted Disease (STD) and Pregnancy Recommendations[24]**

Condition	Diagnosis	Treatment
Gonorrhea/ Chlamydia	Culture all sites; urethral swab (males) Reculture in 2 weeks if not treated	Ceftriaxone sodium 125 mg IM plus azithromycin 1 g po or doxycycline 100 mg po bid × 7 days
Syphilis	RPR or VDRL; repeat in 6, 12, 24 weeks if NR	No prophylaxis; treat if positive
HIV	HIV baseline; repeat in 6, 12, 24 weeks if negative	Consider zidovudine (AZT) 200 mg po tid and lamivudine 150 mg po bid for 4 weeks[6]
Hepatitis B	Hepatitis B surface antigen	Hepatitis B vaccination; complete HBV series in 1 to 2 and 4 to 6 months
Trichomonas	Wet preparation; repeat in 2 weeks if untreated	Metronidazole 2 g po
Pregnancy	Serum β-hCG; repeat in 2 weeks if negative	Ethinyl estradiol/norgestrel 2 tabs initially, repeat in 12 hours

RPR or Venereal Disease Research Laboratory (VDRL) = serologic test for syphilis; HIV = human immunodeficiency virus; HBV = hepatitis B virus; β-hCG = human chorionic gonadotropin; NR = nonreactive.

removed affect of the *controlled style*.[6,25] The emotional sequelae of sexual assault are significant and can be long-lasting even if physical signs are limited. Not only does the assault victim require special attention, the victim's spouse, family, and close friends also need support and counseling. The care a patient initially receives influences recovery.[26] Up to one third of victims develop posttraumatic stress disorder and one third experience a major depressive episode within a year of the assault.[6] Sexual assault may also be a risk factor for somatization, panic disorder, obsessive-compulsive disorder, somatiform disorders, eating disorders, drug or alcohol abuse, and dependence and dissociative disorders.[27]

Male victims commonly report sexual dysfunction, ranging from long periods of abstinence to periods of promiscuity, as well as difficulty during intercourse. Men may also question their sexual orientation following an assault.[28]

Personal characteristics of the victim, characteristics of the sexual assault, and the victim's social support system influence the posttraumatic response. More severe responses are seen in patients with a history of severe psychiatric symptoms, previous sexual violation, and concurrent life stresses. The single most important factor in recovery is the victim's social support system.[29]

Table 29.3. **Rape Trauma Syndrome: Psychological Sequelae**

Acute phase—may last days to weeks
  Disbelief, numbness, humiliation, feelings of violation
    Controlled style—subdued feelings, slow, soft speech
    Expressed style—emotional lability, expressed anxiety, fear, shame, guilt
Reorganized phase
  Outward adjustment stage
    Deals with practical, usual matters
    Denies feelings about rape
    Experiences flashbacks
  Personal integration stage
    Depression, inability to stop thinking about rape
  Recovery stage
    Return to normal functioning

Rape Trauma Syndrome

The rape trauma syndrome is applicable to all sexual assault victims and is outlined in Table 29.3. The acute disorganization phase can last a few days to several weeks. The second recognization or reorganization phase lasts weeks to years.[6,25]

Follow-Up

Referrals for counseling should be made before the patient leaves the emergency room. Victims also need a follow-up appointment in 1 to 2 weeks to ensure adequate healing of injuries; to repeat serologies, cultures, and pregnancy testing; to complete hepatitis vaccinations; and to treat other medical conditions. Reexamination in a couple of days may reveal bruising that may not become visible for at least 48 hours.[7]

Prevention

Family physicians have a special opportunity to counsel patients, adolescents in particular, to reduce their risk of sexual assault. Effective communication regarding dating expectations can prevent unplanned or unsupervised activity where sexual assault may occur. Both sexes should be warned about the relationship of alcohol and drugs to sexual assault. Low self-esteem, self-destructive behavior, eating disorders, sleep disturbance, regressive behavior, acting out, or abrupt behavioral change may indicate undisclosed sexual assault.[18] Many college campuses are initiating mixed-gender date sexual assault workshops to increase awareness, promote shared responsibility, and facilitate discussion. These workshops, along with programs targeted for individual female and male audiences, have shown some success in modifying attitudes and increasing awareness.[10]

The family physician should support community campaigns to dispel common myths regarding rape. Common misperceptions include that victims are in someway responsible for the assault or that they could have done more to avert it.

Conclusion

Sexual assault is a violent, not a sexual, act. It is a pervasive crime with physical and psychological impact. Family physicians must be prepared to recognize and assess victims of sexual assault. One study of medical schools in the United States and Canada found that 58% of curricula did not include formal teaching on adult domestic violence and sexual assault.[30] The physician's role involves history taking, physical examination, collection of legal evidence, injury treatment, prevention of sexually transmitted diseases and pregnancy, psychological support, and follow-up counseling. The initial care given to victims, with the attention of the family physician to both medical and psychological aspects of treatment, positively influences recovery.

References

1. Rennison CM, Welchans S. Bureau of Justice Statistics special report, intimate partner violence. NCJ-178247. 2000. Publications published by U.S. Dept. of Justice, National Criminal Justice. Found at http://www.ojp.usdoj.gov.bjs/welcome.html or http://www.usdoj.gov or http://www.ncjrs.org or ordered from: United States Department of Justice, 950 Pennsylvania Ave. NW, Washington, D.C. 20530-0001.
2. Tjaden P, Thoennes, N. Full report of the prevalence, incidence, and consequences of violence against women. Findings from the National Violence Against Women Survey. NCJ 183781. November 2000.
3. Feldhaus KM, Houry D, Kaminsky R. Lifetime sexual assault prevalence rates and reporting practices in an emergency department population. Ann Emerg Med 2000;36(1):23–7.
4. Greenfeld LA. Bureau of Justice Statistics. An analysis of data on rape and sexual assault: sex offenses and offenders. NCJ-163392. 1997.
5. Bureau of Justice Statistics. Criminal victimization in United States, 1999 statistical tables from National Crime Victimization Survey. NCJ-184938. 2001.
6. Linden JA. Sexual assault. Domestic violence in the emergency department. Emerg Med Clin North Am 1999;17(3):685–97.
7. Riggs N, Houry D, Long G, Markovchick V, Feldhaus KM. Analysis of 1,076 cases of sexual assault. Ann Emerg Med 2000; 35(4):358–62.
8. Male rape. Nurs Times 1993;89(6):18–19.
9. Whatley MA. For better or worse: the case of marital rape. Violence Victims 1993;8(1):29–39.
10. Rickert VI, Wiemann CM. Date rape among adolescents and young adults. J Pediatr Adolesc Gynecol 1998;11:167–75.
11. Rohypnol information sheet. http://danenet.wicip.org, 2/18/01.
12. Schwartz RH, Milteer R, LeBeau MA. Drug-facilitated sexual assault ("date rape"). South Med J 2000;93(6):558–61.
13. Kalra M, Wood E, Desmarais S, Verberg N, Senn C. Exploring negative dating experiences and beliefs about rape among younger and older women. Arch Sex Behav 1998;27(2):145–53.
14. Beebe DK, Gulledge KM, Lee CM, Replogle W. Prevalence of sexual assault among women patients seen in family practice clinics. Fam Pract Res J 1994;14:223–8.
15. American College of Emergency Physicians. Management of the patient with the complaint of sexual assault. Ann Emerg Med 1995;25:728–9.
16. Bechtel K, Podrazik M. Evaluation of the adolescent rape victim. Adolescent gynecology part II: the sexually active adolescent. Pediatr Clin North Am 1999;46(4):809–23.
17. Kobernick ME, Seifert S, Sanders AB. Emergency department management of the sexual assault victim. J Emerg Med 1985;2: 205–14.
18. AMA Guidelines: strategies for treatment and prevention of sexual assault. Chicago: AMA, 1995.
19. Tintinalli JE, Kelen GD, Stapczynski JS, eds. Emergency medicine: a comprehensive study guide, 5th ed. New York: McGraw-Hill, 2000.
20. Collins KA, Rao PN, Hayworth R, et al. Identification of sperm and non-sperm male cells in cervicovaginal smears using fluorescence in situ hybridization: applications in alleged sexual assault cases. J Forensic Sci 1994;39:1347–55.
21. Hochbaum SR. The evaluation and treatment of the sexually assaulted patient. Emerg Med Clin North Am 1987;5:601–22.
22. McGregor JA. Risk of STD in female victim of sexual assault. Med Aspects Hum Sex 1985;19:30–42.
23. Babl FE, Cooper ER, Damon B, Louie T, Kharasch S, Harris J. HIV postexposure prophylaxis for children and adolescents. Am J Emerg Med 2000;18(3):282–7.
24. Centers for Disease Control and Prevention. 1998 guidelines for treatment of sexually transmitted diseases. MMWR. Jan 23 1998;47(RR-1):1–118.
25. Burgess AW, Holmstrom LL. Rape trauma syndrome. Am J Psychiatry 1974;131:981–6.
26. Martin CA, Warfield MC, Braen GR. Physician's management of the psychological aspects of rape. JAMA 1983;249:501–3.
27. Butterfield MI, Panzer PG, Forneris CA. Victimization of women and its impact on assessment and treatment in the psychiatric emergency setting. Emergency psychiatry. Psychiatr Clin North Am 1999;22(4):875–96.
28. Mezey G, King M. The effects of sexual assault on men: a survey of 22 victims. Psychol Med 1989;19:205–9.
29. Moscarello R. Psychological management of victims of sexual assault. Can J Psychiatry 1990;35:25–30.
30. Williams L, Forster G, Petrak F. Rape attitudes amongst British medical students. Med Educ 1999;33:24–7.

30
Family Stress and Counseling

Thomas L. Campbell, David Seaburn, and Susan H. McDaniel

Patients often present to their family physician with symptoms and problems that are largely related to stress experienced in the family context. Less often, patients identify family stress as a source of the symptoms they are experiencing. The challenge for the family physician is to accurately assess the role that family stress plays in a patient's symptoms and decide what interventions are most appropriate and effective. The physician needs to use a biopsychosocial approach, with particular attention to the role family may play in the patient's problems, assess the family dynamics that may contribute to the patient's difficulties, and decide if the problem is appropriate for primary care counseling.

This chapter presents basic principles and guidelines for identifying family stress, assessing family functioning, and intervening with families. Marital stress and marital problems are used as an example of how to deal with family stress. The common problems that families face and the principles of treating these problems are discussed. A case vignette illustrates how marital stress may present and be managed in a clinical setting. Chapter 4 discusses many of the principles underlying this approach and how to interview families in clinical practice.

Dimensions of Family Stress

There are many types of family stress that patients experience. Family stress can occur within the family or result from outside events affecting the family. It can occur with normative transitions or be the result of nonnormative crises. Intrafamily stress may result from acute events, such as the serious illness or death of a family member, or from longstanding interpersonal difficulties, such as marital conflicts or chronic parent–child problems. External stresses, such as loss of employment, natural disasters, or forced relocations, may result in family members' feeling they lost a sense of control over their lives. Some family stressors are a normal part of

the family life cycle, such as the illness or death of an elderly family member. Desired life cycle events, such as marriage and childbirth, can also be stressful and result in emotional distress and health problems.[1,2] Nonnormative crises that occur out of phase or sequence in the life cycle, such as an unwanted pregnancy or the illness of a child, can be particularly stressful.

The family physician should be alert to the unique issues that particular family stressors present and to special approaches to helping families cope. Some of these issues are discussed in other chapters in the book, including death and bereavement, substance abuse, physical and sexual abuse, and mental health problems. Marital problems (or problems in any committed relationship), ranging from marital dissatisfaction and conflict to separation and divorce, are common and often seen in family practice. These problems are presented to the physician in many forms, including acute physical or psychological symptoms, exacerbation of a chronic illness, or problems with children. The challenge of handling marital problems in the office illustrates most of the challenges of dealing with other forms of family stress. The physician must see both members of the couple and use special skills to interview the couple in conflict and deal with secrets between family members. The physician frequently must resist the pull to take sides in a conflict. Finally, serious or chronic marital problems usually require referral to a family therapist and ongoing collaboration.

Research has clearly demonstrated that stress has a significant negative impact on health and that the family is the most common source of stress in individuals' lives.[3] Chapter 4 reviews current research on the impact of family stress on health. Many retrospective and prospective studies have shown that an increase in stressful life events precedes the development of a wide range of diseases. The two most stressful life events are the loss of one's spouse by death or by divorce, and both of these events are associated with significantly increased morbidity and mortality. On the other hand, family support has a strongly positive influence on health and can buffer the impact of stress.[4–7] By recognizing family stress and the ways in which it can affect an individual's health, the family physician has an opportunity to prevent some of these adverse outcomes.

Principles for Dealing with Family Stress

There are some basic principles for treating problems related to family stress. These principles are relevant for the full range of family difficulties, but for illustrative purposes are applied to a couple dealing with physical complaints and marital discord.

Because family stress often presents in an individual as physical symptoms, the first principle is that it is important for the physician to understand the family context of every patient's problem.[8,9] Patients seldom come to their physician with a complaint about family stress or a family problem. They usually present with a physical symptom related to the psychosocial problem. The patient may be aware only of the physical symptom and not connect it to family stress or may consider a physical symptom as the more appropriate "ticket" to see the doctor. These physical symptoms may represent some type of somatization for which there are no physiologic abnormalities, ranging from simple stress-related symptoms (e.g., headaches, fatigue, difficulty concentrating) to full-blown somatization disorder. These symptoms may also be the result of stress-related illnesses (e.g., peptic ulcer disease or irritable bowel syndrome) or exacerbation of an underlying chronic disease related to poor compliance with medical treatment. Physical symptoms can be associated with or caused by psychiatric problems related to family stress, such as depression, substance abuse, and physical or sexual abuse. The physician should be alert to all these possibilities.

Two techniques are helpful for detecting family stress or other psychosocial problems in medical patients. The first is to be aware of "red flags" indicating psychosocial factors that may play an important role.[10] A more detailed psychosocial assessment may then be helpful. These flags include common stress-related symptoms such as headaches, unexplained or inconsistent physical symptoms, a change in the patient's affect or the manner in which the clinical history is presented, and who accompanies the patient to the visit.

The second approach is to have a basic understanding of the family context of every patient visit. This step may be as simple as reviewing the chart to determine who is in the family (especially if it is a family chart[11]) or by asking the patient who is at home. This information provides not only a genogram[12] but also the family structure. Knowing family members' ages allows the physician to determine what developmental issues the family may be coping with.[2] Other simple questions are useful for assessing the family context: "How has this problem affected you and your family? What does your family think about the problem you are having? Have there been any recent changes or stresses at home that

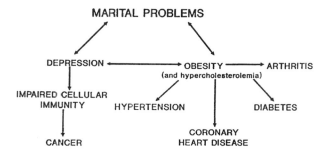

Fig. 30.1. Relations between marital problems, depression, and health problems.

you have had to deal with?" By looking for red flags and asking one or two family-oriented questions, the physician can begin to assess the situation effectively and efficiently.

The following case illustrates a common pattern of problems seen in family practice: marital stress, depression, and obesity with its associated medical problems (Figure 30.1).

Margaret Schafer is 56 years old and suffers from obesity and mild hypertension. She has been Dr. C.'s patient for several years, seeing him every 6 months to monitor her blood pressure and to attempt weight reduction. On her most recent visit, she complained of frequent headaches, pain in her knees, and feeling tired most of the time. On examination, Dr. C. noted that she had gained 20 pounds since her last visit and was spilling glucose in her urine.

Dr. C. inquired more about her mood and learned that she was moderately depressed, had frequent crying spells, and had lost interest in her work and hobbies. She was not suicidal but felt helpless to change her situation. When asked how these problems were affecting her relationship with her husband, Mrs. Schafer gave a long litany of complaints about him, saying that he ignored her and her problems, refused to help out with household jobs, and was spending more and more time at his job. They had not had sexual intercourse in over a year.

Research has shown that these three problems—marital distress, depression, and obesity—affect each other and are difficult to treat independently of each other.[13,14] For example, epidemiologic studies have shown that women in distressed marriages are 20 times more likely to be depressed than happily married women.[15] Other studies have demonstrated that treating depressed patients who have marital problems with antidepressant medication or individual psychotherapy is ineffective if the partner is not involved and the marital problems are not addressed.[14,16] In this case, Dr. C. suspected depression from the clinical presentation and the patient's affect. He inquired about her marriage because of the strong association of depression and marital difficulties. By doing so, Dr. C. was able to place the patient's symptoms in the larger context of the marriage.

The second principle is that the biopsychosocial approach is essential when dealing with family stress and for avoiding a split between biomedical and psychosocial problems. Partly because of our culture and medical training, there is a tendency to diagnose problems as either physical or emotional and to focus exclusively on one aspect of the problem or the other. It is particularly a problem with somatizing patients in which serious disease is commonly ruled out, and the psychological problems are then sought. Most problems have some physical and psychological components that are best assessed simultaneously. In addition, most problems have an interpersonal as well as a psychological or intrapsychic component. For example, depression is often caused or exacerbated by relationship problems, and these problems may worsen as a result of the depression. The biopsychosocial approach allows the physician to choose the most relevant levels or systems for intervention. To return to the Schafer case:

At a follow up visit 1 week later, Dr. C. reviewed Mrs. Schafer's laboratory results and discussed his assessment with her. He explained that she was suffering from a major depression and that it had caused her to gain additional weight, which had precipitated diabetes. He prescribed an oral hypoglycemic and an antidepressant, fluoxetine (Prozac). He also suggested that the depression and the martial problems influence each other negatively and that the combination of the two was affecting her physical health as well.

In this case, Dr. C. thought it was important to intervene at three levels: treat the medical complications from her obesity, start her on an antidepressant, and begin discussing her marital problems.

The third principle is that it is important for the physician to maintain an alliance with each family member and to avoid taking sides in any conflict. In our society when problems develop, whether they are riots in our cities or emotional difficulties, we tend to look for someone to blame. Similarly, when there are family conflicts, family members may see someone else as the problem or the one to blame and then try to get others to validate their view. Thus patients may present to the physician with complaints about another family member, such as "My husband drinks too much," "I think my wife is having an affair," or "Our son won't listen to us any more." They are usually looking for the physician's support and suggestions for how the family member should change. The physician's usual instinct is to listen to patients' story, empathize with them, and support or validate their assessment of the problem, inadvertently taking the patients' side in the problem or conflict. Taking any side, that of the patient or of another party, is rarely helpful when there are family conflicts. In fact, it can make it more difficult for the patient to resolve the problems. If the physician accepts and agrees with the patient's view of an interpersonal problem, the patient may use the physician's comments against the other person ("My doctor said you are wrong"), which makes it less likely that patients will change their own behavior ("I am not the problem") and more difficult for the physician to engage the other family member in counseling to resolve the problem.

An alternative, more effective way to view family conflicts is that they are a result of problematic interpersonal relationships in which each person involved has some responsibility and some opportunity for improving the situation. Taking this approach, the physician avoids taking sides or blaming anyone for family problems but works to establish a therapeutic relationship with the patient and each person involved in the problem. In practice, this approach means listening to the patient's story and acknowledging and empathizing with the stress it is causing without validating the patient's assessment as to what the problem is or who is to blame. As early as possible the physician can explain that with a family problem it is helpful to involve the other relevant family members. To listen repeatedly to a patient complain about another family member can be similar to only prescribing pain medication for a peptic ulcer; it may make the patient feel better acutely but does not deal with the underlying problems. In this case, Dr. C. recognized the risk of listening too long to his patient's complaints about her husband:

Mrs. Schafer agreed with Dr. C.'s assessment of her marital problems and said she thought her husband's "workaholism" was making her more depressed and causing her to eat more. Dr. C. gently interrupted her new complaints about her husband and explained that he thought it was important to address the couple's problems, and he would be willing to try and help them. She said she wasn't sure how Dr. C. could help, but she would appreciate anything he could do. Dr. C. said he would be glad to work with and support both of them in making whatever changes were necessary.

The fourth principle is that to adequately assess and treat significant family problems, it is necessary to convene other relevant family members. It is often difficult to assess or treat these family problems by seeing the patient alone. When there is family or marital distress, it is most efficient to bring the other relevant family members in for an assessment session. Often a simple invitation (e.g., "I'd like your husband to join you for the next visit") is all that is necessary. Family members often accompany patients to doctor visits and are in the waiting room, but if the problems are long-standing or particularly conflictual, it may take more time and effort to convene the couple or family. The other family member may be reluctant to come in, fearing that the physician will blame him or her for the problem. The patient may even say this to the family member ("Dr. C. thinks you are causing my headaches, so he wants you to come for my next appointment"). Patients may also be reluctant to bring the other family member in, knowing that the physician will hear another side of the story or fearing what changes they will have to make. The patient may say that the family member either cannot come in (due to work, lack of child care or transportation) or refuses to come in (is not interested in the problem, refuses counseling). It is important not to accept at face value the patient's word that the family member refuses to come in.

If it seems likely that the family member will attend a meeting, it is often sufficient to ask the patient to invite the family member in. The patient can be "coached" with specific instructions as to what to say to the family member. If there is some uncertainty about how the patient will present an invitation to the family member, it can be helpful to write a brief letter, in the presence of the patient, inviting the family member. The patient can then deliver the note. This method ensures that the patient does not distort the physician's message. If there seems to be major resistance to the family member's coming in, calling the family member directly, with the patient's permission (ideally with the patient present), can be effective. Family members are more likely to come in if they are told how they can help with the patient's problems or concerns and if the physician does not seem to blame the family members or immediately suggest that they need therapy.

If the patient refuses to involve the family member, the physician can acknowledge that there is a family problem but that the patient is not ready or able to deal with it at this time. Involving family members is a process that can take time. It is analogous to the patient who has an elevated cholesterol level but is not yet willing or able to make dietary changes. If the physician is unable to engage the family member in treatment, the patient can be referred to a family therapist who can spend more time and effort with the patient to try to move the other family member into counseling. In the case of Mrs. Schafer, further discussion made clear her cautiousness about inviting her husband in. Dr. C. had to be sensitive to her reluctance without giving up the importance of such a visit:

Dr. C. explained to Mrs. Schafer that he did not know whether she or her husband would decide to change, but he thought it important for him to meet with both of them together to learn more about the problems they were having and how it was affecting her depression. Mrs. Schafer immediately claimed that her husband would never come in for a joint appointment, that he avoided doctors, and he would never agree to counseling. Moreover, she explained, he could not get time off from his job during the day. Dr. C. suggested that she think more about it, and they could discuss it at her next visit.

Sensing that getting Mrs. Schafer's husband into the office would be difficult, at the next visit Dr. C. asked her if she objected to him calling Mr. Schafer directly to explain the importance of his participation. She reluctantly agreed and gave Dr. C. her husband's phone number at work. Mr. Schafer was surprised to receive the call, but said he shared Dr. C.'s concern about his wife's health and her mood swings. Over the past few months, he said she had become so irritable that he felt he had to avoid her to keep from being yelled at. Dr. C. asked if he would be willing to join his wife at her next medical visit in 2 weeks to share his thoughts about her health and any problems that resulted. Mr. Schafer cautiously agreed to accompany his wife if Dr. C. thought he might be helpful.

In this situation, Mrs. Schafer wanted to complain more about her husband and his insensitivity but was reluctant to have him come in for a session. Dr. C. recognized that the only way to evaluate the marital problems accurately was to see the couple together and not blame either person for the problems. It is common for the reluctant partner to be willing to participate in a couple's session as a resource who can be helpful, not as someone to be blamed for the patient's problems.

Occasionally, the physician faces an acute crisis in which the safety of a family member is in jeopardy, such as physical abuse or family violence. In that case, the physician may need to intervene on behalf of the individual patient to establish safety. Such interventions, though, should not be seen as taking sides but as addressing an acute crisis in a direct manner. It is still important for the physician to think about the problem as a complex interaction of many relational factors. It enables the physician to continue treating the couple or family after the crisis. By maintaining an alliance with both partners, the physician may be able to avert future crises. When the physician is successful in convening a family meeting or conference, it is useful to organize the session ahead of time.

The fifth principle is that when assessing a family or couple, it is important to have a specific plan for conducting a family conference. The general goals of conducting a family or couple conference are to join with the family, establish specific goals, facilitate discussions, identify resources and supports, and establish a plan that the family can agree to. The

details of conducting a family conference are discussed in Chapter 4 and outlined in Table 30.1.

Dr. C. scheduled a 45-minute appointment to meet with the Schafers during an afternoon he normally devotes to counseling. He began by thanking Mr. Schafer for joining his wife for the appointment and by explaining how helpful it was when a spouse was willing to participate in the partner's medical care. He spent 5 minutes learning more about Mr. Schafer, his work, and his interests. He then inquired about the rest of the family and began constructing a genogram (Fig. 30.2). He turned to Mrs. Schafer and asked how she was doing. Then he asked her husband how he thought she was doing. This quickly

Table 30.1 **Steps for Conducting a Family Conference**

Preconference tasks
Set the stage
    Choose your contact person
    Establish a rationale
    Establish who will attend
    Set the appointment
Review the genogram
    Prepare the genogram
    Note the family's life cycle stage
Develop hypotheses
    Set goals for the interview
    Develop tentative hypotheses about the family and its
        concerns
    Develop a strategy for conducting the interview

Phases of a family conference
Phase 1: socialize
    Greet the family
    Orient the family to the room
    Join with each family member
Phase 2: set the goals (approximately 5 minutes)
    Solicit goals for the session from each person who wishes
        to speak
    Make each goal clear, concise, and realistic
    Add any other necessary goals
    Prioritize the goals
Phase 3: Discuss the problem or issue(s) (approximately 15
    minutes)
    Solicit each person's point of view
    Encourage the family to ask questions
    Ask how the family dealt with similar past problems
Phase 4: Identify resources (approximately 10 minutes)
    Identify family strengths
    Identify medical resources
    Identify community resources
Phase 5: Establish a plan (approximately 10 minutes)
    Solicit the family's plan
    Contact with the family regarding their concerns, including
        referral or reappointment if necessary
    Ask for any remaining questions about the plan
    Conclude the family conference

Postconference tasks
Revise the genogram
Revise the preconference hypotheses
Write up a conference report, including
    Attendance
    Problem list
    Assessment of family functioning
    Family strengths and resources
    Treatment plan

Source: McDaniel et al,[1] with permission.

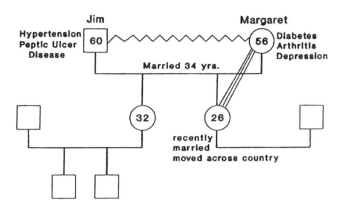

Fig. 30.2. Genogram of the Schafer family.

erupted into an argument about their relationship, which Dr. C interrupted. He explained that he could see that Mrs. Schafer's medical problems had caused significant stress for both of them and their relationship, and he wanted to hear from each of them about those problems.

One at a time, Dr. C. had Mr. and Mrs. Schafer describe their views of the marital problems, blocking any interruptions by the other. He inquired more generally about the history of their relationship and their family, focusing on their achievements, especially the raising of two children, who were now adults. This history revealed that the couple had a stable relationship without major difficulties until 2 years ago, when their daughter, to whom Mrs. Schafer had been close, married and moved across the country. Since then, the couple had been having an increasing number of arguments, and Mr. Schafer was spending more time at work.

The sixth principle is that when treating family or other relationship problems, the goal of treatment is to help the family members decide how they want to deal with the problem, not to fix or cure the problem for them. Physicians are trained in the treatment of acute medical problems, in which a diagnosis is made and a specific treatment is instituted or prescribed. The goal is to cure the disease or treat the symptoms. When this approach is applied to psychosocial difficulties, a number of problems develop. First, the physician may be overwhelmed by the responsibility for curing these difficulties and may avoid identifying them for fear of "opening Pandora's box." Second, these problems are rarely amenable to quick fixes or cures but are usually lifelong problems that require considerable effort to overcome. Lastly, the responsibility for change must lie with the patient and family. The physician's responsibility is to make treatment options available to the patient in a manner that is acceptable to the patient and family.

Toward the end of the 45-minute session with the Schafers, Dr. C. gave the couple the following assessment: "I can see that you are both experiencing a tremendous amount of stress. Part of your difficulty results from normal stresses experienced by couples when their last child leaves home and moves away, especially when the parents are as close to the child as you are to your daughter. I think these stresses have been complicated by Mrs. Schafer's health problems, which are stressful on their own, and by Mr. Schafer's work demands. With all that you are having to cope with, it is not surprising that some of this has come between you and you are having some problems in your relationship."

After soliciting the couple's reaction and general agreement with

his assessment, Dr. C. made a recommendation: "I am very concerned about the problems you are having, particularly because of their impact on Mrs. Schafer's health. I am also concerned about their effect on your health, Mr. Schafer, and wonder if you would consider coming in for a general checkup. [Mr. Schafer nods]. If the two of you have found this session helpful, I would be willing to meet with you both for four or five sessions to see if I can help you sort out some of these problems and reduce the amount of stress you are both experiencing. Then I would see either of you separately for your medical problems. What do you both think?"

The seventh principle is that early on, physicians must decide if they can deal with the family problem via primary care family counseling or if a referral to a family therapist is necessary. Deciding whether the family physician can treat a family or marital problem with primary care counseling depends on the interests, expertise, and time availability of the physician. Obviously, a physician who does not have the interest, time, or additional training in family counseling should refer these problems to a skilled therapist. But many family physicians find these problems interesting, challenging, and enriching to their practice, and want to counsel families in their practice.[17]

Table 30.2 shows the types of problems that can be usually managed by primary care counseling and those that usually require referral to a mental health professional. Marital or couple's problems can usually be managed by the family physician in the following cases: (1) The problem is situational and has a recent onset. These areas include difficulty related to recent changes or life cycle transitions, such as coping with a new baby, recent illness, and death in the family. (2) The problem is specific rather than general. The more clearly a couple can define the problem, the more likely it is that brief office counseling can be effective. Vague concerns about "communication problems" or being "unhappy with the relationship" are likely to be more difficult to treat. (3) The couple has a good relationship and is motivated to change. Couples who have a long-standing history of difficulties or

Table 30.2. **When to Treat and When to Refer Family Problems to a Family Therapist**

Problems commonly seen during primary care counseling
    Adjustment to the diagnosis of a new illness
    Other adjustment or situational disorders
    Crises of limited severity or duration
    Behavioral problems
    Mild depressive reactions
    Mild anxiety reactions
    Uncomplicated grief reactions

Problems commonly referred to a mental health specialist
    Suicidal or homicidal ideation, intent, or behavior
    Psychotic behavior
    Sexual or physical abuse
    Substance abuse
    Somatic fixation
    Moderate to severe marital and sexual problems
    Multiproblem family situations
    Problems resistant to change during primary care counseling

Source: McDaniel et al,[1] with permission.

in which one partner seems uninterested in counseling should be referred to a marital therapist.

In general, primary care couples counseling should be short term with the focus on problem solving. A specific contract with the goals and format of counseling can be negotiated with the couple. This contract includes the number of sessions (usually four to eight), the frequency of visits (weekly to monthly), and the length of visits (30 to 45 minutes). The couple should decide together what changes they want to make during counseling, and these goals are used to determine whether progress is being made. If significant progress has not been made at the end of the agreed-on number of visits, the couple should be referred to a marital therapist.

The use of a quid pro quo technique can be effective for short-term marital counseling. With this approach the couple identifies the behaviors they would like each other to change. Each partner then agrees to try a new behavior in exchange for a new behavior the other partner tries. In this way the couple builds trust and begins to have their needs met. It is often useful to have the couple carry out specific tasks between counseling visits and to give feedback to each other about any progress.

With the Schafers, Dr. C.'s initial assessment was that their marital problems were not chronic, their relationship had been healthy in the past, and that a trial of primary care family counseling was reasonable. The couple agreed, and at the next visit they negotiated a specific contract to meet for six 45-minute sessions 2 weeks apart, focusing on how they could reduce the number of arguments they had about household chores and find more activities they could enjoy together.

During these sessions, Mr. Schafer agreed to spend less time at work and to assume responsibility for several household chores without his wife asking or reminding him. In return, Mrs. Schafer agreed not to nag her husband about being away at work or completing chores. She also agreed to mention her knee pain to him only once a day. During her subsequent medical visits with Dr. C., Mrs. Schafer would begin to complain about her husband, but Dr. C. set a firm rule that any discussion about her husband or marital problems had to take place during the conjoint sessions.

Although there was initially some progress in reducing their arguments, both Mr. and Mrs. Schafer were critical of the other not living up to his or her agreements. During the course of treatment, Mrs. Schafer revealed for the first time that as a teenager, she had been sexually abused by her uncle. She said that she had never really enjoyed her sexual relationship with her husband who in recent years had developed intermittent problems with erectile dysfunction. She also raised concerns that her husband drank too much, particularly after their arguments. After one argument when he had been drinking, she said he tried to hit her in the face with his fist. Thus there were many signals that Dr. C. needed to collaborate with a family therapist.

The eighth principle is that it is helpful for the family physician to establish a collaborative relationship with a family therapist with whom the physician can consult or to whom patients can be referred. Many family and marital problems are too chronic, complex, or time-consuming for the family physician to counsel. These problems necessitate referral to a marriage and family therapist. Few family physicians have been trained as family therapists. This specialty training takes several years of supervised training after residency. Family therapists share many of the same perspectives and philosophies on patient care as family physicians and are ideal collaborators for mental health problems. Some therapists have been trained specifically to help patients and families cope with health problems, a field called medical family therapy.[17] Unlike medical specialists, whom family physicians meet and work alongside in the hospital, there are no easy ways to find skilled therapists in one's community. The most frequently used method for finding a good therapist is to ask respected colleagues whom they use and why. The American Association of Marriage and Family Therapy, the accrediting organization for family therapists, has a Web site (*www.aamft.org*) that lists certified family therapists by city. The Collaborative Family Healthcare Association is dedicated to developing and promoting collaborative models of health care and provides consultation through its Web site (*www.cfha.org*). Perhaps the most useful way to find a good and trusted therapist in the community is to arrange face-to-face meetings with several recommended therapists to learn about how the therapists interact, their theoretic orientations, and their interests and experience in interfacing with the medical system.[1]

When referring a patient, couple, or family to a therapist, it is helpful to consult the therapist early in the process to share ideas and strategies and clarify the consultation or referral question.[18] If the referral is the physician's idea rather the patient's, it is often necessary to maximize the patient motivation to see the therapist. Using the patient's language and understanding of the problem can help "pitch" the referral. Referral for an "evaluation" or "consultation" is usually more acceptable than for "family therapy." Some patients hear a referral for "family therapy" as meaning that their family is bad or in some way responsible for the current problem. Having the patient make the appointment with the therapist while still in the physician's office can also help facilitate the referral. With reluctant, difficult, or somatizing patients, a joint session with the therapist may be helpful for facilitating a referral. The timing of a referral to a therapist is important. With some patients and families, it takes months or years to reach an agreement about a therapy referral.

Once the couple or family has gone for consultation or for ongoing therapy, it is important that referring physicians communicate regularly with the therapist and let the patient and family know that they will continue to see the patient and collaborate with the therapist.[18]

After the fourth session of couples counseling, in which drinking and potential violence were discussed, Dr. C. spoke about the case with a family therapy colleague, Dr. M., who agreed that a referral for marital therapy was indicated. At the next couple's session, Dr. C. explained his concerns to the Schafers and said that he wanted to involve a colleague with more expertise in marital counseling in the treatment. The couple agreed to meet with Dr. C. and Dr. M. for the next session at Dr. M.'s office several blocks away.

At that session, Dr. C. introduced the family therapist, Dr. M., to the couple and gave his assessment of the case including his opinion that they deserved marital counseling from a specialist. After discussing it together as a group, the couple agreed to see Dr. M. for a series of marital therapy sessions while Dr. C. would continue to see each of them individually for their medical problems. (Mr. Schafer had been diagnosed with mild hypertension and ulcer symptoms.) Dr. C. also agreed to continue to prescribe Mrs. Schafer's antidepressant and to communicate regularly with Dr. M. to coordinate their overall health care.

Conclusion

Family stress-related problems are best treated with a family approach that is firmly grounded in the biopsychosocial model. Recognizing that relationship problems may be a significant factor in a patient's somatic complaints is one of the most important tasks of the physician when working with patients who are in a committed relationship. The physician who recognizes the importance of relational dynamics to patient health can either help couples use their strengths to make changes or, as in many cases, refer couples to a marital or family therapist. Of all professionals, no one is more advantageously positioned to recognize problems and help couples than their family physician.

References

1. McDaniel S, Campbell T, Seaburn D. Family-oriented primary care: a manual for medical providers. New York: Springer-Verlag, 1990.
2. Carter B, McGoldrick M, eds. The expanded family life cycle: individual, family and social perspectives, 3rd ed. New York: Gardner, 1999.
3. Campbell TL. Family's impact on health: a critical review. Fam Syst Med 1986;4:135–8.
4. Osterweis M, Soloman F, Green M, eds. Bereavement: reactions, consequences, and care. Washington, DC: National Academy Press, 1984.
5. Kiecolt-Glaser JK, Fisher LD, Ogrocki P, Stout JC, Speicher CE, Glaser R. Marital quality, marital disruption, and immune function. Psychosom Med 1987;49:13–34.
6. Uchino BN, Cacioppo JT, Kiecolt-Glaser JK. The relationship between social support and physiological processes: a review with emphasis on underlying mechanisms and implications for health. Psychol Bull 1996;119:448–531.
7. House JS, Landis KR, Umberson D. Social relationships and health. Science 1988;241:540–5.
8. Campbell TL, Patterson JM. The effectiveness of family interventions in the treatment of physical illness. J Marital Fam Ther 1995;21:545–84.
9. Doherty WA, Campbell TL. Families and health. Beverly Hills, CA: Sage, 1988.
10. Doherty WJ, Baird MA. Family therapy and family medicine: toward the primary care of families. New York: Guilford, 1983.
11. Farley ES. Is it worthwhile to file by family folders in family practice? An affirmative view. J Fam Pract 1990;30:697–700.
12. McGoldrick M, Gerson S, Shellenberger S. Genograms: assessment and intervention. New York: Norton, 1999.
13. Hooley JM, Orley J, Teasdale JD. Levels of expressed emotion and relapse in depressed patients. Br J Psychiatry 1986;148:642–7.
14. Rounsaville BJ, Prusoff BA, Weissman MM. The course of marital disputes in depressed women: a 48-month follow-up study. Compr Psychiatry 1980;21:111–9.
15. Weissman MM. Advances in psychiatric epidemiology: rates and risks for major depression. Am J Public Health 1987;77:445–51.
16. O'Leary DK, Beach SRH. Marital therapy: a viable treatment for depression and marital discord. Am J Psychiatry 1990;147:183–6.
17. McDaniel SH, Hepworth J, Doherty WJ. Medical family therapy. New York: Guilford, 1992.
18. Seaburn DB, Gawinski BA, Gunn W, Lorenz A. Models of collaboration: a guide for family therapists practicing with health care professionals. New York: Basic Books, 1996.

31
Anxiety Disorders

Deborah S. McPherson

Anxiety disorders are among the most frequently occurring mental disorders in the general population. They encompass a group of conditions that share pathologic anxiety as a principal disturbance of mood with resultant effects on thought, behavior, and physiologic activity. This category of disorders includes panic disorder with agoraphobia, generalized anxiety disorder, social anxiety disorder, obsessive-compulsive disorder, and posttraumatic stress disorder.

Panic Disorder with Agoraphobia

Panic disorder is a common, chronic, and potentially disabling psychiatric condition that frequently presents in the primary care setting. The disorder is characterized by the experience of two or more unexpected panic attacks followed by persistent concern about future attacks or change in behavior to avoid panic attacks. Panic attacks are characterized as discrete episodes of intense fear or discomfort associated with numerous somatic and cognitive symptoms (Table 31.1). Symptoms occur abruptly and reach their maximum intensity within 10 to 15 minutes. Episodes rarely persist longer than 30 minutes.[1] By definition, panic attacks are not caused by any underlying medical condition, due to the effects of a drug or substance, or attributable to another psychiatric disorder (Table 31.2).

Panic attacks are common, with 15% of respondents in the National Comorbidity Survey reporting at least one in their lifetime; 3% of respondents reported a panic attack in the month preceding the survey.[2] Panic disorder has a lifetime prevalence of 2% to 4% in adults and occurs twice as often in women as in men. In half of the patients, agoraphobia is also present. In these cases, patients avoid situations or places where help may be unavailable or escape difficult if a panic attack occurs. Symptoms can become so severe that patients are almost totally disabled. Patients are unable to predict when

attacks will occur, although certain situations may be associated with the attacks, such as driving a car or using public transportation. The disorder usually begins in late adolescence to middle adulthood and is infrequent after age 50. Early onset carries a greater risk of comorbidity, chronicity, and impairment. Between 50% and 65% of patients with panic disorder have had at least one episode of depression, and 20% to 30% suffer from alcoholism or substance abuse.[3] About 20% of patients have attempted suicide at least once.[4]

Differential Diagnosis

Because of the associated somatic symptoms, patients with panic disorder frequently present to the family physician's office. Unfortunately, the diagnosis can be missed because the symptoms mimic cardiopulmonary, gastrointestinal, and neurologic illnesses. Medical conditions that should be excluded are coronary artery disease, mitral valve prolapse, hypoglycemia, thyroid dysfunction, asthma, and partial complex seizures. In addition, many over-the-counter medications, herbal therapies, caffeine, and alcohol may precipitate or exacerbate symptoms of panic disorder. A careful history and physical examination and appropriate laboratory studies, when indicated, are sufficient to identify an underlying medical disorder.[5]

Management

Treatment of panic disorder consists of counseling and pharmacotherapy in conjunction with cognitive behavioral therapy (CBT). Because of the chronic nature of this disorder, patients should recognize that sustained improvement requires long-term adherence to the prescribed regimen.

Behavioral Therapy

Cognitive-behavior therapy treatment may be used alone or in conjunction with pharmacotherapy. In CBT, exposure ex-

Table 31.1. Common Symptoms of Panic Attacks

Autonomic
  Sweating
  Chills
  Hot flushes
Cardiopulmonary
  Chest pain
  Palpitations
  Shortness of breath
  Tachycardia
Gastrointestinal
  Choking
  Nausea
Neurologic
  Dizziness
  Paresthesias
  Trembling
Psychiatric
  Depersonalization
  Derealization
  Intense fear

Table 31.2. Diagnostic Criteria for Panic Disorder with Agoraphobia

A. Both 1 and 2
  1. Recurrent unexpected panic attacks
  2. At least one of the attacks has been followed by 1 month (or more) of one (or more) of the following:
    a. Persistent concern about having additional attacks
    b. Worry about the implications of the attack or its consequences (e.g., losing control, having a heart attack, "going crazy")
    c. Significant change in behavior related to the attacks
B. Presence of agoraphobia
C. Panic attacks are not due to the direct physiologic effects of a substance (e.g., drug abuse, medication) or a general medical condition (e.g., hyperthyroidism)
D. Panic attacks are not better accounted for by another mental disorder, such as social phobia (e.g., occurring on exposure to feared social situations), specific phobia (e.g., on exposure to a specific phobic situation), obsessive-compulsive disorder (e.g., on exposure to dirt in someone with an obsession about contamination), posttraumatic stress disorder (e.g., in response to stimuli associated with a severe stressor), or separation anxiety disorder (e.g., in response to being away from home or close relatives)

Source: American Psychiatric Association,[1] with permission.

ercises are used to desensitize the patient to situations that provoke panic attacks and to assist patients in learning symptom management skills. Systematic desensitization is especially effective when coupled with family and physician support. Exposure to phobic situations should be encouraged. Family members frequently adapt to the agoraphobic's fears, so successful treatment often changes family dynamics. Cognitive restructuring is also emphasized to change the patient's thought process during panic attacks. Response rates of up to 60% have been demonstrated using CBT alone.[6]

Pharmacologic Therapy

Four classes of medication may be used in the treatment of panic disorder. All four are effective, but they differ in terms of safety and tolerability as well as their activity in treating comorbid conditions. Overall, pharmacotherapy is effective in the majority of patients with panic disorder, but should be maintained for at least 12 months to minimize the risk of recurrence.

Selective serotonin reuptake inhibitors (SSRIs) are considered first-line therapy for panic disorder because of their efficacy and low side-effect profile, especially among patients with comorbid depression or suicidal risk factors. Reduction of frequency and severity of panic attacks is appreciated as early as the second week of therapy. In all agents in this class, up to 80% improvement in frequency has been reported. SSRIs have been shown to be equally effective in both men and women and in patients with or without agoraphobia in clinical trials. Currently, only sertraline (Zoloft) and paroxetine (Paxil) are approved by the Food and Drug Administration (FDA) for the treatment of panic disorder. Because pharmacokinetic properties vary within the class, patients who fail to respond to one agent should be given a trial of another. Side

Table 31.3. Medications Used in Panic Disorder

Class	Starting dose	Recommended dose
Selective serotonin reuptake inhibitors (SSRIs)		
Citalopram (Celexa)	10 mg	20–60 mg/day
Fluoxetine (Prozac)	5–10 mg qd	20–80 mg/day
Fluvoxamine (Luvox)	25–50 mg qd	50–300 mg/day
Paroxetine (Paxil)	10 mg qd	40–60 mg/day
Sertraline (Zoloft)	25 mg qd	50–200 mg/day
Benzodiazepines		
Alprazolam (Xanax)	0.25–0.5 mg tid	2–10 mg/day
Clonazepam (Klonopin)	0.25 mg bid	1–4 mg/day
Monoamine oxidase inhibitors (MAOIs)		
Phenelzine (Nardil)	15 mg tid	60–90 mg/day
Tricyclic antidepressants (TCAs)		
Desipramine (Norpramin)	10 mg qd	25–300 mg/day
Imipramine (Tofranil)	10 mg qd	50–300 mg/day
Nortriptyline (Pamelor)	10 mg qd	25–150 mg/day

effects include nausea, diarrhea, insomnia, and sexual dysfunction. Initial agitation may also occur during titration, especially with fluoxetine.[7] Recommended starting and therapeutic doses of medications used in the treatment of panic disorder are given in Table 31.3.[8]

If treatment is effective and panic attacks have been eliminated after 12 to 18 months, dose reduction can begin over the next 4 to 6 months. Treatment with SSRIs may continue indefinitely as tolerated if any symptoms persist, the patient retains comorbid psychiatric conditions, has a history of prior relapse, or is experiencing significant stress and is concerned about relapse.

Until recently, the tricyclic antidepressants (TCAs) were considered first-line therapy in panic disorder. Within this class, imipramine (Tofranil) at 50 to 300 mg/day, nortriptyline (Pamelor) at 25 to 150 mg/day, and desipramine (Norpramin) at 25 to 300 mg/day have demonstrated effectiveness.[9] Important disadvantages of TCAs include the potential for orthostatic hypotension and direct cardiac effects that can lead to potentially fatal arrhythmias in overdosage. TCAs have a relatively slow onset of action and initial worsening of anxiety may occur during dose titration.[10]

Monoamine oxidase inhibitors (MAOIs) have been successfully used in the treatment of panic disorder for many years. The most commonly used agent is phenelzine (Nardil), although tranylcypromine (Parnate) is also effective. In recent years, these medications have given way to more effective and safer products as first-line treatment. The MAOIs require a strict adherence to a tyrosine free diet to prevent hypertensive crisis and have the potential for serious drug–drug interactions with many over-the-counter preparations. Side effects include orthostatic hypotension, insomnia, weight gain, and sexual dysfunction. The recommended starting dose of phenelzine (Nardil) is 15 mg tid with a gradual increase to the lowest effective total dose between 60 and 90 mg/day.

Benzodiazepines are effective in the treatment on panic disorder, are generally well tolerated, and have a rapid onset of action. Because of their ability to potentiate the effects of alcohol and their potential for physical dependence, however, their utility is limited to treating acutely distressed patients until a more appropriate agent reaches maximal effectiveness. Both alprazolam (Xanax) given at 0.25 to 0.5 mg tid to a maximum dose of 10 mg/day and clonazepam (Klonopin) given at 0.25 mg bid to a maximum dose of 4 mg/day are approved by the FDA in the treatment of panic disorder. Benzodiazepines may cause sedation, poor coordination, and memory impairment. Withdrawal symptoms may become evident between doses in the form of rebound anxiety. While these medications are considered short acting in younger adults, they should be used judiciously in elderly patients.

Patients with panic disorder are frequently seen by family physicians and present no immediate need for referral. Family physicians may consider home visits for the treatment of agoraphobic patients until they are able to return to a more active lifestyle. Referral is appropriate when first- or second-line pharmacotherapy is ineffective or for patients who are suffering from comorbid substance abuse or who are actively suicidal.

Generalized Anxiety Disorder

Generalized anxiety disorder (GAD) is characterized by unrealistic and excessive worry about life circumstances in disproportion to actual problems. Patients with GAD may have extended periods of time when they're not consumed by their worries, but report feeling anxious most of the time. Symptoms are typically associated with three different categories: excessive physiologic arousal such as muscle tension, irritability, and insomnia; distorted cognitive processes including poor concentration and unrealistic assessment of problems; and poor coping strategies such as avoidance, procrastination, and poor problem-solving skills. Symptoms must be present for at least 6 months and must adversely impact the patient's life (Table 31.4).[1]

Lifetime prevalence of GAD is 4.1% to 6.6%, but in patients presenting to physicians' offices the prevalence is twice the rate found in the general community.[11] As with panic disorder, GAD is more common in women, with an onset typically in the early 20s. The condition tends to be chronic, with periods of exacerbation and remission, although symptoms can be intensified by stressful life events. Patients rarely seek

Table 31.4. **Diagnostic Criteria for Generalized Anxiety Disorder**

A. Excessive anxiety and worry (apprehensive expectation), occurring more days than not for at least 6 months, about a number of events or activities (such as work or school performance).
B. The person finds it difficult to control the worry.
C. The anxiety and worry are associated with three (or more) of the following six symptoms (with at least some symptoms present for more days than not for the past 7 months). Note: Only one item is required in children.
   1. Restlessness or feeling keyed up or on edge
   2. Being easily fatigued
   3. Difficulty concentrating or mind going blank
   4. Irritability
   5. Muscle tension
   6. Sleep disturbance (difficulty falling or staying asleep, or restless unsatisfying sleep)
D. The focus of the anxiety and worry is not confined to features of an axis I disorder, e.g., the anxiety or worry is not about having a panic attack (as in panic disorder), being embarrassed in public (as in social phobia), being contaminated (as in obsessive-compulsive disorder), being away from home or close relatives (as in separation anxiety disorder), gaining weight (as in anorexia nervosa), having multiple physical complaints (as in somatization disorder), or having a serious illness (as in hypochondriasis); and the anxiety and worry do not occur exclusively during posttraumatic stress disorder.
E. The anxiety, worry, or physical symptoms cause clinically significant distress or impairment in social, occupational, or other important areas of functioning.
F. The disturbance is not due to the direct physiologic effects of a substance (e.g., drug of abuse, medication), or a general medical condition (e.g., hyperthyroidism) and does not occur exclusively during a mood disorder, a psychotic disorder, or a pervasive developmental disorder.

Source: American Psychiatric Association,[1] with permission.

psychiatric help, but often present to their family physician with multiple nonspecific complaints.

Diagnosis

Because the difference between normal anxiety and GAD is sometimes unclear and GAD frequently presents with comorbid psychiatric disorders, the diagnosis can be challenging. More than 70% of GAD patients have had at least one panic attack. Depression is very common, with a 67% lifetime prevalence of major depressive episodes.[12] Patients with persistent anxiety, worry, or multiple nonspecific complaints should first be evaluated for an underlying medical condition. Medical disorders frequently associated with anxiety include hyperthyroidism, Cushing's disease, mitral valve prolapse, carcinoid syndrome and pheochromocytoma. Additionally, medications such as corticosteroids, digoxin, thyroxine, and theophylline may cause anxiety. Patients should also be asked about any herbal products or over-the-counter medications they might be using as well as their use of alcohol, nicotine, caffeine, or illicit drugs.[13] Because of the significant overlap of symptoms and comorbidity with other psychiatric illness, GAD should be considered a diagnosis of exclusion. Unlike panic disorder, the anxiety experienced in GAD is usually specific and chronic. GAD may be contrasted with major depression on the basis of the neurovegetative symptoms frequently seen in depression. Restlessness and motor tension are more commonly found in cases of GAD. Somatization disorder should also be considered in the differential diagnosis. In this disorder, multiple chronic physical complaints occur, which involve several organ systems. While GAD patients often present with mainly somatic complaints, they are usually much more limited in scope than in somatization disorder.[14]

Management

Behavioral Therapy

Mild anxiety should be treated initially with counseling. Patients should be advised to discontinue all stimulants including caffeine and nicotine as well as to participate in a regular exercise program most days of the week.[15] Biofeedback, progressive relaxation, and stress management may be used in individual and group settings and may include family participation. Family members should be included as much as possible to help the patient develop problem-solving skills and to provide an alternative perspective on the patient's problems.[16] Cognitive-behavior therapy may also be helpful in identifying and redirecting anxious thoughts.[17]

Pharmacologic Therapy

In patients with significant impairment of daily function, use of benzodiazepines should be considered. A favorable response is likely if significant depression is lacking, the patient is aware of the psychological basis for their anxiety, and there has been a prior favorable response to benzodiazepines. Results are usually seen within 1 week with development of tolerance to the sedation, impaired concentration, and amnesic effects of these medications within several weeks.[18] Benzodiazepines act primarily by decreasing vigilance and eliminating somatic symptoms such as muscle tension rather than by decreasing anxiety. These agents should be used cautiously in elderly patients, beginning with the lowest therapeutic dose available of lorazepam (Ativan), oxazepam (Serax) or temazepam (Restoril), because of their favorable method of metabolism by conjugation.[19] Several alternatives are available as listed in Table 31.3. All benzodiazepine therapy can lead to physical dependence. Withdrawal symptoms include irritability, anxiety, and insomnia, and tend to be more severe at higher doses or in patients with a prior history of substance abuse. After 6 to 8 weeks of therapy, medication may be gradually discontinued. Reduction of the dose by 25% or less per week minimizes withdrawal symptoms. Rebound anxiety may occur at the end of the tapering process, but typically persists for less than 72 hours.

Buspirone (BuSpar) may also be considered as first-line therapy for chronic anxiety. Unlike benzodiazepines, symptomatic relief of anxiety with buspirone may require 2 to 3 weeks of treatment. The initial dosage of buspirone is 5 mg tid with titration to symptom relief or to a maximum dose of 20 mg tid. Dosage should be increased by 5 mg per day every 2 to 3 days to avoid symptoms of headache or dizziness.[20] In patients taking benzodiazepines during the initial period, tapering of the benzodiazepine should not begin until the patient reaches a daily dose of 20 to 40 mg of buspirone. Side effects associated with buspirone include dizziness, nausea, headache, nervousness, and light-headedness.

Venlafaxine extended release (Effexor XR) is a serotonin-norepinephrine reuptake inhibitor (SNRI) that has been studied specifically in the treatment of GAD. In randomized, double-blind, placebo-controlled trials, venlafaxine was shown to significantly reduce symptoms of anxious mood, tension, irritability, restlessness, and startle response in patients with anxiety. Currently, venlafaxine extended-release is the only FDA approved treatment for GAD. The recommended starting dosage is 75 mg/day with an increase of 75 mg/day at 4-day intervals to a maximum of 225 mg/day. Reduced dosages should be used in patients with renal impairment.[21] The most common side effects include asthenia, sweating, nausea, constipation, anorexia, dry mouth, and blurred vision. Modest yet sustained elevations in blood pressure have also been reported.

Point of Referral

Indications for referral include difficulty establishing a psychiatric diagnosis in patients with comorbid psychiatric illnesses, and the patient's failure to respond to standard treatment. Referral to a mental health professional should occur for CBT either as primary therapy or in addition to pharmacologic therapy prescribed by the family physician.

Social Anxiety Disorder

Social anxiety disorder, or social phobia, is described as an intense, irrational, and persistent fear of being scrutinized or negatively evaluated by others (Table 31.5).[1] Most commonly, patients report fear of public speaking or performance, but the disorder can encompass any social interaction and may

Table 31.5. **Diagnostic Criteria for Social Phobia**

A. A marked and persistent fear of one or more social or performance situations in which the person is exposed to unfamiliar people or to possible scrutiny by others. The individual fears that he or she will act in a way (or show anxiety symptoms) that will be humiliating or embarrassing. Note: In children, there must be evidence of the capacity for age-appropriate social relationships with familiar people and the anxiety must occur in peer settings. not just in interactions with adults.

B. Exposure to the feared social situation almost invariable provokes anxiety, which may take the form of a situationally bound or situationally predisposed panic attack. Note: In children, the anxiety may be expressed by crying, tantrums, freezing, or shrinking away from social situations with unfamiliar people.

C. The person recognized that the fear is excessive or unreasonable. Note: In children, this feature may be absent.

D. The feared social or performance situations are avoided or else are endured with intense anxiety or distress.

E. The avoidance, anxious anticipation, or distress in the feared social or performance situation(s) interferes significantly with the person's normal routine, occupation (academic) functioning or social activities or relationships, or there is marked distress about having the phobia.

F. In individuals under 18 years of age, the duration is at least 6 months.

G. The fear or avoidance is not due to the direct physiologic effects of a substance (e.g., a drug of abuse, a medication) or a general medical condition and is not better accounted for by another mental disorder (e.g., panic disorder with or without agoraphobia, separation anxiety disorder, body dysmorphic disorder, a pervasive developmental disorder or schizoid personality disorder).

H. If a general medical condition or another mental disorder is present, the fear in criterion A is unrelated to it (e.g., the fear is not of stuttering, trembling in Parkinson's disease, or exhibiting abnormal eating behavior in anorexia nervosa or bulimia nervosa.)

Specify if:
   Generalized: If the fears include most social situations (also consider the additional diagnosis of avoidant personality disorder).

Source: American Psychiatric Association,[1] with permission.

be generalized as well as specific. Exposure to the feared situation almost always induces anxiety, and anticipation of the event or situation interferes significantly with the patient's normal routine or relationships. The patient is usually aware that the fear is irrational and excessive, but this awareness does not reduce the physical and psychological symptoms associated with the disorder. These symptoms may include diaphoresis, blushing, tachycardia, trembling, and halting or rapid speech. Fears of fainting and loss of bowel or bladder function are also common.

Left untreated, social anxiety disorder is chronic and may result in severe disability. Avoidance of social situations may reduce symptoms but has no impact on the underlying psychological distress. Significant academic and occupational limitations can occur as a result of the disorder. Patients are frequently unable to complete their education and may remain

in less rewarding careers as a result of their persistent fears and anxiety.[22]

The lifetime prevalence of social anxiety disorder has been estimated at about 13%. Social phobia is slightly more common in women and usually begins in childhood or adolescence. Rarely does onset occur after age 25; however, symptoms may become more apparent as new social and occupational situations arise throughout adulthood.[23] About half of the patients report an association of the onset of their phobia with a specific experience, with the remainder reporting social anxiety for most of their lives.[24-26] Because patients are typically unwilling to acknowledge their fears in an interview format, brief screening questions can be used to improve the detection of social anxiety disorder. In a recent study of 9375 patients, the following yes-or-no statements were found to be 89% sensitive in detecting social phobia: (1) "Being embarrassed or looking stupid is among my worst fears"; (2) "Fear of embarrassment causes me to avoid doing things or speaking to people"; (3) "I avoid activities in which I am the center of attention."[27]

Complications and Comorbidity

Depression, addiction, and suicide are frequently associated with social anxiety disorder. The lifetime risk of depression is increased by four times, and nearly one fifth of patients presenting with social phobia also abuse alcohol.[25] Longitudinal data suggest that social anxiety disorder preexists in 70% of cases of substance abuse, emphasizing the importance of early detection and treatment of this disorder.[26]

Management

Behavioral Therapy

The most effective therapy in treating social phobia is focused on reducing anxiety by reducing avoidance behavior. Components of CBT include anxiety management techniques, improvement in social coping skills, cognitive restructuring, and finally gradual exposure. Treatment may require up to 24 sessions and can be conducted individually or in groups. Up to 75% of patients have demonstrated benefit from CBT, even after discontinuing sessions. Relapse rates are significantly higher following discontinuation of effective pharmacotherapy, supporting the consideration of CBT as initial treatment in appropriate patients.[28]

Pharmacologic Therapy

Selective serotonin reuptake inhibitors (SSRIs) are considered an appropriate first-line therapy for generalized social anxiety disorder. Controlled trials of paroxetine (Paxil), fluvoxamine (Luvox), and sertraline (Zoloft) have demonstrated acute treatment improvement rates in 50% to 75% of patients.[29] A recent open trial of citalopram (Celexa) has shown effectiveness as well.[30] As a class, these agents provide the benefit of an antidepressant, are non–habit-forming, and have a relatively low side-effect profile. Because of their delayed onset of action, the SSRIs are not appropriate for acute anxiety episodes. Common adverse reactions include nausea, dry mouth, headache, and sexual dysfunction. SSRIs should not be used within 2 weeks of MAOIs because of the potential for serious or fatal interactions.

Benzodiazepines have long been effectively used in the treatment of acute social phobia because of their rapid onset and tolerability. Improvement rates of 40% to 80% have been demonstrated in controlled studies of alprazolam (Xanax) and clonazepam (Klonopin).[31] Benzodiazepines should be used cautiously in patients with a history of substance abuse because of their ability to produce physical dependence. With the introduction of effective long-term treatments, benzodiazepines are frequently used in low doses for initial symptom relief in combination with SSRIs and CBT.

Controlled clinical trials demonstrate that approximately two third of patients with generalized social anxiety disorder will achieve improvement with MAOIs. The typical recommendation for treatment is phenelzine (Nardil), 45 to 90 mg per day.[32] Careful consideration should be given to dietary restrictions and risks associated with the use of MAOIs. Strict adherence to a low tyramine diet is required to prevent potentially fatal hypertensive reactions. Many over-the-counter medications are contraindicated in patients using MAOIs, including several antihistamines and decongestants. Common adverse effects include weight gain, sedation, postural hypotension, and sexual dysfunction.

While controlled trials using beta-blockers for generalized social phobia have shown little effectiveness, these agents are clinically effective in low doses episodically for performance anxiety.[33] Typically, propranolol (Inderal) 10 to 40 mg is used. These agents are contraindicated in patients with asthma, sinus bradycardia, second- or third-degree heart block, congestive heart failure, and cardiogenic shock.

Obsessive-Compulsive Disorder

Obsessions are recurrent, intrusive thoughts, impulses, or images that are perceived as inappropriate, grotesque, or forbidden (Table 31.6).[1] Obsessions are uncontrollable, and patients often feel they will unwillingly act upon these impulses. Common themes include contamination, self-doubt, need for order or symmetry, or loss of control of violent or sexual impulses.

Compulsions are repetitive behaviors or thoughts that reduce the anxiety accompanying the obsessions. They may include physical behaviors such as checking locks or hand washing or mental acts such as counting or praying. Patients are frequently aware that their behavior is excessive and irrational.

Obsessive-compulsive disorder (OCD) occurs equally in men and women, although the onset is frequently earlier in men. While once considered rare, OCD is now recognized as relatively common with a lifetime prevalence of 2.5%.[34] Age of onset is usually during late adolescence or early adulthood, although some childhood presentations have been reported. Presentation in late adulthood is rare and should prompt an investigation for an organic cause. The onset may be insidious or acute; however, the disorder is usually chronic. Even in pa-

Table 31.6. Diagnostic Criteria for Obsessive-Compulsive Disorder

A. Obsessions or compulsions

Obsessions as defined by 1, 2, 3, and 4:
1. Recurrent and persistent thoughts, impulses, or images that are experienced, at some time during the disturbance, as intrusive and inappropriate and that cause marked anxiety or distress.
2. The thoughts, impulses, or images are not simply excessive worries about real-life problems.
3. The person attempts to ignore or suppress such thoughts, impulses, or images or to neutralize them with some other thought or action.
4. The person recognizes that the obsessional thoughts, impulses, or images are a product of his or her own mind (not imposed from without, as in thought insertion).

Compulsions as defined by 1 and 2:
1. Repetitive behaviors (e.g., hand-washing, ordering, checking) or mental acts (e.g., praying, counting, repeating words silently) that the person feels driven to perform in response to an obsession, or according to rules that must be applied rigidly.
2. The behaviors or mental acts are aimed at preventing or reducing distress or preventing some dreaded event or situation; however, these behaviors or mental acts either are not connected in a realistic way with what they are designed to neutralize or prevent or are clearly excessive.

B. At some point during the course of the disorder, the person has recognized that the obsessions or compulsions are excessive or unreasonable. Note: This does not apply to children.

C. The obsessions or compulsions cause marked distress, are time-consuming (take more than 1 hour a day), or significantly interfere with the person's normal routine, occupational (or academic) functioning, or usual social activities or relationships.

D. If another axis I disorder is present, the content of the obsessions or compulsions is not restricted to it (e.g., preoccupation with food in the presence of an eating disorder; hair pulling in the presence of trichotillomania; concern with appearance in the presence of body dysmorphic disorder; preoccupation with having a serious illness in the presence of hypochondriasis; preoccupation with sexual urges or fantasies in the presence of paraphilia; or guilty ruminations in the presence of major depressive disorder).

E. The disturbance is not due to the direct physiologic effects of a substance (e.g., a drug of abuse, a medication) or a general medical condition.

Specify if:
With poor insight: If, for most of the time during the current episode, the person does not recognize that the obsessions and compulsions are excessive or unreasonable.

Source: American Psychiatric Association,[1] with permission.

tients receiving appropriate treatment, elimination of symptoms is uncommon. Prognosis is most favorable when the onset is mild, the disorder begins in adulthood, obsessions are more prominent than compulsions, and treatment is sought promptly.

Because of the nature of the disorder, patients may present as a result of a secondary physical symptoms such as extremely dry skin from repeated hand washings. A supportive, nonthreatening approach is recommended because the patient's embarrassment and fears concerning the compulsive behavior cause reluctance to disclose the source of symptoms. Useful screening questions include: "Do you ever find that certain thoughts and images keep coming into your head even though you try to keep them out? Do these thoughts make sense or do they seem absurd or silly? Do you sometimes feel that you must do certain things over and over even though you don't want to? Does this seem reasonable or does this seem excessive?" Affirmative answers to these questions may prompt further evaluation for OCD.

Differential Diagnosis

Depressive disorders, GAD, and hypochondriasis should be considered when symptoms resembling OCD occur. Of significance in diagnosing OCD is the patient's perception of the obsessive thinking. In patients with depression or GAD, excessive worries may resemble obsessive thinking, but the patient considers these ruminations to be realistic and appropriate. In OCD, the patient usually recognizes the obsessions as absurd. Hypochondriasis is more similar to OCD because of the unrealistic nature of the obsessions with disease; however, the patient rarely experiences compulsions. Physical disorders that may present with symptoms similar to OCD include encephalitis, diabetes insipidus, head trauma, Huntington's chorea, and some brain tumors.

Management

Behavioral Therapy

The basis of behavioral therapy for OCD involves increasing exposure to the feared object or obsession while preventing patients from performing their usual rituals. Therapy is usually continued for 8 to 10 weeks and may involve family members, especially if the family is supporting the patient's disorder by assisting in the compulsive behavior. Although the exposure technique can be difficult for both the patient and the family, 80% to 90% of patients with OCD are improved after behavior therapy.[35]

Pharmacologic Therapy

Patients with a purely obsessional disorder, comorbid depression, or an inability to comply with behavioral therapy often have improvement with pharmacologic therapy. SSRIs have demonstrated effectiveness in treating OCD with significantly fewer side effects than TCAs. Their ease of use and relative safety have improved the opportunity for treatment of OCD by family physicians. In general, higher doses of SSRIs must be used to treat OCD than in the treatment of depression. Fluoxetine (Prozac) at 40 to 80 mg/day, paroxetine (Paxil) at 20 to 60 mg/day, sertraline (Zoloft) at 50 to 200 mg/day, and fluvoxamine (Luvox) up to 300 mg/day, have all been demonstrated to be effective to some extent in OCD patients.[36] Because fluvoxamine is dosed twice daily, this agent presents an increased risk of serotonin withdrawal due to incorrect dosing over that of the remaining agents in this class. Side effects associated with SSRIs include nausea, diarrhea, insomnia, and sexual dysfunction.

Clomipramine (Anafranil), a TCA, has been shown to be effective in OCD in doses from 150 to 250 mg/day. While therapy must often continue for at least a year, the dose may be reduced once improvement in the obsessive symptoms is established. TCA side effects are dose dependent and include seizures, weight gain, sedation, anticholinergic effects, impotence, and cardiac conduction delays. Regardless of the choice of therapy, termination of pharmacotherapy will usually result in the return of symptoms.

Posttraumatic Stress Disorder

Posttraumatic stress disorder (PTSD) is characterized by a cluster of symptoms that occur following experience of a profound trauma such as rape, combat, natural disaster, or sudden violent death of a friend or family member (Table 31.7).[1] Four categories of criteria are required to accurately diagnose PTSD. A traumatic event occurred in which the patient witnessed or experienced actual or threatened death or serious injury and responded with intense fear, helplessness or horror. Upon exposure to memory cues, the event is reexperienced through intrusive flashbacks, recollections, or nightmares. The patient avoids trauma-related stimuli and feels emotionally numb or disassociated. The patient has increased arousal indicated by irritability, difficulty sleeping, hypervigilance, difficulty concentrating, or increased startle response. In addition, these symptoms must persist for more than 1 month and significantly interfere with the patient's occupation and/or social life.[1]

PTSD is the fifth most prevalent psychiatric disorder, with a lifetime prevalence of 8% to 12%. Although often associated with war, it is estimated that more than 50% of people will experience a traumatic event severe enough to cause PTSD at some time in their lives. Of those exposed to such an event, 20% will develop PTSD.[37] Symptoms usually begin within 3 months of the traumatic event. Having had a psychiatric disorder prior to the trauma or a family history of psychiatric disorders increases the risk of developing PTSD. Developing PTSD also increases the risk of subsequent psychiatric problems. Up to 80% of patients with PTSD have a comorbid psychiatric disorder. The most common comorbidities include depression, dysthymia, GAD, substance abuse, panic disorder, bipolar disorder, phobias, and dissociative disorders.[38] In a recent study, the risk for a major depressive episode increased by 5.7-fold in men and 3.4-fold in women compared to individuals without this disorder. Risk for mania increased by 15.5-fold in men and 4.1-fold in women. Additionally, patients with PTSD were six times more likely to attempt suicide. Notably, these risks return to normal levels when patients achieve remission of their PTSD symptoms.[39]

Diagnosis

The diagnosis of PTSD during an office visit can be challenging. Patients frequently do not offer information about traumatic events or typical PTSD symptoms. In addition, depression and substance abuse may obscure the underlying dis-

Table 31.7. **Diagnostic Criteria for Posttraumatic Stress Disorder**

A. The person has been exposed to a traumatic event in which both of the following were present:
  1. The person experienced, witnessed, or was confronted with an event or events that involved actual or threatened death or serious injury, or a threat to the physical integrity of self or others.
  2. The person's response involved intense fear, helplessness, or horror. Note: In children, this may be expressed instead by disorganized or agitated behavior.
B. The traumatic event is persistently reexperienced in one (or more) of the following ways:
  1. Recurrent and intrusive distressing recollections of the event, including images, thoughts, or perceptions. Note: In young children repetitive play may occur in which themes or aspects of the trauma are expressed.
  2. Recurrent distressing dreams of the event. Note: In children there may be frightening dreams without recognizable content.
  3. Acting or feeling as if the traumatic event were recurring (includes a sense of reliving the event that occurs on awaking or when intoxicated). Note: In young children trauma-specific reenactment may occur.
  4. Intense psychological distress at exposure to internal or external cues that symbolize or resemble an aspect of the traumatic event.
  5. Physiologic reactivity on exposure to internal or external cues that symbolize or resemble an aspect of the traumatic event.
C. Persistent avoidance of stimuli associated with the trauma and numbing of general responsiveness (not present before the trauma), as indicated by three (or more) of the following:
  1. Efforts to avoid thought, feelings, or conversations associated with the trauma
  2. Efforts to avoid activities, place, or people that arouse recollections of the trauma
  3. Inability to recall an important aspect of the trauma
  4. Markedly diminished interest or participation in significant activities.
  5. Feeling of detachment or estrangement from others
  6. Restricted range of affect (e.g., unable to have loving feelings)
  7. Sense of foreshortened future (e.g., does not expect to have a career, marriage, children, or a normal life span)
D. Persistent symptoms of increased arousal (not present before the trauma), as indicated by two (or more) of the following:
  1. Difficulty falling or staying asleep
  2. Irritability or outbursts of anger
  3. Difficulty concentrating
  4. Hypervigilance
  5. Exaggerated startle response
E. Duration of the disturbance (symptoms in criteria B, C, and D) is more than 1 month.
F. The disturbance causes clinically significant distress or impairment in social, occupational, or other important area of functioning.

Specify if:
  Acute: if duration of symptoms is less than 3 months
  Chronic: if duration of symptoms is 3 months or more

Specify if: *With delayed onset* if onset of symptoms is at least 6 months after the stressor

Source: American Psychiatric Association,[1] with permission.

---

order. It is essential to approach the patient with an empathetic and nonjudgmental attitude to elicit a history of trauma. In the case of adult trauma, questions may be asked directly, such as, "Have you ever been physically attacked or threatened? Have you ever been in a severe accident or disaster?" Childhood trauma often requires an approach that established normality. "Many persons are troubled by frightening events from their childhood. Have you ever had thoughts like this?"[40]

Management

The treatment of PTSD is complicated because of the wide range of symptoms and likelihood of predisposing factors and comorbid conditions. In general, the goals of treatment are to reduce symptoms, improve coping mechanisms, reduce disability, and lower comorbidity. These goals can be achieved through patient education, pharmacotherapy and psychotherapy.

Behavioral Therapy

Individual or group therapy plays an important role in the treatment plan of PTSD. CBT or exposure therapy, which uses repeated, detailed imagining of the trauma in a controlled environment, can help patients learn to cope with their anxiety through desensitization. Other effective skills gained through behavioral therapy include cognitive restructuring, anger management, and relapse prevention. Group therapy often enables patients to benefit from empathy provided by other survivors while directly confronting their grief and anxiety. PTSD can have devastating effects on family members as well, so family therapy is often warranted.[41]

Pharmacologic Therapy

While behavioral therapy is indicated for all patients with PTSD, appropriate pharmacologic therapy can reduce symptoms associated with reexperiencing, avoidance, and hypervigilance. In addition, effective treatment of coexisting conditions improves the success of behavioral therapy. SSRIs have demonstrated the broadest range of efficacy and lowest side effect profile in the treatment of PTSD. Sertraline (Zoloft) is the only SSRI approved by the FDA specifically for the treatment of PTSD.[42] Fluvoxamine (Luvox) has effectiveness in reducing obsessional thoughts and eliminating insomnia.[43] TCAs and MAOIs have historically been used in the treatment of PTSD, but have essentially been replaced by the use of SSRIs. Because of the frequent use of alcohol and other contraindicated substances by patients with PTSD, MAOI and benzodiazepine use is discouraged. Trazodone (Desyrel) at doses of 50 to 200 mg has a unique role in promoting sleep through sedative properties and suppression of rapid eye movement sleep, thereby reducing the nightmares associated with PTSD.[44] Antiadrenergic agents are often effective in reducing nightmares, hypervigilance, startle reactions, and outbursts of rage. Clonidine (Catapres), 0.2 mg tid, titrated from 0.1 mg at bedtime is typically used. Propranolol (Inderal) in doses of 60 to 640 mg/day and guanfacine (Tenex) 1 to 2 mg/day at bedtime may also be considered. Blood pressure should be checked periodically with long-term use of these agents because of the potential for hypotension.[45]

Referral

Family physicians are trained to initiate counseling and begin first-line pharmacotherapy. If symptoms persist despite use of a combination of an SSRI, trazodone, and clonidine, psychiatric consultation should be obtained before sedative or hypnotic agents are used. In most cases, PTSD patients require referral to a mental health professional for psychotherapy.

References

1. American Psychiatric Association. Diagnostic and statistical manual of mental disorders, 4th ed. Washington, DC: American Psychiatric Association, 1994;411–7.
2. Eaton WW, Kessler RC, Wittchen HU, Magee WJ. Panic and panic disorder in the United States. Am J Psychiatry 1994;151: 413–20.
3. Marshall JR. Alcohol and substance abuse in panic disorder. J Clin Psychiatry 1997;58(suppl 2):46–9.
4. Gorman J. Recent developments in understanding panic disorder leading to improved treatment strategies. Primary Psychiatry 1996;3:31–8.
5. Roy-Byrne PP, Stein MB, Russo J. Panic disorder in the primary care setting: comorbidity, disability, service utilization, and treatment. J Clin Psychiatry 1999;60:492–9.
6. Liebowitz MR. Panic disorder as a chronic illness. J Clin Psychiatry 1997;58(suppl 13):5–8.
7. Nutt DJ. Antidepressants in panic disorder: clinical and preclinical mechanisms. J Clin Psychiatry 1998;59(suppl 8):24–8.
8. Vanin JR, Vanin SK. Blocking the cycle of panic disorder: ways to gain control of the fear of fear. Postgrad Med 1999;105: 141–6.
9. Saeed SA, Bruce TJ. Panic disorder: effective treatment options. Am Fam Physician 1998;57:2405–12.
10. Mavissakalian MR, Perel JM. Imipramine treatment of panic disorder with agoraphobia. J Psychiatry 1995;152:673–82.
11. Schweizer E, Rickels K. Strategies for treatment of generalized anxiety in the primary care setting. J Clin Psychiatry 1997; 58(suppl 3):76–80.
12. Rickels K, Schweizer E. The clinical course and long-term management of generalized anxiety disorder. J Clin Psychopharmacol 1990;10:101–8.
13. Wise MG, Griffies WS. A combined treatment approach to anxiety in the medically ill. J Clin Psychiatry 1995;56(suppl 2): 14–19.
14. Noyes R, Woodman C, Garvey MJ, et al. Generalized anxiety disorder vs. panic disorder. Distinguishing characteristics and patterns of comorbidity. J Nerv Ment Dis 1992;180:369–79.
15. Taylor CB, Sallis JF, Needle R. Relation of physical activity and exercise to mental health. Public Health Rep 1985;100: 195–202.
16. Mathews A. Why worry? The cognitive function of anxiety. Behav Res Ther 1990;28:455–68.
17. Butler G, Fennell M, Robson P, Gelder M. Comparison of behavior therapy and cognitive behavior therapy in the treatment of generalized anxiety disorder. J Consult Clin Psychol 1991;59: 167–75.
18. Schweizer E. Generalized anxiety disorder. Longitudinal course and pharmacologic treatment. Psychiatr Clin North Am 1995; 18:843–57.
19. Shorr RI, Robin DW. Rational use of benzodiazepines in the elderly. Drugs Aging 1994;4:9–20.
20. Davidson JR, DuPont RL, Hedges D, Haskins JT. Efficacy, safety and tolerability of venlafaxine extended release and buspirone in outpatients with generalized anxiety disorder. J Clin Psychiatry 1999;60(8):528–35.
21. Silverstone PH, Ravindran A. Once-daily venlafaxine extended release (XR) compared with fluoxetine in outpatients with depression and anxiety: Venlafaxine XR 360 Study Group. J Clin Psychiatry 1999;60(1):22–8.
22. Schneier FR, Johnson J, Hornig CD, Liebowitz MR, Weissman MM. Social phobia: comorbidity and morbidity in an epidemiological sample. Arch Gen Psychiatry 1992;49:282–8.
23. Kessler RC, McGonagle DK, Zhao S, et al. Lifetime and 12-month prevalence of DSM-III-R psychiatric disorders in the United States. Results from the National Comorbidity Survey. Arch Gen Psychiatry 1994;51:8–19.
24. Ost LG, Hugdahl K. Acquisition of phobias and anxiety response patterns in clinical patients. Behav Res Ther 1981;19:439–47.
25. Schneier FR, Martin LY, Liebowitz MR, Gorman JM, Fyer AJ. Alcohol abuse in social phobia. J Anx Disord 1989;3:15–23.
26. Kushner MG, Sher KJ, Beitman BD. The relation between alcohol problems and the anxiety disorders. Am J Psychiatry 1990; 147:685–95.
27. Bruce TJ, Saeed SA. Social anxiety disorder: a common, underrecognized mental disorder. Am Fam Physician 1999;60: 2311–22.
28. Juster HR, Heimberg RG. Social phobia: longitudinal course and long-term outcome of cognitive-behavioral treatment. Psychiatr Clin North Am 1995;18:821–42.
29. Stein MB, Liebowitz MR, Lydiard RB, Pitts CD, Bushnell W, Gergel I. Paroxetine treatment of generalized social phobia (social anxiety disorder): a randomized controlled trial. JAMA 1998;280:708–13.
30. Bouwer C, Stein DJ. Use of the selective serotonin reuptake inhibitor citalopram in the treatment of generalized social phobia. J Affect Disord 1998;49:79–82.
31. Davidson JR, Potts N, Richichi E, Krishnan R, Ford SM, Smith R. Treatment of social phobia with clonazepam and placebo. J Clin Psychopharmacol 1993;13:423–8.
32. Versiani M, Nardi AE, Mundim FD, Alves AB, Liebowitz MR, Amrein R. Pharmacotherapy of social phobia. A controlled study with moclobemide and phenelzine. Br J Psychiatry 1992;161: 353–60.
33. Turner SM, Beidel DC, Jacob RD. Social phobia: a comparison of behavior therapy and atenolol. J Consult Clin Psychol 1994; 62:350–8.
34. Karno M, Golding JM, Sorenson SB, Burnam MA. The epidemiology of obsessive-compulsive disorder in five US communities. Arch Gen Psychiatry 1988;45:1094–9.
35. Abramowitz JS. Effectiveness of psychological and pharmacological treatments for obsessive-compulsive disorder: a quantitative review. J Consult Clin Psychol 1997;65:44–52.
36. Greist JH, Jefferson JW, Kobak KA, Katzelnick DJ, Serlin RC. Efficacy and tolerability of serotonin transport inhibitors in

obsessive-compulsive disorder. A meta-analysis. Arch Gen Psychiatry 1995;52:53–60.

37. Kessler RC, Sonnega A, Bromet E. Posttraumatic stress disorder in the National Comorbidity Study. Arch Gen Psychiatry 195;52:1048–60.

38. Brady KT. Posttraumatic stress disorder and comorbidity: recognizing the many faces of PTSD. J Clin Psychiatry 1997; 58(suppl 9):12–5.

39. Kessler RC. Posttraumatic stress disorder: the burden to the individual and to society. J Clin Psychiatry 2000;61(suppl 5):4–12.

40. Blank AS Jr. Clinical detection, diagnosis, and differential diagnosis of post-traumatic stress disorder. Psychiatr Clin North Am 1994;17:351–83.

41. Foa EB, Heast-Ikeda D, Perry KJ. Evaluation of a brief cognitive-behavioral program for the prevention of chronic PTSD in recent assault victims. J Consult Clin Psychol 1995;63:948–55.

42. Brady KT, Sonne SC, Roberts JM. Sertraline treatment of comorbid posttraumatic stress disorder and alcohol dependence. J Clin Psychiatry 1995;56:502–5.

43. Marmar CR, Schoenfeld F, Weiss DS, et al. Open trial of fluvoxamine treatment for combat-related posttraumatic stress disorder. J Clin Psychiatry 1996;57(suppl 8):66–72.

44. Friedman MJ. Current and future drug treatment for posttraumatic stress disorder patients. Psychiatr Ann 1998;28:461–8.

45. Silver JM, Sandberg DP, Hales RE. New approaches in the pharmacotherapy of PTSD. J Clin Psychiatry 1990;51(suppl 10):33–8.

32
Depression

Rupert R. Goetz, Scott A. Fields, and William L. Toffler

Depression in primary care settings has been a particular focus of recent attention.[1,2] To effectively treat patients with the many common presentations of depression, family physicians need a systematic understanding of the types of depressive disorders. We first explore diagnostic and therapeutic concepts, highlighting the structure behind the current understanding of these disorders. Then we discuss the application of these concepts to the process of evaluation and treatment of patients, including special populations.

Epidemiology

Almost half of all office visits resulting in a mental disorder diagnosis are to nonpsychiatrists, mostly physicians in primary care. Patients seen in this setting may be in an earlier, less organized stage of illness. Table 32.1 summarizes the prevalence of depressive disorders. Generally, women are at higher risk than men, as are patients with other medical or psychiatric conditions.

Etiology

Mechanisms of depression in three main areas have been investigated: biologic abnormalities, psychological causes, and social factors. These areas are summarized in the biopsychosocial model of Engel.[3] The ultimate causes of these disorders remain unclear. Clinically, etiologic differentiation and specific biologic tests remain limited in their usefulness. Genetic factors may play a role in increased susceptibility. First-degree relatives of a patient with depressive disorder have about a 25% to 30% likelihood of major depression or bipolar disorder. Twin studies have shown concordance for major depression of 50% for monozygotic twins and 25% for dizygotic twins.[4] The variation in risk makes unlikely a single depressive disorder gene with predictable penetrance for specific disorders.

Psychological factors have long been considered important in depression. Cognitive-behavioral theory holds that cognitive distortions, activated by a stressor, lead some individuals to unrealistically negative and demeaning views of themselves, the world, and the future. Some theories of depression place a high value on the patient's function within society. That is, patients cannot be understood outside their social context.

Diagnosis

The *Diagnostic and Statistical Manual of Mental Disorders*, 4th edition, revised (DSM-IV) divides mood disorders into 10 categories: major depression; bipolar I; bipolar II; dysthymic; cyclothymic; those due to general medical conditions; those due to substance abuse; and depressive, bipolar, and mood disorders not otherwise specified.[5]

Diagnostic Criteria

A *major depressive disorder* requires the patient to have a major depressive episode (Table 32.2), and there should never have been a manic, hypomanic, or mixed episode. Symptoms should cause significant impairment and not be due to substances or bereavement. Either depressed mood or loss of interest or pleasure is required. Once the diagnosis is made, the severity (mild, moderate, severe), result of treatment (partial or full remission), and presence or absence of psychotic features are noted.

Dysthymia is used to describe a specific disorder rather than a "mild depression." It is diagnosed when two of six criteria (Table 32.3) are met over a period of 2 years, uninterrupted by more than a 2-month period and not initiated by a major depression.

Bipolar disorders are divided into types I and II, the former characterized by at least one manic (Table 32.4) or mixed

Table 32.1. **Epidemiology of Depressive Disorders in the General Population**

Disorder	Current prevalence (%)	Lifetime prevalence (%)
Major depression	3–6	10–20
Dysthymia	1	2–3
Bipolar disorder	<0.5	0.5–1.0

episode, the latter by at least one hypomanic episode and major depressive episodes. Mania is distinguished from hypomania by the longer duration and presence of marked impairment in social or occupational functioning or the need for admission to a hospital because of danger to self or others. A mixed episode is defined as fitting criteria for major depressive and manic episodes together for 1 week.

Analogous to dysthymia, *cyclothymia* is a disorder characterized by hypomanic and depressed episodes over 2 years, never without depressive symptoms for longer than 2 months. Mood disorders caused by general medical conditions and substance-induced mood disorders are now included within the group of depressive disorders, and atypical disorders are divided into three "not otherwise specified" categories.

In family practice and other primary care settings, depressed patients usually present with physical complaints. Depression may co-occur with medical problems such as chronic pain or human immunodeficiency syndrome (HIV), or with substance abuse. Thus, an organic basis for the disturbance must first be ruled out. The condition should also not be attributable to a primary psychotic disorder. Depressive disorders can be linked in a diagnostic algorithm (Fig. 32.1). The important role of early detection of medical disorders and a possible manic episode is emphasized by its placement near the top of the sequence. There is a spectrum of disease that

Table 32.2. **DSM-IV Diagnostic Criteria for a Major Depressive Episode**

A. Five of the following nine symptoms are present for at least 2 weeks
 1. Depressed mood
 2. Diminished interest or pleasure
 3. Significant appetite or weight change
 4. Sleep disturbance (insomnia or hypersomnia)
 5. Psychomotor agitation or retardation
 6. Fatigue or loss of energy
 7. Feelings of worthlessness or inappropriate guilt
 8. Diminished ability to think or concentrate
 9. Recurrent thoughts of death or suicide
B. Not a mixed episode
C. Causes significant distress or impairs function
D. Not attributable to medical condition or substance abuse
E. Not attributable to bereavement

Note: A mnemonic may be useful to recall these criteria: Depression is worth seriously memorizing extremely gruesome criteria, sorry (DIWSMEGCS). These initials stand for: Depressed mood, Interest, Weight, Sleep, Motor activity, Energy, Guilt, Concentration, and Suicide.[6]

Source: Adapted from American Psychiatric Association,[5] with permission.

Table 32.3. **DSM-IV Diagnostic Criteria for Dysthymic Disorder**

A. Depressed mood for at least 2 years
B. Two of the following six symptoms
 1. Poor appetite or overeating
 2. Insomnia or hypersomnia
 3. Low energy or fatigue
 4. Low self-esteem
 5. Poor concentration or difficulty making decisions
 6. Feelings of hopelessness
C. Never interrupted for more than 2 months at a time
D. No major depression during the first 2 years
E. Never had a manic episode
F. Not superimposed on a psychotic disorder
G. Not attributable to medical conditions or substance abuse
H. Causes significant distress or impairment

Source: Adapted from American Psychiatric Association,[5] with permission.

should be considered. While the criteria for diagnosing major depression are well defined by DSM-IV, subthreshold depressive symptoms have a significant impact on patients' ability to function and quality of life. Depression has also been associated with other adverse outcomes such as increased medical morbidity and mortality.

Related Diagnoses

Several other disorders present with dysphoria as the chief complaint or prominent feature. They should be considered as part of a differential diagnosis (Fig. 32.2).

Cognitive Disorders

Cognitive mood disorders may include both depressed and manic presentations together with indications of an underlying medical disorder in the physical, mental status, or laboratory examination. In particular, abnormalities in cognitive testing, such as disorientation, memory deficits, and attention and concentration difficulties should raise the concern of a cognitive disorder.

Table 32.4. **DSM-IV Diagnostic Criteria for Manic Episode**

A. Distinct period of elevated, expansive or irritable mood for 1 week
B. Three of the following seven symptoms (four if the mood is only irritable)
 1. Inflated self-esteem or grandiosity
 2. Decreased need for sleep
 3. More talkative than usual or pressure to keep talking
 4. Flight of ideas or experience of racing thoughts
 5. Distractibility
 6. Increased goal directed activity or psychomotor agitation
 7. Excessive involvement with pleasurable activities with potential painful consequences
C. Not a mixed episode
D. Disturbance causes marked impairment
E. Not based on medical conditions or substance abuse

Source: Adapted from American Psychiatric Association,[5] with permission.

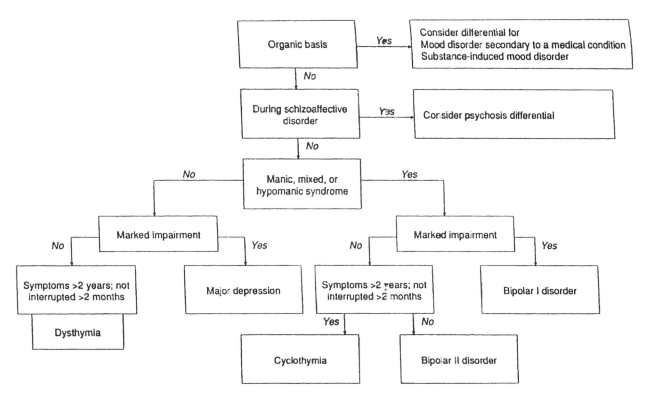

Fig. 32.1. Differential diagnostic algorithm of depressive disorders.

Delirium and dementia may have prominent depressive symptoms. Delirium, characterized by inability to sustain attention, is more likely in elderly or medically ill patients. It is often acute in onset and shows fluctuation. Dementia begins insidiously. Affective lability, periods of apathy, and concentration and memory problems are prominent. Differentiation from the "pseudo-dementia of depression" may be difficult, and treatment may have to be directed at a depressive disorder to clarify the diagnosis. Alcohol and drug abuse and dependence disorders fall into the category of substance-related mental disorders (see Chapters 59 and 60). The classification of the psychiatric disorders induced by substances into each category emphasizes the importance of distinguishing them as a first priority.

Psychotic Disorders

Psychotic disorders are characterized by loss of reality contact. When the depressive symptoms meeting criteria for a major depressive episode or for mania are present as well, a diagnosis of a schizoaffective disorder is made. Differentiation from the depressive disorders with psychotic features is possible when there is a 2-week history of psychosis in the absence of depressive symptoms. Occasionally, treatment for both disorders over time is required to clarify the underlying diagnosis.

Anxiety Disorders

Anxiety disorders, in particular panic and posttraumatic stress disorder, may have severe dysphoria as the presenting complaint. The prominence of anxiety and vegetative signs characteristic of depression may help define the diagnosis (see Chapter 31).

Somatoform Disorders

With somatoform disorders, such as chronic pain (somatoform pain disorder) and hypochondriasis, a patient who meets criteria for the depressive disorder should be assigned this diagnosis in addition to the somatoform diagnosis (see Chapter 34).

Personality Disorders

Personality disorders are characterized by long-standing, pervasive, maladaptive personality traits; they therefore also often include significant dysphoria. The presence of a personality disorder should not obviate the diagnosis of a major depressive disorder. However, a patient who has suffered from intense constant distress since adolescence is much less likely to respond to biologic treatments than a patient with major depression alone.

Bereavement

Grief, though intense, must be seen within its cultural context. The duration may be variable, though morbid preoccupation with worthlessness, prolonged and marked functional impairment, and marked psychomotor retardation may raise the concern that the patient is suffering from a major depression (see Chapter 62).

Evaluation

A clear series of diagnostic and therapeutic steps allows differentiation of disorders and logical treatment choice. Formal screening tools, such as the Beck Depression Inventory[7] or

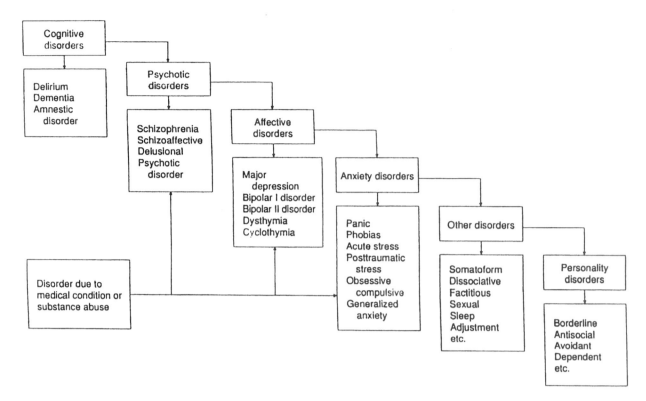

Fig. 32.2. Implied differential diagnostic cascade of psychiatric disorders.

simple screening questions about loss of interest or pleasure may be helpful in identifying whom to evaluate.

1. History: A thorough evaluation should include safety, current history and review of systems, prior episodes of depression (including psychosis, suicide ideation and attempts), treatments, prior medical problems, childhood and developmental difficulties, and family and social histories. The question of suicidal risk is the initial overriding concern. Together with this consideration the degree of the patient's competence to participate in treatment planning must be assessed.[8] History of a previous manic episodes must be investigated. Vegetative signs, including changes in sleep, appetite, weight, and sexual functioning, should be explored because of their relevance for medication choice.

2. Mental status examination: The general appearance of the patient must be noted. Abnormalities in the patient's cognitive function should raise the suspicion of an organic etiology. Loose associations, flight of ideas, or loss of reality contact point toward psychosis. Abnormal emotional states are the hallmark of depressive disorders. Irritability and euphoria may speak for mania. Rating scales such as the Mini-Mental Status Examination or the Beck Depression Inventory may be helpful for objectifying this examination.

3. Laboratory evaluation: Laboratory workup of depression should include basic chemistries, complete blood count, and thyroid studies. Patients evaluated for depression are at increased risk for physical disorders.

4. Consultation: Each family physician must define when to refer a patient. Physician variables regarding consultation include experience with particular drugs, comfort with psychotherapeutic modalities, and availability of reliable consultants. Patient variables include trust in the physician, openness to referral, specific diagnostic characteristics such as psychosis, or treatment failure. Admission of a suicidal patient or treatment with electroconvulsive therapy (ECT) generally requires psychiatric consultation.

Treatment Principles

The patient's safety must be established. Voluntary or involuntary hospitalization must be offered when such safety is in doubt. No-harm contracts may be useful for assessing the risk to the patient; they cannot replace a comprehensive plan. Biologic, psychological, and social interventions must be prioritized. A return visit for more extended evaluation and treatment planning may be necessary.

In the context of depression, several rules based on diagnostic considerations or documented clinical confidence have been formulated to guide treatment[9]:

1. Treat medical disorders that underlie the depression first.
2. Address alcohol and drug abuse before attempting other interventions.
3. When a patient meets criteria for major depression, make the diagnosis and provide medical treatment.
4. When a patient does not fully meet these criteria, psy-

chotherapy alone or a treatment trial with antidepressants may be reasonable.

5. A 6-week treatment period at full, recommended strength may be considered an adequate medication treatment trial.
6. In the presence of psychosocial issues, psychotherapy should be provided in addition to biologic treatments.
7. The effect of treatment should be monitored, and patients who fail follow-up appointments should be actively reengaged in treatment.

When a patient does not respond to the initial treatment strategy, the history is reviewed for hidden alcohol or drug abuse, unrecognized underlying medical problems, or subtle psychotic symptoms. Patient compliance and determination of antidepressant blood levels are considered. The treatment plan is reviewed and revised as appropriate. Strategies used when there has been no response include changing to another antidepressant, such as tricyclics, or augmentation with lithium or thyroid.

Treatment

Biologic Therapies

Differentiation of unipolar from bipolar depressive disorders is crucial because the basic treatment strategies differ. The mainstay of therapy for major depression is the antidepressant, although mood stabilizers and neuroleptics are used adjunctively. Conversely, the main treatment for bipolar disorders is a mood stabilizer, and adjunctive use of neuroleptics and antidepressants may be required.

When major depression is present, treatment with antidepressants should (and in some cases of dysthymia may) be offered. The compounds differ little in their antidepressant efficacy, but their side-effect profiles are diverse (Table 32.5). Choice is dictated by the desire to achieve or avoid certain side effects. Obviously, cost is also an important consideration, highlighted by managed care. Use of antidepressants in patients with bipolar disorders may increase the number of cycles per year and may provoke a manic episode.

Selective Serotonin Reuptake Inhibitors (SSRIs)

The SSRI antidepressants (e.g., citalopram, fluoxetine, fluvoxamine, paroxetine, and sertraline) with almost exclusive serotonin activity have favorable side-effect profiles. Due to ease of use (often once-a-day dosing), they have become a frequent first choice, despite their cost. They have low sedative and anticholinergic properties. There is also a very low risk of death from overdose. They are activating and should be given during the day. This activation may trigger agitation, anxiety, and restlessness (akathisia), which can be disconcerting to the patient. Resulting or primary sleep difficulties may require addition of a medication such as diphenhydramine or a sedating antidepressant, such as trazodone.

Interactions with other medications can lead to dangerous side effects. These are most often mediated through effects on the cytochrome P-450 hepatic isoenzymes. Different antidepressants affect differing subsystems, thus current drug interaction tables should be used when prescribing them with other medications.

Tricyclic and Related Antidepressants

These classic antidepressants include, for example, amitriptyline, imipramine, nortriptyline, and desipramine (from most sedating to least). They are well studied, effective, and generally the least inexpensive. These drugs are also known as serotonin-norepinephrine reuptake inhibitors. Newer preparations include clomipramine and venlafaxine. These preparations may be especially helpful if the SSRIs are ineffective.

Once a medication is chosen, a low starting dose is generally initiated. Incremental increases are made until the expected target range is reached, a clinical response is noted, or unacceptable side effects occur. Such dosage increases are often tolerated every 3 or 4 days. Full therapeutic effects on their mood and energy can be expected after approximately 4 weeks, yet sleep may improve within a few days. The patient may experience increased energy before mood and depressive thought patterns are reversed. Thus the early treatment phase is potentially more dangerous for a patient with suicidal thoughts. Because beneficial effects and side effects vary greatly in individual patients, frequent visits, initially weekly or even more often, are required until the depression has been alleviated.

When the patient has achieved remission of the depression, the medication should be continued for a minimum of 4 to 5 months. In cases of recurring or severe depression, continued medication for a longer period, possibly years, may be best. Once the decision to stop treatment has been made, dosage should be reduced slowly over several weeks while observing for any signs of relapse for several months.

Other Antidepressants

Newer medications include bupropion, mirtazapine, nefazodone, trazodone, and venlafaxine. Bupropion may cause fewer sexual side effects, yet it must be taken in several daily doses. Mirtazapine may be useful in depression with anxiety or insomnia. Nefazodone and venlafaxine may combine the usefulness of the two prior drugs, and trazodone's sedation may make it particularly useful when sleep is impaired. Monoamine oxidase inhibitors are rarely used and have largely been supplanted SSRIs. The risk of a hypertensive crisis can be avoided by excluding foods high in tyramine.

Mood Stabilizers

Lithium is one of the most effective mood stabilizers also used to augment antidepressants. It has antidepressant properties for the bipolar patient with depression as well as antimanic properties for the patient with elevated mood; it works best when used prophylactically. It is excreted renally, so changes in fluid balance or dietary salt intake can dramatically affect the lithium level and produce toxicity. Side effects include gastrointestinal disturbances, hypothyroidism, and nephrogenic diabetes insipidus. Carbamazepine, gabapentin, topiramate, and valproate represent alternatives to lithium in bipolar disorders.

Table 32.5. **Effects and Side Effects of Common Antidepressants**

Generic and trade names	Chemical type	Mean $t_{1/2}$ (hours)	Seda-tion	Anticho-linergic	Ortho-stasis	Usual dosage[a] (mg/day)	Cost[b] ($/month)	Watch for
Amitriptyline Elavil Endep	Tricyclic tertiary amine	35	+++	+++	+++	75–300	5.30 47.99 44.36	
Amoxapine Asendin	Dibenzoxapine	8	++	+++	+	100–300	180.81	EPS
Bupropion Wellbutrin	Aminoketone	15	+	+	+	75–450	67.60	Seizures, agitation
Citalopram Celexa	SSRI	35	+/−	0	0	20–60	69.99	Baseline liver function and thyroid tests
Clomipramine Anafranil	Tricyclic tertiary amine	25	+++	+++	++	75–200	98.10	
Desipramine Norpramin Pertofrane	Tricyclic secondary amine	20	+	+	+	75–200	53.36 105.62	
Doxepin Sinequan Adapin	Tricyclic tertiary amine	15	+++	++	++	75–200	16.94 57.27 48.20	
Fluoxetine Prozac	SSRI	100	0	0	0	20–60	64.75	Insomnia, anxiety
Fluvoxamine Luvox	SSRI	15	+	0	0	50–300	69.99	Avoid with cisapride, diazepam, pimozide, and MAOIs
Imipramine Tofranil Janimine	Tricyclic tertiary amine	20	++	++	+++	75–200	5.40 88.94	
Maprotiline Ludiomil	Tetracyclic	25	++	++	++	75–225[c]	64.37 81.15	Seizures, rash
Nefazodone Serzone	SSRI	5	+/−	+/−	0	200–600	49.68	Headache, nausea
Mirtazapine Remeron	Piperazino-azepine	30	+	+	+	15–45	69.99	Agranulocytosis
Nortriptyline Pamelor Aventyl	Tricyclic secondary amine	35	+	+	+	50–150	60.51 78.43 74.92	
Paroxetine Paxil	SSRI	20	+/−	+/−	0	20–50	54.60	Headache, nausea
Protriptyline Vivactil	Tricyclic secondary amine	80	+	+++	++	15–40	83.82	
Sertraline Zoloft	SSRI	25	+/−	0	0	50–200	58.23	
Trazodone Desyrel	Triazolo-pyridine	7	+++	+/−	++	100–400	34.37 99.02	Priapism
Trimipramine Surmontil	Tricyclic tertiary amine	20	+++	++	++	75–200	67.74	
Venlafaxine Effexor	Phenethylamine	7	0	0	0	75–300	59.96	Headache, nausea

Treat the elderly with approximately half the recommended dosage of each of these medications.

+++ = marked; ++ = moderate; + = mild; +/− = equivocal; 0 = none.

SSRI = selective serotonin reuptake inhibitor; EPS = extrapyramidal symptoms; MAOI = monoamine oxidase inhibitor.

[a]Dosage: usual daily maintenance dose.

[b]Based on wholesale price listings, 1995.

[c]Maprotiline: ceiling dose due to possible seizures.

Psychological Therapies

When asked, significant numbers of patients requiring treatment for depression prefer psychotherapy to medications. For mild cases of major depression, interpersonal and cognitive-behavioral treatments should be used first. Combination of psychotherapy with antidepressants may be particularly indicated in patients maintained on medications, patients with severe neurotic character problems, and in the context of marital conflict.[10] There may be significant differences in the usefulness of these therapies for the short-term versus the long-term treatment of depression. Particularly when both biologic and psychological treatments are suggested, clear agreements, possibly contractual, are necessary between collaborating providers specifying who is responsible for care.

Electroconvulsive Therapy

Psychiatric referral for ECT remains a useful, effective option for treatment of severe depression and mania. Studies have shown it to be as effective or superior to other antidepressant treatments. It is contraindicated in a patient with recent stroke, space-occupying intracranial lesions, or recent myocardial infarction. There are no scientifically valid studies showing longer-term memory loss or disturbances in the ability to learn new information. Maintenance antidepressant treatment should follow to prevent relapse.

Social Treatments

Implications of the depression for marital, family, job, and social functioning must be considered and addressed. The patient's support network must be explored. Expectations regarding length of complete or partial disability should be discussed early. Social work interventions can hasten full recovery, which may otherwise be delayed or even made impossible.

Special Populations

Children

Social withdrawal, poor school performance, a phobia, aggression, self-deprecation, and somatic complaints may herald depression, in which case standardized testing of children may be helpful (see Chapter 19). Biologic treatments are generally considered to be effective for major depression in children and adolescents. The dosage of medications must take into consideration the lower fat/muscle ratio, which leads to a decreased volume for distribution of the drug. The relatively larger liver in children leads to more rapid metabolism of the tricyclic agents than in adults. Prepubertal children can have more dramatic swings in blood levels; therefore, doses should be divided three times daily, a practice that can likely be discontinued in the adolescent. Psychotherapy is frequently necessary, at times with inclusion of the whole family in treatment.

Elderly Population

Distinction between somatic (vegetative) symptoms of depression and physical problems is a common problem in the elderly (see Chapters 23 and 24). Vague somatic discomforts may herald depression. Psychotic symptoms may be subtle and focus on somatic complaints. When symptoms of cognitive impairment accompany depression, three main disorders must be distinguished: delirium, pseudodementia of depression, and depression in dementia. Delirium is characterized by its course, but the latter two diagnoses may be more difficult to delineate. A family history of depressive disorder, concern about the deficits, and an inability to try hard at cognitive tasks all speak for depression.

A treatment trial with antidepressants to influence the reversible portion of the patient's dysfunction may be helpful. Side effects require particular attention. Of most concern are excess sedation, cardiac arrhythmias, orthostatic hypotension, and anticholinergic syndromes. Medications are usually begun at half the normal dosages for the average adult patient, and changes are made less frequently. Side effects should be monitored carefully and levels determined when questions arise. ECT may be useful in elderly patients with refractory depression, psychotic symptoms, medication intolerance, or medical compromise, as rapid progression to severe nutritional depletion is not uncommon.

References

1. Cole S, Raju M, Barrett J. The MacArthur Foundation depression education program for primary care physicians (section 9: participant's monograph). Gen Hosp Psychiatry 2000;22:334–46.
2. Webb MR, Dietrich AJ, Katon W, Schwenk TL. Diagnosis and management of depression. Am Fam Physician 2000; (monograph no. 2):1–19.
3. Engel G. The need for a new medical model: a challenge for biomedicine. Science 1977;196:129–36.
4. Torgersen S. Genetic factors in moderately severe and mild affective disorders. Arch Gen Psychiatry 1986;43:222–6.
5. American Psychiatric Association. Diagnostic and statistical manual of mental disorders, 4th ed., rev. Washington, DC: APA, 2000.
6. Andreasen NC, Black DW. Introductory textbook of psychiatry. Washington, DC: American Psychiatric Press, 1990;191.
7. Beck AT, Ward CH, Mendelson M, Mock J, Erbaugh J. An inventory for measuring depression. Arch Gen Psychiatry 1961;4:561–7.
8. Gutheil TG, Bursztajn H, Brodsky A. The multidimensional assessment of dangerousness: confidence assessment in patient care and liability prevention. Bull Am Acad Psychiatr Law 1986;14:123–9.
9. American Psychiatric Association. Practice guidelines for the treatment of patients with major depressive disorders (revised). Am J Psychiatry 2000;157(suppl):1–45.
10. Scott WC. Treatment of depression by primary care physicians: psychotherapeutic treatments for depression. In: Informational report of the Council on Scientific Affairs, American Medical Association. Chicago: AMA, 1991.

33
The Suicidal Patient

Marc Tunzi and George Saba

Suicide is the eighth leading cause of death in the United States, accounting for more than 30,000 fatalities and leaving nearly 200,000 family survivors yearly.[1] Among the young (those 15 to 24 years old), suicide is the third-leading cause of death, having tripled in incidence over the past 40 years.[1,2] Suicide *rates* are highest in the elderly (age 65 years and older), however, and they are continuing to rise, especially for those 75 years of age and older.[1,3]

The rate of attempted suicide is estimated to be between 10 and 50 times the rate of completed suicide[4,5]; because many attempts go unreported, statistics are inaccurate. Reports do suggest, however, that nearly 10% of all adults have contemplated suicide, and 2% to 3% have attempted suicide at some point in their lives.[1,4]

Major Risk Factors

Suicide risk factors comprise five major categories. Table 33.1 lists specific risk factors by primary category, although many overlap. Similarly, most suicide victims exhibit several risk factors that overlap and contribute synergistically to their specific suicidal ideation and behavior.

Psychiatric disorders comprise the most significant risk factor for suicide,[5,6] with estimates suggesting that more than 90% of suicide victims suffer from them. Depression is the most common diagnosis, but the lifetime risk of suicide in patients with schizophrenia or chronic alcoholism is approximately 15% (see Chapters 32, 35, and 59).

Demographic, environmental, and social risk factors are the most diverse and difficult to discuss. Differences between male and female suicide completion rates are generally attributed to men having greater intent and using more lethal means, especially firearms, which account for nearly 60% of all suicide deaths.[4–6] Social isolation is a common thread among many of the environmental and social risk factors. The role of physical illness is especially concerning: 50% to 80%

of suicide victims have seen a physician shortly before their death,[6] most of them seeking care for medical problems not obviously related to increased suicide risk.

Biochemical factors are the newest determinants of suicide risk and promise to be clinically useful in the future. Research has shown that brainstem and cerebrospinal fluid levels of the serotonin metabolite 5-hydroxyindoleacetic acid (5-HIAA) are lower in patients with well-planned and highly lethal suicide attempts compared to patients with low lethality attempts, irrespective of psychiatric diagnosis.[7]

Young Versus Old Individuals

Knowing the particular characteristics of suicide in the young and the elderly may help assess individuals from these two special populations. Unlike older persons, few young suicide patients have a confirmed diagnosis of mental illness, though a psychiatric disorder is still the most important risk factor when known. Consequently, assessment of familial and psychological risk factors is often more clinically useful. Important risk factors in young persons include substance abuse, family dysfunction and conflict, a history of physical or sexual abuse, relationship problems (particularly with parents and boyfriends/girlfriends), and school-related problems.[2,8,9] Feelings of extreme hopelessness and helplessness, rejection, and humiliation, coupled with a high degree of impulsivity, are common (see Chapter 22). The young are also at greater risk for "copycat" or "cluster" suicides triggered by recent personal or media exposure to the suicide of others.

Important risk factors for the elderly, in contrast, include chronic alcoholism, depression, and physical illness.[3,10] The recent loss of a spouse, whether by divorce or death, is a particularly strong precipitant of suicide among older persons. Older suicide victims are also much more likely to have visited a health care provider shortly before their death. The elderly make fewer suicide attempts than the young, but because their attempts are more premeditated and the means more lethal, rates are higher.

Table 33.1. **Major Risk Factors for Suicide**

Psychiatric disorders
  Depression
  Manic-depressive disorder
  Schizophrenia
  Alcohol and substance abuse
Personality and psychological factors
  Previous suicide attempt
  Antisocial personality traits/disorder
  Borderline personality traits/disorder
  Impulsivity
  Anger/aggression
  Hopelessness
  Worthlessness/humiliation
  Guilt/need for punishment
  Rigidity
Demographic, environmental, and social factors
  Male > female ~ 4:1
  Whites > Blacks ~ 1.5:1.0
  Native Americans
  Mainstream > ethnic/minority groups
  Protestants > Catholics, Jews
  Immigrants
  Inmates
  Single > married
  Physical illness
  Divorce/separation/death of spouse
  Loss of other important relationship
  Unemployment
  Recent personal or media exposure to suicide
Family history and genetic factors
  Previous suicide of an immediate family member
  Family history of psychiatric and psychological problems
Biochemical factors
  Low cerebrospinal fluid levels of the serotonin metabolite
    5-HIAA

Data are from refs. 4–10.

Attempted Versus Completed Suicide

Although the major risk factors for attempted suicide and completed suicide are the same, there are some differences between the two groups.[1,4,5] Demographically, men complete suicide more often (Table 33.1), but women attempt it three to seven times more often. Approximately 40% of suicide attempters have made a previous attempt, about 1% of attempters complete suicide within the following year, and between 2% and 10% complete it sometime in the future. Psychologically, suicide attempts are seen more as an impulsive cry for help related to chronic psychosocial problems than as an act of premeditated hopelessness or anger related to true psychiatric or medical illness. Consequently, attempters tend to use less lethal means (e.g., overdosing and "cutting") than completers.

Evaluation

Predicting suicide for a specific patient is difficult.[11] Because risk factors overlap, because they identify populations at risk (not individuals), and because suicide occurs infrequently in the general population, current assessment tools lack sensitivity and specificity.[12,13] A continuous doctor–patient rela-

tionship that enables the physician to notice changes in appearance and self-care and changes in behavioral, cognitive, and emotional functioning may be the most accurate assessment tool.

Physicians automatically assess many suicide risk factors as part of the complete history that forms the database for all family practice patients; assessing others may require some degree of suspicion. If a patient is even remotely suspected to be suicidal, further inquiry is essential. Some physicians hesitate to raise the topic of suicide for fear it may precipitate a patient's attempt. In fact, the opposite is true: by routinely and appropriately asking about suicide, physicians can identify real risks and prevent future crises.

Questions that help assess suicidal ideation include the following:

1. Do you want to die? Have you thought about dying? Have you considered hurting yourself?
2. Do you have a plan for hurting or killing yourself? Do you have the means to carry out this plan? If not, how would you obtain the means?
3. Have you taken any medications, alcohol, or drugs today? Have you had problems with alcohol or drugs in the past? Have other people thought so?
4. Have you ever tried to hurt or kill yourself before?
5. Has anyone in your family or any of your friends ever taken their life?
6. Have you lost interest in life? What problems in your life would be solved by killing yourself? Do you feel hopeless about your life? Do you feel hopeless about these problems ever being solved?
7. Have you begun to give away your belongings? Have you made plans for your loved ones?
8. What would happen if you successfully killed yourself? Would anything happen to you after you died? Who would be upset and who would be relieved if you killed yourself?

In addition to assessing patients individually, family and close friends should also be interviewed.[14] Suicidal patients may feel isolated and may resist involving others in their problem, but they are rarely without significant emotional contact with one or more people. Family physicians must observe local mental health laws regarding confidentiality but must also strongly encourage patients to authorize family involvement in their care. Physicians should not simply agree to forgo informing family or close friends if a patient is truly suicidal.

Once a patient is evaluated to be seriously considering suicide, an assessment of the acuity of the situation is necessary to determine appropriate treatment.[15] One validated tool to assess acuity is the SAD PERSONS scale[16] based on the number of major risk factors a patient possesses. The acronym refers to *s*ex (male); *a*ge (<19 or >45); *d*epression (diagnosis of); *p*revious attempt(s); *e*thanol or other substance abuse; *r*ational thinking impaired (psychosis, delusions, hallucinations); *s*ocial supports lacking; *o*rganized plan for suicide; *n*o significant other (single, separated, divorced, widowed); and *s*ickness (physical illness). One point is scored for each factor present. A score of 7 to 10 suggests hospitalization is warranted, and a score of 4 to 6 suggests outpatient treatment is an appropriate clinical action.

Another means to assess acuity—and begin treatment—is a "no-harm contract."[17,18] This contract asks patients to contact their physician if they have a desire to harm or kill themselves and addresses several issues: How will they contact their physician? Will they agree to speak with another physician or call a suicide hotline if their physician is unavailable? Will they agree to come, or have someone bring them, to the emergency room? Often patients' response to the no-harm contract can help their physician assess the seriousness of their suicidal ideation and help determine if it is safe for them to leave the office.

Management

Initial management plans must reduce the immediate precipitating causes of a patient's suicidal ideation and involve the patient's family and close friends to create a context for change. Physicians should address the following issues:

1. What problems led the patient to feel that suicide was an acceptable alternative? What circumstances seem hopeless?
2. What are the barriers and risks to other ways of handling the problems?
3. Will the patient accept the possibility that professional treatment can help overcome these barriers and risks and lead to new ways to handle the problems?
4. Who will be involved in the treatment (family? counselors?), and what will be their roles?
5. What will be the ground rules (e.g., regarding "no shows," arriving late for appointments) for participation in the treatment?
6. What concurrent medical care (e.g., substance abuse treatment) might be necessary?
7. What medications, if any, will be used and how will their use be monitored?

The goal of treatment is to introduce new problem-solving patterns and help patients implement them in their own lives and interpersonal relationships. Although suicide risk must be continuously reevaluated during treatment, focusing exclusively on this issue prevents the opportunities for change that can improve the well-being of the patient and possibly the entire family for many generations.

Deciding whether patients can be treated safely at home or need hospitalization depends principally on whether their family and friends can provide a 24-hour "suicide watch" in place of a professional nursing "sitter." If patients are permitted to return home, they and their physician must mutually develop a specific plan for follow-up and treatment. Obvious means of harming oneself (e.g., firearms, ropes, drugs and alcohol, certain medications) must be removed from the home, and patients must agree to return to the office the next day. Telephone contact is not adequate follow-up for suicidal patients. Overall case management, possibly including home visits by a nurse or case worker, should also be arranged.[12]

If social support is unavailable, if patients refuse to involve others, or if outpatient management is assessed to be too risky, patients must be hospitalized. Patients who do not consent voluntarily must be involuntarily committed. Family physicians must know local laws regarding committal and must develop an office protocol for managing such admissions. Nursing and clerical staff, for example, must know how to describe a patient's appearance and how to contact security or police, contact local mental health officials, contact a patient's family, and manage others in the waiting room who witness conflicts. Family physicians should remain actively involved in the hospitalization to facilitate subsequent outpatient care and successful reintegration into the community.

Patients, families, and physicians alike must remain alert about a return of suicidal ideation during treatment. As patients improve and again try to face their problems, they may feel even more discouraged and hopeless than before. Furthermore, as possible psychomotor retardation declines with the use of antidepressant medications, patients may finally have the physical energy to successfully attempt suicide. Continuing treatment and discussing this possibility with everyone is critical.

Underlying medical and psychiatric conditions must also be treated. Such treatment should begin immediately or may be deferred for a brief time until the patient is stable. Interventions range from chronic illness support groups to medications for particular illnesses. Lithium prophylaxis has been specifically shown to decrease suicide potential in patients with bipolar disease and is being studied in patients with other mood disorders.[19]

Prevention

Suicide prevention efforts are as varied and overlapping as the risk factors they address and include both community-oriented and patient-oriented measures.[20,21] Some community-oriented measures are as follows:

1. Improving gun control to decrease the most common lethal means.
2. Improving community suicide education to help individuals learn more about when and how to reach emergency help such as crisis centers and hotlines.
3. Improving "gatekeeper" training so community members (teachers, clergy, police, adolescent peer counselors, senior citizen advocates) and health care providers become more aware of suicide risk factors and referral strategies.
4. Improving access to, and the quality of, community mental health services.

Patient-oriented measures include the following:

1. Screening for the presence of guns in all homes.
2. Screening for a history of mental illness and substance abuse in all patients.
3. Screening for suicidal ideation in individuals who have experienced recent divorce or loss, serious physical illness, unemployment, or other environmental or social risk factor (Table 33.1).

4. Screening for suicide risk factors and mental illness in the family members of suicidal patients.

Physician Suicide

Physicians commit suicide at least as often as the general population; in fact, female physicians have higher suicide rates than women in general.[22] Most physicians who commit suicide have a chronic physical or mental health disorder, and most are successful on their first attempt. Many have a history of drug or alcohol problems; others have experienced personal humiliation from financial losses or a malpractice suit. The family physician's behavioral assessment skills and ability to communicate with other physicians can be of great help in identifying and supporting colleagues at risk.

Suicide in the Family Physician's Practice

The "premature" death of a patient is often difficult for physicians to accept; death by suicide may be even more troubling. When a patient commits suicide, the physician's clinical responsibilities include reaching out to the patient's family, reaching out to other staff and colleagues who knew and worked with the patient, and not discussing fault or assessing blame. Legal responsibilities may include notifying the local coroner's office of the death, carefully reviewing and maintaining the confidentiality of the patient's medical record, avoiding casual discussion of the case in nonprivileged settings (e.g., the hallway, nurses' station, doctors' lounge), and consulting an attorney if necessary.

Personally, physicians must reach out to their own family and friends for support and not replicate the same kind of social and emotional isolation that affected their patient. Colleagues of a physician who has lost a patient to suicide should be supportive, acknowledging that the physician may experience the same denial, anger, guilt, shame, and sense of inadequacy as the victim's family and friends. Professional counseling should be considered and encouraged, as appropriate.

References

1. McIntosh JL. U.S.A. suicide: 1998 official final data. American Association of Suicidology. Available at *www.suicidology.org*.
2. Centers for Disease Control. Suicide among children, adolescents, and young adults—United States, 1980–1992. MMWR 1995;44:289–91.
3. Centers for Disease Control. Suicide among older persons—United States, 1980–1992. MMWR 1996;45:3–6.
4. Roy A. Psychiatric emergencies: suicide. In: Sadock B, Sadock V, eds. Kaplan and Sadock's comprehensive textbook of psychiatry, 7th ed. Baltimore: Williams & Wilkins, 2000;2031–40.
5. Moscicki EK. Identification of suicide risk factors using epidemiologic studies. Psychiatr Clin North Am 1997;20:499–517.
6. Blumenthal SJ. An overview and synopsis of risk factors, assessment, and treatment of suicidal patients over the life cycle. In: Blumenthal SJ, Kupfer DJ, eds. Suicide over the life cycle. Washington, DC: American Psychiatric Press, 1990;685–733.
7. Arango V, Underwood MD, Mann JJ. Biologic alterations in the brainstem of suicides. Psychiatr Clin North Am 1997;20:581–93.
8. Brent DA, Perper JA, Moritz G, et al. Psychiatric risk factors for adolescent suicide: a case-control study. J Am Acad Child Adolesc Psychiatry 1993;32:521–9.
9. Gould MS, Fisher P, Parides M, Flory M, Shaffer D. Psychosocial risk factors of child and adolescent completed suicide. Arch Gen Psychiatry 1996;53:1155–62.
10. Carney SS, Rich CL, Burke PA, Fowler RC. Suicide over 60: the San Diego study. J Am Geriatr Soc 1994;2:174–80.
11. Kleespies PM, Dettmer EL. An evidence-based approach to evaluating and managing suicidal emergencies. J Clin Psychol 2000;56:1109–30.
12. Rudd MD, Joiner TE, Jobes DA, King CA. The outpatient treatment of suicidality: an integration of science and recognition of its limitations. Professional Psychol: Res Pract 1999;30:437–46.
13. Chiles JA, Strosahl K. The suicidal patient: principles of assessment, treatment, and case management. Washington, DC: American Psychiatric Press, 1995.
14. Magne-Ingevar U, Ojehagen A. Significant others of suicide attempters: their views at the time of the acute psychiatric consultation. Soc Psychiatry Psychiatr Epidemiol 1999;34:73–9.
15. Cochrane-Brink KA, Lofchy JS, Sakinofsky I. Clinical rating scales in suicide risk assessment. Gen Hosp Psychiatry 2000;22:445–51.
16. Patterson WM, Dohn HH, Bird J, Patterson GA. The evaluation of suicidal patients: the SAD PERSONS scale. Psychosomatics 1983;24:343–9.
17. Stanford EJ, Goetz RR, Bloom JD. The no harm contract in the emergency assessment of suicidal risk. J Clin Psychiatry 1994;55:344–8.
18. Kelly KT, Knudson MP. Are no-suicide contracts effective in preventing suicide in suicidal patients seen by primary care physicians? Arch Fam Med 2000;9:1119–21.
19. Baldessarini RJ, Jamison KR. Effects of medical interventions on suicidal behavior. J Clin Psychiatry 1999;60(suppl 2):117–22.
20. Potter LB, Powell KE, Kachur SP. Suicide prevention from a public health perspective. Suicide Life Threaten Behav 1995;25:82–91.
21. The Center for Mental Health Services. National strategy for suicide prevention. Available at *www.mentalhealth.org/suicideprevention*.
22. American Medical Association Council of Scientific Affairs. Results and implications of the AMA-APA physician mortality project. JAMA 1987;257:2949–53.

34
Somatoform Disorders and Related Syndromes

Margaret E. McCahill

Patients with somatic complaints and no objective findings suffer greatly and are a challenge to their physicians, their families, and their health care insurance companies. It is estimated that 25% to 75% of visits to primary care physicians are due to psychosocial problems with somatic presentations.[1–3] These patients may consume half of the physician's time, and although usually given a different diagnosis, those who meet the diagnostic criteria for somatization disorder alone represent 5% of patients seen in the outpatient setting, making it the fourth most common problem seen in family practice.[3]

Disorders on the somatoform spectrum are chronic, relapsing conditions. Although not curable, somatoform disorders are readily manageable, providing welcome comfort to the patient and family and satisfaction to the family physician. Recent recommendations for therapy give the patient, family, and physician more hope for improvement in the patient's health status. It is, moreover, the most cost-effective care possible.

Background and Impact

The problem presented by patients with somatic complaints and no apparent cause has been recognized since antiquity. In 1859 Paul Briquet wrote a treatise on hysteria in which he noted, "No illness is more difficult to cure than hysteria. . . . Half of hysterical women recover only when advancing age dulls their sensitivities. . . . They may spend a year or more in bed, completely incapacitated."[4] Patients who suffer a somatoform disorder are convinced that they have a serious physical ailment and generally refuse to see a mental health professional. The impact of the somatoform disorder on the patient's quality of life is enormous: These patients report that they spend 4.9 to 7.0 days in bed per month, compared to patients with major medical problems, who average 1 day or

less in bed each month[5–7]; they average 2.2 days in the hospital annually, compared to the national average of 0.9 days[7]; their health care costs have been estimated to be nine times as much as those of the general population[8]; and 82% of them stop work because of perceived health problems.[8]

The *Diagnostic and Statistical Manual of Mental Disorders*, 4th edition, text revision (DSM-IV-TR)[9] lists the diagnostic criteria for the following somatoform disorders: body dysmorphic disorder, conversion disorder, hypochondriasis, pain disorder, somatization disorder, somatoform disorder not otherwise specified, and undifferentiated somatoform disorder. It is important to note that patients with somatoform disorders do not intentionally cause their symptoms (as with factitious disorders), and they do not develop symptoms intentionally for secondary gain, as with malingering. Although factitious disorders and malingering have different psychodynamics, they are mentioned here in a discussion of the somatoform spectrum because they are in the same differential diagnosis for patients with somatic complaints and no objective findings.

The somatoform disorders should be considered a spectrum, with some patients having a subsyndromal form and some meeting the full criteria for a particular disorder. A patient may appear to meet criteria for one disorder at one point in time and a different disorder at another time. This is especially true for hypochondriasis, pain disorder, somatization disorder, and subsyndromal somatization (diagnosed as undifferentiated somatoform disorder or somatoform disorder not otherwise specified), which are the most common somatoform disorders treated by the family physician. Distinguishing the latter four disorders from each other can be challenging at times, but their management is similar, allowing the physician to consider them as a spectrum and still optimally manage them.

Somatoform disorders are generally underdiagnosed, with few outpatients formally assigned the diagnosis. In a study of general hospital patients, none of the 19 patients found with the diagnostic criteria for somatization disorder were so diagnosed.[10] When making a somatoform spectrum diagnosis, it is critical to ensure that organic pathology has not been overlooked as the cause of the patient's symptoms.

Several classic medical illnesses can masquerade as diverse medical and psychiatric syndromes, including multiple sclerosis, central nervous system (CNS) syphilis, tuberculosis, lupus erythematosus, acute intermittent porphyria, brain tumors, thyroid and parathyroid disorders, myasthenia gravis, and human immunodeficiency virus (HIV) disease, which have joined the list of disorders that can present with multiple, diffuse symptoms (see Chapter 42). Whenever a somatoform disorder diagnosis is considered, it is essential that the patient receive a thorough medical history and physical examination, and that prior medical records and tests are reviewed. This thorough overview by the family physician and the continuity of care with that physician are essential to the correct diagnosis and management of somatoform disorders.

Somatoform Spectrum

The family physician only occasionally encounters a patient with true conversion disorder (CD) or with body dysmorphic disorder (BDD). These two conditions are important to recognize, as they are a part of the somatoform spectrum, but they are not usually managed in the primary care setting exclusively. If symptoms of either of these conditions persist, a psychiatric consultation is likely to be sought.

Conversion Disorder

A patient with CD unintentionally develops symptoms or deficits affecting voluntary motor or sensory function that suggest a neurologic or other medical condition but that cannot be explained by a medical condition, effects of a substance, or as a culturally sanctioned behavior.[9] Examples include paralysis of an extremity, pseudoseizure, pseudocyesis, complaints of blindness, aphonia, and sensory complaints that do not follow neurologic parameters. True CD is uncommon, and because many of the organic causes of conversion symptoms may take years to declare themselves, it has been suggested that a diagnosis of CD be considered tentative.[9] When CD occurs, it is usually seen in a rural setting in a patient with little formal education and of low socioeconomic status; it may also be more common among military personnel.[11] A single episode is usually short but may be prolonged if secondary gain is involved. Most conversion symptoms are transient and respond to supportive treatment; 90% are resolved by the time of hospital discharge.[12] Somatization disorder requires a conversion symptom as one of its diagnostic criteria, creating a connection between these two diagnoses within the somatoform spectrum. It has been suggested that "it is more useful to conceive of conversion phenomena as symptoms rather than as a psychiatric disorder per se."[12] Telling patients that their symptoms are thought to be psychogenic often results in worsening of symptoms.

It is more helpful to explain that, based on a thorough medical evaluation, the symptom (e.g., weakness, blindness, seizure) should resolve quickly. Psychiatric consultation should be sought if symptoms persist.

Body Dysmorphic Disorder

Patients with BDD have a loathing for or a preoccupation with an imagined defect in their appearance or excessive concern about a slight physical anomaly. This preoccupation causes significant distress or impairment in social, occupational, or other areas of function.[9] Comorbid conditions are often found with BDD, such as depression, delusional disorder, social phobia, and obsessive-compulsive disorder.[9] It has been estimated that 12% to 14% of patients seeking treatment by a dermatologist have BDD.[13] Family studies suggest that BDD is part of the familial spectrum of obsessive-compulsive disorder,[14] and thus treatment for BDD may include antiobsessional medications. In a recent open-label study, 63% of 30 BDD patients improved with fluvoxamine treatment, including both delusional and nondelusional patients.[15] While further studies will be needed to establish evidence-based treatment, if the physician notes the presence of depression or other obsessive-compulsive features, a trial of an antidepressant or antiobsessional medication may be indicated. Examples include clomipramine (Anafranil), fluoxetine (Prozac), fluvoxamine (Luvox), or paroxetine (Paxil). Some long-term follow-up studies of patients with BDD have shown that those who had cosmetic surgery often had later emergence of even more severe psychopathology.[11] If the patient with BDD has persistent symptoms, psychiatric consultation should be considered.

Disorders Commonly Managed in Family Medicine

Somatization Disorder

The DSM-IV-TR diagnostic criteria for somatization disorder (SD) are listed in Table 34.1. This relatively common disorder is seen in 0.2% to 2.0% of American women and fewer than 0.2% of American men.[9,16] The disorder tends to run in families, with both genetic and environmental factors implicated.[9,16] Several screening tests have been proposed to assist in the diagnosis of SD in the primary care setting.[17,18]

Somatization disorder is a chronic condition, and patients are usually not amenable to psychiatric treatment initially. If patients believe that their complaints are not taken seriously, they usually go to another physician, increasing the likelihood of unnecessary procedures. An important goal in the management of SD is to gradually increase the patient's insight regarding the psychiatric basis of the complaints over months or years of work with the patient, such that referral for psychotherapy is possible. When the patient engages in psychotherapy, health care costs can be reduced, mainly because the rate of hospitalization decreases.[11] Cognitive-behavioral therapy (CBT) has shown particular promise in the treatment of SD and related syndromes, and the improvement in phys-

Table 34.1. **Diagnostic Criteria for Somatization Disorder (DSM Code 300.81)**

A. A history of many physical complaints beginning before age 30 years that occur over a period of several years and result in treatment being sought or significant impairment in social, occupational, or other important areas of functioning.

B. Each of the following criteria must have been met, with individual symptoms occurring at any time during the course of the disturbance.
   1. *Four pain symptoms:* a history of pain related to at least four different sites or functions (e.g., head, abdomen, back, joints, extremities, chest, rectum, during menstruation, during sexual intercourse, or during urination).
   2. *Two gastrointestinal symptoms:* a history of at least two gastrointestinal symptoms other than pain (e.g., nausea, bloating, vomiting other than during pregnancy, diarrhea, or intolerance of several different foods).
   3. *One sexual symptom:* a history of at least one sexual or reproductive symptom other than pain (e.g., sexual indifference, erectile or ejaculatory dysfunction, irregular menses, excessive menstrual bleeding, vomiting throughout pregnancy).
   4. *One pseudoneurologic symptom:* a history of at least one symptom or deficit suggesting a neurologic condition not limited to pain (conversion symptoms such as impaired coordination or balance, paralysis or localized weakness, difficulty swallowing or lump in throat, aphonia, urinary retention, hallucinations, loss of touch or pain sensation, double vision, blindness, deafness, seizures; dissociative symptoms such as amnesia; or loss of consciousness other than fainting).

C. Either 1 or 2
   1. After appropriate investigation, each of the symptoms in criterion B cannot be fully explained by a known general medical condition or the direct effects of a substance (e.g., drug of abuse, a medication)
   2. When there is a related general medical condition, the physical complaints or resulting social or occupational impairment are in excess of what would be expected from the history, physical examination, or laboratory findings.

D. The symptoms are not intentionally produced or feigned (as in factitious disorder or malingering).

Source: American Psychiatric Association,[9] with permission.

ical complaints may be seen even if psychological distress is not ameliorated.[19]

Pain Disorder

The DSM-IV-TR diagnostic criteria for pain disorder (PD) are listed in Table 34.2. The symptom of pain and its consequent disability is the focus in PD. The patient with PD is focused on the intensity of the pain itself, whereas the hypochondriac patient focuses on the fear of the catastrophic implications of the pain.[9] PD is common, with 10% to 15%

of adults per year in the United States having some form of work disability due to back pain alone.[9]

The clinical course of PD is affected by age, sex, ethnic factors, personality factors, the learned behavior of "painsmanship," and by many other variables, including secondary gain and disability entitlement. PD patients should be evaluated for the presence of comorbid conditions, such as depression, anxiety disorders, or any other psychiatric disorder. The best management of chronic pain syndromes is early intervention after an injury, with treatment aimed at prompt restoration of normal function. A patient who has already de-

Table 34.2. **Diagnostic Criteria for Pain Disorder (DSM Codes 307.80 and 307.89)**

A. Pain in one or more anatomic sites is the predominant focus of the clinical presentation and is of sufficient severity to warrant clinical attention.

B. The pain causes clinically significant distress or impairment in social, occupational, or other important areas of functioning.

C. Psychological factors are judged to have an important role in the onset, severity, exacerbation, or maintenance of the pain.

D. The symptom or deficit is not intentionally produced or feigned (as in factitious disorder or malingering).

E. The pain is not better accounted for by a mood, anxiety, or psychotic disorder and does not meet criteria for dyspareunia.

Code is as follows:
   307.80, pain disorder associated with psychological factors
   307.89, pain disorder associated with both psychological factors and a general medical condition

For both of above, specify if:
   Acute: duration < 6months
   Chronic: duration ≥6 months

Note: The following is not considered to be a mental disorder and is included here to facilitate differential diagnosis: pain disorder associated with a general medical condition—a general medical condition has a major role in the onset, severity, exacerbation, or maintenance of the pain. (If psychological factors are present, they are not judged to have a major role in the onset, severity, exacerbation, or maintenance of the pain.) The diagnostic code for the pain is selected based on the associated general medical condition if one has been established or on the anatomic location of the pain if the underlying general medical condition is not yet clearly established.

Source: American Psychiatric Association,[9] with permission.

veloped a lifestyle of chronic pain has a poor prognosis. The treatment of chronic pain syndromes includes a wide variety of treatment modalities, including medicinal, somatic, and psychotherapeutic approaches[1,16,20] (see Chapter 61). A structured review of evidence-based data on the use of antidepressant medications in chronic pain syndromes (both those with and those without a significant psychogenic basis) supports the use of antidepressant therapy.[21]

After thorough evaluation of the patient with PD, it is helpful to assure the patient that it appears all appropriate interventions have been done, acknowledge the patient's suffering, and explain that the immediate treatment goal is rehabilitation and not necessarily to be pain-free. Rehabilitation requires a treatment plan, which might include medications, physical therapy, biofeedback, pain control programs, and in some cases psychotherapy.[11] As in other somatoform spectrum disorders, CBT may be of benefit.

Hypochondriasis

The DSM-IV-TR diagnostic criteria for hypochondriasis are listed in Table 34.3. The patient with hypochondriasis has the intense fear of having a serious disease; the fear causes impairment in function, and this fear persists despite all reassurance to the contrary. The estimated prevalence of hypochondriasis is 2% to 7% in primary care outpatients.[9]

Hypochondriasis can begin at any age and is seen in both sexes equally. It may fluctuate, and it may become chronic, although an estimated one third to one half of all patients recover significantly.[11] Hypochondriasis may be the primary symptom of major depression, and studies have shown that almost half of patients with transient hypochondriasis had an anxiety or depressive disorder; 75% had at least one axis I diagnosis[22] (a psychiatric clinical disorder or other condition that is the focus of clinical attention). Those with hypochondriasis have real symptoms. As with all somatoform disorders, patients with hypochondriasis require thorough evaluation by the family physician to exclude serious illness, but hypochondriac patients are not reassured by the absence of pathology on testing. It is often helpful to present normal test results with a statement that although it is reassuring that the test results show no serious disease, regularly scheduled visits will be continued to monitor any new signs of illness (not

symptoms) in the future. Some patients with hypochondriasis have been given diagnoses of chronic fatigue, malaise, and others. The World Health Organization–sponsored International Classification of Diseases and Related Health Problems (ICD-10) includes a diagnosis of neurasthenia (literally, a lack of nerve energy), which is rarely made in the United States but is often used in other countries for patients with hypochondriasis.[11,23] The etiologic theory for hypochondriasis with the most support is the amplification hypothesis, which proposes that hypochondriasis is the result of a catastrophic overinterpretation of normal bodily sensations.[11] Management of the hypochondriac patient is similar to that for pain disorder and somatization disorder.

Undifferentiated Somatoform Disorder and Somatoform Disorder Not Otherwise Specified

The patient with undifferentiated somatoform disorder (USD) has impairment due to one or more unexplained physical complaints of at least 6 months duration, and the symptoms seem to be temporally related to a stressor.[11] A subset of patients with USD are said to have subsyndromal somatization disorder, or the somatizing syndrome (also called abridged somatization disorder), which requires a lifetime history of four unexplained symptoms for men and six for women.[11,24] USD has a 30 times greater prevalence than somatization disorder, with a female predominance and a lifetime prevalence of 4% to 11%. The course is chronic and relapsing, and USD patients show excessive health care utilization, but the degree of impairment is less that that seen with somatization disorder.[11] Somatoform disorder not otherwise specified (SD NOS) is a residual category for patients whose symptoms do not quite fit the other diagnoses on the somatoform spectrum.[9]

Management of the Somatoform Disorders

Most of the disorders on the somatoform spectrum are managed almost exclusively in the primary care realm. The family physician typically manages the following disorders without psychiatric consultation, except for unusually challenging patients: hypochondriasis, pain disorder, somatization disorder, undiffer-

---

Table 34.3. **Diagnostic Criteria for Hypochondriasis (DSM Code 300.7)**

A. Preoccupation with fears of having, or the idea that one has, a serious disease based on the person's misinterpretations of bodily symptoms.

B. The preoccupation persists despite appropriate medical evaluation and reassurance.

C. The belief in criterion A is not of delusional intensity (as in delusional disorder, somatic type) and is not restricted to a circumscribed concern about appearance (as in body dysmorphic disorder).

D. The preoccupation causes clinically significant distress or impairment in social, occupational, or other important areas of functioning.

E. The duration of the disturbance is at least 6 months.

F. The preoccupation is not better accounted for by generalized anxiety disorder, obsessive-compulsive disorder, panic disorder, a major depressive episode, separation anxiety, or another somatoform disorder.

Specify if:

With poor insight: if, for most of the time during the current episode, the person does not recognize that the concern about having a serious illness is excessive or unreasonable.

Source: American Psychiatric Association,[9] with permission.

entiated somatoform disorder (including those with somatizing syndrome), and SD NOS. The management principles for all five of these disorders are similar. The first step requires a thorough medical history, physical examination, and review of prior medical records and results of tests and procedures. It is important to acknowledge patients' suffering and the disability that they experience. It often takes several visits to the family physician to establish patients' trust that their complaints are taken seriously and that the physician is knowledgeable about diagnosis and treatment. For many patients it is helpful to have a diagnostic label that enables them to work cooperatively with the physician.[25] For example, a diagnosis of hypochondriasis is rarely given to patients directly, but it might be explained that they have a syndrome that causes a person to experience a distressing amplification of bodily functions and sensations.

After the thorough medical evaluation and the assessment or diagnosis is presented to the patient, a solid therapeutic alliance is established, which is the most essential ingredient for successful management of somatizing patients. The somatizing patient is then scheduled to see the family physician at regular intervals, the length of which depends on how well the patient's illness is compensated. A somatizing patient who is severely decompensated may require brief weekly visits, whereas a patient who is doing well may be scheduled for an office visit every 4 to 6 weeks.[11] It is important that the visits be scheduled regularly, regardless of the development of new symptoms. To tell a somatizing patient to "return when you need to" invites the development of new symptoms as a new entitlement to see the physician, possibly generating new diagnostic procedures. Specialty consultations should be limited and must be carefully handled such that the patient does not experience them as rejection by the family physician. The number of tests and procedures are limited to those indicated by the development of new physical findings, and the use of medications is minimized.[16] The physician avoids giving direct advice, with the patient being encouraged to develop problem-solving skills.[26] In addition to these general principles, the pain disorder patient needs encouragement to understand that the goal is to restore maximal function, not necessarily total relief of all pain.

As noted above in the discussion of the individual syndromes, antidepressant or antiobsessional medication (often the same medication) is often prescribed. A review of the treatment recommendations of consultation-liaison psychiatrists regarding the somatoform disorders revealed that they recommended antidepressants in 40% of patients, anxiolytics in 18%, sedatives in 18%, antipsychotics in 10%, and psychological treatment (CBT or other) for 76% of patients.[27] A review of 31 controlled trials showed that CBT is often of great benefit, at times even for those who have limited insight, and even for those who do not seem to have improvement in their psychological symptoms.[19]

Somatization in Children and Adolescents

Somatization is common in youths, with the most common complaints being headache (10–30% of children and adolescents), recurrent abdominal pain (10–25%), chest pain (7–15%), and fatigue (33–50% of adolescents).[28] Pseudoneurologic symptoms are rare in children and adolescents, and a cause other than somatization should be sought. There appear to be no gender differences in the presentation of somatization until late adolescence, when female predominance emerges. There is some association between pediatric somatization and perceived adverse life events; for example, the death of a family member may precipitate symptoms in the child similar to those of the family member who died.[28] Several studies have associated somatization with sexual abuse, particularly somatic complaints involving genitourinary or gastrointestinal symptoms or pseudoseizures in children.[28] Somatization is one of the most common ways for a psychiatric disorder to present during childhood and adolescence, especially anxiety disorders and major depression. The family physician should carefully evaluate youths who somatize to exclude serious medical illness, psychiatric illness, adverse life events, and maltreatment.[28]

Factitious Disorders

The essential element for the diagnosis of factitious disorder (FD) is *intentional* production of physical or psychological symptoms, with the hope of having psychological needs met by assuming a sick role.[9] Secondary gain is not apparent, which distinguishes FD from malingering. FD is more common in women, and it seems to occur more frequently among health care workers than other occupational groups.[11] Patients with FD often have disrupted interpersonal relationships, and personality disorders are frequent. They may give dramatic, vague, inconsistent histories, and if challenged, they usually leave treatment against medical advice, only to present with the same symptoms at another facility soon thereafter.[9]

Factitious disorder in children and adolescents is an uncommon but critical problem that is often unrecognized for an extended (and therefore dangerous) period of time.[29] The mean duration of symptoms is almost 16 months before detection, and the most common presentations of FD in children are fever, ketoacidosis, purpura, and infections.[29] Children with FD may have been the victims of FD by proxy when they were younger, and they may become the adult patient with FD if not treated. Recognition of the FD is essential for the immediate safety of the child, as well as beginning treatment aimed at prevention of FD and other disorders in adulthood.

Factitious Disorder by Proxy

Listed in DSM-IV-TR under factitious disorder not otherwise specified is the diagnosis factitious disorder by proxy. In this disorder, the perpetrator (usually the mother of a young child), is intentionally causing a physical or psychological symptom or illness in the victim so the perpetrator can assume the sick role by proxy.[9] Dependent adults could also be victims. The most frequently seen symptoms are bleeding (44%), CNS symptoms (seizures, ataxia, impaired consciousness) (approximately 50%), diarrhea and vomiting (21%), fever (10%), and rash (9%).[30] It is important to recognize this entity as a dangerous form of abuse and to secure the victim's safety. It has been noted that Munchausen syndrome by proxy was responsible for 14% of children with failure to thrive, and that the *mortality rate was 9%*.[31] Discovery of FD by proxy would be an indication to immediately notify authorities involved in protecting children or dependent adults from abuse (see Chapters 26 and 27). Emergency hospitalization may be necessary to ensure the safety of the victim until authorities can intervene.

Factitious Disorder by Internet

Widespread access to the Internet and the abundance of Web sites dedicated to specific medical conditions bring a wealth of information to patients, with some of that information valid and very useful, and some of it invalid and without substance. With the availability of Internet chat rooms, patients can join in "virtual support group" sessions for nearly any malady. Since the Internet is largely unproctored and unjuried, it presents an easily accessible medium in which anyone may assume the patient role, obtaining attention, sympathy, and sometimes control and favor from others. Several cases of "Munchausen by Internet" have been reported,[32] and this may become a larger challenge for physicians in the future.

Clinical Course

The course of FD is usually chronic, and morbidity is high. Data are lacking on mortality, but case reports document that some patients die of their behavior (e.g., fatal factitious hypoglycemia), and suicides have occurred.[30] No specific treatment is considered effective. Several controversial approaches to the patient have been advocated, including direct confrontation or "blacklisting" the patient (neither of which is recommended), behavioral modification, prolonged inpatient psychiatric hospitalization, and individual and group psychotherapy.[1,30,33,34] A gentler method, treatment without confrontation, uses inexact interpretations of the patient's behavior in which the patient's symptoms are partially explained; it stops short of actually confronting the factitious behavior. For example, telling patients that it seems their feeling about the psychological issue might be adversely affecting the healing of a chronic wound lets them know that the physician is aware of what's going on but avoids open confrontation and allows patients to save face.[35]

Malingering

Malingering is not considered a medical or psychiatric disorder but is presented here in the differential diagnosis of patients with somatic symptoms and no objective findings. The individual presents with intentional symptoms and perhaps signs of physical or psychological disorders motivated by clear secondary gain. Malingering should be suspected with any combination of the following[9]:

1. Medicolegal context of presentation
2. Marked discrepancy between the person's claimed symptoms and findings
3. Lack of cooperation during the evaluation and noncompliance with treatment
4. Presence of antisocial personality disorder

Sometimes neuropsychological testing can be helpful in discerning the malingerer from the litigant chronic pain patient.[36] It is crucial to be certain that medical and psychiatric disorders do not coexist with malingering. Beyond this step, several authors agree that there is no treatment as such for malingering.[1,20,33] It has been suggested that the individual be presented with a diagnosis of malingering only indirectly; physicians can subtly imply that they are aware of the simulation of illness,[20] and that the symptoms are not consistent with serious disease.[1] Depriving the individual of the usual benefits of the sick role and in some settings (e.g., military) discussing the natural consequences of continued illness often result in rapid recovery.[20] Although rare, a case of fatal result of reporting malingering was described in which a 39-year-old man shot and killed two of four orthopedic surgeons who labeled him a malingerer, wounded a third, and then killed himself using a homemade bomb.[37] Hence, careful conveyance of a diagnosis of malingering might be important to the well-being of both the physician and the individual who malingers.

Conclusion

When managing the patient with a disorder on the somatoform spectrum, it is essential that the family physician modify the treatment goals from "curing" to "caring." It is not possible to eliminate the patient's distress, but careful management with continuity over an extended time allows the patient to settle into a comfortable therapeutic alliance with the physician that allows monitoring the patient's status; most patients demonstrate gradual improvement in function in this setting. The patient may not perceive this improvement or express gratitude and is unlikely to develop insight into the problem. The primary therapeutic modality for the treatment of all of the somatoform disorders has been shown to be "the physician," administered via the doctor–patient relationship.[20] One study demonstrated the first intervention that improved the physical functioning and decreased the health care utilization of somatizing patients.[7] The intervention consisted of a standardized psychiatric consultation letter addressed to the primary care physician, verifying the diagnosis of a somatoform disorder, explaining what it is, and making specific treatment recommendations. The recommendations included (1) frequently scheduled visits with a brief physical examination performed at each visit (during visits the physician looks for signs of disease rather than taking the complaints at face value); (2) avoidance of "as needed" visits; (3) avoidance of diagnostic procedures, hospitalization, surgery, and laboratory tests unless absolutely necessary; and (4) the physician being discouraged from communicating any message that "it's all in your head."[7] This approach, which summarizes the commonly given advice from consultation/liaison psychiatrists, and what is presented in this chapter, has resulted in a decrease in the number of days in bed per month, an improvement in patients' physical functioning (which endured 2 years after the intervention), and a decrease in annual medical care charges of 32.9% during the first year after the intervention.[7] The family physician should also prescribe medication (typically antidepressants or antiobsessional medications) as indicated, and encourage the patient's engagement in psychotherapy (especially cognitive-behavioral therapy) to the extent that the patient will agree.[13–15,19,21,27]

The family physician comes to know well the patient's usual pattern of complaints, listens for a time during each visit, and then shifts the focus of the visit to how the patient is dealing with various life issues. The goal during those frequently scheduled visits is to listen carefully for changes, then proceed with additional medical workup and treatment only if that change is substantiated by clinical findings to suggest new disease. The patient sometimes needs explanations from the physician that allow the patient to "give up" symptoms without losing face. Family physicians manage somatoform spectrum disorders on a daily basis, and as continuity of care is provided over the years for these patients, great professional satisfaction can come from seeing the patient and family enjoy optimum health made possible by the skillful, therapeutic application of the physician–patient relationship.

References

1. Purcell TB. The somatic patient. Emerg Med Clin North Am 1991;9:137–59.
2. Kaplan C, Lipkin M, Gordon GH. Somatization in primary care: patients with unexplained and vexing medical complaints. J Gen Intern Med 1988;3:177–90.
3. Rasmussen NH, Avant RF. Somatization disorder in family practice. Am Fam Physician 1989;40:206–14.
4. Murphy GE. The clinical management of hysteria. JAMA 1982;247:2559–64.
5. Smith GR. Toward more effective recognition and management of somatization disorder. J Fam Pract 1987;25:551–2.
6. Smith GR. The course of somatization and its effects on utilization of health care resources. Psychosomatics 1994;35:263–7.
7. Smith GR, Rost K, Kashner TM. A trial of the effect of a standardized psychiatric consultation on health outcomes and costs in somatizing patients. Arch Gen Psychiatry 1995;52:238–43.
8. Smith GR, Monson RA, Ray DC. Patients with multiple unexplained symptoms: their characteristics, functional health, and health care utilization. Arch Intern Med 1986;146:69–72.
9. American Psychiatric Association. Diagnostic and statistical manual of mental disorders, 4th ed., text revision. Washington, DC: American Psychiatric Association, 2000;485–511, 513–17, 739–40, 781–3.
10. DeGruy F, Crider J, Hashimi DK, et al. Somatization disorder in a university hospital. J Fam Pract 1987;25:579–84.
11. Guggenheim FG, Smith GR. Somatoform disorders. In: Kaplan HI, Sadock BJ, eds. Comprehensive textbook of psychiatry/VI, 6th ed. Baltimore: Williams & Wilkins, 1995;1251–70.
12. Ford CV, Folks DG. Conversion disorders: an overview. Psychosomatics 1985;26:371–83.
13. Phillips KA, Dufresne RG Jr, Wilkel CS, Vittorio CC. Rate of body dysmorphic disorder in dermatology patients. J Am Acad Dermatol 2000;42(3):436–41.
14. Bienvenu OJ, Samuels JF, Riddle MA, et al. The relationship of obsessive-compulsive disorder to possible spectrum disorders: results from a family study. Biol Psychiatry 2000;48(4):287–93.
15. Phillips KA, McElroy SL, Dwight MM, et al. Delusionality and response to open-label fluvoxamine in body dysmorphic disorder. J Clin Psychiatry 2001;62(2):87–91.
16. Cloninger CR. Somatoform and dissociative disorders. In: Winokur G, Clayton PJ, eds. The medical basis of psychiatry, 2nd ed. Philadelphia: WB Saunders, 1994;169–92.
17. Othmer E, DeSouza C. A screening test for somatization disorder (hysteria.) Am J Psychiatry 1985;142:1146–9.
18. Goldberg RJ, Novack DH, Gask L. The recognition and management of somatization: what is needed in primary care training. Psychosomatics 1992;33:55–61.
19. Kroenke K, Swindle R. Cognitive-behavioral therapy for somatization and symptom syndromes: a critical review of controlled clinical trials. Psychother Psychosom 2000;69(4):205–15.
20. Ford CV. The somatizing disorders: illness as a way of life. New York: Elsevier, 1983.
21. Fishbain D. Evidence-based data on pain relief with antidepressants. Ann Med 2000;32(5):305–16.
22. Barsky AJ, Cleary PD, Sarnie MK, Klerman GL. The course of transient hypochondriasis. Am J Psychiatry 1993;150:484–8.
23. Bankier B, Aigner M, Bach M. Clinical validity of ICD-10 neurasthenia. Psychopathology 2001;34(3):134–9.
24. Ford CV. Dimensions of somatization and hypochondriasis. Neurol Clin 1995;13:241–53.
25. McCahill ME. Somatoform and related disorders: delivery of diagnosis as first step. Am Fam Physician 1995;52:193–204.
26. Stuart MR, Lieberman JA. The fifteen minute hour: applied psychotherapy for the primary care physician, 2nd ed. Westport, CT: Praeger, 1993.
27. Smith GC, Clarke DM, Handrinos D, Dunsis A, McKenzie DP. Consultation-liaison psychiatrists' management of somatoform disorders. Psychosomatics 2000;41(6):481–9.
28. Campo JV, Fritsch SL. Somatization in children and adolescents. J Am Acad Child Adolesc Psychiatry 1994;33:1223–35.
29. Libow JA. Child and adolescent illness falsification. Pediatrics 2000;105(2):336–42.
30. Taylor S, Hyler SE. Update on factitious disorders. Int J Psychiatry Med 1993;23:81–94.
31. Rosenberg DA. Web of deceit: a literature review of Munchausen syndrome by proxy. Child Abuse Negl 1987;11:547–63.
32. Feldman MD. Munchausen by internet: detecting factitious illness and crisis on the internet. South Med J 2000;93(7):669–72.
33. Stern TA. Malingering, factitious illness, and somatization. In: Hyman SE, Tesar GE, eds. Manual of psychiatric emergencies, 3rd ed. Boston: Little, Brown, 1994;265–73.
34. Yates WR. Other psychiatric syndromes: adjustment disorder, factitious disorder, illicit steroid abuse. In: Winokur G, Clayton PJ, eds. The medical basis of psychiatry, 2nd ed. Philadelphia: WB Saunders, 1994;276–80.
35. Eisendrath SJ. Factitious physical disorders: treatment without confrontation. Psychosomatics 1989;30:383–7.
36. Meyers JE, Diep A. Assessment of malingering in chronic pain patients using neuropsychological tests. Appl Neuropsychol 2000;7(3):133–9.
37. Gorman WF. Legal neurology and malingering: cases and techniques. St. Louis: Warren Green, 1993;139–69.

35
Selected Behavioral and Psychiatric Problems

Michael K. Magill and Leonard J. Haas

The disorders discussed in this chapter comprise a diverse group of problems, appearing on axes I and II of the *Diagnostic and Statistical Manual of Mental Disorders*, 4th edition (DSM-IV).[1] They require different diagnostic and management strategies and represent differing degrees of prevalence in the typical family physician's practice. However, they have several aspects in common. First, patients with any of the disorders discussed in this chapter require careful attention to history and a sophisticated understanding of communication styles and interpersonal needs. Each condition demands extraordinary efforts from the family physician to maintain a productive doctor–patient relationship. Second, major progress has occurred in recent years regarding the genetic and neurobiologic contributions to etiology of each of these problems. Third, the diagnostic boundaries between these and other conditions are recognized as less distinct than once thought. Finally, medical management of each is becoming increasingly directed at specific symptom complexes, independent of diagnosis.

Caring for patients and their families with these disorders can be demanding but also rewarding. Care of these patients provides the family physician with opportunities to practice the highest art of medicine.

Eating Disorders

Anorexia nervosa and bulimia nervosa, the most prevalent eating disorders, are commonly found in primary care populations among adolescent and young adult female patients. Anorexia is characterized by refusal to maintain a minimally normal body weight. Bulimia is not characterized by underweight or overweight but by repeated episodes of binge eating followed by inappropriate compensatory behavior (e.g., vomiting, laxative abuse, fasting, or excessive exercise). Estimates of prevalence are 5% for anorexia and 2% for bulimia

in the general population. Prevalence is likely to be much higher among patients in weight-loss programs. Patients are 90% female. Female athletes may be at increased risk.[2]

Patients are often reluctant to reveal symptoms; they come for treatment of other conditions or under pressure from family members. Typically practitioners do not routinely assess patients for these problems.[3] Family systems problems predominate, especially in adolescent patients, and distorted body image is prominent as well. Although anorexia and bulimia occur at similar rates in a variety of cultures, they appear to be more common among urbanized populations and in cultures that equate thinness with attractiveness. Preoccupation with weight and body image are both predisposing factors and prominent in the clinical picture. Concomitant disorders include anxiety, depression, substance abuse, borderline personality disorder, and avoidant personality disorder. There is equivocal evidence of a relationship between childhood sexual abuse and eating disorders.[4] Obsessive-compulsive disorder is not related to eating disorders even though the behavior appears compulsive.

These disorders have common features. There is significant overlap in the degree of guilt and shame about the disordered eating patterns and similar intense anxiety about gaining weight. There may be similar distortions in body image (it tends to be more common in anorexia), and there may be bingeing and purging with both conditions. There are also common family conflicts when the patient lives with parents; eating and discussions of food and weight may become volatile issues in family discussions, and normal family meal times may be completely disrupted. The family physician can be quite helpful in providing brief family counseling in such situations.

Treatment is primarily symptom-focused. Key symptoms of concern include weight loss, which may lead to malnourishment; purging, which may lead to metabolic complications; emotional distress, which may lead to various forms of personal acting out; and family discord, which may precipitate or worsen episodes of the disorders. Unlike other addictive or habit problems, food cannot be avoided; thus, recovery from disordered eating requires developing a healthier relationship to food and to one's own body. The weight, cardiac, and metabolic status of the eating-disordered patient should be key factors in deciding whether psychiatric hospitalization, medical hospitalization, or outpatient treatment should be attempted (note that most bulimic patients do not require hospitalization).

Anorexia Nervosa

The prevalence of anorexia nervosa among females during late adolescence and young adulthood is estimated at 0.5% to 1.0%. The incidence of this disorder appears to have increased in recent decades. The prevalence of such threshold conditions may be as high as 10% in college-age women.[5] The onset of illness is often associated with a stressful life event, such as leaving home for college. The course of anorexia is highly variable, with some patients recovering completely after one episode and others becoming chronically ill and requiring hospitalization to treat the starvation and malnourishment.

Diagnosis

Diagnostic criteria include body weight below a minimally normal level or, during childhood or early adolescence, failure to make expected weight gains. The strict diagnostic guidelines promulgated by the World Health Organization–sponsored International Classification of Diseases and Related Health Problems (ICD-10) establish a body mass index (BMI), calculated as weight in kilograms divided by height in square meters, equal to or below 1.75 kg/m.[2] Some patients feel globally overweight, whereas others recognize that they are thin but are overly concerned that certain parts of their bodies are "too fat." It is rare for the patient to complain of weight loss per se. There is often considerable denial about the underweight or the medical implications of the malnourishment.

Despite the syndrome's name, actual loss of appetite is rare. The patient is typically intensely afraid of gaining weight and exhibits a significant disturbance in the perception of the shape or size of her body. Amenorrhea is present among pubescent girls.

Two subtypes of anorexia are identified: (1) the restricting subtype, which involves weight loss through dieting, fasting, or excessive exercise but not binge eating or purging on a regular basis; and (2) the binge eating/purging type, which involves regular binge eating, purging, or both. Usually purging involves self-induced vomiting or misuse of laxatives, diuretics, or enemas. The behaviors usually occur at least weekly.

Patients are usually secretive about their eating habits, and weight loss may be the predominant symptom. Careful history taking, rapport building with the patient, and information from family members may help to establish the diagnosis. Age of onset is typically late adolescence. The personality style is often overcontrolled and rigid, with an unexpressive temperament. There is extreme hesitance or embarrassment about discussing the symptoms.

Depressive symptoms, social withdrawal, irritability, insomnia, and decreased libido may also be associated with anorexia. Obsessive-compulsive features are often prominent, taking the form of preoccupation with food, collecting recipes, and hoarding food. The binge/purge subtype is sometimes associated with other impulse control problems (e.g., substance abuse, sexual overactivity). Other features occasionally associated with anorexia include concern about eating in public. Abnormal laboratory findings related to the semistarvation as well as the induced vomiting and abuse of laxatives and diuretics can be present. Gastrointestinal (GI) disorders are common in eating-disordered patients.[6]

Differential Diagnosis

The differential diagnosis of anorexia includes other possible causes of significant weight loss, especially if the presentation is atypical (e.g., onset after age 40). Several conditions [e.g., GI disease, brain tumor, occult malignancies, acquired immunodeficiency syndrome (AIDS)] may trigger serious weight loss, but the distorted body image and desire for further weight loss is typically not present. Inflammatory bowel disease, peptic acid diseases, and intestinal motility disorders also may mimic eating disorders.[1] Superior mesenteric artery syndrome can be distinguished from anorexia, although it can also develop in anorexic patients. Other psychiatric problems that involve weight loss, distorted body image, shame regarding weight, or odd eating patterns include major depression, schizophrenia, social phobia, obsessive-compulsive disorder, and body dysmorphic disorder.

Risk Factors and Complicating Factors

There is high comorbidity between anorexia and depression especially among adolescent girls. The mortality rate due to anorexia is between 15% and 18%[7]; mortality from eating disorders is about equally divided between medical complications (electrolyte disturbances, acute kidney failure, cardiac complications) and suicide.[8]

Management

Treatment approaches include psychosocial, individual, and group approaches. Family therapy has shown promise, especially when maternal expectations are driving the disordered eating.[9] Cognitive-behavioral approaches in which the distorted beliefs about body image and the effects of gaining weight are explored has also been shown to be helpful, as has use of the primary care relationship in a few studies. Referral is often necessary. Inpatient hospitalization is variable in effectiveness. Professional attitudes may be a problem regarding this disorder as well, as providers sometimes view these patients as less likable and as responsible for their own illness.[10] Anorexia patients show a high rate of relapse, so long-term strategies are necessary. If the family physician believes that the patient cannot be trusted or there is evidence of deception and failure to make treatment gains after several weeks, referral should be considered.

Nutritional rehabilitation should be a treatment objective

for patients who suffer from disordered eating. For the anorexic patient, psychotherapy and pharmacotherapy are best initiated after weight gain has begun. In general, patients who weigh less than approximately 85% of their healthy weight have considerable difficulty gaining weight without being enrolled in a highly structured program. Patients who weigh less than 75% of their healthy weight will likely require inpatient hospitalization—either medical or psychiatric. It is also helpful to determine at what weight the patient's disorder has become unstable in the past. The recently developed treatment guidelines for eating disorders from the American Psychiatric Association provide greater detail on these decisions. It is important to recognize that helping a patient with anorexia to change creates extreme anxiety. Gaining weight is exactly that of which they are most frightened. It is important to help them recognize that the doctor does not simply wish to make them fat.

Drug Therapy

Zinc supplementation may be useful for helping the patient to gain weight.[11] Antidepressants, particularly selective serotonin retuptake inhibitors (SSRIs), in combination with cognitive-behavioral psychotherapy, are effective.[12]

Bulimia

Bulimia is characterized by binge eating, a sense of helplessness during the binge about controlling what is eaten, and attempts to compensate for the overeating by vomiting or purging. Symptoms must last at least 3 months and occur at least twice a week. Prevalence is about 1% to 3% among adolescents and young adult women. Patients are 90% female. Although binge eating typically includes sweet or high-calorie foods, the binge is characterized more by abnormal craving and sense of control than by the type of food eaten. There is considerable shame and secrecy about the binges, which are usually triggered by interpersonal stress, negative moods, or intense hunger following excessive dieting. Vomiting as a method of purging is characteristic of 80% to 90% of bulimia patients; approximately 30% misuse laxatives and (more rarely) enemas. Diabetic patients with bulimia may reduce or omit insulin doses as a method of weight control.

Bulimia patients have an increased frequency of depressive symptoms or mood disorders, as well as anxiety. It is estimated that 33% of bulimic patients also qualify for a diagnosis of substance abuse or dependence, and similar proportions meet the criteria for one or more personality disorders.

Common physical findings include loss of dental enamel especially from lingual surfaces of the front teeth. The teeth may become chipped and appear ragged and "moth-eaten." GI complaints are common among obese bulimia patients. Clearly if the patient complains of GI distress, an eating disorder would not be the first diagnostic consideration; however, after other medical conditions have been ruled out, bulimia should be considered as well.

Differential Diagnosis

Occasional guilt-driven purging after overeating indicates a subthreshold eating disorder. Subthreshold conditions may be risk factors for bulimia, depending on the level of guilt.[13] The research diagnosis of "binge eating disorder" appears to have extremely high prevalence, approximating 30%, among obese patients.[11]

Management

Desipramine (24 weeks) or an SSRI (commonly fluoxetine[14]) in combination with cognitive-behavioral therapy has been shown to be effective.[15] If purging is present, attempting to help the patient gain cognitive control over this maladaptive compensatory habit is important.

Personality Disorders

In contrast to axis I disorders, which are either time-limited or episodic and highly symptomatic, personality disorders (axis II) are more enduring, ingrained, pervasive, and inflexible. Personality disorders are defined as recurrent patterns of interpersonal difficulty that cause the patient (and those with whom the patient interacts) undue distress and impairment. Such patients may experience a range of negative emotional states (e.g., anger, fear, loneliness) but do not attribute these uncomfortable feelings to their own actions. Instead, the patient blames others (parents, family, employers, the environment) for the difficulties. Most individuals with personality disorders do not present to primary care providers for the personality disorder per se.

The presence of a personality disorder complicates the management and treatment of almost any medical problem.[16] Patients with personality disorders are hospitalized for medical problems significantly more often than controls (38% versus 17%).[17] These disorders can affect the doctor–patient relationship, make it difficult to manage a medical condition, or result in confusing requests for medical services. Prevalence rates for axis II disorders in community samples range from 6% to 13%.[18]

Personality disorders are likely to result both from genetic factors ("nature") and experiences during development ("nurture"),[19] resulting in multiple neurotransmitter abnormalities in patients diagnosed with these disorders.[20] Personality-disordered patients may be usefully considered to have a biologic predisposition to certain altered thoughts, affect, and behavior, and may have also been raised in a skewed environment in which they developed problematic ways of behaving and relating to others. Such patients arrive at the office of the primary care physician having experienced, for some or all of their life, a repetitive series of baffling, hurtful, frustrating encounters with people who mattered to them. Having limited interpersonal options at their command, they resort to their characteristic ways of influencing others, expressing their discomfort, establishing their authority, or finding their optimal degree of intimacy. All of these maneuvers may have disastrous consequences for the doctor–patient encounter, and each style of enacting a particular personality disorder may respond better or worse to certain physician behaviors. A key therapeutic task, as Balint[21] put it, is determining "What kind of doctor does this patient need?"

Diagnosis

The DSM-IV describes various personality disorders, clustered into these categories: cluster A, odd-eccentric disorders (paranoid, schizoid, schizotypal); cluster B, dramatic-emotional disorders (antisocial, borderline, histrionic, narcissistic); and cluster C, anxious-fearful disorders (avoidant, dependent, obsessive-compulsive). Recent thinking about personality disorders highlights the somewhat artificial distinction between axis I and axis II disorders and focuses on the continuity of symptoms. Each cluster appears to be associated with certain axis I comorbidities. The diagnostic index of suspicion is raised by the doctor's own discomfort, high levels of frustration with the course of care, and complaints about the patient from the office staff. A more formal diagnosis may be established by careful history taking or the use of one of several psychological or psychiatric diagnostic tools.[22]

Differential diagnosis requires confirmation of long-term patterns of functioning and ruling out of substance use disorders (SUDs) as the underlying cause of the disordered behavior (although SUD frequently coexists with personality disorders).[23] A variety of medical conditions may cause personality changes and should be considered as well, including tumors, head trauma, cerebrovascular disease, Huntington's disease, epilepsy, central nervous system (CNS) infections, endocrine conditions, autoimmune conditions, and chronic toxicity such as lead poisoning.

Cluster A Disorders

Cluster A includes paranoid, schizoid, and schizotypal personality disorders. Patients often experience mistrust or interpersonal aversion. Therefore, these individuals do not typically self-refer for treatment and are often resistant to psychiatric referrals.[17] There are moderately strong relationships between cluster A personality disorders and schizophrenia. It has been suggested that these disorders reflect a psychobiologic disturbance in the processing of sensory stimuli.[24]

Paranoid Personality Disorder

Paranoid personality disorder (PPD) patients are suspicious and mistrustful. They refuse responsibility for their own feelings and are often hostile, irritable, and angry.[18] Muscular tension, inability to relax, and the need to scan the environment for clues may be evident on examination. Affect is often humorless and serious. Pathologic jealousy is often present. Psychotherapy is the treatment of choice. Antianxiety agents such as diazepam may be helpful for agitation and anxiety.

The prevalence estimate for PPD is 0.5% to 2.5% in the general population[1]; the prevalence may be lower in a primary care population, as these patients tend to avoid care until their problems are advanced. PPD patients may appear business-like but have an underlying expectation of harm or trickery by the clinician. There is some evidence that PPD is genetically linked to paranoid schizophrenia or delusional disorder.[25]

Schizoid Personality Disorder

Schizoid personality disorder (SPD) is characterized by a lifelong pattern of social withdrawal. These individuals are often seen by others as eccentric, isolated, or lonely. Prevalence may be as high as 7.5% in the general population. Patients tend to select solitary jobs. It is difficult for them to tolerate eye contact during office visits, and spontaneous conversation is avoided. They may be fascinated with inanimate objects or metaphysical constructs. They give the impression of being cold and aloof, quiet, distant, seclusive, and unsociable. They seem to have little need for sexual activity or intimacy with others. SPD patients may appear eager for medical visits to end, may give limited information in response to questions, and may delay coming for medical visits until their problems are severe. Psychotherapy appears to be the treatment of choice.

Schizotypal Personality Disorder

The prevalence of schizotypal personality disorder (SzPD) is 3% in the general population,[25] but the prevalence may be lower in a primary care population, as these patients have difficulty with physical examinations and with direct communication with the physician. There is fairly strong evidence of SzPD being genetically linked to the schizophrenic spectrum.[25] Patients have peculiar patterns of thinking, acting, and appearance. They are highly sensitive to others' feelings, especially negative feelings, and they may be superstitious. The presenting picture of this disorder is easily confused with that of schizophrenia. Reports of suicide rates as high as 10% among SzPD patients are also reported in the literature.[26] Antipsychotic and antidepressant medication may be useful for symptomatic relief.

Cluster B Disorders

Cluster B includes histrionic, narcissistic, antisocial, and borderline personality disorders. Patients with cluster B disorders can be manipulative and drug seeking or disability-claim seeking, but these disorders are extremely diverse. Borderline personality disorders are the most common cluster B disorders in the general population and the most commonly encountered in primary care, perhaps because these patients experience the greatest distress and impairment.

Histrionic Personality Disorder.

The prevalence of histrionic personality disorder is estimated at 2% to 3% and is more frequently diagnosed in women.[1] Patients may attempt to forget unacceptable feelings, ideas, or appointments with medical providers, and they may minimize the seriousness of their health problems. Essential features include dramatic, extroverted behavior by an excitable, emotional person. There may be remarkable forgetfulness of emotionally important material. Attention-seeking behavior is common, as are exaggeration and overdramatization. Temper tantrums, tears, and accusations may be displayed if the patient is not the center of attention or is not receiving praise or approval. Seductive behavior is common despite the fact that sexual dysfunctions are common as well.

Narcissistic Personality Disorder

The prevalence of narcissistic personality disorder is estimated at less than 1% in the general population[1]; the prevalence may be lower in a primary care population, as admitting medical problems is incompatible with the patient's inflated sense of self and grandiose feelings of uniqueness. These patients cannot handle criticism, may be ambitious, and may have a sense of entitlement. Empathy is foreign to them and interpersonal exploitiveness common. There is less impulsivity than is seen with the borderline, histrionic, and antisocial disorders. Lithium and antidepressants may be of some use in symptom management.

Antisocial Personality Disorder

The prevalence of antisocial personality disorder is 3% among men and 1% among women; onset is usually before age 15.[1] The prevalence may be higher in a primary care population, as these patients are among the disability-compensation and drug seekers. There is usually a family history of antisocial disorders. Neurologic findings often show soft signs and abnormal electroencephalographic (EEG) results. Initial presentation may be normal, even charming and ingratiating. However, the history usually reveals lying, truancy, runaways, thefts, fights, substance abuse, and so on. There is a lack of anxiety or depression that seems incongruous. Suicide threats and somatic preoccupations may be common but may lack realism. During adulthood, promiscuity, spousal abuse, child abuse, and drunken driving are common events. There is rarely remorse for these actions. The patient may seem to lack a conscience. Symptoms of antisocial personality disorder may be secondary to premorbid alcohol or other substance abuse. With age, somatization disorder may become more prevalent. Pharmacotherapy is of limited use, especially in light of the drug abuse often present in this patient group.

Borderline Personality Disorder

The essential characteristic of borderline personality disorder (BPD) is instability of affect, mood, behavior, object relations, and self-image. In the ICD-10, BPD is called "emotionally unstable personality disorder." The disorder is twice as common in women as in men, and in the general population the prevalence estimate is 2%.[1] The prevalence may be higher in a primary care population, as these patients seem attracted to medical settings. Evidence for an important genetic component to the etiology of BPD has grown in recent years.[19,27] BPD patients tend to give primary care providers the most difficulty, and ironically family physicians and other primary care physicians may be more likely to see them than other specialists. These patients are often demanding of their physicians and difficult to refer to psychotherapists. BPD overlaps heavily with multiple other psychiatric syndromes, including other personality disorders, major depression, substance use disorders, posttraumatic stress disorder, and somatization disorders.[23,28–30]

In contrast to such disorders as depression, which can be diagnosed from symptoms and mental status examination, the diagnosis of BPD relies heavily on observing the patient's style of interaction with providers and family. Nowlis[31] noted that one informal indicator of BPD is a relationship with the provider that always seems fragile, stormy, or inappropriate. Patients may also be exquisitely sensitive to loss or change

in the health care team, as they are to any changes in the family structure. For this reason referrals elicit fear of abandonment and rejection in BPD patients. Dividing the staff and polarizing them into good and bad is also characteristic of BPD. BPD underlies many cases of Munchausen syndrome and false accusations of providers' sexual improprieties.

Patients with BPD often complain about chronic feelings of emptiness, boredom, and loneliness, and despite the presence of many other affective states they are depressed most of the time. Life seems to be an almost constant state of crisis for these patients. Mood swings are common, and "micropsychotic episodes" or suicidal behaviors may require brief hospitalizations. Patients with BPD may engage in self-mutilation or other forms of self-destructive behavior.

Physicians must maintain appropriate time and financial boundaries and a professional and objective attitude with BPD patients. This care involves limit setting but not harshness. Developing a sturdy, workable treatment relationship is one of the most difficult aspects of caring for BPD patients. Both extremes of constant availability and harsh limit setting are destructive to the working alliance. A team approach is needed that typically includes family practice, social work, psychology, psychiatry, and perhaps family therapy. Skillful handling of the transition between providers (e.g., when residents graduate or coverage changes and care must be transferred) is important. Although it is helpful for the provider to understand the conditions that give rise to BPD, it is not always helpful to try to explain them to the patient. Fragile borderline patients often experience an explanation as criticism. It is far more useful simply to acknowledge the patient's current situation and distress without interpretation of reasons for it.[32] Caring for BPD patients may prompt providers to seek their own sources of support within the professional community, such as Balint groups, psychotherapy, or team conferences.

Cluster C Disorders

Cluster C includes avoidant, dependent, and obsessive-compulsive personality disorders. Dependent and obsessive-compulsive personality disorders are most common.[33] Cluster C is heavily comorbid with axis I depression and anxiety disorders. Medical help is more frequently sought by these patients because of the prominence of worry.

Avoidant Personality Disorder

The prevalence estimate for avoidant personality disorder is 0.5% to 1.0% in the general population.[1] The prevalence may be lower in a primary care population, as these patients may be afraid to ask questions and delay seeking medical attention. A key feature of the disorder is extreme sensitivity to rejection coupled with a strong desire for companionship. These patients are commonly referred to as having an inferiority complex. The ICD-10 classifies the condition as "anxious personality disorder." Because social inhibition is present, the disorder may be difficult to distinguish from social phobia. There is also a strong overlap with dependent personality disorder. Individual and group therapy are indicated, as are social skills training and assertiveness training. Symptoms of anxiety and depression may be treated with pharmacotherapy.

Dependent Personality Disorder

The prevalence of dependent personality disorder is unknown in the general population,[1] but the prevalence may be higher in a primary care population, as these patients may attempt to get the physician to make decisions for them, have endless questions (which prolongs their visits and gives them more of a sense of being cared for), and are noncompliant (i.e., have difficulty with self-care responsibilities). A pattern of dependent and submissive behavior is present, as is extreme difficulty making decisions without excessive amounts of advice and reassurance. These patients may tolerate abusive or otherwise difficult partners for long periods so as not to be alone. It may be difficult to distinguish this disorder from schizoid and schizotypal disorders. Antianxiety and antidepressant medication may be helpful for symptom relief. Psychotherapy is usually indicated.

Obsessive-Compulsive Personality Disorder

The prevalence estimate for obsessive-compulsive personality disorder is 1% in the general population.[1] The prevalence may be higher in a primary care population, as these patients may seek multiple opinions about the diagnosis and may meticulously document their symptoms. Key features include emotional constrictions, stubbornness, and indecisiveness. There is also pervasive perfectionism and inflexibility. These patients are preoccupied with rules, regulations, neatness, and details. They are often formal, serious, and humorless. They do show eagerness to please those whom they see as powerful. Disruptions in the routine precipitate substantial anxiety. There may not be the specific obsession or compulsion present in the axis I obsessive-compulsive disorder, although these traits may occur during the course of the axis II disorder. Late-onset depressive disorders are common features of the later course. SSRIs and clomipramine may be useful treatment.

Management

While personality traits are not altered by psychotropic medications, advances in understanding of the neurochemistry of these problems and positive results of recent therapeutic trials suggest that medications targeted to specific symptom complexes are useful for many patients with personality disorders. Borderline personality disorder provides a model for this approach to treatment.[34,35] Target symptoms are in the areas of cognitive, affective, and behavioral dysfunction. Low-dose (high-potency) neuroleptics (e.g., haloperidol, perphenazine, or trifluoperazine) are helpful for cognitive problems such as mild thought disorders, suspiciousness, paranoid ideation, and dissociation. Affective symptoms, including depressed, angry, anxious or labile moods may be helped with SSRIs, monoamine oxidase inhibitors (MAOIs), or mood-stabilizing drugs such as valproate, lithium, and carbamazepine. Impulsive dyscontrol may respond to SSRIs, low-dose neuroleptics, or mood stabilizers. Alprazolam, however, may increase impulsivity, and amitriptyline may increase suicide

threats; therefore, these should be avoided.[30] Suicide potential must be kept in mind, and consideration given to limiting prescriptions to sublethal amounts of medication. In this regard, evidence for the specific "antisuidical" effect of lithium carbonate is important.[36] Also of recent note is the rather remarkable antihostility and antiaggression effect of the SSRIs.[24,36] It is also important to note that pharmacotherapy occurs in the context of the doctor–patient relationship; the meaning of prescribing medication may differ depending on the patient. In some cases patients believe that medication means the physician no longer wants to talk to them; this should be carefully clarified. In general, long-term medication management of the personality-disordered patient may require a referral, keeping in mind that many axis II patients rapidly become noncompliant with complex medication regimens.[37]

The personality-disordered patient does not respond well to being accused of having a personality disorder, although the patient may respond well to being diagnosed with a personality disorder and being helped to cope with the symptoms. New data about the underlying genetic and neurobiologic abnormalities of BPD provide a physiologic explanation useful to patients. Indeed, patients may be strangely reassured when told that their lapses, misperceptions, and judgment errors may be caused by a neuropsychological deficit. It may be much easier to see oneself as flawed (but able to develop coping tools) rather than to see oneself as (1) dumb, bad, or manipulative, or (2) the victim of developmental failures.[38]

Several authors have suggested detailed management strategies for difficult patients, many if not all of whom are likely to be personality disordered.[39,40] Principles of management include the following:

1. Assume that the disorder is a true symptom and not a deliberate attempt to infuriate the physician.
2. Assume that the disorder can be managed; it is chronic and sometimes unremitting (especially without long-term psychotherapy) but is amenable to structured intervention.
3. Be consistent in implementing the chosen approach.
4. Develop a collaborative relationship with patients (e.g., ask for feedback on how they feel about their medical care); assure them that you understand their perspective.

Nowlis[31] noted, regarding treatment of borderline individuals (but the point is more generally valid), that successful treatment may involve "maturation of the providers as well as the patient."

Vaillant[41] noted that all of us display more mature defenses when we believe we are understood, which in turn suggests that understanding these difficult patients may be an avenue toward improving the ability to manage them in primary care. This is echoed in Livesley's[32] more recent recommendation that "the most appropriate stance for treating BPD is to be empathetic, supportive, and validating," and "to recognize the legitimacy of patients' experience." Yet this can be very difficult, given the tendency for health care providers to react with strong emotions, often negative, to patients with BPD and other PDs. Although family physicians must know their

Table 35.1. **Personality-Disordered Patient in the Medical Setting**

Major personality trait	Likely DSM-IV axis II disorder(s)	Meaning of illness to patient	Helpful physician response style
Dependent and overdemanding	Dependent PD, borderline PD,	Abandonment and rejection	Balanced approach combining empathic recognition of patient's need for reassurance and anxiety about being alone with limit-setting, clarity, consistency, and structure
Orderly and compulsive	Obsessive-compulsive PD	Loss of control	Respect for patient's need to be as much in control as possible; provide complete information, including test results, as quickly as possible; engage patient's participation in treatment planning, scheduling
Dramatizing	Histrionic PD	Threat to physical intactness and attractiveness	Respectful and professional manner, without abbreviating time spent with the patient
Self-sacrificing (self-defeating style)	Dependent PD, passive-aggressive PD, depressive PD	Combination of prospect of pain and of kindness from others	Spend adequate time to hear detailed symptomatology, anticipate ambivalence/lack of enthusiasm on improvement
Self-important	Narcissistic PD	Threat of having to rely on others; prospect of being cared for by inferiors (threat of being dismissed, demeaned)	Nondefensive acceptance of "less experienced" status; readiness to call in the experts
Detached	Schizoid PD, schizotypal PD, avoidant PD	Too-intense close contact with others; threat to privacy	Respect patient's need for privacy and distance; insist on adequate time for necessary medical care
Suspicious	Paranoid PD	Vulnerability; threat of being harmed by strangers	Inform patient about hospital procedures; provide exact details of medical procedures (especially risks and benefits); acknowledge validity of tension, guardedness
Manipulative	Antisocial PD	Chance to work hidden agenda (e.g., escaping criminal justice system, maintaining drug dependence)	Provide only clearly medically indicated treatments; request psychiatric consult if malingering likely

Source: Adapted from Oldham,[18] with permission.
PD = personality disorder.

own limits in how many difficult patients can be managed, long-term primary care management may work well when supplemented by appropriate and prompt referral to specialists during times of change or flare-up of symptoms. Oldham[18] updated the guide provided by Kahana and Bibring[42] as adapted in Table 35.1.

Schizophrenia

Epidemiology

Approximately 1% of the population suffers from schizophrenia. Of patients with schizophrenia, 29% see a general medical physician within any given year, and 14% are cared for exclusively by general medical care providers.[43] About 1% of primary care patients have psychotic disorders,[44] most of them being schizophrenic.

Diagnosis

The criteria for diagnosis of schizophrenia are listed in Table 35.2. Hallucinations, delusions, loose associations, and flat affect are among the "positive," or classic, psychotic symptoms of schizophrenia. They are typical of the acute or active phase of the illness. Although most criteria for schizophrenia emphasize the presence of psychosis, this may not be an essential feature of the illness,[45] and the diagnostic boundaries

Table 35.2. **Differential Diagnosis of Psychotic Disorders**

Part I: Consideration of other problems

Step 1: Consider other problems	Diagnostic categories	Organ system	Specific examples

General medical condition	Delirium, dementia or psychotic
	  disorder due to general medical
	  condition
	Dementia of Alzheimer's type
	Vascular dementia
		Neurologic
		Endocrine
		Metabolic
		Neoplasm, epilepsy
		Fluid/electrolyte
		Hepatic/renal failure
		Autoimmune
			CNS infection
			Hyper- or hypothyroidism
			  parathyroidism
			Hypoxia, hypoglycemia

Substance abuse	Alcohol or other substance
	  intoxication or withdrawal
	Alcohol or other substance-induced
	  persisting dementia		

Other mental disorders	Bipolar disorder Major depressive disorder		

Part II: Consideration of psychotic disorders

Step 2: Consider psychotic disorder	Diagnosis	Criteria
If: sudden onset (<1 month)	Brief psychotic disorder	Sudden onset Duration >1 day and <1 month

If: multiple psychotic symptoms	Schizophrenia	Of 6 months duration, at least 1 month of "active phase"
		  (positive and/or negative symptoms) significant
		  impairment

Schizophreniform disorder	Schizoaffective disorder	Duration 1–6 months
		Significant concomitant mood disturbance, 2 weeks with
		  delusions or hallucinations but without mood
		  disturbance

If: delusions (not bizarre), no
  other psychotic symptoms
	Delusional disorder	Nonbizarre delusions for 1 month; behavior
		  and function not obviously disordered

The table shows steps to diagnosis of a psychotic disorder presenting with symptoms such as delusions, hallucinations, disorganized speech or behavior, "negative symptoms" (flat affect, limited speech, reduced goal-directed activity, anhedonia), or catatonia.

are not clear between schizophrenia, schizoaffective disorder, and bipolar illness.

The "negative" symptoms of schizophrenia, such as social isolation and withdrawal, impairment of social role function, odd beliefs or magical thinking, marked loss of initiative or interests, and circumstantial or impoverished speech, are more typical of the prodromal and residual phases of the illness. Negative symptoms and cognitive impairment are often the most disabling symptoms of chronic schizophrenia.

Drug Therapy

Drug therapy is the mainstay of treatment for schizophrenia.[46,47] Treatment varies by the phase of the disease. Medication should be begun as promptly as possible after diagnosis, since early treatment and prevention of relapses leads to improved long-term outcome. Although if medication treatment could be initiated before the first psychotic episode, outcomes might be improved, medication is not usually initiated during the prodromal phase of the illness, as the diagnosis cannot be made definitively. With acute exacerbation of the positive symptoms that characterize the active phase, relatively high doses of medication are often used to obtain initial control of symptoms. During the residual phase negative symptoms tend to predominate, and lower doses of medica-

tions are used. Evidence-based guidelines for treatment of schizophrenia are now available.[48] Unfortunately, many patients are undertreated relative to these guidelines.[49]

Antipsychotic drugs are generally divided into low-potency (high daily dose) and high-potency (low daily dose) neuroleptics, and atypical antipsychotic agents. The low- and high-potency agents are of similar efficacy, especially against the "positive" symptoms of schizophrenia. They differ in their side-effect profiles. Low-potency drugs tend to cause more sedation and hypotension; high-potency drugs cause more extrapyramidal effects.

Although commonly used antipsychotic (neuroleptic) drugs more effectively control the positive than the negative symptoms of the disease, newer atypical antipsychotic drugs are changing the picture. These agents add blockade of 5-hydroxytryptamine (5-HT) (serotonin) receptors to dopaminergic receptor blockade. This is thought to be the mechanism whereby these newer agents improve negative symptoms in addition to the positive symptoms of schizophrenia.

Clozapine (Clozaril), the first atypical antipsychotic, showed improved effectiveness in treatment of both positive and negative symptoms, but severe side effects (particularly agranulocytosis) limit its use to patients who have failed to improve despite trials at least two other agents.[48]

The atypical agent risperidone (Risperdal) is rapidly becoming a first-line treatment for schizophrenia because it improves both positive and negative symptoms and shows a safer side-effect profile. Other atypical antipsychotics include olanzapine (Zyprexa), quetiapine (Seroquel), and ziprasidone (Geodon). Schizophrenic patients often become depressed, in which case treatment with the usual antidepressant medications is appropriate.

Medication Side Effects

Short-term side effects of the older neuroleptics include sedation, orthostatic hypotension, and anticholinergic symptoms such as dry mouth, blurred vision, and urinary retention. Galactorrhea and amenorrhea may occur. The most troublesome common side effects of neuroleptics reflect neuroleptic blockade of dopaminergic receptors in the extrapyramidal nigrostriatal system. The most common acute extrapyramidal side effect is dystonia, characterized by intermittent or sustained muscle spasms of a variety of facial or truncal muscle groups. Dystonia is reversible with administration of anticholinergics.

Subacute side effects include akathisia and parkinsonian-like symptoms. Akathisia, a subjective sensation of motor restlessness, occurs within days to weeks of starting a neuroleptic agent. It is often reversible with change to a low-potency agent or reduction in dose of the neuroleptic. β-adrenergic blocking medication such as propranolol may also be helpful.[46]

Parkinsonian-like symptoms, including resting tremor, bradykinesia, rigidity, and postural instability, may occur within weeks to months of beginning therapy. These symptoms usually respond to antiparkinsonian drugs such as benztropine, trihexyphenidyl, diphenhydramine, and amantadine.[46] Many clinicians start antiparkinsonian drugs simultaneously with high-potency neuroleptics, as this regimen has been found to reduce the likelihood of major parkinsonian-like symptoms.[47]

Because they are generally irreversible, delayed extrapyramidal side effects of neuroleptics are the most feared. Not all late dyskinesias are drug induced, however; up to 23% of schizophrenic patients never treated with neuroleptics exhibit movement disorder.[50] Neuroleptic-induced syndromes include tardive dyskinesia, in which patients experience involuntary facial and tongue movements, rhythmic trunk movements, and choreoathetoid movements of the extremities. There is no effective treatment for tardive dyskinesia. Tardive dystonia and tardive akathisia represent the late onset of these symptoms. Perioral tremor ("rabbit syndrome") may be reversible with antiparkinsonian drugs.[46] Patients and their families should be made aware of the risk of these late syndromes, and informed consent for treatment must be documented in the patient's medical record.

Atypical antipsychotics seldom cause extrapyramidal side effects, except for risperidone in relatively high doses greater than 3 mg per day,[51] and have not been reported to cause tardive dyskinesia. Clozapine and olanzapine can cause anticholinergic effects, sedation, and orthostatic hypotension. Risperidone does not cause anticholinergic effects. Clozapine

should be reserved for patients for whom at least two other agents prove ineffective. Because of the 1% to 2% incidence of agranulocytosis, patients taking clozapine must have a complete blood count performed once per week for the first 6 months of therapy, once every 2 weeks thereafter. Clozapine also causes seizures in 3.5% of patients.

Neuroleptic malignant syndrome (NMS) is an uncommon but dangerous complication of treatment with neuroleptic medications. NMS is characterized by muscular rigidity, fever, and altered mental status. Although patients generally recover with appropriate treatment, up to 20% fatality has been reported.

The development of NMS has been reported in as many as 12% of patients treated with neuroleptics, but the true incidence is likely around 0.07% to 0.15%.[52] Patients with psychomotor agitation or dehydration may be at increased risk of NMS, as may those who have had previous episodes of NMS, rapid increases in the neuroleptic dose, or parenteral administration of the drug.[53]

Management of NMS begins with cessation of the neuroleptic agents. Patients should receive intensive supportive medical care; monitoring for complications such as aspiration, thromboembolic disease, and renal failure; and maintenance of hydration and respiratory and cardiac functions.[53] Although there are no controlled clinical data regarding pharmacologic treatment, patients may be given dopamine agonists to reverse the effect of dopamine blockade, including bromocriptine, levodopa/carbidopa (Sinemet), and amantadine. Dantrolene may also be given to reduce muscle contractility.[52]

Psychotherapy and Family Involvement

Insight-oriented psychotherapy is generally not appropriate for patients with schizophrenia, as it does not reduce symptoms and in fact may exacerbate them.[54] But it is often possible to establish a helpful therapeutic alliance with such patients as part of their ongoing care. Patients with schizophrenia commonly experience paranoid ideation, demoralization, stigmatization, denial of illness, and fear. The physician can use specific strategies to help maintain an effective relationship despite these problems. Such problems include "sharing" paranoid patients' mistrust of others, supporting demoralized patients via appreciative or approving comments, helping to normalize the experiences of stigmatized patients, and offering alternative viewpoints to patients who deny their illness.[55] Simple medication compliance training may create a "virtuous circle" by enhancing medication compliance which, in turn, enhances function.[56] Other therapeutic approaches showing variable results include psychosocial skills training and cognitive-behavioral therapy.[56]

Whereas family dynamics were previously believed to contribute to the development of schizophrenia, it is no longer thought to be the case. Families are often considerably stressed by the presence of an affected family member, and physician support and counsel are important parts of management. The family should be educated about the condition, medications, and early recognition of relapse. They should be reassured that they did not cause the illness and instructed about access to community support groups. Family interventions have been shown to reduce relapse rates substantially for patients with schizophrenia, especially in families that demonstrate high levels of critical expressed emotion,[57] although trials of family intervention in the United States show equivocal results[56] (see also Chapter 4).

Indications for Referral or Consultation

Family physicians' level of involvement in ongoing management of schizophrenia varies widely depending on their knowledge level and comfort, the availability of mental health professionals, and patients' insurance status. Psychiatric consultation should be sought to confirm a diagnosis, assist with or provide hospital management of acute exacerbations, and deal with refractory or complicated cases.

References

1. American Psychiatric Association. Diagnostic and statistical manual of mental disorders, 4th ed. Washington, DC: American Psychiatric Press, 1995.
2. Nattiv A, Agostini R, Drinkwater B, Yeager K. The female athlete triad: the interrelatedness of disordered eating, amenorrhea, and osteoporosis. Clin Sports Med 1994;13:405–18.
3. Wilfley D, Grilo C. Eating disorders: a women's health problem in primary care. Nurse Pract Forum 1994;5:34–45.
4. Kinzl J, Traweger C, Guenther V, Biebl W. Family background and sexual abuse associated with eating disorders. Am J Psychiatry. 1994;151:1127–31.
5. Haller E. Eating disorders: a review and update. West J Med 1992;157:658–62.
6. McClain C, Humphries L, Hill K, Nickl N. Gastrointestinal and nutritional aspects of eating disorders. J Am Coll Nutr 1993; 12:466–74.
7. Siddiqui A, Ramsay B, Leonard J. The cutaneous signs of eating disorders. Acta Derm Venereol 1994;74:68–9.
8. Palmer T. Anorexia nervosa, bulimia nervosa: causal theories and treatment. Nurse Pract 1990;15:12–18,21.
9. Woodside D. Anorexia nervosa and bulimia nervosa in children and adolescents. Curr Opin Pediatr 1993;5:415–18.
10. Fleming J, Szmukler G. Attitudes of medical professionals towards patients with eating disorders. Aust NZ J Psychiatry 1992;26:433–6.
11. Birmingham C, Goldner E, Bakan R. Controlled trial of zinc supplementation in anorexia nervosa. Int J Eat Disord 1994;15: 251–5.
12. Yanovski S. Bulimia nervosa: the role of the family physician. Am Fam Physician 1991;44:1231–8.
13. Herzog D, Hopkins J, Burns C. A follow-up study of 33 subdiagnostic eating disordered women. Int J Eat Disord 1993;14: 261–7.
14. Goldstein D, Wilson M, Thompson B, Potman J, Rampy A. Longterm fluoxetine treatment of bulimia nervosa. Br J Psychiatry 1995;166:660–6.
15. Agras W, Rossiter E, Arnow B, et al. Pharmacologic and cognitive-behavioral treatment for bulimia nervosa: a controlled comparison. Am J Psychiatry 1992;149:82–7.
16. Searight H. Borderline personality disorder: diagnosis and management in primary care. J Fam Pract 1992;34:605–12.
17. Reich J, Boerstler H, Yates W, et al. Utilization of medical resources in persons with DSM-III personal disorders in a community sample. Int J Psychiatry Med 1986;19:1–9.
18. Oldham J. Personality disorders: current perspectives. JAMA 1994;272:1770–1.
19. Torgersen S. Genetics of patients with borderline personality disorder. Psychiatr Clin North Am 2000;23(1):1–9.
20. Gurvits I, Koenigsberg H, Siever L. Neurotransmitter dysfunction in patients with borderline personality disorder. Psychiatr Clin North Am 2000;23(1):27–40.
21. Balint M. The doctor, his patient, and the illness, rev. ed. New York: International Universities Press, 1955.
22. Kaplan H, Satlock B. Comprehensive textbook of psychiatry, 5th ed. Baltimore: Williams & Wilkins, 1995.
23. Trull T, Sher K, Minks-Brown C, Durbin J, Burr R. Borderline personality disorder and substance use disorders: a review and integration. Clin Psychol Rev 2000;20(2):235–53.
24. Kapfhammer HP, Hippius H. Special feature: pharmacotherapy in personality disorders. J Pers Disord 1998;12(3):277–88.
25. Wiseman M. The epidemiology of personality disorders:a 1990 update. J Pers Disord 1990;7:44–62.
26. McGlashan T. Schizotypal personality disorder: Chestnut Lodge followup study VI; longterm followup perspectives. Arch Gen Psychiatry 1986;43:329.
27. Silk K. Overview of biologic factors. Psychiatr Clin North Am 2000;23(1):61–75.
28. Koenigsberg H, Anwunah I, New A, Mitropoulou V, Schopick F, Siever L. Relationship between depression and borderline personality disorder. Depress Anxiety 1999;10(4):158–67.
29. Hollander E. Managing aggressive behavior in patients with obsessive-compulsive disorder and borderline personality disorder. J Clin Psychiatry 1999;60(suppl 15):38–44.
30. Kjellander C, Bongar B, King A. Suicidality in borderline personality disorders. Crisis 1998;19(3):125–35.
31. Nowlis D. Borderline personality disorders in primary care. J Fam Pract 1990;30:329–35.
32. Livesley W. A practical approach to the treatment of patients with borderline personality disorder. Psychiatr Clin North Am 2000;23(1):211–32.
33. Zimmerman M, Coryell W. Diagnosing personality disorders in the community. Arch Gen Psychiatry 1990;47:525–31.
34. Soloff P. Psychopharmacology of borderline personality disorder. Psychiatr Clin North Am 2000;23(1):169–92.
35. Hirschfeld R. Pharmacotherapy of borderline personality disorder. J Clin Psychiatry 1997;58(suppl 14):48–52.
36. Soloff PH. Algorithms for pharmacological treatment of personality dimensions: symptom-specific treatments for cognitive-perceptual, affective, and impulsive-behavioral dysregulation. Bull Menninger Clin 1998;62(2):195–214.
37. Pare' MF, Rosenbluth M. Personality disorders in primary care. Prim Care 1999;26(2):243–78.
38. O'Leary K. Neuropsychological testing results. Psychiatr Clin North Am 2000;23(1):56.
39. Linehan M, Armstrong H, Swariz A, Allmon D, Herd H. Cognitive-behavioral treatment of chronically parasuicidal borderline patients. Arch Gen Psychiatry 1991;48:1060–4.
40. Millon T. Disorders of personality: DSM-IV and beyond, 2nd ed. New York: Wiley, 1996.
41. Vaillant G. Ego mechanisms of defense and personality psychopathology. J Abnorm Psychol 1994;103:44–50.
42. Kahana R, Bibring G, eds. Personality types in medical management. In Zinberg N, ed. Psychiatry and medical practice in a general hospital. New York: International Universities Press, 1964.
43. Regier D, Burke J, Manderscheid R, Burns B. The chronically mentally ill in primary care. Psychol Med 1985;15:265–73.
44. Regier D, Narrow W, Rae D, et al. The de facto US mental and addictive disorders service system: epidemiologic catchment area prospective 1-year prevalance rates of disorders and services. Arch Gen Psychiatry 1993;50:85–94.
45. Tsuang M, Stone W, Faraone S. Toward reformulating the

diagnosis of schizophrenia. Am J Psychiatry 2000;157(7): 1041–50.

46. Martin R. Outpatient management of schizophrenia. Am Fam Physician 1991;43:921–33.

47. Kane J. Schizophrenia. N Engl J Med 1996;334:34–41.

48. Lehman A, Steinwachs D. At issue: translating research into practice: the schizophrenia patient outcomes research team (PORT) treatment recommendations. Schizophr Bull 1998; 24(1):1–10.

49. Lehman A, Steinwachs D. Patterns of usual care for schizophrenia: initial results from the schizophrenia patient outcomes research team (PORT) client survey. Schizophr Bull 1998;24(1): 11–20.

50. Fenton W, Wyatt R, McGlashan T. Risk factors for spontaneous dyskinesia in schizophrenia. Arch Gen Psychiatry 1994;51: 643–50.

51. Amadio P, Cross L, P Amadio J. New drugs for schizophrenia:

an update for family physicians. Am Fam Physician 1997;56(4): 1149–59.

52. Buckley P, Hutchinson M. Neuroleptic malignant syndrome (editorial). J Neurol Neurosurg Psychiatry 1995;58:271–3.

53. Caroff S, Mann S. Neuroleptic malignant syndrome. Med Clin North Am 1993;77:185–202.

54. Mueser K, Berenbaum H. Psychodynamic treatment of schizophrenia: is there a future? (editorial) Psychol Med 1990;20: 253–62.

55. Weiden P, Havens L. Psychotherapeutic management techniques in treatment of outpatients with schizophrenia. Hosp Community Psychiatry 1994;45:549–55.

56. Hemsley D, Murray R. Commentary: psychological and social treatments for schizophrenia: not just old remedies. Schizophr Bull 2000;26(1):145–51.

57. Tarrier N, Barroclough C. Family interventions for schizophrenia. Behav Modif 1990;14:408–40.

36
Allergic Rhinitis

Etan C. Milgrom

Allergic disease annually affects about 50 million Americans or about 20% of the total U.S. population.[1] Allergic rhinitis alone affects about 25 million Americans annually, at a cost of $3 billion in 1990. The cost for sinusitis was estimated at $700 million in 1995.[2] In recent quality of life studies, children with allergic rhinitis exhibited low self-esteem and decreased concentration abilities and school performance, and therefore this condition warrants special attention.

History

The most important component in the workup of the allergic patient is the history. A careful history can help the astute clinician detect different triggers in the patient's environment that are inducing the patient's symptoms. To obtain an adequate allergy history, the clinician needs to first recognize typical allergy symptoms and be aware of the different types of allergens present in the community.

Allergens

The common allergens known to provoke immunoglobulin E (IgE)-mediated symptoms, can be divided into two groups: (1) seasonal allergens, including grass, trees, and weed pollens; and (2) perennial allergens, including house dust mites, cockroach, animal allergens (animal dander, saliva, and urine) and mold spores.[3]

The grass, tree, and weed pollens are classified as seasonal because they are generated at different times of the year in different regions of the country. Grass pollens are released during the spring, tree pollens in spring and early summer, and weed pollens in early fall. Patients with specific pollen allergies will usually manifest their symptoms during the season in which the offending allergen is released. Ragweed hay fever is a notorious example of this on the East Coast during the month of September.

The perennial allergens are present year round except in cold climate conditions where mold spores are smothered by falling snow. House dust mites are ubiquitous microscopic organisms that proliferate in warm (65–80°F) humid environments. They feed off of desquamated human skin; their waste products are the true sensitizing antigens.[4] High levels of mite antigen are found in mattresses, box springs, pillows, carpet, upholstered furniture, clothes, and stuffed animals. Mold spores are found both indoors (*Penicillium* and *Aspergillus*) and outdoors [*Alternaria* and *Hormodendrum* (*Cladosporium*)]. They are found in high numbers in moist, humid, damp, shaded areas (basements, bathrooms, areas with overgrown vegetation, standing water or poor soil drainage, compost heaps, etc.). Animal dander is typically a sensitizing antigen, but it is the protein in animal saliva and urine that is the actual allergen. Household pets are a constant source of allergenic stimulation. Cockroach antigens are also proving to be a perennial sensitizing antigen.

Atopy

Atopy is inherited. Any family member who suffers from one or more of the "allergic triad" (i.e., allergic rhinitis, asthma, and atopic dermatitis) carries the genetic makeup for allergic disease. If both parents of the patient have allergic problems, then the patient carries a 70% chance of having allergic problems as well. One parent alone with allergic problems gives the patient at least a 30% chance of suffering from some form of allergic disease. Even if both parents do not have an allergic predisposition, the patient still has a 10% probability of developing true allergic disease.

Physical Exam

There are several physical findings in allergic rhinitis that are suggestive of atopy, but none is pathognomonic. A nasal crease secondary to repeated rubbing of the nose typically suggests allergic rhinitis. "Allergic shiners" (black-eye appearance suborbitally) are thought to be caused by venous stasis produced by chronic allergic congestion. Excessive mouth breathing secondary to chronic nasal congestion can lead to orofacial dental deformities and malocclusion. The nasal turbinates usually appear pale, bluish, and boggy, and are coated with clear mucus. Physical findings related to other allergic disorders, especially those found in atopic dermatitis and asthma, are further evidence of an atopic predisposition.

Laboratory Evaluation of Allergic Disease

The laboratory workup of the allergic patient is not particularly helpful. The IgE level is elevated in only one third of allergic patients. Peripheral eosinophilia is more diagnostic in parasitic disease than allergic disease. The nasal smear, if performed properly, can be of assistance in the diagnosis of allergic rhinitis.[5] Interpretation of the smear can be attained by quantitating an eosinophil to neutrophil ratio (E/N). An E/N ratio of greater than 1 is suggestive of allergic rhinitis.[6]

Skin Testing and Radioallergosorbent Testing

Skin testing is the "gold standard" diagnostic procedure in the workup of allergic disease. Skin testing can be performed by either the prick or scratch method. Antigen extracts (premade by several companies) are placed in droplet form on the skin and the skin is pricked or scratched with a needle directly through the extract droplet.[7] This will allow exposed specific serum IgE to bind to its counterantigen and cause the immediate degranulation of mast cells, producing a wheal and flare reaction within 15 to 20 minutes of the initial prick or scratch. It is preferable to perform these tests on the patient's arm so that the patient can also view the results. All skin tests should be performed with a positive histamine and negative diluent control. Positive skin tests need to be correlated with a history of exposure to the antigens involved. Skin testing should be performed by clinicians well trained in this area.

In vitro radioallergosorbent tests (RAST) have been developed during the past 20 years to help identify IgE-mediated disease. The patient's serum, containing allergen-specific IgE, is allowed to interact with allergen that is bound to a solid phase. The specific IgE that binds to the allergen is detected by adding labeled anti-IgE antibody to the solid phase.[8] RAST can be a helpful adjunct tool in the evaluation of allergic disorders, especially in patients with severe atopic dermatitis who have no disease-free skin available to perform skin testing and in patients who exhibit significant dermatographism during skin testing.

Skin testing, if performed properly, remains the most sensitive and specific testing mode for identifying antigen-specific IgE-mediated disease.[9] The average cost per allergen for skin testing is $3 to $5 and for RAST is $10 to $20.[10] Skin testing can be an effective educational tool for patients. Nothing replaces the educational value of a wheal and flare reaction that occurs right before patients' eyes. This leads to a better understanding of their disease and ultimately to improved compliance and therapeutic outcome.

Differential Diagnosis

Rhinitis, or inflammation of the nasal mucosa, may be subdivided into nonimmunologic and immunologic causes. A careful history and specific IgE workup will identify most allergic rhinitises.

Vasomotor rhinitis is by far the most common nonimmunologic, noninfectious chronic rhinitis. Patients with this disorder complain of perennial symptoms of nasal congestion, rhinorrhea, anosmia, and postnasal drip without itching or eye involvement. Symptoms are precipitated by cholinergic stimuli such as alcohol, temperature/humidity changes, and nonspecific irritants (smog, odors, smoke). These patients, unlike those suffering from allergic rhinitis, exhibit no evidence of atopy. They have normal IgE; negative skin, intradermal, and RAST tests; and no eosinophils on nasal or peripheral smear.[11] Treatment involves avoidance of provoking nonallergic stimuli, antihistamines/decongestants, and the use of topical intranasal steroids and topical anticholinergics (ipratropium). It is clear from several studies that the parasympathetic nervous system plays a vital role in inducing hypersecretion of the nasal mucosa in several disease states. Ipratropium bromide therapy should be considered when treating unresponsive rhinorrhea.[12] It is available in nasal-spray form. The recommended dose of ipratropium bromide in this format is two puffs per nares four times a day.

Nasal polyps are grape-like, gelatinous gray translucent growths that commonly originate in the anterior ethmoid sinuses. Their etiology is unknown. They typically occur as a triad with asthma and aspirin sensitivity. Polyps predominate in middle-age asthmatic patients and seldom occur in children or adolescents with atopic dermatitis, allergic rhinitis, or IgE-mediated asthma. Patients with nasal polyposis often exhibit perennial nasal stuffiness, anosmia, associated sinusitis, asthma, and/or aspirin (acetylsalicylic acid)/nonsteroidal antiinflammatory drug (ASA-NSAID) intolerance. The diagnosis can be made by careful nasal exam, sinus x-rays, computed tomography (CT) scan, or rhinolaryngoscopy. Treatment includes intranasal and/or systemic steroids; avoidance of ASA, NSAIDs, and tartrazine; and lastly surgical polypectomy/intranasal ethmoidectomy.

Rhinitis medicamentosa is a rhinitis that involves overuse of over-the-counter vasoconstricting nasal sprays. These patients exhibit tachyphylaxis along with rebound erythema, rhinorrhea, congestion, and edema of the nasal mucosa. Therapy includes avoidance of topical vasoconstrictors, followed by administration of topical steroids, and, in severe cases, systemic steroids.

Foreign-body rhinitis is very common in children. Children with this problem classically present with a unilateral, purulent, foul-smelling nasal discharge. The foreign body, or rhinolith, needs to be carefully removed.

Nasal tumors, such as inverted papillomas or carcinoma of the nasopharynx, are relatively rare but need to be considered in the differential diagnosis.

A severe deviated septum can induce a compensatory turbinate hypertrophy in the contralateral nasal passage and lead to chronic rhinitis. This usually needs to be corrected surgically.

Signs of nasal itching accompany hormonally induced rhinitis, and symptoms of hyperthyroidism or hypothyroidism are usually present. Birth control pills, as well as other medications (methyldopa, hydralazine), are also known to induce nasal congestion.

Complications of Allergic Rhinitis

Serous otitis media and chronic sinusitis are the most common and best-understood complications. Serous otitis media more commonly occurs in children because of the horizontal orientation of the eustachian tube in early childhood. Excessive mucosal edema and secretions that obstruct the eustachian tube opening in the posterior pharynx can exacerbate it. Chronic serous otitis media may lead to hearing loss, resulting in possible delayed speech and cognitive development.

Chronic sinusitis usually occurs as a result of inflammatory processes in the nasal mucosa that extend into the paranasal sinuses and obstruct the sinus ostia. Mucosal edema and secretions also damage ciliary function and interrupt the normal sinus drainage. Patients typically present with prominent postnasal drip, purulent discharge, sinus pain over facial surfaces, nocturnal cough, low-grade fever, or nasal stuffiness. Sinus disease is one of the most prevalent chronic diseases, causing widespread morbidity and economic hardship, and yet it is one of the most difficult diseases to diagnose with objective criteria.

Management of Allergic Rhinitis

The management of allergic rhinitis involves four major steps: good patient education, institution of appropriate environmental control measures, pharmacologic therapy, and immunotherapy for carefully selected patients.[13]

Patient Education

The importance of patient education cannot be overemphasized. Good patient education not only fosters a stronger physician–patient relationship, but also provides a framework for better understanding of disease processes and ultimately leads to improved compliance and therapeutic responses. Proper patient education takes time and effort and demands a team approach. Time needs to be spent teaching patients about different aspects of their disease and should be followed up with written information to reinforce what has been learned.

Environmental Control

To minimize allergic symptoms, an attempt should be made to identify the inciting causes in each patient.[14] By identifying the specific triggers, patients can receive educational information on ways to avoid or minimize exposure to these agents, and, it is hoped, reduce their symptoms. As previously mentioned, these triggers can be identified by a careful history and by correlating the history with either skin testing or RAST testing.

Once the antigens have been identified, an attempt should be made to avoid or minimize exposure to those antigens that cause clinical symptoms. The seasonal antigens (grass, trees, and weed pollens) are difficult to avoid, as patients often have multiple sensitivities and pollens are too scattered to be properly eliminated. If sensitivity to pollen is significant, it is recommended that the affected patient remain indoors with the windows shut during the midday and afternoon when the pollen count is highest. During the ragweed season, which peaks in September, patients can choose to vacation in ragweed-free areas.

The perennial allergens are easier to avoid because they are more contained. Although animals may not be difficult to avoid physically, many patients have an emotional attachment that cannot be broken. At a minimum, it should be recommended that the animal stay out of the patient's bedroom and even outdoors, if possible. House dust mite sensitivity has been shown to play a major role in allergic disease. Of utmost importance in mite-sensitive patients is covering the mattress, box spring, and pillows with plastic airtight covers. It is also important to wash bedding in water heated to at least 130°F weekly and avoid sleeping or lying on upholstered furniture.

Pharmacologic Therapy

There are four classes of medications that are useful in the treatment of allergic rhinitis: (1) antihistamines (topical and oral), (2) decongestants (topical and oral), (3) cromolyn sodium (topical only), and (4) corticosteroids (topical and oral). Each has its own specific use, but all are more beneficial if used as a prophylactic maintenance medication and not in the acute setting.

Antihistamines

Antihistamines are histamine receptor blockers that can alleviate the nasal itching, rhinorrhea, and sneezing caused by histamine release. Approximately 30 million Americans per year rely on H1 antihistamines for allergic symptomatic relief. The traditional first-generation antihistamines, many of which are available over the counter, are known to cross the blood-brain barrier and produce sedation 10% to 25% of the time.[15] The newer, second-generation antihistamines [i.e., loratadine (Claritin), fexofenadine (Allegra), and cetirizine (Zyrtec)] are less sedating because they are more lipophilic, making them less likely to cross the blood–brain barrier.[16] The topical antihistamine is in the form of an azelastine nasal spray (Astelin) which can be applied directly to the nares 2 sprays per nostril 2 times per day as needed.

Decongestants

Decongestants are α-adrenergic agents that decrease swelling in the nasal mucosa by inducing vasoconstriction, thereby reducing edema and rhinorrhea. They can be administered by either the oral or topical route. Each method has significant side effects that can be avoided if used properly.

Oral Decongestants. Pseudoephedrine hydrochloride and phenylpropanolamine [recently implicated in possibly causing strokes and removed from the market by the Food and Drug Administration (FDA) in 2001] are the two most commonly prescribed decongestants. They function better when prescribed in combination with antihistamines because together they provide more comprehensive relief of symptoms. Because they are sympathomimetic agents, their potential side effects include nervousness, irritability, and insomnia, which may be countered when combined with some of the more sedating antihistamines. Nonetheless, they should be given cautiously to patients with concomitant heart disease, seizure disorders, and hypertension (especially those on β-adrenergic blocking agents).

Topical Decongestants. The three main topical decongestants include one short-acting decongestant [phenylephrine hydrochloride (Dristan, Neo-Synephrine)] and two long-acting decongestants [oxymetazoline (Afrin), Dristan 12-hour spray, and xylometazoline (Otrivin)]. They are very effective in obtaining prompt relief of congestion in the early stages of therapy. Although they have a minimal systemic side-effect profile, their continued use and abuse can lead to rebound congestion, which demands more frequent dosing of the identical medication used for relief of symptoms and results in rhinitis medicamentosa. To avoid this complication, topical decongestants should not be used longer than 2 to 3 days during a particular treatment period.

Topical Ophthalmic Decongestants. The ophthalmic decongestants [phenylephrine (Neo-Synephrine), naphazoline (Naphcon, Opcon), and oxymetazoline) are very effective in alleviating the conjunctival injection and irritation of allergic conjunctivitis/rhinits. When prescribed in combination with antihistamines [antazoline (Vasocon-A) or pheniramine maleate (Naphcon-A, Opcon-A)], the itchiness can be alleviated as well.

Cromolyn Sodium

Cromolyn sodium is a mast cell stabilizer that blocks the release and action of mediators produced by mast cells. It inhibits both the early and late phase of the allergic response, reduces airway hyperreactivity, has a minimal side-effect profile, and is the safest long-term maintenance drug available in allergic therapy.

Cromolyn is not effective for acute allergic therapy, is expensive, and cannot be used on a PRN basis. For proper use of cromolyn, it is recommended to commence therapy at four-times-a-day dosing for the first month, then gradually taper to three times a day and two times a day if allergic control is maintained. It is important to note that the effects of cromolyn may not be appreciated until 2 to 3 weeks into therapy. In allergic rhinitis, cromolyn reduces sneezing, itching, and rhinorhea as long as it is used properly. It can also be useful

prior to the onset of and through an anticipated pollen season to diminish allergic symptomatology.

Nedocromil sodium is another cromolyn agent that is touted to be more potent and longer acting than cromolyn. Like cromolyn, it has a similar low side-effect profile including a foul taste.

Corticosteroids

Nasal corticosteroids are very effective in relieving nasal congestion, rhinorrhea, sneezing, and itchiness.[17] Because the nasal corticosteroids are rapidly metabolized, they have very few systemic side-effect risks. Local irritative side effects of the nasal steroid are attributed to the freon propellants and the lower pH solutions (Nasalide). With the advent of aqueous pumps and aerosol delivery systems, this side effect was significantly diminished.

Nasal steroids begin to take effect within 2 to 4 days after administration and should be prescribed early in the course of therapy. They are usually administered twice a day and tapered to once a day when symptom control is maintained. Patients need to be taught to spray laterally in the nasal passage, away from the septum to avoid perforating it. Systemic steroids are very effective in the management of severe, recurrent, recalcitrant allergic rhinitis.

The bioavailability of nasal steroids is the primary factor in causing growth suppression and other systemic adverse events. The majority of nasal steroids are swallowed so that the systemic bioavailability is determined from the gastrointestinal (GI) tract and the degree of first-pass hepatic inactivation. The absorption of the fraction that is deposited on the nasal mucosa varies from drug to drug and is influenced by bioavailability and solubility characteristics. Fluticasone propionate and mometasone furoate have the least bioavailability of all the nasal steroids and clearly have the least potential to cause systemic side effects, such as bone growth retardation in children.[18]

Immunotherapy

Immunotherapy is a very effective form of treatment in the management of allergic rhinitis if the appropriate patients are chosen to receive it.[19] Management of allergic rhinitis should begin with the implementation of appropriate environmental control measures (to avoid sensitization by specific allergens), and followed by pharmacotherapy directed at controlling allergic inflammatory reactions and patient's allergic symptoms. If these two measures are unsuccessful, i.e., poor control is maintained, medications are used in excess to achieve desired control, or symptom control is obtained at the expense of too many intolerable side effects, then immunotherapy should be employed. To achieve the best results with immunotherapy and to minimize the significant complicating risks of anaphylaxis, immunotherapy should be administered in consultation with a physician who has had expert training in this area. If performed properly, immunotherapy has an 85% to 90% success rate in improving the symptoms of allergic rhinitis. During the initial months of immunotherapy, patients may need to continue to use their medications for symptom control until the immunotherapy takes effect.

The mechanism of action of immunotherapy is not completely understood. The overwhelming evidence seems to suggest that immunotherapy stimulates the production of IgG antibodies against offending antigens and inhibits the allergic reaction from taking place. As immunotherapy is administered, the level of antigen-specific IgA and IgG in nasal secretions increases and the blood IgE level during seasonal exposure diminishes.

Proper administration of immunotherapy involves first identifying the appropriate antigens to place in the immunotherapy solutions. The allergy mixtures are injected subcutaneously once or twice a week, initially with a very dilute solution and slowly increased with each injection until a maintenance dose is reached. The maintenance dose is determined by the degree of local reaction to the injection site. The maintenance dose is usually reached within 4 to 6 months. The interval between injections can be increased by 1 week every 1 to 2 months, and usually within 18 to 24 months it can be given once every 4 to 6 weeks as long as symptoms are reduced. Any form of a systemic reaction, i.e., total body itching, wheezing, urticaria, anaphylaxis, etc., should alert the physician to back off to the previous injection dose. Emergency resuscitation equipment should always be available whenever administering immunotherapy.

Immunotherapy, if performed properly, can significantly reduce the symptoms of allergic rhinitis. Unlike pharmacotherapy, it actually modifies the immune system. The process is a long and tedious one, but when it is effective, patients are very appreciative because it allows them to become symptom free and less dependent on their medication.

References

1. Smith JM. Epidemiology and natural history of asthma, allergic rhinitis and atopic dermatitis (eczema). In: Middleton E, Reed CE, Ellis EF, et al, eds. Allergy: principles and practices, 3rd ed. St. Louis: CV Mosby, 1988;891–929.
2. Smith JM. The epidemiology of allergic rhinitis. NES Allergy Proc 1982;3(3):383–8.
3. Plant M, Pierce JH, Watson CJ, Hanley-Hyde J, Nordan RP, Paul WE. Mast cell lines produce lymphokines in response to cross-linkage of FceRI or to calcium ionophores. Nature 1989; 339:65–8.
4. Lichtenstein LM, Histamine releasing factors and IgE heterogeneity. J Allergy Clin Immunol 1988;81:814–20.
5. Meltzer EO, Orgel HA, Rogenes PR, Field EA. Nasal cytology in patients with allergic rhinitis: effects of intranasal fluticasone propionate. J Allergy Clin Immunol 1994;94(4):708–15.
6. Mullarkev ME, Hill JS, Webb DR. J Allergy Clin Iummunol 1980;65:123.
7. Meltzer EO, Jalowayskl AR. Nasal cytology in clinical practice. Am J Rhinol 1988;212:47.
8. Zeiss CR. Immunology of IgE mediated and other immediate hypersensitivity states. In: Patterson R, ed. Allergic disease: diagnosis and management, 4th ed. Philadelphia: JB Lippincott, 1993;33–47.
9. Milgrom EC: Skin testing vs RAST in the allergic patient. Intern Med Alert 1992;14(3):19–20.
10. Lawlor GJ, Fischer TJ, Adelman DC. Manual of allergy and immunology, 3rd ed. Boston: Little, Brown, 1994;29–39.
11. Baroody FM, Cruz PA, Lichtenstein LM, Kagey-Sobotka A, Proud D, Naclerio RM. J Allergy Clin Immunol 1992;89:1065–75.
12. Milgrom EC. Who'll stop the rhinorrhea? Intern Med Alert 1992;14(17):129–30.
13. Dykewicz MS, Fineman S, Skoner DP, et al. Diagnosis and management of rhinitis: complete guidelines of the Joint Task Force on Practice Parameters in Allergy, Asthma and Immunology. Ann Allergy Asthma Immunol 1998;81:478–518.
14. Corren J, Stoloff. Seasonal allergic rhinitis: an update. Leawood KS: American Academy of Family Physicians, CME Production Department, 1998;1–15.
15. Vurman E, Van Veggel LMA, Uiterwijk M, et al. Seasonal allergic rhinitis and antihistamine effects on children's learning. Ann Allergy 1993;71:121–6.
16. Virant FS. Audio forum on rhinorrhea in the child. Scientific Exchange, January 1998.
17. Meltzer EO. The pharmacological basis for the treatment of perennial allergic rhinitis and non-allergic rhinitis with topical corticosteroids. Allergy 1997;52(suppl 36):33–40.
18. Allen DB. Systemic effects of intranasal steroids. J Allergy Clin Immunol 2000;106(suppl):S179–90.
19. Ferguson BJ. Allergic rhinitis—option for pharmacotherapy and immunotherapy. Postgrad Med 1997;101:117–20.

37
Anaphylaxis and Anaphylactoid Reactions

Judith A. Fisher and Robert A. Baldor

Anaphylaxis is a severe, life-threatening allergic reaction. Recognition of symptoms and rapid initiation of appropriate therapy is imperative to ensure an optimal outcome. There are approximately 2000 deaths from anaphylactic reactions in the United States annually.[1] Fortunately, fatal reactions are unusual among hospitalized patients. One study reported about one case of anaphylaxis per 5000 admissions but only one death per 400,000 admissions.[2] Anaphylaxis reactions occur when the immune system is challenged by an antigen to which it had been previously sensitized, triggering a massive and inappropriate outpouring of inflammatory mediators.

The first anaphylactic reaction was believed to have been described in the year 2640 B.C. when Pharaoh Menes was killed by a wasp sting. However, it was not until 1902 that the term was coined by researchers attempting to find an antidote for poisoning by the *Actinaria* jellyfish. During the course of this research several dogs died shortly after the administration of a second small dose of the antidote. Richet coined the term *anaphylaxis* from the Greek *ana*, meaning backward, and *phylaxis*, meaning protection, reflecting the opposite effect expected from his experiment.[3] He eventually received a Nobel Prize for this work.

Pathophysiology

Anaphylaxis is an immunoglobulin E (IgE)-mediated response that releases antiinflammatory substances from circulating basophils and tissue mast cells. The primary substances released are histamines, tryptases, cytokines, prostaglandins, and platelet-activating factors. In addition, this response initiates the synthesis of arachidonic acid metabolite.[4] Anaphylactoid reactions result in the release of the same substances from basophils and mast cells, but are not an IgE-mediated event. Anaphylactoid reactions do not require a previous antigen exposure with sensitization of the patient; rather, they are immediate. Activation is triggered directly (seen with reactions to exercise, opiates, and radiocontrast medium) or via direct activation of the complement pathway from changes in arachidonic acid metabolism (aspirin sensitivity).[5] The presentation and treatment of the subsequent inflammatory clinical response is the same for both anaphylactoid and anaphylactic types of reactions.

Clinical Presentation

Clinical presentation is variable. While reactions are often seen as rapid, catastrophic events (typically within 1 hour of exposure), they may occur up to a day or two later. Patients present with a variety of symptoms: hives, urticaria, nausea, vomiting, diarrhea, abdominal pain, hypotension, arrhythmias, wheezing, and angioedemia.[6] Angioedema frequently involves the neck and tongue, causing severe swelling that can result in a life-threatening blockage of the airway. Hypotension causes syncope, and patients may complain of a feeling of "impending doom" or a metallic taste in the mouth.[5] A patient who is having such a reaction may be thought to be experiencing a vasovagal reaction. However, patients who have fainted respond quickly by being laid flat, and their hypotension is due to bradycardia. Those undergoing an anaphylactic reaction will be tachycardic as the body attempts to correct the hypotension induced by vasodilation.[6]

Diagnosis and Management

Patients with an anaphylactic reaction should be approached in three stages. The first stage is an immediate assessment and stabilization. The second is ongoing monitoring and treatment for a relapse or a delayed reaction. Finally, once patients are over the reaction, they must be considered for prophylactic measures to prevent a recurrent attack. Such measures include searches for trigger events and possible desensitization therapy.

Initial Evaluation and Management

Severe reactions are true emergencies and even mild reactions should prompt active monitoring. Emergency airway, breathing, and circulation (ABC) evaluation should be carried out. Oxygen should be administered, and if the airway is compromised, the patient should be intubated, although an emergency tracheotomy may be required in the setting of significant laryngoedema. If pulseless, start cardiopulmonary resuscitation (CPR). Intravenous (IV) access must be attained immediately and epinephrine administered as soon as possible and repeated every 3 to 5 minutes as needed. One study demonstrated less mortality if epinephrine was administered within 30 minutes of the insult.[7] The cardiac rhythm should be monitored continuously. For children with difficult IV access, administering epinephrine via a large-bore needle inserted through the anterior tibia into the interosseous space should be considered. Epinephrine can also be given subcutaneously (SC); however, in the face of an anaphylactic reaction, absorption is variable. IV fluid should be administered by a rapid bolus.[5,8] Less severe

reactions can be treated with intramuscular (IM) epinephrine and antihistamines, and bronchospasm can be treated with nebulized β-agonist (Table 37.1).

Secondary Evaluation and Management

Once patients have gone through an initial assessment and stabilization, it is crucial that they continue to be observed, usually in the hospital. A quarter of the patients will have persistent symptoms, and will require ongoing aggressive therapy (Table 37.2). These symptoms frequently will last up to a day. Another quarter of patients will have a relapse, or biphasic reaction after the initial successfully treated reaction, with symptoms returning 8 to 12 hours after the initial event. Patients on beta-blockers and angiotensin-converting enzyme (ACE) inhibitors may require higher doses of adrenaline as these drugs may block some of the adrenaline's beneficial effect.[6]

Prevention

Once patients have recovered from their anaphylactic reaction, treatment is not yet complete. The risk of a subsequent reaction is likely again if the patient is challenged by the trig-

Table 37.1. **Initial Evaluation and Management of Anaphylaxis**

System	History	Physical evidence	Evaluation and management[a]
			For all reactions:
General	Weakness Lightheadedness Faintness	Altered level of consciousness	1. Assess and support ABC. 2. Administer epinephrine 1:10,000 solution 0.1–0.5 mg SC q 3–5 min × 3 doses. 3. Administer Ringer's lactate or normal saline solution through a 14- to 16-gauge needle: 0.5–1.0 L over 15–20 minutes to support vital signs.
Skin	Feeling warm Rash Redness Itching	Urticaria Flushing Diffuse erythema Angioedema Scratching	4. Administer diphenhydramine hydrochloride 1 mg/kg IM or PO (max. dose 50–75 mg) q4h. 5. Administer either 250 mg Solu-Medrol IV or prednisone 1–2 mg/kg PO.
Gastro-intestinal	Abdominal cramps Nausea Vomiting Diarrhea	Hyperperistalsis Vomiting Diarrhea	6. If beta-blockers or ACE inhibitors have been taken administer: (a) glucagon 5–15 μg/min IV; (b) atropine sulfate 0.5–1.0 mg IV.
			If respiratory system is involved:
Respiratory	Watery nose or eyes Throat tightness Choking Wheezing Hoarseness Swelling: mouth, throat, tongue	Rhinorrhea Choking Wheezing Stridor Dysphonia Hoarseness Edema of tongue, oropharynx, or larynx	7. Administer oxygen via mask or nasal cannula. 8. Nebulize albuterol 0.5 mL of 0.5% solution in 2.5 mL normal saline or metaproterenol sulfate 0.3 mL of 0.5% solution in 2.5 mL of normal saline as often as necessary to keep the airways open. 9. Administer aminophylline 5–6 mEq/kg to load, then 2–3 mEq/kg q6h PO or IV.
			If cardiovascular system is involved:
Cardiovascular	Chest pain Palpitations	Hypotension Cardiac arrhythmia	10 Administer dopamine 2–50 μg/kg/min IV. 11. Administer as many units of albumin as necessary to support the circulation. 12. Place a MAST suit. 13. Alternate tourniquets.

ABC = airway, breathing, cardiovascular system; ACE = angiotensin-converting enzyme; MAST = military antishock trousers.
[a]These steps apply to all cases of anaphylaxis regardless of the system affected.

Table 37.2. **Secondary Evaluation and Management of Anaphylaxis**

Differential diagnosis	Repeat history	Repeat physical examination	Management
Vasovagal reaction	Exposure to known allergen	HEENT: purulence, edema,	Minimal laboratory
Scromboid poisoning	Aphylaxis in the past	conjunctivitis, rhinorrhea,	investigation:
secondary to tuna,	Atopy	pale or swollen nasal,	CBC and differential
bluefish, or mackerel	Family history plus allergies	oropharyngeal, and	Chest radiography
Ingestion of aged cheeses	or anaphylaxis	laryngeal mucous	Electrocardiography
Hyperventilation	What was patient doing/	membranes	Elderly: cardiac enzymes
Cardiac shock	eating just prior to onset	Skin: flushing, swelling,	ABGs
Arrhythmia	of symptoms	rash	At 1 hour after the onset:
Ischemia	What was patient doing/	Pulmonary: tracheal	spot urine sample for
Septic shock	eating 1, 2, and 3 hours	wheeze, stridor	histamine, serum tryptase
ARDS	prior to onset of symptoms	Cardiac: irregular heart	
Cold-induced urticaria	Medication usage	rate, tachycardia	
Hereditary angioneurotic		Abdomen: increased bowel	
edema		sounds, tenderness, and	
Insulin reactions		swelling	
Systemic mastocytosis			
Factitious stridor			
Hysterical reaction			
Pheochromocytoma			
Carcinoid syndrome			

Source: Data were compiled from multiple sources including Yunginger,[1] Stoloff and Greenberger,[38] Saryan and O'Laughlin,[41] and Cohn et al.[42]

ARDS = adult respiratory distress syndrome; HEENT = head, eyes, ears, nose, throat; CBC = complete blood count; ABGs = arterial blood gases.

gering antigen. Therefore, an aggressive search for the trigger should be undertaken. The patient should be prescribed self-administered epinephrine and advised to keep an antihistamine on hand. The patient's family members should be educated about the signs and symptoms of anaphylaxis and instructed in how to give epinephrine to the patient. Two commercial products that can be prescribed are the Ana Kit and the Epi Pen. Individuals should wear a MedicAlert bracelet (*www.medicalert.org*; 888-633-4298). The patient should undergo allergy testing with either skin tests or seroimmunoassay via the radioallergosorbent testing (RAST).

Anaphylactic Triggers

There are a multitude of anaphylactic triggers. The most common is penicillin, with reactions occurring in one of every 10,000 patients. It contributes to a quarter of all anaphylactic deaths.[1] Next is radiocontrast medium reactions, followed by stings and bites from insects.[6] Many foods trigger reactions (see Chapter 94), and peanuts have recently been highlighted as they are used in numerous processed foods and represent a hidden threat for sensitive individuals.[5] Some recent studies have suggested that foods are the most common anaphylactic triggers outside of the hospital, accounting for as many reactions as insects and drugs combined.[5]

Food

Up to 2% of adults have food allergies; however, the incidence of anaphylaxis is unknown. What is known is that individuals with food-induced anaphylaxis usually have a history of reactions to peanuts, tree nuts, fish, or shellfish, and

are likely to have a history of asthma.[9] One prospective study found that 8% of children under age 3 are allergic to at least one food.[7] Reaction to cow's milk is frequently seen in children, likely because it is one of the first foreign antigens to which they are exposed. This is followed closely by egg allergy. These allergies are usually outgrown.[8] The most common food allergens in children are peanuts, tree nuts (walnuts, cashews, hazelnuts, almonds), cow's milk, soy, and eggs.[10] In addition to this list, adults are most often affected by shellfish, cereal grains, celery, and fruits[11]; additives such as sulfites, monosodium glutamate, tartrazine, and benzoates[12]; spices such as coriander[13]; and sunflower seeds.[14]

Once the trigger(s) are identified, patients and their caregivers must be taught to read food labels and ask questions of restaurant personnel. The day-to-day investigation process necessary for the patient to avoid the food trigger(s) is tedious and may feel demeaning, but it is absolutely necessary. Stores, bakeries, and restaurants must make an effort to have available lists of ingredients for all of their products. Although allergists can provide some desensitization with immunotherapy, avoidance is still the cornerstone of preventing food-induced anaphylaxis.

Insect Sting

About 0.4% to 4.0% of the population is allergic to the venom of one or more stinging insects.[15] Wasps, honeybees, hornets, yellowjackets, fire ants, and mosquitoes are the most common culprits (see Chapter 47). Insect sting anaphylaxis is classified as type I (dermal reactions only)—urticaria or angioedema; type II (non–life-threatening systemic reactions)—bronchospasm, abdominal cramps, dyspnea, and dermal reactions; and type III (life-threatening reactions)—shock, hypotension, loss of consciousness, severe respiratory distress, and upper airway edema. Only 56% of individuals with a history of insect sting reaction have a second reaction when stung again by the same type of insect.[16] In these individuals, the natural history of insect sting reactions shows that re-sting reactions are similar to the original reactions. Thus, an individual with a type I reaction is most likely to have a type I reaction with a re-sting.[16] Children under 16 years of age are least likely to experience re-sting reactions. Once it is discovered that the anaphylactic reaction is due to an insect sting, the sting location should be found, a tourniquet applied proximal to the sting site, the stinger dug out with a surgical blade (using forceps may only serve to release further venom from the venom sac), and epinephrine 1:1000 solution 0.005 mL/kg injected intradermally at the site of the sting (maximum dose 0.15–0.25 mL).

Follow-up of these patients includes (1) testing for a true allergy (skin testing is most sensitive; RAST has a false-negative rate of 20%[17]); (2) avoidance of perfumes and strong scents, and nests and congregation points for insects (e.g., trash bags, picnic areas, leaf piles, and sweet-smelling bushes); (3) wearing long sleeves, pants, and shoes when outdoors; (4) carrying injectable epinephrine at all times; and (5) possibly venom immune therapy (VIT).

Because the natural history of insect sting reactions shows that the re-sting reactions are similar to the original reactions, most clinicians do not suggest that individuals with a type I reaction undergo VIT. It is controversial whether VIT should be recommended for type II reactions. Type II reactors with chronic health problems, the elderly, and those on ACE inhibitors or beta-blockers are candidates for VIT. For all other type II reactors one should consider the cost-benefit issues. Immunotherapy is definitely indicated for type III reactions.

Exercise

Exercise-induced anaphylaxis (EIA) occurs within 5 to 8 minutes of the onset of exercise. EIA is a worsening of exercise-induced asthma (see Chapter 51). EIA often occurs when certain foods or medications are consumed prior to exercise. The prevalence is unknown, but it has been on the rise since exercise became more fashionable during the 1970s. The usual patient profile includes a history of atopy, positive family history, and female sex.

Treatment is similar to that for generic anaphylaxis. Preventive management includes (1) avoiding food or medication triggers if known—patient can safely exercise 4 to 6 hours after eating; (2) exercising in pairs; (3) carrying epinephrine—each member of a pair should know how to inject; (4) avoiding exercise when the weather is humid or cold; (5) stopping exercise at the onset of pruritus or urticaria; and (6) using cromolyn sodium prior to exercise.[18–20]

Latex

A recent concern is the growing number of latex allergies, particularly among health care workers. First reported in Germany in 1927[21] and initially described as a curiosity in the United States,[22] latex allergy has become a public health hazard since the Centers for Disease Control (CDC) issued recommendations for universal precautions in 1987.[23] Anaphylactic reactions are triggered by natural latex allergens in rubber gloves derived from the rubber tree (*Hevea brasiliensis*). Latex particles adhere to the cornstarch powder used to coat these gloves and may trigger allergic reactions in the sensitized individual, who, although avoiding physical contact, may inhale the airborne particles of powder.[24] Cross-reactivity reactions have occurred in latex-sensitized individuals exposed to foods that are believed to share similar antigenic structure to the rubber plant such as bananas, chestnuts, kiwi, avocado, and tomato.[25] The federal government has recently issued workplace and product labeling guidelines to ensure a safer environment for patients and health care workers.[26,27] When treating anaphylaxis secondary to a latex allergy, vigilance must be exercised to avoid additional contact with latex allergens from IV tubing and catheters during resuscitation efforts.[24]

Persons most affected are medical and dental personnel, individuals who have undergone multiple surgical or diagnostic procedures, and rubber workers. Although many of these reactions occur in the medical arena, something as simple as blowing up a balloon may trigger anaphylaxis in a latex-sensitized individual.

Latex-sensitive patients should wear a MedicAlert bracelet and be taught to question the ingredients of all products. These individuals must use lambskin condoms and nonrubberized diaphragms for sexual encounters. Doctors' offices, hospitals, and surgical personnel must be alerted and have nonlatex products available for use.[28]

Anesthesia

Anesthesia anaphylaxis occurs in 1:5000 to 1:20,000 individuals during anesthesia. In 80% of the cases the agent is one of the neuromuscular blocking drugs, although many other agents have been described including local anesthetics used by dentists.[29,30] These reactions are more common in females and in individuals with autoimmune disorders.[31] Skin prick testing and intradermal testing are available for high-risk individuals prior to surgery.

Other Drugs

Many drugs have been reported to cause anaphylactic reactions, the most common of which is penicillin; however, it is often withheld unnecessarily.[1,32] Points of note are (1) penicillin anaphylaxis occurs mainly if administered parenterally; (2) before diagnosing a penicillin allergy, the physician should see the patient to be sure that the skin rash is urticaria or angioedema and not just a maculopapular eruption; (3) if skin testing is conducted with penicilloyl-polylysine (PPL) and a minor determinant mixture (MDM), a negative test indicates that all β-lactam antibiotics are safe. If a patient is skin test positive, and penicillin is indicated for treatment, the patient can be desensitized (done in a hospital giving small oral doses every 15 to 30 minutes until therapeutic levels are reached).

Transfusion Reactions

An anaphylactic transfusion reaction is immunoglobulin A (IgA)-mediated. It is often immediate and does not have to be preceded by a history of blood transfusion or pregnancy. To definitively diagnose an IgA-mediated transfusion reaction, blood is obtained immediately and submitted to a passive hemagglutination assay (PHA).[33] The literature has reported one case of an anaphylactoid reaction with anti-IgA antibodies in an IgA-deficient individual.[34] Such individuals must be transfused with IgA-deficient blood.

Vaccines

In Canada, anaphylaxis was reported to occur in 1 per 1 million doses of administered vaccines at all ages. Atopic individuals are not thought to be at a greater risk than others. All doctors' offices and clinics where vaccine is administered should be prepared with the necessary equipment and training to treat an anaphylactic reaction. Physicians should know how vaccines are produced, whether made in chick embryos, sterilized with antibiotics, or stabilized with preservatives (see Chapter 7). An individual who is allergic to any component of this process should be desensitized and vaccinated in the hospital setting.[35]

Idiopathic Anaphylaxis

There are many known triggers to an anaphylactic or anaphylactoid reaction, yet 20,000 to 50,000 patients in the United States carry the diagnosis of idiopathic anaphylaxis (IA).[36] IA is a diagnosis of exclusion, when after extensive evaluation no known substance can be found to trigger the reaction. IA is insidious in that the patient has no warning and no trigger to avoid. Patients who carry a diagnosis of IA are treated prophylactically with sympathomimetic amines, glucocorticoids, antihistamines, or aminophylline to suppress episodes of anaphylaxis. These patients appear to go into remission in equal numbers regardless of whether they are treated with glucocorticoids. Therefore, remission of IA is not steroid dependent.[37]

Anaphylactoid Triggers

Radiocontrast Media

Over a million diagnostic procedures in the United States annually involve the use of radiocontrast material: 1% to 2% of patients have an anaphylactic reaction, and 1:10,000 patients die.[38] Anaphylactoid reactions are neither dose-related nor always immediate. Pretreatment orally with corticosteroids, diphenhydramine, and ephedrine decreases the reaction rate to 5% (Table 37.3). A reported 16% to 44% of patients with a history of anaphylactoid reaction to radiocontrast media react. Patients with atopy have a twofold increase in reactivity when compared to nonatopic individuals. It is important for the family physician to notify the radiographer so a nonionic contrast medium can be used.[39]

Table 37.3. **Pretreatment Regiment for Adults Allergic to Radiocontrast Dye**

Drug	Hours prior to procedure	Dose (mg)
Prednisone	13	50
Prednisone	7	50
Prednisone	1	50
Ephedrine	1	25
Diphenhydramine HCl	1	50

All drugs are given orally.

Hemodialysis

Anaphylactoid reactions can occur during hemodialysis. One study showed 21 severe reactions among 260,000 treatments, most commonly in individuals on ACE inhibitor drugs and when negatively charged membranes were used for dialysis.[40] It is thought that the same reaction could occur with any extracorporeal membrane device.

References

1. Yunginger JW. Anaphylaxis. Ann Allergy 1992;69(2):87.
2. Kaufman DW. An epidemiologic study of severe anaphylactic and anaphylactoid reactions among hospital patients: methods and overall risks. The International Collaborative Study of Severe Anaphylaxis. Epidemiology 1998;9(2):141–6.
3. Ring J, Behrendt H. Anaphylaxis and anaphylactoid reactions. Clin Rev Allergy Immunol 1999;17:387–99.
4. Busse WW, Lemanske RF. Advances in immunology—asthma. N Engl J Med 2001;344(5):350–62.
5. Murrart T, Bihar D. Anaphylaxis and anaphylactoid reactions. Int J C in Pract 2000;54(5):322–8.
6. Atkinson, TP, Kaliner MA. Anaphylaxis. Clin Allergy 1992; 76(4):841.
7. Sampson HA, Mendelson L, Rosen JP. Fatal and near-fatal anaphylactic reactions to food in children and adolescents. N Engl J Med 1992;327:380–4.
8. Kagy L, Blaiss M. Anaphylaxis in children. Pediatr Ann 1998;27(11):727–34.
9. Burks WA, Jones SM, Wheeler JG, Sampson HA, Anaphylaxis and food hypersensitivity. Immunol Allergy Clin North Am 1999;19(3):533–52.
10. Kanerva SB. Anaphylaxis is caused by banana. Allergy 1993; 48:215–16.
11. Celestin J, Heiner DC. Food induced anaphylaxis. West J Med 1993;158:610–11.
12. Tarlo SM, Sussman GL. Asthma and anaphylactoid reactions to food additives. Can Fam Physician 1993;39:1119–23.
13. Bock SA. Anaphylaxis to coriander: a sleuthing story. J Allergy Clin Immunol 1993;91:1232–3.
14. Axelsson IGK, Ihre E, Zetterstrom O. Anaphylactic reactions to sunflower seed. Allergy 1994;49:517–20.
15. Moffitt JE, Yates AB, Stafford CT. Allergy to insect stings. Postgrad Med 1993;93:197–207.
16. Reisman RE. Natural history of insect sting allergy: relationship of severity of symptoms of initial sting anaphylaxis to re-sting reactions. J Allergy Clin Immunol 1992;90:335–9.
17. Sobotka AK, Adkinson NF Jr, Valentine MD, et al. Allergy to insect stings. IV. Diagnosis by radioallergosorbent test (R.A.S.T.). J Immunol 1978;121:2477–84.
18. Hough DO, Dec KL. Exercise-induced asthma and anaphylaxis. Sports Med 1994;18:162–72.

19. Nichols AW. Exercise-induced anaphylaxis and urticaria. Clin Sports Med 1992;11:303–12.

20. Briner WW, Sheffer AL. Exercise-induced anaphylaxis. Med Sci Sports Exerc 1992;24:849–50.

21. Ebo DG, Stevens WJ, DeClerck LS. Latex anaphylaxis. Acta Clin Belg 1995;50(2):87–93.

22. Kokoszka J, Nelson R. Latex anaphylaxis. Dis Colon Rectum 1993;36:868–72.

23. Steiner DJ, Schwager RG. Epidemiology, diagnosis, precautions, and policies of intraoperative anaphylaxis to latex. J Am Col Surg 1995;180:754–61.

24. Reddy S. Latex allergy. Am Fam Physician 1998;57(1):93–100.

25. Blanco C, Carrillo T, Casillo R, Quirate J, Cuevas M. Latex allergy: clinical features and cross-reactivity with fruits. Ann Allergy 1994;73:309–14.

26. National Institute for Occupational Safety and Health. Preventing allergic reactions to natural rubber latex in the workplace. NIOSH publication no. 97-135. Washington, DC: United States Department of Health and Human Services, Centers for Disease Control and Prevention, 1997.

27. Food and Drug Administration. Latex-containing devices: user labeling. Document no. fr24;N96-46. Fed Reg June 24,1996; 61(122):32617–21. (*www.access.gpo.gov*).

28. Young MA, Meyers M, McCulloch LD, et al. Latex allergy. AORN J 1992;56:488–502.

29. Fisher M, Baldo BA. Anaphylaxis during anesthesia: current aspects of diagnosis and prevention. Eur J Anesthesiol 1994;11: 263–84.

30. Hodgson TA, Shirlaw PJ, Challacombe SJ. Skin testing after anaphylactoid reactions to dental local aesthetics. Oral Surg Oral Med Oral Pathol 1993;75:706–11.

31. Assem EK. Highlights of controversial issues in anesthetic reactions. Monogr Allergy 1992;30:1–14.

32. Miles AM, Bain B. Penicillin anaphylaxis: a review of sensitization treatment, and prevention. J Assoc Acad Minority Physicians 1992;3(2):81–6.

33. Sandler SG, Mallory D, Malamut D, et al. IgA anaphylactic transfusion reactions. Transfus Med Rev 1995;9(1):1–8.

34. Kumar ND, Sharma S, Sethi S, et al. Anaphylactoid transfusion reaction with anti-IgA antibodies in an IgA deficient patient: a case report. Indian J Pathol Microbiol 1993;36:282–4.

35. Thibodeau JL. Office management of childhood vaccine-related anaphylaxis. Can Fam Physician 1994;40:1602–10.

36. Patterson R, Hogan MB, Yarnold PR, et al. Idiopathic anaphylaxis. Arch Intern Med 1995;155:869–71.

37. Kahn DA, Yocum MW. Clinical course of idiopathic anaphylaxis. Ann Allergy 1994;73:370–4.

38. Stoloff R, Greenberger PA. Anaphylaxis. Allergy Proc 1993;14: 133–4.

39. Wittbrodt ET, Spinler SA. Prevention of anaphylactoid reactions in high-risk patients receiving radiographic contrast media. Ann Pharmacol 1994;28:236–41.

40. Schaeffer RM, Horl WH. Anaphylactoid reactions during hemodialysis. Clin Nephrol 1994;42(suppl 1):S44–7.

41. Saryan JA, O'Laughlin MD. Anaphylaxis in children. Pediatr Ann 1992;21:590–8.

42. Cohn JR, Cohn JB, Fellin F, et al. Systemic anaphylaxis from low dose methotrexate. Ann Allergy 1993;70:384–5.

38

Epstein-Barr Virus Infection and Infectious Mononucleosis

James A. McSherry

First detected in African Burkitt's lymphoma cells in 1964,[1] the Epstein-Barr virus (EBV) was identified as the cause of infectious mononucleosis (IM) in 1968 when a laboratory worker developed antibodies to the virus during an episode of IM.[2] Large-scale seroepidemiologic studies subsequently confirmed the role of EBV in IM.[2] EBV has also been implicated as an etiologic factor in undifferentiated nasopharyngeal carcinoma, non-Hodgkin's lymphoma and oral hairy leukoplakia in immunocompromised individuals, and other malignant conditions.

Background

EBV is a double-stranded DNA herpes virus with a 30- to 60-nm diameter core, a 98- to 100-nm diameter nucleocapsid of icosahedral symmetry, and a lipoprotein envelope with a diameter of 120 to 250 nm and glycoprotein projections.[3] EBV is B lymphotropic. The major EBV envelope glycoprotein is gp350 and this binds to the CD21 viral receptor on the B-cell surface to facilitate entry of the virus into the cell.[4] The EBV genome encodes approximately 100 proteins and becomes incorporated within infected B cells (immortalization), making them capable of continuous proliferation, although spontaneous activation of these latently infected cells is rare. Individuals with X-linked agammaglobulinemia cannot be infected with EBV since they lack mature B cells.[5]

In primary EBV infection, the proliferation of infected B cells is controlled by natural killer cells and CD4+ and CD8+ T cells.[6] Most of the symptoms of IM can be attributed to this response to infection, whereas the hematologic abnormalities are the result of polyclonal antibodies produced by the infected B cells themselves.

Nasopharyngeal carcinoma has a peak prevalence of 50 per 100,000 persons per year in southern China, and virtually all poorly differentiated carcinomas contain EBV genomes in the transformed epithelial cells. Measurement of EBV-specific antibody titers after therapy for nasopharyngeal carcinoma has prognostic value as a declining or constant level indicates a good prognosis and vice versa.[7]

Burkitt's lymphoma was first described in equatorial Africa and usually presents as a jaw tumor. It is strongly associated geographically with *Plasmodium falciparum* malaria and the malaria is presumed to inhibit T-cell activity, thus enhancing EBV-infected cell proliferation. Almost all African Burkitt's lymphoma cases are associated with EBV infection, whereas only 20% of cases occurring in the United States are EBV associated and, in any case, tend to present as abdominal tumors. EBV DNA can be found in the Hodgkin's and Reed-Sternberg cells of approximately 50% of patients with Hodgkin's disease in the United States.[8]

Individuals infected with the human immunodeficiency virus (HIV) have many times more circulating EBV-infected cells than healthy persons, and T-cell suppression of EBV-infected B cells is less effective.[9] There is evidence that increasing EBV viral load and decreased numbers of EBV-cytotoxic T cells precede EBV-associated non-Hodgkin's lymphoma development in HIV-infected patients.[10]

Oral hairy cell leukoplakia is a nonmalignant hyperplastic lesion affecting the epithelial cells of the lateral borders of the tongue. Distinctive in appearance from candidiasis, oral hairy cell leukoplakia presents as raised, white, corrugated lesions in immunosuppressed individuals, primarily those infected with HIV, but also in some transplant recipients. Lesions may contain multiple strains of EBV.

Epidemiology

Infectious mononucleosis is the self-limiting clinical expression of symptomatic primary EBV infection and occurs mainly in young adults in the developed world. Asymptomatic infections are common, and the ratio of clinical to subclinical infections is approximately 1:3. Most adults are EBV seropositive. Seroepidemiologic studies in the United States show that 50% of students are immune to EBV at college entry; another 12% are infected each year, but only 3% develop a clinical illness. This pattern of increasing prevalence in young people in association with widening opportunities for socialization has led some commentators to liken IM to a sexually transmitted disease, "the kissing disease." The primary infection, usually asymptomatic, is common during childhood in lower socioeconomic groups, especially in underdeveloped countries where more than 80% of infants are seropositive by age 18 months.[11,12]

EBV is mainly spread by contact with saliva, as the virus replicates in oropharyngeal cells and virus shedding may persist for many months after infection. Oscultation may well be an efficient means of transmitting EBV from person to person, but coughing and inhalation of infected fomites clearly have an additional significant role to play, especially when large groups including susceptibles gather together in classrooms and college lecture halls. Sexual transmission and transmission by blood transfusion and shared use of needles and syringes are also possible. The incubation period is 30 to 50 days. IM is not particularly contagious because most contacts of known cases are already immune, and epidemics are therefore rare.

Clinical Presentation

Prodromal Illness

Infectious mononucleosis is usually preceded by a prodromal illness lasting 5 to 10 days. Patients complain of headache, malaise, fatigue, decreased exercise tolerance, anorexia, and night sweats. An enlarging spleen may cause left lower anterior chest wall pain. Clinical examination is usually normal or yields nonspecific findings during this phase. Bacterial sinusitis may result from posterior choanal obstruction due to adenoidal hypertrophy. Prescription of ampicillin or amoxicillin at this stage runs the risk of provoking an intensely pruritic, generalized erythematous rash.

Acute Symptoms

Ninety percent of patients with IM experience the acute anginose form of the disease (angina actually means "throat inflammation"). Patients present with fever, malaise, sore throat, and painful neck glands. Clinical findings during the acute phase include high fever, exudative tonsillitis and generalized lymphadenopathy (98–100% of patients), splenomegaly (75%), palatine petechiae (50%), periorbital edema (33%), and hepatomegaly (20%).[13] Small numbers of patients present with jaundice or an erythematous maculopapular skin rash. Some patients with acute IM exude a characteristic, pungent odor. Ten percent of IM patients have the typhoidal variety, where the disease is slower in onset, the symptoms less florid, and the appearance of typical hematologic and serologic signs is delayed.

Convalescence

Acute IM symptoms usually lessen within 2 weeks and resolve completely within 4 weeks. Convalescence is usually complete within 3 months of acute symptom onset, although 6% of patients report persistence of symptoms such as depressed mood, tiring easily, and impaired concentration a year after clinical recovery.[14] Mononucleosis-type infections may occur more than once, but are generally caused by sequential infections with different pathogens rather than reactivated EBV infections, although EBV can be reactivated in immunosuppressed patients.

Diagnosis

Infectious mononucleosis can be diagnosed with confidence when patients have a compatible illness and laboratory tests show the following: relative and absolute lymphocytosis on differential white blood cell count from a peripheral blood smear; lymphocyte atypia (Downey lymphocytes) of more than 20%; and heterophile antibody titers of at least 1:56 by the traditional Paul-Bunnell-Davidsohn test or a positive rapid slide assay.[15]

Hematologic Signs

Leukopenia, neutropenia, thrombocytopenia, and even neutrophil leukocytosis often precede the characteristic atypical lymphocytosis (T cells responding to infected B cells). Blood counts should be repeated if they are initially uncharacteristic and the patient's condition continues to suggest IM.

Heterophile Antibodies

Heterophile antibodies are acute-phase reactants produced by infected B cells and directed against erythrocyte antigens of a variety of nonhuman species. They can be detected by a rapid slide test. Present in 90% of IM patients at some point in the illness, they usually disappear after 3 to 4 months. Forty percent of patients with IM produce detectable levels of heterophile antibodies by the end of the first week of acute symptoms, and more than 80% produce high titers during the second week.

A slide test is unreliable as the sole diagnostic test for IM in patients with sore throats because of low negative predictive value in undifferentiated cases. The laboratory should be asked to obtain a blood sample for a complete blood count (CBC) and a slide test, but to perform the slide test only if the CBC suggests IM. This practice is cost-effective and spares a sick person an extra trip to the laboratory.

Repeated testing to assess progress is pointless once IM has been confirmed, as the patient's condition is the best guide to progress. False-positive tests for heterophile antibody have been reported as a result of technical error and in the presence of leukemia, rubella, malaria, malignant lymphoma, pancreatic carcinoma, hepatitis B, and other unknown causes.

EBV Antibody Testing

Tests for specific EBV serologic markers are unnecessary when patients satisfy clinical and hematologic criteria and are heterophile antibody positive. Ten percent of patients with IM never produce heterophile antibody, and testing for specific EBV antibodies may be indicated in these cases. Three EBV serologic tests are commonly used when available: (1) viral capsid antigen (VCA) immunoglobulins G and M (IgG and IgM); (2) early antigen (EA), diffuse (D) and restricted (R); and (3) EBV nuclear antigen (EBNA).

The VCA antibodies appear early in IM; VCA IgG persists for life, whereas VCA IgM disappears within 6 months. EA antibodies appear after VCA antibodies and remain elevated for about 6 months, whereas EBNA appears relatively late in the illness and persists lifelong. The presence of VCA IgM and EA(D) antibodies in significant titers suggests acute infection, and elevated levels of VCA IgG and EBNA antibodies indicate past infection.

Throat Cultures

Concurrent streptococcal pharyngitis is a recognized complication of IM, and throat culture for bacterial pathogens should be performed at the patient's first assessment (see Chapter 40). EBV culture is impractical in the everyday world of family medicine.

Differential Diagnosis

Severe pharyngitis can be caused by herpes simplex, group A β-hemolytic streptococci, Vincent's angina, and diphtheria. Each can be distinguished from IM by its clinical appearance and the absence of extrapharyngeal signs, atypical lymphocytosis, or a positive test for heterophile antibody. Infections caused by cytomegalovirus, *Toxoplasmosis gondii*, and *Bartonella henselae* often produce a systemic illness clinically indistinguishable from IM and featuring an atypical lymphocytosis. Sometimes referred to as "pseudomononucleosis" or the "mononucleosis syndrome," tests for heterophile and EBV-specific antibodies are negative, whereas serologic tests for other organisms assist in defining the correct etiologic agent.

Complications

Infectious mononucleosis is not always a benign illness, and its potential complications can involve any organ system. Transient impairment of liver function is common in uncomplicated IM, but routine liver function testing is unnecessary unless the diagnosis is in doubt or the patient is jaundiced. Spontaneous rupture of the spleen is a rarity in the developed world, but when it does happen IM is the commonest cause.

One to two percent of patients develop a neurologic syndrome: meningoencephalitis, transverse myelitis, Guillain-Barré syndrome, autonomic and peripheral neuropathies, cranial nerve palsies, and optic neuritis. Peritonsillar abscess occurs in 1% of cases, and tonsillar enlargement can be so extreme that upper airway obstruction results. Viral pneumonia affects 5% of patients; 6% of patients have electrocardiographic changes; and pericarditis, myocarditis, cardiomy-

opathy, and genital ulcers have been reported (see Chapters 82 and 84).

Hemolytic anemia mediated by anti-IgM cold agglutinins, thrombocytopenia, granulocytopenia, and interstitial nephritis can occur, the result of polyclonal antibody production by EBV-activated B cells, as is the appearance of heterophile antibodies themselves. The presence of clinically insignificant cold agglutinins can be inferred when the CBC shows a reduced number of red blood cells (RBCs), and an elevated mean corpuscular volume when RBC clumps are misread by an automated counter as single cells of large volume.

Six cases of "chronic infectious mononucleosis" have been described.[16] Chronic active EBV infection has the following three defining characteristics: a severe illness lasting longer than 6 months that began as a primary EBV infection or is associated with abnormal EBV antibody titers; histologic evidence of organ disease, e.g., pneumonitis, hepatitis, uveitis, or bone marrow hyperplasia; and the finding of EBV antigens or DNA in tissue.

Duncan's disease is a rare familial X-linked lymphoproliferative disorder wherein fatal IM is associated with agammaglobulinemia and lymphoma.

Management

There is no specific therapy for IM except supportive care to the extent required by individual patients. Attention should be paid to hydration, and simple analgesics/antipyretics such as acetaminophen should be allowed as required. Antibiotics are prescribed only to treat bacterial complications. Ampicillin and amoxicillin should always be avoided in patients with IM or symptoms suggestive of IM because of the risk of producing a generalized, intensely pruritic, maculopapular, erythematous rash. This reaction is a temporary intolerance to aminopenicillins, not an allergy; and later use is not contraindicated.

Corticosteroids are effective therapy for such serious complications as impending upper airway obstruction, hemolytic anemia, and severe thrombocytopenia, but are not indicated for routine management of uncomplicated IM. Specific antiviral therapies do not appear to be beneficial in IM. A meta-analysis of five randomized controlled trials involving 339 patients with acute IM treated with acyclovir showed no significant advantage in the treated group whether treated orally or intravenously.[17] A multicenter, double-blind, placebo-controlled trial found that the combination of acyclovir and prednisolone in acute IM reduced oropharyngeal shedding of EBV without having any significant effect on illness duration, symptom severity, or return to work or school.[18] Acyclovir is recommended as therapy for oral hairy leukoplakia in immunocompromised patients because of its beneficial effect on oropharyngeal shedding of EB virus.

All patients with IM should be advised to refrain from contact sports until splenic involution is complete, although there is no harm for most patients in resuming physical exercise to the degree tolerated when they feel well enough to do so.

Prevention

There have been a number of developments since a vaccine derived from EBV gp350 was first used successfully to protect cottontop tamarins against lymphomagenic doses of EBV.[19] A small-scale trial of immunization of nine seronegative children using vaccinia virus expressing gp350 produced neutralizing antibody responses to EBV in all recipients, six of whom remained uninfected by EB virus 16 months later in comparison to universal infection of an unimmunized control group. A phase 1 clinical trial using recombinant gp350 protein has been completed.[21] Emerging technologies seem to be at a point where vaccine prevention trials are not far off for infectious mononucleosis, posttransplant lymphoproliferative disease, nasopharyngeal cancer, and Hodgkin's disease, although the challenges posed by Burkitt's lymphoma justify greater caution.[22]

Family and Community Issues

For the family, the main concern is care of a sick member. Isolation is unnecessary, as most adults are already immune, and the long incubation period means that family and friends have been exposed to the index case for several weeks by the time the disease becomes apparent. Secondary cases are rare within households.

Infectious mononucleosis is rare during pregnancy because of the small number of susceptible women. There is no evidence that primary EBV infection or reactivation of latent infection during pregnancy has any adverse effect on the fetus.[23]

References

1. Epstein MA, Achong BG, Barr YM. Virus particles in cultured lymphoblasts from Burkitt's lymphoma. Lancet 1964;1:702–3.
2. Henle G, Henle W, Diehl V. Relation of Burkitt's tumour associated herpes-type virus to infectious mononucleosis. Proc Natl Acad Sci USA 1968;101:94–101.
3. Cohen JI. Molecular biology of Epstein-Barr virus and its mechanism of B-cell transformation. Ann Intern Med 1993;118: 48–50.
4. Fingeroth JD, Weis JJ, Tedder TF, Strominger JL, Biro PA, Pearson DT. Epstein-Barr virus receptor of human B lymphocytes in the C3d receptor CR2. Proc Natl Acad Sci USA 1984;81:4510–4.
5. Faulkner GC, Burrows SR, Khanna R, Moss DJ, Bird AG, Crawford DH. X-linked agammaglobulinemia patients are not infected with Epstein-Barr virus: implications for biology of the virus. J Virol 1999;73:1555–64.
6. Rickinson AB, Moss DJ. Human cytoxic T lymphocyte responses to Epstein-Barr virus infection. Annu Rev Immunol 1997;15:405–31.
7. Halprin J, Scott AL, Jacobson LJ, et al. Enzyme-linked immunosorbent assay of antibodies to Epstein-Barr virus nuclear and early antigens in patients with infectious mononucleosis and nasopharyngeal carcinoma. Ann Intern Med 1986;104:331–7.
8. Weiss LM, Movahed LA, Warnke RA, Sklar J. Detection of Epstein-Barr viral genomes in Reed-Sternberg cells of Hodgkin's disease. N Engl J Med 1989;320:502–6.
9. Bircx DL, Redfield RR, Tosato G. Defective regulation of Epstein-Barr virus infection in patients with acquired immunodeficiency syndrome (AIDS) or AIDS-related disorders. N Engl J Med 1986;314:874–9.
10. Kersten MJ, Klein MR, Holwerds AM, Miedema P, van Oers MH. Epstein-Barr virus-specific cytotoxic T cell responses in HIV-1 infection: different kinetics in patients responding to opportunistic infection or non-Hodgkin's lymphoma. J Clin Invest 1997;99:1525–33.
11. Biggar RJ, Henle W, Fleisher G, Bocker J, Lennette ET, Henle G. Primary Epstein-Barr virus infections in African infants. I. Decline of monoclonal antibodies and time of infection. Int J Cancer 1978;22:239–43.
12. Biggar RJ, Henle G, Bocker J, Lennette ET, Fleisher G, Henle W. Primary Epstein-Barr virus infections in African infants. II. Clinical and serological observations. Int J Cancer 1978;22: 244–50.
13. Hoagland RJ. Clinical manifestations. In: Glade PR, ed., Infectious mononucleosis. Orlando, FL: Grune & Stratton, 1967;52–60.
14. Lambore S, McSherry J, Kraus A. Acute and chronic symptoms of mononucleosis. J Fam Pract 1991;33:33–7.
15. Hoagland RJ. General features of infectious mononucleosis. In: Glade PR, editor. Infectious mononucleosis. Philadelphia: Lippincott, 1973;3–4.
16. Straus SE. The chronic mononucleosis syndrome. J Infect Dis 1988;157:405–12.
17. Torre D, Tambini R. Acyclovir for treatment of infectious mononucleosis: a meta-analysis. Scand J Infect Dis 1999;31: 543–7.
18. Tynell E, Aurelius E, Brandell A, et al. Acyclovir and prednisolone treatment of acute infectious mononucleosis: a multicenter, double-blind, placebo-controlled study. J Infect Dis 1996;174(2):324–31.
19. Morgan AJ, Allison AC, Finerty S, et al. Validation of first-generation Epstein-Barr virus vaccine preparation suitable for human use. J Med Virol 1989;29:74–8.
20. Gu S-Y, Huang T-M, Ruan I, et al. First EBV vaccine trial in humans using recombinant vaccinia virus expressing the major membrane antigen. Dev Biol Scand 1995;84:171–7.
21. Jackman WT, Mann KA, Hoffman HJ, Spaete RR. Expression of Epstein-Barr virus gp 350 as a single chain glycoprotein for EBV subunit vaccine. Vaccine 1999;17:660–8.
22. Khanna R, Moss DJ, Burrows SR. Vaccine strategies against Epstein-Barr virus associated diseases: lessons from studies on cytotoxic T-cell-mediated immune regulation.
23. Durbin WA, Sullivan JL. Epstein-Barr virus infections. Pediatr Rev 1994(2);15:63–8.

39
Viral Infections of the Respiratory Tract

George L. Kirkpatrick

Viral infections of the respiratory tract are responsible for large amounts of time lost from the workplace and significant morbidity and mortality in the very young and the very old. The worldwide pandemic of influenza in 1918 was alone responsible for nearly 30 million deaths in excess of those expected for influenza. Viral respiratory infections are the most frequent illnesses in human beings. The most frequent causes of respiratory infections are adenoviruses, influenza viruses, parainfluenza viruses, respiratory syncytial viruses, and rhinoviruses. Frequency and severity of infection are increased in the very young and the elderly, worsened by crowding and inhaling pollutants, and influenced by anatomic, metabolic, genetic, and immunologic disorders. Respiratory infections are the leading cause of death in children under age 5 living in underdeveloped countries.[1]

Viruses Involved with Upper Respiratory Tract Infections

Table 39.1 compares the results of studies over the past 15 years detailing the prevalence rates of the common respiratory viruses. These prevalence rates include data from various parts of the world, and all age groups. Prevalence rates as high as 35% reflect the reason why these viruses are such common causes of disease.[2–13]

Viral Identification and Specimen Collection

Three techniques are commonly utilized to obtain specimens for viral identification. Nasopharyngeal swabs are sterile swabs inserted 3 to 4 cm into one nostril, left in place about 5 seconds, then removed and placed in a culturette containing modified Stuart's medium for transport to the lab. (One such system is the Becton Dickinson Microbiology Systems Mini-Tip Culturette, San Diego, CA.) Nasopharyngeal wash specimens are

collected according to the method described by Hall and Douglas.[14] A 1-ounce rubber ear syringe (Davol, Inc., Cranston, RI) is loaded with 3 to 5 mL of sterile phosphate-buffered saline. With the patient's head tipped back about 70 degrees, the bulb tip is inserted until it occludes the nostril. With one complete squeeze and release, the nasal wash is collected in the bulb. The bulb contents are then emptied into a sterile screw-top tube for transport to the lab. Nasopharyngeal aspirate specimens are collected using a pediatric suction catherer (Safe-T-Vac, Kendall Healthcare Products, Mansfield, MA). Normal saline, 2 to 3 mL, is instilled into a nostril and the specimen is aspirated moments later into a sterile specimen trap.

Laboratory Testing

The standard to which laboratory tests for viral identification are compared is viral culture on monkey kidney, human lung laryngeal epidermoid carcinoma (Hep-2), and human embryonal diploid lung cell tissue culture. These cultures are studied daily for evidence of cytopathic effect. Cultures may become positive in several days to several weeks. Sensitivity of viral culture ranges from 7% to 94%. Specificity is very high. The Bartels viral respiratory screening and identification kit is an indirect fluorescence antibody procedure that contains monoclonal antibodies for seven respiratory viruses. This type of test has sensitivity of 84% to 88% and results are available in less than 24 hours after specimen collection.[15] Several laboratories are developing rapid reverse-transcription polymerase chain reaction (RT-PCR) tests (Prodesse, Inc., Milwaukee, WI) that improve sensitivity and shorten reporting time for respiratory virus identification. Sensitivities for rhinoviruses improved from 8% for tissue culture methods to 56% for the RT-PCR method.[8,16] Tests based on the reaction between viral neuraminidase from influenza viruses and a chromogenic substrate (Z Statflu Test, Zymetx, Oklahoma City, OK, USA) are available to detect influenza types A and

Table 39.1. **Prevalence Rates of the Common Respiratory Viruses**

	Flu A	Flu B	Para	Adeno	RSV	Rhino	Corona	Flu A & B
Croatia study[2]			2.3		7.6	33.6		0.6
Indian hospital study[3]			5	3	5			6
Nursing home study[4]			2		12	9.4		
COPD study[5]			8	0.7	3.1	6	5	4.2
Hospitalized colds[6]						12.5	4.7	
Cost-effective study[7]	5.9	1.2		0.35	18			
Early detection study[8]	1.8		2.7	4.5	12.8	35.8		
Pediatric inpatients, Taiwan[9]	5.5	2.6	2.0	4.0	1.7	12.7		
Chronically ill patients[10]	7.2	0.1	7.5	1.1	10.3	4.2	2.5	
Hospitalized Korean children[11]	4.8	1.3	6.5	3.9	11.8			
Hospitalized German children[12]	7.0	1.3	2.8	7.7	12.6			
Children in Jordan[13]		4.0	2.0	14.0				

COPD = chronic obstructive pulmonary disease; RSV = respiratory syncytial virus.

B. Sensitivity approaches 78% and specificity nears 91% for this method with turnaround times of a few hours using throat swab specimens.[17]

Respiratory Syncytial Virus

Respiratory syncytial virus (RSV), a single-stranded RNA paramyxovirus, is the leading cause of pneumonia and bronchiolitis in infants and children. Virtually 100% of young children are infected with RSV by age 3. Two antigenically distinct groups of RSV (A and B) are recognized. Community outbreaks of RSV usually appear during the winter and spring in temperate climates. The diagnosis of RSV in the acute setting is usually made by viral culture of nasopharyngeal secretions. A rapid diagnostic test (Abbott test pack RSV; Directigen RSV by Becton Dickinson) employing antigen detection in nasal secretions is 95% sensitive and 99% specific. Results are available in an hour.

The spectrum of illness associated with RSV is broad, ranging from mild nasal congestion to high fever and respiratory distress. What seems to begin as a simple cold may suddenly become a life-threatening illness. Modes of spread are primarily via large-droplet inoculation (requiring close contact) and self-inoculation via contaminated fomites or skin. RSV is recoverable from countertops for up to 6 hours from the time of contamination, from rubber gloves for up to 90 minutes, and from skin for up to 20 minutes. Viral shedding of RSV in infants is a prolonged process averaging 7 days. Strategies for controlling spread of RSV should be aimed at interrupting hand carriage of the virus and self-inoculation of the eyes and nose. Masks commonly employed for respiratory viruses have not been shown to be an effective measure for curtailing RSV outbreaks on pediatric wards. Hand washing is probably the single most important infection control measure for RSV.

Influenza Viruses

Influenza, considered a benign disease today, has ravaged human populations recently enough that there are still those living who can recall the 1918 worldwide pandemic, called the "Spanish flu." This particular influenza began as an ordinary attack of influenza and rapidly developed into severe pneumonia. Within hours, the patients had mahogany-colored spots over the cheekbones and cyanosis began to spread over the face. Death shortly overcame them as they struggled for air and suffocated. It is important to realize that although worldwide 30 million deaths were attributed to influenza, 97% of people who were infected had a 3-day course of fever and malaise and recovered. Of the 3% who died, most died of pneumonia. A small subset died very rapidly of massive pulmonary edema and hemorrhage. Influenza pandemics occur about every 7 to 11 years. They are always associated with extensive morbidity and a marked increase in mortality.

Type A influenza is an RNA virus with a negative-sense segmented genome. It undergoes continuous antigenic drift because it has no proofreading mechanism, and is prone to mutate during replication. Influenza virus is chimeric, existing in wild bird and swine reservoirs, with minor antigenic drifts making the same virus infectious among birds, humans, or swine.[18]

In addition to the predominant influenza virus that invades an area each season, many types, subtypes, or variants are identified during each epidemic period. During the early stage of an epidemic, a disproportionate number of cases involve school-age children, 10 to 19 years old. Later in the epidemic, more cases are diagnosed in younger children and adults. The age shift suggests that the early spread of influenza viruses in a community is concentrated among schoolchildren.

Parainfluenza Viruses

Parainfluenza is a single-stranded RNA virus of which four serotypes and two subtypes are recognized (parainfluenza types 1, 2, 3, 4A, and 4B). Bronchiolitis, croup, and pneumonia occur with all parainfluenza types. In children under 1 year of age, bronchiolitis is associated mostly with type 2. In older children, croup is most commonly associated with types 1 and 2. Immunosuppression, chronic cardiac, or pulmonary diseases are associated with increased risk of parainfluenza infection.[19] Most persons have been infected with parainfluenza virus by age 5. Immunity to parainfluenza is incomplete, and, as with RSV, reinfection occurs throughout life and probably plays a major role in the spread of virus to the young infant.

Parainfluenza types 1 and 2 tend to peak during the autumn of the year, whereas parainfluenza type 3 shows an increased prevalence during late spring. Adult infection results in mild upper respiratory tract symptoms, although pneumonia occasionally occurs. Outbreaks of parainfluenza types 1 and 3 have been reported from long-term-care facilities.[20] Illness is characterized by fever, sore throat, rhinorrhea, and cough. The rate of pneumonia is relatively high.

Most studies suggest direct person-to-person transmission. Parainfluenza is stable in small-particle aerosols at the low humidity found in hospitals. Outbreaks tend to proceed more slowly than influenza or other aerosol-spread infections.[21] Infection control policies should emphasize hand washing and isolation of patients.

Rhinoviruses

Rhinovirus is a non-enveloped, 30-nm, RNA virus with over 100 serotypes. It only replicates in primates. It is characterized by a single positive stranded genome not only acting as a template for RNA synthesis, but also encoding for a single polypeptide necessary for viral replication. It belongs to the picornavirus family, a diverse group of viral pathogens that together are the most common causes of infection in human beings. Within the picornavirus family are found the rhinoviruses, the enteroviruses, and the hepatoviruses (including hepatitis A). Rhinovirus infection is transmitted by direct contact with the eye or nasal mucous membrane. The most efficient modes of spread are hand-to-hand contact or contact with a contaminated surface followed by inoculation of the nose or conjunctiva. Rhinoviruses remain infectious for as long as 3 hours on nonporous surfaces. Transmission can be decreased by hand washing and disinfecting environmental surfaces. After deposition on nasal mucosa, the virus binds to intercellular adhesion molecule type 1 (ICAM-1) receptors on epithelial cells, initiating a cascade of inflammatory responses. Viral replication occurs in the nose, and viral shedding continues for up to 3 weeks. The cascade of interleukin-6, -8, and -16, histamine, bradykinin, and cytokines recruit neutrophils and produce the rhinorrhea, vascongestion, sinus congestion, sore throat, cough, wheezing, and middle ear inflammation.[22,23]

There is now evidence that direct invasion of the lower respiratory tract does occur, causing bronchitis and possibly triggering asthma attacks and exacerbation of chronic obstructive pulmonary disease (COPD). New antirhinoviral treatments are being tested. Intranasal interferon prevents infection, but provides no therapeutic benefit. Oral pleconaril shows therapeutic promise. Intranasal tremacamra and AG7088 are under investigation.[24,25] For the time being, treatment is mostly symptomatic, with antibiotics and steroids showing no benefit.

Coronaviruses

Coronaviruses, members of the Coronaviridae family, are single-stranded RNA viruses first identified in 1962. They do not appear to replicate in any animal models and are almost impossible to isolate in standard tissue cultures. Acute and convalescent sera for enzyme immunoassay will identify the two common subtypes, 229E and OC43. The enzyme-linked immunosorbent assay (ELISA) has been used to identify coronaviruses in nasal secretions.[26] A 1997 study of frail older persons by Falsey and McCann[27] found 37 (8%) of 451 serologies positive for coronavirus 229E over 44 months. It was noted that illnesses were indistinguishable from RSV and influenza virus infections. Lower respiratory complications, such as pneumonia, occurred in one fourth of the infected residents.

Epidemics occur during late fall through early spring. Clinical symptoms usually include nasal congestion, headache, cough, sore throat, malaise, and low-grade fever similar to rhinoviral infections. Coronavirus infections have been associated with lower respiratory tract illnesses, including pneumonia and bronchiolitis in young children. Coronavirus is the second most frequent virus associated with asthma exacerbations; rhinovirus is the most frequent. Interferon-α, tremacamra, and pleconaril have shown promise in prevention and treatment of these infections.

Adenoviruses

Adenoviruses are double-stranded DNA viruses. There are 51 serotypes divided into six subgenera (A–F) that exhibit distinctly different organ tropisms. Adenoviruses cause a broad spectrum of diseases, including conjunctivitis, keratoconjunctivitis, pharyngoconjunctival fever, pharyngitis, tonsillitis, coryza, pneumonia, heart disease, hepatitis, nephritis, and gastroenteritis. All ages are affected, but the majority of illness occurs in children younger than 6 years old. Military recruits in the United States from 1971 to 1995 received adenovirus vaccine to types 4 and 7. Since vaccine production ceased in 1995, an average of 4555 cases of adenoviral respiratory disease occur annually on military bases, costing about $2.6 million per year.[28] Adenovirus is ubiquitous, found everywhere during all seasons of the year, with annual peaks of activity in midsummer and midwinter. Transmission can occur by aerosolized droplets, fomites, hand carriage, fecal-oral, and by contact with contaminated lake water while swimming. The virus can be isolated for prolonged periods from respiratory secretions, conjunctival secretions, and stools of infected patients. Adenoviruses are identified by cytopathic effect in tissue cultures from nasopharyngeal specimens. They are also detected by indirect fluorescence antibody procedures (e.g., Bartels, Issaquah, WA, Viral Respiratory Screening and Identification Kit) using monoclonal antibodies. Newer RT-PCR testing (Taqman PCR, Glaxo Wellcome, Research Triangle Park, NC) can provide very accurate results in 6 to 12 hours, and primers are available for all adenovirus serotypes.[18]

Disease Presentations

Common Cold

The common cold, a disease of antiquity, is characterized by objective signs and subjective symptoms that are usually self-limited. Symptoms that occur with common colds include sneezing, watering of the eyes, nasal stuffiness, nasal obstruction, postnasal discharge, sore throat, hoarseness, cough, and sputum production. The common cold is a clinical diagnosis and lacks specificity because other ailments such as allergies and early symptoms of more serious illnesses mimic common cold symptoms. In the United States colds account for 23 million lost days of work and 26 million lost school days per year.

Diagnosis

Rhinoviruses and coronaviruses are the most common causes of the common cold, with RSV and adenoviruses producing a similar set of signs and symptoms especially in adults. Mild cases of influenza and parainfluenza infection can be mistaken for the common cold. Because there are now a number of specific (as well as nonspecific and symptomatic) treatments for these viruses, it has become prudent medicine to undertake identification of the infecting virus, especially in more severe cases. Direct and indirect immunofluorescent staining techniques with virus-specific monoclonal antibodies (e.g., Chemicon International, Inc., Temecula, CA) or RT-PCR tests (e.g., Taqman PCR, Glaxo Wellcome) are well tested throughout the world and provide virus identification in a matter of hours almost anywhere.

Management

There are as many ways to manage the common cold as there are physicians. Gwaltney and Park[29] tested the therapeutic efficacy of clemastine fumarate, a second-generation antihistamine, and found reduction in total volume of rhinorrhea and number of sneezes in their patients challenged with rhinovirus. First-generation antihistamines reduce rhinorrhea and sneezing, and nonsteroidal antiinflammatory drugs reduce coughing, headache, malaise, and myalgias.

Intranasal steroid sprays reduce symptoms, but have little effect on duration of illness. Steroids may lengthen the period of viral shedding. Renewed interest in herbal and homeopathic remedies has produced clinical trials designed as randomized double-blind, placebo-controlled, multicenter studies mostly focused on symptom relief.[30] Jackson and Lesho[31] conducted a meta-analysis of 10 clinical trials on the use of zinc gluconate lozenges for treatment of the common cold. They concluded that evidence for effectiveness of zinc lozenges in reducing the duration of common colds is still lacking. Similar negative results have been reported from studies using heated, humidified air (steam) for cold treatment. Recent improved understanding of the pathophysiology of rhinoviral colds has focused attention on the neutrophilic inflammatory reaction, chemotaxis regulation, cytokinesis, and upregulation of immunocompetent cells. Pleconaril 200 mg twice a day for 7 days decreases signs and symptoms as well as reducing viral shedding.[32] Tremacamra, a synthetic ICAM-1 glycoprotein acts as an antiadhesion molecule when sprayed into the nostrils. Tremacamra produces a significant decrease in symptoms.[33] Rest, adequate hydration, and time to recover should be stressed during management of the com-

mon cold. In the future, antirhinovirus drugs and interferon may reach development levels where alleviation of symptoms or prevention of infection exceeds side effects.

Complications and Sequelae

When the diagnosis of the common cold is accurate, complications and sequelae are minimal. Complications generally result from assuming the cold symptoms are caused by rhinovirus or coronavirus, when in fact influenza, RSV, adenovirus, or a bacterial pathogen are responsible. Complications also occur in immunocompromised patients where rhinovirus can cause fatal pneumonia. Sequelae include asthma triggered by the rhinoviral-induced airway inflammation, and otitis media precipitated by viral-induced eustachian tube dysfunction with altered middle ear pressure.

Hand washing is the most important way to prevent transmission of these viruses. With rhinoviruses and RSV, direct contact with a contaminated surface followed by inoculation of the nose or conjunctiva can result in infection. Use of masks and gloves and isolation of infected persons is the most effective way to limit the spread of cold viruses.

Influenza

Influenza has one of the more characteristic sets of clinical findings. The onset is usually sudden, with shivering, sweating, headache, aching in the orbits, and general malaise and misery. Cough is often found early in the course, aggravating headaches and causing generalized aching. The onset is generally explosive, with fever in adults ranging up to 102°F. In children the fever may be higher than 102°F, and sore throat may be an early sign. The most consistent signs are the presence of polymyalgias, weakness, and malaise.

Diagnosis

Not surprisingly, the diagnosis of influenza is more accurate during epidemics and less accurate during nonepidemic periods. Influenza in the United States usually occurs during December, January, and February. Successful presumptive diagnosis requires appropriate clinical symptomatology at the right time of the year and a knowledge of the pattern of influenza illness around the world. Virologic studies, including cultures from throat swabs and nasopharyngeal washings, cells from nasopharyngeal washings stained with monoclonal antibody fluorescence stains, and complement fixation studies on paired serum samples can confirm the diagnosis. The Zstatflu test (Zymetx, Oklahoma City, OK, USA) is a rapid detection kit for both type A and type B influenza. It is based on the reaction between influenza neuraminidase and a chromogenic substrate. Throat swab or nasopharyngeal swab specimens will generate results in a few hours. There are several rapid flu A and flu B tests available currently that report results in less than an hour.

Management

Because several new effective medications are now readily available for treatment of influenza, virologic testing to confirm the diagnosis and type the virus is important. Amantadine (Symmetrel) 100 mg twice a day, is effective treatment for influenza type A, but not type B. Patients with compromised renal function should reduce the dose to 100 mg once a day. The dose in children up to age 10 is 3 mg/pound/day as a single dose. More recently, rimantadine (Flumadine) in the same doses offers the same good results with fewer side effects. Within the past 2 years, two neuraminidase inhibitors, zanamivir (Relenza) and oseltamivir (Tamiflu), have been approved for use and are widely available to treat both types of influenza. Zanamivir is inhaled as 10 mg twice a day. Oseltamivir is taken orally as 75 mg twice a day for adults and 2 mg/kg twice a day for children, used daily for 5 days. Because of the severity of the myalgias and headache associated with influenza, aspirin and nonsteroidal antiinflammatory drugs (NSAIDs) may not suffice and a narcotic-containing product is frequently indicated.

Complications and Sequelae

Most statistical methods for assessing excess morbidity and mortality are based on an index of influenza complicated by pneumonia, which may produce an underestimation of the serious morbidity and mortality. During an influenza outbreak, there is usually an increased death rate among the elderly mostly due to pneumonia and cardiovascular disease. Influenza itself can cause severe and rapidly evolving viral pneumonia with multiorgan failure. Children under 5 years of age have the highest rates of hospitalization for acute upper and lower respiratory tract disease when infected with influenza. Pandemic strains of extreme virulence such as the 1918 influenza can cause far-reaching complications. The 1918 Spanish flu caused 5 million cases of encephalitis lethargica (of von Economo) with symptoms of acute encephalitis with or without death and postencephalitic Parkinson's disease. The 1957 pandemic produced a small number of people with massive pulmonary edema and hemorrhage with rapid death as was seen commonly in 1918. Even in the years where the circulating influenza strains are mild, there is a rise in the number of cases of otitis media, bronchitis, asthma, and exacerbation of COPD.

Control and Prevention

Influenza vaccine is produced on the recommendation of the Food and Drug Administration (FDA) Vaccines and Related Biologicals Advisory Committee. Antigenic choices are based on (1) the viruses that have been seen during the previous year, (2) the viruses that are being seen in other parts of the world during the current year, and (3) the estimated antibody response in persons previously infected or vaccinated to these viruses. The current strategy is to immunize high-risk groups (the elderly and children with underlying conditions including heart, pulmonary, malignant, and some metabolic diseases). Unfortunately, the level of acceptance by patients and the overall delivery of vaccines to high-risk children has been consistently poor. This approach leaves most of the population unvaccinated, which produces a large "at-risk" population to be infected. Another approach to the control of influenza is to immunize all schoolchildren, children in day care, college students, military personnel, and employees of large companies. These groups have the highest susceptibil-

ity and, because of the nature of their activities, are the principal vectors of influenza virus in the community. They are also an accessible population with a structured environment that permits effective distribution of influenza vaccine. Efforts should also be directed toward immunizing as many high-risk patients as possible or to start them on chemotherapy at the first evidence of an epidemic.

Bronchitis

Diagnosis

Bronchitis is an inflammation of the major and minor bronchial branches. It is characterized by a cough that is frequently productive of sputum, depending on the inflammatory cause. Bacterial causes of bronchitis generally produce purulent-looking sputum. Viral causes of bronchitis more commonly produce either clear sputum or a nonproductive cough. On physical examination, a patient with bronchitis has a noticeable cough, but the lungs are usually normal to auscultation. Rales, dullness to percussion, egophony, and other lower respiratory findings are usually absent. Cigarette smoking, other air pollutants, and chemical exposures that cause bronchial irritation may prolong an episode of bronchitis. Systemic lupus erythematosus is a cause of persistent bronchitis in a small number of affected patients.[34]

Spectrum of Infection

Acute lower respiratory tract illness in previously well adults is usually labeled acute bronchitis and treated with antibiotics before establishing the etiology. An English study of 638 patients over 1 year identified pathogens in 55% of cases; viruses were identified as 28% of the pathogens. Outcome did not relate to pathogens. Most patients improved without antibiotics in spite of the pathogen identified.[35] Viral causes of acute bronchitis tend to be more common with influenza (types A and B), parainfluenza of all four serotypes, and RSV. RSV and parainfluenza viruses are found more commonly in the young population, and coronaviruses and adenoviruses occur in older patients. Influenza causes bronchitis at all ages. Increases in frequency of bronchitis as a reason for adult hospital admissions usually occur during influenza epidemics. RSV is a significant problem in elderly populations in nursing homes. Falsey and Walsh[36] found attack rates of up to 10% per year in nursing home patients, with up to 20% going on to pneumonia, and 5% dying.

Spasmodic Croup and Laryngotracheobronchitis

Though croup is a frightening family experience, especially for parents of very young children, it is a self-limited illness. There are two variations of croup presentation, episodic (spasmodic) croup and laryngotracheobronchitis (LTB). Episodic croup presents as the sudden onset without warning of inspiratory stridor, cough, and hoarseness. The young child has not been overtly ill, but is suddenly crouping. There is minimal or no fever and no other respiratory symptoms. LTB has early warning signs of respiratory infection for several days that gradually lead to cough and inspiratory stridor. Cool night air or a steamed bathroom will usually break episodic croup, and it does not tend to recur in the same time period. At most, one treatment of aerosolized racemic epinephrine (0.25–0.5 mL of a 2.25% solution in 3 mL of normal saline) will break the attack. On the other hand, LTB may break with one epinephrine treatment, improve, and then worsen again.

On occasion, LTB will become severe enough to warrant admission for repeated aerosol treatments or a croup tent with mist and oxygen. Steroids are effective in improving the outcome of croup when given within 6 hours of symptom onset. Prednisolone (Pediapred or Prelone) 5 to 60 mg po divided bid can be continued for several days. Steroids given prior to a racemic epinephrine treatment may reduce the likelihood of rebound return of crouping as the epinephrine wears off. Physicians should look for the coexistence of underlying illnesses and reassure the family that croup is a manageable illness. Munoz and Glasso[37] reported that 70% of croup cases were caused by parainfluenza viruses. Children under 15 years of age are more likely to croup with parainfluenza types 1 and 2. Croup has peak incidence at age 2 years, and is more common in the fall and winter months. Croup is not commonly associated with rhinovirus infections, but is associated with coronavirus infections. Adenovirus is a common cause of croup in children and occurs sporadically throughout the year, being most common during the winter and spring.

Bronchiolitis

Bronchiolitis is an acute viral respiratory disease generally found in children younger than 2 years old. The typical clinical presentation is an upper respiratory infection with cough that progresses to a more severe cough and tachypnea. Respirations become rapid and shallow with a prolonged expiratory phase. Because the infants are not able to breathe well, they are also unable to suck or drink and can become dehydrated.

Diagnosis

Physical findings include intercostal retractions and nasal flaring, which suggest pneumonia. A chest roentgenogram shows only hyperinflation with no infiltrates. Tight expiratory sounds (not entirely typical of wheezes found with asthma) are usually present, as are some rhonchi. Rales and dullness to percussion suggest the coexistence of pneumonia. Bronchiolitis is most commonly caused by RSV, occurring predominantly during the winter and spring. Parainfluenza viruses, particularly types 1 and 2, can cause bronchiolitis during early winter. The most severe cases of bronchiolitis are usually caused by influenza viruses, especially type A. The virus involved can be identified by culture of nasopharyngeal secretions or by RT-PCR or immunofluorescent assay.

Management

Management of bronchiolitis depends on the progression of signs and symptoms. Hospitalization may be necessary to correct hypoxemia or dehydration. If fever is significant, pneumonia must be ruled out. Cases that appear to be recurrent bronchiolitis may be asthma, even if the child is younger than 1 year old.

Outpatient treatment is generally supportive, with careful attention to hydration. If hospitalization becomes necessary to correct hypoxemia or dehydration, treatment is focused on oxygenation, mist, and mechanically clearing the upper airway. There is no effective antiviral agent to treat RSV and parainfluenza viruses. Ribavirin (Virazole) has shown variable effectiveness in the most severe cases of bronchiolitis, especially respirator-dependent infants. Steroids are of no proven value; however, the tight airway that reminds one of asthma may respond to both steroids and bronchodilators such as albuterol.

Infants who are at highest risk of developing severe bronchiolitis (preterm birth, bronchopulmonary dysplasia, immunocompromise and other underlying chronic diseases) can be protected during the winter season by prophylaxis with human RSV immunoglobulin or monoclonal antibodies (Palivizumab).

Complications and Sequelae

The most serious complication of bronchiolitis is respiratory failure requiring ventilatory assistance. It is best managed with continuous positive airway pressure and oxygen. RSV accounts for an estimated 90,000 hospitalizations and 4500 deaths per year in children under 16 years of age in the United States. Mortality rates in institutionalized elderly can reach 20%.

Bronchiolitis caused by RSV is strongly associated with postinfection wheezing for as long as 10 years. Careful studies have shown rates of asthma from 23% to 30% several years after hospitalization as an infant for RSV bronchiolitis.

Pharyngoconjunctival Fever

Pharyngoconjunctival fever is an upper respiratory illness that affects teenagers and adults. It manifests as pharyngitis, cough, fever, headache, myalgias, malaise, and particularly conjunctivitis. This syndrome is caused by adenovirus, particularly serotypes 3 and 7, which are frequently found in natural bodies of water and reservoirs. Symptoms may be similar to those of influenza. Conjunctivitis is generally not present with influenza but is always found with pharyngoconjunctival fever and usually at an early stage. There is a spring and summer seasonal prevalence. It can be diagnosed by viral cultures of nasopharyngeal and throat swabs and the recently developed immunofluorescent and RT-PCR tests. Management of pharyngoconjunctival fever is symptomatic. There is no indication for systemic antibiotic treatment or ophthalmic antibiotics. There are no long-term complications or sequelae. Recovery is generally within 1 week.

Laryngitis

There are six distinct causes of laryngitis, the most common being viral infections of the upper respiratory tract. Vocal cord tumors can cause laryngitis; allergies are a frequent cause, and strain of the vocal cords caused by long periods of loud talking produces laryngitis. A fairly frequent cause of laryngitis is hard coughing associated with an upper or lower respiratory tract infection. The least frequent cause is a bacterial infection of the throat. Most of the causes of laryngitis are obvious. Viral laryngitis is difficult to distinguish from the less frequent bacterial laryngitis, which might require antibiotic treatment. Children over age 2 and adults rarely have sig-

Table 39.2. **Patterns of Viral Illness in Children and Elderly Patients**

Virus	Signs and Symptoms		
	Young children	Adults	Elderly
Respiratory syncytial virus	Wheezing, bronchiolitis, pneumonia, bronchitis	Nasal congestion and cough	Nasal congestion, cough, fever, pneumonia, wheezing, bronchitis
Influenza	Sore throat, high fever, myalgias, bronchitis, croup, bronchiolitis, rhinorrhea, otitis media	Fever, headache, myalgias, malaise, cough, weakness, bronchitis, laryngitis	Bronchitis, low-grade fever, sore throat, pneumonia
Parainfluenza	Croup, bronchitis, pneumonia, sore throat, bronchiolitis	Common cold, laryngitis	Rhinorrhea, sore throat, cough, pneumonia, fever
Rhinoviruses	Sore throat, rhinorrhea	Rhinorrhea, sneezing, cough, sore throat, laryngitis	Rhinorrhea, cough, sneezing
Coronaviruses	Croup, sore throat	Common cold, malaise, headache, sore throat, low-grade fever	Exacerbation of chronic pulmonary disease, pneumonia, bronchitis
Adenoviruses	Croup, sore throat	Coryza, sore throat, pneumonia, pharyngoconjunctival fever, keratoconjunctivitis, laryngitis	Bronchitis rarely

nificant swelling of the throat that would put them at risk of airway obstruction. Children under age 2 are more likely to develop airway obstruction. Viral causes of laryngitis include the parainfluenza viruses, rhinoviruses, adenoviruses, and the influenza viruses. Voice rest has the greatest impact on recovery. Patients who are able to gargle with warm, weak saltwater solution sometimes find it soothing. Patients should be told that laryngitis is not a serious disease and that adequate time to recover is the only therapy in most cases.

Viral Respiratory Tract Infections in Very Young and Very Old Patients

Patients younger than age 2 present some special problems. Perhaps as many as two thirds of pediatric emergency room visits for respiratory infections are inappropriate. Parents frequently need only reassurance that their child is not seriously ill. Although most viral respiratory infections in children appear to be self-limited and without complications, they are among the leading causes of death in the youngest children. Table 39.2 details the patterns of viral illness found in young children, adults, and elderly patients. The institutionalized elderly represent a subgroup of older people who are prone to excess morbidity and mortality from respiratory tract infections. Each year many elderly persons living in long-term-care facilities become ill with respiratory illnesses that are mistakenly attributed to bacterial pneumonia or influenza. The respiratory tract viruses listed in Table 39.2 (particularly RSV, parainfluenza virus, and influenza virus) are a significant cause of disease in this high-risk population. RSV ranks second to influenza as the most common cause of serious viral respiratory infections in long-term-care facility patients. The pattern of reported outbreaks of RSV in a long-term-care facility is

usually a steady trickle of cases over several months—distinctly different from outbreaks of influenza, which tend to be explosive. Parainfluenza virus is a common cause of croup and bronchitis in young children; however, because full immunity does not develop, reinfection is common in the older population. In the institutionalized elderly, parainfluenza presents as rhinorrhea, pharyngitis, cough, and pneumonia.

References

1. Denny FW. The clinical impact of human respiratory virus infections. Am J Respir Crit Care Med 1995;Oct. 152(4PT2):54–12.
2. Milinaric G. Epidemiological picture of respiratory viral infections in Croatia. Acta Med Iugosl 1991;45:203–11.
3. Jain A. An Indian hospital study of viral causes of acute respiratory infection in children. J Med Microbiol 1991;35:219–23.
4. Falsey AR, Treanor JJ. Viral respiratory infections in the institutionalized elderly; clinical and epidemiology findings. J Am Geriatr Soc 1992;40:115–19.
5. Greenberg SB, Allen M. Respiratory viral infections in adults with and without chronic obstructive pulmonary disease. Am J Respir Crit Care Med 2000;162:167–73.
6. El-Sahly HM, Atmar RL. Spectrum of clinical illness in hospitalized patients with "common cold" virus infections. Clin Infect Dis 2000;31:96–100.
7. Barenfanger J, Drake C. Clinical and financial benefits of rapid detection of respiratory viruses: an outcomes study. J Clin Microbiol 2000;38:2824–8.
8. Steininger C, Aberle SW. Early detection of acute rhinovirus infections by a rapid reverse transcription–PCR assay. J Clin Microbiol 2001;39:129–33.
9. Tsai HP, Kuo PH. Respiratory viral infections among pediatric inpatients and outpatients in Taiwan from 1997 to 1999. J Clin Microbiol 2001;39:111–18.
10. Glezen WP, Greenberg SB. Impact of respiratory virus infections on persons with chronic underlying conditions. JAMA 2000;283:499–505.
11. Kim MR, Lee HR. Epidemiology of acute viral respiratory tract infections in Korean children. J Infect 2000;41:152–8.

12. Weigl JA, Puppe W. Epidemiological investigation of nine respiratory pathogens in hospitalized children in Germany using multiplex reverse-transcriptase polymerase chain reaction. Eur J Clin Microbiol Infect Dis 2000;19:336–43.
13. Nasrallah GK, Meqdam MM. Prevalence of parainfluenza and influenza viruses amongst children with upper respiratory tract infection. Saudi Med J 2000;21:1024–9.
14. Hall CB, Douglas RG. Clinically useful method for the isolation of respiratory syncytial virus. J Infect Dis 1975;131:1–5.
15. Irmen KE, Kelleher JJ. Use of monoclonal antibodies for rapid diagnosis of respiratory viruses in a community hospital. Clin Diagn Lab Immunol 2000;7:396–403.
16. Kehl SC, Henrickson KJ. Evaluation of the hexaplex assay for detection of respiratory viruses in children. J Clin Microbiol 2001;39:1696–701.
17. Shimizu H. The rapid detection kit based on neuraminidase activity of influenza virus. Nippon Rinsho 2000;58:2234–7.
18. Munoz FM, Glasso GJ. Current research on influenza and other respiratory viruses. Antiviral Res 2000;46:91–124.
19. Laurichesse H, Dedman D. Epidemiological features of parainfluenza virus infections: laboratory surveillance in England and Wales, 1975–1997. Eur J Epidemiol 1999;15:475–84.
20. Todd FJ, Drinka PJ. A serious outbreak of parainfluenza type 3 on a nursing unit. J Am Geriatr Soc 2000;48:1216–8.
21. Graman PS, Hall CB. Epidemiology and control of nosocomial viral infections. Infect Dis Clin North Am 1989;3:815–41.
22. Mygina N. The common cold as a trigger of asthma. Monaldi Arch Chest Dis 2000;55:478–83.
23. Van Kempen MJ, Bachert C. An update on the pathophysiology of rhinovirus upper respiratory tract infection. Rhinology 1999;37:97–103.
24. Hayden FG. Influenza virus and rhinovirus-related otitis media: potential for antiviral intervention. Vaccine 2000;19(suppl): 566–70.
25. Rotbart HA. Antiviral therapy for enteroviruses and rhinoviruses. Antivir Chem Chemother 2000;11:261–71.
26. Isaacs D, Flowers D. Epidemiology of coronavirus respiratory infections. Arch Dis Child 1983;58:500–3.
27. Falsey AR, McCann RM. The "common cold" in frail older persons: impact of rhinovirus and coronavirus in a senior day care center. J Am Geriatr Soc 1997;45:706–11.
28. Hyer RN, Howell MR. Cost-effectiveness analysis of reacquiring and using adenovirus types 4 and 7 vaccines in naval recruits. Am J Trop Med Hyg 2000;62:613–8.
29. Gwaltney JM Jr, Park J. Randomized controlled trial of clemastine fumarate for treatment of experimental rhinovirus colds. Clin Infect Dis 1996;22:656–62.
30. Henneicke-Von Zepelin H. Efficacy and safety of a fixed combination phytomedicine in the treatment of the common cold: results of a randomized, double blind, placebo controlled, multicentre study. Curr Med Res Opin 1999;15:214–27.
31. Jackson JL, Lesho E. Zinc and the common cold: a meta-analysis revisited. J Nutr 2000;130(55 suppl):15125–55.
32. Schiff GM, Sherwood JR. Clinical activity of pleconaril in an experimentally induced coxsackievirus A21 respiratory infection. J Infect Dis 2000;181:2000–26.
33. Meddiratta PK, Sharma KK. A review on recent development of common cold therapeutic agents. Indian J Med Sci 2000;54: 485–90.
34. Raz E, Bursztyn M. Severe recurrent lupus laryngitis. Am J Med 1992;92:109–10.
35. Macfarlane J, Holmes W. Prospective study of the incidence, aetiology and outcome of adult lower respiratory tract illness in the community. Thorax 2001;56:109–14.
36. Falsey AR, Walsh EE. Respiratory syncytial virus infection in adults. Clin Microbiol Rev 2000;13:371–84.
37. Munoz FM, Glasso GJ. Current research on influenza and other respiratory viruses Antiviral Res 2000;46(2):91–124.

40
Sinusitis and Pharyngitis

Paul Evans and William F. Miser

Sinusitis

Sinusitis, or rhinosinusitis, is a common problem, with 25 million office visits per year in the United States and over $7 billion in direct costs.[1] It is primarily caused by ostial obstruction of the anterior ethmoid and middle meatal complex due to retained secretions, edema, or polyps. Barotrauma, nasal cannulation, or ciliary transport defects can also precipitate infection.[2] Most sinusitis is handled well at the primary care level; there appear to be few discernible differences in technical efficiency between generalists and specialists in its treatment.[3]

Classification and Diagnosis

There are four classification categories, all of which have similar signs and symptoms but varying durations and recurrence rates. Signs and symptoms associated with sinusitis include major and minor types. Two or more major, or one major and two or more minor, or nasal purulence typify all rhinosinusitis classifications. Major symptoms include facial pain and pressure, nasal obstruction, nasal or postnasal discharge, hyposmia, and fever (in acute sinusitis). Minor signs and symptoms include headache, fever (other than acute sinusitis), halitosis, fatigue, dental pain, cough, and ear fullness or pain.[4,5] *Acute sinusitis* lasts up to 4 weeks. *Subacute sinusitis* lasts 4 to <12 weeks and resolves completely after treatment. *Recurrent acute sinusitis* has four or more episodes per year, each lasting a week or longer, with clearing between episodes. *Chronic sinusitis* lasts 12 weeks or longer.

Clinical Presentation

Pain is localized by sinus involvement: frontal sinus pain in the lower forehead, maxillary sinus in the cheek and upper teeth, ethmoidal sinus in the retro-orbital and lateral aspect of the nose, sphenoid sinus in the skull vertex.[6] Maxillary sinuses are most commonly infected, followed by ethmoidal, sphenoidal, and frontal sinuses.[7] Sneezing, watery rhinorrhea, and conjunctivitis may be seen in sinusitis associated with an allergy.

Physical Findings

Examination reveals nasal mucosal erythema and edema with purulent nasal discharge. Palpatory or percussive tenderness over the involved sinuses, particularly the frontal and maxillary sinuses, is common. Drainage from the maxillary and frontal sinuses may be seen at the middle meatus. The ethmoids drain from either the middle meatus (anterior ethmoid) or superior meatus (posterior ethmoid). The sphenoid drains into the superior meatus.[8]

Diagnostic Imaging and Laboratory Studies

Definitive diagnosis is based on clinical presentation. No imaging studies or laboratory studies are recommended for the routine diagnosis of uncomplicated sinusitis.[1] In unusual or recurrent cases, plain sinus radiographs may show air-fluid levels, mucosal thickening, and anatomic abnormalities that predispose to the condition. Views specific to each sinus are the Caldwell (frontal), Waters (maxillary), lateral (sphenoid), and submentovertical (ethmoid).[9] Computed tomography (CT) is more sensitive and may better reveal pathology, with focused sinus CT now a cost-competitive alternative to plain films.[10,11] The severity of symptoms does not correlate with severity of CT findings.[12]

Microbiology

Bacterial pathogens responsible for acute sinusitis commonly include *Streptococcus pneumoniae, Haemophilus influenzae,* group A streptococci, and *Moraxella catarrhalis.* Less commonly *Staphylococcus aureus, Streptococcus pyogenes, My-*

coplasma pneumoniae, and *Chlamydia pneumoniae* are seen. Anaerobic organisms include *Peptostreptococcus, Corynebacterium, Bacteroides,* and *Veillonella*.[13,14] Adenovirus, parainfluenza, rhinovirus, and influenza virus may cause or exacerbate sinusitis. *Aspergillus fumigatus* and *Mucormycosis* can cause sinusitis, especially in those who are immunocompromised.[9] The immunocompromised patient also has a higher susceptibility to common pathogens.[15]

Nonmicrobiologic Causes

Sinusitis may be a complication of allergic rhinitis, foreign bodies, deviated nasal septum, nasal packing, dental procedures, facial fractures, tumors, barotraumas, and nasal polyps. The cause appears to be stasis of normal physiologic sinus drainage.[16] Prolonged nasal intubation may also be associated with sinusitis (presumably by the same mechanism) with subsequent infection by *S. aureus, Enterobacter, Pseudomonas aeruginosa, Bacteroides fragilis, Bacteroides melaninogenicus,* and *Candida* sp.[2]

Treatment

Initial treatment of acute sinusitis is controversial. Almost two thirds of primary care patients with an upper respiratory infection (URI) expect antibiotics.[17] Since viruses frequently cause acute sinusitis, some authors advocate no antibiotic treatment if the condition is not severe, wanes in 5 to 7 days, and resolves in 10 days ("watchful waiting").[18] If symptoms persist, antibiotics, decongestants, and nonpharmacologic measures should be used to maintain adequate sinus drainage.

Antibiotics (Table 40.1)[19]

For patients with no antibiotics use in the prior 30 days and in areas where drug-resistant *Streptococcus pneumoniae* (DRSP) is ≤ 30%, use either amoxicillin, amoxicillin-clavulanate, cefdinir, cefpodoxime, or cefuroximine axetil. If DSRP is ≥ 30%, use either amoxicillin-clavulanate or a fluoroquinolone. If the first regimen fails, use amoxicillin-clavulanate plus extra amoxicillin, or cefpodoxime in mild to moderate disease; and use gatifloxacin, levofloxacin, or moxifloxacin in severe disease. The duration of treatment is 10 days. In hospitalized patients with nasotracheal and or nasogastric tubes, remove tubes if possible and use imipenem 0.5 g q6h or meropenem 1.0 g q8h. Alternately, use an antipseudomonal penicillin (e.g., piperacillin) or ceftazidime plus vancomycin or cefepime 2.0 g q12h. Antibiotics are usually ineffective for chronic sinusitis, but if an acute exacerbation occurs, use one of the acute regimens above. Otorhinolaryngology consultation is appropriate.[20]

Decongestants

Normal saline nasal sprays and steam may increase sinus drainage.[21] Oxymetazoline 0.05% topical nasal spray inhibits nitric oxide synthetase with resulting decrease in inflammation; it should be used for no more than 3 to 4 days. Guaifenesin preparations maintain sinus drainage by thinning secretions and thus decreasing stasis.[22]

Nasal Steroids

The addition of intranasal corticosteroids to antibiotics reduces symptoms of acute sinusitis vs. antibiotics alone. With allergic sinusitis, nasal steroids shrink edematous mucosa and allow ostial openings to increase. A two or three times per day dosage is commonly used.[23]

Nonpharmacologic

Increasing oral fluids, local steam inhalation, and application of heat or cold have had some success in reducing discomfort.[11]

Complications

Mucocele and osteomyelitis are rare complications of sinusitis. Mucoceles, treated surgically, may be identified by radiography or sinus CT. Osteomyelitis, a serious infection of the surrounding bone, requires prolonged parenteral antibiotics and debridement of necrotic osseous structures with later cosmetic reconstruction.[9] Meningitis, cavernous sinus thrombosis, brain abscess, or hematogenous spread may also occur. Orbital infections occur more commonly in children.[24]

Chronic Recurrent Sinusitis

More than 32 million cases of chronic sinusitis occur annually in the United States.[25] Predisposing factors include anatomic abnormalities, polyps, allergic rhinitis, ciliary dysmotility, foreign bodies, chronic irritants, adenoidal hypertrophy, nasal decongestant spray abuse (rhinitis medicamentosa), smoking, swimming, chronic viral URIs, and immunocompromised states. Pathogens are those above with an increase in *Bacteroides* sp., *Peptostreptococcus,* and *Fusobacterium*. Parasitic sinusitis by microsporidium, cryptosporidium acanthamoeba species has been reported in acquired immunodeficiency syndrome (AIDS) patients.[26] Treatment is aimed at resolving predisposing factors, but acute sinusitis is treated with organism specific antibiotics.[20] Endoscopically guided microswab cultures from the middle meatus correlate 80% to 85% with results of more painful antral puncture in antibiotic failures.[27]

Surgical Management

When antibiotic management fails, surgical management is indicated. Chronic sinusitis patients have significant decrements in bodily pain and social functioning. Surgery reduces symptoms and medication use.[28] Functional endoscopic sinus surgery is a minimally invasive technique used to restore sinus ventilation and normal function. Improvement in symptoms have been reported in up to 90%.[29]

Sinusitis in Children

Sinusitis affects 10% of school-age children, and 21% to 30% of adolescents.[30] Chronic rhinosinusitis may affect quality of life more severely than juvenile rheumatoid arthritis, asthma, or other chronic childhood illnesses.[31] The differential diagnosis includes allergy, immunodeficiency [immunoglobulin A (IgA) is most common], cystic fibrosis, ciliary disorders

Table 40.1. **Antibiotics for Rhinosinusitis[20] and for GABHS Pharyngitis[51]**

Antibiotic	Dosage[a] Adults (mg)	Children (mg/kg/day)	Dosing frequency[b]	Cost[c]
Rhinosinusitis				
Oral administration				
Suggested primary regimen				
Trimethoprim-sulfamethoxazole	160/300	8/40	bid	$
Amoxicillin-clavulanate	875/125	45/6.4	bid	$$$$–$$$$$
Cefaclor	500	40	tid	$$$$
Second-line treatment				
Clarithromycin extended release	1000	15	qd	$$$$
Amoxicillin	500	40	tid	$–$$
Cefuroxime axetil	250	30	bid	$$–$$$
Cefpodoxime-proxetil	200	10	bid	$$$$
Cefdinir	600	14	qd	$$$$$
Levofloxacin	500	*	qd	$$$$$
Moxifloxacin	400	*	qd	$$$$$
Gatifloxacin	400	*	qd	$$$$$
Parenteral administration				
Imipenem	500	15–25	q6h	$$$$$
Meropenem	1000	60–120	q8h	$$$$$
Ceftazidime	1000–2000	50	q8h	$$$$$
Vancomycin	15 mg/kg	40–60	q12q/q6h	$$$$$
Gatifloxacin	400	*	qd	$$$$$
Cefepime	2000	150	q12h/q8h	$$$$$
GABHS pharyngitis				
Suggested primary regimen				
Benzathine penicillin G				
<60 pounds, 27 kg	600,000 U IM	Same	Once	$
≥60 pounds, 27 kg	1,200,000 U IM	Same	Once	$–$$
Benzathine/procaine PCN	900,000/300,000 U IM	Same	Once	$
Penicillin VK	500 mg total	250 mg total	bid	$
Penicillin-allergic				
Erythromycin estolate	Not advised	20–40	bid–qid	$$
Erythromycin ethylsuccinate	400	40	bid–qid	$
Second-line treatment				
Amoxicillin	500	40	tid	$–$$
Amoxicillin-clavulanate	500–875	40	bid–tid	$$$$–$$$$
Cephalexin	500	25–50	bid	$–$$
Cefadroxil	1000	30	qd	$$–$$$$$
Cefaclor	250	20–30	tid	$$$$
Cefuroxime axetil	125	15	bid	$$–$$$
Cefixime	200	8	qd	$$$–$$$$$
Clarithromycin	250	—	bid	$$$$$
Azithromycin (5 days)	500 mg day 1 250 mg days 2–5	12	qd	$$–$$$

[a]Unless otherwise indicated, antibiotic is given orally for 10 days.

[b]qd = once a day; bid = twice a day; tid = three times a day; qid = four times daily.

[c]Cost for therapeutic course based on average wholesale price from 2000 Drugs Topics Red Book; prices for generic drugs were used when available; $ = 0–15 dollars; $$ = 16–30 dollars, $$$ = 31–45 dollars, $$$$ = 46–60 dollars, $$$$$ = greater than 60 dollars.

*Fluoroquinolones not recommended under 18 years of age except in cystic fibrosis.

(e.g., primary ciliary dyskinesia), and gastroesophageal reflux.[32] Maxillary and ethmoidal sinuses are the primary sites of infection in infants. The sphenoid sinus develops later during the third to fifth year of life and the frontal sinus during the sixth to tenth year.

Childhood sinusitis may be a challenge to diagnose. Common symptoms include fever over 39°C, periorbital edema, facial pain, and daytime cough.[24] Periorbital cellulitis is seen in infants with ethmoidal sinus disease. If a URI is severe or persists beyond 10 days in a child, suspect sinusitis. In young children, sinusitis may present only with cough and persistent rhinorrhea. Low-dose, high-resolution CT is recommended when available.[33] The radiographic diagnosis of sinusitis is based on air-fluid levels, mucosal thickening of 4 mm or more, or sinus opacification. Organisms in antral cultures include *S. pneumoniae, M. catarrhalis,* and *H. influenzae.*[34] In July 1998, the Food and Drug Administration (FDA) approved amoxicillin-clavulanate, cefprozil, cefuroxime, clarithromycin, loracarbef, levofloxacin, and trovafloxin for childhood sinusitis treatment. Quinolones are not established as safe for those younger than 18 years old. Amoxicillin is the initial antibiotic of choice. Trimethoprim-sulfamethoxazole, amoxicillin-clavulanate, cefaclor, and cefuroxime axetil are useful alternatives if β-lactamase–producing organisms are suspected. All antibiotics are given for 10 days. Antihistamines may impair ciliary clearing mechanisms and thicken secretions. If oral antibiotics are unsuccessful, parenteral antibiotics such as imipenem, ceftazadime, and cefepime have been recommended (Table 40.1).[24]

Pharyngitis

Sore throat is the third most common presenting complaint in family practice, with an annual cost of $37.5 million for antibiotics.[35] The challenge for family physicians is to determine, in a cost-effective manner, which patients need antibiotics.[35,36]

Epidemiology

The infectious causes of a sore throat are listed in Table 40.2. Although viruses are the most common infectious agents, Group A β-hemolytic *Streptococcus* (GABHS) is most important because of potential sequelae. GABHS can be isolated by throat culture in 30% to 40% of children and 5% to 10% of adults with sore throat, with the highest prevalence found in children age 5 to 15 years.[37,38] Groups C and G streptococci, *Mycoplasma pneumoniae,* and *Chlamydia pneumoniae* (TWAR agent) occur most commonly in adolescent and young adults, and usually have no serious sequelae.[38] Rare bacterial causes include *Corynebacterium diphtheria, Neisseria gonorrhoeae* (especially in those who practice fellatio), *N. meningitidis, Treponema pallidum,* and tuberculosis. In 20% to 65% of patients, no infectious pathogen can be found. Noninfectious causes to consider are postnasal drip, low-humidity in the environment, irritant exposure to cigarette smoke or smog, and malignant disease (e.g., leukemia, lymphoma, or squamous cell carcinoma). GABHS pharyngitis is seen most frequently in late winter and early spring, while other infectious agents occur year round. All are spread by close contact or by droplets. A higher incidence of disease occurs in schools, day-care centers, and dormitories.

Clinical Presentation

The classic features of GABHS pharyngitis are sudden onset of severe sore throat, moderate fever (39°–40.5°C), headache, anorexia, nausea, vomiting, abdominal pain, malaise, tonsillopharyngeal erythema, patchy and discrete tonsillar or pharyngeal exudate, soft palate petechiae, and tender cervical adenopathy.[35] The majority of patients have mild disease, with overlap of these features and those of vi-

Table 40.2. **Infectious Causes of Pharyngitis**[*35,36]

Primary bacterial pathogens (30% in children age 5–11 years old, 15% in adolescents, 5% in adults)	Group A β-hemolytic streptococci (GABHS) Group B, C, and G streptococci *Neisseria gonorrhoeae* (uncommon) *Corynebacterium diphtheriae* (rare) *Treponema pallidum* (unusual) Tuberculosis (unusual)
Possible bacterial pathogens (5–10%, primarily in young adults)	*Arcanobacterium haemolyticum* *Chlamydia pneumoniae* (TWAR) *Chlamydia trachomatis* *Mycoplasma pneumoniae*
Probable bacterial co-pathogens (all age groups)	*Staphylococcus aureus* *Haemophilus influenzae* *Klebsiella pneumoniae rhinoscleromatis* *Moraxella (Branhamella) catarrhalis* *Bacteroides melaninogenicus* *Bacteroides oralis* *Bacteroides fragilis* *Fusobacterium* species Peptostreptococci
Viruses (15–40% in children, 30–80% in adults)	Rhinovirus (100 types)—most common Coronavirus (three or more types) Adenovirus—types 3, 4, 7, 14, and 21 Herpes simplex virus—types 1 and 2 Parainfluenza virus—types 1–4 Influenzavirus—types A and B Coxsackievirus A—types 2, 4–6, 8, 10 Epstein-Barr virus Cytomegalovirus Human immunodeficiency virus type 1
Fungal (uncommon in immuno-competent patient)	*Candida albicans*

*No pathogen is isolated in 20–65% (avg. 30%) of cases of sore throat.

ral pharyngitis. Scarlet fever produces a fine, blanching, sandpaper-texture rash, circumoral pallor, and hyperpigmentation in the skin creases. Although highly suggestive of GABHS, it also may be caused by *Arcanobacterium haemolyticum.* Exudative pharyngitis/tonsillitis, anterior cervical adenopathy, fever, and lack of other URI symptoms such as cough and rhinorrhea are most predictive of a positive GABHS culture, with a probability of occurrence of 56% when all four are present.[35]

Groups C and G streptococcus and *A. haemolyticum* produce tonsillopharyngitis indistinguishable from GABHS, but rarely have sequelae.[36] The tonsillo-pharyngitis of *M. pneumoniae* and *C. pneumoniae* is similar to GABHS infection, but is usually accompanied by a cough.[38] Membranous pharyngitis with a gangrenous exudative appearance is found in Vincent's angina or diphtheria. Herpangina (caused by the Coxsackie A virus) is characterized by a severe sore throat, fever, and 1- to 2-mm pharyngeal vesicles that subsequently ulcerate and resolve within 5 days. Hand-foot-and-mouth disease (caused by

Coxsackie A-16 virus) presents as pharyngitis accompanied by vesicles on the palmar and plantar surfaces. Patients with aphthous stomatitis have a sore throat and round, painful oral lesions that resolve within 2 weeks. Herpes simplex virus causes fever, oral fetor, submaxillary adenopathy, and gingivostomatitis. Symptoms of infectious mononucleosis include sore throat, anterior and posterior adenopathy, a gray pseudomembranous pharyngitis, and palatine petechiae. Acute retroviral syndrome due to primary infection of human immunodeficiency virus (HIV) presents as fever, nonexudative pharyngitis, lymph-adenopathy, and systemic symptoms such as fatigue, myalgias, and arthralgias.[36]

Diagnosis

Since no single element of the history or physical exam is diagnostic for GABHS, the standard for diagnosis is a properly processed and interpreted throat culture on sheep blood agar.[36] For best results, use a Dacron swab and thoroughly swab both tonsils and posterior pharyngeal wall, avoiding the tongue. Since it takes 24 to 48 hours to obtain definitive results from a throat culture, streptococcal rapid antigen-detection tests were developed that can provide answers within minutes. Most are highly specific (90–96%), but not as sensitive (80–90%) as throat cultures.[36,38] If a rapid antigen test is positive, one can almost be certain that GABHS is present. If the test is negative in clinically suspicious situations, national advisory committees recommend obtaining a confirmatory throat culture.[36] Recently, newer tests using optical immunoassay and chemiluminescent DNA probes have sensitivities similar to that of throat cultures, and may one day become the standard method for diagnosis.[1,36]

Complications of GABHS Tonsillopharyngitis

Suppurative complications include peritonsillar abscess (PTA), retropharyngeal abscess, and cervical lymphadenitis. Peritonsillar abscess occurs in fewer than 1% of patients treated with appropriate antibiotics.[39] It is seen most frequently in teenagers and young adults, and is rare in children. Symptoms include a severe unilateral sore throat, dysphagia, rancid breath, trismus, drooling from a partially opened mouth, and a muffled "hot potato" voice. There is generalized erythema of the pharynx and tonsils, with a deeper dusky redness overlying the involved area, swelling of the anterior pillar and soft palate above the tonsil, and uvular deviation to the opposite side.[40] Diagnostic ultrasound [41] or CT scan [42] helps distinguish between peritonsillar cellulitis and abscess. Treatment includes intravenous penicillin and needle aspiration.[40] Tonsillectomy is indicated when needle aspiration fails and in those with recurrent PTA.[43]

Once the leading cause of death in children and adolescents in the United States, acute rheumatic fever (ARF) now occurs infrequently, with a reported annual incidence of 1 case per 1,000,000 untreated patients with GABHS pharyngitis.[35] Symptoms begin 2 weeks after the pharyngitis with polyarthritis and cardiac valvulitis. Acute glomerulonephritis may occur 10 days after GABHS pharyngitis, and presents as anasarca, hypertension, hematuria, and proteinuria. It generally is a self-limited condition and almost never has permanent sequelae, and antibiotics do not prevent its occurrence.[37]

Treatment

Since a small but significant portion of patients with GABHS pharyngitis will develop complications, many physicians treat all patients who have a sore throat with antibiotics. However, treating all patients as if they had GABHS infection means overtreating at least 70% of children and 90% of adult patients. Treating GABHS pharyngitis accomplishes four goals[36]: (1) patients clinically improve quicker; (2) they become noninfectious sooner, thus preventing transmission of infection; (3) suppurative complications such as PTA are avoided; and (4) ARF is prevented. Children who complete 24 hours of antibiotics can be considered noninfectious, and if they feel better, may return to school. Although patients clinically respond within 1 to 2 days of antibiotics, treatment for 10 days remains the optimal duration to prevent ARF. Patient compliance issues should be addressed; up to 80% do not complete a 10-day course.[39]

Penicillin remains the drug of choice for treating GABHS pharyngitis because it is effective in preventing ARF, inexpensive, and relatively safe (Table 40.1).[36] Penicillin-resistant GABHS has yet to be identified. Even when started as late as 9 days after the onset of pharyngitis, penicillin effectively prevents primary attacks of ARF. Intramuscular benzathine penicillin is the definitive treatment but is infrequently used because injections are painful. Amoxicillin offers a low-cost, better-tasting alternative to penicillin, and one recent study suggested that a single daily dose for 10 days had similar efficacy.[44]

For those allergic to penicillin, erythromycin is the antibiotic of choice. Clarithromycin and azithromycin have a susceptibility pattern similar to that of erythromycin, but with less gastrointestinal distress, and may be administered once or twice a day. Azithromycin as a 5-day treatment regimen for GABHS pharyngitis is attractive, but its cost and the potential rapid development of streptococcal resistance of macrolides make this a second-line antibiotic.[36] Cephalosporins are more expensive, may hasten the development of resistant bacteria, and should not be used in patients with a history of immediate (anaphylactic) hypersensitivity to penicillin.[38] Recent evidence suggests that a 5-day course of nonpenicillin antibiotics is just as effective as a 10-day course of oral penicillin, but further studies are needed before this is accepted as the standard of care.[45]

The same antibiotic treatment choices exist for groups C and G streptococci and *A. haemolyticum*.[36] Both *M. pneumoniae* and *C. pneumoniae* are sensitive to tetracycline and erythromycin. Treatment for diphtheria includes antitoxin and erythromycin 20 to 25 mg/kg every 12 hours intravenously for 7 to 14 days. Vincent's angina is treated with penicillin, tetracycline, and oral oxidizing agents such as hydrogen peroxide to improve oral hygiene. Treatment of viral pharyngitis with antivirals is not indicated. An oral rinse consisting of corticosteroids (Kenalog suspension) and topical tetracycline (250 mg/50 cc water) may hasten recovery in those patients with aphthous stomatitis. Therapy for infectious mononucleosis is supportive and may include penicillin (avoid amoxicillin and ampicillin) for simultaneous GABHS infection, and steroids for respiratory obstruction.

Ibuprofen 400 mg every 6 hours is superior to acetaminophen in alleviating throat pain.[39] Available suspension analgesics include ibuprofen 100 mg/5 cc, naproxen 125 mg/5 cc, acetaminophen with codeine elixir, and acetaminophen with hydrocodone elixir.[39] Avoid aspirin in children and teenagers because of the risk of Reye's syndrome. Warm liquids are an effective adjuvant treatment. Patients with severe inflammatory symptoms may benefit from corticosteroids, given as a short course of oral prednisone or a single 10-mg injection of dexamethasone.[39]

Cost-Benefit Treatment Strategy

The most important task when evaluating a sore throat is to determine whether or not the patient has GABHS. Although national guidelines exist,[46] consensus on the most cost-effective approach remains elusive. A rational policy should be based on the incidence of GABHS in the population, cost containment, avoidance of adverse outcomes, reducing unnecessary use of antibiotics, and patient priorities. When the probability of GABHS is greater than 20%, treating all patients with pharyngitis without testing may be rational.[47] Otherwise, those individuals who may have GABHS based on clinical findings should have a rapid antigen test or throat culture performed.[46] In those cases where rapid antigen tests are negative and a confirmatory throat culture is pending, presumptive antibiotic use should be based on severity of illness, risk of transmission to others, need to return to school or work, and the patient's willingness to accept risks of unnecessary use of antibiotics should the culture return negative.

Treatment Failures and Chronic Carriers

Posttreatment throat cultures are indicated only in those who remain symptomatic after completion of antibiotics, who develop recurrent symptoms within 6 weeks, or who have had rheumatic fever and are at high risk for recurrence.[46] Reasons for treatment failures include poor compliance, β-lactamase–producing bacteria, and recurrent exposure to a family member who harbors GABHS ("ping-pong" infections).[48] The family pet is an unlikely reservoir for GABHS.[49] A chronic GABHS carrier is asymptomatic with a positive throat culture. As many as 50% of school-age children are GABHS carriers, are rarely contagious, and are at little risk for developing GABHS complications.[50] Indications to eradicate GABHS from the chronic carrier include a personal or family history of ARF and "ping-pong" spread occurring within a family.[50] The treatment for those who fail an adequate course of oral penicillin is a single injection of benzathine penicillin (Table 40.1). If this fails, clindamycin 20 to 30 mg/kg/day (up to 450 mg per day) may be given in three divided doses for 10 days.[46]

Tonsillectomy

Tonsillectomy is indicated in those who have recurrent peritonsillar abscesses or respiratory obstruction.[43] The American Academy of Otolaryngology and Head and Neck Surgery considers four or more infections of the tonsils per year, despite adequate medical therapy, to be sufficient indication for tonsillectomy, although the benefit of decreased frequency of GABHS tonsillitis may only last for 2 years.

References

1. Stewart M, Siff J, Cydulka R. Evaluation of the patient with sore throat, earache, and sinusitis: an evidence-based approach. Em Med Clin North Am 1999;17(1):153–87.
2. Linden B, Aguilar E, Allen S. Sinusitis in the nasotracheally intubated patient. Arch Otolaryngol Head Neck Surg 1988;114:860–1.
3. Ozcan Y, Jiang H, Pai C. Do primary care physicians or specialists provide more efficient care? Health Serv Manag Res 2000;13(2):90–6.
4. Lanza D, Kennedy D. Adult rhinosinusitis defined. Otolaryngol Head Neck Surg 1997;117:S1–7.
5. Hadley J, Schafer S. Clinical evaluation of rhinosinusitis: history and physical examination. Otolaryngol Head Neck Surg 1997;117:S8–11.
6. Kormos WA. Approach to the patient with sinusitis. In Goroll AH, May LA, Mulley AG, eds. Primary care medicine 4th ed. Philadelphia: JB Lippincott; 2000:1127–8.
7. Way L. Current surgical diagnosis and treatment, 10th ed. East Norwalk, CT: Appleton & Lange, 1994.
8. Ferguson B. Acute and chronic sinusitis—how to ease symptoms and locate the cause. Postgrad Med 1995;97(5):45–57.
9. Tierney L, McPhee S, Papadakis M. Current medical diagnosis and treatment, 34th ed. East Norwalk, CT: Appleton & Lange, 1995.
10. Burke T, Guertler A, Timmons J. Comparisons of sinus x-rays with CT scans in acute sinusitis. Acad Emerg Med 1994;1(3):235–9.
11. Hopp R, Cooperstock M. Evaluation and treatment of sinusitis: aspects for the managed care environment. JAOA 1996;96(4 suppl):S6–10.
12. Bhattacharyya T, Piccinillo J, Wippold F. Relationship between patient-based description of sinusitis and paranasal sinus CT findings. Arch Otolaryngol Head Neck Surg 1997;123:1189–92.
13. Sanford J, Gilbert D, Sande M. Sanford's guide to antimicrobial therapy, 26th ed. Dallas: Antimicrobial Therapy, 1996.
14. Nord C. The role of anaerobic bacteria in recurrent episodes of sinusitis and tonsillitis. Clin Infect Dis 1995;20:1512–24.
15. Decker C. Sinusitis in the immunocompromised host. Curr Infect Dis Rep 1999;1(1):27–32.
16. Kormos WA. Approach to the patient with sinusitis. In Goroll AH, May LA, Mulley AG, eds. Primary care medicine 4th ed. Philadelphia: JB Lippincott; 2000:1127.
17. Ray N. Healthcare expenditures for sinusitis in 1996: contributions of asthma, rhinitis, and other airway disorders. J Allergy Clin Immunol 1999;103(3 pt 1):408–14.
18. Snow V, Mottur-Pilson C JMJH. Princples of appropriate antibiotic use for acute sinusitis in adults. Ann Intern Med 2001;134:495–7.
19. Holten K, Onusko E. Appropriate prescribing of oral beta-lactam antibiotics. Am Fam Physician 2000;62:611–20.
20. Gilbert D, Moelleering R, Sande M. The Sanford's guide to an-

timicrobial therapy, 31st ed. Dallas,TX: Antimicrobial Therapy. 2001.

21. Taccariello M, Parikh A, Darby Y, Scadding G. Nasal douching as a valuable adjunct in the management of chronic rhinosinusitis. Rhinology 1999;37(1):29–32.

22. Malm L. Pharmacological background to decongesting and anti-inflammatory treatment of rhinitis and sinusitis. Acta Otolaryngol Suppl (Stockh) 1994;515:53–5.

23. Naclerio R. Allergic rhinitis. N Engl J Med 1991;325:860–9.

24. Parsons DS, Wilder BE. Rhinitis and sinusitis (acute and chronic). In: Burg TD, Ingelfinger JR, Wald ER, Polin RA, eds. Current pediatric therapy 16th ed. Philadelphia: WB Saunders, 1999:506–7.

25. Mellen I. Chronic sinusitis: clinical and pathophysiological aspects. Acta Otolaryngol Suppl (Stockh) 1994:515:45–8.

26. Dunand V, Hammer S, Rossi R, et al. Parasitic sinusitis and otitis in patients infected with human immunodeficiency virus: report of five cases and review. Clin Infect Dis 1997;25(2): 267–72.

27. Osguthorp J. Adult rhinosinusitis: diagnosis and management. Am Fam Physician 2001;63:69–76.

28. Metson R, Gliklich R. Clinical outcomes in patients with chronic sinusitis. Laryngoscope 2000;110(3 pt 3):24–8.

29. Slack R, Bates G. Functional endoscopic sinus surgery. Am Fam Physician 1998;58:707–18.

30. Deda G, Caksen H, Ocal A. Headache etiology in children: a retrospective study of 125 cases. Pediatr Int 2000;42:668–73.

31. Cunningham J, Chiu E, Landgraf J, Gliklich R. The health impact of chronic recurrent rhinosinusitis in children. Arch Otolaryngol Head Neck Surg 2000;126(11):1363–8.

32. Lasley M, Shapiro G. Rhinitis and sinusitis in children. Immunol Allerg Clin North Am 1999;19:437–52.

33. Konen E, Faibel M, Kleinbaum Y, et al. The value of the occipitomental (Waters') view in diagnosis of sinusitis: a comparative study with computed tomography. Clin Radiol 2000;55: 856–60.

34. Diaz I, Bamberger D. Acute sinusitis. Semin Respir Infect 1995;10:14–20.

35. Ebell M, Smith M, Barry H, Ives K, Carey M. Does this patient have strep throat? JAMA 2000;284:2912–8.

36. Bisno A. Acute pharyngitis. N Engl J Med 2001;344:205–11.

37. Kiselica D. Group A beta-hemolytic streptococcal pharyngitis: current clinical concepts. Am Fam Physician 1994;49(5):1147–54.

38. Pichichero M. Group A streptococcal tonsillopharyngitis: cost-effective diagnosis and treatment. Ann Emerg Med 1995;25(3): 390–403.

39. Kline J, Runge J. Streptococcal pharyngitis: a review of pathophysiology, diagnosis, and management. J Emerg Med 1994; 12(5):665–80.

40. Epperly T, Wood T. New trends in the management of peritonsillar abscess. Am Fam Physician 1990;42:102–12.

41. Ahmed K, Jones A, Shah K, Smethurst A. The role of ultrasound in the management of peritonsillar abscess. J Laryngol Otol 1994;108:610–2.

42. Patel K, Ahmad S, O'Leary G, Michel M. The role of computed tomography in the management of peritonsillar abscess. Otolaryngol Head Neck Surg 1992;107:727–32.

43. Richardson M. Sore throat, tonsillitis, and adenoiditis. Med Clin North Am 1999;83(1):75–83.

44. Gerber M, Tanz R. New approaches to the treatment of group A streptococcal pharyngitis. Curr Opin Pediatr 2001;13(1):51–5.

45. Adam D, Scholz H, Helmerking M. Short-course antibiotic treatment of 4782 culture-proven cases of group A streptococcal tonsillopharyngitis and incidence of poststreptococcal sequelae. Clin Infect Dis 2000;182:509–16.

46. Bisno A, Gerber M, Gwaltney J, Kaplan E, Schwartz R. Diagnosis and management of group A streptococcal pharyngitis: a practice guideline. Clin Infect Dis 1997;25:574–83.

47. Green S. Acute pharyngitis: the case for empiric antimicrobial therapy. Ann Emerg Med 1995;25(3):404–6.

48. Pinchichero M, Casey J, Mayes T, et al. Penicillin failure in streptococcal tonsillopharyngitis: causes and remedies. Pediatr Infect Dis J 2000;19:917–23.

49. Wilson K, Maroney S, Gander R. The family pet as an unlikely source of group A beta-hemolytic streptococcal infection in humans. Pediatr Infect Dis J 1995;14:372–5.

50. Gerber M. Treatment failures and carriers: perception or problems? Pediatr Infect Dis J 1994;13:576–9.

51. Hayes C, Williamson H. Management of group A beta-hemolytic streptococcal pharyngitis. Am Fam Physician 2001; 63:1557–64.

41
Sexually Transmitted Diseases

Donald R. Koester

Sexually transmitted diseases (STDs) continue to cause significant health problems. In the United States, more than 65 million people have an incurable sexually transmitted disease, with an additional 15 million people contracting one or more STDs each year.[1] Except for the human immunodeficiency virus (HIV), the most common STDs seen in the United States are chlamydia, gonorrhea, syphilis, genital herpes, human papillomavirus (HPV), hepatitis B, trichomoniasis, and bacterial vaginosis. While some STDs have declined in recent years, others such as gonorrhea, genital herpes, and HPV have increased.[2] Teenagers and young adults continue to practice behaviors putting them at high risk for STDs. These facts illustrate the importance of family physicians' being well informed about the treatment and prevention of STDs.

Chlamydia Infection

Chlamydia trachomatis infection is the most commonly reported infectious disease in the United States.[2] Approximately three million individuals contract chlamydia each year, with millions of cases undetected and untreated.[1] Women with untreated chlamydia are at risk to develop pelvic inflammatory disease (PID) and are three to five times more likely to contract HIV when exposed.[2] In some areas more than 5% of teenage males and 5% to 10% of teenage females are infected with chlamydia.[3] Continued sexual activity by untreated asymptomatic individuals contributes to the transmission of chlamydial infections.

Clinical Presentation

Fifty percent of men are asymptomatic. Symptomatic men have urethritis, epididymitis, proctitis, or conjunctivitis. Seventy-five percent of women are asymptomatic. Women with symptoms have dysuria with sterile pyuria (acute urethral syndrome), cervicitis with or without vaginal discharge, PID, proctitis, or conjunctivitis.[2]

Diagnosis

The gold standard for the diagnosis of chlamydial infection has been culture, which has specificity approaching 100%. However, cultures are technically difficult and require 3 to 7 days to obtain results. Culture is recommended for a specimen from the nasopharynx in infants, the rectum in all patients, the vagina in prepubertal girls, in situations where documentation of a true positive is necessary, and in medicolegal cases.[4] Nonculture tests are available and provide a more rapid diagnosis. These include the direct fluorescent antibody (DFA), the enzyme immunoassay (EIA), the nonamplified DNA probe, the ligase chain reaction (LCR), the polymerase chain reaction (PCR), and transcription-mediated amplification (TMA) tests. The LCR and PCR tests are reported to be more sensitive than culture and can be performed on first voided urine.[5]

Proper specimen collection is important when evaluating a patient for chlamydia.[6] Obtain samples for Gram stain, Papanicolaou (Pap) smear, and *Neisseria gonorrhoeae* culture before collecting specimens for chlamydial testing. Sources for specimen collection include the endocervix, urethra, rectum, or conjunctiva as clinically indicated in women, and the urethra, rectum, or conjunctiva as clinically indicated in men. In women, exocervical mucus must be carefully removed prior to endocervical specimen collection. Collect endocervical specimens by inserting the appropriate swab 1 to 2 cm into the endocervical canal and rotating it for 10 to 30 seconds.[7] Care must be taken to avoid contact with the vaginal side walls when removing the swab. Collect urethral specimens by inserting the swab 1 to 2 cm into the urethra in women and 2 to 4 cm in men. Rotate the swab for at least one revolution and place it in the appropriate transport medium or use it to prepare a slide.

Treatment

Treatment of uncomplicated urethral, endocervical, and rectal *C. trachomatis* infection is with:

Azithromycin (Zithromax) 1 g po once or
Doxycycline (Doryx, Monodox, Vibramycin, Vibra-Tab) 100 mg po twice a day for 7 days

Alternative regimens include:

Erythromycin base (E-Mycin, ERYC, Ery-Tab, PCE) 500 mg po four times a day for 7 days or
Erythromycin ethylsuccinate (EES) 800 mg po four times a day for 7 days or
Ofloxacin (Floxin) 300 mg po twice a day for 7 days[6]

Pregnant women should not be treated with quinolones or tetracyclines. Adolescents ≤18 years of age should not be treated with quinolones. Consider a test of cure 3 weeks after treatment with erythromycin. A test of cure is not necessary if symptoms resolve and treatment was with azithromycin or doxycycline.

The treatment of *C. trachomatis* infection in pregnant women is with:

Erythromycin base (E-Mycin, ERYC, Ery-Tab, PCE) 500 mg po four times a day for 7 days or
Amoxicillin (Amoxil) 500 mg po three times a day for 7 to 10 days

Alternative regimens include:

Erythromycin base (E-Mycin, ERYC, Ery-Tab, PCE) 250 mg po four times a day for 14 days or
Erythromycin ethylsuccinate (EES) 800 mg po four times a day for 7 days or
Erythromycin ethylsuccinate (EES) 400 mg po four times a day for 14 days or
Azithromycin (Zithromax) 1 g po once[6]

While some experts state the safety and efficacy of azithromycin in pregnant women has not been established, others feel it is the drug of choice for treatment of chlamydia in pregnancy.[8] Repeat testing 3 weeks after completion of treatment is recommended with these regimens.[6]

Prevention

Patient education is important to prevent chlamydial infection. Encourage patients to adopt behavioral changes that reduce the risk of acquiring or transmitting the disease (see Chapter 7). These behaviors include delaying the age of first intercourse, decreasing the number of sex partners, practicing careful partner selection, and using barrier contraception (condoms). States that identify and treat asymptomatic individuals through screening programs show decreases in chlamydial infections.[9] During annual examinations, screen sexually active women 20 to 24 years of age who use barrier contraception inconsistently or who have new or multiple sex partners. Screen all sexually active adolescents during annual examinations.[6] Sexually active adolescent boys can be screened for urethritis with a leukocyte esterase (LE) dipstick test. A positive LE test suggests infection but requires specific testing for *C. trachomatis* and *N. gonorrhoeae*. Instruct patients to abstain from intercourse for 7 days after single-dose treatment or until a full 7-day course of treatment is completed. Evaluate and treat the last sex partner, or any sex partners within 60 days prior to the onset of symptoms or diagnosis of chlamydial infection in the patient.[6]

Gonorrhea

Gonorrhea is a bacterial STD caused by the gram-negative diplococcus *N. gonorrhoeae*. This STD continues to be a major cause of PID and can enhance transmission of HIV.[2,10] While rates of gonorrhea declined until the late 1990s, between 1997 and 1999 gonorrhea infections increased by 9%.[9] The highest rates for gonorrhea are in 15- to 19-year-old females and 20- to 24-year-old males.[2]

Clinical Presentation

Men can be asymptomatic or have urethritis, epididymitis, proctitis, or pharyngitis. Women are more likely to be asymptomatic than men. Symptomatic women have dysuria, cervicitis with purulent vaginal discharge, PID, proctitis, or pharyngitis. Symptoms usually begin 2 to 5 days after acquiring the infection, but can take as long as 30 days to appear. Untreated infection increases the risk of transmission to sex partners and the development of complications. Complications in men with untreated infections include prostatitis, epididymitis, and urethral stricture. Women with untreated infections can develop salpingitis or perihepatitis. Both sexes can develop disseminated gonococcal infection with fever, petechial or pustular acral skin lesions, asymmetrical polyarthralgia, tenosynovitis, or septic arthritis. Rare complications of gonorrhea include hepatitis, endocarditis, myocarditis, and meningitis.[11]

Diagnosis

Gram stain and culture remain the primary means to diagnose gonorrhea.[12] Nonculture tests are also available and include the antigen detection test, direct specimen nucleic acid probe, and nucleic acid amplification tests such as PCR and LCR. The presence of a mucopurulent endocervical or urethral discharge with a history of sexual exposure to a person infected with *N. gonorrhoeae* is suggestive of the diagnosis. A presumptive diagnosis is made if two of three of the following are present: gram-negative intracellular diplococci on microscopic examination of urethral or endocervical discharge, growth of *N. gonorrhoeae* on culture medium, and/or detection of *N. gonorrhoeae* by nonculture laboratory testing. Definitive testing is required for medicolegal purposes. This is accomplished by isolation of *N. gonorrhoeae* from sites of exposure and confirmation of isolates by biochemical, enzymatic, serologic, or nucleic acid testing.[13]

For diagnostic testing, collect a sample of urethral exudate from men with a dry cotton or calcium alginate swab. If no exudate can be expressed, obtain a sample using the same technique as described for the diagnosis of chlamydia. Culture or perform nonculture testing on symptomatic patients with negative Gram stains. In women collect a specimen from the endocervix for culture or nonculture testing. Men and women who practice oral or rectal intercourse are at risk for pharyngeal and rectal infections. In these patients collect specimens from the pharynx and rectum as clinically indicated for culture.

Treatment

The treatment of uncomplicated urethral, cervical, rectal, or pharyngeal infection is with:

Cefixime (Suprax) 400 mg po once (for urethral, cervical, and rectal infections) or

Ceftriaxone (Rocephin) 125 mg IM once (for urethral, cervical, rectal, and pharyngeal infections) or

Ciprofloxacin (Cipro) 500 mg po once (for urethral, cervical, rectal, and pharyngeal infections) or

Ofloxacin (Floxin) 400 mg po once (for urethral, cervical, rectal, and pharyngeal infections)[6]

Alternative regimens for the treatment of urethral, cervical, and rectal infections include:

Spectinomycin (Trobicin) 2 g IM once (recommended for individuals who cannot tolerate cephalosporins or quinolones) or

Ceftizoxime (Cefizox) 500 mg IM once or

Cefotaxime (Claforan) 500 mg IM once or

Cefotetan (Cefotan) 1 g IM once or

Cefoxitin (Mefoxin) 2 g IM once with probenecid 1 g po or

Norfloxacin (Noroxin) 800 mg po once or

Enoxacin (Penetrex) 400 mg po once or

Lomefloxacin (Maxaquin) 400 mg po once or

Azithromycin (Zithromax) 2 g po once (may cause gastrointestinal side effects limiting its use)[6]

When treating gonorrhea, include treatment for possible co-infection by *C. trachomatis* with:

Azithromycin (Zithromax) 1 g po once or

Doxycycline (Doryx, Monodox, Vibramycin, Vibra-Tab) 100 mg po twice a day for 7 days[6]

Pregnant women should not be treated with quinolones or tetracyclines. Adolescents ≤18 years of age should not be treated with quinolones. Treatment of complicated infections including disseminated gonococcal infection, meningitis, endocarditis, and infection in children is beyond the scope of this chapter.

A test-of-cure culture is not necessary after treatment following the Centers for Disease Control and Prevention (CDC) recommended regimens. Patients with persistent symptoms following treatment for gonorrhea should be cultured and any gonococci isolated evaluated for antimicrobial sensitivity.

Consider infection with *C. trachomatis* or other organisms in patients who continue to experience symptoms of urethritis, cervicitis, or proctitis after appropriate treatment.[6]

Prevention

Patient education as previously described plays an important role in the prevention of gonorrhea. Instruct patients to refer sex partners for evaluation and treatment if the last sexual contact with the infected person was within 60 days of symptom onset or diagnosis. Evaluate the most recent sex partner if the last sexual contact was greater than 60 days. Patients must abstain from sexual contact until therapy is completed and the patient and partners are asymptomatic.[6]

Pelvic Inflammatory Disease

Pelvic inflammatory disease (PID) is inflammation of the upper female genital tract including endometritis, salpingitis, tubo-ovarian abscess, and pelvic peritonitis. STDs including *N. gonorrhoeae* and *C. trachomatis* are frequently involved but normal vaginal flora can also cause PID.[6] Ten to 20 percent of women with untreated gonorrhea and chlamydia develop PID.[2] Approximately one fourth of women with PID suffer one or more serious sequelae, including infertility, ectopic pregnancy, or chronic pelvic pain[14] (see Chapters 13, 61, and 102).

Clinical Presentation

The diagnosis of PID is difficult because patients present with a wide range of symptomatology. Women can be asymptomatic, have mild or nonspecific symptoms such as abnormal bleeding, dyspareunia, or vaginal discharge, or have severe symptoms with peritoneal signs. The most common symptom is dull, constant lower abdominal pain for less than 2 weeks.[15]

Diagnosis

According to the CDC, minimum criteria for the diagnosis of PID are lower abdominal tenderness, adnexal tenderness, and cervical motion tenderness. If all three are present and no other cause established, begin empiric treatment for PID. Women with more severe clinical signs require further diagnostic evaluation. Additional criteria that increase the specificity of the minimum criteria include an oral temperature over 38.3°C (101°F), abnormal cervical or vaginal discharge, elevated erythrocyte sedimentation rate, elevated C-reactive protein, and laboratory documentation of cervical infection with *N. gonorrhoeae* or *C. trachomatis*. Definitive criteria for the diagnosis of PID includes histopathologic evidence of endometritis on endometrial biopsy, transvaginal sonography or other imaging studies showing thickened, fluid-filled fallopian tubes or tubo-ovarian complex, and laparoscopic abnormalities consistent with PID.[6]

Treatment

Hospitalize patients with PID when surgical emergencies cannot be excluded, the patient is pregnant, is unable to follow outpatient treatment, has nausea and vomiting or high fever, is immunodeficient, tubo-abscess is suspected, or there is no response to oral medication.[6]

The parenteral treatment for PID is with:

Regimen A
Cefotetan (Cefotan) 2 g IV q12h or
Cefoxitin (Mefoxin) 2 g IV q6h plus
Doxycycline (Doryx, Monodox, Vibramycin, Vibra-Tab) 100 mg IV or po q12h

Continue parenteral therapy for 24 to 48 hours after clinical improvement. Continue doxycycline 100 mg po twice a day for a total of 14 days treatment. If tubo-ovarian abscess is present, consider the addition of clindamycin or metronidazole with doxycycline for better anaerobic coverage.[6]

Regimen B
Clindamycin (Cleocin) 900 mg IV q8h plus
Gentamicin (Garamycin) 2 mg/kg IV as a loading dose followed by 1.5 mg/kg q8h

Continue parenteral therapy for 24 hours after clinical improvement. Continue doxycycline 100 mg po twice a day or clindamycin 450 mg po four times a day for a total of 14 days treatment. If tubo-ovarian abscess is present, consider using clindamycin rather than doxycycline for continued treatment for better anaerobic coverage.[6]

With both regimens, consider additional diagnostic testing in patients who do not show marked clinical improvement after 3 days of treatment.

Other cephalosporins such as ceftizoxime (Cefizox), cefotaxime (Claforan), or ceftriaxone (Rocephin) may be utilized in appropriate doses in place of cefoxitin or cefotetan. However, clinical data for these agents are limited, and they are less active than cefoxitin or cefotetan against anaerobic bacteria.[6]

Alternative parenteral regimens include:

Ofloxacin (Floxin) 400 mg IV q12h plus
Metronidazole (Flagyl) 500 mg IV q8h or
Ampicillin/sulbactam (Unasyn) 3 g IV q6h plus
Doxycycline (Doryx, Monodox, Vibramycin, Vibra-Tab) 100 mg IV or po q12h or
Ciprofloxacin (Cipro) 200 mg IV q12h plus
Doxycycline (Doryx, Monodox, Vibramycin, Vibra-Tab) 100 mg IV or po q12h plus
Metronidazole (Flagyl) 500 mg IV q8h[6]

Oral treatment for PID is with:

Regimen A
Ofloxacin (Floxin) 400 mg po twice a day for 14 days plus
Metronidazole (Flagyl) 500 mg po twice a day for 14 days

Regimen B
Ceftriaxone (Rocephin) 250 mg IM or
Cefoxitin (Mefoxin) 2 g IM plus probenecid (Benemid) 1 g po concurrently or

Other parenteral third-generation cephalosporin such as ceftizoxime (Cefizox) or cefotaxime (Claforan) plus
Doxycycline (Doryx, Monodox, Vibramycin, Vibra-Tab) 100 mg po twice a day for 14 days[6]

Alternative oral regimens include amoxicillin/clavulanate (Augmentin) 875 mg/125 mg po plus doxycycline 100 mg po both twice a day for 14 days. Azithromycin (Zithromax) has been evaluated by some clinical trials as treatment for upper tract disease, but the CDC states data are insufficient to recommend it for treatment of PID.[6]

Reexamine patients for clinical improvement within 72 hours of initiating treatment. Treat patients not responding to oral therapy with parenteral antibiotics.[6]

Prevention

Retest patients for gonorrhea and chlamydia 4 to 6 weeks after completing treatment for PID. If PCR or LCR is used, delay reevaluation for at least 1 month. Examine and treat sex partners who have had sexual contact with the patient within 60 days of onset of symptoms. Treat sex partners of women with PID empirically for gonorrhea and chlamydia to reduce the risk of reinfection. Patient education as previously described is also essential.[6]

Syphilis

Syphilis is caused by the spirochete *Treponema pallidum*. The infection is transmitted by contact with infectious mucocutaneous lesions primarily through sexual contact, although indirect evidence suggests syphilis may be spread by the practice of sharing needles among intravenous drug users.[16] The reported rate of syphilis in the United States is at its lowest level since reporting began in 1941.[2] However, the genital ulcers of syphilis increase the risk of transmission of HIV, making it an STD of continued significance.

Clinical Presentation
Primary Syphilis

The classic chancre of primary syphilis appears about 21 days after exposure. The chancre is an indurated, painless ulcer usually located on the genitalia but also found at other sites of sexual contact including the cervix, breast, mouth, anus, or vaginal canal. The primary lesion heals spontaneously. Because the chancre is painless the primary stage of syphilis may be undetected.[16]

Secondary Syphilis

Hematogenous spread of *T. pallidum* produces the symptoms of secondary syphilis. Some patients are asymptomatic while others have constitutional symptoms including fever, malaise, and generalized lymphadenopathy. A macular, papular, annular, or follicular rash classically is present on the palms of the hands and soles of the feet. Mucous patches are shallow, painless ulcerations found on mucous membranes. Broad, raised, grayish, papular lesions known as condylomata lata appear on moist body areas such as the genitalia, cervix, scrotum, anus, or inner thighs. Alopecia may also be present. The signs and symptoms of secondary syphilis resolve spontaneously, after which the patient enters the latent stages of syphilis.[16]

Latent Syphilis

The first year of untreated infection is known as early latent syphilis. During this time, infectious mucocutaneous symptoms of secondary syphilis recur in approximately 25% of untreated patients with recurrences taking place up to 5 years after infection.[16,17] Late latent syphilis or syphilis of unknown duration occurs after the first year of untreated infection. During this time the patient has a positive specific treponemal antibody test but usually no other signs or symptoms of disease.

Late (Tertiary) Syphilis

One third of men and women with untreated syphilis go on to develop tertiary syphilis, which includes cardiovascular syphilis, gummatous syphilis, and neurosyphilis. It is important to note that neurosyphilis is not confined only to the tertiary stage.[16] Cardiovascular problems include aortitis, aortic regurgitation, and aortic aneurysm. Gummas are granulomatous-like lesions that infiltrate the skin, soft tissues, bone, liver, and other organ systems.

Neurosyphilis

Neurosyphilis can occur any time after the primary infection. Central nervous system (CNS) involvement by syphilis is often asymptomatic. Historically, 4% to 9% of patients with untreated syphilis develop symptomatic neurosyphilis.[16] Patients with neurosyphilis have a number of clinical syndromes. Meningeal syphilis usually occurs during the first year of infection and is characterized by headache, stiff neck, nausea, and vomiting. Cranial nerve involvement can result in hearing loss, facial weakness, or visual disturbances. Syphilis can also affect the spinal cord, causing meningomyelitis. Meningovascular syphilis occurs 4 to 7 years after infection causing focal CNS ischemia or stroke. General paresis and tabes dorsalis occur later in the course of the disease, often decades after the primary infection. Paretic neurosyphilis causes a chronic progressive dementia. Tabes dorsalis symptoms include sensory ataxia, pain, optic atrophy, and autonomic dysfunction. Other presentations of neurosyphilis include uveitis, retinitis, and optic neuritis.[16]

Diagnosis

Definitive diagnosis of syphilis is by direct detection of *T. pallidum* by examination of a smear or tissue from an active mucosal or cutaneous lesion using darkfield microscopy or DFA testing. Presumptive diagnosis of syphilis is by serology. Nontreponemal tests include the Venereal Disease Research Laboratory (VDRL) test and rapid plasma reagin (RPR) test. These tests are used primarily to screen asymptomatic patients and follow disease activity. Nontreponemal tests should not be used alone to diagnose the disease since false-negative and false-positive tests occur.[18] False-positive nontreponemal tests occur with a variety of chronic conditions, usually at dilutions of less than 1:8. Antibody levels gradually decline in untreated patients, often reaching dilutions of less than 1:4 during late latent stages. In about one fourth of untreated patients the VDRL eventually becomes nonreactive. Specific treponemal tests include the fluorescent treponemal antibody absorption (FTA-ABS), the microhemagglutination *T. pallidum* (MHA-TP), and hemagglutination treponemal tests.[16] These tests are used to confirm a positive screening test and once positive usually remain so for life.[6] Neurosyphilis is diagnosed based on clinical and laboratory findings including cerebrospinal fluid (CSF) examination showing mononuclear pleocytosis, elevated CSF protein, and a positive CSF VDRL. A reactive CSF VDRL is sufficient to diagnose neurosyphilis, but a negative test does not exclude the diagnosis. The CSF VDRL is highly specific, with false positives occurring only with blood contamination of the CSF. Some experts recommend a FTA-ABS on the CSF to diagnose neurosyphilis. This test yields more false-positive tests, but some experts feel a negative test excludes the diagnosis of neurosyphilis.[6] The serum VDRL is negative in up to 25% of patients with late neurosyphilis, but the treponemal tests remain positive.[16]

Treatment

The recommended treatment for primary or secondary syphilis is with benzathine penicillin G (Bicillin LA, Permapen) 2.4 million units IM in one dose. For nonpregnant penicillin allergic patients treatment is with:

Doxycycline (Doryx, Monodox, Vibramycin, Vibra-Tabs) 100 mg po twice a day for 14 days or
Tetracycline (Sumycin, Tetracyn) 500 mg po four times a day for 14 days or
Erythromycin (E-Mycin, ERYC, Ery-Tab, PCE) 500 mg po four times a day for 14 days if compliance and follow-up are certain or
Ceftriaxone (Rocephin) 1 g once a day for 8 to 10 days with careful follow-up[6]

Perform CSF and ocular slit-lamp examinations on patients with neurologic or ophthalmic disease and treat according to the results of these tests. Reexamine treated patients and perform quantitative nontreponemal testing 6 and 12 months after treatment. Patients with signs or symptoms of syphilis or who have a fourfold increase in the nontreponemal titer should be considered treatment failures or reinfected. Reevaluate these patients for HIV. Unless the patient is likely to be reinfected, perform a lumbar puncture to evaluate for neurosyphilis. Failure of the nontreponemal titer to decline fourfold within 6 months after treatment also identifies treatment failure. Reevaluate these patients for HIV and consider performing a CSF examination. At a minimum perform additional clinical and serologic follow-up on these patients and consider retreatment if follow-up cannot be assured. Retreatment is with three weekly intramuscular injections of 2.4 million units of benzathine penicillin G unless CSF findings suggest neurosyphilis.[6]

Treatment of patients with early latent syphilis who have a normal CSF examination (if performed) is with benzathine penicillin G (Bicillin LA, Permapen) 2.4 million units IM once. For nonpregnant penicillin-allergic patients treatment is with:

Doxycycline (Doryx, Monodox, Vibramycin, Vibra-Tab) 100 mg po twice a day for 14 days or
Tetracycline (Sumycin, Tetracyn) 500 mg po four times a day for 14 days

Repeat quantitative nontreponemal testing at 6, 12, and 24 months after treatment. If titers increase fourfold, a titer of ≥1:32 fails to decline at least fourfold within 12 to 24 months, or signs or symptoms of syphilis develop, evaluate the patient for neurosyphilis and re-treat appropriately.[6]

Treatment for patients with late latent syphilis or syphilis of unknown duration who have a normal CSF examination (if performed) is with benzathine penicillin G (Bicillin LA, Permapen) 2.4 million units IM weekly for 3 consecutive weeks. For nonpregnant penicillin-allergic patients treatment is with:

Doxycycline (Doryx, Monodox, Vibramycin, Vibra-Tab) 100 mg po twice a day for 28 days or
Tetracycline (Sumycin, Tetracyn) 500 mg po four times a day for 28 days

Repeat quantitative nontreponemal testing at 6, 12, and 24 months after treatment. If titers increase fourfold, a titer of ≥1:32 fails to decline at least fourfold within 12 to 24 months, or signs or symptoms of syphilis develop, evaluate the patient for neurosyphilis and re-treat appropriately.[6]

Tertiary syphilis includes gummatous and cardiovascular syphilis, but not neurosyphilis. Perform a CSF examination on patients with symptomatic tertiary syphilis before treatment. Some experts recommend treating all patients with cardiovascular syphilis with a neurosyphilis regimen. The complete treatment of cardiovascular and gummatous syphilis is complex and should be done in consultation with experts. Treatment for tertiary syphilis is with benzathine penicillin G (Bicillin LA, Permapen) 2.4 million units IM weekly for 3 consecutive weeks. For nonpregnant penicillin-allergic patients treatment is with:

Doxycycline (Doryx, Monodox, Vibramycin, Vibra-Tab) 100 mg po twice a day for 28 days or
Tetracycline (Sumycin, Tetracyn) 500 mg po four times a day for 28 days

Little information exists on the proper follow-up of treated late syphilis. Clinical response depends on the nature of lesions present.[6]

Neurosyphilis can occur at any stage of syphilis. Perform a CSF evaluation on patients with auditory symptoms, cranial nerve palsies, uveitis, neuroretinitis, optic neuritis, symptoms of meningitis, or other neurologic or ophthalmic symptoms. Treatment for neurosyphilis is with:

Aqueous crystalline penicillin G (Pfizerpen) 3 to 4 million units IV q4h for 10 to 14 days or
Procaine penicillin G (Wycillin) 2.4 million units IM per day plus probenecid 500 mg po four times a day, both for 10 to 14 days

An injection of benzathine penicillin G 2.4 million units IM after completion of neurosyphilis treatment is recommended by many experts. In patients with CSF pleocytosis, reexamine the CSF every 6 months until cell counts are normal. If the cell count does not decrease in 6 months or is not normal by 2 years, consider retreatment.[6]

Prevention

Test all patients with syphilis for HIV (see Chapter 42). Presumptively treat individuals sexually exposed to a person with primary, secondary, or early latent syphilis within 90 days preceding the diagnosis even if seronegative. If the exposure was more than 90 days before the diagnosis, treat presumptively if serologic testing is not immediately available or if follow-up is uncertain. Patients with syphilis of unknown duration and nontreponemal serologic titers ≥1:32 may be considered as having early syphilis for purposes of partner notification and presumptive treatment of sex partners. Evaluate long-term sex partners of patients with late syphilis clinically and serologically and treat appropriately.[6] Educate patients as previously described.

Genital Warts

Human papillomavirus (HPV) primarily affects sexually active young adults. Approximately 20 million individuals in the United States have genital HPV infection, with about 5.5 million people contracting the infection each year. Not all patients with HPV have clinically apparent disease. About 1% of sexually active adults in the United States have genital warts.[2] Some subtypes of HPV are associated with external genital squamous intraepithelial neoplasia and cervical intraepithelial dysplasia, which can lead to squamous cell carcinoma.[2,6] Most HPV infections seem to be cleared by the immune system. A recent study reported 91% of women with new HPV infections had undetectable HPV within 2 years of diagnosis.[19]

Clinical Presentation

HPV causes genital warts or infection with no noticeable symptoms. Warts most often appear on areas that are subject to trauma during sexual contact. Exophytic lesions usually cause no symptoms other than those related to their physical presence, though some patients report itching, burning, pain, or bleeding.[20] Visible warts appear as raised, skin-colored, cauliflower-like growths or smooth, flat papules that may be difficult to visualize without staining or magnification. Lesions are single or multiple. In men warts are found on the penis, scrotum, perianal area, and in the urethra. In women warts are found on the vulva, cervix, perianal area, and in the vagina. HPV lesions are also found on the oral mucosa, larynx, nose, conjunctiva, and anus in some patients.[6]

Diagnosis

Most genital warts are diagnosed by their clinical appearance. Biopsy confirms the diagnosis but is usually not necessary unless the diagnosis is uncertain, the lesions do not respond to treatment as expected, the disease worsens during treatment, the patient is immunocompromised, or warts are pigmented, indurated, fixed, or ulcerated.[6] Subclinical infection is often detected by cytologic or histologic examination of infected tissue. When external warts are present near the anal, vaginal, or urethral orifices, internal warts are possible. Perform anoscopy, urethroscopy, vaginal, and cervical examination, and a Pap smear as clinically indicated in these patients.[21]

Treatment

Untreated genital warts regress spontaneously, grow larger, increase in number, or remain the same. The goal of treatment is to remove exophytic warts and decrease symptoms. Removal of visible warts may or may not decrease infectivity.[6] Treatment can result in wart-free periods but recurrences can occur from reactivation of existing disease or reinfection from a sex partner.[2]

Patient applied treatment for *external genital warts* is with:

Podofilox 0.5% (Condylox) solution or gel for self-treatment applied to warts twice a day for 3 days, followed by 4 days of no therapy; repeated as necessary for four cycles (for genital warts only and safety during pregnancy not established) or
Imiquimod 5% (Aldara) cream applied at bedtime three times a week, treatment area washed with mild soap and water 6 to 10 hours after application, until warts clear or for as long as 16 weeks (safety during pregnancy not established)[6]

Provider-applied treatment for external genital warts is with:

Cryotherapy with liquid nitrogen or cryoprobe, treatments repeated every 1 to 2 weeks, or
Podophyllin resin 10% to 25% in compound tincture of benzoin applied to warts and air dried, washed off in 1 to 4 hours; repeated weekly as necessary (safety during pregnancy not established) or
Trichloroacetic acid (TCA) or bichloracetic acid (BCA) 80% to 90% applied to warts only, powdered with talc or baking soda to remove unreacted acid if an excessive amount is applied; repeated weekly as necessary or
Surgical removal by excision, curettage, or electrosurgery[6]

Alternative treatments include intralesional interferon or laser surgery.[6]

Treatment of *vaginal warts* is with:

Cryotherapy with liquid nitrogen (use of a cryoprobe is not recommended in the vagina because of the risk of vaginal perforation and fistula formation) or

TCA or BCA 80% to 90% applied to warts only, powdered with talc or baking soda to remove unreacted acid if an excessive amount is applied; repeated weekly as necessary or
Podophyllin 10% to 25% in compound tincture of benzoin applied to a treatment area that must be dry before speculum removal; repeated weekly as necessary (not recommended by some experts because of concern of systemic absorption; safety during pregnancy not established)[6]

Treatment of *urethral meatus warts* is with:

Cryotherapy with liquid nitrogen or
Podophyllin 10% to 25% in compound tincture of benzoin applied to a treatment area that must be dry before contact with normal mucosa; repeated weekly as necessary and limited to six applications (safety during pregnancy not established)[6]

Treatment of *anal warts* is with:

Cryotherapy with liquid nitrogen or
TCA or BCA 80% to 90% applied to warts only; powdered with talc or baking soda to remove unreacted acid if an excessive amount is applied; repeated weekly as necessary or
Surgical removal[6]

Treatment of *oral warts* is with:

Cryotherapy with liquid nitrogen or
Surgical removal[6]

Instruct patients to watch for recurrences, especially during the first 3 months after treatment. Women with exophytic cervical warts must have high-grade squamous intraepithelial lesions excluded before treatment. Expert consultation is recommended. Treat warts on the rectal mucosa in consultation with a specialist. Treatment of subclinical HPV infection without exophytic warts is not recommended unless dysplasia is present. When dysplasia is present, treatment is determined by the degree of dysplasia. Counsel women to have regular Pap smears as indicated for women without genital warts.[6]

Prevention

Routine examination of sex partners is not recommended since most partners are already infected with HPV. However, sex partners of patients with genital warts may benefit from an examination to determine the presence of genital warts or other STDs. Since HPV possibly is still present even after treatment, counsel patients they may be infective despite the absence of warts. The use of condoms may reduce the transmission of HPV to uninfected partners.[6]

Herpes Virus Infections

More than one million people in the United States contract genital herpes simplex virus (HSV) each year, with more than 45 million people infected.[2] Most patients are asymptomatic and unaware of their infection. The disease can be transmitted between sex partners and from mothers to newborns. Genital herpes is also thought to enhance the transmission of HIV. HSV is subdivided into HSV-1 and HSV-2, with most symptomatic genital ulcer disease caused by HSV-2.[6] HSV is transmitted by direct contact with secretions or mucosal surfaces contaminated with the virus.[22] After the primary infection, latent infection is established in the dorsal root ganglia of nerve cells. Recurrences cause symptoms ranging from asymptomatic viral shedding to painful ulcers. Symptoms can be treated but the disease has no cure.

Clinical Presentation

Primary Infection

Primary infections with HSV can be severe. These patients experience a prodrome consisting of malaise, fever, headache, myalgias, and genital paresthesias followed by outbreaks of multiple painful vesicles that erode and ulcerate. Atypical nonulcerated presentations of HSV include fissures, furuncles, excoriations, and nonspecific vulvar erythema.[23] Lesions in men occur on the glans, prepuce, and penile shaft while in women lesions are found on the perineum, vulva, and cervix.[24] Men and women who practice anal intercourse can develop HSV proctitis. Complications of primary HSV infection include aseptic meningitis, urinary retention, extragenital cutaneous lesions, cutaneous dissemination, bacterial superinfection, erythema multiforme, spontaneous abortion, pneumonitis, and hepatitis.[2,22]

Recurrent Infections

Recurrent outbreaks of HSV are generally milder, more localized, and of shorter duration than the primary episode. A prodrome consisting of pruritus, itching, and burning occurs 2 to 48 hours before an outbreak of skin lesions. During the prodromal period, patients with no active skin lesions can shed viral particles and thus are potentially infective. Lesions usually recur at the site of the primary infection and healing occurs over a 2-week period. Women can experience vaginal discharge and dysuria with recurrent infections.[22]

Diagnosis

The diagnosis of HSV infection is based on the history, physical findings, and laboratory evaluation. Culture remains the gold standard for the diagnosis of HSV, although 20% to 30% of cultures are negative when infection is present.[22] Cultures are ideally obtained within 7 days of the outbreak for primary HSV and within 2 days for recurrent infections. A specimen from an intact vesicle is desirable since dry, crusted lesions provide low yield. The Tzanck or Pap smear is useful as an adjunct to clinical diagnosis. A specimen from the base of a vesicle or ulcer is collected and stained with Wright, Giemsa, or Papanicolaou stain. Microscopy reveals multinucleated giant cells with HSV infection. However, the Tzanck smear cannot differentiate between HSV and herpes zoster infection and a negative smear does not rule out infection. Alternatives to

culture for the diagnosis of HSV include the immunofluorescence, immunoperoxidase, PCR, and EIA antigen detection tests.[22] Serology cannot distinguish between acute and past infection with HSV.

Treatment

Treatment for the first clinical episode of genital herpes is with:

Acyclovir (Zovirax) 400 mg po three times a day for 7 to 10 days or
Acyclovir (Zovirax) 200 mg po five times a day for 7 to 10 days or
Famciclovir (Famvir) 250 mg po three times a day for 7 to 10 days or
Valacyclovir (Valtrex) 1 g po two times a day for 7 to 10 days[6]

Extend treatment with all regimens if healing is not complete after 10 days of therapy. Treatment studies of first clinical episodes of HSV proctitis, stomatitis, or pharyngitis used acyclovir 400 mg po 5 times a day. Valacyclovir and famciclovir are also probably effective.[6]

Treatment of recurrent episodes of HSV, if instituted during the prodrome or within 1 day of outbreak of lesions, is with:

Acyclovir (Zovirax) 400 mg po three times a day for 5 days or
Acyclovir (Zovirax) 200 mg po five times a day for 5 days or
Acyclovir (Zovirax) 800 mg po two times a day for 5 days or
Valacyclovir (Valtrex) 500 mg po two times a day for 5 days or
Famciclovir (Famvir) 125 mg po two times a day for 5 days[6]

Patients with six or more recurrences per year may benefit from daily suppressive therapy. Suppressive therapy does not decrease viral shedding or eliminate the potential for transmission. Treatment for frequent recurrences with suppressive therapy is with:

Acyclovir (Zovirax) 400 mg po two times a day or
Famciclovir (Famvir) 250 mg po two times a day or
Valacyclovir (Valtrex) 250 mg po two times a day or
Valacyclovir (Valtrex) 500 mg po once a day or
Valacyclovir (Valtrex) 1 g po once a day[6]

After 1 year of suppressive therapy, discuss stopping therapy to reassess the rate of recurrent disease. Many patients have fewer recurrences over time.[6]

Treatment for severe disease or complications requiring hospitalization is with acyclovir (Zovirax) 5 to 10 mg/kg body weight IV q8h for 5 to 7 days or until clinical resolution occurs.[6]

The management of HSV in patients with HIV, pregnant women, and infants is beyond the scope of this chapter.

Prevention

Counseling is an important part of the treatment of patients with HSV. Educate patients about the possibility of recurrence of the disease, asymptomatic viral shedding, and risk of sexual transmission. Advise patients to abstain from sexual activity when active lesions or prodromal symptoms are present and use condoms during sexual contact with new or uninfected partners. Counsel women of childbearing age and men with genital HSV infection regarding the potential for neonatal infection (see Chapter 10). Pregnant women with HSV should inform their health care providers about the infection. Encourage patients to inform their sex partners that they have HSV.[6]

Other Genital Ulcer Disease

Although genital herpes and syphilis are the most common genital ulcer STDs, chancroid, lymphogranuloma venereum (LGV), and granuloma inguinale are also present in the United States. More than one genital ulcer disease is present in 3% to 10% of patients. Chancroid is caused by *Haemophilus ducreyi*, which is endemic in parts of the United States and is a cofactor for HIV transmission. LGV is caused by invasive serovars of *C. trachomatis*. Granuloma inguinale is caused by a gram-negative bacterium *Calymmatobacterium granulomatis*.[6] Because of the rarity of granuloma inguinale in the United States, it will not be discussed in this chapter.

Clinical Presentation

Patients with chancroid present with a small papule or pustule that erodes into an ulcer. One to several ulcers are present initially. The ulcer is typically deep, indurated, and painful with a soft consistency resembling putty.[25]

Patients with LGV classically have one to several genital ulcers. Because the ulcer is not painful and heals spontaneously, it may not be noticed. The most common clinical presentation of LGV is tender inguinal or femoral lymphadenopathy that is usually unilateral. Women and homosexual men can present with proctitis, proctocolitis, and perirectal or perianal lymphatic tissue inflammation with fistulas and strictures.[6]

Diagnosis

Serologic testing for syphilis and evaluation for HSV is indicated in all patients with genital ulcer disease. Specific tests include darkfield examination or immunofluorescence testing for *T. pallidum*, culture or antigen testing for HSV, and culture for *H. ducreyi* (if available). Test patients with syphilis or chancroid for HIV and consider HIV testing in patients with HSV.[6]

Definitive diagnosis of chancroid is made by growth of *H. ducreyi* on special culture medium, but this medium is not commercially available, and its sensitivity is no higher than 80%. PCR, antigen testing, and DNA probe technology are in development but not commercially available.[26] A presumptive diagnosis is made if the patient has one or more painful genital ulcers; there is no evidence of *T. pallidum* by darkfield examination of ulcer exudate or by serologic testing for syphilis; the clinical presentation, appearance of ulcers, and regional lymphadenopathy are typical for chancroid; and testing is negative for HSV.[6]

The diagnosis of LGV is made clinically and by serology. Culture of the aspirate from an involved lymph node for *C. trachomatis* is the most specific test available.[25]

Treatment

Treatment of chancroid is with:

Azithromycin (Zithromax) 1 g po in a single dose or
Ceftriaxone (Rocephin) 250 mg IM in a single dose or
Ciprofloxacin (Cipro) 500 mg po two times a day for 3 days (contraindicated for pregnant and lactating women, children, and adolescents ≤18 years of age) or
Erythromycin base (E-Mycin, ERYC, Ery-Tab, PCE) 500 mg po four times a day for 7 days[6]

Reexamine patients with chancroid in 3 to 7 days. If no improvement is evident, consider whether the diagnosis is correct, co-infection with another STD exists, the patient has HIV, the patient was noncompliant with therapy, or the *H. ducreyi* strain is resistant to the therapy prescribed. Resolution of fluctuant lymphadenopathy is slower than ulcers and may require aspiration or incision and drainage.

Treatment for LGV is with doxycycline (Doryx, Monodox, Vibramycin, Vibra-Tab) 100 mg po two times a day for 21 days. An alternative regimens is with erythromycin base (E-Mycin, ERYC, Ery-Tab, PCE) 500 mg po 4 times a day for 21 days.[6] Follow patients with LGV until signs and symptoms of the disease have resolved. Buboes may require aspiration or incision and drainage.

Prevention

Treat sexual contacts of patients with chancroid even in the absence of clinical disease if the last sexual contact was within 10 days of the onset of symptoms. Retest patients with chancroid for HIV and syphilis 3 months after the diagnosis if initial tests were negative at the time of diagnosis.[6]

Test sexual contacts of patients treated for LGV for chlamydial infection if the last contact was 30 days before onset of symptoms.[6]

Trichomoniasis

Vaginal discharge is common in women with STDs. Three common causes of vaginal discharge are trichomonal vaginitis, candidiasis, and bacterial vaginosis (see Chapter 102). Vaginal discharge with mucopurulent cervicitis can also occur with infections caused by *N. gonorrhoeae* or *C. trachomatis*. Trichomoniasis is caused by the protozoan *Trichomonas vaginalis*. Both women and men can be infected by *T. vaginalis*. While trichomonal infection can be sexually transmitted, there is less certainty with candidiasis and bacterial vaginosis.

Clinical Presentation

Most infected women have a malodorous, yellow-green discharge with vulvar irritation. Most infected men are asymptomatic or have urethritis.[6]

Diagnosis

Trichomoniasis in women is diagnosed by microscopic examination of a fresh sample of the vaginal discharge mixed in one to two drops of normal saline. Motile protozoans are usually easily identified. Culture media are available and useful when signs and symptoms suggest trichomoniasis but no organisms are seen. The diagnosis in men is difficult because fewer organisms are present in infected men than in women. Evaluation of men includes urinalysis and wet mount examination of urethral discharge. A negative microscopic evaluation does not rule out disease. Culture is indicated if clinical suspicion is high for trichomoniasis.[27]

Treatment

Treatment for trichomoniasis is with:

Metronidazole (Flagyl) 2 g po in a single dose (acceptable as treatment in pregnant women according to the CDC) or
Metronidazole (Flagyl) 500 mg po twice a day for 7 days[6]

Some strains of *T. vaginalis* have diminished susceptibility to metronidazole but respond to higher doses. Treat patients with repeated treatment failures with metronidazole (Flagyl) 2 g po once a day for 3 to 5 days.[6]

Prevention

Follow-up is not necessary for women and men whose symptoms resolve after treatment. Treat sex partners and instruct patients to abstain from sexual contact until treatment is completed and symptoms resolved.

Ectoparasitic Infections

Pediculosis pubis and scabies can be sexually transmitted (see Chapter 116). Pediculosis pubis is caused by the louse *Phthirus pubis*. Scabies is caused by the mite *Sarcoptes scabiei*.

Clinical Presentation

Pediculosis is highly contagious, with transmission occurring after one exposure in 95% of cases.[28] Patients with pubic lice usually present with pruritus of the genitalia. Erythematous papules, excoriations, nits on hair shafts, and lice are found on physical examination. Maculae cerulea are blue-gray macules on surrounding skin caused by degradation of blood pigments by louse saliva.

Scabies is highly contagious and transmitted by close physical contact. *S. scabiei* can survive 24 to 36 hours on objects, but fomite spread is less important than direct contact. The major symptom of scabies is severe pruritus, often worse at night. Symptoms begin 3 to 4 weeks after infestation with the first exposure to scabies. Reinfected patients can develop pruritus within 24 hours of reinfestation. Burrows, papules, and nodules are found on the skin. Burrows are classically found on the flexor areas of the wrists, web spaces of the hands, lateral palms, and instep of the feet. Some patients present with lesions on the genitalia. Norwegian scabies is relatively rare but can occur in immunologically compromised patients, including those with HIV. These patients have thick, crusted plaques and subungual debris.[29]

Diagnosis

Confirm the diagnosis of pediculosis by identifying lice or nits with microscopic examination. To diagnose scabies examine a scraping of a nonexcoriated burrow or new papule in mineral oil under microscopy. Multiple scrapings increase the chance of a positive microscopic diagnosis. The presence of mites, eggs, or fecal pellets confirms the diagnosis.

Treatment

Treatment of *pediculosis pubis* is with:

Lindane (Kwell) 1% shampoo applied for 4 minutes and then thoroughly washed off (not recommended for pregnant or lactating women or children <2 years of age) or
Pyrethrins with piperonyl butoxide (Rid) applied to affected areas and washed off after 10 minutes[6]

Do not apply these regimens to the eyes. Treat pediculosis of the eyelashes by applying occlusive ophthalmic ointment to the eyelid margins for 10 days.

Treatment of *scabies* is with:

Permethrin (Elimite) 5% cream applied to all areas of the body from the neck down, washed off after 8 to 14 hours or
Lindane (Kwell) 1% lotion (1 oz) or cream (30 g) applied thinly to all areas of the body from the neck down, washed off thoroughly after 8 hours (not used after a bath, by persons with extensive dermatitis, pregnant or lactating women, or children <2 years of age) or
Sulfur 6% precipitated in ointment applied thinly to all areas nightly for 3 nights, old applications washed off before new applications applied, and thoroughly washed off 24 hours after the last application[6]

Prevention

To prevent the transmission of pediculosis, all bedding and clothing should be machine-washed and machine-dried using the heat cycle, dry-cleaned, or removed from body contact for 72 hours. Recheck patients 1 week after treatment and retreat with an alternative regimen if infection is still present. Treat sex partners from the preceding month.[6]

To prevent the transmission of scabies, all bedding and clothing should be machine-washed and machine-dried using the heat cycle, dry-cleaned, or removed from body contact for 72 hours. Pruritus can persist for several weeks. Some experts recommend re-treatment after 1 week if the patient is still symptomatic. Other experts advise re-treatment only if live mites are demonstrated. Retreat patients with an alternative regimen when there is no response to treatment. Examine and treat sexual contacts and close personal or household contacts within the last month.[6]

Enteric Pathogens

Individuals who practice anal intercourse or whose sexual practices involve oral-fecal contact can develop proctitis, proctocolitis and enteritis (see Chapters 91 and 94). Sexually transmitted proctitis is caused by *N. gonorrhoeae*, *C. trachomatis* (LGV serovars), *T. pallidum*, and HSV. Pathogens involved in proctocolitis include *Campylobacter* spp., *Shigella* spp., *Entamoeba histolytica*, and rarely *C. trachomatis* (LGV serovars). *Giardia lamblia* is the most frequent pathogen identified in otherwise healthy patients with sexually transmitted enteritis. Enteritis can also be a primary effect of HIV. Patients with HIV can also develop infections from pathogens not usually sexually transmitted, including cytomegalovirus, *Mycobacterium avium-intracellulare*, *Salmonella* spp., *Cryptosporidium*, *Microsporidia*, and *Isospora*.[6]

Clinical Presentation

Patients with proctitis have anorectal pain, tenesmus, and rectal discharge. Symptoms of proctocolitis include anorectal pain, tenesmus, rectal discharge, diarrhea, and abdominal cramps. Patients with enteritis present with abdominal cramps and diarrhea without symptoms of proctitis or proctocolitis.

Diagnosis

Perform appropriate diagnostic testing and procedures, such as anoscopy, sigmoidoscopy, stool examination, culture, and evaluation for HSV, *N. gonorrhoeae*, *C. trachomatis*, and *T. pallidum*. Multiple stool specimens are sometimes necessary for the diagnosis of *Giardia*.[6,30]

Treatment

Treatment is based on the specific diagnosis. If anorectal pus is present on physical examination or polymorphonuclear neutrophils (PMNs) found on a Gram stain of anorectal secretions, initiate empiric treatment for sexually transmitted acute proctitis (pending results of other tests) with:

Ceftriaxone (Rocephin) 125 mg IM once (or other agent effective against anal and genital gonorrhea) plus
Doxycycline (Doryx, Monodox, Vibramycin, Vibra-Tab) 100 mg po twice a day for 7 days[6]

Prevention

Follow-up is based on the diagnosis. Counsel patients regarding the mechanism of transmission of their infection. Examine, evaluate, and treat sex partners for diseases diagnosed in the patient.

References

1. Cates W, and the American Social Health Association Panel. Estimates of the incidence and prevalence of sexually transmitted diseases in the United States. Sex Transm Dis 1999; 26(suppl):S2–S7.
2. Centers for Disease Control and Prevention. Tracking the hidden epidemics. Trends in STDs in the United States. Biennial Report: 2000;1–31.
3. Mertz KJ, McQuillan GM, Levine WC, et al. A pilot study of the prevalence of chlamydial infection in a national household survey. Sex Transm Dis 1998;May:229–31.
4. Centers for Disease Control and Prevention. Recommendations for the prevention and management of *Chlamydia trachomatis* infections. MMWR 1993;42 RR-12:1–32.
5. Stamm WE. *Chlamydia trachomatis* infections: progress and problems. J Infect Dis 1999;179(suppl 2):S380–3.
6. Centers for Disease Control and Prevention. 1998 guidelines for treatment of sexually transmitted diseases. MMWR 1998;47: 1–116.
7. Kellogg JA. Impact of variation in endocervical specimen collection and testing techniques on frequency of false-positive and false-negative *Chlamydia* detection results. Am J Clin Pathol 1995;104:554–9.
8. Jackson SL, Soper DE. Sexually transmitted diseases in pregnancy. Obstet Gynecol Clin North Am 1997;24:631-44.
9. Division of STD Prevention. Sexually transmitted disease surveillance, 1999. Atlanta: U.S. Department of Health and Human Services, Centers for Disease Control and Prevention, September 2000.
10. Wasserheit JN. Epidemiological synergy: interrelationships between human immunodeficiency virus infection and other sexually transmitted diseases. Sex Transm Dis 1992;19:61–77.
11. Sparling PF. Gonococcal infections. In: Goldman L, Bennett JC, eds. Cecil textbook of medicine. Philadelphia: WB Saunders, 2000;1742–5.
12. Chernesky M, Morse S, Schachter J. Newly available and future laboratory tests for sexually transmitted diseases (STDs) other than HIV. Sex Transm Dis 1999;26(4 suppl):S8–11.
13. Division of AIDS, STD, and TB Laboratory Research. *Neisseria gonorrhoeae*, 2000. Available at *www.cdc.gov/ncidod/ dastlr/gcdir/NeIdent/Ngon.html*.
14. Hillis SD. PID prevention: clinical and societal stakes. Hosp Pract 1994;29(4)121–30.
15. Ault KA, Faro S. Pelvic inflammatory disease current diagnostic criteria and treatment guidelines. Postgrad Med 1993;93: 85–91.
16. Hook EW, Marra CM. Acquired syphilis in adults. N Engl J Med 1992;326:1060–7.
17. Clark EG, Danbolt N. The Oslo study of the natural course of untreated syphilis: an epidemiologic investigation based on a restudy of the Boeck-Bruusgaard material. Med Clin North Am 1964;48:612–23.
18. Flores JL. Syphilis a tale of twisted treponemes. West J Med 1995;163:552–9.
19. Ho GYF, Bierman R, Beardsley L, Chee JC, Burk RD. Natural history of cervicovaginal papillomavirus infection in young women. N Engl J Med 1998;338(7):423–8.
20. Stone KM. Human papillomavirus infection and genital warts: update on epidemiology and treatment. Clin Infect Dis 1995; 20(suppl 1):S91–7.
21. Heaton CL. Clinical manifestations and modern management of condylomata acuminata: a dermatologic perspective. Am J Obstet Gynecol 1995;172:1344–50.
22. Clark JL, Tatum NO, Noble SL. Management of genital herpes. Am Fam Phys 1995;51:175–81.

23. Koutsky LA, Stevens CE, Holmes KK, et al. Underdiagnosis of genital herpes by current clinical and viral-isolation procedures. N Engl J Med 1992;326:1533–9.

24. Hoffman IF, Schmitz JL. Genital ulcer disease. Postgrad Med 1995;98:67–82.

25. Goens JL, Schwartz RA, De Wolf K. Mucocutaneous manifestations of chancroid, lymphogranuloma venereum and granuloma inguinale. Am Fam Phys 1994;49:415–25.

26. Lewis DA. Diagnostic tests for chancroid. Sex Transm Inf 2000;76:137–141.

27. Krieger JN. Trichomoniasis in men: old issues and new data. Sex Transm Dis 1995;22:83–6.

28. Forsman KE. Pediculosis and scabies. Postgrad Med 1995; 98:89–100.

29. Arlian LG, Runyan RA, Achar S, Estes SA. Survival and infectivity of Sarcoptes scabiei var canis var hominis. J Am Acad Dermatol 1984;11:210–15.

30. Rompalo AM. Diagnosis and treatment of sexually acquired proctitis and proctocolitis: an update. Clin Infect Dis 1999; 28(supl 1):S84–90.

42

Human Immunodeficiency Virus Infection and Acquired Immunodeficiency Syndrome

Steven P. Bromer and Ronald H. Goldschmidt

Care for patients with human immunodeficiency virus (HIV) infection requires excellence in all aspects of family practice. The family physician's roles include providing patient education to prevent uninfected persons from becoming infected, identifying and counseling infected persons, delivering comprehensive medical care, initiating and monitoring antiretroviral (ARV) therapy, providing prophylaxis against opportunistic infections, managing the acquired immunodeficiency syndrome (AIDS), and providing support and care for the family. New manifestations of HIV disease, diagnostic protocols, and drug recommendations for HIV disease change on a regular basis, so familiarity with sources of updated information and guidelines on HIV care is essential[1] (Table 42.1).

The striking benefits of combination antiretroviral therapy, sometimes called highly active antiretroviral therapy (HAART), have changed the implications of HIV disease dramatically.[2] The demonstrated effectiveness of ARV therapy in reducing opportunistic infections and decreasing mortality has made the hope of a normal life span with a high quality of life a real possibility for HIV-positive persons.

Despite substantial progress in the medical management of HIV infection, the AIDS epidemic continues to exact a tremendous toll on families, communities, and society. The World Health Organization estimates that there are more than 40 million people infected with HIV worldwide and more than 3 million deaths annually. In North America as many as 45,000 new infections occur annually.[3] Minority communities in the United States are disproportionately affected and the proportion of women infected continues to increase.[4] Family-centered approaches to prevention and treatment are needed to address the new challenges created by the changing epidemic.

Risk Factors, Risk Reduction, and Patient Education

HIV is usually transmitted from person to person by the passage of blood or body fluids such as semen and vaginal secretions. Urine, sweat, and saliva are not generally considered to be infectious. Persons engaging in unprotected sexual activity and intravenous drug use with needle-sharing account for most cases of HIV infection. The risk of transfusion-related infection is very low and is estimated to be about 1 in every 677,000 units of donated blood.[5] Vertical transmission occurs in 25% of children of infected mothers who are not receiving ARV therapy. Effective ARV therapy decreases this transmission rate dramatically.[6] Casual transmission (in the absence of sexual contact or passage of blood) from person to person does not seem to occur. Transmission from infected patients to health care workers occurs at a rate of approximately 0.3% (one seroconversion for every 333 needlesticks or similar injury) and constitutes an uncommon but important transmission category. The use of timely postexposure prophylaxis with ARV medications can decrease the risk of transmission following a needlestick injury when the source patient is known to be HIV-positive.[7] Universal blood and body fluid precautions are essential for minimizing health care worker risk.

Physicians should assess their patients' risk for HIV infection by obtaining a sexual and drug history. Education about the use of condoms is essential for all persons who do not remain celibate or in a mutually monogamous relationship. Intravenous drug users can be encouraged to enter a drug treatment program. Those who do not abstain from intravenous drug use must be educated about safe needle use through a needle

Table 42.1. **Internet Resources for HIV Management**

www.hivatis.org	Up-to-date Public Health Service guidelines on use of antiretroviral medications, prophylaxis against opportunistic infections and other important management issues in HIV disease
www.cdc.gov	HIV/AIDS and other sexually transmitted disease guidelines from the Center for Disease Control and Prevention
www.hivinsite.ucsf.edu	Comprehensive site with information on treatment, prevention and policy from the University of California at San Francisco
www.hopkins-aids.edu	Comprehensive site with access to resources for treatment, prevention and policy from Johns Hopkins University AIDS Service
www.ucsf.edu/hivcntr	Web site of the National HIV Telephone Consultation Service (Warmline) and the National Clinicians' Post-Exposure Prophylaxis Hotline (PEPline); based in the National HIV/AIDS Clinicians' Consultation Center at San Francisco General Hospital, sponsored by the Health Resources and Services Administration
www.actis.org	A resource of federally and privately funded HIV/AIDS clinical trials; sponsored by the United States Department of Health and Human Services

exchange program or by cleaning their injection equipment with bleach. Physicians' offices should have health education materials about HIV and sexually transmitted diseases openly available for patients and families to read and take with them. HIV-positive patients also need to be counseled about risk reduction both to protect themselves from other infections and to prevent transmission of HIV to their partners.

Counseling and Testing

Counseling and testing for HIV should be offered to all patients who have risk factors for HIV infection. Patients who have unexplained constitutional symptoms should also be offered HIV counseling and testing. Physicians should keep acute HIV infection in the differential diagnosis for patients presenting with a febrile illness who have a recent history of risk activities. Acute HIV infection usually causes a flu-like illness (Table 42.2) with symptoms of fever, myalgia, sore throat, and fatigue. On exam patients may have elevated temperatures, postural hypotension, mucous membrane ulcerations, maculopapular rash, adenopathy, and neurologic signs consistent with aseptic meningitis.[8] Patients with acute HIV infection may benefit from early ARV therapy and need to be counseled about risk reduction to prevent transmission of the virus to others.

Counseling about HIV is the beginning of a critical medical intervention.[9] During the pretest counseling sessions, the

Table 42.2. **Acute Retroviral Syndrome: Associated Signs and Symptoms**

Common symptoms	Fever
	Myalgia
	Fatigue
	Sore throat
	Headache
	Rash
Common signs	Elevated temperature
	Maculopapular rash
	Mucous membrane ulcers (including oral and genital lesions)
	Adenopathy

physician and patient need to discuss the patient's risk of being infected, ongoing activities that put the patient or others at risk, and methods of future risk reduction. Before offering testing, the physician should assess whether the patient appears psychologically and socially prepared for the results and if support from friends and family is available. A discussion of the complications of the HIV antibody testing including false-positive results, false-negative results, possible loss of confidentiality, and family and social disruption precedes obtaining informed consent for testing. The difference between confidential and anonymous testing needs to be discussed. Although confidential testing can be done in the physician's office, it results in charted documentation that can reveal HIV status to health care workers and others who process medical records. To avoid possible breaches of confidentiality and to ensure anonymity, the patient can be referred to an anonymous test site or obtain home testing.

Testing to establish the diagnosis of HIV infection usually requires an enzyme-linked immunosorbent assay (ELISA) screening test followed by either a Western blot (WB) or immunofluorescent antibody (IFA) confirmatory test. A "window period" of several weeks to 3 months exists between the time of infection and seroconversion with the development of specific antibodies against HIV. During this time patients can be viremic and infectious but not have sufficient levels of antibodies to result in positive serologic testing. For seronegative patients with recent at-risk activities, retesting at 3 to 6 months is advised. If there is strong clinical suspicion of recent HIV infection, antigen assays such as a plasma HIV RNA viral load or P24 antigen assay can be checked, but a positive antigen test needs to be interpreted with care because of concerns for false-positive results in these assays. A positive result needs to be confirmed with standard antibody tests in the future. In a few patients, serologic evidence of HIV infection may be delayed beyond 6 months.

All patients should receive their test results during a face-to-face posttest counseling session. For patients testing HIV positive, this session likely marks a turning point in their life. Patients should be told clearly that the test is positive, and that they are infected with HIV. It is important to reassure patients that HIV positivity does not mean they are at risk of becoming ill in the near future. Because HIV infection has a long asymptomatic phase and because of continuing advances in the treatment of HIV, there may be many years before problems arise. Upon hearing an HIV-positive result, however, patients may be in some degree of psychological shock and might not be able to assimilate much information. A commitment to ongoing care should be the focus of the first posttest counseling session. Perhaps the most important intervention that family physicians can make is to provide reassurance that they will remain the patient's personal physician while assembling a multidisciplinary team to help the patient address the challenges of the new diagnosis. At future visits, the family physician can offer to meet with the family and members of the patient's social network to help the patient combat isolation and identify particular challenges faced in coping with the diagnosis. The posttest counseling session is also important for patients who test negative for HIV. These patients need to be counseled about risk reduction and helped to develop specific plans to prevent future exposures.

Medical Management of HIV Disease

Health Care Maintenance

The seropositive patient requires routine health care maintenance and special attention to specific signs, symptoms, and laboratory markers for HIV disease progression. Routine health care maintenance includes a comprehensive history and physical examination with special attention to a history of sexually transmitted diseases and physical findings of skin and oral conditions. Laboratory evaluation includes a routine complete blood count including platelet count, chemistry panel, hepatitis and syphilis serologies, and markers of HIV disease (see below). A chest roentgenogram is required for persons with a history of cardiopulmonary problems but is not required for all HIV-infected persons. Women should have Pap smears performed and repeated at 6 months. Annual influenza vaccination and one-time pneumococcal vaccination should be administered. Hepatitis A and B vaccination is recommended if patients do not have serologic evidence of immunity. Polio vaccination for HIV-infected persons and their family members should be with the inactivated (intramuscular) preparation.

Because HIV infection contributes to an increased risk of progression from latent to active tuberculosis (TB), it is essential to screen all HIV positive patients for TB. A purified protein derivative (PPD) skin test for TB in HIV-infected persons is considered positive for TB infection with a 5-mm (rather than the usual 10-mm) reaction. PPD-negative patients should be screened annually. For HIV-infected persons known to be at high risk for TB (injection drug users, homeless persons, and persons from countries with a high incidence of TB) even a negative tuberculin skin test cannot eliminate the possibility of co-infection with TB. Patients with positive tuberculin skin tests and those with a high risk of TB require a chest roentgenogram to exclude active TB (see Chapter 84). Once active disease has been ruled out, patients should be offered treatment for latent TB with either isoniazid 300 mg daily for 9 months or rifampin 600 mg daily with pyrazinamide 2 g daily for 2 months.[10]

Laboratory Markers of HIV Disease

$CD4^+$ lymphocyte counts and plasma HIV RNA viral load measurements are essential tools in monitoring HIV disease. Depletion of $CD4^+$ lymphocytes is the hallmark of HIV disease and is an important marker of the degree of immunosuppression and predictor of the risk for opportunistic infections. The normal range for $CD4^+$ lymphocyte counts is broad and variable, so multiple measurements are required to detect trends. Viral load testing provides an assessment of viral activity and the patient's ability to control viral replication as well as the effectiveness of antiretroviral medications. The viral load also helps to predict the rate of decline in $CD4^+$ counts, with high viral loads predicting more rapid depletion of $CD4^+$ cells. $CD4^+$ counts and viral loads should be measured three to four times per year, in patients both receiving and not receiving antiviral therapy. In addition, viral load and $CD4^+$ counts should be checked within 2 months of starting a new antiviral regimen and if any significant clinical events occur.

Antiretroviral Therapy

Effective combination ARV therapy is a powerful medical intervention that can control viral replication and preserve immune function for HIV-positive patients, but it does not cure HIV infection. ARV agents can have substantial short-term and long-term side effects and toxicities. In addition, a patient's virus can become resistant to all agents currently in use. Guidelines for antiretroviral therapy change frequently.[1,11]

Prior to prescribing ARV medications, the family physician must assess the patient's ability to adhere to complex treatment regimens. Unlike therapeutics in other chronic diseases, such as diabetes or hypertension, the consequence of nonadherence to HIV medications can be the rapid development of resistance and permanent loss of clinical benefit.[12] Therefore, if a patient is unlikely to adhere to a medication regimen, it is better to postpone starting treatment until more supports are in place to help the patient adhere or other areas of the patient's life are more organized. Involving family members as well as utilizing the resources of case managers, clinical pharmacists, social workers, and other members of the care team can help with adherence issues.

Controversy exists over the best time to begin ARV therapy. The most recent guidelines on the use of antiretroviral agents from the Department of Health and Human Services[12] recommend starting ARV therapy in all patients who are symptomatic from HIV disease regardless of $CD4^+$ count and in asymptomatic patients with $CD4^+$ counts below 200 cells/mm^3. There is controversy about starting antiretroviral therapy in asymptomatic patients with $CD4^+$ counts between 200 and 350, but most experts recommend offering therapy to these patients. The guidelines recommend considering therapy for patients with $CD4^+$ counts between 350 and 500 cells/mm^3 who have high viral loads [greater than 55,000 copies by polymerase chain reaction (PCR) RNA assay or 30,000 copies on branched DNA assay]. Many clinicians would not treat patients with CD4$^+$ counts greater than 350 cells/mm^3 who have viral loads less than 55,000 (PCR RNA) or 30,000 (branched DNA) copies. These patients need regular CD4$^+$ cell counts and viral load testing to monitor disease progression and to assess the need for beginning therapy.

Initial antiviral regimens include at least three drugs, often from several different classes of agents. Common regimens are two nucleoside analogues with either one or two protease inhibitors, two nucleoside analogues with a nonnucleoside analogue, or three nucleoside analogues (Table 42.3). The goal of an initial regimen in patients without prior treatment is suppression of the viral load to undetectable levels and preservation or improvement in CD4 counts. Patients need to have CD4$^+$ counts and viral load testing by 8 weeks after starting a regimen, with the expectation of a log reduction in the pretreatment viral load. Depending on the initial viral load, it may take up to 6 months to achieve undetectable viral loads, so regimens should not be changed in the first few months unless there is clear virologic failure.

Table 42.3. **Common Antiretroviral Medications**

Medication	Dose	Comment and side effects
Nucleoside reverse transcriptase inhibitors (NRTIs)		
Zidovudine (AZT, Retrovir)[a,b]	200 mg tid or 300 mg bid	Anemia, neutropenia, headaches, nausea, malaise
Didanosine, (DDI, Videx, Videx EC)	200 mg bid or 400 mg qd	Need to take on empty stomach; diarrhea, pancreatitis, peripheral neuropathy, lactic acidosis
Zalcitabine (DDC, Hivid)	0.75 mg tid	Peripheral neuropathy, oral ulcers
Stavudine (D4T, Zerit)	20–40 mg bid	Peripheral neuropathy, insomnia, lactic acidosis, lipoatrophy
Lamivudine (3TC, Epivir)[a,b]	150 mg bid	Headache, fatigue, peripheral neuropathy, lactic acidosis
Abacavir (Ziagen)[b]	300 mg bid	Nausea, headache, malaise, hypersensitivity reaction, lactic acidosis, lipoatrophy
Non–nucleoside reverse transcriptase inhibitors (nNRTIs)		
Efavirenz (Sustiva)	600 mg qhs	Dizziness, anxiety, headache, nightmares, hepatitis; avoid during pregnancy; mixed P-450 enzyme inducer and inhibitor
Nevirapine (Viramune)	200 mg qd × 14 days then 200 mg bid	Rash, hepatitis, nausea, vomiting, diarrhea, fatigue, headaches, rare hematologic toxicity; P-450 enzyme inducer.
Delavirdine (Rescriptor)	400 mg tid	Rash, nausea, headache, hepatitis; P-450 enzyme inducer
Protease inhibitors (PIs)		
Nelfinavir (Viracept)	750 mg tid or 1250 mg bid (see dual PI regimens below)	Take with food; diarrhea, hyperlipidemias, abnormal fat accumulation, insulin resistance, hepatitis
Indinivir (Crixivan)	800 mg tid (see dual PI regimens below)	Take on empty stomach; nephrolithiasis, hyperlipidemias, abnormal fat accumulation, insulin resistance, diarrhea and asymptotic hyperbilirubinemia
Ritonavir (Norvir)	600 mg bid (see dual PI regimens below)	Take with food; potent P-450 enzyme inhibitor; nausea, vomiting, diarrhea, anorexia, hepatitis, hyperlipidemias, abnormal fat accumulation, insulin resistance, circumoral paresthesias
Saquinavir soft gel (Fortovase)	1200 mg tid (see dual PI regimens below)	Take with food; headache, confusion, hyperlipidemias, abnormal fat accumulation, insulin resistance, nausea, diarrhea, hepatitis
Amprenavir (Agenerase)	1200 mg bid (see dual PI regimens below)	Take with food; nausea, vomiting, diarrhea, hyperlipidemias, abnormal fat accumulation, oral paresthesias, headache, rash and hepatitis
Dual PI combinations		
Lopinavir/ritonavir (Kaletra)	400 mg/100 mg bid (three capsules); increase to four capsules if also giving efavirenz or nevirapine	Take with food; nausea, diarrhea, rash, headache, hyperlipidemia, insulin resistance
Ritonavir/Indinavir	200 mg/800 mg bid or 400 mg/400 mg bid	OK to take with food; see individual agents
Ritonavir/saquinavir soft gel	400 mg/400 mg bid	See individual agents
Ritonavir/amprenavir	200 mg/600 mg bid	See individual agents

Source: Adapted from Goldschmidt and Dong.[1]

[a]AZT/3TC available as Combivir 300 mg/150 mg.

[b]AZT/3TC/Abacavir available as Trizavir 300 mg/150 mg/300 mg.

Patients failing antiviral regimens or patients with extensive history of antiviral use need special consideration in devising regimens that have the best chance of success. It is essential to obtain a complete history of ARV use, including the chronology of ARV regimens, CD4$^+$ counts and viral loads, as well as the reasons for change or discontinuation of specific medications. Resistance tests that measure either genotypic or phenotypic resistance to antiviral medications may play an important role in helping guide treatment options.[13] Given the complexity of the decisions involved in choosing or changing ARV regimens, it is reasonable for physicians without extensive experience with these medications to consult with colleagues who have more experience or with telephone resources such as the National HIV Telephone Consultation Service (Warmline) at (800) 933-3413 of the Department of Family and Community Medicine at San Francisco General Hospital.

All patients taking ARV therapy need both laboratory and clinical monitoring for adverse medication effects. Complete blood count and a chemistry panel with liver function tests should be included. Because many antiviral medications alter lipid metabolism, fasting lipid levels should be monitored. If lipid abnormalities develop, alternative regimens can be considered or the patient can be treated with lipid-lowering agents. Patients taking protease inhibitors have a higher incidence of hyperglycemia, which can be treated with dietary counseling or antihyperglycemic medications if needed. Often the most troubling side effects for patients are changes in body habitus from loss of subcutaneous adipose tissue in the face and limbs and accumulation of visceral adipose tissue in the abdomen. A very serious toxicity from antiviral medications is the development of potentially fatal lactic acidosis with multisystem organ failure. Patients on antiviral medications with complaints of malaise, dyspnea, and nonspecific gastrointestinal complaints should be evaluated for hyperlactatemia and liver abnormalities.[14] Potentially fatal hypersensitivity reactions to ARV medications can occur and need to be considered especially in patients restarting ARV regimens.

Management of the Immunocompromised Patient

Not all patients are able to benefit from ARV therapy because of intolerance to ARV medications, an inability to adhere to complex regimens, or virologic failure secondary to viral resistance. These patients are at risk of progressive decline in immune function and in developing opportunistic infections and malignancies. In this setting, it is especially important to maintain a close doctor–patient relationship to optimize care and to help address the medical, psychological, and social consequences of illness and disability.

Prophylaxis Against Opportunistic Infections

Preventing *Pneumocystis carinii* pneumonia (PCP) and other opportunistic infections decreases morbidity and mortality in immunocompromised patients.[15,16] When CD4$^+$ lymphocyte counts fall to fewer than 200 cells/mm^3 or when patients develop symptoms of advanced HIV disease, prophylaxis against PCP should be initiated. Prophylaxis has been shown to delay or prevent the development of PCP and improve the survival and health of HIV-infected persons. Trimethoprim-sulfamethoxazole (TMP-SMX), one double-strength tablet daily, is the drug of choice. For patients unable to tolerate TMP-SMX, alternative regimens are available. Prophylaxis against toxoplasmosis is generally provided by standard TMP-SMX regimens for PCP prophylaxis.

Prophylaxis against *Mycobacterium avium* complex (MAC) disease has been recommended for all patients with fewer than 50 CD4$^+$ lymphocytes/mm^3. Azithromycin or clarithromycin are the drugs of choice. Primary prophylaxis against fungal, herpes simplex, herpes zoster, and cytomegalovirus infections is not routinely recommended. Primary and secondary prophylaxis against many opportunistic infections can be discontinued if patients are able to maintain CD4$^+$ counts above the high-risk levels for more than 6 months while on ARV therapy. Recommendations for prophylaxis and discontinuation of prophylaxis change as more data become available. The most recent recommendations can be accessed through the Internet resources listed in Table 42.1.

Clinical Manifestations of AIDS
Nonspecific Symptoms and Signs
Nearly all patients with progressive HIV disease develop weight loss,[17] weakness, malaise, and anorexia. Unexplained fevers are common with advanced HIV disease. Investigation for specific organ system disease and opportunistic infections and malignancies is the first step in evaluating these symptoms and signs. This investigation includes evaluations for pulmonary disease including PCP and disseminated MAC infection.[18] Sepsis caused by bacteria and fungi (including cryptococcal sepsis) can also be identified. When no specific pathogenic process can be found, constitutional symptoms and signs are usually attributed to the HIV infection itself. Fevers can be treated with nonsteroidal antiinflammatory drugs (NSAIDs), but these drugs can be especially nephrotoxic in AIDS patients. Weight loss, especially from loss of muscle mass, needs to be aggressively worked up and treated.[19]

Skin and Oral Cavity
Skin and oral cavity lesions are the most frequent first manifestations of AIDS.[20] A form of seborrheic dermatitis is the most common skin condition found in HIV-infected persons. This condition is readily treated with a combination of low-strength hydrocortisone cream plus ketoconazole cream. Drug rashes can be bothersome and serious. Careful investigation to identify and discontinue the offending drug (including nonprescription drugs the patient may be taking without the physician's knowledge) is essential.

Kaposi's sarcoma (KS) is an AIDS-defining condition. The violaceous to brown lesions can occur anywhere on the body. A biopsy can be required, especially to distinguish KS from bacillary angiomatosis, a bacterial condition that can produce similar lesions. KS does not require treatment unless the lesions are cosmetically bothersome, bulky, or painful, or the patient wishes the lesions to be treated. Other skin conditions include bacterial folliculitis, fungal rashes, and molluscum contagiosum. Herpes zoster infections (shingles) can occur early in HIV disease. Herpes simplex infections of the perioral and perirectal areas can be extensive and persistent. Treatment with oral acyclovir is usually effective, but extensive lesions require intravenous acyclovir. Disseminated herpes simplex and zoster infections usually require intravenous acyclovir treatment.

Oral candidiasis (thrush) is not an AIDS-defining condition. Thrush takes the form of white plaques that can be scraped from the tongue or other areas of the oral mucosa. Oral candidiasis can also present in an inflammatory form with erythema and atrophy but without white plaques. Treatment with topical or systemic antifungal agents is effective. Oral hairy leukoplakia is a viral lesion that appears on the lateral borders of the tongue. Because this condition is asymptomatic and recedes spontaneously, no treatment is required. Other oral conditions include KS, angular cheilitis secondary to candidal infection, and periodontal disease.

Eyes

Cytomegalovirus (CMV) retinitis usually occurs when CD4+ lymphocyte counts are lower than 50 cells/mm^3. Hemorrhages, perivascular exudates, and white, gray, or yellow discoloration of the peripheral retina are characteristic. When CMV retinitis is identified, treatment with ganciclovir (Cytovene) or foscarnet (Foscavir) should be instituted, as progression to blindness can occur rapidly and without warning.[21] Cotton-wool spots are nonspecific signs of ischemia that are frequently noted on funduscopic examination of many AIDS patients. These small white lesions with indistinct margins can come and go and do not threaten vision.

Lymph Nodes and Hematopoietic System

Generalized lymphadenopathy caused by HIV-induced nodal hyperplasia is common and does not require biopsy or specific treatment. Treatable causes of lymphadenopathy, including lymphoma, tuberculosis, fungal infections, and KS, should be considered when suspicious clinical syndromes are present, lymphadenopathy is asymmetric, or prominent hard lymph nodes are present. Biopsy may be required in these instances.

All blood cell lines can be affected by HIV infection. Neutropenia is common, with reductions in the absolute neutrophil count to fewer than 300 to 500 neutrophils/mm^3 frequently occurring in the patient with AIDS. Careful observation, blood cultures, and consideration of empiric antibiotic treatment are required for severe neutropenia. Granulocyte/macrophage-stimulating factors can help raise the neutrophil count to noncritical levels in the presence of drug-induced granulocytopenia. Anemia caused by HIV disease can require transfusions or erythropoietin therapy. Macrocytosis is a normal hematologic response to zidovudine therapy and does not require or respond to treatment. Some patients receiving zidovudine develop anemia with or without macrocytosis, requiring discontinuation of the drug or blood transfusion. Thrombocytopenia can occur early in the course of HIV infection and does not appear to predict disease progression, nor is it a condition that requires treatment. Thrombocytopenia late in the course of HIV disease does not require treatment unless bleeding is present.[22]

Lungs

Pulmonary disease is a significant cause of morbidity and mortality in HIV-infected persons.[23] The symptoms and signs can vary from only minimal shortness of breath or nonproductive cough to severe respiratory distress. The physical examination usually reveals tachypnea. Rales and cough with purulent sputum are not usually present unless bacterial pneumonia or pulmonary tuberculosis is present. Evaluation is based on the findings of the chest radiograph and arterial blood gas measurements. X-ray findings of PCP and other pulmonary processes in AIDS typically show diffuse interstitial infiltrates or alveolar infiltrates. Thoracic and mediastinal lymphadenopathy and pleural effusions, when present, may indicate fungal disease, *Mycobacterium tuberculosis* infection, lymphoma, or pulmonary KS. Pleural effusions do not occur with PCP alone. The chest film is normal in 10% of patients with PCP. A negative high-resolution computed tomography (CT) scan of the chest in these patients can rule out PCP but a positive study is not specific for PCP. Arterial blood gas measurements usually show substantial hypoxemia with hypocarbia. Lactic dehydrogenase levels are frequently elevated in patients with AIDS pulmonary disease but do not provide sufficient information on which to base differential diagnostic decisions. Abnormalities of chest radiographs or arterial blood gases require further diagnostic investigation to establish the pathologic diagnosis.

PCP is one of the most common pulmonary disease in immunocompromised patients with HIV. Examination of pulmonary specimens for *P. carinii* requires sputum induction or bronchoscopy; patients with PCP do not spontaneously expectorate sputum containing *P. carinii* organisms. *P. carinii* cysts can be detected for at least 3 weeks after initiation of therapy. Therefore, patients seriously ill with presumptive PCP should be treated empirically, with diagnostic procedures performed later.

First-line treatment of PCP is with intravenous or oral TMP-SMX. The duration of PCP therapy is 3 weeks. TMP-SMX has the added advantage of treating possible concurrent bacterial pneumonia. Patients with PaO$_2$ less than 70 mm Hg should receive concurrent corticosteroids.[24] Patients with moderate to severe PCP are usually hospitalized to provide monitoring and ensure proper medication administration. Marked clinical worsening after 1 week or failure to respond after 2 weeks of therapy is a reasonable indication for changing to an alternative agent. Patients with mild PCP who have adequate home support services can be treated as outpatients with oral medications. Oral treatment of PCP is with TMP-SMX or with dapsone plus trimethoprim. PCP recurrences can be treated with the same agent that was successful on previous episodes.

Other pulmonary pathogenic processes to be considered include pneumonia (most commonly caused by *Haemophilus influenzae*, *Streptococcus pneumoniae*, *Legionella pneumophila*, and *Mycoplasma pneumoniae*), tuberculosis, MAC, and KS.

Gastrointestinal Tract

Esophagitis with dysphagia, odynophagia, and retrosternal pain can be caused by *Candida albicans*, CMV, or herpes simplex virus. Candidal esophagitis, which is an AIDS-defining disease, is most common. In patients with coexisting oral candidiasis, systemic treatment with fluconazole or ketoconazole should be initiated as an empiric trial. If the patient does not have oral candidiasis or a previous case diagnosis of AIDS, esophagoscopy with biopsies and cultures is advised to establish the diagnosis and direct therapy. Treatment of CMV esophagitis with ganciclovir or foscarnet and of herpes esophagitis with acyclovir is usually effective.

Chronic diarrhea with weight loss can occur in immunocompromised patients. Bacterial cultures and parasite determination should be performed to identify treatable causes such as *Shigella*, *Salmonella*, and *Campylobacter* infections or *Cryptosporidium* or other parasitic infestations. *Clostridium difficile* titers should be determined.

Perianal disease, most commonly caused by herpes simplex virus infections, requires prolonged therapy with oral acyclovir. Extensive perianal disease requires intravenous therapy.

Liver disease can be the result of drug toxicity, hepatitis, or other infections and malignancies. Patients with laboratory findings suggesting a predominantly obstructive pattern (elevated alkaline phosphatase) should undergo ultrasound examination to rule out hepatic masses or biliary tract obstruction. An AIDS-associated cholangiopathy with strictures and papillary stenosis can be identified by upper endoscopy with retrograde cholangiography. Sphincterotomy can effectively palliate symptoms of a biliary tract obstruction. When the ultrasound examination is negative, MAC disease, tuberculosis, fungal diseases, or other infiltrative hepatic processes should be considered (see Chapter 90).

Gynecologic Problems

Women with HIV infection can have severe, persistent vaginal candidiasis (see Chapter 102). Prolonged or repeated antifungal treatment is often necessary. Cervical dysplasia and cancer are also more frequent and more aggressive than in women not infected with HIV. Papanicolaou smears should be examined every 6 months; dysplasia should be evaluated by colposcopy.[25]

Renal and Adrenal Disease

The most common renal problem is drug toxicity. Special attention is required when patients are taking TMP-SMX, NSAIDs, or other drugs known to cause nephrotoxicity. HIV-associated nephropathy with renal failure can occur, most commonly among patients who have been intravenous drug users, hypertensive patients, or those who have coexisting intrinsic renal disease. Adrenal insufficiency, characterized by hypotension and blunted stress response, can occur.

Neurologic Problems

Neurologic problems[26,27] occurring in immunocompromised patients include peripheral neuropathies, myelopathies, and central nervous system (CNS) disorders. The most common CNS disorders is the AIDS dementia complex and is usually a late manifestation of HIV disease. Dementia can present with cognitive impairment, motor disturbances, or behavioral dysfunction. The most typical presentation is confusion, forgetfulness, and lethargy. Predominant features can also include ataxia and clumsiness. Behavioral changes are dominated by apathy, listlessness, and withdrawal. The major cause of the AIDS–dementia complex is HIV infection of the brain. The diagnosis is one of exclusion of other treatable causes of CNS disease. Treatment with effective ARV regimens can improve dementia.

The differential diagnosis of CNS disorders includes cryptococcal meningitis, toxoplasmic encephalitis, CNS lymphoma, and progressive multifocal leukoencephalopathy. Cryptococcal meningitis can present with the AIDS–dementia complex, fever, photophobia, headache, or stiff neck. Serum and cerebrospinal fluid cryptococcal antigen tests are positive more than 90% of the time. Treatment with amphotericin B or fluconazole is usually effective.[28] Toxoplasmic encephalitis[29] can present as the AIDS–dementia complex but also can cause seizures and focal neurologic signs. Empiric treatment is usually given when suspicious lesions on CT or magnetic resonance imaging scans are noted. Failure to respond clinically or radiologically within 2 weeks can be an indication for a brain biopsy to rule out lymphoma and other CNS problems.

Lymphomas

Multisystem lymphomas, including non-Hodgkin's lymphoma,[30] can occur in the thoracic and abdominal lymph nodes, gastrointestinal tract, bone marrow, brain, and other organs. Systemic disease can be treated with combination chemotherapy and/or radiation therapy.

HIV Disease in Children

Infection with HIV can occur transplacentally, at the time of delivery, and with breast-feeding. Because treatment with ARV therapy can greatly reduce the rate of perinatal transmission, all pregnant women at risk for HIV infection should be offered counseling and testing. HIV-infected mothers should be counseled about the benefits of ARV therapy and offered treatment. They should be discouraged from breast-feeding when there are safe alternatives.

The diagnosis of HIV infection in infants is complicated by the presence of maternal antibodies for HIV until the age of 15 months. A definitive diagnosis can usually be made earlier with viral assays. HIV DNA PCR is the preferred assay for detecting infection. Infants born to HIV-positive mothers should be tested within 48 hours of birth. A positive test should be confirmed with a repeat test as soon as possible. If the initial test is negative, follow-up testing should occur at 1 to 2 months and again at 3 to 6 months of age. Infants at risk for HIV infection should be given PCP prophylaxis with TMP-SMX at age 4 to 6 weeks until HIV infection has been ruled in or out.[31]

HIV-infected children should have CD4+ counts with CD4+ percentages and viral load testing every 3 months. Because children have higher CD4$^+$ counts than adults, percentage of CD4$^+$ cells is a better marker of immunosuppression than absolute CD4$^+$ counts. HIV-infected children should receive PCP prophylaxis for the first year of life regardless of CD4$^+$ count, with subsequent prophylaxis based on immune status. HIV-positive children should receive routine diphtheria/pertussis/tetanus (DPT), *H. influenzae* type b (HiB), and inactivated (intramuscular) poliovirus vaccine at standard intervals. Mumps/measles/rubella (MMR) vaccination should be given on schedule unless the child is profoundly immunocompromised. Oral poliovirus vaccine should not be given to HIV-infected children or to household members living with immunocompromised persons. Influenza and pneumococcal vaccines are recommended for children with symptomatic HIV infection.

In children, immunosuppression from AIDS usually presents with constitutional symptoms (e.g., fever and failure to thrive), oral candidiasis, lymphadenopathy, hepato-splenomegaly, and persistent or recurrent bacterial infections. Viral infections can also be severe and persistent. Pulmonary manifestations include PCP and lymphocytic interstitial pneumonitis. Gastrointestinal complications include diarrhea and candidal esophagitis. Neurologic and developmental problems also occur and must be evaluated thoroughly.

ARV therapy in children has been shown to slow disease progression and lower mortality. Therapy should be considered in HIV-infected children with evidence of immunosuppression. As in adults, issues of adherence need to be addressed prior to starting therapy. Families with HIV-positive children need a family-centered approach from a multidisciplinary care team.

References

1. Goldschmidt RH, Dong BJ. Treatment of AIDS and HIV-related conditions: 2001. J Am Board Fam Pract 2001;14:283–309.
2. The Concerned Action on Seroconversion to AIDS and Death in Europe. Survival after introduction of HAART in people with known duration of HIV-1 infection. Lancet 2000;355:1158–9.
3. The World Health Organization. AIDS Epidemic Update: December 2000. Available at *www.who.int*.
4. Centers for Disease Control and Prevention. HIV/AIDS Surveillance Report, 2000. Available at *www.cdc.gov/hiv/stats/hasr1201.htm*.
5. Kleinman S, Busch MP, Korelitz JJ, Schreiber GB. The incidence/window period model and its use to assess the risk of transfusion-transmitted human immunodeficiency virus and hepatitis C virus infection. Transfusion Med Rev 1997;11(3):155–72.
6. Mandelbrot L, Landreau-Mascaro A, Rekacewicz C, et al. Lamivudine-zidovudine combination for prevention of maternal–infant transmission of HIV-1. JAMA 2001;285:2083–93.
7. Centers for Disease Control and Prevention. Updated Public Health Service guidelines for the management of health-care worker exposures to HIV and recommendations for postexposure prophylaxis. MMWR 2001;50:1–52.
8. Schacker T, Collier A, Hughes J, Shea T, Corey L. Clinical and epidemiologic features of primary HIV infection. Ann Intern Med 1996;125:257–64.
9. Goldschmidt RH, Legg JJ. Counseling patients about HIV test—results. J Am Board Fam Pract 1991;4:361–3.
10. Havlir DV, Barnes PF. Tuberculosis in patients with human immunodeficiency virus infection. N Engl J Med 1999;340:367–73.
11. Panel on Clinical Practices for Treatment of HIV Infection. Guidelines for the use of antiretroviral agents in HIV-infected adults and adolescents. 2001. Available at *www.hivatis.org*.
12. Chesney MA, Ickovics J, Hecht FM, Sidipa G, Rabkin J. Adherence: a necessity for successful HIV combination therapy. AIDS 1999;13(suppl A):S271–8.
13. Hirsch MS, Brun-Vezinet F, D'Aquila RT, et al. Antiretroviral drug resistance testing in adult HIV-1 infection. JAMA 2000;283:2417–26.
14. Carr A, Cooper DA. Adverse effects of antiretroviral therapy. Lancet 2000;356:1423–30.
15. Kovacs JA, Masur H. Prophylaxis against opportunistic infections in patients with human immunodeficiency virus infection. N Engl J Med 2000;342:1416–29.
16. Center for Disease Control and Prevention. 1999 USPHA/IDSA guidelines for the prevention of opportunistic infections in persons infected with human immunodeficiency virus. MMWR 1999;43(RR-10):1–67.
17. Grunfeld C, Feingold KR. Metabolic disturbances and wasting in the acquired immunodeficiency syndrome. N Engl J Med 1992;327:329–37.
18. Horsburgh CR Jr. *Mycobacterium avium* complex infection in the acquired immunodeficiency syndrome. N Engl J Med 1991;324:1332–8.
19. Nemechek PM, Polsky B, Gottlieg MS. Treatment guidelines for HIV-associated wasting. Mayo Clin Proc 2000;75(4):386–94.
20. Berger TG, Obuch ML, Goldschmidt RH. Dermatologic manifestations of HIV infection. Am Fam Physician 1990;41:1729–42.
21. Holland GN, Tufail A. New therapies for cytomegalovirus retinitis. N Engl J Med 1995;333:658–9.
22. Glatt AE, Anand A. Thrombocytopenia in patients infected with human immunodeficiency virus: treatment update. Clin Infect Dis 1995;21:415–23.
23. Miller R. HIV-associated respiratory disease. Lancet 1996;348:307–12.
24. Consensus statement on the use of corticosteroids as adjunctive therapy for *Pneumocystis carinii* pneumonia in the acquired immunodeficiency syndrome: the National Institutes of Health–University of California Expert Panel for Corticosteroids as Adjunctive Therapy for *Pneumocystis carinii* pneumonia. N Engl J Med 1990;323:1500–4.
25. Legg JJ. Women and HIV. J Am Board Fam Pract 1993;6:367–77.
26. Simpson DM, Taglati M. Neurologic manifestations of HIV infection. Ann Intern Med 1994;121:769–85.
27. Newton HB. Common neurologic complications of HIV-1 infection and AIDS. Am Fam Physician 1995;51:387–98.
28. Saag MS, Powderly WG, Cloud GA, et al. Comparison of amphotericin B with fluconazole in the treatment of acute AIDS-associated cryptococcal meningitis. N Engl J Med 1992;326:83–9.
29. Luft BJ, Hafner R, Korzun AH, et al. Toxoplasmic encephalitis in patients with the acquired immunodeficiency syndrome. N Engl J Med 1993;329:995–1000.
30. Little RF, Gutierrez M, Jaffe ES, Pau A, Horne M, Wilson W. HIV-associated non-Hodgkin lymphoma: incidence, presentation and prognosis. JAMA 2001;285:1880–5.
31. The Working Group on Antiretroviral Therapy and Medical Management of HIV-Infected Children. Guidelines for the use of antiretroviral agents in pediatric HIV infection. 2000. Available at *www.hivatis.org*.

43
Bacteremia and Sepsis

William J. Curry and Peter R. Lewis

Bacteremia indicates the presence of viable bacteria in the circulatory blood and is usually defined clinically as positive blood cultures.[1] A cascade of local and systemic regulatory mechanisms, both proinflammatory and antiinflammatory, exist to protect against endothelial damage caused by a variety of nonspecific insults including infection. The systemic inflammatory response syndrome (SIRS) denotes clinical response to endothelial damage including two or more of the following: (1) temperature higher than 38°C or lower than 36°C; (2) respiratory rate more than 20 breaths per minute, or a Pco_2 less than 32 mm Hg; (3) pulse higher than 90 beats per minute; or (4) white blood cell count more than $12.0 \times 10^9/L$ or less than $4.0 \times 10^9/L$, or more than 10% immature neutrophils. When the clinical insult is a documented infection, sepsis is present. If counterregulatory mechanisms fail, endothelial damage progresses, leading to severe sepsis (previously the sepsis syndrome), which includes hypotension and hypoperfusion manifested by lactic acidosis, oliguria, or altered mental status. Finally, septic shock occurs when hypotension and hypoperfusion abnormalities persist despite adequate fluid resuscitation.[2,3]

Epidemiology

Despite advances in antimicrobial therapy and circulatory support, sepsis is the 12th leading cause of death in the United States.[4] It is estimated that 400,000 to 700,000 cases of sepsis occur annually; mortality can approach 40% in uncomplicated sepsis, and 80% in severe sepsis and septic shock.[5,6]

The increasing age of the United States population, increased utilization of invasive medical devices, and survival rate improvements in individuals at risk for sepsis (elderly, neonates, and patients with comorbidities such as diabetes mellitus, cancer, or human immunodeficiency virus infection) will cause an increase in sepsis incidence. Increasing antibiotic resistance and increased nosocomial infection rates will also increase sepsis incidence.[7,8]

Gram-negative organisms cause 50% to 60% of sepsis in the intensive care unit. Gram-positive organisms account for 35% to 40% of cases, with fungi, viruses, and protozoa implicated in the remaining cases. As many as 20% of sepsis cases have negative blood cultures. Sites of infection most commonly implicated include genitourinary, gastrointestinal, and respiratory tracts, and the skin.

Genetic factors have been identified that increase susceptibility to and mortality of septic shock. A specific allele within the tumor necrosis factor-α (TNF-α) gene promoter causes enhanced production of TNF-α. Increased levels of this proinflammatory cytokine lead to physiologic and metabolic manifestations of septic shock.[9] Genetic factors affecting host response to infections have not been clearly understood to date, and certainly not controlled for in studies of sepsis and specific treatments.

Pathophysiology

The pathophysiology of sepsis is complex,[7] involving interaction with microbial signals, humoral mediators, mononuclear and polymorphonuclear leukocytes, platelets, lymphocytes, and vascular endothelium. With gram-negative infections, the microbial signal is endotoxin, which prompts a release of proinflammatory mediators that include cytokines such as interleukin-1 (IL-1), IL-6, IL-8, TNF-α, platelet activating factor, and prostaglandins. These mediators eliminate damaged tissues, promote growth of new tissue, and fight pathogens, foreign antigens, and neoplastic cells.[10] As clinical trials that attempted to block the proinflammatory effects of the mediators have been unsuccessful, it has been recognized that antiinflammatory mediators play a critical role in the sepsis cascade as well.[11] To maintain balance after proinflammatory mediators are released, antiinflammatory mediators such as IL-4, IL-10, IL-11, soluble tumor necrosis factor receptors, and transforming growth factor are released. Antiinflammatory effects include alteration in monocyte function, decreased antigen presenting activity, and reduced production of proinflammatory cytokines.[12] When balanced, the human host displays no or mild evidence of systemic signs or symptoms. When a mismatch occurs between proinflammatory and antiinflammatory mechanisms, or in the setting of an excessive infectious insult, sepsis develops.

Sepsis in Adults

Clinical Features

The systemic signs of sepsis include fever, hypothermia, tachycardia, or tachypnea. Oliguria or altered mental status indicates progression to severe sepsis, and persistent hypotension indicates septic shock. Although these signs may occur abruptly, they may also present subtly, particularly in the elderly (see Chapter 24).

Early clues to the diagnosis of sepsis include tachypnea and in older patients disorientation or confusion. Cutaneous manifestations of sepsis may also be helpful in diagnosis. Peripheral cyanosis is a common finding caused by hypoperfusion. A petechial rash may indicate infection with *Neisseria meningitidis* or *Haemophilus influenzae*, or may be associated with a tick-borne illness such as Rocky Mountain spotted fever, Lyme disease, or ehrlichiosis. Erythroderma is seen with toxic shock syndrome caused by *Staphylococcus aureus* or *Streptococcus pyogenes*.

Laboratory findings include respiratory alkalosis secondary to tachypnea followed by lactic acidosis and hypoxemia as sepsis worsens. Positive blood cultures confirm the presence of bacteremia. Leukocytosis with left shift is frequently seen, but neutropenia and thrombocytopenia secondary to increased endothelial adherence and immunologic mechanisms imply a poor prognosis. Hyperglycemia (due to increased gluconeogenesis) is common. In diabetic patients, severe infection may precipitate diabetic ketoacidosis (see Chapter 120). Liver dysfunction due to endothelial damage and hypoperfusion may cause hyperbilirubinemia, transaminasemia, and alkaline phosphatase elevation.[13]

Diagnostic Evaluation

A thorough history and physical examination are the mainstays of diagnosis. Appropriate testing must be individualized, but generally includes a complete blood count, blood chemistry profile, coagulation studies, arterial blood gases, urinalysis and culture, blood cultures, electrocardiogram, and chest radiography. In the septic-appearing patient, an aggressive search for an infectious source is important to guide therapy.

Treatment

Cardiovascular Support

Sepsis and septic shock must be managed aggressively. Patients frequently require care in an intensive care unit. Consultation with intensivists and infectious disease specialists should be considered. Support of the cardiovascular system is of primary initial concern. Volume infusion to restore blood pressure, capillary refill, mental function, and urine output to a minimum of 0.5 mL/kg/h is mandatory. Neither colloids nor crystalloids have been proven superior to the other as a volume expander during septic shock. Adequate oxygen delivery is ensured by providing inspired supplemental oxygen or mechanical ventilation. The benefit of blood transfusion to improve oxygen delivery should be balanced against the inherent risks. Factors such as cardiopulmonary disease, hematocrit, and age should be considered.

Dopamine may be used at low doses (2–5 μg/kg/min) to improve renal perfusion or at a midrange (5–10 μg/kg/min) or higher (10–20 μg/kg/min) rate for inotropic, chronotropic, and vasopressor effects. Pressors may improve or reverse shock but have not been shown to improve overall survival.[14] Invasive monitoring (e.g., Swan-Ganz catheters and intraarterial blood pressures) should be considered for all patients with hypotension, low systemic vascular resistance, and high cardiac output due to septic shock. A mean capillary wedge pressure of 12 to 18 mm Hg is desirable.

Antibiotic Selection

After appropriate culture specimens have been obtained, treatment with empiric broad-spectrum antibiotics to cover suspected pathogens should be started. Antibiotic therapy is not absolutely curative because it cannot prevent damage by previously released endotoxin, TNF-α, and the other mediators.[13] Local antibiotic susceptibility patterns must be considered, and knowledge of previous adverse reactions to antimicrobials is necessary. Table 43.1 lists common site-specific bacterial etiologies of sepsis and suggestions for empiric therapy.[15] Appropriate broad-spectrum antibiotic selection is important. Studies of antibiotic usage have demonstrated inappropriate selection in 22% to 64% of cases.[14]

Antibiotics should be administered intravenously. Increased loading doses to account for an expanded volume of distribution in the septic patient may be required. Dosage adjustments must be made in response to antibiotic levels, renal and hepatic function, cultures and sensitivities of offending organisms, and clinical response. Agents that cross the blood–brain barrier are necessary at high doses to treat meningitis and other central nervous system (CNS) infections. Multiply resistant organisms such as methicillin resistant *S. aureus* or *Pseudomonas* require therapy with more than one antibiotic. A minimum of 10 to 14 days of appropriate coverage is recommended, although depending on clinical response, continuation of therapy may not require hospitalization for the entire treatment period. The use of a quality standard in the form of a therapeutic pathway or algorithm for the treatment of sepsis and bacteremia can lead to improved treatment and decreased mortality.[14]

Adjunctive Therapy

Attempts to modify cytokine (mediator) release and action have had limited success to date. No new agent has been brought to market, indicative of difficulties in developing treatments for a heterogeneous patient population. In gram-negative sepsis, the use of steroids or naloxone has not shown

Table 43.1. **Common Etiologic Agents and Empiric Therapy for Patients with Bacteremia/Sepsis**

Source	Organisms	Empiric therapy
Pneumonia		
Community acquired	*Streptococcus pneumoniae* *Haemophilus influenzae* *Klebsiella pneumoniae* *Legionella*	Cefuroxime ± macrolide
Nosocomial	*Pseudomonas aeruginosa* *Staphylococcus aureus* *K. pneumoniae* *Enterobacter*	Aminoglycoside + ceftazidime *or* Vancomycin + antipseudomonal penicillin
Urinary tract infection	*Escherichia coli* *P. aeruginosa* *Klebsiella* *Proteus* *Serratia*	Ceftriaxone *or* Ampicillin + gentamicin *or* Quinolones
Intraabdominal infection	*Bacteroides* *Enterococcus* *E. coli* *Klebsiella* *Enterobacter*	Clindamycin + aminoglycoside *or* Clindamycin + aztreonam *or* Imipenem
Pelvic infection	*Bacteroides* *E. coli* *Neisseria gonorrhoeae* *Enterobacter* *Klebsiella* *Chlamydia*	Clindamycin + gentamicin *or* Cefoxitin
CNS infection	*S. pneumoniae*, community acquired Gram-negative bacilli, nosocomial *Neisseria meningitidis* *Listeria*	Cefotaxime *or* Ceftriaxone *or* Vancomycin + ceftriaxone

consistent clinical benefit. Initial studies of the use of antibodies to endotoxin have demonstrated a small benefit in some patient subgroup populations. Because these agents are expensive, the widespread addition of monoclonal antibody therapy for sepsis would significantly increase health care costs with marginal overall clinical benefit.[12]

Studies are ongoing for other agents.[16] Soluble TNF receptor (a naturally occurring antagonist to TNF-α) is being considered as an adjunct to therapy after initial protection was demonstrated in experimental models.[13] Interleukin-1 receptor antagonist (IL-1ra) improves outcome in patients with septic shock. Clinical trials of cyclooxygenase and nitrous oxide inhibitors, granulocyte colony-stimulating factor, recombinant human activated protein C, nuclear factor κB, and extracorporeal adsorbents are under way.[17–19]

Sepsis in Infants and Children

Bacteremia and sepsis represent significant causes of morbidity and mortality among newborns and young children. However, the rates in industrialized nations are declining in large measure due to improvements in neonatal care, including intrapartum chemoprophylaxis against group B streptococcus (GBS), and higher immunization rates against *H. influenzae* type B (HiB), and *Streptococcus pneumoniae*. Bacteremia is more likely to be occult in infants and children, compared with adults. Infants and children who are bacteremic may be clinically well, and suitable for management as outpatients, or clinically ill or even septic upon their presentation, and require hospitalization for definitive evaluation and treatment. Risk factors for bacteremia and its complications (pneumonia, septic arthritis, osteomyelitis, meningitis, sepsis, and death) among newborns and young children include prematurity, prolonged hospitalization and intensive level of care, immunosuppression, and lack of immunization.

Epidemiology

Newborn sepsis occurs in 1 to 10/1000 live births[20]; attack rates are higher in premature and very low birth weight infants. Newborn deaths in the United States due to sepsis declined by 25% between 1979 and 1994; nearly half of the deaths occurred in those born prematurely.[21] Among term newborns, GBS is the number one cause of sepsis and death, followed by *Escherichia coli* (Table 43.2).[22]

Bacterial sepsis in premature neonates requiring prolonged hospitalization may be due to nosocomial pathogens such as coagulase-negative *Staphylococcus* and *Pseudomonas*. Another class of infectious agent producing sepsis in the critically ill premature infant is yeast and fungi, in particular *Candida* species. For both premature and term newborns the case fatality rate is higher for sepsis caused by gram-negative pathogens.

In general, the rates of bacteremia and the risk of serious sequelae, including death, due to bacteremia decline following the newborn period. GBS remains the most common cause of bacteremia and sepsis through the first month of life in term neonates. From 3 months of age onward, the most common cause of bacteremia, meningitis, and death in children is *S. pneumoniae*; peak attack rates occur between 6 and 24 months of age. In the era of universal vaccination against HiB, upward of 80% of episodes of bacteremia in this age group is due to *S. pneumoniae*.[23] Chief among the remaining isolates are *Neisseria meningitidis* and *Salmonella* spp. Although much less common than pneumococcal bacteremia, morbidity and mortality is much higher for meningococcal bacteremia.

Clinical and Diagnostic Features

Newborns, and young children with bacteremia may present with very nonspecific symptoms (e.g., poor feeding or irritability) and/or signs (e.g., fever), and an absence of localizing features. In general, the more premature the neonate, or younger the child, the greater the potential for devastating consequences from unrecognized bacteremia.

Risk factor appraisal begins during pregnancy, labor, and delivery. Premature rupture of membranes, premature delivery, maternal GBS colonization or chorioamnionitis at delivery, and prolonged rupture of membranes greater than 18 hours in term pregnancy increase the risk for bacteremia and sepsis. Other risk factors during the newborn and early childhood period include congenital anomalies (e.g., genitourinary), the postoperative state, known exposure to a subject with bacterial invasive disease, crowding such as may occur in day-care centers, and African-American race. Nearly half of neonates with early-onset (less than 7 days of age) GBS sepsis have no risk factors other than maternal GBS colonization.[22]

Physical examination commences with detailed observation of appearance and behavior. Even systematic infant observation scales have limited sensitivity in detecting serious bacterial infection[24] and should therefore guide, not determine, patient management. Vital sign abnormalities may represent the only clinical clues to the presence of bacteremia or sepsis. Such newborns and young children may be tachypneic, tachycardic, and/or febrile; hypotension, despite adequate fluid resuscitation, is an ominous sign and may be indicative of septic shock. Pediatric fever assessment warrants special comment. Whereas hypothermia or temperature instability may be an indicator of bacteremia or sepsis in the neonate, most infants and young children presenting with serious bacterial infection will have elevated temperature. Temperature thresholds for increasing the clinician's suspicion for bacteremia include 38°C (100.4°F) in infants younger than 3 months of age, and 39°C (102.2°F) in those 3 months of age or older.

Clinicians should be guided by their observations and vital signs during the child's examination and diligently search for localizing features such as rales, a warm and erythematous joint, or petechial rash. It should be noted that a nonfocal physical examination does not exclude the possibility of a serious bacterial infection. In one study, 26% of young children presenting with fever, white blood cell (WBC) count ≥20,000/mm³, and an absence of respiratory findings on initial physical examination had radiographic evidence of pneumonia,[25] a certain percentage of which were complicated by bacteremia and/or sepsis.

Following the history and physical examination, the clinician must determine the scope of testing utilized to assist di-

Table 43.2. **Common Pathogens and Antibiotic Regimens in Children with Bacteremia and Sepsis**

Age group or population	Pathogens	Antibiotic regimen(s)
Newborn		
Term	GBS, *E. coli* (and other gram-neg. enterics), *Listeria*, *S. aureus*	Ampicillin plus cefotaxime or aminoglycoside or ceftriaxone
Preterm	As for term newborns, plus nosocomial	As above and below
Postnatal to 3 months	As above for term neonate	As above for term neonate
Three months to 3 years	*S. pneumonia*, *S. aureus*, GABHS, *Salmonella* sp., *N. meningitides*, HiB (unvaccinated)	Semisynthetic antistaphylococcal penicillin plus cefotaxime or ceftriaxone
Immunocompromised	As for immunocompetent plus nosocomial	Extended-spectrum penicillin plus aminoglycoside
Nosocomial	Coagulase-negative staphylococcus, *S. aureus*, enterococcus, *Enterobacter* sp., *Pseudomonas*, *Candida* sp.	Nafcillin plus ceftazidime or cefotaxime Extended-spectrum penicillin plus aminoglycoside Vancomycin for methicillin–resistant *S. aureus* Amphotericin B for *Candida* sp.
Septic shock	*N. meningitidis*, GBS, *E. coli* (and other gram-neg. enterics), *Pseudomonas*, *S. pneumoniae*, *S. aureus*	As above for nosocomial, vancomycin if catheter related

GBS = group B streptococcus; *S. aureus* = *Staphylococcus aureus*; GABHS = group A β-hemolytic streptococcus; HiB = *Haemophilus influenzae* type b; *E. coli* = *Escherichia coli*; *S. pneumonia* = *Streptococcus pneumoniae*; *N. meningitidis* = *Neisseria meningitidis*.

agnosis and management. Selecting appropriate laboratory and radiology testing is more straightforward for the ill or frankly septic-appearing newborn or young child. Greater practice variation and debate exist concerning the necessary diagnostic testing of the well-appearing child older than 1 month of age presenting with fever alone.

An elevated WBC count, although having a low positive predictive value for serious bacterial infection, may be indicative of bacteremia. Neutropenia may be a marker of sepsis, particularly in the premature neonate. Whereas some protocols for the evaluation of well-appearing children older than 3 months of age presenting with fever base the decision to collect a blood culture on the WBC count, a culture should routinely be obtained in the neonate or infant younger than 1 month of age presenting with fever. Lumbar puncture for cerebrospinal fluid (CSF) analysis and culture is routinely performed in neonates and young infants suspected of having bacteremia and sepsis; it is less commonly required in older ($\geq$3 months of age), well-appearing, immunocompetent infants presenting with fever alone. Urinalysis with culture and chest x-ray are less likely to be a part of the septic workup in the immediate newborn period, whereas urinalysis, in particular, may assist in the evaluation of the young child presenting with fever.

Stool WBC measurement and culture may be indicated when diarrhea is present. Gram stain and culture of other potentially infected body fluid (e.g., joint synovial fluid) that may represent a source for or metastatic focus of bacteremia will be guided by the history and clinical examination. Blood chemistries, coagulation studies, and blood gas measurements may be required in the ill or septic-appearing patient. Hypoglycemia and hyperbilirubinemia may herald bacteremia and sepsis in the newborn.

Management

Even with the addition of selected diagnostic testing to a thorough risk factor assessment, history, and physical examination, serious bacterial infection may remain occult upon initial examination. For example, 3% to 6% of cases of occult pneumococcal bacteremia are complicated by meningitis, resulting in death 8% to 15% of the time.[26] This emphasizes the importance of serial reassessment as the cardinal feature of patient management. Reevaluation of the infant older than 1 month of age presenting with fever alone as a potential marker of bacteremia may safely occur in the outpatient setting, if follow-up and means of communication of blood culture results are deemed reliable. For the newborn or infant younger than 1 month of age, reassessment should occur in the inpatient setting. Careful inpatient observation of term neonates born to mothers receiving intrapartum antibiotic prophylaxis against GBS is warranted through the first 48 hours of life; 90% of cases of GBS sepsis display signs and symptoms within the first 12 hours of life.

For obviously ill-appearing neonates and young children, prompt attention to supportive care (airway management, fluid resuscitation, and nutritional support) is warranted. Empiric intravenous antibiotics should be selected based on likely pathogens and known susceptibility patterns (Table 43.2). Of increasing concern is the rise of pneumococcal strains resistant to penicillin and ceftriaxone, and *E. coli* resistance to ampicillin. Systemic antifungal therapy is required if fungal sepsis is documented or suspected. If indwelling central venous or umbilical catheters are identified as a source of infection, they should be removed, and, as necessary, replaced. In rare cases, such as necrotizing fasciitis due to group A β-hemolytic *streptococcus*, surgical debridement or abscess incision and drainage becomes a necessary component of sepsis management.

Optimal management of the well-appearing infant or young child with suspected or documented bacteremia is uncertain.[26,27] At the time of initial evaluation in the outpatient or emergency department setting, some practice guidelines advocate the use of empiric oral (typically amoxicillin) or parenteral (typically ceftriaxone) antibiotic therapy. It is unclear, in the era of the vastly predominant pneumococcal bacteremia, that empiric antibiotic therapy decreases the incidence of complications, and, if it does, whether parenteral therapy is superior to oral therapy.[28,29]

For the child being managed as an outpatient who proves to have documented bacteremia, prompt reevaluation is essential. Added or repeat diagnostic testing may be indicated. Ill-appearing patients, and those with more virulent pathogens (e.g., *Neisseria*), should be hospitalized and receive appropriate parenteral antibiotics and supportive care. The majority of patients will have pneumococcal bacteremia, be well appearing on follow-up, and be suitable for outpatient antibiotic therapy if compliance and follow-up are assured.[29]

Bacteremia in Special Populations

Immune suppression increases the risk of bacteremia and sepsis for pediatric and adult patients alike. Immunosuppression may be a function of age as demonstrated by the increased incidence of bacteremia and its complications in premature neonates and geriatric adults. Pediatric and adult immunosuppressed populations include patients receiving chronic steroids, cancer patients receiving chemotherapy when neutropenic, solid-organ transplant recipients on chronic immunosuppressive therapy, HIV-infected patients with low CD4 counts, and sickle cell and other asplenic individuals. These subpopulations of patients experience more frequent hospitalizations and invasive testing, treatment, and monitoring. Therefore, they are at heightened risk for colonization and infection with nosocomial and multiple drug-resistant pathogens. Patients with central-venous catheters are at increased risk for bacteremia and sepsis due to coagulase-negative staphylococci, *S. aureus*, and *Candida* sp. Neutropenic children and adults have increased susceptibility to gram-negative organisms such as *Pseudomonas* and gram-positive organisms such as *S. aureus* and *Streptococcus viridans*.

While these patients may experience bacteremia with uncommon pathogens and nonbacterial sepsis particularly when hospitalized, in the outpatient setting they are still more likely to experience bacteremia and sepsis due to common pathogens such as *S. pneumoniae*. Asplenic patients (functional or surgical) are at increased risk for serious bacterial infection with *S. pneumoniae* and other encapsulated organisms such as HIB and *Neisseria*.

Prevention

Primary prevention of bacteremia and sepsis in children and adults begins with reducing the incidence of disease states that carry an increased risk of bacteremia and sepsis such as cancer, AIDS, and neonatal prematurity. Added methods of prevention include optimal nutrition (e.g., breast-feeding in infancy and enteral feedings in intensive care unit patients), limitation of invasive testing and treatment, avoidance of inappropriate hospitalization, attention to hand washing and antiseptic techniques, judicious use of antibiotics, chemoprophylaxis, immune-modulation, and immunization.

Examples of effective chemoprophylaxis shown to decrease bacteremia and sepsis include intrapartum antibiotics for GBS and penicillin for children with sickle cell disease (SCD). It should be noted that some authorities believe that intrapartum antibiotics for GBS may increase the rate of neonatal gram-negative sepsis, and the future role of penicillin for children with SCD in the dawning era of effective pediatric pneumococcal vaccination (see below) remains uncertain. Routine antibiotic prophylaxis in the afebrile neutropenic patient is not advised.

Immune-modulating agents such as granulocyte colony-stimulating factor (G-CSF) are being evaluated as prophylactic agents in the prevention of bacteremia and sepsis within special populations such as very low birth weight premature neonates and cancer patients with neutropenia.

Vaccination remains one of the most effective available resources to prevent bacteremia and sepsis in children and adults as witnessed by the plummeting rate of invasive HiB disease in children. Preliminary data regarding the newly licensed pneumococcal seven-valent conjugate vaccine for universal childhood immunization indicate that it provides protection against more than 80% of the strains responsible for invasive disease in children younger than age 5, including, importantly, drug-resistant ones. It is hoped that universal pneumococcal childhood vaccination will make invasive pneumococcal disease vaccine-preventable. Finally, whereas young children and older adults are appropriately targeted for receipt of pneumococcal conjugate and polysaccharide vaccines, respectively, it should be noted that patients between the ages of 2 and 64 years may well have an indication for pneumococcal vaccination that should not be overlooked.[30]

Family Issues

Illness in one member of a family has the potential to change the structure and function of the family unit (see Chapter 4). Additional family members, particularly the very young and old, may become afflicted with the same serious bacterial illness (e.g., meningitis). Unexpected severe illness may overwhelm the capacity of the family to adapt, especially when infants and children are affected and die. Regular physician contact and communication with the patient and family members regarding the patient's illness, treatment, and prognosis represent an essential component of effective patient care.

References

1. Bone RC. Sepsis, the sepsis syndrome, multi-organ failure: a plea for comparable definitions. Ann Intern Med 1991;114:332–3.
2. Rangel-Frausto MS, Pittet D, Costigan M, Hwang T, Davis CS, Wenzel RP. The natural history of the systemic inflammatory response syndrome (SIRS). JAMA 1995;273:117–23.
3. American College of Chest Physicians–Society of Critical Care Medicine Consensus Conference. Definitions for sepsis and organ failure and guidelines for the use of innovative therapies in sepsis. Crit Care Med 1992;20:864–75.
4. National Vital Statistics Report 2000;48(11):63–65.
5. Linde-Zwirble WT, Angus DC, Carcillo J, Lidicker J, Clermont G, Pinsky MR. Age-specific incidence and outcome of sepsis in the US. Crit Care Med 1999;27(suppl 1):A33.
6. Patterson RL, Webster NR. Sepsis and the systemic inflammatory response syndrome. J R Coll Surg Edinb 2000;45:178–82.
7. Opal SM, Cohen J. Clinical gram-positive sepsis: does it fundamentally differ from gram-negative sepsis? Crit Care Med 1999;27:1608–16.
8. Bone RC. The pathogens of sepsis. Ann Intern Med 1991;115:457–69.
9. Miro JP, Carion A, Grall R. Association of TNF2, a TNF-x promoter polymorphism with septic shock susceptibility and mortality: a multicenter study. JAMA 1999;282:561–8.
10. Dinarello CA, Gelfand JA, Wolff SM. Anticytokine strategies in the treatment of the systemic inflammatory response syndrome. JAMA 1993;269:1829–35.
11. Bone RC. Immunologic dissonance: a continuing evolution in our understanding of the systemic inflammatory response syndrome (SIRS) and the multiple organ dysfunction syndrome (MODS). Ann Intern Med 1996;125(8):680–7.
12. Munoz C, Carlett J, Ritting C. Dysregulation of in vitro cytokine production by monocytes during sepsis. J Clin Invest 1991;88:1747–54.
13. Rachow EC, Astiz ME. Pathophysiology and treatment of septic shock. JAMA 1991;226:548–59.
14. Gross PA, Barrett TL, Dellinger EP, et al. Quality standard for the treatment of bacteremia. Clin Infect Dis 1994;18:428–30.
15. The choice of antibacterial drugs. Med Let 1999;41:95–104.
16. Barriere SL, Ognibene FP, Summer WR, Young LS. Septic shock: beyond antibiotics. Patient Care 1991;25:95–109.
17. Bernard GR, Vincent JL, Laterre PF, et al. Efficacy and safety of recombinant human activated protein c for severe sepsis. N Engl J Med 2001;344(10):699–709.
18. Christman JW, Lancaster LH, Blackwell TS. Nuclear factor kappa B: a pivotal role in the systemic inflammatory response syndrome and new target for therapy. Intensive Care Med 1998;24:1131–8.
19. Jabur BL, Pereira BJG. Extracorporeal adsorbent-based strategies in sepsis. Am J Kidney Dis 1997;30(5):S44–S56.
20. Perez EM, Weisman LE. Novel approaches to the prevention and therapy of neonatal bacterial sepsis. Clin Perinatol 1997;24(1):213–29.
21. Stoll BJ, Holman RC, Schuchat A. Decline in sepsis-associated neonatal and infant deaths in the United States, 1979 through 1994. Pediatrics 1998 Aug [cited 2001 March 1];102(2). Available at *www.pediatrics.org/cgi/content/full/102/2/e18*.

22. Schuchat A, Zywicki SS, Dinsmoor MJ, et al. Risk factors and opportunities for prevention of early-onset neonatal sepsis: a multicenter case-control study. Pediatrics 2000;105(1):21–6.

23. Lee GM, Harper MB. Risk of bacteremia for febrile young children in the post-Haemophilus influenzae type b era. Arch Pediatr Adolesc Med 1998;152:624–8.

24. Baker MD, Avner JR, Bell LM. Failure of infant observation scales in detecting serious illness in febrile, 4- to 8-week-old infants. Pediatrics 1990;85(6):1040–3.

25. Bachur R, Perry H, Harper MB. Occult pneumonias: empiric chest radiographs in febrile children with leukocytosis. Ann Emerg Med 1999;33(2):166–73.

26. Kuppermann N. Occult bacteremia in young febrile children. Pediatr Clin North Am 1999;46(6):1073–109.

27. Kramer MS, Shapiro ED. Management of the young febrile child: a commentary on recent practice guidelines. Pediatrics 1997;100(1):128–34.

28. Rothrock SG, Green SM, Harper MB, Clark MC, McIlmail DP, Bachur R. Parental vs oral antibiotics in the prevention of serious bacterial infections in children with streptococcus pneumoniae occult bacteremia: a meta-analysis. Acad Emerg Med 1998;5(12):1230–1.

29. Bachur R, Harper MB. Reevaluation of outpatients with streptococcus pneumoniae bacteremia. Pediatrics 2000;105(3):502–9.

30. Robinson KA, Baughman W, Rothrock G, et al. Epidemiology of invasive streptococcus pneumoniae infections in the United States, 1995–1998. Opportunities for prevention in the conjugate vaccine era. JAMA 2001;285(13):1729–35.

44
Selected Infectious Diseases

Richard I. Haddy and Richard D. Clover

Infectious diseases that family physicians deal with less commonly but should be cognizant of include toxoplasmosis, trichinosis, psittacosis, giardiasis, Lyme disease, Rocky Mountain spotted fever, and illness caused by hantavirus. All of these diseases have the potential for causing severe morbidity and mortality in humans. In the case of Rocky Mountain spotted fever, early diagnosis and treatment may be lifesaving.

Toxoplasmosis

Family physicians are treating more cases of acquired immunodeficiency syndrome (AIDS) and are involved in the care of immunosuppressed cancer patients, and toxoplasmosis may affect these patients. For this reason and because of its continuing disease-causing role in children and infants, toxoplasmosis is a disease that is becoming more important to family physicians.

Etiology and Epidemiology

Toxoplasma gondii is an obligate intracellular protozoan parasite of the subphylum Apicomplexa, class Sporozoasida, and order Eucoccidiorida. The term *toxoplasmosis* describes the clinical disease caused by this parasite. Toxoplasma infection is generally asymptomatic in immunocompetent patients.

T. gondii is distributed worldwide; birds, cats, and other domesticated animals serve as reservoirs. The definitive hosts are cats. *T. gondii* has four life forms: the oocyst (spread in the feces of the cat), the tachyzoite (the invasive form), the tissue cyst, and the slower-growing, dormant form of *T. gondii*, the bradyzoite.[1] The presence of cats appears to be of primary importance in transmission of the infection to humans; 3% to 70%, depending on the geographic location and population group, of humans who reach adulthood in the United States will be infected with toxoplasma. The two major routes of transmission of toxoplasma to humans are oral and congenital. Transmission may also occur, however, by organ transplantation.

T. gondii may actively invade and infect virtually all cell types. The risk of toxoplasmic encephalitis in human immunodeficiency virus (HIV)-infected patients increases as the CD4+ count falls, and up to half of HIV-infected, toxoplasma-seropositive humans will develop toxoplasmic encephalitis.

Clinical Features

Clinically, toxoplasmosis is divided into four categories: (1) acquired disease in immunocompetent patients, (2) acquired or reactivated disease in immunodeficient patients, (3) ocular, and (4) congenital. The clinical manifestations are usually nonspecific and a large differential diagnosis must be considered.

Acute Acquired Toxoplasma Infection in the Immunocompetent Patient

In the immunocompetent patient the clinical course is mild and self-limited. Symptoms usually resolve within a few months. Only 10% to 20% of cases of toxoplasma infection in the adult are symptomatic. It may present simply as asymptomatic cervical lymphadenopathy. There may also be malaise, fever, myalgias, night sweats, sore throat, a maculopapular rash, and hepatosplenomegaly, and a few atypical lymphocytes may be present on blood count. Unilateral chorioretinitis may occur.

Acute Toxoplasmosis in the Immunodeficient Patient

Toxoplasmosis in immunocompromised patients may be due to either newly acquired or reactivated infection. Toxoplasmosis in AIDS patients commonly presents as toxoplasmic encephalitis. Toxoplasmic encephalitis is the most frequent of focal central nervous system lesions in AIDS. Hemiparesis and abnormalities of speech are the most common major initial signs. A wide range of other clinical findings such as weakness, altered mental state, cerebellar signs, sensory abnormalities, movement disorders, and meningismus are seen in toxoplasmic encephalitis. Psychiatric symptoms often seen are apparent psychosis, dementia, anxiety, and agitation. Magnetic resonance imaging (MRI) scanning with gadolinium contrast is the most sensitive radiologic procedure to demonstrate cerebral brain lesions.

Pulmonary disease with toxoplasmosis has been noted in patients with AIDS.

Ocular Toxoplasmosis in the Immunocompetent Patient

Typical symptoms of ocular toxoplasmosis are blurred vision, scotoma, photophobia, eye pain, and possibly epiphora. Symptoms may improve and then relapse.

Toxoplasma chorioretinitis results from congenital infection. However, patients are usually asymptomatic until their second or third decade of life. The characteristic lesion is a focal necrotizing retinitis.

Congenital Toxoplasmosis

Signs and symptoms of congenital toxoplasmosis are varied, nonspecific, and may present at various times after birth. Signs include pneumonitis, rash, anemia, jaundice, chorioretinitis, strabismus, blindness, seizures, psychomotor or mental retardation, hydrocephalus, diarrhea, hypothermia, and microcephaly.

Congenital toxoplasmosis is caused by acute infection, usually asymptomatic, acquired by the mother during pregnancy. Signs may occur in the newborn if the outcome of the pregnancy is not spontaneous abortion or stillbirth.

Laboratory Diagnosis

Isolation of the organism from the placenta is usually diagnostic of congenital toxoplasmosis. Demonstration of tachyzoites in smears of body fluid or in tissue sections establishes the diagnosis of acute toxoplasma infection. The diagnosis of toxoplasmosis, however, is usually made by serology.

Acute Acquired Toxoplasma Infection in the Immunocompetent Patient

A test for immunoglobulin G (IgG) [e.g., the Sabin-Feldman dye test, enzyme-linked immunosorbent assay (ELISA), immunoassay (IA), and the agglutination test] and immunoglobulin M (IgM) (e.g., IgM-ELISA or IgM-immunosorbent assay) are used for initial evaluation of these patients. Acute infection is supported by documented seroconversion of IgG or IgM antibodies or a greater than two-tube rise in antibody titer.

Toxoplasmosis in the Immunodeficient Patient

In an ill, immunocompromised patient, no single immunologic test will definitively diagnose toxoplasmosis. A definitive diagnosis will rest on histologic demonstration of tachyzoites or detection of specific T. gondii DNA by polymerase chain reaction in infected tissues.

Ocular Toxoplasmosis

Toxoplasma chorioretinitis may be diagnosed when the IgG antibody titer is positive and a characteristic retinal lesion is noted. High antibody titers in the aqueous humor may also be useful in the diagnosis of active disease.

Congenital Toxoplasmosis

The diagnosis of toxoplasmosis in the newborn is made by detecting IgA or IgM in serum obtained at the time of the birth. Detection of IgM antibody is made by the double-sandwich IgM ELISA test. Amniotic fluid assessment using polymerase chain reaction is now used for diagnosing fetal T. gondii infection in utero.[1]

Toxoplasma Infection in Pregnancy

Maternal serum is tested for specific IgG and IgM. If both are negative, this excludes current infection. If IgG is present and IgM is not, this would indicate chronic maternal infection and minimal risk of congenital infection.

Treatment

Acute Acquired Toxoplasma Infection in the Immunocompetent Patient

Immunocompetent adult patients are not treated unless gastrointestinal disease is obvious or symptoms are severe.

Acute Toxoplasmosis in the Immunodeficient Patient

Acutely ill, immunodeficient patients should be treated until 4 to 6 weeks after resolution of all signs and symptoms. Immunodeficient patients with chronic asymptomatic infection are not treated. Brain biopsy is recommended in toxoplasmic encephalitis patients who deteriorate during treatment by 7 days or who do not improve clinically by 10 days of empirical therapy. AIDS patients with toxoplasmosis are prescribed pyrimethamine (200 mg loading dose and 50 to 75 mg daily) combined with sulfadiazine (1 to 1.5 g po q6h) and folinic acid (10 to 20 mg daily). Clinical response is seen in 60% to 95% in patients with toxoplasmic encephalitis. Pyrimethamine combined with clindamycin (600 mg IV or po q6h) is of comparable efficacy. When the illness is in remission, pyrimethamine 25 mg per day plus sulfadiazine 500 mg po qid is used as a maintenance regimen. The main adverse affect of pyrimethamine is dose-related bone marrow suppression, the risk of which may be decreased by concomitant administration of folinic acid.

Prophylaxis against T. gondii is recommended in AIDS patients with a CD4[+] count below 100 per cubic mm.[2] Trimethoprim/sulfamethoxazole (which is also the drug of choice for prophylaxis against Pneumocystis carinii pneumonia) is commonly used, but pyrimethamine/dapsone, roxithromycin, and Fansidar are also effective.

Anticonvulsants are used in patients with toxoplasmic encephalitis who have had seizures.

Ocular Toxoplasmosis

Pyrimethamine, sulfadiazine, and folinic acid are administered orally for 1 month. A favorable clinical response can be expected within 10 days. Systemic corticosteroids are also used during the active phase of inflammation.

Acute Acquired Toxoplasmosis in Pregnant Women

Cases of acute maternal infection receive immediate treatment with spiramycin 1 g po tid until the fetus can be assessed for congenital infection. Clarithromycin (500 mg bid) and azithromycin (500 mg on day 1 followed by 250 mg daily) may be considered alternatives.[1,3] If fetal infection is established, therapy with pyrimethamine, sulfadiazine, and folinic acid should be started (if the pregnancy is past the first trimester) and alternated every 3 weeks with spiramycin until delivery.[1]

Congenital Infection

In the first year of life, continuous sulfadiazine (50 mg/kg bid), pyrimethamine (2 mg/kg/day for 2 days, then 1 mg/kg/day for 2 to 6 months, then 1 mg/kg/day three times a week), and folinic acid (from 5 mg three times weekly up to 20 mg/day) is administered for a minimum of 12 months.

Prevention

Cat feces should be completely avoided. Hands should be washed with soap after handling vegetables or raw meat, and eggs should not be eaten raw. Unpasteurized milk should be avoided. Cysts in meat are made noninfectious by heating to 66°C or smoking or curing it.

Pregnant women should avoid exposure to cat feces and should not eat raw eggs or raw meat.

Trichinosis

Trichinosis is often part of a large differential diagnosis in a patient with a nonspecific or undiagnosed infectious illness. It is for this reason—and because approximately 100 cases are still reported to the Centers for Disease Control and Prevention yearly—that family physicians should be cognizant of this disease.

Etiology and Epidemiology

Trichinella spiralis is the species of intestinal nematode that has been recognized for many years as the cause of trichinosis. However, a total of five species and three phenotypes that have the potential for causing disease have been described in this genus. *T. spiralis* has a worldwide distribution and has pigs and rats as its common host; *T. pseudospiralis* is common in birds and rats; *T. nelsoni* is common in hyenas in tropical Africa; *T. britovi* is seen in arctic foxes and wolves; *T. nativa* is seen in arctic bears and walruses; T5 is common in arctic bears; T6 is common in bears, wolverines, and pumas; and T8 is commonly seen in panthers and hyenas.

Most swine in the United States are fed grain and therefore are generally uninfected. However, the small proportion of swine fed garbage may become infected.

Viable larvae in inadequately cooked meats are ingested, passed into the small intestine, and attach to the mucosa at the bases of the intestinal villi. They then develop into adult worms that mate and produce more larvae, which seed the skeletal muscles via the blood stream.

Clinical Features

Most infections are subclinical. However, infection with a heavy load of larvae may lead to the typical features of diarrhea, periorbital edema, myositis, and fever. Diarrhea is the most common symptom, and the patient may complain of abdominal discomfort and vomiting. Some degree of fever may present in the second week after infection. The patient may complain of myalgias (often initially in the extraocular muscles), swollen muscles, and weakness. A maculopapular rash may be observed. Systemic symptoms begin to subside 2 to 3 weeks after infection, although fatigue and weakness may persist long after this. If history reveals the recent consumption of uncooked meat, especially pork, the likelihood of the diagnosis of trichinosis is further established. Occasionally a patient dies. This is usually from myocarditis but may also be from encephalitis or severe pneumonia.

The differential diagnosis in a patient with trichinosis is large and may include influenza, dermatomyositis, and viral gastroenteritis.

Laboratory Diagnosis

Eosinophilia is often found around the second week of illness and may reach very high levels. If muscles are involved to a large extent, serum creatine phosphokinase and lactic dehydrogenase may be elevated. Organism-specific antibodies are not detectable until 3 weeks or longer after infection. A bentonite flocculation antibody titer of 1:5 or more—or a fourfold rise in titer—may help establish the diagnosis of trichinosis. Specific antibodies may also be measured by immunofluorescence or ELISA. If the diagnosis is still in doubt, muscle biopsy may be obtained from a tender, swollen muscle.

Treatment

Unfortunately, most experts still feel that the treatment for trichinosis is unsatisfactory. For mild cases, the mainstays of treatment may be bed rest and salicylates. The main antihelmintic drugs used against trichinosis are mebendazole (200 to 400 mg po tid × 3 days, then 400 to 500 mg tid for 10 days) and thiabendazole (50 mg/kg/day in divided doses for 7 days), but most reports of success with these medications are anecdotal. Jarisch-Herxheimer–like reactions have been reported with these drugs in severe infestations due to massive release of antigenic substances.[4] Corticosteroids may be used in severely ill patients, but evidence of their efficacy is, again, anecdotal.

Prevention

The mainstay of prevention of trichinosis is the proper cooking of meats. Meats should be cooked until there is no trace of pink fluid or flesh. The thermal death point for trichinella larvae is 55°C. Exposure to freezing temperatures of −15°C or lower for 3 weeks also sterilizes meat in most instances.[4]

Psittacosis

Psittacosis is an uncommon infectious disease that usually manifests itself as pneumonia. However, it may cause significant morbidity and even death if not properly diagnosed and treated. It is most commonly acquired from birds.

Etiology and Epidemiology

Psittacosis is caused by the bacterium *Chlamydia psittaci*, which is one of the three species of the genus *Chlamydia*. The other two are *C. pneumoniae* and *C. trachomatis*, both of which cause disease in humans.

C. psittaci commonly infects birds and animals. Human infection, therefore, is most common in pet owners, pet shop employees, veterinarians, poultry farmers, and workers in slaughterhouses and processing plants. Cases in humans may occur individually or as outbreaks. Most commonly, however, patients with psittacosis have had some contact with birds, usually as a pet; 5% to 8% of birds carry *C. psittaci*. While infected birds may be obviously sick, about 10% become chronic asymptomatic carriers. The infection is usually spread by the respiratory route. Saliva, lacrimation, feces, and urine in affected birds all are infective. The disease has also been transmitted from infected cows, goats, sheep, cats, and other mammals.

Clinical Features

Psittacosis is a systemic infection that commonly presents as an atypical pneumonia. The incubation period is 5 to 15 days. Clinical manifestations may be very nonspecific, and several syndromes may result from the infection. Also, the infection may be entirely subclinical. The infection may present as a nonspecific viral illness with fever and malaise, or it may present as a mononucleosis-like syndrome with fever, pharyngitis, lymphadenopathy, and hepatosplenomegaly. Another form of presentation is with fever, bradycardia, malaise, and splenomegaly. Finally, the illness may present as an atypical pneumonia with fever, headache, and nonproductive cough. The chest x-ray often shows abnormalities out of proportion to that of physical findings.

The most common symptoms are fever and cough, though cough may appear late in the illness. The next most common symptoms are headache and myalgias.

The most frequent signs are fever, pharyngeal erythema, rales, and hepatomegaly. Splenomegaly may occur at the end of the first week of the illness.

Many end organs may be involved in psittacosis. As discussed previously, the most commonly involved organ in humans is the lung. There are several possible complications involving the heart, including myocarditis, pericarditis, and endocarditis. Rarely, embolism to major arteries is noted, though the exact mechanism for these emboli is unknown. Hepatitis may develop, occasionally with jaundice.

There are several neurologic sequelae that may develop, including meningitis.[5] Lumbar puncture may reveal a few white cells (usually, predominately lymphocytes) or be normal. Other neurologic consequences that may ensue include cerebellar signs, encephalitis, cranial nerve palsies, transverse myelitis, and seizures.

Various dermatologic signs may develop. The most characteristic of these is Horder's spots, a pink maculopapular rash. Other dermatologic phenomena include erythema nodosum, erythema multiforme, erythema marginatum, subungual splinter hemorrhages, and common urticaria.

Acute glomerulonephritis may develop, which may result in acute tubular necrosis. In severe cases, disseminated intravascular coagulation may occur.

Second infections have been documented to occur after the first. Helpful clues to the diagnosis of psittacosis are splenomegaly, bradycardia, rashes, and hemoptysis.

Laboratory Diagnosis

The leukocyte count is normal or slightly elevated and most patients have a left shift. Many patients have mildly elevated liver function tests.

The chest x-ray is abnormal in the majority of the patients and the most frequent finding is consolidation in a single lower lobe. However, virtually any x-ray abnormality of the lung fields may be found. Small asymptomatic pleural effusions are noted in up to half the cases.

C. psittaci may be cultured from the patient's sputum or blood, but this is dangerous because laboratory personnel have been infected by working with this organism. The diagnosis is best made by demonstrating high titers of complement-fixing antibodies in the serum. A case is considered confirmed if a clinical illness compatible with psittacosis is noted with a fourfold or greater change in complement-fixation titer to at least 1:32. The diagnosis is considered presumptive in a patient with a compatible illness and a complement-fixation titer of at least 1:32 in a single specimen.[6]

Treatment

Clinical response to treatment is often noted within 24 hours. The drug of choice is tetracycline 500 mg po qid or doxycycline 100 mg po bid for 10 to 21 days. Erythromycin is the alternate treatment of choice, but anecdotal experience suggests that it may be less efficacious than tetracycline. The mortality rate for treated patients is about 1% but rises to 20% in untreated patients. Patients with endocarditis generally require valve replacement.

Prevention

Prevention involves appropriate antibiotics for infected birds and antibiotic prophylaxis for imported birds. If possible, the source of infection (usually groups of birds) should be identified and quarantined.

Giardiasis

Giardia lamblia is a common worldwide cause of diarrhea. It is the most prevalent enteric parasite in the United States and Canada.

Etiology and Epidemiology

G. lamblia is a flagellated enteric protozoan and an aerotolerant anaerobe. The genus *Giardia* comes under the class Zoomastogiphorea, the order Diplomonadida, and the family Hexamitidae.

G. lamblia has two stages in its life cycle: the trophozoite (the active living stage) and the cyst. The trophozoite has a flat ventral service, which contains a sucking or adhesive disk. It also has two nuclei, giving it a face-like image, and four pairs of posterially directed flagellae for locomotion. *G. lamblia* cysts are thin-walled, smooth, and oval-shaped. Trophozoite division may occur as the cyst matures.

G. lamblia are acquired orally in one of three different ways: (1) ingestion of contaminated water, (2) person to person, and (3) food-borne transmission. Waterborne outbreaks occur when untreated surface water is used. Outbreaks have also occurred when water is used that has been treated by faulty purification systems or by inadequate chlorination and without flocculation, sedimentation, and filtration. The second most common mode of transmission is person to person. This commonly occurs in groups with poor oral-fecal hygiene, such as children in day-care centers, institutionalized persons, and sexually active homosexual males. Food-borne transmission has been indicated by *Giardia* outbreaks from restaurant food and in corporate office settings.

Infection with *G. lamblia* has been documented in many mammalian species.

Infection occurs after oral ingestion of cysts, which are excysted following exposure to gastric acid and pancreatic enzymes. The trophozoites then colonize and multiply in the upper small bowel. *Giardia* attaches to the brush border of the bowel either by a suction or clasping mechanism. It has been suggested that chronic infection occurs when the host fails to develop IgA against specific *Giardia* antigens.[7]

Clinical Features

Infection with *G. lamblia* may be asymptomatic, may manifest itself as a self-limited diarrhea, or may exhibit itself as a syndrome with chronic diarrhea, malabsorption, and weight loss. Most people infected with *Giardia* cysts will be asymptomatic.

In the acute diarrheal syndrome there is an incubation period of 1 to 2 weeks followed by the acute onset of diarrhea, abdominal cramps, and flatulence. The patient may also complain of nausea, excessive belching, and fatigue. Stools are characteristically frequent and watery but may then become greasy and foul smelling. Gross blood is usually absent. Patients often delay coming to the physician, and significant weight loss by this time is not uncommon. Rare features of *G. lamblia* infection are reactive arthritis,[8] urticaria, and biliary tract disease. Post-*Giardia* lactose intolerance occurs in 20% to 40% of patients and sometimes lasts several weeks after treatment.

Laboratory Diagnosis

The diagnosis of giardiasis is most commonly made by identification of the cysts or, occasionally, trophozoites in fecal specimens. Stool samples can be concentrated by the formalin-ethyl acetate or zinc sulfate methods and then stained by the trichrome or iron hematoxylin methods. At least three different stool specimens should be examined by this method. *Giardia* antigens may be detected in feces by enzyme immunoassay or indirect or direct immunofluorescence using monoclonal antibodies and direct fluorescent assays.[9]

If the results of stool examinations are persistently negative in patients highly suspicious for giardiasis, direct examination of small intestinal contents must be undertaken. This may be done with the string test, in which the patent swallows a capsule on the end of a string. The string moves to the jejunum, the trophozoites attach, and in 4 to 12 hours the string is withdrawn and inspected microscopically. Occasionally, esophagogastroduodenoscopy with duodenal aspiration or biopsy may be necessary.

Treatment

Most patients respond to a single course of metronidazole 250 mg tid for 5 days. Quinacrine, formerly the treatment of choice, is now no longer commercially available because of potentially severe side effects. The most common side effects of metronidazole are nausea and a disulfiram-like reaction, and the patient should be warned not to ingest alcohol 24 hours before starting or after finishing the medication. Furazolidone (100 mg qid × 7 to 10 days or 6 to 8 mg/kg/day) is probably less effective than metronidazole but is commonly used to treat children. Paromomycin (25 to 30 mg/kg/day in three doses × 7 days) is a nonabsorbable aminoglycoside. It is probably less effective than the other agents but is commonly used for the treatment of pregnant women. Tinidazole (2 g × 1 dose) is also widely used for giardiasis but has not yet received approval in the United States.

Prevention

In addition to chlorination, public water should be subjected to flocculation, sedimentation, and filtration. For persons traveling to wilderness areas, water should be generally boiled for at least 10 minutes. Uncooked foods that have been washed and prepared in contaminated water should be avoided.[7] During outbreaks in day-care centers, strict hand washing, appropriate disposal of soiled diapers, and treatment of symptomatic children should be undertaken. If this fails to control the outbreak, consideration should be given to treating all infected children. Venereal transmission of *G. lamblia* can be decreased by avoidance of oral-anal sex.

Lyme Disease

Lyme disease is the most common tick-borne disease in the United States.[10] It has become a disease of importance for the family physicians because patients with this illness may present to them, and a diagnosis of actual Lyme disease may present a true challenge.

Description of Pathogen and Epidemiology

Lyme disease is caused by the tick-transmitted, flagellated spirochete *Borrelia burgdorferi*. The vectors of the disease are the ticks *Ixodes scapularis* in the eastern and upper midwestern United States and *I. pacificus* in the West. *I. scapularis* larvae and nymphs generally feed on rodents, usually white-footed mice, and adults generally feed on larger animals, mainly deer, which are abundant in endemic areas of New England. Human disease occurs when humans intervene in the ecology of these ticks, *B. burgdorferi*, rodents, and larger mammals. It is thought that ticks must be attached to the skin for at least 24 hours for transmission of the organism to occur. While Lyme disease occurs in other countries, in the United States it occurs mainly in three areas: the Mid-Atlantic, from Massachusetts to Maryland; North Central, especially Wisconsin and Minnesota; and the Northwest, principally northern California. Most illness occurs between May and November with peak onset in midsummer.

It should be kept in mind that *Ixodes* ticks may be infected with other pathogens capable of causing human disease, including *Ehrlichia, Babesia*, other *Borrelia* species, and viruses.[10,11] Coinfection with *B. burgdorferi* and one of these other pathogens has been documented.

Clinical Features

Lyme disease is difficult to diagnose and is probably over-diagnosed. The most difficult problem is distinguishing features of this disease from chronic fatigue syndrome, fibromyalgia, chronic pain syndromes, anxiety, depression, or other states of psychological stress. Similar to syphilis, Lyme disease occurs in early (erythema migrans) and late forms.

Erythema migrans (EM) begins as a red macule or papule at the site of the tick bite. The area of redness expands around the center with partial clearing in the center. The full lesion averages 15 cm in diameter. The thigh, axilla, and groin are common sites for the lesion, although the lesion can be located virtually anywhere on the body. About 50% of the patients develop other annular secondary lesions within several days of onset of the initial skin lesion. Some patients develop a nonspecific macular rash along with these lesions, and EM usually fades within 3 to 4 weeks. EM is generally accompanied by regional lymphadenopathy and flu-like symptoms such as headache, myalgias, fatigue, fever, and chills.

Arthritis

Within a few weeks to months of onset of the disease, most patients have joint symptoms ranging from migratory joint pain to frank arthritic swelling and erosive synovitis. The most common presentation is that of acute monoarthritis of the knee. Typically, the patient may have attacks of arthritis, separated by complete remissions, which last from a few weeks to months. Recent research suggests that an autoimmune, self-perpetuating process is involved in patients with chronic Lyme arthritis.[10,12]

Neurologic Disease

Symptoms of meningeal irritation may occur early in the illness when EM is present. After several weeks to several months, the common pattern is of symptoms of meningitis and headache with superimposed facial palsy or peripheral radiculopathies (encephalomyelitis). In patients with meningitis, the cerebrospinal fluid rarely has more than 100 cells/mm^3, most of which are lymphocytes. The patient may develop a chronic encephalopathy, which may affect mood, memory, or sleep. These symptoms may be subtle. They usually begin years after the onset of the disease but sometimes occur within months.

Lyme Carditis

A small percentage of patients with Lyme disease have cardiac involvement within the first several weeks of the illness. The most common manifestation is varying degrees of atrioventricular block, including first-degree atrioventricular block, Wenckebach phenomenon, or complete heart block. The period of heart involvement is usually brief (a matter of days), and insertion of a permanent pacemaker is usually unnecessary. The diagnosis of Lyme disease should be considered in an otherwise healthy patient in a Lyme disease endemic area who develops atrioventricular heart block.

Other features of cardiac involvement are pericarditis, myocarditis, and ventricular tachycardia.

Laboratory Diagnosis

The organism may be cultured from the edge of an erythema migrans lesion by biopsy and subsequent inoculation on Barbour-Stoenner-Kelly medium. However, since this is difficult to do, diagnosis is usually confirmed by serologic testing. Serologic testing early in the infection is not sensitive because the immune response in this disease develops slowly. However, later in the illness serologic testing can be performed with a high degree of sensitivity and specificity. The most commonly used serologic method is ELISA with equivocal or positive tests followed by a confirmatory Western immunoblot. Most other laboratory abnormalities in this disease are nonspecific. Serologic testing only confirms a logically made clinical diagnosis. A false-positive ELISA test may occur as a result of cross-reacting antibodies in patients with other infections and noninfectious inflammatory diseases.

Treatment

Most stages of manifestations of Lyme disease can be treated with oral antibiotic therapy. Early in the illness doxycycline 100 mg twice daily or amoxicillin 500 mg three times daily (30–50 mg/kg/day in children) for 2 to 3 weeks is probably adequate. Another antibiotic that is considered effective against the organism is cefuroxime axetil. Four weeks of oral antibiotic therapy for arthritis and 3 weeks for carditis are also probably adequate.

In patients with a neurologic involvement, intravenous antibiotic therapy is considered necessary. Ceftriaxone 2 g per day (in children 50–100 mg/kg/day) for 3 to 4 weeks is commonly used, but cefotaxime 2 g every 8 hours (in children 90–180 mg/kg/day) or penicillin G 5 million units every 6 hours (in children 300,000 U/kg/day) is also considered effective.

Prevention

Recommended protective measures against tick bites include wearing long pants, long sleeve shirts, and light-colored clothing, and tucking pants into socks. Also recommended are using tick repellants on clothing and exposed skin and performing regular complete body checks.[10]

Antibiotic prophylaxis for tick bites is not recommended because of potential adverse drug reactions.

A subunit recombinant vaccine against *Borrelia bugdorferi* (LYMRix) had been shown to be safe and effacious in humans.[10,13,14] However, as of early 2002 the vaccine has been withdrawn from the market.

Rocky Mountain Spotted Fever

Knowledge of Rocky Mountain spotted fever (RMSF) is important for the family physician because patients with RMSF may present to the family physician and because it has a high mortality rate if undiagnosed or if diagnosed late.

Description of the Pathogen and Epidemiology

Rocky Mountain spotted fever is a member of the "spotted fevers" group of illnesses caused by closely related rickettsiae transmitted by ticks and mites. The spotted fevers are in turn part of a larger group of rickettsial infections.

The etiologic agent, *Rickettsia rickettsii*, is an obligatory intracellular gram-negative bacterium. It is transmitted in the eastern states by the American dog tick, *Dermacentor variabilis*, which is both the vector and the main reservoir. It is transmitted by the Rocky Mountain wood tick, *D. andersoni*, in the western states. Only adult *Dermacentor* ticks feed on humans, but the disease may also be transmitted when the tick is removed and crushed between the fingers, when one may be exposed to infective tick hemolymph. Ticks become infected by feeding on the blood of infected animals, through fertilization, or by transovarial passage. Ticks transmit the organism to humans during feeding. The organisms in turn invade the endothelial and smooth muscle cells of blood vessels and cause generalized vascular injury.

While at one time the disease was thought to exist only in the Rocky Mountain states, at present the disease incidence is higher in the south Atlantic states and the south-central states. RMSF is most commonly seen during the late spring and summer.

Clinical Features

The incubation period of RMSF is 2 to 14 days. The initial diagnosis of RMSF is based on clinical manifestations. Early diagnosis may be difficult but is important because of the relatively high mortality associated with the disease if not treated in a timely fashion. In RMSF the early manifestations of the disease are fatigue, myalgias, spiking fever, and headache, which is usually quite severe. Gastrointestinal involvement may be marked and may include abdominal pain, nausea, vomiting, or diarrhea. The rash appears 3 to 5 days after the onset of fever. It usually starts on the ankles and feet and moves to the wrists and hands and then to the trunk and head. The rash starts out red and macular, and blanches to pressure. It may become papular and darker red and is usually edematous. Within 2 to 3 days it may become petechial and purpuric. Ten percent or more of patients with the disease may not have a rash (Rocky Mountain "spotless" fever), and this happens more often in older patients. The rash is less likely to be recognized in African-American patients.[15] In a small number of patients, the rash may progress to skin necrosis or gangrene of the digits or limbs, occasionally requiring amputation. Meningismus, encephalitis, focal neurologic deficits, deafness, seizures, and coma may ensue, and neurologic involvement may indicate a poor prognosis. Acute renal failure from hypovolemic hypotension may ensue in severe RMSF. Pulmonary involvement may be manifested by cough, pulmonary infiltrates on chest x-rays, pleural effusion, frank pulmonary edema, and adult respiratory distress syndrome.[16] Hyponatremia is observed in more than half of the patients.

The disease is easily confused with measles in unimmunized patients. In RMSF, however, the rash is more edematous. The rash often starts on the face with measles, while it almost never does in RMSF. The rhinorrhea, cough, and conjunctivitis that are typical of measles are unusual in RMSF. The rashes of both diseases may be petechial at one point, but the rash of meningococcemia usually becomes purulent and necrotic quite early.[17] Most patients with meningococcemia also have meningitis, and meningeal signs are often marked.

Laboratory Diagnosis

The diagnosis of RMSF is largely clinical, since serology, the usual method for confirmation of the diagnosis, is retrospective. Acute and convalescent serum should be drawn on patients suspected of RMSF. Indirect fluorescent antibody (IFA) is the most sensitive and specific serologic test for RMSF, and the diagnostic titers for indirect immunofluorescence are 1:64 (between 7 and 10 days after onset of illness) or a fourfold rise between acute and convalescent sera.[15]

Treatment

RMSF is treated with oral tetracycline 25 to 50 mg/kg/day or chloramphenicol 50 to 75 mg/kg/day given in four divided doses for 7 days. There is some evidence in favor of tetracycline being the drug of choice.[15,18] Doxycycline 100 mg every 12 hours for 7 days is also quite effective. The drugs should generally be continued for 2 days after the patient has been afebrile. Tetracycline or chloramphenicol should be given intravenously in patients with marked nausea and vomiting or if otherwise severely ill. Tetracycline is contraindicated in pregnant women. The organism is also susceptible to rifampin, ciprofloxacin, and pefloxacin. Fluid and electrolyte maintenance is often important in managing this illness because of increased vascular permeability. Without treatment, death may occur within 8 to 15 days in 20% of patients. The disease is considered more lethal in the elderly and in men. Early fatalities from fulminant RMSF have been noted in African-American men with glucose-6-phosphate dehydrogenase (G6PD) deficiency.

Prevention

Preventive measures include use of protective clothing, tick repellants, and regular, frequent checks of the entire body for ticks while in endemic areas. Carefully and completely remove ticks with forceps and steady upward traction, and then wash the site with soap and water.

Hantaviruses

Hantaviruses came to light in the United States in 1993 when a genotype of the virus, the Sin Nombre virus, was responsible for an outbreak of illness with severe pulmonary features in the southwestern United States. Family physicians should be aware of this pathogen because of its known presence now in the United States, because diagnosis may be difficult, and because of its potential to cause high mortality.

Description of the Pathogen and Epidemiology

It has been estimated that there are thousands of hospitalized cases of hantavirus annually, most of which occur in the People's Republic of China. Hantaviruses are one of five genuses within the Bunyaviridae family. It is the only one of the genuses that is not transmitted via an arthropod vector. They are RNA viruses, roughly spherical, with a diameter of 100 nm. They have been recognized in many different rodent populations throughout the world. There are over 20 recognized sero/genotypes and each hantavirus is specific to a different rodent host. A species of rodent is persistently affected with a genotype of hantavirus and secretes active virus for prolonged periods of time, while the virus does not appear to detrimentally affect the rodent. The virus is transmitted among rodents and to humans via respiratory secretions, urine, and occasionally bites. Patients with occupations that put them into contact with rodents, such as animal trappers, forestry workers, farmers, and military personnel, are at highest risk for infection. Accordingly, men are more often infected than women.

Clinical Features

Asymptomatic or mild infections probably outnumber symptomatic infections in humans. When the virus presents clinically, however, there are two common clinical presentations of illness: hemorrhagic fever with renal syndrome (HFRS) and hantavirus pulmonary syndrome (HPS).

The most severe form of HFRS is caused by Hantaan virus in eastern Asia and Dobrava virus in Europe. One could think of HFRS as a classic triad of fever, hemorrhagic features, and renal failure. The first phase is a febrile period accompanied by headache and myalgia and lasts 2 to 7 days. The second phase is a hypotensive one with thrombocytopenia, petechial hemorrhages, and proteinuria. The third phase is an oliguric phase that lasts from 3 to 7 days after the blood pressure returns to normal. The fourth phase, the diuresis phase, may last for several weeks. The fifth phase is the convalescent phase with the patient often not feeling back to normal for several months. The mortality rate is 5% to 10% with deaths due to shock, multiorgan hypoperfusion, and uremia.

HFRS caused by Plumula virus in Europe or the Seoul virus in Southeast Asia causes a much milder form of HFRS with lower morbidity and mortality.

HPS has been recognized in North America since 1993 with the initial outbreak in the southwestern United States. Cases have also been seen in South America, but HPS thus far has been described only in the Americas.[19] The hantavirus genotype responsible for this illness is named Sin Nombre and its host is *Peromyscus maniculatus*, a sigmodontine rodent. The illness generally progresses through three stages. In the short prodromal phase there is fever, headache, and myalgia. The second stage, the cardiopulmonary phase, is characterized by severe respiratory insufficiency caused by noncardiogenic pulmonary edema and hypotension. There also may be rhabdomyolysis in this stage. The third stage is the convalescent stage, which may be prolonged. The mortality rate is about 50%. Unlike HFRS, renal involvement is not marked. However, some note that leukocytosis and hemoconcentration occur as they do in HFRS.

Vascular dysfunction is apparently the main abnormality in both HFRS and HPS, and there is evidence that immune mechanisms are responsible for this as opposed to direct viral cytopathology. The principal histopathologic findings in fatal cases of HFRS are hemorrhagic necrosis of the renal medulla with widespread tubular degeneration.

Laboratory Diagnosis

Isolating hantaviruses from human specimens is very difficult and may take several weeks. Therefore, hantavirus infections are best diagnosed by serologic means. Indirect immunofluorescence with native virus can detect both IgM and IgG and is the most commonly used serologic test for hantavirus infection. Enzyme immunoassays with both native and recombinant antigens have also been developed for detecting hantavirus infection. For research purposes, the plaque reduction neutralization test is the gold standard and can be used to differentiate between infections caused by different hantaviruses.

Treatment

The mainstay of therapy in severe hantavirus infections is general supportive therapy. Management of fluid and electrolytes are elements of treatment as is support of intravascular volume. Renal dialysis in the face of acute renal failure may be lifesaving. Close monitoring and intensive care are usually needed in HPS, and cardiovascular support with vasopressor and inotropic agents may be necessary. Heparin and platelet infusions may be necessary for disseminated intravascular coagulation.

Clinical trials of intravenous ribavirin in the People's Republic of China have shown that this can significantly reduce the mortality in HFRS if given in the first 5 days after onset of the illness.[20]

Prevention

Potentially the most effective means of control of hantavirus is by application of simple rodent-proofing measures in dwellings and other measures to limit human contact with rodents and their excrement. All laboratory work involving growth of hantaviruses in cell cultures or animals should be conducted in biosafety level III conditions.[21]

References

1. Beazley DM, Egerman RS. Toxoplasmosis. Semin Perinatol 1998;22:332–38.
2. Lynfield R, Guerina NG. Toxoplasmosis. Pediatr Rev 1997;18: 1–17.
3. Alger LS. Toxoplasmosis and parvovirus B19. Infect Dis Clin North Am 1997;11:55–75.
4. Clausen MR, Meyer CN, Krantz T, et al. Trichinella infection and clinical disease. Q J Med 1996;89:631–6.
5. Hughes P, Chidley K, Cowie J. Neurological complications in psittacosis: a case report and literature review. Respir Med 1996;89:637–8.
6. Schlossberg D. Chlamydia psittaci (psittacosis). In: Mandell GL, Douglas RG Jr, Dolin R, eds. Mandell, Douglas, and Bennett's principles and practice of infectious diseases, 4th ed. New York: Churchill Livingstone, 1995;1693–6.
7. Hill DR. Giardia lamblia. In: Mandell GL, Douglas RG Jr, Dolin R, eds. Mandell, Douglas, and Bennett's principles and practice of infectious diseases, 4th ed. New York: Churchill Livingstone, 1995;2487–93.
8. Letts M, Davidson D, Lalonde F. Synovitis secondary to giardiasis in children. Am J Orthop 1998;27:451–4.
9. Ortega YR, Adam RD. Giardia: overview and update. Clin Infect Dis 1997;25:545–50.
10. Evans J. Lyme disease. Curr Opin Rheumatol 1999;11:281–8.
11. Katavolos P, Armstrong PM, Dawson JE, Telford SR. Duration of tick attachment required for transmission of granulocytic ehrlichosis. J Infect Dis 1998;177:1422–5.
12. Gross DM, Forsthuber T, Tary-Lehman M, et al. Identification of LFA-1 as a candidate autoantigen in treatment-resistant Lyme arthritis. Science 1998;281:703–6.
13. Steere AC, Sikand VK, Meurice F, et al. Vaccination against Lyme disease with recombinant *Borrelia burgdorferi* outer-surface lipoprotein A with adjuvant. N Engl J Med 1998;339: 209–15.
14. Lapp T. AAP issues recommendations on the prevention and treatment of Lyme disease. Am Fam Physician 2000;61:3463–4.
15. Thorner AR, Walker DH, Petri WA Jr. Rocky Mountain spotted fever. Clin Infect Dis 1998;27:1353–60.
16. Walker DH. Rocky Mountain spotted fever: a seasonal alert. Clin Infect Dis 1995;20:111–7.
17. Riley HD Jr. When to suspect Rocky Mountain spotted fever. Diagnosis 1987;May:22–38.
18. Dalton MJ, Clarke MJ, Holman RC, et al. National surveillance for Rocky Mountain spotted fever, 1981–1992: epidemiologic summary and evaluation of risk factors for fatal outcome. Am J Trop Med Hyg 1995;52:405–13.
19. Hart CA, Bennett M. Hantavirus infections: epidemiology and pathogenesis. Microbes Infect 1999;1:1229–37.
20. Huggins JW, Hsiang CM. Cosgriff TM, et al. Prospective, double-blind, concurrent, placebo-controlled clinical trial of intravenous ribavirin therapy of hemorrhagic fever with renal syndrome. J Infect Dis 1994;164:1119–27.
21. McCaughey C, Hart CA. Hantaviruses. J Med Microbiol 2000: 49:587–99.

45
Occupational Health Care

James E. Lessenger

Occupational medicine addresses the health of employees in the workplace. The concept of what is "occupational" has evolved from treating obvious injuries to a broader definition. The World Health Organization has proposed four categories of occupational disease syndromes related to the workplace: (1) diseases only occupational in origin, (2) diseases in which occupation is one of the causal factors, (3) diseases in which occupation is a contributing factor in complex situations, and (4) diseases in which occupation may aggravate preexisting disease.[1–3]

There is a distinction made between occupational injury and illness. The Occupational Safety and Health Administration (OSHA) defines an occupational injury as a physical injury, such as a laceration, fracture, or sprain, resulting from a single accident or exposure in the work environment. An occupational illness is any abnormal condition or disorder other than an injury caused by exposure to environmental factors associated with employment.[4]

Need for Services

The passage of the Occupational Safety and Hazard Act of 1970 was a watershed event for occupational medicine. The act and similar legislation created the Environmental Protection Agency, OSHA, and the National Institute for Occupational Safety and Health. These organizations, in turn, spawned research and regulation mandating medical surveillance of workers and, consequently, increasing the need for occupational medicine services.[5]

Several additional factors contributed to the increased need for occupational medicine services. Unions demanded hazard monitoring, improved injury treatment, and more prevention measures. Insurance carriers encouraged prevention and preplacement examination to avoid placing at-risk employees in jobs with a greater risk of injury. Concerns about fraud placed a greater burden on physicians for careful documentation of the mechanism of injury in workplace accidents. Management sought services to limit liability and decrease absenteeism. Employees took a greater interest in their own health and welfare in the workplace as they learned about hazardous exposures through the media.[6]

The Concept of Hazards

By approaching risk analysis from the standpoint of hazards, a more comprehensive evaluation can prevent injuries from recurring (Table 45.1). For example, when physicians walk into a warehouse they are confronted with a busy environment full of noise, forklifts scurrying around, and people walking. Possible hazards include auditory damage from the noise, vibratory injury from driving the forklifts, and trauma from being struck by a vehicle.[4–6]

Core Content of Occupational Medicine

Treatment of Industrial Injuries and Illness

The majority of workplace injuries and illness can be treated by the family physician in the office. Table 45.2 lists the industrial injuries most commonly seen in a family practice.[7] The American College of Occupational and Environmental Medicine published protocols for treatment that are helpful in plotting the treatment regimen of the injured employee. It is also useful to hand out copies so the patient is informed of the treatment plan.[8]

When a physician treats an industrial injury or illness, the insurance company, attorneys, consultants, government agencies, and perhaps the patient may review the chart. The history of how the injury occurred, preferably in the patient's

Table 45.1. **Workplace Hazards (Representative List)**[3–7]

Type	Example	Disease or condition
Traumatic		
Slips and falls	Wet floors	Traumatic injuries
Crush injuries	Poor maintenance	
Explosive	Improper design	
Flying objects	Poor safety plan	
Lacerations	Inadequate equipment	
Sprains	Improper warnings	
Toxic		
Chemicals		
Inorganic	Asbestos	Mesothelioma
Organic pesticides	Organophosphates	Organic brain disease
Heavy metals	Lead, battery workers	Wrist drop
Radiation		
Ionizing	Radiation burns	Keloids
		Leukemias
Nonionizing	Welding flash burns	Keratoconjunctivitis
Physical environment		
Acoustic trauma	Unshielded machines	Deafness
Vibration	Pneumatic hammers	Carpal tunnel syndrome
Heat	Miners	Heat exhaustion
Cold exposure	Professional mountain climbers	Hypothermia
Shift work	Aircraft crews	Frostbite-impaired judgment
Barotrauma	Caisson accidents, professional divers	Caisson disease (bends)
Repetitive motion	Packing houses	Carpal tunnel syndrome
Personal environment		
Air pollution	Sand blasting	Pneumoconiosis
Water pollution	Trail maintenance	Giardiasis
	Crews drinking stream water	
Hazardous waste	Solvents	Neuropathies
Cigarette smoking	Restaurant workers	Bronchitis
Reproductive hazards	Operating room staffs, anesthetic gases	Decreased sperm counts, miscarriages
Infectious		
Blood-borne exposure	Needle sticks	Hepatitis B
Travel exposures	Endemic areas	Malaria
Special environments	Search and rescue	Tick-borne infections
Animal bites	Veterinarians	Brucellosis, rabies

own words, needs to be legibly recorded, the injury accurately described, and a clear diagnosis given. Treatment must be carefully documented and work status, return visits, treatment modalities, and other parts of the treatment plan listed. When the injury is resolved, it is mandatory to close the case. Evidence of fraud must be carefully documented and reported.[8]

There are a myriad of emotions a patient feels about an injury that entails the loss of one's job, status, and income, such as feelings of insecurity, and attacks on one's self-image as the breadwinner and provider. It is important to reassure the patient about the prognosis of the injury, plot out the treatment plan, and explain what results can be reasonably expected.[9]

Modified duty or returning the injured employee to a less demanding job decreases the patient's expenses and shortens the recovery time. It is important for the physician to understand the work environment the employee will return to and, if possible, to observe the actual workplace. It is helpful if the physician and employer have agreed in advance on what modified positions are available and what tasks they will en-

tail. A call to the employer can also help coordinate modified duty and return the employee to the workplace. Duty instructions need to be clearly transmitted to the employer in writing, but need not be complicated.[9]

Preplacement and Fitness-for-Duty Examinations

Preplacement Examinations

These examinations determine if the prospective employee meets the essential requirements to perform the job task. The Americans with Disabilities Act (ADA) has created a tougher standard for preplacement exams, but the basic concept is for the physician to match the employee and the job. This may mean creating accommodations for the employee who is not able to do tasks as originally assigned.[10,11]

Apart from decisions of employability, the preplacement physician examination establishes a baseline for long-term hazard monitoring, especially in industries were there is exposure to hazardous materials, loud noises, and vibration.

The first step in a preplacement examination program is to

Table 45.2. **Industrial Injuries Commonly Seen in a Family Practice**[7]

Diagnosis	Percent
Lacerations, all sites	14.0
Contusions, all sites	14.0
Lumbar strain	13.0
Strains, sprains	12.0
Eye injuries, all types	8.0
Low back pain	6.0
Dermatitis, all types	4.0
Tenosynovitis, forearm	3.0
Fractures, all sites	2.0
Pesticide exposure	2.0
Cellulitis, all sites	2.0
Thoracic strain	2.0
Cervical strain	2.0
Hernias, all sites	2.0
Epicondylitis, elbow	1.3
Burns, all sites	1.0
Insect bite	1.0
Abrasions, all sites	1.0
Inhalation pneumonitis	1.0
Carpal tunnel syndrome	1.0
Rotator cuff tear	0.6
Nonconcussive head trauma	0.6
Posttraumatic arthritis	0.5
Abdominal muscle strain	0.5
Herniated nucleus pulposus	0.5
Infectious diseases	0.5
Crush injury, finger	0.5
Internal derangement, knee	0.5
Ganglion cyst	0.4
Chemical toxic poisoning	0.4
Concussion	0.4
Torsion of the testicle	0.2
Cubital tunnel syndrome	0.2
Chest wall strain	0.1
Dislocated joint	0.1
Chemical sinusitis	0.1
Adhesive capsulitis, shoulder	0.1
Bursitis hip	0.1
Traumatic Morton's neuroma	0.1
Metal fume fever	0.1
Dog bite	0.1
Anxiety, stress	0.1
Heat exhaustion	0.1
Basal cell carcinoma, face	0.1
Cardiovascular disease	0.1
Other	0.2

determine what tasks the employee will be required to perform. Next, the essential physical requirements of the tasks are delineated and an examination designed to determine if the candidate can perform those tasks. The preplacement physical is a directed examination to determine if the applicant can meet the essential requirements. Special tests, such as x-rays or pulmonary function tests, or a review of past medical records may be necessary to answer the question.[12,13]

There are five possible results from the preplacement examination: (1) no medical contraindication to performing the job; (2) no medical contraindication with accommodations; (3) based on a probability of substantial harm, the employee could pose a direct threat to self or others; (4) medical hold, pending additional data; and (5) further testing required to fully evaluate the ability or risk. To place the applicant in the third category, the disqualifying physical finding must be certain, current, severe, of long duration, objective, and result in specific outcomes that could put the employee or others at risk for accident or illness.[13,14]

The medical hold gives the applicant an opportunity to seek care for correctable conditions such as hypertension and poor visual acuity. The alternative of requiring further testing provides the opportunity to monitor applicants with diabetes, seizure disorders, and similar diseases for proof of control.[13–15]

Typically, for applicants of public safety jobs such as police, fire, bus drivers, truck drivers, dispatchers, and the like, there are industry or government standards to which the examination results of the applicant can be compared.[13]

Routine-screening back x-rays are not predictive of back injury. They are expensive and expose the applicant to needless radiation, especially if the applicant is pregnant. Back x-rays are useful on a case-by-case basis for evaluating the suitability of an applicant, but a well-done examination and review of medical records usually provides more information.[14,15]

Fitness-for-Duty Examinations

These examinations evaluate workers to determine if they can remain at or return to a job task. Employees may develop a physical or mental defect that prevents them from doing the jobs in which they are already working, or they may be returning to the workplace after a physical or mental illness. As in preplacement examinations, the basic demands of the job must be defined and employees examined to determine if they meet those demands.[16,17]

One must consider the requirements of the ADA; it is appropriate to give the employee an opportunity to correct conditions, if practical. Further, it may be necessary to obtain medical records and a psychiatric or medical consultation in making a determination. Workers who carry firearms, usually peace officers, not only must be in sound mental condition, but also must be able to safely discharge their weapons when necessary while protecting themselves and the public.[16]

Executive Health Maintenance Examinations

The executive health examination can be tailored to meet the company's requirements and integrated with periodic assessments. It is important to have a clear idea of why the examination is being performed and how the results will be used. If the examination will be used to decide on retention or promotion, clear-cut criteria for selection that meet the basic requirements of the job need to be defined in advance. Further, test results and examination findings need to be transmitted to the employee in a clear, understandable manner. Reports sent to the company personnel department must not violate patient confidentiality.[17]

The annual examination is a good opportunity to assess the executive's risk of cardiovascular and other diseases and to detect alcoholism, drug abuse, and domestic violence. The executive health physical examination can be a portal for entry into treatment and prevention services.

Periodic Health Assessment of Workers

Mandated Examinations

These examinations include U.S. Department of Transportation and state motor vehicle examinations of drivers of trucks, buses, and other vehicles in commerce; Federal Aviation Administration (FAA) examinations of aircrews; and specialized examinations of hazardous materials handlers and public safety personnel such as police and firefighters. These examinations include both an overall evaluation of the health of the employee and specific emphasis on body systems and senses required for the job. For example, truck drivers hauling hazardous chemicals need perfectly corrected vision, use of both hands and both legs, and no illness that may result in a sudden loss of consciousness such as uncontrolled insulin-dependent diabetes or a seizure disorder.[16–18]

Hazard-Monitoring Examinations

These examinations are typically required by federal or state regulations. Examples include cholinesterase testing of pesticide applicators, hearing testing of machine operators, pulmonary testing of foundry workers, vision testing of computer terminal users, and blood lead testing of battery handlers and lead foundry workers. These examinations are valuable to establish a baseline level of organ function when an employee begins the job. They are most helpful when trended over time, integrated with preplacement examinations and periodic health assessments and evaluated using standardized protocols.

Postexposure hazard monitoring of employees exposed to an environmental insult measures the extent of injury and is especially helpful if trended over time. For example, hepatorenal function studies, serial pulmonary function studies, semen analysis, and hearing and sight examinations may be necessary after certain chemical or physical insults in the workplace.[7–9,17]

OSHA and other agencies have requirements about testing equipment, operator qualifications, periodicity of examinations, record keeping, reporting results, and actions necessary if results are abnormal. Before beginning a hazard monitoring program it is vital to obtain exact information from the agencies and employer as to which examinations are required and how they should be administered.

Drug Testing

Drug testing can be ordered by an employer as part of the preplacement exam, randomly, or "for cause." Preplacement exams are required before the employee is hired. Random testing is designed to prevent drug use. For-cause tests are ordered by an employer when a specific incident has occurred, such as a traffic accident or injury at the workplace. For-cause testing also applies to employees in whom the employer has identified behaviors or appearances suggestive of drug or alcohol intoxication. Drug testing is specifically exempted from the ADA.[19–21]

Drug testing can be regulated or nonregulated. Regulated tests are required by government codes to be performed upon certain public safety personnel. Regulated testing requires a physician acting as the medical review officer (MRO) to receive all positive results and determine if there is a reason-

able medical explanation such as prescription pharmaceuticals. MROs are usually certified and may set up the entire drug collection process. Physicians may also function as substance abuse professionals (SAPs) to evaluate employees for the necessity or effectiveness of rehabilitation in employee assistance programs (EAPs).[19–21]

Unregulated testing may vary from dipstick tests done in the bathroom of the employer's personnel office to tests collected under the supervision of a physician, analyzed in a certified laboratory, and reviewed by an MRO. There is a wide range in quality in nonregulated testing, but in the last 5 years the standards applied to regulated testing have become the standard of care for nonregulated testing as well.[19–21]

Drug testing is just one tool in a broader company drug policy that may include drug rehabilitation as an alternative to job termination. The policy typically includes a statement that must be signed by each employee and contains contact phone numbers for an EAP. Within the context of a company program, the physician often monitors employees who are in EAPs for compliance.[19–21]

Immunizations

Immunizations are location, job, or injury specific. Location-specific immunizations are for employees who travel to various parts of the world. Job-specific immunizations include hepatitis B immunizations for health care workers and brucellosis and rabies vaccines for veterinarians. Injury-specific immunizations include tetanus vaccine for lacerations and abrasions, and hepatitis B immunoglobulin prophylaxis for blood-borne exposures. Record keeping is vital, and it is important to provide the employee with an individual immunization record. Immunization advice is constantly changing and the best source of information is the Center for Disease Control and Prevention (www.cdc.gov)[22] (also see Chapter 7).

In the best of all worlds, the results of all examinations, immunizations, and testing would be integrated into the same file and observed for trends over successive years. Several commercially available computer programs serve this purpose. Federal laws require records of physicals and hazard monitoring in the workplace be kept by the employer for 30 years, thus placing a burden on the physician to maintain the records for that length of time or to find a suitable repository. State record retention times vary considerably. Employers should purchase equipment that meets OSHA specifications.[6]

Work-Site Visits to Familiarize Physicians with the Work Environment to Assist in Return-to-Work Modified Duty Orders

These visits help ensure that the employee will recover and the injury will not exacerbate. Under the best of circumstances, the physician will have visited the plant in advance and determined which duties could be modified to prevent common injuries. Postaccident, a physician's visit to the work site can assist an employee's return to work in difficult cases.

Postaccident Investigations and Reenactments

These visits document how an injury actually occurred. A change in equipment or industrial process may be possible based on the information obtained in an investigation. Frequently, an employer may question if an accident really occurred and a reenactment can resolve inconsistencies in accounts.[22,23]

The Safety Checklist

The site visit is an opportunity to prevent injuries by monitoring hazards using a safety checklist to assure they are properly controlled.

Consultation and Counseling Programs for Employees

"Right-to-Know" Laws

These laws at the federal and state levels have placed the burden on employers to warn their employees of the hazards they may face in the workplace and their potential health consequences. The physician may be involved in implementing these laws, either by creating the explanatory documents or by explaining hazards to the employees. Many employers find it less expensive to purchase "right-to-know" documents and have people in the personnel department or the medical consultant distribute and explain them to their employees. If physicians embark upon this task, they should research the material well, as many of the employees will have done their homework on the Internet before consulting with the physicians.[24]

Answering Employee Questions and Concerns About a Hazard Exposure

This task is becoming common due to the increasing number of reports in the media of toxic problems and public concern. The family physician is in a unique position to hear these concerns and either allay the fears or take the necessary action to act on what may be an unacceptable exposure. There is also a tremendous amount of information available to consumers in libraries and on the Internet, and the physician may have to do a lot of research to answer these questions fully.

Employee Assistance Programs (or Plans) (EAPs)

These programs were originally created to decrease the large number of lost workdays due to alcohol and drug abuse. However, psychiatric illness, marital problems, grief, suicide, depression, and sexual difficulties have joined the list of problems handled by EAPs. With the threat of loss of employment as a strong incentive for the employee to cooperate, it is possible for the physician to refer an identified problem employee to an EAP. In organizing a program, issues such as identification, confidentiality, reports to management, treatment modalities, and cost must be addressed.[25]

Wellness Programs

These programs are attractive to employers as a mechanism to increase productivity and employee morale and decrease lost workdays through illness. Programs may focus on exercise, smoking cessation, hypertension control, cardiovascular conditioning, weight reduction, or a combination of these goals.[26]

Pesticides

Tons of pesticides are used throughout the world in home, office, industrial, and agricultural applications. New techniques in integrated pest management may decrease the dependence on chemicals in the future. Growth regulators, nutrients, and buffers are sometimes considered in this class of chemicals because they are often used together. Pesticides using engineered viruses and bacteria have entered the market and it remains to be seen if they produce injuries.

Pesticides comprise hundreds of chemicals mixed into thousands of formulations targeted at a specific pest, crop, or structure. These chemicals are used in gaseous forms as fumigants; in liquid form as mists and sprays applied by aircraft, spraying rigs, hand-held sprayers, and injection into irrigation water; and in solid form as powders, granules, and pellets for distribution by hand, aircraft, and ground machines. The range of chemicals includes organophosphates, elements, organochlorides, carbamates, dipyridyls, chlorophenoxy, anticoagulants, and hydrocarbons.[27,28]

A person's presence in an area where pesticides are used does not necessarily mean there will be exposure, and exposure does not necessarily mean there will be adequate contact to produce the physiologic changes of poisoning. Poisoning may not automatically lead to impairment or disability.[27,28]

Outpatient Care

Persons who are exposed must leave the area immediately and stay away until it is safe. Clothing should be removed and be treated like hazardous waste. Each exposed person should bathe thoroughly, with careful attention to the hair. If exposed, the eyes need to be aggressively irrigated. Emergency care should be instituted as soon as practical, but care providers must be careful not to expose themselves to the chemical.[27,28]

Diagnosis

The history may be the only positive data. If there is any doubt as to the identity of the offending agent, contact the employer or applicator for the name of the formulation and the material safety data sheet (MSDS). Question the employee on how the exposure occurred, with emphasis on the exact mechanism of exposure, the cause-and-effect relationship of exposure and symptoms, previous exposures and poisoning, and drug or alcohol problems.

Symptoms and signs may vary by the formulation the person was exposed to, the length and concentration of exposure, and decontamination. Nausea, vomiting, fatigue, and vertigo are common reactions to most poisonings but may also represent other diseases. The classic symptoms of salivation, lacrimation, urination, and diarrhea—the SLUD syndrome seen in organophosphate poisoning—may not be seen in low-concentration poisoning of short duration, although the person may have fatigue and vertigo.[29]

The physical examination may reveal subtle findings. Rashes should be carefully described and secondary changes caused by scratching and treatment documented. Halogenated hydrocarbons can produce chloracne, often confused with acne vulgaris.[30] Inhalation of dusts, mists, and gases may cause bronchospasm. Nausea, vomiting, diarrhea, and abdominal pain occur as a result of eating contaminated food or by ingestion in attempted suicides and homicides. Acute or delayed polyneuropathy and chronic lapses in concentration and memory can result from exposure to organophosphates and halogenated hydrocarbons. Sprays or mists to the eyes can cause problems ranging from simple conjunctivitis to corneal opacities.[31,32]

Laboratory tests are of limited usefulness. Tests of urine and blood pesticide levels are costly, must be performed as close to the time of exposure as possible, may take weeks to produce results, and may be negative even in well-documented exposures.[31] Blood, liver, and renal test results may be clouded by the presence of other diseases and may be abnormal in only the most severe poisoning cases. Cholinesterase (ChE) activity tests are useful only in organophosphate and carbamate poisoning, and are most effective when used in a monitoring program for applicators where baselines have been established. A person can have a 60% drop in ChE activity levels and still stay in normal ranges. A postexposure series of tests demonstrating recovery may be the only laboratory response elicited. ChE activity levels can also be affected by cocaine use and medications.[29]

Whenever possible, physicians should learn the name of the chemical and its properties before embarking on nonemergency treatment. Sources include the MSDS, reference texts, poison control centers, telephone numbers on the pesticide container, TOXLINE, and MEDLINE.

Treatment

Mild poisonings cause few symptoms, and vital signs remain normal. Moderate poisonings cause more severe symptoms and objective signs, but again vital signs remain normal. Severe poisonings result in multiple complaints, objective signs, and unstable vital signs. Some pesticides may exhibit delayed onset of symptoms and signs.

Mild and moderate poisonings can usually be evaluated and followed on an outpatient basis. They rarely need any treatment other than reassurance, antiemetics for nausea and vomiting, and steroids for rash.

Severe poisonings will usually require hospitalization and intensive physiologic support. Decontamination should not be ignored in the hospital setting and gastrointestinal (GI) lavage may be needed in cases of ingestion. Antidotes such as atropine are rare. They may not be needed and should not be attempted unless the pesticide is identified. Forced diuresis, exchange transfusion, and chelation are replete with complications and should only be considered when the patient's condition is severe, on an inpatient basis, and when the specific agent is identified.

Atropine is useful in organophosphate and carbamate poisoning when bradycardia causes hypotension or when secretions threaten respiration. The dose is 0.5 to 2.0 mg IV every 20 to 30 minutes. There have been numerous reports of persons who were brought near death by inappropriate atropine administration. Atropine may require serial administrations over several days in severe cases.[28–30]

In jurisdictions where required, reports must be made to the appropriate agencies. Serial examinations to follow chronic problems may be necessary, especially with neurologic and respiratory involvement. Work, impairment and disability status must be documented. The possibility of fraud must be considered and documented if discovered.[33]

Building-Related Illness (Sick-Building Syndrome)

Defects in building construction, design, or maintenance may lead to conditions where people who live or work in buildings develop illnesses, or think they have developed illnesses, related to exposure to toxicants within the building. Sick-building syndrome (SBS) is a subcategory of building-related illness (BRI) used to denote a self-limiting mild illness of short duration.[34]

Etiology

Buildings of all types, especially modern ones, can produce illness through one or a combination of factors: inadequate ventilation and temperature control, contaminants, microbial agents, noise, and mass psychogenic hysteria. Illness can be magnified by litigation, secondary gain, inadequate medical or industrial hygiene investigation, and incomplete or misleading reports by the building owner or by the news media.[35]

Inadequate ventilation decreases the amount of air circulation and raises the levels of carbon monoxide in the building air. Increased levels may exist throughout the entire building or in isolated pockets of poor air circulation and high occupancy density. The temperature may be too high or too low for the comfort or safety of the workers. Buildings with low humidity may produce respiratory mucosal irritation due to dryness. High humidity may predispose to mold growth. Hot and cold surfaces and draft may also affect perceptions of indoor air quality.[34–36]

Contaminants may be intrinsic or extrinsic to the building. Building materials intrinsic to the building include fiberboard, insulation materials, or construction materials that produce volatile organic compounds, formaldehyde, odors or dusts. Extrinsic materials such as furniture, carpets, plants, or equipment import volatile organic compounds, formaldehyde, dusts, odors, or other materials.[37]

The health effects of indoor-air microorganisms may be divided into five categories: (1) irritative symptoms, (2) respiratory infections, (3) allergic diseases, (4) alveolitis and organic dust toxic syndrome, and (5) other chronic pulmonary diseases such as chronic bronchitis.[38]

Microbial agents are viruses spread through human contact among occupants; bacteria spread in contaminated water or air conditioning systems; or fungi (molds). Legionnaires' disease can be spread through heating, air conditioning, and ventilation (HVAC) systems with improper sanitation. Viruses, especially the influenza virus, may transmit though a closed building filled with workers. Molds are ubiquitous throughout any building. However, in certain conditions of heat and humidity, molds may grow on cellulose in construction materials or in other areas where nutrients are available. Fungus can cause disease through the allergic response, mycoses, irritation, and mycotoxicosis.[38–40]

Toxigenic species of *Aspergillus, Stachybotrys,* and *Penicillium* have been associated with BRI. Dried, their parts may cause alveolitis or hypersensitive reactions. Most dangerous, however, are the mycotoxins produced by these species. For example, *Stachybotrys chartarum* conidia produce a mycotoxin that inhibits RNA, DNA, and protein synthesis, and produce a syndrome mimicking radiation poisoning. Rashes, epilation, leukopenia, diarrhea, visual disturbances, and immune impairment are common in persons exposed to the mycotoxin of this mold.[38,40]

Noise can produce headache and other symptoms attributed to other causes of BRI. Poor acoustics, noise-producing equipment (dot matrix printers), or poor office design may result in as much noise as in a factory.[41]

Factors contributing to mass psychogenic hysteria include job stress, dissatisfaction with a supervisor, job monotony, repetitive work, and lack of influence in management. Other factors include the observation or rumors of illness in a coworker attributable to real or imagined BRI.[42]

Sick-building syndrome has been attributed by some authorities to causes not associated with BRI, such as ventilation, microorganisms, or contaminants. Some authorities have suggested this self-limiting disorder is related to levels of substances below the levels of detection, individual susceptibility, or large numbers of people working in close proximity.[35]

Diagnosis

The diagnosis is often made on clinical-epidemiologic-industrial hygiene grounds. Symptoms include dry, itching or irritated eyes, sore or dry throat, stuffy or runny nose, sinus congestion, cough, wheezing, shortness of breath, chest tightness, headache, unusual tiredness, fatigue, difficulty remembering or concentrating, dizziness or light-headedness, dry or itchy skin, and a rash. Signs may include a rash around the neck and on the chest, conjunctivitis, and wheezing. Epidemiologic studies may include cluster analysis and cohort studies. Industrial hygiene studies may include air sampling techniques, swab and wipe samples, and cultures.[43,44]

A precise diagnosis may require an intense review of the clinical course, past medical records, industrial hygiene reports, and a careful physical examination. Laboratory testing includes hypersensitive panels and IgG and IgE studies to *Stachybotrys* or other molds that may have been discovered in the building.[45]

Treatment

Treatment includes steroids, bronchodilators, and psychotherapy, depending on the causative agent, the body's immune reaction, and the presenting clinical picture. Removal from exposure, that is, removal from the building until remediation of the exposure, is the first step.[46]

References

1. Collins G. Examining the "occupational" in occupational medicine. J Occup Med 1984;26:509–12.
2. World Health Organization. Early detection of health impairment in occupational exposures to health hazards. Technical report series No. 571. Geneva: WHO, 1975.
3. Lessenger JE. Occupational medicine: an overview for the family physician. Fam Pract Recert 2000;22:81–96.
4. Dickerson OB, Zens C, eds. Occupational medicine, 3rd ed. Chicago: Mosby-Year Book, 1994.
5. Rom WN, ed. Environmental and occupational medicine. Philadelphia: Lippincott Williams & Wilkins, 1998.
6. LaDou J, ed. Occupational and environmental medicine, 2nd ed. Stanford, CT: Lange, 1997.
7. Lessenger JE, Giebel HN. An analysis of 2846 industrial illnesses and injuries seen in a family practice. Fam Pract Res J 1992;12:271–81.
8. Harris JS. Occupational medicine practice guidelines. Boston: OEM Press, 1997.
9. Schuman SH, Mohr LJ, Simpson WM. A clinical guide to the occupational and environmental medicine patient in a busy family practice: the two-task, four-prototype approach in the SC/EHAP initiative. J Occup Environ Med 1997;39:1191–4.
10. Equal Employment Opportunity Commission. Technical assistance manual on the employment of the Americans with Disabilities Act. Washington: EEOC, 1992.
11. Harber PH, Hsu P, Chen W. An "atomic" approach to dis/ability assessment. J Occup Environ Med 1996;38:359–66.
12. Halperin WE, Ratcliffe J, Frazier TM, Wilson L, Becker SP, Schulte PA. Medical screening in the workplace: proposed principles. J Occup Med 1986;28:547–52.
13. Schilling RSF. The role of medical examination in protecting worker health. J Occup Med 1986;28:553–7.
14. Himmelstein J, Andersson GBJ. Low back pain: risk evaluation and preplacement screening. Occup Med State of the Art Rev 1988;3:255–69.
15. Cohen JE, Goel V, Frank JW, Gibson ES. Predicting risk of back injuries, work absenteeism, and chronic disability. J Occup Environ Med 1994;36:1093–9.
16. Wyman DO. Evaluating patients for return to work. Am Fam Physician 1999;59:844–8.
17. Rothstein MA. Medical screening of workers. Washington, DC: Bureau of National Affairs, 1986.
18. Kakaiya R, Fulkerson P. Medical evaluation for driver qualification for patients with cardiovascular disorders. J Am Board Fam Pract 2000;13:261–7.
19. Council on Social Issues, American College of Occupational Medicine. Drug screening in the workplace: ethical guidelines. J Occup Med 1991;33:651–2.
20. Vogl WF, Bush DM. Medical review officer manual for federal workplace drug testing programs, Center for Substance Abuse Prevention technical report no. 15. Washington, DC: Department of Health and Human Services, 1997.
21. El Sohly M, Jones AB. Drug testing in the workplace: could a positive test for one of the mandated drugs be for reasons other than illicit use of a drug? J Anal Toxicol 1995;19:450–8.
22. Herzstein JA, Bunn WB, Fleming LE, Harrington JM, Jeyaratnam J, Gardner IR. International occupational and environmental medicine. St. Louis: Mosby, 1998.
23. Lessenger JE. Case report: fraudulent pesticide injury: value of the work site visit. J Agromed 1996;3:27–32.
24. Greenberg MI, Hamilton RJ, Phillips SD. Occupational, industrial and environmental toxicology. St Louis: Mosby, 1997.
25. Lloyd GG, Doyle Y, Grance C. Medical implications of employee assistance programmes. Occup Med (Lond) 1999;49:193–5.

26. Guidotti TL, Cowell JWF, Jamieson GG. Occupational health services: a practical approach. Chicago: American Medical Association, 1989.
27. Lessenger JE, Riley N. Neurotoxicities and behavioral changes in a 12-year old male exposed to dicofol, an organochloride pesticide. J Toxicol Environ Health 1991;33:255–61.
28. Lessenger JE. The office evaluation of the pesticide injured worker. J Am Board Fam Pract 1993;6:33–41.
29. Lessenger JE, Reese BE. Rational use of cholinesterase testing in pesticide poisoning. J Am Board Fam Pract 1999;12:307–14.
30. Lessenger JE. A rash and chemical burns in a cowboy exposed to permethrin. J Agromed 1995;2:25–8.
31. Lessenger JE, Estock MD, Younglove T. An analysis of 190 cases of suspected pesticide poisoning. J Am Board Fam Pract 1995;8:278–82.
32. Lessenger JE. Case report: multiple system illness in a woman exposed to aluminum phosphide. J Agromed 1999;6:25–31.
33. Lessenger JE. Case report: fraudulent pesticide injury: value of the work site visit. J Agromed 1996;3:27–32.
34. Menzies D, Bourbeau J. Building-related illnesses. N Engl J Med 1997;337:1524–31.
35. Redlich CA, Sparer J, Cullen MR. Sick-building syndrome. Lancet 1997;349:1013–16.
36. Crawford JO, Bolas SM. Sick building syndrome, work factors and occupational stress. Scand J Work Environ Health 1996; 22:243–50.
37. Oliver LC, Shackleton BW. The indoor air we breathe. Public Health Rep 1999;113:398–409.
38. Husman T. Health effects of indoor-air microorganisms. Scand J Work Environ Health 1996;22:5–13.
39. Rowan NJ, Johnstone CM, McLean RC, Anderson JG, Clarke JA. Prediction of toxigenic fungal growth in buildings by using a novel modelling system. Appl Environ Microbiol 1999;65: 4814–21.
40. Sudakin DL. Toxigenic fungi in a water-damaged building: an intervention study. Am J Ind Med 1998;34:183–90.
41. Yassi A, Pollock N, Tran N, Cheang M. Risk to hearing from a rock concert. Can Fam Physician 1993;39:1045–50.
42. Ford CV. Somatization and fashionable diagnoses: illness as a way of life. Scand J Work Environ Health 1997;23(suppl 3):7–16.
43. Linz DH, Pinney SM, Keller JD, White M, Buncher CR. Cluster analysis applied to building-related illness. J Occup Environ Health 1998;40:165–71.
44. Hodgson MJ, Morey P, Leung W-Y, et al. Building-associated pulmonary disease from exposure to *Stachybotrys chartarum* and *Aspergillus versicolor*. J Occup Environ Health 1998;40: 241–49.
45. Johanning E, Biagini R, Hull D, Morey P, Jarvis B, Landsbergis P. Health and immunology study following exposure to toxigenic fungi (*Stachybotrys chartarum*) in a water-damaged office environment. Int Arch Occup Environ Health 1996;68: 207–18.
46. Flappan SM, Portnoy J, Jomes P, Barnes C. Infant pulmonary hemorrhage in a suburban home with water damage and mold (*Stachybotrys atra*). Environ Health Perspec 1999;107:927–30.

46
Problems Related to Physical Agents

James E. Lessenger

Heat Injuries

Military personnel, athletes, the young, the elderly, and persons with emphysema, diabetes, or heart, neurovascular, or kidney disease are particularly susceptible to heat. Workers in the fields of mining, drilling, transportation, and construction are also at risk. Drugs such as amphetamines, cocaine, and anticholinergics decrease sweating, placing people at increased risk. Good conditioning, proper clothing, adequate rest, avoidance of the sun, and drinking lots of water (not sodas, tea, or coffee) will decrease risk. Acclimatization by graded increasing activity in warm environments under controlled conditions can be particularly useful in athletes, military recruits, and miners. Special precautions to protect the elderly and other persons at risk during heat waves may be necessary, particularly if there is also high humidity.

Heat Exhaustion
Pathogenesis

Heat emergencies occur when the body is unable to adequately dissipate heat resulting from the metabolic and environmental sources. The hypothalamus controls thermoregulation by reducing vasoconstriction, increasing blood flow to the skin. Dissipation of heat occurs through radiation, conduction, convection, and evaporation of sweat. At environmental temperatures above 35°C (95°F) most body heat is lost through sweating, which becomes inefficient when humidity rises above 75%. Doppler studies of patients with heatstroke and heat exhaustion demonstrate changes reflecting a hyperdynamic circulation with tachycardia and high cardiac output. Relative hypovolemia is more pronounced in patients with heatstroke compared to patients with heat exhaustion. Signs of peripheral vasoconstriction are more often present in heatstroke, while patients with heat exhaustion more often demonstrated peripheral vasodilation.

Clinical Presentation

Typically, there is a history of heavy exertion in heat with inadequate water intake. Symptoms of heat injuries include headache, dizziness, nausea, vomiting, muscle weakness, visual disturbances, and flushing. Clinical findings include profuse sweating, warm moist pale skin, and tachycardia. Laboratory analysis will usually demonstrate dehydration, metabolic acidosis, increased glucose and ferritin, and a mild increase in creatine kinase, aspartate transaminase, and lactate dehydrogenase.

Treatment

In the field, the goal is to decrease the core temperature and rehydrate by loosening clothing, moistening the face, removing the injured person to the shade, providing rest, and giving oral fluids until the person urinates. In the hospital, findings of hemoconcentration, hypernatremia, and azotemia are common and treatment should commence before laboratory results are available. An air-conditioned emergency room should cool the patient adequately, but moist cool towels on the forehead and around the flank may be necessary. Hypoglycemia may be present and require correction.[1–4]

Heat Stroke
Pathogenesis

As the core body temperature rises and heat dissipation mechanisms fail, metabolic demand increases and energy stores fail. Cellular enzyme systems fail, cell membrane permeability increases, and shock follows. People with exertional heat stroke have high blood flow to exercising muscles, which overloads the body's cooling mechanisms. In the elderly, severe heat exposure during heat waves leads to progressive dehydration.

Clinical Presentation

Usually, there is a history of acute changes of mental status change after exertion in hot weather. Examination of the patient demonstrates tachycardia, hypotension, and tachypnea. Core temperature is usually at least 40.5°C (105°F) but may lower with cooling during examination. Neurologic signs include irritability, confusion, ataxia, seizures, decorticate posturing, and coma. In the elderly, coma may be the presenting condition. The skin is usually dry and hot due to vasoconstriction. Cardiovascular collapse and disseminated intravascular coagulation may progress in severe and advanced cases. A complete blood count, liver and renal panels, cardiac isoenzymes, and arterial blood bases are needed to assess the extent of dehydration and acid–base balance. Coagulation studies may be abnormal and urine analysis may demonstrate concentration and urine myoglobin.

Differential Diagnosis

Illegal and prescription drug overdose, homicidal or suicidal poisoning, stroke, and myocardial infarction may mimic heatstroke.

Treatment

In the field, it is critical to decrease core temperature by removing unnecessary clothing, spraying the face with lukewarm water, augmenting airflow, and providing oral fluids, if the person is conscious. During transport, oxygen and respirator support may be necessary. Intravenous diazepam may be necessary to control seizures. In the hospital, cardiopulmonary status needs to be quickly evaluated and maintained. Immediate venous access must be achieved and volume depletion corrected with dextrose/normal saline or dextrose/half-normal saline. Core temperature and urine output must be monitored. Evaporative cooling through sprayed lukewarm water and fans may be necessary to decrease the temperature, but care must be taken to avoid overcooling. Shivering, which increases body temperature, should be avoided and diazepam (Valium), 2 to 5 mg given orally or intramuscularly, may be needed. Hypoglycemia, if present, must be corrected. Blood coagulation disturbances may need correction with fresh frozen plasma and platelets.

Long-Term Complications

Renal, hepatic, myocardial, and cerebral complications such as coma, stupor, or stroke may be transitory or long term, depending on the age of the person, preexisting conditioning, and the depth of the heatstroke.[1–3]

Cold Injuries

Occupations with exposure to cold, winter athletic activities, outdoor youth outings, and winter military operations present greater risk of cold injuries. Alcoholics, the elderly, disabled persons, troops in combat, and people with diabetes and heart disease are more susceptible. Medications, especially cardiac and antipsychotic, reduce cold tolerance. Alcoholic drinks increase heat loss from the body due to vasodilation.

Careful attention to the early warning signs of shivering, poor coordination, and lethargy can allow identification of the problem before it advances. Multiple layers of clothing, removal of wet clothing, warm fluids, and shelter can be lifesaving. Altitude and cold acclimation as well as general fitness is important, especially in industries such as logging and mining. In the elderly and those taking cardiac and antihypertensive medications, altitude acclimation is particular important.

Hypothermia
Pathogenesis

Metabolism is the source of body heat in cold environments. Moisture and perspiration increase heat loss through convection and evaporation. Reduction of core temperature below 35°C (95°F) can occur in air temperatures up to 18.3°C (65°F) and water temperatures up to 22.2°C (72°F). Maintenance and restoration of the core temperature is the key to prevention and treatment.

Clinical Presentation

Typically, there is a history of exposure to cold ambient temperatures, inadequate clothing, preexisting medical conditions, medications, or drug abuse. Early symptoms include drowsiness, slurred speech, impaired coordination, weakness, and lethargy. The patient may have puffy, cool skin.

Late symptoms include lethargy, stupor, unconsciousness, and diminished reflexes. The person may have weak or absent pulse, hypotension, slow respiratory rate, and decreased esophageal or rectal temperature of 25° to 35°C (77°–95°F). The complete blood count, chemistries, thyroid studies, arterial blood gases, electrocardiogram (J wave at QRS-ST) and chest radiograph may demonstrate dysrhythmias, dehydration, or pneumonia.

Treatment

In the field, rewarming can be accomplished with electric blankets, sleeping bags, radiant heaters, or heated stones in sleeping bags. Warm (not hot) fluids given slowly and a change to warm, dry clothing can accelerate recovery. Alcoholic drinks are contraindicated because they cause vasodilation and increase heat loss.

In the emergency department, the patient should be rewarmed slowly over a period of 2 to 3 hours to avoid rewarming shock. Rehydration and correction of acid-base and electrolyte imbalances need to be carried out concomitant with rewarming. Inhaled warm oxygen, if available, may be helpful. Peritoneal dialysis with lactated Ringer's at 43°C exchanged at a rate of 10 to 12 L/h may be needed in severe cases. Warm baths, if used, should be maintained at 40° to 42°C.

Frostbite
Pathogenesis

As the skin temperature drops due to exposure or contact with extremely cold surfaces such as snow, perfusion slows, allowing for crystal formation in the extremities, ears, and nose. At 15°C there is tissue damage due to thrombosis and ischemia. At −3°C there is actual freezing of tissue. There are marked similarities in the inflammatory processes to those seen in thermal burns and ischemia/reperfusion injury. Recently, frostbite has been seen in the close application of unpadded chemical ice packs to orthopedically injured extremities.

Clinical Presentation

In mild cases, numbness, prickling, and itching of the skin may be present. In severe cases there may be paresthesia, stiffness, and pale white edematous skin. As the skin thaws, severe pain typically results, followed by chronic paresthesia in severe cases.

Differential Diagnosis

Frostbite may mimic vibration-induced white finger disease (common in construction industries where pneumatic hammers are used) and Raynaud's phenomenon (see Chapter 113).

Treatment

Replacement of wet clothing with dry and warm clothing will accelerate recovery. Rewarming can be accomplished by contact with warm skin or cloth, but massaging and rubbing is best avoided. In severe cases the physician must decide if refreezing is likely before rewarming because repeated cycles of freezing and thawing will rupture more cells and extend injury. Slow rewarming is accomplished by placing the extremity in water at 40° to 42°C until thawed (it will hurt) and leaving clothing open to the air. Eventual amputations and grafts may be needed.

Chilblains

Pathogenesis

Prolonged dry cold exposure causes capillary breakdown and extravasation of fluids.

Clinical Presentation

Typically, there are red, pruritic skin lesions associated with edema that may progress to ulcerations with eventual scarring.

Treatment

Elevation of the extremity, gentle rewarming, and exposure to warm room temperature usually restores capillary function. Skin massage is contraindicated.

Immersion Foot (Trench Foot, Shelter Leg)

Pathogenesis

Prolonged immersion in cold water causes capillary breakdown, edema, and ischemia.

Diagnosis

In the ischemic (immediate) phase, feet are cold, swollen, and waxen in appearance. In the hyperemic phase (2 to 3 days after exposure), there is intense pain, swelling, redness, blistering, lymphangitis, and ecchymosis. In the posthyperemic phase (10 to 30 days), there are paresthesias, temperature sensitivity, and hyperhidrosis. In severe cases, cellulitis, gangrene, and thrombophlebitis may be present.

Treatment

The patient must be thoroughly dried and slowly warmed with attention to general nutrition. Treatment of bacterial and fungal infections may be difficult and require repeated therapies.[4–6]

Ionizing Radiation Injuries

Particulate radiation consists of electrons, protons, neutrons, alpha particles, and other subatomic particles. Natural background radiation comes from cosmic rays, thorium, radium, and other radionuclides in the earth's crust and potassium 40, carbon 14, and other naturally occurring radioactive elements in the body.

The rad is the standard unit of absorbed dose (1 rad = 100 erg/kg tissue). One rem is that dose of any radiation that produces a biologic effect equivalent to 1 rad of x- or y-rays. Collectively, a person living at sea level may receive about 80 mrem per year. Persons living at high altitude or near deposits of radioactive ores receive twice that amount.

Man-made sources account for an estimated 106 mrem per person per year from global fallout, nuclear power, diagnostic procedures, radiopharmaceuticals, smoke detectors, color television sets, phosphate fertilizers, and instrument dials. The average chest x-ray exposure is 10 mrem; the average barium enema exposes one to 500 to 800 mrem.

Radiation loses energy as it penetrates tissue and interacts with atoms in its path. The removal of electrons from atoms results in the formation of ions and reactive radicals. These, in turn, cause damage to molecules through breakage of chemical bonds. Molecular injury may result in DNA, enzyme, or structural damage.

The biologic consequences of exposure to ionizing radiation include gene mutation, chromosome aberrations, malignant transformation, and cell death. Cellular damage may occur in somatic or germ cells. Genetic effects are a result of damage to germ cells, while somatic effects may be seen acutely, chronically, or delayed. Rapidly dividing germ and bone marrow cells are more acutely susceptible.[7,8]

Acute and Chronic Radiation Sickness

Nuclear Attack

At 8:15 A.M. local time on August 6, 1945, a uranium atomic bomb was detonated 580 m over Hiroshima, Japan. Initial radiation was composed of gamma rays and neutrons spread out at detonation. Residual radiation consisted of products of nuclear fission that fell to the earth as "death ash" or "black rain" and radiation caused by the bombardment of the ground and concrete buildings by neutrons.

Acute effects included fever, bloody diarrhea, weakness, exhaustion, vomiting, hemoptysis, hematemesis, hematuria, nose bleeds, and subcutaneous hemorrhage. Pathologic examination revealed destruction of bone marrow, leukopenia, anemia, and decrease of platelets in direct proportion to how close the person was to the hypocenter. Many deaths in this period were due to sepsis and destruction of endocrine function.

Subacute effects were mainly to the bone marrow and endocrine system. Hemorrhaging, epilation, sepsis, adrenal dysfunction, and aspermia occurred in severity proportional to the distance from the hypocenter. Death from pneumonia was common. Recovery was marked by regrowth of hair and skin and healing of infections.

Late effects over a period of 50 years included increases in malignant tumors (especially leukemias of all types, cataracts, chromosome aberrations, somatic cell mutations, mental retardation, growth retardation, and functional abnormalities to organs, especially glands. There was no increase in leukemia, sterility or congenital abnormalities in children born to survivors more than 9 months after the attack.[9]

Nuclear Accident

During the overnight hours of April 25 to 26, 1986, reactor 4 of the Chernobyl nuclear plant in the Ukraine exploded and released an estimated 300 MCi (megacuries) of radioactive substances, including 40 MCi of iodine 131 and 100 MCi of short-lived radioiodines. There were 143 cases of acute radiation syndrome similar to those seen in Hiroshima. There were 34 deaths, primarily in firefighters who received massive doses of radiation and died of radiation burns, sepsis, and multiorgan failure. Survivors demonstrated chronic leukopenia, lens opacities, and other problems similar to those of the Hiroshima survivors.[10]

Tens of thousands of persons were exposed to various amounts of radionucleotide, primarily I 131. The radioactive debris spread throughout Belarus, northern Ukraine, western Russia, parts of eastern Europe, and Scandinavia. The threat of thyroid cancer from the I 131 was immediately recognized and 16 million people were given potassium iodine to prevent the uptake of I 131 by the thyroid. Nevertheless, thousands of children in Belarus and northern Ukraine developed thyroid cancer. The problem was probably exacerbated by a chronic iodine deficiency that hastened the uptake of the I 131. Epidemiologic studies documented an increased incidence of all cancers, including leukemias of all types within the former Soviet Union, but not Europe. Children who had been exposed in utero demonstrated extremity agenesis and mental retardation. Chromosomal aberrations in the exposed populations have been reported, but their long-term consequences remain to be seen.[11–13]

Prevention

Limitation of the use of medical x-rays and nuclear medicine studies is prudent. Proper handling of radioactive materials, shielding of workers and the public, protective clothing, and proper handling procedures are critical to prevent exposure. In the event of a spill, evacuation and isolation of the problem are essential and a detailed advanced safety plan may be lifesaving.[14]

Treatment

The exposed person must decontaminated immediately. Contaminated body parts should be isolated with plastic wraps. Clothing constitutes contaminated material and needs to be disposed of as nuclear waste. Burns and trauma are treated in the usual manner, concurrent with decontamination. In the event of I 131 release, iodine supplements should be given as soon as possible, especially to children. Cataracts usually require lens implants. Leukopenia may require antibiotic prophylaxis and treatment and perhaps bone marrow transplants. Cancers induced by radiation are indistinguishable from those occurring naturally and are treated using standard protocols. Acute radiation sickness may require aggressive supportive medical care including cardiopulmonary assist, intravenous fluids, antibiotics, and antiemetics.[15]

Nonionizing Radiation Injuries

Radiofrequency (RF) and Microwave (MW) Radiation

Radiofrequency and microwave radiation causes molecular ionization by vibration and rotation of molecules, particularly those with asymmetric charges. The risk of injury increases with increased radiation intensity and proximity of the source.

Injuries are typically seen in employees working with or maintaining equipment used in sealing plastics, physiotherapy, and radio communications. Injuries are characterized by protein denaturation and tissue necrosis at the site of exposure. There is an inflammatory reaction usually followed by scar formation. Nonthermal effects include cataracts.

The exposed body part feels hot with a clicking or buzzing sensation and a sunburned appearance. Other symptoms include irritability, headache, pain, watery eyes, dysphagia, anorexia, abdominal cramps, and nausea.

Infrared Radiation

Exposures to infrared radiation (wavelengths of 750 to 3 million nm) occur in welders, glassmakers, and bakers of consumer products. Thermal injury to the skin is common but the cornea, iris, and lens are most susceptible. Eye and skin shielding is the major protection.

Visible Radiation

Visible light (wavelengths of 400 to 750 nm) causes damage via structural, thermal, and photochemical light-induced reactions. The eye is the most sensitive organ. Sources of injury are sunlight, high-intensity lamps, lasers, flashbulbs, spotlights, and welding.

Ultraviolet (UV) Radiation

The longer wavelengths of ultraviolet radiation (wavelengths from 100 to 400 nm) are more biologically active. Eye injuries from thermal action and skin damage from photochemical reactions are most common. Injuries are found in welding, and using specialized photo imaging equipment and germicidal units.[16–19]

Lasers

Electrical energy is applied to a crystal or gas to produce a coherent, monochromatic, and highly collimated light in a narrow beam and in the same plane of polarization. The resulting light beam (laser) can be of extremely high intensity and is usually in the UV range.

Lasers cause damage, primarily to the eye and skin, by photochemical and mechanical mechanisms, especially coagulation of retinal proteins. The increased temperatures may cause explosive vaporization of cells. In the eye, retinal burns and corneal injuries are most common, and thermal burns predominate on the skin.[20]

Treatment of Nonionizing Radiation Injuries

Photokeratoconjunctivitis (Welder's Flash)

Symptoms of severe pain, photophobia, tearing, and the sensation of sand in the eyes follow exposure by 6 to 12 hours. A single short exposure may provoke symptoms, but increases in duration and intensity shorten the latency period and increase the symptoms. The eyelids may be red and swollen, and examination of the eye may be normal or reveal punctuate staining of the cornea. The problem is typically bilateral. Treatment is symptomatic with cold packs, eye patches, mild sedation, and dark rooms. Ophthalmic anesthetics are discouraged.

Skin lesions vary from erythema to frank bullae formation. These are usually treated similarly to sunburn and there may be a resultant "toughening" of the skin. Extensive burns may produce systemic responses such as shock. Phototoxic and photoallergic reactions commonly occur with medications, bacteriostatic agents, and perfumes. Premalignant and malignant skin lesions including actinic keratosis, keratoacanthoma, and Hutchinson's melanosis are common. Progression to basal cell carcinoma, squamous cell carcinoma, and malignant melanoma is common. The risk is greater in fair-skinned people.[21]

Prevention of Nonionizing Radiation Injuries

Training of workers, supervisors, and users in the proper use of equipment and safety measures, with instructions and labels followed carefully, is essential. Shielding of equipment to prevent emissions, proper maintenance, adjustment of equipment, safety clothing, sun blocking creams, and, most importantly, safety glasses are essential.[16,20,21]

Electrical Injury

Outdoor risks include lightning strikes and hanging wires after disasters. Home risks include faulty appliances, children who place fingers into sockets, frayed wires, and home repair of appliances. Occupational risks affect electricians, high-voltage repair workers, and maintenance personnel.

Prevention strategies include training to avoid dangling live wires, taking cover during lightning storms, proper repair of equipment, shielding of equipment and use of protective tools and clothing.[22,23]

Pathogenesis

Alternating current produces more injury than direct current because it causes muscle tetanization. Current as low as 60 to 80 mA will cause ventricular fibrillation. The greater the voltage and longer the duration, the greater the damage. Shocks exceeding 10,000 volts will usually throw the person off the cable or machine when touched or grabbed, causing blunt trauma.

Electric current follows the course of least resistance, usually through water-laden tissues. Therefore, the vascular system is most at risk, and bone is least at risk. Circular or elliptical thermal burns may occur at entrance and exit sites, and tissue necrosis and thrombosis may occur in muscles and vessels. Muscle destruction may result in necrosis and myoglobulinuria, with the potential of renal compromise. Depolarization of peripheral nerves and the brain may produce tetany and seizures. Renal and liver damage may occur as a consequence of electrocution and blunt trauma may result from falling or being thrown.[22,23]

Clinical Findings

Burns, blunt trauma, and ventricular fibrillation may be present. An electrocardiogram (ECG) should be performed to look for changes in cardiac conduction. Tetany of the diaphragm may lead to respiratory arrest. The patient may be postictal from seizures. Renal and hepatic function may be impaired.[22–24]

Treatment

Careful attention to live wires will protect rescuers from injury. Cardiopulmonary resuscitation is performed in the standard fashion. In the hospital, massive muscle necrosis may necessitate close renal observation, and lactated Ringer's or saline solution may be necessary to maintain urine output. Cardiac dysrhythmias are treated in the usual manner. Burns and tissue destruction may require aggressive debridement and grafts.[24,25]

Inhalation Injury

Pathogenesis

The sheer volume of inspired air makes the lungs a sensitive organ for environmental damage. Inhalation of toxic substances produces disease depending on the phase (liquid, particulate, or gaseous), temperature, duration of exposure, density, and inherent toxicity of the substance and on the health of the individual. Defense mechanisms against inhalation or inspiration of gases or dusts include the nose, pharynx, and larynx, which block entry, removal by the mucous blanket and cilia, and alveolar macrophages. Only a small number of particles penetrate into the distal bronchioles and persist in the interstitium. Highly soluble gases such as ozone, ammonia, and sulfur dioxide can be readily removed by the upper airways, but only at low concentrations. Large particles fail to enter the airways while small ones are easily expired. Particles of a critical density and "dynamic radius" remain in the bronchioles to cause pathologic changes.

Toxic injury can cause cell degeneration and necrosis, leading to sloughing of the airway. Acute alveolar injury is also accompanied by a massive pulmonary edema created by the extravasation of fluids from damaged capillaries. In the alveoli, type I pneumocytes are most susceptible, followed by secretory cells and brush cells. Repair begins with a fibrin meshwork containing necrotic cellular debris and neutrophilic infiltrate. Smaller airways follow the same sequence as larger airways. The cycle of destruction and repair causes fibrosis in the upper airways, lower airways, and alveoli depending on the parameters of exposure.[26,27]

Population at Risk

People may be exposed to toxic gases in disasters such as earthquakes and explosions, but occupational exposure is most common, especially in foundries, chemical plants, agriculture and welding operations. Firefighters and emergency medical technicians (EMTs) are especially at risk as first responders.[25,27]

Prevention

Shielding and proper ventilation can prevent employee exposure by removing the agent. Protective equipment at the workplace with attention to a properly fitted mask and correct filter canister can prevent short- and long-term problems. Conditioning and health maintenance prevent fatigue that can lead to injury. Isolation of disasters and evacuation is crucial before clouds engulf large numbers of people.[26–28]

Agents Causing Toxic Lung Injury

Phosgene and chlorine cause intense airway irritation. Oxides of nitrogen liberated by anaerobic microbial fermentation in silos cause alveolar injury with pulmonary edema and hyaline membrane dysfunction. In industry, oxides of nitrogen are used in metals production, with welders in confined spaces particularly at risk. Sulfur dioxide and sulfuric acid cause acute bronchitis, bronchiolitis, and alveolar injury. Cadmium and metal fume fever in machinists and welders cause alveolar damage as well as systemic symptoms such as fever and malaise. Paraquat, a herbicide used to spray marijuana patches in the 1970s, cause intense lung necrosis and fibrosis. Ozone causes damage to bronchial columnar cells and alveoli. Butylate hydroxytoluene, used in food production, can cause alveolar injury.[26,27]

Products of combustion are a special problem. Burning materials aerosolize large amounts of particulates and release hot gases, which can be chemically transformed. Large amounts of hot carbon monoxide, hydrogen cyanide, nitrogen dioxide, and aldehydes enter the respiratory tract, causing burns to upper airways and intense tissue necrosis and pulmonary edema to lower airways.

Transient hypoxemia has been found in firefighters exposed to polyvinyl chloride and other pulmonary irritants. This is thought to be due to a breakdown in the oxygen-carrying capacity of the alveolar membranes.[26]

Clinical Findings

Mild cases may present with transient shortness of breath and vertigo. More severe exposures will present with respiratory distress, pulmonary edema, and burns around the mouth and nose. Changes in chest radiographs and blood gases may be evident.

Treatment

Mild cases of inhalation injury may require only observation and oxygen. Moderate cases may require antibiotics, steroids, and bronchodilators. More severe cases will require intense pulmonary support, intubation, respirators, and medications in an intensive care unit with specialist backup. Early bronchoscopy may be necessary to assess damage and monitor treatment.[29,30]

Long-Term Complications

Obstruction and restrictive pulmonary disease with air trapping and bronchiectasis are commonly found after severe inhalation injuries.[30]

Acoustic Trauma (Noise)

Noise accounts for about one fifth of all hearing loss. Sound or noise is a form of energy transmitted through air in the form of waves. The decibel (dB) is an arbitrary sound-pressure measurement used to express intensity of sound. Frequency, expressed as the hertz (Hz), is given in cycles per second and expresses pitches or tones. Typical noise generators are impact or shear among solids (machinery), fluid jets (jet engines), pressure pulses (sirens), and secondary excitation (sounding boards).[31] An interaction between noise and chemical exposures in the workplace can accelerate hearing loss.

There are two main mechanisms for measuring acoustic trauma. The dosimeter measures instantaneous or fluctuating noise levels over time, and the audiogram measures noise effects on the ear.[32]

Exposure is measured by the dose concept (i.e., intensity multiplied by time). In industry, two measurements of dose are used to evaluate risk: the time weighted average (TWA), a measure of exposure over the workday (85 dB), and the permissible exposure limit (PEL), the maximum noise level a person can be exposed to at any given time (95 dB).[32]

Population at Risk

Noise-induced hearing loss is of particular interest in industry, but natural disasters, inadvertent exposure to loud noises such as a gunshot, and deliberate exposure to loud noises such as rock bands, can cause temporary or permanent damage. Temporary noise damage causes a temporary threshold shift (TTS) in hearing, while permanent damage causes a permanent threshold shift (PTS).[32,33]

Prevention

Prevention is targeted at avoidance, equipment engineering controls, and personal protective equipment. Avoidance of noise is accomplished by keeping unauthorized people out of areas of high noise exposure such as areas near airports. Individuals can protect themselves by avoiding sound that causes pain or ringing in the ears such as rock bands. Engineering controls include the design of equipment low in noise production or which shields workers and bystanders. Personal protective measures include ear muffs and plugs, which are especially important at firing ranges.

Treatment

Audiologic monitoring identifies workers who may have a TTS or incipient PTS so that programs can be implemented to limit exposure. Other causes of deafness such as infections and tumors need to be identified and treated appropriately. Permanent loss may necessitate rehabilitation in the form of hearing aids or training of the deaf.[34,35]

References

1. Donoghue AM, Sinclair MJ, Bates GP. Heat exhaustion in a deep underground metalliferous mine. Occup Environ Med 2000; 57:165–74.
2. Semenza JC, McCullough JE, Flanders WD, McGeehin MA, Lumpkin JR. Excess hospital admissions during the July 1995 heat wave in Chicago. Am J Prev Med 1999;16:269–77.
3. Shahid MS, Hatle L, Mansour H, Mimish L. Echocardiographic and Doppler study of patients with heatstroke and heat exhaustion. Int J Card Imaging 1999;15:279–85.
4. Bracker MD. Environmental and thermal injury. Clin Sports Med 1992;11:419–36.
5. Smith JH, ed. Committee on Sports Medicine. Sports medicine: health care for young athletes. Evanston: American Academy of Pediatrics, 1983.
6. Murphy JV, Banwell PE, Roberts AH, McGrouther DA. Frostbite: pathogenesis and treatment. J Trauma 2000;48:171–8.
7. Mottet NK. Environmental pathology. New York: Oxford University Press, 1985.
8. Wright EG. Inducible genomic instability: new insights into the biological effects of ionizing radiation. Med Confl Surviv 2000;16:117–30.
9. Shigematsu I, Ito C, Kamada N, Akiyama M, Sasaki H. Effects of A-bomb radiation on the human body. Switzerland: Harwood Academic, 1995.
10. Robbins J. Lessons from Chernobyl: the event, the aftermath fallout: radioactive, political, social. Thyroid 1997;7:189–92.
11. Krissenko N. Overview of 1993 research activities in Belarus related to the Chernobyl accident. Stem Cells 1997;15(suppl 2): 207–10.
12. Sali D, Cardis E, Sztanyik L, et al. Cancer consequences of the Chernobyl accident in Europe outside the former USSR: a review. Int J Cancer 1996;67:343–52.
13. van Hoff J, Averkin YI, Hilchenko EI, Prudyvus IS. Epidemiology of childhood cancer in Belarus: review of data 1978–1994, and discussion of the new Belarusian Childhood Cancer Registry. Stem Cells 1997;15(suppl 2):231–41.
14. Recommendations of the International Commission on Radiological Protection. International Commission on Radiological Protection (IARP) publication 26. Oxford: Pergamon Press, 1977.
15. International Atomic Energy Agency. What the general practitioner (MD) should know about medical handling of overexposed individuals. IAEA-TEC DOC-366. Vienna: IAEA, 1986.
16. Meyer-Rochow VB. Risks, especially for the eye, emanating from the rise of solar UV-radiation in the Arctic and Antarctic regions. Int J Circumpolar Health 2000;59:38–51.
17. Krutman J. Ultraviolet A radiation-induced biological effects in human skin: relevance for photoimaging and photodermatosis. J Dermatol Sci 2000;23(suppl 1):S22–6.
18. Beers GJ. Biological effects of weak electromagnetic fields from 0 Hz to 200 Hz: a survey of the literature with special emphasis on possible magnetic resonance effects. Magn Reson Imaging 1989;7:309–31.
19. Lin RS, Dischinger PC, Conde J, Farrell KP. Occupational exposure to electromagnetic fields and the occurrence of brain tumors. J Occup Med 1985;27:413–9.
20. Barbanel CS, Ducatman AM, Garston MJ, Fuller T. Lazer hazards in research laboratories. J Occup Med 1993;35:369–74.
21. Michaelson SM. Influence of power frequency electric and magnetic fields on human health. Ann NY Acad Sci 1987;502: 55–75.
22. Fish R. Electric shock, part I: physics and pathophysiology. J Emerg Med 1993;11:309–12.
23. Fish R. Electric shock, part II: nature and mechanisms of injury. J Emerg Med 1993;11:393–6.
24. Fish R. Electric shock, part III: deliberately applied electric shocks and the treatment of electric injuries. J Emerg Med 1993; 11:599–603.
25. Fontanarosa PB. Electrical shock and lightning strike. Ann Emerg Med 1993;22(2 pt 2):378–87.
26. Kimmel EC, Still KR. Acute lung injury, acute respiratory distress syndrome and inhalation injury: an overview. Drug Chem Toxicol 1999;22:91–128.
27. Verdon ME. Common clinical presentations of occupational respiratory disorders. Am Fam Physician 1995;52:939–46.
28. Lee-Chiong TL. Smoke inhalation injury. Postgrad Med 1999; 105:55–62.
29. Macklem PT. The pathophysiology of chronic bronchitis and emphysema. Med Clinic North Am 1973;57:669–79.
30. Lentz CW, Peterson HD. Smoke inhalation is a multilevel insult to the pulmonary system. Curr Opin Pulmon Med 1997;3: 221–6.
31. Arslan E, Orzan E. Audiological management of noise induced hearing loss. Scand Audio Suppl 1998;48:131–45.
32. Morata TC. Assessing occupational hearing loss: beyond noise exposures. Scand Audio Suppl 1998;49:111–6.
33. Yassi A, Pollock N, Tran N, Cheang M. Risk to hearing from rock concert. Can Fam Physician 1993;39:1045–50.
34. Chen JT, Chiang HC, Chen SS. Effects of aircraft noise on hearing and auditory pathway function of airport employees. J Occup Med 1992;34:613–9.
35. May JJ. Occupational hearing loss. Am J Ind Med 2000;37: 112–6.

47
Bites and Stings

Laeth S. Nasir

Bites and stings account for a small but significant number of patients seen in the primary care setting. Family physicians can provide the patient, family, and community with anticipatory guidance regarding common hazards and appropriate care if a bite or sting does occur.

Mammalian Bites

Most mammalian bites are from dogs or cats. Children are the most frequent victims of dog bites.[1] Most of the dogs involved are known to the victim and were considered friendly prior to the biting episode. Injuries inflicted by cats tend to involve the hand and upper limb.

Clinical Presentation

Significant dog bites tend to be lacerations, often with crushing or tearing of tissue. Bites are most often sustained on the extremities, head, and neck. In children, dog bites may penetrate the skull. Because of their needle-like teeth, cat and rodent bites are usually puncture wounds, often involving tendons or joint spaces. A multitude of organisms reside in the mouths of all higher primates. For this reason, these bites are notoriously predisposed to infection. Human bite wounds most commonly result from conflict or contact sports. Potentially the most serious human bite wound is the "clenched-fist" injury. This injury is sustained when the victim strikes an adversary in the mouth with a clenched fist and suffers a laceration inflicted by the other's teeth. Microorganisms may be inoculated into the deep tissues of the hand, resulting in a devastating infection.

Diagnosis

All bites are examined meticulously for foreign bodies and devitalized tissue. Radiographs are considered if there is the possibility of fracture or a retained foreign body. The med-ical record should include information regarding the site, depth, and circumstances of the biting episode, as well as a sketch of the injury.

A clenched-fist injury should be examined after reproducing the position of the hand when the injury occurred. Otherwise, penetration of the wound into the deep tissues of the hand may not be appreciated.

Management

All mammalian bites should undergo copious irrigation with sterile saline. A 19-gauge or larger needle on a syringe is often used to generate a high pressure stream. Careful debridement of all devitalized tissue is necessary (see Chapter 49). Further management depends on classifying the wound as high risk or low risk for infection. There is general agreement that high-risk bites are those involving the hands or feet, injuries older than 6 to 12 hours, deep puncture wounds, crush injuries, human bites, cat bites, and bites sustained by elderly or immunocompromised individuals. Bites involving deep structures such as bones, joints, or tendons are also at high risk of infection. Individuals with high-risk bites should have their wounds debrided, packed, and reevaluated in 72 hours to consider delayed primary closure. Prophylactic antibiotics should be administered. In practice, many bites otherwise considered high risk are primarily repaired if functional or cosmetic considerations strongly warrant it. Deep puncture wounds, bites of the hand, and wounds that present late should never be closed primarily.[2] Bite wounds involving the deep tissues of the hand should be surgically debrided, packed, immobilized in the position of function, and elevated. These injuries require intravenous antibiotic therapy. Low-risk wounds may be sutured immediately; antibiotic prophylaxis is not required. Cultures of an uninfected wound are not useful.

Human bites may transmit hepatitis B and C as well as herpes simplex virus. Prophylaxis against hepatitis B may be achieved by administering hepatitis B immune globulin (HBIg) 0.06 mL/kg and hepatitis B vaccine. The potential for human immunodeficiency virus (HIV) transmission by human bites is thought to be low, although there are case reports of transmission by this route.[3–5] The need for tetanus and rabies vaccination should be assessed.

Prophylactic Antibiotics

Patients with high-risk wounds should receive a 3- to 5-day course of prophylactic antibiotics. Amoxicillin-clavulanate (Augmentin) 875 mg bid is an appealing agent for prophylaxis of human and animal bite wounds. Its spectrum of activity includes *Pasteurella multocida*, *Staphylococcus aureus*, streptococci, *Eikenella corrodens*, and β-lactamase-producing oral anaerobes. Penicillin-allergic patients may receive cefuroxime 500 mg bid or doxycycline 100 mg bid.

Established Infections

For established infections, empiric treatment with ampicillin-sulbactam (Unasyn) 1.5 to 3.0 g IV q6h, cefuroxime (Zinacef) 0.75 to 1.5 g IV q8h, or clindamycin 600 to 900 mg IV q8h and ciprofloxacin 200 to 400 mg IV q12h may be good empiric choices.

Rabies Prophylaxis

Rabies is a uniformly fatal condition. Therefore, a high index of suspicion for this infection must be maintained after any mammalian bite. Bats and other wild mammals are currently the major source of rabies in the United States. Assessment of risk involves a thorough history and physical examination. A break in the skin from teeth or claws of an infected animal or contact with saliva on mucous membranes or broken skin constitutes exposure. The decision to apply prophylaxis is then guided by the specific situation and animal species. In general, bats, skunks, raccoons, woodchucks, foxes, and other wild carnivores should be regarded as rabid and immunoprophylaxis administered. If the animal is captured, it should be killed immediately and the head sent under refrigeration to an appropriately equipped laboratory for fluorescent antibody examination. If the test is negative, the vaccination series may be discontinued. Domestic dogs, cats, and ferrets that are otherwise healthy should be confined and observed for a period of 10 days. If they remain asymptomatic, prophylaxis is unnecessary. The management of all other exposures, from either wild or domestic mammals, should be decided after consultation with the local health department.

Early, thorough wound cleansing is necessary to reduce the viral inoculum. Wounds are flushed with soap and water. Suturing the wound is avoided if possible. Human rabies immune globulin (HRIg) is administered in a dose of 20 U/kg body weight to both adults and children. This dose should not be exceeded, as passive antibody may interfere with response to the active vaccine. Half of the dose is infiltrated around the wound, if feasible, and the rest given intramuscularly in the gluteal area. Active immunization is accomplished by human diploid cell vaccine (HDCV) or rabies vaccine adsorbed (RVA), the first dose given simultaneously with HRIg with repeat doses on days 3, 7, 14, and 28. The active vaccine is administered intramuscularly in the deltoid. In infants it is given in the anterolateral thigh.[6]

Prevention

The role of education in the prevention of these injuries cannot be overemphasized. Dog bites are reported to be among the top 12 causes of nonfatal injury in the United States.[1] Situations reported to be potentially dangerous include approaching dogs immediately after entering their territory, waking a dog from sleep, and teasing or playing with a dog until it becomes overexcited.[7] Male dogs and dogs that have not been neutered are more likely to bite.[1,8]

Family and Community Issues

Most dog bites are preventable. Parents should be counseled never to leave a child alone with a dog, and children should be taught never to approach an unfamiliar dog. They should also be warned of the danger of startling animals. Children should learn to recognize signs of distress in familiar animals and be warned not to disturb them when they are exhibiting this behavior.

Spider Bites

In North America two species of spider account for most medical problems after bites. The brown recluse spider (*Loxosceles reclusa*) is found primarily in the south-central regions of the United States but may be transported anywhere. It is a small (1–2 cm) tan to dark brown spider with a violin-shaped pattern on the back. It produces a venom containing sphingomyelinase D, which causes endothelial swelling, platelet aggregation, and thrombosis. The black widow spider (*Lactrodectus mactans*) is a shiny black color with a red hourglass-shaped marking on the ventral abdomen. Black widow venom contains α-latrotoxin, a potent neurotoxin.

Clinical Presentation

Brown recluse spider bites are painless or only mildly painful. Within 2 to 8 hours, though, severe local pain may occur. An erythematous or cyanotic macule ("volcano lesion") may appear at the site of the bite often followed by a deep necrotic ulcer, which may take months to heal. Systemic absorption of toxin may lead to fever, malaise, vomiting, skin rash, and jaundice. Hemolysis and disseminated intravascular coagulation (DIC) may occur. Desquamation of the extremities, petechiae, and skin rashes may appear as late as 3 weeks after the bite.[9]

Black widow spider bites are often painless, but 20 minutes to several hours later localized pain, cramps, and fasciculations may occur. Progression to pain and rigidity in the abdomen, shoulders, and back often follows. Autonomic signs such as nausea, vomiting, fever, dizziness, hypertension, and sialorrhea may occur.

Diagnosis

Often the diagnosis of a spider bite is made presumptively by the victim. One study found that 90% of suspected spider bites were actually bites from other insects or manifestations of disease states.[10] For this reason, it has been suggested that in the absence of conclusive evidence as to the identity of the culprit such bites be labeled "arthropod bite, vector unknown" in the medical record.[11]

Management

For most spider bites wound care, ensuring current tetanus immunization status, and monitoring for infection are the only interventions required. Local symptoms are controlled through the use of ice, analgesics, and antihistamines.

Severe systemic symptoms due to brown recluse spider bites may require treatment with enteral or parenteral corticosteroids. Dapsone, 50 to 100 mg po daily for 10 days, may abort or ameliorate the development of skin lesions.

If available, specific antivenin (Antivenin; Merck, West Point, PA) may be the management option of choice for all significant envenomations due to black widow spiders[12–14] (Table 47.1). Parenteral narcotics, intravenous diazepam, or methocarbamol are useful for muscle cramps, as are prolonged hot baths. Calcium gluconate 10% solution, 0.1 to 0.2 ml/kg IV, with cardiac monitoring may provide transient relief of symptoms.

Prevention

Clearing away debris, plugging openings into houses, wearing gloves and long pants, using insecticides, and avoiding heavily infested areas are the major preventive steps that can be taken to avoid bites.

Hymenoptera Stings

Stings by bees, wasps, hornets, and ants are common in most climates. Their shared manifestation is the production of localized dermal wheal-and-flare reactions. Full-blown anaphylaxis occurs in a subset of individuals. Domestic honeybees are relatively nonaggressive in defense of their colony. In contrast, Africanized bees ("killer bees") endemic to parts of Arizona, Texas, and New Mexico, engage in massive stinging attacks that are often fatal. Fire ants are endemic to many southern states, and their bites are sustained by a large proportion of the population in infested areas each year.

Clinical Presentation

Wheal-and-flare dermal lesions are the most common presentation. The fire ant often makes a series of stings, leading to a characteristic semicircular pattern of sterile pustular lesions. Systemic toxicity may develop in the adult if more than approximately 50 bee stings are sustained simultaneously. Generalized edema, dizziness, weakness, and vomiting may be followed by DIC, rhabdomyolysis, and acute tubular necrosis.

Management

The lesion is examined for the presence of a stinger. If one is present, it is promptly removed. Squeezing the venom sac is avoided

Applying ice to the lesion reduces pain. Topical steroid preparations and oral antihistamines may be used for local reactions. Calamine lotion and cool, moist dressings are useful. Treatment of massive envenomation is identical to that for anaphylaxis, and it may be difficult to differentiate between the two conditions.

Prevention

Individuals at risk should avoid perfumes and brightly colored clothing while outdoors. People who clear vegetation and discarded junk are at increased risk of being stung. Individuals with a history of anaphylaxis after stings should be offered desensitizing immunotherapy. They should also carry an anaphylaxis self-treatment kit (Ana-Kit or Epi-Pen injectors).

Snakebite

There are two families of poisonous snakes in the United States. Elapidae, or coral snakes, are found in the South. Brightly colored with black, red, and yellow rings, they produce a neurotoxic venom. They rarely bite humans. Crotalidae, or pit vipers, which include rattlesnakes, cottonmouths, and copperheads, are distinguished by heat-sensing organs, or "pits," in the area between the eye and the nostril. Crotalid toxin primarily causes hemolysis, hemorrhage, and local soft tissue damage, although a few Mojave rattlesnakes produce a neurotoxic venom.[9]

Clinical Presentation

Patients presenting after snakebite may display extreme anxiety, and it is important not to mistake it as evidence of envenomation. Local tissue changes include pain, edema, bullae, and ecchymosis. DIC and acute renal failure may occur. Coral snake envenomation may result in bulbar and respiratory paralysis.

Table 47.1. **Antivenins**

Antivenin	Indication	Dosage
Antivenin (Crotalidae) (Wyeth Laboratories)	Pit viper envenomation	See text
Antivenin (*Micrurus fulvius*) (Wyeth Laboratories)	Coral snake envenomation	Asymptomatic: 3–5 vials Symptomatic: 6–10 or more vials
Antivenin (*Lacrodectus mactans*) (Merck)	Black widow spider envenomation	1–2 Vials IM (IV in severe cases)
Scorpion antivenin (available through Arizona State University[a])	Bark scorpion envenomation	1–2 Vials IV

[a]Not FDA-approved. Available to Arizona physicians only.

Diagnosis

All patients who have sustained a venomous snakebite should undergo a complete evaluation regardless of the initial presentation, as effects can occur unpredictably for up to 12 hours after the bite. In addition to the history and physical examination, a complete blood count, DIC screen, creatine phosphokinase assay, electrocardiogram, and urinalysis are recommended, and may be repeated at intervals. Serial circumferential measurements of the affected extremity should be performed to monitor swelling. Consideration should be given to prophylactic endotracheal intubation in patients having sustained a bite of the face or head.[9]

Management

Intensive supportive care is indicated. Antivenin is the only specific treatment available (Table 47.1). Its use for crotalid snakebites is recommended only if there is clinical evidence of envenomation.[9] Clinical assessment of the snakebite severity guides the amount of antivenin administered. Several objective scoring systems are in use.[15,16] For minimal envenomations, up to 10 vials of antivenin are used and for moderate envenomation 10 to 20 vials.[9] For severe cases, 20 or more vials of antivenin may be necessary. In children these doses may have to be increased by as much as 50%. Specific antivenin should be administered to anyone sustaining a bite from a coral snake, regardless of initial presentation, as symptoms may progress rapidly once they appear. Antivenin administration is associated with anaphylaxis and serum sickness in a significant percentage of patients.

Prevention

Prevention is practiced by avoiding infested areas and high-risk behaviors, such as turning over logs and stones in the wild. Boots and long trousers provide significant protection from snakebite. Carrying a light while walking at night is an effective snake repellent.

Other Arthropods

Many other arthropods, including mosquitoes and ticks, target humans among their hosts. In the United States mosquitoes transmit a number of arboviral encephalitides. Tick-borne diseases include Lyme disease, typhus, babesiosis, Rocky Mountain spotted fever, and ehrlichiosis (see Chapter 44). Scorpions native to the United States are not significantly toxic except for the bark scorpion (*Centruroides exilicauda*) endemic to Arizona and New Mexico.

Clinical Presentation

The most common presentation of a tick bite is discovery of an attached tick. Ticks have a barbed feeding organ, or hypostome, through which they suck blood. This feeding mechanism is buried under the skin of the host, making removal of the tick difficult. Patients may also present with sequelae

of a tick bite, such as erythema migrans. Rarely, injection of a neurotoxin by a female *Dermacentor andersoni* or *Dermacentor variabilis* tick results in a rapidly ascending motor paralysis known as "tick paralysis."

Most scorpion stings result in localized pain and swelling only. Systemic toxicity presents with localized numbness and paresthesias, followed by nausea, vomiting, dyspnea, and sialorrhea. Hypertension, involuntary motor activity, and seizures may occur.

Diagnosis

Ticks may attach anywhere but are often found at the hairline or on the scalp. Tick bites may induce persistent granulomas or ulcers at the site of attachment. Tick paralysis often presents with flaccid paralysis. Bulbar paralysis and respiratory depression may occur. Cerebrospinal fluid examination is unremarkable.

Management

An attached tick is removed by grasping it as close to the host's skin as possible with tweezers or protected fingers. Steady traction should be applied to detach the tick. Pulling too hard decapitates it and leaves the mouth parts embedded in the skin. Tick paralysis resolves spontaneously after removal of the tick.

Patients who display evidence of systemic toxicity from scorpion stings require supportive care. Beta-blockers are used for management of severe hypertension. Specific antivenin is available for severe envenomations.

Prevention

Protective clothing should be worn when traveling in infested areas to avoid tick and mosquito bites. Individuals at risk should be counseled to carry out a visual inspection of the entire body twice daily to detect and remove any attached ticks. An insect repellent containing diethyltoluamide (DEET) should be applied to all exposed skin. Permethrin 0.5% spray (Nix, Elimite) applied to clothing provides further protection. A new vaccine against Lyme disease has recently been approved by the Food and Drug Administration (FDA) for individuals between 15 and 70 years of age. The recommended schedule is three doses, given immediately and at 1 month and 12 months. It is recommended that the third dose be given in March for maximum efficacy during transmission season. The American Academy of Family Physicians (AAFP) recommends that the vaccine be considered for individuals at moderate to high risk of exposure to Lyme disease. It is unknown whether booster doses will be required in the future.[17–19] (also see Chapter 44).

Marine Animal Stings

In the United States stingrays and coelenterates (sea anemones, jellyfish, corals) cause most of the significant human envenomations.

Clinical Presentation

Most commonly the victim steps on a stingray hidden under the sand and is envenomated by a spine on the dorsum of the creature's tail. Stingray venom contains serotonin and proteolytic enzymes. The victim often experiences immediate pain and swelling of the affected extremity. Nausea, vomiting, weakness, diaphoresis, cramps, and dyspnea may occur.

Coelenterates have thousands of stinging organs called nematocysts on their tentacles. Contact with these organs triggers the sting, which penetrates the skin and releases toxin.

Diagnosis

Wounds inflicted by stingrays are often jagged and edematous. Pieces of the dorsal spine may be embedded in the wound or surrounding tissue.

Coelenterate stings present with a stinging or burning sensation involving the affected area. Erythema and papules appear in a linear distribution. Systemic symptoms include headache, nausea, muscle pain, spasm, and tachycardia. Massive envenomations have led to death.

Management

After soaking the stingray-induced wound in hot (45°C) water for up to 90 minutes to deactivate the toxin, the wound is carefully irrigated and debrided. It is then packed and reevaluated at 72 hours for delayed primary closure. Tetanus vaccination status is assessed and updated if necessary.

Soaking areas affected by coelenterate stings in 50% vinegar solution helps to alleviate pain. Any adherent tentacles are removed with gloved hands, and the affected areas may be shaved with a razor or sharp knife to remove any remaining nematocysts. A steroid-containing cream may be applied.

Prevention

Individuals should consider wearing sandals or shoes when wading in areas where stingrays or coelenterates are found. Stingrays and other marine animals must be avoided, even when apparently lifeless.

References

1. Sacks JJ, Lockwood R, Hornreich J, Sattin RW. Fatal dog attacks, 1989–1994. Pediatrics 1996;97:891–5.
2. Griego RD, Rosen T, Orengo IF, Wolf JE. Dog, cat, and human bites: a review. J Am Acad Dermatol 1995;33:1019–29.
3. Infectious bite treated as bloodborne transmission. AIDS Alert 1995;10:155.
4. Pretty IA, Anderson GS, Sweet DJ. Human bites and the risk of human immunodeficiency virus transmission. Am J Forensic Med Pathol 1999;20:232–9.
5. Richman KM, Rickman LS. The potential for transmission of human immunodeficiency virus through human bites. J Acquir Immune Defic Syndr 1993;6:402–6.
6. Human rabies prevention—United States, 1999. Recommendations of the Advisory Committee on Immunization Practices (ACIP). MMWR 1999;48:1–21.
7. Shewell PC, Nancarrow JD. Dogs that bite. BMJ 1991;303:1512–3.
8. Gershman KA, Sacks JJ, Wright JC. Which dogs bite? A case-control study of risk factors. Pediatrics 1994;93:913–7.
9. Walter FG, Bilden EF, Gibly RL. Envenomations. Crit Care Clin 1999;15:353–86, ix.
10. Russell FE, Gertsch WJ. For those who treat spider or suspected spider bites. Toxicol 1983;21:337–9.
11. Blackman JR. Spider bites. J Am Board Fam Pract 1995;8:288–94.
12. Miller TA. Treatment of black widow spider envenomation. J Am Board Fam Pract 1995;8:503.
13. White J. Envenoming and antivenom use in Australia. Toxicon 1998;35:1483–92.
14. Woestman R, Perkin R, Van Stralen D. The black widow: is she deadly to children? Pediatr Emerg Care 1996;12:360–4.
15. Dart RC, McNally J. Efficacy, safety, and use of snake antivenoms in the United States. Ann Emerg Med 2001;37:181–8.
16. Dart RC, Hurlbut KM, Garcia R, Boren J. Validation of a severity score for the assessment of crotalid snakebite. Ann Emerg Med 1996;27:321–6.
17. Hu LT, Klempner MS. Update on the prevention, diagnosis, and treatment of Lyme disease. Adv Intern Med 2001;46:247–75.
18. Shadick NA, Liang MH, Phillips CB, Fossel K, Kuntz KM. The cost-effectiveness of vaccination against Lyme disease. Arch Intern Med 2001;161:554–61.
19. Smith DL. Complying with AAP Lyme disease recommendations. Am Fam Physician 2001;63:635.

48
Poisoning

Lars C. Larsen and Stephen H. Fuller

More than 2.2 million poison exposures were reported to United States poison centers in 1999,[1] at least 75% of which were by intentional or accidental ingestion. This chapter provides primary care clinicians with sufficient information to diagnose and comprehensively manage common oral poisonings associated with significant morbidity and mortality. Ingestions of acetaminophen, cyclic antidepressants, aspirin/salicylates, and benzodiazepines are discussed.

General Treatment Measures

When presented with a patient who has ingested toxic amounts of a substance, gastric decontamination should be considered if the ingested substance is highly toxic or if the amounts ingested are sufficient to cause harm to the patient. Activated charcoal is the most effective method of gastrointestinal decontamination and is used with or without gastric emptying. When indicated, gastric emptying by lavage is generally preferable to ipecac-induced emesis. However, gastric emptying should not be routinely used in all cases of toxic ingestion. The doses of these treatments are described in Table 48.1, with additional information provided in the following discussion.

Activated Charcoal
Indications

Administration of activated charcoal is the most effective method used to prevent absorption of ingested drugs and chemicals from the gastrointestinal (GI) tract. It is not effective for treating ingestions of corrosive agents, cyanide, iron, ethanol, ethylene glycol, methanol, lead, lithium, or organic solvents. Multiple dosing has been shown to be effective for ingestions of theophylline, phenobarbital, carbamazepine, dapsone, and quinine. It is possibly effective for ingestions of salicylates, tri-

cyclic antidepressants, digoxin, digitoxin, piroxicam, phenytoin, dextropropoxyphene, disopyramide, nadolol, phenylbutazone, and sotalol.[2] Dosing information is outlined in Table 48.1. If a patient is to receive ipecac, activated charcoal should be withheld until ipecac-induced vomiting has stopped (usually 1 to 2 hours after the last ipecac dose). Activated charcoal should never be given before ipecac therapy. Absolute contraindications to the use of activated charcoal include patients with an unprotected airway, intestinal obstruction, or a dysfunctional gastrointestinal tract.

Dosing and Administration

The initial dose of activated charcoal is usually about 5 to 10 times the amount of ingested substance or 1 to 2 g/kg (Table 48.1). This protocol results in adult doses of 50 to 100 g of activated charcoal and pediatric doses of 10 to 25 g. Multiple-dose therapy is usually administered until the patient passes a charcoal stool. A level measuring tablespoon contains about 5 to 6 g of activated charcoal. Activated charcoal is commercially available as a powder to be mixed with water or a ready-made suspension with or without the cathartic sorbitol. Although cathartics were once recommended, they are no longer considered the standard of practice; they may be used with multiple dosing if the patient has not produced a stool after two to three doses of charcoal. The powder form is mixed with tap water to form a slurry (which contains 15 to 120 g of ingredient depending on the strength); the slurry must be shaken vigorously, as charcoal does not mix well in water. This process can be avoided by using a ready-made suspension containing 25 to 50 g in 120- to 240-mL containers. The poor taste of the slurry or suspension can be improved by using the cherry-flavored products or by adding small amounts of fruit juice or chocolate; milk products should be avoided because they decrease the adsorptive properties of the activated charcoal.

Table 48.1. **Dosing and Administration of Ipecac and Charcoal**

Treatment	Age (years)	Dose (mL)	Frequency	Comments
Ipecac	0.5–1 1–12 >12	5–10 15 30	Repeat in 20–30 minutes if first dose unsuccessful [give with 0.5 glass (<1 year) to 1 glass (≥1 year) of water]	Do not give >2 hours after ingestion; *do not give after charcoal; do not use ipecac fluid extract*
Activated charcoal (Liqui-Char, CharcoAid, Actidose)	All	1–2 g/kg (initial dose)	Single dose (most substances); repeat (1 g/kg q4h) until charcoal stool: for theophylline, phenobarbital, carbamazepine, dapsone, and quinine	If ipecac used, should wait until ipecac-induced emesis stops (usually 1–2 hours after last dose of ipecac); use cathartic with first dose

Cathartics

Cathartics can be used in combination with activated charcoal to decrease GI transit time and further decrease toxin absorption. Sorbitol and magnesium citrate (or sulfate) are considered the cathartics of choice; irritant cathartics such as cascara, senna, phenolphthalein, and bisacodyl are not recommended. Sorbitol (adults and children receive 4 mL/kg of a 35% solution) is the treatment of choice because it works faster than the magnesium salts. Magnesium citrate (adult dose 200 mL, children's dose 5 mL/kg) is an alternative. Cathartics may be administered after the first dose of activated charcoal but should not be repeated when multiple doses of activated charcoal are used.

Gastric Lavage

Indications

Gastric lavage is the preferred method for gastric emptying in patients with potentially life-threatening ingestions treated in emergency room settings.[3] Lavage is most effective if performed within 1 hour of the toxic ingestion.

Contraindications

Patients who have ingested acidic or alkaline substances are not considered candidates for gastric lavage. Lavage should not be used in patients who have ingested low-viscosity hydrocarbons (kerosene, gasoline, paint thinner), strychnine, or acids or alkalis because of the potential of aspiration. However, lavage is indicated for ingested aromatic or halogenated hydrocarbons and hydrocarbons containing pesticides, camphor, or heavy metals. Risk of hemorrhage or gastrointestinal perforation should also be considered prior to lavage. The passing of a lavage tube may induce vomiting or retching, which may result in aspiration of the hydrocarbon substance. Aspiration can be prevented by endotracheal intubation with a cuffed tube to protect the trachea prior to gastric lavage.

Administration

Conscious patients should drink a glass of water before the gastric tube is passed. Remove all foreign materials (e.g., dentures) from the patient's mouth prior to inserting the gastric tube. A large-diameter orogastric hose [36 to 40 French (F)] is used for adults and one of 24 to 28 F in children. After confirming tube placement, remove the stomach contents using an irrigating syringe. When the stomach contents have been removed and sent to the laboratory for toxicologic examination, begin lavage by administering 100- to 300-mL aliquots of fluid (warm water or 0.45% saline) until the lavage return is continuously clear for at least 2 L or a total of 10 to 20 L has been administered. At the conclusion of the lavage, activated charcoal 1 mg/kg is administered (followed by a cathartic, if used).

Ipecac

Indications

Ipecac syrup has traditionally been used for acute oral drug overdose and oral poisonings managed at home.[4] If possible, individuals attempting to manage an acute poisoning at home should contact a regional poison control center or an emergency facility prior to the administration of ipecac. The potential for serious toxicity and inability to be seen at a health care facility within 1 hour of ingestion may be justifications for its use. However, the mean recovery of ingested substances is 28% (range 25–50%) if given within 1 hour of ingestion, and ipecac appears to add no benefit compared to activated charcoal alone in terms of clinical deterioration and hospital admission. If ipecac is used, it is most effective if emesis is induced within 1 hour after a toxic ingestion; emesis after 1 hour may recover less than 20% of the ingested substance. Emesis usually occurs within 30 minutes, with the emetic effects lasting for up to 2 hours. If the first dose is not successful administer a second dose within 30 minutes of the first dose (maximum is two doses). If the second dose is not successful begin administration of activated charcoal if it is applicable to the ingested substance (see Table 48.1 for dosing and frequency). Once the patient vomits, save the emesis contents for analysis. If emesis occurs and a decision is made to administer activated charcoal, the charcoal must be given after the cessation of vomiting.

Contraindications

Ipecac should not be used in patients who have ingested acids or alkalis because of the potential of aspiration. The use of ipecac in patients ingesting hydrocarbons is usually not recommended (same exceptions as with gastric lavage). Ipecac syrup should not be confused with ipecac fluid extract, which is 14 times more potent than ipecac syrup. Ipecac should not be used in patients with an impaired sensorium or seizures, those who lack a gag reflex, infants younger than 6 months of age, when gagging where vagal stimulation may cause bradycardia (patients taking calcium channel blockers, beta-blockers, clonidine, digitalis), those with coagulation defects, or following ingestion of substances that cause rapid changes in sensorium.

Adverse Effects

When ipecac syrup is used in the recommended doses, patients experience common adverse effects such as vomiting, diarrhea, and drowsiness. Other complications, such as Mallory-Weiss tears, aspiration, and bradycardia have occurred.

Acetaminophen

Acetaminophen overdoses account for large numbers of patients seen in emergency rooms and primary care physician offices. Data from the 1999 Annual Report of the American Association of Poison Control Centers (AAPCC) Toxic Exposure Surveillance System (TESS) documented more than 104,400 ingestions of acetaminophen-containing medications that necessitated poison control center contacts in 1999.[1] Children under the age of 6 years accounted for 38% of these exposures; about 39% of the poisoned were age 20 years or older. There were 177 deaths for all ages among those who took acetaminophen and combination products.

Pharmacokinetics

Acetaminophen (APAP) is rapidly and completely absorbed from the GI tract following ingestion of a therapeutic dose. Peak plasma levels occur approximately 0.5 to 1.0 hour after ingestion of therapeutic amounts of immediate-release products but may be delayed 2 to 4 hours after large ingestions. Peak levels may occur even later after ingestion of toxic amounts of extended-release products (e.g., Tylenol Arthritis Extended Relief Caplets) or products containing diphenhydramine which slow gastric motility (Extra-Strength Tylenol PM).[5,6] Once absorbed, acetaminophen is distributed throughout the body water. Protein binding is less than 50%.

Acetaminophen is metabolized in the liver (96%) with only 2% to 4% excreted unchanged in the urine.[7] Metabolism of therapeutic doses via glucuronidation and sulfation results in the formation of benign metabolites (90–95%). Oxidation through the cytochrome P-450 enzyme system (CYP 3A4 and CYP 2E1) results in the formation of the toxic metabolite *N*-acetyl-*p*-benzoquinonimine (NAPQI) (5–10%). NAPQI is rapidly conjugated with glutathione to form a nontoxic metabolite. The metabolites are excreted in the urine along with the small amount of unchanged drug.

Acetaminophen metabolism in children younger than 6 years of age appears to differ from that in older children and adults, as evidenced by lower levels of hepatotoxicity with toxic plasma levels from single doses. Although young children have more CYP 3A4 enzyme than adults and may form more NAPQI, they have a greater activity of glutathione replacement and can eliminate NAPQI more readily.[8] Once ap-proximately 70% of glutathione stores are depleted, levels of NAPQI increase, resulting in hepatocyte destruction. Acetyl-cysteine (Mucomyst), the treatment of choice for toxic acetaminophen ingestions, exerts its protective effect by replacing the depleted glutathione stores and increasing acetaminophen metabolism through benign pathways.

Several risk factors result in increased NAPQI formation and hepatotoxicity, the first being large ingestions of APAP. "Toxic" doses are considered to be >7.5 grams in adults and >150 mg/kg in children. However, supratherapeutic doses (>50–75 mg/kg/day) for 1 to 5 days in children have been shown to cause hepatotoxicity and death. This occurs more often in children ≤2 years of age who have not eaten for a prolonged period. This also can occur in a febrile child with viral gastroenteritis who is not eating and has received several doses of APAP to lower the fever. Parents using adult-strength APAP products instead of the child products may further increase this risk.[9]

Risk factors seen in adults include malnutrition, long-term use of acetaminophen, and chronic alcohol consumption, which also deplete glutathione stores. Medications that induce the CYP 3A4 enzyme (carbamazepine, phenobarbital, phenytoin, rifampin) will further increase the formation of NAPQI. All risk factors must be considered in the prevention and treatment of APAP poisoning.

Clinical Presentation

The clinical course of acetaminophen toxicity consists of four stages.[10] Stage 1 is seen within the first 24 hours after ingestion, and in older children and adults it consists of nausea, vomiting, diaphoresis, and malaise. Children under 6 years of age seem to vomit earlier and at lower serum acetaminophen levels. Hepatic enzymes are usually not elevated unless there are other causes of hepatic dysfunction. Severe symptoms including coma indicate extremely large ingestions or co-ingestants.

Stage 2 occurs 24 to 48 hours after ingestion and is characterized by the appearance of laboratory abnormalities indicating hepatic damage and necrosis. The aspartate transaminase [AST, serum glutamic-oxaloacetic transaminase (SGOT)], alanine transaminase [ALT, serum glutamic-pyruvic transaminase (SGPT)], and bilirubin levels begin to rise; with severe toxicity the prothrombin time (PT) is increased. The nausea, vomiting, diaphoresis, and malaise encountered during stage 1 typically subside, although complaints of right upper quadrant pain may be encountered.

Stage 3 is seen 3 to 4 days after ingestion and reflects maximal hepatic damage. Nausea, vomiting, and malaise reappear and with severe poisonings may be accompanied by jaundice, confusion, somnolence, and coma. Renal, pancreatic, and cardiac damage may also occur. Peak AST, ALT, bilirubin, and PT values occur during this stage. Although AST levels over 1000 IU/L are diagnostic for acetaminophen-induced hepatotoxicity, levels as high as 30,000 IU/L may be found with severe poisonings. Bilirubin levels exceeding 4 mg/dL, and PT values more than 2.2 times control are indicative of serious hepatotoxicity.

Stage 4 occurs in survivors 7 to 8 days after ingestion and represents resolution of the hepatic damage. Clinical signs of hepatic dysfunction and enzyme abnormalities have nearly or completely resolved. Permanent hepatic damage is infrequent.

Infrequently, patients suffer hepatic damage following ingestion of "nontoxic" amounts of acetaminophen (see Pharmacokinetics, above) and may present initially at any stage of toxicity. Abnormally high hepatic transaminase levels for the clinical situation are often seen. At risk are those who regularly drink large amounts of alcohol, take acetaminophen long-term, are malnourished, or take other drugs that affect hepatic metabolism.

Despite the potential for hepatotoxicity, fewer than 1% of adult patients develop fulminant hepatic failure, and it is almost never seen in children under 6 years of age. In fact, hepatic abnormalities are seen in fewer than 5% of children under 6 years of age who have toxic plasma acetaminophen levels.

Diagnosis

The patient's history of medication ingestion is often inaccurate, may fail to identify potentially toxic ingestions, and may omit co-ingestants. The absence of specific clinical signs and symptoms can also be misleading, particularly early in stage 2 when laboratory findings that indicate hepatic damage are minimal and the clinical symptoms seen in stage 1 are abating. A high level of suspicion is helpful particularly in those who are malnourished, consume alcohol on a chronic basis, and are on CYP 3A4 enzyme-inducing medications.

Therefore, plasma acetaminophen levels should be obtained 4 hours (possibly at 2 hours if ingestion of a liquid with APAP only) or longer after ingestion from all patients with known or suspected acetaminophen overdoses. Acetaminophen levels should also be obtained for *all* ingestions undertaken as a suicide attempt given the risk of co-ingestion of various substances including acetaminophen. The plasma level is then plotted on the Rumack-Matthew nomogram (Fig. 48.1) and a decision made regarding the need for treatment.

Management

Treatment of acetaminophen poisoning embodies three principles: preventing absorption of ingested acetaminophen from the GI tract, appropriate use of the antidote *N*-acetylcysteine (NAC), and supportive care. Preventing absorption from the

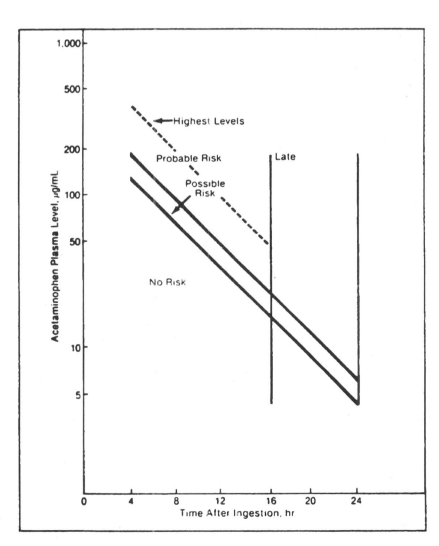

Fig. 48.1. Rumack-Matthew nomogram. (From Rumack et al,[10] with permission.)

GI tract is described under General Treatment Measures, above. Activated charcoal should be given in most cases of acute poisoning, within 1 hour of acetaminophen ingestion for best results and preferably at least 1 hour before NAC administration. Untreated patients seen within 1 hour of ingestion are candidates for gastric lavage. The value of emptying the stomach with ipecac is doubtful, and aggressive use of ipecac may cause prolonged vomiting, thereby expelling the oral NAC as well. If a patient has consumed ipecac, activated charcoal should be given not less than 1.0 to 1.5 hours after ipecac administration (and only if vomiting has stopped) because of the risk of aspiration.

Plasma acetaminophen concentrations should be measured 4 hours or more after ingestion in all patients. A full course of NAC treatment is indicated for initial levels in the "possible risk" or higher ranges on the Rumack-Matthew nomogram (Fig. 48.1) regardless of the type of acetaminophen ingested (immediate- or extended-release products). If the concentration is below the possible-risk level and the ingested acetaminophen is known to be an immediate-release product, further evaluation and treatment are unnecessary. If the type of acetaminophen ingested is unknown or includes an extended-release product, it is recommended that a second acetaminophen level be determined 4 to 6 hours after the first level. If the second level is higher than the first level or is close to the possible-risk level on the nomogram, it is prudent to measure additional acetaminophen levels every 2 hours until the levels stabilize or decline. A full course of NAC treatment should be given if a repeat concentration is in the possible-risk or higher ranges on the nomogram. If the concentration remains below the possible-risk level, treatment is not indicated.

For optimal therapeutic effect, NAC should be given within 8 hours of the toxic ingestion (simultaneously with activated charcoal if necessary to achieve treatment during this period).[11] If serum levels are not immediately available 8 to 16 hours after ingestion, NAC is given empirically. If the initial and repeat (when indicated) serum concentrations return at nontoxic levels, the NAC may be discontinued in most cases. Possible exceptions include patients at risk for hepatic damage at normal or slightly elevated serum concentrations, including those who regularly drink large amounts of alcohol and those who are severely malnourished. NAC therapy may be effective up to 36 hours or more after ingestion, particularly in patients with fulminant hepatic failure.[7,12]

N-acetylcysteine is given orally in a loading dose of 140 mg/kg, followed by 70 mg/kg every 4 hours for 17 additional doses. Although activated charcoal adsorbs NAC in vitro, it appears to have a small effect on NAC in vivo, and there are no data showing that activated charcoal inhibits the antidotal efficacy of NAC. Therefore, most information supports the immediate use of activated charcoal with administration of NAC 1 hour afterward. If the patient vomits within 1 hour of administration of any dose, the dose is repeated. NAC has an odor similar to that of rotten eggs and can be diluted in fruit juices or carbonated beverages to a concentration of approximately 5% to prevent nausea and vomiting. Placement of a nasogastric tube may be necessary in cases of refractory vomiting.

Intravenous NAC has been used extensively for treatment of acetaminophen poisoning in Great Britain and Canada, but it is not approved for use in the United States. Intravenous regimens commonly used include a 20-hour regimen with a loading dose of 150 mg/kg over 15 minutes followed by 50 mg/kg over 4 hours, then 100 mg/kg over the next 16 hours, or a 48-hour regimen with a loading dose of 140 mg/kg followed by 70 mg/kg every 4 hours for 12 doses.[7,13] Intravenous administration of oral NAC through millipore filters has been described for situations when intravenous preparations of NAC are not available.[14]

Supportive care is often necessary after gastrointestinal decontamination and administering NAC. AST, ALT, bilirubin, PT, complete blood count (CBC), and creatinine values are followed daily until improvement is noted. Treatment for hepatic insufficiency is initiated as indicated.

Cyclic Antidepressants

The 1999 AAPCC TESS identified antidepressants as the poison category associated with the second largest number of deaths that year, after analgesics. Antidepressant poisonings were responsible for the third highest percentage of deaths among categorical exposures, following only stimulants/street drugs and cardiovascular drugs.[1] Cyclic antidepressants (CAs) accounted for only 20% of antidepressant exposures, but 67% of deaths. Conversely, selective serotonin reuptake inhibitors (SSRIs) represented 41% of exposures and 14% of deaths. The SSRIs are as efficacious as CAs for treatment of depression and are considered first-line therapies for social anxiety disorder, obsessive-compulsive disorder, and panic disorder.[15–18] Despite their low safety profile, CAs continue to be indicated in selected patients for a variety of conditions, including depression, enuresis, and chronic pain (Table 48.2) (see Chapters 21, 32, and 61).

Table 48.2. **Cyclic Antidepressants**

Generic name	Brand name
Tricyclics	
Amitriptyline	Elavil
	Endep
Amoxapine	Asendin
Clomipramine	Anafranil
Desipramine	Norpramin
Doxepin	Adapin
	Sinequan
Imipramine	Tofranil
Nortriptyline	Pamelor
Protriptyline	Vivactil
Trimipramine	Surmontil
Tetracyclic	
Maprotiline	Ludiomil
Selective serotonin reuptake inhibitors (SSRIs)	
Fluoxetine	Prozac
Paroxetine	Paxil
Sertraline	Zoloft
Fluvoxamine	Luvox
Citalopram	Celexa

Pharmacokinetics

Cyclic antidepressants are rapidly and completely absorbed when therapeutic amounts are ingested, with peak plasma levels occurring 2 to 6 hours after therapeutic doses. In overdose situations, the severe anticholinergic effects of the CAs result in delayed gastric emptying. Once absorbed, CAs are highly protein-bound to plasma proteins (>90%) and tissue proteins.[19] The remaining unbound compounds readily accumulate in various body tissues (myocardium, liver, brain) at 5 to 30 times the plasma concentration. The fraction of unbound drug increases as the plasma pH decreases, allowing the antidepressants to accumulate in the tissues and produce toxic effects.

Metabolism of CAs occurs primarily in the liver (90–95%) and results in the formation of active and inactive metabolites. Metabolites are excreted in the urine and stool. Less than 5% of CAs or their active metabolites is excreted unchanged. Because of enterohepatic recirculation and variations in metabolism, the normal half-life for therapeutic doses of CAs ranges from 18 to 36 hours. With overdoses the combination of delayed gastric emptying and enterohepatic recirculation leads to increased serum concentrations of CA with half-lives prolonged to >80 hours. Plasma drug levels also vary greatly regardless of the dose ingested.

Metabolism of CAs may be affected by patient age and concurrent medications. Consequently, elderly patients typically have a prolonged CA half-life, whereas the converse occurs in children. CA half-lives are shortened by co-ingestions of ethanol, barbiturates, lithium, and tobacco and are prolonged by steroids, oral contraceptives, and phenothiazines, and benzodiazepines.

The SSRIs are almost exclusively eliminated by hepatic metabolism, with all SSRIs (except paroxetine) having active metabolites contributing to serotonergic activity. SSRIs can inhibit hepatic enzymes CYP 3A4 and CYP 2D6 increasing the serum concentrations of several medications (alprazolam, tricyclic antdepressants, propoxyphene, venlafaxine, trazodone) that can further increase toxicity in overdose situations.[20]

Clinical Presentation

Overdoses of CAs affect the parasympathetic, cardiovascular, and central nervous (CNS) systems. Clinical signs and symptoms are the result of several pharmacologic actions including neurotransmitter reuptake inhibition of norepinephrine, dopamine, and serotonin, α-adrenergic blockade, anticholinergic effects, and blockade of myocardial fast sodium channels producing the quinidine-like effect on the myocardium.[21] The signs and symptoms of CA overdose are summarized in Table 48.3, with most fatal overdoses resulting from cardiac complications. CA overdose should be suspected in any patient (child or adult) who presents with signs of anticholinergic poisoning, seizures, coma, hypotension, respiratory depression, or arrhythmias.[22]

Signs and symptoms of an overdose are variable and may change rapidly. Findings resulting from the anticholinergic effects (dilated pupils, dry mouth, hyperpyrexia, blurred vision, CNS excitability) are typically the first to appear. Depending on the time since ingestion, however, patients may present as asymptomatic, have mild to moderate anticholinergic effects, or exhibit signs of severe toxicity including seizures, coma, arrhythmias, and cardiac arrest. Symptoms rapidly progress, with seizures and ventricular arrhythmias typically occurring within 6 hours after ingestion.[23]

Sinus tachycardia is frequently present with serious CA overdoses but is a nonspecific finding. A limb-lead electrocardiographic (ECG) QRS interval of more than 0.10 second is more specific and is considered a sign of potentially serious toxicity.[21,23] A rightward shift in the terminal 40-millisecond QRS frontal plane axis and R wave ≥3 mm in lead AVR are also commonly associated with CA toxicity and considered to be a more significant predictor for seizures or dysrhythmias.[21,24]

Cyclic antidepressants have a low therapeutic index (median toxic dose divided by median effective dose). Whereas doses of 1 to 4 mg/kg may be therapeutic, overdoses as small as 20 mg/kg may be fatal. For example, ingestion of four 100-mg tablets could be fatal if ingested by a 20-kg child, and in-

Table 48.3. **Signs and Symptoms of Cyclic Antidepressant Overdose**

Central nervous system
Sedation
Restlessness
Confusion
Ataxia
Nystagmus
Dysarthria
Hallucinations
Myoclonus
Seizures
Respiratory depression
Respiratory arrest
Coma

Additional anticholinergic effects
Mydriasis (dilated pupils)
Blurred vision
Dry mouth
Hyperpyrexia
Hypoactive bowel sounds
Urinary retention

Cardiovascular system
Sinus tachycardia
Prolonged QRS, PR, QTc intervals
Rightward-terminal 40-ms frontal plane axis deviation of QRS
Bundle branch block (especially RBBB)
Second- or third-degree AV block
Intraventricular conduction delays
Arrhythmias (atrial and ventricular)
Hypotension
Congestive heart failure
Cardiac arrest

Miscellaneous effects
Adult respiratory distress syndrome
Renal tubular acidosis
Metabolic acidosis

RBBB = right bundle branch block; AV = atrioventricular.

gestion of a 2-week supply of 100 mg tablets can be fatal for an adult.

Overdoses of SSRIs are considered much less lethal than CA and the actual fatality rate due to SSRIs overdose alone is not clear due to the effects of co-ingestants in many patients. The toxic effects of SSRI overdose stem from the effects of excess serotonin (5-hydroxytryptamine, 5-HT) on multiple receptors. Stimulation of 5-HT$_1$, 5-HT$_2$, and 5-HT$_3$ receptors, as well as the resulting inhibition of dopamine release, produces many of the symptoms seen in toxic situations.[20]

Patients can experience minor symptoms such as drowsiness, nausea, vomiting, and/or tremors when ingesting doses 50 to 75 times the normal daily dose of SSRIs. Higher doses (150 times the normal daily dose) can result in severe toxicity or death. Patients may experience "serotonin syndrome" if they present with three or more of the following: mental status changes, diaphoresis, myoclonus, diarrhea, fever, hyperreflexia, tremor, or incoordination. Patients can also experience tachycardia, QT prolongation, and seizures. Many patients experiencing toxicity have co-ingested ethanol, benzodiazepines, or serotonergic agents (dextromethorphan, tricyclic antidepressants).[15,20]

Diagnosis

A comprehensive history and physical examination (Table 48.3) should alert the clinician to the possibility of CA overdose. The diagnosis can be confirmed by blood or urine screens for the presence of CAs or SSRIs. Although plasma levels are useful for confirming the diagnosis, they are of little help in predicting serious toxicity.

Co-ingestions of other drugs and the presence of preexisting heart disease must be considered when evaluating patients for CA or SSRI overdose. Each may complicate the clinical presentation and result in a delay in diagnosis.

Management

Treatment of CA poisoning embodies four general principles: preventing absorption of ingested CA from the GI tract, supportive (especially circulatory and respiratory) care, seizure management, and control of arrhythmias. Absorption from the GI tract should be prevented via gastric lavage and use of activated charcoal, as described above (see General Treatment Measures). Ipecac is contraindicated because vomiting may delay charcoal administration or cause aspiration of vomitus in patients with rapidly changing sensoriums.

Asymptomatic patients without signs of CA overdose and with QRS intervals of less than 0.10 second, no QT prolongation, and no deviation of the terminal portion of the QRS (R wave <3 mm in AVR) may be transferred for psychiatric management after being closely observed in the emergency room for a minimum of 6 hours. Patients showing initial signs and symptoms of CA toxicity and patients with QRS or QT prolongation, or deviation of the R wave in AVR should be admitted to the intensive care unit (ICU) and monitored until signs and symptoms of toxicity (including ECG abnormalities) resolve. Patients with refractory or prolonged signs

of toxicity should remain in the ICU until 24 hours after resolution of all toxic manifestations.

Aggressive supportive care is essential for managing CA poisoning. Patients with depressed mental status should be evaluated for other possible etiologies. Where appropriate, the patient is intubated with a cuffed endotracheal tube to secure the airway and prevent impending respiratory failure or aspiration. Intravenous access should be established and isotonic fluids administered to correct hypotension and restore effective blood volume. If signs of cardiotoxicity are present (QRS ≥0.10 second, R in AVR ≥3 mm, QT prolongation, right bundle branch block, wide-complex tachycardia), intravenous NaHCO$_3$ boluses of 1 to 2 mEq/kg given over 1 to 2 minutes can be used until signs of cardiotoxicity and the hypotension improve. An infusion of 150 mEq of NaHCO$_3$ in 1 L of 5% dextrose in water is then given to maintain an arterial pH of 7.45 to 7.55.[25] Patients unable to tolerate large amounts of intravenous sodium may be treated with mechanical ventilation, although this is not as effective as NaHCO$_3$ administration.

Hypotension refractory to crystalloid and sodium bicarbonate therapy may be treated with vasopressors such as norepinephrine or dopamine.[25,26] Dopamine may be less effective than norepinephrine in treating refractory hypotension from CA overdoses when given at the usual doses, but use at a high dosage (up to 30 μg/kg/min) may improve the response rate in resistant cases. Dobutamine can be used to treat hypotension associated with myocardial depression but causes hypotension in some patients.

Seizures may be treated immediately with intravenous diazepam (Valium) 0.15 mg/kg at 15- to 20-minute intervals until seizures are controlled or to a total dose of 30 to 40 mg. This regimen is followed by treatment with an anticonvulsant with a longer half-life, such as phenobarbital. Although recommended as second-line therapy, phenobarbital can cause respiratory depression and acidosis and must be used with caution.[27] Phenytoin (Dilantin) should be avoided because of potential cardiotoxicity. Although physostigmine has been advocated for the treatment of anticholinergic CNS effects, it has considerable cardiac and CNS toxicity and should not be used in CA overdoses.

Arrhythmias induced by CAs are treated by sodium bicarbonate therapy and alkalinization of the plasma to pH 7.45 to 7.55, the use of antiarrhythmics, and cardioversion when necessary. If serious ventricular arrhythmias persist following alkalinization and other supportive measures, lidocaine is the initial drug of choice[25,28] (see Chapter 77). The use of class IA (quinidine, procainamide, disopyramide) and IC (flecainide, encainide, propafenone) antiarrhythmic agents are contraindicated because they also inhibit the myocardial fast sodium channels and worsen the cardiotoxicity.

Treatment of SSRI intoxication includes gastric decontamination (activated charcoal) and supportive care for seizures or cardiovascular manifestations as necessary. Treatment for serotonin syndrome includes supportive therapy, cooling blankets, ice packs or ice water enemas, and the use of dantrolene and cyproheptadine in a manner similar to that used in treating neuroleptic malignant syndrome.

Aspirin/Salicylates

Poisoning by ingestion of oral salicylate-containing medications remains a serious problem in the United States. According to U.S. poison control center data, there were more than 16,300 exposures to aspirin and combination products containing aspirin that necessitated poison control center contacts in 1999.[1] Approximately 28% of exposures were in children younger than 6 years of age, 32% in those 6 to 19 years, and 40% in adults older than 19 years. There were 51 deaths in all categories of exposure.

Pharmacokinetics

Salicylates are rapidly absorbed from the stomach, jejunum, and small intestine. Peak plasma salicylate concentrations are achieved 0.5 to 2.0 hours after ingestion of immediate-release preparations and usually 4 to 6 hours or more after ingestion of extended-release enteric-coated tablets.[29] With large ingestions, absorption and subsequent peak plasma levels may be delayed as much as 8 to 12 hours because of decreased gastric emptying. In addition, large ingestions are often absorbed more slowly because clumps of aspirin tablets form concretions in the stomach resulting in salicylate in the stomach long after ingestion. Consequently, peak levels may occur 24 hours or more after ingestion of large amounts of extended-release tablets.

Following absorption of therapeutic doses, aspirin is rapidly hydrolyzed to salicylic acid, and both compounds are highly protein-bound (80–90%) to albumin. Distribution throughout body fluids is extensive and largely dependent on the amount of salicylate ingested and the pH of the body fluids. The amount of pharmacologically active free salicylate increases as salicylate levels increase above the therapeutic range.

Free salicylate exists in either ionized or nonionized form, the nonionized form being able to readily diffuse into body tissues. Decreased body fluid or tissue pH results in increased relative amounts of the nonionized salicylate, allowing greater tissue penetration. Consequently, large overdoses (with greater amounts of free salicylate) in conditions associated with metabolic acidosis (dehydration, chronic or large salicylate overdoses, sepsis) often result in large tissue and CNS concentrations and hence greater toxicity. Also, alkalinizing the urine increases the concentration of ionized form in the urine, thereby reducing the amount of salicylate that is reabsorbed.

After therapeutic doses, salicylic acid is eliminated unchanged in the urine (5–10%) or as one of five metabolites (90–95%). At higher doses metabolic pathways are saturated, resulting in exponential increases in plasma salicylate levels. For example, an increase in daily aspirin dose from 65 to 100 mg/kg increases the serum concentration 300%.[30]

Clinical Presentation

The actions of salicylates that account for most of the signs and symptoms seen with poisonings include the following: (1) direct stimulation of the CNS respiratory center, producing respiratory alkalosis and initial compensatory renal excretion of HCO_3; (2) uncoupling of oxidative phosphorylation with increased catabolism, increased oxygen utilization, and increased CO_2 production, an action that can result in metabolic acidosis and hyperpyrexia (tissue glycolysis and utilization of glucose are also increased); (3) inhibition of Krebs cycle dehydrogenases, leading to increased amounts of pyruvic acid and lactic acid; (4) stimulation of gluconeogenesis; (5) increased lipolysis and lipid metabolism with formation of ketones, acetoacetic acid, β-hydroxybutyric acid, and acetone; (6) inhibition of aminotransferases, resulting in increased plasma amino acids and aminoaciduria; (7) irritation of the gastric mucosa and stimulation of the chemoreceptor trigger zone, with subsequent nausea and vomiting; and (8) altered coagulation and hemostasis via cyclooxygenase inhibition and decreased platelet aggregation, increased capillary fragility, thrombocytopenia, and hypoprothrombinemia.

The predominant clinical effects of salicylate poisoning can be grouped into two general categories: acid-base and fluid-electrolyte abnormalities. Approximate guidelines correlating the amount of salicylate ingested to the symptoms produced are as follows:

<150 mg/kg—minimal symptoms
150–300 mg/kg—moderate symptoms
300–500 mg/kg—severe symptoms
>500 mg/kg—potentially fatal

Minimal symptoms include mild to moderate hyperpnea, sometimes with lethargy. Moderate symptoms are characterized by severe hyperpnea and CNS signs including lethargy, excitability, or both. Severe symptoms include severe hyperpnea, semicoma, coma, and convulsions.[31]

Signs and symptoms, which usually begin within 3 to 8 hours of ingestion, include nausea and vomiting, hyperpnea, and respiratory alkalosis. The respiratory alkalosis typically persists but is accompanied by progressive metabolic acidosis as the severity and duration of the poisoning increases. Additional findings may include tinnitus, disorientation, and hyperpyrexia. Cumulative GI, renal, pulmonary, and skin losses of fluids can be massive and may result in hypovolemia, oliguria, and renal failure. Hypernatremia, hyponatremia, and hypokalemia are frequently seen. Initial hyperglycemia may be followed by hypoglycemia caused by depletion of tissue glucose stores. Signs of CNS hypoglycemia, including lethargy, coma, and seizures, may occur despite normal plasma glucose levels.[32] Unexpected bleeding and hepatotoxicity are uncommon.

The progression of signs and symptoms is increased in young children, with large ingestions, with illnesses that include dehydration, and with chronic exposures. Also, use of therapeutic doses of salicylates for conditions accompanied by dehydration and acidosis may result in greater tissue (i.e., CNS) concentrations and increased morbidity and mortality, despite relatively low blood salicylate concentrations.

The clinical presentation of patients with chronic salicylate intoxication may differ from that of patients with acute intoxication. Potential differences include a more gradual onset of symptoms, an advanced stage of intoxication at initial presentation, and a predominance of neurologic symptoms particularly in the elderly.[33] Neurologic findings may include confusion, agitation, stupor, paranoia, and bizarre behavior. Chronic salicylism has been misdiagnosed as sepsis, alcohol withdrawal, myocardial infarction, organic psychosis, and dementia.

Salicylate-induced noncardiogenic pulmonary edema and the adult respiratory distress syndrome are complications of salicylate ingestion, particularly chronic ingestions.[34] Risk factors include increased age, cigarette smoking, and concurrent medical illnesses. Chronic salicylate intoxication has also been associated with development of a pseudosepsis syndrome characterized by hyperthermia, leukocytosis, hypotension with decreased systemic vascular resistance, and multiple organ failure.[35]

Diagnosis

A history of salicylate ingestion helps confirm the clinical impression, but documentation of toxic serum salicylate levels is essential for establishing the diagnosis. The Done nomogram (Fig. 48.2) is used to assess the significance of serum salicylate levels following acute ingestions.[31] Blood salicylate levels should be determined 6 hours or more after the acute ingestion. By plotting the serum level at a given time after ingestion, it is possible to predict the severity of the poisoning and the expected symptoms. This nomogram is most useful for acute ingestions and may underestimate the severity of poisonings after chronic exposures, in patients with illnesses accompanied by dehydration and acidosis, in cases of ingestion of enteric-coated or sustained-release products, and

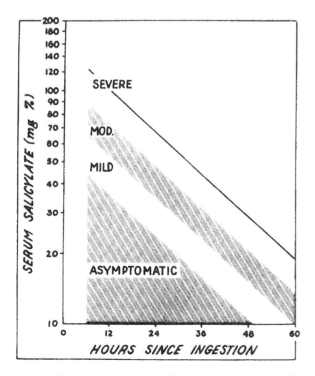

Fig. 48.2. Done nomogram. (From Done AK. *Pediatrics* 1960;26:800–7, with permission.)

in those with indeterminate times of ingestion. Therefore serial serum salicylate levels every 1 to 2 hours after the initial salicylate level have been recommended until levels decline and the patient's condition stabilizes.[36]

Management

Treatment of salicylate poisoning encompasses three principles: preventing absorption of ingested salicylate from the GI tract; treating any fluid, electrolyte, or metabolic derangements; and enhancing elimination of salicylate from the body. Careful monitoring of the acid–base status, including prevention of worsening acidosis (respiratory or metabolic), is essential. Preventing absorption from the GI tract (described under General Treatment Measures, above) includes emesis and/or gastric lavage (depending on the necessity for gastric emptying), and administering activated charcoal to increase elimination.

Fluid resuscitation is initially directed toward restoring an effective blood volume. If hypotension is present, an isotonic solution should be given intravenously until the patient is no longer orthostatic. If hyperglycemia is not a problem, the solution should contain at least 5% dextrose. If dextrose is not desired, normal saline or a mixture of 0.45% NaCl with one ampule of sodium bicarbonate (total 50 mEq $NaHCO_3$) at 10 to 15 mL/kg/h for 1 to 2 hours may be used, depending on the presence and degree of acidosis. Subsequent fluid management is directed toward alkalinizing the urine, preventing CNS hypoglycemia, and treating electrolyte and fluid abnormalities.

An effective alkaline diuresis (urine pH >7.5) to enhance salicylate excretion should be attempted once the patient is no longer orthostatic and urine output has been established. Superiority of a single method to achieve this has not been established. An initial bolus of $NaHCO_3$, 2 mEq/kg intravenously, followed by an infusion of 1000 cc of dextrose 5% in water (D_5W) plus three ampules of $NaHCO_3$ (50 mEq $NaHCO_3$/ampule) at 1.5 to 2 times maintenance rate has been effective. Potassium should be added to the IV as needed for potassium levels below 4.0 mEq/L. Frequent monitoring of serum electrolytes and glucose is essential. The urine pH should be checked hourly until stable at >7.5. Arterial blood gases should be monitored 2 to 4 hours into treatment to ensure the blood pH is *no more than* 7.5. Alkalinization can be discontinued when the serum salicylate level is within the therapeutic range.

Hemodialysis is indicated for unresponsive or worsening acidosis, acute and chronic poisonings with salicylate levels of >100 mg/dL and 40 to 60 mg/dL respectively, renal or hepatic failure, noncardiac pulmonary edema, and persistent, severe CNS symptoms.[31,36] Additional supportive care may be necessary depending on the severity of the poisoning and the patient's response to therapy.

Benzodiazepines

Benzodiazepines are widely prescribed for a variety of conditions, including acute anxiety, convulsions, neuromuscular disorders, panic attacks, insomnia, alcohol withdrawal, and induction of anesthesia. They are commonly used in inpatient

Table 48.4. **Commonly Prescribed Benzodiazepines**

Generic name	Brand name
Alprazolam	Xanax
Chlordiazepoxide	Librium
Clonazepam	Klonopin
Clorazepate dipotassium	Tranxene
Diazepam	Valium
Estazolam	ProSom
Flurazepam	Dalmane
Lorazepam	Ativan
Midazolam	Versed
Oxazepam	Serax
Quazepam	Doral
Temazepam	Restoril
Triazolam	Halcion

and outpatient settings to produce conscious sedation for minor surgical procedures. U.S. Poison Control Center data from 1999 indicate that benzodiazepines accounted for 56% of sedative exposures and 59% of sedative deaths (65 of 110 total deaths) at the 64 reporting centers.[1] More than 76% of exposures were in persons over 19 years of age, and approximately 70% of all exposures were intentional (see Chapter 33). Because this information does not include poisonings seen in other health care facilities, it is likely that the total number of benzodiazepine overdoses in the United States was considerably greater. Commonly used benzodiazepines are listed in Table 48.4.

Pharmacokinetics

Most benzodiazepines are rapidly and completely absorbed following an oral dose. Peak plasma levels occur 0.5 to 3.0 hours after ingestion of therapeutic doses but may be delayed after large overdoses or when co-ingested with alcohol or antacids. Once absorbed, benzodiazepines are extensively bound to serum proteins (70–99%), with the unbound drug being the active form. Conditions associated with hypoalbuminemia (e.g., cirrhosis) result in a greater proportion of unbound drug and may cause an increased frequency of side effects.

Benzodiazepines have a large volume of distribution in the body, with concentrations in the brain, liver, and spleen being greater than unbound drug concentrations in the blood. The duration of action depends on the rate and extent of tissue distribution (lipid solubility) as well as the rate of elimination.

Benzodiazepines are metabolized in the liver primarily by the CYP 3A4 enzyme pathway and to a minor extent the CYP 2C9 pathway resulting in the formation of active and inactive metabolites. Depending on the benzodiazepine ingested, metabolism may be prolonged by advanced age, cirrhosis, and the coadministration of various medications. These include macrolide antibiotics (clarithromycin, erythromycin), calcium channel blockers (diltiazem, verapamil), antifungal agents (fluconazole, itraconazole, ketoconazole), antidepressants (fluoxetine, fluvoxamine, nefazodone), protease inhibitors, and omeprazole. In addition, concomitant ingestion of grapefruit juice and acute alcohol ingestion can increase benzodiazepine serum concentrations.[37,38] Although differences exist among benzodiazepines, excretion of metabolites and small amounts of unchanged drug (<1% of the total dose) occurs primarily in the urine.

Clinical Presentation

Benzodiazepines exert their clinical effects by increasing neurotransmission in γ-aminobutyric (GABA)ergic synapses in the CNS. Specific benzodiazepine receptors, associated with GABAergic pathways, are found predominantly in the cerebral cortex, limbic structures, and cerebellum.[39,40] Because the major CNS inhibitory effect is mediated via GABAergic pathways, benzodiazepine stimulation causes several physiologic effects, including sedation, anxiolysis, striated muscle relaxation, and anterograde amnesia.

Benzodiazepines have a high margin of safety, and overdoses usually produce only mild to moderate signs of toxicity, including ataxia, dysarthria, drowsiness, and lethargy. However, severe overdoses can cause coma, hypotension, hypothermia, and respiratory distress requiring endotracheal intubation and assisted ventilation or in select cases, administration of flumazenil.[41,42] Such complications are rare in benzodiazepine-only ingestions but occur much more frequently with co-ingestions of other drugs that cause CNS depression (especially alcohol) (see Chapter 59). CNS depression is worsened in the elderly, in those taking large amounts, in patients with chronic diseases, and in those taking medications that impair hepatic benzodiazepine metabolism. Deaths caused by benzodiazepine-only overdoses are rare.

Diagnosis

A complete history and physical examination are important for determining the diagnosis and type of ingested medication. The diagnosis should be confirmed in all patients by blood or urine screens for the presence of benzodiazepines. It is important to screen routinely for the presence of co-ingestants, particularly in comatose patients. Quantitative determinations of blood benzodiazepine levels are not useful for the management of benzodiazepine overdoses because blood concentrations do not correlate well with clinical manifestations.[43,44]

Management

Treatment of benzodiazepine overdoses consists of patient stabilization, preventing absorption of ingested benzodiazepines from the GI tract, and supportive care including airway support and mechanical ventilation when necessary. Administration of the antidote flumazenil may be useful in selected patients, but is not recommended for routine use in patients with possible mixed drug overdoses or unknown medical histories.[45,46] Preventing absorption from the GI tract is described above (see General Treatment Measures).

Patients are initially assessed for complications from CNS depression. Vital signs are evaluated and the adequacy of the airway and respiratory status ensured. Patients with respiratory depression and hypoxia or hypoventilation are intubated and placed on mechanical ventilation. Comatose patients and others with severe overdoses are examined for evidence of aspiration, hypotension, and hypothermia. Once stabilized, selected patients with benzodiazepine overdose (documented by drug screen or reliable history) who are comatose or have severe CNS depression may be treated with flumazenil (Romazicon). Flumazenil should be avoided in patients suspected of co-ingesting cyclic antidepressants, those with a history of benzodiazepine dependence, or those with a history of seizure disorders treated with benzodiazepines.[46–48] The risks of lethal dysrhythmias, benzodiazepine withdrawal, or seizures outweigh the potential benefits of treatment in these cases.

Flumazenil is a competitive inhibitor of CNS benzodiazepine receptor sites and reverses benzodiazepine-induced CNS depression. Recommended doses for benzodiazepine overdoses in adults are 0.2 mg IV over 30 seconds; if no response, give 0.3 mg IV over 30 seconds. Additional doses of 0.5 mg may be given at 1-minute intervals as needed up to a total dose of 3 mg. Patients occasionally require a total dose of 5 mg for optimal response, but the requirement for higher dosages may indicate CNS depression due to the presence of co-ingestants.[49] Comatose patients typically awaken within minutes of intravenous administration. The duration of action is approximately 1 hour (it may be shorter) and is related to the doses of benzodiazepine ingested and flumazenil administered.[39] Resedation may be observed in cases with prolonged CNS depression and can be treated with repeat 0.2 mg IV boluses (given over 30–60 seconds) as required, to no more than 3 mg in 1 hour. Patients who fail to respond to a maximum dose of flumazenil (5 mg within 5 minutes) should be evaluated for co-ingestants and other causes of CNS depression. Flumazenil is not approved for treatment of overdoses in children. For reversal of conscious sedation in children, 0.01 mg/kg (up to 0.2 mg) may be given intravenously over 15 seconds. If there is no response after 45 seconds, 0.01 mg/kg (up to 0.2 mg) may be given every 60 seconds (up to four doses) as needed to a maximum total dose of 0.05 mg/kg (or 1.0 mg, whichever is lower).

The stomach may be evacuated by gastric lavage (regardless of flumazenil administration) if the time since ingestion is less than 1 hour, particularly in mixed drug ingestions. Activated charcoal should be administered in most cases and is effective when used as the sole treatment. The use of ipecac should be avoided.

Forced diuresis or efforts to remove the drugs by "cleansing" the vascular compartment (hemodialysis and hemoperfusion) are ineffective and are not indicated for management of overdoses. Antibiotics and corticosteroids are not used except for specific indications.

Supportive care is provided as needed. Hypotension can be managed with crystalloid solutions initially and vasopressors thereafter, as indicated. Treatment of poisoning by co-ingestants is targeted to the specific overdose agents.

References

1. Litovitz TL, Klein-Schwartz W, White S, et al. 1999 annual report of the American Association of Poison Control Centers toxic exposure surveillance system. Am J Emerg Med 2000;18:517–74.
2. American Academy of Clinical Toxicology; European Association of Poisons Centres and Clinical Toxicologists. Position statement and practice guidelines on the use of multidose activated charcoal in the treatment of acute poisoning. Clin Toxicol 1999;37:731–51.
3. American Academy of Clinical Toxicology; European Association of Poisons Centres and Clinical Toxicologists. Position statement: gastric lavage. Clin Toxicol 1997;35:711–19.
4. Shannon M. Ingestion of toxic substances by children. N Engl J Med 2000;342:186–91.
5. Professional product information: Tylenol. McNeil Consumer Healthcare 2000.
6. Cetaruk EW, Dart RC, Hurlbut KM, Horowitz RS, Shih R. Tylenol Extended Relief overdose. Ann Emerg Med 1997;30:104–8.
7. Zed PJ, Krenzelok EP. Treatment of acetaminophen overdose. Am J Health Syst Pharm 1999;56:1081–93.
8. Peterson RG, Rumack BH. Pharmacokinetics of acetaminophen in children. Pediatrics 1978;62(suppl):877–9.
9. Kearns GL, Leeder JS, Wasserman GS. Acetaminophen intoxication during treatment: what you don't know can hurt you. Clin Pediatr 2000;39:133–44.
10. Rumack BH, Peterson RC, Koch GC, Amara IA. Acetaminophen overdose. Arch Intern Med 1981;141:380–5.
11. Smilkstein MJ, Knapp GL, Kulig KW, Rumack BH. Efficacy of oral N-acetylcysteine in the treatment of acetaminophen overdose. N Engl J Med 1988;319:1557–62.
12. Jones AL. Mechanism of action and value of NAC in the treatment of early and late acetaminophen poisonings: a critical review. Clin Toxicol 1998;36(4):277–85.
13. Tucker JR. Late-presenting acute acetaminophen toxicity and the role of N-acetylcysteine. Pediatr Emerg Care 1998;14:424–6.
14. Yip L, Dart RC, Hurlbut KM. Intravenous administration of oral N-acetylcysteine. Crit Care Med 1998;26:40–3.
15. Barbey JT, Roose SP. SSRI safety in overdose. J Clin Psychiatry 1998;59(suppl 15):42–8.
16. Liebowitz MR. Update on the diagnosis and treatment of social anxiety disorder. J Clin Psychiatry 1999;60(suppl 18):22–6.
17. Hollander E, Kaplan A, Allen A, Cartwright C. Pharmacotherapy for obsessive-compulsive disorder. Psychiatric Clin North Am 2000;23:643–56.
18. Sheehan DV. Current concepts in the treatment of panic disorder. J Clin Psychiatry 1999;60(suppl 18):16–21.
19. Jarvis MR. Clinical pharmacokinetics of tricyclic antidepressant overdose. Psychopharmacol Bull 1991;27(4):541–50.
20. Goeringer KE, Raymon MS, Christian GD, Logan BK. Postmortem forensic toxicology of selective serotonin reuptake inhibitors: a review of pharmacology and report of 168 cases. J Forensic Sci 2000;45:633–48.
21. Harrigan RA, Brady WJ. ECG abnormalities in tricyclic antidepressant ingestion. Am J Emerg Med 1999;17:387–93.
22. Biggs JT, Spiker DG, Petit JM, Ziegler VE. Tricyclic antidepressant overdose—incidence of symptoms. JAMA 1977;238:135–8.
23. Boehnert MT, Lovejoy FH. Value of the QRS duration versus the serum drug level in predicting seizures and ventricular arrhythmias after an acute overdose in tricyclic antidepressants. N Engl J Med 1985;313:474–9.
24. Liebelt EL, Francis PD, Woolf AD. ECG lead AVR versus QRS interval in predicting seizures and arrhythmias in acute tricyclic antidepressant toxicity. Ann Emerg Med 1995;26:195–201.
25. Shanon M. Toxicology reviews: targeted management strategies for cardiovascular toxicity from tricyclic antidepressant overdose: the pivotal role for alkalinization and sodium loading. Pediatr Emerg Care 1998;14:293–8.
26. Buchman AL, Dauer J, Geiderman J. The use of vasoactive agents in the treatment of refractory hypotension seen in tri-

cyclic antidepressant overdose. J Clin Psychopharmacol 1990; 10:409–13.

27. Newton EH, Shih RD, Hoffman RS. Cyclic antidepressant overdose: a review of current management strategies. Am J Emerg Med 1994;12:376–9.

28. Marshall JB, Forker AD. Cardiovascular effects of tricyclic antidepressant drugs: therapeutic usage, overdose, and management of complications. Am Heart J 1982;103:401–14.

29. Needs CJ, Brooks PM. Clinical pharmacokinetics of the salicylates. Clin Pharm 1985;10:164–77.

30. Paulus HE, Siegel M, Morgan E, et al. Variations in serum concentrations and half-life of salicylate in patients with rheumatoid arthritis. Arthritis Rheum 1971;14:527–32.

31. Temple AR. Acute and chronic effects of aspirin toxicity and their treatment. Arch Intern Med 1981;141:364–9.

32. Thurston JH, Pollock PG, Warren SK, Jones EM. Reduced brain glucose with normal plasma glucose in salicylate poisoning. J Clin Invest 1970;11:2139–45.

33. Durnas C, Cusack BJ. Salicylate intoxication in the elderly—recognition and recommendations on how to prevent it. Drugs Aging 1992;2:20–34.

34. Gonzolez ER, Cole T, Grimes MM, Fink RA, Fowler AA. Recurrent ARDS in a 39-year-old woman with migraine headaches. Chest 1998;114:919–22.

35. Leatherman JW, Schmitz PG. Fever, hyperdynamic shock, and multiple-system organ failure: a pseudo-sepsis syndrome associated with chronic salicylate intoxication. Chest 1991;100:1391–6.

36. Yip L, Dart RC, Gabow PA. Concepts and controversies in salicylate toxicity. Emerg Med Clin North Am 1994;12:351–64.

37. Landrum EL. Update: clinically significant cytochrome P-450 drug interactions. Pharmacotherapy 1998;18(1):84–112.

38. Slaughter RL, Edwards DJ. Recent advances: the cytochrome P450 enzymes. Ann Pharmacother 1995;29:619–24.

39. Votey SR, Bosse GM, Bayer MJ. Flumazenil: a new benzodiazepine antagonist. Ann Emerg Med 1991;20:181–8.

40. Ghoneim MM, Mewaldt SP. Benzodiazepines and human memory: a review. Anesthesiology 1990;72:926–38.

41. Hojer J, Baehrendtz S, Gustafsson L. Benzodiazepine poisoning: experience of 702 admissions to an intensive care unit during a 14 year period. J Intern Med 1989;226:117–22.

42. Wiley CC, Wiley JF. Pediatric benzodiazepine ingestion resulting in hospitalization. J Toxicol Clin Toxicol 1998;36;227–31.

43. Jatlow F, Dobular K, Bailey D. Serum diazepam concentrations in overdose—their significance. Am J Clin Pathol 1979;72: 571–7.

44. Divoll M, Greenblatt DJ, Lacasse Y, Shader RI. Benzodiazepine overdosage: plasma concentrations and clinical outcome. Psychopharmacology 1981;73:381–3.

45. Vernon DD, Gleich MC. Poisoning and drug overdose. Crit Care Clin 1997;13:647–67.

46. Goldfrank LR. Fulmazenil: a pharmacologic antidote with limited medical toxicology utility, or . . . an antidote in search of an overdose. Acad Emerg Med 1997;4:935–6.

47. Bayer MJ, Danzl D, Gay GR, et al. Treatment of benzodiazepine overdose with flumazenil—the flumazenil in benzodiazepine intoxication multicenter study group. Clin Ther 1992;14:978–95.

48. Hoffman RS, Goldfrank LR. The poisoned patient with altered consciousness—controversies in the use of a "coma cocktail." JAMA 1995;274:562–9.

49. Spivey WH, Roberts JR, Derlet RW. A clinical trial of escalating doses of flumazenil for reversal of suspected benzodiazepine overdose in the emergency department. Ann Emerg Med 1993; 22:1813–21.

49
Care of Acute Lacerations

Bryan J. Campbell and Douglas J. Campbell

The optimum management of lacerations requires knowledge of skin anatomy and the physiology of wound healing. Such knowledge facilitates proper management of wounds of varying depth and complexity. By understanding the healing process, the family physician can maximize the options for repair and minimize the dangers of dehiscence and infection. The goals of primary closure are to stop bleeding, prevent infection, preserve function, and restore appearance. The patient always benefits from a physician who treats the patient gently, handles the tissue carefully, understands anatomy, and appreciates the healing process.[1,2]

Skin Anatomy

Figure 49.1 represents a model of the skin and the underlying tissue down to structures such as bone or muscle. Two additional features of skin anatomy that affect the repair of injuries are cleavage lines and wrinkles. Lines of cleavage are also known as Langer's lines. These lines (see Fig. 117.1) are formed by the collagen bundles that lie parallel in the dermis. An incision or repair along these lines lessens disruption of collagen bundles and decreases new collagen formation and therefore causes less scarring. Wrinkle lines are not always consistent with Langer's lines. If a laceration is not in an area of apparent wrinkling, following the basic outline of Langer's lines results in the best repair.

Wound Healing

Phase One: Inflammatory Phase

The substrate, or inflammatory, phase occurs during the first 5 to 6 days after injury. Leukocytes, histamines, prostaglandins, and fibrinogen, delivered to the injury site via blood and lymphatic channels, attempt to neutralize bacteria and foreign material. The amount of inflammation present in a wound is related to the presence of necrotic tissue, which is increased by dead space and impaired circulation. Specific measures that reduce the inflammatory response include debridement, removal of foreign material, cleaning, control of bleeding, and precise tissue coaptation.

Phase Two: Fibroblastic Phase

The fibroblastic, or collagen, phase occupies days 6 though 20 after injury. Fibroblasts enter the wound rapidly and begin collagen synthesis, which binds the wound together. As the collagen content rises, the wound strength increases until the supporting ligature can be removed. Compromise of the vascular supply can inhibit the development of collagen synthesis and interfere with healing.

Phase Three: Maturation (Remodeling) Phase

The wound continues to undergo remodeling for 18 to 24 months, during which time collagen synthesis continues and retraction occurs. Normally during this time the scar becomes softer and less conspicuous. The prominent color of the scar gradually fades, resulting in a hue consistent with the surrounding skin. Aberrations of the maturation process can result in an unsightly scar such as a keloid. Such scars are due to a combination of inherited tendencies and extrinsic factors of the wound. Proper technique in wound care and repair minimizes the extrinsic contribution to keloid formation. If it is necessary to revise an unsightly scar, the ideal delay is 18 months or more after the initial repair.

Anesthesia

Under most circumstances it is preferable to anesthetize the wound prior to preparation for closure. Before applying anesthesia, the wound is inspected using a slow, gentle, aseptic technique to ascertain the extent of injury including an assessment of the neurovascular supply. At this time a decision

Fig. 49.1. Model of skin and subcutaneous tissue.

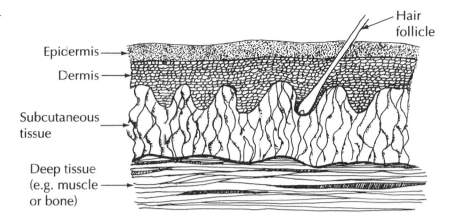

Epidermis

Dermis

Subcutaneous tissue

Deep tissue (e.g. muscle or bone)

Hair follicle

is made to refer the patient if the complexity of the wound warrants consultation.

Topical Agents

When appropriate, topical anesthesia is ideal, as pain can be relieved without causing more discomfort or anxiety. Small lacerations may be closed without additional medications.

PAC (Pontocaine/Adrenaline/Cocaine) and TAC (Tetracaine/Adrenaline/Cocaine)

Pontocaine or tetracaine 2%/aqueous epinephrine (adrenaline) 1:1000/cocaine (PAC) is the most commonly used topical agent.[3,4] It may be prepared in a 100-mL volume by mixing 25 mL of 2% tetracaine, 50 mL of 1:1000 aqueous epinephrine, 11.8 g of cocaine, and sterile normal saline to a volume of 100 mL.

Placing a saturated pledget over the wound for 5 to 15 minutes often provides adequate local anesthesia. Blanching of the skin beyond the margin of the wound allows an estimation of adequate anesthesia. Further anesthesia may be applied by injection if necessary.

Emla

Emla is a commercially available preparation of 2.5% lidocaine/ 2.5% prilocaine in a buffered vehicle. It is squeezed onto the skin surface and covered with an occlusive dressing. Its efficacy is similar to that of TAC, but it takes nearly twice as long to anesthetize the skin (30 minutes). The same guideline of skin blanching applies to the use of Emla.

Ethyl Chloride

A highly volatile fluid, ethyl chloride comes in commercially prepared glass bottles with a sprayer lid. This fluid can be sprayed onto the skin surface by inverting the bottle and pressing the lid. The flammable fluid chills the skin rapidly. The agent may be applied until skin frosting occurs. It provides brief anesthesia, allowing immediate placement of a needle without causing additional pain.

Injectable Agents

Lidocaine

Lidocaine produces moderate duration of anesthesia (about 1–2 hours) when used in a 1% or 2% solution. When mixed with 1:100,000 aqueous epinephrine, the anesthetic effect is prolonged (2–6 hours), and there is a local vasoconstrictive effect. Any anesthetic mixed with epinephrine should be used with caution on fingers, toes, ears, nose, or the penis to avoid risk of ischemia and subsequent necrosis. Occasional toxicity occurs with lidocaine, but most reactions are due to inadvertent intravascular injection. Manifestations of toxicity include tinnitus, numbness, confusion, and rarely progression to coma. True allergic reactions are unusual.

It is possible to reduce the discomfort of lidocaine injection by buffering the solution with the addition of sterile sodium bicarbonate.[5–8] A solution of 9 mL of lidocaine plus 1 mL of sodium bicarbonate (44 mEq/50 mL) is less painful to inject but provides the same level of anesthesia as the unbuffered solution. It is also possible to buffer other injectable agents including those with epinephrine. However, epinephrine is unstable at a pH above 5.5 and is commercially prepared in solutions below that pH. Therefore, any buffered local anesthetic with epinephrine must be used within a short time of preparation.[9] Warming a buffered solution to body temperature provides additional reduction of the pain of injection. Buffering also appears to increase the antibacterial properties of anesthetic solutions.[10]

Additional Agents

Mepivacaine (Carbocaine) produces longer anesthesia than lidocaine (about 45–90 minutes). It is not used with epinephrine. Reactions are similar to those seen with lidocaine. Procaine (Novocain) works quickly but has a short duration (usually less than 30–45 minutes). It has a wide safety margin and may be used with epinephrine. Bupivacaine (Marcaine) is the longest-acting local anesthetic (approximately 6–8 hours). It is often used for nerve blocks or may be mixed with lidocaine for problems that take longer to repair. It is also useful for injecting into a wound to provide postprocedural pain relief. It may be mixed with epinephrine and is available in 0.25%, 0.50%, and 0.75% solutions.

Diphenhydramine

Diphenhydramine (Benadryl) may also be used as an injectable anesthetic.[11] It is somewhat more painful to inject than lidocaine but has an efficacy similar to that of lidocaine. Diphenhydramine may be prepared in a 0.5% solution by mixing a 1-mL vial of 50 mg diphenhydramine with 9 mL of saline. This solution is useful when a patient claims an allergy to all injectable anesthetics.

Anesthetic Methods

Infiltration Blocks

Infiltration blocks are useful for most laceration repairs. The wound is infiltrated by multiple injections into the skin and subcutaneous tissue. Using a long needle and a fan technique decreases the number of injection sites and therefore decreases the pain to the patient. Using a 27-gauge or smaller needle to inject through the open wound margin also minimizes the patient's discomfort, as does moving from an anesthetized area slowly toward the unanesthetized tissue.

Field Blocks

Field blocks result in similar pain control but may distort the wound margin less and are useful where accurate wound approximation is necessary (e.g., the vermillion border). The area around the wound is injected in a series of wheals completely around the wound, thereby blocking the cutaneous nerve supply to the laceration. This technique is more time-consuming but produces longer-lasting anesthesia. Another option to reduce the initial pain of the injection is to produce a small wheal using buffered sterile water and then injecting the anesthetic through the wheal. The buffered water has a brief anesthetic action.

Nerve Blocks

Nerve blocks are most commonly effected by injecting a nerve proximal to the injury site. The most frequent use of this technique is the digital block performed by injecting anesthetic into the webbing between the digits at the metacarpophalangeal joint on each side of the digit (Fig. 49.2). Mouth and

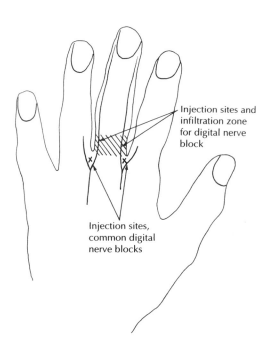

Fig. 49.2. Digital nerve block.

tongue lacerations are repairable using dental blocks. It is useful to receive practical instruction in such blocks from a dental colleague.

Sedation

The Task Force on Sedation and Analgesia by Non-Anesthesiologists[12] provides excellent protocols for sedative use by family physicians. Under adequate observation sedative agents can help the doctor deal with difficult patients. For all agents described herein, it is imperative that there be appropriate monitoring and that adequate resuscitation equipment be readily available. The welfare of the patient is of prime concern, and such medications should not be used solely for the provider's convenience.

Ketamine

Ketamine is a phencyclidine derivative. It provides a dissociative state resulting in a trance-like condition and may provide amnesia for the procedure. Ketamine can be administered by many routes, but the most practical for laceration repair is the oral method. It usually results in significant analgesia without hypotension, decreased heart rate, or decreased respiratory drive. The use of proper monitoring and the availability of resuscitation equipment is mandatory. Oral ketamine can be prepared by adding 2.5 mL of ketamine hydrochloride injection (100 mg/mL) to 7.5 mL of flavored syrup. It is then given at a dose of 10 mg/kg. Sedation occurs over 20 to 45 minutes after ingestion. The most common side effects include nystagmus, random extremity movements, and vomiting during the recovery stage.[13]

Midazolam (Versed)

Midazolam is a benzodiazepine with typical class effects of hypnosis, amnesia, and anxiety reduction. It is readily absorbed and has a short elimination half-life. It may be given as a single dose via the nasal, oral, rectal, or parenteral route. The rectal route is useful when the patient is combative. A cooperative patient prefers oral or nasal administration (oral dose 0.5 mg/kg; nasal dose 0.25 mg/kg, by nasal drops). Injectable midazolam is used to make a solution that may be given orally or nasally. The drug should be made into a 5 mg/mL solution. For oral use it may be added to punch or apple juice to improve the taste. The maximum dose for children by any route is 8 mg.

For rectal administration, a 6-French (F) feeding tube is attached to an angiocath connected to a 5-mL syringe. The lubricated catheter is then inserted into the rectum and the drug injected followed by a syringe full of air to propel the medication into the rectum. The tube is then withdrawn and the patient's buttocks are held together for approximately 1 minute. The dose is 0.45 mg/kg by this route. The medication may begin to work as soon as 10 minutes after administration. Side effects may be delayed, so the patient should be observed for at least an hour as the duration of a single dose lasts about an hour. Some burning can occur when the nasal route is used. Inconsolable agitation may appear regardless of the route of administration. This side effect of agitated crying resolves after several hours. Vomiting may also occur.[12,14,15]

Fentanyl

Fentanyl is a powerful synthetic opioid that produces rapid, short-lasting sedation and analgesia. Like other opioids, its effects are reversible, and it has limited cardiovascular effects. Although it can be given in many forms, oral transmucosal fentanyl citrate (OTFC) is available commercially in a lollipop (Fentanyl Oralet). This drug, commonly used as an preanesthetic medication, is available in three dosage forms (200, 300, and 400 mg). The dose for adults is 5 mg/kg to a maximum of 400 mg regardless of weight. Pediatric dosages begin at 5 mg/kg to a maximum of 15 mg/kg or 400 mg (whichever is less). Children weighing less than 15 kg should not receive fentanyl. OTFC effects are apparent 5 to 10 minutes after sucking the Oralet. The maximum effect is usually achieved about 30 minutes after use, but effects may persist for several hours. Side effects are common but usually minor. About half of patients develop transient pruritus, 15% notice dizziness, and at least one third develop vomiting. The most dangerous effect is hypoventilation, which can be fatal.[12,16,17] Oversedation or respiratory depression responds to naloxone.

Nitrous Oxide

Nitrous oxide is a rapid-acting anesthetic that works within 3 to 5 minutes with a similar duration after cessation of administration.[18] Commercial equipment is available to deliver a mixture of nitrous oxide and oxygen at various ratios (usually 30–50% N_2O/50–70% O_2). Side effects include nausea in about 10% to 15% of patients with occasional emesis. The efficacy of nitrous oxide is known to be variable. Although some patients object to the use of the mask, many patients prefer using a specially designed self-administration mask. Nitrous oxide can cause expansion of gas-filled body pockets, and for that reason it should not be used in patients with head injuries, pneumothoraces, bowel obstructions, or middle ear effusions.

Wound Preparation

Proper preparation of a wound can improve the success of aesthetically acceptable healing. The wound should be closed as soon as possible, although most lacerations heal well if closed within 24 hours after the injury. After anesthesia, proper cleansing should be accomplished by wiping, scrubbing, and irrigating with normal saline using a large syringe with or without a 22-gauge needle, which produces enough velocity to clean most wounds. Antiseptic soaps such as hexachlorophene (pHisoHex), chlorhexidine gluconate (Hibiclens), or povidone-iodine (Betadine) can also be used, but one should be aware that all of these cleansing agents with the exception of normal saline will delay wound healing to some extent by destroying fibroblasts and leukocytes as well as bacteria. Sterile scrub brushes may be useful for cleaning grossly contaminated lesions.

After washing and irrigation, the area is draped with sterile towels to create a clean field. The wound is then explored using sterile technique to confirm the depth of injury, ascertain whether injury to underlying tissue has occurred, rule out the presence of any foreign body, and determine the adequacy of anesthesia. After examination, debridement is performed if necessary.

Debridement is the process of converting an irregular dirty wound to a clean one with smooth edges. Wound margins that are crushed, mangled, or devitalized are excised unless it is unwise to do so. Tissue in areas such as the lip or eyelid should be removed with extreme caution. It is pointless to increase the deformity when a somewhat imperfect scar can provide a more functional result. If a considerable amount of tissue has been crushed, initial removal of all the damaged tissue may result in undesirable function (such as would occur if the skin over a joint was removed). Such injuries should be closed loosely using subcutaneous absorbable sutures. The scar can be revised later if necessary.

The initial incision is made with a scalpel followed by excision with a pair of sharp tissue scissors. The edges should be perpendicular to the skin surface or even slightly undercut to facilitate eversion of the skin margins (Fig. 49.3). In hairy areas incisions should parallel the hair shafts to minimize the likelihood of hairless areas around the healed wound (Fig. 49.4).

After debridement the skin edges are held together to see if it is possible to approximate them with minimal tension. Generally, it is necessary to undermine the skin to achieve greater mobility of the surface by releasing some of the subcutaneous skin attachments that prevent the skin from sliding (Fig. 49.5). This step takes place in the subcutaneous layer and can be done with a scalpel or scissors. The wound is then undermined circumferentially about 4 to 5 mm from the edge of the margin. The undermining should be equal across the wound and widest where the skin needs to move the most, usually the center of the cut.

Hemostasis can be accomplished most easily by simple pressure on the wound site for 5 to 10 minutes. If pressure is

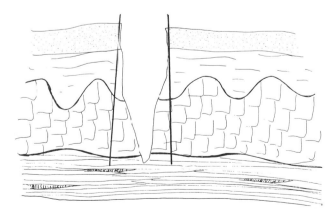

Fig. 49.3. Slight undercutting of the wound edges facilitates slight eversion of the wound edge.

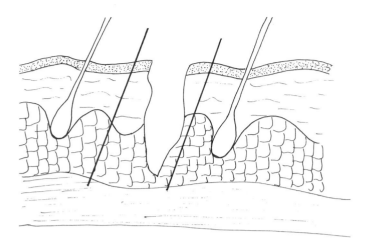

Fig. 49.4. Parallel debridement in a hairy area avoids damaging hair follicles.

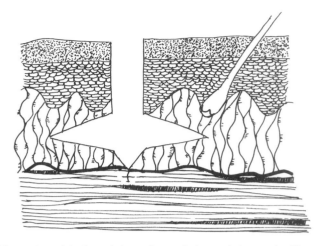

Fig. 49.5. Undermining the subdermal layer facilitates closure.

unsuccessful, bleeders may be carefully cauterized or ligated. Cautery or ligation can hinder healing if large amounts of tissue are damaged. Small vessels can be controlled with absorbable suture if necessary, but large arterial bleeders may need to be controlled with permanent ligature if it is possible to do so without compromising the distal circulation. If oozing persists, the wound is closed with a drain (e.g., a sterile rubber band or Penrose drain) left in the wound several days. An overlying pressure dressing minimizes bleeding. Advancing the drain every other day permits healing with minimal hematoma formation.

Wound Closure

Suture options are listed in Table 49.1. Absorbable materials are gradually broken down and absorbed by tissue; nonabsorbable sutures are made from chemicals that are encapsulated by the body and thus isolated from tissue. Monofilament sutures are less irritating to tissue but are more difficult to handle and require more knots than braided sutures. Stitches placed through the epidermis are done with nonabsorbable materials to minimize the tissue reactivity that occurs with absorbable stitches. Reverse cutting needles in a three-eighths

Table 49.1. **Common Suture Materials**

Suture	Advantages	Disadvantages
Absorbable		
Catgut	Inexpensive	Low tensile strength
		Strength lasts 4–5 days
		High tissue reactivity
Chromic catgut	Inexpensive	Moderate tensile strength and reactivity
Polyglycolic acid (Dexon)	Low tissue reactivity	Moderately difficult to handle
Polyglactic acid (Vicryl)	Easy handling	Occasional "spitting" of suture due to
	Good tensile strength	absorption delay
Polyglyconate (Maxon)	Easy handling	Expensive
	Good tensile strength	
Nonabsorbable		
Silk	Handles well	Low tensile strength
	Moderately inexpensive	High tissue reactivity
		Increased infection rate
Nylon (Ethilon, Dermilon)	High tensile strength	Difficult to handle; slippery, so many knots needed
	Minimal tissue reactivity	
	Inexpensive	
Polypropylene (Proline SurgiPro)	No tissue reaction	Expensive
	Stretches, accommodates swelling	
Braided polyester (Mersilene, Ethiflex)	Handles well	Tissue drag if uncoated
	Knots secure	Expensive
Polybutester (Novofil)	Elastic, accommodates swelling and retraction	Expensive

Fig. 49.6. Layer closure showing sutures in the epidermis, at the dermal–epidermal junction, and at the dermal–fat junction.

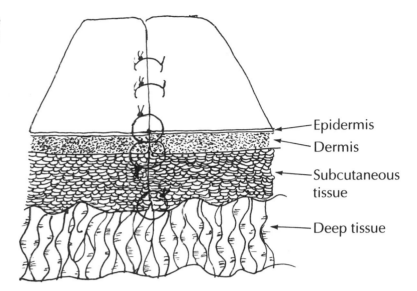

— Epidermis

— Dermis

— Subcutaneous tissue

— Deep tissue

or one-half circle design are available in various sizes for each type of suture.

A well-closed wound has three characteristics: the margins are approximated without tension, the tissue layers are accurately aligned, and dead space is eliminated. Deep stitches are placed in layers that hold the suture, such as the fat–fascial junction or the derma–fat junction. A buried knot technique is the preferred method for placing deep sutures. Deep sutures provide most of the strength of the repair, and skin sutures approximate the skin margins and improve the cosmetic result (Fig. 49.6).

Suture Techniques[19–21]

Simple Interrupted Stitch

A simple interrupted stitch is placed by passing the needle through the skin surface at right angles, placing the suture as wide as it is deep. The goal is to place sutures that slightly evert the edge of the wound (Fig. 49.7). This maneuver pro-

duces a slightly raised scar that recedes during the remodeling stage of healing and leaves a smooth scar. The opposite margin is approximated using a mirror image of the first placement. Following the natural radius of the curved needle places the suture in such a way as to evert the wound margin. It can be modified to correctly approximate the margins when the wound edges are asymmetric[1] (Fig. 49.8). Occasionally a wound exhibits excessively everted margins. By reversing the usual approach and taking a stitch that is wider at the top than at the base, the wound can be inverted, improving the cosmetic appearance (Fig. 49.9). A useful general rule is that the entrance and exit points should be 2 mm from the margin for facial wounds but may be farther apart on other surfaces.[1,2] The open-loop knot (Fig. 49.10) avoids placing the suture under excessive tension and facilitates removal of the stitch. The first throw of the knot with two loops ("surgeon's knot") is placed with just enough tension to approximate the wound

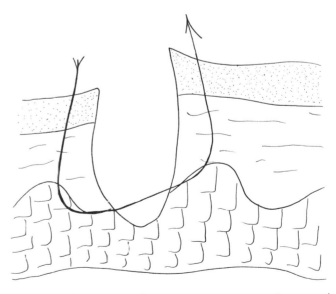

Fig. 49.7. Simple interrupted suture with placement to facilitate wound eversion.

Fig. 49.8. Placement of suture in an asymmetric wound.

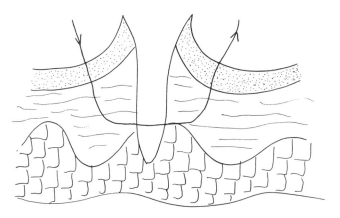

Fig. 49.9. Suture placement in a wound with everted edges.

margin. The second throw, a single loop, is tied, leaving a little space so no additional tension is place on the first loop. Subsequent throws can be tightened snugly without increasing tension on the wound edge. Pulling all the knots to the same side of the wound makes suture removal easier and improves the aesthetics of the repair. As a rule of thumb one should put at least the same number of knots of a monofilament suture as the size of the ligature (e.g., five knots with 5-0 suture).

Vertical or Horizontal Mattress Suture

The vertical mattress suture promotes eversion and is useful where thick layers are encountered or tension exists. Two techniques may be used. The classic method first places the deep stitch and closes with the superficial stitch (Fig. 49.11). The short-hand method[22] is performed by placing the shallow stitch first, pulling up on the suture (tenting the skin), and then placing the deeper stitch. Horizontal mattress sutures also have the advantage of needing fewer knots to cover the same area.

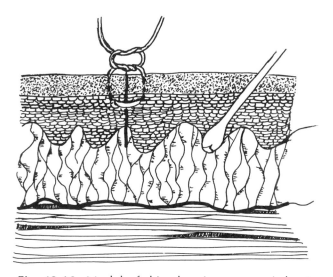

Fig. 49.10. Model of skin showing surgeon's knot.

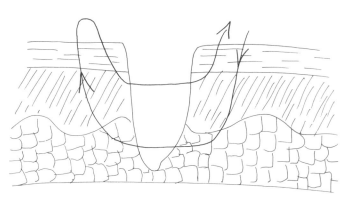

Fig. 49.11. Vertical mattress suture.

Intracuticular Running Suture

The intracuticular running suture, utilizing a nonabsorbable suture, can be used where there is minimal skin tension. It results in minimal scarring without suture marks. Controlled tissue apposition is difficult with this method, but it is a popular technique because of the cosmetic result. The suture ends do not need to be tied but can be taped in place under slight tension (Fig. 49.12).

Three-Point Mattress Suture

The three-point or corner stitch is used to minimize the possibility of vascular necrosis of the tip of a V-shaped wound.

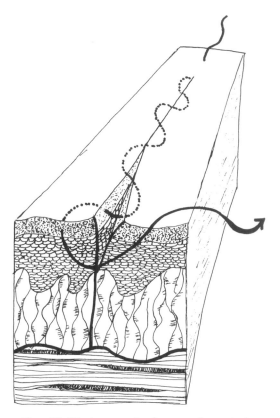

Fig. 49.12. Intracuticular running stitch.

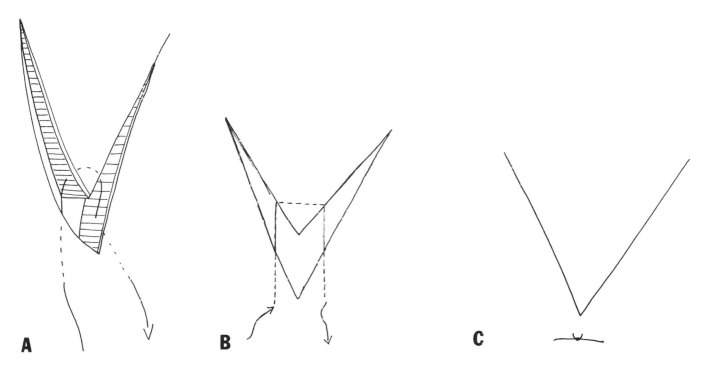

A   **B**   **C**

Fig. 49.13. Three-point stitch. (A) Three-dimensional view showing suture placement. (B) Schematic view. (C) Finished stitch.

The needle is inserted into the skin of the wound edge on one side of the wound opposite the flap near the apex of the wound (Fig. 49.13A,B). The suture is placed at the mid-dermis level, brought across the wound, and placed transversely at the same level through the apex of the flap. It is then brought across the wound and returned at the same level on the opposite side of the V parallel to the point of entry. The suture is then tied, drawing the tip of the wound into position without compromising the blood supply (Fig. 49.13C). This method can also be used for stellate injuries where multiple tips can be approximated in purse-string fashion.

Running or Continuous Stitch

The running stitch is useful in situations where speed is important (e.g., a field emergency) because individual knots do not have to be tied. It is appropriate for use on scalp lacerations especially, because it is good for hemostasis. The continuous method does not allow fine control of wound margins (Fig. 49.14).

Specific Circumstances

Lacerations Across a Landmark

Lacerations that involve prominent anatomic features or landmarks, such as the vermilion border of the lip or the eyebrow, require special consideration. Commonly a laceration is closed from one end to the other, but in special situations it is advisable to place a retention stitch (a simple or vertical mattress stitch) to reapproximate the landmark border accu-

rately. The remainder of the wound can then be closed by an appropriate method. If the retention stitch is under significant tension when the repair seems complete, it should be removed and replaced.

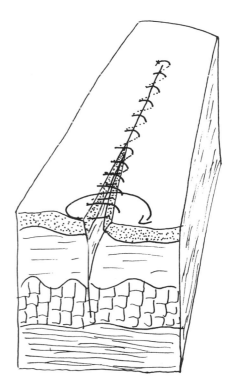

Fig. 49.14. Running stitch.

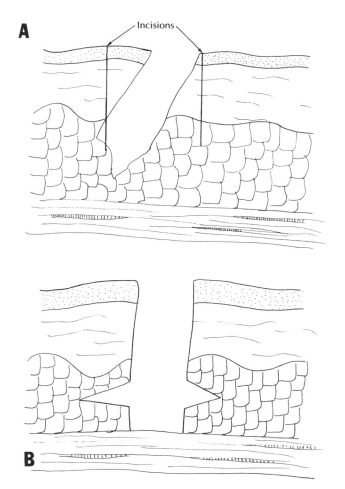

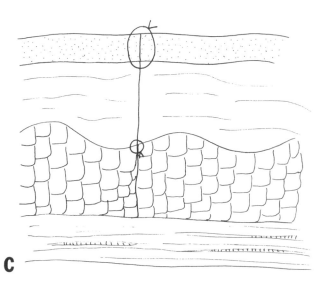

Fig. 49.15. Closure of beveled wound. (A) Squaring beveled edges. (B) Undermining the fat layer. (C) Layered closure.

Beveled Lacerations

A frequently seen injury, the beveled laceration, tempts the physician to close it as it is; but the undercut flap may not heal well owing to disruption of the blood supply. The margins of the wound should be modified, as shown in Figure 49.15. The edges are squared, undermined, and closed in layers.

Dog Ears

Dog ears, a common problem, results from wound closure where the sides of the laceration are unequal. One side bunches up, and a mound of skin occurs. It also occurs when an elliptical wound is closed in the center, leaving excess tissue at each end. To correct the problem, the dog ear is tented up with a skin hook, and a linear incision is made along one side. The excess triangle is then grasped at the tip and a second linear incision is made (Fig. 49.16). This maneuver allows closure in a single line.

Complex Lacerations

A wound may occur with unequal sides with a hump of tissue on one side. This lump of tissue may be excised using the technique described above for removal of dog ears. The triangular defect is then closed using a modification of the three-point mattress suture, the four-point technique shown in Figure 49.17. The resulting closure forms a T-shaped repair.

Finger Injuries

Amputated Fingertip

If the area of the fingertip amputation is less than 1 cm^2, the wound can be handled by careful cleansing, proper dressings, and subsequent healing by secondary intention. If the wound is larger, the complexity of treatment increases. If the amputation is beveled dorsally and distally, a conservative approach without suturing or grafting usually results in good healing. An unfavorable angle requires more extensive repair.[23] Referral to a plastic or hand surgeon may be warranted.

Nail Bed Injuries

Nail bed injuries can be managed by saving the nail and reapproximating nail matrix lacerations with fine absorbable sutures. It may be necessary to remove the nail to repair an underlying nail bed tear. The nail may then be replaced and held in position with several sutures, allowing the nail to act as a splint.

Alternatives to Suturing

Suturing has been an effective method for closing wounds for centuries, but options for skin suturing are now available. They may even represent more cost-effective methods of wound closure.

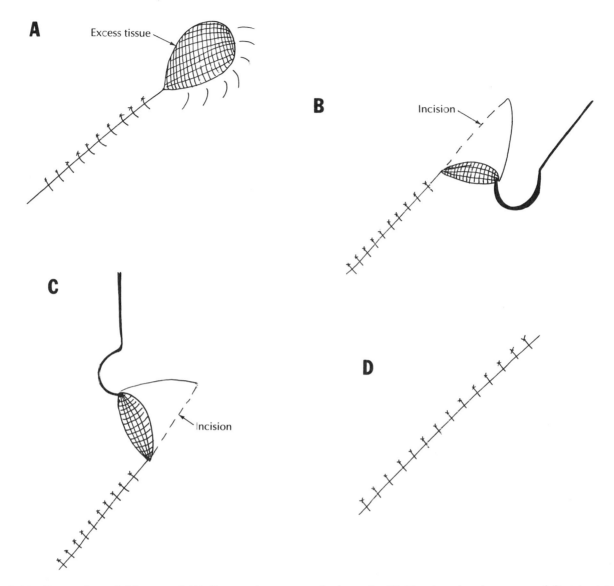

Fig. 49.16. Correction of "dog ear." (A) Excess tissue at end of repair. (B) Tenting the dog ear and first incision. (C) Pulling flap across initial incision and position of second incision. (D) Appearance of final closure.

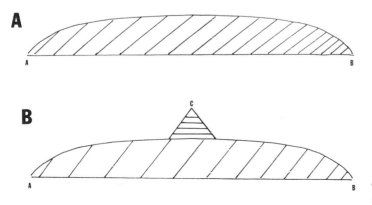

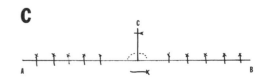

Fig. 49.17. Unequal wound closure. (A) Sides of laceration are unequal. (B) Excise triangle of tissue on longer side. (C) T-closure showing four-point suture.

Staples

One option is the use of skin staples, which have been used for years in the operating room as the final closure for a variety of incisions. Typically, staples are used on the skin in wounds that would be closed in a straight line. The skin is closed with staples after other layers are closed by suturing. The most significant advantage to the use of staples is the decreased time necessary to close the skin. An assistant may be required to position the skin properly.[24]

Adhesives

The most commonly used tissue glues are related to cyanoacrylate ester known as Super Glue. Tissue glues for superficial wounds have the advantage of rapid closure, minimal physical and emotional trauma to the patient, and absence of a foreign body in the wound.[25,26] They may also be less expensive to use than traditional methods of closure.

Histoacryl Blue, a.k.a. Dermabond, has been commercially available in Canada since 1975, and in the United States since 1998. It is a safe alternative to suturing.[27–29] Hemostasis must be achieved before applying the glue. Because some chemicals used for hemostasis such as Monsel's solution will prevent the adhesive from bonding to the skin, care must be taken to avoid skin edges. Layered closure may be accomplished using deep, absorbable sutures combined with surface adhesive. Surface sutures combined with adhesive should be avoided because the adhesive will bond to the suture material and may make removing the suture difficult. Only wounds that are under no tension are appropriate for adhesive, such as those on the face and the forearm. Even wounds such as on the foot are generally inappropriate because as soon as the patient steps on the foot, pressure is generated across the wound edges. After hemostasis and cleansing have been achieved, the wound must be approximated using gloved fingers (vinyl is preferred to latex because it also not bond as well to the adhesive), metal instruments (preferred because metal also does not bond as tightly to the adhesive as plastic), Steri-strips, or specially manufactured closure devices for use with the adhesive. With the wound edges approximated, a layer of adhesive is applied to the top of the wound and allowed to polymerize. Two more subsequent layers should be applied and allowed to polymerize over the top

of the first layer. Some other precautions: Because the adhesive is a very thin, runny liquid, gravity should be utilized to keep the liquid from running into eyes, the wound itself, or other undesirable areas. If adhesive does get on the cornea in spite of appropriate precautions, it does not cause damage and may be left to come off within a few days. Other methods to control the spread of the adhesive include sponges lightly moistened with saline or use of Vaseline around the area. The patient should be instructed to keep the wound dry for 7 to 10 days because moisture weakens the bonding strength. The wound can either be left open to air, or covered with a clean bandage. Petroleum-based products should also be avoided on the adhesive because of a weakening effect.

Postrepair Management

Most wounds should be protected during the first 1 to 2 days after repair. Frequently a commercial bandage may be used; but when the wound is still oozing, a pressure dressing is applied.

Table 49.2. Instructions for Patients

1. Keep wound dressings clean and dry. Protect dressings from moisture when bathing.
2. If the dressing gets wet, remove it and reapply a clean, dry dressing.
3. Remove the dressing after 2 days and reapply every 2 days unless instructed otherwise.
4. If any of the following signs appears, contact your physician or clinic immediately:
   A. Wound becomes red, warm, swollen, or tender.
   B. Wound begins to drain.
   C. Red streaks appear near the wound or up the arm or leg.
   D. Tender lumps appear in the armpit or groin.
   E. Chills or fever occur.
5. Because of your particular injury the doctor would like your wound check in _____ days.
6. Please return for removal of your stitches in _____ days.
7. You received the following vaccinations:
   A. Tetanus toxoid _____
   B. DT (diphtheria/tetanus) _____
   C. DPT (diphtheria/pertussis/tetanus) _____

Table 49.3. Guide to Tetanus Prophylaxis During Routine Wound Management

History of adsorbed tetanus toxoid (doses)	Clean, minor wounds		All other wounds[a]	
	Td[b]	TIg	Td[b]	TIg
Unknown or <3	Yes	No	Yes	Yes
≥Three[c]	No[d]	No	No[e]	No

[a]Such as, but not limited to, wounds contaminated with dirt, feces, soil, and saliva; puncture wounds; avulsions; and wounds resulting from missiles, crushing, burns, and frostbite.

[b]For children <7 years old; DPT (DT if pertussis vaccine is contraindicated) is preferred to tetanus toxoid alone. For persons ≥7 years of age Td is preferred to tetanus toxoid alone.

[c]If only three doses of *fluid* toxoid have been received, a fourth dose of toxoid, preferably an adsorbed toxoid, is given.

[d]Yes, if >10 years since last dose.

[e]Yes, if >5 years since last dose. (More frequent boosters are not needed and can accentuate side effects.)

Td = tetanus-diphtheria toxoid; TIg = tetanus immune globulin; DPT = diphtheria/pertussis/tetanus.

The initial layer is a nonstick gauze dressing available in sterile packages, such as Adaptic, Telfa, or Xeroderm. A gauze pad is then placed and held in place by roller gauze, elastic wrap, or elastic tape. Dressings are removed and the wound reexamined at 48 to 72 hours. If a drain has been placed, it should be advanced every 24 to 48 hours. If the wound is under significant tension, additional support can be achieved by using Steri-Strips or bulky supportive dressings, including splints that are commercially available or custom-made from plaster or fiberglass.

Most wounds can be left open after the first 24 to 48 hours. It is important to remove wet dressings from a repair because the skin maceration that results from them may prolong healing and increase the risk of infection. Initial epithelialization takes place during the first 24 hours, and thereafter it is permissible to wash the wound briefly. Lacerations on the scalp and face may be impractical to bandage.

Wounds should be reexamined for infection or hematoma formation after 2 to 3 days if there is any concern at the time of repair. Contaminated wounds and wounds that have been open longer than 24 hours have a greater likelihood of infection.

Timing of suture removal should be individualized, based on wound location, the mechanical stress placed on the repair, and the tension of the closure. Facial sutures should be removed within 3 to 5 days to minimize the possibility of suture tracks. Supporting the repair with Steri-Strips may decrease the likelihood of dehiscence. In skin areas that are not highly mobile (e.g., the back or extremities) sutures are left in place for 7 to 10 days. On fingers, palms, soles, and over joints, the sutures remain in place at least 10 to 14 days and sometimes longer. Table 49.2 is a sample instruction sheet for patients.

Concurrent Therapy

Preventing infection is an important aspect of laceration treatment. Puncture wounds and bites usually should not be closed because the risk of infection negates the advantage of closure. Dog bites can usually be safely closed, however. Sometimes a gaping puncture wound on the face requires closure for cosmetic reasons despite the risk of infection.

Antibiotic Usage

Antibiotic prophylaxis is probably not helpful in most circumstances unless given in sufficient quantity to obtain good tissue levels while the wound is still open. If extensive repair is necessary, intravenous antibiotics should be started during wound closure. Animal and human bite wounds are often treated by post-closure antibiotics. The efficacy of this practice remains controversial, but antibiotics are often given because of the extensive contamination that occurs with bite wounds, especially those from cats. Amoxicillin-clavulanate covers the typical bacteria of bite wounds. Doxycycline and ceftriaxone are alternative medications.[29]

Tetanus Prophylaxis

Tetanus prophylaxis is a crucial part of the care of the lacerated patient; it is imperative that the immunization status of the patient be documented. Patients most likely to be inadequately immunized are the elderly, who may have never received a primary series. Table 49.3 is a summary of the guide published by the Centers for Disease Control and Prevention. Whenever passive immunity is required, human tetanus immune globulin (TIg) is preferred. The usual dose of TIg is 500 units IM. Tetanus toxoid and TIg should be given through separate needles at separate sites.[30,31]

References

1. Brietenbach KL, Bergera JJ. Principles and techniques of primary wound closure. Prim Care 1986;13:411–31.
2. Snell G. Laceration repair. In: Pfenninger JL, Fowler GC, eds. Procedures for primary care physicians. St. Louis: Mosby, 1994;12–19.
3. Bonadio WA, Wagner V. Efficacy of TAC topical anesthetic for repair of pediatric lacerations. Am J Dis Child 1988;142:203–5.
4. Hegenbarth MA, Altieri MF, Hawk WH, Green A, Ochsenschlager DW, O'Donnell R. Comparison of topical tetracaine, adrenaline, and cocaine anesthesia with lidocaine infiltration for repair of lacerations in children. Ann Emerg Med 1990;19:63–7.
5. Matsumoto AH, Reifsnyder AC, Hartwell GD, Angle JF, Selby JB, Tegtmeyer CJ. Reducing the discomfort of lidocaine administration through pH buffering. J Vasc Interv Radiol 1994;5:171–5.
6. Bartfield JM, Ford DT, Homer PJ. Buffered versus plain lidocaine for digital nerve blocks. Ann Emerg Med 1993;22:216–19.
7. Mader TJ, Playe SJ, Garb JL. Reducing the pain of local anesthetic infiltration: warming and buffering have a synergistic effect. Ann Emerg Med 1994;23:550–4.
8. Brogan BX Jr, Giarrusso E, Hollander JE, Cassara G, Mararnga MC, Thode HC. Comparison of plain, warmed, and buffered lidocaine for anesthesia of traumatic wounds. Ann Emerg Med 1995;26:121–5.
9. Murakami CS, Odland PB, Ross BK. Buffered local anesthetics and epinephrine degradation. J Dermatol Surg Oncol 1994;20:192–5.
10. Thompson KD, Welykyj S, Massa MC. Antibacterial activity of lidocaine in combination with a bicarbonate buffer. J Dermatol Surg Oncol 1993;19:216–20.
11. Ernst AA, Marvez-Valls E, Mall G, Patterson J, Xie X, Weiss SJ. 1% lidocaine versus 0.5% diphenhydramine for local anesthesia in minor laceration repair. Ann Emerg Med 1994;23:1328–32.
12. Task Force on Sedation and Analgesia by Non-Anesthesiologists. Practical guidelines for sedation and analgesia by nonanesthesiologists. Anesthesiology 1996;84:459–71.
13. Qureshi FA, Mellis PT, McFadden MA. Efficacy of oral ketamine for providing sedation and analgesia to children requiring laceration repair. Pediatr Emerg Care 1995;11:93–7.
14. Connors K, Terndrup TE. Nasal versus oral midazolam for sedation of anxious children undergoing laceration repair. Ann Emerg Med 1994;24:1074–9.
15. Shane SA, Fuchs SM, Khine H. Efficacy of rectal midazolam for the sedation of preschool children undergoing laceration repair. Ann Emerg Med 1994;24:1065–73.
16. Schutzman SA, Burg J, Liebelt E, et al. Oral transmucosal fentanyl citrate for the premedication of children undergoing laceration repair. Ann Emerg Med 1994;24:1059–64.
17. Clinical considerations in the use of fentanyl Oralet. North Chicago, IL: Abbott Laboratories, 1995;1–16.
18. Gamis AS, Knapp JF, Glenski JA. Nitrous oxide analgesia in a pediatric emergency department. Ann Emerg Med 1989;18:177–81.

19. Moy RL, Lee A, Zolka A. Commonly used suture materials in skin surgery. Am Fam Physician 1991;44:2123–8.

20. Epperson WJ. Suture selection. In: Pfenninger JL, Fowler GC, eds. Procedures for primary care physicians. St. Louis: Mosby, 1994;3–6.

21. Moy RL, Waldman B, Hein DW. A review of sutures and suturing techniques. J Dermatol Surg Oncol 1992;18:785–95.

22. Jones JS, Gartner M, Drew G, Pack S. The shorthand vertical mattress stitch: evaluation of a new suture technique. Am J Emerg Med 1993;11:483–5.

23. Ditmars DM Jr. Finger tip and nail bed injuries. Occup Med 1989;4:449–61.

24. Edlich RF, Thacker JG, Silloway RF, Morgan RF, Rodeheaver GT. Scientific basis of skin staple closure. In: Haval Mutaz B, ed. Advances in plastic and reconstructive surgery. Chicago: Year Book, 1986;233–71.

25. Osmond MH, Klassen TP, Quinn JV. Economic comparison of a tissue adhesive and suturing in the repair of pediatric facial lacerations. J Pediatr 1995;126(6):892–5.

26. Quinn JV, Drzewiecki A, Li MM, et al. A randomized, controlled trial comparing tissue adhesive with suturing in the repair of pediatric facial lacerations. Ann Emerg Med 1993;22:1130–5.

27. Applebaum JS, Zalut T, Applebaum D. The use of tissue adhesive for traumatic laceration repair in the emergency department. Ann Emerg Med 1993;22:1190–2.

28. Fisher AA. Reactions to cyanoacrylate adhesives: "instant glue." Cutis 1995:18–22,46,58.

29. Lewis KT, Stiles M. Management of cat and dog bites. Am Fam Physician 1995;52:479–85.

30. Centers for Disease Control. Tetanus prophylaxis during routine wound management. MMWR 1991;40(RR-10):1–28.

31. Richardson JP, Knight AL. The management and prevention of tetanus. J Emerg Med 1993;11:737–42.

50
Selected Injuries

Allan V. Abbott

Unintentional injuries remain the fifth leading cause of death in the United States. Table 50.1 lists these deaths according to cause and frequency.[1]

Near-Drowning

Drowning is the third leading cause of accidental death in the United States, accounting for about 4,000 deaths annually. *Near-drowning* is defined as survival after an episode of suffocation and cerebral hypoxia in a liquid medium, whereas *submersion injury* (*drowning*) is death within 24 hours of such an episode. *Secondary drowning* is death from complications that occur more than 24 hours after the submersion. *Immersion syndrome* is sudden death after contact with cold water.[2]

Most near-drownings and drownings occur among inadequately supervised children younger than 4 years of age in swimming pools, ocean surf, bathtubs, or hot tubs. In small children, drowning is more common than toxic ingestions and firearm injuries. Boys and young men between the ages of 15 and 24 and the elderly over age 75, especially if unable to swim, are also at risk because of alcohol or drug use while swimming, infirmity, or associated trauma or seizures.

Clinical Presentation

The usual submerged drowning victim at first holds his or her breath and becomes anoxic and panics, then swallows or gasps and aspirates water, loses consciousness, and dies in cardiac arrest. Approximately 10% of victims have acute laryngospasm that results in dry drowning, because there is no aspiration of water into the lungs and death typically occurs owing to profound obstructive asphyxia.[2]

The duration of hypoxia that can be tolerated depends on the individual's age and health, the water temperature, and the promptness and effectiveness of the resuscitation. Young victims usually recover if the submersion is less than 3 minutes, or up to 10 minutes if the water is cold (0°–15°C) (32°–59°F). Survival has been reported after 15 to 20 minutes of submersion and up to 40 minutes in cold water.[3]

With near-drowning the clinical presentation depends on the stage at which the drowning sequence was interrupted. Aspiration of water leads to varying degrees of pulmonary edema and can result in adult respiratory distress syndrome as late as 72 hours after the near-drowning. There may be shortness of breath, rales, rhonchi, or wheezing. Chest radiographs may initially show pulmonary edema or appear misleadingly normal. Severe pulmonary edema can develop slowly in a patient who initially has no pulmonary signs or symptoms. Hypothermia due to submersion in cold water often leads to bradycardia or atrial fibrillation. Hypoxia leads to cerebral damage with subsequent cerebral edema. Internal injuries should be suspected with falls into the water and boating accidents; cervical spine and head injuries are particularly common. Severe acidosis and electrolyte disturbances can occur. Subsequent intravascular hemolysis, disseminated intravascular coagulation, and renal failure are uncommon but possible.

Management

Immediate Management

Aggressive emergency resuscitation is the most important factor influencing outcome.[4] Airway protection and respiratory support should begin immediately, even before removal from the water. Advanced cardiopulmonary life support (ACLS) is begun immediately as indicated by the circulatory status and cardiac rhythm. Maneuvers to promote postural drainage, such as that advocated by Heimlich et al,[5] are controversial, with most experts discouraging their use because of interruption of cardiopulmonary resuscitation, loss of airway control, aspiration, and aggravation of possible cervical spine injuries.[6] Oxygen at 100% is administered to all near-drowning victims as soon it is available.

Table 50.1. **Deaths Due to Unintentional Injuries—United States, 1999[1]**

Type of injury	Deaths per year
All unintentional injuries	96,900
Motor vehicle accidents	41,300
Falls	17,100
Drowning	4,000
Suffocation by ingested object	3,200
Fires and burns	3,100
Firearms	700
Poisoning by gas and vapors	500
All other	16,500

Hospital Management

The initial appearance of near-drowning patients who are conscious may be deceptively normal. Therefore, virtually all near-drowning patients should be admitted for observation, oxygen, and supportive care. If they remain asymptomatic and if chest films and arterial blood gas assays remain normal, they may be discharged after 8 hours, or after 24 hours if there was any aspiration. A large-bore intravenous line should be positioned. The rectal temperature is measured; and if the patient is hypothermic ($<35°C$, $<95°F$), rewarming is begun (see Hypothermia in Chapter 46). Most serious cases are reflected in lactic acidosis and electrolyte disturbances, and treatment is guided by monitoring the arterial blood gases and serum electrolytes.

Patients are monitored for respiratory and central nervous system (CNS) function. Indications for endotracheal intubation in hospitalized patients include (1) protection of the airway in nearly comatose patients, (2) neurologic deterioration, (3) copious secretions or gross aspiration of particulate matter, and (4) inability to maintain a PaO_2 of 60 to 90 mm Hg. Positive end-expiratory pressure (PEEP) is helpful with a pulmonary injury to recruit gas exchange in spaces and to prevent terminal airway closure. A nasogastric tube is placed to remove excess swallowed water and air.

Bronchospasm can be managed with β-adrenergic aerosols. Early therapeutic bronchoscopy should be considered if particulate matter such as vomitus or mud have been aspirated. Most centers currently employ supportive care and do not use prophylactic antibiotics, barbiturates, steroids, hypothermia, hyperventilation, intracranial pressure monitoring, or neuromuscular blockade routinely.[2]

Survival after near-drowning and cerebral anoxia can be predicted by neurologic examination 24 hours after the drowning incident. The absence of spontaneous, purposeful movements and normal brainstem function after 24 hours suggests severe neurologic deficits or death. Satisfactory recovery can be expected in presence of spontaneous, purposeful movements and normal brainstem function.[6]

Children who are involved in bathtub near-drownings may have suffered from abuse or neglect. In these cases the medical evaluation should include a social work consultation and a search for accompanying injuries.[7]

Prevention

Physicians should counsel parents that most drownings of small children can be prevented if pools and hot tubs are surrounded by a fence of at least 55 inches in height with locked or self-closing, self-latching gates, if pool safety covers are in place, and if house door-opening alarms are used.[3]

Adults should provide immediate supervision at all times when children have access to pools. Children should always wear life jackets while in boats. Adults should be trained in basic cardiopulmonary resuscitation. Also, swimming must be avoided while under the influence of alcohol or psychoactive drugs.

Barotrauma

Barotrauma—injury caused by barometric pressure changes—usually results from diving under water, ascending into the atmosphere, or mechanical respiratory support. As one ascends into the atmosphere, the atmospheric pressure decreases gradually; at 5500 m (18,000 feet) it reaches a pressure of about one half that at sea level. In contrast, when one descends into water, the pressure of the water increases more rapidly, with a doubling of pressure every 10 m (33 feet) below the surface. Barotrauma resulting from changes in atmospheric pressure occurs commonly to the ear and sinuses. Among divers, barotrauma results in ear and sinus injuries, decompression sickness, and air embolism. Pulmonary barotrauma can result from diving or mechanical ventilation.

Ear and Sinus Barotrauma

Barotrauma can affect the external ear canal, middle ear, inner ear, and sinuses. It is sometimes referred to as the "squeeze" when the ambient pressures are greater than the pressures within the body cavities; it is called "reverse squeeze" under the opposite conditions.

External Barotitis

Ear canal squeeze occurs when divers descend with ear canals plugged with earplugs or cerumen. The diver experiences pain and bloody drainage as the pressure in the middle ear exceeds that within the canal. On examination of the tympanic membrane, petechiae, hemorrhagic blebs, and rupture may be seen.[8]

Barotitis Media

Barotitis media is the most common ear injury resulting from pressure. The eustachian tube provides the only route for air to enter or exit the middle ear. The normally functioning eustachian tube acts as a one-way valve, allowing excess pressures to vent passively from the middle ear while allowing air to enter only with active swallowing, yawning, or autoinflation (the patient holds nose and mouth shut, blows to puff cheeks, and swallows with cheeks puffed).[8] When eustachian tube function is impaired by mucosal inflammation due to upper respiratory infection (URI), allergy, or trauma, the active movement of air into the inner ear is usually impaired first, with passive venting being impaired later in more severe cases. Thus a person with a URI flying in an airplane usually finds that ear pressures adjust on ascent, but pain increases during descent if swallowing or autoinflation maneuvers fail to "pop" the ears. Commercial airliners maintain cabin pressure equal to about 6000 to 8000 feet, so severe middle ear barotrauma is unlikely.

Divers who do not achieve middle ear pressure equalization experience pain on descent. Inward bulging to the tympanic membrane, hemorrhage, and edema develop, with rupture of the tympanic membrane if descent continues.[8]

Inner Ear Barotrauma

If pressure is great enough, the oval or round window can rupture, with a sudden onset of sensorineural hearing loss, severe vertigo, tinnitus, nystagmus, and fullness in the affected ear.[9,10]

Sinus Barotrauma

The frontal and maxillary sinuses may be "squeezed" when mucosal inflammation due to URI or other condition blocks the sinus ostia. It usually occurs in divers during descent, resulting in pain and epistaxis from the area of the sinus.[9]

Management

When barotitis involves a ruptured tympanic membrane, treatment includes keeping the ear dry, giving analgesics as needed, and prohibiting swimming or flying until the tympanic membrane heals spontaneously. Decongestants and antihistamines are usually recommended. Antibiotics have been suggested but are of uncertain value. Patients should not dive or fly until they have movement of the tympanic membrane on autoinflation during otoscope examination by the physician. Patients with inner ear barotrauma should be referred to an otolaryngologist. Sinus barotrauma can be treated with decongestant nasal sprays, such as phenylephrine 0.5% (Neo-Synephrine), and oral decongestants, such as pseudoephedrine (Sudafed), which shrink the nasal mucosa to help open and drain the affected sinuses.[9] Patients with recurrent sinus barotrauma or sinus barotraumas that is resistant to medical treatment should be referred to an otolaryngologist.[11]

Decompression Sickness/Pulmonary Barotrauma

Decompression sickness ("the bends") most often occurs after divers descend and remain deeper than 10 m (33 feet). As divers increase underwater depth time, nitrogen gradually dissolves in the blood and tissues. If ascent is rapid, this nitrogen can become insoluble, forming bubbles in the bloodstream and the tissues. Decompression sickness usually manifests immediately or shortly after the dive but may occur as long as 12 hours later. Most commonly, the victim experiences steady or throbbing pain in the shoulders or elbows with some relief on "bending" the affected joint. The skin may become pruritic, with rashes and purplish mottling. Cerebral effects include headache, fatigue, inappropriate behavior, seizures, hemiplegia, and visual disturbances. Pulmonary effects include substernal pain, cough, and dyspnea.[10,12]

Pulmonary barotrauma is a risk during scuba diving and mechanical ventilation, especially when peak airway pressures are more than 70 cm H_2O. A scuba diver breathing compressed air, who ascends from depth without exhaling, runs a risk of pulmonary trauma as a result of overdistention of the lungs. Overinflated alveoli can rupture and allow air to escape into the interstitium, pleural cavity, or pulmonary vessels. Slow leakage from alveoli may produce subcutaneous or mediastinal emphysema. Subcutaneous emphysema may present as neck fullness and crepitance, dysphagia, and change in voice quality. Mediastinal emphysema may present with chest pain and dyspnea. Pneumothorax occurs in as many as 15% of patients on mechanical ventilators and is difficult to recognize on portable chest radiographs.[13]

If air enters the pulmonary vessels, the symptoms of air embolism are immediate as bubbles disseminate throughout the circulation. The CNS is most frequently affected, with neurologic manifestations consistent with acute stroke. Unconsciousness, stupor, focal paralysis, sensory loss, blindness, and aphasia may be seen. Acute coronary occlusion and cardiac arrest can occur.

Treatment

Immediate recompression therapy in a compression chamber is essential for both decompression sickness and air embolization. Family physicians should know the location of the nearest recompression chamber. Until recompression is possible, the patient should remain in a horizontal position breathing oxygen with monitoring of respiratory and circulatory status, and should receive oral or isotonic intravenous fluids. The most common treatment error is failure to recompress mild or questionable cases. Dramatic recoveries from decompression sickness have occurred even after recompression was delayed for 1 week.[14] Pneumothorax is treated with a chest tube. Subcutaneous and mediastinal emphysema can be treated symptomatically unless the emphysema hinders breathing or the circulation.[10]

Prevention

To prevent barotitis, scuba divers and individuals flying in aircraft should have normally functioning eustachian tubes and be able to "clear their ears" by swallowing, yawning, or performing an autoinflation maneuver. The physician can confirm this functioning by observing each tympanic membrane with an otoscope while the patient performs an autoinflation maneuver. Each tympanic membrane visibly moves or "pops" as air enters the middle ear through the eustachian tube. Individuals with a URI who must fly should be advised to use oral decongestants before flying and a decongestant nasal spray before descent to help avoid the mild but painful middle ear barotrauma on descent. Scuba divers undergo thorough training in the prevention of all types of barotrauma as part of their scuba certification. Individuals who dive without this training are at great risk for barotrauma. Pressure-targeted ventilation that limits peak ventilator pressures to 35 cm H_2O or less can help prevent barotrauma due to mechanical ventilation.[13]

Burns

Burns are the fifth leading cause of accidental deaths, with 3100 related deaths in the United States annually.[1] Of all age groups, children have the highest incidence of burn injuries: more than half occur in preschoolers, with most resulting from hot liquids, especially hot tap water from heaters set above 54°C (129°F).[15]

Most burned patients have minor injuries that can be adequately treated on an outpatient basis. Family physicians must be able to recognize and initiate emergency care for more severe burns and inhalation injuries that require hospitalization. Severe burns can cause rapid derangements of fluids and electrolytes and can lead to sepsis. For these reasons and for the prevention management of cosmetic and functional sequelae, surgical consultation is often required.

Pathophysiology

Management of burn injuries requires an understanding of the etiology and pathophysiology of the injury. In addition to the depth and extent of the burn, several special conditions may warrant hospitalization.

The skin normally prevents fluid loss, regulates heat, and protects against infection. As skin is burned it undergoes coagulation necrosis, with cell death and loss of vascularity. Next to the dead tissues is a layer of injured cells in which the circulation is impaired. There is increased capillary permeability and rapid edema development with rapid loss of fluid and heat. This injured tissue can be damaged further by improper care, which may allow drying, trauma, or infection. Gram-positive and, in a few days, gram-negative bacteria grow rapidly on the burned surface.

Partial-thickness burns leak and sequester serous exudate, which forms a yellow, sticky eschar. During healing, scarring and contractures occur wherever the dermis is devitalized.[16]

Causes

The severity of the burn is determined by the type of burning agent, the temperature, and the duration of exposure.

Temperatures less than 45°C (113°F) rarely cause cell damage, yet temperatures of 50°C (122°F) can cause burns depending on the duration of exposure. Brief flash burns and scalds tend to cause relatively superficial injury, yet flash burns can be partial-thickness burns and scalds can be full-thickness burns. Burns from flames and from adherent substances cause deeper burns. Electrical injuries may appear to be minor, yet deep tissue damage may become evident in several days, often manifesting as red urine caused by the release of myoglobin from damaged muscle. The skin of elderly patients and the very young is thin and subject to greater injury.[17]

Classification

Treatment and hospitalization decisions depend on classification of burns according to the extent of the skin burned and the depth and location of the burn. The total area of the burn can be approximated in adults using the "rule of nines," although this surface area rule varies in the young age group (Fig. 50.1).[18] Small burns can be compared to the size of the patient's hand, which is about 1% of the total skin area.

Burns are traditionally classified according to depth as first, second, or third degree; however, these terms are being replaced by superficial, superficial partial-thickness, deep partial-thickness, and full-thickness. Burn depth is rarely uniform and may be difficult to determine initially and require reevaluation after a few days.[19]

Superficial Burns (First Degree)

Superficial burns involve only the superficial epidermis, appear erythematous, and blanch with pressure. Mild sunburn is an example with uneventful healing and some delayed peeling. The protective functions of the skin are maintained.

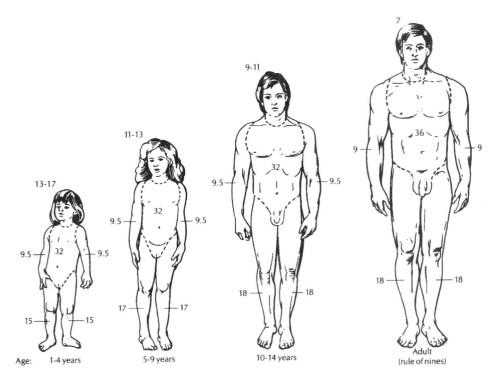

Fig. 50.1. Assessment of the percent of the total surface area. (Lund CC, Browder NC. The estimate of areas of burns. Surg Gynecol Obstet 1944;79:352–8.)

Superficial and Deep Partial-Thickness Burns (Second Degree)

Superficial partial-thickness burns spare the deeper dermis components, including hair follicles and the sweat and sebaceous glands, and are either superficial or deep. These burns form bullae and are red, painful, and weeping. They blanch with pressure, and the superficial skin is sometimes wiped away. These burns heal in about 2 to 3 weeks with little or no scarring. Deep partial-thickness burns are mottled with red elements (dermal vessels) or are waxy-white and dry and do not blanch with pressure. They may be nearly painless, with sensation only to pressure. These burns may take a month or more to heal and usually form scars. They may progress to full-thickness burns if not properly treated and take 3 weeks or more to heal.

Full-Thickness Burns (Third Degree)

Full-thickness burns appear dry, white, or charred and inelastic. They are painless and avascular, and thrombosed vessels may be visible. A dry eschar covers the burn and may cause constriction of underlying structures. Healing occurs only from the edges by epithelial migration with scarring and contracture.[15]

Hospitalization

Decisions regarding hospitalization can be made according to guidelines from the American Burn Association.[20] (Table 50.2). Family physicians should consider surgical consultation anytime there is doubt about the depth of burns or need for hospitalization. Because inhalation injury occurs frequently in large fires and is a common cause of death, the physician must be alert for the presence of associated signs: facial burns, singed nasal hair, sooty mucus, hoarseness, or cough. Initial physical examination, chest roentgenograms, and blood gas measurements may be helpful but may also be normal in the presence of inhalation injury.

Burn Management

Severe Burns

Immediately after the burn, the victim's clothing and any hot substances remaining in contact with the skin are removed, and the victim is covered with a dry, sterile sheet. Copious irrigation with water is indicated for chemical injuries. Cool compresses (not ice) can be used to relieve the pain of small burns but can cause hypothermia if used for large burns. Breathing is assessed immediately and oxygen administered if there is any distress or suspicion of carbon monoxide inhalation.[21]

Airway. Early endotracheal intubation is warranted at the first indication of inhalation injury. All patients with inhalation injury should be placed on humidified oxygen. Steroids are warranted only in the presence of bronchospasm. Bronchoscopy can confirm large airway injury, and lung scans can detect small airway damage.

Fluids. Patients with burns of more than 15% to 20% of the surface area require intravenous fluid replacement. Lactated Ringer's solution at a rate of 4 mL/kg per percent of burned area during the first 24 hours is the most common fluid replacement regimen used in the United States, with half of this amount given during the first 8 hours after the burn. Many other fluid regimens have been used, but all must be administered with close monitoring of renal output and cardiovascular status.

Pain Management. Narcotics and benzodiazepines are used initially for relief of pain and anxiety *with caution* because they can exacerbate the hypotension that may follow a major burn. Immediate administration of narcotics may also interfere with evaluation of other associated trauma. After intravenous fluids have been administered and fluid status has stabilized, narcotic doses can be increased. Inhaled or intravenous anesthesia may be needed for the severe pain of early dressing changes.[22]

Consultation. Consultation with a surgical burn specialist is appropriate for all severe burns, small burns that are deep partial-thickness or deeper, and those located on the face, eyes, ears, or neck or in areas of critical function including the hands, elbows, popliteal fossae, or feet. Major complications including sepsis and hypermetabolism, and subsequent major burn management is best handled in major burn centers.[23]

Minor Burns

Minor burns, those not requiring hospitalization, are by far the most common type of burn managed by the family physician. Partial-thickness burns contain portions of epithelium that must be protected from further damage so epithelialization can occur.

Local Care. For all burns, the clothing and any hot or caustic materials are removed immediately; and cool saline-soaked

---

Table 50.2. **Burns Requiring Hospitalization**[20]

Moderate burns (require hospitalization)
Partial-thickness burns on 15–25% of total body surface area (2–10% in children or elderly)
Full-thickness burns on 2–10% of body surface
Suspected inhalation injury
Suspected high-voltage (200 volts) electrical burns (may appear mild initially)
Circumferential burn (decompressive escharotomy may be needed)

Major burns (consider referral to burn center)
Partial-thickness burns on >25% body surface (>20% in children or elderly)
Full-thickness burns on >10% of body
Burns with inhalation injury, major trauma, or other poor risk condition such as diabetes or immunodeficiency that increase risk of infection
High-voltage (200 volts) electrical burns (may appear mild initially)
All but minimal burns to face, eyes, feet, hands, perineum, or genitalia where cosmetic or functional impairment is likely
Burns from caustic chemicals such as hydrofluoric acid (may appear mild initially)

gauze is applied. The ideal temperature for those compresses is 12°C (54°F), which avoids hypothermia while relieving pain and increasing circulation for up to 3 hours after the burn. Burns are cleaned with saline or mild soapy water; the use of chlorhexidine gluconate (Hibiclens) or half-strength povidone-iodine (Betadine) is now discouraged because these agents may inhibit healing. Cytotoxic cleansing agents such as hydrogen peroxide should be avoided. Necrotic skin is carefully removed using aseptic technique; whirlpool debridement is often well tolerated by patients. The yellow eschar of partial-thickness burns should not be removed initially. Blisters may be left intact but are removed if they appear to contain cloudy fluid, if broken or if they cover possible full-thickness burns.

Topical chemoprophylaxis is used for all but superficial burns to prevent infection. Silver sulfadiazine (Silvadene) cream, classically the most commonly used topical agent, is applied to the burn in a thickness of about 1 to 2 mm and is then covered with a loose-fitting dressing such as soft gauze. Silver sulfadiazine should not be used on the face, on patients with sulfonamide sensitivity, or in pregnant patients. Bacitracin (Baciguent) ointment is a good alternative. Systemic antibiotics are used only with a proved burn infection. Oral nonsteroidal antiinflammatory drugs, acetaminophen with codeine, and rarely narcotics, can be given for pain.[15]

An alternative to topical chemoprophylaxis and dressing changes for superficial partial-thickness burns (not deeper burns) is the use of synthetic dressings such as Duoderm, Opsite, or Biobrane.[24] These expensive dressings are applied to fresh, clean, moist burns and are left in place until the burn heals or until the dressing separates in about 1 to 2 weeks. In many cases these dressings are easy to use, promote fast healing, decrease infection, do not limit activity, reduce pain, and are acceptable to the patient overall. Immunity to tetanus should be ensured, as burns are readily subject to tetanus infections.[25] (See Table 49.3.)

Follow-Up Care. Patients should bathe daily and gently wash off completely and reapply the silver sulfadiazine. Dressings should remain intact under any circumstances where the burns might become dirty but may be removed at home when the burns can be protected. The physician should recheck partial-thickness burns daily, and patients should be alert to signs of impaired circulation caused by a tight dressing and to signs of infection such as chills or fever. The physician should remain alert for hypertrophic scarring and contractures and refer these patients to a burn specialist. Depending upon depth, 6 to 24 months may be required for complete healing; during this period the healing skin should be protected from sun exposure and lubricated with moisturizing cream.[26]

Sunburn

Superficial burns resulting from sunburn are common in fair-skinned individuals and frequently come to the attention of the family physician. The skin appears red, blanches with light pressure, and is tender and painful. Skin lubricants such as Eucerin may improve comfort. The use of topical anesthetic sprays should be limited because they may sensitize the skin to the anesthetics. Topical steroids have little effect; but with extensive sunburns, constitutional symptoms may be improved with oral prednisone at a daily dose of 20 mg for 2 to 3 days.

Prevention

Prevention of most burns takes place in the home by the family. Water heaters should be set to a temperature below 51°C (124°F) to avoid scalds. Smoke detectors should be installed and checked regularly. Electrical outlets should be covered to protect children from electrical injury, and chemicals and caustic agents must be stored away from the reach of children. In the kitchen, hot pot handles should be turned away from children, and all foods should be temperature-tested before being offered to children. Oily rags must be discarded and flammables stored properly. Finally, sunscreens should be used to prevent sunburn, and sun exposure should be avoided between 10 A.M. and 4 P.M.

As many as one in five burns of young children are the result of abusive acts, so abuse must be considered when a child has more than two burn sites, burns at various stages of healing, and burns that follow a particular pattern (e.g., "stocking-glove" distribution).[27] When abuse is suspected, evaluation of previous medical records, checking with protective services, and hospital admission should be considered (see Chapter 27).

Aspirated or Swallowed Foreign Body

Pathophysiology

More deaths in the United States result from suffocation by foreign bodies than from burns or from firearms accidents. Children younger than 3 years of age have a natural tendency to place objects in their mouths, putting them at high risk of choking injury. In children younger than 1 year, asphyxiation is an important cause of unintentional death. The foreign bodies most often aspirated are food, including nuts, vegetable or fruit pieces, seeds, and popcorn. Small items such as pen caps, beads, or crayons may be aspirated by small children. Balloons pose a high risk for aspiration and asphyxiation to children of any age. Items that may become lodged in the cricopharyngeus or esophagus include coins, pieces of food, pieces of toys or hardware, batteries, glass, chicken bones, etc.[28]

Large objects in the esophagus can cause airway obstruction. The gastrointestinal (GI) tract can become obstructed or perforated; mediastinitis, cardiac tamponade, paraesophageal abscess, or aortotracheoesophageal fistula can occur. Perforation may be the result of direct mechanical erosion (bones), or chemical corrosion (button batteries).[29]

Most pediatric obstructions occur in the proximal esophagus, and most obstructions in adults occur at the distal esophagus in those with a history of esophageal disease. Most swallowed foreign bodies that pass through the esophagus continue through the entire GI tract without difficulty, but 10% to 20%

require some intervention and about 1% require surgery. Objects larger than 3 to 5 cm may have difficulty passing the duodenal loop in the region of the ligament of Treitz.

Clinical Manifestations

The most frequent symptom of aspirated foreign body is a sudden onset of choking and intractable cough with or without vomiting. Other presenting symptoms may be cough, fever, breathlessness, and wheezing. Some patients will be asymptomatic and many, especially older adults, are misdiagnosed as having other pulmonary diseases. On chest radiograph a pneumonic patch or atelectasis may be present in adults, and air trapping is more common in children. Older adults predisposed to aspiration include those with stroke or other central nervous system disease or major underlying lung disease.[30]

A swallowed foreign body can be painful and can provoke great anxiety. Foreign bodies in the esophagus usually cause dysphagia, especially with solid foods, and occasionally dyspnea due to compression of the larynx. Patients may be unable to swallow their own secretions. The initial period may be symptom-free, with symptoms of esophageal obstruction developing later as the result of edema and inflammation. Increasing pain, fever, and shock suggest perforation.[31]

Management

When aspirated foreign body is suspected or diagnosed on chest radiograph, bronchoscopy is indicated. Success of foreign body removal by bronchoscopy depends on the experience of the bronchoscopist.

Because most ingested foreign bodies pass without problems, evaluation and treatment are often expectant. When patients complain of a sticking sensation in their throat (as is often the case when a fish bone is swallowed), direct or indirect laryngoscopy permits direct visualization and removal with forceps. Esophagogastroscopy is preferred for removal of most foreign bodies lodged in the esophagus or stomach. Radiopaque foreign bodies can be easily diagnosed with standard radiographs of the neck, chest, or abdomen. An esophagram can be used to locate nonopaque objects. The physical examination is repeated to detect signs of obstruction or early peritonitis with perforation. The progress of the object through the GI tract can be monitored with repeat abdominal films. If a foreign body remains in one position distal to the pylorus for longer than 5 days, surgical removal should be considered.

Food Impaction

The typical patient with an esophageal food impaction is elderly, usually a denture wearer. The history is usually that the patient swallowed a bolus of meat and feels that it is caught "halfway down." Complete occlusion is evident when the patient cannot swallow water and regurgitates. The airway is usually uninvolved, and the patient speaks and breathes without difficulty. Endoscopic removal is preferred. The use of proteolytic enzymes, such as aqueous solution of papain (e.g., Adolph's meat tenderizer) is not recommended owing to the risk of perforation. When endoscopy is not available, intra-

venous glucagon (1.0 mg) has been suggested to relax the esophageal smooth muscle. If the food bolus has not passed in 20 minutes, an additional 2.0 mg is given intravenously. An esophagram should be obtained to ensure passage of the impaction.

Coin Ingestion

Half of the children with coins lodged in their esophagus are asymptomatic; therefore, radiographs are obtained for all children suspected of swallowing coins. Endoscopy is the preferred and safest method of coin removal. If endoscopy is not available, a Foley catheter can be passed down the esophagus beyond the object. The balloon is then inflated, and as the catheter is slowly withdrawn the coin is withdrawn with it. There is a high incidence of aspiration with this technique in small children younger than 5 years of age. Coins have been observed to remain in the stomach for 2 to 3 months before spontaneous passage.[32]

Battery Ingestion

Most batteries pass uneventfully through the GI tract within 48 to 72 hours. However, a button battery lodged in the esophagus is an emergency. These batteries contain 45% potassium hydroxide, which is erosive to the esophagus and especially hazardous. Button batteries should be removed endoscopically from the esophagus or if they remain in the stomach longer than 24 hours.[29]

Ingestion of Sharp Objects

Children who have swallowed a sharp object yet are asymptomatic can be managed on an expectant basis.[31] Progression of the sharp object should be documented by serial radiographs. If it is not seen to progress past the stomach and perforation is suspected, a water-soluble contrast radiograph is obtained. Perforation requires prompt surgical intervention. Close observation or hospitalization is recommended for children who have swallowed open safety pins or long, sharp objects such as sewing needles.

Prevention

Young children should not have access to small objects such as toys with small detachable parts, coins, pins, etc. Children younger than 3 years should not be given food in forms that could be aspirated; nuts, popcorn, vegetable chunks, etc. should be avoided. Care should be taken to avoid aspiration when feeding older adults who have stroke or other serious debilitating disease. If metered dose inhalers are carried in bags or pockets without their safety caps on, foreign bodies may enter their mechanism and be expelled forcefully into the bronchial tree. The ensuing symptoms are often difficult to distinguish from those of an acute attack of asthma.

Fishhook Removal

There are four basic strategies for removing a barbed fishhook when it has accidentally penetrated a person's skin. Sterile technique, local cleansing, and local anesthesia are appropriate with

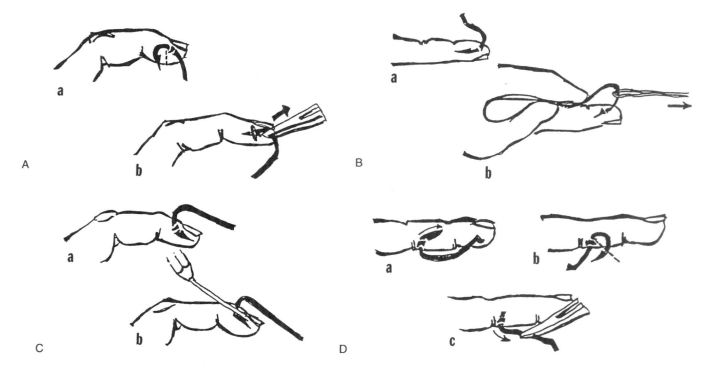

Fig. 50.2. Fishhook removal. (A) Simple retrograde pull. (B) String-yank technique. (C) Needle-cover technique. (D) Push and cut technique.

all the techniques. Fishhook injuries are tetanus prone, and antibiotics should be given when the wound is particularly dirty or when infection is already evident. Fishhook injuries to the eye or orbit should be referred to an ophthalmologist.[33]

Simple Retrograde Pull

If the hook has a small barb or is not embedded deeply, the hook can be held close to the skin with a needle holder or hemostat and withdrawn along its entry path (Fig. 50.2A). A small 1- to 2-mm incision may be needed to help the barb pass through the dermis.

String-Yank Technique

This technique (Fig. 50.2B) does not involve any incisions or surgical equipment and may be tried in the field. A strong suture or fishing line is passed around the bend of the hook, and both ends are held together with one hand while the hook is stabilized and gently depressed against the skin with the other. A sharp pull is applied to the suture in the direction parallel to the shank of the hook.

Needle-Cover Technique

The needle-cover technique (Fig. 50.2C) is often useful when the barb is large. The hook is held in a needle holder or hemostat, and a 16- or 18-gauge hypodermic needle is introduced through the entry wound and advanced along the hook's bend until the barb can be sheathed within the lumen of the needle. The hook and needle are then gently withdrawn to-

gether. It is my experience that, with practice, this technique is usually successful.

Advance and Cut Technique

This method is nearly always successful but causes additional trauma to the surrounding tissue (Fig. 50.2D). The middle of the shank is firmly grasped with a needle holder and the hook tip is advanced out through the skin. The exposed point of the hook is removed with wire cutters, and the hook shank is withdrawn from the wound in a retrograde manner.

References

1. Injury Facts, 2000 edition. Itasca, IL: National Safety Council, 2000.
2. Ramesh CS. Near drowning. Crit Care Clin 1999;15:281–96.
3. Levin DL, Morriss FC, Toro LO, Brink LW, Turner GR. Drowning and near-drowning. Pediatr Clin North Am 1993;40:321–6.
4. Christensen DW, Jansen P, Perkin RM. Outcome and acute care hospital costs after warm water near drowning in children. Pediatrics 1997;99:715–21.
5. Heimlich H, Hoffman K, Canestri F. Food choking and drowning deaths prevented by external subdiaphragmatic compression. Ann Thorac Surg 1975;20:188–95.
6. Bratton SL, Jardine DS, Morray JP. Serial neurologic examinations after near-drowning and outcome. Arch Pediatr Adolesc Med 1994;148:167–70.
7. Lavelle JM, Shaw KN, Seidl T, Ludwig S. Ten-year review of pediatric near-drownings: evaluation for child abuse and neglect. Ann Emerg Med 1995;25:344–8.
8. James JR. Dysbarism: the medical problems from high and low

atmospheric pressure. J R Coll Physicians Lond 1993;27: 367–74.

9. Jerrard DA. Diving medicine. Emerg Med Clin North Am 1992; 10:329–38.

10. Moon RE. Treatment of diving emergencies. Crit Care Clin 1999;15:429–49.

11. Parell JG, Becker GD. Neurological consequences of scuba diving with chronic sinusitis. Laryngoscope 2000;110:1358–60.

12. Melamed Y, Shupak A, Bitterman H. Current concepts: medical problems associated with underwater diving. N Engl J Med 1992;326:30–5.

13. Marcy TW. Barotrauma: detection, recognition, and management. Chest 1993;104:578–84.

14. Boettger ML. Scuba diving emergencies: pulmonary overpressure accidents and decompression sickness. Ann Emerg Med 1983;12:563–7.

15. Feller I. Burn epidemiology: focus on youngsters and the aged. Burn Care Rehabil 1982;3:285.

16. Griglak MJ. Thermal injury. Emerg Med Clin North Am 1992; 10:369–83.

17. Carvajal HF. Burns in children and adolescents: initial management as the first step in successful rehabilitation. Pediatrician 1991;17:237–43.

18. Lund CC, Browder NC. The estimate of areas of burns. Surg Gynecol Obstet 1944;79:352–8.

19. Clark J. Burns. Br Med Bull 1999;55:885–94.

20. Joint Committee of the American Burn Association and the American College of Surgeons Committee on Trauma. Assessment and initial care of burn patients. Chicago: ACS, 1986.

21. Robertson C, Fenton O. ABC of major trauma: management of severe burns. BMJ 1990;301:282–6.

22. Henry DB, Foster RL. Burn pain management in children. Pediatr Cln North Am 2000;47:681–98.

23. Nguyen TT, Gilpin DA, Meyer NA, Herndon DN. Current treatment of severely burned patients. Ann Surg 1996;223:14–25.

24. Wyatt D, McGowan DS, Najarian MP. Comparison of a hydrocolloid dressing and silver sulfadiazine in the outpatient management of second-degree burns. J Trauma 1990;30:857–65.

25. Smith DJ. Burn wounds: infection and healing. Am J Surg 1994;167:46S–8S.

26. Morgan ED, Scott CB, Barker J. Ambulatory management of burns. Am Fam Physician 2000;62:2016–26.

27. Rosenberg NM, Marino D. Frequency of suspected abuse/neglect in burn patients. Pediatr Emerg Care 1989;5:219–21.

28. Rimell FL, Thome A, Stoll S, et al. Characteristics of objects that cause choking in children. JAMA 1995;274:1763–6.

29. Litovitz T, Schmitz BE. Ingestion of cylindrical and button batteries, an analysis of 2382 cases. Pediatrics 1992;89:727.

30. Baharloo F, Veyckemans F, Francis C, et al. Tracheobronchial foreign bodies: presentation and management in children and adults. Chest 1999;115:1357–62.

31. Paul RI Jaffe DM. Sharp object ingestions in children: illustrative case and literature review. Pediatr Emerg Care 1988;4:245.

32. Caravati EM, Bennett DL, McElwee NE. Pediatric coin ingestion: a prospective study on the utility of routine roentgenograms. Am J Dis Child 1989;143:549.

33. Gammons M, Jackson S. Fishhook removal. Am Fam Physician 2001;63:2231–6.

51

Medical Problems of the Athlete

Jeffrey L. Tanji

Background

Medical conditions in athletes and physically active individuals encompass a broad spectrum of problems commonly seen by the family physician. The diagnosis, management, and attitudinal approach toward these patients might reasonably be assumed to be the same as for any other patient; in fact, however, it is not always the case. Some medical conditions are improved with exercise, others may be exacerbated with certain types of activity, and for others the interaction of medication and physical activity may require a tailor-made design for the intensity, duration, and frequency of exercise. This chapter examines in some detail the medical problems associated with asthma, the athlete's heart, hypertension, diabetes mellitus, anemia and other blood disorders, pregnancy, and medical problems specific to the exercising woman.

Exercise Has Proven Health Benefit, but Few Follow the Guidelines

Strong scientific evidence continues to build showing the positive impact of physical activity (whether leisure time or work-related) on health and longevity.[1–5] There is a remarkable consistency to these studies highlighted by the 1996 Report of the U.S. Surgeon General on Physical Activity and Health.[6] This report summarized the findings of both national and international researchers who felt that the maintenance of a regularly scheduled program of physical activity was one of the most important ways to maintain health and to promote longevity. The report calls for an exercise program of either 30 to 45 minutes of low-intensity (walking) aerobic exercise 5 to 6 days per week, or a vigorous exercise program of 20 minutes three times a week. It was further emphasized that

the exercise could be achieved by a leisure-time program of recreation (a fitness program), by exercise at work (job demands), or in activities of daily living (walking instead of driving). The exercise need not be achieved in a continuous 30 to 45 bout of training, but can be interspersed in smaller increments throughout the day.

Unfortunately, in spite of the clarity of studies and reports emphasizing the positive impact of exercise, a report of the Centers for Disease Control and Prevention (CDC) highlighted the remarkable absence of exercise in the lives of Americans.[7] In a telephone survey conducted by the CDC in 43 states, only 25.4% of Americans met the current national guidelines for exercise. Nearly 30% of the population was fully sedentary. Researchers speculate that television viewing, the convenience of the automobile, and the demands of a high-stress job contribute to this deficiency. Further, it appears that the population understands the need and importance of exercise; in spite of this knowledge, the exercise is not being done. Several models to motivate patients to exercise using the physician as catalyst have proven to be useful in research trials.[1] Unfortunately, they have not resulted in changing exercise behavior on a national level.

Newer Findings on the Benefit of Exercise

It has been well established over the past two decades that both physical fitness level and amount of physical activity, if sufficient, result in reduced mortality and cardiovascular morbidity. These landmark studies include the Aerobics Center Longitudinal Study,[5] the Multiple Risk Factor Intervention Trial,[3] the Lipid Research Clinics Study,[4] and the Harvard Alumni Study.[2] Several studies have shown that sufficient exercise can reduce cancer rates for colon, breast, and ovarian cancer.[8–10] Exercise can result in decreased morbidity in the elderly associated with injuries from falls and trauma.[1–13] Regular physical exercise can improve the signs and symptoms of generalized anxiety disorder and depression.[14–16]

Men and women in the Aerobics Center Longitudinal Study, a well-regarded longitudinal cohort study of several thousand subjects, showed that colon cancer rates were significantly reduced among those subjects who achieved a reasonable level of physical fitness as measured by duration on a modified Balke exercise treadmill test protocol.[8]

Frisch et al[9] demonstrated reduced rates of breast, uterine, and ovarian cancer among physically active women. Thune et al,[10] in a large epidemiologic study in Norway, also found breast cancer rates to be lower in women who were regular exercisers.

For those over 65 years of age, exercise programs have been strongly associated with maintenance of functional capacity (activities of daily living), the ability to live independently, and reduced risk of falls—one of the leading causes of morbidity in that population.[11,12] While it has been well established that regular exercise prevents osteoporosis, many believe that it is the strength, flexibility, and balance training, not the aerobic component, that results in overall long-term health benefit in this population.[13]

Regularly scheduled exercise programs have been demonstrated to improve the signs and symptoms of depression and generalized anxiety disorder.[14–16] On the other hand, exercise programs have been shown to enhance self-esteem by objective measures and to enhance a sense of self-control and well-being.

The clinically relevant point for family physicians is to understand that overwhelming evidence shows the health benefit of exercise beyond even cardiovascular factors, but for unknown reasons many Americans do not exercise.

Asthma

Asthma is a common medical condition that affects 12% to 15% of the general population of the United States[17] (see Chapter 83). Approximately 80% of patients with asthma are prone to exacerbation of asthmatic symptoms during exercise. What is new and current is the understanding that seasonal allergic rhinitis, far more common than asthma, may be part of the same disease as asthma to the upper respiratory tract. Because of this relationship, up to 70% of patients with only the diagnosis of allergic rhinitis may demonstrate signs and symptoms of exercise-induced asthma, while never having the symptoms of asthma at rest. So the family physician must be mindful of asking about shortness of breath in the patient population with allergic rhinitis, not only asthma.

Physical activity need not be limited with asthma, in contrast to popular beliefs.[18] Studies continue to demonstrate the benefit of exercise in those with asthma, and also show that exercise is well tolerated and can result in the benefit of reduced severity of symptoms.[19]

Physical conditioning plays a role in improving aerobic capacity, increasing the ventilatory threshold—the respiratory level where it is not the drive for oxygen consumption but rather the drive to blow off excess carbon dioxide that increases the respiratory rate. During exercise, it is common to have asthmatic episodes at or just above the ventilatory threshold. Therefore, exercise that raises this threshold can result in reduction of asthmatic attacks.

The best exercise for patients with asthma is aerobic exercise of low intensity and long duration[17], for example, a walking program with a speed below the level where one becomes short of breath. It is also well known that symptoms of asthma are exacerbated in cold, dry climates. Patients with asthma who participate in Nordic and downhill skiing must be mindful of the risk of an asthmatic attack because of environmental conditions. On the other hand, water-based activities such as swimming and water polo, where the athlete is exposed to warm, moist environmental conditions, tends to decrease the chance of an episode of shortness of breath.

There is an emerging role for using both antihistamines and nasal corticosteroids, common treatments for allergic rhinitis, in the patient with exercise-induced asthma, given the newer concept that these two diseases are closely related. The standard treatment continues to be oral β-agonist inhalers and oral corticosteroid inhalers.

Athletic Heart Syndrome

The athletic heart syndrome is a constellation of clinical variants of cardiac structure and function present in physically active individuals.[20,21] These changes, originally thought to result as a consequence of heart disease associated with "overexertion," are now thought to represent changes that occur as a result of normal physiologic responses to training. The family physician should understand that the prevalence of cardiac disease in the athletic population is low, and although the precise risk for cardiovascular disease in that population is not known, the risk is low. However, because death and disease in this population is uncommon, when it does occur it often, like airplane accidents, captures the headlines in the news media. When it occurs in a community and a physician is involved, it stimulates an assessment of what is known and what is assumed in dealing with cardiac disease in the athletic population.

The physician is often put in a difficult position during preparticipation evaluations for sport competition. On the one hand, he or she is ordinarily expected to clear a physically active young person to participate in sport. This does occur over 99% of the time. At the same time, the physician is asked to be responsible for not allowing an individual at risk to participate. When this occurs, there is often much emotion involved by the athlete, the athlete's family, the team, and even the doctor. Even more emotion is involved when an athlete at risk is allowed to participate and a morbidity or mortality subsequently occurs. Of all of the areas where a physician is asked to render a medical judgment about allowing an athlete to play or not, the most serious and the most risky area is in the realm of cardiovascular disease. Fortunately for the physician, nationally published guidelines—the Bethesda Conference: Recommendations for Determining Eligibility for Competition in

Athletes with Cardiovascular Abnormalities[22]—have been published. This is a large document, developed by a multidisciplinary task force, that serves as a resource to support the decisions of the individual physician working with athletes.

Specific Findings in the Athlete's Heart

The structural and anatomic changes that occur in the heart as a result of sustained athletic training include increased left ventricular mass (about 45% greater mass than controls), increased left ventricular wall thickness (15–20% greater), and a 10% increase in left ventricular end diastolic volume.[22] Functionally, the heart adapts to exercise training with bradycardia. The cause of this bradycardia is unclear, but is not solely the result of increased vagal tone.

For the family physician, the key clinical point is to be aware that these physiologic changes occur normally as an adaptation to work in the physically active individual and should not always be misconstrued as being pathologic. The negative consequences of always worrying about pathology in this group are unnecessary invasive testing and the emotional trauma of altering a physically active to a sedentary lifestyle with the fear of chronic cardiac disease.

The significant historical questions to ask the athlete include a history of syncope, a family history of sudden death, or the history of a heart murmur. These three historical questions are very important in the screening process for athletic participation and in the decision-making process for further cardiac testing. If an athlete gives a history of syncope, the next key question is whether or not the syncopal episode occurred during a bout of exercise or at rest. If the syncope occurred during exercise, while in the process of exertion, the history is ominous. All experts in the field would recommend follow-up testing including an echocardiogram and an exercise treadmill test. If the syncope occurred at rest, for example when an athlete is sitting or lying down, and then changes to a standing position quickly, the syncope is considered to be vasovagal or benign. Vasovagal symptoms are very common in well-conditioned endurance athletes, perhaps as an adaptation to training. If it is unclear whether the syncope is vasovagal or not, a tilt table test can be used to firm up the diagnosis.

On physical examination bradycardia (heart rate of 30–60 beats per minute) is common. A physiologically split S2 is often present. The third heart sound, S3, can be found as the result of rapid ventricular filling, and less frequently a fourth heart sound, S4, may be auscultated. A benign systolic flow murmur is present in 30% to 50% of athletes. Generally this murmur is early to mid-systolic and tends to soften in intensity when listening to the patient in the sitting position. The presence of a holosystolic, late systolic, or diastolic murmur always requires further evaluation to rule of significant disease. The murmur of hypertrophic cardiomyopathy classically increases in volume during standing or a Valsalva maneuver, as benign murmurs soften while standing.

The resting 12-lead electrocardiogram in the athlete is often "abnormal." These abnormalities fall into three general categories:

1. Changes in the ST segment and T wave as a result of alterations in repolarization
2. Abnormalities of rate and rhythm
3. Abnormalities attributable to cardiac chamber enlargement

Alterations in repolarization manifest in elevation, depression, inversion or early take-off of the T wave. These changes are most problematic to the family physician who must decide whether they are normal or abnormal. Early repolarization, defined as ST segment elevation greater than 0.5 mm in two consecutive leads (often in precordial leads), is believed to be benign. Deep T wave inversion of the lateral precordial leads associated with a symmetric contour of the T wave, ST segment depression, the absence of a normal septal Q wave, or an abnormal QT interval can represent cardiac pathology and warrants further workup.

The association of bradycardia with the athletic heart syndrome is almost universally benign. Sinus bradycardia, often associated with sinus arrhythmia, is the most common finding in athletes. When the heart rate decreases below 50 beats/minute, it is not unusual to find a second-degree atrioventricular (AV) block (AV Mobitz type I). First-degree AV block may also be present as a result of AV conduction delay. AV junctional escape beats or rhythms may also occur. Supraventricular tachycardia or ventricular tachycardia are not generally thought to be associated with the athletic heart syndrome and should be evaluated. Other findings of rate and rhythm associated with pathology and warranting workup include:

1. Bradycardia or high-grade AV block in an individual not involved with endurance training
2. Sinus pauses greater than 3 seconds
3. Complete heart block
4. Syncope or near syncope during strenuous exercise

Sudden Death in the Athlete

Sudden death in the athlete under the age of 30 is associated with hypertrophic cardiomyopathy (HCM) in 50% of instances. Although a rare condition affecting less than 1 in 1000 individuals, it is the leading cause of cardiac death in the young, physically active population.[23] This disease, felt to be strongly heritable, is a genetic condition where abnormal fibrous tissue invades and thickens the interventricular septum of the patient. This abnormal tissue is felt to be arrhythmogenic, and associated with sudden death. The distinction between athletic heart syndrome and HCM is probably the single most important clinical decision during cardiac evaluation of an athlete. The diagnosis of HCM is made by echocardiographic measurement of the interventricular septum. A width in excess of 15 mm is considered to be diagnostic, 13 to 14 mm is in the "gray zone," and 12 mm of width or less is considered to be normal. At a few academic centers, cardiac catheter-guided interventricular biopsies can be performed, and the finding of more irregular tissue architecture is considered to be a poor prognostic sign. Electrophysiologic study (EPS) testing with programmed electrical stimulation has also been done in an attempt to provoke abnormal cardiac rhythms in controlled settings. The use of cardiac biopsy and EPS testing is still in an experimental phase. If the athlete presents with a history of syncope or a family history of sudden cardiac death in a relative, echocardiographic testing is indicated, and if the interventricular septal wall thickness exceeds 15 mm, by definition the athlete has HCM and should not be allowed to compete. Some experts point to the physical finding of an enhanced systolic murmur on Valsalva maneuver as indicative of the presence of HCM, but in general clinical practice the echocardiogram is the definitive test to diagnose this condition.

Hypertension

Hypertension is a prevalent condition affecting an estimated 58 million adults in the United States. In spite of numerous advances in the area of cardiovascular health, this area of disease continues for the fifth consecutive decade to be the leading cause of death in Americans. Family physicians see 95% of patients with primary, or essential, hypertension. Of these patients, 80% have mild hypertension. Physical activity and exercise, along with diet, continue to be the first step in the treatment of this condition[24,25] (see Chapter 75).

Overwhelming evidence in both animal and human studies clearly demonstrates the benefit of an aerobic exercise program on the control of blood pressure for the mildly hypertensive population.[24] Exercise, along with pharmacotherapy, is used in the treatment of moderate to severe hypertension.

Low-intensity aerobic exercise, for example a walking program that puts the heart at 50% to 65% of its maximal heart rate, is felt to be optimal for the management of hypertension. At this intensity of exercise, relaxation of total peripheral resistance allows blood pressure values to decrease slightly, resulting in a therapeutic antihypertensive effect. The blood pressure–lowering effect of a walking program has further shown benefit in vascular changes as measured in quantitative measurements of corneal blood flow in mildly hypertensive patients.[26] Higher intensity aerobic exercise is not contraindicated in the hypertensive population, but for the purpose of blood pressure control, it may not have the same therapeutic benefit as lower intensity exercise.

Heavy-load resistance training, for example maximal leg or bench press exercises, is contraindicated in the hypertensive athlete. Dramatically high blood pressure values have been measured in normotensives and hypertensives who lift maximal weights.[27] Low-weight, high-repetition weight training programs are safe, and appear to actually help control blood pressure in mildly hypertensive populations.

Large population studies now demonstrate that the finding of an abnormally high blood pressure measurement in a young, normotensive patient is predictive of the development of hypertension later in life.[25]

Diabetes Mellitus

Diabetes mellitus is a common condition affecting nearly 5% of the American population. Young athletes and physically active individuals with type I or II diabetes mellitus may be advised to safely participate in sports with medical supervision.[28] It is well known that physical exercise is associated with an insulin-independent uptake of glucose resulting in enhanced glycemic control in both type I and type II diabetes mellitus. The risk of severe hypoglycemia is greatest during the hours immediately following strenuous physical activity rather than in the midst of such activity. Hypoglycemia may occur 6 to 14 hours postexercise as the result of depletion of glycogen stores. Close monitoring of glycemic control as well as the prudent adjustment of insulin and caloric intake following vigorous physical activity can prevent these episodes (see Chapter 120).

For the type I diabetic, there are four challenges to be addressed associated with a regular exercise program.[29] First, exercise potentiates the effect of insulin by independently lowering blood glucose. Second, patients with type I diabetes mellitus may have too little circulating insulin during exercise, which leads to potentiation of ketogenesis. Third, exercise of high intensity can stimulate the sympathetic nervous system, in turn raising blood glucose. Fourth, exercise is known to have a "carryover" effect, where insulin sensitivity is increased throughout the day, and a risk for hypoglycemia can occur. Based on these issues, there are a number of practical strategies that a family physician can use to manage these challenges. Eating should be encouraged 1 to 3 hours before the bout of exercise to slightly raise blood glucose levels at the time of exercise. Frequent carbohydrate feedings during prolonged exercise periods can maintain blood glucose levels, and adequate fluid levels must be maintained in the postexercise period where increased insulin sensitivity can cause hypoglycemia. With frequent monitoring as the exercise program is developed, insulin requirements will decrease, but the athlete can stay on top of the needed adjustments.

For the type II diabetic there are a series of different concerns. Recent data from the CDC continue to address the importance of exercise for not only the management of blood glucose control, but also the management of obesity.[28] There is a clear association between a sedentary lifestyle and the development of type II diabetes. In the Nurses Health Study[30] and the Physicians Health Study,[31] those who exercised at least once a week were a third less likely to develop type II diabetes mellitus. In the Finnish Diabetes Prevention Study,[32] those who were randomized into an exercise program had a significant decrease in the development of type II diabetes. Currently, a randomized clinical trial, the U.S. Diabetes Prevention Program,[33] is in data collection, and the results are expected to be presented in 2003.

The fear of allowing a diabetic to play in organized sport in the latter part of the 20th century has given way to a more favorable view of the role of exercise in type I and II diabetes mellitus. Athletic participation is now encouraged. A regular exercise program is considered to be a part of the foundation for glycemic control, and virtually no one disagrees with the statement that the benefit of exercise outweighs the risks of involvement.

The insulin pump, now a common form of treatment for type I diabetes mellitus, can easily be titrated to allow for regular bouts of exercise, and provide a more precise method to control hour-to-hour glycemic fluctuations. However, close physician supervision is essential, and a cohesive team of the patient, doctor, and family is essential to prevent morbidity.

The family physician must be mindful of the risk of accelerated cardiovascular disease in the diabetic patient, and use prudent cardiac screening in the diabetic athlete.

Anemia

The most common blood abnormality associated with athletes is a slightly low hemoglobin level as a result of increased plasma volume and a normal or slightly increased red blood cell mass, resulting in the term *sports anemia*. But this terminology is a misnomer. The expansion of plasma volume associated with regular aerobic exercise represents a beneficial adaptation to the loss of plasma volume that can occur daily as a consequence of dehydration associated with exercise. On a regular basis, plasma volume can be reduced by 5% to 15% during dehydration. During exercise and muscle contraction, plasma volume pushes fluid into tissues as the result of increased capillary pressure. As plasma volume decreases, the body adapts by releasing renin, aldosterone, and vasopressin, which results in an increase in resting plasma volume. The hemoglobin and hematocrit are temporarily diluted, but exercise performance and oxygen-carrying capacity are not compromised.

Of the clinical causes of anemia, iron deficiency anemia is the most common (also see Chapter 125). In menstruating women, the prevalence of iron deficiency can reach 10% to 20% and the risk of anemia secondary to iron loss is directly related. Other subtle causes of iron loss can include GI loss, urinary tract loss, and possibly even trace loss through perspiration.

Hemolytic anemia may be seen in athletes, and the mechanism to explain this remains controversial. At first, in the 1970s, this hemolysis was thought to be associated with destruction of red blood cells (RBCs) with the "foot strike" of runners and was called "foot strike hemolysis." More recently, even cardiac valve turbulence has been listed as a cause of possible hemolysis in the athlete.[34]

The clinical evaluation of anemia in the athlete is no different than for the nonathlete (see Chapter 125).

The Woman Athlete

There are gender-specific benefits to exercise, and it is very important to family physicians to be aware of these factors in order to provide timely and relevant advice. These benefits include, but are not limited to, the following:

1. Increased bone mineral density and decreased risk of fractures
2. Diminished symptoms associated with the menstrual cycle
3. Amelioration of symptoms associated with pregnancy

We have known for a long time that weight-bearing exercise lowers the risk of osteoporosis and fractures by main-

taining bone mineral density in the postmenopausal woman.[35] Current research in data collection seeks to find specific recommendations about such exercise for women. Newer studies show that insulin-like growth factor-1 produced by osteoblasts mediates the anabolic growth of bone.[36] This factor was present in much higher quantities in the serum of competing female gymnasts and may be a mediating factor in the maintenance of healthy bone.

Research shows that a regular exercise program can ameliorate negatively perceived symptoms of the menstrual cycle.[37] Premenstrual syndrome is a common condition affecting women cyclically and includes symptoms of low back pain, pelvic pain, headache, anxiety, depression, and fatigue.

Exercise and Pregnancy

According to Clapp,[38] the benefits of exercise during pregnancy include the following:

1. Increases or maintains aerobic fitness
2. Increases cardiopulmonary reserve
3. Reduces the risk of gestational diabetes
4. Promotes less symptomatic labor
5. Promotes faster recovery from labor
6. Reduces the risk of post-dates deliveries
7. Improves psychological factors during pregnancy
8. Promotes muscle tone
9. Improves sleep
10. Prevents low back pain
11. Prevents excessive weight gain associated with pregnancy

A large population-based study at Kaiser Hospital system[39] showed significantly lower adverse symptoms of pregnancy associated with regular aerobic exercise during the preterm state.

Current guidelines from the American College of Obstetricians and Gynecologists[40] recommend the following advice about exercise for women during pregnancy:

1. Regular, three times a week aerobic exercise is better than intermittent exercise
2. Avoid exercises where you lie flat on your back after the 12th week of pregnancy
3. Do not exercise to the point of exhaustion
4. Make sure you do not overheat; drink plenty of fluids
5. Avoid activities that require precise balance
6. Avoid activities that have the potential for abdominal trauma

Specific types of exercise that are recommended include walking, swimming, cycling (stationary late in pregnancy), and low-impact aerobics.

References

1. Harris SS, Caspersen CJ, DeFriese GH, Estes EH. Physical activity counseling for healthy adults as a primary preventive in-

tervention in the clinical setting: report for the US Preventive Services Task Force. JAMA 1989;261:3590–8.

2. Paffenbarger RS Jr, Hyde RT, Wang AL, Hsieh CC. Physical activity, all cause mortality and longevity of college alumni. N Engl J Med 1986;314:605–13.

3. Leon AS, Connett J, Jacobs DR Jr, Rauraman R. Leisure time physical activity levels and risk of coronary heart disease and risk of coronary heart disease and death: the Multiple Risk Factor Intervention Trial. JAMA 1987;258:2388–95.

4. Ekelund RS, Haskell WL, Johnson JL, et al. Physical fitness as a predictor of cardiovascular mortality in North American men. N Engl J Med 1986;314:605–13.

5. Blair SN, Kohl HW, Paffenbarger RS Jr, et al. Physical fitness and all-cause mortality. JAMA 1989;262:2395–2401.

6. Centers for Disease Control and Prevention. The 1996 Surgeon General's Report on Physical Activity and Health (S/N 017-023-03196-5). CDC, 1996.

7. Centers for Disease Control and Prevention. CDC Report on Physical Inactivity. MMWR CDC, December 25, 1998.

8. Kohl HW, LaPorte RE, Blair SN. Physical activity and cancer: an epidemiological perspective. Sports Med 1988;6:222–37.

9. Frisch RE, Wyshad G, Albright NL, et al. Lower lifetime occurrence of breast cancer and cancers of the reproductive system among former college athletes. Am J Clin Nutr 1987;45:328–35.

10. Thune I, Brenn T, Lund E, et al. Physical activity and risk of breast cancer. N Engl J Med 1997;336:1269–75.

11. Fiatrone M, Marks E, Ryan N, et al. High intensity strength training in nonagenarians: effects on skeletal muscle. JAMA 1990;263:3029–34.

12. Fiatrone M, O'Neill E, Ryan N, et al. Exercise training and nutritional supplementation for physical frailty in very elderly people. N Engl J Med 1994;330:1769–75.

13. McCartney N, Hicks A, Martin J, et al. Long-term resistance training in the elderly: effects on dynamic strength, exercise capacity, muscle and bone. J Gerontol 1995;50:B97–104.

14. Camacho TC, Roberts FE, Lazarus NB, et al. Physical activity and depression: evidence from Alameda County study. Am J Epidemiol 1991;134:220–31.

15. Emery C, Gatz M. Psychological and cognitive effects of an exercise program for community residing older adults. Gerontology 1990;30:184–92.

16. North TC, McCullagh P, Tran ZV. Effect of exercise on depression. Exerc Sport Sci Rev 1990;18:379–415.

17. McCarthy P. Wheezing or breezing through exercise-induced asthma. Phys Sport Med 1989;17(7):125–30.

18. Varray AL, Mercier JG, Terral CM, et al. Individualized aerobic and high intensity training for asthmatic children in an exercise readaptation program: is training always helpful for better adaptation to exercise? Chest 1991;99:579–86.

19. Ram FSF, Robinson SM, Black PN. Physical training for asthma. Cochrane rev abstracts. Oxford: Cochrane Library, issue 2, 2001.

20. Huston TP, Puffer JC, Rodney WM. The athletic heart syndrome. N Engl J Med 1985;312:24–32.

21. Bryan G, Ward A. Rippe JM. Athletic heart syndrome. Clin Sports Med 1992;11:291–302.

22. 26th Bethesda Conference. Recommendations for determining eligibility for competition in athletes with cardiovascular abnormalities. J Am Coll Cardiol 1994;24:845–99.

23. Maron BJ, Isner JM, McKenna WJ. Hypertrophic cardiomyopathy, myocarditis and mitral valve prolapse. 26th Bethesda Conference. J Am Coll Cardiol 1994;880–5.

24. Tanji JL. Exercise and the hypertensive athlete. Clin Sports Med 1992;11:291–302.

25. Townsend RR. The young athlete with high blood pressure. J Clin Hypertens 2000;2(6):413–14.

26. Tanji JL. Exercise and hypertension. Proceedings of the American Medical Society for Sports Medicine annual meeting, 1999.

27. MacDougall JD, Tuxen D, Sale DG, et al. Arterial blood pressure response to heavy resistance exercise. J Appl Physiol 1983;58:785–90.

28. Mokdad AH, Ford ES, Bowman BA, et al. Diabetes trends in the US 1990–1998. Diabetes Care 2000;23:1278–83.

29. Bloomgarden ZT. Exercise and diabetes: weighing the pros and cons. 17th International Diabetes Federation Congress, November 5, 2000, Mexico City.

30. Manson JE, Rimm EB, Stampfer MJ, et al. Physical activity and incidence of non–insulin dependent diabetes in women. Lancet 1991;338:774–8.

31. Manson JE, Nathan DM, Krolewski AS, et al. A prospective study of exercise and the incidence of diabetes among US male physicians. JAMA 1992;268:63–7.

32. Uusitupa M, Louheranta A, Lindstrom J, et al. The Finnish Diabetes Prevention Study. Br J Nutr 2000;83(suppl 1):S137–42.

33. Fujimoto WY. Background and recruitment data for the US Diabetes Prevention Program. Diabetes Care 2000;23(suppl 2):B11–13

34. Koskolou MD, Roach RC, Calbet JA, et al. Cardiovascular responses to dynamic exercise with acute anemia in humans. Am J Physiol 1997;273:H787–93.

35. Prince RL, Smith M, Dick IM, et al. Prevention of postmenopausal osteoporosis: a comparative study of exercise, calcium supplementation and hormone replacement therapy. N Engl J Med 1991;325:1189–95.

36. Nattiv A. Female athlete triad: an update. Proceedings of the American Medical Society for Sports Medicine annual meeting, 1997.

37. Lebrun CM. Effects of the menstrual cycle and birth control pill on athletic performance. In: Agostini R, ed. Medical and orthopedic issues of active and athletic women. Philadelphia: Hanley and Belfus, 1994;78–91.

38. Clapp JF. Exercise in pregnancy. Fetal Med Rev 1990;2:89–101.

39. Sternfield B, Quesenberry CP Jr, Eskenazi B, et al. Exercise during pregnancy and pregnancy outcome. Med Sci Sports Exerc 1995;27:634–40.

40. American College of Obstetricians and Gynecologists. Exercise during pregnancy and the postnatal period. ACOG technical bulletin 189, 1994.

52
Athletic Injuries

Michael L. Tuggy and Cora Collette Breuner

Family physicians routinely treat many athletic injuries in their clinical practice. The benefits of long-term exercise in the prevention of common illnesses such as cardiovascular disease, osteoporosis, and falls in the elderly are well established. With the increased interest in fitness in the general population, the number of people resuming more active exercise as they age is increasing. Injuries sustained in childhood or adolescence may have long-term effects that can hamper later attempts at physical activity.[1] For all ages of patients, proper training and prevention can lead to lifelong participation in athletic activities.

Most sports injuries are related to overuse injuries and often are not brought to the attention of the family physician until the symptoms are advanced. Traumatic injuries are more readily diagnosed, but may have more serious long-term sequelae for the life of the athlete. Sport selection has a great impact on risk of injury. The adolescent athlete is probably at highest risk for injury due to sport selection, presence of immature growth cartilage at the growth plates and joint surfaces, and lack of experience.[2] High-risk sports selected by young adults also have higher degrees of risk, which can be modified to lessen injury rates by training and education. Table 52.1 lists common sports activities and their relative injury rates.

Mechanisms of Injury

Direct trauma is a common mechanism that leads to injury. Deceleration injuries are the most common form of serious injury, resulting in significant blunt trauma or joint injury. The athlete's momentum, enhanced by self-generated speed, gravity, and equipment, is translated into energy when impact occurs. This energy is then absorbed by the body in the form of blunt trauma, torsion of joints, or transfer of stress within the skeleton.

Collision sports, such as football or rugby, and high-velocity sports, such as alpine skiing, have much higher rates of significant musculoskeletal injury due to the combination of speed and mass effect on impact. Factors that affect the extent of injury include tensile strength of the ligaments and tendons of affected joints, bony strength, flexibility, and ability of the athlete to reduce the impact. This is where appropriate conditioning for a sport reduces injury risk. Not only are endurance and strength training important, but also practicing falls or recovery from falls can help the athlete diffuse the energy of the fall or impact. Athletes should be encouraged to use the appropriate safety equipment and to train comprehensively for their sport.

Overuse injuries comprise the most common form of sports injuries seen by the family physician. These injuries are induced by repetitive motion leading to microscopic disruption of a bone–tendon or bone–synovium interface. This microtrauma initiates an inflammatory response. If the inflammatory response is not modulated by a rest phase or is excessive due to mechanical factors, then degradation of the tendon or bone may occur. Predisposing factors that lead to overuse injuries include poor flexibility, imbalance of strength of opposing muscle groups, mechanical deformity (e.g., pes planus), inadequate rest between exercise periods, and faulty equipment.[3] Adolescent athletes are especially vulnerable to such injuries, especially in areas where growth cartilage is present in the epiphyseal or apophyseal attachments of major muscle groups. Elderly athletes also are at higher risk because of preexisting degenerative joint disease (DJD) and poor flexibility.

Overuse injuries can be classified in four stages. Stage 1 injuries are symptomatic only during vigorous exercise and stage 2 during moderate exercise. Stage 3 injuries are symptomatic during minimal exercise, and the symptoms usually last up to 24 hours after exercise has ceased. Stage 4 injuries are painful at rest with no exercise to exacerbate the symptoms. Most overuse injuries are seen at later stages by physicians (stage 3 or

Table 52.1. **Common Sports Injuries and Injury Rates**

Sports activity	Common injuries	Injury rate (per 1000 exposures)
Running	Tibial periostitis, stress fracture Metatarsal stress fractures	14
Football	ACL/MCL tears Shoulder dislocation/ separation Ankle sprain	13
Wrestling	Shoulder dislocation MCL, LCL tears	12
Gymnastics	Spondylolysis/ spondylolisthesis Ankle sprains	10
Alpine/telemark skiing	ACL/MCL tears Skier's thumb Shoulder dislocation	9
Basketball	Ankle sprains Shoulder dislocation/ separation	4
Baseball	Lateral epicondylitis Rotator cuff tear	4
Cross-country skiing	Ankle sprains Lateral epicondylitis	3

ACL = anterior cruciate ligament; LCL = lateral collateral ligament; MCL = medial collateral ligament.

4) and require significant alteration in training schedules to allow healing of the injury. Progressive inflammation from overuse can eventually lead to tendon disruption, periostitis (stress reaction), true stress fractures, or cartilaginous degeneration. Early periostitis may only appear as a "fluffiness" of the cortical margin with compensatory cortical thickening underlying it (Fig. 52.1). In more advanced cases, the margin is clearly blurred and the cortex significantly thickened. If symptoms suggest a significant stress reaction but x-rays are negative, then a bone scan is indicated. True stress fractures can be visualized on plain film while stress reactions (periostitis) are best seen on bone scan. Because stress fractures are inflammatory in nature, the complication rates due to delayed or nonunion are higher than those with traumatic fractures.[4] The results of improper treatment of these injuries can be severe, resulting in permanent degenerative changes or deformity. The primary care provider plays an important role not only in diagnosing the injury early (and thus shortening the rehabilitation period) but also in stressing prevention with proper training guidance and timely intervention.

Traumatic Injuries

Physicians providing coverage for athletic events must recognize high-risk situations for serious injuries and evaluate the safety of the sports environment. Asking the following questions when first evaluating a patient with a traumatic injury helps suggest the correct diagnosis and focus the physi-

cal examination: During what sport did the injury occur? How did the injury occur? Where does it hurt? What aggravates the pain? Did other symptoms accompany the injury? Did swelling occur and if so, how soon? How old is the athlete? Has the athlete been injured before? Once these questions are answered, the physician should then perform a focused musculoskeletal and neurovascular exam.

Ankle Injuries

Ankle injuries are ubiquitous and constitute the most common acute musculoskeletal injury, affecting the entire spectrum of grade school to professional athletes. It is estimated that 1 million people present with ankle injuries each year, with an average cost of $300 to $900 for diagnosis and rehabilitation requiring 36 to 72 days for complete rehabilitation. Basketball players have the highest rate of ankle injuries, followed by football players and cross-country runners.[5] Eighty-five percent of athletes with ankle sprains have inversion injuries. The most common structures injured with inversion are the three lateral ligaments that support the ankle joint: the anterior and posterior talofibular ligaments, and the calcaneofibular ligament (Fig. 52.2). The other primary mechanism of ankle sprains is eversion, accounting for 15% of ankle injuries. In general, these are more severe than inversion injuries because of a higher rate of fractures and disruptions of the ankle mortise, leading to instability. The deltoid ligament is the most common ligament to be injured in eversion injuries. Fifteen percent of all complete ligament tears are associated with avulsion fractures of the tibia, fibula, talus, or the base of the fifth metatarsal. Epiphyseal growth plate injuries may be present in the young athlete who sustains an ankle injury. Clinical evidence for an epiphyseal injury of the distal fibula or tibia is bony tenderness about two finger breadths proximal to the tip of the malleolus.[6]

Diagnosis

The examination in the immediate postinjury period may be limited by swelling, pain, and muscle spasm. Inspection should focus on an obvious deformity and vascular integrity. Ankle x-rays are necessary only if there is inability to bear weight for four steps both immediately and in the emergency department, or if there is bony tenderness at the posterior edge or tip of either malleoli.[7] The patient should be reexamined after the swelling has subsided, as the second examination may be more useful in pinpointing areas of tenderness. A pain-free passive and active range of motion of the ankle should be determined in all aspects of movement. The anterior drawer test should be used to assess for joint instability. A positive test, which entails the palpable and visible displacement of the foot more than 4 mm out of the mortise, is consistent with a tear of the anterior talofibular ligament and the anterior joint capsule.[8] Injuries to the lateral ligament complex are assigned grades 1, 2, or 3 depending on the amount of effusion and functional disability.

Management

Immediate treatment is applied according to the RICE (rest, ice, compression, and elevation) protocol.

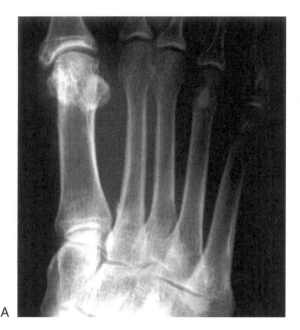

A

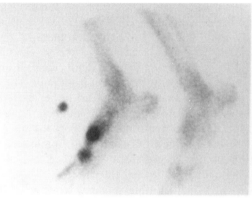

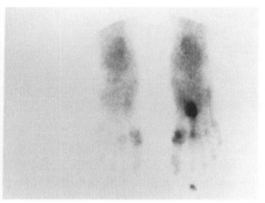

B

Fig. 52.1. (A) Periostitis of the proximal second metatarsal characterized by thickening of the cortex and "fluffy" appearance of the medial margin of the cortex. (B) The confirmatory bone scan identified two areas of significant inflammation of the second metatarsal.

Rest. The athlete can exercise as long as the swelling and pain are not worse within 24 hours. Exercise should include simple weight bearing. If there is pain with walking, crutches are required with appropriate instructions on use until the athlete is able to walk without pain.

Ice. Ice should be applied directly to the ankle for 20 minutes at a time every 2 hours, if possible, during the first 1 to 2 days. Icing should continue until the swelling has stopped.

Compression. Compression can be applied in the form of a horseshoe felt adhesive (0.625 cm). An elastic wrap will do but is not optimal. The compression dressing is worn for 2 to 3 days. Air stirrup braces are recommended to allow dorsiflexion and plantar flexion and effectively eliminate inversion and eversion. For grade 3 sprains, casting for 10 to 14 days may be an option.

Elevation. The leg should be elevated as much as possible until the swelling has stabilized.

Orthopedic Referral

Indications for orthopedic referral include the following factors: fracture, dislocation, evidence of neurovascular com-

promise, penetrating wound into the joint space, and grade 3 sprain with tendon rupture. All patients with ankle injuries should begin early rehabilitation exercises, including passive range of motion and graduated strength training immediately after the injury.

Overview of Knee Injuries

It has been estimated that during each week of the fall football season at least 6000 high school and college players injure their knees, 10% of whom require surgery.[9] Even more discouraging are the results of a 20-year follow-up study of men who had sustained a knee injury in high school. The investigators found that 39% of the men continued to have significant symptoms, 50% of whom had radiographic abnormalities.[9] Knee braces, while popular, have not been proven to be effective in preventing knee ligament injuries. The best time to evaluate the knee is immediately after the injury. Within an hour of a knee injury, protective muscle spasm can prevent a reliable assessment of the joint instability. The following day there may be enough joint effusion to preclude a satisfactory examination. When evaluating knee injuries, compare the injured knee to the uninjured knee. The Pittsburgh Decision Rules delineate evidence-based

Fig. 52.2. Lateral view of major ankle ligaments and structures.

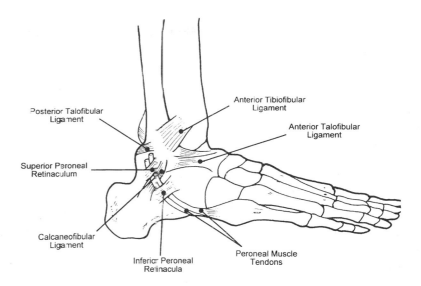

guidelines for when radiographs should be obtained. In general, any sports injury that involves a fall or torsional stress to the knee resulting in an effusion would mandate a knee radiograph. Knee radiographs are necessary to rule out tibial eminence fractures, epiphyseal fractures, and osteochondral fractures. Finally, an evaluation of the neurovascular status of the leg and foot is mandatory.

Meniscus Injuries

Meniscus injuries can occur from twisting or rotation of the knee along with deep flexion and hyperextension. Symptoms include pain, recurrent effusions, clicking, and with associated limited range of motion. Meniscus flaps may become entrapped within the joint space, resulting in locking or the knee "giving out."

Diagnosis

Classically, meniscus tears are characterized by tenderness or pain over the medial or lateral joint line either in hyperflexion or hyperextension. This should be differentiated from tenderness along the entire medial collateral ligament elicited when that ligament is sprained. When the lower leg is rotated with the knee flexed about 90 degrees, pain during external rotation indicates a medial meniscus injury (McMurray's test).

Management

After a meniscus injury, the athlete should follow the RICE protocol. Crutch usage should be insisted upon to avoid weight bearing until the pain and edema have diminished. In most athletes, an orthopedic referral should be considered for arthroscopy in order to repair the damaged meniscus. Plan for follow-up to initiate a rehabilitative program and return to sports.

Medial Collateral Ligament (MCL) Sprain

The MCL ligament is the medial stabilizer of the knee and it is usually injured by an excessive valgus stress of the knee.

The resulting stress can result in a first-, second-, or third-degree sprain. MCL tears are often associated with medial meniscus injury. Lateral collateral ligament tears are unusual and are caused by an inwardly directed blow (varus force) to the inside of the knee.

Diagnosis

The player is usually able to bear some weight on the leg immediately after the injury. Medial knee pain is usually felt at the time of the injury and the knee may feel "wobbly" while the player walks afterward. The examination will reveal acute tenderness somewhere over the course of the MCL usually at or above the joint line. The integrity of the MCL is assessed by applying a valgus stress to the knee while holding the tibia about a third of the way down and forcing it gently laterally while holding the distal femur in place. A patient with a partial (grade 1 or 2) tear of a collateral ligament will have marked discomfort with valgus and varus testing. The athlete with a complete (grade 3) tear of a collateral ligament may have surprisingly little pain on testing but remarkably increased laxity of the ligament. Swelling, ecchymosis over the ligament or a joint effusion, usually develops within several hours of the injury.

Management

A grade 1 sprain is treated with the RICE protocol. Running should be restricted until the athlete is pain free in knee flexion. Generally in 5 to 10 days there will be complete recovery, and with physician clearance, the player can resume full activity. The management of more serious sprains should be directed by an orthopedist.

Anterior Cruciate Ligament (ACL) Injury

This is the most frequent and most severe ligament injury to the knee. It usually occurs not with a direct blow to the knee, but rather from torsional stress coupled with a deceleration injury. These injuries are seen when an athlete changes direction while running and the knee suddenly "gives out."

Diagnosis

A "pop" is often felt during the injury. The player falls on the field in extreme pain and is unable to continue participating. A bloody effusion will develop in 60% to 70% of athletes within the next 24 hours. One of three tests can be employed to test for ACL insufficiency: the anterior drawer, the Lachman maneuver, or the pivot shift test. The *anterior drawer test* should be performed with the knee in 30 degrees of flexion. The injured leg is externally rotated slightly to relax the hamstrings and adductor muscles. The examiner kneels lateral to the injured leg, stabilizes the femur with one hand, and directs a gentle but firm upward force with the other hand on the proximal tibia. If the tibia moves anteriorly, then the ACL has been torn. The *Lachman test* is performed with the hamstrings relaxed and the knee placed in 15 to 20 degrees of flexion. With one hand on the femur just above the knee to stabilize it, the tibia is pulled forward with the opposite hand placed over the tibial tuberosity. If the ACL is intact, the tibia comes to a firm stop. If the ligament is torn the tibia continues forward sluggishly. A *pivot shift test* is performed with the ankle and leg held under the examiner's arm. The leg is abducted and the knee extended. Place the knee in internal rotation with gentle valgus stress to the knee. The hands are placed under the proximal tibia while the knee is flexed to about 25 degrees. If the lateral tibial condyle rotates anteriorly (subluxes forward) during the flexion maneuver, then the test is positive.

Posterior cruciate ligament injuries are usually caused by a direct blow to the upper anterior tibia or posterior forces applied to the tibia while the knee is in flexion. This might apply to a karate player who is kicked in the area of the tibial tuberosity while the foot is firmly on the ground, or to someone who falls forward onto a flexed knee. Posterior cruciate ligament tears are detected by posterior displacement of the tibial tuberosity (the *sag sign*) when the leg is held by the heel with the hip and knee flexed.

Management

Initial management of ACL tears follows the RICE protocolalong with immobilization and crutches, with instructions on their use. The rehabilitation requires the early initiation of quadriceps contractions to prevent atrophy and promote strengthening. Protective bracing with a hinged knee brace may be appropriate for certain athletes. Referral to an orthopedist should be made acutely if there is evidence on x-ray of an avulsion fracture of the ACL attachments or subacutely for possible arthroscopic repair if there is joint laxity.

Patellar Dislocation

This injury can result from a blow to the patella or when an athlete changes direction and then straightens the leg. It is most common in athletes with significant valgus deformity of the knee joint and in adolescents.

Diagnosis

The dislocation usually occurs laterally, but the medial joint capsule and retinaculum may also be torn, sometimes simulating or actually associated with a medial collateral ligament sprain. The dislocation usually reduces spontaneously and the athlete will have a painful swollen knee due to hemarthrosis and tenderness at the medial capsule. Lateral pressure on the patella while gently extending the knee will be met with obvious anxiety and resistance.

Management

If there is no obvious evidence of fracture, an attempted reduction of the dislocation can be made by first extending the knee. It can be helpful to massage the hamstring muscle and ask the athlete to relax it. As the patient allows more knee extension, exert gentle midline pressure directed to the lateral aspect of the patella. The patella should relocate in seconds to minutes. Difficulty with this maneuver suggests a fracture or displaced chondral fragment; the next step would be to splint the knee and refer to an emergency room for radiographs and reduction. Postreduction management follows the RICE protocol, with crutch use for those who can't bear weight. The leg should be elevated while the edema persists, with immediate quadriceps strengthening exercises to prevent atrophy.

Neck Injuries

Injuries to the head and neck are the most frequent catastrophic sports injury. The four common school sports with the highest risk of head and spine injury are football, gymnastics, ice hockey, and wrestling. Nonschool sports risks far outweigh those from organized sports. Common causes of head injuries in this group are trampoline use, cycling, and snow sports.[10] Fortunately, many neck injuries are minimal strains, diagnosed after a quick history and physical examination. Axial loading is the most common mechanism for serious neck injury. Classic examples include the football player "spearing" or tackling head first, and the hockey player sliding head first into the boards. Axial loading can produce spinal fracture, dislocation, and quadriplegia at very low impact velocities—lower than for skull fractures. Extension spinal injuries are more serious than flexion injuries. With extension spine injury (whiplash), the anterior elements are disrupted and the posterior elements are compressed. In flexion injury, the anterior elements are compressed, causing anterior vertebral body fracture, chip fracture, and occasionally anterior dislocation.

Diagnosis

When an athlete is unconscious and motionless, an initial assessment is mandatory. Athletes with focal neurologic deficits or marked neck pain should be suspected of having cervical spine injury until cleared by x-ray examination.

Management

The ABC (airway, breathing, and circulation) of emergency care apply, along with neck stabilization and initiation of emergency transport. Cervical spine injury is assumed until proven otherwise. Proper stabilization precautions must be carried out while the athlete is removed from the playing field or injury site. If the athlete is wearing a helmet, it should not be removed until arrival in the emergency room.

Closed Head Injuries

The definition of concussion by the Neurosurgical Committee on Head Injuries is "a clinical syndrome characterized by immediate and transient posttraumatic impairment of neural function, such as the alteration of consciousness disturbance of vision, equilibrium, etc., due to brainstem involvement."[11] There is also a complication of concussion called a " second-impact syndrome" in which fatal intracerebral edema is precipitated by a second blow to the head of an athlete who has persisting symptoms from an earlier concussion.[12] Fortunately, this syndrome is rare. If athletes have any persisting symptoms from any degree of concussion, they should not be allowed to play. Postconcussion syndrome consists of headache (especially with exertion), labyrinthine disturbance, fatigue, irritability, and impaired memory and concentration. These symptoms can persist for weeks or even months. Both football and snowboarding are common sports associated with closed head injuries.

Epidural hematoma results when the middle meningeal artery, which is embedded in a bony groove in the skull, tears as a result of a skull fracture, crossing this groove. Because the bleeding in this instance is arterial, accumulation of clot continues under high pressure and, as a result, serious brain injury can occur. Subdural hematomas are caused by the shearing forces applied to the bridging arachnoid veins that surround the brain.

Diagnosis

Reviewing the recognition and classification of concussion can simplify its management (Table 52.2). The classic description of an epidural hematoma is that of loss of consciousness in a variable period, followed by recovery of consciousness after which the patient is lucid. This is followed by the onset of increasingly severe headache; decreased level of consciousness; dilation of one pupil, usually on the same side as the clot; and decerebrate posturing and weakness, usually on the side opposite the hematoma. Patients with acute subdural hematoma are more likely to have a prolonged lucid interval following their injury and are less likely to be unconscious at admission than patients with epidural hematomas.

Management

Patients with closed head injuries need a thorough neurologic evaluation, usually including a computed axial tomography (CAT) scan or magnetic resonance imaging (MRI). Return to competition should be deferred until all symptoms have abated and the guidelines described in Table 52.2 have been followed. Adequate head protection in skiers, snowboarders, and football players is an appropriate prevention measure and should be mandatory if the patient has a history of a previous concussion.

Shoulder Dislocation

Shoulder dislocation may occur when sufficient impact tears the anterior joint capsule of the glenohumeral joint, resulting in a slippage of the humeral head out of the glenoid fossa. In anterior glenohumeral dislocation there are two mechanisms of injury: a fall onto an outstretched hand, or a collision with a player or object with the shoulder abducted to 90 degrees and externally rotated. While the shoulder may dislocate posteriorly, an anterior-inferior dislocation is the most common. Careful examination to rule out humeral neck fracture is important before reduction of the shoulder in the field. Small avulsion fractures can occur at the attachment of the supraspinatus tendon (Fig. 52.3), but this injury will not preclude immediate reduction of the shoulder.

Diagnosis

Athletes who have anterior shoulder dislocation will often state that the shoulder has "popped out" and complain of excruciating pain. The athlete is unable to rotate the arm and has a hollow region just inferior to the acromion with an anterior bulge caused by the forward displacement of the humeral head. Subluxation of the shoulder may occur when the humerus slips out of the glenohumeral socket and then spontaneously relocates. Posterior subluxations are seen more commonly in athletes who use repetitive overhand motion such as swimmers and baseball and tennis players.

Management

Anterior dislocation is the only shoulder injury that requires prompt manipulation. The Rockwood technique involves an assistant who applies a long, folded towel around the ipsilateral axilla crossing the upper anterior/posterior chest. Gentle traction is applied while the physician applies in-line traction at 45 degrees abduction on the injured extremity. Traction is gradually increased over several minutes. Successful reduction will manifest as a "thunk" when the humerus relocates

Table 52.2. **Grading of Head Injuries and Management**

Grade of concussion	Symptoms	Management
1	Brief confusion, <30 min, no LOC	No head imaging required unless focal deficit appears or LOC develops; may return to activity with head protection in 7 days
2	Prolonged amnesia or confusion, >30 min, no LOC	No head imaging required unless focal deficit appears or LOC develops; may return to activity with head protection in 21 days
3a	LOC <5 min; amnesia, confusion common	Computed tomography or magnetic resonance imaging recommended to rule out hemorrhage; no further sports activity with risk of head injury for remainder of season; helmet use
3b	LOC ≥5 min	in the future is strongly recommended

LOC = loss of consciousness.

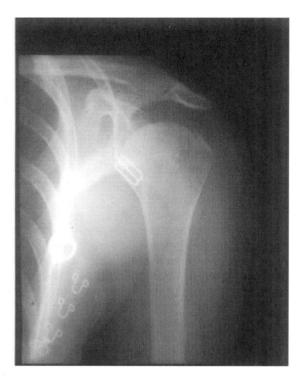

Fig. 52.3. Small avulsion fracture of the proximal humerus in a skier who sustained a shoulder dislocation.

in the glenoid cavity. If started immediately, the dislocation should be reducible in 2 to 3 minutes. Postreduction radiographs are required. With the Stimson technique, the patient lies prone on a flat surface with the arm hanging down. A 5-pound weight is tied to the distal forearm. The reduction will usually take place within 20 minutes.[13] Scapular manipulation in a similar position has also been described as another method to relocate the shoulder with minimal traction.[13] If these attempts at early reduction are unsuccessful, reduction using analgesia or anesthesia can be attempted in the emergency room. In the patient who dislocates for the first time, the shoulder should be immobilized for 2 to 3 weeks. Rehabilitation may reduce the rate of recurrence with goals being the restoration of full shoulder abduction and strengthening of the rotator cuff muscles.[14]

Acromioclavicular (AC) Separation

Acromioclavicular separation may be caused by a direct blow to the lateral aspect of the shoulder or a fall on an outstretched arm. AC separations are classified as grades 1, 2, or 3 as determined by the involvement of the AC and/or the coracoclavicular ligaments.

Diagnosis

There will be discrete tenderness at the AC joint. In grade 1 AC separation, there is tenderness to palpation at the AC joint but no visible defect. Grade 2 or grade 3 AC separation will cause a visible gap between the acromion and the clavicle. A grade 2 separation involves a partial tear of the AC ligaments;

a grade 3 separation is due to a complete tear of the AC ligaments. When a grade 2 or 3 separation is suspected, a radiograph should be obtained of both shoulders to rule out fracture and to delineate the grade of separation. With grade 2 injuries, the clavicle is elevated by one half the width of the AC joint due to the disruption of the AC joint. With grade 3 injuries both the AC and coracoclavicular ligaments are disrupted with resultant dislocation of the AC joint and superior migration of the clavicle.

Management

Initial management of AC separations requires the shoulder to be immobilized in a sling. The extent of medical intervention is determined by the grade of the injury. Those with grade 1 and 2 injuries may be treated conservatively with sling immobilization for 7 to 14 days. When symptoms subside, controlled remobilization and strengthening of the shoulder should begin. There is ongoing controversy regarding conservative versus operative management of the grade 3 injury. An orthopedic referral should be made for these athletes.

Brachial Plexus Injury

A brachial plexus injury, or "burner" or "stinger," is a temporary dysfunction of the neural structures in the brachial plexus after a blow to the head, neck, or shoulder. Burners are reported in football, wrestling, ice hockey, skiing, motocross, soccer, hiking and equestrian sports.[15] Several mechanisms probably contribute to injuries to the brachial plexus, usually involving lateral flexion of the cervical spine with concomitant depression of one of the shoulders. Lateral flexion with rotation and extension of the cervical spine toward the symptomatic side causes a direct compression of the nerve roots, while lateral flexion with shoulder depression causes a traction injury to the nerves.[16]

Diagnosis

Typically the player experiences a sharp burning pain in the shoulder with paresthesia or dysesthesia radiating into the arm and hand. The patient may have associated sensory deficits, decreased reflexes, and weakness of the deltoid, biceps, supraspinatus, or infraspinatus muscles.

Management

If the neurologic findings return to normal within a few minutes, the athlete may return to play. In 5% to 10% of patients, signs and symptoms will persist requiring referral to either a neurologist or a physiatrist.

Thumb and Finger Injuries

Extensor injuries of the distal phalangeal joints occur when there is avulsion of the extensor tendon from the distal phalanx with and without a fracture. This results in a "mallet "or "drop" finger. Proximal phalangeal joint injuries occur when there is avulsion of the central slip of the distal phalanx, resulting in a flexion "boutonniere" deformity. Metacarpophalangeal (MCP) joint sprain of the thumb ("gamekeeper's" thumb) is caused by a fall on an outstretched hand, causing forced abduction to the thumb.

Diagnosis

The distal or proximal phalanx is flexed and lacks active extension in extensor tendon ruptures. It is imperative that any distal interphalangeal (DIP) injury be evaluated for full extension to avoid missing a extensor tendon rupture. Gamekeeper's thumb causes pain and swelling over the ulnar aspect of the MCP joint and is made worse by abducting or extending the thumb. Complete tears of the ulnar collateral ligament are demonstrated by marked laxity in full extension.

Management

An x-ray should be obtained in all of the above injuries to rule out intraarticular fractures or avulsions that require orthopedic referral. In extensor tendon injuries, continued splinting of the distal finger joint in extension for at least 6 weeks is necessary. The treatment for a gamekeeper's thumb requires a thumb spica cast or splint protection for 4 to 6 weeks. During activity, the thumb can be protected by taping it to the index finger to prevent excessive abduction. A complete tear of the ulnar collateral ligament requires orthopedic referral for surgical repair.[17] Minor sprains can be rehabilitated in 3 to 4 weeks.

Specific Overuse Injuries

Shoulder Impingement Syndromes

Overuse injuries of the shoulder are most commonly seen in swimming, throwing, or racquet sports. Swimmers almost uniformly develop symptoms of this injury to varying degrees, especially those swimmers who regularly perform the butterfly stroke. Repetitive motions that abduct and retract the arm followed by antegrade (overhand) rotation of the glenohumeral joint can lead to impingement of the subacromial bursa and the supraspinatus tendon. Early in the course, only the subacromial bursa may be inflamed, but with progressive injury supraspinatus tendonitis develops and may become calcified. Other muscles that make up the rotator cuff can also be strained with this motion and eventually can lead to rotator cuff tears.

Diagnosis

Patients with impingement will complain of pain with abduction to varying degrees and especially with attempts to raise the arm above the level of the shoulder. The pain radiates deep from the subacromial space to the deltoid region and may be vague and not well localized. Palpation of the subacromial bursa under the coracoacromial ligament will often elicit pain deep to the acromion, as will internal rotation of the arm when abducted at 90 degrees with the elbow also flexed at 90 degrees. A second maneuver to detect impingement is to extend the arm forward so it is parallel to the ground and then internally rotate and abduct the arm across the chest while stabilizing the shoulder with the examiner's hand. Both

maneuvers narrow the subacromial space to elicit symptoms. The "painful arc"—pain only within a limited range of abduction—may indicate an advanced calcific tendonitis of the supraspinatus tendon. Radiographic imaging may be useful if this finding is present, as calcific tendonitis may require more invasive treatment.

Management

Modification of shoulder activity and antiinflammatory measures [the RICE protocol, nonsteroidal antiinflammatory drugs (NSAIDs)] are instituted early. Swimmers will need to alter the strokes during their training periods and reduce the distance that they swim to the point that the pain is decreasing daily. Rehabilitation exercises should consist of both aggressive shoulder stretching to lengthen the coracoacromial ligament and improve range of motion. The use of an upper arm counterforce brace will alter the fulcrum of the biceps in such a way as to depress the humeral head further. Strength training of the supraspinatus and biceps internal and external rotator muscles should be performed to aid in depressing the humeral head when stressed, thus increasing the subacromial space. In advanced calcific tendonitis, steroid injection into the subacromial bursa or surgical removal of the calcific tendon may be required.[18]

Tennis Elbow (Lateral Epicondylitis)

Lateral epicondylitis is characterized by point tenderness of the lateral epicondyle at the attachment of the extensor carpi radialis brevis. The most common sports that cause this syndrome are tennis, racquetball, and cross-country skiing.[19] The mechanism of injury in all of the sports is the repetitive extension of the wrist against resistance. Adolescent or preadolescent athletes are at highest risk of significant injury if the growth plate that underlies the lateral epicondyle is not yet closed. If the inflammation of the epicondyle is not arrested, the soft growth cartilage can fracture and rotate the bony attachment of the extensor ligaments, requiring surgical reimplantation of the epicondyle. Without surgery, a permanent deformity of the elbow will result.

Diagnosis

Patients will complain of pain with active extension of the wrist localized to the upper forearm and lateral epicondyle. There is usually marked tenderness of the epicondyle itself. Pain with grasping a weighted cup (Canard's test) or with resisted dorsiflexion is also diagnostic. X-ray studies are not necessary but may show calcific changes to the extensor aponeurosis in chronic cases. Comparison views of the unaffected elbow may be helpful in the adolescent in whom a stress fracture is suspected and the growth plate is not yet closed. Stress fractures of the lateral epicondyle are best diagnosed with a technetium-99 (Te-99) bone scan.

Management

Rest, NSAIDs, and ice to the area are the initial treatment modalities. Modification of the gripped object (racquet or ski pole) with a thicker grip will reduce the stress on the extensors. A counterforce brace worn over the belly of the forearm extensors or a volar cock-up splint can be used to relieve symptoms and alter the dynamic fulcrum of the muscles. Steroid injections superficial to the aponeurosis can be used in more refractory cases but should be limited to three injections.[20] Steroids should not be used in patients who may have a stress fracture or if the growth plates have not yet closed. Gradual return to the sport may begin immediately in grade 1 or 2 injuries, or as soon as the tenderness has resolved in higher grade injuries.

Lumbar Spondylolysis/Spondylolisthesis

Spondylolysis (fracture of the pars interarticularis) of the vertebrae results from repeated forced hyperextension of the spine. Spondylolisthesis (slippage of one vertebrae over another) may result from the facet joint degeneration induced by spondylolysis. Young preadolescent gymnasts are at highest risk for developing spondylolysis but it can also be seen in weight lifters, runners, swimmers who perform the butterfly stroke, divers, and football players.[21] In one large study, up to 10% of adolescent female gymnasts had spondylolysis.[22] Spondylolisthesis usually occurs in older teens and develops primarily at the L5-S1 joint. Their prognosis is worse than those with isolated spondylolysis.

Diagnosis

The athlete usually complains of unilateral back pain that worsens with rotation of the trunk. There is usually regional spasm of the paraspinous musculature and the hamstrings. Pain from spondylolisthesis may cause radicular symptoms in the L5-S1 distribution. Lateral and anteroposterior (AP) x-rays of the spine may not reveal pars interarticularis pathology so oblique films should be added. Even if the x-rays are normal, if the diagnosis is suspected, restriction of the activity is necessary until repeat films are done in 4 to 6 weeks. A Te-99 bone scan is a sensitive test for detecting pars interarticularis fractures or stress reactions.

Management

Rest is essential in both of these conditions. Bone scans can be used to follow the healing process but costs may be prohibitive. Resolution of symptoms is an adequate indicator of healing. The athlete may continue to train in sports that do not result in hyperextension or rotation of the spine (e.g., cycling, stair-climbing) as long as the back symptoms are improving. Referral to a physical therapist for neutral spine stability exercises is warranted.

Low-grade spondylolisthesis can be managed conservatively by restriction of activity until the pain has resolved. Serial x-rays every 4 to 6 months can monitor progression in athletes who returned to their sport after the symptoms resolved. High-grade spondylolisthesis (>25% displacement of the vertebral body) can also be managed conservatively, but the patient must be permanently restricted from contact or collision sports. Bracing or surgical repair of spondylolisthesis may be required if pain is severe or persistent nerve root irritation is present.[23]

Retropatellar (Patellofemoral) Pain Syndrome

Retropatellar pain syndrome (RPPS) is most commonly found in patients participating in running, hiking, or cycling. The symptoms probably represent the majority of knee pain complaints in athletes. Retropatellar pain is caused by the repetitive glide of the patella over the femoral condyles, which can lead to inflammation of the retropatellar synovium or the cartilage itself. The glide of the patella is usually laterally displaced in athletes who have recurrent symptoms. Factors that increase this friction are instability of the knee from previous injury, valgus deformity of the knee, deficient vastus medialis obliquus muscle strength, patella alta, or recent increase in running program. Relative valgus stress on the knee is created in patients with abnormal Q angles, pes planus, femoral anteversion, or external tibial torsion causing lateral displacement of the patella. If progressive, RPPS can progress to chondromalacia patellae with destruction of the retropatellar cartilage.

Diagnosis

Patients with RPPS present with vague retropatellar or peripatellar pain, which is usually most significant several hours after exercise. Walking downhill or downstairs, bending at the knees, and kneeling exacerbates pain symptoms. In more advanced cases, pain can be constant, occur during and after exercise. Oddly, patients often experience pain if the knee is not moved enough; i.e., if left flexed for several minutes, pain will develop. The examination of the knee should first include inspection of the patient's entire leg, feet, and hips to assess for a significant Q angle, torsional deformities, leg length discrepancy, or pes planus. On palpation of the knee, the lateral posterior margins of the patella should be palpated with the patella deviated laterally to detect tenderness of the retropatellar surface. This should also be repeated on the medial aspect of the patella with medial deviation. Effusions are usually absent in RPPS. A compression test of the patella is performed with the patient relaxing and then flexing the quadriceps group while the patella is displaced distally by the examiner. Fine crepitus with this test may indicate synovial inflammation but it is not specific. Coarse crepitus or popping with significant pain is indicative of chondromalacia. Sunrise views of the knees may reveal radiographic evidence of retropatellar degeneration, but usually these findings are present only in advanced cases and are not necessary for diagnosis.[24]

Management

For athletes with symptoms only at higher training levels, reduction of the exacerbating activity and NSAID use are the first steps. If the patient has a grade 3 or 4 injury, then cessation of the exacerbating activity for 2 to 4 weeks until the pain is no longer present at rest is necessary. Selective strengthening of the vastus medialis obliquus (VMO), orthotics, and alteration of mechanical forces when pedaling (for cyclists) can also relieve symptoms. Lateral deviation of the foot while extending the knee allows more medial tracking of the patella during exercise and forces the VMO to perform more of the quadriceps function. Stretching to reduce both hamstring and quadriceps tension is an important component of the rehabilitation of RPPS. As with all overuse injuries, a graduated increase in exercise duration at a rate of 10% per week, with relative rest periods every 3 to 4 weeks, may prevent recurrence of the symptoms.

Tibial Periostitis ("Shin Splints")

Tibial periostitis is the most common overuse injury in recreational runners and is often confused with other lower leg pain syndromes.[25] Any pain in the tibial area is often labeled "shin splints" but must be differentiated from anterior compartment syndrome, patellar tendonitis, or a simple muscular strain. The primary cause of tibial periostitis is mechanical; the attachment of a calf muscle is strained due to the pounding of running on a mechanically deficient foot. A recent increase in duration of running often triggers shin splints if the increase is too rapid and there is no rest phase. Over 4 to 8 weeks after such increases in training, this condition progresses to involve the bone by disrupting the periosteum and cortex.

Diagnosis

Most patients with this syndrome have pes planus, which results in tibialis posterior tendonitis initially. Their pain is localized to the lower third of the medial aspect of the tibia. Patients with pes cavus have anterior tibialis tendonitis with pain localized laterally on the middle or upper tibia. If other calf flexors are involved, the pain may be deep in the calf, resembling a deep vein thrombosis (DVT). Homans' sign may be positive in these patients because the posterior aspect of the tibia is inflamed. If point tenderness is present, x-ray studies are indicated, with careful attention being paid to subtle changes in the cortical margin in the area of pain.

Management

Table 52.3 delineates rehabilitation strategies for this injury. The importance of adequate rest and graduated resumption of exercise with cycled rest phases cannot be overemphasized.[26] Aggressive stretching of the calf muscles, twice daily icing the affected area, and NSAIDs are essential adjuncts to adjustments in the training program. Corrective arch supports for either pes planus or pes cavus are necessary if these conditions are present. Combining strength training with resumption of running will enhance tendon healing and adaptive cortical thickening.

Jones' Fractures (Proximal Fifth Metatarsal Fractures)

Overuse injuries of the foot can occur in multiple sites including the metatarsal, tarsal, and sesamoid bones. Jones' and sesamoid bone fractures have very high rates of nonunion (50–90%).[27] These stress fractures must be detected and treated early to prevent this complication. Jones' fractures are primarily seen in distance runners, especially in those with a recent increase in activity. There is usually a history of antecedent pain for several weeks at the attachment of the peroneus brevis tendon to the proximal fifth metatarsal.

Diagnosis

Pain and tenderness at the site are universal. Inversion of the ankle, causing stress of the peroneus brevis tendon, or attempts to evert the foot against stress also localize pain to the proximal head of the fifth metatarsal. Radiographs may show evidence of cortical thickening, sclerotic changes within the medullary bone, or a true fracture line. The more proximal the fracture, the higher the risk of delayed union. If the radiographs are negative, but if there is significant tenderness, then a bone scan should be performed because of the high rate of false-negative radiographs for this fracture.

Management

All athletes with evidence of stress fracture on bone scan or sclerotic changes on x-ray should be referred for possible screw placement.[28] If there is evidence only of a periosteal reaction, without visible fracture or medullary sclerosis, the foot should be placed in a non–weight-bearing short leg cast for 4 to 6 weeks and follow-up films obtained when pain-free to ensure that healing has been complete. Despite appropriate care, avascular necrosis may occur, requiring grafting of the bone. After the fracture is healed, the athlete may gradually return to the activity, with close follow-up to prevent recurrence of symptoms.[29]

Table 52.3. **Overuse Injuries: Staging and Rehabilitation**

Stage	Symptoms	Rehabilitation
1	Pain with maximal exertion, resolves after event; nonfocal exam	Decrease activity to 50–70%, ice, NSAIDs for 7 days; every other day training
2	Pain with minimal exertion, resolves in <24 hours; minimal tenderness	Decrease activity to 50%, ice, NSAIDs for 10-14 days; every other day training
3	Pain despite rest, not resolved within 48 hours; tender on exam, mild swelling of tendon	Stop activity 2–4 weeks or until pain free; ice, NSAIDs; resume training at 50%, increase by 10% per week; every 4 weeks reduce to 50%
4	Continual pain, stress fracture, point tenderness and swelling	Immobilize if indicated; rest 4–6 weeks until pain free; ice, NSAIDs; resume training at 50%, increase by 10% per week; every 4 weeks reduce to 50%

NSAID = nonsteroidal antiinflammatory drug.

Prevention of Injuries

The primary focus of injury prevention stems from understanding the mechanisms of injury. In contact or collision sports, appropriate protective equipment is essential in reducing the severity of injuries sustained by the participants. Wearing protective helmets substantially reduces risk of head injuries in many collision sports. In sports where the risk of falls is prominent, use of wrist guards and knee pads can reduce injuries to these joints. Alpine skiers must use releasable bindings that are adjusted appropriately for their weight and skill level to reduce the risk of ligamentous knee injuries. Overuse injuries can be prevented by developing graded training programs that allow time for compensatory changes in tendons and bones to prevent inflammation. Orthotics and focused training of muscle groups can correct mechanical problems that could lead to overuse injuries.

The second aspect of injury prevention is maximizing the strength, proprioceptive skills, and the flexibility of the athlete. Appropriate off-season and preseason training of athletes, coaches, and trainers can substantially reduce injuries during the regular season.

References

1. Cook PC, Leit ME. Issues in the pediatric athlete. Orthop Clin North Am 1995;26:453–64.
2. Patel DR. Sports injuries in adolescents. Med Clin North Am 2000;84:983–1007.
3. Brody DM. Running injuries. Clin Sym 1987;39:23–5.
4. Hulkko A, Orava S. Stress fractures in athletes. Int J Sports Med 1987;8:221–6.
5. Clanton TO, Porter DA Primary care of foot and ankle injuries in the athlete. Clin Sports Med 1997;16:435–66.
6. Brostrom L. Sprained ankles, I. Anatomic lesions in recent sprains. Acta Chir Scand 1964;128:483–95.
7. Stiell IG. Decision rules for the use of radiography in acute ankle injuries. JAMA 1993;269:1127–32.
8. Perlman M, Leveille D, DeLeonibus J, et al. Inversion lateral ankle trauma: differential diagnosis, review of the literature and prospective study. J Foot Surg 1987;26:95–135.
9. Dyment PG. Athletic injuries. Pediatr Rev 1989;10(10):1–13.
10. Proctor MR, Cantu RC. Head and spine injuries in young athletes. Clin Sports Med 2000;19:693–715.
11. Committee on Head Injury Nomenclature of the Congress of Neurological Surgeons. Glossary of head injury including some definitions of injury to the cervical spine. Clin Neurosurg 1966;12:386.
12. Cantu RC. Second impact syndrome. Physician Sports Med 1992;20:55–66.
13. Hergengroeder AC. Acute shoulder, knee and ankle injuries. Part 1: diagnosis and management. Adolesc Health Update 1996;8(2):1–8.
14. Blake R, Hoffman J. Emergency department evaluation and treatment of the shoulder and humerus. Emerg Med Clin North Am 1999;17:859–76.
15. Aronen JC, Regan K. Decreasing the incidence of recurrence of first time anterior shoulder dislocations with rehabilitation. Am J Sports Med 1984;12:283–91.
16. Archambault JL. Brachial plexus stretch injury. J Am Coll Health 1983;31(6):256–60.
17. Vereschagin KS, Weins JJ, Fanton GS, Dillingham MF. Burners, don't overlook or underestimate them. Phys Sportsmed 1991;19(9):96–106.
18. Kahler DM, McLue FC. Metacarpophalangeal and proximal interphalangeal joint injuries of the hand, including the thumb. Clin Sports Med 1992;11:5–76.
19. Smith DL, Campbell SM. Painful shoulder syndromes: diagnosis and management. J Gen Intern Med 1992;7:328–39.
20. Safran MR. Elbow injuries in athletes: a review. Clin Orthop 1995;310:257–77.
21. Mehlhoff TL, Bennett B. The elbow. In: Mellion MB, Walsh WM, Shelton GL, eds. The team physician handbook. Philadelphia: Hanley & Belfus, 1990. p. 334–345.
22. Wilhite J, Huurman WW. The thoracic and lumbar spine. In: Mellion MB, Walsh WM, Shelton GL, eds. The team physician handbook. Philadelphia: Hanley & Belfus, 1990. p. 374–400.
23. Jackson DW, Wiltse LL. Low back pain in young athletes. Phys Sportsmed 1974;2:53–60.
24. Smith JA, Hu SS. Disorders of the pediatric and adolescent spine. Orthop Clin North Am 1999;30:487–99.
25. Davidson K. Patellofemoral pain syndrome. Am Fam Physician 1993;48:1254–62.
26. Batt ME. Shin splints—a review of terminology. Clin J Sports Med 1995;5:53–7.
27. Stanitski CL. Common injuries in preadolescent and adolescent athletes. Sports Med 1989;7:32–41.
28. Orava S, Hulkko A. Delayed unions and nonunions of stress fractures in athletes. Am J Sports Med 1988;16:378–82.
29. Lawrence SJ, Bolte MJ. Jones fractures and related fractures of the fifth metatarsal. Foot Ankle 1993;14:358–65.

53
Care of the Obese Patient

Michael T. Railey

An estimated 97 million adults in the United States are overweight or obese. Obesity is the most common nutritional disease of the Western world.[1] The number of overweight Americans has increased from 20% to 34% over the last 10 to 12 years, with one half of adults overweight and one of three obese.[2] Twenty-five percent of children and adolescents are also considered obese.[2,3] In the United States, the prevalence of obesity is highest among African-American women (48.6%) and Mexican-American women (46.7%).[2] The reasons for this are multifactorial and strongly imply that effective treatments will have to include management plans that encompass cultural awareness. Management of obesity is individualized, complicated, and often frustrating for both patient and physician.[4] Obesity is associated with numerous health risks. Excess body weight increases the risk of developing cardiovascular disease, hypertension, diabetes, and many other diseases[5–8] (Table 53.1). The direct health care costs of treating obesity and its related diseases have been estimated to be $45.8 billion per year.[1,9,10] Indirect costs due to loss of income amounts to another $23 billion annually.[9]

Etiology

Obesity is a very complex and heterogeneous disease; its pathogenesis involves genetic influences combined with an imbalance between caloric intake and energy output. Other elements that play an additional role in the development of obesity include race, age, gender, and environmental and psychosocial factors. More specific evidence is rapidly accumulating, in the study of the genetic components of obesity. Researchers have identified an appetite suppressor released from fat cells called leptin.[11] Further interest has focused on the *Ob* or "obesity" gene and its subtypes.[11] The current model for a clinical approach to this difficult-to-treat condition is that of a chronic disease with a definite genetic influence requiring treatment on multiple levels, predominantly directed at environmental and behavioral changes.

Diagnosis

The measurement of height and weight should be a part of every comprehensive patient visit. Initially, the Hamwi principle can be used to estimate ideal body weight (IBW) in screening for endogenous obesity.[9] IBW is estimated using this principle (Table 53.2). When IBW is exceeded, body mass index (BMI) should also be calculated or determined using Figure 53.1; this value is recorded in the permanent medical record for future reference.[5] The calculation can be made by dividing the patient's weight in kilograms by the square of the height in inches as a BMI greater than or equal to 30. Morbid obesity is considered a BMI of 40 or more.[12]

Deposits of fat in the upper body leading to particular configurations also put an individual at higher risk for metabolic abnormalities and the ravages of the obesity syndrome.[5] Sometimes referred to as "apple or pear" configurations, the waist to hip ratio (WHR) has been the most widely accepted practical method of classifying body fat distribution.[13] Measuring the smallest circumference below the rib cage and above the navel as the waist circumference, and the widest circumference at the posterior of the buttocks over the greater trocanters as the hip circumference, a ratio (waist to hip) is obtained. A WHR of 0.95 or less for men and 0.85 or less in women are the normal cutoff points.[1,5,13] Elevated measurements indicate increased risk for associated illnesses (see Table 53.1).[5,9,13]

There are rare secondary causes of obesity, which must be considered prior to constructing a treatment plan. These secondary causes include hypothalamic obesity due to trauma, malignancy, inflammatory disease, Cushing syndrome, growth hormone deficiency, hypogonadism, hypothyroidism, polycystic ovary syndrome, pseudohypoparathyroidism, and insulinoma.[9] These potential causes are uncommon but should be considered as a part of the differential diagnosis. In each case, history, physical exam, and laboratory testing can be used to rule out these disorders.

Table 53.1. Health Complications of Obesity

Hypertension
Diabetes
Cancer (breast, possibly colon, others)
Dyslipidemias
Arthritis
Depression
Cholelithiasis
Coronary Artery Disease
Obstructive sleep apnea

Table 53.2. Determination of Ideal Body Weight

Men: 106 lbs for 5 feet in height plus 6 lbs for each
   additional inch
Women: 100 lbs for 5 feet in height plus 5 lbs for each
   additional inch
Light frame: reduce estimate by 10%
Heavy frame: add 10%

Multiple autosomal-recessive defects have been described in association with human obesity. Dysmorphic mutations associated with human obesity include Prader-Willi, Cohen, Carpenter, Bardet-Biedl, and Alström syndromes.[9]

Medications occasionally are implicated in the genesis of obesity. These include phenothiazines, steroids, lithium, antiserotoninergic compounds, neuroleptics, and tricyclic antidepressants.[9]

Constructing a Treatment Plan[14–18]

Once a patient has been determined to be overweight or obese (having ruled out secondary causes), a treatment plan must be formulated. This should be discussed in detail with the pa-

tient. Obesity, especially in a society where beauty and thinness is held in high esteem, is difficult to manage and often accompanied with bouts of depression and extreme frustration for patients.[4] Depending on the staging of the patient, a nutritional consultation can be extremely important in getting off to a good start. The approach to management must be multilevel, and include detailed instruction and planning for exercise along with reduced-intake meal planning to create the necessary caloric deficit. In some instances, medications are useful either in the beginning of the treatment plan or as a continuous supplemental tool to maintain consistent progress to goal.

The family physician must probe for any emotional and psychological issues that serve to impede or contribute to blocking weight loss attempts. Personal family problems, marital dysfunction, and financial worries can be at the root of inconsistent weight management. Any significant social mores such as varied concepts of what constitutes beauty and idiosyncrasies common to specific populations should be

Height (Feet and Inches)

Weight(Pounds)	5'0"	5'1"	5'2"	5'3"	5'4"	5'5"	5'6"	5'7"	5'8"	5'9"	5'10"	5'12"	6'0"	6'1"	6'2"	6'3"	6'4"
100	20	19	18	18	17	17	16	16	15	15	14	14	14	13	13	12	12
105	21	20	19	19	18	17	17	16	16	15	15	15	14	14	13	13	13
110	21	21	20	19	19	18	18	17	17	16	16	15	15	15	14	14	13
115	22	22	21	20	20	19	19	18	17	17	17	16	16	15	15	14	14
120	23	23	22	21	21	20	19	19	18	18	17	17	16	16	15	15	15
125	24	24	23	22	22	21	20	20	19	18	18	17	17	16	16	16	15
130	25	25	24	23	22	22	21	21	20	19	19	18	18	17	17	16	16
135	26	26	25	24	23	22	22	21	21	20	19	19	18	18	17	17	16
140	27	26	26	25	24	23	23	22	21	21	20	20	19	18	18	17	17
145	28	27	27	26	25	24	23	23	22	21	21	20	20	19	19	18	18
150	29	28	27	27	26	25	24	23	23	22	22	21	20	20	19	19	18
155	30	29	28	27	27	26	25	24	24	23	22	22	21	20	20	19	19
160	31	30	29	28	27	27	26	25	24	24	23	22	22	21	21	20	19
165	32	31	30	29	28	27	27	26	25	24	24	23	22	22	21	21	20
170	33	32	31	30	29	28	27	27	26	25	24	24	23	22	22	21	21
175	34	33	32	31	30	29	28	27	27	26	25	24	24	23	22	22	21
180	35	34	33	32	31	30	29	28	27	27	26	25	24	24	23	22	22
185	36	35	34	33	32	31	30	29	28	27	27	26	25	24	24	23	23
190	37	36	35	34	33	32	31	30	29	28	27	26	26	25	24	24	23
195	38	37	36	35	33	32	31	31	30	29	28	27	26	26	25	24	24
200	39	38	37	35	34	33	32	31	30	30	29	28	27	26	26	25	24
205	40	39	37	36	35	34	33	32	31	30	29	29	28	27	26	26	25
210	41	40	38	37	36	35	34	33	32	31	30	29	28	28	27	26	26
215	42	41	39	38	37	36	35	34	33	32	31	30	29	28	28	27	26
220	43	42	40	39	38	37	36	35	34	33	32	31	30	29	28	27	27
225	44	43	41	40	39	37	36	35	34	33	32	31	31	30	29	28	27
230	45	43	42	41	39	38	37	36	35	34	33	32	31	30	30	29	28
235	46	44	43	42	40	39	38	37	36	35	34	33	32	31	30	29	29
240	47	45	44	43	41	40	39	38	36	35	34	33	32	31	31	30	29
245	48	46	45	43	42	41	40	38	37	36	35	34	33	32	31	31	30
250	49	47	46	44	43	42	40	39	38	37	36	35	34	33	32	31	30

Fig. 53.1. Determination of body mass index.

taken into account in counseling. Obese patients are surprisingly frequently unaware of modifying factors in their lives that influence their success in losing weight.[17,18] These factors include personal health belief systems, such as believing extra weight is attractive to some persons; race; nutritional habits; and hair care issues, such as avoiding perspiration to protect chemical treatments.[15] If necessary, supportive psychotherapy or referral for counseling might be necessary, and should not be overlooked.

Exercise

Developing a pattern of routine exercise is one of the most difficult areas of change for the overweight patient. Many patients have lost or never had an appreciation of exercise for fun and energy production.[15,18] They instead envision the drudgery of work and depletion of their energy in association with exercising. Exercise then becomes an unpleasant task, and pleasure is not taken in the process. Long-term success is in many respects dependent on changing these erroneous concepts.[1,5,19] The patient who becomes "addicted" to an exercise regime invariably enjoys a better outcome even if weight loss goals are incompletely realized, due to improved self-esteem (also see Chapter 8). Chronically overweight patients frequently overestimate the amount and quality of effective calorie burning exercise that they accomplish while underestimating the amount of food taken in.[15] This is a deadly self-deceit, which must be uncovered and brought into the patient's consciousness to increase the opportunity for success.[18] If the clinical history is not taken meticulously, the patient will continue believing misinformation about how much exercise is necessary for effective negative calorie balance.

A minimum of 4 or 5 days per week should be exercise days,[5,12] with each session lasting for at least 20 to 30 minutes. The patient's pulse should reach 60% to 80% of the age-specific target heart rate maximum as a goal.[14,15] Physicians should give overweight patients—in writing, on a prescription pad—an "exercise prescription," including suggested length of time for activities and the target pulse, which is calculated by subtracting their age from 220 and multiplying by 0.6 and 0.8 to get a range. Patient education charts and handouts with calorie-burning equivalents are very helpful to teach the concept of caloric deficit through increasing activity and decreasing intake. Encouraging incorporation of more walking, climbing stairs, and manual activities into daily routine is also beneficial.[1,14,16] It is critical for the patient to understand that temperature and weather changes must not deter efforts to maintain exercise. Many patients believe that pleasant weather is the only time to exercise.[15,18]

Food Intake

Many physicians refer patients for dietary counseling to determine and resolve the difficult problem of what and how much to eat. Another relatively simple approach that primary care physicians can incorporate into their practice is to determine by dietary history an estimate of the calories consumed daily, and then to assist the patient in diminishing 500 calories per day from that starting point.[5,16] This sets a goal of approxi-

mately a 3500-calorie deficit per week, leading minimally to a 1 pound per week weight loss calorie deficit. Many patients have difficulty in ascertaining exactly how much of each type of food on a percentage basis they should eat. Keeping daily total fat under 30% is a fair approximation of a more healthy diet. Generally the normal healthy diet has 30% to 35% fat, 15% protein, and about 50% carbohydrate (combined simple and complex). Measuring exact quantities of food often leads to "burn out" over the long haul. Changing habits by reducing excessive quantities of the wrong types of foods in large amounts frequently leads to better compliance.[15]

Medications

Overweight patients often inquire about the use of medications to enhance weight loss. These agents can be very helpful, but should not be considered the primary solution. Consider medications for patients who have a BMI >30, or for those with a BMI >27 and a condition such as arthritis, diabetes, or hypertension. Be aware of the contraindications. The following medications are currently thought to be useful as adjuncts for weight loss. The patient should be warned that behavioral and lifestyle changes must accompany any medications if success is to be realized. The development of tolerance to these medications is also very common, and physicians must be prepared with new plans and encouragement when plateaus are reached. In all cases, cessation of the drug has been shown to result in rapid reaccumulation of weight if lifestyle changes are not accomplished and maintained.[1,20]

Sibutramine (Meridia)

This drug suppresses appetite by blocking reuptake of norepinephrine and serotonin. Long-term safety is unknown. The medication has been associated with blood pressure elevation, dry mouth insomnia, headache, and constipation. The usual dosage is 10 to 15 mg daily.[1,20] One approach is to try 10 mg for 60 days, and then 15 mg for another 60 days. If satisfactory weight loss is not achieved after this regime, the likelihood of success is very low.

Orlistat (Xenical)

Orlistat has been used safely in studies for up to 2 years. Patients have been found to lose weight with slow regain. Chemically, tetrahydrolipstatin is a lipase inhibitor and it decreases absorption of dietary fat. Use of this medication is contraindicated if the patient has a chronic malabsorption syndrome.[20] Adverse gastrointestinal effects are oily spotting, flatus, increased defecation, and fecal incontinence. The usual dose is 120 mg three times a day, taken with the three main meals.[1]

Phentermine (Adipex-P, Ionamin)

This medication stimulates release of norepinephrine and is given before meals to reduce appetite. The usual starting dose is 24 to 37.5 mg daily given either in divided doses or a single dose. Drugs from this group tend to produce more adverse effects than sibutramine.[20] These include dry mouth, gastrointestinal (GI) discomfort, nervousness, dizziness, hypertension, insomnia, tachycardia, agitated states, and libidinous changes.[1,20,21] This class of drugs also includes diethylpropion (Tenuate) and phendimetrazine (Bontril). Their contraindications and side effects are similar to those of phentermine.

Surgical Options

There is a place for surgical or bariatric treatment for obesity,[1] which should be reserved for patients who are clinically severely obese with a BMI $\geq$40 kg/m^2. Patients with a BMI >30 and one or more comorbid risk factors, such as diabetes, hypertension, arthritis, hyperlipidemia, or sleep apnea; and have been resistant to nonsurgical therapy are also considered candidates. Individuals who have made only minimal effort to lose weight by exercising and reducing intake should not be routinely referred for bariatric surgery for their convenience.

Currently, for those patients who appropriately qualify, the most successful procedures have been the Roux-en-Y gastric bypass or vertical banded gastroplasty procedures.[1] These surgeries have resulted in a 40% to 70% loss of excess body weight. The gastric bypass procedure is more effective than gastroplasty alone.[1] In experienced hands at most large medical centers, perioperative mortality is less than 1%. Many of these patients become independent of antihypertensive and diabetic medications. Improvements in the symptoms of degenerative arthritis can be anticipated. Risks include anastomotic leaks, wound infections, stomal stenosis, and incisional hernia.[1,14,16] Postoperative metabolic complications include vitamin and mineral deficiencies, especially iron and vitamin B$_{12}$. Some patients experience chronic nausea, vomiting, dumping syndrome, or constipation.[1]

Fad Diets

A fad diet is a weight loss scheme that touts a rapid result with very little effort. Many of these diets work for short periods of time, but usually have drawbacks of craving, nutritional inadequacy, or difficulty in maintenance. The successful diet always results in diminished overall total daily calories while simultaneously providing appropriate nutrients, vitamins, and minerals. Each diet should be analyzed individually for adequate amounts of protein, carbohydrate, fat, and fluid content. If necessary, seek a certified dietary consultation to evaluate diets or dietary supplements. Caution patients about the use of diets that include appetite-suppressant additives or over-the-counter food supplements, which could prove to be metabolically dangerous,[1,20,21] especially with comorbid conditions such as hypertension. Many of these supplements have caffeine, guarana, and or ma huang (ephedrine) to make the patient feel energetic about the program. There are no easy "fad" diet answers to the difficult problem of obesity.

Summary

Obesity is a serious chronic disease fraught with frustration, low self-esteem, multiple setbacks, and a poor prognosis for most patients.[5] Success must be measured individually, and patients must remain under continuous periodic medical attention to detect psychological, personal, and behavioral influences that can lead them back to previous bad habits. Restraint in eating, evaluation, therapy for emotional problems, continuous exercise, and lifestyle changes are the only interventions that can result in permanent weight loss.[9,11,21] In some cases personal and or genetic influences are so powerful that surgery is the only option left. Physicians treating these patients must take special care to remain encouraging and nonjudgmental in managing this tremendous medical problem that affects a large segment of society.

References

1. Obesity. June 2001. Available at *www.dynamicmedical.com*.
2. Kuczmarski RJ, Flegal KM, Campbell SM, et al. Increasing prevalence of overweight among US adults: The National Health and Nutrition Examination Survey, Phase 1, 1988–1991. JAMA 1994;272:205–11.
3. Flegal KM, Carroll MD, Kuczmarski RJ, et al. Overweight and obesity in the United States—prevalence and trends, 1960–1994. Int J Obes Relat Metab Disord 1998;22:39–47.
4. Martin LF, Hunter SM, Lauve RM, et al. Severe obesity: expensive to society, frustrating to treat, but important to confront. South Med J 1995;88:895–902.
5. Pi Sunyer FX. Medical hazards of obesity. Ann Intern Med 1993;119:655–60.
6. Gibbs WW. Gaining on fat. Sci Am 1996;275:88–94.
7. Bray GA. Complications of obesity. Ann Intern Med 1985;103: 1052–62.
8. McGinnis JM, Foege WH. Actual causes of death in the United States. JAMA 1993;270:2207–12.
9. Chan S, Blackburn GL. Helping patients reverse the health risks of obesity. J Clin Outc Manage 1997;4(3)37–50.
10. Wolf AM, Colditz GA. The cost of obesity: The U.S. Perspective. Pharmacoeconomics 1994;5(1 suppl):34–7.
11. Rippe JM, Yanovski SZ. Obesity—a chronic disease. Patient Care 1998;October 15:29–62.
12. NIH Consensus Statement, Physical Activity and Cardiovascular Health, vol 13, No. 3 Dec. 18–20, 1995.
13. Egger G. The case for using waist to hip ratio measurements in routine medical checks. Med J Aust 1992;156:280–5.
14. Guidance for treatment of adult obesity. Available at *www. shapeup.org*.
15. Railey MT. Evaluation and treatment of obesity. Prim Care Rep 1997;3(14):125–32.
16. Shikora SA, Saltzman E. Revisiting obesity: current treatment strategies. Hosp Med 1998;11:41–9.
17. Walcott-McQuigg JA, Sullivan J, Dan A, Logan B. Psychosocial factors influencing weight control behavior of African-American women. West J Nurs Res 1995;17:502–20.
18. Railey MT. Parameters of obesity in African-American Women. Nat Med Assoc 2000;92(10):481–4.
19. Report of the Secretary Task Force on Black and Minority Health. Executive summary, vol. 1, DHHS pub. 85-487367 (Q63). Washington, DC: U.S. Department of Health and Human Services, 1985.
20. Allison DB, Anderson JW, Aronne LJ, Campfield LA, Vash PD. Taking advantage of antiobesity medications. Patient Care 2000; 11:34–62.
21. Agrawal M, Worzniak M, Diamond L. Managing obesity like any other chronic condition. Postgrad Med 2000;108(1):75–82.

54
Home Care

David B. Graham

The adage that "a picture is worth a thousand words" holds especially true for the provision of medical care in the home. A single home visit can be worth countless hours of patient contact in the office. McWhinney[1] describes the family physician who works in the home as a "practicing ecologist," one who studies living things in their environmental home. Home care has always been an essential part of health care delivery and remains equally important in the technology-driven world of 21st century medicine.

Trends in Home Care

The Aging U.S. Population

As the population of the United States ages, there is a dramatic increase in the number of patients who are elderly and frail. Currently, 13% of the U.S. population is over 65 years old, which is estimated to rise to over 20% by 2025.[2] However, home care in the U.S. is far behind other industrialized nations. In England and Wales in 1992, home visits averaged 229 per 1000 patient-years, and those over 85 years old received 3009 visits per 1000 patient-years.[3] By contrast, in 1993 the U.S. average was 26.6 visits per 1000 patient-years, representing a mere 0.2% of all Medicare reimbursement to physicians.[4]

Explosive Growth in the Home Health Industry

While physician home visits remain low, the home health care industry is booming.[2,5–7] From 1989 to 1995, the number of home health agencies, both for-profit and not-for-profit, grew by over 50%, and Medicare spending for home health services rose sixfold,[6] now standing at over $22 billion per year.[2] Over 90% of all physician home visits are to elderly patients,[4] and those over 65 years of age represent 48% of total hospital inpatient charges.[8] Home care helps minimize hospital costs; however, it identifies additional problems and the need for more services, thereby increasing the total health care bill.[1,2,4–6] Additionally, Welch et al[6] found that the majority of home health care is for long-term management of chronic conditions; only 22% of visits were within 30 days of discharge.

Medicare Reimbursement for Home Care Services

In January 1998, the Health Care Financing Administration (HCFA) added six new common procedural terminology (CPT) codes for home care[5,9,10] (Table 54.1). HCFA also increased reimbursement for care plan oversight (CPO),[10,11] allowing physicians to bill for time spent on indirect patient management and for the certification of home health services[1] (Table 54._). These changes make home care financially feasible for the busy family physician.[4,5,9,12,13]

Specifics of a Home Care Practice

Physicians Who Make Home Care Visits

In the 1930s, home care represented 40% of all U.S. physician–patient interactions. After World War II, this fell to 10% in the 1950s and to 0.6% in the 1980s.[4] Family physicians do the majority of home care,[2,4,13–15] making about 21.2 home visits per year in 1991[1,13]; however, 35% made no home visits that year.[1] Statistically, the home care physician was a male family physician with a longer time in solo or small group practice, caring for chronic illnesses,[14] living in the Northeast,[15] and making frequent home health agency referrals.[13] This situation is changing.

Patient Selection

The range of patients and problems cared for in the home is broad and challenging. Meyer and Gibbons[4] described typical patients receiving home visits as over 82 years old, sicker,

Table 54.1. **CPT Codes for Home Care Services and HCPCS Codes for Care Plan Oversight**

Home care services

New patient	History	Exam	MDM	Time (minutes)
99341	PF	PF	SF	20
99342	ExPF	ExPF	LC	30
99343	D	D	MC	50
99344	Comp	Comp	MC	60
99345	Comp	Comp	HC	90

Note: patient 99345 is typically unstable and requires immediate physician attention.

Established patient	History	Exam	MDM	Time (minutes)
99347	PF	PF	SF	15
99348	ExPF	ExPF	LC	30
99349	D	D	MC	40
99350	Comp	Comp	MC-HC	72.5

Note: patient 99350 may be unstable and requires immediate physician attention.

Care plan oversight (CPO)

New HCPCS code	Former CPT code	Level of service
G0179	N/A	Recertification of home care
G0180	N/A	Certification of home care services
G0181	99375	>30 minutes (home health)
G0182	99378	>30 minutes (hospice)

CPT = current procedural terminology; MDM = medical decision making; PF = problem focused; ExPF = expanded problem focused; D = detailed; Comp = comprehensive; SF = straight forward; LC = low complexity; MC = moderate complexity; HC = high complexity; HCFA = Health Care Financing Administration; HCPCS = HCFA Common Procedure Coding System.

Source: Current Procedural Terminology (CPT) 2001,[10] with permission. See this document for full details and explanations of documentation requirements.

and more likely to be hospitalized or to die within the next year. However, family physicians should consider all age groups in their home care profile[2–5,16] (Table 54.2). Common home care diagnoses include hypertension, congestive heart failure, diabetes mellitus, chronic obstructive pulmonary disease, osteoarthritis, and cerebrovascular disease.[3,4] Home visits can be categorized as urgent/emergent, continuity/ongoing care, or consult/comprehensive assessment.[2,5,12] One must be proactive and schedule regular visits rather than simply react to acute needs.[1,5] Patient preference is a hallmark of family medicine, and many patients prefer the reassurance and comfort of a professional coming to the home.[7]

Table 54.2. **Potential Home Care Patients**

Elderly and infirm
Disabled—physically and mentally
Extreme difficulty traveling to the office
Hospice care/terminally ill
Patients receiving home health nursing
Management of chronic illness
Acute care to avoid emergency room visits
New baby/postpartum checkup
Patient, family, or teen in distress
Adolescents at risk (behavioral and medical)
Wound care and management
Comprehensive evaluation
　After hospital discharge
　Medication management
　Noncompliance
　Tenuous health status
　Excessive utilization of medical services
Safety evaluation
　Uncertain quality of caregiver
　Suspected child or elder abuse
　Suspected addiction/alcoholism

Source: Adapted from AAHCP,[5] with permission.

Home Health Care Team

The multidisciplinary approach to home care includes nurses, pharmacists, dietitians, home aides, physical, speech and occupational therapists, social workers, and mental health counselors.[2,5,12] It is essential to have a designated coordinator who can answer calls, establish visit schedules, plan routes, relay information between team members, and coordinate referrals.[5] Weekly or monthly meetings help facilitate communication and improve care.[5,7]

Benefits of Home Care

Home care provides distinct benefits to both patients and family physicians: improved quality of patient care, increased patient satisfaction, and increased personal satisfaction.[1,2,4,5,12,15] Other benefits include improved continuity, less money spent on transportation, increased support for family caregivers, prevention of falls, and treatment of depression.[1,2,5,7,12] However, outcomes data are either scarce or conflicting,[17] and there is a distinct need for studies measuring the benefits of home care.[7,17] Most physicians cite the lack of training as the primary barrier to increased home care; other barriers include poor

Table 54.3. **Black Bag for the 21st Century: Equipment and Supplies for the Family Physician's Home Care Bag**

Equipment
Patient's chart
Street map
Stethoscope
Sphygmomanometer—three sizes
Penlight
Handheld otoscope/ophthalmoscope
Tongue blades
Sterile cotton-tipped applicators
Ear speculums
Gloves
Lubricant
Hemoocult cards and developer
Tuning fork
Bandage scissors
Tape measure
Personal data assistant (Palm, Visor, etc.) or laptop computer
    with modem
Drug interaction program
Cellular telephone
Dictaphone
Prescription pads
Home health agency/referral numbers
Laboratory and radiology requisition forms
Home visit progress notes
Reflex hammer
Chart forms and surveys
Pulse oximeter
Peak flow meter
Blood glucose monitor
Scale

Sterilized supplies—multiple of each
Hemostats
Scissors
Forceps
Scalpel (#15, #11)
Syringes (3, 5, 10 cc)
Needles (18 G, 22 G, 27 G 1.5 in, 30 G 1.0 in)
Alcohol, Betadine wipes, and swabs
Suture removal kits

Dressings and supplies
Sterile gauze—multiple sizes
Nonstick dressings
Petrolatum gauze
Triple antibiotic ointment
Tape
Rapid Strep test kit
Culture swabs
Urine/specimen cup

reimbursement, perceptions of inefficiency, lack of time, and lack of technical support.[1,2,5–7,9,11,13,16] With a systematic approach and proper planning, these barriers are easily overcome.

The Home Care Visit

Equipment and Supplies

The family physician's "black bag" of the 21st century contains many basic tools that have not changed in 50 years[18]; however, several pieces of equipment are new. In 1950, Dr.

William Gordon described the physician's home care bag as "a container of equipment and medications which when combined with the knowledge of the physician gives relief to the suffering and often is the difference between life and death."[18] An extensive set of supplies may be included to assure the family physician greater preparedness (Table 54.3). Family physicians today must be cautious because of those seeking to steal narcotics and may choose to carry a less conspicuous case.

Small supplies of certain medicines may prove helpful in acute emergencies; however, these would only be used to stabilize a patient while awaiting the arrival of the home health or hospice team member with a more comprehensive formulary or while anticipating transport to an acute care facility.[18] Maps, chart forms, and evaluation tools such as the Geriatric Depression Scale (GDS),[19] Folstein mini-mental status exam (MMSE),[20] and measures of activities of daily living (ADL)[21] and instrumental ADLs[22] should also be included in the home care kit (see Chapters 23, 25, and 32). The family physician's black bag must be continuously reevaluated, adding or removing items as space and usefulness dictate.

Logistics

One can maximize productivity by clustering visits in geographic areas.[5,9,12] An employee, acting as both chauffeur and medical assistant, can draw blood, perform electrocardiograms (ECGs), and phone in prescriptions, leaving the physician free to make phone calls, coordinate care, and dictate notes en route to the next home.[2,5,9,12] Directions to the patient's home and telephone numbers for home health agencies and family contacts should be on the front of the chart.[2,5,12] A confirmatory telephone call helps to assure that key family members and support persons will be present.[2,5] Patient records are always confidential and should be locked in the trunk or somewhere out of sight.[5]

Comprehensive Assessment

There are many models available for comprehensive assessment in home care.[2,5,12] Unwin and Jerant[2] have adopted a mnemonic to guide them through each visit (Table 54.4). Others advocate using preprinted forms to direct the home visit, to document their assessment, and to assure accurate coding for billing purposes[2,5,12] (Figure 54.1). The observations and

Table 54.4. **The INHOMESSS Mnemonic: A Model for Home Care Assessments**

*I*mmobility
*N*utritional
*H*ome environment
*O*ther people
*M*edications
*E*xamination
*S*afety
*S*piritual
*S*ervices

Source: Unwin, BK, Jerant, AF. The home visit. Am Fam Physician 1999;60(5), with permission.

Home Visit Progress Note

Date: _____

Provider: _____

Patient's Name: _____

Insurance: changed Y N _____

Address: changed Y N _____

Primary home health contact:

Telephone number: changed Y N _____

Name: _____

Primary family caregiver/support: _____

Phone: _____

Address _____

Pager/Emergency: _____

Phone _____

Person requesting visit: _____

Reason for Visit: _____

Physical Exam: General:

HPI:

Height: _____ Weight: _____ BMI: _____

BP: _____ HR: _____ RR: _____ Temp: _____

HEENT:

LUNGS:

CV:

ABD:

PMSFHx: changes Y   N

GU/GI:

details:

EXT:

NEURO:

LYMPH:

SKIN:

ROS:

OTHER:

ADL/IADL	Home Environment	Medications	Support-frequency
Ambulation	Neighborhood	Chart updated Y N	Family visits
Assist device	Cleanliness (smells)	Pill box Y N	Friends
Supports/Rails	Phone (contact #s)	Who fills it?	Pastor
Falls	Furniture	Vitamins	HH nurse
Bathing	Bed		HH aide
Toileting	Kitchen	Herbals	Meals
Grooming	Food & nutrition		
Dressing	Bathroom	New meds?	Advance Directive
Feeding	Lighting & electric cords	Rx by whom?	
	Heating & A/C		
Finances	Rugs & Stairs	OTC meds	
Managed by whom?	Fire detection & suppression		
	Water: City, Well, Temp	Alcohol & drugs	

Assessment/Plan:

1.

2.

3.

4.

Problem List: updated Y N

Referrals:

Additional dictation: Y N

Billing/Coding: History _____   Exam _____   MDM _____   Time _____

New	99341	99342	99343	99344	99345
Established	99347	99348	99349	99350	

Signature: _____

Fig. 54.1. Sample progress note for home care visits.

---

information gleaned from home care begin on the street.[2,5,12] The proximity to the local pharmacy, grocery store, and other shopping is valuable information when assessing the home care patient. Great insight regarding ADLs and financial stability can come from comparing the patient's home to others in the neighborhood.[2,5]

Mailing an information packet in advance may increase efficiency, especially for the new patient visit. This packet should have chart forms for the patient and caregivers to complete that include demographics; past hospitalizations; medical, surgical, and family histories; medications with doses; and advance directive forms.[5] A complete review of this information puts the physician several steps ahead on arrival. Specific measures of function such as the GDS,[19] MMSE,[20] and ADLs[21,22] should be administered at the first visit and multiple times thereafter to assess the patient's level of stability and overall safety in the home. The best measure of patients' ADLs, however, is watching them perform these activities in the home.

Entering the patient's home is an act of humility that gives patients greater control over their care.[1] Witnessing family values, represented by memorabilia on the walls, and observing the patient–caregiver interactions add further insight into the patient's needs. When assessing nutritional status, nothing compares to a simple glance in the cupboards and refrigerator.[2,5] A thorough analysis of the patient's pill bottles and medicine cabinet is essential and often reveals inconsistent dosing habits and many herbal products not previously discussed. A drug interaction program on one's hand-held or laptop computer is invaluable. As the family physician's experience grows, surveying the home for hazards will become second nature. Performing the physical examination, whether on the sofa or at the patient's bedside, is comforting, therapeutic, and shows respect for the individual.[1] The family physician should review the patient's overall management plan and coordinate with the home health agency and other service providers at each visit. A methodical approach to each visit ensures quality and improves patient care skills.

Documentation and Billing

Effective documentation and coding ensures timely reimbursement and provides medical-legal protection.[5,9,11] In a 1992 study, physicians making many home health referrals spent over 4.5 additional hours per week on the phone and on paperwork managing their home care patients.[23] Using the care plan oversight CPT codes (Table 54.1) to bill for this time helps the home care physician remain financially stable.[11] Preprinted forms (Fig. 54.1) also provide an easy tracking system for quality improvement, a necessary component of all practices.[2,5,11,12]

Ancillary Services

No longer is the home isolated from the realm of modern medical technologies. Home services now include intravenous therapy, ECG monitoring, home oxygen, laboratory services, diagnostic radiography, echocardiography, and more.[5,9,12] However, these broad services have limited availability in the rural areas where home care is more commonly practiced.[4,14] The home care physician must also coordinate community-based resources such as meals on wheels providers, adult daycare programs, and religious support groups. As times have changed, physicians rely more heavily on technologic advances and have turned away from the home as a primary venue for meaningful care.[1,16] Despite these technologic advances, most home care is still conventional clinical medicine and nursing.[1] A practice that has internal organization and efficiency will promote itself and allow the physician more time to care for patients in the home.[5,9,12]

Integrating Home Care into the Practice

Financial Considerations

A practice that includes home visits "demands meticulous care, accurate documentation, and frequent review of records."[11] The first step is to develop a business plan and to examine the local medical culture with specific attention to potential referral base and overall payer mix.[5,9] When choosing home care alone, one may need to join an existing home care agency or seek funding support from a hospital or charitable foundation.[5,9] When adding home care to an existing office practice, one must define a scope of practice and set specific limits with regard to the number of visits per day, geographic coverage area, availability for urgent care, and maintaining continuity within the office.[2,5,11,12] It is advisable that family physicians start with 1 or 2 half-days per month dedicated to home care. As the volume of home care grows, so will the demands on support staff. Higher complexity of visits and increased coding levels make home care more financially successful.[2,5,9] However, the volume and acuity of the visits must be sufficient to absorb increased overhead costs.[5,9]

Support Agencies and Organizations

Many nationwide organizations can support the family physician who is embarking on the path of home care visits. The American Academy of Home Care Physicians is an excellent resource and has links to other organizations through *www.aahcp.org*.[24] Most major metropolitan areas have several practices that are dedicated to home care alone.

Implications for Training

The single most common barrier to the expansion of home care is lack of training. Of the 130 U.S. and Canadian medical schools, only 15% offer lectures in home care, and only 22% require at least one home visit in the clinical training years.[25] A study of residency training programs found only 68% offering any teaching in home care with only 25% requiring home visits.[26] Adequate and supportive training is one the greatest determinants of physicians choosing to practice in the home.[1,14,15]

The Future of Home Care by Family Physicians

The changes and challenges of medical care in the 21st century will surely be extreme. One way that family physicians can maintain their firm grasp of patient-centered care is to return to the home. Continuity of care, understanding family dynamics, cultivating family relationships, emphasizing quality of life, and responding to patient preferences are all pillars upon which family medicine is built. Providing home care responds to patient's needs in all of these areas. Typically reserved for frail and infirm elderly patients, home care can be an exciting and rewarding adjunct to obstetrical, pediatric, and adolescent care as well. Home care improves patient satisfaction, builds strong relationships and offers personal rewards to the physicians who practice it. Family physicians should strongly consider home care as a valuable addition to their practices.

References

1. McWhinney IR. The doctor, the patient, and the home: returning to our roots. J Am Board Fam Pract 1997;10:430–5.
2. Unwin BK, Jerant AF. The home visit. Am Fam Physician 1999; 60:1481–8.
3. Aylin P, Majeed AF, Cook DG. Home visiting by general practitioners in England and Wales. BMJ 1996;313:207–10.
4. Meyer GS, Gibbons RV. House calls to the elderly—a vanishing practice among physicians. N Engl J Med 1997;337: 1815–20.
5. American Academy of Home Care Physicians (AAHCP). Making house calls a part of your practice. Edgewood, MD: AAHCP, 2000;39.
6. Welch HG, Wennberg DE, Welch WP. The use of Medicare home health care services. N Engl J Med 1996;335:324–9.
7. Campion EW. New hope for home care? [editorial]. N Engl J Med 1995;333:1213–4.
8. Freid TR, van Doorn C, O'Leary JR, Tinetti ME, Drickamer MA. Older persons' preferences for home vs hospital care in the treatment of acute illness. Arch Intern Med 2000;160:1501–6.
9. Preston SH. The bottom-line case for making house calls. Med Econ 2000;77(4):114–21.
10. Current Procedural Terminology (CPT) 2001, standard edition. Chicago: American Medical Association, 2000;23–24,26–27.
11. American Academy of Home Care Physicians. Making home care work in your practice. Edgewood, MD: American Academy of Home Care Physicians, 2001;1–18.
12. Giovino JM. House calls: taking the practice to the patient. Fam Pract Manag 2000;7:49–54.
13. Keenan JM, Boling PA, Schwartzberg JG, et al. A national survey of the home visiting practice and attitudes of family physicians and internists. Arch Intern Med 1992;152:2025–32.
14. Boling PA, Retchin SM, Ellis J, Pancoast SA. Factors associated with the frequency of house calls by primary care physicians. J Gen Intern Med 1991;6:335–40.
15. Adelman AM, Fredman L, Knight AL. House call practices: a comparison by specialty. J Fam Pract 1994;39:39–44.
16. Saultz JW. Continuity of care. In: Saultz JW, ed. Textbook of family medicine. New York: McGraw-Hill, 2000;62–3.
17. Masters PA. Review: evidence is unclear that preventive home visits for elderly persons in the community improve mortality or health outcomes. ACP J Club 2000;133:59.
18. Taylor RB. AFP 50 years ago: the doctor's bag—what should be in it [commentary]. Am Fam Physician 1999;61:2323–6.
19. Yesavage JA, Brink TL, Rose TL, et al. Development and validation of a geriatric depression screening scale: a preliminary report. J Psychiatr Res 1982–83;17:37–49.
20. Folstein MF, Folstein SE, McHugh PR. Mini-mental state: a practical method for grading the cognitive state of patients for the clinician. J Psychiatr Res 1975;12:186–98.
21. Katz S, Downs TD, Cash HR, Grotz RC. Progress in development of the index of ADLs. Gerontologist 1970;10:20–30.
22. Lawton MP, Brody EM. Assessment of older people: self-maintaining and instrumental activities of daily living. Gerontologist 1969;9:179–86.
23. Boling PA, Keenan JM, Swartzberg J, Retchin SM, Olson L, Schneiderman M. Reported home health agency referrals by internists and family physicians. J Am Geriatr Soc 1992;40: 1241–9.
24. Links to home care web pages, American Academy of Home Care Physicians, 2001. Available at *www.aahcp.org*.
25. Knight SR, Musliner M, Boling PA. Medical schools and home care [correspondence]. N Engl J Med 1994;331:1098–9.
26. Stoltz CM, Smith LG, Boal JH. Home care training in internal medicine residencies: a national survey. Acad Med 2001;76: 181–3.

55
Care of the Patient with Fatigue

John Saultz

Everyone experiences fatigue periodically as a result of hard physical labor or loss of sleep. Fatigue, loss of energy, and lassitude are also common symptoms experienced by patients with any of a large number of diseases. A patient who complains of fatigue presents a difficult problem for the family physician because there are many possible explanations for it. The subjective nature of the complaint and the potential seriousness of some of the diseases in the differential diagnosis compound this difficulty.

Background

Fatigue is common in the general population and is present in at least 20% of the patients who visit a family physician.[1–4] Community-based surveys indicate that as many as 50% of the population report fatigue if asked.[2,3] In the United States, fatigue is responsible for at least 10 million office visits and up to $300 million in health costs each year.[5] Valdini and colleagues[6] determined that 58% of family practice patients with a chief complaint of fatigue were still fatigued 1 year after the initial visit. But, in the absence of identifiable underlying organic diseases, 19 studies examining the prognosis of chronic fatigue found only three deaths among 2075 patients.[7] Chronic fatigue lasting over 6 months has a population prevalence of 1775/100,000 to 6321/100,000.[1] Fatigue consistently ranks among the most common presenting complaints to family physicians regardless of practice setting or culture. A systematic, organized, efficient evaluation of these patients represents an essential skill for all family physicians.

Although fatigue is common and often persistent, many chronically fatigued patients defy diagnostic categorization. For centuries physicians have been perplexed by the diagnostic difficulties inherent in evaluating patients with chronic fatigue. Clinical syndromes have been defined to explain chronic fatigue including terms such as febricula, neurasthe-

nia, nervous exhaustion, Da Costa syndrome, chronic brucellosis, hypoglycemia, total allergy syndrome, chronic candidiasis, and chronic Epstein-Barr virus infection.[8] In 1987 the United States Centers for Disease Control (CDC) established a clinical definition for the chronic fatigue syndrome (CFS).[9] It was hoped that such categorization would facilitate clinical investigation of the causes and most successful treatments for this problem. But the case definition did not clearly identify a clinically useful subset of chronically fatigued patients, and the definition was revised in 1994.[10] This chapter reviews a contextual, biopsychosocial differential diagnosis of fatigue and outlines a practical approach to evaluating and helping patients who complain of fatigue

Clinical Presentation

What are the characteristics of patients who complain of fatigue to the family physician? There is a bimodal distribution of patient age, with a peak between the ages of 15 and 24 and a second peak at 60-plus years. Women complain of fatigue to the physician at least twice as often as men.[3–6,9,11,12] This excess may be explained by a higher incidence of fatigue in women, that women are more likely to tell the physician about fatigue, or that physicians are more sensitive to the ways in which women complain about fatigue. Fatigued patients tend to score lower than nonfatigued patients on tests that measure physical activity. They also score significantly higher than control patients on standardized instruments measuring anxiety and depression, and have a higher lifetime likelihood of being diagnosed with these disorders.[5,13,14]

It is useful to consider the clinical presentation of fatigue in different contexts depending on how the patient describes the problem. Some patients experience fatigue as part of a larger symptom complex in which the fatigue is identified only on detailed history or review of systems by the physician. Other patients present with a chief complaint of fatigue. A third group of patients presents to the physician specifically with questions about CFS. Patients rarely report acute fatigue to the physician when they have an understanding of why the fatigue is present. For example, a patient who is experiencing a common viral illness usually expects fatigue to be part of the symptom complex and is less likely to be concerned enough to complain about fatigue to the physician. Such patients would not present to the family physician complaining of fatigue but would admit to fatigue on a review of systems. Thus fatigue is a secondary symptom to these patients.

Most studies that have addressed fatigue in family practice have examined only those patients in whom fatigue was the chief or primary complaint. Such a complaint generally causes the physician to consider a long differential diagnosis of diseases that may cause fatigue as a primary symptom. In this clinical situation, the ability to address a broad differential diagnosis in a cost-efficient manner is essential. CFS has received substantial publicity in the lay press. For this reason, a number of patients present to the family physician with questions about this disorder. It is important for the family physician to understand the diagnostic criteria of CFS and to be familiar with the latest research in this area.

Diagnosis

Few patient problems illustrate the inadequacies of the biomedical model of diagnosis more clearly than does fatigue. A diagnostic model that examines the patient's complaint and attempts to determine its cause and then apply a treatment regimen to that cause is called an "epidemiologic model." The traditional biomedical model of diagnosis is largely an epidemiologic model. A contextual model of diagnosis, instead of attempting to identify cause, attempts to identify associated symptoms and factors that make the patient's complaint easier to understand and manage.[15] Contextual diagnosis can include a biomedical approach to the patient but necessarily also includes family, community, and sociocultural considerations. What follows is a contextual approach to diagnosis when a patient complains of fatigue as a secondary concern or chief complaint, or has concerns about CFS.

Fatigue as a Secondary Symptom

Many of the most common problems seen by family physicians are problems associated with fatigue. Chronic medical conditions such as diabetes, commonly prescribed medications such as antihypertensives, acute illnesses such as viral hepatitis, physiologic changes such as pregnancy, and stressful life situations such as divorce may be associated with fatigue. In these situations, fatigue often is identified as a secondary symptom and, from a diagnostic point of view, may be relatively unimportant. From a contextual point of view, however, the family physician is interested in the degree to which the patient's fatigue is interfering with job performance, family relationships, physical activity, or sexual activity. The contextual approach requires the physician to be as interested in the effects of symptoms as in their cause. Thus when fatigue is a secondary symptom, its importance may rest with its effect on the patient's lifestyle and coping skills for the underlying illness.

Fatigue as a Presenting Complaint

Few clinical situations more fully exercise the skills of a family physician than the patient who presents with a chief complaint of unexplained fatigue. Table 55.1 lists some of the medical and psychosocial problems associated with a chief complaint of fatigue. Evaluation of such a patient begins with a careful, comprehensive medical history, which includes a detailed psychosocial history including symptoms of depression, sleep disorders, anxiety disorders, substance abuse, and the marital and sexual experience.

The most common causes of fatigue as a presenting complaint to a family physician are depression, life stress, chronic medical illnesses, and medication reactions. The history must also include information about the other symptoms of such illnesses as those listed in Table 55.1.

The complete medical history is followed by a careful physical examination. Areas of particular importance on the physical examination are the thyroid gland, cardiovascular system, rectum, pelvis, and mental status (for associated signs of depression or anxiety disorders).

Table 55.1. **Diagnoses Associated with Fatigue**

Infectious diseases	Vascular disorders
Viral syndromes	Atherosclerotic heart disease
Mononucleosis	Valvular heart disease
Hepatitis	Congestive heart failure
Pharyngitis	Cardiomyopathy
Endocarditis	Congenital heart disorders
Urinary tract infections	
HIV infection	**Pulmonary conditions**
Tuberculosis	Asthma/COPD
	Allergic disorders
Toxins and drug effects	Restrictive lung diseases
Medication side effects	
Alcohol and drug abuse	**Miscellaneous conditions**
Chronic poisoning	Anemia
	Pregnancy
Endocrine and metabolic	Systemic lupus erythematosus
problems	Iron deficiency
Electrolyte disturbance	Renal failure
Hypothyroidism	Chronic liver disease
Hypoglycemia	Multiple sclerosis
Diabetes	Sleep disorders including sleep
Hyperthyroidism	apnea
Starvation or dieting	
Obesity	**Psychosocial problems**
Adrenal insufficiency	Depression
	Anxiety disorders
Neoplastic conditions	Adjustment reaction
Occult malignancy	Situational life stress
Leukemia and lymphoma	Alcohol and drug abuse
Carcinoma of the colon	Sexual dysfunction
	Spouse abuse, child abuse, or
	other family violence
	Occupational stress and professional burnout syndrome

HIV = human immunodeficiency virus; COPD = chronic obstructive pulmonary disease.

Laboratory evaluation of the patient who presents with chronic fatigue, though important to consider, is unlikely to be helpful in most cases. Sugarman and Berg[16] found that laboratory testing was helpful in securing a diagnosis in only nine of 118 fatigued patients in a university family practice clinic. An appropriate laboratory evaluation is directed by the history and physical examination. For most patients, testing includes a complete blood count, a serum chemistry profile, an erythrocyte sedimentation rate (as a screen for inflammatory disorders), and thyroid-stimulating hormone level (as a screen for hypothyroidism). Other laboratory tests, including a chest radiograph, electrocardiogram, urinalysis, and tuberculin skin testing, may be indicated, depending on the results of the history and physical examination.

Patients without a readily apparent explanation for their fatigue should also be evaluated with a careful family assessment. Such an assessment may include convening a family meeting, preparing a family genogram, or using other family assessment instruments. An assessment of the occupational history, living environment, and social and financial circumstances should also be included in the complete evaluation of patients with fatigue.

Chronic Fatigue Syndrome

The CDC's definition of CFS is outlined in Table 55.2.[10] The purpose of establishing these diagnostic criteria was to identify a subgroup of fatigued patients to direct future research studies. Research projects have since focused on learning more about patients who meet these criteria. Because of obvious similarities to infectious mononucleosis, a number of studies have searched for an association with viral infections. Although these investigations continue, there is no good evidence to link CFS and viral infections.[17–20] Other research has examined the immune function of patients with CFS. Although measurable immune abnormalities have been associated with CFS, no consistent pattern has been delineated from

Table 55.2. **Case Definition: Chronic Fatigue Syndrome and Idiopathic Chronic Fatigue**

Prolonged fatigue is self-reported, persistent fatigue lasting 1 month or longer. Chronic fatigue is self-reported persistent or relapsing fatigue lasting 6 or more consecutive months.

A case of *chronic fatigue syndrome* is defined as chronic fatigue that is not explained by medical conditions that adequately explain the fatigue (see below) with the presence of the following:

1. clinically evaluated, unexplained, persistent or relapsing chronic fatigue that is of new or definite onset, is not the result of ongoing exertion, is not substantially relieved by rest, and results in substantial reduction in previous levels of occupational, educational, social, or personal activities; and
2. the concurrent occurrence of four or more of the following symptoms, all of which must have persisted or recurred during 6 or more consecutive months and must not have predated the fatigue:
    self-reported impairment in short-term memory or concentration severe enough to cause substantial reduction in previous levels of occupational, educational, social, or personal activities
    sore throat
    tender cervical or axillary lymph nodes
    muscle pain
    multijoint pain without joint swelling or redness
    headaches of a new type, pattern, or severity
    unrefreshing sleep
    postexertional malaise lasting more than 24 hours

A case of *idiopathic chronic fatigue* is defined as clinically evaluated, unexplained chronic fatigue that fails to meet the criteria for chronic fatigue syndrome.

The following conditions exclude the patient from being classified as unexplained chronic fatigue:

Any active medical condition that may explain chronic fatigue including medication side effects
Any previously diagnosed medical condition whose resolution has not been documented beyond a reasonable doubt and whose continued activity may explain chronic fatigue
Any past or current diagnosis of a major depressive disorder with psychotic or melancholic features, bipolar affective disorder, schizophrenia of any subtype, delusional disorders of any subtype, dementias of any subtype, or bulimia nervosa
Alcohol or substance abuse within 2 years before the onset of chronic fatigue or at any time afterward
Severe obesity defined as a body mass index equal to or greater than 45

The following conditions do not exclude the patient from being classified as unexplained chronic fatigue:

Any condition defined primarily by symptoms that cannot be confirmed by diagnostic laboratory tests, including fibromyalgia, anxiety disorders, somatoform disorders, nonpsychotic or nonmelancholic depression, neurasthenia, and multiple chemical sensitivity disorder
Any condition under specific treatment sufficient to alleviate all symptoms related to that condition and for which the adequacy of treatment has been documented
Any condition, such as Lyme disease or syphilis, that was treated with definitive therapy before development of symptomatic sequelae
Any isolated and explained physical examination finding or laboratory or imagining test abnormality that is insufficient to strongly suggest the existence of an exclusionary condition

study to study.[17,19,20] Another area of ongoing research has been an attempt to associate connective tissue and autoimmune diseases with CFS. Only a few patients have abnormal autoantibodies, and no association with autoimmune diseases has been clearly established.[21] More recent studies have examined the hypothesis that abnormalities of the central nervous system or changes in the regulation of the hypothalamic-pituitary-adrenal axis might explain chronic fatigue. At this time, evidence of a clinically useful association is inconclusive.[18,19,22,23] Finally, studies have examined the relationship between chronic fatigue and psychiatric disorders. These studies suggest that depression alone is insufficient to explain most cases of chronic or persistent fatigue.[19,22] Several recent studies have raised questions about the degree of diagnostic overlap between chronic fatigue and other conditions such as fibromyalgia and irritable bowel syndrome. Clinically important fatigue is present in over 75% of patients with fibromyalgia and many patients with chronic fatigue have demonstrable trigger points on musculoskeletal exam. Some authors suggest that the family of functional somatic syndromes may in fact be different manifestations of the same process.[24–26] It now seems clear that patients with CFS are not a homogeneous group and are not different from other patients with chronic fatigue in most respects.

It is also clear that chronic fatigue is much more common than CFS. Fewer than 5% of patients who present with chronic fatigue to a family physician ultimately fulfill the diagnostic criteria for CFS.[1,11] Patients who present to the family physician concerned about CFS represent a complex challenge. Some patients are simply looking for information, a need that can be met by discussing questions and providing educational resources. Many patients who are concerned about CFS do not satisfy the criteria listed in Table 55.2 sufficiently to qualify for this diagnosis. These patients require a contextual diagnostic approach from the physician.

Evaluation of the chronic fatigue patient should begin with a comprehensive history and physical examination. Most patients have previously seen other physicians for this problem, and copies of previous medical records from these physicians should be obtained. At the initial visit it is imperative that the physician discuss in detail the way in which chronic fatigue has affected and changed the patient's life. A careful family assessment should be completed, including convening the family whenever possible. Although chronic fatigue patients have a high prevalence of depression, anxiety disorders, somatization disorders, and family dysfunction, patients may not be receptive to discussing psychosocial issues early in the process of caring for this problem. Because biomedical evaluation is unlikely to yield a definitive diagnosis, a complete biopsychosocial evaluation beginning at the initial visit is crucial. Patients should be seen frequently, and the laboratory evaluation should include those studies described above for the patient with a chief complaint of chronic fatigue. At the present time there is little justification for extensive immunologic or autoimmune diagnostic testing. Focused laboratory tests should be ordered when indicated from the history and physical examination.

Management

In an epidemiologic model, management of the problem begins after the correct diagnosis has been determined. With a contextual approach, management begins at the time of initial contact between the patient and physician. Caring for patients with a primary complaint of fatigue requires a contextual approach, which means that the physician's diagnostic inquiry must include the broadest possible scope. The physician begins at the initial visit to assist the patient in delineating ways to cope with the symptoms more effectively. What follows are the basic principles of a systemic management plan for a patient with a primary complaint of chronic fatigue.

1. The physician must be as interested and concerned about the effects of the patient's fatigue as about its cause. Delineating the effects of the symptom on the patient's life is an important step in understanding the symptom and managing the problem.
2. The physician should explain to the patient at the initial visit that the most common causes of fatigue as a presenting complaint are depression and psychosocial problems. The physician should ascertain what this information means to the patient and whether the patient thinks that psychosocial issues may play a role in the fatigue.
3. The physician should discuss the other common causes of fatigue with the patient at the initial visit and ask the patient to think about these possibilities between the initial and first follow-up visit. At the first follow-up visit the physician can then inquire as to whether the patient has had an opportunity to consider possible explanations for the fatigue and if there is new insight into the problem.
4. The physician should continue to return to the discussion of family, occupational, psychosexual, and substance abuse issues at each of the follow-up visits. This can take place while a detailed biomedical evaluation of the patient's symptoms is progressing. Even if fatigue is being caused by a physical disorder, there are important effects on family and job.
5. The physician can consider convening the family to explore the attitudes and ideas of other family members. This point is especially important if the patient has a spouse or significant other.
6. The physician should be able to discuss professional burnout, career dissatisfaction, and other issues that are outside the usual biomedical model of thinking about patient problems. It may be helpful to provide patients with copies of articles about fatigue. Some studies suggest that cognitive-behavioral therapy may be beneficial for patients with chronic fatigue.[27]
7. If the physician believes that a psychosocial problem is of primary importance to the patient's condition but the patient is unwilling to accept this explanation, the biomedical workup should be paced slowly and scheduled across several follow-up visits. This will allow the doctor–patient rapport to deepen and discussions about psychosocial concerns to continue.

8. The physician should refer the patient to a consultant only for a well-specified purpose. It is essential to communicate with consultants in advance and to avoid using consultants who lack sophistication about psychosocial issues.

9. Prolonged rest is more likely to harm than help patients with chronic fatigue. A gradual program of activity has resulted in improved functional status in some studies.

10. Tricyclic or selective serotonin reuptake inhibitor antidepressants may benefit some patients, particularly those with disturbed sleep patterns. When used, these medications should be started in low doses and their therapeutic effect should be carefully monitored.[28,29]

Summary

Acute fatigue may be a presenting complaint for a large number of important diseases. Fatigue has a large biomedical differential diagnosis and requires a broad contextual approach to optimize diagnosis and management. Although few presenting complaints are more challenging, few patient problems more urgently require the broad contextual diagnostic approach that can best be provided by the family physician.

References

1. Buchwald D, Umali P, Umali J, Kith P, Pearlman T, Komaroff AL. Chronic fatigue and the chronic fatigue syndrome: prevalence in a Pacific Northwest health care system. Ann Intern Med 1995;123:81–8.
2. Kroenke K, Wood DR, Mangelsdorff D, Meier NJ, Powell JB. Chronic fatigue in primary care. JAMA 1988;260:929–34.
3. Pawlikowska T, Chalder T, Hirsch SR, et al. Population based study of fatigue and psychological distress. BMJ 1994;308: 763–6.
4. Shahar E, Lederer J. Asthenic symptoms in a rural family practice. J Fam Pract 1990;31:257–62.
5. Kirk J, Douglass R, Nelson E, et al. Chief complaint of fatigue: a prospective study. J Fam Pract 1990;30:33–41.
6. Valdini AF, Steinhardt S, Valicenti J, Jaffe A. A one-year follow-up of fatigued patients. J Fam Pract 1988;26:33–8.
7. Joyce J, Hotopf M, Wessely S. The prognosis of chronic fatigue and chronic fatigue syndrome: a systematic review. Q J Med 1997;90:223–33.
8. Straus SE. History of chronic fatigue syndrome. Rev Infect Dis 1991;13(suppl 1):S2–S7.
9. Holmes GP, Kaplan JE, Gantz NM, et al. Chronic fatigue syndrome: a working case definition. Ann Intern Med 1988;108: 387–9.
10. Fukuda K, Straus SE, Hickie I, Sharpe M, Dobbins JG, Komaroff AL. The chronic fatigue syndrome: a comprehensive approach to its definition and study. Ann Intern Med 1994;121: 953–9.
11. Manu F, Lane TJ, Matthews DA. The frequency of the chronic fatigue syndrome in patients with symptoms of persistent fatigue. Ann Intern Med 1988;109:554–6.
12. Morrison JD. Fatigue as a presenting complaint in family practice. J Fam Pract 1980;10:795–801.
13. Cathebras PJ, Robbins JM, Kirmayer LJ, Hayton BC. Fatigue in primary care: prevalence, psychiatric comorbidity, illness behavior, and outcome. J Gen Intern Med 1992;7:276–86.
14. Kroenke K, Spitzer RL, Williams JB, et al. Physical symptoms in primary care. Predictors of psychiatric disorders and functional impairment. Arch Fam Med 1994;3:774–9.
15. Saultz JW. Contextual care. In: Saultz JW, ed. Textbook of family medicine. New York: McGraw-Hill, 2000;135–59.
16. Sugarman JR, Berg AD. Evaluation of fatigue in a family practice. J Fam Pract 1984;19:643–7.
17. Glaser R, Kiecolt-Glaser JK. Stress-associated immune modulation: relevance to viral infections and chronic fatigue syndrome. Am J Med 1998;105:35S–42S.
18. Johnson SK, DeLuca J, Natelson BH. Chronic fatigue syndrome: reviewing the research findings. Ann Behav Med 1999;21: 258–71.
19. Komaroff AL, Buchwald DS. Chronic fatigue syndrome: an update. Annu Rev Med 1998;49:1–13.
20. Mawle AC. Chronic fatigue syndrome. Immunol Invest 1997; 26:269–73.
21. Buchwald DS, Komaroff AL. Review of laboratory findings for patients with chronic fatigue syndrome. Rev Infect Dis 1991;13(suppl 1):S12–S18.
22. Demitrack MA. Chronic fatigue syndrome and fibromyalgia. Dilemmas in diagnosis and clinical management. Psychiatr Clin North Am 1998;21:671–92.
23. Demitrack MA, Crofford LJ. Evidence for and pathophysiologic implications of hypothalamic-pituitary-adrenal axis dysregulation in fibromyalgia and chronic fatigue syndrome. Ann NY Acad Sci 1998;840:684–97.
24. Bennet R. Fibromyalgia, chronic fatigue syndrome, and myofascial pain. Curr Opin Rheumatol 1998;10:95–103.
25. Goldenberg DL. Fibromyalgia, chronic fatigue syndrome, and myofascial pain syndrome. Curr Opin Rheumatol 1997;9: 135–43.
26. Wessely S, Nimnuan C, Sharpe M. Functional somatic syndromes: one or many? Lancet 1999;354:936–9.
27. Butler S, Chalder T, Ron M, Wessely S. Cognitive behaviour therapy in chronic fatigue syndrome. J Neurol Neurosurg Psychiatry 1991;54:153–8.
28. Brunello N, Akiskal H, Boyer P, et al. Dysthymia: clinical picture, extent of overlap with chronic fatigue syndrome, neuropharmacological considerations, and new therapeutic vistas. J Affect Disord 1999;52:275–90.
29. O'Malley PG, Jackson JL, Santoro J, Tomkins G, Balden E, Kroenke K. Antidepressant therapy for unexplained symptoms and symptom syndromes. J Fam Pract 1999;48:980–90.

56
Care of the Patient with a Sleep Disorder

Thomas A. Johnson, Jr. and James J. Deckert

Sleep is a periodically recurring physiologic state of lessened responsiveness from which one can be readily awakened. The quality and quantity of sleep vary with age. Newborns sleep an average of 16 hours each day in randomly fragmented fashion. As an individual matures, sleep usually coalesces into a single prolonged nighttime period, with an average length of 7 to 8 hours in adults. A few individuals function well with as little as 4 hours per day, whereas others require 10 hours or more.

Sleep architecture also evolves with age. Slow wave sleep (SWS), the stage of deepest sleep, is maximal in young children and decreases gradually through midlife.[1] Older adults often take longer to fall asleep, take daytime naps, and experience more frequent awakenings. A wide variety of disorders can interfere with normal sleep patterns.

Insomnia

Insomnia can be clinically defined as any difficulty falling or staying asleep that results in impaired daytime functioning. Inadequate sleep can result in fatigue, decreased concentration, and irritability. Insomnia can be classified as acute or chronic.

Acute insomnia is difficulty sleeping that lasts 1 month or less. The cause is generally some situational stress readily identified or even anticipated by the patient. Examinations, funerals, vacations, and illnesses are examples of stresses that frequently precipitate acute insomnia. Patients often tolerate this brief disruption without bringing it to the attention of their physician.

In contrast, chronic insomnia is a significant health problem, often frustrating to patients and their physicians. The etiology is often multifactorial. Underlying causes cover a spectrum of behavioral, psychiatric, and medical disorders (Table 56.1). It is essential that the physician clarify, as much as possible, the cause of insomnia before attempting treatment.

Evaluation

Patients often seek physician advice regarding insomnia. However, more than half of patients with concerns about sleep fail to discuss the problem with their doctor.[2] Incorporating a brief sleep history into the review of systems is helpful in detecting these individuals. If the history is consistent with chronic insomnia, the following areas need to be explored.

Drugs

A review of the patient's drug use is essential. Alcohol, often self-prescribed to induce sleep, can produce abnormal sleep architecture and early awakening. Caffeine has a long half-life (8–14 hours) and can interfere with sleep onset long after consumption. Nicotine, through smoking or administered as a drug, can produce enough arousal to interfere with sleep initiation. A variety of over-the-counter and prescription drugs can cause insomnia (Table 56.1). If discontinuation of the offending medication is not feasible, a change in the timing of administration may be helpful.

Psychiatric Disorders

Psychiatric disorders, particularly depression and anxiety, are common causes of sleep disturbance. Screening questions for these disorders can generally uncover the diagnosis. Referral to a psychiatrist is sometimes appropriate if more severe psychiatric disorder, such as schizophrenia, is suspected.

Medical Disorders

A variety of medical problems can cause insomnia (Table 56.1). Occult medical problems are a particularly common etiology of sleep disruption in the elderly. A complete history, physical exam, and appropriate laboratory testing should be conducted to rule out suspected medical causes.

Primary Sleep Disorders

Poor sleep hygiene frequently contributes to insomnia, but it is seldom the sole cause. The rules of good sleep hygiene are

Table 56.1. **Causes of Insomnia**

Drug-induced insomnia
Nonprescription: alcohol, decongestants, caffeine, nicotine (smoking)
Prescription: amphetamines, stimulating tricyclics, thyroid hormones, β-agonists, aminophyllines, beta-blockers, steroids,
    diuretics, sedatives (withdrawal), serotonin reuptake inhbitors, oral contraceptives

Psychiatric disease
Affective disorders: depression, bipolar disorder, dysthymic disorders
Anxiety disorders: generalized anxiety disorders, panic disorder, posttraumatic stress
Schizophrenia

Medical problems
Gastrointestinal: reflux esophagitis, peptic ulcer disease, inflammatory bowel disease
Cardiac: angina, paroxysmal nocturnal dyspnea
Genitourinary: pregnancy, urinary tract infection, benign prostatic hypertrophy, uremia
Respiratory: chronic obstructive pulmonary disease, asthma
Endocrine: hyperthyroidism, diabetes, Cushing syndrome, Addison syndrome, menopause
Skin: pruritus
Central nervous system: dementia, delirium, seizure disorder
Musculoskeletal: arthritis, fibromyalgia
Pain from any source

Primary sleep disorders
Poor sleep hygiene
Primary insomnia
Circadian rhythm disturbance
Sleep apnea
Periodic limb movements and restless legs syndrome

listed in Table 56.2. Patients can initially be evaluated by history, but a more accurate assessment is obtained by utilizing a sleep diary to record details of the sleep pattern over a period of 1 to 2 weeks.

Circadian rhythm disturbance is also common. Patients whose jobs require shift work or excessive plane travel are often unable to fall asleep on schedule. These individuals should be questioned regarding drug use, as they often aggravate their sleep disturbance by excessive use of caffeine, nicotine, alcohol, and sedatives. Another type of circadian rhythm disturbance is delayed sleep-phase syndrome. This syndrome consists of early night insomnia with chronically late bedtimes and arising times. Delayed sleep-phase syndrome is particularly common in adolescents. In contrast, older individuals often complain of early morning waking with a tendency to fall asleep too early in the evening. This is designated advanced sleep-phase syndrome. Jet lag, perhaps the most common circadian rhythm disturbance, is discussed in Chapter 9.

Table 56.2. **Rules of Good Sleep Hygiene**

Maintain regular bedtime and time of arising.
Avoid naps.
Exercise regularly, but avoid exercise just prior to bedtime.
Control sleep environment to avoid temperature extremes and
    excessive noise.
Provide for a wind-down time of at least 30 minutes of non-
    stressful activities prior to bedtime.
Reserve the bedroom for sleep and sexual activity only,
    eliminating stimulating activities such as watching
    television, reading, paying bills, making phone calls.
Go to bed only when ready for sleep and leave if unable to
    sleep after 30 minutes.

Finally, primary insomnia is the diagnosis of exclusion and should be reserved for patients in whom known secondary causes have been ruled out or treated.

Treatment

The easiest, most effective treatment for insomnia is specific to an identified cause. A change in drug use or treatment of an underlying psychiatric/medical disorder often results in a dramatic improvement in sleep pattern. Nonspecific treatment for primary insomnia is generally less effective.

Nonpharmacologic Measures

A number of nonpharmacologic interventions have been found helpful in treating insomnia. These interventions include sleep hygiene education, cognitive therapy, sleep restriction, relaxation techniques, and light therapy.

Sleep Hygiene Education. Education regarding the rules of good sleep hygiene (Table 56.2) is helpful for most patients with insomnia. A sleep diary is valuable for identifying needed improvements and monitoring progress. The physician can help the patient select changes and can provide follow-up to encourage compliance.

Cognitive-Behavioral Therapy. Cognitive-behavioral therapy is a training program designed to correct misconceptions about sleep that may be adversely affecting a patient's sleep pattern. In some individuals, for example, concerns about amount of sleep needed or exaggerated fears about the effect of insomnia may generate excessive anxiety. This anxiety, in turn, interferes with their ability to initiate and maintain sleep. The goal of therapy is to diminish the anxiety surrounding sleep by changing the patient's understanding and attitude about the problem.[3]

Sleep Restriction Therapy. Sleep restriction therapy is a technique used to improve sleep efficiency. This approach is most useful for patients who spend an excessive amount of sleepless time in bed. Patients are instructed to limit the amount of time they spend in bed to the average amount of time they actually spend sleeping based on their sleep diary. Initially this practice results in some degree of sleep deprivation, but it helps to consolidate the sleep pattern. The patient is then instructed to gradually increase time in bed while maintaining sleep efficiency at more than 85% (i.e., more than 85% of time in bed is spent sleeping).

Relaxation Techniques. A wide variety of relaxation techniques may be useful for treating insomnia. Common approaches include progressive muscle relaxation, abdominal breathing, meditation, self-hypnosis, biofeedback, and imagery. All of these techniques are about equally effective, so choice is based on the therapist's experience and patient preference. Relaxation works best in patients with primary insomnia and those with associated anxiety disorders. Referral to a behaviorist is generally required unless the physician is skilled in teaching these techniques.

Light Therapy. Light therapy consists of exposing patients to bright light to manipulate their biologic clock. Exposure during the evening tends to cause a phase delay (i.e., delays sleep onset), whereas early morning exposure causes a phase advance (i.e., promotes earlier sleep onset). Light therapy is most useful for circadian rhythm disturbances.

Pharmacologic Therapy

Prescription Drugs. Hypnotic drugs are clearly useful for the treatment of transient insomnia. Prescribing a short-acting hypnotic can minimize sleep disruption during a stressful period and improve daytime functioning.

The role of hypnotics in chronic insomnia is more controversial. Although hypnotics are widely used for these patients, most published guidelines caution against using drugs in this setting. If a drug is prescribed for chronic insomnia, it should be prescribed in the lowest effective dose to minimize side effects. Recent studies suggest intermittent use of a short-acting hypnotic (i.e., 3 to 5 nights per week) may be the safest, most efficacious approach.[4,5]

The most commonly used hypnotics are the benzodiazepines and benzodiazepine receptor agonists (Table 56.3). The critical difference among these drugs is their duration of action. Short-acting drugs such as zolpidem (Ambien) produce minimal daytime sedation, but they are more likely to result in early awakening. Conversely, long-acting drugs such as flurazepam (Dalmane) reliably produce a full night's sleep at the cost of increased daytime drowsiness and potential accumulation effects.[6]

The newest hypnotic available in this class is zaleplon (Sonata). This drug is a pyrazolopyrimidine that binds selectively to benzodiazepine receptors. Zaleplon (Sonata) has an extremely short half-life, resulting in a duration of action of approximately 4 hours.[6] This brief duration of action allows PRN administration during the night, after the patient has experienced difficulty falling asleep.

The choice of hypnotic depends on the patient's specific needs. Individuals who have difficulty initiating sleep would be good candidates for a short-acting drug. Patients with symptoms of daytime anxiety or early awakening may do better with an intermediate- or long-acting drug.

A number of older prescription hypnotics such as barbiturates, chloral hydrate, and meprobamate are still available. These drugs are not recommended due to their relatively high toxicity and the increased risk of dependence.[6]

Some patients are not good candidates for hypnotic drugs. These drugs are relatively contraindicated in patients with known drug abuse potential, including those with a history of alcohol dependence. Patients taking other central nervous system (CNS) depressants, such as pain relievers or antidepressants, should be dosed carefully with an awareness of possible drug potentiation. Hypnotics should be avoided if sleep apnea is suspected. Pregnancy is a contraindication owing to possible effects on the fetus. Individuals who must function well when awakened during the night (e.g., physicians, firemen) should be warned of possible impairment. Finally, hypnotics must be used with caution in the elderly. Older patients are more likely to exhibit side effects, such as confusion, amnesia, and dizziness. They are also at risk for secondary complications including hip fracture.[7] Because of age-related prolongation of half-life, long-acting drugs are more likely to accumulate to toxic levels and should seldom be used in this age group.

Sedating antidepressants are often prescribed for insomnia. Trazodone (Desyrel) in doses of 25 to 150 mg at bedtime is widely used. However, in the nondepressed patient, there is lit-

Table 56.3. **Selected Hypnotics**

Drug	Duration of action	Half-life (hours)	Usual daily dosage (mg)
Zaleplon (Sonata)	Ultra-short	1	5–10
Zolpidem (Ambien)	Short	2.4	5–10
Triazolam (Halcion)	Short	1.5–5.5	0.125–0.250
Estazolam (ProSom)	Intermediate	10–24	1–2
Temazepam (Restoril)	Intermediate	8–10	15–30
Flurazepam (Dalmane)	Long	47–100	15–30
Quazepam (Doral)	Long	39	7.5–15.0

tle data to support this approach. The clearest indications for treating insomnia with antidepressants are in patients with underlying depression or in those with a history of substance abuse.

Nonprescription Drugs. Two antihistamines are currently approved and marketed as "sleep-aids": diphenhydramine (Nytol) and doxylamine (Unisom). These drugs are long acting and only modestly effective. They can produce daytime drowsiness, impair performance, and have a high incidence of anticholinergic side effects such as dry mouth and urinary retention.

Melatonin is an over-the-counter hormone preparation that has attracted considerable public attention for its proposed hypnotic properties. Although secreted by the pineal gland during nighttime hours, it is not clear that melatonin supplementation induces or maintains sleep. There are few controlled studies, the therapeutic results are mixed, and long-term safety has not been established. The most convincing trials have demonstrated efficacy in blind patients and others with circadian rhythm disturbances.[8] Despite its possible benefits and apparent short-term safety, melatonin probably should not be recommended to most patients until better studies are conducted.

Herbal therapy is increasingly used by those seeking "natural" alternatives (see Chapter 128). Valerian root, kava, chamomile, passionflower, lemon balm, and lavender are among the herbal options marketed for insomnia. Of these, valerian root is the best studied and is mildly effective in bedtime doses of 200 to 900 mg. However, as with most herbal products, the optimal dose is uncertain and purity/safety is a major concern.

Narcolepsy

Narcolepsy is a relatively uncommon sleep disorder that typically presents in adolescence or early adulthood. The illness is characterized by excessive daytime sleepiness with a tendency to fall asleep uncontrollably even during stimulating activities. These irresistible sleep episodes generally last 10 to 30 minutes and sometimes occur suddenly, without warning. This sudden onset can put the patient at risk while participating in dangerous activities such as working or driving. The other major symptom of narcolepsy is cataplexy. Cataplexy occurs in about two thirds of patients with narcolepsy and consists of a sudden loss of muscle tone precipitated by an emotion such as laughter or surprise. When present, cataplexy is considered pathognomonic for the disorder. Other associated symptoms can include sleep paralysis and hypnagogic hallucinations.

Evaluation of patients suspected of having narcolepsy is complex and generally requires referral to a sleep laboratory. This evaluation, which should include a multiple sleep latency test (MSLT), can frequently confirm the diagnosis. Confirmation is important, as treatment includes potent CNS stimulants with addictive potential and black-market value. Narcolepsy is sometimes feigned to obtain these drugs.

Behavioral therapy consists chiefly of optimizing sleep hygiene and scheduling daytime naps. Drug therapy focuses on administration of stimulants for control of daytime sleepiness. Stimulants typically used include methylphenidate (Ritalin), dextroamphetamine (Dexedrine), and modafinil (Provigil).[9] Cataplexy may respond to antidepressants, including tricyclics and selective serotonin reuptake inhibitors (SSRIs).

Sleep Apnea

Sleep apnea consists of repeated episodes of complete (apnea) or partial (hypopnea) pharyngeal obstructions during sleep. These physiologic events plus the symptom of daytime somnolence characterize the obstructive sleep apnea syndrome (OSAS). This important syndrome is common, dangerous, and underdiagnosed. Approximately 2% to 4% of middle-aged adults have OSAS.[10] Sleep apnea is typically a disease of middle age and beyond. Also children can develop sleep apnea, typically from adenotonsillar hypertrophy. Although pregnant women often snore, overt OSAS is uncommon.

The recurrent arousals and associated episodes of transient hypertension followed the next day by daytime somnolence of OSAS often results in significant increased risk of traffic accidents, poor job and social performance, as well as cardiovascular and cerebrovascular disease. There is a 37% death rate over 8 years of diagnosis seen in untreated OSAS.[11]

There is significant overlap between hypertension and sleep apnea. Approximately 30% of middle-aged men with primary hypertension have OSAS, and more than 40% of patients with OSAS have daytime hypertension. Also, the treatment of OSAS frequently reduces daytime systemic blood pressure.[12] It is, therefore, important to inquire about sleep apnea symptoms in patients with hypertension.

Diagnosis

Apnea is defined as cessation of airflow for at least 10 seconds. This is typically associated with what is called sleep fragmentation as measured by electroencephalographic (EEG) arousal during an overnight polysomnogram and a 2% to 4% decline in oxygen saturation during the apneic episode. An hypopnea is a reduction in airflow that results in an arousal and/or oxygen desaturation.

An overnight polysomnographic study is the best way to diagnose this syndrome. It should be performed for (1) patients who habitually snore and report daytime sleepiness and (2) those who habitually snore and have observed apnea (regardless of daytime symptoms). Snoring is generally the first symptom of sleep apnea. It is produced by vibration of soft tissues within the upper airway. The polysomnogram report will include a measure of the respiratory disturbance index (RDI), which is the number of abnormal breathing events per hour of sleep.

The characteristic nocturnal symptom pattern is loud snoring or brief gasps that alternate with 20 to 30 seconds of silence. These apnea events are noted by 75% of bed partners. Snoring intensity increases with weight gain and sedative or heavy alcohol intake, all of which lead to flaccidity of the pharyngeal tissues. Also, the pharyngeal trauma resulting from the repeated vibrations of untreated OSAS causes further pharyngeal changes, resulting in worsening of the syndrome in that patient. Half of patients toss and turn at night. About a quarter have choking or dyspnea and also about a quarter have nocturia four to seven times a night.[13]

The daytime fatigue may be subtle or dangerous, such as falling asleep while driving. It is important for the physician to look for subtle symptoms of driving while tired, such as excessive need for coffee. There are often reductions in dexterity, judgment, memory, and concentration. Patients sometimes report irritability, anxiety, aggressiveness, depression, decreased libido, and erectile dysfunction.

Treatment

The goals of treatment are to establish normal nocturnal oxygenation and ventilation, abolish snoring, and eliminate disruption of sleep due to upper airway closure. Any decision to treat should be based on daytime symptoms and cardiopulmonary function, rather than the RDI. Patients need to avoid factors that increase the severity of upper airway obstruction (e.g., sleep deprivation, heavy alcohol use especially near bedtime, sedatives, and obesity).

Continuous Positive Airway Pressure

Most patients will also need nasally applied continuous positive airway pressure (CPAP). This is the "gold standard" of treatment of OSAS. It provides a pneumatic splint for the collapsed pharyngeal airway of sleep apnea. CPAP quickly corrects the anatomy of the airway, improves sleep efficiency, and reduces the cardiovascular risk and daytime somnolence found in this syndrome.

Oral Appliances

Oral appliances can effectively treat snoring and mild to moderate OSAS. There are many appliances that can change the three-dimensional configuration of the airway. Patients often prefer them instead of CPAP, but they are not uniformly effective.

Surgical Therapy

Surgical therapy is invasive and not uniformly effective. There are several surgical options. Nasal reconstruction is the most commonly used. Very rarely, even tracheostomy is needed for patients with morbid obesity with severe hypoxemia. Tonsillectomy is typically curative for children with sleep apnea from adenotonsillar hypertrophy.

Restless Legs Syndrome

Patients with restless legs syndrome (RLS) have dysesthetic sensations at rest. These sensations are described as "pins and needles" or as "creepy, crawly" sensations. There is an almost irresistible urge to move the legs trying to find relief. Symptoms are usually worse later in the day and at bedtime. They sometimes awaken the patient from sleep. The sleep disruption that sometimes occurs can cause daytime somnolence.

RLS is a common disorder. Epidemiologic studies have indicated that 2% to 15% of the population may experience RLS symptoms.[14] Primary RLS is a central nervous system disorder with a high familial incidence. Secondary causes of RLS

are also important. Iron deficiency, even without anemia, as demonstrated by a low serum ferritin level (<50 μg/L) can cause RLS. Up to 19% of women during pregnancy develop RLS. It usually subsides within a few weeks postpartum. Spinal cord and peripheral nerve lesions as well as uremia and certain medications, including tricyclic antidepressants, as well as selective serotonin reuptake antagonists, lithium, and dopamine antagonists can also cause RLS.

Diagnosis

A sleep study is not usually indicated in the workup of RLS. Laboratory tests include serum ferritin and serum chemistry tests to rule out uremia, diabetes, and hypothyroidism.

Treatment

Nonpharmacologic treatment includes reduction in caffeine and alcohol intake and cessation of smoking. Drug treatment of RLS can be challenging. L-dopa with carbidopa (Sinemet one-half to one 25/100 mg tablet before bedtime can be helpful. Sometimes a middle of the night dose is needed. Dopamine agonists such as pergolide (Permax) and pramipexole (Mirapex) are also useful. Mirapex is better tolerated and used in doses of 0.375 to 1.5 mg per night. This class of drugs is highly effective, but the role of their long-term use is unknown.[15] They can cause severe nausea and more importantly, sleepiness, which has been reported to be severe enough to cause automobile accidents.[16] They need careful dosing to optimize symptom control and minimize side effects. Opioids including codeine, hydrocodone, oxycodone, propoxyphene, and tramadol can be used intermittently or continuously. Tolerance and dependance can occur. Benzodiazepines such as clonazepam and temazepam are helpful when other medications are not tolerated. Anticonvulsants such as carbamazepine and gabapentin are considered when dopamine agonists have failed. They are most helpful with coexisting peripheral neuropathy.[17]

Augmentation is a worsening of RLS symptoms in the course of therapy. Typically, symptoms can occur earlier in the day than before therapy began. It can occur at any time in the course of RLS therapy. Augmentation has been reported with dopamine agonists and may occur with other medications.[17]

Periodic Movements During Sleep

Almost all patients with RLS also have stereotyped repetitive movements during sleep. These are called periodic leg movements during sleep (PLMS). These movements consist of extensions of the big toe and dorsiflexions of the ankle with occasional flexions of the knee and hip. They last about 0.5 to 5.0 seconds, recur about every 20 seconds, and cluster into episodes lasting minutes or hours.

References

1. Cauter EV, Leproult R, Plat L. Age-related changes in slow wave sleep and REM sleep and relationship with growth hormone and cortisol levels in healthy men. JAMA 2000;284:861–8.
2. National Heart, Lung and Blood Institute Working Group on Insomnia. Insomnia: assessment and management in primary care. Am Fam Physician 1999;59:3029–38.

3. Edinger JD, Wohlegemuth WK, Radtke RA, Marsh GR, Quillian RE. Cognitive behavioral therapy for treatment of chronic primary insomnia. JAMA 2001;285:1856–64.

4. Walsh JK, Roth T, Randazzo A, et al. Eight weeks of non-nightly use of zolpidem for primary insomnia. Sleep 2000;23:1087–96.

5. Roth T. New trends in insomnia management. J Psychopharmacol 1999;13:S37–40.

6. Medical Letter consultants. Hypnotic Drugs. Med Lett Drugs Ther 2000;42:71–2.

7. Ancoli-Israel S. Insomnia in the elderly: a review for the primary care practitioner. Sleep 2000;23:S23–30.

8. Sack RI, Brandes RW, Kendall AR, Lewy AJ. Entrainment of free-running circadian rhythms by melatonin in blind people. N Engl J Med 2000;343:1070–7.

9. Medical Letter consultants. Modafinil for narcolepsy. Med Lett Drugs Ther 1999;41:30–1.

10. Young T, Palta M, Dempsey J, et al. The occurrence of sleep-disordered breathing among middle-aged adults. N Engl J Med 1993;328:1230–5.

11. He J, Meier H, Kryger MR, et al. Mortality and apnea index in obstructive sleep apnea: experience in 385 male patients. Chest 1988;94:9–14.

12. Fletcher EC. The relationship between systemic hypertension and obstructive sleep apnea: facts and theory. Am J Med 1995;98:118–28.

13. Hoffstein V, Szalai JP. Predictive value of clinical features in diagnosing obstructive sleep apnea. Sleep 1993;16:118–22.

14. Lavigne GJ, Montplaisir JY. Restless legs syndrome and sleep bruxism: prevalence and association among Canadians. Sleep 1994;17(8):739–43.

15. Montplaisir J, Nicolas A, Denesle R, et al. Restless legs syndrome improved by pramipexole. A double blind randomized trial. Neurology 1999;52:938–43.

16. Frucht S, Rogers JD, Greene PE, et al. Falling asleep at the wheel: motor vehicle mishaps in persons taking pramipexole and ropinirole. Neurology 1999;52:1908–10.

17. National Center on Sleep Disorder Research, NHLBI, NIH. Restless legs syndrome. Detection and management in primary care. NIH publication no. 00-3788, March 2000.

57
Medical Care of the Surgical Patient

Mel P. Daly

Family physicians are frequently called on for consultations and medical management of patients who require surgical procedures. Advances in surgical techniques and anesthesia have significantly reduced the risk of death and serious morbidity from intraoperative and postoperative complications.[1] Factors that increase the risk for adverse outcomes have been more clearly defined, and interventions to address and treat known risk factors before surgery have contributed to declines in morbidity and mortality. Notwithstanding these advances, up to 20% of all surgical patients have at least one perioperative complication. Most surgical morbidity and mortality occurs as a result of cardiac (5%), pulmonary (10%), or infectious complications (15%).[2]

There are 25 million patients who undergo noncardiac surgery in the United States annually. Up to 7 million of them have cardiac disease or are at risk of developing cardiac disease during the operative period. About 50,000 patients sustain perioperative myocardial infarctions (MIs); 50% die as a result of their MI. Whereas cardiac problems are the major cause of mortality, most morbidity results from pulmonary complications, sepsis, or renal failure. Overall risk is related to individual patient factors (coexistent medical illness, age, pathology requiring surgery) and the type and urgency of the surgical procedure.[3]

The goal of the medical consultant is to identify prohibitive or potentially treatable risk factors so that the patient can be taken to the operating room in the best possible condition within the time available. Prior to surgery, patients, families, and surgeons should be aware of the potential medical risks of the procedure and if this risk can be reduced by preoperative interventions. It is imperative that family physicians become involved in the medical care of their patients during this most physiologically stressful time of their life.

Preoperative Assessment

History

The preoperative medical history should be comprehensive and focus on uncovering factors that may affect outcome. Previous surgery or anesthetic mishaps should be documented. It is important to take a menstrual history to prevent elective surgery on a pregnant woman inadvertently. For pediatric patients, particular attention must be paid to recent or current infectious conditions to ensure that they are infection free at the time of surgery. Seriously chronically ill pediatric patients with congenital anatomic anomalies (especially those children with cardiac disease) should be referred to specialists, when appropriate, prior to surgery.

A list of prescription and nonprescription medications should be obtained. Cardiac medications (digoxin, antiarrhythmic agents), antihypertensives (beta-blockers and alpha-blockers), major tranquilizers, and monoamine oxidase inhibitors can result in life-threatening arrhythmias. All currently taken medications should be documented and strategies developed for their use before, during, and after surgery. Patients should be asked about their use of corticosteroids within the previous 6 months to a year, as there are reports of patients failing to mount an adequate intraoperative stress response to surgery as a result of iatrogenic hypothalamic-pituitary-adrenal axis suppression.[4] All patients should be asked about their use of alcohol, cigarettes, and recreational drugs.

A major determinant of outcome for patients undergoing noncardiac operations is baseline functional capability. This is especially true for older patients, and patients with cardiac and pulmonary conditions. All patients should be asked about their daily routines and how well they are able to perform activities of daily living. Patients who can climb a flight of stairs without difficulty or who can mow their lawn, play golf without a cart, or do housework are likely to have good physiologic reserve and will usually tolerate most surgical procedures. For older patients, this assessment is also likely to be useful in predicting how much help will be required after surgery that will result in functional impairment after discharge (e.g., hip or knee replacement surgery, or trauma surgery).

Physical Examination

A comprehensive physical examination is always indicated. Anesthesiologists appreciate knowing about a deviated nasal septum, loose teeth, and the patient's ability to open his or her mouth. The examiner should pay particular attention to the cardiac and pulmonary systems. The heart rhythm, presence of significant murmurs, and added sounds (particularly an S_3) should be noted. It is important to note signs of congestive heart failure (rales, jugular venous pressure, edema) and aortic stenosis (murmur, pulse pressure). A careful respiratory examination, observing for lung expansion and diaphragmatic excursion and listening for wheezing or rhonchi, may identify the presence and severity of emphysema, asthma, or chronic obstructive lung disease. Patients with rheumatoid arthritis have a high incidence of atlantoaxial joint involvement and may be at risk of spinal cord compression with hyperextension during intubation. Range of motion should be tested and cervical spine radiographs considered. A mental status examination should be done for all elderly patients prior to surgery, because of the high incidence of postanesthesia delirium among elderly surgical patients.

Laboratory Testing

Many studies cite the lack of data supporting the routine use of laboratory testing before surgery. Many screening tests are ordered, but few are abnormal and rarely is surgery or anesthesia changed as a result.[5] This is especially true for patients who are to have low-risk surgical procedures (e.g., cataract surgery, breast biopsy, podiatric procedures, outpatient procedures, hernia repair).[6] Thus, routine preoperative laboratory testing is not justified; selective testing should be done instead if there are specific clinical indications. From a primary care perspective, routine testing may be indicated if a broader focus on long-term, otherwise neglected health care needs is appropriate. In many instances surgery is necessary and may be the only reason for someone to see a physician. This may present an opportunity for primary care assessment and maintenance.

It has been estimated that it costs in excess of $2 million for screening tests to identify an abnormal prothrombin time if it is not suspected by the history and physical examination. It is unusual to detect renal abnormalities on preoperative laboratory testing unless there is a suspicion based on risk factors for renal insufficiency (e.g., diabetes mellitus, hypertension, use of nephrotoxic medications). Similar data have revealed low yields for detecting abnormal results by doing a routine complete blood count (CBC), urinalysis, and liver function tests in asymptomatic patients. Thus laboratory testing must relate to the medical history, the proposed surgical procedure, and the potential for morbidity and mortality.[7]

In most centers patients are required to have a CBC prior to surgery, yet a strong argument can be made not to obtain this test, especially for men under age 60, as the incidence of anemia is low. Surgeons are unwilling to operate without knowing their patient's hemoglobin level, prothrombin time (international normalized ratio, INR), and partial thromboplastin time (PTT) because of potential bleeding risks; however, there is little indication for doing these tests unless there is a specific indication.

There is a high incidence of unsuspected abnormal electrocardiograms (ECGs) among presurgical patients, yet whether it changes the anesthesiologist's approach to surgery has not been studied. Because most deaths after surgery result from cardiac complications, it is worthwhile to order an ECG prior to surgery for people over age 40. After age 70, a measure of renal function (blood urea nitrogen, creatinine) is indicated because of age- and disease-related changes in creatinine clearance.

The likelihood of finding abnormal laboratory tests is increased in patients with underlying pathologic conditions and those taking prescription medications. Patients who have a history of bleeding disorders or bruiseability/excessive bleeding or who are currently taking anticoagulant medications should have a prothrombin time, INR, PTT, and platelet count determined. Those with renal disease should have their renal function measured, and patients with diabetes or who are currently taking corticosteroids should have serum electrolyte and glucose levels determined. Patients taking digitalis should have serum digoxin and potassium levels measured. Previously ordered laboratory tests rarely need to be repeated; tests done up to 4 months prior to surgery that were normal are rarely abnormal on repeat testing and usually do not affect anesthesia or surgical outcomes. Thus it is reasonable to accept laboratory testing and ECGs done within 4 months of elective surgery.[8]

Preoperative Report

Surgery should be postponed if a patient's medical condition can be improved and surgery safely delayed (elective and semielective procedures). If, in the opinion of the medical consultant surgery ought to be postponed, it should first be communicated to the surgeon. The written preoperative report should identify medical conditions that place the patient at increased risk of adverse outcomes and make suggestions about how risk may be reduced in the time available.

It is tempting to make recommendations about the type and route of anesthesia. There is, however, little evidence to suggest that the type or route of anesthesia is important for predicting adverse outcomes.[9] General anesthetic agents are myocardial suppressants and peripheral vasodilators. Spinal anesthesia induces a sympathectomy at the level at which it is administered and causes levels of hypotension similar to those seen with general anesthetic agents. Furthermore, spinal anesthesia induces motor muscle paralysis that may interfere with forced expiration. Patients may have a heightened level of anxiety because they are awake, which increases myocardial oxygen demand. There is a greater likelihood of aspiration pneumonitis among patients given spinal anesthesia because the airway is unprotected. Occasionally, particularly in elderly patients, it is not possible to administer spinal anesthesia because of thoracolumbar spondylosis. Thus if a patient is "cleared" for spinal anesthesia and the anesthesiologist is technically unable to administer spinal anesthesia, general anesthesia may be the only option.

Assessment of Risk

The risk of mortality or morbidity is low and is individualized and related to the presence and severity of comorbid medical illnesses (especially cardiac and pulmonary pathology), the surgical procedure, and whether the procedure is emergent or elective. The risk of an adverse outcome can be estimated in a number of ways. The American Society of Anesthesiologists (ASA) physical status classification, first described during the 1950s, is widely used today.[10] Patients are classified based on their physical health status to somewhat qualitatively determined classes, ranging from class 1 (healthy) to class 5 (moribund). In large studies describing outcomes of thousands of operations, the ASA classification system has proved useful for predicting risk of complications and death. Limitations of the ASA system are that assignment of risk is subject to observer bias, and the inherent risk of the surgical procedure is not considered. Emergency operations are associated with a two- to fourfold risk of adverse outcomes when compared to elective surgery. True surgical emergencies (perforated organ, peritonitis, trauma, aortic aneurysm) rarely allow time for a comprehensive preoperative medical evaluation. In most other instances, the risk of adverse outcomes can be estimated by assessing clinical predictors in the context of the hemodynamic physiologic stress (alterations in heart rate, blood pressure, volume, hemoglobin, oxygenation, thrombogenicity) of the proposed operation. Major surgery can be long (intrathoracic, vascular, or neurosurgical procedures) and associated with a greater likelihood of adverse outcomes. Moderate-risk operations include extremity operations lasting 2 hours or longer (e.g., orthopedic surgery), and surgery that is less likely to result in adverse medical outcomes includes distal extremity operations, hernia repair, thoracoscopy, and transurethral resection of the prostate (Table 57.1).

Another commonly used risk assessment instrument is the Goldman Cardiac Risk Index, which was first published during the late 1970s and has been widely used subsequently.[11] More than 1000 patients admitted to Massachusetts General Hospital for surgical procedures underwent comprehensive preoperative physical assessments and were followed postoperatively to identify major cardiac complications and death. A multivariate discriminate risk analysis identified factors significantly associated with these outcomes, and each risk factor was assigned a weighted point score based on its relative association with adverse outcomes. Based on point scores, patients were retrospectively assigned to a level of risk associated with serious cardiac complications (ventricular tachycardia, death, MI, pulmonary edema) (class I, 0.7%, to class IV, 22.0%) and mortality (class I, 0.2%, to class IV, 50.0%). Factors not found to increase the risk of serious cardiovascular morbidity and mortality were controlled hypertension, the presence of an S_4, diabetes mellitus, hyperlipidemia, and stable angina pectoris. The latter was defined as angina that had not changed over the previous year in patients able to ambulate a distance of two blocks. Some of these factors (congestive heart failure and general medical condition) are potentially reversible preoperatively.

Lower reinfarction rates for patients operated on within 6 months of the original MI have been reported more recently and reflect an increased awareness of risk and more experience using invasive hemodynamic monitoring, pressors, and beta-blockers.[12] Perhaps more important for estimating the risk of reinfarction is the extent of prior myocardial damage and whether the patient has myocardium that is at risk because of coronary artery stenosis. Patients who have had non–Q-wave MIs may be at a greater risk of reinfarction than patients who have survived a transmural infarction. These patients frequently have borderline zones of potential ischemia that may be in jeopardy during anesthesia. Symptom-linked exercise testing to assess the extent of previous damage and identify at-risk myocardium is indicated in all patients who have had recent MIs requiring noncardiac surgery.

More recently published cardiac risk indices have taken these and other factors into consideration. Subsequent modifications (Table 57.2) of the Goldman Risk Index and includes point ratings for unstable angina (class III angina after one to

---

Table 57.1. **Surgical Procedure Risk**

High risk (reported cardiac risk $\geq 5\%$)
  Coronary artery bypass graft surgery
  Pneumonectomy
  Trauma surgery
  Neurosurgery
  Major vascular procedure
  Ruptured abdominal viscus
  Emergency surgery
  Anticipated prolonged surgery, with hemodynamic
    instability

Moderate risk (reported cardiac risk usually $\leq 5\%$)
  Abdominal surgery (open cholecystectomy, colon resection,
    etc.)
  Orthopedic surgery
  Urogynecologic surgery (prostatectomy, hysterectomy,
    cesarean section)
  Splenectomy
  Cancer staging procedures
  Peripheral vascular procedures (endarterectomy, femoral-
    popliteal bypass)
  Prostate surgery

Low risk (generally <1%)
  Cataract surgery
  Podiatry procedures
  Endoscopy and biopsy
  Breast biopsy
  Mastectomy
  Herniorrhaphy
  Vasectomy
  Appendectomy
  Dermatologic procedures

Source: Modified from Eagle et al,[16] with permission.

Table 57.2. Cardiac Risk Assessment (Modified Multifactorial Risk Index)

Criteria, Points
Coronary artery disease, 10
Myocardial infarction ≤6 months
Myocardial infarction >6 months
Canadian Cardiovascular Society angina
Class 3, 10
Class 4, 20
Unstable angina within 3 months, 10
Alveolar pulmonary edema
Within 1 week, 10
Ever, 5
Valvular disease
Critical aortic stenosis, 20
Arrhythmias
Sinus plus atrial premature beats or rhythm other than sinus on preoperative ECG, 5
More than 5 PVCs/min at any time prior to surgery, 5
Medical status, 5
Poor general medical status
PO_2 <60 or PCO_2 >50
K <3.0 or HCO_3 <20 mEq/L
BUN >50 mg/dL or creatinine >3 mg/dL
Abnormal SGOT
Chronic liver disease
Bedridden due to noncardiac cause
Age >70 years, 5
Operation: emergency, 10

Source: Modified from American College of Physicians,[17] with permission.

ECG = electrocardiogram; PVCs = premature ventricular contractions; BUN = blood urea nitrogen; SGOT = serum glutamate oxolic acid.

two blocks of ambulation; class IV angina at rest) and critical aortic stenosis.[13] Each of the published cardiac risk indices has been studied and shown to accurately predict the risk (class III or IV) of having an adverse cardiac outcome (pooled data: 16% for class III and 56% for class IV). A higher than expected serious complication rate for class I and II patients has been reported among those operated on for abdominal aortic aneurysms, probably reflecting a high incidence of asymptomatic cardiac disease among these patients, resulting in their being misclassified as low-risk class I patients.[14]

Cardiac Risk

Coronary Artery Disease

Patients with a history of a documented MI have a greatly increased likelihood of having an intra- or postoperative cardiac complications (see Chapter 76). This is especially true for patients who have sustained their infarction within 3 months of their noncardiac surgery. Patients who have sustained a recent MI and who have evidence of residual ischemic risk (unstable or severe angina, poorly controlled ischemic-

mediated congestive heart failure, or severe valvular heart disease) should be considered at prohibitively high risk for adverse perioperative cardiac complications. These patients should be referred to cardiologists for further evaluation and potential cardiac surgical interventions prior to considering noncardiac elective surgery.[15]

Patients with mild angina, prior MI (older than 1 month), history of congestive heart failure, diabetes mellitus, and elderly patients should be classified at intermediate risk for having perioperative cardiac-related complications. Patients with underlying peripheral vascular disease should also be considered at intermediate risk because of the high incidence of coexisting cardiac pathology (often "silent").[16] Patients without cardiac disease have a low incidence of postoperative MI and other cardiac complications (Table 57.3).

An important component of the preoperative cardiac evaluation for all patients is an assessment of how well a patient can perform functional activities. This may be helpful in deciding whether further cardiac testing is necessary, especially for intermediate-risk patients who are scheduled to have major surgery. Patients who can participate in strenuous activities such as running, playing basketball, or long-distance swimming have excellent functional reserve capacity, while sedentary patients who have difficulty carrying groceries up a flight of stairs have poor functional capacity. Patients with

Table 57.3. Clinical Predictors of Increased Perioperative Cardiac Risk

High risk
  Recent myocardial infarction (within 1 month)
  Congestive heart failure (unstable)
  Valvular heart disease (esp. aortic stenosis)
  Unstable angina
  Significant cardiac arrhythmias (ventricular tachycardia with ischemia, supraventricular arrhythmias with uncontrolled ventricular response)

Intermediate risk
  History of myocardial infarction
  Stable congestive heart failure
  Stable/mild angina pectoris
  Diabetes mellitus
  Age over 70 years
  Rhythm other than normal sinus rhythm on the preoperative ECG
  Uncontrolled hypertension
  Peripheral vascular disease
  Mitral valve prolapse ± regurgitation

Low risk
  Age over 70 years
  Controlled hypertension
  History of cerebrovascular disease
  Cardiac murmur
  "Minor" ECG abnormalities (premature atrial contractions, nonspecific STT changes)
  Controlled atrial fibrillation
  History of stroke
  Low functional capacity

STT = serial thrombin time.

Source: Modified from Eagle et al,[16] with permission.

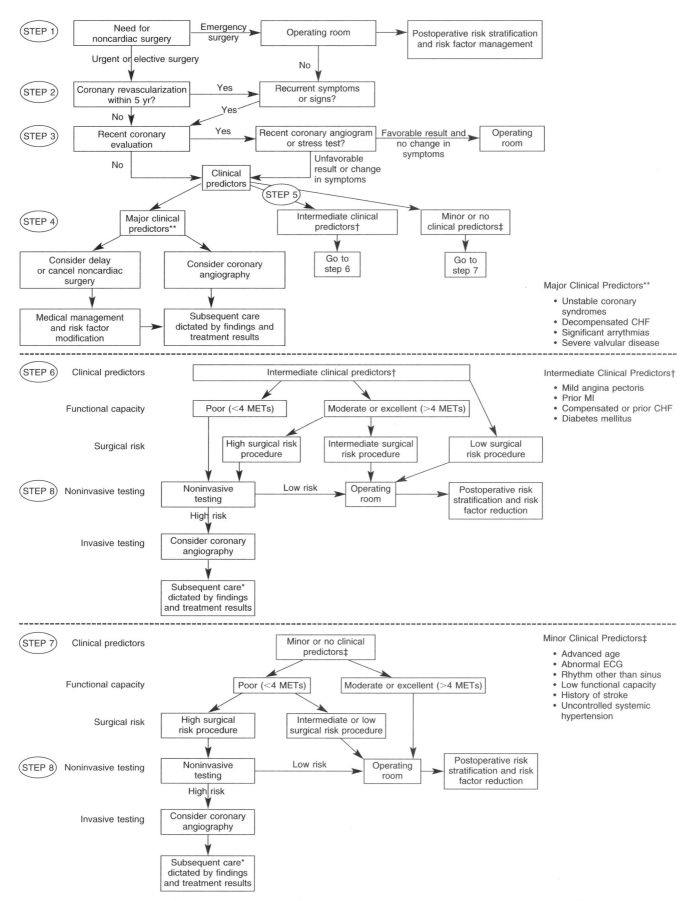

Fig. 57.1. Stepwise approach to preoperative cardiac assessment. Steps are discussed in text. *Subsequent care may include cancellation or delay of surgery, coronary revascularization followed by cardiac surgery, or intensified care. (From Eagle et al,[16] with permission.)

excellent functional capacity usually can tolerate major surgery, while patients with poor functional capacity are at much greater risk for adverse outcomes. Patients with moderate functional capacity should be further evaluated if they have intermediate- or high-risk clinical profiles or if they are to have major surgery.

Further testing and recommendations about how best to proceed can be made by carefully evaluating the preoperative clinical risk profile, functional capacity, and the proposed procedure. This is outlined by the American College of Cardiology/American Heart Association (ACC/AHA) Task Force, which suggests a progressive stepwise approach to preoperative cardiac assessment (Fig. 57.1).

The goal of the preoperative assessment is to evaluate not only the risk of the immediate surgery but also the long-term cardiac risk. Thus this may be an ideal time to consider further testing (noninvasive or invasive) if this is likely to improve outcome. Noninvasive testing (see below) should be considered for patients who are at intermediate clinical risk and are to undergo a major procedure. Exercise stress testing, echocardiography (resting, stress), or perfusion imaging (dipyridamole, dobutamine) can further assist in stratifying risk; however, there is as yet no evidence that this type of testing improves perioperative care. Invasive testing (arteriography) should be reserved for high-risk patients with suspected left main disease, triple vessel disease, or unstable angina in whom angioplasty or coronary artery bypass grafting would be indicated. Patients at low risk should have no further testing.[17]

The peak time of occurrence of postoperative MI is 3 to 6 days after surgery; it is due to increased activity, pain, and shifts of third-space fluid. Most postoperative MIs are "silent," perhaps accounting for the high mortality (up to 50%) among patients who sustain postoperative MIs. Patients who have had previous coronary artery bypass graft (CABG) surgery have a low incidence of infarction when subjected to further noncardiac procedures.[18] The restenosis rate after CABG surgery (native or saphenous graft) increases with time after the original surgery. This is also true for patients who have had percutaneous transluminal coronary angioplasty (PTCA). Asymptomatic patients who have undergone coronary artery bypass grafting within the last 5 years and patients who have had coronary evaluation (cardiac stress testing) within the last 2 years and are clinically stable require no further cardiac testing prior to noncardiac surgery.[16]

Surgical stress can lead to increased circulating levels of catecholamines that can result in arrhythmias and atherosclerotic plaque rupture. One study suggests that the use of beta-blockers can reduce the incidence of perioperative myocardial ischemia, and over time (6 months to 2 years) the incidence of MI, congestive heart failure, and death.[19] While these data are less than conclusive, it seems prudent that all patients (unless there is a contraindication) with an intermediate or high risk for cardiac complications should be given therapeutic doses of beta-blockers prior to surgery.[20]

In certain situations, preoperative intensive care, intraoperative infusion of nitroglycerine, transesophageal echocardiographic monitoring, perioperative use of pulmonary artery catheterization, and surveillance for perioperative MI may be indicated.

Congestive Heart Failure

The presence of preoperative congestive heart failure (CHF) has repeatedly been shown to be associated with a risk of postoperative CHF (see Chapter 79). Ideally, patients who present with CHF should be hemodynamically stable for a period of about 2 weeks before surgery.[21] Invasive (Swan-Ganz catheter) monitoring and treatment may be indicated for patients who have CHF and require emergent or urgent major surgical procedures. Patients with low left ventricular ejection fractions (EFs) are more likely to develop postoperative CHF, whereas those with EFs of 50% or more have low complication rates, even if they have had a history of CHF. The presence of jugular venous distention, current pulmonary edema, or an S_3 gallop places a patient at risk for perioperative cardiac complications. If possible, surgery is postponed until the CHF has been treated with a goal of euvolemia for a period of 2 weeks or more prior to surgery.

Hypertension

Poorly controlled hypertension is associated with perioperative cardiac complications, blood pressure lability, and renal failure (see Chapter 75). Severe hypertension may occur especially during induction of anesthesia, intubation, and emergence from anesthesia. Diastolic blood pressure readings of more than 120 mm Hg and systolic blood pressures of more than 200 mm Hg are associated with a greater likelihood of adverse cardiac outcomes.[22] Patients with well-controlled hypertension are not at increased risk during surgery. Patients taking antihypertensive medications such as beta-blockers, angiotensin-converting enzyme (ACE) inhibitors, clonidine, and calcium channel blockers show attenuated blood pressure responses to intubation and induction of anesthesia. Of greater importance for patients with mild to moderate hypertension is the effect of anesthesia on mean arterial blood pressure (MAP) levels. Large reductions in MAP (>30% for more than 10 minutes) are associated with a greater likelihood of intraoperative MI, CHF, and renal insufficiency. The goal of treatment prior to surgery is to achieve consistent systolic blood pressure readings below 170 mm Hg and diastolic blood pressures below 110 mm Hg.

Cardiac Arrhythmias

The significance of cardiac arrhythmias identified preoperatively is somewhat controversial (see Chapter 77), as it has become clear that the presence of nonsustained premature ventricular contractions (PVCs) is not a risk factor for ventricular tachycardia or sudden death unless associated with underlying cardiac ischemia (suggesting the presence of severe coronary artery disease).[23] Prophylaxis with antiarrhythmic medications is indicated for patients with sustained ventricular tachycardia, especially if they have had a recent MI. Atrial fibrillation is an important rhythm during the perioperative period, because when the ventricular response rate is rapid, the ability to increase cardiac output is compromised. This situation occurs because of reduced left ventricular filling volume as a result of a shorter diastolic filling time and loss of the presystolic "atrial kick." New-onset atrial fibrillation, particularly in patients with fixed outflow tract obstruction (aortic stenosis, asymmetric septal hypertrophy) may result in severe CHF and an inability to increase cardiac output. Thus control of the ventricular rate becomes important during anesthesia to allow adequate end-diastolic filling volumes and cardiac output. There is a higher incidence of atrial fibrillation during anesthesia in patients who undergo long surgical procedures, those with thoracic or neurosurgical procedures, and the elderly. Digoxin, beta-blockers, or calcium channel blockers should be continued up to and including the day of surgery. Most patients undergoing anesthesia (especially those with a history of arrhythmias) develop some kind of arrhythmia on induction of anesthesia, usually isolated occasional ectopic ventricular or atrial beats. Supraventricular arrhythmias may exacerbate underlying cardiac disease by increasing myocardial oxygen demand. These arrhythmias may also be a manifestation of noncardiac problems such as electrolyte abnormalities, or infection.

It is rare that patients need to have a pacemaker inserted prior to a major surgical procedure.[24] Placement of a pacemaker should be considered in patients who have long sinus pauses, high-grade second-degree heart block, or complete heart block. There is no indication for pacemaker placement in patients with first-degree atrioventricular (AV) block or asymptomatic bifascicular block, as these patients rarely develop complete heart block. The use of the electrocautery machine during surgery may interfere with "demand" pacemaker function; if the earth lead is placed away from the pacemaker magnet and the surgeon administers short bursts of electrocautery, this effect is reduced. However, it may be necessary to convert the pacemaker function to the fixed-rate mode when "demand" pacemaker responses are suboptimal.

Valvular Heart Disease

Valvular heart disease (especially hemodynamically significant aortic stenosis) is associated with an increased risk for perioperative mortality[25] (see Chapter 78). Severe and symptomatic aortic stenosis may require valve replacement or valvuloplasty if high-risk noncardiac surgery is to be done safely. Mitral stenosis is not associated with increased mortality, but these patients are sensitive to preload volume changes especially when tachycardia results in a reduction in diastolic filling time. Patients with aortic regurgitation and mitral regurgitation are less sensitive to volume changes but require adequate left ventricular contractility, as regurgitation takes place during both diastole and systole. Bradycardia is less well tolerated because of increased potential for regurgitation during prolonged diastole. Prosthetic valves increase the risk of bacterial endocarditis and thrombotic complications. Asymmetric septal hypertrophy may be difficult to manage perioperatively because the degree of outflow tract obstruction is variable. Certain medications exacerbate outflow tract obstruction; diuretics and nitrates reduce preload and intravascular volume; inotropes may increase obstruction because of increased contractility; and tachycardia may cause similar effects because of decreased diastolic filling time.

Peripheral Vascular Disease

There is a high incidence of occult coronary artery disease among patients with peripheral vascular disease (PVD) (see Chapter 76). Up to 60% have severe coronary artery disease; many have no clinical symptoms and frequently have normal ECGs. Patients with PVD have a high incidence of postoperative mortality, mostly because of intraoperative and postoperative MIs.[26] Additional cardiac testing should be considered for patients with PVD scheduled for major surgery.[27] Exercise stress testing (EST), if positive, can identify patients at increased risk of having a cardiac event, but the positive predictive value is low. The negative predictive value is high (i.e., a negative test makes it unlikely that a patient will develop a postoperative cardiac complication). Many patients cannot tolerate EST because of intermittent claudication, deconditioning, rest ischemia, or amputations. Furthermore, many patients with PVD have ECG changes of the left bundle branch block or left ventricular hypertrophy, or they are currently taking digoxin, making exercise test ECG readings uninterpretable.

Evidence has suggested that perioperative ECG monitoring may be useful in patients with PVD.[28] Preoperative ischemia and silent ischemia are good predictors of perioperative and postoperative ischemia and cardiac events. Furthermore, patients without signs of ischemia preoperatively are unlikely to have ischemic events. Again, the positive predictive value of silent ischemia is low because few patients with PVD and positive tests develop postoperative cardiac complications.

Perhaps even more useful is chemical stress testing using nuclear medicine imaging or echocardiography.[29] Dipyridamole is a coronary vasodilator; hence, stenotic arteries do not dilate, and infarcted areas remain unperfused. In normal hearts thallium is evenly distributed throughout the myocardium, with no distribution distal to stenosed arteries. These areas show up as "cold spots" on thallium imaging studies. If thallium redistributes on delayed imaging (4 hours later) to a previously imaged "cold spot," it may be an indication of underperfused myocardium. Thus redistribution on late imaging with thallium may be an important factor for determining the risk of intraoperative ischemia in a patient with PVD. The advantages of dipyridamole thallium testing are that patients do not have to exercise and increase their target heart rate, and there are few complications associated with infusing dipyridamole.

When dipyridamole thallium scintigraphy results are considered in conjunction with important clinical parameters (angina, CHF, Q wave on ECG, diabetes mellitus, PVCs), they add significant weight when predicting adverse outcomes for patients with PVD.[30] Risk stratification may be further enhanced by quantifying the number of areas on thallium imaging that show evidence of redistribution on delayed imaging studies.

A strategy for patients with PVD scheduled for a major vascular procedure may be to conduct a noninvasive stress test, which if negative suggests that surgery can proceed without further testing.[31] If the imaging study shows evidence of thallium redistribution, the size of the defect should be measured. If in the opinion of the radiologist or cardiologist the defect is small, the risk is low; but if it is moderate to large, the patient may be a candidate for cardiac catheterization and revascularization before having major noncardiac surgery. If the patient is not a candidate for coronary artery revascularization, the previously planned surgery or an alternative surgical procedure should be considered. If the patient is a candidate for coronary vascularization, coronary angiography may be indicated.

Table 57.4. **Relative Risk for Further Investigation Versus Proceeding with Noncardiac Surgery in Patients with PVD**

No revascularization prior to noncardiac surgery
Risk of noncardiac procedure
Long-term outcome

Revascularization prior to noncardiac surgery
Risk of cardiac catherization (1% risk)
Risk of CABG/PTCA (6–10%)
Risk of delaying surgery
Risk of surgery after revascularization (2–3%)
Long-term outcome
Perioperative risk without revascularization must be ≥15% for CABG or PTCA to be of benefit.

PVD = peripheral vascular disease; CABG = coronary artery bypass grafting; PTCA = percutaneous transluminal coronary angioplasty.

It is important to consider the cumulative and relative risks of having these procedures[32] (Table 57.4). The risk of mortality from coronary angiography is about 1%, and the risk for CABG or PTCA in a patient with PVD is in the range of 6% to 10%. The risk of delaying noncardiac surgery for testing depends on the reason for the delay and the urgency of the proposed procedure (e.g., a limb that is ischemic or in jeopardy). The risk of mortality for noncardiac surgery after a revascularization procedure is still in the range of 2% to 3%, together with unknown long-term risks of morbidity and mortality. Thus the potential risk of death by further investigating and treating patients with PVD is in the range of about 10% to 15%. If the risk of the noncardiac procedure without further testing is less, it may be appropriate to proceed with surgery and inform the patient, anesthesiologist, and surgeon of the increased risk.[33]

Medications

In general, all medications should be continued up to the day of surgery. Monoamine oxidase inhibitors interfere with autonomic function and may cause perioperative hypertension and hypotension. These agents may prolong neuromuscular blockade, inhibit hepatic enzymes, and prolong the action of narcotic drugs. If possible, the medication is discontinued a few weeks before surgery. Beta-blockers and clonidine should be continued until the day of surgery, as there is a possibility of postwithdrawal rebound hypertension. The surgeon should order antibiotic prophylaxis. Most surgeons prefer first-generation cephalosporins (usually cefazolin), starting with the preanesthetic dose and continuing for 24 hours.

Management of anticoagulants may be problematic during the perioperative period. For patients taking Coumadin, the risk of discontinuing anticoagulation must be assessed. For patients with metallic heart valves, Coumadin discontinuation is risky, although continuing Coumadin up to the time of surgery is contraindicated. If it is reasonable to discontinue the Coumadin, it is stopped 3 days before surgery and then reinstituted after surgery. If it is necessary to anticoagulate the patient up to surgery, Coumadin can be stopped 3 days before the operation and the patient treated with intravenous heparin. The heparin infusion is stopped 6 hours before surgery, and Coumadin is reinstituted after surgery. Alternatively, low molecular weight heparin (LMWH) may be used in doses of ~1 mg/hr every 12 hours adjusted to renal function for 3 days prior to surgery with the last dose administered 12 hours prior to the operation. LMWH or Coumadin may then be reinstituted after surgery. Aspirin, which irreversibly inhibits cyclooxygenase and affects platelet adhesiveness, should be discontinued 7 days before surgery. Other nonsteroidal and nonsalicylate products may be continued up to surgery.

Patients who are at risk for bacterial endocarditis (patients with prosthetic heart valves, previous endocarditis, congenital malformations, hypertrophic cardiomyopathy, and mitral valve prolapse with mitral regurgitation) should receive prophylactic antibiotic coverage (Table 57.5). Bacterial endocarditis prophylaxis is recommended for cardiac conditions that are high (prosthetic valves) or intermediate risk (mitral valve prolapse with regurgitation), for developing endocarditis; and for procedures that may result in bacteremia. Simpli-

Table 57.5. **Bacterial Endocarditis Prophylaxis**

Oral, respiratory tract, esophageal procedures
Standard regimen: amoxicillin 2 g orally, 1 hour before the procedure (children, 50 mg/kg)
Unable to take oral medications: ampicillin 2 g given IV or IM within 30 minutes of the procedure (children, 50 mg/kg)
Penicillin allergic: Clindamycin 600 mg orally 1 hour before the procedure (children, 20 mg/kg); cephalexin or cefadroxil 2 g orally 1 hour before the procedure (children, 50 mg/kg)
Penicillin allergic unable to take oral medicine: clindamycin 600 mg, IV within 30 minutes of the procedure (children, 20 mg/kg); cephazolin 1 g IV within 30 minutes of the procedure (children, 25 mg/kg)

Genitourinary, gastrointestinal procedures
High-risk patients: ampicillin 2 g (children 50 mg/kg) plus gentamicin (1.5 mg/kg for adults and children not to exceed 120 mg) IV or IM within 30 minutes of the procedure; 6 hours later ampicillin 1 g (children, 25 mg/kg) or amoxicillin 1 g (children, 25 mg/kg) orally
High-risk (penicillin allergic): vancomycin 1 g (children, 20 mg/kg) IV over 2 hours, plus gentamicin 1.5 mg/kg (adults and children, not to exceed 120 mg) IM or IV, within 30 minutes of the procedure
Moderate-risk patients: amoxicillin 2 g (children, 50 mg/kg) one hour before the procedure; ampicillin 2 g (children, 50 mg/kg) 1 hour before the procedure
Moderate-risk (penicillin allergic): vancomycin 1 g (children 20 mg/kg) over 1 to 2 hours, completing 30 minutes or more before the procedure

Source: American Heart Association World Wide Web Site, *http://www.americanheart.org/Heart_and_Stroke_A_Z_Guide/bend.html* ©2000, Copyright American Heart Association. Reprinted with permission.

fied prophylaxis regimens are recommended for dental, gastrointestinal, and genitourinal procedures. There is no need to institute endocarditis prophylaxis for patients with atrial septal defects, post-CABG patients, or patients with pacemakers.[34]

Pulmonary System

Pulmonary complications are the most common reasons for morbidity among patients undergoing noncardiac surgery (25–50% of major surgical procedures). Pneumonia, lobar collapse, pneumonitis, atelectasis, and respiratory failure can occur. These complications frequently result in prolonged hospital stays and increased mortality.

A number of reproducible physiologic changes occur with general anesthesia that place patients (especially those with underlying pulmonary disease) at risk of developing a respiratory complication. Predictable changes occur in patterns of ventilation, lung volumes, gas exchange, and pulmonary defense mechanisms.[35] These changes occur as a result of the procedure itself, the anesthesia, altered sensorium, analgesia, immobility, restrictive bandages, and relative immobility. General anesthesia results in a 20% decrease in tidal volume, but a compensatory increase in respiratory rate occurs, such that the minute ventilation changes minimally. Lung compliance decreases by 33%, and sighing is abolished by the effects of narcotic medications. Total lung capacity and all subdivisions of lung volumes decrease. Vital capacity decreases by half and lasts for 2 weeks after general anesthesia. Most importantly, functional residual capacity (FRC) decreases by up to 40% after upper abdominal and thoracic procedures. Closing volume (CV, the volume at which airway flow stops during expiration) increases significantly. Under normal circumstances FRC is about 50% and CV is about 30% of total lung capacity, and when these volumes decrease because of general anesthesia the lungs become subject to airway closure, atelactasis, and pneumonia.[36]

General anesthesia results in relative hypoxia because of ventilation-perfusion mismatches. Nondependent areas of lung are relatively overventilated and underperfused (dead space), whereas dependent parts of the lung are relatively perfused and underventilated (shunts). Normal pulmonary defense mechanisms (cough and ciliary action) are also impaired during general anesthesia.

Factors that further increase the likelihood of developing pulmonary complications (Table 57.6) include the site of the incision (thoracic and upper abdominal incisions), supine position, prolonged anesthesia (>3 hours), a history of productive cough, cigarette smoking, and fluid overload. Obesity, defined as weighing more than 30% over ideal body weight, is associated with an increased work of breathing, reduced lung volumes, and hypercapnia; all are associated with an increased risk of complications.

The limits of pulmonary operability have never been clearly defined. There are no studies that demonstrate the level of forced expiratory volume in 1 second (FEV_1) below which a person is at increased risk, nor is there consensus about indications for preoperative pulmonary function testing.[37] An FEV_1 of less than 2 L is associated with an increased risk of

Table 57.6. **Major Risks for Adverse Pulmonary Outcomes**

Forced expiratory volume in 1 second (FEV_1) <1 L
Maximum voluntary ventilation <50% of predicted
PCO_2 >90 mm Hg
PCO_2 <50 mm Hg
Relative hypoxemia
Upper abdominal and intrathoracic procedures
Prolonged anesthesia (>3 hours)
Cigarette abuse
Obesity (>30% above ideal body weight)
Chronic obstructive pulmonary disease
American Society of Anesthesiologists (ASA) class IV
Age >70 years

pulmonary complications, and patients with an FEV_1 value as low as 1 L may be more likely to require ventilator support and develop pulmonary complications.

There are no clear guidelines for estimating potential risk of developing pulmonary complications prior to surgery. Chest radiographs may be useful in high-risk patients. There are no clear indications for ordering pulmonary function tests. These tests may help in defining the severity of underlying pulmonary disease, and thus may help estimate the potential risk for complications. For patients who are to have cardiac surgery, pneumonectomy, or esophagectomy, more sophisticated testing such as quantitative ventilation-perfusion scanning, diffusing capacity studies, and estimation of maximum oxygen consumption during exercise may be indicated.

For patients with pulmonary disease, it may be possible to reduce complications by instructing them to stop cigarette smoking at least 8 weeks before surgery,[38] which results in enhanced mucociliary transport mechanisms, reduced secretions, less bronchospasm, and reduced levels of circulating carboxyl hemoglobin. Optimal bronchodilation prior to surgery may require home or inpatient nebulizer treatments and use of steroids for patients with asthma. Incentive spirometry has been shown to reduce the incidence of pulmonary complications and the length of hospital stay. Emphasis is placed on general conditioning, nutrition, and psychological preparation if a person is likely to spend some time in the intensive care unit after surgery. Anesthesiologists are aware of the need to minimize anesthesia time, use intermittent hyperinflation, and control secretions. Postoperatively, patients should be encouraged to get out of bed early, take deep breaths, use the incentive spirometer, and cough. Narcotic and analgesic medications should be administered in doses titrated to obtain analgesic effects without clouding the sensorium. Because cardiac and pulmonary complications occur for up to 7 days after surgery, medical consultants should closely monitor patients during this stressful time.

Hematologic System

See Chapters 125 and 126.

Hemoglobin and Hematocrit

The optimal levels of hemoglobin and hematocrit for surgery traditionally have been ≥10 g/dL and 30%, respectively. Consensus conference reports have now recognized the increasing evidence of the safety of transfused blood products and the excellent outcomes of surgery on anemic patients; it is therefore concluded that no single criterion can be used to support preoperative blood transfusion.[39] There is good evidence that surgical procedures can be done in patients with hemoglobin levels above 8 g/dL and in patients with hemoglobin levels as low as 6 g/dL if blood loss is less than 500 mL. The risks associated with blood transfusion are low; there is a less than 1% risk of transfusion mortality associated with the human immunodeficiency virus (HIV) and a less than 0.3% risk of acquiring hepatitis C (since testing became available during the 1990s); the risk of hemolytic reactions or congestive cardiac failure is also low.

Higher hemoglobin levels are advisable for older patients, those likely to experience significant blood loss, and patients with coronary artery or cerebrovascular disease. Lower levels of hemoglobin are acceptable for patients with chronic anemia with compensated intravascular volumes. When possible, transfusion is done preoperatively, as transfusion reaction signs may be obliterated under general anesthesia. The more widespread use of autologous blood, cell savers, and erythropoietin has greatly reduced the need for transfusion with banked blood.[40] The hematocrit level for optimal oxygen delivery to tissues and rheology is around 45%. Patients with polycythemia and erythrocytosis are more likely to bleed or have blood clots and should be phlebotomized to hematocrits of around 45% to 50% before elective surgery.

Platelets

Patients with thrombocytopenia rarely bleed until platelet counts are below 100,000 cells/μL, and the risk of bleeding is procedure-dependent for patients with platelet counts between 50,000 and 100,000/μL.[41] Platelet counts below 50,000/μL are associated with an increased risk of bleeding. Qualitative platelet functioning can be impaired even when platelet counts are normal. Medications including nonsteroidal antiinflammatory drugs (NSAIDs), aspirin, tricyclic antidepressants, alcohol, and even beta-blockers can impair platelet adhesion. Patients with uremia, liver disease, alcoholism, and leukemia may also develop qualitative platelet disorders. For these patients it may be useful to determine the bleeding time prior to surgery.

Coagulation Disorders

Coagulation disorders are rare, as a loss of 80% of clotting factor levels is required to prolong the prothrombin time (PT) or partial thromboplastin time (PTT). The most common disorder affecting clotting factor production is severe liver disease. Patients with prolonged PTs and PTTs can be managed intraoperatively with transfusions of fresh frozen plasma and whole blood. For patients with known or suspected acquired factor deficiency, a hematologist should be consulted for further investigation, recommendations, and treatment perioperatively.

Deep Venous Thrombosis

All surgical patients are at risk for developing deep venous thrombosis (DVT) (see Chapter 81). This risk is increased for elderly patients, the obese, cigarette smokers, cancer patients, patients who are having long procedures, those with previous venous disease, and those with a history of CHF. The risk of developing a postoperative DVT depends on the type of surgical procedure and the presence of risk factors. The optimal modality for DVT prophylaxis is controversial. LMWH (40 mg/day or 30 mg q12h) significantly reduces the incidence of DVT and pulmonary embolism in patients undergoing general surgical procedures, such as urologic or gynecologic surgery, surgery for elective hip or knee replacement or hip fracture, and other orthopedic procedures including trauma surgery. LMWH in doses of 40 mg per day or 30 mg every 12 hours significantly reduces the incidence of postoperative DVT.[42] It is unclear if LMWH is superior to warfarin (Coumadin) for prophylaxis of DVT for major surgical procedures, including orthopedic surgery. LMWH is expensive and not without side effects (thrombocytopenia, bleeding). Dosing of LMWH must be adjusted according to creatinine clearance. Elderly patients should be carefully monitored for bleeding complications. LMWH prophylaxis is not recommended for patients who are to have neurosurgical procedures or spinal anesthesia, because of an increased risk of bleeding that may compromise neurologic functioning.[43] Neurosurgical patients or patients undergoing spinal cord surgical procedures should have prophylaxis with intermittent compression or elastic stockings, as there is no risk for hemorrhagic complications. A decision to institute pharmacologic prophylaxis should be made by the neurosurgeon.

Multicenter trials comparing warfarin and LMWH are currently under way. Consensus conference opinion supports the use of LMWH (30 mg enoxaparin SC q12h), heparin (5000 IU SC q12h), or warfarin (10 mg po on the night of surgery followed by 5 mg po qhs, titrating the dose to achieve an international normalized ratio of 2–3) for prophylaxis of DVT for general surgery and orthopedic surgical patients. The optimal duration of DVT prophylaxis is controversial. Some would recommend that LMWH or warfarin be continued for 6 weeks to 2 months after surgery. At a minimum DVT prophylaxis should be continued until the patient is ambulatory for functional distances.

Liver Disease

For patients with liver disease, the likelihood of developing complications is related to the degree of hepatic compromise[44] (see Chapter 90). Patients with acute viral hepatitis and elevated liver enzyme levels, determined by liver function tests (LFTs), should not have surgery until about 4 weeks after the LFTs are normalized. Most surgical procedures cause elevated LFTs because of hypoxia, hypercarbia, traction, reduced blood flow, and portal hypotension induced by anesthetic agents. The major perioperative complications in patients with liver disease are bleeding, infection, and renal insufficiency (especially in patients with obstructive jaundice secondary to malignant disease). Patients with liver disease are likely to have a poor prognosis if they have hypoalbuminemia, a prolonged prothrombin time, ascites, esophageal varices, or encephalopathy. These patients should be managed aggressively with the help of a gastroenterologist using mannitol, lactulose, hyperalimentation, fresh frozen plasma, vitamin K, spironolactone, and other diuretics.

Endocrine Disorders

The most common endocrine disorder encountered during the perioperative period is diabetes mellitus (see Chapter 120). Surgical mortality for patients with diabetes is greater among those who have concomitant cardiac disease, those who are having peripheral vascular surgery, and those with end-organ damage (autonomic neuropathy or nephropathy) as a result of their diabetes. Autonomic cardiac neuropathy may result in reduced ability to perceive postoperative chest pain, and these patients may be unable to mount an adequate cardiac response to the myocardial suppression due to anesthesia. Patients with diabetes are more likely to develop urinary retention, gastric retention, and pulmonary aspiration. Surgery places an additional strain on the diabetic patient, resulting in wide swings in blood glucose levels, volume shifts, electrolyte abnormalities (most frequently hypo- and hyperkalemia), and changes in acid–base status.[45]

The goal of management is to control blood glucose levels throughout the period of surgical stress. A number of opposing factors are involved. Usually patients are not eating well, which reduces the requirement for insulin, and they are inactive, increasing insulin requirements. During surgery there is an outpouring of catecholamines, glucagon, and cortisol, which dramatically increase insulin requirements. The net effect is the frequently encountered hyperglycemia during surgery. In general, the goal is to keep the blood glucose level below 250 mg/dL. For patients who are insulin-dependent, one half to two thirds of their intermediate-acting insulin should be administered on the morning of surgery and fingerstick glucose levels monitored every 2 hours during surgery, with sliding-scale regular insulin coverage. For patients with "brittle" diabetes, better control may be achieved by starting an insulin infusion a few hours before surgery. The usual rate of infusion is 2 units of insulin per hour, but this dosage can be adjusted depending on the serum glucose levels. To avoid hypoglycemia, a dextrose infusion is administered simultaneously in the other arm. The infusion rates are adjusted based on fingerstick glucose levels. For patients with diabetes taking oral hypoglycemic agents, the oral agent is stopped on the day before surgery and the patient managed with sliding-scale insulin similarly to the patient with insulin-dependent diabetes.

Steroid Use

Patients who are currently taking corticosteroids may be at risk of hypothalamic-pituitary-adrenal axis insufficiency when faced with the stress of surgery. Published case reports describe cardiovascular collapse among patients with steroid-related adrenal insufficiency. Patients who are currently taking steroids, who have used long-acting steroids, or who have taken steroids for more than a week during the previous year may be at increased risk of iatrogenic axis suppression. Consideration should be given to treating these patients with "stress-dose" intravenous steroids during surgery. One critical review of the literature on stress-dose steroids reported that few studies fulfilled the diagnostic criteria for iatrogenic adrenal insufficiency.[46] Furthermore, studies of renal allograft patients who had adrenal functioning testing reported that patients who had been taking prednisone for long periods had normal adrenal responses to adrenocorticotropic hormone (ACTH) stimulation, suggesting that adrenal function was preserved. For patients who are at risk for adrenal axis suppression, it may be useful to assess adrenal gland function. If the patient's cortisol level doubles over a fasting level 1 hour after administering 250 μg of ACTH intravenously or intramuscularly, or if any cortisol level is in the range of 17 to 20 μg/dL, adrenal function is likely to be intact. If it is decided to treat the patient empirically with stress-dose steroids, hydrocortisone sodium succinate (Solu-Cortef) or equivalent 100 mg IV q6h should be given for 24 hours, tapering the dose by 50% until the patient can take the usual dose of steroids.

Renal System

New-onset renal insufficiency during the perioperative period is associated with significant morbidity and mortality (see Chapter 97). A meta-analysis study reported that the only consistent predictors of postoperative acute tubular necrosis were preoperative elevations of creatinine and blood urea nitrogen (BUN) and patients having a major vascular procedure.[47] Patients who are volume-depleted, elderly, septic, or having a major procedure are at increased risk for developing perioperative acute tubular necrosis. Morbidity and mortality result from sepsis, coagulopathy, and volume and electrolyte disturbances. Anesthesiologists have a heightened level of concern about avoiding this complication, especially in patients with a suspected creatinine clearance of less than 50%. Patients on chronic hemodialysis or peritoneal dialysis can be operated on safely, but dialysis should be completed 6 hours or more before surgery because of the anticoagulant effects of heparin added to the dialysate.

Nutrition

Protein-calorie undernutrition results in increased surgical morbidity and mortality. Surgery may transform mild undernutrition into severe malnutrition, which if it occurs is associated with impaired wound healing, immunodeficiencies, and a reduced ability to resist infection. Older patients are especially at risk for undernutrition after surgery because of co-existent chronic medical illnesses (e.g., congestive heart failure, chronic lung disease), functional impairments, coexistent dementia/postoperative delirium, and surgery-related factors (e.g., nil per mouth, liquid diet).

Patients who have multiple trauma or pancreatitis or who are unable to eat for 7 to 10 days are most likely to develop perioperative malnutrition. The Veterans Administration Parenteral Nutrition Cooperative Study found that mortality and complication rates among patients who received total parenteral nutrition (TPN) were similar to those who did not.[48] The authors concluded that TPN should be considered for severely malnourished patients or those whose gastrointestinal tract was to be rested for 7 to 10 days if previously normally nourished or for 5 days in previously malnourished patients. The exact optimal duration of nutritional support is not well established; however, low-risk nutritional supplementation (oral supplements) make intuitive sense for all perioperative patients until adequate nutritional intake is established.

Conclusion

Family physicians are increasingly being requested to participate in the care of patients during the perioperative period. In general, surgical and anesthesia outcomes have greatly improved, even among elderly patients in good medical condition. There remain, however, categories of patients who are at high risk for adverse outcomes, especially those with comorbid cardiovascular disease, those having peripheral vascular surgery, and those at risk for developing pulmonary complications, sepsis, or renal failure. The medical care of the surgical patient is highly individualized, with a goal of bringing the person to the operating room in the best condition possible and then not abandoning the patient after surgery.

References

1. Milamed DR, Hedley-Whyte J. Contributions of the surgical sciences to a reduction of the mortality rate in the United States for the period 1968 to 1988. Ann Surg 1994;219:94–102.
2. Khuri SF, Daley J, Henderson W, et al. The National Veterans Administration Surgical Risk Study: risk adjustment for the comparative assessment of the quality of surgical care. J Am Coll Surg 1995;180:519–31.
3. King MS. Preoperative evaluation. Am Fam Physician 2000;62:387–93.
4. Adrenal dysfunction and steroid use. In: Adler AG, Merli GJ, McElwain GE, Martin JH, eds. Medical evaluation of the surgical patient. Philadelphia: WB Saunders, 1985;101–17.
5. MacPherson, DS. Preoperative laboratory testing: should any tests be "routine" before surgery? Med Clin North Am 1993;77:289–306.
6. More preoperative assessment by physicians and less by laboratory tests [editorial]. N Engl J Med 2000;342:204–5.
7. Fischer S. Cost-effective preoperative evaluation and testing. Chest 1999;115(suppl 5):96S–100S.
8. MacPherson DS, Snow R, Lofgren RP. Preoperative screening: value of previous tests. Ann Intern Med 1990;113:969–73.
9. Farrow SC, Fowkes FGR, Lunn JN, et al. Epidemiology in anesthesia. II. Factors affecting mortality in hospital. Br J Anaesth 1982;54:811–7.
10. Dripps RD. A new classification of physical status. Anesthesiology 1963;24:111.
11. Goldman L. Cardiac risks and complications of non-cardiac surgery. Ann Intern Med 1983;98:504–13.
12. Belzberg H, Rivkind AI. Preoperative cardiac preparation. Chest 1999;115(suppl 5):82S–95S.
13. Detsky AS, Abrams HB, McLaughlin JR. Predicting cardiac complications in patients undergoing noncardiac surgery. J Gen Intern Med 1986;1:211–9.
14. Jeffrey CC, Kunsman J, Cullen DJ, Brewster DC. A prospective evaluation of cardiac risk index. Anesthesiology 1983;58:462–4.
15. Hollenberg SM. Preoperative cardiac risk assessment. Chest 1999;115(Suppl 5):51S–7S.
16. Eagle KA, Brundage BH, Chaitman BR, et al. Guidelines for perioperative cardiovascular evaluation for noncardiac surgery; report of the American College of Cardiology/American Heart Association Task Force on Practice Guidelines (Committee on Perioperative Cardiovascular Evaluation for Noncardiac Surgery). J Am Coll Cardiol 1996;27:910–48.
17. American College of Physicians. Clinical guideline, Part I. Guidelines for assessing and managing the perioperative risk from coronary artery disease associated with major noncardiac surgery. Ann Intern Med 1997;127:309–12.
18. Crawford ES, Morris GC, Howell JF, Flynn WF, Moorhead DT. Operative risk in patients with previous coronary artery bypass. Ann Thorac Surg 1978;26:215–21.
19. Mangano DT, Layug EL, Wallace A, Tateo I. Effect of atenolol on mortality and cardiovascular morbidity after noncardiac surgery. N Engl J Med 1996;335:1713–20.
20. Higham H, Handa A, Hands LJ, et al. Slowing the heart saves lives: advantage of perioperative beta-blockade. Br J Surg 2000;87(12):1736–7.
21. Weitz HH. Non-cardiac surgery in the elderly patient with cardiovascular disease. Clin Geriatr Med 1990;6:511–29.
22. Wolfsthal SD. Is blood pressure control necessary before surgery? Med Clin North Am 1993;77:349–63.
23. O'Kelly B, Browner WS, Massie B, Tubau J, Ngo L, Mangano DT. Ventricular arrhythmias in patients undergoing noncardiac surgery. JAMA 1992;268:217–21.
24. Weitz HH, Goldman L. Non-cardiac surgery in the patient with heart disease. Med Clin North Am 1987;71:413–32.
25. O'Keefe JH, Shub C, Rettke SR. Risk of non-cardiac surgical procedures in patients with aortic stenosis. Mayo Clin Proc 1989;64:400–5.
26. Wong T, Detsky AS. Having peripheral vascular surgery. Ann Intern Med 1992;116:743–53.
27. Fleisher LA, Barash PG. Preoperative evaluation of the cardiac patient for noncardiac surgery. Yale J Biol Med 1993;66:385–95.
28. Mangano DT, Hollenberg M, Fegert G, et al. Perioperative myocardial ischemia in patients undergoing noncardiac surgery. I. Incidence and severity during the 4 day perioperative period. J Am Coll Cardiol 1991;17:843–50.
29. Botvinick EH, Dae MW. Dipyridamole perfusion scintigraphy. Semin Nucl Med 1991;21:242–65.
30. Lette J, Waters D, Cerino M, Picard M, Champagne P, Lapointe J. Preoperative coronary artery disease risk stratification based on dipyridamole imaging and a simple three-step, three-segment model for patients undergoing noncardiac vascular surgery or major general surgery. Am J Cardiol 1992;69:1553–8.
31. Fleisher LA, Barash PG. Preoperative cardiac evaluation for noncardiac surgery: a functional approach. Anesth Analg 1992;74:586–98.
32. Potyk DK. Cardiac evaluation and risk reduction in patients undergoing major vascular operations. West J Med 1994;161:50–6.
33. Goldman L. Cardiac risk for vascular surgery (editorial comment). J Am Coll Cardiol 1996;27(4):799–802.
34. Dajani AS, Taubert KA, Wilson W, et al. Prevention of bacterial endocarditis. Recommendations of the American Heart Association. JAMA 1997;277:1794–801.
35. Tisi GM. Preoperative identification and evaluation of a patient with lung disease. Med Clin North Am 1987;71:399–412.
36. Ferguson MK. Preoperative assessment of pulmonary risk. Chest 1999;115(suppl 5):58S–63S.
37. Zibrak JD, O'Donnell CR. Indications for preoperative pulmonary function testing. Clin Chest Med 1993;14:227–36.
38. Warner MA, Offord KP, Warner ME, Lennon RI, Conover MA, Jansson-Schumacher U. Role of preoperative cessation of smoking and other factors in postoperative pulmonary complications:

488   Mel P. Daly

a blinded prospective study of coronary artery bypass patients. Mayo Clin Proc 1989;64:609–16.

39. Carson JL, Willett LR. Is a hemoglobin of 10 g/dl required for surgery? Med Clin North Am 1993;77:335–47.

40. Konishi T, Ohbayashi T, Kaneko T, Ohki T, Saitou Y, Yamato Y. Preoperative use of erythropoietin for cardiovascular operations in anemia. Ann Thorac Surg 1993;56:101–3.

41. Hematology. In: Adler AA, Merli GJ, McElwain GE, Martin JH, eds. Medical evaluation of the surgical patient. Philadelphia: WB Saunders, 1985;44–50.

42. Ament PW, Bertolino JG. Enoxaparin in the prevention of deep venous thrombosis. Am Fam Physician 1994;50:1763–8.

43. Clagett GP, Anderson FA, Geerts W, et al. Prevention of venous thromboembolism. Chest 1998;114(suppl 5):531S–60S.

44. Brown FH, Shiau YF, Richter GC. Anesthesia and surgery in the patient with liver disease. In: Goldmann DR, Brown FH, Levy WK, et al, eds. Medical care of the surgical patient: a problem-oriented approach to management. Philadelphia: Lippincott, 1982;326–42.

45. Ockert DBM, Hugo JM. Diabetic complications with special anaesthetic risk. S Afr J Surg 1992;30:90–4.

46. Salem M, Tainsh RE, Bromberg J, Loriaux DL, Chernow B. Perioperative glucocorticoid coverage: a reassessment 42 years after emergence of a problem. Ann Surg 1994;219:416–25.

47. Novis BK, Roizen MF, Aronson S, Thisted RA. Association of preoperative risk factors with postoperative acute renal failure. Anesth Analg 1994;78:143–9.

48. Buzby GP. Overview of randomized clinical trials of total parenteral nutrition for malnourished surgical patients. World J Surg 1993;17:173–7.

58
Counseling the Patient with Sexual Concerns

Charles E. Driscoll and Jacquelyn S. Driscoll

In the last few years, a remarkable change has occurred in the typical family physician's practice relative to issues of sexuality. Sildenafil (Viagra) made its entry into pharmacies in 1998, and suddenly there appeared to be a good reason for men to discuss sexual concerns that were previously covert and presumed to be "unfixable." A number of drugs now under development for women could be available in the next 2 years (e.g., Femprox Cream, Vasofem). Family physicians are challenged to gain a better understanding of sexual medicine to meet their patients' increasingly overt demands for assistance with sexual concerns.

The current societal milieu in the United States provides a strong push for family doctors to deliver sexual health care and counseling. The publicly reported sexual indiscretions of very visible people have forced parents to face up to the task of talking about sex with their children. Many who are unprepared will ask their family physician for information. Other issues that physicians will discover affecting their patients are listed in Table 58.1. Family physicians must keep current with the changing social environment to diagnose and manage health and emotional problems that may originate in the realm of sexuality.

The principal goals are to achieve a general understanding of sexual anatomy and physiology, elicit a sexual history from patients of all ages, explain the concept of safe sex, and recognize opportunities to provide anticipatory guidance for the age-specific eras of a person's life.

Sexual History Taking: A Must for All Patients

For the patient to feel comfortable when discussing sexuality issues, the physician must first create an atmosphere of permissibility for the story to unfold. A straightforward approach lets the patient know the subject is a routine part of medical practice. Using patient education materials about sexuality and genital or breast conditions tells the patient that it is all right to talk about sex. Language, body postures, and facial expressions that are congruent with messages of permission convey a feeling of comfort about discussing the subject of sex.

Collecting the Necessary Data

The daily work of a family physician includes common encounters that deal directly with issues of sexuality (e.g., contraception, obstetrics, routine physicals with genital and rectal examinations, breast pain, vaginitis, urinary tract infection, and prostate disease); to ignore a sexual history in these instances is poor medical practice. Less obvious are medication-related problems, chronic disease and disability, emotional maladjustments, and the aftereffects of surgery that may be dealt with perfunctorily without looking beneath the surface to determine how a patient's sexuality is affected. These silent problems are discovered by taking a sexual history as a matter of routine, inquiring first by general queries and moving on to seek the details of any positive responses. Table 58.2 outlines a series of questions that will uncover most sexual problems, identify high-risk sexual behaviors, and find knowledge gaps that could easily be corrected by patient education or prevented by anticipatory guidance. Advanced questioning techniques can be found in an excellent guidebook by Ross and Channon-Little.[1] A drug history (prescription, recreational, and alcohol) is an essential part of investigating any sexual concern, as medication side effects commonly cause problems with sexual performance. Certain nonspecific complaints (e.g., back pain, genital pain, fatigue, unhappiness, or "stress") serve as "tickets for admission" to the doctor's office and disguise underlying sexual distress. Usually, there is a subconscious hope that the real reason for the visit (i.e., sexual difficulties) will be discussed.

Table 58.1. **Recent Issues in Sexuality Affecting Patients**

Societal issues	Reflections in medical practice
"Oral sex is not really sex"—a dangerous gap in sex education arose. We need to do more than prevent pregnancy.	Since 1988, the percent of boys ages 15–19 who have had oral sex from a female has risen from 13% to 49.5%. Oral gonorrhea, oral herpes, and an oral wart virus are on the rise.
Sildenafil marketed—the term "Viagra-vation" is coined to reflect stress on the spouses.	Sexual partners may not be equally enthusiastic about the return of sexual activity; extramarital affairs used by some men for experimentation with the drug. Relationships are strained or broken.
Rohypnol, GHB, and other designer "love" drugs gain in popularity.	Unwanted sexual intercourse, sometimes with multiple partners, and "date rape" occur. Severe psychological manifestations are seen. Educate for prevention.
Availability of RU486 and emergency contraception.	Less consequences encourage irresponsible sexual behavior.
More talk and joking about sex appear on TV; there are fewer messages about safe sex and risk.	In the 1999–2000 television season, ~75% of programs featured sexual content. Sex outside of a committed relationship is being normalized.
Cybersex and Internet pornography are greatly increasing.	Sexual addiction is a recognized result; spouses are "cheating" on each other online. Prurience and paraphilias are nurtured.

Counseling About "Safer Sex"

Using a format similar to that for sexual history taking, Table 58.3 shows how to progress comfortably into a discussion of "safer sex" techniques. Americans do not seem particularly concerned about keeping themselves from becoming infected, as evidenced from the continued rising incidence of most sexually transmitted diseases (STDs), including human immunodeficiency virus (HIV) infection (see Chapter 41). When talking with the patient, physicians should impart general information about the viral and bacterial nature of STDs, and explain that no sexual activity with another person can be guaranteed to be 100% safe, and that there are recommended techniques to make sex between two people safer.

Table 58.2. **Sexual History Taking**

Openers
"I need to ask some questions about your lifestyle that will help me to take better care of you. It might include information about your use of seat belts, tobacco, alcohol, exercise habits, and sexual activity."

First approaches
"How satisfactory is your sexual functioning?"
"What concerns (questions) do you have about sex?"

Next level questions (*use when patient is sexually active and comfortable with questioning*)
"How many different sexual partners have you had?"
"Have you ever had sex in exchange for money (drugs)?"
"Do you have sex with men, women, or both?"
"Do you or your sexual partners use intravenous drugs?"

Diagnostic level questions (*use when sexual problem is presented by the patient*)
"How has sex changed for you?"
"What happens when you . . . ?"
"How do you feel when you . . . ?"
"What does your partner (say/do/feel) when you . . . ?"
"How would you (your partner) like it to be different?"
"What is your explanation for this problem?"
"Has anything sexual been done to make you uncomfortable?"

Physical Examination of Patients with Sexual Complaints

Patients with sexual concerns must undergo a focused physical examination before counseling can take place. The purpose of the examination is to detect physical problems that may be causing a secondary sexual symptom or dysfunction. A general physical examination is used to detect chronic illness (e.g., diabetes). The breasts are examined for galactorrhea and a normal erectile response of the nipple during palpation. A chaperon is needed when examining opposite-gender patients with a sexual complaint in order to avoid the psychological phenomenon of transference, where the physician becomes the object of a patient's sexual feelings or fantasies.

Children

When examining young children, have the child seated facing you, straddling the parent's lap. Alternatives are to place the child supine in the frog-leg position, in the knee-chest position, or in the lateral decubitus position on the examination table and do the inspection from behind. Examine the female child for gaping of the vaginal introitus (normal is ≤4 mm), perihymenal erythema, swelling or petechiae, and hymenal transections, which may signal abuse. If a vaginal examination of a small child is necessary to check for vaginitis or a foreign body, use an otoscope or nasal speculum after carefully explaining to the child and parent what is to be done. Check the penis of the male child for circumferential red marks indicating toilet training abuse. Take note of secondary sex characteristic development, and in adolescents record Tanner staging for sexual maturity (see Chapter 22, Figs. 22.1, 22.2).

Women

Examine the vulva for lesions and palpate for tenderness or thickening. Retract the clitoral hood to ensure it is free of adhesions that may cause pain with engorgement. Minimal

Table 58.3. **Counseling for "Safer Sex"**

Opener

"Even though much has been written about the term *safe sex,* most people are still somewhat confused about it. This subject is important for everyone to know about."

First approaches

"How did you learn about the term *safe sex?*"

"Tell me your understanding of the term *safe sex.*"

(*If patient verbalizes an accurate understanding, the discussion may end here.*)

Next level: teaching safer sex options (*use when patient seems comfortable with line of discussion*)

"Massage, hugging, rubbing, dry kissing, masturbation, and hand-to-genital touching are the safest sexual practices."

"Latex condoms and a spermicide containing nonoxynol-9 should be used for intercourse."

"Intercourse between monogamous partners is safest. Multiple partners increase the risk. Enjoy more time with fewer partners."

"Oral sex on a man wearing a male condom or a woman wearing a female condom is probably safe."

"Any exchange of bodily fluids (e.g., blood, semen) carries a higher risk for transmission of sexually transmitted disease. Any type of unprotected sex should be avoided."

"Sex exchanged for money or drugs carries a very high risk for infection."

"Sex under the influence of alcohol or drugs clouds your judgment and raises the risk of behaviors that lead to infection."

Diagnostic level: individualizing the concern

"Which behaviors have you engaged in that might have increased your personal risk of sexually transmitted diseases?"

"What questions do you have about the term *safe sex?*"

touching of the vulva may trigger a strong spasmodic contraction of the bulbocavernosus muscles, preventing further internal examination of the vagina (vaginismus). If this occurs, discontinue the examination and teach the patient how to use a finger or vaginal dilators to progressively overcome the resistance to penetration. Try to discover if the problem is primary (the woman has never been able to allow intromission) or secondary (usually developing after genital injury, abuse, or infection); the latter condition is easier for the family physician to treat, whereas patients with the former condition take considerable skill and time and should probably be referred to a sex therapist. The bulbocavernosus reflex is an anal "wink" in response to gentle squeezing of the clitoris. If present, this reflex indicates that the sacral nerves (S2–4) responsible for the neurologic component of the human sexual response are intact. (Only 70% of normal females have a bulbocavernosus reflex, so its absence requires clinical correlation and does not necessarily denote pathology.)

A vaginal speculum examination is followed by digital bimanual palpation of the vagina, uterus, fallopian tubes, and ovaries. When prior trauma or childbirth has occurred, look for gaps in submucosal tissue integrity, tender areas, or areas of anesthesia along the vaginal walls. Palpate the urethra and note whether a discharge can be expressed. Test for vaginal muscle tone by asking the patient to squeeze the examining finger with her vaginal muscles. The rectovaginal examination should be a part of all investigations for a sexual problem to detect nodularity in the cul de sac, which may indicate endometriosis. When the complaint involves burning or itching and the vaginal wet preparation is unremarkable, a colposcopic examination with 5% acetic acid staining may reveal occult human papilloma virus (HPV) infection (see Chapter 102).

Men

If the man is uncircumcised, have him retract his foreskin to permit examination of the glans and meatus. Palpate the penile shaft, testicles, perineal body, and perianal tissues. Look for testicular atrophy. Elicit the bulbocavernosus reflex by squeezing the glans, and the cremaster reflex by lightly stroking the upper, inner thigh. Perform a rectal examination to check for tone and to palpate the prostate. When a man complains of a "crooked" erection, it may indicate Peyronie's disease; to confirm it have him take a home Polaroid photograph of the erection problem. Unexplained genital skin lesions or irritative symptoms should prompt androscopy with 5% acetic acid staining.

Life Cycle Approach to Sexuality

Equipped with the skills of sexual history taking and the physical examination, the physician is prepared to deal with most sexual problems presented by patients (e.g., erectile dysfunction, painful intercourse, misinformation, psychosexual dysfunction, premature ejaculation).[2] Most sexual problems result from misinformation the patient has acquired; anticipatory guidance by the physician throughout the life cycle does much to avert this problem. Before the physician attempts to assist patients with sexual concerns, an accurate knowledge base is needed. The books by Berman and Berman[3] and Masters et al[4] are a good place to start. These books may also be recommended to patients.

Sexuality Issues: Infancy and Childhood

Ultrasonographic studies have shown that our awareness of sexual feelings begins even before birth, as fetuses in utero can be observed repeatedly touching the genital area to produce reflex erections of the male penis. After birth, male infants develop firm erections while nursing, and clitoral erection and vaginal lubrication occur in female infants. Babies are highly responsive to skin touching, and arousal signs may occur during diapering, bathing, or play. Parents who observe these signs of sexual arousal should be told that they are reflex responses and in no way indicate hypersexuality or any conscious appreciation of the sexual nature of their responses. As the child gets older, happy expressions can be seen on the baby's face as genital self-stimulation takes place. Parents with more sexually repressive backgrounds may express alarm, disgust, or fear that their child is a masturbator. It is appropriate to provide reassurance that it is normal infant behavior and that it will disappear if ignored.

During early childhood up to age 6, genital play is common and progresses from self-exploration to playing "doctor" with other children of the same and opposite sex. A natural curiosity is present, and in the 3- to 4-year-old interest in bathroom functions and "bathroom talk" increases. The child also begins to pick up cues that overt sexual play is not acceptable. Sex education should begin when the child starts asking questions by giving answers in a matter-of-fact tone of voice, answering only what is asked to avoid information overload, teaching values and feelings as well as anatomy, and using correct terminology for body parts. At school entry most children begin to develop a great deal of modesty, and the openness to sex play begins to regress. Encourage parents to be gentle and consistent in their approach to explaining what is and is not socially acceptable. There is a time and place for sexual talk and play. Children are less likely to think of it as "dirty" if they are encouraged to appreciate sex as a private subject.

A word of caution is needed about children who are sexually aggressive toward other children, especially those who act as if they are trying to have intercourse or oral-genital contact. This behavior is far beyond the natural development of sexual curiosity and usually is a "red flag" for prior sexual abuse of the child by a parent or family member. Other unnatural childhood behaviors include seeking sexual contact with adults, physical force or coercion used during sex play, genital mutilation, and compulsive sexual behaviors.

The sexual experiences of older children take place more in private than under the awareness of their parents. Parents must respect their children's privacy in the bathroom and bedroom. Sexual arousal begins to become more deliberate than accidental and occurs differently between the sexes. Boys tend to talk to each other in groups, seek to look at nudity in magazines, show their genitalia to each other, and engage in masturbation. Girls are more private and personal, gazing at their own developing body in the mirror and talking discreetly with a special girlfriend. Parents who discover sex play in their children need to understand it as a part of normal development, and should react calmly and matter-of-factly set limits. Potential harm to later sexual adjustment can result when parents react with anger, shame, and punishment. Early in the course of routine well-child visits, physicians can use the handout "Sexuality in Childhood and Adolescence" (Table 58.4) to stimulate parents to think and talk about their responsibility for sex education of their children.

Sexuality Issues: Adolescents

According to a Boston study,[5] teenagers want their physicians to talk to them about sex and give them the facts about how to avoid HIV and other STDs. While most of the students studied wanted their physician to give information about sex, they were uncomfortable initiating the discussion. It appears that it is up to the physician to initiate the discussion. The foremost concern of teenagers is whether their bodies and emotions are normal, whereas parents and society are more concerned about safety from pregnancy, HIV, and other STDs. It seems, then, that rapport with the teen for more in-depth education about

the latter agenda is best reached by comments during sports physical examinations or routine examinations that reassure them their bodies are developing according to a normal schedule of events. Also, acknowledging the struggles with which all teens deal (e.g., developing independence while still needing parents, peer group pressures, personal identity) is an empathic rapport builder. Self-image problems are intertwined with a sense of one's sexuality, so be alert to detect eating disorders that typically have their emergence during the teenage years. Normalizing body image and nurturing self-esteem will be a positive influence on the teen's ability to make proper choices concerning sexuality.

When the teen appears comfortable with this area of discussion, move toward imparting information that enables the teenager to learn responsible sexual behavior (see Chapter 22). A discussion can be opened about safer sex and contraceptive use. If a teenager is sexually active, it is proper and ethical to protect that confidentiality from the parents in order to keep the trust of the teen to promote healthier and safer sex practices. Parental consent is unnecessary for provision of sex education, care for STDs, contraception, or pregnancy care.

Finally, a caveat is needed about language used with sexually active teens. The prevalence of homosexuality is about 5% to 6% among teens, and the topic is difficult for them to discuss. Assuming that every sexually active person is heterosexual is a common error made by health care professionals. Try to use gender-neutral language and talk about the "sexual partner" rather than the "boyfriend" or "girlfriend" so as not to destroy the rapport and respect you have worked so hard to build.

Sexuality Issues: Adults

Men and women in their twenties through forties experience the highest monthly frequency of sexual encounters, a larger number of sexual partners, and wider experimentation with a variety of sexual experiences. The younger years, marked by the excitement of activities of mating and childbearing, are followed by periods of stress on the sexual relationship that result from child rearing, career conflicts, and sometimes attraction to sex outside the marriage, and that result, ultimately, in divorce in one third of marriages. The threat of acquired immunodeficiency syndrome (AIDS) has placed some constraints on casual sex and multiple partners; however, the rate of sexual activity outside a marital relationship is higher now than it ever has been. Some younger couples choose cohabitation rather than marriage as a means to reduce the fear of STDs. As the desire for more permanence in the relationship increases and couples enter into marriage, many present to their physician for HIV/STD testing to ensure that past encounters have been without consequence. Although more sophisticated in their knowledge than teens, young adults are still very much in need of sound advice about safety and health in sexual matters.

Sexual Patterns

Early marriage is marked by more frequent intercourse, on average three or four times weekly; as the couple and the re-

Table 58.4. **Sexuality in Childhood and Adolescence**

Childhood[a]

Normal developmental issues

Children are capable of sexual response at birth.

Babies respond to nursing, touch, diapering, and bathing by reflex sexual arousal.

Nursing mother may have normal sexual feelings in the breast or genitalia when feeding.

Normal children of 2–3 years of age touch their own genitals for pleasure and show affection to others.

Sex education should begin when the child's curiosity about sex becomes apparent.

By school age, overt sexual play normally decreases as modesty increases.

Older boys and girls develop differently in terms of gaining sex experiences and information.

Common concerns (if you cannot answer these questions, discuss them with your doctor)

How much information do you give children about sex and when to start giving it?

Can a parent be too tolerant of children's sex talk or play?

Are body changes progressing in the proper way?

Are there effects of magazines, television, and movies on a child's learning about sex?

Should the child see the parents nude?

How do you teach children to protect themselves against sexual abuse?

Adolescence[b]

Normal developmental issues

Sexual maturation occurs in girls before boys and for girls starts with breast growth, followed by pubic hair growth, a growth spurt in height, and menstruation; for boys it starts with testicular growth followed by pubic hair growth, an increase in penis size, and growth spurt.

Rising hormone levels activate sexual arousals, wet dreams, and stimulate sexual activities that include masturbation and sexual intercourse.

More than half of teenagers are sexually experienced before graduating from high school.

Isolated same-sex encounters are not uncommon for boys and girls in their teens, but it does not imply homosexual tendencies.

Teenagers are generally unwilling to admit to ignorance about sexual matters.

Common concerns (if you cannot answer these questions, discuss them with your doctor)

What are the effects of magazines, television, and movies on teen sexual behavior?

Does sex education encourage sexual behavior or merely alter it?

How do I encourage the teen to act "grown up" without condoning adult sexual behavior?

Are we seeing equality of the sexes or the old "double standard" about contraception use?

How accurate are the teens' sources of sexual information?

[a]Reading suggestions for parents and children:

Eyre L, Eyre RM. *How to Talk to Your Child About Sex: It's Best to Start Early, But It's Never Too Late—A Step By Step Guide for Every Age.* New York: Golden Books, 1998.

Johnson TC. *Understanding Your Child's Sexual Behavior.* Oakland: New Harbinger, 1999.

Mayle P. *Where Did I Come From? A Guide for Children and Parents.* Secaucus, NJ: Carol Publishing Group, 1999.

[b]Reading suggestions for adolescents and their parents:

Westheimer RK. *Sex for Dummies,* 2nd ed. Foster City, CA: IDG Books Worldwide, 2001.

Madaras L, Saavedra D. *The What's Happening to My Body? Book for Boys. The New Growing Up Guide for Parents and Sons.* New York: New Market Press, 2000.

Madaras L, Madaras A. *The What's Happening to My Body? Book for Girls. The New Growing Up Guide for Parents and Daughters.* New York: New Market Press, 2000.

Hein K, DiGeronimo TF. *AIDS: Trading Fears for Facts. A Guide for Young People,* 3rd ed. Yonkers, NY: Consumer Reports Books, 1993.

lationship age, intercourse frequency decreases to an average of twice weekly after the first decade and to once a week after the second decade. Sexual activity by a married couple commonly takes on a predictable pattern and rhythm over time, occurring in such a familiar pattern that the intercourse act has been called a couple's "sexual signature." It is a matter of comfort for most sexual partners. Some men and women, however, wish for more variety, and this desire has been postulated as a major reason for extramarital sexual affairs. In 1953 Kinsey's research revealed that one half of married men and one fourth of married women have affairs. Sub-

sequent studies have found both higher and lower rates, depending on the population studied. A family physician will treat at least one in four married persons in the practice who is or has been involved in extramarital sexual relations. This underscores the fact that no person is above consideration for taking a sexual history and counseling for safer sex.

Sexual Dysfunction

Most couples have a problem with sexual functioning at some time in their life together. Some problems are simple and transitory (e.g. erectile failure after a night of heavy drinking),

Table 58.5. **Suggestions for Enhancing Sexual Satisfaction**

Always remember that good sex begins while your clothes are still on. (*Expression of tenderness and affection, verbal and nonverbal, kindles desire.*)
Take time to think about yourself as a sexual being. (*Sex is not an isolated activity but rather, a part of your total personhood.*)
Take responsibility for your own sensual and sexual pleasure. (*Your partner should not have to guess what you want; say what makes you happy.*)
Talk about sex with your partner. (*Most problems can be corrected by a few words, discreetly and softly spoken.*)
Make regular time for togetherness with your partner. (*Plan for private, quality time together inside and outside the bedroom.*)
Do not let sex become routine. (*Avoid boredom with too much of the same thing; try new things.*)
Fantasy is one of the best aphrodisiacs you can find. (*Daydreaming can bring variety to the sexual relationship.*)
Working at sex does not work. (*Do not focus on the mechanics or become too pressured; allow spontaneity to prevail.*)
Do not carry anger into your bedroom. (*Adrenaline is incompatible with arousal; sex should not be a power struggle.*)
Realize that good sex is not just a matter of pushing the right buttons. (*Emotional content is more important than mechanics.*)
Keep some romance in your life. (*Continue the courtship with unexpected surprises and kindness.*)
Do not make sex too serious. (*Experience sex with joy and fun, not a march toward a goal.*)
Don't always wait to be "in the mood" before agreeing to have sex. (*Your sexual enjoyment may rise when you least expect it.*)
If you do not always "see eye to eye" on what you enjoy sexually, it will not destroy things. (*Not everyone shares the same feelings about a particular act, but compromise may work.*)
If sexual problems occur, realize you are like most people. If the problems persist over time, get help. (*If difficulties persist for several months despite attempts to improve them, seek assistance.*)
Keep your sexual expectations realistic. (*Every orgasm is not "atomic"; sex has its ups and downs.*)

Source: Masters et al,[4] with permission.

but others are deep-rooted and need intensive treatment (e.g., sexual aversion disorder). The majority of sexual problems are now thought to originate with an organic etiology with subsequent psychological overlay; a minority are strictly psychological. A useful classification for both male and female sexual dysfunction sorts conditions into four categories: hypoactive sexual desire disorder, sexual arousal disorder, orgasmic disorder, and sexual pain disorders.[3] Most of the problems uncovered by family physicians lend themselves to straight talk, education, and a few specific suggestions.

The chances for success of simple therapy offered by the physician can be predicted by assessing the three C's—chronicity, communication, and commitment—of a relationship disorder. If there is a long-standing, chronic problem, poor or no communication, and a lack of commitment by both parties to change, referral is advisable because any success that occurs takes a large investment of a therapist's time and is outside the usual scope of practice for a family physician. Masters et al[4] listed 16 suggestions for people who are dis-

satisfied with their sex lives. This advice, presented in Table 58.5, may be helpful to pass on to couples who do not yet need referral to a sex therapist. As another avenue of education for those who are computer literate, Table 58.6 presents reputable Web sites that can be recommended.

Normal Variations in Sexuality

Some events in a person's life are so predictably associated with a change in sexual practice or enjoyment that they should be acknowledged to the patient during the routine course of care, and anticipatory guidance should be given to make more satisfying adjustments. The appearance of urinary tract infections in adolescence is associated with the onset of sexual activity in over 85% of cases; therefore, safe sex and contraceptive counseling can be initiated. Urinary infection and vaginitis after all-night lovemaking are common enough to have the nickname "honeymoon cystitis," so the woman seeking contraception before beginning marital sexual activity can be told to use a water-soluble vaginal lubricant, clean the per-

Table 58.6. **Reliable Internet Resources for Physicians and Patients**

Web site URL (http://www.-)	Resources available
medicalsexuality.org	*Journal of Medical Aspects of Human Sexuality*; free journal and links available
familydoctor.org	Many patient education items on sexuality subjects
aasect.org	American Association of Sex Educators, Counselors and Teachers; find certified sex therapists
glma.org	Gay and Lesbian Medical Association; health issues and counseling
hivatis.org	HIV/AIDS Treatment Information Service; prevention counseling
indiana.edu/~kinsey/	The Kinsey Institute; links to sexology resources and journals
hisandherhealth.com/index.shtml	Medical/sexual health views; numerous links
siecus.org	Sexuality Information and Education Council of the U.S.
sexuality.org	Society for Human Sexuality; review before recommending
umkc.edu/sites/hsw/index.html	University of Missouri site; sex education and issues
newshe.com	Drs. Laura and Jennifer Berman provide women's information
sexualhealth.com	Sexuality information for persons with disability/illness

ineum after intercourse with a warm washcloth, and empty the bladder after sex. A pregnancy can bring with it some of the best sex (i.e., no fear of pregnancy) and some of the worst (i.e., fear of harming the baby may lead to anorgasmia or aversion to sex). Women and their partners can be instructed on the safety and enjoyment of sex throughout pregnancy, using different sexual positions for comfort, and when to avoid sex (active infection, vaginal bleeding, fluid draining from the vagina, blowing air into the vagina, or uterine contractions for more than 20 minutes after orgasm) (see Chapter 11). The lactating mother can be taught to use vaginal lubricants to compensate for the estrogen-deficient dry vagina and to expect milk letdown when orgasmic. The patient with herpes simplex of the genitalia or lip can be instructed to use a vaginal sheath (female condom) to prevent transmission or secondary infection (see Chapters 41, 116).

Sexual Care for Homosexuals and Bisexuals

We should keep in mind that when caring for gay and lesbian patients it is specific behaviors that predispose them to HIV or STDs, not their sexual orientation. These men and women have a right to the same respect and compassionate care given to heterosexuals, and the health care profession must be careful not to discriminate against them. Most homosexuals believe that their health care is enhanced by a nonjudgmental physician who is trusted to be aware of their sexual orientation. Specific sexual behaviors that may lead to disease are oral-anal contact, receptive anal intercourse, and the use of sexual enhancer drugs. Probably the most significant health risk for gays and lesbians, however, is that they avoid routine wellness care and thereby deny themselves access to procedures such as mammograms, sigmoidoscopy, and other cancer screening tests.[6] Homosexuals have higher alcohol and tobacco usage and a greater incidence of eating disorders. If their homosexuality is disclosed, it predisposes them to a risk of violence from other social sectors. The best sexual care that can be given to homosexuals is more a matter of attention to their holistic health care than to their sexual orientation.

Sexuality Issues: Seniors

Aging alone does not change sexual interest or diminish responsiveness; however, society portrays sex as a thing of youth and usually dismisses the idea that seniors have any

---

Table 58.7. **Sexuality in Adults and Seniors**

Adults[a]

Normal developmental issues
  Sexual lifestyle is usually chosen during young adulthood.
  Experiencing sexual attraction within a loving relationship requires letting go of shyness and building self-esteem.
  Deciding to marry and experience changing sexual patterns with career stress and children.
  Keeping the romance alive within a marriage.
  Marital affairs, divorce, remarriage, and blended families.

Common concerns (if you cannot answer these questions, discuss them with your doctor)
  How does one learn to solve conflicts within the sexual relationship?
  What information is needed about infertility, contraception, and disease prevention?
  How do I match partner satisfaction and self-satisfaction in the sexual relationship?
  How and when do I get help for a sexual problem?

Seniors[b]

Normal developmental issues
  Declining frequency of sexual encounters; unavailability of partners.
  Lifestyle and sexual orientation may still be evolving.
  Combating an ageist viewpoint that "old people don't have sex."
  Understanding and accepting normal age-related changes in sexual functioning.
  Human contact and intimacy becoming more important than orgasms.
  Declining health status.

Common concerns (if you cannot answer these questions, discuss them with your doctor)
  How do I overcome a lack of privacy while living with adult children or in a nursing home?
  Is there a normal loss of sexual feelings?
  Does a continued risk for sexually transmitted diseases exist?
  Is there a female and male menopause?
  What is the potential for help or harm to the sexual response cycle from medications?

[a]Reading suggestions for adults:

  Barbach L. *For Each Other: Sharing Sexual Intimacy.* New York: Signet: Doubleday, 1984.

  Heiman JR, LoPiccolo J. *Becoming Orgasmic: A Sexual and Personal Growth Program for Women.* New York: Prentice-Hall, 1988.

  Zilbergeld B. *The New Male Sexuality,* revised edition. New York: Doubleday, 1999.

[b]Reading suggestions for seniors:

  Butler RN, Lewis MI. *Love and Sex After 60,* revised edition. Thorndike, ME: G. K. Hall, 1996.

  Doress-Worters PB, Siegal DL. *Ourselves Growing Older.* New York: Simon & Schuster, 1994.

sexual activity unless it is lecherous or comical. Although menopause and physiologic changes alter the sexual pattern, older patients who have a well-developed sex life maintain their satisfaction with sexual feelings (see Chapters 23 and 24). For men, the erection requires more tactile stimulation and may not be as firm and upwardly angled, and the force and amount of ejaculate diminish. The refractory period increases, causing a lengthening of time between erectile capability. For women, the vaginal barrel thins and diminishes in size; reduction in muscle tension leads to a decrease in the intensity of orgasms; and lubrication is slower and less in amount, making injury during intercourse a potential problem. The physician can provide enough education about the normal progression of these matters so the patients do not believe their sexuality is vanishing. Encourage modification of positions for comfort and use of lubrication, and ask couples to work harder at touching and arousal. If there are no contraindications to use of the drug (e.g., hypersensitivity or concurrent use of nitrate medications), Sildenafil may be of some benefit. Those who want to be sexually active can then maintain their enjoyment.

When disease or disability occurs in concert with aging, more modifications are called for to make things work. Groups such as the American Cancer Society, Arthritis Foundation, American Heart Association, and others offer educational materials for patients interested in learning ways of coping with their illness so as to maintain sexual activity. Most patients are uninformed and embarrassed about bringing up these issues; therefore, the responsibility to anticipate and counsel falls to the family physician. Particular attention to the side effects of medication is necessary so patients do not assume that a sudden failing of sexual capabilities is a normal part of the aging process. Drugs proven to alter sexual function include antihypertensives (diuretics, beta-blockers, calcium channel blockers), antidepressants [selective serotonin reuptake inhibitors (SSRIs), trazodone, tricyclics], anxiolytics (benzodiazepines), antipsychotics, antiparkinsonian drugs, anticonvulsants [phenytoin, carbamazepine (Tegretol)], antiulcer drugs (H_2 receptor antagonists), digoxin, gemfibrozil, antiinflammatories, anticancer drugs, and drugs of abuse (alcohol, cocaine, nicotine, narcotics).[7]

The sexual life cycles of the members of families afford the sensitive and caring physician many opportunities to practice preventive health care.[8] By sensing the "teachable moment," putting a patient at ease about discussing sex, and delivering factual information within a proper doctor–patient professional relationship, the family physician does a great deal to enhance the individual's life as well as meet the broader societal goal of improving community health. Tables 58.4 and 58.7 offer suggestions and information regarding sexuality that can be adapted as handouts for use in a family physician's practice.

References

1. Ross MW, Channon-Little LD. Discussing sexuality—a guide for health practitioners. Australia: MacLennan & Petty, 1991.
2. Bachmann GA, Coleman E, Driscoll CE, Renshaw DC. Patients with sexual dysfunction: your guidance makes a difference. Patient Care 1999;33:99–123.
3. Berman J, Berman L. For women only. New York: Henry Holt, 2001.
4. Masters W, Johnson V, Kolodny R. Masters and Johnson on sex and human loving, 2nd ed. Boston: Little, Brown, 1986;452–61.
5. Rawitscher LA, Saitz R, Friedman LS. Adolescents' preferences regarding human immunodeficiency virus (HIV)-related physician counseling and HIV testing. Pediatrics 1995;96:52–8.
6. Harrison AE. Primary care of lesbian and gay patients: educating ourselves and our students. Fam Med 1996;28:10–23.
7. Tomlinson J, Milgrom EC. Taking a sexual history. West J Med 1999;170:284–6.
8. Alexander E, Allison AL. Sexual medicine: home study self-assessment program. Monograph, edition no. 201. Kansas City, MO: American Academy of Family Physicians, 1996.

59
Care of the Alcoholic Patient

Gerald M. Cross, Kenneth A. Hirsch, and John P. Allen

The abuse of alcohol is one of the major health problems in our society. Individuals with alcohol problems are disproportionately represented in the primary care population. In that setting, 11% to 20% of patients meet diagnostic criteria for alcohol dependence or abuse.[1] The family physician's role in the care of patients with alcohol problems may include screening, brief intervention, identification of affected family members, pharmacotherapy, detoxification, treatment of associated medical problems, and referral for consultation and rehabilitation.[2]

Background

Prevalence

Misuse of alcohol has a dramatic impact on many facets of life. The economic burden to society of alcohol abuse exceeds that of either illicit drugs or tobacco. The annual cost to U.S. society associated with alcohol abuse has been estimated as $184.6 billion for 1998. The major economic impact of alcohol abuse is on productivity losses due to alcohol-related illness and premature death. Over $26 billion of the total cost of alcohol abuse derives from treatment and prevention.[3] Annually, more than 100,000 deaths are believed to be alcohol-related.

Approximately 7.4% of Americans meet the diagnostic criteria for alcohol abuse or alcoholism (Table 59.1).[2] Their medical care costs up to three times more than that of the general population.[4] Fifty percent of all alcohol is consumed by 10% of the drinking population. More people drink heavily in the 21- to 34-year age group, and the fewest people drink heavily in the over 65 age group.[5]

Specific Populations
Ethnicity

Employment status, ethnicity, age, and gender influence the severity of alcohol abuse and treatment outcome. African-American men have only a slightly higher incidence of drug and alcohol disorders than do Caucasian men.[6] Among these two groups employment status was a better predictor of the severity of alcohol problems than was race.[7] American-Hispanic teenagers drink more heavily than either their African-American or Caucasian age peers, and Hispanic men suffer more alcohol-related problems than either African-American or Caucasian men. Alcohol abuse is a particularly serious problem for Native Americans. Although drinking behavior varies widely from tribe to tribe, most Native-American families are affected by alcoholism. Accidents, liver disease, homicide, and suicide, all of which may be alcohol related, rank among the top 10 causes of Native-American mortality.[6] Asian Americans have the lowest level of alcohol consumption and the lowest frequency of alcohol-related problems of any ethnic group in the United States. Within this group, drinking seems to be more socially controlled. Genetic factors may also diminish the risk of alcohol problems in this group.

Age

Overall, the earlier the age when drinking begins, the greater the long-term risk of alcohol abuse. Those who begin drinking during pre- and early adolescence are more likely to develop an alcohol disorder.[8] Many children and adolescents fall into this group. Among high school seniors, 80% report that they have already used alcohol, and 33% report having been drunk in the past 30 days.[3] Compared to parental influence, peer group norms more strongly influence the adolescent's drinking behavior. An adolescent's involvement with alcohol and tobacco serves as a predictor of subsequent experimentation with other illicit drugs.[9] Alcohol-associated violence and vehicular accidents have become the leading cause of death for America's youth.[9] Suicide victims often have a positive blood alcohol concentration (BAC). Unlike older patients, adolescents usually present psychosocial rather than

Table 59.1. **Definitions**

Adult children of alcoholics (ACOA): This group has an increased risk for alcohol problems and may have personality traits such as perfectionistic attitude with low self-esteem.

Alcohol: Refers to ethanol.

Alcohol abuse: *Diagnostic and Statistical Manual of Mental Disorders* (DSM) category for individuals who suffer adverse consequences of drinking that are not sufficient to meet the definition for alcohol dependence.

Alcohol dependence: A group of cognitive, behavioral, and physiologic symptoms defined by the DSM. It encompasses individuals who are unable to control their drinking despite the adverse consequences of drinking.

Alcoholic: Used as the equivalent of the DSM diagnosis of alcohol dependence.

Binge drinking: Five or more drinks at a single setting.

Blackout: Anterograde amnesia associated with drinking.

Co-dependent: Usually a nonalcoholic family member who suffers as a result of the alcoholic's behavior and who attempts to control that behavior.

Cross-tolerance: Tolerance often carries over to other drugs of the same class.

Enabler: A spouse, friend, coworker, physician, or other individual who makes excuses for the alcoholic's behavior so the alcoholic does not have to face the consequences of his or her drinking.

Heavy drinking: Fourteen or more drinks per week.

Kindling: Phenomenon of progressively increased neuroexcitation during repeated withdrawals.

One drink: Equivalent to 12 ounces regular beer, 5–6 ounces wine, or 1.5 ounces "hard liquor."

Tolerance: The individual requires larger amounts of alcohol to produce the same effect. It is partially due to accelerated liver metabolism of alcohol and cellular resistance to alcohol's effects.

physical signs of alcohol abuse. Elderly people typically drink less alcohol than do young people. Reduced consumption among older individuals may be due to health problems, decreased income, or changes in metabolism and the distribution of alcohol (higher BAC for equivalent amount of alcohol consumed). The combined use of medications and alcohol is a particular risk for elderly patients. Alcohol interacts with medications and can alter the effects of medication, especially in this age group (Table 59.2) (see Chapter 22).

Gender

Men and women have differences in the way they absorb and metabolize alcohol. After consuming the same amount of alcohol, women reach a higher blood alcohol concentration, probably due to their smaller amount of body water and due to a lower activity of the enzyme alcohol dehydrogenase (ADH). These differences make women more susceptible to alcohol-induced liver and heart damage.[10] Women also experience a modest dose-response relationship between breast cancer and alcohol consumption.[3] Alcohol metabolism alters the balance of reproductive hormones, decreasing testosterone levels in men and increasing estradiol levels in women.

Throughout all age groups, men are two to five times more likely to be "problem drinkers" than are women. Although women drink less alcohol than men, they and their children are often the victims of family members who abuse alcohol.[6] Women who enter the labor force tend to drink somewhat more alcohol than other women.[11]

Etiology

Several models have been proposed to explain alcoholism.[12] Historically, the moral model has influenced Western culture. This model views alcoholism as a character weakness and recommends willpower as the solution for alcohol problems. Some proponents of this model remain, and the United States

Supreme Court once labeled alcoholism "willful misconduct." The learning model provides another view of alcoholism, describing it as a maladaptive habit. The model contends that new learning can reverse the habit. Although this model is generally consistent with a goal of complete abstinence, it raises the unfortunate belief that the alcohol-dependent patient can someday resume drinking safely.

Today a modified or developmental disease model provides a widely accepted explanation of alcoholism.[13] Alcoholism is viewed as a complex disorder influenced by environmental and genetic influences. The goal of treatment is complete abstinence. Although not without criticism, the disease model has the advantage that it avoids blame and supports treatment. As with other diseases, biopsychosocial factors (ethnicity, age, gender, environment, genetics) and personal choices can affect the onset and outcome of alcoholism. Related to this is the concept of problematic alcohol use developing as a consequence of depression, e.g., self-medication. To the extent that this is valid for a given patient, treatment for depression as an independent disease entity becomes crucial (see Chapter 32).

Evidence that a significant portion of our vulnerability to alcoholism is genetic has greatly influenced the direction of alcohol research and established a biologic basis of alcoholism.[3] Twin and adoption studies suggest a genetic predisposition to alcoholism and pattern of alcohol consumption. A study of Finnish twins[14] revealed that the quantity of alcohol consumed over a period of 6 years was influenced more by heredity than by environmental factors. The genetic predisposition to alcohol abuse may also be related to alcohol sensitivity due to genetic variants in metabolism of acetaldehyde, as is found in the Chinese Han people. A variant form of the enzyme aldehyde dehydrogenase-2 (ALDH2) has a dominant inheritance pattern and results in slower clearing of acetaldehyde.[13] This sensitivity to alcohol results in rapid flushing, which may protect against heavy or frequent use.[15] Attention has focused on serotonin (5-hydroxytryptamine, 5-HT) dys-

Table 59.2. **Selected Alcohol–Drug and Alcohol–Herbal Interactions**

Anesthetics	
Propofol (Diprivan)	Increased dose required to produce unconsciousness in chronic drinkers
Enflurane (Ethrane)	Greater risk of liver damage in chronic drinkers
Halothane (Fluothane)	Greater risk of liver damage in chronic drinkers
Antibiotics	
Furazolidone (Furoxone)	Increased risk of nausea, vomiting, headache, and convulsions with acute alcohol consumption
Griseofulvin (Grisactin)	Increased risk of nausea, vomiting, headache, and convulsions with acute alcohol consumption
Metronidazole (Flagyl)	Disulfiram-like reaction; increased risk of nausea, vomiting, headache, and convulsions with acute alcohol consumption
Isoniazid	Decreased availability in the bloodstream with acute alcohol consumption
Rifampin	Decreased availability in the bloodstream with chronic alcohol consumption
Anticoagulants	
Warfarin (Coumadin)	Increased risk of hemorrhages due to increased warfarin availability with acute alcohol consumption; chronic alcohol consumption decreases warfarin availability
Antidepressants	
Amitriptyline (Elavil)	Alcohol increases sedative effect
Monoamine oxidase (MAO) inhibitors	Tyramine found in some beers and wine may produce a dangerous rise in blood pressure
Antidiabetic	
Tolbutamide (Orinase)	Increased availability with acute alcohol consumption and decreased availability with chronic consumption
Antihistamines	
Diphenhydramine (Benadryl)	Increased sedation with acute alcohol consumption
Antipsychotic	
Chlorpromazine (Thorazine)	Increased sedation with acute alcohol consumption; possible liver damage with chronic alcohol consumption
Antiseizure	
Phenytoin (Dilantin)	Increased availability with acute alcohol consumption; chronic drinking decreases availability
Cardiovascular	
Nitroglycerin	Vasodilation; acute alcohol consumption may cause fainting upon standing up
Propranolol (Inderal)	Chronic alcohol consumption decreases availability
Disulfiram	Aldehyde dehydrogenase inhibition produces nausea, vomiting, and potentially shock in the presence of alcohol
Humulus lupulus (Hops)	May potentiate other sedative medications
Narcotics	Increased sedative effect with alcohol
Nonnarcotic pain relievers	
Aspirin	Increased risk of gastric bleeding with alcohol; aspirin may heighten the effects of alcohol
Acetaminophen (Tylenol)	Chronic alcohol consumption increases the risk of liver damage
Oenotherabiennis (evening primrose oil)	Caution if used in patients taking drugs that may lower seizure threshold
Piper methysticum (Kava-Kava)	May potentiate benzodiazepines, alcohol and other central nervous system depressants.
Sedative/hypnotics	
Benzodiazepines	Increased sedation with alcohol; increased risk of accidents, especially in older patients
Barbiturates	Acute alcohol consumption prolongs sedative effects; chronic alcohol use decreases availability of barbiturates due to enzyme activation
Valerian officinalis (Valerian)	May potentiate sedatives and barbiturates

function as part of the biologic basis of alcoholism. 5-HT modulates impulse control and mood. Substantial evidence points to defects in 5-HT neurotransmission in alcoholics, generally indicating that alcoholics have decreased 5-HT neurotransmission.[16] Predisposition toward alcoholism is clearly not predestination for alcoholism, but a family history of alcoholism does increase the vulnerability to developing it. As with atherosclerosis and other diseases, individuals with a positive family history for alcoholism can modify their behavior to decrease their risk of alcohol dependence. Early tolerance may be a marker for a genetically related increased risk of alcoholism.[17]

Physiology

Alcohol is absorbed through the gastrointestinal tract, largely metabolized in the liver, and goes on to affect every organ system. Alcohol absorption is increased when concentrated drinks are taken on an empty stomach. Food (especially fat) in the stomach slows alcohol absorption by dilution and by delayed emptying into the small intestine where absorption is faster. Alcohol passes through the liver before it reaches the circulatory system. High concentrations of alcohol exceed the metabolic capacity of the liver, allowing more alcohol to reach the blood and brain. Typically, after one standard drink (12 ounces of beer, 5 ounces of wine, or 1.5 ounces of 80-proof distilled spirit), the BAC will peak within 30 to 45 minutes.

Alcohol metabolism proceeds at a constant rate (zero-order kinetics). Alcohol is first metabolized to acetaldehyde. The ADH enzyme carries out most of this metabolic step, but there are genetic variations in its activity. With chronic exposure to alcohol, the microsomal ethanol-oxidizing system (MEOS), another metabolic pathway for alcohol, may accelerate the rate of metabolism. Although individuals vary greatly in their ability to metabolize alcohol, an average man can metabolize about 10 mL of absolute alcohol (or one drink) per hour.

Acetaldehyde is subsequently metabolized to acetate owing to the action of aldehyde dehydrogenase. Disulfiram (Antabuse) inhibits several enzymes that metabolize acetaldehyde. In the presence of alcohol, disulfiram causes acetaldehyde to accumulate, leading to flushing, tachycardia, nausea, vomiting, and later a drop in blood pressure. These signs and symptoms are referred to as the disulfiram-ethanol reaction.

About 5% to 10% of alcohol is released unchanged in breath and urine. Alcohol in alveolar air correlates directly with the arterial BAC, whereas levels in urine correlate with the current level of intoxication only if the bladder is emptied and the subsequent urine is tested.

Alcohol interacts with both water and lipids, allowing it to penetrate and disorder cell membranes. There is no blood–brain barrier to alcohol. Because of the brain's vascularity, the concentration of alcohol in the brain may in fact exceed the level in the venous peripheral blood until the alcohol equilibrates in total body water. Until this balance is reached, the blood alcohol concentration may be less than the cerebrospinal fluid (CSF) concentration.[18] The placenta is unable to protect the fetus from exposure to alcohol in the mother's blood. Similarly, breast milk conveys some of the alcohol in the mother's blood to the infant.

Clinical Presentation

Mental Status

In the emergency room, intoxicated patients often present with a history of recent drinking and demonstrate socially inappropriate behavior, impaired judgment, and altered consciousness. Hospitalized patients who show mental status impairment combined with sympathetic signs should be evaluated for withdrawal from alcohol, other sedative-hypnotics, or both. These patients may have anterograde amnesia, referred to as a blackout. Head trauma should be ruled out by both examination and by the patient's own report. Serial mental status examinations using a standardized format such as the Mini-Mental Status Examination are needed until substantial cognitive clearing is demonstrated. Alcoholics may present with frank delirium (altered consciousness, impaired attention, sleep–wake cycle disturbance, cognitive disorganization, dysperceptions), dementia (intellectual decline and personality changes resulting in social impairment), or both. Fluctuation in the patient's level of functioning argues for delirium, which should be considered a medical emergency until the etiology is clearly identified. To differentiate between delirium and a psychotic disorder, a generally valid guideline is that the predominance of visual or tactile hallucinations suggests an organic etiology (e.g., delirium), whereas predominantly auditory hallucinations are more suggestive of a psychotic disorder.

Many alcoholics appear anxious or depressed, conditions that often resolve after detoxification. Sometimes clinical depression coexists with or underlies alcoholism. If depression does not diminish within several weeks of drinking cessation, treatment with an antidepressant is recommended. Treatment of primary depression may reduce the risk of a return to drinking because of continued depression, and if treatment is with a serotonergic agent, craving for alcohol (and other drugs) may be reduced, further promoting abstinence.

Brain

Chronic alcoholics lose both gray and white matter volumes. Neuronal damage may result from increased levels of reactive oxygen species and lipid peroxidation products, exceeding the capacity of the body's normal nucleotide excision repair of damaged DNA.[19] Organic brain syndromes among alcohol-dependent patients can usually be categorized as Wernicke-Korsakoff syndrome or alcoholic dementia. Wernicke's disease includes a triad of signs: confusion, ocular disturbances, and ataxia, caused by thiamine deficiency. Korsakoff's psychosis may be the chronic phase of Wernicke's disease. It includes impaired recent memory and the inability to learn new information. Confabulation, or making up details to fill in gaps in memory, has been associated with Korsakoff's psychosis. Alcoholic dementia includes total intellectual decline with dysphasia, apraxia, and cerebral atrophy. This condition may be difficult to distinguish from Alzheimer's disease (see Chapter 25). The long-term effect of alcohol on the brain, even after prolonged abstinence, is demonstrated by the extreme rapidity with which tolerance is redeveloped if the patient returns to drinking.

Neurotransmitter function constitutes an important area of alcohol research. Broadly summarized, it appears that withdrawal phenomena are mediated by dopaminergic pathways, pleasure from alcohol and drugs (and other stimuli) by opioid pathways, and craving by serotonergic pathways. This hypothesis has given rise to potential treatment options (discussed under Management, below).

Liver

Alcohol is hepatotoxic even in the presence of adequate nutrition. A single weekend of heavy drinking may be all that is necessary to produce a fatty liver. This may represent a stress reaction, as the adrenals contribute to the mobilization of fatty acids while the liver is occupied metabolizing alcohol. Continued drinking may produce alcoholic hepatitis. Whereas the fatty liver is asymptomatic, alcoholic hepatitis produces jaundice, fever, and loss of appetite. The size of the liver may increase, and enzyme levels may be elevated. Liver biopsy may reveal polymorphonuclear leukocytes and necrosis near the central vein. A typical, but nonspecific, feature of hepatocytes damaged by alcohol is the Mallory body, a hyaline inclusion. These effects on the liver may be due to the combination of a hepatic hypermetabolic state following alcohol exposure and inadequate oxygenation. Necrosis appears where the oxygen tension is lowest. Whereas fatty liver and alcoholic hepatitis are reversible, cirrhosis is not. It develops after continued necrosis and scar formation. The cirrhotic liver tends to be small and hard. Histologic findings of fatty liver, alcoholic hepatitis, and cirrhosis can be found concurrently in the same patient.[20] Although the risk of cirrhosis is a function of the amount of alcohol consumed, individual susceptibility also plays a role, and only about 10% of heavy drinkers develop clinically apparent cirrhosis (see Chapter 90).

The high prevalence of hepatitis C in the substance abusing population complicates the medical status of patients, their efforts at abstinence, and their psychiatric status (the latter adversely impacted by interferon treatment).

Pancreas

Acute pancreatitis seems to occur randomly among heavily drinking men.[21] The combination of heavy alcohol consumption, increased amylase, upper abdominal pain, nausea, and vomiting suggest the diagnosis, but it can be confirmed only at laparotomy or autopsy. The absence of an elevated amylase level does not rule out the diagnosis. Some alcoholics have an increased amylase level in the absence of pancreatitis due to amylase from the salivary glands. Radiographic findings may include a sentinel loop. Acute hemorrhagic pancreatitis can be fatal. Acute pancreatitis may be a separate entity or the early stage of chronic alcoholic pancreatitis. Seventy-five percent of cases of chronic pancreatitis in the United States are related to alcohol abuse.[21] Deep epigastric pain radiating to the back following alcohol ingestion or a heavy meal is the characteristic presentation. There may be few physical findings. Amylase levels may be normal. Ultrasonography, computed tomography, and endoscopic retrograde pancreatography are useful tests for confirming the diagnosis. Relief of pain and abstinence from alcohol are the foundation for the treatment of chronic alcoholic pancreatitis. Abstinence may allow the patient to avoid more severe disease but does not necessarily normalize pancreatic function (see Chapter 89).

Prenatal Effects

Alcohol consumption during the first trimester is associated with multiple fetal anomalies. Exposure during the second and third trimesters is associated with growth retardation and neurobehavioral changes such as sleep disturbances and decreased attentiveness. Moderate to heavy drinking pregnant women experience a two- to fourfold increase in the incidence of second trimester spontaneous abortions. Fetal alcohol syndrome (FAS) describes a set of fetal abnormalities associated with alcohol consumption during pregnancy. The prevalence of FAS in the United States ranges from 0.5 to 3.0 per 1000 live births, and higher in some populations.[3] Criteria for FAS are prenatal or postnatal growth retardation (or both), central nervous system (CNS) involvement, and specific craniofacial dysmorphic features (microcephaly, hypoplastic maxilla, thinned upper lip, short upturned nose, and short palpebral fissure). Facial features associated with FAS tend to disappear during adulthood. Until recently, infants of alcoholic mothers who partially meet the criteria were diagnosed as having fetal alcohol effect (FAE). The Institute of Medicine of the National Academy of Sciences has classified prenatal alcohol exposure into five categories. Three categories represent children who have all or some of the FAS facial features. The other two categories do not have FAS facial features: alcohol-related neurodevelopmental disorder (ARND) and alcohol-related birth defects (ARBDs). Magnetic resonance imaging (MRI) scans of children with FAS show proportionally reduced basal ganglia, a smaller corpus callosum and cerebellum. The peak BAC contributes more to the development of FAS than does the amount consumed.[6] The more severe morphologic defects occur with more extreme levels of alcohol consumption. There is substantial individual variation in susceptibility to alcohol's effect on the fetus. Not all women who drink heavily deliver FAS infants, but no ethnic or racial group is invulnerable to the teratogenic effect of alcohol.[22] In light of the severity of the risk of FAS, it is not yet possible to recommend that any level of alcohol consumption is safe for a pregnant woman (see Chapter 11).

Cardiac Effects: Risk Versus Benefit

Advice to patients should include a discussion of the potential risks and benefits associated with alcohol consumption. Caucasian-American men who report drinking fewer than three drinks per day were found to be less likely to die over a 12-year follow-up period than men who reported complete abstinence. Meta-analysis found that the lowest overall mortality for men was associated with an alcohol consumption of 10 g (less than one drink) per day for men and less for women. At 20 g of alcohol per day (between one and two drinks) women had an overall mortality significantly higher than abstainers.[3] The improved outcome is primarily associated with reduced coronary artery disease. Some risks of alcohol consumption may occur at moderate levels of consumption, including hemorrhagic stroke, vehicular accidents, harmful interactions with more than 100 medications and alternative medications, a 50% increase in breast cancer among women drinking three to nine drinks per week, and decreased intelligence quotient (IQ) of children born to mothers reporting as few as two drinks per day while pregnant. Heavy alcohol consumption over a period of years is associated with heart failure secondary to cardiomyopathy and susceptibility to a variety of other illnesses including tuberculosis (TB) and human immunodeficiency virus (HIV). Binge drinking has been associated with cardiac dysrhythmias, especially atrial fibrillation (see Chapter 77).

Physicians should inform their patients about these known trade-offs. Individuals who have a very low risk of heart disease are unlikely to experience reduced mortality from moderate drinking. The reverse appears to be true for those with a high risk of heart disease. Individuals with a family history of alcoholism should be frankly discouraged from drinking. The National Institute of Alcohol Abuse and Alcoholism recommends that people 65 and older limit their alcohol consumption to one drink per day.

Diagnosis

Alcoholics may be difficult to identify, and collateral information is often critical for evaluating the patient's history. Alcoholics often minimize alcohol's impact on their life, but collateral information from family and friends typically reveals personal and marital problems related to drinking. During any routine medical examination all adolescents and adults should be asked about alcohol use. No single symptom or test can diagnose alcoholism, although the screening tests described below[23,24] are useful. Screening may itself be beneficial by drawing the patient's attention to problems related to drinking, and it may promote self-monitoring and behavioral change.[25] The diagnostic criteria in the *Diagnostic and Statistical Manual of Mental Disorders*, 4th edition (DSM-IV)[26] (Table 59.3). defines alcohol abuse as recurrent problems in one or more of the four areas of functioning; dependence is defined by the presence of at least three of seven specific areas of dysfunction.

Screening

A variety of self-report instruments are available to screen for alcohol problems.[27] Administration times generally range from less than a minute to about 5 minutes. Perhaps the most common measure is the CAGE, an acronym for the key word in each of four questions related to drinking[28]:

1. Have you ever felt you should *C*ut down on your drinking?
2. Have people *A*nnoyed you by criticizing your drinking?
3. Have you ever felt *G*uilty about your drinking?
4. Have you ever had a drink first thing in the morning to steady your nerves or to get rid of a hangover (*E*ye-opener)?

Despite its popularity and brevity, the CAGE has certain limitations. In particular, it focuses on emotional reactions to drinking and asks about lifetime occurrence of symptoms rather than recent events.

The Michigan Alcoholism Screening Test (MAST)[29] and variants are also commonly used in primary care settings. This family of instruments has been criticized for focusing too heavily on late-stage symptoms such as liver pathology and delirium tremens. Furthermore, as with the CAGE, the questions on the MAST do not specify when the symptoms occurred, thus causing individuals with earlier, resolved problems to still score positively. Nevertheless, the CAGE, the MAST, and similar scales have fairly high validity.

A newer measure, the Alcohol Use Disorders Identification Test (AUDIT)[30] merits particular attention from primary care physicians (Table 59.4). Its advantages are brevity (approximately 2 minutes), focus on the preceding year, and item sampling from several domains (intake, level of dependence, and adverse consequences of drinking). The

---

Table 59.3. **Diagnosis of Alcohol Use Disorders**

Alcohol abuse
For a diagnosis of alcohol abuse the patient must show one or more of the following, related to alcohol, on a recurrent basis:
1. Failure to fulfill major role obligations
2. Use in physically hazardous situations
3. Legal problems
4. Continued use despite having persistent or recurrent social or interpersonal problems related to alcohol use

Alcohol dependence
For a diagnosis of alcohol dependence at least three of these seven criteria must be met:
1. Clinically significant tolerance[a]
2. Clinically significant withdrawal
3. Recurrent failure of intent
4. Recurrent failure of control
5. Preoccupation with alcohol
6. Predominance of alcohol-related activities
7. Continued alcohol use despite knowledge that the drinking contributes to a psychological, physical, social, or other problem

[a]It is noteworthy that tolerance to some effects of alcohol (e.g., gait, coordination) does not necessarily suggest tolerance to all effects. Certain effects, especially impaired social judgment, may demonstrate little or no tolerance.

Source: American Psychiatric Association,[5] with permission.

Table 59.4. **Alcohol Use Disorders Identification Test (AUDIT) Questionnaire**

1. How often do you have a drink containing alcohol?
   - (0) Never
   - (1) Monthly or less
   - (2) Two to four times a month
   - (3) Two or three times a week
   - (4) Four or more times a week
2. How many drinks containing alcohol do you have on a typical day when you are drinking?
   - (0) 1 or 2
   - (1) 3 or 4
   - (2) 5 or 6
   - (3) 7 or 9
   - (4) 10 or more
3. How often do you have six or more drinks on one occasion?
   - (0) Never
   - (1) Less than monthly
   - (2) Monthly
   - (3) Weekly
   - (4) Daily or almost daily
4. How often during the last year have you found that you were not able to stop drinking once you had started?
   - (0) Never
   - (1) Less than monthly
   - (2) Monthly
   - (3) Weekly
   - (4) Daily or almost daily
5. How often during the last year have you failed to do what was normally expected from you because of drinking?
   - (0) Never
   - (1) Less than monthly
   - (2) Monthly
   - (3) Weekly
   - (4) Daily or almost daily
6. How often during the last year have you needed a first drink in the morning to get yourself going after a heavy drinking session?
   - (0) Never
   - (1) Less than monthly
   - (2) Monthly
   - (3) Weekly
   - (4) Daily or almost daily
7. How often during the last year have you had a feeling of guilt or remorse after drinking?
   - (0) Never
   - (1) Less than monthly
   - (2) Monthly
   - (3) Weekly
   - (4) Daily or almost daily
8. How often during the last year have you been unable to remember what happened the night before because you had been drinking?
   - (0) Never
   - (1) Less than monthly
   - (2) Monthly
   - (3) Weekly
   - (4) Daily or almost daily
9. Have you or someone else been injured as a result of your drinking?
   - (0) No
   - (2) Yes, but not in the last year
   - (4) Yes, during the last year
10. Has a relative, friend, doctor, or other health worker been concerned about your drinking or suggested that you should cut down?
    - (0) No
    - (2) Yes, but not in the last year
    - (4) Yes, during the last year

Numbers in parentheses are scoring weights. The usual cutoff for the AUDIT to be scored as positive is 8 points.

AUDIT can be embedded in a general health risk appraisal survey dealing with other medical concerns such as smoking, diet, and nutrition. In a recent review contrasting it with other self-report alcohol screening measures, the AUDIT tended to perform best. A cutoff score of 6 points for females may be preferable to the more common research cutoff of 8.[31]

History

The history should include what the patient drinks, how much, how often, when alcohol was last drunk, and if the patient has used any other drugs or medications. Patients in denial minimize their drinking history. It is therefore important to review the history with the patient's family members or friends. The focus should not be on whether the individual has a problem with alcohol, but rather on the consequences of drinking (e.g., legal, financial, medical, social difficulties). Asking if others believe the patient has a problem or that drinking contributes to a social problem may be more effective than direct questions about the patient's drinking. It is important to inquire about previous withdrawal history, as successive withdrawals tend to become more severe.

Laboratory Tests

Laboratory tests can be used for screening and to support the diagnosis. Such tests might include measuring the BAC, a urine drug screen, bilirubin assay, prothrombin time, assays of liver-associated enzymes, electrolytes, and a complete blood count. Elevation of the bilirubin, liver-associated enzymes, and prothrombin time suggests the presence of liver dysfunction. Increased mean corpuscular volume (MCV) and mean corpuscular hemoglobin (MCH) and a decreased red blood cell (RBC) count suggest that the patient has been drinking heavily for weeks or months. MCV changes may persist for months.

The half-life of γ-glutamyltransferase (GGT) is approximately 26 days, and an elevated GGT level may be one of the most sensitive laboratory screening tests for alcoholism. An elevated carbohydrate-deficient transferrin (CDT) level is the most sensitive indicator of relapse to drinking in a purportedly abstinent patient.[23] Unlike the other biochemical markers, a rise in CDT does not seem to reflect organ damage, but rather recent heavy (five drinks or more per day) consumption of alcohol. (CDT was recently approved by the Food and Drug Administration as an indicator of excessive drinking, the first alcohol biomarker so approved.) An elevated aspartate transferase/alanine transferase (AST/ALT) ratio (e.g., 2:1 or higher) has been interpreted as evidence of liver disease secondary to drinking alcohol, whereas a reversed ratio (e.g. 1:2) has been seen as evidence of hepatitis due to other causes. This "rule" may not hold true for all populations. The simultaneous use of CDT and GGT assays to screen for excessive alcohol consumption seems reasonably sensitive (75%) and specific (85%). Ultimately, the diagnosis of alcohol dependence must meet the criteria established by the DSM-IV.[26]

Management

Intervention

The physician should give clear directions to the patient to reduce alcohol consumption, usually in the context of health, social, or family problems.[2] The goal is to present information about the illness in a manner that can be understood and accepted by the alcoholic. A more formal intervention may include gathering friends, family members, and even the employer to firmly confront the alcoholic's behavior. The goal of this type of intervention is to obtain the alcoholic's agreement to enter treatment that same day. To be successful, this procedure often requires hours of preparation before the intervention takes place. Some treatment programs assist the physician and family in preparing the intervention. The intervention is a powerful tool that often succeeds in getting the alcoholic patient into treatment. Patients entering treatment as a result of intervention often do as well as those who enter voluntarily.

Comprehensive Assessment

The American Society of Addiction Medicine (ASAM) has released the second version of the patient placement criteria (PPC-II), a tool to help the clinician utilize the data from a comprehensive assessment to determine the appropriate level of care for a particular patient. Although alcoholism is a primary illness, it is often accompanied by a variety of medical problems (Table 59.5).

Supportive Therapy During Withdrawal

Alcohol withdrawal produces adrenergic arousal. To compensate, the patient's room should be quiet and evenly lit to allow constant reorientation to surroundings. Dimming the room lights at night mimics diurnal variation and supports orientation. Staff members should present a pleasant, nonthreatening attitude. Restraints are rarely necessary with proper sedation. Patients may be allowed to eat and drink when they feel ready. Intravenous fluids are usually not necessary for uncomplicated alcohol withdrawal. The medical staff can promote long-term recovery by directing the patient to a rehabilitation program immediately following detoxification. Indeed, some aspects of rehabilitation can be started on the detoxification unit by providing books and tapes, an introduction to an Alcoholics Anonymous (AA) sponsor, and attendance at an AA meeting as soon as the patient is physically able.

Detoxification

Monitored detoxification safely transports the patient through withdrawal. Rehabilitation is the goal; detoxification is a step toward that goal. Detoxification may be done on an inpatient or outpatient basis depending on the clinical presentation and history of the patient. In the context of managed care pressures, outpatient or ambulatory detoxification is becoming more commonplace and appears to work well for many pa-

Table 59.5. **Summary of Alcohol Effects**

Organ	Acute effect (up to months)	Chronic effects (years)
Breast	Portion of blood alcohol content in breast milk	?Increased risk of breast cancer Male breast enlargement
Cardiovascular system	Moderate blood pressure increase "Holiday heart" syndrome[a]	Hypertension
Central nervous system (CNS)	Impaired motor coordination Sleep apnea	Depression Dementia Peripheral neuropathy Widening of frontal cortical sulci Distal symmetric polyneuropathy Hemorrhagic stroke
Endocrine system	Increased plasma corticosteroids Increased plasma catecholamines	Low testosterone Testicular atrophy Amenorrhea, anovulation
Fetal development	Fetal alcohol syndrome	
Gastrointestinal system	Delayed gastric emptying Gastroesophageal reflux Injures the gastric mucosa Loss of enzymes (disaccharidases) Worsen preexisting peptic ulcers	Esophageal carcinoma Chronic atrophic gastritis ?Gastric carcinoma[b] Esophageal inflammation
Hematopoietic system		Megaloblastic anemia Decreased platelet function
Immune system		Increased risk of infections Decreased production of polymorphonuclear leukocytes Decreased cell-mediated immunity Decreased T lymphocytes Impaired phagocytosis
Liver	Fat deposition Liver enlargement Alcoholic hepatitis	Cirrhosis Hepatocellular carcinoma[c]
Muscular system	Increased chance of muscle injury Sudden muscle necrosis	Chronic alcoholic myopathy
Nutritional system	Interferes with vitamin metabolism Inhibits gluconeogenesis Indirect loss of calcium and potassium Loss of magnesium, zinc, and phosphorus Thiamine deficiency	Folate deficiency Thiamine deficiency Alcoholic ketoacidosis Decreased serum calcium Wernicke-Korsakoff syndrome
Other malignancies		Squamous cell carcinoma of the head and neck
Pancreas	Acute pancreatitis	Chronic pancreatitis Pseudocyst formation
Pulmonary system	Increased cough and sputum production	Pneumonia

[a]Holiday heart syndrome refers to atrial or ventricular dysrhythmias following days of heavy drinking.
[b]Smoking may also contribute to the development of gastrointestinal carcinoma.
[c]May be secondary to hepatitis B virus.

tients.[32] Once detoxified, an alcoholic may still not function well cognitively for days, weeks, or months.

Withdrawal Syndrome

Alcohol withdrawal consists of signs and symptoms ranging from hangover to delirium tremens. The severity depends on the patient's age, physical condition, prior withdrawals, and amount of alcohol consumed. Withdrawal begins as the blood alcohol level falls and includes anxiety, restlessness, insomnia, and nausea. About 24 hours after the last drink (sometimes days longer) the patient may have increased blood pressure and pulse, a low-grade fever, and tremors that increase with the withdrawal severity. Hand tremors may be the most reliable early sign of alcohol withdrawal unless the tremors

are reduced by beta-blockers or other medication. Patients in withdrawal may also have tachycardia and dry mouth, which may be misinterpreted as volume depletion. During withdrawal, total body water is more likely to be normal, and plasma volume is likely to be increased.[33] Transient hallucinations may occur that involve any sense, but visual hallucinations are more common. Typically, 2 days after the last drink (but occasionally up to 10 days after the last drink) one or more grand mal seizures occur. Seizures occur in about 5% of untreated withdrawal patients; 30% to 40% of patients with seizures proceed to delirium tremens, typically during the third to fifth day of withdrawal, if adequate treatment is not provided. Delirium tremens is characterized by severe autonomic hyperactivity (e.g., tachycardia, hypertension, fever, diaphoresis, tremor), electrolyte disturbances, hyperreflexia, confusion, disorientation, and clouding of consciousness. Dysperceptions, especially visual and tactile hallucinations, are common, usually without the insight that accompanies hallucinations of milder withdrawal. Delusions are likewise common. Psychomotor activity may fluctuate widely during the course of the delirium, and the patient frequently demonstrates affective lability. Delirium tremens typically persist for 3 to 5 days. Medical management is directed at patient safety, as pharmacologic intervention has not been demonstrated to shorten the duration of the delirium. The physician should be aware that in a debilitated or elderly patient a delirium of any etiology may persist for weeks beyond resolution of the cause of the delirium. Delirium tremens may be fatal, especially in debilitated or elderly patients.

Adolescents often do not develop the classic signs of physical withdrawal seen in adults. They do exhibit the usual behavioral and emotional aspects of dependence. Elderly patients usually have more severe withdrawal than young patients. The rehabilitation progress of elderly patients may be delayed owing to the slower metabolism of medications used to control their alcohol withdrawal.

Pharmacotherapy

The physician should assess the patient's risk of withdrawal before treatment begins. The Clinical Institute Withdrawal Assessment (CIWA)-Ar scale may be used as an adjunct to assess the patient's risk for severe withdrawal.[34] A decision to allow the patient to go through withdrawal without the benefit of medication should be carried out only with informed consent.

Oral multivitamin supplementation, including thiamine, folic acid, and pyridoxine, should be given when the patient can tolerate oral fluids. If intravenous fluids containing dextrose are needed, 100 mg thiamine should be added to each liter of intravenous fluid administered to the patient. A normal magnesium level does not necessarily mean that magnesium supplementation is unnecessary. Serum magnesium levels do not correlate with CSF magnesium levels. Adequate levels of magnesium help prevent cardiac dysrhythmia and seizures. If the clinical history and examination suggest that the patient is at risk for serious withdrawal or is nutritionally compromised, $MgSO_4$ 2 g IM (deep) up to every 8 hours for 2 to 3 days may be administered.

The pharmacologic basis for detoxification traditionally has been the use of cross-tolerant medication to control alcohol withdrawal. Usually the agent chosen is a benzodiazepine or a barbiturate with a longer biologic half-life than alcohol. Residual symptoms are treated with adjunctive medications (e.g., antiemetic for nausea). Pharmacotherapy is justified to prevent or treat signs and symptoms of withdrawal and possibly to curb alcoholic dementia and kindling.[35] The "kindling" hypothesis suggests that repeated subthreshold (for seizures) stimulation of the CNS during withdrawal increases the risk of subsequent withdrawal seizures. All protocols for the treatment of withdrawal should be modified according to patient needs. Individuals with physical dependence on more than one drug should first be withdrawn from the drug that produces the most dangerous withdrawal. In practice, it may mean withdrawing the patient from sedative-hypnotics (e.g., alcohol) first while medically delaying withdrawal from opiates.

An appropriate benzodiazepine for the treatment of alcohol withdrawal can be selected based on the patient's age and hepatic function. Diazepam is preferred if the patient is under 55 years of age and has a well-functioning liver. Oxazepam is appropriate for older patients and those with liver dysfunction. Diazepam is administered 10 to 20 mg po every hour until the patient's symptoms are relieved and the patient is sedated. Further doses may be unnecessary. Total dosage should not exceed 60 mg without further evaluation by the physician, but doses in excess of 120 mg within 24 hours are not uncommon in the heavy drinker. Patients who are tolerant of alcohol are similarly tolerant of other sedative-hypnotics. Intramuscular chlordiazepoxide is less desirable because of erratic uptake, prolonged metabolism, and delayed onset. Patients requiring high-dose withdrawal pharmacotherapy should be in a monitored bed.

Oxazepam (15–30 mg) may also be given orally every hour until the patient's symptoms are relieved or the patient becomes drowsy. Unlike the diazepam regimen, the cumulative dose of oxazepam necessary to initially relieve the patient's symptoms is repeated every 6 to 8 hours for the remainder of the first day of treatment. The dose is then reduced by 25% on each subsequent day. Most patients complete the regimen by the fifth day.

Phenobarbital remains a reliable, effective medication for the treatment of alcohol withdrawal, for mixed sedative-hypnotic withdrawal, and for seizure prophylaxis when used by experienced clinicians as part of an established protocol. It is easily absorbed. Phenobarbital's effectiveness has been reported to be superior to that of diazepam for delirium tremens.[36] Nervousness or nausea may be treated with promethazine (Phenergan) or hydroxyzine (Atarax, Vistaril). Until recently there was scant literature supporting the use of anticonvulsants in withdrawal treatment, except in the case of an independent seizure disorder. Research supports the clinical efficacy of some agents.[37] For delirious, hallucinating, and combative patients, haloperidol is the agent of choice, in combination with the above withdrawal agents. Haloperidol is safe in oral, intramuscular, and intravenous doses of 70 to 80 mg/day for monitored patients; higher doses are not uncommon. Usually, a dose of just 5 mg orally or intramuscularly two to four times a day is sufficient. The potential of haloperidol to lower seizure threshold is controlled by concomitant administration of an anticonvulsant.

Complications

Seizures are one of the most common complications of alcohol withdrawal. If a seizure occurs, diazepam 5 to 10 mg IV is given until the seizures are controlled or the patient is drowsy but responsive. Causes other than withdrawal should be determined if seizures are associated with head trauma, are not preceded by tremulousness, are focal in nature, or a residual neurologic defect is present (see Chapter 64).

The combination of liver dysfunction and poor vitamin K absorption can contribute to systemic bleeding. In these circumstances, minor head trauma can lead to a subdural hematoma. This diagnosis should be considered if the patient does not recover as expected.[37] The differential diagnosis for seizures also includes infection and metabolic disturbances.

Keeping the patient in the program during withdrawal is one of the most difficult challenges facing the clinician. Alcoholic patients often have a strong but unrecognized compulsion to leave treatment and return to drinking. Patients who receive adequate medication for withdrawal are less likely to leave "against medical advice." From the first day of treatment, the detoxification unit staff should repeatedly educate the patient that rehabilitation is the treatment goal, not just detoxification. Patients whose urge to leave treatment persists can often be encouraged by concerned family members to persevere.

Rehabilitation

Treatment approaches involving the family tend to be more effective than individual-focused treatment for alcoholics. The family can be used to motivate the patient to enter and stay in treatment. The family can set a common goal, participate in education, and reduce emotional distress. Rehabilitation can be accomplished on an inpatient or outpatient basis or in a partial hospitalization program. Inpatient rehabilitation is preferred for patients who require nursing care or continuous observation, and for those who need an opportunity to progress in an environment that is free of violence and drugs. The severity of alcohol dependence and the absence of an adequate social support system may also justify inpatient treatment. Patients without convenient and reliable transportation may have a better chance of success in an inpatient program. Patients should be individually assessed and given the appropriate level of treatment from the start. The ASAM PPC-II[23] is currently being validated, and it may be used to guide the family physician to select the most appropriate level of treatment for a specific patient. The "first fail" philosophy, which requires patients to fail the least intensive treatment program before they can receive more intensive treatment, may not be cost-effective and is not consistent with quality medical care.

Physical evaluation, psychological assessment, and education of the patient and the patient's family are the foundation of rehabilitation programs. Typically, it is accomplished with group and individual therapy, classes, a family program, and a relapse prevention program. Many programs ascribe to the 12 steps of Alcoholics Anonymous as the philosophic basis of their programs. The long-term success of patients treated in such programs varies,[38] but when there is employer and family support the results can be outstanding.[39]

Continuing Care

An aftercare plan specific to the patient's needs should be created. The family physician should be familiar with this and encourage compliance with the plan. Physicians should generally avoid giving aftercare patients mood-altering medications, as these drugs may increase the chance of relapse. As previously indicated, antidepressants and the opioid antagonists may constitute an exception to this general recommen-

dation. Alcoholism is sometimes associated with a wide range of psychiatric disorders; most notable are mood or affective disorders, anxiety disorders (especially posttraumatic stress disorder), mania, and schizophrenia. When coexisting with another psychiatric disorder, both that disorder and the alcoholism may be exacerbated; both must be treated. Potentially addictive medications should be avoided when treating coexisting psychiatric disorders in alcoholic patients, but rapidly acting benzodiazepines should be specifically avoided. In the event that hospitalization is needed for a condition requiring pain medication or anesthesia, the patient is given medications as necessary, but mood-altering medications are discontinued while the patient is still in the hospital.

Current evidence indicates that serotonin reuptake inhibitors can reduce drinking by heavy drinkers whether or not they are depressed, but the magnitude of the decrease is not dramatic. Placebo-controlled trials showed that naltrexone (ReVia) 50 mg/day could benefit alcoholics in terms of relapse prevention. Naltrexone reduced the number of drinking days and craving for alcohol. Compared to the serotonergic drugs, the opioid antagonists seem to produce more consistent reductions in alcohol consumption.[16] Some aftercare plans include disulfiram in an effort to prevent relapse. If disulfiram is prescribed, specific procedures to ensure compliance are needed. The family physician should educate the patient about food, medications, and cosmetics that contain alcohol and might produce a disulfiram-alcohol reaction. Relapses do occur, and the physician should use such occasions to refocus the continuing care plan for the patient and family.

Prevention

Physicians can play a major role in the prevention and treatment of alcohol-related problems. Training for this role should begin in medical school. Interested faculty members should be offered fellowship training in the study of addiction. Curricula and tests ought to include alcohol-related topics. Medical students and residents should play an integral role on the team that cares for patients in addiction treatment centers. This kind of physician training can support community initiatives for education and social policy changes to prevent alcohol abuse.

Of all the proposed methods to prevent alcohol abuse, education is the least controversial. The most effective educational efforts probably occur during or before adolescence. After that, peer influence becomes more important than parental influence. The physician can support parental norms by teaching adolescents to be comfortable standing up for what they believe. Counseling that delays the onset of drinking until age 15 or later may reduce alcohol related problems.[8] Such "anticipatory guidance" teaches adolescents respect for their own beliefs. The physician can also identify adolescent patients at particularly high risk for alcoholism due to their family backgrounds, peer associations, difficulties in school, or problems with impulse control. These adolescents need specific education concerning the risks of drinking alcohol during pregnancy or while driving.

Social policy changes can support education in preventing alcohol abuse. Several decades ago the price of a beer was a quarter while the price of a soft drink was a nickel. This 5:1 ratio of alcoholic beverage cost to soft drink cost has been lost. The main reason for the change is that taxation on alcoholic beverages has not kept pace with inflation. Today there is near parity in price for these beverages. Social policies that restrict the consumption of alcohol-containing beverages seem to reduce per-capita consumption of alcohol.[40]

Family and Community Issues

Alcohol-related motor vehicle accidents cause more than 20,000 deaths each year. This toll disproportionately affects young Americans. Nearly half of the violent deaths (accidents, suicide, homicide) among males under age 34 are alcohol-related.[6]

Risks of an automobile accident increase sharply as the BAC rises. Heightened risk begins near 0.04% BAC, and the risk of an accident is doubled at 0.06% BAC. A driver with a BAC of 0.08%, a common legal limit, is six times as likely to have an accident than a sober driver.[18] Raising the drinking age from 18 to 21 years results in decreased alcohol use among high school seniors and an overall decrease in alcohol-related traffic accidents.[41] Raising the legal drinking age has been associated with decreased death rates from automobile accidents, unintentional injuries, and suicide among adolescents and young adults.[42] The single most important deterrent that enhances traffic safety is license suspension.[43] For those convicted of a driving under the influence (DUI) offense, an education program successfully completed may be beneficial; however, the repeat offender also benefits from treatment, including involvement with AA.[44]

Ethical Issues and Physician Responsibilities

Households in which chemicals are abused are at substantially greater risk for both physical and sexual abuse. Neither the victim nor the perpetrator of abuse is likely to speak freely. The victim may experience fear of more severe abuse or even death, abandonment by the abuser, or the shame of being discovered to be a victim. The abuser is fearful of being caught and punished; losing family, job, and freedom; and being publicly humiliated. Honest disclosure by the patient and honest reporting by the physician are also limited by a frequently overlooked factor: in the managed care environment, it is not unusual that payment for services may be denied if the injury has resulted from intoxication. The likelihood of honest disclosure is increased if the physician offers support, hope, and understanding.

There are legal guidelines that govern the physician's actions in the event of threatened suicide or assault, but danger to others may also take the form of an intoxicated patient planning to drive home from the emergency room. Ordinarily, intoxicated patients cannot be legally restrained unless they can be committed under state law, except by police. If a patient is thought to be impaired, it becomes the provider's duty to persuade the patient not to drive, to use a taxi, to call a friend, and as a last resort to contact the police and inform them of the situation. Public safety may take precedence over the patient's right to confidentiality, and failure to notify appropriate authorities of a threat to public safety exposes the physician to liability. This caution may apply especially for employees of the U.S. Department of Transportation. Legal counsel is recommended before notification, as this area is in flux.

Ethical guidelines for physicians and other health care professionals clearly stipulate the responsibility to report an impaired health care provider. The treatment success rate for impaired physicians is among the highest of any patient group. Utilizing intervention services through the licensure board or impaired provider programs allows the impaired provider to maintain professional status, employment, and self-respect by receiving treatment. It also protects the public.

References

1. Bradley K. The primary care practitioner's role in the prevention and management of alcohol problems. Alcohol Health Res World 1994;18(2):97–104.
2. Barry K, Fleming M. The family physician. Alcohol Health Res World 1994;18(2):105–9.
3. U.S. Department of Health and Human Services. The tenth special report to the U.S. Congress on alcohol and health. Rockville, MD: Public Health Service, National Institutes of Health, National Institute on Alcohol Abuse and Alcoholism, 2000;xiii, 14–17,30,273,283–295,364,365.
4. Blose J, Holder H. Injury-related medical care utilization in a problem drinking population. Am J Public Health 1991;81:1571–5.
5. American Psychiatric Association. Diagnostic and statistical manual of mental disorders. 3rd rev. ed. Washington, DC: American Psychiatric Press, 1987;173.
6. U.S. Department of Health and Human Services. The seventh special report to the U.S. Congress on alcohol and health. Rockville, MD: Public Health Service, Alcohol, Drug Abuse, and Mental Health Administration, 1990:ix,xv,xxii,xxiv,26,27, 33–36,46,119,123,141.
7. Conigliaro J, Maisto SA, McNeil M, et al. Does race make a difference among primary care patients with alcohol problems who agree to enroll in a study of brief interventions? Am J Addict 2000;9(4):321–30.
8. DeWit DJ, Adlaf EA, Offord DR, et al. Age at first alcohol use: a risk factor for the development of alcohol disorders. Am J Psychiatry 2000;157:745–50.
9. Smith D. Social and economic consequences of addiction in America. Commonwealth 1996;90(5):1–4.
10. National Institute on Alcohol Abuse and Alcoholism. Publication no. 35 PH371, January, 1997.
11. Parker DA, Harford TC. Gender-role attitudes, job competition and alcohol consumption among women and men. Alcohol Clin Exp Res 1992;16:159–65.
12. Brower K, Blow F, Beresford T. Treatment implications of chemical dependency models: an integrative approach. J Subst Abuse Treat 1989;6:147–57.
13. Devor E. A developmental-genetic model of alcoholism: implications for genetic research. J Consult Clin Psychol 1994;62: 1108–15.
14. Kaprio J, Viken R, Koskenvuo M, Romanov K, Rose R. Consistency and change in patterns of social drinking: a 6-year fol-

low-up of the Finnish Twin Cohort. Alcohol Clin Exp Res 1992; 16:234–40.

15. Wall T, Ehlers C. Acute effects of alcohol on P300 in Asians with different ALDH2 genotypes. Alcohol Clin Exp Res 1995; 19:617–22.

16. Kranzler H, Anton R. Implications of recent neuropsychopharmacologic research for understanding the etiology and development of alcoholism. J Consult Clin Psychol 1994;62:1116–26.

17. Schuckit MA, Edenberg HJ, Kalmijn J, et al. A genome-wide search for genes that relate to a low level of response to alcohol. Alcohol Clin Exp Res 2001;25(3):323–9.

18. Goldstein DB. Pharmacology of alcohol. New York: Oxford University Press, 1983:80.

19. Brooks PJ. Brain atrophy and neuronal loss in alcoholism: a role for DNA damage? Neurochem Int 2000;37(5–6):403–12.

20. Maddrey W. Alcoholic hepatitis: clinico-pathologic features and therapy. Semin Liver Dis 1988;8:91–102.

21. Geokas M. Ethanol and the pancreas. Med Clin North Am 1984;68:60–7.

22. Day N, Richardson G. Prenatal alcohol exposure: a continuum of effects. Semin Perinatol 1991;15:272–9.

23. Allen JP, Litten RZ. The role of laboratory tests in alcoholism treatment. J Subst Abuse Treat 2001;81:85.

24. Alexander D, Gwyther R. Alcoholism in adolescents and their families. Pediatr Clin North Am 1995;42:217–30.

25. Allen J, Maisto S, Connors G. Self-report screening tests for alcohol problems in primary care. Arch Intern Med 1995;155: 1726–30.

26. Diagnostic and statistical manual of mental disorders, 4th ed. Washington, DC: American Psychiatric Association, 1994;176–83.

27. Connors GJ. Screening for alcohol problems. In: Assessing alcohol problems: a guide for clinicians and researchers. Washington, DC: DHHS, 1995;17–29.

28. Ewing JA. Detecting alcoholism, the CAGE questionnaire. JAMA 1984;252:1905–7.

29. Selzer ML. The Michigan alcoholism screening test: the quest for a new diagnostic instrument. Am J Psychiatry 1971;127: 1653–8.

30. U.S. Department of Health and Human Services. Assessing alcohol problem. Rockville, MD: DHHS, 1995: series 4:11, 22, 260. NIH publ. no. 95-3745.

31. Allen JP, Litten RZ, Fertig JB, Babor T. A review of research on the Alcohol Use Disorders Identification Test (AUDIT). Alcohol Clin Exp Res 1997;21(4):613–19.

32. Soyka M, Horak M. Ambulatory detoxification of alcoholic patients—evaluation of a model project (article in German). Gesundheitswesen 2000 Jan;62(1):15–20.

33. Mander A, Young A, Merrick M, et al. Fluid balance, vasopressin and withdrawal symptoms during detoxification from alcohol. Drug Alcohol Depend 1987;24:233–7.

34. Foy A, March S, Drinkwater V. Use of an objective clinical scale in the assessment and management of alcohol withdrawal in a large general hospital. Alcohol Clin Exp Res 1988;12:360–4.

35. Nutt D, Glue P. Neuropharmacological and clinical aspects of alcohol withdrawal. Ann Med 1990;22:275–81.

36. Kramp P, Rafaelsen O. Delirium tremens: a double blind comparison of diazepam and barbital treatment. Acta Psychiatr Scand 1978;58:174–90.

37. Koranyi E, Ravindran A, Seguin J. Alcohol withdrawal concealing symptoms of subdural hematoma—a caveat. Psychiatr J Univ Ottawa 1990;15:15–17.

38. Vaillant G. A summing up: the natural history of alcoholism. Cambridge: Harvard University Press, 1983;307–16.

39. Cross G, Morgan C. Mooney A, Martin C, Rafter J. Alcoholism treatment: a ten-year follow-up study. Alcohol Clin Exp Res 1990;14:169–73.

40. Hoadley J, Fuch B. Holder H. The effect of alcohol beverage restrictions on consumption: a 25 year longitudinal analysis. Am J Drug Alcohol Abuse 1984;10:375–401.

41. O'Malley P, Wagenaar A. Effects of minimum drinking age laws on alcohol use, related behaviors and traffic crash involvement among American youth: 1976–1987. J Stud Alcohol 1991;52: 478–91.

42. Jones N, Pieper C, Robertson L. The effect of legal drinking age on fatal injuries of adolescents and young adults. Am J Public Health 1992;82:112–15.

43. Mann R, Vingilis E, Gavin D, Adlaf E, Anglin L. Sentence severity and the drinking driver: relationships with traffic safety outcome. Accid Anal Prev 1991;23:483–91.

44. Green R, French J, Haberman P, Holland P. The effects of combining sanction and rehabilitation for driving under the influence: an evaluation of the New Jersey Countermeasures Program. Accid Anal Prev 1991;23:543–55.

60
Care of the Patient Who Misuses Drugs

Jerome E. Schulz

Patients who misuse drugs are commonly seen by family physicians in the clinic, emergency room, and hospital. Almost all patients who misuse illicit drugs also misuse alcohol and tobacco, and those medical complications are discussed elsewhere in this book (see Chapters 8, 59, and 83).

Acute Medical Treatment

Cocaine

Although the illicit use of cocaine declined during the early 1980s, its misuse increased dramatically in 1985 with the marketing of "crack" cocaine. Crack is a highly addictive form of cocaine readily accessible at a low cost (as inexpensive as $5 to $10). Crack cocaine misuse has changed cocaine from a drug of the rich and affluent to a drug anyone can afford (including adolescents and children). Cocaine continues to be one of the most commonly reported illicit drugs causing emergency room visits. The age of the average cocaine user has dropped substantially, and the number of female cocaine abusers has risen since the mid-1980s. The use of cocaine has declined over the past 5 years.

Cocaine hydrochloride is water-soluble and can be injected intravenously or inhaled intranasally (snorted). Cocaine hydrochloride cannot be smoked because it decomposes. If it is dissolved in ether and distilled, the base form of cocaine (freebase) is reprecipitated, and this substance can be smoked. "Crack" cocaine is produced by dissolving cocaine hydrochloride in sodium bicarbonate and distilling off the water. It then forms "rocks," which can be smoked. The term *crack* comes from the noise the rocks make as they are heated and smoked.

Effects

Cocaine causes euphoria, talkativeness, increased energy, and increased confidence. Rapid euphoria is followed by a let-down characterized by depression, irritability, restlessness, and a generalized feeling of uneasiness and discomfort. When misusers start feeling letdown, they use more cocaine, which results in blood levels that frequently cause medical complications and can be lethal. Alcohol is frequently used with cocaine and forms cocaethylene, which produces prolonged symptoms and toxicity.[1] The most frequent presenting complaints for patients misusing cocaine are listed in Table 60.1. Physical findings suggestive of cocaine misuse include agitation, dehydration, malnutrition, tachycardia, elevated blood pressure, rhinorrhea, singed eyebrows (from crack or freebase smoking), coughing, wheezing, poor dentition, and a generally unkempt appearance.

Complications

The three primary cardiovascular complications of cocaine abuse are hypertension, myocardial ischemia, and cardiac arrhythmias. Cardiac toxicity can occur with all three routes of administration (intranasal, intravenous, and inhaled). In individuals who are sensitive to cocaine or who have coronary artery disease, cardiac symptoms can occur with relatively low doses of cocaine. Cocaine's effect on the heart appears to be caused by blocking the reuptake of norepinephrine at the neuronal synapses. The norepinephrine excess produces an increased heart rate and increased blood pressure; simultaneous coronary vasospasm decreases the myocardial oxygen supply. The increased cardiac work load with decreased oxygenation causes chest pains in one half to two thirds of heavy cocaine users. Cocaine also enhances platelet aggregation and in situ thrombus formation.[2]

Hypertension usually responds to diazepam 5 to 10 mg IV repeated for three doses if needed.[3] If the blood pressure does not respond, give an α-adrenergic blocker such as phentolamine, or a direct vasodilator such as nitrates, hydralazine, or nitroprusside intravenously.[4] Beta-blocking agents should not be used because in conjunction with cocaine they increase

Table 60.1. **Chief Complaints and Presenting Problems—Cocaine**

Chest pain
Cardiac arrhythmias
New-onset seizures
Recurrent sinusitis
Anxiety problems
Cough
Chronic nasal problems
Headache
Sleep disorders
Family dysfunction
Weight loss
Obstetrical complications

vasoconstriction, increase the blood pressure, decrease left ventricular function, and can cause a paroxysmal increase in heart rate.

Cocaine causes myocardial ischemia and chest pain (see Chapter 76). Cocaine misuse should be suspected in any young patient who presents with chest pain. The risk of an acute myocardial infarction increases dramatically after the use of cocaine.[5] A positive urine drug screen for benzoylecgonine (a metabolite of cocaine) confirms the presence of cocaine.

Electrocardiographic (ECG) changes of ischemia are common, but occasionally are not present even with an acute myocardial infarction caused by cocaine. It is impossible to clinically differentiate patients with cocaine-induced chest pain and those experiencing a myocardial infarction.[6] Patients frequently do not admit they have been using cocaine.[7] If patients are "coming down" from a cocaine binge, they may have significant chest pain but do not report it.[8]

The evaluation of cocaine misusers with chest pain is also complicated by increased serum creatine kinase containing M and B subunits caused by cocaine-induced rhabdomyolysis.[9] Cardiac troponin I is more specific for the diagnosis of myocardial infarction in patients with cocaine-associated ischemia.

Nitroglycerin relieves the coronary spasm caused by cocaine, and it should be used as the initial treatment.[10] Phentolamine can be used if the chest pain persists. Thrombolytic therapy appears to be safe for cocaine-associated myocardial infarction after the blood pressure is normal unless a subarachnoid hemorrhage or aortic dissection is suspected.[11] Calcium channel blocking agents should be used cautiously because animal studies have shown they increase cocaine's cardiac toxicity. Patients with cocaine-induced myocardial infarction should not be treated with beta-blocking agents. Chronic cocaine misuse causes myocardial fibrosis and congestive heart failure.[12]

The most common arrhythmia associated with cocaine misuse is tachycardia, but it usually resolves spontaneously as the drug is metabolized or with use of an anxiolytic agent. Cocaine-induced wide complex dysrhythmias associated with acidosis need to be treated aggressively with sodium bicarbonate.[13] Both acidosis and hyperthermia (which should be treated aggressively with rapid cooling to prevent rhabdomyolysis and subsequent renal failure) are associated with a poor prognosis

in cocaine intoxication.[14] Because cocaine has properties similar to those of type I antiarrhythmic agents (procainamide and quinidine), the potential exists for increased toxicity if these agents are used to treat cocaine-induced arrhythmias.[15] If patients state that they have a feeling of "impending doom," cardiovascular collapse may be imminent. Initial euphoria rapidly changes to irritability with hallucinations. After an initial elevation of the pulse and blood pressure, the patient may experience a rapid fall in blood pressure and develop life-threatening cardiac arrhythmias. Other cardiovascular complications caused by cocaine misuse are aortic rupture, subacute and acute endocarditis (for injection drug users), pneumopericardium, and left ventricular hypertrophy.

Smugglers may swallow large bags of cocaine to prevent detection ("body packing"). Rupture of the bags causes severe cocaine intoxication, which can be treated with activated charcoal (50–100 g in adults) and a cathartic along with all the treatments described above. The term *body stuffing* describes the ingestion of cocaine packets to hide the evidence when confronted by the police. This usually involves lesser quantities of cocaine but it can lead to more toxicity because the cocaine is poorly wrapped. Frequently it does not show up on x-ray.[16]

Seizures are common with cocaine misuse. Cocaine decreases the seizure threshold and increases the body temperature, which makes an individual more susceptible to seizures. The increased body temperature is caused by vasoconstriction and increased muscle activity. Seizures may also be a terminal event in severe overdose patients. Children passively exposed to cocaine in crack houses or small confined areas where crack is being smoked may have seizures. Cocaine and cocaethylene can also be ingested by breast-feeding infants. A urine toxicology screen for benzoylecgonine should be considered for all children presenting with their first seizure.[17] Intravenous diazepam is the treatment of choice for seizures caused by cocaine (see Chapter 64).

Subarachnoid hemorrhages occur with cocaine misuse. They are caused by ruptured aneurysms or arteriovenous malformations secondary to the marked elevation in the blood pressure from cocaine. Cerebral infarction associated with cocaine misuse may be caused by vasoconstriction and increased platelet aggregation caused by cocaine. A urine toxicology screen should be obtained on any young person presenting with stroke symptoms. There are reported cases of cerebral infarction in infants born to mothers who misused cocaine during pregnancy.[18] Cocaine misuse should be considered in patients who have a sudden onset of severe new headaches, which may precede a cerebral vascular accident (see Chapter 65).

Serious obstetric complications, including abruptio placentae, spontaneous abortions, premature labor, and stillbirths, are increased in cocaine-misusing pregnant women.[19] Intrauterine exposure to cocaine causes fetal atrial and ventricular arrhythmias, congestive heart failure, cardiorespiratory arrest, and fetal death.[20] Newborn infants may demonstrate signs of cocaine withdrawal, including irritability, tremulousness, and poor eating. Maternal–infant bonding is poor. Although long-term effects are not clear, cocaine babies may have developmental delays and attention-deficit disorders.[21]

The most common psychiatric symptoms of cocaine misuse are paranoia, anxiety, and depression. Paranoia occurs in 80% to 90% of heavy cocaine misusers, and these patients are at high risk to develop a psychosis. The psychosis (similar to an amphetamine psychosis) may seem to be an acute schizophrenic episode, but it clears within 12 to 24 hours. Hallucinations called "snow lights" (flashing visual hallucinations) and "coke bugs" (tactile and visual hallucinations) are common with cocaine misuse. Patients experience withdrawal symptoms when they stop using cocaine. Initially, they become lethargic and somnolent. Depression is common after cocaine cessation, and patients frequently experience severe anhedonia that may last several months (antidepressants such as desipramine may help).

Smoking cocaine can cause a cough with black sputum production and dyspnea. Hemoptysis and spontaneous pneumothorax are common in crack addicts. Pulmonary edema (noncardiac) may be an acute hypersensitivity reaction. Patients with "crack lung syndrome" have fever, marked bronchospasm, infiltrates, eosinophilia, marked pruritus, and increased immunoglobulin E (IgE). Bronchiolitis obliterans and organizing pneumonia (BOOP) has been reported in crack cocaine users. Both crack lung and BOOP may respond to high-dose systemic steroids.[22] Asthma can be exacerbated by smoking crack cocaine. Pollutants in crack can also cause bronchitis and tracheitis.

Severe rhabdomyolysis is rare, but mild cases are seen in one third of the patients seen in emergency rooms for cocaine overdoses. In severe cases, 15% of patients die with renal hepatic failure and disseminated intravascular coagulation.[23] The prognosis worsens with increased temperature, seizures, and hypotension. Rhabdomyolysis is an acute medical emergency and requires intensive treatment to prevent death. Initial treatment should focus on preventing renal damage and establishing diuresis. Hyperthermia should be treated aggressively with cooling to prevent rhabdomyolysis. Muscle activity should be decreased and seizures prevented to limit rhabdomyolysis.

Almost all patients who snort cocaine have chronic sinusitis. They may have unilateral inflammation of the nose (cocaine addicts frequently snort in one nostril at a time so only one nostril is inflamed). Chronic rhinitis, perforations of the nasal septum, and abscessed teeth are common in cocaine snorters. Patients who misuse cocaine frequently engage in high-risk sexual behaviors that expose them to sexually transmitted diseases and human immunodeficiency virus (HIV) disease.

Opiate Intoxication

Heroin is the most commonly misused opiate. Over the past 10 years, emergency room (ER) visits due to heroin overdose have dramatically increased. The 2000 DAWN survey showed the largest increase in 12- to 17-year-old youths in whom ER visits have quadrupled.[24] In the 1999 Household Inventory Survey, 2.3% of eighth graders had used heroin at some time in their lives. Most new heroin abusers are snorting and smoking the drug. Recently the abuse of OxyContin has reached epidemic levels. Opiate overdoses occur in new users, in older users who have stopped using and lost their drug tolerance, whenever the purity of the street drug in-creases, and whenever a more potent opiate (e.g., fentanyl) is substituted for heroin. The recent purity of the drug has increased and the average price has decreased by two thirds. Before the drug is sold on the streets, pure heroin is adulterated (cut) with quinine, lactose, mannitol, dextrose, or talc, and will sell for as little as $10 (a dime bag). A history of heroin abuse is usually available from patients, their friends or family, or the hospital record.

The presenting signs and symptoms of opiate overdose are stupor, miosis, hypotension, bradycardia, and decreased bowel sounds. Frequently needle marks or tracks are present. In more severe cases, respiratory depression with apnea and pulmonary edema can occur. Seizures are seen with meperidine and propoxyphene overdoses. A urine toxicology screen detects most opiates except fentanyl.

Naloxone (Narcan) is the primary treatment for opiate overdose. An initial intravenous dose of 0.4 to 0.8 mg usually reverses the opiate effects. This dose can be repeated every 2 to 3 minutes up to a total dose of 10 to 20 mg. The goal in treatment is to reverse the respiratory depression, not to get the patient awake and alert, which may precipitate an acute withdrawal syndrome and make the patient hostile and potentially violent. Higher doses of naloxone are needed for codeine, propoxyphene, and pentazocine overdoses. Patients with pulmonary edema should be intubated. Positive end-expiratory pressure ventilation is used if necessary. Diuretics and digitalis are not effective therapies to treat opiate-induced pulmonary edema. In high dosages, naloxone has been reported to cause pulmonary edema, convulsions, and asystole in about 1% of treated patients.[25] The half-life of naloxone is shorter than that of most opiates, so patients may need to be treated with repeated doses of naloxone. For propoxyphene and methadone overdoses, an intravenous drip of naloxone (0.2–0.8 mg/h) can be used. Some authors advocate discharging heroin overdose patients without hospital admission if they are stable (usually after 8–12 hours of observation).[26] Patients who have attempted suicide, used other potentiating drugs, or for whom there is a question about the opiate used should be admitted for observation.

Pregnant heroin addicts or pregnant patients on methadone present a special problem. Because there is an increased risk of serious complications to the fetus, pregnant women should not be withdrawn from opiates. They should be maintained on methadone through the pregnancy. Hyperactivity, irritability, hyperreflexia, yawning, tachypnea, tremors and myoclonic seizures, poor sleep patterns, vomiting, and diarrhea characterize the neonatal withdrawal syndrome. Every attempt should be made to modify the infant's environment to reduce external stimuli. Phenobarbital and paregoric are used to treat withdrawing newborns.[27]

In the future, family physicians may be allowed to provide long-term maintenance therapy (methadone and buprenorphine) to heroin addicts.[28]

Amphetamines

Emergency room visits for amphetamine misuse have increased. The introduction of "ice" to the drug scene may account for this increase. Ice (Hawaiian ice) is methamphetamine made in the Far East and smuggled through Hawaii into the continental United States. *Crack* and *crank* are two street terms that are commonly confused. Crank is a street name for methamphetamine that can be taken as pills, injected, or snorted. Crack is freebase cocaine. The effects and complications of amphetamine misuse are similar to those of cocaine except amphetamines have a longer half-life.

Agitation is the most common presenting symptom of amphetamine misuse. Hallucinations, suicidal ideation, delusions, and confusion may be present. Cardiac symptoms include chest pain, palpitations, and myocardial infarction. Intracranial hemorrhagic strokes in young patients (15–45 years old) are associated with amphetamine abuse.[29] Acute signs of amphetamine intoxication include an elevation in the blood pressure and pulse, dilated pupils, tremor, cardiac arrhythmias, and increased reflexes. The long-term effects of amphetamine abuse include impaired concentration, abrupt mood changes, weight loss, paranoid delusions, and violence. Amphetamine psychosis is a combination of paranoid delusions with hallucinations; it can be treated with benzodiazepines.

Marijuana

Marijuana is the most commonly abused illicit drug. Its use has recently increased in adolescents, and the perception of marijuana's harmful effects has decreased.[30] In the 1999 National Institute of Drug Abuse (NIDA) Household Survey, which is available through the NIDA Web site, an estimated 14.8 million people (6.7% of the population) used marijuana in the month prior to the interview. Marijuana is a mixture of compounds, with the most psychoactive being Δ9-tetrahydrocannabinol (THC). Hashish, which is more potent than regular marijuana, refers to a dried resin made from the flower tops of the cannabis plant. Sinsemilla is a seedless form of marijuana that is approximately twice as potent as hashish. Marijuana is smoked in "joints," "bowls" (miniature pipes), or "bongs" (water- or air-cooled smoking devices that enable the smoker to inhale more drug with less irritation). Marijuana smoke has a pungent odor that can be identified on the clothes of chronic marijuana misusers.

Patients smoke marijuana to achieve a state of euphoria and relaxation. Users become less inhibited and laugh spontaneously. Marijuana may be "laced" with other drugs, such as cocaine, phencyclidine (PCP), or other hallucinogens, causing bizarre reactions. Marijuana is highly lipophilic, with a half-life of approximately 3 days. Impaired concentration, judgment, and coordination can last up to 2 days after using marijuana.

Chronic marijuana smoking leads to dependence with increased tolerance and withdrawal symptoms when the drug is stopped. Withdrawal symptoms include irritability, drowsiness, increased sleeping, and increased intake of high carbohydrate foods ("marijuana munchies"). Depression, paranoia, and anxiety are common effects of chronic marijuana misuse. Long-term abuse of marijuana may cause permanent cognitive impairment especially in patients who start abusing the drug at a young age.[31] Marijuana may impair the immune system and promote tumor growth,[32] a particularly important point when caring for HIV-positive patients.

The most common physical signs of marijuana misuse are tachycardia and conjunctival irritation (which may be masked in experienced users by using eyedrops). Urine testing is the most effective laboratory method for screening patients suspected of marijuana misuse. In daily misusers, urine toxicology screens may remain positive for several weeks. After a single misuse episode the urine test is positive for 3 to 4 days. When an adolescent is experiencing deterioration in school performance or a marked change in personality or behavior, a urine drug screen for marijuana should be done before formal psychological or psychiatric testing (see Chapter 22).

Designer/Club Drugs

Designer drugs are compounds that are chemically altered derivatives of federally controlled substances. They are changed slightly to produce special mood-altering effects. Contaminant by-products cause many of the complications of designer drugs produced in basement laboratories. The best known designer drug is ecstasy (3,4-methylenedioxymethamphetamine, MDMA), which is commonly used at "rave" parties. MDMA's use by teenagers has increased significantly in the past 5 years.[33] MDMA, which is ingested orally, causes euphoria, increased self-esteem, enhanced communication skills, and an elevated mood. Adverse effects include jaw clenching, tachycardia, panic attacks, nausea and vomiting, nystagmus, inhibited ejaculation, and urinary urgency. The letdown after taking MDMA, which lasts 1 to 3 days, is characterized by drowsiness, muscle aches, jaw soreness, depression, and difficulty concentrating. As more of the drug is ingested, the toxic effects increase and the euphoric effects decrease. Recent evidence shows that chronic MDMA abuse can cause permanent brain damage.[34]

Other commonly abused club drugs are γ-hydroxybutyric acid (GHB), flunitrazepam (Rohypnol), and ketamine. GHB is used primarily by adolescents and young adults at nightclubs or raves and by body builders as a muscle builder. Emergency room mentions of GHB increased from 55 in 1994 to 2,973 in 1999.[24] It is usually combined with alcohol to cause relaxation, intoxication and euphoria.[35] It has increasingly been involved in overdoses causing severe respiratory depression and death. Withdrawal symptoms occur and GHB is one of the "date rapes" drugs because it causes amnesia. GHB's effect is short acting (about 4 hours) and overdoses can be treated with respiratory support.

Ketamine (Special K, Vitamin K and K) is an anesthetic that causes a dream-like state, loss of inhibitions, and hallucinations. It can be injected, snorted, or smoked with marijuana. In high doses it causes delirium, amnesia (making it another "date rape" drug), elevated blood pressure, depression, and potentially fatal respiratory depression. Rohypnol (roofies, rophies, roche, or the forget-me pill), the third "date rape" drug,[36] is a benzodiazepine used in Europe and Latin America as a sedative/hypnotic. It is usually ingested orally with alcohol. Rohypnol has a long half-life, so overdoses need prolonged respiratory support. Flumazenil (a benzodiazepine antagonist) has been used in severe overdose patients (0.02 mg/kg in children and 0.2 mg in adults and repeat 0.3 mg up to a total dose of 3 mg).

Hallucinogens

Hallucinogens are defined as drugs that produce visual, auditory, tactile, and in some cases olfactory hallucinations. Lysergic acid diethylamide (LSD) is the most potent, most common hallucinogen. It is referred to as acid, dots, cubes, window pane, or blotter. LSD can cause bizarre behavior that begins a few minutes after ingestion, peaks in about 3 to 4 hours, and lasts up to 12 hours. Paranoia, depression, anxiety, acute psychosis, combative behavior, and panic attacks are associated with "bad trips." Patients experiencing adverse reactions to hallucinogens can be confused with patients having a schizophrenic reaction. Patients toxic from hallucinogens (1) have no history of mental illness, (2) tell you they have ingested the drug, and (3) have visual instead of auditory hallucinations. On physical examination, patients have pronounced pupillary dilation, tachycardia, sweating, and fever. Patients diagnosed with LSD intoxication need to be carefully screened for other problems such as hypoglycemia, head trauma, drug withdrawal, electrolyte abnormalities, endocrine disease, central nervous system (CNS) infection, hypoxia, and toxic reactions to other street or prescription drugs. Frequently patients can be "talked down" in a quiet setting. If necessary for severe agitation, a benzodiazepine can be used.[38] Patients may have chronic effects from LSD that include flashbacks, psychoses, depressive reactions, and chronic personality changes.

Phencyclidine

The complications of phencyclidine (PCP) misuse are still seen in emergency rooms. PCP intoxication is a frequently missed diagnosis, and physicians must be aware of the potential toxicity of PCP and its presenting signs and symptoms. PCP can be an adulterant, and patients may not know they took the drug. PCP can be smoked with cocaine (spacebasing). In low doses PCP causes euphoria and sedation. Increasing doses can cause hypertension, muscle rigidity, seizures, and coma. The presence of nystagmus, rapidly changing behaviors, and muscle rigidity help distinguish PCP intoxication from stimulant and hallucinogen overdoses. A urine drug screen helps diagnose PCP intoxication.

The treatment of PCP intoxication depends on the stage of intoxication. Mild intoxication can be treated with quiet observation and a benzodiazepine for combative behavior. Benadryl can be given for dystonic reactions. Physical restraints should be avoided because they increase the risk of rhabdomyolysis. Activated charcoal helps eliminate the drug and prevents reabsorption. Propranolol can be given intravenously for severe hypertension and tachycardia (contraindicated if the patient has used cocaine with PCP). Patients should be catheterized to prevent urine retention. Furosemide (Lasix) can increase urine flow and PCP excretion. The toxic effects of PCP can last up to 24 hours.

Volatile Substances

Volatile substance misuse (gasoline, airplane glue, cleaning agents, Freon, typewriter fluid, and lighter fluid) is common among early adolescent boys in large urban areas and on North American Indian reservations.[39] The agents are used to "get high," and they cause euphoria, light-headedness, a state of excitation, and frequently hallucinations. They are inexpensive and readily available. Volatile substances are sniffed, "bagged" (inhaling the substance from a plastic or paper bag), and "huffed" (inhaling the vapors by holding a piece of cloth soaked in the volatile substance against the mouth and nose).

Volatile substances are rapidly absorbed into the bloodstream, are highly lipid-soluble, and produce marked CNS effects (depression most commonly). They frequently cause nausea and vomiting. Tolerance and dependence (with withdrawal symptoms) can develop. In the emergency room, solvent misuse frequently can be mistaken for acute psychiatric problems because of the altered mental state and hallucinations. Solvent abuse should be suspected in teenagers who suddenly collapse while partying. Chronic abuse causes permanent damage to the brain (toluene), liver (chlorinated hydrocarbons, chloroform, trichloroethane, and trichloroethylene), heart, kidneys, and bone marrow (benzene).

Airplane glue causes peripheral neuropathies, tremors, and ataxia. Gasoline causes coughing and wheezing secondary to irritation to the respiratory tract and frequently intense hallucinations. Anemia, cardiac arrhythmias, and confusion are also seen with gasoline intoxication, and renal toxicity can be detected by proteinuria. Freon is cardiotoxic and causes arrhythmias. Typewriter fluid (trichloroethylene) causes neuropathies, headache, cardiac arrhythmias, renal and hepatic dysfunction, and diffuse CNS symptoms.

When teenagers present with confusion, physicians must be sensitive to the smell of solvents on the clothes or breath of patients. Unusual burns are indicative of solvent abuse. Laboratory tests may show an abnormal blood count, and urinalysis may reveal protein or blood in the urine. Liver function tests may be elevated. With chronic solvent abuse, the chest radiograph may reveal an enlarged heart. Supportive care for acute inhalant toxicity usually allows symptoms to clear within 4 to 6 hours. Benzodiazepines are indicated for seizures, and haloperidol (Haldol) can be used for extreme agitation. Cardiac monitoring is frequently necessary.

Care of Patients in Recovery

Overview

Little has been written about the care of patients after they recover from drug and alcohol addiction. Because many medical problems resolve as patients abstain from illicit drugs and alcohol, it is reasonable to wait a few months before treating less severe medical problems. Patients in recovery must be screened to ensure their continued abstinence from drugs and alcohol. A few brief questions can help with the assessment (Table 60.2). Patients in active recovery programs answer

Table 60.2. **Recovery Assessment Questions**

Are you attending aftercare or recovery meetings?
When was the last time you attended a meeting?
Do you have a sponsor, and when did you last contact him or her?
What step are you working on (if patient is in a 12-step program)?

these questions in a straightforward manner. If family members are present, ask them how the patient is doing. Positive support of patients, even if they have relapsed, is imperative. Physicians should emphasize the need to have accurate current drug misuse information to prevent serious side effects with prescription medications.

Any medication has the potential to cause a relapse, especially mood-altering medications. Prescription medications can cause a relapse by lowering patients' resistance or by patients becoming addicted to the prescribed medication. The following guidelines are for patients with a history of drug and alcohol addiction[40]:

1. Whenever possible, use nonpharmacologic treatments. Encourage patients to exercise, meditate, and change their diet; use acupuncture or biofeedback before prescribing medications.
2. Avoid benzodiazepines and narcotics. If they are necessary, patients should be carefully monitored with regularly scheduled follow-up visits.
3. Be cautious about prescribing "cue stimuli" medications, such as inhalants in former intranasal cocaine addicts.
4. Use "alternate" drugs, such as antidepressants for chronic pain or buspirone (BuSpar) for anxiety, because they have less addiction potential.
5. Choose medications with side effects that may be beneficial, such as beta-blocking drugs to treat hypertension because they decrease anxiety, which is common during early recovery.
6. Beware of increased drug sensitivity secondary to damage caused by patients' previous drug and alcohol misuse. Patients need a thorough evaluation focusing on specific complications from their previous addiction. Injection drug users must be assessed for hepatitis and HIV disease.
7. Before prescribing medications, wait for normal resolution of medical problems associated with withdrawal and early recovery, such as hypertension, depression, hyperglycemia and tachycardia.
8. Anticipate the normal changes (insomnia, anxiety, depression, and some sexual dysfunction) that occur during recovery and counsel patients about them so the patients are less likely to be concerned or to seek medications.

Treatment of Specific Diseases

The treatment of many common diseases can be complicated in patients with a history of drug/alcohol addiction. Most injection drug abusers have HIV disease (up to 90% in some areas) and frequently they abuse alcohol. Antiviral drugs that cause liver or pancreatic problems need to be avoided or used very cautiously. The dose of methadone in methadone maintenance patients may have to be altered after beginning antiviral therapy. Several antiviral drugs have side effects that mimic the narcotic withdrawal syndrome, making it difficult to differentiate drug side effects from narcotic withdrawal. Ritonavir formulations contain alcohol and cause a severe reaction in patients taking disulfiram. The alcohol may cause a relapse.

In managing acute and chronic pain in patients in recovery, every effort should be made to avoid narcotic medications by using nonsteroidal antiinflammatory drugs. If narcotics are needed, they should be prescribed for a limited period and with a fixed-dose schedule instead of "as needed."

Medications for upper respiratory infections frequently contain drugs that can jeopardize patients in recovery. Most cough syrups contain alcohol and codeine, and they should be avoided in patients in recovery. Several over-the-counter cough suppressants are available that do not contain alcohol. Pseudoephedrine is a stimulant, and it is potentially dangerous in former cocaine addicts.

Care of Patients Who Continue to Misuse Drugs

Treating patients for any medical problem while they misuse drugs and alcohol is difficult. The primary goal should be to help patients with their drug and alcohol misuse. A physician's caring nonjudgmental recommendation to abstain can be effective, especially if the recommendation is connected to the patient's present medical problem. Studies have shown that brief interventions by primary care physicians can decrease alcohol consumption.[41] Patients should be encouraged to enter a drug and alcohol treatment program. Most patients can be treated as outpatients unless they have significant medical or psychiatric problems. Detoxification may require a brief hospitalization. If a physician is uncomfortable treating patients who continue to misuse drugs, patients should be referred to another physician. To prevent a serious or potentially fatal reaction caused by concurrent drug or alcohol misuse, physicians must be extremely cautious when prescribing any medication to patients misusing drugs or alcohol. Poor medication compliance is a major problem with patients who continue to misuse drugs and alcohol.

References

1. Farre M, De La Torre R, Gonzalez M, Roset PN, Menoyo E, Cami J. Cocaine and alcohol interactions in humans: neuroendocrine effects and cocaethylene metabolism. J Pharmacol Exp Ther 1997;283:164–76.
2. Heesch CM, Wilhelm CR, Ristic J, Adnane J, Bontepo FA, Wagner WR. Cocaine activates platelets and increases the formation of circulating platelet containing microaggregates in humans. Heart 2000;83:688–95.
3. Goldfrank LR, Hoffman RS. The cardiovascular effects of cocaine. Ann Emerg Med 1991;20:165–75.

4. Nolan AG. Recreational drug misuse: issues for the cardiologist. Heart 2000;83:627–33.

5. Mittleman MA, Mintzer D, Maclure M, Tofler GH, Sherwood JB, Muller JE. Triggering of myocardial infarction by cocaine. Circulation 1999;99:2737–41.

6. Hollander JE, Hoffman RS, Gennis P, et al. Prospective multi-center evaluation of cocaine-associated chest pain. Acad Emerg Med 1994;1:330–9.

7. McNagny SD, Parker RM. High prevalence of recent cocaine use and the unreliability of patient self-report in an inner-city walk-in clinic. JAMA 1992;267:1106–8.

8. Trabulsy ME. Cocaine washed out syndrome in a patient with acute myocardial infarction. Am J Emerg Med 1995;13:538–9.

9. Rubin RB, Neugarten J. Cocaine-induced rhabdomyolysis masquerading as myocardial ischemia. Am J Med 1989;86:551–3.

10. Brogan WC, Lange RA, Kim AS, Moliterno DJ, Hillis LD. Alleviation of cocaine-induced coronary vasoconstriction by nitroglycerin. J Am Coll Cardiol 1991;18:581–6.

11. Hollander JE, Burstein JL, Hoffman RS, Shih RD, Wilson LD. Cocaine-associated myocardial infarction. Chest 1995;107:1237–41.

12. Hogya PT, Wolfson AB. Chronic cocaine abuse associated with dilated cardiomyopathy. Am J Emerg Med 1991;8:203–4.

13. Kerns W, Garvey L, Owens J. Cocaine-induced wide complex dysrhythmia. J Emerg Med 1997;15(3):321–9.

14. Stevens DC, Campbell JP, Carter JE, Waston WA. Acid-base abnormalities associated with cocaine toxicity in emergency department patients. Clin Toxicol 1994;32:31–9.

15. Om A, Ellahham S, DiSciascio G. Management of cocaine-induced cardiovascular complications. Am Heart J 1993;125:469–75.

16. June R, Aks SE, Keys N, Wahl M. Medical outcome of cocaine bodystuffers. J Emerg Med 2000;18(2):221–4.

17. Mott SH, Packer RJ, Soldin SJ. Neurologic manifestations of cocaine exposure in childhood. Pediatrics 1994;93:557–60.

18. Chasnoff IJ, Bussey ME, Savich R, Stack CM. Perinatal cerebral infarction and maternal cocaine use. J Pediatr 1986;108:456–9.

19. Cohen HR, Green JR, Crombleholm WR. Peripartum cocaine use: estimating risk of adverse pregnancy outcome. Int J Gynecol Obstet 1991;35:51–4.

20. Frassica JJ, Orav EJ, Walsh EP, Lipshultz SE. Arrhythmias in children prenatally exposed to cocaine. Arch Pediatr Adolesc Med 1994;148:1163–9.

21. Arendt R, Angelopoulos J, Salvator A, Singer L. Motor development of cocaine-exposed children at age two years. Pediatrics 1999;103:86–92.

22. Haim DY, Lippmann ML, Goldberg SK, Walkenstein MD. The pulmonary complications of crack cocaine. Chest 1995;107:233–49.

23. Roth D, Alarcon FJ, Fernandez JA, Preston RA, Bourgoignie JJ. Acute rhabdomyolysis associated with cocaine intoxication. N Engl J Med 1988;319:673–7.

24. DAWN Report 2000. Substance Abuse and Mental Health Services Administration. Available at www.samhsa.gov.

25. Osterwalder JJ. Naloxone—for intoxication with intravenous heroin and heroin mixtures—harmless of hazardous? J Toxicol Clin Toxicol 1996;34(4):409–16.

26. Smith DA, Leake L, Loflin JR, Yealy DM. Is admission after intravenous heroin overdose necessary? Ann Emerg Med 1992;21:1326–30.

27. Levy M, Spino M. Neonatal withdrawal syndrome: associated drugs and pharmacological management. Pharmacotherapy 1993;13:202–11.

28. O'Connor PG, Fiellin DA. Pharmacologic treatment of heroin-dependent patients. Ann Intern Med 2000;133:40–54.

29. Buxton N, McConachie NS. Amphetamine abuse and intracranial haemorrhage. J R Soc Med 2000;93:472–7.

30. Mathias R. Student's use of marijuana, other illicit drugs, and cigarettes continued to rise in 1995. NIDA Notes 1996;Jan/Feb. Vol III(1). Available online http://165.112.61/NIDAHome.html under NIDA Notes Newsletter.

31. Solwij N. Do cognitive impairments recover following cessation of cannabis use? Life Sci 1995;56:2119–26.

32. Zhu LX, Sharma S, Stolina M, et al. Delta-9-tetrahydrocannabinol inhibits antitumor immunity by a CB2 receptor-mediated, cytokine dependent pathway. J Immunol 2000;165(1):373–80.

33. Zickler P. Annual survey finds increasing teen use of ecstasy, steroids. NIDA Notes 2001;16(2). Available online http://165.112.61/NIDAHome.html under NIDA Notes Newsletter.

34. Statement of the director of the National Institute of Drug Abuse. U.S. Senate caucus on international narcotics control. Available at www.drugabuse.gov/Testimony/7-25-00Testimony.html.

35. Nicholson KL, Balster RL. GHB: a new and novel drug of abuse. Drug Alcohol Depend 2001;63:1–22.

36. Waltzman ML. Flunitrazepam: A review of "roofies". Pediatr Emerg Care 1999;15(1):59–60.

37. Nicholson KL, Balster RL. GHB: a new and novel drug of abuse. Drug Alcohol Depend 2001;63:1–22.

38. Blaho K, Merigian K, Winbery S, Geraci SA, Smartt C. Clinical pharmacology of lysergic acid diethylamine: case reports and review of the treatment of intoxication. Am J Ther 1997;4:211–21.

39. Kurtzman TL, Otsuka K, Wahl R. Inhalant abuse by adolescents. J Adolesc Health 2001;28:170–80.

40. Schulz JE. The integration of medical management with recovery. J Psychoactive Drugs 1997;29(3):233–7.

41. Fleming MF, Barry RL, Manwell LB, Johnson, London R. Brief physicians' advice for problem alcohol drinkers: a randomized controlled trial in community based primary care practice. JAMA 1997;277:1039–45.

61
Care of the Patient with Chronic Pain

Carole Nistler

Chronic pain is pain that persists beyond the usual healing time for tissue injury. It is often defined as pain lasting longer than 3 to 6 months.[1–3] It may or may not represent continuing tissue pathology. Family physicians encounter many nonmalignant disease states that involve chronic pain, such as headache, trigeminal neuralgia, neck injury, low back problems, arthritis, and peripheral neuropathy.

The management of chronic pain is challenging because a patient's symptoms may not be confirmed by physical examinations, laboratory tests, or diagnostic procedures. Chronic pain represents a complex interaction of physical, psychological, social, and spiritual factors.

Physiology of Pain and Pain Management

The experience of pain is initiated by stimulation of nociceptors located in skin, subcutaneous tissue, viscera, muscle, periosteum, joints, and so on. Interneurons located in the dorsal horn of the spinal cord control whether impulses transmitted from the nociceptors are subsequently transmitted to the rest of the central nervous system (CNS). Interference with pain transmission at the level of the interneuron in the dorsal horn may explain the effectiveness of peripheral stimuli in modifying pain perception, e.g., massage, acupuncture, transcutaneous external nerve stimulation (TENS), and capsaicin cream.

Descending control of the pain response from the CNS can be activated by arousal, attention, and emotional stress, and, via descending pathways and receptors, they can also modify the pain experience. CNS modification of pain transmission explains the effectiveness of cognitive-behavioral therapies such as biofeedback training, visualization, and music therapy.[2,4]

The action of specific neurotransmitters involved in CNS control of pain perception can be modified by a growing number of adjunctive agents used in pain management. Baclofen (Lioresal), benzodiazepines, and the many antiepileptic drugs such as carbamazepine (Tegretol) work by binding to γ-aminobutyric acid (GABA) receptors in the dorsal horn.[4]

Opioid analgesics modulate the pain response by binding to opioid receptors located in the dorsal horn and other areas of the spinal cord and brain. Opioid receptors are classified as mu, kappa, or sigma. Opioid drugs that bind primarily to mu-opioid receptors produce analgesia, euphoria, respiratory depression, and bradycardia. These agents are known as mu-opioids or pure mu-agonists and include codeine, hydrocodone, morphine, oxycodone, and hydromorphone. Opioids of the agonist-antagonist type have a primarily kappa-agonist analgesic effect, but a mu-receptor antagonist effect, thereby producing limited analgesia.[4,5]

The physiology underlying the use of nonsteroidal antiinflammatory drugs (NSAIDs) for pain control relate to their ability to inhibit prostaglandin synthesis at sites of tissue injury. This produces both an analgesic and antiinflammatory effect. NSAIDs act on the cyclooxygenase (COX) enzyme system that produces prostaglandins. COX enzymes are classified into two isoforms—COX-1 isoforms found in the gastrointestinal tract, renal tract, and platelets, and COX-2 sites found in areas of inflammation and in the CNS. Selective COX-2 inhibitor drugs have been developed to provide the analgesic benefit of an NSAID with fewer gastrointestinal and bleeding diathesis side effects.[6]

Therapeutic Choices

The World Health Organization (WHO)[7] has promoted a three-step approach to cancer pain management that is also widely recommended and used for chronic noncancer pain.[2,8] The WHO approach recommends first the use of nonopioid drugs starting with acetaminophen and then the NSAIDs; second, for continued uncontrolled pain of a mild to moderate nature, the addition of a weak opioid; and third, for continued uncontrolled pain of a moderate to severe nature, the substitution of a stronger opioid. While it provides a useful guideline, the strict application of the WHO approach to chronic noncancer pain is problematic for several reasons: (1) growing concern regarding the significant morbidity and mortality related to long-term NSAID use, (2) controversy regarding the safety and efficacy of opioids in noncancer pain, and (3) the development of new antiepileptic drugs and other agents that may provide safer alternatives to opioids for certain types of chronic pain.

Clinicians must individualize pain management regimens per patient. The goals of therapy are not only to reduce or control pain, but also to improve daily functioning, physical capabilities, sleep function, and mood.[7] These goals will determine the need for and choice of pharmacologic agents.

Nonpharmacologic therapies can enhance pain control and improve daily functioning. Adjunctive therapies to consider include cognitive-behavioral training, occupational therapy, vocational training, physical therapy, and individual or family therapy.[2,9] Availability of these resources is dependent on practice setting. Pain management clinics may provide many of these services in one coordinated setting. They are also of-ten the source of anesthetic or neurosurgical procedures for pain management.

Nonopioid Analgesics

The nonopioid analgesics—acetaminophen and NSAIDs—are frequently used, although not without safety concerns, for almost all types of chronic pain. These drugs are effective alone for mild to moderate pain and have a synergistic effect when used in combination with opioids for severe pain. They are nonaddictive, antipyretic, and, except for acetaminophen, have an antiinflammatory effect. The nonopioid drugs have an analgesic ceiling—dosage increases beyond recommended levels do not produce further analgesia (Table 61.1).

Acetaminophen

Acetaminophen (Tylenol, others) is recommended for noninflammatory osteoarthritis and other causes of mild to moderate pain. It is safe for patients with renal insufficiency, although liver toxicity can occur in cases of overdose or chronic alcoholism. Some chronic pain patients may require maximum doses of 4 g per day for at least 1 week to determine effectiveness.[10]

Table 61.1. **Selected Nonopioid Analgesics[6,9–12]**

Drug name	Usual dose	Maximum dose	Comments
Acetaminophen (Tylenol, others)	500–1000 mg po q4–6h	4000 mg/d	Recommended for noninflammatory osteoarthritis. May require maximum dose for 1 week for chronic pain trial. Avoid with chronic alcoholism.
Salsalate (Disalcid others)	1000 mg po q8–12h	3000 mg/d	Nonacetylated salicylates produce similar analgesia to, but less gastropathy than aspirin. Minimal antiplatelet activity.
Ibuprofen (Motrin, others)	400–800 mg po q4–6h	3200 mg/d	NSAIDs in recommended doses usually provide superior analgesia compared with aspirin, but do not produce the same analgesic effect in all patients. Major adverse effects are:
Naproxen (Naprosyn, others)	500 mg po q12h	1250 mg/d	1. Elevated blood pressure especially in the elderly and in conjunction with beta-blockers or angiotensin-converting enzyme inhibitors
Indomethacin (Indocin)	25–50 mg po q8h or SR-75 mg po q12h	200 mg/d	2. Fluid retention in patients with congestive heart failure
Ketoralac (Toradol, others)	10 mg po q4–6h	40 mg/d	3. Acute renal failure or renal insufficiency 4. Drowsiness and confusion
	Pts <65 years: 30 mg IM/IV q6h	120 mg/d	5. Reversible inhibition of platelet aggregation
	Pts ≥65 years: 15 mg IM/IV q6h	60 mg/d 60 mg/d	6. Anaphylaxis in aspirin-sensitive patients 7. Peptic ulcer disease, regardless of mode of administration, especially in the first month of therapy.
Diclofenac (Cataflam, Voltaren)	50 mg po q8h or SR-75 mg po q12h	150 mg/d	
Nabumetone (Relafen)	1000–1500 mg po qd	1500 mg/d	
Celecoxib (Celebrex)	100–200 mg po q12h	400 mg/d	Selective COX-2 inhibitors and NSAIDs have demonstrated decreased gastrointestinal complications compared with nonselective NSAIDs. They do not inhibit platelet aggregation.
Rofecoxib (Vioxx)	25–50 mg po q24h	50 mg/d	

COX = cyclooxygenase; NSAID = nonsteroidal antiinflammatory drug; SR = sustained release.

Nonacetylated Salicylates

Salsalate (Disalcid and others) and choline magnesium trisalicylate (Trilisate and others) produce analgesic levels similar to aspirin but with less gastropathy and less inhibition of platelet function than aspirin.[11] Nonacetylated salicylates have not been shown to reduce the risk of gastropathy compared to other NSAIDs.

NSAIDs

NSAIDs produce superior analgesia compared with aspirin when given in recommended doses.[11] However, their analgesic effectiveness varies per patient so that several drugs may need to be tried before some patients will report a response. NSAIDs have multiple adverse effects as listed in Table 61.1.[6] Gastrointestinal toxicity is the most frequently reported adverse effect[12] and can lead to significant morbidity and mortality.

Risk factors for NSAID-related gastropathy are (1) age older than 65 years, (2) previous history of peptic ulcer disease (PUD), (3) high doses or multiple types of NSAIDs, (4) concomitant glucocorticoid use, and (5) duration of treatment less than 3 months. The greatest risk of NSAID-related PUD occurs within the first month of therapy.[6]

Recommended methods to reduce the risk of gastropathy are the following[6,12]: (1) Use alternative drugs, if possible. (2) Use the lowest effective dose possible and discontinue, if possible. (3) For patients with two or more risk factors, use concomitant misoprostol (Cytotec), a synthetic prostaglandin analogue that has been shown to decrease gastrointestinal complications of NSAID use by 40%. The recommended dose of misoprostol is 200 μg four times daily but lower doses of 200 μg twice daily may be effective and may help to limit side effects of abdominal cramping and diarrhea. (4) Histamine-2 blockers, e.g., ranitidine (Zantac) or famotidine (Pepcid), have been shown to reduce the incidence of gastric and duodenal ulcers when given prophylactically to patients on chronic NSAID therapy, but the studies are not definitive. (5) Proton pump inhibitors, e.g., omeprazole (Prilosec), also may be effective as preventive agents for NSAID-related gastropathy but add significant cost. (6) Selective COX-2 inhibitor NSAIDs, e.g., celecoxib (Celebrex) and rofecoxib (Vioxx), cause fewer gastrointestinal complications than nonselective agents. They also do not inhibit platelet aggregation and can be used for patients on warfarin. They can cause all of the other adverse effects associated with NSAIDs. They are not more effective analgesics than nonselective NSAIDs.

Sucralfate (Carafate) and buffered aspirin provide no benefit in the prevention of NSAID-related gastropathy. While enteric-coating of aspirin or naproxen would seem to reduce the risk of topical gastric damage by transferring absorption to the small intestine, there are insufficient data to suggest an overall reduction in gastrointestinal complications.

Opioid Analgesics

The use of opioid analgesics for chronic noncancer pain remains controversial. A recent survey of primary care physicians indicated that, while most physicians are willing to prescribe low potency opioids on an as-needed basis for chronic noncancer pain, a significant portion are unwilling to use higher potency opioids on an around-the-clock basis.[13]

Rationale

The rationale for the use of opioids to alleviate chronic pain is based on the recognition that some patients do not respond to or cannot tolerate other therapy. Physicians' concerns about chronic use of opioids center around three clinical issues: (1) efficacy, (2) safety, and (3) risk of addiction. Available studies of opioid use in noncancer patients suggest the following conclusions regarding these concerns[3,5,14]: (1) Efficacy. Opioids are effective for many types of chronic noncancer pain. Unlike nonopioids, there is no ceiling analgesic effect so that opioids can be titrated up to achieve adequate analgesia. Unfortunately, studies do not demonstrate that this improved analgesic effect is associated with improved daily functioning. (2) Safety: Gastrointestinal and CNS side effects are usually not a problem with long-term opioid use because of the rapid development of tolerance to most of these side effects including nausea, vomiting, cognitive impairment, respiratory depression, and sedation. Constipation can usually be managed with prophylactic use of stool softeners and fiber laxatives. Unlike NSAIDs, there is no known direct organ damage associated with long-term opioid use. (3) Risk of addiction: The risk of inducing opioid addiction among patients with legitimate chronic pain is minimal, although not absent. Long-term opioid therapy often induces *physical dependence*, which is the occurrence of withdrawal symptoms after cessation, and may induce *tolerance*, which is the need for increasing doses to achieve the same analgesic effect. Neither of these physiologic phenomena cause *addiction*, which is a pattern of compulsive behaviors centered around the desire for, acquisition of, and use of the drug. Additional caution and more extensive evaluation are warranted before using chronic opioids for patients with a history of chemical dependency.

There are also legal and regulatory disincentives to prescribing chronic opioid therapy,[3,5,14,15] including diversion of drugs for nonmedical uses, diversion of drugs for treatment of narcotics withdrawal, and physicians' fears of licensing or regulatory scrutiny and sanctions for prescribing controlled substances.

Indications/Contraindications

Opioids should be considered for patients with chronic pain who are refractory to other treatments and who have shown responsiveness to opioids.[5] Relative contraindications to starting chronic opioid therapy are a history of substance abuse, drug-seeking behaviors, personality disorders, hepatic insufficiency, renal insufficiency, severe respiratory disease with impaired respiratory drive, preexisting constipation or urinary retention, suicidal tendency, or cognitive impairment.[16]

Guidelines for Therapy

Patients should be educated regarding the goals of therapy; the potential for side effects; the meaning and risks of developing physical dependence, tolerance, and addiction; and the method and schedule for monitoring their use of the drug. A "one physician–one pharmacy" policy should be considered. A patient contract documenting the patient's understanding of these issues should be kept in the medical record.[3,5,15]

Specific Opioids

Table 61.2 lists the commonly used opioid analgesics. Tramadol (Ultram) is an opioid agonist that also blocks norepinephrine and serotonin reuptake. Its effectiveness and side effects are similar to those of weak opioids and may be minimized by gradual titration up to the recommended dose.[10] Physical dependence has been reported but abuse potential is low; therefore, tramadol is not scheduled as a controlled substance.[17] Tramadol may increase the risk of seizures among patients who are at risk for seizures or who are also taking selective serotonin reuptake inhibitors (SSRIs), tricyclic antidepressants (TCAs), opioids, monoamine oxidase inhibitors (MAOIs), or neuroleptics.[4,10]

Meperidine (Demerol) is poorly absorbed orally and cannot be used for patients with impaired renal function or those taking MAOIs because of the risk of seizures and other CNS toxicity.[16] The agonist-antagonist group of opioids—pentazocine (Talwin), butorphanol (Stadol), nalbuphine (Nubain), and buprenorphine (Buprenex)—have moderate to strong analgesic potential, but unlike morphine and the other pure agonist drugs, they exhibit an analgesic ceiling. They offer no advantage in analgesic effect or avoidance of side effects. If given to a patient already on a pure agonist drug such as morphine, they precipitate withdrawal symptoms.[5]

Propoxyphene (Darvon, Darvocet) is a nonopiate narcotic that binds to opioid receptors but is no more effective than acetaminophen and causes significant side effects including nausea, vomiting, constipation, dizziness, cardiac toxicity, and chemical dependency.[10]

Fentanyl is the only opioid available transdermally (Duragesic). It is also available as an oral lozenge (Actiq) for acute pain and in parenteral form (Sublimaze). Because of its slow onset of action, the fentanyl patch is appropriate for patients already on opioids who have constant pain with few pain breakthrough episodes. Individual dosing varies greatly owing to differences in skin absorption.[16]

Dosing

Patients with only episodic pain do well with intermittent dosing of opioids. Those with more frequent or continuous symptoms should be given doses around the clock, with rescue doses for sudden exacerbations of pain. Patients with relatively steady pain who are on longer-acting opioids also require occasional rescue doses in the form of shorter-acting agents. Patients in whom sedation may be particularly hazardous because of their occupations can be started at lower than recommended doses of opioids and be titrated upward to build tolerance to the sedative effects. Patients who develop persistent side effects to one opioid may do better with another. The dosages of some products are limited by being placed in combination with acetaminophen or aspirin.[5,16]

Discontinuation

Discontinuation of opioids should be considered in the event that the underlying cause of the pain is resolved, other pain management strategies are providing sufficient pain relief, if unacceptable side effects develop, or if abuse behavior occurs. Discontinuation of chronic opioid therapy can be achieved without precipitating withdrawal symptoms by gradually tapering the dose over 1 to 4 weeks. Clonidine (oral dose 0.05–0.2 mg every 6 hours) can be used to inhibit withdrawal symptoms during opioid tapering. Dosing should be adjusted based on the patient's blood pressure and level of sedation induced by clonidine. Benzodiazepines may also be used to reduce irritability and anxiety during opioid withdrawal.[5,15]

Table 61.2. **Selected Opioid Analgesics**[8,11]

Drug name	Usual dose	Equianalgesic dose to 10 mg oral morphine	Comments
Tramadol (Ultram)	50 mg po tid–qid	—	Slow titration to effective dose may limit side effects.
Codeine (Tylenol #2, #3, #4, others)	30–60 mg po q3–4h	70 mg po	Available in combination with nonopioids, as single agent, as an elixir and injectable.
Hydrocodone (Vicodin, Lortab)	5–10 mg po q3–4h	10 mg po	Only available in combination with nonopioids.
Oxycodone (Percocet, others)	5–10 mg po q3–4h	5–10 mg po	Usually in combination with nonopioids, also as an elixir and as 12-hour sustained-release OxyContin.
Morphine	20–60 mg po q3–4h	—	Also available as rectal suppository.
	Sustained-release (MS Contin) 15–60 mg po q12h	—	
	10 mg IM/IV q3–6h	3 mg IM/IV	
Fentanyl (Duragesic)	25–100 μg/h patch q72h	—	Maximum dose of transdermal patch is 300 μg/hr.

Adjuvant Agents

Antidepressants

Although their mechanism is unknown, TCAs are effective in the treatment of neuropathic pain such as diabetic neuropathy or postherpetic neuralgia.[9,14] Amitriptyline (Elavil) is commonly used in low initial doses of 10 to 25 mg at bedtime with gradual upward titration as needed and as tolerated. There are less data supporting the use of SSRIs for chronic neuropathic pain, but SSRIs do not produce the anticholinergic side effects and cardiac conduction abnormalities associated with TCAs and are effective in treating the depression, insomnia, and anxiety associated with chronic pain.

Antiepileptics

Traditional antiepileptic drugs (AEDs) such as carbamazepine (Tegretol), phenytoin (Dilantin), and valproate (Depakote) are effective for many types of neuropathic pain, but their use may be limited by side effects and drug interactions. Of the newer AEDs, initial research shows gabapentin (Neurontin) is a safe, effective drug for neuropathic pain with few drug interactions.[4,9,14] Its onset of analgesic effect may be more rapid than TCAs and it may be opioid sparing. Its mechanism of action is unknown. Dosing begins at 100 to 300 mg daily, increasing to 900 mg daily in 3 days with an additional increase of 100 to 300 mg every week until therapeutic effect is achieved. Most reports suggest dosages for chronic neuropathic pain are 1800 to 3600 mg daily in three to four divided doses.

Baclofen

Baclofen (Lioresal) is a GABA analogue that, by binding to GABA receptors in the spinal cord, alters CNS control of pain.[14] It is used for neuropathic pain, particularly trigeminal neuralgia. The usual daily dose is 20 to 60 mg divided into three to four doses. Side effects are sedation, weakness, dizziness, nausea, and confusion.

Capsaicin

Capsaicin (Zostrix Cream), derived from jalapeno peppers, is a topical agent useful for osteoarthritis localized to a few joints.[10] Its mechanism of action is depletion of substance P in peripheral nociceptors. It is available over the counter, may be applied two to four times daily, and has no serious side effects. Application site burning or stinging reduces with continued use.

References

1. Newberger PE, Sallan SE. Chronic pain: principles of management. J Pediatr 1981;98(2):180–9.
2. Russo CM, Brosse WG. Chronic pain. Annu Rev Med 1998;49:123–33.
3. Barnsworth B. Risk-benefit assessment of opioids in chronic noncancer pain. Drug Safety 1999;21(4):283–96.
4. Hanson HC. Treatment of chronic pain with antiepileptic drugs: a new era. South Med J 1999;92(7):642–9.
5. Savage SR. Opioid use in the management of chronic pain. Med Clin North Am 1999;83(3):761–86.
6. Brooks P. Use and benefits of nonsteroidal anti-inflammatory drugs. Am J Med 1998;104(3A):9S–13S.
7. World Health Organization. Cancer pain relief and palliative care: report of a WHO expert committee. Geneva, Switzerland: World Health Organization, 1990.
8. Montauk SL. Treating chronic pain. Am Fam Physician 1997;55(4):1151–60.
9. Marcus D. Treatment of nonmalignant chronic pain. Am Fam Physician 2000;61(5):1331–8.
10. Schnitzer TJ. Non-NSAID pharmacologic treatment options for the management of chronic pain. Am J Med 1998;105(1B):45S–52S.
11. Drugs for pain. Med Lett 2000;42(1085):73–8.
12. Ament PW, Childers RS. Prophylaxis and treatment of NSAID-induced gastropathy. Am Fam Physician 1997;55(4):1323–32.
13. Potter M, Schafer S, et al. Opioids for chronic nonmalignant pain. J Fam Pract 2001;50(2):145–51.
14. Pappagallo M. Aggressive pharmacologic treatment of pain. Rheum Dis Clin North Am 1999;25(1):193–213.
15. Longo LP, Parran T. Addiction: part II. Identification and management of the drug-seeking patient. Am Fam Physician 2000;61(8):2401–8.
16. Brown RL, Fleming M. Chronic opioid analgesic therapy for chronic low back pain. J Am Board Fam Pract 1996;9(3):191–204.
17. Cicero TJ, Adams EH. A postmarketing surveillance program to monitor Ultram abuse in the United States. Drug Alcohol Depend 1999;57(1):7–22.

62
Care of the Dying Patient

Frank S. Celestino

Family physicians have traditionally prided themselves on comprehensive and continuous provision of care throughout the human life cycle. When managing the terminal phases of illness, however, most clinicians have had little formal education directed at the experience of human suffering and dying.[1,2] For many physicians the task and challenge of caring for a dying patient can seem overwhelming. The aging of the United States population, the development and widespread use of life-prolonging technologies, the ascendence of managed care emphasizing the central role of the primary care physician, media attention, the growing discomfort with futile treatment, the public's interest in physician-assisted suicide and the demand for better palliation have all fueled a growing need for physicians to master the art and science of helping patients achieve death with dignity.[3–5] This need has led to a series of major initiatives to improve palliative care education for both clinicians and the public, including the Education for Physicians in End-of-Life Care Project of the American Medical Association, the Faculty Scholars in End-of-Life Care Program of the Department of Veteran Affairs, the Improving Residency Training in End-of-Life Care Program of the American Board of Internal Medicine, the Project on Death in America of the Soros Foundation, and the Last Acts Program of the Robert Wood Johnson Foundation.[3,6]

This chapter reviews the key components of a comprehensive care program for terminally ill patients (Table 62.1).[7–9] The focus is on optimum care of patients who experience prolonged but predictable dying. Classically, these individuals have had disseminated cancer. It is now recognized that a much broader array of dying patients—those with acquired immunodeficiency syndrome, end-stage renal or cardiac disease, emphysema, and degenerative neurologic diseases—deserve such comprehensive palliative care. For a more detailed discussion of the topics covered in this chapter, the reader can consult two recent theme issues that exhaustively review the cultural, spiritual, political, ethical, economic, social, and medical aspects of terminal care.[10,11]

Cultural Context of Dying and Suffering

The last 50 years have witnessed the increasing medicalization of death in the United States, with most patients now dying in hospitals instead of at home.[3,9–12] The Council on Scientific Affairs of the American Medical Association (AMA)[9] has emphasized that "in the current system of care, many dying patients suffer needlessly, burden their families, and die isolated from families and community." The AMA council and others[3,6] have cited the advance directives movement, the rising public enthusiasm for euthanasia and physician-assisted suicide, the popularity of the hospice, sensationalized court cases, and the establishment of organizations such as Americans for Better Care of the Dying and the Hemlock Society as evidence of increasing uneasiness with medicine's response to dying. They call for acceptance of dying as a normal part of the human life cycle, expanded research into terminal care, educational programs for all health professionals, and better reimbursement for terminal care.[5,6]

Communication of Diagnosis, Therapy Plans, and Prognosis

Several recent reviews have highlighted a number of sources of communication difficulties with dying patients, including social factors, patient and family barriers, and issues specific to physicians.[13–17] Buckman[13] addressed two specific tasks of communication in terminal care: breaking bad news and engaging in therapeutic dialogue. His six-step protocol is a useful paradigm for all health care practitioners: (1) getting started, which includes such issues as location, eye contact, personal touch, timing, and participants; (2) finding out how much the patient already knows and understands; (3) learning how much the patient wants to know; (4) sharing appropriate amounts of information, with attention to aligning and

Table 62.1. **Components of a Comprehensive Care Plan for Dying Patients**

Compassionate and professional communication of diagnosis, treatment options, and prognosis
Psychosocial support of the patient and family
  Includes developing an understanding of the cultural and religious (spiritual) meaning of suffering and death for the patient and family
  Emphasizes continuity to allay fears of abandonment
Implementation of a comprehensive, evidence-based palliative care program
  Multidisciplinary in nature (physicians, nurses, clergy, social workers, pharmacists, nutritionists, lawyers, patient advocates)
  Hospice involvement
  Establishment and clarification of advance care directives (living wills, durable power of attorney for health care, autopsy and organ donation wishes, dying in hospital versus at home), and attitudes toward physician-assisted suicide
  Pain management (WHO and ACS guidelines)
  Nonpain symptom treatment (including behavioral/psychiatric issues)
  Nutritional support
Acknowledgment and management of financial and reimbursement issues
Bereavement management

WHO = World Health Organization; ACS = American Cancer Society.

educating; (5) responding to the patient's and family's feelings; and (6) planning ongoing care and follow-through.

There is usually no reason to provide detailed answers to questions the patient has not yet asked. The concept of gradualism—revealing the total truth in small doses as the illness unfolds—allows the patient the opportunity to develop appropriate coping strategies. However, it is important not to use euphemisms (such as swelling or lump), but to acknowledge the presence of cancer when confirmation is in hand. One must also realize that many patients do not hear the bad news accurately when it is first presented, and reexplanation is often needed.

Not only has the primacy of patient autonomy in modern medicine encouraged truth telling, but studies reveal that patients greatly prefer open, honest communication.[13–17] Overall, the drive for disclosure must be counterbalanced by the realization that the terminally ill patient struggles to maintain a sense of hope in the face of an increasingly ominous medical situation. Clinicians must continue to nurture hope in their dying patients through appropriate optimism around aspects of treatment, achievable goals, and prognosis, combined with timely praise for the patient and family's efforts to achieve spiritual healing and death with dignity. When physicians apply good communication skills (including attending to both verbal and nonverbal signals, exploring incongruent affect, and empathically eliciting patients' perspectives) and actively work to reduce barriers to mutual understanding, patients experience a reduction in both physical and psychological aspects of suffering.

One of the most difficult tasks is predicting how long the patient will live. With improved computing and statistical tools, more accurate objective estimates of survival are often available.[18] Despite these advances prognostication for many patients remains an imperfect science. One approach is to provide a conservative estimate that allows the patient and family to feel proud about "beating the odds" and exceeding expectations.

Psychosocial Support of the Patient and Family

One of the greatest challenges facing clinicians is to adequately address the multitude of psychosocial needs of dying patients and their families.[19] Kubler-Ross was one of the first to study and popularize the notion that terminally ill individuals often experience predictable stages of emotional adaptation and response to the dying process.[20] The five stages were characterized as shock and denial, anger, bargaining, depression, and acceptance. Although duration of these stages and the intensity and sequencing with which they are experienced are highly variable from one individual to the next, accurate recognition of the patient's psychological stage allows the clinician to optimize communication, support, and empathy to meet new needs as they arise.

In addition to the needs delineated in Table 62.1, and the desire for truth telling and a sense of hopefulness, dying patients above almost all else want assurance that the physician (and others) will not abandon them.[21] There is often great fear of dying alone in an environment separated from loved ones and worry about being repulsive to others because of loss of control over bodily functions. Terminally ill patients often seek physical expressions of caring, such as touching, hugging, and kissing. Regardless of their formal involvement with organized religion, they also often seek closure on the spiritual issues of their lives. Many individuals find great solace in life review: the pleasures, pains, accomplishments, and regrets. Most desire some input into making decisions about their care. The above list of concerns applies as much to the family as to the patient. Although in many circumstances family members are critical to the success of terminal care, one must recognize not only caregiver depression and burnout but also dysfunctional family relationships that impede successful physician management.

An often underappreciated aspect of successful supportive care is developing understanding of the symbolic meaning of suffering and dying for the individual patient. Experiences of illness and death and beliefs about the appropriate role of healers are profoundly influenced by a patient's cultural[22] and religious[19,22,23] background. Efforts to use racial or ethnic background alone as predictors of beliefs or behaviors may lead to stereotyping of patients and culturally insensitive care for the dying. Koenig and Gates-Williams[24] provide a protocol to assess the impact of culture. They recommend assessing, in addition to ethnicity, (1) the vocabulary most appropriate for discussing the illness and death; (2) who has decision-making power—the patient or the larger family unit; (3) the relevance of religious beliefs (death, afterlife, miracles, sin);

(4) the attitude toward dead bodies; (5) issues of age, gender, and power relationships within both the family and the health care team; and (6) the patient's political and historical context (e.g., poverty, immigrant status, past discrimination) (also see Chapter 3).

Comprehensive Palliative Care

At some point in the course of a chronic illness, it becomes clear that further therapeutic efforts directed at cure or stabilization are futile. Emphasis then shifts from curative to palliative care with an enhanced focus on optimal function and quality of life. According to the World Health Organization (WHO), palliative care "affirms life, regards dying as a normal process, neither hastens nor postpones death, provides relief from pain and other distressing symptoms, integrates the psychological and spiritual aspects of care, offers a support system to help patients live as actively as possible until death and provides support to help the family cope during the patient's illness and in their own bereavement."[25]

Hospice

In the United States, palliative care is most effectively provided by the now more than 2000 hospice organizations that coordinate the provision of high-quality interdisciplinary care to patients and families much more effectively and efficiently than most physicians could do on their own.[26] The first hospice was opened in South London by Dr. Cicely Saunders in 1967, with the concept first appearing in America by 1974. Philosophically, the objectives of hospice and palliative care are the same. Hospice care, which is provided regardless of ability to pay, has grown from an alternative health care movement to an accepted part of the American health care system, with Medicare reimbursement beginning in 1982. Hospice organizations provide a highly qualified, specially trained interdisciplinary team of professionals (nurses, pharmacists, counselors, pastoral care, patient care coordinators, volunteers) who work together to meet the physiologic, psychological, social, spiritual, and economic needs of patients and families facing terminal illness.[26] Classically, more than 80% of hospice patients have had disseminated cancer, but in recent years patients with chronic diseases that are deemed inevitably terminal within 6 months have become eligible as well. The hospice team collaborates continuously with the patient's attending physician (who must certify the terminal condition), to develop and maintain a patient-centered, individualized plan of care. Hospice medical services and consultation are available 24 hours a day, 7 days a week, though minute-to-minute personal care of the patient by the hospice team is not feasible and must be provided by family or volunteers. Hospice care, though aimed at allowing the patient to remain at home if desired, continues uninterrupted should the patient need acute hospital care or a hospice inpatient unit.

Advance Directives

Because it is now possible to keep sick patients alive longer at greater cost with lesser quality of life, patients and physicians have welcomed the emphasis on advance directives planning. *Advance directive* is an "umbrella" term that refers to any directive for health care made in advance of serious, cognition-impairing illness that robs the patient of decision-making capability.

Two general types of directive are widely recognized.[27] With the instructional type the patient specifies in writing certain circumstances and, in advance, declines or accepts specific treatments. The second type involves appointment of a health care agent, a person to whom is delegated all authority about medical decisions. Each type of directive has its strengths and drawbacks, and they should be seen as complementary, not competitive.

The advance directives movement seems to fit well with an emphasis on patient autonomy and the economic reality of needing to conserve health costs. Unfortunately, studies have revealed that advance directives may make little difference in the way patients are treated at the end of life and reduce costs only modestly.[28,29] Similar drawbacks have applied to the Patient Self-Determination Act, which when implemented in 1991 was designed to encourage competent adults to complete advance directives and to help identify those patients who previously had executed such documents on admission to acute or long-term facilities. Nonetheless, in practice the discussions among physician, patient, and family leading up to establishment of a formal directive are often of greater importance than the documents themselves. When a terminally ill patient calmly discusses foreseeable events and choices leading up to death, the effect on anxious family members can be dramatic and salutary. Such discussions ideally occur relatively early after a terminal illness is diagnosed so as to avoid a crisis situation in which the patient becomes incapacitated and the family must assume responsibility for clinical decisions in the absence of knowledge about their loved one's preferences. State statutes vary widely regarding living wills and health care proxies as well as the authority granted to close friends or family members in the common situation where an incapacitated person has left no advance directives.

Physicians must realize that most dying patients at some point contemplate suicide and that a small but significant number, in one way or another, will ask their physicians to help hasten death[30,31] (see Chapter 23). With the publicity surrounding doctor-aided suicides in Michigan and the onslaught of state and federal judicial and legislative activity concerning physician-assisted suicide (PAS), clinicians caring for dying patients must explore their own moral stance in this challenging area so as to deal more effectively with patient suffering. Fortunately, approval of PAS in Oregon (and the Netherlands) has greatly stimulated clinicians' interest in palliative care, especially when abuses of the PAS process are uncovered.[31]

Inherent in any discussion of advance directives is the concept of the loss of "decision-making capacity." This catchphrase obscures the fact that in common practice decisional capacity is difficult to assess. The elements of capacity seem straightforward: Can the person indicate a choice and do so free of coercion? Can the person manipulate relevant information meaningfully and understand the consequences of choosing each of the options? Searight[32] published a helpful, clinically relevant interview framework for assessing patient medical decision-making capacity. Such approaches verify that early dementia does not by itself usually prevent patients from participating in advance directives discussions.

Pain Management

Symptom management, especially achieving pain relief (see Chapter 61), remains the first priority for the attending physician and palliative care team.[3,7–9,25,33–35] Without effective control of pain and other sources of physical distress, quality of life for the dying patient is unacceptable, and progress on the psychological work of dying is aborted. The very prospect of pain induces fear in the patient, and frustration, anxiety, fatigue, insomnia, boredom, and anger contribute to a lowered threshold for pain. Thus treatment of the entire patient contributes to pain control.

Despite decades of evidence that physicians can and should be successful in controlling cancer pain, studies continue to reveal undertreatment and multiple barriers to effective cancer pain management.[6,33–35] Physicians have been guilty of inadequate knowledge of pain therapies, poor pain assessment, overconcern about controlled substances' regulations, and fear of patient addiction and tolerance. On the other hand, patients may be reluctant to report pain accurately. The health care system also presents impediments by giving cancer pain treatment low priority and inadequate reimbursement, along with restrictive regulation of controlled substances.

Pain during terminal illness and with cancer may be of two types: (1) nociceptive (somatic/visceral) and (2) neuropathic.[25,33–35] Somatic/visceral pain arises from direct stimulation of afferent nerves due to tumor infiltration of skin, soft tissue, or viscera. Somatic pain is often described as dull or aching and is well localized. Bone and soft tissue metastases are examples of somatic pain. Visceral pain tends to be poorly localized and is often referred to dermatomal sites distant from the source of the pain.

Neuropathic pain results from injury to some element of the nervous system because of the direct effect of the tumor or as a result of cancer therapy (surgery, irradiation, or chemotherapy). Examples include brachial or lumbosacral plexus invasion, spinal nerve root compression, or neuropathic complications of drugs such as vincristine. Neuropathic pain is described as sharp, shooting, shock-like, or burning and is often associated with dysesthesias. Unlike somatic/visceral pain, neuropathic pain may be relatively less responsive to opioids, whereas antidepressants, anticonvulsants, or local anesthetics may have good efficacy (also see Chapter 61).

An optimum pain management program includes assessing the pathophysiology of the patient's pain, taking a pain history, noting response to prior therapies, discussing the patient's goals for pain control, assessing psychosocial contributors to pain, and frequently reevaluating the patient after changes in treatment. Use of visual analogue or other pain scales is particularly useful for initial assessment and follow-up. This technique is in keeping with the new Joint Commission on Accreditation of Healthcare Organizations (JCAHO) standards of pain assessment, which encourage viewing pain as a vital sign.

Classically, the management of pain in terminally ill patients has involved multiple modalities: analgesic drugs, psychosocial and emotional support, palliative irradiation and surgery, and anesthesia-related techniques, such as nerve blocks, which can be both diagnostic and therapeutic.[33–35] Sometimes chemotherapy, radiopharmaceuticals, or hormonal therapies are of some help with cancer pain.

Analgesics are the mainstay for management of cancer and terminal illness pain. Traditionally, they have been classified into three broad categories: nonopioids (aspirin, acetaminophen, nonsteroidal antiinflammatory agents), opioids (with morphine the prototype), and adjuvant analgesics (antidepressants, anticonvulsants, local anesthetics, capsaicin, corticosteroids, and neuroleptics).

Because patients with advanced disease often have mixed types of pain, drugs from different classes are often combined to achieve optimal pain relief. This concept, together with the principle of using the simplest dosing schedule and the least-invasive modalities first, form the basis for WHO's "analgesic ladder" approach to pain management.[25] This approach, which has been validated in clinical trials worldwide and championed by other agencies,[25] recommends nonopioids for mild to moderate pain (step 1), adding opioids (including tramadol) for persistent or increasing pain (step 2), and finally increasing the opioid potency or dose as the pain escalates (step 3). At each step, adjuvant medications are considered based on the underlying causes of the pain. The ladder-based protocol should not be seen as rigid, as therapy must always be individualized, with doses and intervals carefully adjusted to provide optimal relief of pain with minimal side effects.

Although many opioid analgesics exist, morphine remains the gold standard. Morphine has a simple metabolic route with no accumulation of clinically significant active metabolites. There are a wide variety of preparations, making it easy to titrate or change routes of administration. When switching narcotics or routes of administration, physicians must be familiar with the well-publicized charts of equianalgesic dosing equivalents.[33–35]

Regardless of the choice of specific drug, doses should be given on a regular schedule, by the clock, to maintain steady blood levels. Additional rescue doses can be superimposed as needed on the baseline regimen. Transdermal fentanyl has been another option for achieving steady-state blood levels.

There is no ceiling effect for morphine dosing. The hallmark of tolerance development is shortening of the duration of analgesic action. Physical dependence is expected, and addiction is rare. Sharp increases in dosage requirements usually imply worsening of the underlying disease. Opioid side effects—constipation, nausea, vomiting, mental clouding, sedation, respiratory depression—are watched for vigilantly, anticipated, and prevented if possible. Constipation is so pervasive an issue that all patients on opioids should be started on a bowel management regimen that may include fluid, fiber, stool softeners, laxatives, enemas, or lactulose.

Regarding adjuvants, corticosteroids provide a range of effects, including mood elevation, antiinflammatory activity, antiemetic effects, appetite stimulation (helpful with cachexia), and reduction of cerebral and spinal cord edema. They may be helpful for bone and nerve pain. Megestrol may also stimulate appetite. Antidepressants in lower doses (e.g., 10–100 mg of the prototype amitriptyline) and anticonvulsants (especially gabapentin) help alleviate neuropathic pain and provide innate analgesia as well as potentiation of opioids. In standard doses the antidepressants are mood elevating, with particularly promising results achieved with the newer selective serotonin reuptake inhibitors. Psychostimulants (e.g., methylphenidate) may be useful for reducing opioid-induced respiratory depression and sedation when dosage adjustment is not feasible. Bisphosphonates and radiopharmaceuticals can be helpful with bone pain.

Physical and psychosocial modalities can be used with drugs to manage pain during all phases of treatment. Physical modalities include cutaneous stimulation, heat, cold, massage, pressure, gentle exercise, repositioning, biofeedback, transcutaneous electrical nerve stimulation, aroma therapy, acupuncture, and even immobilization (casting). A variety of cognitive-behavioral interventions can also be employed: relaxation, guided imagery, distraction, reframing, psychotherapy, and support groups.

Nonpain Symptom Management

Dying patients struggle with numerous losses and fears that are exacerbated by debilitating and often demeaning nonpain symptoms, including nausea, vomiting, anorexia, diarrhea, bowel impaction, depression, anxiety, delirium, cough, dyspnea, visceral or bladder spasms, hiccups, decubiti, and xerostomia. To preclude unnecessary suffering, clinicians must utilize diverse methods to optimize palliative care and provide a relatively symptom-free death.[3,7–9,36] Morphine is of particular help with dyspnea.[33] The key is to search for reversible causes of these diverse symptom complexes before resorting to medication management, which in extreme cases of unrelieved suffering can include legally and morally sanctioned "terminal" sedation (the so-called double-effect phenomenon).[7–9,36]

Anorexia with decreased intake is distressing to families. In addition, concerns about providing adequate nutrition and hydration have arisen on both a moral and symptom relief basis. Studies have revealed that hunger is a rare symptom, and that thirst and dry mouth are usually easily managed with local mouth care and sips.[10,11,37] Thus food and fluid administration are now thought not to play a significant role in providing comfort to terminally ill patients, nor is such provision thought to be morally mandated (though the symbolic meaning of feeding efforts should not be overlooked). Interestingly, force feeding and total parenteral nutrition tend to shorten survival, and tube feedings do not decrease aspiration risk.[37]

Bereavement and Grief

Most family members suffer psychologically during the dying of a loved one and then go through an expected process of bereavement. A multitude of feelings—shock, disbelief, a general numbing of all affect, protest, relief, guilt, anguish, emotional lability, tearfulness—accompany the first days to weeks of grieving, eventually giving way to less intense feelings that in normal circumstances are largely resolved within 1 year. The mourning period is a time of physical vulnerability, with bereaved persons likely to suffer impaired immune status and behavioral problems.[38]

The family physician is often best situated to provide ongoing bereavement services. The 13-month bereavement support offered by hospice agencies and community grief support groups can be utilized. Key tasks for the physician providing care to the bereaved include validating and normalizing feelings, not medicating emotions simply because they are intense, assessing the progress of the family's grief work, identifying and intervening in abnormal grief, and using age-appropriate models and interactional styles.[38] Short-acting benzodiazepines can be helpful during the first 1 to 2 weeks if family members need relief from sleeplessness and extreme tearfulness.

Special Needs of Dying Children

Although most of the previously mentioned principles of comprehensive terminal care apply equally well to dying children, several additional considerations should be emphasized.[39,40] Communication must include age and developmentally appropriate vocabulary. Although most children do not develop an accurate understanding of dying until age 7 to 8, those as young as 4 to 5 recognize that they are gravely ill. Physicians should openly discuss with parents what role they wish to play in discussions of diagnosis, prognosis, and death.

Multidisciplinary hospice involvement may be even more important for children than adults. Likewise, studies have verified that most terminally ill children, as well as their families, fare better when the caring and dying occur at home.[39,40] Clinicians must remain cognizant of sibling issues such as feelings of neglect or jealousy. Siblings may need reassurance that they are not in some way responsible for the child's dying. In general, siblings should be encouraged to participate in the care of their dying loved one.

Conclusion

The challenge in providing terminal care is to form an accurate understanding of the needs and preferences of the dying patient and to fit the delivery of care to those needs. The fundamental rule is that good care involves giving patients options and some sense of control. Physicians must realize that patients' needs are shaped in unusual ways by factors (cultural and religious) that fall outside the comfortable biomedical domain.

References

1. Billings JA, Block S. Palliative care in undergraduate medical education. JAMA 1997;278:733–8.
2. Rabow MW, Hardie GE, Fair JM, McPhee SJ. End-of-life care content in 50 textbooks from multiple specialties. JAMA 2000; 283:771–8.

3. Cassell CK, Field MJ, eds. Approaching death: improving care at the end of life. Washington, DC: National Academy Press, 1997.
4. Block SD, Bernier GM, Crawley LM, for the National Consensus Conference on Medical Education for Care Near the End of Life. Incorporating palliative care into primary care education. J Gen Intern Med 1998;13:768–73.
5. Mularski RA. Educational agenda for interdisciplinary end of life curricula. Crit Care Med 2001;29(2 suppl):N16–23.
6. Emmanuel LL, von Gunten CF, Ferris FD. Gaps in end-of-life care. Arch Fam Med 2000;9:1176–80.
7. Task Force on Palliative Care. Precepts of palliative care. J Palliat Med 1998;1:109–12.
8. Cassell CK, Foley KM, eds. Principles for care of patients at the end of life: an emerging consensus among the specialties of medicine. New York: Millbank Memorial Fund, 1999.
9. Council on Scientific Affairs, American Medical Association. Good care of the dying patient. JAMA 1996;275:474–8.
10. Winker MA, Flanagin A, eds. Theme issue: end-of-life care. JAMA 2000;284:2413–528.
11. Matzo ML, Lynn J, eds. Death and dying. Clin Geriatr Med 2000;16:211–398.
12. Fox EJ. Predominance of the curative model of medical care. JAMA 1999;278:761–3.
13. Buckman R. How to break bad news: a guide for health care professionals. Baltimore: Johns Hopkins University Press, 1992.
14. Siegler EL, Levin BW. Physician–older patient communication at the end of life. Clin Geriatr Med 2000;16:175–204.
15. von Gunten CF, Ferris FD, Emanuell LL. Ensuring competency in end of life care—communication and relational skills. JAMA 2000;284:3051–7.
16. Balaban RB. A physician's guide to talking about end of life care. J Gen Intern Med 2000;15:195–200.
17. Quill TE. Initiating end of life discussions with seriously ill patients: addressing the "elephant in the room." JAMA 2000;284:2502–7.
18. Christakis NA. Death foretold: prophecy and prognosis in medical care. Chicago: University of Chicago Press, 2000.
19. Block SD. Psychological considerations, growth, and transcendence at the end of life—the art of the possible. JAMA 2001;285:2898–905.
20. Kubler-Ross E. On death and dying. New York: Macmillan, 1969.
21. Singer PA, Martin DK, Kelner M. Quality end of life care: patient perspectives. JAMA 1999;281:163–8.
22. Vincent JL. Cultural differences in end of life care. Crit Care Med 2001;29(2 suppl):N52–5.
23. Daaleman TP, VandeCreek L. Placing religion and spirituality in end of life care. JAMA 2000;284:2514–7.
24. Koenig BA, Gates-Williams J. Understanding cultural differences in caring for dying patients. West J Med 1995;163:244–9.
25. Jadad AR, Bowman GP. The WHO analgesic ladder for cancer pain management. JAMA 1995;274:1870–3.
26. Lynn J. Serving patients who may die soon—the role of hospice and other services. JAMA 2001;285:925–32.
27. Fischer GS, Arnold RM, Tulsky JA. Talking to the older adult about advance directives. Clin Geriatr Med 2000;16:239–54.
28. Lynn J. Rethinking fundamental assumptions: SUPPORT's implications for future reform. J Am Geriatr Soc 2000;48:S214–21.
29. Emanuel EJ. Cost savings at the end of life: what do the data show? JAMA 1996;275:1907–14.
30. Emanuell LL. Facing requests for physician-assisted suicide— toward a practical and principled clinical skill set. JAMA 1998; 280:643–7.
31. Nuland SB. Physician-assisted suicide and euthanasia in practice. N Engl J Med 2000;342:583–4.
32. Searight HR. Assessing patient competence for medical decision making. Am Fam Physician 1992;45:751–9.
33. Cherny NI. The management of cancer pain. CA 2000;50: 70–116.
34. Abrahm JL. Advances in pain management for older adult patients. Clin Geriatr Med 2000;16:269–311.
35. Chang HM. Cancer pain management. Med Clin North Am 1999;83:711–36.
36. Bruera E, Neumann CM. Management of specific symptom complexes in patients receiving palliative care. Can Med Assoc J 1998;158:1717–26.
37. Huang Z, Ahronheim C. Nutrition and hydration in terminally ill patients: an update. Clin Geriatr Med 2000;16:313–25.
38. Casarett D, Kutner JS, Abrahm J, for the ACP-ASIM End of Life Consensus Panel. Life after death—a practical approach to grief and bereavement. Ann Intern Med 2001;134:208–15.
39. Masri C, Farrell CA, Lacroix J, Rocker G, Shesnie SD. Decision-making and end of life care in critically-ill children. J Palliat Care 2000;16(suppl):S45–52.
40. American Academy of Pediatrics Committee on Bioethics and Committee on Hospital Care. Palliative care for children. Pediatrics 2000;106:351–7.

63
Headache

Anne D. Walling

Headache is an almost universal experience, afflicting patients of any age or characteristic, although it is reported to be particularly frequent in young adults. Nearly 60% of men and 76% of women aged 12 to 29 years report at least one headache within any 4-week period.[1] The societal costs of headache are enormous but can be estimated only indirectly in terms of days lost from work or school, expenditures on medical services, and consumption of nonprescription medications. The total burden of suffering due to this symptom, including disruption of relationships and loss of normal activities, is incalculable. Although headache is the principal reason for more than 50 million physician office visits and 2.5 million emergency room visits per year, it is important to realize that most headache episodes are not brought to medical attention. Over 20% of those headache patients who do seek medical attention are dissatisfied with the care provided, making headache the leading diagnosis associated with patient dissatisfaction.[2]

Headache is a symptom, not a diagnosis. Numerous conditions can produce cephalic pain (see Classification of Headaches, below) as part of a localized or systemic process; thus headache may be a prominent symptom in the child with fever, the adult with sinusitis, or the elderly patient with temporal arteritis. The pathophysiology of "primary" headaches, such as migraine and cluster headaches, is a controversial, rapidly developing area with the principal developments focused on the role of neurotransmitters, endothelial cells, and whether neuronal tissue can itself generate pain.[3,4]

Whatever the etiology, each headache episode is interpreted by the individual patient in terms of experience, culture, and belief systems (see Chapter 3). Thus a relatively minor degree of pain may prompt one patient to seek emergency care and comprehensive neurologic assessment, whereas a patient with extensive personal or family experience of recurrent headache may cope with several days of incapacitating symptoms without seeking medical assistance. Patients and physi-

cians tend to be uncomfortable with the diagnosis and management of headache. In addition to extensive patient dissatisfaction,[5] headache is frequently identified as a "heart-sink" condition by physicians (i.e., the patient evokes "an overwhelming mixture of exasperation, defeat, and sometimes plain dislike"[6]). The reasons for this situation include the recurrent nature of most headache syndromes, the potential for secondary gain and iatrogenic complications (particularly overuse of narcotic analgesics), and fear of missing a potentially serious but rare intracranial lesion. The effective management of headaches requires the development of a therapeutic alliance between the physician and patient based on objectivity and mutual respect.[7] Most chronic headaches are recurrent and cannot be completely cured. Physicians can, however, greatly help patients to understand their condition, develop effective strategies to reduce the number and severity of attacks, and follow healthy lifestyles not skewed by the presence or fear of headache.

Clinical Approach to the Headache Patient

With so many potential causes and complicating circumstances, a systematic approach to the headache patient is essential for objective, effective, efficient management. It can be achieved in four stages:

1. Clarification of the reasons for the consultation
2. Diagnosis (classification) of the headache
3. Negotiation of management
4. Follow-up

Not infrequently, a significant headache history is discovered on systematic inquiry of a patient presenting for other reasons. The clinical approach to these patients reverses "clarification" to identify why the patient has avoided seeking medical help for headache symptoms.

Clarification of the Reasons for Consultation

Those headaches that lead to medical consultation have particular significance. It is important to have patients articulate their beliefs about the symptoms and expectations of treatment.[7] Reasons for consultation range from fear of cancer to seeking validation that current use of nonprescription medication is appropriate. Headache is frequently used as a "ticket of admission" symptom by the patient who wishes to discuss other medical or social problems. In practice, a change in the coping ability of the patient, family, or coworkers is as frequent a cause of consultation as any change in the severity or type of headache. Patients may also consult when they learn new information, particularly concerning situations in which a severe illness in a friend or relative presented as headache. Recent public advertising campaigns by drug companies have led to patients consulting physicians specifically to request the newer medications.

All headache patients should be asked directly what type of headache they believe they have and what causes it. These issues must be addressed during the management even if they are inaccurate. Patients should also be asked about expectations of management. Successful management avoids dependence by emphasizing the patients' role in reducing the frequency and severity of headaches and increasing their ability to cope with a recurrent condition.

Background information from relatives and friends may give useful insights. Disruptive headaches lead to highly charged situations, and the physician must remain objective and avoid becoming triangulated between the patient and others. With good listening and a few directed questions, the background to the consultation can be clarified and the groundwork laid for accurate diagnosis and successful management. This short time is well invested. In headache patients presenting to family physicians, "listening" time makes a significantly greater contribution to the diagnosis and management than time spent on the physical examination or other investigation,[8] although all are appropriate.

Classification of Headaches

The 1988 International Classification of Headaches[9] established diagnostic criteria for 13 major types of headache with approximately 70 subtypes (Table 63.1). A useful grouping for family practice uses five categories.

1. Migraine (all types)
2. Cluster headaches
3. Tension/stress (or muscle contraction) headaches
4. Headaches secondary to other pathology
5. Specific headache syndromes (e.g., cough headache)

These categories are broad with considerable overlap. "Mixed headaches," where the clinical picture contains elements of more

Table 63.1. **Headache Types**

Primary headaches
Migraine
    Without aura
    With aura (several types)
    Ophthalmoplegic
    Retinal
    Childhood syndromes
    Complicated migraine
    Other
Tension type
    Episodic
    Chronic
    Other
Cluster
    Episodic
    Chronic
    Chronic paroxysmal hemicrania
    Other
Miscellaneous
    "Ice-pick"
    External compression
    Cold stimulus (including ice cream)
    Cough
    Exertional
    Coital

Secondary headaches
Associated with
    Head trauma
    Vascular disorders
    Intracranial disorders
    Substance use or withdrawal (including medication side effects)
    Systemic infections
    Metabolic disorders
    Structural disorder of head or neck
    Neuralgia syndromes

Unclassifiable headaches

than one headache category, are common. Individual patients may also describe more than one type of headache; for example, migraineurs experience tension headaches on occasion.

Diagnosis

The diagnosis of headache syndromes (Table 63.2) requires systematic clinical reasoning based on the history augmented by physical examination and judicious use of investigations or consultation to establish the most probable etiology for the pain. A particular feature is the potential to use the diagnostic process to increase patients' understanding and prepare them to take responsibility for long-term management in cooperation with the physician.

Tension headaches are by far the most prevalent type of cephalic pain encountered in family practice,[8,10] probably followed by headaches secondary to other causes. The medical literature, research efforts, and therapeutic innovations focus on migraine and other interesting primary headache syndromes, but all headache patients deserve a competent assessment and appropriate, individualized treatment for their symptoms.

Table 63.2. **Diagnostic Criteria for Common Primary Headaches**

Headache	Duration	Characteristics	Associated symptoms	Other

Migraine	4–72 hours	At least two:
		Unilateral
		Pulsating
		Moderate to severe
		Aggravated by activity
			At least one:
			Nausea/vomiting
			Photophobia and
			  phonophobia
				No neurologic source for
				  symptoms
				Multiple types (Table 63.1)
				At least five attacks for
				  diagnosis

Cluster	Individual attacks:
	  15–180 minutes
	Cluster episodes: 1–8
	  attacks/day for 7
	  days to 1 year or
	  longer
		Unilateral orbital/
		  temporal stabbing
		Severe to very severe
			At least one:
			Conjunctival
			  injection
			Lacrimation
			Nasal congestion
			Rhinorrhea
			Sweating
			Miosis
			Ptosis
			Eyelid edema
				No neurologic source for
				  symptoms
				At least five attacks for
				  diagnosis

Tension/stress	Individual headaches:
	  30 minutes to 7 days
	Headaches <15 days/month
	  or <180/year
		At least two:
		Pressure/tightness
		Bilateral
		Mild to moderate
		Not aggravated by
		  activity
			No nausea
			Photophobia and
			  phonophobia: absent
			  or only one present,
			  not both
				No neurologic source for
				  symptoms
				At least 10 episodes for
				  diagnosis

History

Headache diagnoses depend on the medical history. An open-ended approach, such as "Tell me about your headaches," followed by specific questions to elucidate essential features usually indicates which of the diagnostic categories is most probable. The history should address the criteria shown in Table 63.2 and clarify the following:

1. *Characteristics:* nature of pain, location, radiation in head, intensity, exacerbating and relieving factors or techniques, associated symptoms and signs.
2. *Pattern:* usual duration and frequency of episodes, precipitating factors, description of a typical episode, change in pattern over time, prodromes and precipitating factors, postheadache symptoms.
3. *Personal history:* age at onset, medical history (including medication, alcohol, and substance use) with special emphasis on secondary causes of headache, such as depression or trauma; environmental and occupational exposure history (see Chapters 32 and 45).
4. *Investigations and treatments:* previous diagnoses and supporting evidence, patient's degree of confidence in these diagnoses, patient's beliefs and concerns about diagnosis and potential treatments; previous treatments and degree of success; side effects of any investigations and treatments; patient preferences for treatment; current use of prescription and nonprescription medications.
5. *Family history:* headache, other conditions, family attitudes to headache.

The headache profile that emerges from the history has a high probability of correctly classifying the headache[7,8,10,11] without further investigation. It is important, however, to complete the usual review of systems to uncover additional data.

Throughout the history-taking process, the physician forms a general impression of the patient. Although subjective, this should correlate with the headache profile and is particularly useful for assessing psychological components of the situation, including which management strategies are most likely to be successfully implemented and followed by the patient. By the end of the history taking, the physician should have the answer to two questions: Which of the five headache groups best fits the story? and Is this diagnosis likely in this particular patient?

Physical Examination

The physical examination continues the dual processes of confirming a specific diagnosis and laying the groundwork for successful management. Unless the consultation coincides with an attack, many migraine, cluster, and other headache patients can be expected to have no abnormal findings on physical examination. Some authors recommend that only a targeted examination be performed, focusing on the most probable cause of the secondary headache elicited from the history,[8] whereas others emphasize the importance of complete physical and neurologic examination of every headache patient.[11] The time devoted to a complete examination may be a wise investment, as it documents both positive and negative physical findings, contributes to the therapeutic alliance, and in many instances is therapeutic. Any physical examination targets the most probable diagnoses based on the symptoms presented by the patient and the physician's knowledge of conditions relevant to the individual.

Other Investigations

A logical test strategy is guided by the most probable diagnosis (or diagnoses) suggested by the history and physical examination. Targeted laboratory and radiologic investigations are most useful for confirming the underlying cause of secondary headaches. Tests are often performed to relieve either physician or patient distress and uncertainty. If the patient or family insists on tests the physician does not believe appropriate, the contributions and limitations of the test in question should be reviewed. Similarly, the physician experiencing the WHIMS (what have I missed syndrome) must review the data and attempt to make a rational decision as to the potential contribution of additional testing.

Most of the debate over the appropriate role of testing currently involves radiologic investigation, specifically computed tomography (CT) and magnetic resonance imaging (MRI). The role of these modalities is limited by the rarity in family practice of headaches caused by intracranial lesions. Serious intracranial pathology was the cause of only 0.4% of new headaches presented to primary care physicians in two studies.[8,12] When deciding to refer a patient for advanced radiologic investigation, the family physician must seriously consider the potential benefits versus the potential radiation exposure (for CT), patient distress (MRI), and cost. As the investigations have different and often complementary abilities, one must also have a clear concept of what type of intracranial lesion is being sought and its likely location. CT is very sensitive to acute hemorrhage and certain enhancing solid lesions; MRI provides better resolution in the posterior fossa and superior detection of gliosis, infection, posttraumatic changes, and certain tumors.[13] Discussions with a neurologist or radiologist may be useful in this difficult area.

Recent guidelines developed by a consortium including the American Academy of Family physicians (available at www.aafp.org) recommend neuroimaging in migraine only if the result is likely to change clinical management and the patient has a significant risk of a relevant abnormality.[14] An exception may be made if patients are excessively worried about the potential etiology of headaches. This is in general agreement with the National Institutes of Health (NIH) Consensus Development Panel which recommended CT investigation of patients whose headaches were "severe, constant, unusual, or associated with neurological symptoms."[15] This recommendation can be problematic in practice, however, as more than half of the patients describe their headaches as severe.[8] The other elements of the NIH recommendations, particularly the presence of neurologic signs, are more useful. The final decision to refer for CT or MRI remains a clinical judgment based on the characteristics of the patient, the symptom complex, and risk factors for intracranial pathology.

Negotiation of Management

Migraine, cluster, tension/stress, and many secondary headaches are recurrent; hence the emphasis is on enabling the patient to successfully manage a lifestyle that includes headaches. The physician who sets a goal of abolishing headaches is being unrealistic in almost all cases.[7,8] More appropriate goals are effective treatment of individual headache episodes and minimizing the number and severity of these episodes. Most headache patients are open to the concept that they carry a vulnerability to headaches and are willing to learn how to manage this tendency. Patients who strongly resist this management approach are often highly dependent personalities who may have drug-seeking behavior or may change to another chronic pain symptom complex when offered aggressive treatment of headaches. The complete management plan includes patient education, treatment plans for both prophylaxis and acute management, and follow-up.

Patient education is essential for the patient and family to manage headaches. They must understand the type of headache and its treatment and natural history. In addition to providing information, the physician must address hidden concerns. Many myths and beliefs are associated with headaches, and patients are empowered to deal with their headaches once these beliefs are addressed. Patients may be embarrassed by their fears; for example, almost all migraine patients have feared cerebral hemorrhage during a severe attack.

Patient education and treatment overlap as the patient and family become responsible for identifying and managing situations that precipitate or exacerbate headache. These situations range from avoiding foods that trigger migraine attacks to practicing conflict resolution. Stress is implicated in almost all headaches; even the pain of secondary headaches is less easy to manage in stressful situations.

There are few "absolutes" in the pharmacologic treatment of headaches, and the large number of choices can be bewildering to both physicians and patients. In general, first-line analgesics and symptomatic treatment are effective, and narcotic use should be avoided. A common mistake is to appear tentative about therapy. The exasperated physician who uses phrases such as, "We'll try this," may convey the message that the medication is not expected to work. Conversely, implying to patients that one has selected a medication specific to their situation, and based on an understanding of the headache literature, recruits the placebo effect and is much more likely to succeed. Patients gather information about headaches and their treatment from a wide variety of sources, including news media and the experience of friends. Patient knowledge and opinions of specific treatments should be established before issuing a prescription.

Nonpharmacologic advice is a powerful factor in building the placebo effect and therapeutic alliance. Physicians gather experiences from many patients and can pass on tips for headache management, such as Lamaze-type breathing exercises for tension headaches, cold washcloth over the eyes during a migraine attack, and vigorous exercise at the start of migraine, cluster, or tension headaches. Including such information in the overall treatment plan enhances the physician's credibility and reinforces the message that headache management is not solely dependent on medications. Formal therapies such as relaxation therapy, thermal biofeedback, and cognitive-behavior therapy can be effective in individual migraine patients.[16]

Follow-Up

With the exception of headaches secondary to acute self-limiting conditions, headaches tend to be a recurrent problem. Unless follow-up is well managed, the patient returns only at times of severe symptoms or exasperation at the failure of treatment. This pattern implies the risk of emergency visits at difficult times and consultation complicated by hostility or disappointment. In practice, patients manage well if given scheduled appointments, particularly if they are combined with the expectation that the patient will come to the consultation well prepared (i.e., with information on the number, pattern, response to treatment, and any other relevant information about headaches since the last visit). Some authors recommend that patients keep a formal headache diary.[8]

Clinical Types of Headache

Migraine

Migraine-type headaches are estimated to affect more than 23 million Americans, approximately 17% of women and 6% of men.[17] Although all epidemiologic studies are complicated by differences in definitions and design, migraine is more common in women at all ages and has a peak prevalence during young adulthood. Up to 30% of women aged 21 to 34 report at least one migraine-type headache per year.[18]

Up to 90% of migraine patients have a first-degree relative, usually a parent, also affected by migraine.[18] Perhaps because of familiarity with the condition, significant numbers of migraine sufferers (approximately 50%) do not seek medical assistance. Several classifications of migraine have been suggested. As shown in Table 63.2, the current international classification[9] is based on clinical features, particularly the presence of aura. In practice, it is seldom useful to subclassify migraine.

Patients in the "classic" subgroup (approximately 20% of all migraineurs) experience a characteristic aura before the onset of migraine head pain. This aura may take several forms, but visual effects such as scotomas, zigzag lines, photopsia, or visual distortions are the most common. A much larger proportion of patients describe prodromal symptoms, which may be visceral, such as diarrhea or nausea, but are more commonly alterations in mood or behavior. Food cravings, mild euphoria (conversely, yawning), and heightened sensory perception, particularly of smell, are surprisingly common.

The headache of migraine is severe, usually unilateral, described as "throbbing" or "pulsating," and aggravated by movement. The pain usually takes 30 minutes to 3 hours to reach maximum intensity, and it may last several hours. The eye and temple are the most frequent centers of pain, but occipital involvement is common. Each patient describes a characteristic group of associated symptoms among which nausea predominates. Either nausea or both photophobia and phonophobia are required for diagnosis along with the characteristic headache. During attacks, migraine patients avoid movement and sensory stimuli, especially light. They may use pressure and either heat or cold over the areas of maximal pain. The attack usually terminates with sleep. Vomiting appears to shorten attacks, and some patients admit to self-induced vomiting, although this phenomenon is not widely described in the literature. Many patients report a "hangover" on waking after a migraine, but others report complete freedom from symptoms and a sense of euphoria. The cause of migraine remains unknown; research indicates that migraine begins in neurons as a biochemical process, and that vascular phenomena are secondary effects.[19,20]

The treatment of migraine typifies the approach of enabling patients to manage their own condition. A bewildering variety of therapies is available, and management should be individualized. The treatment plan has three aspects: avoidance of precipitants, aggressive treatment of attacks, and prophylactic therapy if indicated. Patients and their families can usually identify triggers of migraine attacks. The role of specific foods has probably been exaggerated,[21] although red wine and cheese continue to have a significant reputation as migraine triggers. Disturbance in daily routine, particularly missed meals, excessive sleeping, and relaxation after periods of stress, are notorious precipitants of migraine attacks. Certain women correlate migraines with the onset of menstruation each month, but the effect of oral contraception and postmenopausal hormone replacement are unpredictable. Migraines commonly disappear during pregnancy.

Patients should be encouraged to recognize their own aura or prodrome, as early treatment is most efficacious. Whatever treatment strategy is followed, early use of metoclopramide helps reduce nausea and counteract delayed gastric emptying. The multiple medications used for migraine may be categorized into four groups:

1. Symptom control: principally analgesics, with or without adjunctive antiemetics or sedatives
2. Ergotamines: based on the theory that migraine pain is due to cerebral vasodilation
3. Serotonin (5-hydroxytryptamine, 5-HT) receptor agonists: new class of agents (prototype is sumatriptan) based on etiology
4. Prophylactic agents: large, diverse group of medications reported to reduce the frequency of attacks (Table 63.3).

A common problem in migraine treatment is subtherapeutic dosage of medication or failure to absorb medication because of vomiting and gastric stasis.

The choice of specific medications and route of delivery must be individualized. Factors contributing to the decision include the migraine characteristics (particularly the likelihood of vomiting), patient factors such as associated medical problems, and medication issues including efficacy, speed of onset, side effects, cost, and acceptability.[17] The headache consortium guidelines stress the balance between adequate, effective treatment and the avoidance of iatrogenic effects from inappropriate medication use.[22] Patients frequently appreciate having more than one agent or combination of agents (e.g., ergotamine, analgesic, or a triptan drug) when they need to "keep going" and a combination analgesic and sedative for "backup" or situations when they can "crash." Many patients also report that a particular agent appears to work well for several months, but then they need to change it.

Narcotics have almost no place in migraine therapy. Even in the emergency room situation, controlled studies have shown that adequate analgesia, use of injections of antiemet-

Table 63.3. **Pharmacologic Treatment of Primary Headaches**

Headache type	Acute attack[a]		Prophylactic therapy	
	Dose	Comment	Dose (per day)	Comment
Migraine				

	Ergotamines
	  Inhalation (0.36 mg/dose)
	  Oral, sublingual (1–2 mg)
	  Rectal IM or IV (0.5–1 mg)
		Many formulations and combination drugs available
		Side effects: nausea, vasoconstriction
			Beta-blockers
			  Propranolol (40–240 mg)
			  Nadolol (80–240 mg)
			  Timolol (20–30 mg)
			  Atenolol (50–100 mg)
			  Metoprolol (50–300 mg)
				Dosage individualized; side effects are fatigue, GI upset; contraindicated with asthma, heart failure

	Analgesics
	  Aspirin (650–1000 mg
	  Acetaminophen (<100 mg)
	  Ibuprofen (<600 mg)
	  Naproxen (<550 mg)
	  Ketorolac (30–60 mg IM)
		Many analgesics and NSAIDs effective
		Dosage individualized
		Combinations available with sedatives and antiemetics
		Side effects: mainly gastric upset
			Amitriptyline (25–150 mg hs)
			
			Sodium valproate (800–1500 mg)
			
			Phenelzine (Nardil) (30–75 mg)
				Sedation, weight gain, dry mouth; synergistic with beta-blockers
				Not in liver disease
				
				Insomnia, hypotension; interacts with tyramine in food

	5-HT agonists
	  Sumatriptan 6 mg SC
	   25–100 mg oral,
	   5–20 mg nasal
	  Zolmitriptan 2.5–5 mg
	  Naratriptan (1–2.5 mg
	
	  Rizatriptan 5–10 mg
		Not given if cerebrovascular, cardiovascular disease risk or hypertensive
		Headache may recur
		Expensive
			Verapamil (240 mg)
			
			Serotonin-receptor antagonists
			
			Methysergide (2–10 mg)
				Constipation; not in conduction block
				
				Pending FDA approval; sedation, weight gain
				
				Vasoconstriction, fibrosis

Cluster	Oxygen 100% 8–10 mL/min for 10 minutes Ergotamine 1–2 mg orally Ergotamine 0.36 mg/puff × 1–3 Lidocaine 4% 1 mL into nostril Methoxyflurane inhale 10 drops		Prednisone 10–80 mg daily Lithium 300–900 mg daily Indomethacin 120 mg daily Nifedipine 40–120 mg daily	
Tension-stress	Analgesics and NSAIDs (as for migraine but at lower dosages)		Amitriptyline (50–100 mg hs) Imipramine (25–75 mg)	

[a]Treatment must be of rapid onset. (1) All therapy should be started at first sign of attack but triptans are not advised during aura. (2) Other symptomatic relief may be added, especially antiemetics and sedative. (3) Encourage patients to find abortive therapy (e.g., caffeine, exercise, cold ± pressure over the site of pain) to use in addition to above. (4) Narcotics are rarely necessary for migraine.

5-HT = 5-hydroxytryptamine (serotonin); NSAID = nonsteroidal antiinflammatory drug.

AAFP treatment guidelines are available at *http://www.aafp.org/afp/20001115/practice.html.*

ics, or injectable ergotamines are superior to narcotics.[18] The migraine patient who demands narcotics or claims allergies to alternative treatments may be a drug abuser. Rarely, patients develop dehydration and "status migrainosus" when the attack lasts several days. These patients may require hospitalization and steroids in addition to fluids and aggressive therapy based on antiemetics plus a triptan drug or ergotamine preparation.

The introduction of the triptans has dramatically changed migraine management,[23] but the experience for individual patients may be unpredictable. Whereas many patients experience dramatic relief, others find triptan use limited by nausea, return of headache 3 to 6 hours after initial clearing, and an unpleasant autonomic reaction of flushing, nausea, hyperventilation, and panic attack as the medication is absorbed. A European study found comparable pain relief but fewer side

effects when a combination of aspirin and antiemetic was compared to sumatriptan.[24] As with all migraine treatment, the importance of working with the patient to achieve optimal results from the many options cannot be overstressed. For some patients the triptans are wonder drugs, but for others an expensive disappointment. The headache consortium concluded there was good clinical evidence of effectiveness for several drugs[25] (Table 63.3).

If patients find normal life disrupted by the frequency and severity of migraine attacks, prophylactic treatment should be considered.[16] Beta-blockers are the most widely studied agents. Those without intrinsic sympathomimetic activity (e.g., propranolol, nadolol, atenolol, metoprolol) are effective, but the dosage at which individual patients benefit must be established by clinical trial. Amitriptyline appears to prevent migraine at lower dosages than that used for treatment of depression. Beta-blockers and amitriptyline are synergistic if used together. Many other drugs have been recommended, but the studies are often small and difficult to interpret because of the placebo effect and patient selection. Verapamil appears to have some prophylactic effect, but there is little evidence to support the use of other calcium channel blocking agents. Studies indicate that the anticonvulsant medication valproic acid can be prophylactic for migraine, and interest is growing in the use of fluoxetine and other selective serotonin reuptake inhibitors for this indication.[26] A serotonin agonist, pizotifen, and a calcium-channel blocker, flunarizine, are widely used in other countries[20] but are not yet approved for use in the United States. Conversely, methysergide, which has largely fallen out of use in the United States because of the fear of retroperitoneal fibrosis, is returning to use in other countries at low dosages plus monitoring for side effects and scheduled "drug holidays."[21]

The choice of any prophylactic agent must balance potential benefit against issues of compliance, side effects, and cost.[16,26] Migraine patients can usually be assisted to find regimens that enable them to minimize attacks and deal effectively with those that do occur. They may be comforted by knowing that the condition tends to wane with age, has been associated with lower rates of cerebrovascular and ischemic heart disease than expected,[19] and has afflicted a galaxy of famous people.[18]

Cluster Headaches

The cluster headache, a rare but dramatic form, occurs predominantly in middle-aged men. The estimated prevalence is 69 per 100,000 adults with a 6:1 male preponderance.[18]

The headache is severe, unilateral, centered around the eye or temple, and accompanied by lacrimation, rhinorrhea, red eye, and other autonomic signs on the same side as the headache. Symptoms develop rapidly, reach peak intensity within 10 to 15 minutes, and last up to 2 hours. During the attack the patient is frantic with pain and may be suspected of intoxication, drug-induced behavior, or hysteria.[8] This behavior, including talk of suicide because of the severity of the pain, is characteristic, but patients may be too embarrassed to volunteer this information. The diagnosis is based on the description of attacks, especially their severity, and is confirmed by the unique time pattern described by the patient. During a cluster period, which typically lasts 4 to 8 weeks, the patient experiences attacks at the same time or times of day with bizarre regularity. Approximately half of these attacks awaken the patient and are particularly frequent around 1 A.M. Most patients experience one or two cluster periods per year and are completely free from symptoms at other times. About 10% of patients develop chronic symptoms, with daily attacks over several years. During a cluster period, drinking alcohol or taking vasodilators almost inevitably precipitates an attack. It is speculated that the cluster headache is due to a disorder of serotonin metabolism or circadian rhythm (or both), but the cause remains unknown.[18]

Management strategies aim to provide relief from individual attacks and prophylactically to suppress cluster episodes

(Table 63.3). Acute treatment must be of rapid onset and able to be administered by the patient or family. Conventional analgesics do not act quickly enough to provide relief, and all the current treatments of acute cluster headaches are difficult to administer to a patient who is restless and distracted with pain. Inhalation of oxygen is the traditional treatment, and inhalation or instillation of local anesthetics into the nostril on the affected side may also be effective. The only ergotamines likely to be effective during the acute attack are those delivered by inhaler or injection. European studies indicate that self-administered injections of sumatriptan are effective.[27]

The mainstay of cluster headache management is to suppress headaches during a cluster period. As shown in Table 63.3, several drugs are effective. Drugs may also be used in combination (e.g., verapamil 80 mg qid with ergotamine 2 mg hs).[28] Treatment should be initiated as soon as a cluster period begins and continued for a few days beyond the expected duration of the cluster. Only the previous experience of each patient can be used to judge the duration of therapy. Each patient has a set length for the cluster period as well as a tendency to repeat the same time and symptom pattern of individual headaches. It is particularly important in the age group usually affected by cluster headaches to monitor prophylactic drugs such as lithium, prednisone, ergotamine, indomethacin, calcium channel blockers, and methysergide for side effects.

Tension-Stress (Muscle Contraction) Headaches

Tension-stress headaches are the most frequent of all headaches encountered in clinical practice.[10,18] In one study of family practice consultations, they accounted for 70% of all new headache patients.[8] These patients represent a select sample of all tension headache patients, as most sufferers are believed to manage their symptoms using simple analgesics or other strategies. Although physicians are familiar with the condition, it is difficult to define it because it presents in myriad forms and is known by several names. The formal definition (Table 63.2) contains both positive and negative criteria, but a common problem is to diagnose tension headaches only after searching for more interesting etiologies for the symptoms.

The etiology and pathophysiology of tension headaches are poorly understood. Stress, psychological abnormalities, muscle contraction, and abnormalities of neurotransmitters have been implicated.[29,30] The clinical syndrome may represent more than one entry, and in many cases there is considerable overlap with migraine.[19]

As with migraine, more than 70% of tension headaches occur in women, and a substantial proportion of patients (40%) give a family history of similar symptoms. Tension headaches, however, tend to have their onset at an older age (70% after 20 years) and to produce symptoms daily or on several days per week, rather than occur as episodic attacks.

The clinical picture is characterized by long periods (up to several years) of almost daily headaches that vary in intensity throughout the day. Most patients keep going with daily activities, but going to bed early is characteristic. The pain is described in many ways, among which "pressure," "tight band," and "aching" predominate. Patients usually express exhaustion, and the patient's affect and body language convey weariness and frustration. Sleep disturbances are common.

Physical examination may be negative or may reveal tightness and tenderness of the muscles of the occipital area, posterior neck, and shoulders. Physical examination is important to rule out secondary headache and to assist in establishing the therapeutic relationship. Attempts to treat the headaches with analgesics before establishing patient confidence in the diagnosis risk failure despite escalating use of analgesics including narcotics.

The treatment of tension headaches is frequently unsatisfactory. Success depends on treatment of any underlying condition (particularly depression), patient education about the nature of the condition, and the control of symptoms without creating dependence or other adverse effects (see Chapters 31 and 32). Tension headache patients frequently take large quantities of analgesics, leading to gastrointestinal and other complications, or they use combination medicines containing sedatives. A wise investment during the history is to clarify all medication use, including nonprescription medication, and to explore previous encounters with physicians. Patients may have already been investigated extensively, and prior medical experiences color expectations and evaluation of management approaches.

Acute episodes of headache are best managed by first-line analgesics, such as acetaminophen, aspirin, or ibuprofen. Narcotics and combination drugs, especially those that contain barbiturates or caffeine, should be avoided. Nonsteroidal antiinflammatory drugs (NSAIDs) may be more effective than other analgesics,[10] especially if prescribed on a regular schedule for several days rather than on an as-needed basis. It is useful to teach the patient and family simple massage and relaxation techniques and to explore methods to resolve conflicts and enhance self-esteem. Not all patients require extensive counseling or biofeedback. The most significant predictor of symptom resolution after 1 year has been shown to be patient confidence that the problem had been fully discussed with a physician.[8] In addition to treating underlying depression, amitriptyline and other antidepressants raise pain thresholds and play a significant role in enabling patients to manage symptoms. The effective dosage may be lower than that required for depressive illnesses.

Secondary Headaches

Headache is part of the clinical picture of many conditions. Particularly in children, frontal headache is a common accompaniment of fever. In all age groups, almost any condition of the head and neck and several systemic conditions can present as headache. A careful history combined with physical examination and other investigations where appropriate can almost always differentiate secondary from primary headache.[3]

There is particular concern in family practice not to miss the rare but serious intracranial condition, especially brain tumor. The symptoms of an intracranial lesion depend on its size, location, and displacement effect on other tissues. No single characteristic headache picture can therefore be given. Suspicion should be raised about headaches of recent onset that appear to become steadily more severe, do not fit any of the primary classifications, and do not respond to first-line treatment. Close follow-up and repeated physical examinations may detect the earliest neurologic abnormalities, but if there is a high degree of suspicion, early radiologic investigation or specialist consultation should be obtained. With intracranial vascular lesions, the first symptom may be a catastrophic hemorrhage.

A growing area of concern for family physicians is "rebound" headache, sometimes called chronic daily headache, which may represent up to 30% of headache consultations.[30] These patients have headaches at least 15 days per month. These patients initially have tension, migraine, or secondary headaches but inappropriate and/or excessive use of medications sets up a vicious cycle in which the treatment itself exacerbates and perpetuates headache. Drug-rebound headaches occur with analgesics, ergotamines, and triptans. In addition, headache may be an adverse effect of several drugs, including NSAIDs.[31]

Specific Headache Syndromes

The literature describes several specific primary headache syndromes that are uncommon but may be encountered in practice (e.g., cough headache) (Table 63.1). These syndromes are more common in men and are characterized by the severity of the pain and the potential for confusion with serious intracranial conditions. Despite the dramatic history, the conditions are generally benign and many respond to indomethacin.[18] Neuroimaging may be necessary to confirm the diagnosis. Explanation, reassurance, and symptom control are usually effective.

References

1. Diamond S, Feinberg DT. The classification, diagnosis and treatment of headaches. Med Times 1990;118:15–27.
2. Lake AE. Psychological impact: the personal burden of migraine. Am J Manag Care 1999;5:S111–21.
3. Olesen J. Understanding the biologic basis of migraine. N Engl J Med 1994;331:1713–4.
4. Thomsen LL, Olesen J. Human models of headache. In: Olsen J, Tfelt-Hansen P, Welch KMA, eds. The headaches, 2nd ed. Philadelphia: Lippincott Williams & Wilkins, 1999;203–9.
5. Silberstein SD. Office management of benign headache. Postgrad Med 1996;93:223–40.
6. O'Dowd TC. Five years of heartsink patients in general practice. BMJ 1988;297:528–30.
7. Graham JR. Headaches. In: Noble J, ed. Textbook of primary care medicine, 2nd ed. St. Louis: Mosby, 1996;1283–319.
8. McWhinney IR. A textbook of family medicine. New York: Oxford University Press, 1989.
9. Headache Classification Committee of the International Headache Society. Classification and diagnostic criteria for all headache disorders, cranial neuralgias and facial pain. Cephalgia 1988;8(S7):1–96.
10. Clough C. Non-migrainous headaches [editorial]. BMJ 1989;299:70–2.

536   Anne D. Walling

11. Diamond S, Dalessio DJ, eds. The practicing physician's approach to headache, 5th ed. Baltimore: Williams & Wilkins, 1992.
12. Becker L, Iverson DC, Reed FM, et al. Patients with new headache in primary care: a report from ASPN. J Fam Pract 1988;27:41–7.
13. Prager JM, Mikulis DJ. The radiology of headache. Med Clin North Am 1991;75:525–44.
14. Morey SS. Practice guidelines. Headache consortium releases guidelines for use of CT or MRI in migraine work-up. Am Fam Physician 2000;62:1699–702.
15. NIH Consensus Development Panel. Computer tomographic scanning of the brain. In: Proceedings from NIH Consensus Development Conference, NIH, Bethesda. Washington DC: Government Printing Office, 1982;4:2.
16. Morey SS. Guidelines on migraine: part 4. General principles of preventive therapy Am Fam Physician 2000;62:2359–60, 2363.
17. Silberstein SD, Lipton RB. Overview of diagnosis and treatment of migraine. Neurology 1994;44(suppl 7):S6–16.
18. Raskin NH. Headache, 2nd ed. New York: Churchill Livingstone, 1988.
19. Blau J. Migraine: theories of pathogenesis. Lancet 1992;339:1202–7.
20. Smith R. Chronic headaches in family practice. J Am Board Fam Pract 1992;5:589–99.
21. Lance JW. Treatment of migraine. Lancet 1992;393:1207–9.
22. Morey SS. Practice guidelines. Guidelines on migraine: part 2.

General principles of drug therapy. Am Fam Physician 2000;62:1915–7.
23. Cady RK, Shealy CN. Recent advances in migraine management. J Fam Pract 1993;36:85–91.
24. Tfelt-Hansen P, Henry P, Mulder LJ, et al. The effectiveness of combined oral lysine acetylsalicylate and metoclopramide compared with oral sumatriptan for migraine. Lancet 1995;346:923–6.
25. Morey SS. Practice guidelines. Guidelines on migraine: part 3. Recommendations for individual drugs. Am Fam Physician 2000;62:2145–51.
26. Morey SS. Practice guidelines. Guidelines on migraine: part 5. Recommendations for specific prophylactic drugs. Am Fam Physician 2000;62:2535–9.
27. Walling AD. Cluster headaches. Am Fam Physician 1993;47:1457–63.
28. Kudrow L. Diagnosis and treatment of cluster headache. Med Clin North Am 1991;75:579–94.
29. Olesen J, Schoenen. Synthesis of tension-type headache mechanisms. In: Olesen J, Tfelt-Hansen P, Welch KMA, eds. The headaches, 2nd ed. Philadelphia: Lippincott Williams & Wilkins, 1999;615–8.
30. Rapoport A, Strang P, Gutterman DL, et al. Analgesic rebound headache in clinical practice: data from a physician survey. Headache 1996;36:1419.
31. Walling AD. Headache. Monograph, Edition No 265, Home Study Self-Assessment Program. Leawood, KS. AAFP June 2001.

64
Seizure Disorders

Donald B. Middleton

Approximately 10% of the population in the United States suffers a seizure at some point in life and between 1% and 3% develop epilepsy.[1–3] Because seizures are so commonly encountered, the family physician must be proficient in their management. If the disorder is recurrent and unprovoked, the patient has epilepsy. The annual incidence of epilepsy is roughly 50 per 100,000 and the prevalence is 5 to 10 per 1000.[3,4] Epilepsy incidence is high in children ages 0 to 9 years, plateaus in the 10- to 39-year-old population, drops to a low in 40- to 59-year-olds, and peaks in the elderly.[3,4] Because of a 3% risk of febrile seizures, nonepileptic seizures peak during childhood.[5] Although two initial seizures within 24 hours may suggest a diagnosis of epilepsy, the prognosis is the same as for a single seizure. On the other hand, a single seizure in the presence of a significant lesion on neuroimaging or a diagnostic electroencephalogram (EEG) qualifies as epilepsy.[6] Most nonepileptic seizures are clonic-tonic, whereas the most common form of epilepsy is the complex partial seizure.

Background

A seizure is a spontaneous, transient burst of abnormal, usually time-limited, involuntary brain activity. Table 64.1 lists possible causes. Pathologic changes in the brain that induce convulsions include anoxic degeneration, focal neuronal loss, neoplasia, and sclerosis.[4] Idiopathic hippocampal sclerosis is the major finding with complex partial seizures of temporal lobe origin. Although the majority of seizures are provoked responses to central nervous system (CNS) stressors like fever or are reflex responses to certain stimuli like a pulsating light, close to 30% of all seizure disorders, the primary epilepsies, have a specific genetic inheritance pattern, such as the autosomal-dominant pattern of tuberous sclerosis. Studies of monozygotic twins demonstrating a 90% concordance rate for epilepsy and EEG abnormalities in other family members support this genetic link.[7] Specific chromosomal loci are linked to some syndromes.[8] Although heredity plays its greatest role in epilepsy with onset before age 5 years, a seizure occurring prior to age 10 years or after age 30 years is still most commonly a reaction to a noxious stimulus or acquired pathology.[8]

Secondary epilepsies or seizures usually have identifiable acquired causes. For example, 30% of patients with intracranial hematomas, 15% of those with depressed skull fracture, and up to 5% of those hospitalized for abnormalities of consciousness develop chronic epilepsy. With head trauma the overall 5-year risk of epilepsy is about 2%, but early-onset seizures following impact are almost never a sign of impending epilepsy.[9] About 40% of people with brain tumors seize. An extremely common cause of convulsions, drugs known to induce seizures are listed in Table 64.2. Sleep cycle plays a pivotal role in some people. About 20% of patients have seizures only during hours of sleep, making diagnosis difficult, whereas 40% have seizures only during periods of alertness. Although supported historically, linking seizures to the menstrual cycle (catamenial) has proven to be difficult.[8] Overall during childhood, 68% of epilepsy is idiopathic, 20% congenital, 5% traumatic, 4% postinfection, and 1% each vascular, neoplastic, or degenerative. For adults, 55% is idiopathic, 16% vascular, 11% neoplastic, 10% traumatic, 3% congenital, 3% degenerative, and 2% postinfection.[9,10] Nonepileptic seizures are most commonly due to infection, fever, metabolic derangement, trauma, stroke, drugs, cardiovascular causes, or tumor, or are idiopathic.

Classification

Classification of seizure disorders is critical to effective treatment and accurate prognosis (Table 64.3). Generalized seizures arise simultaneously from both cerebral hemispheres,

Table 64.1. **Categories of Seizure Etiologies with Examples**

Reactive seizures

Transient stress or injury in the normal population: sleep deprivation, fever, metabolic disturbance (e.g., hypoglycemia from fasting), drug withdrawal or ingestion

Reflex epilepsy—visual: photic stimulation, patterns, video games, television, specific images; auditory: music, specific sound; somatosensory: touch, tooth brushing, water immersion; psychic: calculation, reading, startle, intense focus; motor: swallowing, eye movement

Primary epilepsy: genetic factors

Low seizure threshold, often exacerbated by stress, infection, drugs

Specific genetic abnormality with seizures: autosomal-dominant inheritance for typical absence (petit mal) seizure, Down syndrome

Structural abnormality: neurofibromatosis, hippocampal sclerosis, tuberous sclerosis, Sturge-Weber syndrome

Metabolic abnormality: phenylketonuria, Tay-Sachs, mitochondrial encephalomyelopathy; biotinidase deficiency; glycogen or lipid storage diseases

Cryptogenic: unknown causes

Idiopathic epilepsy syndromes

Secondary acquired epilepsy or seizures

Congenital lesions: porencephalic cyst, cerebral atrophy or dysplasia, ganglioglioma, hamartoma

Head trauma: skull fracture; epidural, subdural, intracranial hematoma or effusion; contusion, concussion, birth trauma

Infection: meningitis, encephalitis; HIV, TORCHS agents, Lyme disease, shigellosis, tuberculosis, abscess, tetanus toxin, parasites

Brain tumor: primary, metastatic; granulomas; lymphoma, leukemia

Cerebrovascular diseases: arteriovenous malformation, hypertensive crisis, stroke, cerebral arteritis, cavernous hemangioma, subarachnoid hemorrhage, venous sinus thrombosis, unruptured intracranial aneurysm; cardiac arrhythmia or arrest; syncope; encephalomalacia

Systemic toxins or drugs (see Table 64.2): alcohol, cocaine; heavy metals (lead); immunization (DTaP); carbon monoxide; maternal drug use (neonates); venom (black widow spider, scorpion)

Metabolic disorder: hypoglycemia, hyperglycemia, hyponatremia, hypomagnesemia, hypocalcemia, hyperosmolality; renal failure, liver failure; porphyria; pyridoxine deficiency; acute respiratory alkalosis; Whipple's disease

Collagen vascular disease: systemic lupus erythematosus, polyarteritis nodosa, Behçet's syndrome

Demyelinating or degenerative disease: multiple sclerosis, subacute sclerosing panencephalitis, Alzheimer's disease

Blood dyscrasia: sickle cell disease, thrombotic thrombocytopenic purpura

Other: dementia, eclampsia, allergic disorders (anaphylaxis)

HIV = human immunodeficiency virus; TORCHS = toxoplasmosis, other virus, rubella, cytomegalovirus, herpesvirus, syphilis; DTaP = diphtheria/tetanus/acellular pertussis.

whereas partial seizures (localization-related) are at least initially localized to part of one hemisphere. Partial seizures can be limited to (1) any motor group, commonly the face or upper extremity since these body parts have the largest neuronal representation; (2) any sensory complaint; or (3) any psychic symptom. If consciousness is preserved, the partial seizure is termed *simple*; if consciousness is altered, it is called *complex*. Partial seizures may generalize to tonic-clonic seizures; in fact the aura preceding a generalized seizure is a partial seizure. Automatisms are purposeless disorders of behavior and occur in at least 50% of complex partial convulsions. In addition to this overall general classification of seizures is a

Table 64.2. **Drugs that Can Cause or Worsen Seizures**

Cold remedies: phenylpropanolamine, ephedrine, antihistamines including over-the-counter agents

Asthma treatments: terbutaline, theophylline, aminophylline, high-dose steroids

Antibiotics: penicillin, ceftazidime, imipenem, isoniazid, quinolones, cycloserine, metronidazole, mefloquine, acyclovir, ganciclovir, others

Drugs of abuse: alcohol, phencyclidine, amphetamine, cocaine (crack), lysergic acid diethylamide (LSD), marijuana overdose

Chemotherapeutic agents: methotrexate, bischloroethylnitrosourea (carmustine) (BCNU), asparaginase, ornithine-ketoacid transaminase-3 (OKT3), tacrolimus (FK-506)

Agents for mental illness: haloperidol, trifluoperazine, chlorpromazine; amitriptyline, maprotiline, imipramine, doxepin, fluoxetine; methylphenidate; bupropion; lithium; flumazenil (in benzodiazepine-dependency)

Anesthetics and pain medications: ketamine, halothane, enflurane, methohexital; local anesthetic (lidocaine); meperidine, fentanyl, tramadol; general anesthesia

Antidiabetic medications: insulin; oral antidiabetic medications (all currently available agents)

Household products: insect repellants, lindane (benzene hexachloride), insecticides

Other: cyclosporine, interferons, strychnine, some beta-blockers, atropine eye drops; "health" and "diet" preparations, immunizations (DTaP), radiographic contrast agents

Withdrawal seizures: alcohol, barbiturates, antiepileptic drugs, amphetamines, opiates, benzodiazepines (especially alprazolam), baclofen, allopurinol

Table 64.3. **Classification of Epileptic Seizures**

Generalized seizures
Convulsive (grand mal)
   Tonic
   Clonic
   Tonic-clonic
Nonconvulsive
   Absence (petit mal)
   Atypical absence
   Myoclonic
   Atonic

Partial (localization-related) seizures
Simple (consciousness unimpaired)
   Motor
   Somatosensory or special sensory
   Autonomic
   Psychic
Complex (consciousness impaired)
   Simple progressing to loss of consciousness
   Loss of consciousness at onset
Evolving to secondary generalized tonic-clonic seizures

Unclassified seizures
   Neonatal seizures
   Infantile spasms
   Other syndrome related seizures

Source: Commission on Classification and Terminology. Proposal for revised clinical and electrocardiographic classification of epileptic seizures. Epilepsia 1981;22:491–501, with permission.

classification of the epilepsies and epileptic syndromes that further defines epilepsy by whether it is idiopathic (primary), symptomatic (secondary), or cryptogenic (unknown).[4,6] Examples of these disorders are infantile spasms, juvenile myoclonic epilepsy, and Lennox-Gastaut syndrome, which can encompass both partial and generalized seizures. Their classification, treatments, and prognoses are covered in detail elsewhere.[4,6–8,11,12]

Clinical Manifestations

Generalized Seizures

Major motor seizures are usually easily recognized. The sudden onset of tonic muscular contractions, apnea, cyanosis, and rolled-back eyes usually evolves into generalized clonus. A short, high-pitched cry precedes and a sigh follows some generalized seizures. Although micturition and defecation are common, either can occur with other diagnoses. Chewing that traumatizes the tongue is most suggestive of a seizure. Convulsions (motor system) usually last 1 to 2 minutes but may continue for as long as 15 minutes without indicating status. The commonly encountered Todd's postictal paralysis, drowsiness, headache, and hyperreflexia, any of which may persist up to 24 hours, reflect a general "switching off" of CNS function while neurons recover from the seizure activity.

Specific generalized epilepsy syndromes during childhood include the Lennox-Gastaut syndrome, which includes two or more types of seizure. Behavioral problems and mental re-

tardation are usual with this syndrome. Half the cases have structural lesions. Another more common example, juvenile myoclonic epilepsy, usually afflicts persons aged 8 to 20 years, accounts for 5% of childhood epilepsy, and is linked to a specific chromosome locus.[4] It presents with early morning myoclonic jerks while performing simple daily tasks such as brushing the hair. Later it may evolve into tonic-clonic epilepsy that requires lifelong treatment.[12] Photic stimulation tends to precipitate these seizures. Other forms of generalized seizures are more difficult to recognize. Atonic seizures or drop attacks usually start during childhood and range from a simple head drop for a few seconds to total collapse with serious injury. Patients revive almost immediately without postictal symptoms. About 10% of epileptic children have typical absence spells (petit mal), which are brief (10–30 seconds) losses of consciousness without motor activity, except perhaps lip smacking or eyelid blinking and are characterized by an unresponsive, blank facial stare. Most importantly patients have no aura or postictal change and rarely suffer loss of body tone. Absence spells develop at 5 to 10 years of age and are rare after age 30. Hyperventilation precipitates these sometimes difficult to recognize seizures. Another 10% have atypical absence spells that usually have some motor activity of the face and extremities, last longer than 30 seconds, and create postictal confusion. Additionally, onset and cessation may be less abrupt than with typical absence spells. All of these seizure types may occur hundreds of times a day.[7,8,12]

Partial Seizures

Partial seizures can present with any of a multitude of symptoms (Table 64.4). Most simple partial seizures (SPSs) last only 10 to 30 seconds but may be followed by events such as temporary postictal paralysis. An example of a motor SPS, jacksonian march is the orderly, progressive spread of localized clonic activity (e.g., from the thumb up the arm to in-

Table 64.4. **Findings in Partial Seizures**

Simple (40% of cases): consciousness maintained
  Autonomic: pallor, flushing, sweating, cardiac arrhythmia, hypertension, micturition, piloerection, nausea, dizziness, salivation, swallowing, apnea, epigastric rising sensation (like a roller coaster), pupillary dilatation
  Motor: version (head or eye turning), focal (movement or paralysis), postural change, eyelid twitching, speech dysfunction, jacksonian march, gelastic (laughing), fencer's posture, paralysis, hemiballismus, cursive (running)
  Sensory: smells, visual changes (flashes, hallucinations, macro- or micropsis), auditory distortions, tastes, dizziness; paresthesias, chest discomfort, headache, abdominal pain
  Psychic: delusions, fear, anger, déjà vu, jamais vu, daydreams, depersonalization

Complex (60% of cases): consciousness altered
  Stare, unresponsiveness, dystonic positioning of arm, hand or head
  Automatisms: chewing, lip movement, vocalizations, fumbling or picking gestures, aimless walking, undressing, emotional outbursts, repetitive movements
  Amnesia, transient aphasia, fugue state

volve an entire side of the body) without loss of consciousness. Gelastic epilepsy presents as inappropriate laughter in nonhumorous situations; uncinate fits present with olfactory auras. Benign partial epilepsy with centrotemporal spikes (BECTS), also known as rolandic epilepsy, is an inherited disorder that affects about 15% of children with epilepsy, with its onset usually between age 2 and 14 years. Nocturnal guttural noises, dysphasias, paresthesias about the face, and tonic face or arm contractions that may generalize characterize BECTS. Neurologic evaluation is normal. About 20% of these children have only one seizure, whereas another 25% are shackled by repetitive convulsions unless treated. These seizures cease during adolescence. A last example of SPS is the continuous partial epilepsy that can incapacitate patients with brain tumors, cerebral anoxia, stroke, or Rasmussen encephalitis following a febrile illness. It may lead to hemiplegia, aphasia, or other permanent neurologic loss.

Complex partial seizures (CPSs) usually last 1 to 2 minutes. Automatisms occur in 50% to 75% of CPS cases. Temporal lobe (psychomotor) epilepsy is associated with an aura such as vague abdominal pain, psychiatric dysfunction, or memory loss.[7,12] Seizures arising from the temporal lobe may be SPSs with illusions, smells, or epigastric distress in an alert patient or CPSs with automatisms, amnesia, and postictal confusion. Either form may generalize into a tonic-clonic convulsion.

In childhood epilepsy 21% of seizures are CPS, 19% generalized tonic-clonic, 12% absence, 11% SPS, 11% other generalized, 7% simultaneous multiple types, 14% myoclonic, and 5% other.[7,10,13] In adult epilepsy 39% of seizures are CPS, 25% generalized tonic-clonic, 21% SPS, 9% other, 4% other generalized, and 2% myoclonic.[7,10,13] Most nonepileptic seizures are motor convulsions. In addition to the disorder brought about by the seizure itself, complications of seizures are often significant: oral lacerations, dislocations and fractures (vertebral, jaw, humeral, skull), burns, drowning, aspiration pneumonia, arrhythmia, pulmonary edema, myocardial infarction, and death. Trauma from observers trying to suppress the seizure is also problematic. Death can be related to the seizure itself, due to accident, caused by pulmonary or cardiac complications, or due to suicide. Sudden, expected death occurs in 1 to 2 cases per 1000 per year.[6]

Diagnosis

Specific attention to the details of the history is the *only* critical diagnostic maneuver, but because of the patient's amnesia for the event, details may be difficult to ascertain. Questioning witnesses greatly enhances historical accuracy especially if home videos of spells are available. The patient's age, presenting complaint, birth history, childhood illnesses, family history, habits, and psychological stresses should be recorded. Determining the exact events before, during, and after the convulsion offers the best chance of achieving an accurate diagnosis. For example specifics regarding the aura can serve to localize a lesion in the brain.[14] Any subsequent motor activity, the body parts involved, the exact sensory ab-

normality, the progression of the seizure, the time of day of the event, the length of the event, the rate of recurrence, associated problems, and the postictal state all serve to enhance recognition of a specific seizure disorder.

Drugs, especially alcohol, frequently enhance seizure activity. Hence, a careful drug history is essential (see Table 64.2). Unfortunately, over-the-counter agents such as antihistamines are often at fault. The careful clinician will uncover all agents being taken, therapeutic or otherwise, and peruse a reference resource for the possibility of drug-induced convulsions. Simple drug avoidance is then curative. Careful prescribing after checking whether a particular pharmaceutical can worsen seizure disorders is paramount.

Complementing a good general physical examination is the special attention accorded to the neurologic examination and to the stigmata of congenital infection and chromosomal disorders. For example, close inspection of the skin may reveal the port-wine stain of Sturge-Weber syndrome or a melanoma suggesting metastasis as the cause of the seizures.

Although routine laboratory studies offer limited help in epilepsy, some basic investigations are mandatory for a nonepileptic seizure. Serum electrolytes, glucose, calcium, magnesium, and complete blood count (CBC) are routine, but a lumbar puncture is indicated only if meningitis, encephalitis, or CNS trauma is possible. As an aid to diagnosis, serum prolactin or creatinine phosphokinase levels can be high up to 30 minutes after a seizure.[4] When drug abuse or withdrawal is suspected, especially in cases of unexplained first seizures, a drug and toxin screen is appropriate.[5] In some instances other evaluations are helpful: (1) assessment of renal, liver or cardiopulmonary function; (2) a search for lead, mercury, or carbon monoxide poisoning; (3) tests for metabolic derangements such as thyrotoxicosis and porphyria, or amino acid disorders such as phenylketonuria; or (4) measurement of blood gases for pH alteration or oxygen deficiency. A chest radiograph may reveal a tumor in a smoker, or an electrocardiogram (ECG) or Holter monitor an arrhythmia in a patient with episodic unconsciousness or a family history of sudden death. Wood's lamp examination of the skin helps to eliminate tuberous sclerosis, and ophthalmologic evaluation can diagnose a phakoma or infectious disease.

EEG provides a diagnosis in 30% to 50% of first-time epileptic patients, but with repeated testing up to 90% of epilepsy can be categorized.[1,15] The EEG serves to identify a specific seizure entity such as the classical three per second spike and wave pattern of absence spells or the repeating spike localized over the rolandic fissure found in BECTS. This invaluable tool also can localize a lesion in the brain, as with the abnormal spiking discharge found over a frontal lobe brain tumor. Unfortunately, up to 2% of normal children without seizures have a genetic trait causing epileptiform spikes on their EEGs, limiting EEG accuracy.[6] If a patient is thought to have epilepsy clinically, an abnormal EEG has over a 95% positive predictive value.[15] However, one third of suspect individuals with a negative EEG will still eventually prove to be epileptic.[4] The accuracy of the EEG can be enhanced through sleep deprivation, hyperventilation, and photic stimulation. A 24-hour ambulatory EEG monitor can reveal a seizure frequency much greater than expected from observer reports.[16]

Although magnetic resonance imaging (MRI) is preferred to computed tomography (CT) because of accuracy for small lesions such as lacunar infarcts, both are useful adjuncts to identify structural lesions like CNS bleeding. In general, persons with partial seizures (except BECTS), with abnormal neurologic examinations, or with focal EEGs, and those over 18 years old require a CNS imaging evaluation to exclude pathologic lesions.[14,17,18] In childhood seizures, MRI may reveal an etiology (sometimes correctable) in the face of an abnormal neurologic examination (55%), status epilepticus (SE) (27%), or partial seizures (15%).[17] Other fruitful evaluations in selected cases include cerebral angiography and positron emission tomography (PET) scans prior to surgery, video EEG to identify nonepileptic seizure of psychogenic origin (formerly called pseudoseizure), and psychometric studies to identify focal cognitive defects and psychological disease. In young women, especially prior to treatment, a pregnancy test may prove helpful.[19]

Differential Entities

Many conditions that look like seizures are not.[8,12] In infants, gastroesophageal reflux, shuddering, and benign myoclonus mimic convulsions. Toddlers with breath-holding spells (both cyanotic and pallid) are particularly difficult to segregate from those with seizures. Concussion, hyperventilation, rage, drug reactions, startle response, and diseases such as tetanus can all produce seizure-like activity. One entity, episodic dyscontrol, consists of inappropriate violent and destructive behavior in otherwise normal patients, some of whom have an abnormal EEG. In adults syncope is the greatest deceiver because it may in fact be accompanied by seizure activity secondary to poor cerebral oxygenation. Psychogenic seizures, panic disorder, alcoholic blackouts, transient global amnesia, and hyperventilation syndrome are particularly common confounding problems in adults.

Behavior dysfunction, especially depression, accounts for a great deal of confusion. About 20% of cases referred to seizure evaluation clinics are psychogenic seizures best diagnosed through video EEG and often difficult to distinguish from frontal lobe epilepsy.[4,19] Psychogenic seizures can coexist with true epilepsy and carry a risk of suicide.[4,6] Psychiatric consultation may help. Of course many seizure disorders have ineluctable psychological consequences, including depression, that may themselves require treatment.[20,21]

Neurologic disease can be camouflaged as a seizure disorder. Shuddering attacks, hereditary chin tremble, familial choreoathetosis, Tourette's syndrome, migraine, narcolepsy, transient ischemic attacks, extrapyramidal disorders, dyssomnias (sleep walking, night terrors, partial cataplexy, sleep apnea), benign paroxysmal vertigo, and tics all masquerade as seizures. Multiple sclerosis, parkinsonism, and carcinoid may simulate epilepsy.[7,8,22,23] However, persons with these conditions usually have normal EEGs and in general will not improve with antiepileptic drugs (AEDs).[24,25]

Management

During the seizure the patient should be turned onto one side, clothing and jewelry around the neck should be loosened and eyeglasses removed. No attempt should be made to insert anything into the mouth. Medical help may be needed if a seizure persists longer than 3 to 5 minutes. Initial medical management includes correction of all identifiable seizure etiologies. Unless a patient remains ill, is at high risk, or lives without adequate supervision, hospitalization is not necessary. Because of amnesia for the event, many appreciate a description of what transpired. For any discharged patient follow-up plans need to be definitive.

Persons with one or several seizures related to a single event like hypoglycemia usually require no further evaluation or treatment aimed specifically at seizure control. Individuals with first-time unexplained seizures have a recurrence risk of less than 50%, and less than 25% develop epilepsy.[4,6] The EEG and seizure etiology are the most important prognostic factors, but time since last seizure, age, and seizure type are also predictive. In the 5% to 10% of the population who have one unprovoked seizure, only 30% ever go to see a physician. About 10% of these patients develop epilepsy. In contradistinction, 80% of those with a second unprovoked seizure develop epilepsy.[7] High-risk factors are brain injury, a stroke, cancer, or an abnormal EEG. A low-risk profile includes a normal EEG, negative family history, normal physical examination, lack of head trauma, and a normal head CT scan or MRI.

Whether all persons with unprovoked convulsions need AED treatment is controversial. Many medications have considerable side effects including worsening of seizures, organ damage, or even death, so delaying treatment until a second episode is justifiable.[26] Additionally, treatment does not guarantee success, as 20% to 30% of patients on AEDs still suffer from some seizures, and the effects of these drugs on long-term prognosis are unknown.[27]

The major drugs utilized in the treatment of seizure disorders are listed in Table 64.5. Although some drugs like ethosuximide or phenytoin can be given quickly to reach therapeutic levels, others are best introduced slowly and raised to the lowest dose that prevents seizures but does not produce major side effects (Table 64.6). The many deleterious effects of these medications are reviewed in various pharmaceutical references such as the *Hospital Formulary*.[28] Side effects are less frequent once a drug has been used for several months. Because most anticonvulsants have numerous drug interactions (Table 64.7), reviewing a standard reference prior to prescription is advisable.[28]

In general, a single agent pushed to the point of seizure control or to just short of toxicity is superior to multiple-drug therapy.[23,27,29] AED levels and blood tests for toxicity guide dosage changes but are not critical.[29,30] At least for the first 3 to 6 months of treatment, prudence dictates close monitoring of hepatic function and CBCs. Thereafter, semiannual or annual checks may be satisfactory. Given in tandem, AEDs may augment each other's toxicity. For example, because of intestinal and liver toxicity, valproate mixes poorly with other

Table 64.5. **Commonly Prescribed Antiepileptic Drugs and Indications**

Drug (trade name)	Route	$T_{1/2}$ (hours)	Adult (mg) SD	Adult (mg) UDD	Pediatric (mg/kg) SD	Pediatric (mg/kg) UDD[a]	# DD	TL (μg/mL)
Phenytoin[b] (Dilantin)	PO IV	12–48	15–20 mg/kg, max 1500	200–700	15–20, max 1500	5–15	1–3	10–20
Fosphenytoin[c] (Cerebyx)	IV IM	12–48	15–30 mg/kg, max 2250	300–1000	15–30	6–9	1–3	10–20 (Phenytoin)
Valproic acid[d] (Depakene)	PO PR	4–12	500	1000–2500	10–15	30–60	2–4	50–120
Divalproex (Depakote)	PO	4–18	500	1000–2500	10–15	30–60	1–3	50–120
Valproate[e] (Depacon)	IV	4–18	500	1000–2500	10–15	30–60	1–3	50–120
Carbamezapine (Tegretol)	PO	8–17	200	400–2000	5–10	10–30	2–4	6–12
Oxcarbazepine (Trileptal)	PO	10–17	300	600–2400	8–10	600–1800 mg	2	6–12
Ethosuximide (Zarontin)	PO	30–60	500	750–2000	10–20	10–40	2	40–100
Primidone (Mysoline)	PO	5–15 (Primidone)	250	250–1500	10	10–30	3–4	5–12 (Primidone)
Phenobarbital (Luminal)	PO IV (IM rare)	40–140	300–800	60–300	4 PO 10–20 IV	4–8	2–3	20–30
Gabapentin (Neurontin)	PO	4–10	300	900–3600	10–15	10–50	3–4	≥2
Lamotrigine (Lamictal	PO	15–60	50–100	100–400	0.15–0.6	1–5	1–2	2–4
Clonazepam (Klonopin)	PO	20–50	1	1.5–2	0.01–0.03	0.05–0.2	2–3	20–80 ng/mL
Topiramate (Topamax)	PO	20–30	50	400–1600	1–3	5–9	1–2	NE
Tiagabine (Gabitril)	PO	7–9	4	4–56	4 mg	4–32 mg	2–4	Up to 550 ng/mL
Levetiracetam (Keppra)	PO	6–10	500	500–3000	NR	NR	2	NE
Zonisamide (Zonegran)	PO	50–70	100	300–800	NR	NR	1–2	Estimate 20

$T_{1/2}$ = half life; SD = starting dose; UDD = usual daily dose; #DD = number doses daily; TL = therapeutic level; GM = grand mal; PM = petit mal; SPS = simple partial seizure; CPS = complex partial seizure; MYO = myoclonic seizure; FS = febrile seizure; MIX = mixed disorder; FL = first line; A = alternative; AO = adjunctive only; X = limited use; C = capsule; T = tablet; CSP = sprinkles; I = injection; S = syrup; V = vial; B = bottle; T(DR) = delayed release; CT = chewable tablet; XR or ER = extended release; E = elixir; PI = powder for injection; SE = status epilepticus; NR = not recommended; NE = not established; NA = not available.

[a]Limit is adult maximal dose.

[b]Phenytoin: May be given IV at ≤50 mg/min rate.

[c]Fosphenytoin: Usually ordered as phenytoin equivalent (PE) at 3/2 of listed doses (75 mg fosphenytoin = 50 mg phenytoin); given IV at ≤150 mg/min rate.

[d]Valproic acid: rectal route—dilute 1 to 1 with water, retention enema 17–20 mg/kg initial dose, then 10–15 mg/kg, q8h.

[e]Valproate: Given IV at ≤20 mg/min.

Other drugs: clorazepate (Tranxene-T), ethotoin (Peganone), methsuximide (Celontin).

Source: (1) Lacy CF, Armstrong LL, Goldman MP, Lance LL. Drug information handbook, 9th ed. Hudson, OH: Lexi-Corp, 2001–2002. (2) Red book update, May 2001. Montvale, NJ: Medical Economics, 2001.

Dosage forms (mg)	Seizure type							Special uses	Average cost ($) month	
	GM	PM	SPS	CPS	MY	FS	MIX		Brand	Generic
100 C; 30, 100 C (XR); 50CT; 30/5 mL, 125/5 mL, (5, 240 mL B); 50 mL I (2, 5 mL V)	FL		FL	FL			A	Frequently used for post trauma or stroke prophylaxis; oral liquids unreliable; nonlinear dose to serum level curve	30	26
75/mL I (2, 10 mL V)	X		X	X			X	For SE or unconscious state		
250 C; 250/5 mL S (5, 50, 480 mL B)	FL	FL	FL	FL	FL	FL	FL		217	83
125, 250, 500 T (DR); 500T (ER)	FL	FL	FL	FL	FL	FL	FL		107	NA
100 mg/mL I (5 mL V)	X		X	X			X	For unconscious state		
200, 300 C(XR); 200 T; 100 CT; 100, 200, 400 T(XR); 100/5 mL S	FL		FL	FL			A		65	48
150, 300, 600 T	A		FL	FL			A	Children age 4 yrs and older and adults	105	NA
250 C; 250/5 mL S (473 mL B)		FL						Useful for akinetic seizures	93	NA
250/5 mL S (240 mL B); 50, 250 T	A		A	A			A	Limited use due to behavior changes	138	65
16 C; 8, 15, 16, 32 60, 65, 100 T; 15/5, 20/5 mL E; 30, 60, 65, 130/mL I; 120 PI	A		A	A			A	Limited use due to behavior changes	10	5
100, 300, 400 C; 600, 800 T; 100/mL liquid mix available			AO	AO			AC	Age 12 yrs and older, not necessary to monitor level	139	NA
25, 100, 150, 200 T; 2, 5, 25 CT;	FL	A	FL	FL	A		A	Lower dose if on valproic acid; age 2 yrs and older	189	NA
0.5, 1, 2 T		A			A		A	Useful for alkinetic seizures	62	54
15, 25 CSP; 25, 100, 200 T	A		AO	AO	AO		AC	Age 2 yrs and older	222	NA
4, 12, 16, 20 T			AO	AO			AC	Age 12 yrs and older	130	NA
250, 500, 750 T			AO	AO				Age 16 yrs and older	110	NA
100 C			AO	AO				Age 16 yrs and older	165	NA

AEDs, especially in young children. Also, multiple seizure and nonseizure drugs affect serum levels of AEDs (Table 64.7). For example, carbamazepine levels are influenced by diltiazem, erythromycin, phenytoin, and phenobarbital, among others. Phenytoin interacts with a host of drugs. Therefore, before adding any agent to a patient's regimen, a careful review of drug interactions (hand-held computer systems have useful programs) is warranted. Only 10% of patients with poor seizure control on one drug achieve good control on two or more drugs, but failure to respond to any one drug does not preclude good response to a different agent.[29] Hence, drugs should be tried in series rather than parallel.[27,29] Shifting from one drug to another is best accomplished by simultaneous tapering of the old agent and initiation of the new drug. Some AEDs such as gabapentin should only be utilized as adjunctive medications.

Drugs of Choice

Primary generalized seizures regardless of type are best treated with valproate, which provides effective monotherapy in 80% of cases.[23,27] Divalproex produces fewer gastrointestinal side effects. For tonic-clonic seizures lamotrigine, carbamazepine, or phenytoin are also good selections. Phenytoin is by far the most cost-efficient drug available. For absence spells if valproate cannot be tolerated or if no other seizure type coexists, ethosuximide is an ideal choice. Lamotrigine can be added to or substituted for any of these drugs if con-

Table 64.6. **Major Antiepileptic Side Effects**

Carbamazepine/oxcarbazepine	Gastrointestinal upset, sleepiness, blurred vision, hepatic failure, bone marrow toxicity, diplopia, allergic rash, nausea; impaired task performance; hyponatremia
Clonazepam/clorazepate	Sleepiness, irritability, depression, salivation, hyperactivity, ataxia, withdrawal seizures, anorexia
Ethosuximide/methsuximide	Abdominal pain, rash, hepatic failure, leukopenia, nausea, bone marrow failure, drowsiness, hiccups, dystonia, abnormal behavior
Gabapentin	Sleepiness, fatigue, ataxia, dizziness, gastrointestinal upset
Lamotrigine	Rash, dizziness, tremor, ataxia, diplopia, headache, gastrointestinal upset; Stevens-Johnson syndrome
Levetiracetam	Sedation, fatigue, incoordination, psychosis, anemia, leukocytopenia
Phenobarbital	Sedation, depression, mental dullness, hyperactivity, rash; irritability, sleep disturbance in children; osteomalacia
Phenytoin	Gastrointestinal upset, nystagmus, hirsutism, acne, gingival hyperplasia, dysarthria, fatigue, ataxia, hepatic failure, bone marrow toxicity, rash, hypotension, lymphadenopathy, anemia (folate deficiency), neuropathy; inattention, dullness; osteomalacia; facial coarsening
Primidone	Similar to phenobarbital plus aggression
Tiagabine	Confusion, sedation, depression, dizziness, psychosis, paresthesia, language or speech dysfunction, gastrointestinal upset
Topiramate	Psychomotor slowness, sedation, fatigue, abulia, paresthesia, renal stones
Valproate/divalproex	Gastrointestinal upset, tremor, hepatic failure, weight change (usually gain), hair loss, pancreatitis, thrombocytopenia, edema
Zonisamide	Sedation, dizziness, confusion, headache, anorexia, renal stones

trol is inadequate. Juvenile myoclonic epilepsy usually responds dramatically to valproate. Unfortunately, myoclonic seizures responding poorly to valproate also respond poorly to other agents and may be difficult to control. Clonazepam can be tried. Because of drug-related personality disorders, primidone and phenobarbital are last choices or best avoided for chronic therapy.

Partial seizures are best treated with carbamazepine or

Table 64.7. **Common Antiepileptic Drug (AED) Interactions**

Carbamazepine/oxcarbazepine	*Variable effect:* phenytoin, phenobarbital, valproic acid, primidone; theophylline; lithium *Toxicity increased:* verapamil, diltiazem; isoniazid, clarithromycin, erythromycin; fluoxetine, monoamine oxidase inhibitors; propoxyphene; cimetidine; danazol *Decreased effect:* doxycycline, haloperidol, warfarin, oral contraceptives, corticosteroids; cyclosporine; imipramine; mebendazole; methadone; thyroid hormone
Clonazepam/clorazepate	*Toxicity increased:* valproic acid (coadministration contraindicated) *Serum level decreased:* phenytoin, barbiturate, primidone
Ethosuximide/methsuximide	*Toxicity increased:* most other AEDs
Gabapentin	None known
Lamotrigine	*Increased serum level:* valproic acid *Decreased serum level:* phenobarbital, phenytoin, carbamazepine
Levetiracetam	None known
Phenobarbital/primidone	*Variable effect:* phenytoin *Toxicity increased:* clorazepate, valproic acid; monoamine oxidase inhibitors; disulfiram; chloramphenicol *Decreased effect:* warfarin; corticosteroids, oral contraceptive, tricyclic antidepressant; griseofulvin, doxycycline; verapamil, nifedipine
Phenytoin	*Decreased effect:* carbamazepine, amiodarone, rifampin, folic acid, barbiturates, chronic alcohol use, theophylline, chemotherapy *Increased effect:* isoniazid, ticlopidine, fluconazole, trimethoprim, nifedipine, omeprazole, fluoroquinolones, selective serotonin reuptake inhibitors (SSRIs), metronidazole, cimetidine *Variable effect:* valproic acid *Effect on other drugs:* warfarin, lithium, acetaminophen, oral contraceptives, thyroid hormone, multiple others
Tiagabine	*Level decreased:* phenytoin, carbamazepine, phenobarbital
Topiramate	*Level decreased:* phenytoin, carbamazepine, phenobarbital
Valproic acid	*Toxicity increased:* clonazepam (coadministration contraindicated), phenytoin, phenobarbital; monoamine oxidase inhibitors, warfarin
Zonisamide	*Level decreased:* phenytoin, carbamazepine, phenobarbital

phenytoin.[8,27,31] Valproate is an effective alternative especially for secondarily generalized epilepsy. Gabapentin and lamotrigine are excellent adjunctive drugs, but primidone and phenobarbital are less desirable due to their side effects. However, despite its adverse effects on mentation, phenobarbital is inexpensive and useful in neonatal seizures, status epilepticus, and other special situations. Unlike valproate, phenytoin and phenobarbital may lessen the efficacy of birth control pills.

Eventually at least 60% of patients become seizure-free. To discontinue therapy after a 2- to 5-year treatment period, the anticonvulsant dose is slowly tapered to zero over a 3- to 6-month period. A normal examination, few seizures of one type before treatment, absence of seizures for at least a 24-month period, normal EEGs, normal intelligence quotient (IQ), growth into adulthood, and absence of a structural brain lesion predict success when medication is stopped. Roughly 20% will have a recurrence. In adults who may lose driving privileges or jobs if convulsions recur, the decision to end treatment is more difficult.[32] Certainly a recently abnormal EEG would make one reluctant to cease treatment.

BECTS is best treated with carbamazepine until at least 2 years of seizure-free time or the child is 16 years old when treatment is tapered. Juvenile myoclonus usually requires lifelong valproate therapy. Prophylaxis of alcohol withdrawal seizures is frustratingly ineffective. Although phenytoin is often prescribed for posttrauma seizure prophylaxis, it is probably not efficacious.[33] If given, it should be stopped after a 6- to 12-month seizure-free period or if proven ineffective.

During pregnancy, 50% of women experience no change in seizure frequency, 30% have an increase, and 20% a decrease. Close follow-up and frequent serum drug-level monitoring are prudent. Although anticonvulsants increase the risk of fetal malformation, especially cleft lip and palate and cardiac defects by 1% to 2%, valproate may carry the highest risk overall.[19,34] Folic acid (1 to 4 mg/day) should be given throughout pregnancy to combat neural tube defects. Nondangerous seizures such as typical absence spells and SPS may not require treatment during pregnancy. Vitamin K (10 mg/day) is indicated during the last month of pregnancy.[19] Some sources also recommend vitamin D supplementation.[19]

The *Hospital Formulary* lists other rarely used drugs.[28] Highly toxic, felbamate should not be used in primary care settings. Specific indications for other agents include magnesium sulfate for pregnancy, acetazolamide (250–500 mg/d) for menstrual epilepsy, and adrenocorticotropic hormone (ACTH) or vigabatrin (Sabril) for infantile spasms.[4,6] Recent reviews detail promising AEDs.[35,36] In difficult cases, referral to a neurologist or an epilepsy center should offer a better chance of seizure control than would random drug selection.

Surgical and Avoidance Therapy

Up to 20% of epilepsy may prove to be refractory to standard AEDs, overwhelming the already handicapped or interfering with daily living in otherwise normal persons. Currently treatment options include epilepsy surgery with 80% seizure-free outcomes for temporal lobe resection or corpus callosum

severing[3,37]; vagus nerve stimulation with a 50% seizure reduction in about 40% of patients[3]; an increasing array of new AEDs[35]; and the ketogenic diet, which reduces seizure episodes by roughly 50%.[16,38]

Avoidance of epileptogenic stimuli is crucial for the control of reflex seizures. All patients require adequate sleep, nutrition, exercise, and stress reduction, and consideration for annual influenza vaccination. Alcohol or sedative drug ingestion and unattended swimming or tree climbing are examples of activities best avoided.

Family Issues

Seizure disorders create obvious problems for daily living. State laws prohibit driving for variable periods after even a single seizure, limiting access to work and altering home duties.[32] Seizures occasionally lead to significant trauma or death. Despite these hazards, only 25% of untreated patients overall are incapacitated by seizures.[8] Many with a single, untreated seizure never have a recurrence. The physician must weigh treatment difficulties such as drug side effects against the need to control convulsions. To serve the patient's best interests, a close relationship should be cultivated to allow mutually agreed-upon therapy and testing.

The clinician should reassure all patients that epilepsy is not the usual cause per se of lower IQ, mental dysfunction, or brain damage. Although most can lead normal lives, a recurrently abnormal EEG, atypical seizures, or an already abnormally functioning CNS signal a poor prognosis. Vigilance for the development of secondary depression is warranted.[21,22]

Families and other caregivers, especially day care center workers, need some seizure management information to outline what to do for a seizure. General information is available from various epilepsy foundations and medical specialty boards. Useful Web sites are *www.aesnet.org* (American Epilepsy Society) and *www.efa.org* (Epilepsy Foundation of America). Vocational rehabilitation and help with medical expenses are often paramount. Guides to office record keeping are available.[39]

Specific Situations

At contrasting ends of the spectrum of seizure management are febrile convulsions and status epilepticus. The treatment of these entities and neonatal seizures serves as a framework for dealing with acute seizures.

Status Epilepticus (SE)

Background

Any seizure or series of recurrent convulsions uninterrupted by a period of consciousness for more than 30 minutes is termed SE. Although usually secondary to generalized tonic-clonic seizures, absence or any type of partial seizure can also cause SE.

Approximately 50,000 individuals in the United States experience SE annually. About 20% of children with epilepsy and 5% with febrile convulsions have SE at least once.[40] SE is most common in adults with street drug overdose, inadequate AED levels, intracranial hemorrhage, anoxic encephalopathy, or brain tumors.[41] The adult population at greatest risk is over age 60 years.[41]

Patients with SE are at risk, albeit low, of residual damage, often hemiparesis. Evidence suggests that intensive treatment that halts seizures within 1 hour results in a marked reduction in postictal morbidity.[42] Death is usually related to the underlying problem producing the SE complicated by circulatory collapse, fever, or renal failure often from rhabdomyolysis.

Clinical Presentation

Persistent generalized tonic-clonic convulsions are readily recognized as SE. In myoclonic SE despite the irregular bilateral motor jerks, normal consciousness is preserved; in absence SE, the mentally confused patient can demonstrate normal motor activity; in Lennox-Gastaut SE, young children have minor motor dysfunction plus mental confusion; and in atonic SE, a limp, unconscious child has mild occasional clonic jerks. Prolonged focal seizures with preserved consciousness suggest simple partial SE. Focal encephalitis, trauma, stroke, or drug-related illness is likely. Complex partial SE produces prolonged mental confusion coupled with psychomotor or psychosensory disturbances, ranging from minor speech arrest to automatisms to total unresponsiveness that may persist for days.

Diagnosis

The recognition of SE is based on clinical suspicion and typical EEG findings.[15] A diligent search for a correctable cause (AED concentrations, screening for drugs of abuse, etc., as in Table 64.8) is often rewarding.

Management

Immediate stabilization of vital signs includes airway maintenance with nasal oxygen or intubation as required, ECG monitoring, and blood pressure control. Termination of the seizure within minutes is usually not mandatory. After blood studies are drawn, adolescents and adults should be given 100 mg of thiamine and 50 mL of 50% (children 2 to 4 mL/kg of 25%) glucose IV as well as naloxone (Narcan) (0.4 to 2 mg for adults, 0.1 mg/kg up to 2 mg for children repeated every 2 to 3 minutes) where appropriate. An immediate EEG will confirm the diagnosis, and continuous EEG recording may aid in guiding medication dosage. Neuroimaging studies are ordered as appropriate to the history.

SE can be controlled with lorazepam (Ativan), 0.1 mg/kg (maximum 4 mg) IV push at less than 2 mg/min. This drug is successful in stopping 80% of SE episodes within a 2- to 3-minute period.[40,41] A second dose can be given after 10 minutes. If lorazepam is not available, diazepam (Valium) can be substituted at a dose of 5 to 10 mg (pediatric dose 0.5 mg/kg maximum 20 mg) IV push at less than 5 mg/min. For poorly controlled SE phenytoin 20 mg/kg IV push at less than 50 mg/min while monitoring blood pressure (BP) and ECG is often effective. An additional 10 mg/kg can be given. Fosphenytoin, a water-soluble phenytoin prodrug, is less irritating for intramuscular or intravenous injection, given at 1.5 mg per 1 mg of phenytoin equivalency, but infused at a faster rate of 150 mg/min. If benzodiazepines have not been given, phenobarbital 20 mg/kg IV push at less than 100 mg/min may be substituted. Serum drug levels of anticonvulsants determine adequacy of treatment. Propofol (Diprivan) 1 mg/kg given over 5 minutes is used in refractory SE. Special treatments are pyridoxine, 50 mg IV for children under age 18 months, hypertonic saline for severe hyponatremia, and physostigmine for tricyclic antidepressant overdose. Some cases require general anesthesia, paraldehyde, valproic acid, calcium channel blockers, neuromuscular blockers, or continuous IV infusions of midazolam, lorazepam, or pentobarbital. These drugs for SE are reviewed elsewhere.[4–8,12,23,25,26,40,41] Later control of seizures depends on the underlying cause.

Family Issues

Although patients usually exhibit amnesia for the event, SE can be an intensely upsetting experience for family members, especially if the victim is a child. The rare death of a patient is devastating, but normally, survival without permanent sequelae is expected.[42] Reassurance to the family is appropriate.

Febrile Convulsions

Febrile convulsions are the most common seizure disorder of childhood, affecting about 3% of all children between the ages of 6 months and 5 years.[5,8] The chance of developing epilepsy is 3%. However, children with at least two of the following have a 15% chance of eventual epilepsy[12]: (1) family history of epilepsy, (2) abnormal neurologic or development status prior to the seizure, and (3) focal or atypical seizures lasting more than 15 minutes.

Clinical Presentation and Diagnosis

In the usual patient a rapidly rising temperature is followed by a generalized tonic-clonic seizure persisting several seconds or minutes. A common scenario is the young toddler with a mild viral infection who lies down for an afternoon

---

Table 64.8. **Etiologies of Status Epilepticus**

Idiopathic
Anoxic encephalopathy: especially postcardiopulmonary arrest
Infection: febrile convulsions, meningitis, encephalitis
Metabolic: drug withdrawal (anticonvulsant, alcohol, sedative), sleep deprivation, inborn errors of metabolism, drug intoxication (cocaine, phencyclidine, amphetamine, theophylline, tricyclic antidepressants), toxins (lead), Reye's syndrome, hypoglycemia, electrolyte disturbance (hypomagnesemia, hypocalcemia, hyponatremia, acidosis, hyperkalemia)
Anatomic: congenital malformations (schizencephaly, lissencephaly), cerebral palsy
Neoplasm: especially frontal lobe
Cerebrovascular disease: intracranial hemorrhage, stroke, vasculitis
Trauma

nap only to be found later seizing by a worried parent. Postictal drowsiness lasts several minutes to hours. Underlying viral illnesses such as roseola or acute bacterial disease such as otitis media are usual (see Chapter 18). Seizures are multiple in about one third of cases. In any suspicious or atypical situation the specter of meningitis is raised. Age under 9 months, focal seizures, seizures in the office or emergency department, or suggestive physical findings may necessitate a lumbar puncture. Other tests are of dubious value.

Management

Warm baths and acetaminophen, 10 to 15 mg/kg, every 4 hours, or ibuprofen 5 to 10 mg/kg every 6 hours help to control fever. Hospitalization is needed only if seizures are prolonged beyond 30 minutes or are recurrent or complicated, follow-up care is inadequate, or parents are overly frightened. Begun at the onset of fever, oral or rectal valproate 20 mg/kg every 8 hours or diazepam, 0.5 mg/kg, every 8 hours for 1 to 3 days or until the patient is afebrile for 24 hours can control febrile seizures.[8,12] Only children with many recurrences at a young age, with persistent neurologic abnormality, or with overly distressed parents should be considered for daily drug treatment. IV lorazepam is the drug of choice for prolonged febrile seizures.

Family Issues

A major responsibility for the physician is to calm the parents of a seizing child and to reassure them that the usual febrile seizure is benign and does not indicate brain damage. A warning about the risk of recurrence, either immediate or in the distant future, is appropriate. After a febrile seizure, 50% of patients younger than 1 year have recurrences, whereas only 20% of patients over age 3 years do so.

Neonatal Seizures

During the first month of life, tonic-clonic activity is unusual, so that seizures are difficult to recognize.[12,43] Focal rhythmic twitching, especially of the face or arms, and brief jerks of the body or distal muscle groups are typical. Rigid posturing, fixed eye deviation, nystagmus, apnea, chewing, excessive salivation, or skin color changes typify subtle convulsive disorders.[43]

Hypoxemic encephalopathy often from birth or intrauterine stroke are the most common seizure etiologies. True seizures are often difficult to control and cannot be altered with gentle restraint. Neonatal myoclonic jerks, clonic seizures, jitteriness, irritability or lethargy in the nursery or within a few weeks of discharge are clues to maternal drug addiction. Appropriate agents for drug withdrawal include phenytoin, phenobarbital, chlorpromazine, methadone and paregoric. Table 64.9 presents a few critical evaluations for the assessment of neonatal seizures. Definitive diagnosis depends on neurologic consultation and EEG tracings. Appropriate prenatal care can greatly diminish the risk of neonatal seizures. Parents can be reassured that controlled seizures with correctable cause such as hypoglycemia usually do not leave permanent neurologic dysfunction. Other abnormalities are unlikely to be corrected. Diligent inquiry in a quest for a familial disease is warranted.[43]

Table 64.9. **Evaluation of Neonatal Seizures**

History
Maternal drug use: cocaine, heroin, barbiturates,
 benzodiazepines
Maternal infection: TORCHS titers, IgM level
Family history: inborn errors of metabolism, chromosomal
 deficiencies
Birthing distress: hypoxic encephalopathy, trauma

Examination: special areas of interest
Eye: chorioretinitis, coloboma
Skin: hypopigmented areas, crusted vesicular lesions,
 abnormal creases, port-wine strain
Body odor
Head shape
Neurologic system: focal defects
Constellations consistent with chromosomal disorders: ear
 position and shape, abnormal hands, feet or eyes

Laboratory assessment
Blood: cultures; CBC; glucose, calcium, magnesium,
 electrolytes, BUN; glycine, ammonia, lactate; karyotype:
 long-chain fatty acid levels
Lumbar puncture: cultures, cell count, xanthochromia, glucose,
 protein, glycine, VDRL
Other: MRI, CT scan, chest radiograph

BUN = blood urea nitrogen; CBC = complete blood count;
CT = computed tomography; IgM = immunoglobulin-M;
MRI = magnetic resonance imaging; TORCHS = toxoplasmosis, other virus, rubella, cytomegalovirus, herpesvirus, syphilis;
VDRL = Venereal Disease Research Laboratory.

References

1. Scheuer ML, Pedley TA. The evaluation and treatment of seizures N Engl J Med 1990;323:1468–74.
2. Cascino GD, Sharbrough FW. Symposium on epilepsy. Foreword. Mayo Clinic Proc 1996;71:403–4.
3. Tatum IV WO, Benbadis SR, Vale Fl. The neurosurgical treatment of epilepsy. Arch Fam Med 2000;9:1142–6.
4. Leppik IE. Contemporary diagnosis and management of the patient with epilepsy, 5th ed. Handbooks in Health Care, Newton, Pa. 2000;1–221.
5. Bradford JC, Kyriakedes CG. Evaluation of the patient with seizures an evidence based approach. Emerg Med Clin North Am 1999;17:203–20.
6. Guberman AH, Bruni J. Essentials of clinical epilepsy, 2nd ed. Boston: Butterworth Heinemann, 1999;1–199.
7. Pedley TA. The epilepsies. In: Goldman L, Bennett JC, eds. Cecil textbook of medicine, 21st ed. Philadelphia: WB Saunders, 2000;2151–63.
8. Forster FM, Booker HE. The epilepsies and convulsive disorders. In Joynt RJ, ed. Clinical neurology. Philadelphia: Lippincott—Raven, 1995;3:1–68.
9. Annegers JF, Rocca WA, Hauser WA. Causes of epilepsy: contributions of the Rochester epidemiology project. Mayo Clin Proc 1996;71:570–5.
10. Hauser WA, Annegers JF, Kurland LT. Incidence of epilepsy and unprovoked seizures in Rochester, Minnesota: 1935–1984. Epilepsia 1993;34:453–68.
11. Mosewick RK, So EL. A clinical approach to the classification of seizures and epileptic syndromes. Mayo Clin Proc 1996;71:405–14.
12. Haslam RHA. Seizures in childhood. Conditions that mimic

seizures. In: Behrman RE, Kliegman RM, Jensen HB, eds. Nelson textbook of pediatrics, 16th ed. Philadelphia: WB Saunders, 2000;1813–22.

13. Hauser WA, Annegers JF, Rocca WA. Descriptive epidemiology of epilepsy: contribution of population-based studies from Rochester, Minnesota. Mayo Clin Proc 1996;71:576–86.

14. Palmini A, Gloor P. The localizing value of auras in partial seizures: a prospective and retrospective study. Neurology 1992; 42:801–8.

15. Westmoreland BF. Epileptiform electroencephalographic patterns. Mayo Clin Proc 1996;71:501–11.

16. Freeman JM, Vining EPG. Seizures decrease rapidly after fasting. Arch Pediatr Adolesc Med 1999;153:946–9.

17. Berg AT, Testa FM, Levy SR, et al. Neuroimaging in children with newly diagnosed epilepsy: a community-based study. Pediatrics 2000;106:527–32.

18. Hirtz D, Ashwal S, Berg A, et al. Practice parameter: evaluating a first nonfebrile seizure in children. Neurology 2000;55: 616–23.

19. Yerby MS. Quality of life, epilepsy advances, and the evolving role of anticonvulsants in women with epilepsy. Neurology 2000;55(suppl 1):S21–9.

20. Chabolla DR, Krahn LE, So EL, Runnans TA. Psychogenic nonepileptic seizures. Mayo Clin Proc 1996;71:493–500.

21. MMWR. Health-related quality of life among persons with epilepsy—Texas, 1998. MMWR 2001;50:24–6,35.

22. Wiegarty P, Seidenberg M, Woodard A, et al. Co-morbid psychiatric disorder in chronic epilepsy: recognition and etiology of depression. Neurology 1999;53(suppl 2):S3–8.

23. Lowenstein DH. Seizures and epilepsy. In: Braunwald E, Fauci AS, Kasper DL, et al. Harrison's principles of internal medicine, 15th ed. New York: McGraw-Hill, 2001;2354–69.

24. Epilepsy in the new millennium. Neurology 2000;55(suppl 3): S1–44.

25. U.S. Dept. of Health and Human Services. Management of newly diagnosed patients with epilepsy: a systematic review of the literature. AHRQ pub. no. 01-E037. Washington, DC: DHHS, February 2001;1–4.

26. Bert AT, Shinnar S. The risk of seizure recurrence following a first unprovoked seizure: a quantitative review. Neurology 1991;41:965–72.

27. Brodie MJ, Dichter MA. Antiepileptic drugs. N Engl J Med 1996;334:168–75.

28. McEvoy GK. AHFS drug information 2002. Bethesda: American Hospital Formulary Service, 2002;28:12:2120–78.

29. Leppik IE. Monotherapy and polypharmacy. Neurology 2000; 55(suppl 3):S25–9.

30. Pellock JM, Willmore LJ. A rational guide to routine blood monitoring in patients receiving antiepileptic drugs. Neurology 1991; 41:961–4.

31. Porter RI, Schmidt D, Treiman DM, Nadi NS. Pharmacologic approaches to the treatment of focal seizures. Past, present, and future. Adv Neurol 1992;57:607–34.

32. Krumholz A, Fisher RS, Lesser RP, Hauser WA. Driving and epilepsy. A review and reappraisal. JAMA 1991;265:622–6.

33. Temkin NR, Dikmen SS, Wilensky AJ, Keihm J, Chabel S, Winn HR. A randomized, double-blind study of phenytoin for the prevention of post-traumatic seizures. N Engl J Med 1990; 323:497–502.

34. Pregnancy and teratogenesis in epilepsy. Neurology 1992; 42(suppl 5):1–160.

35. Willmore LJ. Clinical pharmacology of new antiepileptic drugs. Neurology 2000;55(suppl 3):S17–24.

36. Dicthter MA, Brodie MJ. New antiepileptic drugs. N Engl J Med 1996;334:1583–90.

37. Engel J Jr. Surgery for seizures. N Engl J Med 1996;334:647–52.

38. Vining EPG, Freeman JM, Ballahan-Gil K, et al. A multicenter study of the efficacy of the ketogenic diet. Arch Neurol 1998; 55:1433–7.

39. AAP. Program for renewal of certification in pediatrics. Guides for record review. Seizures 1992;1–12.

40. Sabo-Graham T, Seay AR. Management of status epilepticus in children. Pediatr Rev 1998;19:306–9.

41. Hauser WA. Status epilepticus. Epidemiologic considerations. Neurology, 1990;40(suppl 2):9–13.

42. Dodrille CB, Wilensky AJ. Intellectual impairment as an outcome of status epilepticus. Neurology 1990;40(suppl 2):23–7.

43. Hill A. Neonatal seizures. Pediatr Rev 2000;21:117–21.

65
Cerebrovascular Disease

Michael H. Bross and David C. Campbell

Strokes are the third leading cause of death in the United States, claiming about 160,000 Americans yearly. Each year over 730,000 Americans have a new or recurrent stroke.[1] Two thirds of stroke survivors are impaired neurologically, with over four million Americans suffering from stroke impairments. These stroke survivors have a high risk of subsequent stroke, with about one third having another stroke within 5 years. The costs of strokes, including both medical care and lost productivity, have been estimated to be $30 billion annually.[2]

With the aging of our population, diseases that disproportionately affect the elderly will assume increasing importance. The incidence rate of first-ever stroke rises sharply with age, from 8.72 per 1000 person-years for individuals age 65 to 84 to 17.31 per 1000 person-years for persons 75 years and older.[3] Since women as a group live longer than men, it is not surprising that over 60% of the stroke deaths involve women.

African Americans have higher rates of both stroke incidence and stroke death, nearly double that for whites. African Americans also suffer from more severe impairments after strokes than other racial groups in the United States.[2] This high rate of strokes among African Americans has led to the southeastern United States being referred to as the "stroke belt."

Pathogenesis

Stroke occurs when there is disrupted blood flow to an area of the brain. The brain is perfused by anterior and posterior circulations. The anterior circulation begins with the carotid arteries and perfuses the anterior four fifths of the brain. The internal carotid arteries give off the ophthalmic branch before terminating at the circle of Willis, branching into the anterior and middle cerebral arteries. The posterior circulation supplies only one fifth of the brain and is derived from the vertebral arteries. The vertebral arteries first supply the cerebellum via the posterior inferior cerebellar arteries. The vertebral

arteries then join to form the basilar artery. The basilar artery branches to form the posterior cerebral arteries that supply the occipital lobes.

Arterial and cardiac abnormalities[4] (Fig. 65.1) often develop and lead to ischemic stroke. The most common cause of ischemic stroke is atherosclerosis of large and small arteries. When atherosclerois of an arterial wall leads to thrombus formation, there is partial or complete disruption of blood flow (thrombotic stroke). The thrombus may also dislodge and occlude a more distal artery (embolic stroke). Large artery pathology commonly occurs in the aortic arch, carotids, and major cerebral vessels. Small vessel atherosclerosis may involve intracranial or penetrating arteries, with more focal or limited brain injury occurring (lacunar stroke). The most common cardiac abnormalities leading to stroke are atrial fibrillation, valvular disease (especially mitral stenosis), and poor ejection fraction. These cardiac problems predispose to thrombus formation, with dislodged thrombi (emboli) occluding cerebral vessels. Less common causes of ischemic stroke include drug use, arterial dissection, fibromuscular dysplasia, arteritis, hypercoagulable states, and migraines.

Hemorrhagic strokes comprise approximately 20% of total strokes and are divided into intracerebral and subarachnoid types. Intracerebral hemorrhage is usually caused by hypertensive vascular disease, with bleeding most often into the putamen, thalamus, pons, or cerebellum. Subarachnoid hemorrhage (SAH) is typically the result of leaking from a saccular aneurysm, but may be secondary to an arteriovenous malformation or other vascular abnormality.

Risk Factors

Stroke risk factors[5] (Table 65.1) have tremendous impact and are often additive in any given patient. Although several risk factors cannot be modified, many of the risks are potentially

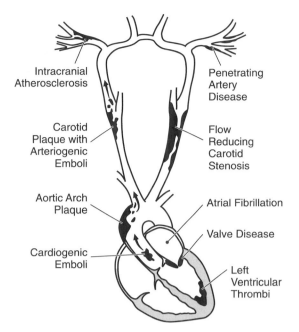

Intracranial
Atherosclerosis

Penetrating
Artery
Disease

Carotid
Plaque with
Arteriogenic
Emboli

Flow
Reducing
Carotid
Stenosis

Aortic Arch
Plaque

Atrial Fibrillation

Valve Disease

Cardiogenic
Emboli

Left
Ventricular
Thrombi

Fig. 65.1. The most frequent sites of arterial and cardiac abnormalities causing ischemic stroke. (From Albers GW, et al,[4] with permission.)

controllable. Recognition of risk factors and implementing effective interventions will lessen the impact of strokes.

Age, gender, race, and family history as risk factors cannot be modified but are important to consider as the individual patient is treated. A patient at high risk for a potentially devastating disease (as a stroke) will warrant more aggressive preventive treatments. The risk of stroke doubles every 10 years after age 55, with the net result of eight times the risk of stroke by age 85. For similar age groupings, men have a 30% greater incidence of stroke than women. The high rate of strokes in African Americans may be secondary to higher rates of several risk factors, including hypertension, diabetes, smoking, poverty, and sickle cell anemia. A family history of

Table 65.1. **The Impact of Stroke Risk Factors**

Male gender	1.3× greater
African-American race	2× greater
Age 65 (vs. 55)	2× greater
Smoking	2× greater
Diabetes	3× greater
Carotid artery disease	3× greater
Peripheral vascular disease	3× greater
Age 75 (vs. 55)	4× greater
Left ventricular hypertrophy	4× greater
Previous heart surgery	4× greater
Atrial fibrillation	6× greater
Other heart disease	6× greater
Blood pressure >140/90	6× greater
Age 85 (vs. 55)	8× greater
Previous transient ischemic attack (TIA)	10× greater
Previous stroke	10× greater

Source: National Stroke Association. Stroke risk factors and their impact, 2001, with permission. Available at *www.stroke.org.*

stroke or transient ischemic attack (TIA) also increases stroke risk.

Several additional risk factors for stroke can be lessened with appropriate interventions. Smoking more than doubles the stroke risk as the result of accelerating atherosclerosis, raising blood pressure, and lowering arterial oxygen. In women, smoking cessation for 2 to 4 years largely decreases the risk of stroke to that of nonsmokers.[6] In men, smoking cessation for 5 years markedly decreases the risk of stroke, but former heavy smokers remain at significant risk for stroke.[7] Cholesterol reduction with the statin drugs reduces stroke rate by almost 30%.[8] Diabetes triples the stroke risk, with accelerated atherosclerosis, hypertension, thrombosis, and hyperlipidemia. For the diabetic patient, tight control of diabetes and lowering low-density lipoprotein (LDL) cholesterol to <100 mg/dL are recommended.[9] In addition, diabetic patients have been found to have a 44% decrease in strokes with tight blood pressure control averaging 144/82.[10]

Carotid artery disease and peripheral vascular disease each triple the stroke risk. With known vascular disease, antiplatelet therapy with aspirin or ticlodipine (Ticlid) has been found to decrease nonfatal strokes by about one third.[11] A newer agent, clopidogrel (Plavix), has been shown to be slightly more effective than aspirin for stroke prevention in patients with vascular disease.[12] In addition, the combination of low-dose aspirin and sustained release dipyridamole (Aggrenox) has been found more effective than aspirin or dipyridamole alone.[13] The surgical treatment of asymptomatic carotid artery disease remains controversial. The Asymptomatic Carotid Atheroslerosis Study compared medical treatment to carotid endarterectomy for the treatment of patients with carotid artery stenosis of 60% or greater. High-risk patients, with respect to surgical risk and projected 5-year survival, were excluded. The study found surgery patients have 5-year risk reduction for ipsilateral stroke of 66% for men and 7% for women. Women suffer higher perioperative complications than men. For surgical benefit to occur, the carotid endarterectomy must be performed with less than 3% perioperative morbidity and mortality.[14] A subsequent analysis of carotid endarterectomy surgery in Ohio found that higher-volume hospitals have a 71% reduction in risk for 30-day stroke or death compared to lower-volume hospitals.[15] The physician must therefore carefully present the risks and benefits of asymptomatic carotid artery surgery to each affected patient.

Hypertension affects over 50 million Americans and is recognized as the most important controllable risk factor. Since hypertension rarely causes symptoms, it is often untreated. Less than 30% of treated hypertensive patients have blood pressure less than 140/90.[16] A prolonged decrease in diastolic blood pressure of only 5 mm Hg has been found to decrease stroke risk by one third.[17] Treatment of isolated systolic blood pressure, 160 mm Hg or more, has been found to decrease nonfatal stroke by 44% in persons 60 and older.[18]

Cardiac disease increases the risk of stroke by several potential mechanisms. Although the direct effect of emboli from the heart is the most recognized risk, the coexistence of atherosclerosis in the heart and cerebral vasculature needs to be recognized. After myocardial infarction, the risk of stroke is estimated to be 8.1% over the following 5 years. Increasing age, lower ejection fraction, and absence of aspirin or anticoagulant treatment are risk factors for stroke. For every 5% decrease in ejection fraction, there is an 18% increase in the risk of stroke.[19] Atrial fibrillation markedly increases stroke risk, with the incidence of stroke averaging about 5% per year. Stroke risk with atrial fibrillation increases with the coexisting risk factors of increasing age, hypertension, diabetes, impaired left ventricular function, mitral stenosis, and a large left atrium. If feasible, cardioversion to a sinus rhythm is recommended. Oral anticoagulation with adjusted-dose warfarin (Coumadin) to achieve a target international normalized ratio (INR) of 2.0 to 3.0 reduces the stroke rate by two thirds for persistent atrial fibrillation.[20,21] It has been found that a combination of low-dose warfarin plus aspirin is not nearly as effective as adjusted-dose warfarin for the prevention of stroke.[22] In summary, atrial fibrillation patients over age 65 and atrial fibrillation patients with one or more additional risk factors (hypertension, diabetes, prior stroke or TIA, mitral stenosis, or impaired left ventricular function) should strongly be considered for warfarin therapy to achieve a target INR of 2.0 to 3.0. Aspirin or other antiplatelet therapy can be substituted for atrial fibrillation patients who cannot tolerate warfarin or are at low risk for stroke.[23]

Previous TIA and previous stroke confer very high risk for future stroke, and is discussed in the following sections.

Cerebrovascular Ischemia

Cerebrovascular ischemia leads to specific signs and symptoms that can help localize the site of brain involvement (Table 65.2). One of the most important factors is to determine whether the anterior or posterior circulation of the brain is involved. Compromise of the anterior cerebral artery leads to contralateral weakness and sensory loss, with the leg more involved. Since the frontal lobe is injured, judgment and insight are often impaired. Middle cerebral artery lesion leads to contralateral weakness and sensory loss, with greater arm and facial involvement. Speech and language are commonly involved with the dominant hemisphere (usually the left hemisphere for right-handed persons). Nondominant hemisphere injuries from the middle cerebral artery commonly lead to symptoms of neglect (the patient does not recognize stimuli to one side of the body). Injury to the posterior circulation of the brain, or vertebrobasilar system, usually affects the brainstem, cerebellum, and occipital lobe. A combination of symptoms usually occurs, including diplopia, vertigo, dysarthria, dysphagia, ataxic gait/limbs, and bilateral or alternating deficits.

Transient Ischemic Attack

Transient ischemic attack is defined as a focal cerebral ischemic event that lasts less than 24 hours and leaves no residual neurologic deficit. The annual incidence rate of TIA, a key predictor of future stroke, rises sharply with age and is 41% of the annual stroke incidence rate.[24] The neurologic

Table 65.2. **Common Clinical Findings with Vascular Lesions**

Anterior cerebral artery
  Contralateral paresis/paralysis/sensory deficits of leg greater than arm
  Confusion, impaired judgment and insight
  Primitive grasp and suck reflexes
  Gait disturbance
  Bowel/bladder incontinence
Middle cerebral artery
  Contralateral paresis/paralysis/sensory deficits of arm and face greater than leg
  Contralateral homonymous hemianopsia
  Speech and language disorder (aphasia) with dominant hemisphere involvement
  Contralateral visual neglect, contralateral sensory neglect, confusion, denial of deficit with nondominant hemisphere involvement
Posterior cerebral artery
  Contralateral homonymous hemianopsia
  Visual hallucinations and trouble recognizing objects (visual agnosia)
Vertebrobasilar artery system
  Diplopia, visual field deficits (homonymous and bilateral)
  Vertigo, syncope
  Dysarthria, dysphagia
  Ataxic gait/limbs
  Bilateral or alternating deficits (sensory and motor)

symptoms of a TIA usually occur suddenly, without warning, and peak within minutes. Most TIAs last less than 6 hours. A full range of neurologic symptoms (Table 65.2) can occur with TIAs, with common symptoms being unilateral weakness, aphasia, unilateral paresthesias, and partial or complete unilateral loss of vision. Vertebrobasilar symptoms include dysarthria, diplopia, ataxia, and vertigo. Hallucinations, tingling, scintillations, and rhythmic shaking of an extremity may occasionally occur and make the diagnosis more difficult. Extremely brief neurologic symptoms that last a few seconds and a sudden loss of consciousness without additional neurologic symptoms are seldom due to a TIA. The lightheadedness associated with sudden change in position is most often due to postural hypotension.

If symptoms suggest a TIA, the physical examination and testing are focused to identify an etiology. Embolic fragments from diseased arteries or the heart are the most common etiologies. Arterial auscultation may reveal bruits in the carotid, aorta, renal, and iliac arteries. Other signs of advanced atherosclerosis may be found with arterial narrowing by funduscopic exam and loss of peripheral pulses. Duplex carotid ultrasound testing is a cost-effective way to screen for significant carotid artery disease, whether or not a carotid bruit is present.[25] Cardiac disease can be detected by listening for the murmur of mitral stenosis or aortic stenosis and the irregularly irregular rhythm of atrial fibrillation. Electrocardiogram readily confirms atrial fibrillation. Transthoracic two-dimensional echocardiography helps to reveal valvular disease and thrombi. Transesophageal echocardiography may be needed to detect small left atrial thrombi, a right to left shunt, and ascending aorta atherosclerosis.

Endarterectomy for symptomatic carotid stenosis is beneficial for patients with ipsilateral high-grade stenosis. The Medical Research Council (MRC) European Carotid Surgery Trial recommends surgery for stenosis 80% or greater.[26] The North American Symptomatic Carotid Endarterectomy Trial found definite benefit with surgery for 70% stenosis or greater and recommended consideration of surgery for 50% to 69% stenosis. To achieve operative benefit with 50% to 69% stenosis, very low endarterectomy risks of <3% for disabling stroke or death must be present.[27]

Chronic atrial fibrillation, mitral stenosis, and thrombi from myocardial injury are best managed with anticoagulation. Warfarin is used to achieve an INR of 2.0 to 3.0.

Ischemic Stroke

Initial Assessment

Symptoms that suggest stroke must be recognized quickly for effective treatment to occur. When blood supply to part of the brain is compromised, the brain tissue that is most directly affected will begin to die within minutes. The brain tissue surrounding the injured area will be hypoperfused. This area of poor perfusion has been termed "ischemic penumbra" and is at high risk for subsequent cellular death. If the stroke is allowed to progress without timely intervention, much of this ischemic penumbra will die and greatly increase the impact of the stroke.

The clinical presentation of a stroke depends on the site of vascular occlusion (Table 65.2). Sudden weakness, confusion, trouble speaking or understanding speech, trouble walking, and vision disturbances are common symptoms. In addition, a severe headache and a sudden decline in consciousness can also indicate stroke. It is important to teach potential patients and their family members to recognize these symptoms and immediately call 911 for timely intervention. Older patients, the highest risk group, are the least knowledgeable about stroke signs.[28]

The prehospital treatment of stroke is first focused on stabilizing airway, breathing, and circulation. Oxygen is administered and an intravenous saline infusion started. Since hypoglycemia can produce many neurologic symptoms, blood glucose is quickly checked. Glucose is given intravenously if hypoglycemia is confirmed. The emergency medical services system should be aware of which local hospitals are equipped to best handle acute stroke and transport to a well-prepared hospital if possible.

Once the patient arrives in the emergency department, pertinent history needs to be obtained. Discerning the time of stroke onset is crucial; information might be provided by any eyewitnesses as well as the patient. If the patient awakens with the symptoms of a stroke, it must be inferred that the symptoms began when the patient fell asleep. Additional key history items include recent trauma, recent signs of illness (temperature, pain, chills, etc.), drug use (alcohol, illicit), medical history, and medications.

Vital signs are checked repeatedly to detect any instability. Elevated blood pressure commonly occurs with an ischemic stroke and may be partially protective, helping perfuse borderline areas. Unless blood pressure consistently exceeds 220 mm Hg systolic or 120 mm Hg diastolic, it should not routinely be treated. Coexisting illnesses, such as myocardial infarction and heart failure, will require more aggressive treatment of blood pressure. In addition, blood pressure should be kept below 180 systolic and 110 diastolic if a thrombolytic agent has been given. Elevation of temperature has been found to be associated with more severe strokes and worse outcomes.[29] Although hypothermic treatment remains controversial, it is prudent to control temperature elevation if possible. The neurologic exam seeks to uncover the most likely site of brain injury, with brief repeated exams to detect changing neurologic status. Cardiovascular exam will detect atrial fibrillation, aortic and mitral murmurs, carotid bruits, and decreased or absent peripheral pulses. If a carotid bruit is heard on the side corresponding to the symptoms, moderate or severe stenosis is more than twice as likely to be present.[25] Ophthalmoscopy will detect signs of long-standing hypertension, chronic diabetes, increased intracranial pressure, and retinal emboli.

Initial diagnostic testing includes an electrocardiogram, pulse oximeter monitoring, complete blood count, prothrombin time (PT) with INR, partial thromboplastin time (PTT), serum electrolytes, glucose, blood urea nitrogen (BUN), and creatinine. Preparations are immediately begun for a non-contrast computed tomography (CT) of the brain. This emergent CT scan is primarily helpful in detecting any bleeding. In addition, local mass effect and ischemia may be seen and help determine the site of injury.

Thrombolytic Treatment

Rapid diagnosis and assessment of stroke is crucial to allow for timely thrombolytic treatment. If thrombolytic treatment with tissue-type plasminogen activator (t-PA) (Activase) is given within 3 hours of symptom onset, it has been shown that partial or total stroke recovery is 1.7 times more likely than in a placebo group.[30] Outcome measures at 3 and 12 months are significantly better.[30,31] In addition to treatment within 3 hours, other inclusion and exclusion criteria must be carefully noted[32] (Table 65.3). It is especially important to exclude bleeding with a CT scan before giving thrombolytic treatment. Since the majority of physicians have difficulty consistently identifying hemorrhage on a CT scan, enhanced training or telemedicine systems may be necessary to widely implement stroke thrombolysis.[33]

Thrombolytic therapy is given at a dose of 0.9 mg/kg, with a 10% bolus and the remainder over 1 hour. Aspirin and anticoagulants are not given for the first 24 hours. If the repeat CT scan at 24 hours shows no evidence of hemorrhage, aspirin or anticoagulants may be started. Blood pressure should be maintained below 180 mm Hg systolic and 110 diastolic. Even with these precautions, intracranial hemorrhage occurs in over 6% of patients with thrombolytic treatment.[30] If the patient exhibits any signs of hemorrhage, such as vomiting or intense headache, thrombolytics/anticoagulants should be held and a CT repeated immediately.

Table 65.3. **Inclusion and Exclusion Criteria for Intravenous Thrombolytic Therapy**

Inclusion criteria
  Ischemic stroke by clinical assessment
  Persistent neurologic deficit beyond an isolated sensory deficit or ataxia
  Cranial computed tomography (CT) negative for hemorrhage
  Initiation of treatment within 3 hours after symptom onset
Exclusion criteria
  Treatment initiated >3 hours after symptoms' onset
  Neurologic deficit is found to be rapidly improving, based on history or observation
  A patient whose CT scan shows hemorrhage or hemorrhagic transformation of an infarct; exercise caution because the risks associated with tissue-type plasminogen activator (t-PA) therapy increase in patients with major early infarct signs revealed by CT (e.g., substantial edema, mass effect, or midline shift); its use should be weighted against the anticipated benefit
  A patient taking oral anticoagulants or with prothrombin time (PT) >15 seconds
  A patient receiving heparin within the preceding 48 hours who has a prolonged partial thromboplastin time (PTT)
  A patient with platelet counts <100,000 per mm³
  A patient with a pretreatment systolic blood pressure >184 mm Hg or diastolic pressure >110 mm Hg or if aggressive treatment is required to reduce blood pressure to the specified limits prior to thrombolytic therapy
  A patient who has had prior stroke or any serious head trauma in the preceding 3 months
  A patient who has had major surgery within the preceding 14 days
  A patient with prior intracranial hemorrhage
  A patient with gastrointestinal tract or urinary tract hemorrhage within the preceding 14 days
  A patient with seizure at the onset of the stroke
  A patient with symptoms suggestive of subarachnoid hemorrhage
  A patient with arterial puncture at a noncompressible site within the previous 7 days

Source: National Stroke Association. Stroke the first hours: guidelines for acute treatment, 2000, with permission. Available at *www.stroke.org.*

Treatment with intravenous thrombolysis should be limited to within 3 hours of symptom onset, since treatment at from 3 to 5 hours of symptom onset results in increased symptomatic intracranial hemorrhage and mortality.[34] Intraarterial thrombolysis may become more widely used in the future, as one study has found benefit with treatment up to 6 hours after symptom onset with intraarterial prourokinase for middle cerebral artery (MCA) occlusion.[35]

Additional Considerations

Most patients present with stroke after the therapeutic window for thrombolysis has passed. Close monitoring reveals any signs of deterioration. It is important to correct electrolyte disturbances, hypoglycemia and hyperglycemia, hypoxia, and volume disturbances. Patients need to be kept NPO until good swallowing reflexes can be demonstrated. A radiologic swallowing study is often necessary before oral feeding is resumed. The complications of immobility can be minimized with appropriate bedding, frequent turning, good nutrition, and early rehabilitation. Deep vein thrombosis (DVT) prophylaxis and aspiration precautions should be used.

Further evaluation is often necessary to determine the likely cause of the stroke and exclude other diagnoses. A magnetic resonance imaging (MRI) head scan with diffusion weighted imaging is very sensitive for ischemia and may demonstrate stroke even when conventional MRI and CT are negative. Carotid duplex ultrasonography will reveal extracranial disease up to the angle of the jaw. MRI angiography may be used in conjunction with ultrasound studies to improve diagnostic sensitivity and specificity.[36] CT and MRI angiography are both effective for evaluation of intracranial vasculature.[37] Cerebral angiography and digital subtraction angiography (angiography using less contrast material) are invasive tests that may be indicated if surgery is being considered. A repeat CT scan with intravenous contrast is often necessary to exclude a tumor or abscess. If the posterior fossa portion of the brain is damaged, MRI provides better visualization than a CT scanning. Suspected central nervous system infection will require a lumbar puncture (after CT scanning). An electroencephalogram (EEG) is indicated if seizures are a consideration. Echocardiography is indicated if heart disease is present or suspected. Transesophageal echocardiography is often helpful to further clarify cardiac abnormalities, such as vegetations and thrombi.

A worsening clinical condition often prompts consideration of heparin therapy. Unfortunately, both intravenous low molecular weight heparin and subcutaneous heparin have failed to reduce recurrent strokes and increase hemorrhagic strokes.[38,39] If the stroke is the result of suspected emboli from atrial fibrillation or a poor ejection fraction, warfarin is recommended but only after the stroke has stabilized.

Early therapy with aspirin after an acute stroke has been shown to decrease future strokes and mortality, with no significant increase in hemorrhagic strokes.[39,40] Since aspirin dosing at 81 or 325 mg daily is more effective than higher doses, a practical approach is to administer one adult aspirin (325 mg) daily.[41]

Hemorrhagic Stroke

Subarachnoid Hemorrhage

A subarachnoid hemorrhage is usually the result of leaking from a ruptured saccular or "berry" aneurysm. An aneurysm forms when there is a weakness, either congenitally or acquired, at an arterial bifurcation. The classic location of these aneurysms is in the circle of Willis. Arteriovenous malformations (AVMs) account for most of the remaining cases of SAH.

Clinically the patient has sudden onset of a severe headache, often described as "the worst headache of my life" or a "thunderclap headache." Nausea, vomiting, photophobia, and meningismus are characteristic. Focal neurologic symptoms, such as ptosis or diplopia, may result from cranial nerve compression. The patient will often lapse into a coma as intracranial pressure rises abruptly.

In some patients, a small leaking from the aneurysm may occur before a catastrophic rupture. This "sentinel leak" characteristically causes severe headache, nausea, and vomiting, and may be mistaken for a migraine headache. Nuccal rigidity may or may not be present. The physician is cautioned to consider a sentinel leak whenever a patient develops a new headache that is excruciating or a different type of headache than ever before (see Chapter 63).

Diagnosis of SAH can be made by CT scan in about 90% of patients by finding blood in the basal cisterns. If the CT scan does not show blood and there is no impending herniation, a lumbar puncture should be performed to reveal cerebrospinal fluid (CSF) blood. A traumatic tap can usually be separated from a SAH, since the blood clears from a traumatic tap by the third tube of CSF. A tube of CSF should be centrifuged immediately to detect xanthochromia (from an earlier bleed).

Once SAH is diagnosed, immediate neurosurgical consultation is recommended. For surgical candidates, cerebral angiography is used to determine the site and size of the bleeding. The timing of angiography and surgery are best determined by the neurosurgeon. Early clipping of a ruptured aneurysm prevents further bleeding but has high mortality if vasospasm has begun. Vasospasm occurs in most SAH patients and produces strokelike symptoms. Nimodipine, a calcium channel blocker, decreases morbidity and mortality from SAH.[42]

Intracerebral Hemorrhage

Intracerebral hemorrhage typically occurs with activity. There is a sudden onset of severe headache, nausea, and vomiting. Focal neurologic deficits, seizures, and mental status changes are common. Blood may extend into the ventricles and subarachnoid space, causing nuccal rigidity. With extensive hemorrhage, patients will lapse into coma. Unfortunately, most patients do not have warning signs. There is usually a history of long-standing hypertension with vascular disease. Other causes of intracranial hemorrhage include trauma, tumor, arteriovenous malformation, and amyloid angiopathy.

Hemorrhage location is categorized as lobar or nonlobar, with nonlobar hemorrhage usually originating in the putamen, thalamus, pons, or cerebellum. Surgical interventions have been disappointing with supratentorial hemorrhage.[43] With large cerebellar hemorrhage or an infarction, rapid brainstem compression can occur. Surgery has been successfully utilized with these cerebellar injuries.[44]

The long-term prognosis of hypertensive intracerebral hemorrhage is reasonably good if the patient survives the acute hospitalization, with a study finding over 90% of survivors ambulatory after an average of 2.5 years.[45] Surviving patients are at increased risk for both ischemic and hemorrhagic stroke, with a slightly higher rate of ischemic stroke than recurrent hemorrhagic stroke.[46] Although antiplatelet therapy remains controversial, additional stroke prevention measures appear warranted.

Strokes in Children and Young Adults

Strokes in children and young adults have some important differences from strokes in older adults. Newborn strokes often present with seizures as the sole manifestation. Perinatal asphyxia and meningitis must be considered. Strokes in children age 1 to 15 are often due to cyanotic heart disease, moyamoya, or a prothrombotic state. The most common prothombotic condition is sickle cell hemoglobinopathy.[47] Young-adult strokes are often the result of a right-to-left atrial shunt, carotid or vertebrobasilar dissection, a hypercoagulable state.[47] A patent foramen ovale (PFO) can be revealed by a transesophageal echocardiogram with a "bubble test." Hypercoagulation can be revealed by testing for protein S deficiency, protein C deficiency, antithrombin III deficiency, and antiphospholipid antibodies. In addition, toxicology studies for drugs of abuse are often warranted.

Recovery and Rehabilitation

The most dramatic improvement following stroke occurs in the first few weeks, and most measurable neurologic recovery occurs in the first 3 months. Reduction of edema, recovery of local circulation, and resolution of metabolic factors are thought to account for the early recovery, while functional reorganization (plasticity) of the central nervous system is responsible for continuing recovery.

An understanding of the anticipated stages of recovery of motor function is important in accessing the progress of an individual patient. Brunnstrom[48] described six sequential stages of recovery in hemiplegia. The clinician may observe some variability at each stage, and must remember that some patients will plateau short of full recovery. Immediately following the acute episode there is a period of flaccidity, and no movement of the limb can be elicited (stage 1). As recovery begins, minimal voluntary movement responses may be present and spasticity begins to develop (stage 2). During this stage, basic limb synergy patterns may be appear as associated reactions. Synergy patterns are primitive movement patterns associated with spasticity. The synergy patterns include both flexion and extension components, and can be seen in both the upper and lower extremities. Typically the strongest components of these patterns include elbow flexion, shoulder adduction, and forearm pronation of the upper extremity, and hip flexion and adduction, knee extension, and ankle plantarflexion of the lower extremity.[49] Associated reactions are abnormal, automatic responses in the involved limb resulting from action occurring in some other part of the body, such as yawning, sneezing, or stretching. In stage 3 the patient gains voluntary control of the movement synergies. Spasticity increases and may be severe. Stage 4 is marked by a decline in spasticity and mastery of some movement combinations that do not follow the paths of either flexion or extension synergy. If progress continues, more difficult movement combinations are mastered in stage 5 and the primitive limb synergies lose their dominance over motor acts. For those who progress to the disappearance of spasticity (stage 6), individual joint movements become possible and coordination improves toward normal.

Rehabilitation should be initiated as soon as possible after the stroke has been diagnosed. If the patient is medically stable, rehabilitation can begin in the hospital within 48 to 72 hours after the stroke has occurred. The rehabilitative process should begin in the hospital, but will continue through some combination of specialized rehabilitation units, outpatient or home therapy, or through stays at long-term-care facilities that provide therapy and skilled nursing care.

The Agency for Health Care Policy and Research of the United States Department of Health and Human Services has published clinical practice guidelines for post-stroke rehabilitation that stress four basic principles of stroke rehabilitation.[50] The first principle involves the importance of a multidisciplinary care team approach to rehabilitation. While the specific rehabilitation professions involved will vary according to the needs of the individual patient, the team will typically include the family physician, a physiatrist, a neurologist, and possibly specialty consultants and psychiatry. Other critical team members include the physical therapist, occupational therapist, rehabilitation nurse, and possibly a recreational therapist, speech and language therapist, social worker, and dietitian. Effective teamwork is challenging and requires clarity of roles and responsibilities, positive leadership, good communication, and strong commitment to the process.

The second basic principle of rehabilitation requires completion and documentation of thorough and consistent ongoing assessment throughout the rehabilitation process. Repeated clinical examinations and use of standardized instruments are key elements of this assessment process, which should monitor neurologic deficits and medical problems as well as physical, cognitive, psychological, and communication disabilities. The validity, sensitivity, and reliability of the assessment tools are critical so that progress can be measured accurately, and adjustments in the rehabilitation program made appropriately.

Continuity of care is the third basic principle of rehabilitation. As noted above the typical patient's rehabilitation will move from the inpatient setting to either a skilled nursing or rehabilitation facility, and, it is hoped, to home and either home or outpatient therapy. The patient's family physician may be the only member of the rehabilitation team to follow the patient from one setting to another. To reduce the risk of gaps in care when the transition from one facility to another takes place, close communication involving the providers and the family is critical. Transfer of all relevant clinical information including the ongoing patient assessments discussed earlier must occur.

The fourth basic principle of rehabilitation is involvement of the patient and the family in rehabilitation decisions. Throughout the rehabilitation process decisions about the determining rehabilitation goals, selection of a rehabilitation settings and interventions, and ultimately decisions about home care or long-term facility placement should involve the patient and their family whenever possible. Once again, the family physician may be the key individual that the family and

patient look to for the information they will need to participate in these decisions.

Once the stroke patient is discharged from the inpatient rehabilitation program, it is recommended that a visit with the primary physician should take place within the first month and at regular intervals during the first year. Continued monitoring of the patient's physical, cognitive, and emotional functioning and integration into the family and social roles is especially important. The family physician should direct the patient toward risk factor reduction. If the patient was on platelet inhibiting therapy with aspirin prior to the stroke, this represents an aspirin failure and use of an alternative agent should be considered.

In addition to working with the rehabilitation team to monitor the patient's physical recovery, the primary physician should also closely monitor the patient's emotional state. Frustration with difficulty in communicating, moving, and functioning will take an emotional toll on the stroke patient. Depression may occur in even mildly impaired patients and is most likely to manifest between 6 months and 2 years after the event. It has been noted that depression is more frequent and more severe in patients with lesions of the left hemisphere compared to patients who had right hemisphere or brainstem lesions, suggesting that the etiology of post-stroke depression may involve more than just the psychological reaction to disability.

References

1. Broderick J, Brott T, Kothari R, et al. The Greater Cincinnati/Northern Kentucky Stroke Study: preliminary first-ever and total incidence rates of stroke among blacks. Stroke 1998;29: 415–21.
2. Brain attack statistics, 2000. Available at *www.stroke.org*.
3. Di Carlo A. Frequency of stroke in Europe: a collaborative study of population-based cohorts. ILSA Working Group and the Neurologic Diseases in the Elderly Research Group. Italian Longitudinal Study on Aging. Neurology 2000;54(11 suppl 5):S28–33.
4. Albers GW, Easton JD, Sacco RL, Teal P. Antithrombotic and thrombolytic therapy for ischemic stroke. Chest 1998;114: 683S–98S.
5. Stroke risk factors and their impact, 2000. Available at *www.stroke.org*.
6. Kawachi I, Colditz GA, Stampfer MJ, et al. Smoking cessation and decreased risk of stroke in women. JAMA 1993;269:232–6.
7. Wannamethee SG, Shaper AG, Whincup PH, Walker M. Smoking cessation and the risk of stroke in middle-aged men. JAMA 1995;274:155–60.
8. Hebert PR, Gaziano JM, Chan KS, Hennekens CH. Cholesterol lowering with statin drugs, risk of stroke, and total mortality. JAMA 1997;278:313–21.
9. Garber AJ. Attenuating cardiovascular risk factors in patients with type 2 diabetes. Am Fam Physician 2000;62:2633–42.
10. UK Prospective Diabetes Study Group. Tight blood pressure control and risk of macrovascular and microvascular complications in type 2 diabetes: UKPDS 38. BMJ 1998;317:703–13.
11. Antiplatelet Trialists' Collaboration. Collaborative overview of randomized trials of antiplatelet therapy—1: prevention of death, myocardial infarction, and stroke by prolonged antiplatelet therapy in various categories of patients. BMJ 1994;308: 81–106.
12. CAPRIE Steering Committee. A randomized, blinded, trial of

clopidogrel versus aspirin in patients at risk of ischaemic events (CAPRIE). Lancet 1996;348:1329–39.

13. Diener HC Cunha L, Forbes C, Sivenius J, Smets P, Lowenthal A. European Stroke Prevention Study 2. Dipyridamole and acetylsalicylic acid in the secondary prevention of stroke. J Neurol Sci 1996;143:1–13.

14. Executive Committee for the Asymptomatic Carotid Atherosclerosis Study. Endarterectomy for asymptomatic carotid artery stenosis. JAMA 1995;273;1421–8.

15. Cebul RD. Indications, outcomes, and provider volumes for carotid endarterectomy. JAMA 1998;279:1282–7.

16. The Sixth Report of the Joint National Committee on Prevention, Detection, Evaluation, and Treatment of High Blood Pressure. Arch Intern Med 1997;157:2413–46.

17. MacMahon S, Rodgers A. Primary and secondary prevention of stroke. Clin Exp Hypertens 1996;18:537–46.

18. Staessen JA, Fagard R, Thijs L, et al. Randomised double-blind comparison of placebo and active treatment for older patients with isolated systolic hypertension. Lancet 1997;350:757–64.

19. Loh E, Sutton MS, Wun CC, et al. Ventricular dysfunction and the risk of stroke after myocardial infarction. N Engl J Med 1997;336:251–7.

20. Hankey GJ. Non-valvular atrial fibrillation and stroke prevention. National Blood Pressure Advisory Committee of the National Heart Foundation. Med J Aust 2001;174:234–9.

21. Atrial Fibrillation Investigators. Risk factors for stroke and efficacy of antithrombotic therapy in atrial fibrillation. Analysis of pooled data from five randomized controlled trials. Arch Intern Med 1994;154:1449–57.

22. Stroke Prevention in Atrial Fibrillation Investigators. Adjusted-dose warfarin versus low-intensity, fixed-dose warfarin plus aspirin for high-risk patients with atrial fibrillation: Stroke Prevention in Atrial fibrillation III randomized clinical trial. Lancet 1996;348:633–8.

23. Singer DE, Go AS. Antithrombotic therapy in atrial fibrillation. Clin Geriatr Med 2001;17:131–47.

24. Brown RD, Petty GW, O'Fallon WM, Wiebers DO, Whisnant JP. Incidence of transient ischemic attack in Rochester, Minnesota, 1985–1989. Stroke 1998;29:2109–13.

25. Hankey GJ, Warlow CP. Symptomatic carotid ischaemic events: safest and most cost effective way of selecting patients for angiography, before carotid endarterectomy. BMJ 1990;300:1485–91.

26. European Carotid Surgery Trialists' Collaborative Group. Randomized trial of endarterectomy for recently symptomatic carotid stenosis: final results of the MRC European Carotid Surgery Trial (ECST). Lancet 1998;351:1379–87.

27. Barnett HJ, Taylor DW, Eliasziw M, et al. Benefit of carotid endarterectomy in patients with symptomatic moderate or severe stenosis. N. Engl J Med 1998;339:1415–25.

28. Pancioli AM, Broderick J, Kothari R, et al. Public perception of stroke warning signs and knowledge of potential risk factors. JAMA 1998;279:1288–92.

29. Reith J, Jorgensen HS, Pedersen PM, et al. Body temperature in acute stroke: relation to stroke severity, infarct size, mortality, and outcome. Lancet 1996;347:422–5.

30. The National Institute of Neurological Disorders and Stroke rt-PA Stroke Study Group. Tissue plasminogen activator for acute ischemic stroke. N Engl J Med 1995;333:1581–7.

31. Kwiatkowski TG, Libman RB, Frankel M, et al. Effects of tissue plasminogen activator for acute ischemic stroke at one year. National Institute of Neurological Disorders and Stroke Recombinant Tissue Plasminogen Activator Stroke Study Group. N Engl J Med 1999;340:1781–7.

32. Stroke the first hours: Guidelines for Acute Treatment, 2000. Available at *www.stroke.org*.

33. Schriger DL, Kalafut M, Starkman S, Krueger M, Saver JL. Cranial computed tomography interpretation in acute stroke. JAMA 1998;279:1293–7.

34. Clark WM, Wissman S, Albers GW, Jhamandas JH, Madden KP, Hamilton S. Recombinant tissue-type plasminogen activator (Alteplase) for ischemic stroke 3 to 5 hours after symptom onset. The Atlantis Study: a randomized controlled trial. JAMA 1999;282:2019–26.

35. Furlan A, Higashida R, Wechsler L, et al. Intra-arterial prourokinase for acute ischemic stroke. The PROACT 11 study: a randomized controlled trial. Prolyse in acute cerebral thromboembolism. JAMA 1999;282:2003–11.

36. Young GR, Humphrey PR, Shaw MD, Nixon TE, Smith ET. Comparison of magnetic resonance angiography, duplex ultrasound, and digital subtraction angiography in assessment extracranial internal carotid stenosis. J Neurol Neurosurg Psychiatry 1994;57:166–78.

37. Shrier DA, Tanaka H, Numaguchi Y, Konno S, Patel U, Shibata D. CT angiography in the evaluation of acute stroke. AJNR 1997;18:1021–3.

38. Publications Committee for the Trial of ORG 10172 in Acute Stroke Treatment (Toast) Investigators. Low molecular weight heparinoid, ORG 10172 (Danaparoid), and outcome after acute ischemic stroke. JAMA 1998;279:1265–72.

39. International Stroke Trial Collaborative Group. The International Stroke Trial (IST): a randomized trial of aspirin, subcutaneous heparin, both, or neither among 19,435 patients with acute ischaemic stroke. Lancet 1997;349:1569–81.

40. CAST (Chinese Acute Stroke Trial) Collaborative Group. CAST: randomized placebo-controlled trial of early aspirin use in 20,000 patients with acute ischaemic stroke. Lancet 1997;349:1641–9.

41. Taylor DW. Low-dose and high-dose acetylsalicylic acid for patients undergoing endarterectomy: a randomized controlled trial. ASA and Carotid Endarterectomy (ACE) Trial Collaborators. Lancet 1999;353:2179–84.

42. Popovic EA, Danks RA, Siu KH. Experience with nimodipine in aneurysmal subarachnoid haemorrhage. Med J Aust 1993;158:91–3.

43. Juvela S, Heiskanen O, Poranen A, Valtonen S, Kuurne T, Kaste M. The treatment of spontaneous intracerebral hemorrhage. A prospective randomized trial of surgical and conservative treatment. J Neurosurg 1989;70:755–8.

44. Heros RC. Surgical treatment of cerebellar infarction. Stroke 1992;23:937–8.

45. Douglas MA, Haerer AF. Long-term prognosis of hypertensive intracerebral hemorrhage. Stroke 1982;13:488–91.

46. Hill MD, Silver FL, Austin PC, Tu JV. Rate of stroke recurrence in patients with primary intracerebral hemorrhage. Stroke 2000;31:123–7.

47. Williams LS, Garg BP, Cohen M, Fleck JD, Biller J. Subtypes of ischemic stroke in children and young adults. Neurology 1997;49:1541–5.

48. Brunnstrom S: Movement therapy in hemiplegia. New York: Harper & Row, 1970.

49. O'Sullivan S. Stroke. In: O'Sullivan S, Schmitz TJ, eds. Physical rehab assessment and treatment. Philadelphia: FA Davis, 1994;327–59.

50. Clinical Practice Guideline Number 16: post-stroke rehabilitation. AHCPR publication no. 95-0662. Rockville, MD: U.S. Department of Health and Human Services, Public Health Service, Agency for Health Care Policy and Research, May 1995.

66
Movement Disorders

Gregory N. Smith

Parkinsonism/Parkinson's Disease

The first recognized description of Parkinson's syndrome (PS) in 1817 by Parkinson included the major criteria of tremor, bradykinesia, gait disturbance, and postural imbalance. Almost 200 years later these clinical findings remain the basis for diagnosis. It is now well recognized that parkinsonism has multiple causes besides idiopathic Parkinson's disease (IPD). The family physician faces the challenge of ruling out other causes based on clinical exam with judicious use of laboratory test or imaging studies. The limited ability of modern diagnostic technology to confirm IPD is counterbalanced by the significant improvements in treatment, especially in early disease. The family physician who chooses to diagnose and treat patients with parkinsonism must recognize the critical clinical distinctions between the various entities to maximize benefit and reduce exposure to nonbeneficial therapy.

PS/IPD Pathology

The anatomic and biochemical pathology of IPD are well known. The "gold standard" for diagnosis of IPD remains the presence of Lewy bodies in the substantia nigra at autopsy. The loss of neurons in this region leads to depletion of the neurotransmitter dopamine. It is the loss of dopamine that eventually results in the neurologic manifestations of the disease. Despite understanding the pathologic basis of the disease, IPD's exact cause is still unknown. Toxic insults producing free radicals and genetic factors have been postulated, but to date evidence to pinpoint specific causes is lacking.

Diagnosis

The diagnosis of parkinsonism requires at least two of the following findings:

Tremor
Bradykinesia
Rigidity

Some advocate the inclusion of postural instability, which is not warranted as it tends to be a late manifestation of IPD and its early presence suggests alternative diagnoses. Two thirds of patients meeting the above criteria have IPD.[1] Distinguishing the other third requires a clinical exam. The accuracy of the clinical examination is 76%, based on autopsy findings of patients diagnosed with IPD.[2] Attempts at more specific diagnosis of IPD would reduce the inclusion of other causes of PS at the cost of excluding bona fide cases of IPD.[3] Close follow-up of patients initially diagnosed as IPD looking for exclusion criteria is an essential component of good care.

The parkinsonism tremor is a resting tremor that is usually asymmetric in the upper extremity. It may begin in a finger, progressing to the classic "pill-rolling" tremor of the hand, and then involve the entire limb. With time, other extremities usually manifest the tremor. Additionally, the chin, lips, tongue, and neck can demonstrate the tremor.[4] Tremor of the head on the neck either up and down or side to side is not consistent with Parkinson's disease.[1] Stress or repetitive activity of the opposite limb may accentuate the tremor, whereas motor activity of the involved extremity diminishes the tremor. Of note is that the frequency of resting tremor decreases as an initial complaint with older age at disease onset.[5]

Bradykinesia is responsible for many of the manifestations of parkinsonism. The "mask facies" and staring so frequently noted are caused by decreased ability to initiate movement. Patients may complain about weakness, fatigue, soft voice or difficulty buttoning clothing or swallowing. This phenomenon causes micrographia. An impaired arm swing while walking suggests the presence of bradykinesia.

Unlike tremor or bradykinesia, which may cause patient-noted symptoms, rigidity is usually detected only during physical examination. Passive movement of an extremity demonstrates increased tone of both flexors and extensors. Early in the disease rigidity is usually asymmetric and can be of either the "lead pipe" or "cogwheeling" type when tremor is superimposed on rigidity. With disease progression rigidity becomes diffuse, and with bradykinesia results in gait disturbances. Shortening stride leading to a shuffling gait with a stooped posture and flexed elbows occurs frequently in the patient with IPD. Initiating ambulation becomes difficult, with the patient frequently marching in place before starting to move forward. The patient also turns in a unique manner, using multiple small steps to turn the entire body as a unit without twisting the torso. Elderly patients are more prone to develop a festinating gait.[5] The patient tends to lean forward involuntarily and take short, quick, running-like steps on the toes or forefoot to avoid falling.

The gait disturbance is a manifestation of the postural instability that occurs in late-stage disease. The "pull-back" test is useful in the office to demonstrate this phenomenon.[6] The examiner stands behind the patient and places his or her hands on the patient's upper arms. After warning the patient, the examiner gently pulls back. The patient with mild to moderate instability catches himself after one or two steps. The examiner must be prepared to catch the patient who has severe instability. The tendency to fall (forward-propulsion/backward-retropulsion) needs to be evaluated to avoid the attendant morbidity associated with falls.

After establishing the presence of parkinsonism, the family physician must then look for clues to causes other than IPD, which ultimately becomes a diagnosis of exclusion. Parkinsonism can be drug induced or caused by multisystem degenerative disorders of the nervous system, metabolic disorders, trauma, toxic exposures, or structural abnormalities of the central nervous system (CNS). Drugs that block dopamine receptors or deplete dopamine can cause parkinsonism. Neuroleptic medications, including phenothiazines, butyrophenones, and thioxanthenes, which block dopamine receptors, are the most common. However, metoclopramide has also been documented to cause the syndrome. Reserpine, which depletes dopamine, can cause the syndrome. In addition to a history of exposure to the offending agent, one should suspect drug-induced parkinsonism with a subacute and bilateral onset, with early onset of tremor. Dyskinesis of the face and mouth frequently accompanies the drug-induced syndrome.[7] Withdrawal of the offending agent should result in resolution in 2 weeks or as long as 6 months.

Risk factors for cerebrovascular disease and an abrupt onset of symptoms suggest the possibility of stroke-induced parkinsonism. CNS imaging reveals infarcts in the area of the basal ganglia or brainstem. Severe carbon monoxide poisoning may damage the globus pallidus, causing the syndrome. The medical history also reveals clues to structural lesions. Patients complaining of an abrupt or subacute onset of Parkinson's complicated by other neurologic symptoms such as paralysis, seizures, or numbness should undergo computed tomography (CT) or magnetic resonance imaging (MRI). The presence of nonparkinsonism focal deficits, e.g., aphasia, abnormal reflexes, and cranial nerve deficits on neurologic exam likewise warrants imaging studies to look for tumors, abscesses, other space-occupying lesions, or hydrocephalus.

A thorough family history is important, as several inherited syndromes are associated with parkinsonism. The one not to miss is Wilson's disease, an autosomal-recessive disorder associated with accumulation of copper in the liver and basal ganglia. Patients with onset of PS under the age of 50, Kayser-Fleischer rings on ocular exam, or abnormal liver function studies should be screened for Wilson's disease as this is potentially curable with chelation.

Of the one third of patients falsely diagnosed with IPD, a significant number have various neurodegenerative disorders. That these may respond to IPD therapy excludes response to levodopa as a diagnostic criterion. However, as distinguishing between IPD and other neurodegenerative disorders early on may be impossible with current clinical techniques, one should not hesitate to start treatment for IPD when clinically indicated. Over time, anti-Parkinson's medications usually fail to work, and other neurologic findings should lead to revision of this diagnosis.

Alzheimer's disease patients frequently develop symptoms and signs of parkinsonism that are usually mild in relation to the dementia. Patients with diffuse Lewy body disease (DLBD), another cause of dementia, may have PS findings. Lack of a PS tremor and declining cognitive function should alert the clinician to these diagnoses. In addition to the mental status examination, a thorough neurologic exam may reveal findings of other neurodegenerative disorders. Patients with progressive supranuclear palsy (PSP) have early onset of postural instability, supranuclear vertical gaze palsy, loss of opticokinetic response, upright posture, labile emotional states, and dystonia. Ataxia, autonomic nervous dysfunction (orthostatic hypotension), and dementia are seen in multiple-system atrophy, previously called Shy-Drager syndrome or olivopontocerebellar atrophy. When one finds unilateral PS with apraxia of one limb, corticobasal degeneration is a more likely diagnosis.

Further diagnostic testing for the patient with IPD is of limited value. Patients with rigidity, bradykinesia, or tremor without other findings on physical examination do not require CT or MRI scans. If one suspects that tumor or stroke is causing the parkinsonism, these studies are useful. The high cost, limited availability, and absence of evidence that positron emission tomography (PET) scans improve patient outcomes limit their use to research at this time.

Therapy

Increased understanding of the neurochemical pathways involved in IPD has led to advances in the pharmacologic treatment during the last 30 years (Table 66.1). Drug therapy improves quality of life, and new drugs may mitigate or delay the onset of late-stage complications. Physical therapy, occupational therapy, and psychological supportive devices have a role in helping patients and their families cope with the disease. A randomized controlled trial has shown that exercise can improve functional measures such as spinal flexibility and physical performance parameters over short-term follow-up.[8] Evidence as to whether physical and occupational therapy have long-term benefit in improving quality of life or reducing falls or the need for additional medications to control other late-stage complications is lacking. Depression, which frequently accompanies IPD, can be treated with antidepressants and counseling.

Table 66.1. **Pharmacologic Treatment of Idiopathic Parkinson Disease**

Class Agent	Starting dose	Maximum dose	Levodopa dose adjustment[a]
Dopamine precursor			
Levodopa/carbidopa (Sinemet, Sinemet CR)	100/25 mg bid–qid	2000/200 mg/day	NA
Dopamine agonists			
Bromocriptine (Parlodel)	1.25 mg bid	30 mg tid	
Pergolide (Permax)	0.05 mg qd	1.5 mg tid	Yes[b]
Pramipexole (Mirapex)	0.125 mg tid	1.5 mg tid	
Ropinirole (Requip)	0.25 mg tid	8 mg tid	
COMT inhibitors			
Entacapone (Comtan)	200 mg/dose	200 mg 8×/day	25%
Tolcapone (Tasmar)	100 mg tid	200 mg tid	25%
MAO inhibitors			
Selegiline (Eldepryl)	2.5 mg bid	5 mg bid	20%
Anticholinergics			
Trihexyphenidyl (Artane)	1 mg qd	10 mg qd	
Benztropine (Cogentin)	0.5 mg qd	6 mg qd	
Miscellaneous			
Amantadine (Symmetrel)	100–200 mg qd	200 mg qd	

[a]Reduction in levodopa dosage when adding agent to levodopa/carbidopa therapy.

[b]No specific dosage reduction recommended.

COMT = catechol-O-methyltransferase.

Pharmacologic treatments are initially aimed at reducing the disabling effects of tremor, rigidity, bradykinesia, and complications of late IPD. In advanced IPD, and possibly related to long-term treatment with levodopa, patients may develop dyskinesias, "wearing off," and the "on-off" phenomenon. Patients may develop stereotypic motor disorders, such as grimacing, that mark the onset of dyskinesias. Rapid wearing off of symptomatic improvement at the end of a dosing interval and rapid fluctuations between marked symptomatology and good control of parkinsonism (on-off phenomenon) are quite disabling and disturbing to patients. The availability of medications acting at different parts of the neurochemical pathway has improved options for both early and late treatment of IPD.

Levodopa, the immediate precursor to dopamine, is still the mainstay of therapy for IPD. It is administered in combination with a decarboxylase inhibitor such as carbidopa to inhibit metabolism of levodopa, thus increasing its availability to the CNS. All three motor manifestations of IPD improve with levodopa. Additionally levodopa therapy improves patient survival.[9] Delaying initiation of levodopa due to unsubstantiated concerns that it may accelerate progress of the disease only prolongs the patient's disability. When initiating levodopa, dose titration allows the clinician to find a dose that provides maximum benefit while avoiding the effects of nausea, som-nolence, and hallucinations. Sustained-release preparations of levodopa/carbidopa allow less frequent dosing and may help to avoid wearing-off episodes later in the disease. Levodopa preparations combining levodopa with other parkinsonian drugs early in therapy may improve patient response at a lower levodopa dose, thereby avoiding side effects. As the disease progresses, other parkinsonian medications are useful adjuncts to levodopa to control late-stage complications.

Dopamine agonists have been used to treat both early and late disease stages. Studies suggest that initial treatment with the agonists pramipexole and ropinirole may delay the onset of dyskinesis or wearing off compared with levodopa.[10] However, patients treated with agonists have a decreased motor response and higher risk of adverse events such as nausea, edema, somnolence, hypotension, and hallucinations than with levodopa.[11,12] Other agonists include bromocriptine and pergolide. Start at a low dose and titrate with close follow-up for side effects when initiating therapy with agonists. With elderly patients, due to the high rate of side effects with initial agonist monotherapy, it may be beneficial to save agonists for treating late-stage complications. Younger patients without comorbidities may survive longer and benefit from a delayed onset of the late-stage phenomenon.[12] When adding agonists to levodopa/carbidopa, one should titrate the dose of levodopa downward.

The monoamine oxidase inhibitor selegiline delays catabolism of dopamine. In early Parkinson's disease (PD) it may help to delay the need to start levodopa therapy. The initial hope that selegiline might be neuroprotective has not been supported by long-term follow-up studies.[13] The initial dose is 2.5 mg in the morning and at noon with maximum dose of 5 mg bid. Decrease levodopa dosage 20% if adding selegiline to treat late-stage wearing off. Anxiety may limit the usefulness of this drug.

Other strategies to inhibit catabolism of levodopa involve blocking catechol-O-methyltransferase (COMT) in the gastrointestinal (GI) tract and periphery. As with carbidopa, this increases levodopa availability to the CNS. Two COMT inhibitors are currently available in the United States—entacapone and tolcapone. Both have been demonstrated to reduce motor fluctuations or the wearing-off phenomenon in late PD treated with levodopa.[14,15] Entacapone is given as a 200-mg dose along with levodopa/carbidopa up to eight times per day. Start tolcapone at 100 mg tid and titrate to a maximum of 600 mg/day. Use caution when patients have preexisting dyskinesia if adding COMT inhibitors to treat motor fluctuations. Reducing levodopa dosage by 25% while initiating COMT inhibitors may prevent or limit worsening of dyskinesia and other levodopa-related side effects. Orthostatic hypotension, especially in patients on antihypertensives, is not uncommon with COMT inhibitors.

In early IPD, amantadine and anticholinergics may be helpful in alleviating symptoms. The anticholinergic benztropine and trihexyphenidyl may help alleviate tremor either as monotherapy or in conjunction with other PD drugs. Anticholinergic side effects—dry mouth, confusion—may limit the usefulness of these drugs. Amantadine can also be used early in the disease to alleviate PD symptoms and is synergistic with levodopa. None of these agents is neuroprotective, and they have no benefit in late stages of IPD.

Patients with severe PD or wearing off, on-off, or dyskinesias that do not respond to sustained-release levodopa preparations, to the addition of dopamine agonists, or to COMT inhibitors may benefit from other therapies. Consultation with neurologists and neurosurgeons can provide alternative delivery systems such as apomorphine infusion pumps or surgical approaches that may alleviate the symptoms of severe IPD or side effects of treatment. It is hoped that in the future, with better understanding of dopamine pathways and specific dopamine receptors, neuroprotective therapy will be available to prevent the long-term deterioration and disability in PD that exacts a heavy toll on patients and their families.

Tremor: Essential Tremor and Other Causes

Tremors are the most common movement disorders with prevalence estimates ranging from 0.3% to 4% for essential tremor (ET).[16] Of more significance, as the U.S. population ages, is the increasing prevalence of tremor with age—9% of people over 80 years. Tremors are involuntary, rhythmical, and periodic oscillations of a body part. They can occur at rest as in Parkinson's, or with voluntary action. Action tremors can occur while maintaining a position, which are postural tremors, or during movement, which are kinetic tremors. The pathology of most tremors is poorly understood, but they are most likely of CNS origin.[17] Although ET is the most common tremor, one can confuse it with other tremors, idiopathic or secondary. Understanding the diagnostic features of each type is essential as the treatment differs.

Diagnosis

ET is a coarse action tremor with a frequency of 4 to 8 cycles/sec. It is not present at rest and usually does not change with activity. It is both postural and kinetic. ET primarily involves a head-on-neck movement, the voice, or the arms. The lower extremities may occasionally be involved. Fifty percent of patients report a family history of tremor due to autosomal-dominant inheritance with variable penetrance. Patients who consume alcohol usually note a diminishment after imbibing. Most importantly, the rest of the neurologic exam is normal. ET must be distinguished from other tremors—physiologic, writing, orthostatic, drug-induced, and other nervous system disorders.

Physiologic tremors are fine tremors that occur normally while maintaining posture. Hyperthyroidism, anxiety, excessive caffeine, and drugs, e.g., sympathomimetic amines, may worsen the tremor. The shaking accompanying stage fright is a classic example of enhanced physiologic tremor.

Writing tremor (WT) occurs while writing or pursuing other fine motor activities. Although WT may occur with ET, it is also seen with dystonia.

Orthostatic tremor occurs when patients assume a standing position, which makes them feel unsteady. Although this tremor primarily involves the lower extremities, it may also involve the upper extremities. Unlike ET, orthostatic tremor diminishes while walking, especially with tandem gait.[16] It does not respond to alcohol. The tremor is absent when the patient's feet are lifted off of the floor. This is the only tremor that has a distinct frequency—16 Hz on electromyography.

Patients taking lithium or tricyclic antidepressants may develop a tremor similar to ET.[18] Reducing dosage or changing the drug resolves the tremor.

Dystonia is a neurologic disorder that can be confused with ET. While ET is symmetric, dystonia is asymmetric and localized to a body part—e.g., spasmodic torticollis. Overlays with ET are not unusual, but dystonia is different.[19] Cerebellar tremors are almost always intention-only and tend to worsen as the patient gets close to completing the action, such as on finger-to-nose testing. Cerebellar lesions such as tumor, stroke, and multiple sclerosis that cause tremor also cause other cerebellar findings, such as gait disturbance, difficulty with rapid alternating movements, and balance difficulties. Other nervous system disorders may have tremor but usually have other manifestations—e.g., fasciculations and weakness with anterior horn cell disease or sensory abnormalities with neuropathies.

A thorough history and physical should establish a specific diagnosis for tremor. In other situations where a tremor of specific origin, such as cerebellar, is suspected, other diagnostic testing, CT scan or MRI, is warranted. Except as noted with orthostatic tremor, the overlap of electromyography (EMG) results limits the usefulness of this modality for diagnosis.

Treatment

Treatment of ET and other tremors is primarily pharmacologic. As different tremors have a distinct response to various drugs, a precise diagnosis should be made prior to treatment. Various agents including beta-blockers, antiseizure medications, benzodiazepines, and dopaminergic agents all have been used to treat tremors. These studies frequently involve small numbers of patients over limited periods of time comparing one medication to placebo. This limits the ability to generalize results to patients who have tremor for a lifetime, as well as to compare different medications. Flexibility with close monitoring of patient response should allow optimizing treatment.

Although alcohol may have a diagnostic (and self-treatment) role in ET, its long-term problems with dependence, tremor rebound, and abuse make it impractical. Propranolol 120 to 240 mg/day either in divided doses or sustained-release preparations[20] is effective in treating ET by decreasing tremor amplitude. Primidone also reduces ET at doses lower than those used to treat seizures, 125 to 250 mg qd.[21] Doses above 250 mg daily do not increase efficacy and increase the likelihood of sedation, nausea, and dizziness. Clonazepam and gabapentin (Neurontin) may be useful when primidone or propranolol fails. Botulism toxin and neurosurgical approaches can be considered in severe cases of ET that fail to respond to pharmacologic treatment. Head-on-neck and voice tremors tend to respond poorly to pharmacotherapy. Botulinum toxin can work well for these patients.

Writing tremor likewise may respond to propranolol and primidone. When writing tremor coexists with dystonia, anticholinergic medications should be considered. Trihexyphenidyl (Artane) starting at 1 mg/day to a maximum of 10 mg/day or benztropine 1 mg/day to a maximum of 6 mg/day may be useful for dystonia. Dystonic patients failing to respond to anticholinergics may benefit from botulinum toxin, which improves both tremor and dystonia.

Orthostatic tremor does not respond to beta-blockade. Primidone and clonazepam alone or in combination can be tried. Clonazepam should be titrated from 0.5 mg tid until relief of tremor, side effects occur, or the maximum daily dosage of 20 mg is reached. Levodopa and gabapentin have also been used in small studies. There is no adequate pharmacologic agent at this time for cerebellar tremors. For tremors accompanying other CNS disorders, treating the underlying cause is warranted.

Diagnosing and treating various tremors will continue to be a significant challenge for family physicians as the population gets older. Patient and family expectations of minimizing the disability and stigmata of tremor need to be addressed. Setting realistic expectations with patients will help the family physician avoid the frustration of coping with less

than a complete response or attendant side effects of the medications.

References

1. Quinn N. Parkinsonism-recognition and differential diagnosis. BMJ 1995;310:447–52.
2. Hughes AJ, Daniel SE, Kilford L, Lees AJ. Accuracy of clinical diagnosis of idiopathic Parkinson's disease: a clinicopathological study of 100 cases. J Neurol Neurosurg Psychiatry 1992;55:181–4.
3. Hughes AJ, Ben-Shlomo Y, Daniel SE, Lees AJ. What features improve the accuracy of clinical diagnosis in Parkinson's disease: a clinicopathological study. Neurology 1992;42:1142–6.
4. Colcher A, Simuni T. Clinical manifestations of Parkinson's disease. Med Clin North Am 1999;83:327–47.
5. Nagayama H, Hamamoto M, Chikako N, Takagi S, Myazaki T, Katayama Y. Initial symptoms of Parkinson's disease with elderly onset. Gerontology 2000;46:129–32.
6. Vitti RJ. Tremor: how to determine if the patient has Parkinson's disease. Geriatrics 1998;53:30–6.
7. Adler CH. Differential diagnosis of Parkinson's disease. Med Clin North Am 1998;83:349–67.
8. Schenkman M, Cutson TM, Kuchibhatla M, et al. Exercise to improve spinal flexibility and function for people with Parkinson's disease: a randomized, controlled trial. J Am Geriatr Soc 1998;46:1207–16.
9. Rajput AH, Vitti RJ, Rajput AH, Offord KP. Timely levodopa administration prolongs survival in Parkinson's disease. Parkinsonism Rel Disord 1997;3:159–65.
10. Halloway R, and the Parkinson Study Group. Pramipexole vs levodopa as initial treatment for Parkinson disease: a randomized controlled trial. JAMA 2000;284:1931–8.
11. Rascol O, Brooks DJ, Lorczyn AD, DeDeyn PP, Clarke CE, Lange AE, for the 056 Study Group. A five-year study of the incidence of dyskinesia in patients with early Parkinson's disease who were treated with ropinirole or levodopa. N Engl J Med 2000;342:1484–91.
12. Tanner CM. Dopamine agonists in early therapy for Parkinson disease promise and problems [editorial]. JAMA 2000;284:1971–3.
13. Shoulson I, and the Parkinson Study Group. DATA TOP: a decade of neuroprotective inquiry. Ann Neurol 1998;44(suppl 1):5160–6.
14. Rinne VK, Larsen JP, Siden A, Worm Peterson J, and the Nomecomt Study Group. Entacapone enhances the response to levodopa in Parkinsonism patients with motor fluctuations. Neurology 1998;51:1309–14.
15. Adler CH, Singer C, Obrien C, et al., for the Tolcapone Fluctuator Study Group III. Randomized, placebo-controlled study of tolcapone in patients with fluctuating Parkinson's disease treated with levodopa carbidopa. Arch Neurol 1998;55:1089–95.
16. Louis ED, Ottman R, Hauser WA. How common is the most common adult movement disorder? Estimates of the prevalence of essential tremor throughout the world. Mov Disord 1998;13(1):5–10.
17. Wills AJ. Essential tremor and related disorders. Br J Hosp Med 1995;54(1):21–6.
18. Hern JEC. Tremor. BMJ 1984;288(7):1072–3.
19. Rehman H. Diagnosis and management of tremor. Arch Intern Med 2000;160:2438–44.
20. Findley LJ. Essential tremor. Br J Hosp Med 1986;35:388–92.
21. Ellias SA. Essential tremor. RI Med J 1993;76:563–6.

67
Disorders of the Peripheral Nervous System

John M. Wilkinson

Disorders of the peripheral nervous system include a wide variety of conditions with diverse etiologies; peripheral nerves may be damaged by many different disease processes, toxic insults, and injuries.[1]

Anatomy and Pathophysiology

The long and often vulnerable axons of the peripheral nervous system may contain motor, sensory, and autonomic fibers, alone or in combination with one another. Motor neurons arise from the anterior horn cells of the spinal cord, exit via the ventral roots, and travel in larger myelinated nerves to their particular muscle fibers. Sensory nerves conveying vibration and joint position sense are made up of large myelinated fibers. Sensory fibers mediating pain and temperature sensation are smaller and conduct impulses less rapidly. The cell bodies of sensory neurons are located in the dorsal root ganglia; the proximal axon enters the spinal cord via the dorsal root, and the distal axon terminates in various sensory receptors. The ventral and dorsal roots unite as they exit the spinal canal and form mixed spinal nerves. The mixed spinal nerve roots unite to form cervical, brachial, and lumbosacral plexi. The plexi then redivide as various individual mixed peripheral nerves. Autonomic fibers, which are smaller and unmyelinated, arise from either the sympathetic ganglia or the parasympathetic nuclei and travel within most peripheral nerves.

Approach to the Patient with Peripheral Neuropathy

Peripheral neuropathies vary widely in their presentation, and the clinician must first recognize when presenting signs or symptoms may represent one of the many disorders of the peripheral nervous system. Specific findings depend on the specific fibers involved, as well as whether the axon itself or only the myelin sheath is affected.[2,3]

Sensory Changes

Early in the course of many peripheral neuropathies, only subjective symptoms of pain or sensory dysfunction are evident. Because there is dermatomal overlap of skin innervation, and because most muscle groups are innervated by fibers from several nerve roots, objective evidence of sensory loss or muscle weakness is more difficult to detect. Symptoms of proximal nerve root disorders occur in a dermatomal distribution. More distal lesions result in pain in the distributions of individual peripheral cutaneous nerves.

Processes affecting primarily small fibers result in pain, burning dysesthesias, impaired pain and temperature sensation, or autonomic dysfunction. If large fibers are damaged, vibratory sense and proprioception are decreased, as are tendon stretch reflexes and muscle strength.

Motor Changes

Motor dysfunction may cause symptoms ranging from mild weakness to complete paralysis. Symptoms are usually most pronounced distally, especially with polyneuropathies, and may be reported as stumbling, tripping, or "clumsiness" of the hands or feet. Denervation of muscles causes eventual atrophy. Decreased tendon stretch reflexes may be the earliest objective sign of motor dysfunction.

Autonomic Changes

Autonomic fibers convey deeper, ill-defined visceral sensation. Autonomic dysfunction, classically seen in association with diabetes, causes symptoms in many organ systems. The overlying skin in involved areas may be cold, smooth, and shiny with decreased sweating. Orthostatic hypotension, as well as gastrointestinal and genitourinary symptoms, may occur.

Classification of Peripheral Neuropathies

Once a particular problem is determined to be a peripheral neuropathy, the primary goal should be the identification of treatable causes or underlying medical conditions; knowing and applying several different classification schemes, as outlined below, helps clinicians determine the most likely etiology. In particular, clinicians should screen for diabetes, alcoholism, and nutritional deficiencies; ask about recent viral illnesses or any new medications; and review the patient's work and hobbies for activities causing repetitive nerve trauma as well as for any potential toxic exposures. Hereditary neuropathies are not uncommon; in previously unrecognized or long-standing distal neuropathies, a detailed family history is often helpful. Neurologic consultation and electrodiagnostic testing often help with the diagnosis.[2,3] Nonetheless, it is not uncommon to be unable to identify a specific etiology for many cases of peripheral neuropathy.[4]

A variety of antibody tests are marketed for the diagnosis of peripheral nerve disorders. At this point, their clinical utility is limited, and they are probably not useful to the family physician.[5]

Anatomic Classification

The peripheral neuropathies fall into three diverse categories with significantly different and rarely overlapping causes: (1) Polyneuropathies are characterized by diffuse, bilateral, usually symmetric damage to peripheral nerves. They often produce a distal, stocking-glove pattern of paresthesias and sensory loss, followed later by decreased tendon reflexes and muscle weakness. (2) Mononeuropathies are caused by damage to single peripheral nerves. This damage is generally due to acute or chronic trauma, although tumor infiltration or infarction of individual nerves occurs occasionally. These same processes may cause more proximal lesions as well. (3) Multiple mononeuropathies occur when a disease process individually affects several peripheral nerves. Recognizing this pattern and diagnosing the underlying condition often present a considerable challenge. Multiple mononeuropathies are relatively less common than other peripheral neuropathies. They generally have a vascular cause (diabetes, vasculitis), although rheumatoid arthritis may cause multiple entrapment neuropathies.

Pathophysiologic Classification

Axonal damage underlies most peripheral neuropathies. Distal or dying-back axonopathy is the common reaction of the peripheral nerves in response to various toxic, metabolic, and nutritional insults. Degeneration begins at the distal ends of the largest and longest axons and advances proximally toward the nerve cell body.

Demyelinating neuropathies primarily damage the investing myelin sheaths, causing segmental or patchy damage. Weakness and decreased tendon stretch reflexes are the most common signs of myelinopathy. Myelinopathies constitute only a small fraction of all peripheral nerve disorders. Within this group, acute inflammatory demyelinating polyradiculoneuropathy (Guillain-Barré syndrome, GBS) occurs most frequently; chronic inflammatory demyelinating polyradiculoneuropathy and certain hereditary neuropathies also primarily affect peripheral nerve myelin.

Temporal Classification

A disorder developing acutely, over a few days, should be assumed to be Guillain-Barré syndrome, particularly if there is predominantly motor involvement. Subacute onset (developing over a few weeks) of a polyneuropathy is most likely due to inflammatory or infiltrative disorders or diabetes. Carcinomatous sensory neuropathy may also evolve over a relatively short time. Chronic inflammatory demyelinating polyradiculoneuropathy and certain metabolic neuropathies may also exhibit a subacute to chronic pattern of evolution. A disorder present for many years, especially if present since childhood, is often a hereditary neuropathy, even in the absence of a positive family history.

Functional Classification

Motor weakness with little sensory loss is the classic presentation of GBS. Diphtheria, Lyme disease, and some toxins may also have predominantly motor involvement. A neuropathy with primarily sensory symptoms and little or late-developing weakness is often associated with diabetes, alcoholism, renal failure, or remote malignancy. Human immunodeficiency virus (HIV), almost all hereditary neuropathies, and occasionally Lyme disease have a mixed sensorimotor pattern of involvement. Less commonly, diabetes and amyloidosis manifest a primarily autonomic peripheral neuropathy.

Cranial Neuropathies

Trigeminal Neuralgia

Trigeminal neuralgia (tic douloureux) is a relatively common, usually idiopathic condition characterized by paroxysmal attacks of severe, lancinating facial pain in the distribution of one of the divisions of the trigeminal nerve. Many patients report trigger points that are particularly sensitive to stimulation by even the simplest of activities, such as chewing on one side, brushing teeth, shaving, or even talking.

Typically, trigeminal neuralgia involves the maxillary or mandibular divisions of the fifth nerve. The ophthalmic division is less commonly involved; pain in this distribution is more likely due to incipient herpes zoster or postherpetic neuralgia.

Most patients respond readily to carbamazepine (Tegretol), 200 to 300 mg three times a day. Starting therapy with a dose of 100 mg at bedtime can minimize side effects; increase the daily dose by 100 mg every 3 days until symptoms are relieved. Phenytoin (Dilantin) 300 to 600 mg/day or baclofen (Lioresal) 5 to 20 mg three times a day are alternatives for patients unable to tolerate carbamazepine; they can also be used as adjunctive therapies, potentiating the effects of carbamazepine. In severe or intractable cases a number of new stereotactic and open neurosurgical approaches have been valuable in providing relief.

Bell's Palsy

Bell's palsy (idiopathic facial paralysis) is relatively common and is characterized by the acute onset of an isolated paralysis of the facial nerve. Its cause is uncertain, but it is presumed to be inflammatory. Bell's palsy may occur in patients of any age. Typically, symptoms develop overnight and the patient first notices a facial droop upon awakening; in other cases, the symptoms may evolve over a few days. Many patients recall sitting in a draft or report a recent viral illness.

The degree of impairment is widely variable, ranging from mild weakness to complete unilateral facial paralysis. Although there are no objective signs of sensory loss, patients may report a vague discomfort or aching behind the ear or around the jaw. Lesions involving more proximal branches of the facial nerve may result in hyperacusis and loss of taste, although the latter is difficult to test. Muscles of the forehead are involved in Bell's palsy; frontal sparing is indicative of a central nervous system (CNS) lesion. Corneal sensation is usually intact, but the patient has difficulty or complete inability to blink or close the eye. Food may be caught in the cheek on the affected side.

Bilateral Bell's palsy is rare; when it occurs it is frequently associated with the early disseminated phase of Lyme disease[6] (see Chapter 44). GBS syndrome, sarcoidosis, and diabetic neuropathy may also initially present with facial paralysis.

The prognosis for those with Bell's palsy, with or without specific treatment, is excellent; almost all patients have spontaneous recovery within 1 to 3 weeks. Older or more severely affected patients may have some residual weakness for several months or even permanently.

The greatest danger with Bell's palsy is to the cornea; careful eye care is of the utmost importance. The eye should be kept moist and lubricated with an ophthalmic ointment or artificial tears. If necessary, protect the eye with a shield or tape the lid shut, particularly during sleep. The use of corticosteroids is controversial, but many clinicians find that a short, 10-day tapering course of prednisone is helpful, especially if started within the first 2 to 3 days.

Mononeuropathies

Mononeuropathies are usually due to entrapment, compression, or other physical injuries, affecting peripheral nerves where they are most anatomically vulnerable (deep to fibrous bands or where they pass through bony openings or arch superficially across bony prominences). Treatment of mononeuropathy is generally conservative, including work and activity modification and the detection and treatment of any underlying conditions. Surgical exploration should be reserved for chronic mononeuropathies that show evidence of weakness and atrophy, with focal conduction block confirmed by electrodiagnostic studies.

Brachial Plexus Neuropathies

Brachial plexopathies may be due to any trauma involving the axilla or causing a violent increase in the angle between the shoulder and head, producing stretching or even tearing of various plexus elements. This injury, the cause of the "burner" or "stinger" syndrome seen in football players, results in temporary numbness, paresthesias, and diffuse weakness of the arm and shoulder (also see Chapter 52). Direct extension of apical lung tumors or compression with a thoracic outlet syndrome may produce severe pain in the shoulder and axilla, often with paresthesias extending into the hand (see Chapter 85). Brachial plexus involvement with breast cancer is not uncommon; it is often difficult to distinguish between metastatic brachial plexopathy and late-onset impairment caused by radiation therapy (see Chapter 107).

Acute idiopathic brachial neuropathy (Parsonage-Turner syndrome) is a poorly understood condition characterized by rapidly progressive pain of the neck and shoulder followed within a few days by weakness and hyporeflexia. This condition is sometimes associated with herpes zoster infection; it may also have an autoimmune basis. Unlike cervical radiculopathy caused by a herniated disk, shoulder and upper arm weakness may be profound. Most cases resolve spontaneously, although narcotic analgesia and supportive measures, including physical therapy, are often required.

Median Neuropathies (Carpal Tunnel Syndrome)

Carpal tunnel syndrome is the most common of all entrapment neuropathies; occasionally more proximal impairment of the median nerve in the forearm is seen, especially in athletes (pronator syndrome, anterior interosseous syndrome).

Any process that encroaches on the median nerve can cause carpal tunnel syndrome. Numbness or intermittent paresthesias in the sensory distribution of the median nerve (palmar surface of thumb, index, and middle fingers; radial half of the ring finger; radial two-thirds of the palm), nocturnal pain, and pain at rest are the classic symptoms of carpal tunnel syndrome. Percussion of the median nerve at the carpal tunnel may cause pain or dysesthesias (positive Tinel sign). Sustained wrist flexion, or sometimes sustained wrist extension, for 60 seconds may produce similar findings (positive Phalen test and positive reverse Phalen test, respectively).

There are many variations in the clinical manifestations of this disorder; only infrequently are all of the typical signs and symptoms found in any one patient. Commonly, patients complain of only nocturnal pain relieved by shaking the hand. About one third of patients have proximal extension of pain into the forearm or even to the shoulder; occasionally, arm pain alone is the only symptom of carpal tunnel syndrome.[7] Severe cases may show weakness of the thumb and thenar atrophy. Carpal tunnel syndrome with negative electromyographic findings is not uncommon.

Although many conditions have been reported to cause carpal tunnel syndrome, often these disorders merely aggravate an underlying neuropathy.[8] For instance, peripheral nerves in patients with diabetes are more prone to compression injures; alternatively, an entrapment may be superimposed on a diabetic neuropathy. Flexor tenosynovitis within the carpal tunnel, whether due to trauma, endocrine factors, pregnancy, or inflammatory conditions, including rheumatoid arthritis, may compress the median nerve. While the role of occupational risk factors is controversial,[9] they must be evaluated in any patient with symptoms of carpal tunnel syndrome (see Chapter 45).

Initial treatment of carpal tunnel syndrome is conservative; in fact, most patients achieve relief without surgical treatment.[10] The wrist may be splinted in a neutral position or at 15 degrees dorsiflexion full-time for 3 weeks and then at night only for an additional 3 weeks. Corticosteroid injection of the flexor tenosynovium under the flexor retinaculum may be effective; more often a positive response merely confirms the diagnosis and only temporarily relieves symptoms. Care should be taken that the median nerve itself is not injected. This procedure may need to be repeated two or three times. If carpal tunnel syndrome is caused by cumulative trauma disorder, the patient's work environment must be modified or even changed completely.

Surgical intervention may be necessary when conservative treatment has failed, when intermittent symptoms are severe, or when there is clear-cut evidence of constant sensory loss, weakness, or thenar atrophy. Pregnant women with carpal tunnel syndrome almost never require operation; symptoms usually resolve completely after delivery.

Ulnar Neuropathies

Ulnar nerve neuropathy typically causes paresthesias in the fourth and fifth fingers, including the dorsoulnar aspect of the hand and forearm. The patient may also have a generalized weakness of grasp and clumsiness of the hand and fingers with fine manipulation, depending on the site of compression. The relatively superficial location of the nerve in the ulnar groove makes it susceptible to compression injuries in patients who continually lean on their elbows or who have had prolonged elbow pressure with a coma or general anesthesia. Progressive valgus deformity occurring many years after a supracondylar humeral fracture may cause stretching of the nerve in the ulnar groove (tardy ulnar palsy).

Cubital tunnel syndrome is caused by entrapment of the ulnar nerve within the cubital tunnel, just distal to the medial epicondyle. Young athletes involved in overhand activities, such as pitching, are particularly prone to this disorder.

Ulnar tunnel syndrome (Guyon's canal syndrome), caused by prolonged pressure on the ulnar part of the palm, occurs with certain occupations and in long-distance bicyclists. It may result in weakness of the intrinsic hand muscles only, without paresthesias.

Radial Neuropathies

Radial nerve injury characteristically leads to wrist-drop and paralysis of finger extension. There may also be weakness of extension of the elbow and weakness with supination of the forearm.

Proximally, the radial nerve is sensitive to pressure in the axilla; improperly fitted crutches may cause a radial neuropathy. A so-called Saturday night palsy has been attributed to a drunken sleep with the arm draped over the back of a chair. Midshaft fractures of the humerus or penetrating wounds to the axilla can also damage the radial nerve.

Posterior interosseus syndrome (radial tunnel syndrome) is a more distal radial neuropathy. Entrapment neuropathy may occur at the level of the supinator muscle in the forearm; it generally involves only the posterior interosseus nerve, which is a purely motor branch of the radial nerve. The patient may nonetheless experience vague aching of the forearm and lateral aspect of the elbow, with weakness of the finger extensors and preservation of wrist dorsiflexion. This condition may be confused with lateral epicondylitis or "tennis elbow."

Lumbosacral Neuropathies

Trauma involving the lumbosacral plexus is much less common than is that of the brachial plexus; lumbosacral neuropathy may occur perioperatively, with pregnancy and childbirth, or from compression by aortic aneurysms or tumors. Vascular lesions associated with diabetes may produce a proximal multiple mononeuropathy of the plexus.

The clinically important branches of the upper, lumbar portion of the plexus include the lateral femoral cutaneous nerve, obturator nerve, and femoral nerve. The lower, sacral portion of the plexus gives rise to the inferior and superior gluteal nerves and the sciatic nerve; the sciatic nerve branches to form the common peroneal and tibial nerves.

Meralgia Paresthetica

Compression neuropathy of the lateral femoral cutaneous nerve of the thigh is relatively common; entrapment may occur where it passes underneath the inguinal ligament or where it pierces the fascia lata. It occurs most frequently in overweight individuals or in diabetics. Compression may also occur as the result of a tight belt compressing the nerve as it passes over the iliac crest. Patients experience increasingly severe numbness, pain, and paresthesias, as well as decreased sensation of the anterolateral thigh; there is no weakness.

Femoral Neuropathy

The femoral nerve mediates extension of the leg at the knee through innervation of the quadriceps muscle. Its sensory distribution includes the anteromedial aspect of the thigh and the medial aspect of the lower leg and foot. The femoral nerve is commonly affected by diabetic vascular mononeuropathy; it may also be compressed by an inguinal hernia or tumor involving the lumbar plexus.

Sciatic Neuropathy

The sciatic nerve arises from the sacral portion of the plexus. It leaves the pelvis through the sciatic notch and passes down the posterior thigh, where it divides into the tibial and peroneal nerves at the level of the popliteal fossa. The sciatic nerve innervates the extensors of the thigh, the hamstrings, and all of the muscles of the lower leg and foot; it also supplies sensation to the perineum, posterior thigh, lateral calf, and foot. Pain and weakness in the distribution of the sciatic nerve are most commonly the result of lumbar disk herniation, although fractures of the pelvis or femur, gunshot wounds to buttock and thigh, or pelvic tumors may damage the sciatic nerve itself (see Chapter 109).

Peroneal Neuropathy

The common peroneal nerve mediates dorsiflexion and eversion of the foot and supplies sensation to the dorsum of the foot and ankle. It is particularly prone to compression at the level of the fibular head, whether due to trauma, sitting cross-legged, improperly applied stirrups at the time of delivery, or an ill-fitting cast. Diabetic, vasculitic, and hereditary neuropathies may also affect the peroneal nerve.

Tibial Neuropathy

The tibial nerve mediates plantar flexion of the foot and supplies sensation to the sole. Most often, compression of the nerve occurs as it passes through the tarsal tunnel at the medial ankle, resulting in burning paresthesias of the sole of the foot, which are aggravated by walking or prolonged standing.

Interdigital Neuralgia

Entrapment neuropathy of an interdigital nerve is a common cause of foot pain. Morton's neuroma, a benign swelling of the nerve, is usually responsible. Unlike metatarsalgia, there is palpable tenderness between the metatarsal heads in the second or third web spaces. Runners, ballet dancers, and women who wear tight shoes and high heels are particularly prone to the development of a neuroma. Conservative measures may be helpful, but surgical resection is often necessary.

Polyneuropathies

Inflammatory Neuropathies

Inflammatory neuropathies are characterized by inflammation directed against the peripheral nerve. The most common causes are herpes zoster neuronitis, Lyme disease, HIV infection, leprosy, diphtheria, and the acute and chronic inflammatory demyelinating polyradiculoneuropathies.

Herpes Zoster

Herpes zoster (shingles) is a neuronopathy caused by the reactivation of latent varicella-zoster virus, often in the face of declining or impaired immunity, resulting in a unilateral vesicular eruption in the distribution of the affected nerve. The virus primarily affects the dorsal root ganglia or sensory ganglia of cranial nerves.

Herpes zoster of the trigeminal nerve usually arises in the ophthalmic division. Vesicles on the tip of the nose may indicate ophthalmic zoster; refer the patient to an ophthalmologist if there is eye pain, redness, or photophobia. Involvement of the geniculate ganglion of the facial nerve may result in an acute facial nerve paralysis, accompanied by an eruption on the ear and within the ear canal (Ramsay Hunt syndrome). Weakness or paralysis, especially of the facial nerves, or disseminated zoster is more likely to occur in elderly individuals or in patients immunocompromised by HIV or malignancy.

High-dose acyclovir (Zovirax) 800 mg five times daily for 7 days, valacyclovir (Valtrex) 1000 mg three times daily for 7 days, or famciclovir (Famvir) 500 mg three times daily for 7 days has been shown to decrease the duration and severity of symptoms if started early. The benefit of these medications in preventing postherpetic neuralgia, which may be particularly debilitating in elderly patients, remains equivocal; nonetheless, start treatment within the first 72 hours in all patients over age 50.[11] For established postherpetic neuralgia, nonspecific measures, including treatment with carbamazepine, phenytoin, tricyclic antidepressants, gabapentin,[12] topical capsaicin 0.075%, or topical lidocaine 5%, have been recommended. There is no good evidence for the efficacy of corticosteroids.[13]

Lyme Disease

In the early disseminated phase of Lyme disease, approximately 10% of patients may present with Bell's palsy (see Chapter 44). As many as one third of that number may have bilateral, although often unequal, symptoms. In later stages patients may present with a neuropathy that resembles a chronic inflammatory demyelinating polyradiculoneuropathy.[14]

Human Immunodeficiency Virus Infection

Secondary opportunistic infections of the peripheral nervous system, primarily by herpes zoster and cytomegalovirus, may occur with HIV infection, although direct infection of the CNS is more common. In addition, HIV infection may trigger acute or chronic inflammatory demyelinating polyradiculoneuropathies during the early or latent stages of infection (see Chapter 42).

A painful sensorimotor polyneuropathy occurs frequently during the late stages of the disease; it may be related to HIV infection of the dorsal root ganglia or to nutritional or toxic factors.[15] Symptomatic relief may be obtained with carbamazepine or amitriptyline.

Leprosy

Although uncommon in the United States, leprosy, or Hansen's disease, remains a frequent cause of treatable peripheral neuropathy throughout much of the world. Always consider leprosy whenever a patient from an endemic area presents with a peripheral neuropathy. As leprosy and its attendant skin lesions progress, increasing anesthesia with the potential for breakdown and injury occurs in the lesion.

Diphtheria

Virtually unheard of today, patients with diphtheria often experience a profound ascending sensorimotor polyneuropathy, similar to acute inflammatory demyelinating polyradiculoneuropathy, beginning some weeks after the initial illness. Classically, prominent cranial nerve involvement often occurred.

Acute Inflammatory Demyelinating Polyradiculoneuropathy (Guillain-Barré Syndrome)

Acute inflammatory demyelinating polyradiculopathy (AIDP), or GBS (also known as acute inflammatory polyneuritis or postinfectious polyneuritis), is a syndrome of symmetric, rapidly progressive, ascending muscle weakness with decreased or absent tendon stretch reflexes; it is an uncommon sequel to several common infections. *Campylobacter jejuni* gastroenteritis is most frequently the antecedent infection; various viral illnesses may also trigger GBS. Serologic testing and measurement of antiganglioside antibodies are not clinically useful. All patients should be hospitalized to carefully monitor respiratory status and ability to handle secretions, for neurologic consultation and electromyographic testing, and to initiate either plasma exchange or intravenous immunoglobulin therapy. While more rapid progression of muscle weakness or evidence of axonal involvement is worrisome, making intubation and respiratory support more likely, the overall prognosis is excellent, with most patients making a full recovery.[16]

Chronic Inflammatory Demyelinating Polyradiculoneuropathy

Chronic inflammatory demyelinating polyradiculoneuropathy (CIDP) is a relatively common neuropathy that is often unrecognized. Clinical and electrophysiologic diagnostic criteria have been established, allowing clinicians to distinguish CIDP from other acquired neuropathies. The usual clinical picture is of a slowly progressive, symmetric motor neuropathy involving both proximal and distal muscles. Sensory symptoms may also be seen. It is important to distinguish CIDP from the hereditary neuropathies as effective therapies are available for CIDP. Prednisone remains an effective, economic, first-line therapy; plasma exchange and intravenous immunoglobulin are also used in more seriously affected patients.[16]

Metabolic Neuropathies

Diabetic Neuropathy

Diabetic neuropathy is the most common polyneuropathy encountered by family physicians. Some form of neuropathy develops in approximately half of all diabetics, although it is most often mild (see Chapter 120). Although neuropathy may occasionally be the presenting feature of diabetes, generally neuropathy is related to increasing duration and severity of the disease.[17] Early recognition of diabetic neuropathy may decrease the incidence of lower extremity complications.[18,19]

Unlike other neuropathies, diabetic neuropathies encompass nearly the full spectrum of peripheral nerve disorders. Most commonly, diabetic patients experience distal, symmetric polyneuropathy with predominantly sensory involvement and mild motor signs. The pain and dysesthesias, particularly of the soles of the feet, may be experienced as severe burning discomfort. Involvement of large myelinated sensory fibers may cause decreased joint position sense, leading to both sensory ataxia and secondary arthropathy (Charcot joints).

Diabetic patients have a much higher frequency of compression and entrapment mononeuropathies than do nondiabetics. Diabetic amyotrophy is a multiple mononeuropathy involving the lumbosacral plexus or motor fibers of the lower extremity; usually preceded by profound weight loss, it may evolve over a period of a few days. Typically, a deep, burning back pain spreads rapidly to the thigh, progressing to significant proximal muscle weakness, which is often bilateral. While the disability may be severe, most patients slowly recover over 6–24 months. More common in diabetics with peripheral vascular disease, diabetic amyotrophy has been thought to be due to small infarcts of proximal nerve trunks;

newer evidence also suggests an inflammatory or immune-mediated etiology.

Some diabetic patients have purely autonomic signs and symptoms. Postural hypotension is most common, but gastrointestinal (diabetic gastroparesis, intestinal hypomotility and constipation, diarrhea) and genitourinary (impotence, atonic bladder) symptoms may also occur. Loss of small pain fibers in the cardiac sympathetic system permits the silent myocardial infarction that is so common in diabetics.

Optimal glycemic control is key for both prevention and treatment. For pain control, tricyclic antidepressants, especially small doses of amitriptyline, 25 to 150 mg at bedtime, may be helpful. Either desipramine or nortriptyline, 75 to 150 mg daily, may be a useful alternative in patients unable to tolerate amitriptyline. Selective serotonin reuptake inhibitors do not offer clear-cut advantages over tricyclics, although they may improve the sleep disturbance, depression, and anxiety that often accompany chronic pain.[20,21] Gabapentin, 300 to 1200 mg three times daily,[22] carbamazepine, or phenytoin may also be used. Mild opioid analgesics, used judiciously, may be helpful. Topical capsaicin 0.075% applied qid may help relieve the pain of diabetic neuropathy. Preliminary studies of exogenously administered recombinant human nerve growth factor have shown some promise for alleviating painful diabetic and HIV-associated polyneuropathy, but larger trials have not confirmed this benefit.[23]

Uremic Neuropathy

Chronic renal failure may cause painful burning paresthesias of the feet (see Chapter 97). Many of these patients have underlying diabetes; it is often difficult to determine whether given symptoms are purely uremic or are caused by a diabetic neuropathy. Uremic neuropathy may respond to proper diet and vitamin supplementation. A more severe distal sensorimotor polyneuropathy associated with more profound renal failure is not diet-dependent. Hemodialysis does not help, but renal transplantation usually rapidly reverses the symptoms of true uremic neuropathy.[24]

Nutritional Neuropathies

The nutritional neuropathies are all related to deficiencies of B vitamins, or rarely, vitamin E. These generally occur in combination with one another, primarily in chronic alcoholics. Patients with anorexia or bulimia, food faddists, or patients with malabsorption may also experience vitamin B deficiencies. The common clinical picture of all the nutritional neuropathies is one of a typical symmetric distal polyneuropathy, with intense burning pain of the soles of the feet.

Alcoholic Neuropathy

The polyneuropathy related to chronic alcoholism is clinically indistinguishable from that due to vitamin deficiencies. Alcohol causes deficiencies by replacing more nutritious foods in the diet, by increasing the requirements for B vitamins (which are needed for its metabolism), and perhaps by impairing vitamin absorption. Alcohol may also have a direct toxic effect on peripheral nerves; in a few patients a neuropathy occurs despite an adequate diet. The prognosis for ultimate, but slow, recovery is good for patients who are able to stop drinking and resume a proper diet with multivitamin supplements (see Chapter 59).

Vitamin B₁ (Thiamine) Deficiency

Thiamine deficiency, or beriberi, is most often seen in chronic alcoholics. Wernicke-Korsakoff encephalopathy often occurs in association with a distal polyneuropathy. Both entities are treated with intramuscular injection of thiamine, 100 mg every 12 hours, followed by 100 mg daily by mouth.

Vitamin B₆ (Pyridoxine) Deficiency

Certain drugs, notably isoniazid and dapsone, interfere with pyridoxine metabolism and may also produce peripheral neuropathies. Inasmuch as these drugs are used to treat leprosy, which itself causes a sensory neuropathy, the clinical picture is potentially confusing. Pyridoxine supplements, 50 mg three times a day, may prevent this complication; however, excessive amounts of pyridoxine (more than 2 g daily) may also cause a severe sensory neuropathy.[25]

Vitamin B₁₂ Deficiency

Vitamin B_{12} deficiency may present initially with vague paresthesias without objective signs. Because hematologic abnormalities may not be apparent until the neurologic complications have become irreversible, it is important to measure serum B_{12} levels in patients being evaluated for distal polyneuropathies.

Hereditary Neuropathies

Hereditary neuropathies are relatively common and underdiagnosed. Because of the slowly progressive, indolent course of these disorders, many patients do not recall other family members being affected, and in some cases they do not even recognize the abnormalities in themselves. The hereditary neuropathies are typically associated with footdrop, high-arched feet (pes cavus), hammer toe deformities, slowly progressive weakness and wasting of peroneal muscle groups, and a high-stepping, slapping gait. Sensory symptoms are much less prominent.

The genetics and pathophysiology of numerous hereditary neuropathies have been elucidated; however, just two types of hereditary motor and sensory neuropathies (HMSN I, HMSN II) represent virtually all forms of this disorder. HMSN I, a demyelinating process with onset during the teenage years, constitutes roughly 10% of the hereditary neuropathies. Nearly all other hereditary neuropathies are HMSN II (formerly called Charcot-Marie-Tooth or peroneal muscle atrophy), a primarily axonal degeneration with secondary demyelination that occurs during the fourth decade of life or later. Specific genetic tests are now available to confirm the diagnosis of many of the hereditary neuropathies.

There is no specific treatment for any of these disorders; genetic counseling, education, and reassurance are often all that is required. The ultimate prognosis is fairly good with a manageable degree of disability. If there is any question about the family history, consider the possibility of CIDP; unlike the hereditary neuropathies, CIDP can be effectively treated.

Toxic Neuropathies

Toxic neuropathies develop over several weeks to months as a result of continued exposure to various drugs, industrial toxins, or heavy metals. A progressive, symmetric, ascending polyneuropathy is most frequently seen with occupational exposures. The most commonly implicated drugs include anticancer agents, particularly cisplatin and *Vinca* alkaloids, antiretroviral drugs (didanosine, zalcitabine, stavudine), as well as isoniazid, dapsone, and amiodarone. Rare cases of arsenic poisoning, either intentional or from insecticide exposure, may cause a delayed-onset progressive polyneuropathy. Chronic lead exposure causes a predominantly motor neuropathy, typically beginning in the upper limbs, with asymmetric radial neuropathy and wrist-drop. A careful review of potential occupational exposures is the key to diagnosis of neuropathy caused by heavy metals and industrial toxins.

The development of a neuropathy is directly related to continued exposure to a particular toxin. The patient with toxic neuropathy often slowly improves when the exposure is discontinued, if not immediately then within several weeks; a neuropathy that continues to progress must be due to some other cause. This has important medicolegal implications for neuropathies that are thought or claimed to be occupationally related.

Vascular Neuropathies

The axon is particularly vulnerable to microinfarction and ischemia. Most vascular neuropathies are caused by diabetes; neuropathies caused by the arteritis of various connective tissue disorders are rare. In patients with rheumatoid arthritis, vasculitic lesions occur far less frequently than do compression and entrapment mononeuropathies. Periarteritis nodosa may cause a multiple mononeuropathy due to vasculitis; an asymmetric sensorimotor polyneuropathy has also been described. Systemic lupus erythematosus can cause cranial neuropathies and multiple mononeuropathies thought to be due to immune complex deposition in nerve fibers; a distal sensorimotor polyneuropathy is less well understood.

Malignancy-Associated Neuropathies

Most peripheral neuropathies associated with malignancy are the result of direct compression by solid tumors or leukemic infiltration. Many drugs used to treat cancer are notable for their neurotoxicity, particularly the *Vinca* alkaloids and cisplatin. Peripheral nerves may also be damaged by radiation therapy; the brachial and lumbosacral plexi are most often affected.

Occasionally, patients with distant, often occult malignancy present with one of the paraneoplastic neurologic syndromes. Although most often involving the CNS, carcinomatous peripheral neuropathies may also occur; they are predominantly associated with small-cell carcinoma of the lung. These syndromes may precede detection of the cancer by several months or even years; their recognition justifies a careful search for occult malignancy.[26]

Dysproteinemic Neuropathies

All patients presenting with peripheral neuropathies of unknown etiology should be screened for monoclonal proteins, using immunoelectrophoresis (IEP) or immunofixation electrophoresis (IFE); serum protein electrophoresis (SPEP) is not as sensitive. Monoclonal gammopathy of undetermined significance (MGUS) is the most common of the dysproteinemias, but myeloma, amyloidosis, cryoglobulinemia, lymphoma, and leukemia must be ruled out.[26]

References

1. Dyck PJ. The causes, classification, and treatment of peripheral neuropathy. N Engl J Med 1982;307:283–5.
2. Poncelet AN. An algorithm for the evaluation of peripheral neuropathy. Am Fam Physician 1998;57:755–64.
3. McKnight JT, Adcock BB. Paresthesias: a practical diagnostic approach. Am Fam Physician 1997;56:2253–64.
4. Barohn RJ. Approach to peripheral neuropathy and neuronopathy. Semin Neurol 1998;18:7–18.
5. Kissel JT. Autoantibody testing in the evaluation of peripheral neuropathy. Semin Neurol 1998;18:83–94.
6. Keane JR. Bilateral seventh nerve palsy: analysis of 43 cases and review of the literature. Neurology 1994;44:1198–202.
7. Spinner RJ, Bachman JW, Amadio PC. The many faces of carpal tunnel syndrome. Mayo Clin Proc 1989;64:829–36.
8. Stevens JC, Beard CM, O'Fallon WM, Kurland LT. Conditions associated with carpal tunnel syndrome. Mayo Clin Proc 1992;67:541–8.
9. Clarke Stevens J, Witt JC, Smith BE, et al. The frequency of carpal tunnel syndrome in computer users at a medical facility. Neurology 2001;56:1568–70.
10. Padua L, Padua R, Aprile I, et al. Multiperspective follow-up of untreated carpal tunnel syndrome: a multicenter study. Neurology 2001;56:1459–66.
11. Beutner KR, Friedman DJ, Forszpaniak C, et al. Valacyclovir compared with acyclovir for improved therapy for herpes zoster in immunocompetent adults. Antimicrob Agents Chemother 1995;39:1546–53.
12. Rowbotham M, Harden N, Stacey B, et al. Gabapentin for the treatment of postherpetic neuralgia: a randomized controlled trial. JAMA 1998;280:1837–42.
13. Stankus SJ, Dlugopolski M, Packer D, et al. Management of herpes zoster (shingles) and postherpetic neuralgia. Am Fam Physician 2000;61:2437–44,2447–8.
14. Finkel MJ. Lyme disease and its neurologic complications. Arch Neurol 1988;45:99.
15. Lange DJ, Britton CB, Younger DS, Hays AP. The neuromuscular manifestations of human immunodeficiency virus infections. Arch Neurol 1988;45:1084–8.
16. Barohn RJ, Saperstein DS. Guillain-Barré syndrome and chronic inflammatory demyelinating polyneuropathy. Semin Neurol 1998;18:49–62.
17. Younger DS, Rosoklija G, Hays AP. Diabetic peripheral neuropathy. Semin Neurol 1998;18:95–104.
18. DCCT Research Group. The effect of intensive treatment of diabetes on the development and progression of long-term complications in insulin-dependent diabetes mellitus. N Engl J Med 1993;329:977–86.
19. Smieja M, Hunt DL, Edelman D, et al. Clinical examination for the detection of protective sensation in the feet of diabetic patients. J Gen Intern Med 1999;14:418–24.
20. Marcus DA. Treatment of nonmalignant chronic pain. Am Fam Physician 2000;61:1331–8,1345–6.
21. McQuay HJ, Tramer M, Nye BA, et al. A systematic review of antidepressants in neuropathic pain. Pain 1996;68:217–27.
22. Backonja M, Beydoun A, Edwards KR, et al. Gabapentin for the symptomatic treatment of painful neuropathy in patients with diabetes mellitus: a randomized controlled trial. JAMA 1998;280:1831–6.
23. Apfel SC, Schwartz S, Adornato BT, et al. Efficacy and safety of recombinant human nerve growth factor in patients with diabetic polyneuropathy: a randomized controlled trial. JAMA 2000;284:2215–21.
24. Fraser CL, Arieff AI. Nervous system complications in uremia. Ann Intern Med 1988;109:143–53.
25. Schaumburg H, Kaplan J, Windebank A, et al. Sensory neuropathy from pyridoxine abuse: a new megavitamin syndrome. N Engl J Med 1983;309:445–8.
26. Amato AA, Collins MP. Neuropathies associated with malignancy. Semin Neurol 1998;18:125–44.

68
Selected Disorders of the Nervous System

G. Anne Cather and Anthony D. Marcucci

Meningitis

Presentation

Meningitis results from the entry of microorganisms into the subarachnoid space with inflammation of the pia and arachnoid layers and adjacent structures. In older children and adults the clinical presentation includes most frequently headache (usually severe), fever, irritability, nuchal rigidity, and pain, and some degree of impaired consciousness. Generalized seizures may occur, and photophobia and eye pain are common complaints. The onset can be acute.

Examination may reveal knee and hip flexion in response to flexion of the neck (Brudzinski sign) or difficulty completely extending the legs (Kernig sign), but these signs may be subtle or absent and should not be relied on for the diagnosis. Acute bacterial meningitis in infants presents initially with nonspecific signs (fever, lethargy, emesis, seizures, fontanel bulging) and later with meningeal signs. The elderly may manifest only fever, lethargy, and confusion. The presence of shaking chills, peripheral leukocytosis, and profound alteration of mental status suggests a bacterial, rather than viral, etiology. Viral meningitis is generally a less severe illness than bacterial meningitis.

Diagnosis
History

A history from available sources can be invaluable in ascertaining whether there are complicating factors such as previous episodes, suspicion of neoplasm, recent trauma, exposure to parasites, venereal disease, immunization history, a neurosurgical procedure, immunosuppression, or known infectious illness. The acute onset of headache requires consideration of subarachnoid hemorrhage.

Physical Findings

Signs of meningeal irritation may be lacking. Careful neurologic examination is required to rule out involvement of deeper brain structures, suggesting encephalitis or mass lesion (tumor, hemorrhage, abscess). Neuroimaging prior to lumbar puncture (LP) is indicated for any focal neurologic finding or papilledema to avoid disastrous herniation.

Cerebrospinal Fluid Examination

Assessment of the cerebrospinal fluid (CSF) should not be delayed, as morbidity and mortality are increased in cases of acute purulent meningitis with diagnosis delay. After computed tomography (CT) or magnetic resonance imaging (MRI) has ruled out a mass in situations involving focal findings (or immediately otherwise), LP should be undertaken. LP is contraindicated in the presence of anticoagulation or other bleeding diatheses, suppurative soft tissue lesions over the lower back, or unevaluated papilledema. Opening pressure is measured in the lateral decubitus position and is normally less than 180 mm H_2O. Four tubes of CSF (several milliliters per tube) are needed for requisite studies that include cell count with differential, protein and glucose levels, Gram stain, and culture. Traditionally tubes 1 and 4 are for cell count (tube 4 is also for cultures); tube 2 is for protein and glucose; and tube 3 is held for specific tests as indicated [bacterial or viral antigen, cryptococcal antigen, polymerase chain reaction (PCR), DNA studies for herpes simplex virus (HSV)]. Normal values are readily obtained from standard references and can be affected with immunocompromised states, hyperglycemia, and prior administration of antibiotics. Additional LPs may be performed later to judge efficacy of therapy.

Blood Tests

Systemic laboratory evaluation should be done immediately, and includes complete blood count (CBC) with differential, electrolytes and glucose assays, and cultures of blood and any other suspected infectious source. Check serum osmolality for the syndrome of inappropriate antidiuretic hormone from central nervous system (CNS) infection.

Course and Prognosis

Bacterial meningitis is usually fatal if not treated. There remains significant mortality, despite treatment, of approximately 5% in cases of *Haemophilus influenzae* and meningococcal meningitis, and 15% to 30% in cases of meningitis due to pneumococcus.[1] Neonatal mortality ranges up to 75%. The prognosis is worse with concomitant disease, delayed treatment, or depressed level of consciousness. Neurologic complications can include hearing loss, seizures, behavioral changes, cognitive impairment, and motor dysfunction. Serious neurologic sequelae occur in at least half of neonates with bacterial meningitis, and residual deficits have been reported in children and adults at varying rates according to the organism.[1] Conversely, viral meningitis is self-limiting, and symptomatic treatment is sufficient in uncomplicated cases. Complete resolution is usual, although malaise and myalgia may persist for weeks.

Treatment

Information about age, coexisting conditions [diabetes, acquired immunodeficiency syndrome (AIDS), alcoholism, prior neurosurgical procedures], and situational circumstances (exposure to ticks, rodents, pigeons) helps narrow down the likely causative agents in acute bacterial meningitis. Antibiotic treatment is begun immediately after cultures are obtained because of potential dire consequences of delayed treatment. Reasonable empiric treatment of pyogenic meningitis in adults consists of ceftriaxone 2 g IV q12h with the addition of vancomycin or rifampin when penicillin resistance is suspected. Steroid usage may be controversial, but is often recommended. In immunocompromised patients, use vancomycin 2–3 g IV divided q6–12h plus ampicillin 2 g IV q4h and ceftazidime 2 g q8h.[1] In a case of uncomplicated viral meningitis with no focal findings and no concomitant conditions, it is often not possible, nor always necessary, to establish the specific agent. Enteroviruses are responsible in the bulk of the cases. Treatment is symptomatic.

Special Considerations

Chronic Meningitis

Meningitis with an insidious symptomatology onset warrants consideration of other organisms. CNS fungal infections are usually opportunistic, and include cryptococcosis, candidiasis, coccidiomycosis, aspergillosis, and mucormycosis. Amphotericin B has variable success in treating these conditions.

Two spirochetal diseases can present as acute meningitis but usually a more chronic nature. *Borrelia burgdorferi* causes the second stage of Lyme disease and *Treponema pallidum* causes syphilitic meningitis.

Tuberculous meningitis does not often present acutely. Cranial nerve involvement and elevated intracranial pressure (ICP) are seen with wide intracranial dispersion of tubercles. The course and treatment with antitubercular agents is usually prolonged. Suspicion of rickettsial meningitis is raised by an appropriate history of travel to an endemic area and skin rash. Serologic testing confirms the diagnosis. Doxycycline is the treatment of choice. Amebic meningoencephalitis can be fulminant in presentation. *Naegleria fowleri* lives in warm, stagnant water, and a history of playing or swimming in farm ponds or similar bodies of water is frequently noted. This condition is generally fatal, with treatment with amphotericin B having limited success.

Cerebral involvement by parasites should be suspected in the context of opportunity for exposure, as in acquired toxoplasmosis, trichinosis, cysticercosis, schistosomiasis, and trypanosomiasis. Neuroimaging can be useful for the diagnosis and for assessing treatment efficacy. Cerebral malaria (*Plasmodium falciparum*) is rapidly fatal if untreated and should be suspected in endemic areas.[2]

Recurrent Meningitis

Recurrent bouts of meningitis should first raise suspicion of a fistula or other congenital defect and a parameningeal focus of infection. Incomplete treatment of CNS infections and immunocompromised states are obvious substrates for recurrence of symptoms. Several noninfectious forms of meningitis discussed below can also present recurrently.

Noninfectious Meningitis

Intermittent leakage of fluid from an intracranial cyst or craniopharyngioma can cause aseptic chemical meningitis. Carcinomatous meningitis can be difficult to confirm, requiring multiple LPs or cisternal taps for recovery of diagnostic cells from the CSF. Autoimmune and collagen vascular diseases can mimic CNS infections. The differential for acute or chronic meningitis includes sarcoidosis, Behçet's disease, systemic lupus erythematosis, and granulomatosus angiitis.[3] Drug-induced causes of sterile meningitis include nonsteroidal antiinflammatory medications and some antibiotics (penicillin, cephalosporins, ciprofloxacin, sulfonamides).[3]

Encephalitis

Presentation

Encephalitis refers to parenchymal inflammation of the CNS (i.e., involvement of the brain itself). Viruses are the primary cause of encephalitis worldwide, although bacteria, fungi, parasites, and noninfectious processes can also be responsible. The clinical syndrome of acute encephalitis consists of a febrile illness with meningeal signs and symptoms as well as evidence of involvement of some part of the brain. The latter may manifest as seizures, impaired level of consciousness, corticospinal tract signs (hemiparesis, deep tendon reflex asymmetry, or Babinski signs), facial weakness, eye movement disturbances, nystagmus, myoclonus, confusion, or any other indication of central involvement. A few of the etiologic entities have distinctive clinical features: frontotemporal signs and symptoms with HSV; psychomotor excitation with bulbar dysfunction and spasm with rabies; or subacute personality changes and dementia with myoclonus in Creutzfeldt-Jakob disease. Other entities having a long latency period after exposure to viral or viral-like particles include subacute sclerosing panencephalitis after measles, late progressive panencephalitis associated with congenital rubella, and the AIDS-dementia complex. Progressive multifocal leukoencephalopathy (PML) evolves in association with chronic neoplastic disease, and paraneoplastic syndromes are associated with intracranial inflammatory changes. Of patients with HSV encephalitis, two thirds occur as a result of reactivation of a latent infection of the trigeminal ganglion, while the remainder is a result of a primary infection. HSV-1 accounts for the majority of the HSV encephalitis cases.[4]

Diagnosis

History

Epidemiologic clues may help identify the etiology of a case of viral encephalitis. Distinctive geographic location and seasonal occurrence is characteristic of the equine and some other viral encephalitides. Association with systemic illnesses can point to specific agents: infectious mononucleosis, chickenpox, mumps, AIDS, *Legionella* species pneumonia, *Mycoplasma* pneumonia, *Listeria* infections, rickettsial diseases, malaria or other protozoal illness, helminth infestation, immunocompromised states with opportunistic infections, and various neoplastic processes

Laboratory Studies

The CSF examination generally shows a lymphocytic pleocytosis with normal glucose and modest elevation of protein. Hemorrhagic processes (as with HSV, *Naegleria*) may yield red blood cells. Recovery of the etiologic agent from CSF is usually difficult or impossible, and serologic testing can be helpful in cases of suspected rickettsia, Lyme disease, syphilis, or HIV. Neuroimaging findings have been characterized for encephalitides of various etiologies.[5] MRI has proved generally more sensitive than CT. Neuroimaging should be done prior to LP to rule out space-occupying lesions and other etiologies of focal neurologic findings. Electroencephalography (EEG) can help localize and confirm cerebral dysfunction. Brain biopsy is rarely indicated.

Characteristic neuroimaging, EEG, and CSF findings help make the diagnosis of HSV. Typically, HSV results in an MRI with medial and temporal lobe lesions, often hemorrhagic, while the EEG shows sharp and slow complexes. PCR-DNA is highly sensitive and specific in detecting HSV in CSF, and has replaced brain biopsy except in rare cases. CSF cultures are usually negative.

Course and Prognosis

Mortality rates among some cases of viral encephalitis are high: varicella 10%, measles 15%, HSV 30%, eastern equine 70%, and rabies and HIV essentially 100%.[2] Residual neuro-logic and neuropsychiatric deficits may occur. Morbidity and mortality from nonviral etiologies depend on associated concomitant factors.

Treatment

Viral Etiologies

Supportive care is important. With the exception of HSV, treatment for viral encephalitis is symptomatic. Maintain appropriate hydration and watch for cerebral edema. Anticonvulsants may be necessary for recurrent seizures. There is no consensus on using steroids in severe cases. HSV encephalitis can be rapidly fatal, and if recovery does occur severe disability can remain. Therefore, urgent treatment with acyclovir 10 mg/kg (500 mg/m^2 for children <12 years) IV infused over 1 hour q8h for 14 to 21 days is recommended.[6] This treatment is undertaken for suspected cases as soon as the initial data have been collected, without waiting for confirmatory results.

Other Etiologies

Guidelines are available for specific therapeutics for several nonviral encephalitides (toxoplasmosis, malaria, cysticercosis, rickettsial fevers, Lyme disease, tuberculosis).[7]

Special Considerations

Immunocompromised Patients

Immunosuppressed patients (organ transplant, chronic illness, AIDS) may develop encephalitis caused by varicella, HSV-1, Epstein-Barr virus, human herpesvirus 6, cytomegalovirus, measles, or enterovirus.[4]

Rabies

There remains no effective treatment for rabies, so aggressive pursuit of the appropriate protocol for possible exposure is mandatory for patient survival. If the status of the animal cannot be established, treatment with rabies vaccine and, if not previously vaccinated, human rabies immune globulin is needed (see Chapter 47).

Brain Abscess

Presentation

Bacteria invade brain parenchyma by means of direct introduction (trauma or surgery), extension from a contiguous suppurative area (paranasal sinus, mastoid, middle ear), or hematogenous spread. An area of damaged brain tissue, albeit microscopic, is required to establish a nidus of infection. Thrombophlebitis or emboli can play a role in creating small areas of infarction. A localized cerebritis develops and becomes necrotic and encapsulated within a few weeks. Presenting features commonly include headache, seizures, obtundation, and focal neurologic signs. Focal findings point to the involved brain area. There may be signs of ICP. Initial fever can resolve with encapsulation of the abscess. The overall development of symptoms may be indolent or relatively rapid. Rupture of an abscess can cause purulent meningitis and formation of daughter abscesses.

Diagnosis

Systemic signs of infection are not always apparent, but an aggressive search for an infectious cause is indicated. Look for sources of local spread (ear or sinus disease, face and skull trauma or surgical procedures, or dental or periodontal infection) and metastatic (hematogenous) origin. The latter commonly occurs with chronic pulmonary infection or congenital heart disease. Differentiation from other space-occupying lesions (tumors), stroke, congenital anomaly, meningoencephalitis, and seizures is required.

Laboratory Studies

Blood and local cultures, CBC, and chest radiographs may or may not be useful but should be done in suspected brain abscess cases. Urgent neuroimaging is indicated prior to LP. Plain head CT is useful, although use of contrast CT or MRI yields more details about edema and inflammation. Imaging can help elucidate infection in contiguous areas.

Aspiration

Surgical aspiration of abscess contents is accomplished stereotactically under CT guidance. This aids specific bacteriologic diagnosis and reduction of increased ICP.

Course and Prognosis

Delay in diagnosis can result in increased morbidity and mortality. Mortality estimates have ranged up to 40% in the past, with poor prognosis associated with extreme age, markedly altered sensorium, size of abscess, acute presentation, metastatic abscesses, cerebellar or deep structure involvement, anaerobic etiology, rupture, and concomitant pulmonary infection.[8] CT scan and MRI have markedly lowered mortality, with MRI the preferred imaging method to detect abscess.[5]

Treatment

Adjunctive Therapy

Successful treatment of a brain abscess usually involves both surgical drainage and prolonged antimicrobial therapy. Early lesions (cerebritis) may respond to antibiotics alone. Increased ICP may need urgent attention (elevation of the head, hyperventilation, fluid restriction, and mannitol) in an intensive care setting. Some recommend seizure prophylaxis. Corticosteroids are not universally recommended.

Specific Therapy

Neurosurgical consultation for aspiration or drainage of a developed abscess is required to relieve pressure symptoms and to isolate the causative organism. If identification of the organism is delayed, empiric antimicrobial treatment strategies based on associated conditions have been suggested.[7,9] High-dose intravenous penicillin with metronidazole is a reasonable initial empiric treatment. Cefotaxime and vancomycin have excellent CNS penetration and should be considered in combination with metronidazole if resistance is suspected.[10] Antibiotics are typically given for weeks with treatment length determined by clinical and radiographic improvement.

Neurosyphilis

Presentation and Course

Syphilis, sometimes known as the "great imitator" due to varied signs and symptoms, is obtained through sexual contact with the spirochete, *T. pallidum* (also see Chapter 41). Neurologic symptoms can occur in the secondary and tertiary phases. Tertiary syphilis is marked by neurologic, cardiovascular (aortitis, aortic aneurysm, aortic regurgitation), dermatologic (gummas), or orthopedic (Charcot's joints) complications if untreated and occurs 2 to 20 years after the initial infection. Earlier presentations (weeks to years after infection) include acute syphilitic meningitis and cerebro- and meningovascular syphilis. Later presentations (years or decades) can include dementia, general paresis, and myeloneuropathy (tabes dorsalis). Neurosyphilis can be initially asymptomatic, although active meningeal inflammation eventually occurs and CSF findings are abnormal.

Acute syphilitic meningitis develops within the first few years of infection. Symptoms are consistent with an aseptic meningitis or meningovasculitis. Headache, meningismus, ocular symptoms (diplopia, decreased vision), otic symptoms (tinnitus, vertigo), and cranial neuropathies are common.[11]

Cerebrovascular syphilis (stroke) tends to occur acutely after a variable latency of months to years, whereas meningovascular syphilis symptoms are more insidious in onset. Most strokes occur in the area referable to the middle cerebral artery.[12] Meningovascular symptoms include headache, vertigo, insomnia, or psychiatric disturbances. The CSF is always abnormal.

Dementia paralytica or general paresis is a frontotemporal encephalitis occurring years after the primary infection. Initial symptoms are similar to those of other dementias until intellectual function declines and prominent psychiatric symptoms appear. Coarse intention tremors and loss of facial and limb muscle tone cause relaxed or expressionless facies. This condition is fatal if untreated.

Myeloneuropathy (tabes dorsalis) is a triad of symptoms (lightning pains, dysuria, ataxia) and a triad of signs (Argyll Robertson pupils, areflexia, loss of proprioception).[13] Other symptoms include visceral crises, optic atrophy, ocular palsy, and Charcot's joints. A progressive ataxia with a wide-based gait and Romberg sign develops.

Diagnosis

Neurosyphilis is diagnosed based on combinations of reactive serologic tests, abnormal CSF, or a reactive Venereal Disease Research Laboratory (VDRL)-CSF with or without symptoms. No single test can be used for diagnosis. There are two serologic test types: nontreponemal tests [VDRL or rapid plasma reagin (RPR)] and treponemal antibody tests [fluorescent treponemal antibody absorption (FTA-ABS) and microhemagglutination assay for antibody to *T. pallidum* (MHA-TP)]. The VDRL-CSF is the standard test for CSF and, when reactive without bloody contamination, is considered diagnostic of neurosyphilis. Some recommend obtaining an FTA-ABS on the CSF since it is highly sensitive, and a negative result would exclude neurosyphilis in a patient with a false-negative VDRL-CSF.[14]

Invasion of the CNS by *T. pallidum* with mild CSF lymphocytic pleocytosis and elevated protein is common among adults with primary or secondary syphilis. Few patients develop neurosyphilis after appropriate treatment. LP is not recommended during primary or secondary syphilis unless there are neurologic symptoms. Perform an LP in any patient with neurologic or ophthalmologic symptoms or who has evidence of active syphilis (aortitis, gumma, iritis), treatment failure, or HIV infection.

Treatment

Antimicrobial Agents

Parenteral penicillin G is the drug of choice for all stages of syphilis and is the only therapy with documented efficacy for neurosyphilis (or for syphilis during pregnancy).[14] Those with penicillin allergy should undergo desensitization and receive penicillin if possible. The recommended regimen is 18 to 24 million units aqueous crystalline penicillin G daily, given as 3 to 4 million units IV q4h for 10 to 14 days. Alternatively, compliant patients may receive a regimen of 2.4 million units of procaine penicillin IM daily plus probenecid 500 mg po qid, both for 10 to 14 days. Some recommend 2.4 million units of benzathine penicillin IM once a week for a total of 3 weeks after the treatment regimen noted.[14]

Follow-up and Response to Therapy

The VDRL-CSF and CSF protein and cell counts are used to follow response to therapy with an LP at 6 and 12 months. Complete normalization of the CSF indicates cure, but it may take place slowly. The VDRL titer falls but may remain positive for more than a year after treatment. If the cell count does not decrease or if it rises, re-treatment should be considered.[15] Relapses may occur up to 2 years after treatment. Persistent deficits and symptoms remain, especially impaired reflexes, abnormal pupillary responses, lightning pains, and sensory ataxia.

Special Considerations

Sexual partners of patients with syphilis should be appropriately evaluated (clinically and serologically) and treated. All pregnant patients should be tested for syphilis during early pregnancy, and those with neurosyphilis should be treated the same as nonpregnant patients. Any child thought to have congenital syphilis or who has neurologic involvement should be treated with aqueous crystalline penicillin G 200,000 to 300,000 units/kg/day IV (given as 50,000 units/kg q4–6h) for 10 days.[15] It is recommended that all patients with syphilis be tested for HIV due to increasing incidence of co-infection. Neurosyphilis should be considered in the differential diagnosis of any person with HIV and neurologic symptoms. The diagnosis of neu-

rosyphilis in a patient with syphilis and HIV can be challenging because serologic tests are positive but the CSF pleocytosis and elevated proteins can be due to either or both.

Brain Tumors

Presentation

There has been a steady increase in the number of primary brain tumors, rising over 25% in the past 20 years.[1,2] There were approximately 17,900 new cases of CNS tumor in 1996. The most common primary cancer types are malignant glioblastoma (>50%) and meningioma. Primary brain tumors are much more common in adults, although the CNS is a common site of childhood malignancy, second only to leukemia. Common primary brain tumors in adults are glioblastoma, meningioma, astrocytoma, and pituitary adenoma, and in children are medulloblastoma, astrocytoma, glioma, ependymoma, craniopharyngioma, and meningioma.

The metastatic tumors, spread hematogenously, account for the majority of adult CNS tumors. Approximately 20% to 40% of cancer patients develop brain metastases, as many as 170,000 new cases per year.[16] This frequency may be increasing due to longer cancer survival rates and better imaging detection. The most common sources are from lung, breast, and skin (melanoma). Malignant melanoma and choriocarcinoma have a predilection for the brain. Other common sources are prostate, kidney, gastrointestinal tract, leukemia, lymphoma, and cancers of the female genital tract. Metastatic distribution also follows the relative weight of and blood flow to an area—80% are to the cerebral hemispheres, 15% to the cerebellum, and 5% to the brainstem.[16] Skull tumors are often metastatic from breast, prostate, or skin. Brainstem metastases are uncommon. Metastases are usually symptomatic. Headache is the most common presenting complaint, and focal weakness is the second most common. Metastases have a poorer prognosis and nearly all untreated patients will die as a direct result of the brain tumor.

About 30% to 40% of adult brain tumors are benign,[17] and the rest are malignant. Tumors can have subtle signs and symptoms and be a challenge to manage due to issues of longer natural history, and maintaining quality of life after treatment. They typically have slow growth rates and are not invasive. The most common benign tumors are meningioma, pituitary adenoma, and vestibular schwannoma (acoustic neuroma). Others include pilocytic and cerebellar astrocytoma, epidermoid cyst, and craniopharyngioma.

Diagnosis

Symptoms and Signs

CNS neoplasm can present with a variety of symptoms from generalized or nonlocalizing to specific or focal. Tumor is often suspected after the development of acute or subacute focal symptoms. Many of the nonlocalizing symptoms are secondary to increased ICP or edema. The most common of these is headache, which can be variable, resembling migraine or muscle contraction headache, and is commonly ipsilateral to the tumor. With increased ICP, the headache may be bifrontal or bioccipital. Other generalized symptoms are seizures, most often seen in slow-growing tumors and in the frontal and parietal lobes; vomiting, which occurs with increased ICP and most consistently with posterior fossa tumors; and altered mental status.

Localizing symptoms and signs depend on the tumor location. Frontal lobe tumors may be silent or present with memory impairment and personality changes. Tumors in the pineal area, third ventricle, or other ventricular or aqueductal areas show signs of obstruction and hydrocephalus (headache, nausea, vomiting). Brainstem tumors often present with cranial nerve neuropathies or long track signs and hydrocephalus. Spinal cord tumors may present with localized back pain or radicular symptoms, sensory loss, ataxia, myelopathy, or sphincter complaints. Common signs include focal weakness or sensory deficits, speech difficulty, aphasia, ataxia, falls, and visual-field defects.

Radiologic Findings

Neuroimaging by either CT or MRI is preferred. Often tumors have characteristic presentations with these modalities. Glioblastoma multiforme and metastatic tumors (renal cell, melanoma, and choriocarcinoma) commonly show hemorrhage. Oligodendrogliomas and meningiomas often have calcifications. Metastatic tumors are often well demarcated and have a zone of surrounding edema. The location of the tumor as seen on MRI or CT can provide a differential diagnosis. Supratentorial hemispheric tumors include astrocytoma, glioblastoma, metastasis, meningioma, and lymphoma. Sellar/suprasellar area tumors are most likely pituitary adenoma, craniopharyngioma, or meningioma. Infratentorial midline tumors are likely medulloblastoma or ependymoma in children, or glioma, schwannoma, meningioma, or metastasis in adults. Cerebellar tumors are often astrocytoma in children and hemangioblastoma, astrocytoma, metastasis, or medulloblastoma in adults. Other helpful imaging modalities include skull x-rays, to evaluate bony metastasis; angiography, to define vascular anatomy; and myelography with CT, to diagnose spinal cord tumors and demonstrate spinal blockage.

Treatment

Treatment depends on the histopathologic type of tumor, the patients' age and general condition, and the tumor size, location, and sensitivity to the method chosen. Current options include surgery (complete excision versus debulking), radiation therapy, chemotherapy, or combinations of some or all of these. Because most malignant tumors have diffuse infiltration, surgery alone is not curative.[18] An acute compressive symptom from spinal cord tumors requires emergent surgery. Radiation therapy (RT) is often not sufficient to control most tumors and is limited by local tissue tolerance. Late CNS effects of RT raise concerns for necrosis, myelopathy, intellectual deterioration, endocrinopathies, and oncogenesis.

Transient worsening of symptoms can occur while receiving therapy. Newer therapies currently being evaluated include whole brain RT, brachytherapy (radioactive seed implants), and radiosurgery (high-dose, focal external beam).[19] Various regimens of chemotherapy are also being evaluated, after surgery and at varying times associated with RT. Future treatments being explored are interstitial chemotherapy, gene therapy, and chemotherapy after bone marrow transplant.

Special Considerations

Steroids

The routine initiation of steroids at the time of tumor diagnosis by imaging is being reconsidered. Although thought to reduce seizure risk and peritumor edema, there are no studies showing brain tumor patients are at increased risk of having seizures. Steroid complications can be concerning; they include hyperglycemia, myopathy, weight gain, insomnia, and predisposition to *Pneumocystis carinii* pneumonia. Additionally, steroics can be oncolytic, as in the case of primary CNS lymphoma (PCNSL), when their use can confound and delay diagnosis. In patients with signs and symptoms of increased ICP, steroids can markedly decrease neurologic symptoms often within 24 hours. Dexamethasone is preferred due to its CNS penetration and lack of mineralocorticoid activity.

Anticonvulsants

Anticonvulsants are often given prophylactically upon tumor diagnosis and before the patient has a seizure. Retrospective data suggest this is not protective and increases the risk for toxicity and poor compliance. Some suggest no anticonvulsants to be given except possibly in patients with metastases from melanomas since there is a high incidence of seizures.

Information Sites Web

The following Web sites offer information about brain cancer: *www.cancersource.com*, *www.cancernet.nci.nih.gov*, *www.cancerpage.com* and *www.abta.org*.

Multiple Sclerosis

Presentation

Multiple sclerosis (MS) is the most common disabling neurologic disease of young adults. The hallmarks of this condition are a variable frequency and duration of attacks and remissions and a variety of CNS symptoms. The initiating event or etiology of MS is unknown but is thought most likely to be due to a viral or viral-like infection, with an autoimmune response to CNS myelin causing the neurologic symptoms. The lesions are thought to be due to inflammation resulting in multifocal loss of myelin (plaque formation), primarily in the brain's white matter. There is a predilection for the optic nerves, periventricular white matter, brainstem, and spinal cord. The clinical manifestations of MS are diverse and the natural history is unpredictable. MS is most common in North America, Europe, Australia, and New Zealand (regions most frequently populated by northern Europeans), with an increasing risk for development in the northern latitudes. This geographic association correlates with the latitude at which the patient lived prior to age 15. There is a familial tendency, and women are twice as likely to be affected as men. Whites are more likely to develop MS than African Americans.

Diagnosis

History and Physical Examination

The diagnosis may be challenging since initial symptoms may not come to medical attention, and the latency period until recurrence may be years.[20,21] A single episode of neurologic symptoms is insufficient for diagnosis. Typical onset is between ages 20 and 40, with a peak incidence at 30.

The most common initial symptoms are weakness in one or more limbs, numbness, optic neuritis, unsteady gait, brainstem symptoms (diplopia, vertigo), and micturition disorders (frequency, urgency, incontinence). Most symptoms are focal. Fatigue is common. Other symptoms include visual acuity impairment, abnormal sensations, incoordination, tremor, mood disorders, spasticity, pain, internuclear ophthalmoplegia, nystagmus, ataxia, impotence, hearing loss, dementia, Lhermitte's sign (passive neck flexion induces an electric-like tingling down the back or anterior thighs), and Uhthoff's phenomenon (worsening of a sign or symptom with increased temperature or exercise).

A number of schemes outline the diagnostic criteria for MS. They have in common a history of remissions and relapses and an examination demonstrating more than one lesion in the CNS. Radiologic and laboratory data help secure the diagnosis. The differential diagnosis includes cerebrovascular disease, vasculitis, metastatic neoplasm, Lyme disease, PML, and primary CNS lymphoma.

Diagnostic Imaging

The imaging method of choice is MRI, and findings are specific. Typical lesions are proximal to the ventricles, infratentorial, and more than 6 mm in size.[22] False-positive results can occur, and a number of normal adults display typical white matter lesions.

Cerebrospinal Fluid

The CSF may reveal a mild pleocytosis, with normal to increased protein levels. Abnormal immunoglobulin G (IgG) oligoclonal bands are present in most patients with definite MS. They are present in other diseases (e.g., syphilis), but can be differentiated by examination.

Course and Prognosis

Multiple sclerosis often follows one of several courses. A relapsing and remitting course with discrete attacks (motor, sensory, cerebellar, or visual) over a several-week period and with resolution within 1 to 2 months occurs in 70% of initial cases. The interval between attacks varies from several months to years. Patients usually return to their baseline function. With time these patients frequently develop progression of their disease and do not return to baseline function. In the primary progressive MS course the patient's condition continually worsens with no periods of stability. If there is a superimposed acute attack or lapse, the term *relapsing pro-*

gressive is used. The so-called stable MS course shows no clinical disease activity over a 12-month period. Patients with mild disability do not have greatly shortened life span, but mortality is definitely increased. Older age at onset, frequency of attacks, incomplete recovery, male gender, and symptoms referable to multiple sites suggest poorer outcome. Death in MS patients typically occurs by one of four means: secondary complications (pneumonia, pulmonary embolism, decubitus infection); non–MS-related problems; suicide; or direct association with an MS attack.[21]

Treatment

General Management

Therapies for MS try to decrease the number and severity of relapses, improve the recovery from exacerbations, and prevent the development progression. Most work has been involved in stopping or reducing the destructive inflammatory damage. No single treatment has been found effective for all patients. Acute attacks are treated with short courses of corticosteroids, typically intravenous methylprednisolone, especially for a presentation of optic neuritis, which seems to respond fairly well. Mild sensory attacks are usually not treated. Although steroids accelerate the time to recovery from a relapse, they do not provide the long-term benefit.[22] Recombinant interferon-β, the first approved, effective treatment for relapsing-remitting MS, decreases the number of relapses and limits new disease activity.[23] Generally there has been a lack of benefit from immune enhancing therapies (azathioprine, cyclosporine, cyclophosphamide, methotrexate, plasma exchange, or immunoglobulin).[24] Promising therapies include the use of monoclonal antibodies (CD6, CD52) and vaccination with Copolymer 1.

Symptomatic Treatment

A number of treatments provide symptomatic relief but do not affect the disease or its progression. Fatigue, a common complaint, is treated with periodic rest, energy conservation, and amantadine. Disability should be addressed on the basis of mobility, bowel and bladder control, sexual function, mood, and mental changes. Walking aids and wheelchairs are to be used as needed. Spasticity, typically in the lower extremities, requires physical therapy and regular passive muscle stretching. Drugs are available to improve muscle spasticity, urinary retention, bladder spasticity, and constipation. Referral to an urologist may be necessary. A constant search for and treatment of urinary tract infections is important. Management of pain and cognitive and emotional dysfunction must also be addressed.

Other Therapy

There are no valid studies to support dietary manipulations, such as fat-free or gluten-free diets or linoleate supplements. Furthermore, there is no evidence to support the efficacy of hyperbaric oxygen or plasmapheresis.

Special Considerations

Support should be geared toward psychological, social, vocational, and marital issues. Depression, cognitive changes, and decreasing activities occur. Studies of depression report variable occurrence. The presence of cognitive deficits also varies, with up to half the patients having some degree of impairment. Most common are defects of recent memory, sustained attention, conceptual-abstract reasoning, and speed of information processing. Rehabilitation is important to make the most use of remaining functions. MS also has a large financial effect on the families. As disabilities increase, work limitations develop; 25% or fewer MS patients are able to maintain their employment throughout the disease course.[25] Stress can play a prominent role in the lives of the patients and their families and divorce is not uncommon. The family physician must serve as an important source of information, support, and hope to MS patients and their families. Reputable Web sites for more information include *www.ninds.nih.gov* and *www.nmss.org*.

References

1. Infections of the nervous system (bacterial, fungal, spirochetal, parasitic and sarcoid). In: Victor M, Ropper AH, eds. Principles of neurology, 7th ed. New York: McGraw-Hill, 2001;734.
2. DeMarcaida JA, Reik L. Disorders that mimic central nervous system infections. Neurol Clin 1999;17(4):901–41.
3. Falcone S, Post MJD. Encephalitis, cerebritis and brain abscess. Neuroimaging Clin North Am 2000;10(2):333–53.
4. Roos KL. Encephalitis. Neurol Clin 1999;17(4):813–33.
5. Anderson M. Management of cerebral infection. J Neurol Neurosurg Psychiatry 1993;56:1243–58.
6. Gilbert DN, Moellering RC, Sande MA, eds. The Sanford guide to antimicrobial therapy, 31st ed. Hyde Park: Antimicrobial Therapy, 2001.
7. Bartlett JG. Pocket book of infectious disease therapy. Philadelphia: Lippincott Williams & Wilkins, 2000.
8. Lerner AJ. The little black book of neurology, 3rd ed. St. Louis: Mosby-Year Book, 1995.
9. Brook I. Brain abscess in children: microbiology and management. J Child Neurol 1995;10:283–8.
10. Tunkel AR, Wispelwey B, Scheld WM. Brain abscess. In: Mandell GL, Bennett JE, Dolin R, eds. Principles and practice of infectious diseases, 5th ed. Philadelphia: Churchill Livingstone, 2000;1023.
11. Johnson PC, Farnie MA. Testing for syphilis. Dermatol Clin 1994;12(1):9–17.
12. Merritt HH. A textbook of neurology, 2nd ed. Philadelphia: Lea & Febiger, 1950.
13. Centers for Disease Control and Prevention. 1998 Guidelines for treatment of sexually transmitted diseases. MMWR 1998; 47(RR-1):28–49.
14. Birnbaum NR, Goldschmidt RH, Buffett WO. Resolving the common dilemmas of syphilis. Am Fam Physician 1999;59(8): 2233–40,2245–6.
15. Young WK, Janus T. Primary neurological tumors. In: Goetz CG, Pappert EJ, eds. Textbook of clinical neurology, 1st ed. Philadelphia: WB Saunders, 1999;933.
16. Patchell RA. Metastatic brain tumors. Neurol Clin 1995;13(4): 915–25.
17. Black FMcL. Benign brain tumors. Neurol Clin 1995;13(4): 927–51.
18. Conrad CA, Milosavljevic VP, Yung WK. Advances in chemotherapy for brain tumors. Neurol Clin 1995;13(4):795–812.
19. Shrieve DC, Loeffler JS. Advances in radiation therapy for brain tumors. Neurol Clin 1995;13(4):773–93.
20. Rolak LA. The diagnosis of multiple sclerosis. Neurol Clin 1996;14:27–43.
21. Weinshenker BG. The natural history of multiple sclerosis. Neurol Clin 1995;13(1):119–46.
22. Becker, CC, Gidal BE, Fleming JO. Immunotherapy in multiple sclerosis, Part 1. Am J Health Syst Pharm 1995;52:1985–2000.
23. Lublin FD, Whitaker JN, Eidelman BH, Miller AE, Arnason BGW, Burks JS. Management of patients receiving interferon beta-1b for multiple sclerosis. Neurology 1996;46:12–18.
24. Compston A. Treatment and management of multiple sclerosis. In: Compston A, Ebers G, Lassman H, McDonald I, Matthews B, Wekerle H, eds. McAlpine's multiple sclerosis, 3rd ed. New York: Churchill Livingstone, 1998;437.
25. Murray TJ. The psychological aspects of multiple sclerosis. Neurol Clin 1995;13:197–223.

69
The Red Eye

Dana W. Peterson

One of the most frequently encountered ocular complaints in the primary care setting is that of a red eye. Most often the cause presents minimal danger to vision, but it is important to be able to recognize serious, vision-threatening pathologic states. Usually the cause can be determined through a focused history and examination performed in the office with relatively few instruments (Table 69.1).

By far the most common cause of the red eye seen in practice is conjunctivitis. Conjunctivitis may have an infectious (bacterial, viral, chlamydial) or a noninfectious (allergic, irritant) etiology. Other, less common causes of the red eye include keratitis, episcleritis, scleritis, anterior uveitis, and acute angle-closure glaucoma.

Conjunctivitis

Bacterial Conjunctivitis

Bacterial conjunctivitis—infection restricted to the conjunctiva—is usually self-limited. In infants and children bacterial infection is the cause of conjunctivitis in approximately 65% of cases and is often associated with otitis media.[1] During the neonatal period, *Staphylococcus aureus, Haemophilus* spp., *Streptococcus pneumoniae*, enterococcus, *Pseudomonas aeruginosa*, and *Neisseria gonorrhoeae* are important pathogens.[2] In infants and children *H. influenzae* is the most common isolate followed by *S. pneumoniae* and *Moraxella catarrhalis*. The most common pathogens isolated from adult cases include *S. aureus*; *Staphylococcus epidermidis*; *Streptococcus, Haemophilus, Acinetobacter*, and *Corynebacterium* species; *S. pneumoniae*; *N. gonorrhoeae*; and *Proteus* or *Morganella morganii*.[3] Gram-negative organisms such as *Proteus, Klebsiella, P. aeruginosa, Moraxella*, and others are more common in immunocompromised patients, neonates, and the elderly.[4]

History

Typically, the presenting complaint is a red, irritated eye with a discharge. Symptoms are often insidious and begin unilaterally, but owing to autoinoculation they often involve both eyes within 2 days. A history of a hyperacute onset, severe inflammation, and discharge should alert the physician to the possibility of gonococcal infection. There is a burning, stinging, or gritty foreign body discomfort that is superficial and distinguished from deep eye pain. Frequently the patient complains that the eyelids are stuck together on waking owing to the discharge drying overnight. There may be visual blurring, as if a film is covering the eye.

Physical Examination

Visual acuity is unaffected. The superficial vessels of both the palpebral and bulbar conjunctiva are injected, giving the eye a redness that is commonly peripheral. A purulent-appearing discharge is present, and often there is crusting of the discharge on the lashes. There may be swelling of the eyelids and edema of the conjunctiva. The cornea appears clear and uninvolved, and the pupil size and reactivity to light is normal.

Laboratory Findings

Most often the history and clinical presentation of acute bacterial conjunctivitis are diagnostic, and cultures of the conjunctival discharge are not necessary. Gram stain and cultures are most useful in cases of suspected gonococcal infection, with infections of the neonate, or when the illness does not respond to appropriate therapy within 24 hours. A Giemsa stain of the discharge showing numerous polymorphonuclear cells may be helpful for differentiating bacterial conjunctivitis from viral or allergic conjunctivitis.

Management

Most cases of acute bacterial conjunctivitis are self-limited and resolve without therapy. Topical antimicrobial therapy is

Table 69.1. **Common Causes of the Red Eye**

Symptoms and signs	Conjunctivitis				Keratitis	Episcleritis	Scleritis	Anterior uveitis	Acute angle-closure glaucoma
	Bacterial	Viral	Chlamydial	Allergic					
Characteristics of eye pain	Superficial, burning gritty	Superficial, burning, gritty	Superficial, scratchy, burning chronic	Superficial, pruritic	Superficial, moderate to severe	Mild superficial scratching or pricking sensation	Severe, deep, periorbital	Moderate, deep, aching	Severe, deep
Photophobia	Absent	Occasional	Absent	Absent	Moderate to severe	Absent to mild	Mild to moderate	Moderate to severe	Mild to moderate
Visual acuity	Unaffected	Unaffected	Unaffected	Unaffected	Unaffected or decreased	Unaffected	Unaffected	Decreased	Decreased
Distribution of redness	Peripheral or diffuse conjunctival injection	Peripheral or diffuse conjunctival injection	Peripheral or diffuse conjunctival injection	Peripheral or diffuse conjunctival injection	Central or diffuse	Localized area of episclera	Localized area of sclera	Central with ciliary flush	Central, perilimbal injection
Discharge	Purulent	Watery	Watery to mucopurulent	Watery or mucoid	Reflex lacrimation to purulent	Reflex lacrimation	Reflex lacrimation	None	None
Pupillary changes	None	None	None	None	None	None	None	Constricted, sluggish, possibly irregular	Semidilated, nonreactive to light
Corneal appearance	Normal	Occasional fluorescein staining with associated keratitis	Scarring and ulceration with trichiasis	Normal	Punctation or ulceration seen with fluorescein staining	Normal	Normal	Normal	Hazy or cloudy with edema
Intraocular pressure	Normal	Normal	Normal	Normal	Normal	Normal	Normal	Normal	Elevated

Table 69.2. **Medications for Treatment of Bacterial Conjunctivitis**

Medication	Formulation	Dosage
Bacteriostatic		
Sulfacetamide sodium 10% (Bleph-10, Sulamyd)	10% solution 10% ointment	Two drops every 2 hours, or a small amount of ointment four times a day and at bedtime
Trimethoprim sulfate and polymyxin B sulfate (Polytrim)	Solution 1 mg; 10,000 units/mL	One drop every 3 hours, six times a day
Erythromycin (Ilotycin)	Ointment 5 mg/g	Apply small amount of ointment one to four times a day
Chloramphenicol (Chloroptic)	0.5% solution 1% ointment	Two drops, or small amount of ointment, every 3 hours for 48 hours; then prolong dosing interval; continue for 48 hours after eye appears normal
Bactericidal		
Gentamicin (Garamycin)	0.3% solution 0.3% ointment	Severe: two drops every hour Mild: two drops every 4 hours, or small amount of ointment two to three times a day
Tobramycin (Tobrex)	0.3% solution 0.3% ointment	Severe: two drops every hour or 0.5 inches of ointment two to three times a day Mild: one to two drops every 2 hours while awake for 2 days, then every 4 hours for 5 days
Norfloxacin (Chibroxin)	0.3% solution	One or two drops four times a day for 7 days
Ciprofloxacin (Ciloxan)	0.3% solution	One or two drops every 2 hours while awake for 2 days, then every 4 hours for 5 days
Ofloxacin (Ocuflox)	0.3% solution	One or two drops every 2–4 hours for 2 days, then four times a day for 5 days
Levofloxacin (Quixin)	0.5% solution	One or two drops every 2 hours while awake for 2 days, then every 4 hours for 5 days

recommended, however, to shorten the course and decrease the frequency of complications, which include keratitis, corneal ulceration, or systemic spread of the infection.[5] Therapy should be initiated with a broad-spectrum topical antimicrobial agent (Table 69.2). Bacteriostatic antibiotics inhibit bacterial growth and rely on host defense mechanisms to ultimately clear the infection. Less severe ocular infections usually respond well to these agents. Bactericidal drugs work to kill the microorganisms and are preferred for severe ocular infections.

Because of the frequent spread of infection, both eyes are treated, with therapy continued for 7 to 10 days. If gonococcal infection is diagnosed, systemic therapy is added to the topical therapy. Warm compresses to the eyes may provide some relief, and patients are instructed in hygienic measures of good hand washing and to avoid sharing towels or pillows. Patients wearing contact lenses are instructed to remove the lenses for the duration of treatment and to properly cleanse the lenses. Solutions for contact lens care and eye makeup should be replaced with new uncontaminated preparations. The eye should not be patched, and steroid eyedrops should not be used.[6]

Viral Conjunctivitis

Conjunctivitis may result from a wide variety of viruses. Adenovirus infection has been reported to cause as much as 20% of conjunctivitis seen in children and is the most common etiology. It typically occurs in epidemics and is more frequent during the autumn months.[7] Adenovirus causes both a conjunctivitis and keratoconjunctivitis. Types 1, 2, 3, and 7 are the cause of pharyngoconjunctival fever, which is characterized by the triad nonpurulent conjunctivitis, pharyngitis,

and fever (see Chapter 18). It is a self-limiting illness that usually runs its course in 7 to 10 days, though it may last several weeks. Two picornaviruses, enterovirus 70 and coxsackievirus A24, cause an acute hemorrhagic conjunctivitis. This illness is characterized by a rapid onset (6–12 hours), severely painful conjunctivitis, and subconjunctival hemorrhage.[8] It has been associated with a polio-like paralysis in approximately 1 per 10,000 patients. Herpes simplex virus may cause conjunctivitis and is the most common viral cause of conjunctivitis in neonates[2] (see Chapter 17). Primary infection and reactivation of the disease may result in keratitis. Measles and rubella classically exhibit conjunctivitis as part of the illness, and conjunctivitis occasionally occurs in patients with Epstein-Barr virus and varicella.

History

The patient typically presents with bilateral onset of redness and irritation of the eyes. There is usually a burning or gritty sensation in the eyes and a profuse watery discharge. Vision is unaffected. Pain and photophobia may be severe in cases with an associated keratitis or with acute hemorrhagic conjunctivitis. Often there are symptoms of pharyngitis and cough, especially with adenoviral infections.

Physical Examination

On physical examination both eyes have diffuse conjunctival injection. Visual acuity testing is normal. A discharge, if present, is clear and watery. Preauricular adenopathy and findings of an acute upper respiratory illness are common with infections caused by adenoviruses. In cases of acute hemorrhagic conjunctivitis, subconjunctival hemorrhages, usually located underneath the superior bulbar conjunctiva, may be present.[8]

Fluorescein staining may reveal a diffuse punctate keratitis with adenoviral or enteroviral infection or a typical dendritic keratitis with herpesvirus infections.

Laboratory Findings

Viral conjunctivitis is usually diagnosed based on the history and physical examination results, though often it is difficult to distinguish between viral and bacterial infections. Antigen detection assays have been developed for adenoviruses, and viral cultures can be obtained from conjunctival swabs but are rarely necessary. A Giemsa-stained smear demonstrating numerous lymphocytes may be helpful for delineating a viral etiology. In cases of suspected herpesvirus infections, a culture and Tzanck preparation of conjunctival scrapings and antigen detection tests (Surecell HSV test kit) may be useful for confirming the diagnosis.

Management

Specific therapy directed toward the treatment of viral conjunctivitis is limited to herpesvirus infections. Viral conjunctivitis is generally self-limited, though it has been shown that topical antibiotics may shorten the course, and recommend treatment with a topical antimicrobial agent to prevent secondary bacterial infection.[9] Patients may find some relief from symptoms with the use of a moisturizing agent for the eyes (Liquifilm Forte, Tears Naturale II, Tears Plus). The use of steroids to decrease inflammation is not recommended.

Viral conjunctivitis is highly contagious, and the patient must be instructed in proper hygienic measures. In adenoviral infections, replicating virus is present in up to 95% of patients 10 days after the onset, and decreases to only 5% by the 16th day.[10] Patients with acute hemorrhagic conjunctivitis should not return to work or school until 14 days after the onset of symptoms. In the physician's office, sterilization of instruments and good hand-washing are important for limiting the iatrogenic spread of the illness. In cases of herpesvirus infections, prompt referral to an ophthalmologist is recommended to determine the extent of infection and to initiate appropriate therapy with systemic and topical antiviral agents.

Chlamydial Conjunctivitis

Chlamydial conjunctivitis is caused by *Chlamydia trachomatis*, an obligate intracellular organism that also commonly causes venereal disease (see Chapter 41). Untreated chlamydial conjunctivitis may progress to trachoma, the leading cause of preventable blindness in the world. During the early stages of the disease, conjunctivitis occurs. Follicles or lymphoid aggregates form on the underside of the upper lid, which over time (typically 20–40 years) can cause scarring, lid distortion (entropion), and turning in of the eyelashes (trichiasis). Chronic irritation of the cornea by the eyelashes can lead to corneal opacification, ulceration, and subsequent blindness.

The World Health Organization estimates that 500 million people worldwide suffer from trachoma, and that 5 to 10 million people are blind as a result of the complications of the disease.[11] Although trachoma is no longer a serious health problem in urban and semiurban areas of industrialized and developing countries, chlamydial infection remains a common cause of neonatal conjunctivitis. The incidence of chlamydial conjunctivitis in neonates is approximately 8.2 per 1000 live births. It has been estimated that 50% of infants born to women with vaginal colonization by *C. trachomatis* develop the illness.[2] Chlamydial conjunctivitis in the adult is most common during the sexually active years. As many as 60% of infected men report associated genitourinary symptoms

History

In the newborn the time of onset may provide a clue to the diagnosis. Chlamydial infection usually begins at 5 to 14 days of life, though it has been reported within 24 hours of delivery.[2] In adolescents and adults the symptoms are usually chronic, bilateral irritation of the eyes. There is no change in vision, and usually a discharge is present. Symptoms of urethritis or a vaginal discharge may be present. An important clue to the diagnosis is a history of chronic conjunctivitis, often unresponsive to topical antimicrobial therapy in association with venereal symptoms.

Physical Examination

Physical findings reveal diffuse bilateral conjunctival injection. Visual acuity is normal. There may be edema of the eyelids and occasionally edema of the bulbar conjunctiva around the cornea (chemosis). A discharge is usually present, and its consistency may range from watery to mucopurulent. Later stages of the disease are characterized by peripheral subepithelial corneal infiltrates (pannus), superior corneal micropannus, and persistent palpebral or bulbar conjunctival follicles. With untreated disease, trichiasis eventually develops with corneal abrasion and ulceration.

Laboratory Findings

Cell culture of conjunctival scrapings is the most sensitive, most specific test for diagnosis, but it is expensive, time-consuming, and not readily accessible to all physicians. Rapid tests using either an enzyme-linked immunosorbent assay (Chlamydiazyme) or direct fluorescent antibody assays (Micro-Trak), have excellent sensitivity and specificity.[2] DNA hybridization assays and polymerase chain reaction tests to identify chlamydial antigens offer new methods for testing.[12] Conjunctival scrapings remain the preferred sample for the rapid tests because the organism remains in the epithelial cells of the conjunctiva.

Management

Topical therapy alone is not always effective and does not eradicate nasopharyngeal colonization. Although prophylaxis of neonates with erythromycin ointment has been effective in preventing conjunctivitis, chlamydial infection in the neonate requires systemic therapy for concurrent infection of the lungs, nasopharynx, throat, and vagina.[13]

In the neonate the therapy of choice is oral erythromycin ethylsuccinate (Eryped 200) 50 mg/kg/day in four divided doses combined with topical tetracycline or sulfacetamide drops or erythromycin ointment four times a day for 2 to 3 weeks.[2] In adults, systemic therapy should be initiated with oral tetracycline (Achromycin V) 250 mg q4h, or doxycycline 100 mg q12h for 2 to 3 weeks. Topical therapy with erythromycin is also recommended.[4] Resistance to erythromycin has been demonstrated, and its use for systemic therapy is best limited to children and pregnant women.[11] Parents of neonates and sexual partners of adults with chlamydial infections should be evaluated and treated.

Allergic Conjunctivitis

Ocular allergies are an important and common cause of the red eye. The most common cause is seasonal allergic conjunctivitis, also known as allergic rhinoconjunctivitis or hayfever. Less common ocular allergies include vernal keratoconjunctivitis, atopic keratoconjunctivitis, giant papillary conjunctivitis, and contact conjunctivitis.[14]

History

The predominant symptom of allergic conjunctivitis is a pruritic sensation in the eye. Symptoms tend to be bilateral from the onset and may be seasonal with associated hayfever symptoms. There may be complaints of a discharge that varies from watery to a stringy mucus accumulation in the eyes. Photophobia is uncommon, as are visual complaints. A personal and family history of atopy may be present. A careful history of topical medications, solutions, and cosmetic use may be helpful for contact conjunctivitis. Giant papillary conjunctivitis is almost always associated with contact lens use.[4]

Physical Examination

Visual acuity testing should be unaffected. The conjunctiva may appear diffusely injected, and there may be edema of the bulbar conjunctiva (chemosis). Edema of the tarsal conjunctiva may give rise to a cobblestone appearance. Frequently there is associated edema of the eyelids and findings of allergic rhinitis. A watery or mucoid discharge is common. The cornea is uninvolved, and the pupils are normal in terms of their size and reactivity to light.

Laboratory Findings

In cases where the diagnosis is uncertain, the most useful test is a Giemsa stain of scrapings of the conjunctiva showing the presence of eosinophils.[15] Eosinophils are not present in the normal conjunctiva, and the presence of even one eosinophil may be indicative of an ocular allergy. Skin testing or radioallergosorbent test (RAST) may be indicated in severe cases associated with systemic allergy symptoms. Skin testing is more sensitive, less expensive, and less time-consuming than the RAST in these cases. Tear assays for immunoglobulin E (IgE), histamine, and tryptase may provide substantiating evidence for the diagnosis but are not commonly employed.

Management

Primary treatment is directed toward the identification and elimination of the specific antigen. Systemic antihistamines may be sufficient for relieving symptoms alone or serve as an adjunct to topical therapy. Topical vasoconstrictor and antihistamine ophthalmic solutions often provide symptomatic relief in those with mild allergic conjunctivitis. Naphazoline HCl with pheniramine maleate (Naphcon-A) two drops q4h is often effective but recommended only for short-term use. Mast cell stabilizers such as cromolyn sodium 4% (Opticrom), lodoxamide tromethamine 0.1% (Alomide), and nedocromil sodium 2% (Alocril), are effective in the relief of mild to moderate symptoms with minimal ocular side effects. Combinations of antihistamine and mast cell stabilizers such as azelastine HCl 0.05% (Optivar), and olopatadine HCl 0.1% (Patanol), provide effective relief and are safe over prolonged use. Levocabastine hydrochloride 0.05% (Livostin), a potent H_1-blocker, and ketorolac tromethamine 0.5% (Acular), a nonsteroidal antiinflammatory drug, effectively relieve itching.[14] Topical corticosteroids are highly effective for the treatment of allergic conjunctivitis, but the side effects of glaucoma and cataracts make them of questionable value; hence they should be utilized only under the supervision of an ophthalmologist.

Other Causes of the Red Eye

Keratitis

Keratitis, an inflammation of the cornea, most often results from infection, though it may be due to corneal irritation by a foreign body or damage by chemicals or ultraviolet light; it may also be a manifestation of a connective tissue disorder (see Chapters 46 and 113). Although several organisms may cause infectious keratitis, microorganisms are rarely able to penetrate the intact corneal epithelium, and infection is usually preceded by factors that have altered the normal defense mechanisms of the outer eye. The primary bacterial pathogens include *S. aureus*, *S. epidermidis*, *Pseudomonas*, *Streptococcus*, and Enterobacteriaceae.[15] Several viruses that cause conjunctivitis may cause associated keratitis. Herpes simplex, varicella-zoster, and Epstein-Barr viruses may result in a necrotizing corneal inflammation via an immunogenic reaction. Various fungal organisms, such as *Fusarium*, *Aspergillus*, and *Curvularia*, and yeasts such as *Candida albicans* have been identified in cases of keratitis. *Acanthamoeba* has been identified as a cause of severe keratitis associated with contact lens wear.[16]

History

The patient with keratitis presents with a complaint of a red eye that is severely painful (owing to the high sensory innervation of the cornea). Corneal ulceration in the visual axis results in symptoms of decreased vision. Complaints of a discharge and photophobia may be present. The patient should be questioned about foreign bodies, abrasions, contact lens wear, the use of topical steroids, or other factors that may have compromised the integrity of the cornea.

Physical Examination

The patient's visual acuity is usually diminished, although with peripheral corneal ulceration outside the visual axis it may be unaffected. With inflammation of the adjacent uveal tract, injection of the vessels is more localized around the cornea. There is a discharge with the consistency ranging from watery with reflex lacrimation to purulent with bacterial ulceration. The pupil may appear normal, but with increasing inflammation there may be associated ciliary muscle spasm resulting in pupillary constriction and photophobia in the affected eye. With advanced infections or with perforation of the cornea, a collection of pus (hypopyon) may be observed in the anterior chamber. The reflection of light may appear irregular over areas of ulceration on the corneal surface. Fluorescein staining of the cornea must be used to visualize any suspected ulceration. Identification of an ulcer with a classic branching or dendritic ulcer pattern is pathognomonic for herpes simplex infection.

Laboratory Findings

Corneal scrapings are necessary to determine the responsible organism in infectious keratitis; it is best performed under slit-lamp examination prior to antimicrobial therapy. Scrapings should be obtained for Gram and Giemsa stains, as well as for bacterial, viral, and fungal culture and sensitivity tests. Antigen detection tests may aid in the diagnosis of herpesvirus infections.

Management

A corneal ulcer is an ophthalmologic emergency, and immediate referral to an ophthalmologist is indicated. The primary care physician may play an important role in the prevention of keratitis through education in hygiene, including the proper use of eye medications, eye protection, and effective disinfection of contact lenses.

Episcleritis

Episcleritis is a localized inflammation of the connective tissue that overlies the sclera just underneath the bulbar conjunctiva. The etiology of episcleritis is unknown, and episcleritis is not regularly associated with any systemic disorder.[17] Patients have reported recent viral infections, hypersensitivity reactions, and contact irritants, and the disorder has been seen in patients with herpes zoster infections, tuberculosis, gout, rheumatoid arthritis, and other autoimmune disorders.[17–19] The condition is most commonly seen in women during their third or fourth decade of life, and it tends to run a benign, self-limited course. It is commonly bilateral and may appear in a simple or a nodular form.

History

The patient usually presents with complaints of a red, watery, uncomfortable eye. Pain, usually not severe, may be characterized as a mild scratchy or pricking sensation. Mild photophobia may be present, but no change in vision is noted. The onset is often acute, with symptoms developing within an hour.

Physical Examination

Visual acuity is unaffected. The involved eye demonstrates an area of localized redness, with engorgement of the superficial episcleral vessels and often edema just below the conjunctiva. The area may be tender to touch. There is no discharge, though reflex lacrimation is often present. Examination with the aid of a slit lamp may be necessary to ensure that the underlying sclera has retained its normal contour and to distinguish the condition from scleritis.

Laboratory Findings

There are no recommended laboratory tests to establish the diagnosis.

Management

Ophthalmologic consultation is recommended to confirm the diagnosis and because of the recurrent nature of the condition. Although the condition is generally self-limiting, episcleritis may run a protracted course and in severe cases may rapidly progress to a necrotizing scleritis.

Scleritis

Scleritis, or inflammation of the scleral tissue, is much more serious than episcleritis. In contrast to episcleritis, approximately 50% of patients with scleritis have an underlying systemic disorder (Table 69.3). The incidence of rheumatoid arthritis in patients presenting with scleritis is 30%; it is the most common connective tissue disorder associated with the condition[17] (see Chapter 113).

History

Pain is the predominant symptom in the patient with scleritis. It is often severe, deep, and periorbital with radiation to the

Table 69.3. **Systemic Diseases Associated with Scleritis and Anterior Uveitis**

Scleritis	Anterior uveitis
Most common	**Most common**
Rheumatoid arthritis	Reiter's syndrome
Juvenile polyarthritis	Ankylosing spondylitis
Systemic lupus erythematosus	Sarcoidosis
Wegener's granulomatosis	Juvenile rheumatoid arthritis
Relapsing polychondritis	Interstitial nephritis
	Crohn's disease
	Ulcerative colitis
Rare	**Rare**
Polyarteritis nodosa	Acute leukemia
Ankylosing spondylitis	Adenoviral infection
Psoriatic arthritis	Behçet's disease
Reiter syndrome	Histoplasmosis
Ulcerative colitis	Kawasaki disease
Crohn's disease	Leprosy
	Leptospirosis
	Lyme disease
	Multiple sclerosis
	Mumps
	Psoriatic arthritis
	Relapsing polychondritis
	Sjögren syndrome
	Syphilis
	Systemic lupus erythematosus
	Toxoplasmosis
	Tuberculosis
	Vogt-Koyanagi-Harada syndrome
	Wegener's granulomatosis

temple and jaw. Frequently the patient is awakened by the pain. There is often marked tearing, and photophobia is common. Symptoms are bilateral in approximately 50% of patients.[18] Most commonly there is no reported change in vision.

Physical Examination

On examination there is intense localized violaceous vascular injection of the sclera that is tender to palpation. Swelling and injection of the sclera may be seen with slit-lamp examination. There is no discharge from the eye, and the cornea and pupil have a normal appearance. Visual acuity is typically unaffected, though certain forms of the disease are sight-threatening.

Laboratory Findings

There are no specific diagnostic laboratory tests for scleritis. Laboratory studies may best be directed toward the associated systemic disease when indicated by the clinical picture. Because of the frequent association of rheumatoid arthritis, rheumatoid factor assay may be useful.

Management

Urgent referral to an ophthalmologist is indicated. Therapy of scleritis should be directed at the underlying disease and may require a rheumatologic workup.

Anterior Uveitis

Anterior uveitis is classified as an inflammation of the iris (iritis) or the anterior ciliary body (cyclitis) or a combination of the two (iridocyclitis). Approximately 50% of patients with anterior uveitis are human leukocyte antigen (HLA)-B27 positive and have a causally related HLA-B27–associated systemic disease. Reiter syndrome and ankylosing spondylitis are the most common systemic illnesses associated with anterior uveitis, and the clinical presentation is highly characteristic[20] (see Chapter 113). Sarcoidosis is the next most common. Juvenile rheumatoid arthritis (JRA) and interstitial nephritis are also frequently associated. A variety of other systemic illnesses are associated less frequently (Table 69.3).[18,20,21]

History

Patients with anterior uveitis typically present with acute onset of a red, painful eye. The pain may initially be superficial but progresses to a deep-seated ache that is sometimes referred to the ocular and periocular regions. Photophobia and decreased vision are common complaints. Symptoms are most commonly unilateral, although each eye may be affected with recurrent episodes. The presence of bilateral symptoms may help to determine an etiologic cause.[22] As the condition is frequently recurrent, there may be a related history. Associated symptoms of systemic disease should be evaluated.

Physical Examination

Initially visual acuity may be unaffected, but it diminishes with increased inflammation in the anterior chamber. The redness becomes most prominent overlying the inflamed uveal tract, resulting in perilimbal vascular congestion (termed a ciliary flush). There is no discharge from the eye, and the cornea

appears clear. The pupil of the affected eye is often constricted owing to spasm of the sphincter, and with chronic recurrent episodes the pupil may become irregular because of the formation of posterior synechiae. Photophobia may be elicited if light is shone in either eye. Occasionally the inflammation is severe enough for inflammatory cells to settle in the anterior chamber, resulting in a hypopyon.

Laboratory Findings

The diagnosis of anterior uveitis is based on clinical findings under slit-lamp examination. Laboratory studies should be directed toward the determination of associated systemic disease based on the clinical history and physical examination, not on an all-encompassing battery of tests.[22] Testing for HLA-B27 is performed in cases of acute-onset unilateral anterior uveitis. In pediatric patients with chronic, bilateral uveitis, an antinuclear antibody test may substantiate a diagnosis of JRA. A chest roentgenogram and serologic tests for syphilis should be considered in every patient whose clinical features defy identification of an associated disease.[23]

Management

Urgent referral to an ophthalmologist is indicated when the diagnosis is suspected. Therapy is directed toward the inflammation and prevention of the complications of synechiae formation and glaucoma. Any associated systemic disease should be treated appropriately.

Acute Angle-Closure Glaucoma

Acute angle-closure glaucoma is characterized by an increase in intraocular pressure that, untreated, results in progressive damage to the optic nerve (see Chapter 71). Patients predisposed to the disease have a reduced angle between the cornea and iris as the result of a shallow anterior chamber. During an acute attack the iris bulges forward to the point of obstructing the normal outflow of aqueous humor from the anterior chamber, resulting in a rapid increase in intraocular pressure. Primary angle-closure glaucoma occurs in 0.6% or less of the general population and affects approximately 6% of all patients with glaucoma.[24] Women are affected three times as often as men, and the incidence increases with advancing age. There are racial differences in the prevalence of angle-closure glaucoma, and though the anatomic features of angle-closure are inherited, the familial incidence of acute angle-closure glaucoma is low.[24]

History

The patient with acute angle-closure glaucoma usually presents with rapidly developing, severe, unilateral eye pain and redness. The pain is typically deep and may be described as a headache. Nausea and vomiting are common owing to vagal stimulation and may be the presenting complaint. Vision is usually decreased, and the patient may see halos around lights due to edema of the cornea. A medication history is important, as certain medications can precipitate an attack.

Physical Examination

The predominant feature is that the pupil of the affected eye is semidilated and does not react to light. If the pupil constricts with light, angle-closure glaucoma is not present.[25] Visual acuity is usually diminished in the affected eye and worsens with increasing corneal edema and pressure on the optic nerve. The vascular injection of the eye may appear more central because of injection of the perilimbal vessels, and the conjunctiva may be edematous. The cornea may appear hazy owing to edema, and the reflection of light off the corneal surface may appear diffuse, losing its sharp borders. A narrow chamber angle and bulging iris may be identified by shining a light across the iris from the temporal side of the patient. In the normal eye the entire iris is illuminated, whereas in an eye with a narrow chamber angle a shadow is cast on the nasal side of the iris. There should be no discharge from the eye. A definitive diagnosis is made by demonstrating increased intraocular pressure through the use of tonometry and finding a narrow chamber angle on slit-lamp examination and gonioscopy.

Laboratory Findings

Laboratory evaluation is not required for the diagnosis of primary angle-closure glaucoma.

Management

Emergent referral to an ophthalmologist is recommended when the diagnosis is suspected. Therapy is initially directed toward lowering the intraocular pressure in preparation for surgery. Once the acute attack is controlled, iridectomy is performed to prevent subsequent attacks. Because of its lower complication rate, laser iridectomy has replaced conventional surgical methods.[24]

Conclusion

The cause of a red eye can usually be determined through systematic evaluation of the patient's history and physical findings (Table 69.1). Decreased vision, deep or severe eye pain, and photophobia are important symptoms when identifying patients with severe ocular pathology. Physical findings of decreased visual acuity, ciliary flush, corneal edema or ulceration, pupillary changes, and increased intraocular pressure are indicative of sight-threatening disorders, and referral to an ophthalmologist is indicated when they are present.

References

1. Weiss A, Brinser JH, Nazar-Stewart V. Acute conjunctivitis in childhood. J Pediatr 1993;122:10–4.
2. O'Hara MA. Ophthalmia neonatorum. Pediatr Clin North Am 1993;40:715–25.
3. Snyder RW, Glasser DB. Antibiotic therapy for ocular infection. West J Med 1994;161:579–84.
4. Bertolini J, Pelucio M. The red eye. Emerg Med Clin North Am 1995;13:561–79.
5. Limberg MB. A review of bacterial keratitis and bacterial conjunctivitis. Am J Ophthalmol 1991;112(suppl):2S–9S.
6. Lavin MJ, Rose GE. Use of steroid eye drops in general practice. BMJ 1986;292:1448–50.
7. Gigliotti F, Williams WT, Hayden FG, Hendley JO. Etiology of acute conjunctivitis in children. J Pediatr 1981;98:531–6.
8. Wright PW, Strauss GH, Langford MP. Acute hemorrhagic conjunctivitis. Am Fam Physician 1992;45:173–8.
9. Leibowitz, HM. The Red Eye. N Engl J Med 2000;343:345–51.
10. Roba LA, Kowalski RP, Romanowski E, et al. How long are patients with epidemic keratoconjunctivitis infectious? Invest Ophthalmol Vis Sci 1993;34:848 (abstract).
11. Tabbara KF. Trachoma: have we advanced in the last 20 years? Int Ophthalmol Clin 1990;30:23–7.
12. Morrow GL, Abbott RL. Conjunctivitis. Am Fam Physician 1998;57:735–46.
13. Whitcher JP. Neonatal ophthalmia: have we advanced in the past 20 years? Int Ophthalmol Clin 1990;30:39–41.
14. Friedlaender MH. Management of ocular allergy. Ann Allergy Asthma Immunol 1995;75:212–22.
15. Butrus SI, Abelson MB. Laboratory evaluation of ocular allergy. Int Ophthalmol Clin 1988;28:324–8.
16. Larkin DFP. Acanthamoeba keratitis. Int Ophthalmol Clin 1991;31:163–72.
17. Hakin KN, Watson PG. Systemic associations of scleritis. Int Ophthalmol Clin 1991;31:111–29.
18. Yanofsky NN. The acute painful eye. Emerg Med Clin North Am 1988;6:21–42.
19. Elkington AR, Khaw PT. The red eye. BMJ 1988;296:1720–4.
20. Rosenbaum JT. Systemic associations of anterior uveitis. Int Ophthalmol Clin 1991;31:131–42.
21. Pavesio CE, Nozik RA. Anterior and intermediate uveitis. Int Ophthalmol Clin 1990;30:244–51.
22. Rosenbaum JT. An algorithm for the systemic evaluation of patients with uveitis: guidelines for the consultant. Semin Arthritis Rheum 1990;19:248–57.
23. Rosenbaum JT, Wernick R. Selection and interpretation of laboratory tests for patients with uveitis. Int Ophthalmol Clin 1990;30:238–43.
24. Greenidge KC. Angle-closure glaucoma. Int Ophthalmol Clin 1990;30:177–86.
25. Richards RD. Glaucoma. Am Fam Physician 1987;35:212–20.

70
Ocular Trauma

Marc W. McKenna

It is estimated that each year there are 2.5 million cases of eye injuries in the United States, many of which are preventable. Injuries range from mild and self-limited to severe. Trauma is the most common cause of monocular blindness in the United States.[1] Worldwide, eye injuries cause blindness in approximately 1.6 million people and unilateral loss of vision in 19 million people.[2] Nearly half of all eye injuries are initially seen by primary care physicians, which makes it essential that family practitioners have the expertise and skills to deal with these problems.[3] This chapter covers four general areas important to every family physician: initial evaluation, common injuries, vision-threatening injuries, and prevention.

Initial Evaluation

The initial evaluation of eye trauma begins with a thorough history, and even with the urgency of the situation, this important step must not be overlooked. The mechanism of injury, the time sequence, and the ocular history, including glasses or contact lens wear, are essential to prompt and appropriate treatment. The patient should be queried concerning change in vision, irritation, pain, discharge, swelling, and bleeding. Any change in vision should be more specifically categorized to include blindness, blurring, floaters, flashes, or field loss. The physical examination must be done systematically and completely to ensure that no area of injury is missed. It should include all of the vital structures and functions of the eye.[4] Many family physicians find it useful to have a preassembled eye tray that is readily available to assist in the evaluation and management of ocular trauma. The eye tray should include a near-vision card, fluorescein strips, a blue cobalt light, lid retractors, cotton-tipped applicators, 25-gauge needle, eye spud, ophthalmoscope, eye patches, protective eye shield, a Schiøtz tonometer, and sterile eye solu-

tion. Table 70.1 lists common medications that should also be included on the eye tray.[5]

Visual Acuity

Assessment of visual acuity is essential to the initial workup of all eye trauma. In the emergency room or the family physician's office, vision in each eye should be recorded using the standard Snellen eye chart at 20 feet. Near-vision cards can be substituted, if necessary. Severe acuity deficits can be recorded as the ability to count fingers, see hand movements, or note a loss of light perception.

Lids and Orbits

The lids and orbits should be examined for swelling, ecchymosis, and deformity. The orbits should be palpated looking for defects, subcutaneous emphysema, or areas of numbness. The lid and lacrimal apparatus are inspected for lacerations. Eversion of the lid is essential for detecting foreign bodies. It can be accomplished with a lid retractor or by using a cotton-tipped applicator stick as a fulcrum to evert the upper lid and enhance inspection of the superior sulcus and tarsal surface. Topical anesthesia can be used prior to this procedure.

Sclera and Conjunctiva

The white of the eye, the sclera and conjunctiva, should be inspected for laceration, hemorrhage, foreign body, and chemosis (swelling). The cornea, the transparent covering over the anterior portion of the eye, should be examined for foreign bodies, cloudiness, and abrasion. Fluorescein staining and topical anesthesia facilitate examination of the cornea.

Ophthalmoscopy

Use of the ophthalmoscope is essential for assessing the anterior and posterior segments of the eye. The anterior cham-

Table 70.1. **Medications for an Eye Tray**

Anesthetics:	proparacaine (Ophthaine) 0.5%
Mydriatics:	phenylephrine (Neo-Synephrine) 2.5%
Cycloplegics:	tropicamide (Mydriacyl) 1%—duration 3 to 6 hours
	cyclopentolate (Cyclogyl) 2%—duration 12 to 24 hours
Antibiotics:	sulfacetamide (Sodium Sulamyd) 10% ointment
	gentamicin (Garamycin) ointment
	ofloxacin (Ocuflox) 0.3% solution

ber, the area between the cornea and the iris, is filled with aqueous humor. It should be inspected for gross blood (hyphema) or pus (hypopyon). The iris should be evaluated for symmetry, a uniform contour, and color change. The lens should be examined for subluxation, dislocation, and traumatic cataract formation. The posterior segment, which includes the vitreous, retina, and optic nerve, is examined for hemorrhage, edema, retinal tears or detachment, and intraocular foreign bodies. Unless contraindicated because of the need to monitor pupillary response in a patient with head trauma, pupillary dilation with a mydriatic eye drop greatly augments the examination with the ophthalmoscope.

Pupils/Extraocular Movements

Also included in the initial evaluation is examination of the pupils and extraocular movements. The pupils should be round, equal, and reactive to light. If unequal, obtaining a history of anisocoria is very important. A dilated pupil resulting from a head injury is a significant warning sign. In cases of trauma or decreased vision, an afferent pupillary defect (Marcus Gunn pupil) should be part of the evaluation. An afferent pupillary defect is a sign of retinal or optic nerve damage. This test measures the pupillary response to direct light versus the indirect consensual pupillary response from light shone into the other eye. Using a "swinging flashlight test," an afferent pupillary defect is present when there is paradoxical dilation of the affected pupil after a light that is being shone into the normal eye is switched and is shone in the injured eye. Extraocular movements should be assessed for entrapment of the extraocular muscles, which can be a sign of a blowout orbital fracture. If there is a concern that acute glaucoma is part of the presenting problem, the intraocular pressure should be measured. It can be done grossly by comparing tactile pressure on both globes. This procedure though is best performed by slit-lamp examination or by using a Schiøtz tonometer. The intraocular pressure should not be measured if there is a suspected rupture of the globe or if there is evidence of an infection.

Common Eye Injuries

Common types of eye trauma are frequently seen in the family physician's office, including injuries that are typically not initially vision-threatening. These injuries are most often evaluated and treated by the family physician.

Corneal Abrasion

Perhaps the most common eye injury seen in the family physician's office is a corneal abrasion.[6] The abrasion can be caused by a myriad of offending objects or projectiles: tree branches, fingers, pieces of paper, contact lenses, and small foreign bodies. The denuded cornea causes photophobia, tearing, pain, and often a foreign-body sensation in the eye. It can be accompanied by blurred vision. Topical anesthesia (proparacaine) is often needed to enable the physician to do a thorough examination.

Fluorescein staining is easy and confirms the diagnosis. The fluorescein strip is lightly wetted, and the lower lid is pulled down. The strip is inserted into the inferior cul-de-sac until the entire eye is stained yellow-orange. The fluorescein is then flushed out of the eye with a sterile eye solution. The abrasion takes up the fluorescein and after irrigation stains blue-green when viewed with a blue cobalt light.

Treatment consists of topical antibiotics, pain control, and, in some cases, a pressure patch over the affected eye. A cycloplegic agent may be instilled into the eye to relieve ciliary spasm and dilate the pupil. Many of these patients require oral analgesia. Topical NSAIDs (ketorolac) are also sometimes used for pain relief.[7] The patient is examined daily with fluorescein staining until the abrasion resolves. The cornea usually reepithelializes within 24 to 48 hours. Vision should return to normal once healing occurs. Topical antibiotics should be continued for 5 to 7 days to prevent infection and for continued lubrication. The major complications of corneal abrasions are recurrent erosions and infection. Recurrent erosion occurs when the new epithelium breaks down days to weeks after the initial event. Treatment of recurrent erosions includes 5% hypertonic saline ointment at bedtime for several months to enhance lubrication and promote healing.

Pressure patching is no longer recommended in the treatment of most corneal abrasions and in fact is contraindicated in abrasions with a high risk of infection.[8] This includes scratches from organic matter (tree branch), a dirty object, or those associated with contact lens wear. If the offending agent is a contact lens, it must be removed before using fluorescein, as soft contacts take up the stain. Topical broad-spectrum antibiotics (aminoglycoside or fluoroquinolone) should be used four times a day and contact lens wear should not be resumed until the eye is completely asymptomatic for 3 to 4 days. The contacts should also be checked for defects, tears, and protein buildups before being reused.[9]

One severe form of corneal injury is a diffuse abrasion caused by ultraviolet light from a sunlamp or welder's arc. With these injuries, large portions of the cornea may be injured. The intense pain requires topical anesthesia to examine the patient. Treatment is similar to that for corneal abrasions but often requires narcotic analgesia at home. As with smaller corneal abrasions, topical anesthetics other than NSAIDs should never be prescribed for home use, and these patients require close follow-up.

Foreign Bodies

Another common eye injury is a foreign body on the surface of the eye. Usually this injury involves particulate matter that flies into the eye. Often multiple foreign bodies are present, so complete examination of the eye is imperative. A penetrating injury must be ruled out. After applying topical anesthesia, loose foreign bodies on the conjunctiva or lid may be irrigated with sterile solution or removed with a moist cotton-tipped applicator. Superficially embedded foreign bodies may be removed with a 25-gauge hypodermic needle or an eye spud. Optimally, this is best done under slit-lamp examination. Metallic foreign bodies, if left in place for more than a few hours, can form a rust ring, which necessitates ophthalmologic referral for slit-lamp examination and removal of the foreign body and rust ring. Removal of a corneal foreign body, by its nature, causes an abrasion, which must then be treated as such with close follow-up. If there is concern that the foreign body is not superficial, immediate consultation with an ophthalmologist is required.

Subconjunctival Hemorrhage and Ecchymosis

Blunt trauma to the eye can be the result of either trivial trauma or high-impact forces, which can cause serious injury. Two common self-limiting injuries are subconjunctival hemorrhage and ecchymosis of the eyelid and surrounding soft tissue (black eye). Again, a history and thorough examination are crucial to rule out more serious pathology. The amount of swelling and ecchymosis can be dramatic because the area is so vascular. Subconjunctival hemorrhage is typically bright red and can extend all the way to the border of the iris and occasionally cover the entire conjunctiva. Chemosis or edema of the conjunctiva can be a sign of scleral rupture and extrusion of the vitreous, which is a harbinger of more serious underlying pathology. If orbital emphysema is present, a careful search, including radiologic studies, for associated orbital or ocular injury should be performed.

Treatment of a subconjunctival hemorrhage consists of watchful waiting. A subconjunctival hemorrhage commonly goes through the stages of changing color to yellow or green and, at times, takes as long as 2 to 3 weeks to resolve. Visual acuity should be normal.

Lid Lacerations

Lid lacerations that are superficial and not involved in the lacrimal apparatus or a lid margin may be repaired with simple suturing (see Chapter 49). Careful attention must be paid to cosmetic appearance and function. Referral is required if these factors are of specific concern. Attention must be given to the type of injury to ensure that there is no associated penetrating trauma. It is particularly important to be aware of high-velocity or sharp, penetrating injuries. If the lid margin or the nasolacrimal ducts are involved, consultation should be sought.

Vision-Threatening Injuries

More serious injuries include those occurrences where vision is imminently threatened and proper treatment is essential. Common vision-threatening injuries include chemical burns, hyphema, penetrating wounds, blowout fractures, and ruptured globes.

Chemical Burns

Chemical burns are common ocular injuries, and the family practitioner must provide prompt treatment in an attempt to prevent permanent vision loss. Chemical burns occur when toxic substances come into direct contact with the eyes often through splashing. Although alkali burns are potentially more devastating than acid burns, each must be treated as a true emergency.

Alkali is found in ammonia-containing products (fertilizers, refrigerators, cleaning solutions), lye-containing products (drain cleaners, magnesium hydroxide, sparklers, flares), and lime products (plaster, mortar). The lipid solubility of alkali, with continued contact, allows deep penetration into the eye. It can cause destruction of the anterior segment. Acid burns are caused by sulfuric acid (battery acids), hydrofluoric acid, and hydrochloric acid. These acids tend to cause superficial damage but in high concentration can lead to blindness.

The initial treatment of all chemical burns is irrigation. This point cannot be emphasized strongly enough. Irrigation should be started as soon as possible, ideally in the field but certainly on initial presentation in the physician's office. The main goal is copious flushing. Neutralizing solutions are of questionable additional benefit; intravenous normal saline is sufficient. Regular intravenous tubing can be used to deliver the irrigation directly to the eye. Clearly, this situation is one where the vision is not checked before starting treatment. Once the patient presents to the office, instill topical anesthesia to the eye(s), pull the eyelids widely apart, and flush. Always inspect and remove particulate matter. Flushing should be continued at least 20 minutes and until the eye's pH has been neutralized. The patient should then have a cycloplegic agent instilled to dilate the eye to relieve ciliary spasm. In addition, a topical antibiotic should be instilled, the eye patched, and referral made to an ophthalmologist for more definitive care.

Hyphema

Hyphema, or bleeding into the anterior chamber, is a serious complication of blunt or penetrating trauma to the eye. The dramatic view of layering of blood in the anterior chamber is often a sign of other associated damage.[10] Such coexisting injuries include lens disruption, glaucoma, iris damage, corneal injury, and retinal tears. The initial treatment is medical to prevent rebleeding. The patient is put at bed rest, the head is elevated and the eye patched. Immediate ophthalmologic consultation is required. Conventional treatment includes cycloplegics and topical steroids. Systemic steroids and antifibrinolytic agents may decrease the incidence of rebleeding. Most uncomplicated hyphemas reabsorb spontaneously and have an excellent prognosis. Occasionally, hyphemas can lead to staining of the cornea and increased intraocular pressure. Poor visual prognostic signs include large hyphemas, injury in a child, rebleeds, and those associated with posterior segment damage. Table 70.2 lists risk factors associated with rebleeds.[11]

Table 70.2. **Risk Factors for Rebleeding of Hyphemas**

Initial visual acuity less than 20/200
Hyphema more than one-third of the anterior chamber
Delayed medical attention of more than 1 day after injury
Elevated intraocular pressure

Blowout Fractures of the Orbit

Orbital fractures can commonly be seen with blunt trauma. The orbit should be palpated for step-offs or crepitus. Rupture into a sinus can cause tissue emphysema, and injury to the inferior orbital nerve causes a dysesthesia below the eye. A blowout fracture constitutes entrapment of orbital fat and an extraocular muscle in the bony fragments. The weakest part of the orbit lies inferiorly and is the most common area for a blowout. The patient presents with diplopia and defective extraocular movements. Diagnosis is confirmed by computed tomography (CT). Immediate surgical decompression of orbital fractures is not essential and is reserved for persistent diplopia, mechanical restriction of gaze, endophthalmos or hypophthalmos, and cosmetic reconstruction.[12] Treatment includes use of oral antibiotics because of the risk of sinus infection and avoidance of nose blowing.

Perforating Wounds/Globe Rupture

Perforating wounds of the eyes with rupture of the globe are devastating injuries and can be missed if one is not observant. The perforation is not obvious on initial presentation in up to 20% of patients with rupture of the globe.[13] The visual acuity may even be intact. Table 70.3 lists situations where a high index of suspicion should be maintained for global rupture. If any one of these situations exists and rupture is suspected, do not pressure-patch the eye or instill topical antibiotics. Avoid manipulation of the globe, place a protective eye shield, and refer immediately to the ophthalmologist. Surgical exploration may well be needed to determine if there is a true rupture. Radiographic studies, either a CT scan or ultrasound, should be done to rule out an intraocular foreign body.

Posterior Segment Injuries

Sudden compression or stretching of the globe following blunt trauma can cause injury to the posterior segments of the eye, including vitreous hemorrhage, retinal detachment, and damage to the optic nerve. The structures of the posterior segment

Table 70.3. **Findings Associated with Ruptured Globe**

History of significant blunt trauma
Penetrating trauma
Projectile object, especially metal on metal
Irregular or oval pupil
Hyphema
Irregular-shaped iris
Traumatic cataract or dislocated lens
Pigmented area on globe consistent with iris prolapse
Conjunctival laceration, especially with dehiscence of tissue
Corneal laceration with leakage of aqueous fluid

are examined using direct ophthalmoscopy, which is most easily performed after dilation of the pupil. If posterior segment injuries are present, a CT scan or ultrasound is usually indicated to better delineate the extent of the trauma.

Vitreous hemorrhage is usually caused be tearing of the retinal vessels. Symptoms range from floaters to profound visual loss. Ophthalmoscopy may reveal a loss of the red reflex or poor visualization of the retina. Patients with vitreous hemorrhage should be seen by an ophthalmologist because of the high association with retinal detachment or the presence of an occult foreign body.[14]

Injury to the globe may also result in retinal detachment or tears.[15] Symptoms include floaters, light flashes, specks, or a black veil across a visual field. On funduscopic exam, a detachment appears as a break in the natural pink color of the retina and appears as a grayish, opaque billowing of the retinal surface. Early recognition of tears is important because the outcome is improved if treatment is started before the macula becomes involved. Surgery within the first 24 hours is sometimes required, so immediate referral is standard. Symptoms of retinal tears may present days to weeks after the initial trauma.

In addition, a contusion to the globe can result in hemorrhage or shearing of the optic nerve. Vision loss may be severe or even total. The patient will have an afferent pupillary defect. Emergency decompression and treatment may be indicated, so immediate consultation is essential.

Prevention of Eye Injuries

Many causes of eye trauma are accidental, and one of the most important roles of a family physician in preventing ocular trauma is anticipatory guidance. The common areas for injury occur in the workplace, at home, during sports activities, and in association with fireworks. A disproportionate number of severe injures occur in those under 15 years of age.[16] The family physician, who is often involved in occupational health or is a team physician, should ensure that proper protective eyewear is required when patients are involved in high-risk activities.

Polycarbonate lenses and frames are the standard for protection during sports, and industrial goggles with side shields are standard for the workplace. Other specific sports, such as hockey, lacrosse, and football, have specifically designed helmets for protection.[17] During health maintenance visits, the family physician should identify those patients with functional vision in only one eye and suggest adequate protection for even low-risk activities. For these patients, participation in high-risk sports where no protective goggles can be worn (wrestling, boxing, and martial arts) should not be allowed.

References

1. Fact Sheet. New York: National Society to Prevent Blindness, 1980.
2. Negrel AD, Thyelfors B. The global impact of eye injuries. Ophthal Epidemiol 1998;5(3):143–69.
3. Shields T, Sloane PD. A comparison of eye problems in primary care and ophthalmology practices. Fam Med 1991;23:544–6.

4. Shingleton BJ, Hersh PS, Kenyon KR, eds. Eye trauma. St. Louis: Mosby Year Book, 1991.

5. Silverman H, Nunez L, Feller D. Treatment of common eye emergencies. Am Fam Physician 1992;45:2279–87.

6. Torok PG, Mader TH. Corneal abrasions: diagnosis and management. Am Fam Physician 1996;53(8):2521–9.

7. Kaiser PK, Pineda RA. A study of topical nonsteroidal anti-inflammatory drops and no pressure patching in the treatment of corneal abrasions. Ophthalmology. 1997;104(8):1353–9.

8. Flynn CA, D'Amico F, Smith G. Should we patch corneal abrasions? A meta-analysis. J Fam Pract 1998;47(4):264–70.

9. Cullen RD, Chang B. The Wills eye manual: office and emergency room diagnosis and treatment of eye disease, 2nd ed. Philadelphia: JB Lippincott, 1994;216–32.

10. MacEwen CJ. Ocular injuries. J R Coll Surg Edinb 1999;44(5): 317–23.

11. Long LP. Secondary hemorrhage in traumatic hyphema. Preventive factors for selective prophylaxis. Ophthalmology 1995; 101:1583–8.

12. Mathog RH. Management of orbital blow-out fractures. In: Weisman RA, Stanley RB Jr, guest eds. Current issues in head and neck trauma, vol 24. Philadelphia: WB Saunders, 1991; 79–91.

13. Shingleton BJ. Eye injuries. N Engl J Med 1991;325:408–13.

14. Catalano R. Eye injuries and prevention. Pediatr Clin North Am 1993;40:827–39.

15. Reichel E. Vitreoretinal emergencies. Am Fam Physician 1995; 52:1415–19.

16. Schein OD, Hibberd PL, Shingleton BJ, et al. The spectrum and burden of ocular injury. Ophthalmology 1988;95:300–5.

17. Stock JG, Cornell FM. Prevention of sports-related eye injury. Am Fam Physician 1991;44:515–20.

Selected Disorders of the Eye

John E. Sutherland and Richard C. Mauer

It is important to identify the ocular symptoms that are serious and require an emergent or urgent examination. These symptoms include recent visual loss, double vision, pain, floaters, flashes, and photophobia. Less serious symptoms, which can be evaluated electively, include vague ocular discomfort, tearing, mucous discharge, burning, eyelid symptoms, or proptosis.

The basic eye examination includes testing for visual acuity with the Snellen chart, modified for small children and mentally handicapped adults through the use of picture cards or tumbling E's. Confrontation visual fields, ocular motility testing, ophthalmoscopy, corneal staining, and the pupillary examination are also essential.

Pupil

Pupils are the most frequently examined part of the eye. As the central opening of the iris, the pupil regulates the amount of light that enters the eye. Normal pupils are round, regular in shape, and nearly equal in size. The pupillary examination is designed primarily to detect neurologic abnormalities that disturb the size of the pupils. Pupillary reflexes include the direct light reflex and the indirect, or consensual, reflex, a response to light falling on the opposite eye. The measurement of pupil size in dim light assesses the motor (efferent) limb of the pupillary reflex arc; the evaluation of pupil response to direct light assesses both the motor and the sensory (afferent) limbs; the swinging light test (testing for the consensual reflex) assesses only the sensory limbs.

Constriction of the pupil to less than 2 mm is called miosis if it does not dilate in the dark. Topical cholinergic stimulating drops and systemic narcotics are the most frequent causes.

Dilatation of the pupil to more than 6 mm is called mydriasis, with failure to constrict to light stimulation. Topical atropine-like drops, trauma, and oculomotor nerve abnormalities are the most common causes.

Anatomic variation in the diameter of the iris is less than 1 mm. It is best to determine this parameter in the dimmest light possible, measuring with the pupil gauge found on the near-vision card. True inequality of pupil size (anisocoria) is caused by drugs, injury, inflammation, angle-closure glaucoma, ischemia, paralysis of the sphincter-pupillae muscle (dilated) and of dilatator pupillae muscles (constricted), Horner syndrome, neuronal lesions (Argyll Robertson pupil), or, most commonly, physiologic variations.[1]

Eyelids

The eyelids, which are anatomically complex, are protective to the cornea, aid in the distribution and the elimination of tears, and limit light entering the eye. Abnormalities can occur in the skin, mucous membranes, glands, and muscles.

Congenital Abnormalities

The most common congenital variation is an epicanthus, which is a vertical skin fold in the medial canthal region; it is normal in persons of Asian ancestry. Asymmetry may simulate an esotropia (pseudostrabismus).

Positional Abnormalities

Entropion

Entropion is inversion of the lid margin. Etiologies are age-related (involutional), cicatricial, spastic, and congenital. Involutional entropion of aging is common, causing misdirected eyelashes (trichiasis) that irritate the eye. Secondary conditions include conjunctivitis, corneal ulcers, keratitis, tearing, and blepharitis. Treatment includes eyelid hygiene, lubricating agents, and topical antibiotics when inflammation is present. Taping or patching can be palliative or temporary, awaiting definitive surgical procedures for symptomatic patients.[2,3]

Ectropion

Eversion of the lid margin, or ectropion, can be age-related, cicatricial, spastic, and allergic. Severe cases may follow Bell's palsy (see Chapter 67). Ocular manifestations include chronic conjunctivitis, keratitis, epiphora, and keratinization of the lid. Treatment options are similar to those for entropion.[2,3]

Blepharoptosis

The etiology of blepharoptosis lies either in the innervation or the structure of the levator palpebrae superioris muscle, leading to a drooping upper eyelid and a narrow palpebral fissure. The congenital type can be unilateral or bilateral. Acquired forms include dehiscence of the levator aponeurosis, neuropathy, intracranial disorders, Horner syndrome, myotonic dystrophy, and myasthenia gravis. Surgical therapy is the only successful management strategy.[2]

Inflammation

Blepharitis

Blepharitis is an inflammatory condition of the lid margin oil glands. It may be infectious, usually due to *Staphylococcus aureus*, involving the eyelash roots, glands, or both. It has been described as "acne" of the eyelids. Individuals who have acne rosacea or seborrheic dermatitis of the scalp and face are particularly vulnerable (see Chapter 115). Symptoms include swelling, redness, debris of the lid and lashes, itching, tearing, a foreign-body sensation, and crusting around the eyes on awakening. Management of blepharitis is primarily lid hygiene using warm compresses with baby shampoo or an eyelid cleansing agent applied with a finger, washcloth, or cotton-tipped applicators. Nightly application of bacitracin, erythromycin, or sulfisoxazole ointment to the lid margins is helpful when there are signs of secondary infection. For severe or recurrent cases systemic therapy with tetracycline (Achromycin), doxycycline (Doryx, Vibramycin), or erythromycin (E.E.S., E-Mycin, Eryc) can be used for several months.[1–3]

Hordeolum

Also known as a stye, an external hordeolum is an inflammation of the ciliary follicles or accessory glands of the anterior lid margin. It is a painful, tender, red mass near the lid margin, often with pustule formation and mild conjunctivitis. An internal hordeolum, which presents in a similar manner, involves an infection of the meibomian gland away from the lid margins.[2,4] Treatment is usually simple for this self-limited condition: intermittent hot, moist compresses plus topical ophthalmic antibiotics such as tobramycin (Tobrex), bacitracin, erythromycin (Ilotycin), gentamicin (Garamycin), or sulfacetamide (Bleph-10, Sulamyd, Sulf-10) to prevent infection of the surrounding lash follicles. One method to hasten drainage of the external hordeolum is to epilate (remove a hair and its root) the lash, which effectively creates a drainage channel. Occasionally an incision or puncture for

drainage and administration of systemic antistaphylococcal antibiotics is necessary.[1]

Chalazion

A chalazion (lipogranuloma) is a chronic granuloma that may follow and be secondary to inflammation of a meibomian gland. During its chronic phase it is a firm, painless nodule up to 8 mm in diameter that lies within the tarsus and over which the skin lid moves freely. It usually begins as an internal hordeolum. Asymptomatic chalazia usually resolve spontaneously within a month. Treatment options for persistent chalazia include an intralesional long-acting corticosteroid injection, which may cause hypopigmentation, or a surgical incision and curettage with a clamp.[1,2,4]

Dermatitis

Dermatitis may be either infectious or of contact etiology. Contact dermatitis is common because of exposure to sensitizing irritants such as neomycin, atropine, cosmetics, lotions, soaps, nickel, thimerosal (often in artificial tears), chloramphenicol, poison ivy, and others. Manifestations include erythema, vesiculation, scaling, edema, and itching. Therapy, most importantly, is removal of the offending agent (see Chapter 115). During the acute stages cool compresses, antihistamines, and topical corticosteroids provide relief. Occasionally, systemic steroids are necessary such as for severe poison ivy dermatitis. The most common infectious etiologies are impetigo, erysipelas, and herpes zoster, with treatment the same as indicated for other locations.[5]

Conjunctiva

Subconjunctival Hemorrhage

Subconjunctival hemorrhage not caused by direct ocular trauma is usually the result of a sudden increase in intrathoracic pressure, as when sneezing, coughing, or straining to evacuate. Rupture of a conjunctival blood vessel causes a bright red, sharply delineated area surrounded by normal-appearing conjunctiva (Fig. 71.1). The blood is located underneath the bulbar conjunctiva and gradually fades in 2 weeks. Usually no cause is found, but it is seen with hypertension and in neonates or their mothers as a result of labor and delivery. No treatment is indicated.[1]

Pingueculum

A pingueculum is an area of nasal or temporal bulbar conjunctiva that contains epithelial hyperplasia, a harmless yellow-white, plaque-like thickening. Occasionally inflammatory discomfort requires a topical vasoconstrictor. Medical treatment is ineffective, and recurrence is common after surgical intervention.

Pterygium

A pterygium is a triangular elevated mass consisting of vascular growth of the conjunctiva, usually nasal, that migrates onto the corneal surface. Environmental factors such as pro-

Tears) containing methylcellulose, polyvinyl alcohol, or 2% sodium hyaluronate four times a day to hourly. Punctal occlusion with a silicone plug or permanent punctual closure via thermal cautery can produce dramatic symptomatic improvement. Severe cases occasionally require patches during the day or acetylcysteine, 10% to 20%, to alter the mucus.

Dacryocystitis

Dacryocystitis is a painful inflammation of the lacrimal sac resulting from congenital or acquired obstruction of the nasolacrimal duct. Even though congenital nasolacrimal duct obstruction occurs commonly in infants, dacryocystitis is rare and is commonly associated with nasolacrimal duct cysts. In adults it is idiopathic or the result of an obstruction from infection, facial trauma, or a dacryolith, rarely neoplasm. The medial lower lid location has a domed mass that is tender and painful, with discharge and tearing. Treatment includes hot packs with topical and systemic antibiotics for penicillinase-producing staphylococcal organisms.

Dacryoadenitis

Dacryoadenitis, an enlargement of the lacrimal gland, may be granulomatous, lymphoid, or infectious in origin. If acute, this lesion is painful, tender, suppurative, and inflamed; if chronic, it may manifest simply as a swollen, hard mass. Treatment of dacryoadenitis is determined by its etiology and ranges from supportive heat therapy and massage to incision and drainage, followed by the use of systemic antibiotics and, if not responsive, by steroids.

Orbit

Preseptal (periorbital) and postseptal (orbital) cellulitis are bacterial infections of the periocular tissue that are serious and potentially vision-threatening and lethal. Preseptal cellulitis involves only the lid structures and periorbital tissues anterior to the orbital septum. Postseptal cellulitis involves tissue behind the septum, which children and adolescents have more commonly than adults. Routes of infection include trauma, bacteremia, upper respiratory infection and sinusitis. Cellulitis should be considered in every patient with swelling of the eye (see Chapter 40). Critical signs include pain, fever, erythema, tenderness, swelling, and conjunctival injection. With postseptal infection, impaired ocular motility, an afferent pupillary defect, proptosis, and visual loss also occur. Cavernous sinus thrombosis may develop. Leukocytosis is usually present, and a peripheral white blood cell count of more than 15,000/mm^3 suggests bacteremia. Sinus radiographs, computed tomography (CT), and orbital ultrasonography are indicated and are often positive in such cases.

Treatment of children age 5 and under has been directed toward the most common pathogen, *Haemophilus influenzae* type B (HiB), although since the introduction of a vaccine for young infants in 1990 there has been about a 90% decrease in the incidence of HiB infections. A bacterial pathogen is identified as the cause of periorbital cellulitis in only 30% of cases.

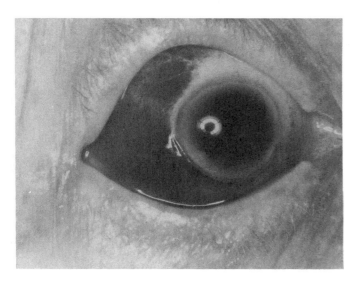

Fig. 71.1. Subjunctival hemorrhage, right eye.

longed sunlight and exposure to heat, wind, and dust contribute to its formation.[6] It may be unsightly and uncomfortable, and it may interfere with vision. Medical treatment is ineffective, and primary excision, with addition of a radiomimetic or chemotherapeutic agent intra- or postoperatively, may be necessary, but recurrence is common.[7]

Lacrimal System

Epiphora

Epiphora is a condition in which tearing occurs because of either hypersecretion or impaired drainage of tears through the lacrimal passages. Causes include muscle weakness, allergy, ectropion, occlusive scarring, glaucoma, dacryocystitis, can-aliculitis, and inflammation.[8] In infancy, it is usually due to congenital nasolacrimal duct obstruction, which has a high rate of spontaneous reservation during the first year. Nasolacrimal duct probing can usually be deferred until after the age of 1 year.[9]

Dry Eye

The tear film is a complex, delicately balanced fluid composed of contributions from a series of glands. Alacrima, decreased or absent tears, occurs with keratoconjunctivitis sicca, associated with the autoimmune systemic complex of Sjögren syndrome, most frequently from rheumatoid arthritis or thyroid diseases (see Chapters 113 and 121). Other causes of dry eye can be blepharospasm, blepharitis, allergies, systemic medications, and toxins.[10] Tear film deficiency also causes nonspecific symptoms of burning, foreign-body sensation, photophobia, itching, and a "gritty" sensation. Physical findings include hyperemia, loss of the usual glossy appearance of the cornea, and a convex tear meniscus less than 0.3 mm in height. The Schirmer and rose bengal test results do not have a significant association with symptoms.[10] Treatment is difficult and lifelong with artificial tears (Lacril, Tears Natural, Thera

If there is an associated local wound, the infection pathogen is most likely *S. aureus* or *Streptococcus pyogenes*.[11]

In older children and adults, treatment must cover staphylococcus, streptococcus, anaerobes, and sometimes fungal infections. Antimicrobial therapy should also provide coverage for the pathogens most commonly associated with sinusitis. A third-generation cephalosporin (Cefizox, Claforan, Rocephin), penicillinase-resistant penicillin (Staphcillin), and clindamycin (Cleocin) intravenously provide excellent coverage for the most likely pathogens.[12] Emergency consultation should be obtained from both an ophthalmologist and an otolaryngologist.

Retina

Various retinal problems are presented to the family physician. Diagnostic criteria are important to direct appropriate referral and care.

Arterial Occlusive Retinal Disease

Central and branch retinal artery occlusions (CRAOs, BRAOs) must be recognized. CRAO is a severe sudden loss of vision due to an embolic or thrombotic occlusion, or obstruction, of the central retinal artery. It is considered an ocular emergency, usually painless, and is always monocular. Occasionally it is preceded by symptoms of amaurosis fugax, lasting 5 to 20 minutes. A cherry red spot is often seen in the central macula (Fig. 71.2). Treatment consists of immediate decompression of the eye by pharmacologic or surgical intervention.

The BRAO is a painless, less severe, more peripheral embolic phenomenon in the retinal arterial circulation, where an immediate blank or dark area is noted in the patient's visual field. It is almost always monocular. Treatment is based on finding the source of the problem. A thorough diagnostic evaluation is needed to rule out carotid plaques, carotid valvular disease, and temporal arteritis.[13]

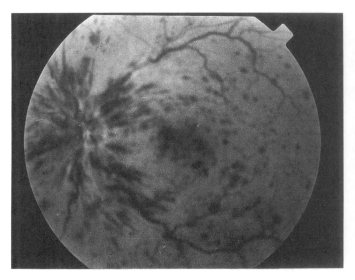

Fig. 71.3. Central retinal vein occlusion.

Venous Occlusive Retinal Disease

Central and branch retinal vein occlusions (CRVOs, BRVOs) must be diagnosed. A CRVO presents as a sudden loss of vision secondary to compression of the venous return by a retinal arterial, causing thrombosis at that location. If an occlusion occurs at the optic nerve head, it is a CRVO; if it is seen more peripherally, it is a BRVO. The CRVO is diagnosed by the presence of flame-shaped and blot hemorrhages throughout the entire retinal field, often obscuring the view of the underlying retina (Fig. 71.3). If it is nonischemic, antiplatelet therapy is used (i.e., aspirin). If it is ischemic, laser photocoagulation is used to prevent conversion to neovascular glaucoma.

A BRVO causes less severe visual loss, often not noticed by the patient. It leads to stasis of the venous flow more peripherally, which if it involves the macula causes central loss of vision. Here again, a flame-shaped hemorrhage is present upon examination. Laser therapy is needed only if macular edema is persistent over 3 months.[14–16]

Retinal Detachment

Several epidemiologic studies have found the annual incidence of retinal detachment at about 1:10,000. The life prevalence is approximately 0.7%, but for people with high myopia it is 5%; it occurs most commonly between the ages of 40 and 80 years. A frequent symptom of detachment is a gray curtain or cloud covering a portion of the visual field. These symptoms may be preceded by a quick flash of light, occurring in an arc-type fashion, across the peripheral field of vision; it lasts for a second or two with a new onset of many small black floaters. On physical examination with a dilated pupil, one sees a corrugated bulbous elevation of the retina. If a detachment can be surgically repaired immediately, prior to a macular detachment, the resulting visual acuity is much better.

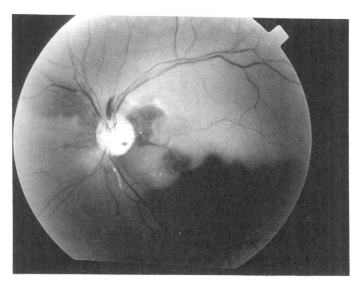

Fig. 71.2. Central retinal artery occlusion.

Diabetic Retinopathy

Early detection of diabetic retinopathy is important. Diabetics should have regular ophthalmologic examinations (see Chapter 120).

Nonproliferative Diabetic Retinopathy

Nonproliferative diabetic retinopathy is graded as mild, moderate, or severe. With the more severe retinopathy, cotton wool spots are present, and dot and blot hemorrhages and lipid accumulation are seen throughout the retina (Fig. 71.4). If there is thickening of the retina in the central macular zone, diabetic macular edema is present and can cause profound visual loss. If macular ischemia is not present, laser can be helpful for stabilizing, and in some cases improving, visual function.

Proliferative Diabetic Retinopathy

Proliferative diabetic retinopathy is diagnosed when a neovascularization is detected at the optic nerve or elsewhere in the retina. It poses a risk of retinal hemorrhage, tractional retinal detachment, fibroglial proliferation, and retinal fibrosis. With a dilated pupil, a lacy network of fine vessels is seen, indicating retinal ischemia (Figs. 71.5 and 71.6). Panretinal photocoagulation (PRP) eliminates the mid-peripheral retina. PRP may cause some night and central vision loss but prevents progressive severe visual loss.[17–20]

Amaurosis Fugax

Amaurosis fugax is the sudden, painless, monocular loss of vision, described as a curtain or a shade being pulled down or up, blanketing the field of vision. It totally resolves in 5 to 30 minutes. A cholesterol plaque in the carotid artery, or rarely, a calcific cardiac valvular condition, is the etiology. Treatment is directed toward anticoagulation or antiplatelet therapy. Based on the patient's risk threshold, surgical intervention, such as carotid endarterectomy,[21] is undertaken.

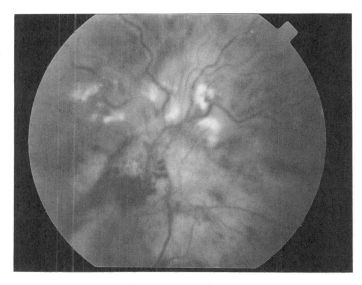

Fig. 71.5. Proliferative diabetic retinopathy.

Ocular Migraine

Ocular migraine is a common condition in individuals over age 40. It presents often as a migraine aura, a fortification scotoma of jagged, multicolored lights that expand in a gradual fashion across the entire field of vision, leaving in its wake a darker or blank scotoma (see Chapter 63). Often associated with the migraine symptoms is a queasy feeling. If the episode lasts longer than 1 hour, the diagnosis is in question. The eye examination at the time is entirely normal. Treatment is optional and is based primarily on the frequency and severity of the visual event. Multiple prophylactic agents, including beta-blockers (Inderal, Tenormin), are effective. Neuroimaging may also be considered if the symptoms are not classic or the duration exceeds 1 hour.[22]

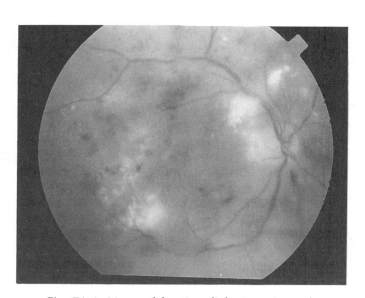

Fig. 71.4. Nonproliferative diabetic retinopathy.

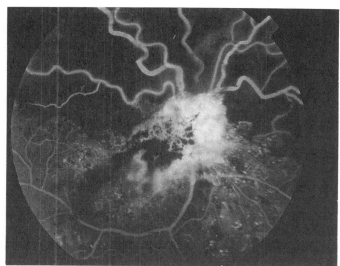

Fig. 71.6. Angiogram of proliferative diabetic retinopathy.

Macular Degeneration

Macular degeneration is an aging phenomenon of the inner retina that results in visual loss due to deterioration of the retinal photoreceptors. There are two types of macular degeneration: dry and wet.

Dry Age-Related Macular Degeneration

Dry age-related macular degeneration presents with slow visual loss in the central field of vision. Often the first signs are reduced reading vision and later scotoma in the central field of vision as the severity increases. There is a loss of photoreceptor function in the central macular zone (Fig. 71.7).

Wet Age-Related Macular Degeneration

Wet age-related macular degeneration presents with sudden visual loss and hemorrhage in the central macular zone. The underlying retinal develops a defect, allowing the choroidal vessels to grow through the retinal pigment epithelium (Fig. 71.8). The patient presents with a dark or distorted spot in the central field of vision. As the hemorrhage progresses, the vision deteriorates further. Any sudden change in vision of a patient with macular degeneration should result in immediate referral to an ophthalmologist, as some cases of wet age-related macular degeneration can be treated by laser therapy, depending on the size and location of the retinal neovascularization.[23]

Retinopathy of Prematurity

Retinopathy of prematurity (ROP) affects thousands of infants each year, but fortunately only a small percentage become blind. When the disease becomes aggressive it is known as "plus disease," and the visual prognosis is reduced. Plus disease is a descriptive term for dilated tortuous vessels in the posterior pole of the eye. ROP can be seen in 85% to 90% of children of low birth weight when exposed to oxygen. The ability to sustain newborns of very low birth weight has brought about a resurgence of ROP despite the tight control of the partial pressure of oxygen, indicating that oxygen is not the only factor in-

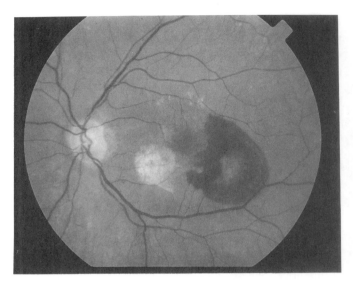

Fig. 71.8. Wet age-related macular degeneration.

volved. ROP is seen classically in infants with a birth weight of less than 1500 g. These infants should be examined 6 weeks after birth. A positive treatment effect was reported in infants found with threshold disease. Follow-up is usually necessary every 2 weeks until there is regression of the ROP. Current treatment includes retinal cryotherapy. If retinal detachment is found, progression to pars plana vitrectomy, membrane peeling, and lensectomy are usually undertaken.[24]

Optic Nerve

Optic Nerve Head Edema (Papilledema)

Optic nerve head edema, or papilledema, is a common end point for several ocular disorders that result in swelling of the optic nerve head and hemorrhage in the surrounding peripapillary retina. Bold vessel margins are often blurred as they cross over the optic nerve, and splinter hemorrhages are present, distinguishing this disorder from pseudopapilledema (Fig. 71.9). The ocular causes of papilledema include the following: optic neuritis, anterior ischemic optic neuropathy (arteritic and nonarteritic), ischemic papillitis as in diabetes, and increased intracranial pressure. When optic nerve head edema is secondary to increased intracranial pressure, it is termed papilledema. Increased intracranial pressure is often differentiated from optic neuritis on the basis of vision, as vision is always impaired with optic neuritis and usually intact with papilledema. Papilledema normally occurs in both eyes but may be asymmetric.

Pseudopapilledema

Pseudopapilledema is a benign, anomalous appearance of the optic nerve head, often seen during a normal eye examination. The optic nerve head has an elevated, lumpy appearance. No nerve fiber layer edema or splinter retinal hemorrhages are seen, as would be seen with true papilledema.

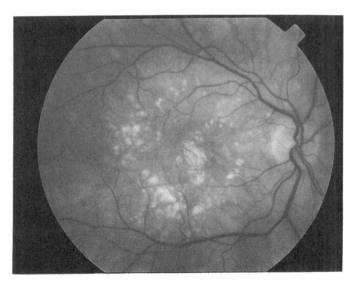

Fig. 71.7. Dry age-related macular degeneration.

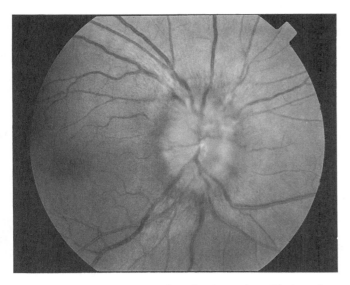

Fig. 71.9. Optic nerve head edema (papilledema).

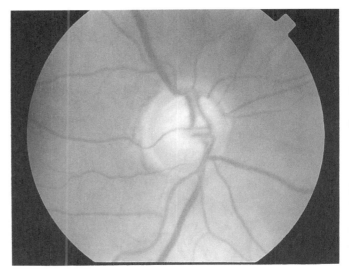

Fig. 71.10. Chronic open-angle glaucoma with loss of axons; note the centrally excavated optic cup.

Lens

Cataracts, or a clouding over of the lens of the eye, is increasingly common among our aged population in the United States. The cataract can be graded in three of the most common varieties, based on the location of the lenticular opacity.

A nuclear sclerotic cataract is hardening of the central nucleus of the lens and leads to gradual yellowing of the nucleus. With further progression, it may turn brown. Frequently this type of cataract is not appreciated at an early stage because of the gradual progression and bilateral aspect of presentation.

Cortical cataract is whitening of the peripheral lens cortex. As the opacity progresses more centrally, more visual deprivation results. Frequently people complain of glare from lights with this type of cataract. Occasionally, double vision is noted, as cortical opacity splits light into different focal points.

Posterior subcapsular cataracts are the most visually disabling and the progression can be rapid. Near vision is more impaired than distance vision. The disorder is often seen in patients on chronic steroids and those with chronic iritis or diabetes.

The diagnosis can be easily made by dilating the pupil and using the red reflex test. Examination indicators are a hazing over with a nuclear sclerotic cataract, a spoke-like defect with a cortical cataract, and a central dark opacity with a posterior subcapsular cataract. Treatment normally is surgical, but if the patient is not a surgical candidate, chronic dilation of the pupil improves the vision in some patients. Visual recovery from surgery is frequently rapid.

Glaucomas

Chronic Open-Angle Glaucoma

Chronic open-angle glaucoma (COAG) is a relatively common disorder whose incidence increases with advancing age. There

is an obstruction of aqueous outflow at the level of the trabecular meshwork. Predisposing factors include a family history of glaucoma, severe blunt trauma to the eye, and possibly high myopia. The incidence of COAG is 10% in those over age 80.

Glaucoma can occur without elevated intraocular pressure, and is diagnosed by observing damage to the optic nerve. Elevated intraocular pressure does tend to raise the risk threshold of developing glaucoma. The diagnosis is based on a triad of findings: increased intraocular pressure, optic nerve head cupping, and visual field defect. A cup/disc ratio of more than 0.60 is often a diagnostic clue, as is asymmetry between the two eyes. When a family history of glaucoma is present, or an enlarged cup-to-disc is seen, referral to an ophthalmologist is indicated (Figs. 71.10 and 71.11).

There are treatment options: pharmacologic lowering of intraocular pressure, laser trabeculoplasty to attempt to increase

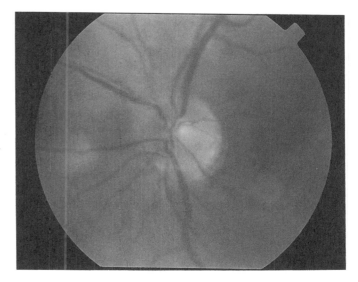

Fig. 71.11. Normal optic nerve with a healthy, nonexcavated optic cup.

the aqueous outflow, or surgical decompression of the eye by trabeculectomy.[25–27]

Angle-Closure Glaucoma

An acute angle-closure glaucoma attack is precipitated by abrupt closure in the aqueous outflow. The iris, with slight dilation, occludes the trabecular meshwork, resulting in progressively increasing pressure within the eye. The acute symptoms include pain, decreased vision, halos around lights, nausea, and vomiting. Examination reveals a cloudy or "steamy" appearance of the cornea, a nonreactive mid-dilated pupil, an area of injection around the limbus, and elevated intraocular pressure. Immediate referral to an ophthalmologist is mandatory. A laser iridotomy is often necessary, and consideration is given to performing a prophylactic laser iridotomy in the uninvolved eye.[28–30]

Oculomotor Motility

Strabismus

Strabismus is commonly defined as a deviation of the visual axis. This ocular misalignment can be found at almost any age. Esodeviation, or esotropia, is present when either one or the other eye is nasally deviated. The cause of most infantile strabismus is unknown. The incidence of strabismus increases with low birth weight, being four times higher in infants weighing 1500 g or less. Maternal cigarette smoking of two packs per day during pregnancy increases the risk about twofold.[31]

Esotropia

Esodeviation that is present before 6 months of age is known as congenital esotropia; if it is found later, it is termed acquired esotropia. The treatment of esotropia is based on first correcting any refractive disorder, patching for amblyopia if present, and, lastly, surgically realigning the eyes. Visual outcome is best when the problem is diagnosed early.[32]

Exotropia

Exodeviation, or exotropia, is the turning out of the eye. It may be diagnosed at any age. At birth most infants have a small degree of exotropia that resolves during the first few months of life. Treatment is similar to that for esotropia, although at surgery the lateral rectus muscle is weakened.[33]

Amblyopia

Amblyopia is defined as a poorly sighted eye secondary to some form of visual deprivation at an early age, normally younger than 6 to 7 years. The earlier it occurs, the more severe is the amblyopia. The most prevalent form of amblyopia is seen in association with strabismus. Treatment for amblyopia must be completed by age 7 or 8.

Strabismus produces amblyopia by preventing stimulation in the fovea of the deviated eye. Occasionally, the diagnosis is made using a red reflex test with a direct ophthalmic scope held about 3 feet from the child's eyes. A difference in the red reflex may indicate a refractive error, amblyopia, or an opacity in the ocular media.

Anisometropia, a difference in the refractive status between the eyes, often causes amblyopia. Fortunately, most cases of anisometropic amblyopia involve only mild defocusing and is often corrected with glasses or, more rarely, contact lenses. Treatment of amblyopia is aimed at restoring the suppressed visual input by occluding the more favored eye with a patch, colored lenses, or pharmacologic intervention.[34]

Optical Defects

Refractive Disorders

A refractive disorder is simply "an eyeball out of focus" because the focal point does not fall on the retina. Technologic advances over the last several years, namely in the form of the excimer laser has produced safe and accurate correction of refractive disorder. Laser-assisted in situ keratomileusis (LASIK) is the most common refractive procedure performed today. In LASIK a corneal flap is fashioned with a mechanical keratome. Once the flap is lifted, the excimer laser is used to abate the underlying corneal stroma in a computer-controlled fashion to connect the "optics" of the eye. Recovery is usually within days to weeks. Complications, although rare, include under- and overcorrections, flap-related mishaps, and infection.[35]

Accommodation Loss, or Presbyopia

Accommodation, the ability to adjust the optic power of the eye, decreases from childhood to about age 75. For example, at age 10 there are 10 diopters of accommodation, and at age 45 there are about 3.5 diopters of accommodation. In the normal human eye, as accommodation occurs the ciliary body contracts, relaxing the zonules (or fibers) to the lens of the eye, and an active increase in lens curvature occurs, increasing the optical power of the eye. As the eye ages, hardening (sclerosis) of the lens reduces the elasticity of the lens capsule and plasticity of the lens core, resulting in a loss of accommodative amplitude. To correct this loss reading glasses are prescribed, progressively increasing in power from age 45 up to age 75.

References

1. Newell FW. Ophthalmology: principles and concepts, 8th ed. St. Louis: Mosby, 1996;149–183.
2. Carter SR. Eyelid disorders: diagnosis and management. Am Fam Physician 1998;57:2695–702.
3. Wishert K. Diagnosing the most frequent eyelid conditions. Practitioner 1998;242:844–50.
4. Leaderman C, Miller M. Hordeola and chalazia. Pediatr Rev 1999;20:283–4.
5. Friedlander MH. Contact dermatitis. In: Fraunfelder FT, Roy FH, eds. Current ocular therapy. Philadelphia: WB Saunders, 2000;144–5.

6. Threlfall TJ. Sun exposure and pterygium of the eye: a dose-response curve. Am J Ophthalmol 1999;128:280–1.

7. Sharma S. Ophthalmic problems: pterygium. Can Fam Physician 1999;45:607–16.

8. Malhotra R, Olver JM. Diagrammatic representation of lacrimal disease. Eye 2000;14:358–63.

9. Maini R, MacEwen CJ, Young JD. The natural history of epiphora in childhood. Eye 1998;12:669–71.

10. Schein OD, Hochberg MC, Munoz B, et al. Dry eye and dry mouth in the elderly. Arch Intern Med 1999;159:1359–63.

11. Ambati BK, Azar N, Stratton L, Schmidt EV. Periorbital and orbital cellulitis before and after the advent of *Haemophilus influenzae* type B vaccination. Ophthalmology 2000;107:1450–3.

12. Barone SR, Aiuto LT. Periorbital and orbital cellulites in the *Haemphilus influenzae* vaccine era. J Pediatr Ophthalmol Strabismus 1997;34:293–6.

13. Brown GC. Retinal arterial obstructive disease. In: Ryan SJ. editor-in-chief. Retina, vol 2: medical retina. St. Louis: Mosby, 1989;403–20.

14. Amirikia A, Scott IU, Murray TG, Flynn HW Jr, Smiddy WE, Feuer WJ. Outcomes of vitreoretinal surgery for complications of branch retinal vein occlusion. Ophthalmology 2001;108(2):372–6.

15. Hattenbach LO, Steinkamp G, Scharrer I, Ohrloff C. Fibrinolytic therapy with low-dose recombinant tissue plasminogen activator in retinal vein occlusion. Ophthalmologica 1998;212(6):394–8.

16. Sperduto RD, Hiller R, Chew E, et al. Risk factors for hemiretinal vein occlusion: comparison with risk factors for central and branch retinal vein occlusion: the eye disease case-control study. Ophthalmology 1999;106(3):439–40.

17. Smiddy WE, Flynn HW Jr. Vitrectomy in the management of diabetic retinopathy. Surv Ophthalmol 1999;43:491–507.

18. Chakrabarti S, Cukiernik M, Hileeto D, Evans T, Chen S. Role of vasoactive factors in the pathogenesis of early changes in diabetic retinopathy. Diabetes Metab Res Rev 2000;16(6):393–407.

19. Antonetti DA, Lieth E, Barber AJ, Gardner TW. Molecular mechanisms of vascular permeability in diabetic retinopathy. Semin Ophthalmol 1999;14(4):240–8.

20. Cunha-Vas JG. Diabetic retinopathy: surrogate outcomes for drug development for diabetic retinopathy. Ophthalmologica 2000;214(6):377–80.

21. Purvin VA. Amaurosis fugax of carotid origin. Focal Points 1992;10(7):1–7.

22. Glaser JS. Topical diagnosis: prechiasmal visual pathways. In: Tasman W, ed. Duane's clinical ophthalmology, rev. ed. Philadelphia: Lippincott, 1991;1–12.

23. Bressler SB. Age-related macular degeneration. Focal Points 1995;12(2 section 2):1–9.

24. Patz A, Palmer EA. Retinopathy of prematurity. In: Ryan SJ, editor-in-chief. Retina, vol 2: medical retina. St. Louis: Mosby, 1989;509–30.

25. Hart WM. The epidemiology of primary open-angle glaucoma and ocular hypertension. In: Ritch R, Shields MB, Krupin T, eds. The glaucomas. St. Louis: Mosby, 1989;789–95.

26. Werner EB. Low-tension glaucoma. In: Ritch R, Shields MB, Krupin T, eds. The glaucomas. St. Louis: Mosby, 1989;797–811.

27. Johnstone MA. Primary open-angle glaucoma: a therapeutic overview. In: Ritch R, Shields MB, Krupin T, eds. The glaucomas. St. Louis: Mosby, 1989;813–21.

28. Lowe RF, Ritch R. Angle-closure glaucoma: mechanisms and epidemiology. In: Ritch R, Shields MB, Krupin T, eds. The glaucomas. St. Louis: Mosby, 1989;825–37.

29. Lowe RF, Ritch R. Angle-closure glaucoma: clinical types. In: Ritch R, Shields MB, Krupin T, eds. The glaucomas. St. Louis: Mosby, 1989;839–53.

30. Ritch R, Lowe RF, Reyes A. Therapeutic overview of angle-closure glaucoma. In: Ritch R, Shields MB, Krupin T, eds. The glaucomas. St. Louis: Mosby, 1989;855–64.

31. Chew E, Remalay NA, Tamboli A, Zhao J, Podgor MJ, Klebanoff M. Risk factors for esotropia and exotropia. Arch Ophthalmol 1994;112:1349–55.

32. Archer SM. Esotropia. Focal Points 1994;12(12 section 3):1–8.

33. Stollers SH, Simon JW, Lininger LL. Bilateral lateral rectus recession for exotropia: a survival analysis. J Pediatr Ophthalmol Strabismus 1994;31:89–92.

34. Lambert SR, Boothe RG. Amblyopia: basic and clinical science perspectives. Focal Points 1994;12(8 section 2):1–7.

35. Updegraff SA, Kritzinger MS. Laser in situ keratomileusis technique. Curr Opin Ophthalmol 2000;11(4):267–72.

72
Otitis Media and Externa

William F. Miser

Otitis Media

Otitis media is the most common reason for medical office visits (over 20 million a year) and for surgery in children in the United States.[1-3] The peak incidence occurs between the ages of 6 and 15 months, with a second peak at age 5 years.[4] Nearly two thirds of children have at least one episode of otitis media by their first birthday, and more than 90% have one by age 2 years.[2,3] The diagnosis of otitis media is the most common reason for antibiotic prescriptions in children.[5] Nearly $5 billion is spent each year in the United States in managing otitis media.[6,7] This cost does not take into account the disruption of child-care arrangements and work schedules, and the generation of parental anxiety and stress.[8] Despite its frequency and associated costs, controversy exists about its proper management.

Definitions

Otitis media refers to inflammation of the middle ear, which is often associated with a middle-ear effusion.[9] *Acute otitis media* (AOM) is an infection of the middle ear with rapid appearance of symptoms and signs such as fever, pain, irritability, and abnormal appearance (erythematous, bulging) of and decreased mobility of the tympanic membrane. *Otitis media with effusion* (OME), also known as "serous otitis media" and/or "glue ear," is a middle-ear effusion without the obvious signs of an acute infection. If this effusion persists for longer than 4 months, it is known as *chronic otitis media with effusion* (COME). *Persistent acute otitis media* is the persistence of symptoms and signs of AOM following at least two courses of antibiotic therapy, whereas *recurrent acute otitis media* is three or more separate episodes of AOM in a 6-month time span, or four or more episodes in a year.[10] *Chronic suppurative otitis media* is an infection of the middle ear resulting in a perforated tympanic membrane with purulent discharge (otorrhea).

Pathophysiology

Dysfunction of the eustachian tube, which allows reflux of bacteria and fluid from the nasopharynx into the middle ear space, contributes to the development of AOM.[3] Children are more prone to AOM because their eustachian tubes are shorter, more flexible, and inefficient at clearing secretions. Over 70% of painful ear episodes develop during a viral upper respiratory infection, which magnifies eustachian tube dysfunction.[3,11] Other major risk factors for AOM include craniofacial abnormalities (e.g., cleft palate), cigarette smoking in the home, exposure to large numbers of children (e.g., day care), and family history of frequent AOM.[12,13] It also appears that prolonged use of a pacifier, especially past age 2 years, increases the risk.[14] Breast-feeding for at least 6 months appears to be protective.[15]

In a recent study of children with AOM, middle ear fluid obtained by tympanocentesis revealed that 41% had a viral cause.[16] The most common virus was respiratory syncytial virus. The most common bacterial causes for AOM were *Streptococcus pneumoniae* (25%), *Haemophilus influenzae* (23%), and *Branhamella catarrhalis* (15%). Both bacteria and viruses were isolated in 65% of children.

Diagnosis

It is commonly accepted that AOM is overdiagnosed in the United States.[8,17] A squirming, uncooperative toddler with an ear canal occluded with cerumen seen by a busy clinician who wants to please anxious parents, often will err on the side of making a diagnosis of AOM based on history alone. Diagnostic uncertainty is as high as 33% to 42%.[18,19]

The diagnosis of AOM is based on a combination of symptoms and physical findings. Typically, symptoms are nonspecific and include fever, earache, tugging or rubbing of the ear, irritability, muffled or diminished hearing, lethargy, anorexia, vomiting, and/or diarrhea.[3] However, these symptoms need not always be present.[20]

An accurate diagnosis of AOM requires a clear and well-illuminated view of the tympanic membrane. Any cerumen obstructing the view should be gently removed with a curette. The use of a cerumenolytic with warm irrigation may be necessary to remove excessive cerumen. The light of the otoscope should work well; bulbs for most otoscopes should be changed every 2 years.[17]

Four characteristics of the tympanic membrane should be evaluated—position, mobility, degree of translucency, and color. The "normal" tympanic membrane is in a neutral position (not retracted or bulging), responds well to positive and negative pressure, and is translucent and pearly gray.[17] Pneumatic otoscopy allows for the evaluation of mobility of the tympanic membrane. If used, the ear speculum should create an air seal against the external auditory canal. A soft rubber sleeve over the speculum usually reduces the discomfort of this exam.[17]

Tympanometry and acoustic reflectometry are tools useful in confirming the presence of a middle ear effusion. Tympanometry is portable and useful in the office by providing information about the actual pressures within the middle ear space.[17] An abnormal, "flat" (type B) tympanogram in infants with acute symptoms strongly suggests AOM, although a normal test is not helpful in ruling out the diagnosis.[3]

Each of the physical findings of the tympanic membrane alone is inadequate to confirm the diagnosis of AOM. In one study, only two thirds of patients with a red tympanic membrane and 16% with a slightly red tympanic membrane had AOM.[3] Erythema of the tympanic membrane can be due to fever, crying, or cerumen removal. However, combining the findings on exam is useful. Typically, a bulging or cloudy tympanic membrane with or without erythema, middle ear effusion, and marked decrease or absence of tympanic membrane mobility is nearly 100% predictive of AOM.[3] Perforation of the tympanic membrane with purulent drainage is also diagnostic of AOM.

To avoid unnecessary antibiotic treatment, it is important to distinguish between AOM and OME, which is sometimes difficult to do. Middle-ear effusion and a decrease in, or absence of, tympanic-membrane mobility characterize both. Both will have a flat (type B) tympanogram and a "plugged ear" feeling with conductive hearing loss. The position of the tympanic membrane in AOM is usually bulging, while it is slightly retracted or in a neutral position in OME. Unlike OME, AOM is often associated with acute symptoms (e.g., ear pain and fever) and signs (erythematous or yellow, bulging tympanic membrane). Visualization of the tympanic membrane in OME often demonstrates "bubbles" or an air-fluid level. Occasionally tympanocentesis is required to determine whether the middle effusion is infected, but there are no consensus guidelines for its routine use in the management of AOM or OME.[17]

Treatment

The management of otitis media is controversial. Results from recent studies have questioned the use of antibiotics and the length of treatment if prescribed, and the role of surgical interventions such as tympanostomy (ventilating) tubes.

Acute Otitis Media

The growing worldwide occurrence of multidrug-resistant bacteria, the uncertainty of diagnosis, and the fact that up to a third of cases of AOM are viral in origin have made popular a "wait and see" approach to the initial prescription of antibiotics, especially in many European countries. In several randomized clinical trials, antibiotics provide only a small benefit.[21–23] The natural course of uncomplicated, untreated AOM is quite favorable. In a recent meta-analysis of over 2000 children with AOM, ear pain resolved spontaneously in two thirds by 24 hours, and in 80% by day 7.[22] This study estimated that 17 children would need to be treated with antibiotics to prevent one child from having some pain after 2 days. Children treated with antibiotics are almost twice as likely to have adverse reactions such as skin rash, vomiting, or diarrhea. Minimizing the use of antibiotics in patients with AOM does not increase the risks of perforation of the tympanic membrane, hearing loss, or contralateral or recurrent AOM.[3]

Most studies do not include children younger than 2 years of age. This group appears to have a higher risk of treatment failure, persistent symptoms, and recurrent AOM.[3] However, a recent trial in this age group found that seven to eight children with AOM need to be treated with antibiotics to improve symptomatic outcome at day 4 in one child.[24] The major benefit of antibiotics was 1 day less of fever, but adverse effects were almost twice as likely compared to placebo, and there were no differences in clinical failure rates at day 11 or in the likelihood of recurrence. The authors conclude that a watchful waiting approach is also justified in this age group.

Some will argue that untreated AOM will increase the risk of mastoiditis or meningitis, although there are insufficient data to suggest that routine antibiotic use makes a difference.[3] Mastoiditis is quite rare; in one study there was only one case among 2202 children with untreated AOM.[22] It is uncertain whether the current rarity is due to widespread antibiotic use or to a change in host defenses or in virulence of the organisms.[3] Further studies will need to be done as the wait and see approach becomes more popular.

In summary, the immediate prescription of antibiotics offers some benefits, but these are balanced by the disadvantages of increased cost, drug resistance, and adverse reactions. A practical approach is to counsel parents about the options, provide pain relief to the child, and write a prescription for antibiotics, to be filled only if the child is no better in 2 to 3 days, sooner if it appears that symptoms are worsening. This watchful waiting has been shown to be feasible and acceptable to most parents, with a 76% reduction in the use of antibiotics.[23]

Antibiotics. If antibiotics are used, amoxicillin is the drug of choice for most children.[13,25] It achieves high levels in the middle ear fluid, is effective against most bacterial pathogens known to cause AOM, is inexpensive, and has a low incidence of side effects (skin rash, nausea, diarrhea). Although there are over a dozen other clinically effective antibiotics approved by the Food and Drug Administration for treating AOM (Table 72.1), none of these more expensive options has

Table 72.1. **Antibiotics for Acute Otitis Media[2,13]**

Antibiotic	Dosage[a] Adults (mg)	Dosage[a] Children (mg/kg/day)	Dosing frequency[b]	Cost[c]
Suggested primary regimen				
Amoxicillin	500	80–90	bid–tid	$–$$
Second-line treatment[d]				
Amoxicillin-clavulanate (Augmentin)	875/125	90/6.4	bid	$$$$–$$$$$
Sulfonamides				
Trimethoprim-sulfamethoxazole (Bactrim, Septra)	160/800	8 (trimethoprim)	bid	$
Erythromycin-sulfisoxazole (Pediazole)	400/1200	50 (erythromycin)	qid	$$
Cephalosporins				
1st generation				
Cefaclor (Ceclor)	500	40	tid	$$$$
2nd generation				
Cefprozil (Cefzil)	250–500	30	bid	$$$$
Cefuroxime axetil (Ceftin)	250	30	bid	$$–$$$
Loracarbef (Lorabid)	200–400	30	bid	$$$–$$$$
3rd generation				
Cefdinir (Omnicef)	600	14	qd–bid	$$$$$
Cefixime (Suprax)	400	8	qd	$$$–$$$$$
Cefpodoxime (Vantin)	200	10	qd–bid	$$$$
Ceftibuten (Cedax)	400	9	qd	$$$$$
Ceftriaxone (IM)[d] (Rocephin)	—	50	qd	$$$$$
Macrolides				
Clarithromycin (Biaxin)	250	15	qd	$$$$$
Azithromycin (Zithromax)	500 mg day 1 250 mg days 2–5	10 mg day 1 5 mg day 2–5	qd	$$–$$$

[a]Do not exceed adult doses in children weighing more than 40 kg. Initial therapy is for 5 days; duration is 10–14 days for treatment failures or recurrence.
[b]qd = once a day; bid = twice a day; tid = three times a day; qid = four times a day.
[c]Cost for therapeutic course based on average wholesale price from 2000 *Drugs Topics Red Book*; prices for generic drugs were used when available; $ = $0–$15; $$ = $16–$30; $$$ = $31–$45; $$$$ = $46–$60; $$$$$ = greater than $60.
[d]See text for further information.

been shown to be more effective for empiric therapy of uncomplicated AOM.[25] Rather, these other antibiotics are good alternatives for those known to be allergic to amoxicillin, to have a more severe clinical course, or to have a treatment failure, defined as no clinical improvement after 2 to 3 days or recurrence of AOM within 2 weeks of therapy.[13] Oral antihistamine-decongestant preparations offer no additional advantage when given with antibiotics, and are no more effective than placebo in decreasing the middle ear effusion.[2]

Amoxicillin is normally given at 40 to 45 mg/kg/day divided into two or three doses daily. There is recent in vitro evidence, and some clinical experience, of increasing penicillin-resistant *Streptococcus pneumoniae*. This resistance is more common in children younger than 2 years of age, especially those in a day-care setting, and in those with recurrent bouts of AOM or who have recently been treated for AOM.[10] As such, a working group of the Centers for Disease Control and Prevention advised a doubling of the amoxicillin dose to 80 to 90 mg/kg/day.[26] For those children who show no improvement with this increased dose in 3 to 5 days, alternatives such as amoxicillin-clavulanate (Augmentin), cefurox-

ime axetil (Ceftin), or intramuscular ceftriaxone (Rocephin) should be tried. Unfortunately, the two former antibiotics rate lowest on palatability and compliance,[27] and the latter requires two to three injections over 2 to 3 days. Although more expensive, third-generation cephalosporins are better tolerated and offer good options for amoxicillin treatment failures. Children with amoxicillin failure who develop a new episode of AOM more than 90 days later may still be treated with amoxicillin as the first choice.[28]

Duration of Therapy. There is strong evidence that 5 days of antibiotic therapy is just as effective as the traditional 10- to 14-day regimen for uncomplicated AOM in children.[29–31] Although the 5-day regimen has a slightly higher risk of treatment failure at a 1-month follow-up compared to the longer course, there appears to be no difference in long-term (2 to 3 months) outcome.[30] A minimum of 17 children would need to be treated with the longer course of antibiotics to avoid one treatment failure.[31] These studies exclude children with underlying disease, a recent bout of AOM, recurrent or chronic OM, craniofacial abnormalities (e.g., cleft palate), or a perforated tympanic membrane. It is recommended that these children be treated with the longer regimen. Most studies also exclude children younger than 2 years of age, although one recent trial demonstrated that the 10-day regimen has a slightly better success rate initially than the 5-day course (92% vs. 84%), with no difference in clinical success 4 to 6 weeks later.[32] In summary, the duration of therapy should be individualized, and most children with uncomplicated AOM can be treated with a shortened 5-day course.

Pain Relief. Analgesia is an important adjunct to therapy. Acetaminophen 10 to 15 mg/kg every 4 to 6 hours or ibuprofen 5 to 10 mg/kg every 6 to 8 hours is effective in relieving pain.[33] Occasionally, codeine is needed for severe pain. Topical analgesia with antipyrine, benzocaine and glycerin (e.g., Auralgan Otic) every 1 to 2 hours effectively relieves pain and congestion within 30 minutes of administration, but should be avoided if the tympanic membrane has ruptured.[33] Occasionally, pain is so severe that referral is needed to an otolaryngologist for relief of pressure with tympanocentesis or myringotomy.

Surgery. As initial therapy, tympanocentesis offers no advantage to antibiotics alone in treating AOM.[34] It should be reserved for those who appear septic, who have persistent AOM unresponsive to multiple courses of antibiotics, or who have a complex anatomic or immunologic abnormality.

Recurrent AOM

About one in five children have recurrent AOM.[8] Antibiotic prophylaxis has been shown to be at least as effective as, if not more effective than, tympanostomy tubes in preventing new episodes.[35] Prophylactic doses are normally half of that required for treatment of AOM. In a large meta-analysis, antibiotic prophylaxis reduced the frequency of new episodes of AOM by 44%.[36] Amoxicillin (20 mg/kg/day in one or two doses) or sulfisoxazole (75 mg/kg/day in one or two doses) is an effective prophylactic antibiotic. In the past, 3 to 6 months of therapy was suggested for prophylaxis. However, because of increasing antimicrobial resistance, it is now recommended that therapy should begin at the first sign of an upper respiratory infection, and should continue for 10 days.[37] In addition to prophylactic antibiotics, it is important to modify known risk factors (e.g., encourage and help parents to quit smoking).

Since *S. pneumoniae* is the leading bacterial cause of otitis media, it is thought that the recent approval of the pneumococcal vaccine Prevnar (Wyeth-Ayerst Labs, Philadelphia, PA) will decrease the occurrence of otitis media. This vaccine is associated with a 6% reduction in the number of episodes of AOM, and a 9% reduction in the frequency of recurrent AOM.[7] Although not as dramatic a decline as hoped, routine vaccination of all children will prevent up to 1.2 million episodes of AOM in the United States each year. Influenza virus vaccination is also recommended for those prone to frequent AOM during the respiratory season.[25]

For those children who have severe and recurrent disease, consider referral to an otolaryngologist for placement of tympanostomy tubes. Concomitant adenoidectomy is commonly performed in the United States, but recent evidence questions its effectiveness, and suggests that it should not be considered as a first surgical intervention in children whose only indication is recurrent AOM.[38]

Chronic Suppurative Otitis Media

Purulent material should be removed by suctioning under direct visualization, or by gently using a cotton swab. Since the tympanic membrane is often ruptured, avoid flushing the ear canal, which may damage the inner ear with resultant hearing loss. Topical treatment with ofloxacin otic solution, 3 mg/mL, five drops twice daily for 10 days, has a similar cure rate to systemic amoxicillin-clavulanate and is better tolerated.[2,39,40]

Chronic Otitis Media with Effusion (COME)

Children who recover from AOM often have a residual middle ear effusion for up to 6 weeks after treatment. In 20% of these children, this effusion persists and there is concern that over time it will result in mild-to-moderate conductive hearing loss with subsequent impairment in language development and academic functioning.[8,41,42]

Initial management for COME is observation. A meta-analysis found that antibiotics offer only a marginal short-term benefit, and no long-term benefit.[36] The use of corticosteroids (prednisone or prenisolone, 1 mg/kg/day in two divided doses for 7 days) has been advised in the past,[8] but a recent study found only marginal short-term benefit in resolution of the effusion, and no long-term benefit in preventing hearing loss.[42]

If the effusion persists for longer than 4 months, the clinical practice guideline developed by the Agency for Health Care Policy and Research recommends a hearing test; if there is evidence of documented bilateral hearing impairment of 20 dB or more, tympanostomy tubes should be considered in children younger than 3 years of age.[43] Myringotomy with insertion of tympanostomy tubes is the most common operation among children beyond the newborn period in the United States.[44] It is thought that surgical resolution of the effusion will restore normal hearing and thereby prevent language and behavioral problems.

However, recent studies have suggested that the benefit from immediate insertion of tympanostomy tubes may not be as great as once thought.[44,45] Compared to watchful waiting, the insertion of tympanostomy tubes improves hearing at 6 months, but this difference disappears by 1 year.[46] In addition, there is relatively little difference in expressive or comprehensive language,[45] developmental behavior,[44] or in quality of life[47] between watchful waiting and insertion of tubes.

Children who undergo placement of tympanostomy tubes require ongoing surveillance. Showering, rinsing the hair, or submersion of the head in plain tap water or in a pool does not promote the entry of water into the middle ear.[48] As such, earplugs are not indicated for routine bathing or swimming, but are needed for deeper swimming or diving. Sequelae of tympanostomy tubes are common but generally transient.[49] Otorrhea occurs in up to 16% in the postoperative period, with 4% experiencing chronic drainage.[50] Cosmetic complications include tympanosclerosis (32%), focal atrophy (25%), and chronic perforation (17%) with long-term use.[50] The clinical implications of these changes are unknown, but this information is useful when counseling parents prior to referral to an otolaryngologist. Clearly, further long-term studies need to be conducted before abandoning the role of tympanostomy tubes in treating COME.

Some children who undergo tympanostomy tube placement for COME also benefit from concomitant adenoidectomy.[41] In one recent study, adenoidectomy or adenotonsillectomy at the time of initial insertion of tympanostomy tubes substantially reduced the likelihood of additional hospitalizations or further surgeries.[1] Eight adjuvant adenoidectomies need to be performed to avoid a single instance of rehospitalization over a 2-year period. For now these surgeries should be reserved for special cases not responding to tympanostomy tube insertion.

Otitis Externa

Otitis externa is an inflammatory process involving the external auditory canal. Cerumen normally acts as a defense against infection by creating an acidic environment that inhibits bacterial and fungal growth, and by preventing water from penetrating to the skin and causing maceration.[51] The most common precipitants for otitis externa are trauma to the ear canal (e.g., mechanical removal of cerumen by cotton swabs or other instruments, insertion of foreign objects such as fingernails or hearing aids), excessive moisture that raises the pH and removes the cerumen (e.g., swimming, diving, high humidity, perspiration), and chronic dermatologic conditions (e.g., eczema, seborrheic dermatitis).[51,52] Because otitis externa is most commonly found in persons involved in water sports, it is also known as "swimmer's ear."

The infectious agents of otitis externa are usually polymicrobial,[53] with *Pseudomonas aeruginosa* (40–60%) and *Staphylococcus aureus* (15–30%) being most common.[40,51,52,54] In about 10% of cases, fungi are involved (*Aspergillus* 80–90%, and *Candida*). Noninfectious causes of external otitis involve skin conditions such as psoriasis, seborrheic dermatitis, atopic dermatitis, lupus erythematosus, acne, and contact dermatitis.

Diagnosis

Patients with otitis externa typically present with ear discomfort varying from mild itching to severe pain associated with gentle traction of the external ear or with chewing. The ear canal is usually tender, erythematous, and swollen, with a foul-smelling discharge. The otorrhea and swelling often obscures the tympanic membrane, making it difficult to exclude an accompanying otitis media with perforation. In younger children, it is important to look for a foreign body that may be the inciting event.

Treatment

The treatment of otitis externa consists of removing the debris and draining the infection, controlling the pain, reestablishing the normal acidic environment, and using topical antimicrobials if needed.[52] If possible, the ear canal should be cleansed by suctioning under direct visualization with a 5- or 7-French Frazier malleable tip attached to low suction.[51] Alternatively, liquid debris may be gently removed using a cot-

Table 72.2. **Topical Agents Commonly Used to Treat Otitis Externa**[40,51,56]

Agent	Advantages	Precautions

2% Acetic acid otic solution (VoSol)
  + Hydrocortisone (VoSol HC Otic)
  + Aluminum acetate (Otic Domeboro)
	Inexpensive; effective against most infections; rarely causes sensitization	Occasionally irritating; possibly ototoxic

Neomycin otic solutions and suspensions
  + Polymyxin B-hydrocortisone (Cortisporin)
  + Hydrocortisone-thonzonium (Coly-Mycin S)
	Effective; generic is inexpensive	May cause contact dermatitis in up to 15% of patients; potentially ototoxic if tympanic membrane ruptured and use is for 14 days or more

Polymyxin B-hydrocortisone (Otobiotic)	Avoids potential dermatitis; also indicated for acute otitis media with perforation	Inactive against *Staphylococcus* and other gram positives

Quinolones
  Otic preparations
  + Ofloxacin 0.3% solution (Floxin Otic)
  + Ciprofloxacin 0.3% and hydrocortisone suspension (Cipro HC Otic)
  Ophthalmic solutions
  + Ofloxacin 0.3% (Ocuflox)
  + Ciprofloxacin 0.3% (Ciloxan)
	Highly effective, no local irritation, no risk of ototoxicity, twice-daily dosing; also indicated for acute otitis media with perforation, and for chronic suppurative otitis media	Expensive, potential development of resistance

Aminoglycoside ophthalmic solutions
  + Gentamicin sulfate 0.3% (Garamycin)
  + Tobramycin sulfate 0.3% (Tobrex)
	Less locally irritating	Potentially ototoxic if tympanic membrane ruptured and use is for 14 days or more; moderately expensive

ton swab with the cotton fluffed out.[51] Hydrogen peroxide may be used to soften thick or crusted debris. Do not flush the ear canal unless the tympanic membrane can be fully seen and found to be without perforation; doing so may damage the inner ear and cause hearing loss, tinnitus, and vertigo. Analgesics such as acetaminophen, a nonsteroidal antiinflammatory, and/or codeine are often required.

The first-line treatment for otitis externa is a topical antibiotic; systemic antibiotics are rarely indicated except when a concomitant acute otitis media is present or if there has been local spread of the infection (see below).[55] Simple acidification of the ear canal with 2% acetic acid is often effective, but a wide variety of other agents is available (Table 72.2). The addition of hydrocortisone may resolve symptoms more quickly by decreasing the edema of the ear canal. The most commonly used topical antibiotic in the United States is polymyxin B-neomycin-hydrocortisone (Cortisporin), although the recently available quinolone preparations have been found to be just as effective and free from ototoxic effects, and applied twice daily as opposed to the four times daily for other preparations.[40,56] Typically three to four drops are placed in the affected ear up to 3 days beyond the cessation of symptoms (usually for 5–7 days), although more severe infections may require up to 14 days of therapy. Warming the bottle of drops in the hands before installation minimizes discomfort.[51] For those times that the ear canal is quite swollen, placing a wick of quarter-inch cotton sterile gauze or using a Pope ear wick facilitates drainage and helps draw the topical medication into the affected canal.[52] This wick can usually be removed within 2 days as the edema resolves. Patients should abstain from water sports such as swimming and diving for at least 7 to 10 days, or until the symptoms have completely resolved.

Prevention

Avoid trauma (e.g., use of cotton swabs or other items used to remove cerumen) to the ear canal. For those prone to developing otitis externa (e.g., swimmers), a hair dryer set on the lowest heat setting can be used to dry the external auditory. Ear drops containing equal portions of white vinegar and rubbing alcohol or an over-the-counter preparation containing acid and alcohol (e.g., Swim Ear) is effective for prophylaxis.[56] Persons who swim frequently should use a barrier to protect their ears from water.

Necrotizing (Malignant) Otitis Externa

Necrotizing otitis externa is a severe form of external otitis with a mortality rate up to 53%.[51] Most often due to *P. aeruginosa* osteomyelitis of the mastoid or temporal bones, it affects elderly patients with diabetes mellitus, and those who are immunocompromised, especially due to human immunodeficiency (HIV) infection. Suspect this condition if pain is constant and disproportionately more severe than the clinical signs would suggest.[52] Examination of the ear canal reveals granulation tissue at the bony cartilaginous junction. Either computed tomography or magnetic resonance imaging confirms the diagnosis. Treatment should be aggressive and include intravenous antipseudomonal antibiotics initially, followed by ofloxacin 400 mg or ciprofloxacin 750 mg orally twice a day for up to 3 months. Consult an otolaryngologist to assist in the care, especially since debridement of granulation or osteitic bones may be needed.

References

1. Coyte P, Croxford R, McIsaac W, Feldman W, Friedberg J. The role of adjuvant adenoidectomy and tonsillectomy in the outcome of the insertion of tympanostomy tubes. N Engl J Med 2001;344:1188–95.
2. Albrant D. APhA drug treatment protocols: management of pediatric acute otitis media. J Am Pharm Assoc 2000;40:599–608.
3. McConaghy JR. The evaluation and treatment of children with acute otitis media. J Fam Pract 2001;50:457–65.
4. Daly K, Giebink G. Clinical epidemiology of otitis media. Pediatr Infect Dis J 2000;19:S31–6.
5. Finkelstein J, Metlay J, Davis R, Rifas-Shiman S, Dowell S, Platt R. Antimicrobial use in defined populations of infants and young children. Arch Pediatr Adolesc Med 2000;154:395–400.
6. Gates G. Cost-effectiveness considerations in otitis media treatment. Otolaryngol Head Neck Surg 1996;114:525–30.
7. Eskola J, Kilpi T, Palmu A, et al. Efficacy of a pneumococcal conjugate vaccine against acute otitis media. N Engl J Med 2001;344:403–9.
8. Berman S. Otitis media in children. N Engl J Med 1995;332:1560–5.
9. O'Neill P. Acute otitis media. BMJ 1999;319:833–5.
10. Pichichero M, Reiner S, Brook I, et al. Controversies in the medical management of persistent and recurrent acute otitis media. Recommendations of a clinical advisory committee. Ann Otol Rhinol Laryngol 2000;183(suppl):1–12.
11. Koivunen P, Konitiokari T, Niemela M, Pokka T, Uhari M. Time to development of acute otitis media during an upper respiratory infection in children. Pediatr Infect Dis J 1999;18:303–5.
12. Uhari M, Mantysaari K, Niemela M. A meta-analytic review of the risk factors for acute otitis media. Clin Infect Dis 1996;22:1079–83.
13. Block S. Strategies for dealing with amoxicillin failure in acute otitis media. Arch Fam Med 1999;8:68–78.
14. Niemela M, Pihakari O, Pokka T, Uhari M, Uhari M. Pacifier as a risk factor for acute otitis media: a randomized, controlled trial of parental counseling. Pediatrics 2000;106:483–8.
15. Heinig M. Host defense benefits of breastfeeding for the infant. Effect of breastfeeding duration and exclusivity. Pediatr Clin North Am 2001;48:105–23.
16. Heikkinen T, Thint M, Chonmaitree T. Prevalence of various respiratory viruses in the middle ear during acute otitis media. N Engl J Med 1999;340:260–4.
17. Pichichero M. Acute otitis media: part I. Improving diagnostic accuracy. Am Fam Physician 2000;61:2051–6.
18. Froom J, Culpepper L, Grob P, et al. Diagnosis and antibiotic treatment of acute otitis media: report from International Primary Care Network. BMJ 1990;300:582–6.
19. Jensen P, Lous J. Criteria, performance and diagnostic problems in diagnosing acute otitis media. Fam Pract 1999;16:262–8.
20. Heikkinen T, Ruuskanen O. Signs and symptoms predicting acute otitis media. Arch Pediatr Adolesc Med 1995;149:26–9.
21. DelMar C, Glasziou P, Hayem M. Are antibiotics indicated as initial treatment for children with acute otitis media? A meta-analysis. BMJ 1997;314:1526–9.
22. Glasziou P, DelMar C, Sanders S. Antibiotics for acute otitis media in children (Cochrane Review). The Cochrane Library, issue 3. Oxford, England: Update Software, 2000.
23. Little P, Gould C, Williamson I, Moore M, Warner G, Dunleavey J. Pragmatic randomized controlled trial of two pre-

scribing strategies for childhood acute otitis media. BMJ 2001; 322:336–42.

24. Damoiseaux R, vanBalen F, Hoes A, Verheij T, deMelker R. Primary care based randomized, double blind trial of amoxicillin versus placebo for acute otitis media in children aged under 2 years. BMJ 2000;320:350–4.

25. Klein J. Clinical implications of antibiotic resistance for management of acute otitis media. Pediatr Infect Dis J 1998;17: 1084–9.

26. Dowell S, Butler J, Giebink G, et al. Acute otitis media—management and surveillance in an era of pneumococcal resistance: a report from the Drug-Resistant *Streptococcus pneumoniae* Therapeutic Working Group (DRSPTWG). Pediatr Infect Dis J 1999;18:1–9.

27. Steele R, Thomas M, Begue R. Compliance issues related to the selection of antibiotic suspensions for children. Pediatr Infect Dis J 2001;20:1–5.

28. Hueston W, Ornstein S, Jenkins R, Wulfman J. Treatment of recurrent otitis media after a previous treatment failure. Which antibiotics work best? J Fam Pract 1999;48:43–6.

29. Pichichero M, Marsocci S, Murphy M, Hoeger W, Francis A, Green J. A prospective observational study of 5-, 7-, and 10-day antibiotic treatment for acute otitis media. Otolaryngol Head Neck Surg 2001;124:318–7.

30. Kozyrskyj A, Hildes-Ripstein E, Longstaffe S, et al. Treatment of acute otitis media with a shortened course of antibiotics—a meta-analysis. JAMA 1998;279:1736–42.

31. Kozyrskyj A, Hildes-Ripstein G, Longstaffe S, et al. Short course antibiotics for acute otitis media. Cochrane Database Syst Rev 2000(2);CD001095.

32. Cohen R, Levy C, Boucherat M, et al. Five vs. ten days of antibiotic therapy for acute otitis media in young children. Pediatr Infect Dis J 2000;19:471–3.

33. Zempsky W, Schechter N. Office-based pain management. The 15-minute consultation. Pediatr Clin North Am 2000;47:601–15.

34. Culpepper L. Tympanocentesis: to tap or not to tap. Am Fam Physician 2000;61:1987,90–2.

35. Bernard P, Stenstrom R, Feldman W, Durieux-Smith A. Randomized, controlled trial comparing long-term sulfonamide therapy to ventilation tubes for otitis media with effusion. Pediatrics 1991;88:215–22.

36. Williams R, Chalmers T, Stange K, Chalmers F, Bowlin S. Use of antibiotics in preventing recurrent acute otitis media and in treating otitis media with effusion: a meta-analytic attempt to resolve the brouhaha. JAMA 1993;270:1344–51.

37. Erramouspe J, Heyneman C. Treatment and prevention of otitis media. Ann Pharmacother 2000;34:1452–68.

38. Paradise J, Bluestone C, Colborn D, et al. Adenoidectomy and adenotonsillectomy for recurrent acute otitis media. Parallel randomized clinical trials in children not previously treated with tympanostomy tubes. JAMA 1999;282:945–53.

39. Acuin J, Smith A, Mackenzie I. Interventions for chronic suppurative otitis media. Cochrane Database Syst Rev 2000(2); CD000473.

40. Morgen N, Berke E. Topical fluoroquinolones for eye and ear. Am Fam Physician 2000;62:1870–6.

41. Gates G. Otitis media—the pharyngeal connection. JAMA 1999;282:987–9.

42. Butler C, vanderVoort J. Steroids for otitis media with effusion—a systematic review. Arch Pediatr Adolesc Med 2001;155:641–7.

43. Stool S, Berg A, Berman S, et al. Managing otitis media with effusion in young children. Quick reference guide for clinicians. AHCPR publication 94-0623. Rockville, MD: Agency for Health Care Policy and Research, Public Health Service, U.S. Department of Health and Human Services, July 1994.

44. Paradise J, Feldman H, Campbell T, et al. Effect of early or delayed insertion of tympanostomy tubes for persistent otitis media on developmental outcomes at the age of three years. N Engl J Med 2001;344:1179–87.

45. Rovers M, Straatman H, Ingels K, vanderWilt Gv, Broek Pv, Zielhuis G. The effect of ventilation tubes on language development in infants with otitis media with effusion: a randomized trial. Pediatrics 2000;106:E42.

46. Rovers M, Straatman H, Ingels K, vanderWilt G, vandenBroek P, Zielhuis G. The effect of short-term ventilation tubes versus watchful waiting on hearing in young children with persistent otitis media with effusion: a randomized trial. Ear Hear 2001; 22:191–9.

47. Rovers M, Krabbe P, Straatman H, Ingels K, vanderWilt G, Zielhuis G. Randomized controlled trial of the effect of ventilation tubes (grommets) on quality of life at age 1–2 years. Arch Dis Child 2001;84:45–9.

48. Morris M. Tympanostomy tubes: types, indications, techniques, and complications. Otolaryngol Clin North Am 1999;32:385–90.

49. Perrin J. Should we operate on children with fluid in the middle ear? N Engl J Med 2001;344:1241–2.

50. Kay D, Nelson M, Rosenfeld R. Meta-analysis of tympanostomy tube sequelae. Otolaryngol Head Neck Surg 2001;124: 374–80.

51. Sander R. Otitis externa: a practical guide to treatment and prevention. Am Fam Physician 2001;63:927–36.

52. Holten K, Gick J. Management of the patient with otitis externa. J Fam Pract 2001;50:353–60.

53. Clark W, Brook I, Bianki D, Thompson D. Microbiology of otitis externa. Otolaryngol Head Neck Surg 1997;116:23–5.

54. Halpern M, Palmer C, Seidlin M. Treatment patterns for otitis externa. J Am Board Fam Pract 1999;12:1–7.

55. Hannley M, Denneny J, Holzer S. Use of ototopical antibiotics in treating 3 common ear diseases. Otolaryngol Head Neck Surg 2000;122:934–40.

56. Schohet J, Scherger J. Which culprit is causing your patient's otorrhea? Postgrad Med 1998;104:50–5.

73
Oral Cavity

William A. Alto and Harry Colt

In May 2000, the surgeon general of the United States issued "Oral Health in America: A Report of the Surgeon General"[1] highlighting the importance of good oral health in the overall well-being of all Americans. Recent research has supported this message with identification of associations between periodontal disease and diabetes mellitus, cardiovascular diseases, and preterm birth. Clues to the timely diagnosis of systemic diseases are often found in the oral cavity. Physicians should play a leading role in the detection and prevention of oral diseases.

Oral Cancer

Approximately 30,000 new cases of oral cancer are diagnosed annually in the United States. Squamous cell cancers represent over 90% of oral malignancies. Salivary gland cancers, melanoma, Kaposi's sarcoma, lymphoma, and metastases are considerably less common.

The primary risk factor for squamous cell cancer is tobacco in any form, whether smoked or chewed. Over 75% of patients with oral squamous cell cancer smoke.[2] There is a dose-response relationship where the degree of risk corresponds to the extent of exposure. Alcohol and age are lesser risk factors. It appears that alcohol can act synergistically with tobacco and augment the risk of oral squamous cell cancer.[3]

Oral cancers are asymptomatic in early stages and may present with white or red patches, ulcers, or nodules, or with lymphadenopathy (submental, submandibular, or cervical). In advanced stages, they can cause bleeding or pain.

White oral lesions without an obvious cause are termed leukoplakia. The prevalence of leukoplakia in the general population ranges from 1% to 5%. The malignant transformation rate is approximately 5% but is considerably higher in smokers and drinkers.[3] Consequently, patients with a white patch in their mouth should have precipitants (tobacco, ill-fitting dentures, cheek biting) discontinued and return for reexami-

nation in 3 weeks. If the white patch persists, they require an oral biopsy to exclude malignancy.

Unexplained red patches are termed erythroplakia. The malignant transformation rate of erythroplakia is much higher, generally over 50%.[3] Patients with unexplained persistent erythroplakia over 3 weeks' duration clearly require biopsy. Persistent mixed red and white lesions (erythroleukoplakia) have intermediate malignant potential and also require biopsy.

Ulcerations can be aphthous, traumatic, infectious, cancerous, or secondary to systemic disease. However, if they are not resolving in 3 weeks, a biopsy is indicated.

When biopsy confirms squamous cell cancer, the treatment generally includes surgery, radiation, or a combination of the two. Prognosis is determined primarily by the time of detection. Overall, the 5-year survival rates are approximately 50%. When recognized early, survival rates are considerably better.

Family physicians, dentists, and other primary care clinicians should contribute to improving public awareness of oral cancer and the principal risk factors of tobacco and alcohol. This may contribute to a lower incidence of squamous cell cancer in their patients and earlier detection with improved survival rates. Family physicians should carefully examine patients' mouths, particularly in those who use tobacco or alcohol or are over age 40.

Aphthous Ulcers

Recurrent aphthous ulcers (RAUs), or canker sores, affect 25% of the general population. They usually first develop during childhood, adolescence, or early adulthood, and recur at variable intervals. There are three common types: RAU minor, RAU major, and herpetiform (clustered) RAU. All three types of aphthous ulcerations are located on the nonkeratinized (soft) oral mucosa, not on the hard palate or gingiva.

RAU minor comprises 80% of recurrent aphthous ulcers.

They are shallow ulcerations usually less than 1 cm in diameter with a gray pseudomembrane and an erythematous halo, which resolve spontaneously within 10 to 14 days.

RAU major consists of deeper, larger irregularly shaped ulcers up to 3 cm in diameter. Healing may take 4 weeks, occasionally leaving scarring.

Herpetiform RAU refers to numerous small clustered ulcerations, several millimeters in size. Although named for their appearance, which is suggestive of a herpes eruption, they are not herpes virus induced. Spontaneous healing takes several weeks.

The pathophysiology and etiology of recurrent aphthous stomatitis are unclear. In recent decades immunologic, infectious, genetic, nutritional, hormonal, stress, and traumatic etiologies have been proposed as precipitants. However, no strong reproducible data support these hypotheses.

Recurrent aphthous stomatitis is diagnosed by history and clinical exam. Rarely a biopsy is needed. When their appearance is atypical, constitutional symptoms are present, or lesions persist longer than 3 weeks, other causes of ulcers must be considered. Behçet's disease, Reiter's syndrome, Crohn's disease, celiac sprue, lichen planus, pemphigus, pemphigoid, erythema multiforme, and drug reactions may all present with oral ulcerations, but these patients usually have additional systemic symptoms or physical findings. Additionally, oral squamous cell cancer may present as an oral ulceration. Consequently, persistent ulcers must be biopsied.

Herpetiform RAU is distinguished from herpetic gingivostomatitis by its location. Primary herpetic gingivostomatitis usually appears on the lips and is associated with systemic symptoms. Secondary herpetic gingivostomatitis occurs on the keratinized hard palate and gingiva. Recurrent aphthous ulcers involve only the soft nonkeratinized mucosa.

Since recurring aphthous stomatitis is self-limited, most exacerbations do not require treatment. However, when treatment is desired, a number of topical treatments have been proposed. Over-the-counter products containing benzocaine, mixtures of equal parts of diphenhydramine and magnesium-containing antacid, and viscous lidocaine (Xylocaine) 2% all provide temporary pain relief but do not hasten healing. Topical corticosteroids (triamcinolone acetonide 0.1%, Kenalog in Orabase) applied two to four times per day or tetracycline "swish and spit" may decrease pain and the duration of symptoms.[4] Amlexanox 5% oral paste is a newer product that has been shown in several double-blind studies to diminish pain and ulcer size.[5] Caustic agents such as silver nitrate and hydrogen peroxide have been used but appear to delay healing and generally should be avoided. Systemic therapies including prednisone, colchicine, lavamisol, and thalidomide have been used in severe cases, but since the disease is self-limited, these agents have the potential to cause more complications than the disease itself.[5]

Cheilitis

Cheilitis is a common painful inflammatory condition of the lips often involving only the angles (angular chelitis). Perlèche (*Candida*-induced angular chelitis), persistent licking of the lips, and the inflammation found in edentulous elderly patients are the most frequent causes of cheilitis. Other causes of cheilitis include allergic contact dermatitis of the lips, which has been attributed to medicaments, lipstick, Chapstick, toothpaste, facial creams, and the nickel mouthpieces of musical instruments.[6] Diagnosis can be secured by skin testing. Treatment is avoidance. Atopic eczema can also affect the lips. Both contact dermatitis and eczema respond to topical corticosteroid ointments. Iron deficiency and other B vitamin deficiencies are rare causes of angular cheilitis or glossitis.

Glossitis

Migratory glossitis (geographic tongue) is a common condition characterized by smooth, erythematous map-like patches of atrophy of filiform papillae on the lateral boarders and dorsum of the tongue. It can change location in hours. The lesions are occasionally painful. Nonlingual erythema migrans is a similar phenomenon involving the buccal mucosa and other mucosal surfaces of the mouth and lips. Biopsy of these lesions shows the presence of inflammation. Symptomatic treatment includes bland foods and topical antihistamines.

Burning mouth syndrome commonly occurs in middle-aged women and affects the tongue and occasionally other mucosal surfaces. The painful areas are normal in appearance but increased sensation to temperature and dysgeusia can be demonstrated. The condition appears to be more common in patients with Parkinson's disease (see Chapter 66). Tricyclic antidepressants are often an effective treatment.

Other causes of glossitis include mineral and vitamin deficiencies. Vitamin B_{12} deficiency may present with a sore tongue or burning mouth.[7] Other B vitamin deficiencies (folic acid, riboflavin, nicotinic acid) may have similar symptoms and signs. Iron deficiency and protein-calorie malnutrition are both associated with a smooth tongue.

Caries

Dental caries along with periodontal disease are the most common oral diseases. By age 18, most American adolescents have several decayed permanent teeth. By age 65, most Americans are missing several teeth, and nearly half are edentulous.[8] Dental decay is caused by the destruction of the protective tooth enamel, often with subsequent degeneration of the inner dentin and pulp. Decay is affected by several factors: (1) high-carbohydrate diet, (2) bacteria, (3) low levels of fluoride, and (4) susceptible tooth surfaces.[9] When carbohydrates are left on the teeth after eating or drinking, bacteria metabolize them and produce acids. These acids slowly demineralize the enamel protecting the tooth and result in caries. Similarly, in adulthood if gum recession due to periodontal disease progresses, the roots of teeth are exposed. The protective layer around the root is demineralized by the acid products of bacterial metabolism, resulting in decay.

The vast majority of caries are preventable with a combination of healthy diet, brushing, flossing, and fluoridation. Decreasing the frequency of high-sugar snacks and meals means less substrate for the bacteria, less acid production, and fewer caries. The most striking example of the effect of carbohydrate solutions on decay is the "nursing-bottle syndrome" in which infants and small children are put to bed with a bottle containing milk or juice. The sugar-rich liquids bathe the teeth, resulting in bacterial proliferation and eventually rapid and extensive decay. In children and adults, brushing helps remove much of the bacteria-rich plaque from smooth surfaces on the teeth. Flossing helps remove plaque from the interdental spaces.

Fluoride is a naturally occurring element that exists in small amounts in water, food, and soil. It protects the teeth by reducing demineralization of the enamel and promoting remineralization.[10] In recent decades in industrialized nations, topical fluorides and fluoridated water systems have become increasingly prevalent, resulting in reduced dental caries rates.[8] Fluoridation of community water systems aims for a fluoride level of 0.7 to 1.2 parts per million (ppm), which has been shown to reduce cavities by up to 60%.[9] Unfortunately, 100 million Americans do not have fluoridated water.

Fluoride supplementation is recommended for children who live in areas with nonfluoridated water systems. However, before initiating supplementation, children and their parents should be asked about other possible sources of fluoride in their diet. These include school fluoride programs, water systems at day care and school, and swallowing of fluoridated toothpaste. If their fluoride intake appears suboptimal, testing the fluoride level of their water source is recommended. The recommended dose of fluoride supplementation depends on the child's age and the fluoride level in their drinking water (Table 73.1).[11]

Fluoride supplementation is inappropriate for children with adequately fluoridated water or adequate fluoride intake. In these instances, supplementation can lead to excessive fluoride ingestion and fluorosis with mottling of the teeth.

Dental sealants are plastic resins that can be painted on the teeth most prone to decay (molars and premolars) and serve as a barrier against acid-induced decay. Presently underutilized, dental sealants are gaining in popularity and are used most commonly at ages 6 to 14, when children are often not following brushing or flossing programs closely.[12] Sealants can reduce decay by 70% and last 4 to 6 years under normal conditions.

Gingival and Periodontal Disease

Gingival lesions can be divided into inflammation caused by plaque and non–plaque-associated disease. The latter can be further separated into gingivitis due to infections, reactions to extrinsic agents, or lesions of presumed autoimmune etiology.

Table 73.1. **Fluoride Supplementation (Milligrams per Day)**

Age	Water fluoride content (ppm)		
	<0.3	0.3–0.6	>0.6
Birth–6 months	0	0	0
>6 months–3 years	0.25	0	0
>3–6 years	0.50	0.25	0
>6–16 years	1.00	0.50	0

Infectious agents that may cause gingivitis or a more generalized stomatitis include bacteria (*Neisseria gonorrhoeae, Streptococcus pyogenes, Treponema pallidum*), virus (herpes simplex types 1 and 2), and fungi (*Candida* sp. and *Histoplasma capsulatum*). The diagnosis can be made by a careful history and knowledge of the typical physical findings such as multiple vesicles or ulcers found in herpes infection or nonadherent white patches with underlying gingival bleeding in human immunodeficiency virus (HIV)-associated candidosis. Culture, biopsy, or blood tests for HIV are occasionally needed. HIV co-infection predisposes to more widespread infectious involvement of the oral mucous membranes.

Acute necrotizing ulcerative gingivitis (Vincent's disease) is a polymicrobial infection characterized by halitosis, gingival bleeding, and painful ulceration of the interdental gums usually found in debilitated tobacco smokers with poor oral hygiene. The treatment is metronidazole (Flagyl, 250 mg tid for 3 days) along with oral debridement, one-half strength hydrogen peroxide mouth rinse, and proper oral care.

Lichen planus is the most common immune-modulated disease of the mouth[13] (also see Chapter 115). Lesions may appear on the skin, the oral mucosa, or both. Oral lichen planus of a reticular, papular, or plaque-like nature is frequently asymptomatic, whereas atopic or ulcerative lesions are painful. The buccal mucosa, gingiva, tongue, and palate, in decreasing order of frequency, are the usual sites of involvement. The most common lesion is a reticular pattern on the buccal mucosa. Diagnosis is made by clinical examination supported by nonspecific histologic findings on biopsy. Lichen planus has been associated with various medications [antimalarials, nonsteroidal antiinflammatory drugs (NSAIDs), diuretics, beta-blockers], infection with hepatitis B or C, systemic diseases (diabetes mellitus, hypertension, lupus erythematosus, graft-versus-host disease), dental restorations, and cinnamon. Treatment is removal of the suspected offending agent and topical, intralesional, or systemic steroids. Bullous lesions occurs on the oral musoca in 10% to 40% of patients with pemphigoid. The skin is usually involved first. Pemphigus vulgaris and systemic lupus erythematosus can occasionally cause a desquamative gingivitis.

Other causes of gingival swelling with or without inflammation include drug-induced (phenytoin, calcium channel blockers, cyclosporine) and pregnancy-associated disease. Both are benefited by improved oral hygiene and resolve when the offending drug is stopped or parturition occurs. Additionally, allergic reactions and trauma from physical or chemical agents can cause gingival injury.

Periodontitis is inflammation of the gingiva and the deeper periodontal membrane. Microbial dental plaque and calculus buildup lead to destruction of the soft tissue and bone that support the teeth, resulting in painless bleeding, halitosis, and increased tooth mobility. Diagnosis is made by dental probing and occasionally by x-rays. Tobacco smoking increases susceptibility to periodontal disease and tissue destruction as does immunosuppression and diabetes mellitus. Although oral bacteria play a part in the disease, systemic antibiotics (doxycycline, Periostat) are at best minimally helpful, and treatment consists of good oral hygiene and dental visits for scaling, polishing, curettage, and occasionally surgery.[14,15] Periodontal disease has been associated with cardiovascular disease and the delivery of low birth weight infants, but a direct cause-effect mechanism has not been identified.[16]

Oral Candidiasis

Candida is part of the normal mouth microflora in approximately 50% of the general population. When this yeast-like fungus overgrows and proliferates, it causes the infection termed oral candidiasis. Anything that alters the environment in the mouth or compromises the immune system may predispose to oral candidiasis. Common predisposing factors include systemic antibiotics and steroids, diabetes, xerostomia, immune deficiency, dental prostheses, and any illness that contributes to a significantly debilitated state (also see Chapter 116).

Oral candidiasis presents in several forms: acute pseudomembranous, hyperplastic, erythematous (atrophic), and *Candida*-associated lesions (angular cheilitis and denture stomatitis).[17,18]

Acute pseudomembranous candidiasis (thrush) is the common cottage cheese–like white patches family physicians are familiar with. The membrane can be scraped off with a tongue depressor or gauze, revealing an erythematous base. It is seen most commonly in infants. The other forms of oral candidiasis are less easily recognized. Hyperplastic candidiasis describes whitish oral plaques due to *Candida* that do not scrape off and resemble leukoplakia. Erythematous candidiasis presents as reddened oral mucosa, often with associated burning. *Candida*-associated lesions include denture stomatitis and angular cheilitis. Denture stomatitis is a subtype of erythematous candidiasis in which the reddened inflamed mucosa lies adjacent to denture material. *Candida* is a cofactor in its development. Angular cheilitis, inflammation at the corners of the mouth, is polymicrobial in origin. However, *Candida* plays a causative role.

The diagnosis of oral candidiasis is usually made by its characteristic clinical appearance and a positive 10% potassium hydroxide preparation on scraping. Potassium hydroxide dissolves the epithelial cells, but the pseudohyphae and budding cells of *Candida* remain. The test is limited by a large number of false positives and negatives. Because *Candida* is commonly found in normal mouths, oral candidiasis cannot be diagnosed by the presence of pseudohyphae on potassium hydroxide preparation alone. When the diagnosis is uncertain, empiric therapy and subsequent response is often used to confirm the diagnosis.

Predisposing factors should be discontinued whenever possible. The treatment of *Candida* depends on the location, extent, type of oral candidiasis, and on underlying medical conditions. Topical antifungals are the first-line therapy and are usually effective in uncomplicated disease. Choice of topical therapy is determined by the need to maximize exposure of *Candida* to the antifungal agent. Nystatin (Mycostatin) is available as a suspension (100,000 U/mL), cream (100,000 U/g), ointment, and troche (200,000 U). Clotrimazole

(Mycelex) troches are more palatable. Infants and younger children are generally treated with nystatin suspension. Patients with oral candidiasis and xerostomia should be treated with solutions. Adolescents and adults often prefer troches, which allow more contact with the area of infection. Angular cheilitis does well with nystatin cream, which can be applied to the corners of the mouth with simultaneous treatment of intraoral infection. Denture stomatitis requires treatment of both the denture and the oral cavity.

When topical therapy fails or patients have extensive disease, systemic options include the imidazole family: fluconazole, ketoconazole, or itraconazole. When imidazoles are used, particularly ketoconazole, consideration of possible interactions with other medications should be considered. Prolonged oral imidazole therapy requires periodic liver function tests.

Temporomandibular Disorders

Temporomandibular disorders (TMDs) are a diverse group of disorders of the muscles of mastication and the temporomandibular joint (TMJ) characterized by pain and/or dysfunction. Most are self-limiting and resolve without treatment.

Patients may complain of clicking, popping, or locking of the jaw accompanied by painful and occasionally limited motion. Examination may demonstrate tenderness of the muscles of mastication and the TMJ along with palpable crepitus and audible clicks (although the latter are found in many asymptomatic individuals). The interincisal opening can be measured and sequentially followed. Panoramic radiography of the jaw may be obtained for screening for other diseases but is usually not helpful in guiding therapy.

An overwhelming majority of patients with TMD are believed to have a complex chronic pain disorder similar to fibromyalgia[19] (see Chapter 114). A variety of psychological, behavioral, and structural factors may contribute to TMD, although an underlying cause remains elusive in most patients. Current opinion is that malocclusion, missing dentition, routine dental procedures, and oral endotracheal intubation are not causes of TMD. Oral habits, such as prolonged gum chewing or persistently holding a tongue stud between the incisors, can strain the TMJ and cause pain. Bruxism probably does not cause but may aggravate preexisting TMD. Degenerative changes in the TMJ found on radiography are common and not symptomatic in most patients.

The differential diagnosis of TMD includes TMJ osteoarthritis (a self-limiting disorder), rheumatoid arthritis with pain and swelling about the joint, acromegaly, tumors, temporal arteritis, and claudication of the masticatory muscles.

Treatment of nonstructural, localized, and chronic TMD and osteoarthritis of the TMJ relies on patient education emphasizing its self-limiting and nonprogressive course. Muscle relaxation techniques, biofeedback, antiinflammatory drugs, low-dose tricyclic antidepressants, and local application of warm compresses may be helpful. A dental splint can be effective adjunctive therapy. Injections of corticosteroids may be necessary in rheumatoid arthritis but are otherwise best avoided. Surgery is generally believed not to be indicated for the treatment of pain alone.

Halitosis

One tenth of the population has a persistent foul-smelling odor emanating from their oral and/or nasal airways. Most patients never report the problem to their medical or dental care provider because halitosis is typically not personally perceived due to olfactory fatigue or adaptation. Usually a parent or spouse demands an evaluation. Paradoxically, patients who bitterly complain of self-recognized halitosis frequently have an unobjectionable breath but do have psychogenic halitosis, often with social phobia.[20]

The etiologies of halitosis range from systemic diseases to abnormalities of the gastrointestinal tract, lungs, upper respiratory tract, and naso- and oropharynx. However, in 85% to 90% of cases its origin is in the mouth.[21] The most common cause is morning breath, a normal event believed to result from the decrease in salivary flow while asleep, which is accentuated by mouth breathing.[20] Dry mouth can also be caused by anticholinergic medications. The oral drying and stasis allow bacteria to multiply. Their metabolic by-products of hydrogen sulfide, methylmercaptan, and other volatile sulfur compounds result in halitosis.

An oral source of halitosis can be confirmed by comparing the exhaled odor from the patient's mouth with that exiting from the nose. Common oral origins of halitosis include the tongue, especially the posterior region. Diagnosis is made by gently scraping the dorsal surface with a plastic spoon and then comparing the spoon's odor with that of the breath. Unclean dentures and those that are worn overnight may have an objectionable odor; this can be demonstrated by placing the dentures in a sealed plastic bag for a time and then smelling the trapped air. Poorly fitting dental appliances, large caries, and the posterior tongue may trap food, resulting in bacterial overgrowth and halitosis. Subgingival plaque and periodontal disease promote bad breath. Diagnosis is suggested by flossing the intradental spaces and then employing the plastic-bag whiff test. Smoker's breath may last for hours. Tonsillar crypts may emit a foul-smelling discharge when infected and enlarged. The discharge can be collected on a tongue depressor.

Nasal causes of halitosis are second in frequency. Sinusitis may have a fetid anaerobic sewer-like odor. Nasal foreign bodies have a ripe, cheesy odor and are usually accompanied by a unilateral nasal discharge. Chronic nasal obstruction from polyps, neoplasms, or granulomatous disease may cause both an odor and mouth breathing, resulting in foul breath from both sites.

Pulmonary sources of halitosis are less common but important since they suggest a significant underlying lung disease or a metabolic disorder. A pulmonary source is suggested by an odor that increases as the breath progresses during a forced expiration. Common lung diseases associated with halitosis are lung abscesses, foreign bodies, bronchiectasis, and empyemas. Radiolucent foreign bodies may be missed by a cursory examination of a chest x-ray.

Hepatic (fishy) and renal failure (urinal), diabetic ketoacidosis (fruity), odor-producing foods (onions, garlic), alcohol, poisons (cyanide), and infections may have halitosis as a presenting symptom. A number of pediatric metabolic disorders may be first suggested by an unusual smelling breath.

Treatment of halitosis should be directed at the suspected source. Fluids and artificial saliva help dry mouth. Routine brushing, flossing, tongue scraping, and antibacterial mouth rinses are usually effective for oral halitosis.

References

1. Oral health in America. a report of the surgeon general, 2000. Available at *www.surgeongeneral.gov*.
2. Scully C, Porter S. Oral cancer. BMJ 2000;321:97–100.
3. Hyde N, Hopper C. Oral cancer: the importance of early referral. Practitioner 1999;243:753–63.
4. McBride D. Management of aphthous ulcers. Am Fam Physician 2000;62(1):149–54.
5. Popovsky J, Camis AC. New and emerging therapies for diseases of the oral cavity. Dermatol Clin 2000;18:113–24.
6. Freeman S, Stephens R. Cheilitis: analysis of 75 cases referred to a contact dermatitis clinic. Am J Contact Derm 1999;10: 198–200.
7. Field EA, Speechoey JA, Rugman FR, Varga E, Tyldesley WR. Oral signs and symptoms in patients with undiagnosed vitamin B12 deficiency. J Oral Pathol Med 1995;24:468–70.
8. Clark M, Albun M, Lloyd R. Preventive dentistry and the family physician. Am Fam Physician 1996;53:6119–26.
9. Kokshin M. Preventive oral health care: a review for family physicians. Am Fam Physician 1994;50:1677–84.
10. Holt R, Roberts G, Sully C. Dental damage, sequla, and prevention. BMJ 2000;320:1717–19.
11. Committee on Nutrition, American Academy of Pediatrics. Fluoride supplementation or children: interim policy recommendations. Pediatrics 1995;95:727.
12. American Dental Association. Available at *www.ada.org*.
13. Holstrup P. Non-plaque-induced gingival lesions. Ann Periodontal 1999;4:20–31.
14. Coventry J, Griffiths G, Scully C, Tonnetti M. ABC of oral health. Periodontal disease. BMJ 2000;321:36–9.
15. Greenstein G, Lamster, I. Efficacy of subantimicrobial dosing with doxycycline. J Am Dent Assoc 2001;132:457–66.
16. Haber J, Wattles J, Crowley M, Mandell R, Joshipura K, Kent RL. Evidence of cigarette smoking as a major risk factor for periodontitis. J Periodont 1993;64:16–23.
17. Epstein J, Polsky B. Oropharyngeal candidiasis: a review of its clinical spectrum and current therapies. Clin Ther 1998;20: 40–57.
18. Rossie K, Guggenheimer J. Oral candidiasis: clinical manifestations, diagnosis, and treatment. Pract Periodontics Aesthet Dent 1997;9:635–41.
19. Goldstein BH. Temporomandibular disorders: a review of current understanding. Oral Surg Oral Med Oral Pathol 1999;88: 379–85.
20. Rosenberg M. Clinical assessment of bad breath: current concepts. J Am Dent Assoc 1996;127:475–82.
21. Johnson BE. Halitosis, or the meaning of bad breath. J Gen Intern Med 1992;7:649–56.

74

Selected Disorders of the Ear, Nose, and Throat

Karen L. Hall and R. Whit Curry, Jr.

Tinnitus

Tinnitus is the sensation of sound that does not originate from stimulation of the hearing apparatus by external sound. Described as an audible noise—which may be clicking, humming, ringing, or buzzing—tinnitus is accompanied by varying levels of distress from annoyance to severe anxiety. Rarely is tinnitus associated with a fatal malady, but the condition may lead to difficulty concentrating, insomnia, feelings of helplessness, and depression. Some patients have voiced thoughts of suicide. Epidemiologic estimates of chronic tinnitus in the population stand at about 1%, and as many as 50% of the population may have suffered tinnitus at one time or another.

Tinnitus may be subjective, heard only by the patient, or objective, heard by the examiner and the patient. Causes are listed in Table 74.1. Although the mechanism is not understood, tinnitus is most often associated with hearing loss. In presbycusis, or age-related hearing loss, the loss of cochlear hair cells and deterioration of the central auditory pathways may cause the perception of tinnitus. The tinnitus associated with conductive hearing loss is usually characterized as a low-pitched, pulsating sound that may be described as more noticeable in the affected ear.

Tinnitus occurs in up to 70% of patients following acoustic trauma such as that experienced at a rock concert or sporting event, and is often associated with a temporary hearing loss (called a temporary threshold shift). Patients must be cautioned that this hearing loss and tinnitus is a warning of damage to their hearing. Upon repetition of the acoustic trauma, permanent threshold shift (hearing loss) may occur.

Drugs and other chemical exposures may be linked to tinnitus. Most well known is the association with aspirin; other offenders are loop diuretics, arsenic, and antimalarials. Tinnitus may also accompany central nervous system (CNS) tumors, atherosclerotic disease, structural defects in the ear, and neurologic conditions such as Ménière's disease (tinnitus, deafness, and vertigo).

The evaluation of tinnitus begins with a historical account: a description of the sounds; questions concerning the onset, timing, and aggravating and alleviating factors; frequency (high or low pitched); and presence of any pulsatile nature to the noise. Other areas for historical information and review of systems include concomitant hearing loss, vertigo, ear pain, drainage, fever or other signs of infection, headaches, other medical problems including heart disease, hypertension, and chronic or previous neurologic disease such as Meniere's disease or multiple sclerosis. Additionally, occupational exposure to noise, head injury, allergy, and drug history may yield vital clues.

The physical examination focuses on the otolaryngologic examination and the neurologic and cardiovascular systems. Historical data may lead to an expanded physical examination. The ear examination should rule out cerumen impaction and other abnormalities such as external otitis, perforation of the tympanic membrane, fluid or pus behind the eardrum, otitis media, and cholesteatoma. The neurologic examination may suggest multiple sclerosis (bilateral internuclear ophthalmoplegia) or other neurologic disease. Bruits over the neck may indicate an objective cause for the tinnitus, or myoclonus of the palate may be observed on the oral examination. The temporomandibular joint should be examined for pain or clicks.

A hearing evaluation is essential. The discovery of bilateral high-frequency loss is often associated with presbycusis or noise-induced hearing loss. A unilateral hearing loss can be associated with CNS pathology and tumors in the cerebellopontine area.

Laboratory tests aim to confirm suspicions arising from the history and physical examination. Patients with suspected neurologic disorders, tumors, or treatable medical and surgical conditions, or if seeking disability compensation, may require referral and further workup by an audiologist and otolaryngologist.

Table 74.1. **Causes of Tinnitus**

Objective (heard by the patient and examiner)
Arteriovenous shunts
Arterial bruits
Carotid stenosis
Venous hum
Stapedial artery abnormalities
Myoclonus of palate, stapedius
Abnormally patent eustachian tube
Temporomandibular joint (TMJ) abnormalities
Transmitted cardiac murmurs

Subjective (heard only by patient)
Hearing loss (noise-induced)
Presbycusis
Cerumen impaction
Acoustic trauma (acute and chronic)
Cholesteatoma
Otosclerosis
Tympanic membrane perforation
Serous otitis
Syphilis
External otitis
Allergy
Anxiety/stress
Zinc deficiency
Closed head injury
Multiple sclerosis
Meniere's disease
Acoustic neuroma
Diabetes
Hypertension
Hypotension
Hyperlipidemia
Salicylates
Antimalarial drugs
Loop diuretics
Tricyclics
Aminoglycosides
Heavy metals (arsenic)

Patients with medical conditions such as hypertension, diabetes, or hyperlipidemia are appropriately treated by their family physician. Despite treatment of underlying medical conditions, tinnitus may not completely resolve.

Most patients with tinnitus have associated hearing loss due to age, repeated acoustic trauma, or occupational (noise-induced) exposure. For these patients various treatments have been used. Noise masking, such as generating "white noise" by setting a radio between two stations on the dial, low-level music, mood music, or environmental sounds such as the ocean may help. During daylight hours, when other noises intrude regularly, tinnitus is less problematic. Hearing aids, because they amplify environmental sound, also serve as maskers.

A variety of strategies and drugs have been used to treat tinnitus. No specific treatment is successful in all cases.[1] In cases of concomitant depression, antidepressants may improve the symptoms. Sedating antidepressants may help with sleep, a time that patients have more trouble with noise intrusion. A review of alprazolam did not support the use of benzodiazepines for tinnitus. Other medications of possible benefit include calcium channel blockers, diuretics, anticon-

vulsants, and anesthetics.[2] Lidocaine infusion has been serendipitously noted to relieve tinnitus in some patients.[3] Cochlear implants and electrical stimulation have been used with some success in debilitating tinnitus.[4,5]

Trials of acupuncture on tinnitus showed no improvement versus placebo,[6] and a trial of one homeopathic preparation demonstrated no benefit.[7] Investigators have attempted behavioral training techniques with an emphasis on coping skills, coupled with relaxation and attention-distraction strategies, with some success.[8] Other investigators have used hypnotherapy with better results in patients with less hearing loss.[9] If chronic tinnitus is not associated with underlying serious disease, the patient can be assured that, although annoying, the tinnitus is not life-threatening.

Hearing Impairment

Human hearing is an elegant and sensitive system. At birth the ear is capable of detecting sound in the range of 20 to 20,000 hertz (Hz). As the ear ages, this range narrows but remains remarkably attuned to the frequency of the human voice at 200 to 4000 Hz.

Hearing impairment may be divided into two basic types: sensorineural and conductive. Conductive hearing loss includes all causes that interfere with the movement of sound through the external auditory canal as it sets up resonance with the tympanic membrane and is amplified and transmitted by the ossicles. Sensorineural hearing loss refers to any sensory defect of the cochlea or acoustic nerve. Hearing impairment is classified as mixed where components of both types of loss are present. Central hearing loss refers to impairment of perception or interpretation of sound at higher cortical levels. Causes of central hearing impairment include stroke, infection, or a tumor affecting the centers of the brain that process acoustic information. Specific syndromes include global aphasia, Wernicke's aphasia, and pure word deafness.

Hearing impairment may be inherited or acquired. Hereditary hearing impairment (HHI) may be secondary to a recognized syndrome or may be an isolated anomaly.[10] The terms *hereditary* and *congenital* are not synonymous. For example, deafness occurs in congenital rubella syndrome, but the cause is infectious rather than genetic. Acquired hearing loss is most often associated with infection, especially following bacterial meningitis and ear infections. Ototoxicity from certain medications also causes acquired hearing loss. As more children are protected against *Haemophilus influenzae*, measles, mumps, and rubella with vaccines, HHI increases in importance in hearing loss in childhood. Likewise, better control and monitoring of ototoxic medications, such as aminoglycosides, decreases hearing loss secondary to the use of these medications.[11]

Pediatric Hearing Impairment

Diagnosis

At birth the human infant reacts to noise with crying, Moro reflex, eye blink, or motor movements, none of which is specific enough to detect the presence of hearing loss. Totally deaf infants exhibit crying and other vocalizations despite their inability to hear. Many studies have demonstrated the early ability of infants to discriminate sounds and process auditory stimuli.[12] Because of the importance of normal hearing to the development of language, intellectual, and social skills, the determination of intact hearing in the infant is vital. In an infant with normal hearing, a loud sound should cause generalized body movement of more than one extremity, even while asleep. Tests using hand clap or bell ring can be used as a rough gauge, but in children at high risk for developing hearing loss, more reliable tests should be used. Transient evoked otoacoustic emissions (TEOEs) are measurable signals generated by the hair cells of the cochlea when stimulated by sound. Using a portable device, TEOEs can be detected in newborns to screen for hearing loss.[13] Children who fail to exhibit TEOEs can then be referred for more extensive testing including auditory brainstem responses. In several studies evaluating TEOE in high-risk newborns, normal newborns, and children up to the age of 12, the failure rate on the initial TEOE was as high as 22%.[14–16] In an extensive screening effort in Rhode Island, the first-screen failure rate was 10% of the 53,121 children screened. Ultimately 111 children were identified as having true hearing loss.[17] Several states now mandate hearing screening in every newborn before hospital discharge. This still leaves unscreened those children born in alternate birthing centers including the home and does not address the issue of hearing loss acquired after the newborn period.

During well-baby visits, specific questions concerning the family and pregnancy history help identify the child at risk for hearing loss. These factors include a family history of hearing loss in blood relatives under 30 years old, pregnancy complicated by ToRCH (toxoplasmosis, rubella, cytomegalovirus, herpes simplex) or other infections accompanied by rash, and exposure to medications such as aminoglycoside antibiotics.

Later in childhood, a variety of conditions can affect hearing, especially otitis media, serous otitis, and bacterial meningitis. Hearing may be significantly impaired in a child with chronic middle ear effusion, leading to delays in intellectual and speech development and ultimately social functioning (see Chapter 72). If a child has had multiple ear infections, chronic nasal congestion or discharge, chronic upper respiratory tract infections or sinusitis, or fits any of the at-risk criteria, screening for hearing loss is warranted (Table 74.2). If parents express concern over their child's hearing, the child should be screened. The "wait and see" approach wastes valuable time in a child's language and intellectual development.

Routine well-baby visits and hospital nursery physical examinations should include evaluation of the general appearance of the infant (as many recognizable congenital syndromes are associated with hearing loss) and examination of the ears, nose, and throat. Signs of chronic otitis, effusion, and allergy (allergic shiners and the allergic salute sign) are important. Because children require sound discrimination to develop normal speech and grammatical patterns, the threshold for impairment should be considered to be 15 dB, rather

Table 74.2. **Risk Factors for Hearing Loss in Infants**

Family history of hearing loss <age 5
Prematurity
Low birth weight
Intensive care nursery admission requiring mechanical ventilation or with neonatal infection
Mechanical ventilation beyond 10 days
Hyperbilirubinemia requiring exchange transfusion
Prenatal TORCH infection (toxoplasmosis, rubella, cytomegalovirus, herpes simplex)
Prenatal syphilis
Presence of minor or major congenital malformations, primarily craniofacial, including abnormalities of the outer ear, low hairline, absent philtrum, or others associated with recognizable syndromes associated with deafness
Low Apgar score (<3 at 5 minutes) or prolonged depression at birth
Bacterial meningitis

than the 25 dB used for adults. For the at-risk infant, referral is required for evaluation, which may include TEOEs or auditory brainstem evoked response (ABR). The ABR uses external scalp electrodes to detect waveforms that occur in predictable patterns following an auditory stimulus. The American Speech-Language-Hearing Association recommends ABRs on all infants defined as being at high risk, including neonatal intensive care unit graduates, who should be tested prior to hospital discharge, with follow-up ABRs at 6-month intervals. Children who are identified with hearing loss require referral for follow-up care and management.

For the older child, audiologic screening may be possible in the office setting using a hand-held audiometry device or office audiometer. To diagnose conductive versus sensorineural hearing loss, Weber and Rinne tests can be used in the child capable of following directions. Although the use of a hand-held pneumatic otoscope is useful for gross evaluation of tympanic membrane compliance, tympanometry provides a more objective, sensitive measure. Several investigators have described tympanogram patterns; widely used are those of Jerger.[18] Assessment of language development can also provide insightful clues about the presence of hearing loss. Assuming the parent has normal speech, one would expect delayed speech, aberrant phonation, and altered grammatical patterns in a child who cannot hear.

Management

In children with conductive hearing loss due to a foreign body, infection, or allergy, treatment of the underlying disorder should ameliorate the hearing problem. Follow-up with office audiology and tympanometry as well as ongoing gross assessment of language development is well within the scope of the family practitioner. If the child with chronic problems does not respond to first-line treatment, such as antibiotics for otitis, referral is appropriate.

When sensorineural hearing loss is detected in the pediatric patient, referral to an otological specialist is necessary. The role of the family physician is timely detection, appropriate referral, and family and patient support.

Adult Hearing Loss

Diagnosis

Hearing impairment in the adult has many causes. Important questions to include in the history are the following: (1) Abrupt or gradual onset? (2) One or both sides affected? (3) Associated with trauma? fever? ear pain? bloody or pustular discharge? (4) Accompanied by dizziness? vertigo? nausea? tinnitus? (5) History of sudden or chronic noise exposure, barotrauma (diving or air travel)? (6) Do family members complain that the patient turns the volume too loud on the television or radio (conductive)? (7) Does noise in the environment make the problem worse (sensorineural)? (8) Does the patient use medications, such as aspirin, antibiotics, diuretics, or cancer treatment?

The ear canal and tympanic membrane should be inspected for signs of infection, old scarring, normal landmarks of the ossicles, and light reflex. Pneumatic otoscopy demonstrates that the tympanic membrane is intact and compliant. Specific tuning-fork tests, the Weber and Rinne, should be done on every patient with suspected hearing loss. Although there is some debate about the optimum frequency tuning fork to use, most recommend the 256-Hz tuning fork.[19] If hearing loss is suspected after the physical examination, pure-tone audiometry can be performed with equipment designed for office use. Tympanometry can also be used in adults to assess the integrity and compliance of the tympanic membrane.

Management

By far the most common cause of conductive hearing loss in adults is cerumen impaction. It can be relieved by curette, suction, or irrigation using warm water or water and peroxide. Occasionally a softening agent such as Cerumenex or Debrox is necessary to facilitate removal. Debrox may be used at home on a monthly or weekly basis to keep wax soft, enabling the natural flow of wax from the ear canal to take place. Prolonged use of Cerumenex may irritate the ear canal, and it should not be prescribed for home use. Advising the patient to refrain from using cotton swabs helps prevent further wax impactions.

Repeated infections and trauma to the tympanic membrane may result in scarring of the drum and decreased compliance, with subsequent conductive hearing loss. Trauma to the ear can lead to conductive loss due to disruption of the drum or dislocation of the ossicles. Urgent referral when acute trauma to the ossicles is suspected is vital for optimal outcome. Small perforations of the drum usually heal spontaneously; larger defects may require surgery.

In adults the most common cause of sensorineural hearing loss is noise-related damage to the cochlea. Treatment is amplification by use of a hearing aid. Prevention is preferable and more cost-effective. Efforts through government regulation have improved noise control in the workplace, but noise associated with recreational, entertainment, and hobby activities impacts the hearing of young and older people alike. Family physicians are in an ideal position to effect change in this area through patient education and local community involvement (see Chapters 45 and 46).

Sudden sensorineural hearing loss has many causes, including viral illness, diabetes, and medications. A concomitant history of dizziness or vertigo, tinnitus, and unilateral hearing loss suggests Meniere's syndrome, which may resolve spontaneously, worsen, or recur after remission. Most causes of sudden sensorineural loss are idiopathic and remit spontaneously.[20] Acoustic neuroma can present as either sudden or gradual hearing loss, with unsteadiness of gait, dizziness, or tinnitus. More advanced presentations may also include ipsilateral facial weakness or hand clumsiness. Computed tomography (CT) and magnetic resonance imaging (MRI) are the imaging techniques of choice. Treatment is surgical, and the prognosis is good if the disorder is diagnosed early.

As the ear ages, changes take place in the hearing organ that result in age-related hearing loss, or presbycusis. Although aging is blamed for most sensorineural hearing loss in the elderly, studies of populations in relatively noise-free environments show less hearing loss than in populations in noisy, industrialized ones. Hearing aid amplification is usually prescribed for presbycusis. Hearing problems may be found in up to 80% of nursing home residents. Proper use of amplification and prompt recognition of cerumen impaction can alleviate confusion, avoid combativeness, and improve the quality of life in this population[21] (see Chapter 24).

Hearing loss is a major problem for people of all ages. The 1980 census indicated that more than 14 million Americans had some type of hearing impairment, and nearly 2 million were considered deaf.[22] Family physicians should work aggressively to detect, evaluate, and appropriately treat or refer the many individuals with hearing loss.

Epistaxis

Nosebleeds are common. More than 60% of the population experience at least one. Epistaxis occurs more often during childhood, and the sexes are affected equally. Physicians generally see the unusually severe episodes because most people successfully treat their nosebleeds without seeking medical care. Epistaxis occasionally presents as a medical emergency.

Epistaxis in children is usually from an anterior site on the nasal septum, generally in Kiesselbach's area (also called Little's area) on the anteroinferior aspect of the nasal septum. Bleeding from this area can be arterial or venous. More serious nosebleeds originate posteriorly and are more often seen in adults. Bleeding from the posterior nose may drain into the pharynx, and patients may present with hematemesis or melena.

Diagnosis

Most nosebleeds are due to low humidity, rhinitis (infectious or allergic), or minor trauma. Low humidity, which dries the nasal mucosa, accounts for the increased frequency of nosebleeds in hot, dry climates and during the winter months. Hypertension is not believed to be an etiologic factor, but rather a stress response, and is often present in adults with posterior epistaxis. Management of such patients is often difficult until blood pressure is controlled. Aspirin or nonsteroidal antiinflammatory drug (NSAID) use prolongs bleeding and is often a factor in refractory epistaxis. For the unusual case, with persistent or recurrent epistaxis, the differential diagnosis includes a hemostatic or platelet disorder (von Willebrand's disease, warfarin administration, alcoholism, chemotherapy, thrombocytopenia), hereditary telangiectasia, tumors, systemic or local infections such as tuberculosis and syphilis, sarcoidosis, and drugs (e.g., inhaled cocaine). In young children foreign bodies may cause epistaxis with a malodorous discharge. The frequency of these disorders is so low that screening patients with simple epistaxis is not recommended unless the history or physical examination is suggestive.[23]

Management

For anterior epistaxis, have the patient lie down with the head elevated, and pinch the nostrils for at least 5 minutes. Assess the amount of blood loss and reassure the patient. Check the blood pressure, hematocrit, and postural vital signs (if significant bleeding is suspected), and don a gown/gloves/mask as universal precautions. Good lighting with a mirror or headlight is critical. Using a small suction tip, the nares should be cleaned of clots and blood. Pledgets containing an anesthetic and vasoconstrictor, such as 4% cocaine or a combination of lidocaine (2–4%) and phenylephrine (0.25–5.0%), are placed on the nasal mucosa at the suspected bleeding site. Sedation with a benzodiazepine is occasionally helpful. The patient is asked to warn of sneezing, which often occurs. The nasal mucosa is then examined, using suction to keep the area dry. Any bleeding point identified can be cauterized with silver nitrate, electrical cautery, or laser coagulation.

One study showed that 65% of patients presenting in an emergency room with epistaxis could be successfully managed with intranasal oxymetazoline as the sole therapy.[24] After bleeding stops, apply petroleum jelly to keep the area moist and advise the patient to avoid picking or blowing the nose for 1 week. Discussion about the importance of humidification, use of a saline nasal spray, and treatment of recurrences at home may prevent unnecessary office visits.

If bleeding is not controlled, anterior packing or endoscopic evaluation is the next consideration. A variety of nasal tampons or balloons are available, and packing of the anterior nasal cavity was described by Randall and Freeman.[25] Endoscopic visualization of the bleeding site and direct cauterization is becoming a more common technique.

Posterior epistaxis is more often a serious problem, frequently seen in elderly individuals and usually associated with hypertension. Aspirin or NSAIDs may be unsuspected contributors. Hospitalization is generally required, and endonasal endoscopy, angiographic embolization, or posterior packing may be needed. Unless one is experienced in posterior packing and its complications, referral is indicated.

Prevention

It is important that parents be made aware that nosebleeds are common in children and usually respond to simple measures such as nose pinching for at least 5 minutes. Parents should be reassured that nosebleed seldom indicates a serious underlying disease. Treatment of infectious and allergic rhinitis, use of humidification, and avoidance of nose picking are worth emphasizing.

Salivary Gland Abnormalities

Saliva is a complex secretion that lubricates the mouth and upper pharynx, modulates the oral flora, aids in initial digestion of food, and facilitates speech and swallowing. Saliva also helps remineralize teeth and buffers gastric acid, thereby protecting the esophagus. High levels of immunoglobulin A (IgA) are present, suggesting a role in host defense. The normal adult produces up to 1.5 L daily. The major salivary glands consist of the parotid glands, submaxillary glands, and sublingual glands. There are minor salivary glands located in the cheeks, lips, and floor of the mouth, tongue, palate, and anterior faucial pillars.

Salivary Gland Swelling

Normal salivary glands should be neither visible nor palpable. Enlargement or swelling mandates investigation. Parotid enlargement eliminates the normal concavity between the mandible and earlobe, giving the patient a "chipmunk" appearance. Lymphadenopathy may be confused with salivary gland enlargement.

The history should probe for recent infection, pain (especially with meals and acidic substances such as lemon juice), recurrent or prior swelling, and dry mouth. Physical examination should include a gloved examination inside the mouth and careful palpation of the jaw and neck. Stensen's duct, the mouth of the parotid duct, should be visualized. If infection is suspected, pressure over the gland may express pus at the orifice.

Ultrasonography is an effective noninvasive technique for evaluating parotid enlargement. When inflammatory disease is suspected, CT scanning is preferred, and if the clinical finding is a mass, MRI usually best evaluates the lesion. Sialography is rarely necessary.[26]

Epidemic mumps, caused by paramyxovirus, is the most common cause of parotid swelling. Sporadically other enteroviruses, including coxsackie A and Epstein-Barr, as well as influenza A, parainfluenza, and lymphocytic choriomeningitis may cause sialoadenitis. Because mumps confers lifelong immunity, infection with these other viruses probably accounts for recurrent attacks in a given individual.

Acute suppurative parotitis most often occurs in elderly individuals who are debilitated by systemic illness or previous surgical procedures. Predisposing factors include dehydration, malnutrition, oral neoplasms, and medications that diminish salivary flow (e.g., diuretics or antihistamines). It may arise from a septic focus in the oral cavity or from a combination of factors. *Staphylococcus aureus* is the most common pathogen, but streptococci and gram-negative bacilli are occasional causative agents. Anaerobic bacteria have also been isolated from patients with parotitis, along with other organisms, including mycobacterium, fungi such as *Candida albicans* and *Actinomyces*, and the bacterium that causes cat-scratch fever. Treatment includes systemic antibiotics and surgical drainage. Parotidectomy is occasionally required.

Noninfectious swelling (sialosis or sialadenosis) is often seen with granulomatous diseases, endocrinopathies such as hypothyroidism, malnutrition, and neurologic disease, and is associated with a variety of medications. Ten to twenty percent of diabetics have asymptomatic parotid swelling with increased fatty infiltration, possibly attempting to compensate for xerostomia (diabetics have one-third less saliva flow). Improvement correlates with better diabetic control[27] (see Chapter 120).

Xerostomia

Dry mouth, or xerostomia, is often a symptom of salivary gland dysfunction. Reduced salivary production is also suggested by difficulty swallowing dry foods without additional fluids, the feeling of dryness in the mouth while eating, complaints that spicy foods and fruit burn the mouth, and foods continually sticking to the teeth. Clinical signs include caries, atrophic candidiasis, and a beefy red, fissured tongue. The three most common causes are medications, therapeutic radiation, and Sjögren's syndrome.

Medications causing xerostomia include sedatives, antipsychotics, antidepressants, antihistamines, and antireflux drugs with anticholinergic effects. Xerostomia has been attributed to more than 400 medications. Therapeutic radiation, often given for ear/nose/throat cancers, may destroy salivary glands. Sjögren's syndrome results from autoimmune destruction of the salivary glands, causing xerostomia and occasionally salivary gland swelling. Sjögren's syndrome may occur without systemic disease or, more commonly, is associated with a major rheumatic disease, such as rheumatoid arthritis, systemic lupus erythematosus, primary biliary cirrhosis, or scleroderma (see Chapter 113). Most of the patients are female. The diagnosis can be confirmed by biopsy of a minor salivary gland and is supported by the presence of the autoantibodies anti–Sjögren's syndrome A (SS-A) and anti–SS-B in serum. Keratoconjunctivitis sicca, from diminished tearing, is often an associated finding.

Treatment of xerostomia is difficult. Artificial lubricants may be used, but many patients find water as effective. Stimulating agents and acupuncture may help if patients still produce some saliva. Chewing gum, citrus-containing beverages, and sugarless hard candies can be tried. Pilocarpine is more effective than artificial saliva for irradiation-induced xerostomia.[28]

Stones

Sialolithiasis, or the formation of salivary stones (sialoliths), usually occurs in the ducts of the submandibular and parotid glands, the submandibular gland being the most common site by far. Pain and swelling are the typical first symptoms, often intensified at mealtimes when salivary flow increases. Because the blockage is rarely complete, symptoms are frequently intermittent. Diagnosis can often be made by inspecting for asymmetry, palpating the gland, milking the gland while observing for salivary flow, finding rock-hard nodules in the ductal area, and obtaining a radiograph.

Ultrasound is a very helpful diagnostic tool. As many as 90% of all stones greater than 2 mm in size can be detected as an echo-dense spot on an ultrasound. Obstructing stones can lead to suppuration requiring antibiotics. Patients presenting with sialolithiasis may benefit from a trial of a conservative management, especially if the stone is small. Hydration, local heat, and massage may help flush the stones out of the duct. In any gland with swelling and sialolithiasis, infection should be assumed and antistaphyloccocol antibiotics administered. Stones not responding to conservative treatment should be surgically removed.[29]

Hoarseness

Family physicians often see patients who complain of hoarseness—a different, raspy, or harsh sound of the voice. It may sound gruff or whispery and worsen as the day goes on owing to vocal fatigue. Singers, preachers, and others who depend on their voice may experience subtle changes, such as a reduction in the high tones of their vocal range.

The normal voice is produced by a coordinated effort of the abdominal, chest, and laryngeal muscles. Sound production begins when the diaphragm and abdominal and chest wall muscles contract, causing airflow across the vocal cords. The laryngeal muscles simultaneously contract, obstructing free exhalation and raising subglottic pressure to about 30 mm Hg. A mucosal "wave" is produced along the free edges of the vocal cords, creating periodic opening and closing of the airway, resulting in rhythmic compressions and refractions of the air column at a frequency we perceive as sound. For the vocal fold mucosa to vibrate properly it must be pliable. Any condition causing edema or swelling of the fold interferes with normal sound production and causes hoarseness. The mucosa is normally moistened by a thin layer of watery mucus secreted from mucous glands in the laryngeal ventricles. The mucus layer cleans the airway, lubricates the mucosa (allowing it to vibrate with less friction against the other mucosa during phonation), and helps to dissipate heat generated during phonation by evaporation. Accordingly, anything interfering with the pliability of the vocal cord mucosa or with the layer of watery mucus constantly being secreted may result in hoarseness.[30]

Acute hoarseness is commonly due to upper respiratory tract infections and the resultant tracheobronchitis frequently accompanying these viral infections (see Chapter 39). This syndrome is readily recognized by the accompanying respiratory tract signs and symptoms. Acute hoarseness due to overuse is also easily diagnosed from the history of singing, speaking, and shouting. For these acute syndromes conservative therapy is appropriate, but it is imperative to follow patients until the normal voice returns.

Hoarseness in children, particularly from ages 3 to 7, may signal early epiglottitis. Boys entering puberty often experience hoarseness and require only reassurance.

Hoarseness that persists or is not associated with overuse or a respiratory tract infection requires investigation and a specific diagnosis. This mandate is particularly important in smokers, in whom minimal or early symptoms should prompt visualization of the vocal cords.

Diagnosis

The history should probe for weight loss, cough, hemoptysis, sore throat, neck or chest pain, wheezing, trouble swallowing, thickening of hair, or cold intolerance. The patient's use of the voice (i.e., singing or shouting) is often important. The medical history should document any chronic disease, especially thyroid or neurologic diseases. Alcohol or drug use should be sought. Allergies and environmental exposures, especially cigarette smoke, may be significant.

A primary consideration is to exclude a vocal cord abnormality. A callus or nodule on the vocal cord is caused by vocal abuse or overuse. It appears at the junction of the anterior one third and posterior two thirds of the vocal cord and is often accompanied by erythema or edema. Benign growths include polyps, caused by chronic irritation of the mucosa, and papillomas, associated with the human papillomavirus (HPV9, HPV11).

Another benign lesion is the contact granuloma, which is usually bilateral and located over the medial arytenoid mucosa in the posterior larynx. This lesion is secondary to a break in the mucoperichondrium and a subsequent reaction to healing. It may be secondary to vocal abuse or to nocturnal acid reflux. Also, benign scarring or webbing of the anterior vocal cords sometimes results in hoarseness.

Cancer may occur anywhere in the larynx but is most common on the vocal folds. Because vocal cord cancer gives rise to symptoms early in its course, it is potentially curable when diagnosed. More than 95% of vocal cord cancers are squamous cell carcinomas. Cigarette smoke is the chief carcinogen responsible for most of the cases.

Additional local causes of hoarseness include trauma, vocal cord paralysis, and spastic dysphonia, a functional disorder of phonation resulting in abrupt interruptions of speech.

Regional disorders producing hoarseness include idiopathic organic tremors, amyotrophic lateral sclerosis, cerebrovascular accidents, and any neurologic deficit that results in paralysis of the diaphragm or loss of coordination of the diaphragm and chest wall musculature. Elderly patients may have hoarseness (presbylaryngeus) simply due to aging. Pulmonary disease of almost any etiology can result in a loss of vocal strength and lung reserve, culminating in hoarseness. Gastroesophageal reflux can also result in hoarseness. Several endocrine disorders may present with hoarseness (see Chapters 120, 121, and 124). Acromegaly results in irreversible laryngeal changes and hoarseness. Hypothyroidism causes vocal cord edema and weakness with resultant hoarseness. Hypoparathyroidism may result in hypocalcemia, and subsequent tetany may cause laryngospasm. Diabetic neuropathy may cause vocal cord weakness or paralysis. Progesterone results in increased vascularity and enlargement of the vocal cords, and it may cause hoarseness during pregnancy or the premenstrual period or when it is prescribed for contraception or gynecologic reasons.

A variety of infectious diseases can involve the larynx. Acute epiglottitis can cause sudden airway obstruction and be life-threatening (see Chapter 18). *Moraxella catarrhalis*, *Streptococcus*, *H. influenzae*, *Neisseria gonorrhoeae*, syphilis, pertussis, and *Brucella* have been demonstrated to cause acute laryngitis. A large number of viruses cause acute laryngitis including herpes, mumps, measles, varicella, variola, influenza A, parainfluenza, echo, coxsackie, and Epstein-Barr viruses. Fungal infections of the larynx are increasing in frequency as we see more individuals immunocompromised by human immunodeficiency virus (HIV) infection or chemotherapy. Pharyngeal candidiasis is common. Blastomycosis, histoplasmosis, and coccidioidomycosis may involve the larynx. Additional agents occasionally infecting the larynx are actinomycosis, tuberculosis, and leprosy.

The autoimmune diseases, such as rheumatoid arthritis, systemic lupus erythematosus, relapsing polychondritis, and scleroderma, may result in hoarseness. Other rare causes are laryngeal amyloidosis, pemphigus, Wegener's granulomatosis, and sarcoidosis.

The history and consideration of the differential diagnosis often yield a provisional diagnosis, but direct examination of the vocal cords is usually indicated for confirmation. The general examination should survey for evidence of hypothyroidism, such as coarse skin or delayed deep tendon reflexes. A complete head and neck examination should emphasize a search for nodes, tracheal deviation, and thyromegaly. The pharyngeal examination and vocal cord visualization may be accomplished with a mirror, telescope, or fiberoptic instrument.[31]

Management

The etiologic diagnosis of hoarseness usually suggests a specific treatment (e.g., voice rest for singer's nodule, antibiotics for bacterial infection). The most important general measure is hydration. Forcing fluids and humidification help restore the watery mucous layer so necessary for effective vocal cord function. Patients must avoid irritants (especially tobacco smoke!) and minimize use of the voice. Referral to an otolaryngologist is appropriate if the vocal cords cannot be visualized, for surgical lesions, or if the family physician is not confident of the diagnosis.

Flexible Fiberoptic Nasolaryngoscopy: Procedure

Flexible fiberoptic nasolaryngoscopy is a procedure family physicians can learn to perform easily in their offices. In addition to visualizing the vocal cords, it often reveals the presence and extent of nasal polyposis or confirms a diagnosis of sinusitis. Postnasal drip, septal deformities, and spurs are easily evaluated, as are the eustachian tube orifices, adenoids, lingual tonsils, hypopharynx, and larynx. Laryngeal mechanics are readily observed while the patient is speaking or singing.

Fig. 74.1. Vocal cords (C, D), epiglottis (D), maxillary orifice (E), and surrounding areas visualized by flexible fiberoptic nasolaryngoscopy. (From Curry,[32] with permission.)

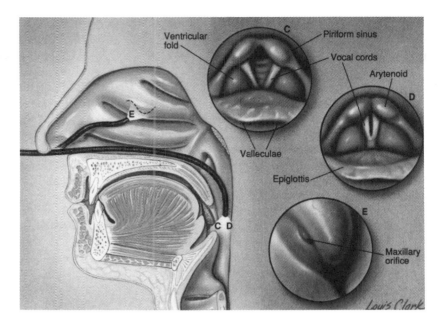

The procedure can be performed with the patient sitting on an examination table. The nasal mucosa is sprayed with a local anesthetic and the instrument advanced underneath the inferior turbinate, over the soft palate, and into the pharynx. With the instrument positioned just above the epiglottis, the valleculae, piriform sinuses, vocal chords, arytenoids, ventricular folds, and nearby structures are visualized (Fig. 74.1). Vocal cord movement is noted during breathing, and while the patient talks, sings, or says "eee." Curry[32] described the procedure in detail.

Foreign Bodies in the Nose and Ear

Discovery of a foreign body in the nose or ear is common in children. Adults present less commonly with foreign bodies in the ear, and most often these are insects, although other materials are occasionally seen, such as cotton from a tipped applicator or rice and birdseed tossed by an overzealous wedding guest.

Foreign bodies can be divided into two general categories: inorganic, such as metal (beads, toy parts, earrings), plastic (buttons, toy parts, beads), or wax (crayon); and organic, such as beans, peas, wood, or organic fiber. Inorganic objects tend to be inert and do not incite an inflammatory response. If they do not cause pain or interference with hearing, inorganic objects in the ear may go undetected for years. Organic objects, on the other hand, absorb water and set up an inflammatory response resulting in ear or nasal discharge. Button batteries used in watches and small electronic devices are especially dangerous whether in the ear, nasal cavity, or swallowed. Button batteries are corrosive, cause extensive tissue necrosis, and should be removed without delay.

Nasal Foreign Body

Children, when bored or perhaps curious, often put small objects in their nasal cavities. They may present immediately because the event was observed or because of symptoms of nasal congestion or upper respiratory tract noise. They may also present later with nasal discharge or congestion. If the object is of long standing, the child may present as a diagnostic dilemma, such as a cold or runny nose that won't go away. Unilateral nasal discharge in a child is nearly always associated with a foreign body. An accompanying foul-smelling discharge or complaint of "terrible breath" by the parent makes a foreign body even more likely. In the nose, organic material sets up an inflammatory response with resultant mucopurulent discharge that may obscure the presence of the foreign body owing to swelling of the turbinates and the presence of a discharge.

The foreign body may be visible in the anterior nasal cavity on gross inspection with a penlight or otoscope. If the object is smooth or small enough and the child is old enough to cooperate, the object may be blown out by occluding the unaffected nostril and asking the child to blow through the nose. Another strategy is a positive pressure technique, which is similar to the nose-blowing method.[33] The parent provides the pressure by giving a puff of air as in the technique of mouth-to-mouth resuscitation. The parent places the child on his or her back and tells the child that the parent is going to give him or her a big kiss. While occluding the unaffected nostril, the parent delivers a puff of air through the child's mouth, which propels the object forward from the child's nose—usually onto the cheek of the parent. The process may need to be repeated once or twice but is less traumatic than repeated attempts with instrumentation. Should the technique fail, instrumentation may be attempted. Neither long-standing foreign bodies nor rough or sharp-edged objects (e.g., jacks or Lego blocks, which may lacerate the mucosa as they are forced out) are as likely to respond to this method.

Another method previously described is a "sneeze" method, where an irritant such as pepper is used to induce a sneeze to help propel the object out.[34]

If the object is irregular in shape, has sharp edges, or is lodged farther up the nasal passage, removal may be more difficult. After gross inspection, the tip of the nose is tilted up and the nasal speculum is used to further inspect the nasal cavity. Lateral films of the head may be needed to characterize the object so that removal can be better planned. Vaseline gauze can be tucked around the object to facilitate removal and lessen the damage done by sharp edges. Cup-shaped forceps can be helpful when removing small, round objects. Regular forceps usually do not work well, because the objects are slippery, difficult to grip, and sometimes end up being propelled farther into the nose as they slip out of the forceps. Another technique is to insert a small Foley catheter beyond the object and withdraw it after inflating the balloon. Because beans, peas, and other organic matter swell as they take up water, prompt removal is usually easier than delayed removal. Once swelling and mucopurulent drainage begin, foreign bodies become lodged more securely, and forceps or other instruments may be required. Always it is important to approach the child gently, realizing often there is only one chance to remove the object without major resistance from the child.

Complications of removal and removal attempts are laceration and bleeding. The most serious complication however, is propelling the object into the airway, leading to aspiration and respiratory compromise. Referral for removal under anesthesia may be necessary.

Foreign Body in the Ear

Foreign bodies in the ear are more common in the pediatric population, but children are not the only ones who put "more than their elbow" in their ears. On inspection with the otoscope, the foreign body may be easily seen or obscured by pustular discharge or may be lodged beyond the isthmus of the canal in the anterior recess. For easily accessible objects, a hook passed over the object, point oriented downward, may be used to rake out the foreign body. Round foreign bodies may require cup-shaped forceps, as regular forceps tend to shoot the object farther into the canal. Many objects can be easily retrieved from the ear by using suction connected to a small-diameter suction tip. Magnetic objects may be removed with a strong magnet if the object is not lodged beyond the bony isthmus of the canal.[35] Inorganic objects may be syringed out using warm water. The stream of water is directed above or past the object with the idea that the backflow of the water flushes out the foreign body as it exits. Use of a water jet device is not recommended because of pain and the possibility of driving the object forcefully into the canal or tympanic membrane. Organic objects should not be syringed. Because of the hygroscopic nature of these objects, a failed attempt at syringing results in a swollen foreign body, which then may occlude the canal and be even more difficult to remove. Cup-shaped forceps and hooks passed over the object may be used in the same fashion as for inert foreign bodies. Using cyanoacrylate glue (superglue) applied to a wood end

of a cotton swab, the glue can be held against the object until it hardens, which does not take long. The swab and object can then be gently removed together.

Adults and children alike may present with insects in the ear, and movement by the insect can cause intense pain. Instilling warm oil can immobilize or kill the insect, which can then be syringed from the canal. If alcohol is used it should be mixed with warm water to prevent precipitating nystagmus and accompanying nausea with possible vomiting. Although not often seen in Western countries, maggots can also become lodged in the ear canal. Prior to syringing, they require treatment with chloroform or ether so they release their hold on the ear canal. Ticks may require referral for removal depending on their position in the canal.

Children with foreign bodies in the ear must be approached gently and calmly. They are often uncooperative, and removal attempts can cause trauma to the ear canal and bleeding even under ideal circumstances. Because trauma to the drum and ossicular chain is also possible during attempts to remove foreign objects, referral for removal under anesthesia may be indicated for the uncooperative child.

References

1. Dobie RA. A review of randomized clinical trials in tinnitus. Laryngoscope 1999;109:202–11.
2. Ciocon JO, Amede F, Lechtenberg C, Astor F. Tinnitus: a stepwise workup to quiet the noise within. Geriatrics 1995;50(2):18–25.
3. Simpson JJ, Davies WE. Recent advances in the pharmacological treatment of tinnitus. Trends Pharmacol Sci 1999;20:12–8.
4. Vernon JA. Masking of tinnitus through a cochlear implant. J Am Acad Audiol 2000;11:293–4.
5. Steenerson RL, Cronin GW. Treatment of tinnitus with electrical stimulation. Otolaryngol Head Neck Surg 1999;121:511–3.
6. Park J, White AR, Ernst E. Efficacy of acupuncture as a treatment for tinnitus: a systematic review. Arch Otolaryngol Head Neck Surg 2000;126:489–92.
7. Simpson JJ, Donaldson I, Davies WE. Use of homeopathy in the treatment of tinnitus. Br J Audiol 1998;32:227–3.
8. Andersson G, Lyttkens L. A meta-analytic review of psychological treatments for tinnitus. Br J Audiol 1999;33:201–10.
9. Mason J, Rogerson D. Client-centered hypnotherapy for tinnitus: who is likely to benefit? Am J Clin Hypn 1995;37:295–9.
10. Jones KL. Smith's recognizable patterns of human malformation, 5th ed. Philadelphia: WB Saunders, 1997.
11. Tomaski SM, Grundfast KM. A stepwise approach to the diagnosis and treatment of hereditary hearing loss. Pediatr Clin North Am 1999;46:35–48.
12. Northern JL, Downs MP. Development of auditory behavior. In: Hearing in children, 4th ed. Baltimore: Williams & Wilkins, 1991;103–36.
13. Francois M, Laccourreye L, Huy E, Narcy P. Hearing impairment in infants after meningitis: detection by transient evoked otoacoustic emissions. J Pediatr 1997;130:712–7.
14. McPherson B, Kei J, Smyth V, Latham S, Loscher J. Feasibility of community-based screening using transient evoked otoacoustic emissions. Public Health 1998;112:147–52.
15. Morlet T, FerberViart C, Putet G, Sevin F, Duclaux R. Auditory screening in high-risk per-term and full-term neonates using transient evoked otoacoustic emissions and brainstem auditory evoked potentials. Int J Pediatr Otorhinolaryngol 1998;45:31–40.

16. Paludetti G, Ottaviani F, Fetoni AR Zuppa AA, Tortorolo G. Transient evoked otoacoustic emissions (TEOEs) in new-borns; normative data. Int J Pediatr Otorhinolaryngol 1999;47:235–41.

17. Vohr BR, Carty LM, Moore PE, Letourneau K. The Rhode Island hearing assessment program: experience with statewide hearing screening (1993–1996). J Pediatr 1998;133:353–7.

18. Martin FN. Auditory tests for site of lesion. In: Introduction to audiology, 4th ed. Englewood Cliffs, NJ: Prentice Hall, 1991; 156–214.

19. Brechtelsbauer DA. Adult hearing loss. Prim Care 1990;17: 249–66.

20. Cowan PF, Chow JM. Sudden sensorineural hearing loss. Am Fam Physician 1988;37:207–10.

21. Palmer C, Adams S, Bourgeois M, Durrant J, Rossi M. Reduction in caregiver identified problem behaviors in patients with Alzheimer's disease post hearing aid fitting. J Sp Lang Hear Res 1999;42:312–28.

22. Keeve JP. Ototoxic drugs and the workplace. Am Fam Physician 1988;38:177–81.

23. Tan LK, Calhoun KH. Epistaxis. Med Clin North Am 1999; 83(1):43–56.

24. Krempl GA, Noorily AD. Use of oxymetazoline in the management of epistaxis. Ann Otol Rhinol Laryngol 1995;104:704–6.

25. Randall DA, Freeman SB. Management of anterior and posterior epistaxis. Am Fam Physician 1991;43:2007–14.

26. Silvers AR. Salivary glands. Radiol Clin North Am 1998; 36(5):941–66,vi.

27. Murrah VA. Diabetes mellitus and associated oral manifestations: a review. J Oral Pathol 1985;14:271–81.

28. Davies AN. A comparison of artificial saliva and pilocarpine in the management of xerostomia in patients with advanced cancer. Palliat Med 1998;12(2):105–11.

29. Williams MF. Sialolithiasis. Otolaryngol Clin North Am 1999; 32(5):819–34.

30. Maragos NE. Hoarseness. Prim Care 1990;7:347–63.

31. Garrett CG. Hoarseness. Med Clin North Am 1999;83(1): 115–23,ix.

32. Curry RW. Flexible fiberoptic nasolaryngoscopy. Fam Pract Recert 1990;12(2):21–36.

33. Backlin S. Positive pressure technique for nasal foreign body removal in children. Ann Emerg Med 1995;25:554–5.

34. Dale BAB, Kerr AIG. Diseases of the external ear. In: Maran AGD, editor. Turner's diseases of the nose, throat and ear, 10th ed. London: Wright, 1988;263–77.

35. Stool SE, McConnel CS. Foreign bodies in pediatric otolaryngology. Clin Pediatr 1973;12:113–6.

75
Hypertension

Stephen A. Brunton

Despite widespread efforts to improve education and enhance public awareness, up to 33% of persons with hypertension remain undiagnosed, and only about 50% of those known to have hypertension are adequately controlled. The percentages of patients who are aware that they have hypertension, who are treated, and who are controlled have increased since the 1970s (Table 75.1). Most have stage 1 hypertension, and controversy still exists concerning the appropriate approach to these patients. Nonpharmacologic therapy is often the first choice, and this approach continues to evolve.[1] Of the 20 to 30 million hypertensives who receive pharmacologic therapy, fewer than 50% adhere to their therapeutic regimen for more than 1 year, and 60% of these patients reduce the dosage of their drug owing to adverse effects. A negative impact on the patient's quality-of-life may occur as a result of just making the diagnosis. Effects such as increased absenteeism, sickness behavior, hypochondria, and decreased self-esteem have been noted in cohorts of previously well individuals who have been told they were hypertensive.[2] A 1987 survey of physicians revealed that they regarded quality-of-life changes to be the primary impediment to effective pharmacologic treatment of hypertension.

The challenge to the clinician is to provide patient education and develop a hypertension regimen that effectively lowers blood pressure or reduces cardiac risk factors, minimizes changes in concomitant disease states, and maintains or improves quality of life. Putting the patient first necessitates integrating the individual patient's lifestyle and current disease states with a thorough understanding of the effect of drug and nondrug therapy on quality of life. This chapter reviews nonpharmacologic and pharmacologic therapy, with special emphasis on individualizing patient regimens to improve adherence.

Detection

The diagnosis of hypertension should not be based on any single measurement but should be established on the basis of at least three readings with an average systolic blood pressure of 140 mm Hg and a diastolic pressure of 90 mm Hg. Mechanisms should be established to standardize the measurement process: (1) The patient should be seated comfortably with the arm positioned at heart level. (2) Caffeine or nicotine should not have been ingested within 30 minutes before measurement. (3) The patient should be seated in a quiet environment for at least 5 minutes. (4) An appropriate sphygmomanometer cuff should be used (i.e., the rubber bladder should encircle at least two-thirds of the arm). (5) Measurement of the diastolic blood pressure should be based on the disappearance of sound (phase V Korotkoff sound). Table 75.2 describes the classification of blood pressure for adults.

Evaluation

Evaluation is directed toward establishing the etiology of hypertension, identifying other cardiovascular risk factors, and evaluating the possibility of target organ damage. Although most hypertension is considered "essential," primary, or idiopathic, it is necessary to eliminate secondary causes of hypertension, including renovascular disease, polycystic renal disease, aortic coarctation, Cushing syndrome, and pheochromocytoma. It is important to ensure that the patient is not on medications that may result in increased blood pressure, such as oral contraceptives, nasal decongestants, appetite suppressants, nonsteroidal antiinflammatory drugs (NSAIDs), steroids, and tricyclic antidepressants.

Medical History

The medical history should include a review of the family history for hypertension and cardiovascular disease, previous measurements of blood pressure, symptoms suggestive of secondary causes of hypertension, and other cardiovascular risk factors including smoking, hyperlipidemia, obesity, and diabetes. Environmental and psychosocial factors that may influence blood pressure control or the ability of the individual to comply with therapy should also be considered.

Table 75.1. **Trends in the Awareness, Treatment, and Control of High Blood Pressure in Adults: United States, 1976–94**[a]

	NHANES II (1976–80)	NHANES III (Phase 1) 1988–91	NHANES III (Phase 2) 1991–94
Awareness	51%	73%	68.4%
Treatment	31%	55%	53.6%
Control[b]	10%	29%	27.4%

[a]Data are for adults age 18 to 74 years with SBP of 140 mm Hg or greater, DBP of 90 mm Hg or greater, or taking antihypertensive medication.

[b]SBP below 140 mm Hg and DBP below 90 mm Hg.

Source: National Institutes of Health.[1]

Physical Examination and Laboratory Tests

The physical examination should include more than one blood pressure measurement in both standing and seated positions with verification in the contralateral arm. (If a discrepancy exists, the higher value is used.) The rest of the physical examination includes (1) an evaluation of the optic fundi with gradation of hypertensive changes; (2) examination of the neck for bruits and thyromegaly; (3) a heart examination to evaluate for hypertrophy, arrhythmias, or additional sounds; (4) abdominal examination to search for evidence of aneurysms or kidney abnormalities; (5) examination of the extremities to check the pulses; and (6) a careful neurologic evaluation.

Some baseline laboratory tests may be helpful for the initial evaluation. They might include urinalysis and serum potassium, blood urea nitrogen, and creatinine levels. A lipid panel may help evaluate cardiovascular risk.

Table 75.2. **Classification of Blood Pressure for Adults Aged 18 Years and Older**[a]

Category	Systolic (mm Hg)	Diastolic (mm Hg)
Optimal[b]	<120	<80
Normal	<130	<85
High normal	130–139	85–89
Hypertension[c]		
Stage 1	140–159	90–99
Stage 2	160–179	100–109
Stage 3	>180	>110

Source: National Institutes of Health.[1]

Note: In addition to classifying stages of hypertension based on average blood pressure levels, the clinician should specify the presence or absence of target organ disease and additional risk factors. For example, a patient with diabetes, a blood pressure of 142/94 mm Hg, and left ventricular hypertrophy should be classified as "stage 1 hypertension with target organ disease (left ventricular hypertrophy) and with another major risk factor (diabetes)." This specificity is important for risk classification and management.

[a]Not taking antihypertensive drugs and not acutely ill. When systolic and diastolic pressures fall into different categories, the higher category should be selected to classify the individual's blood pressure status. For instance, 160/92 mm Hg should be classified as stage 2 and 174/120 mm Hg as stage 3. Isolated systolic hypertension is defined as systolic pressure of 140 mm Hg or more and diastolic pressure of less than 90 mm Hg and staged appropriately (e.g., 170/82 mm Hg is defined as stage 2 isolated systolic hypertension).

[b]Optimal blood pressure with respect to cardiovascular risk is systolic pressure <120 mm Hg and diastolic pressure <80 mm Hg. However, unusually low readings should be evaluated for clinical significance.

[c]Based on the average of two or more readings taken at each of two or more visits after an initial screening.

Treatment

The goal of therapy is not just to bring the blood pressure lower than 140 mm Hg systolic and 90 mm Hg diastolic, but rather to prevent the morbidity and mortality associated with hypertension. As such, the decision to treat hypertension is based on documentation that the blood pressure has remained elevated and on assessment of the risk for that particular patient.

In general, individuals with blood pressure ranges considered borderline high (i.e., systolic of 130 to 139 mm Hg or diastolic of 85 to 89 mm Hg) should have their blood pressures rechecked within 1 year. Blood pressures in the stage 1 range should be confirmed within 2 months by repeated measurements; however, certain lifestyle approaches are appropriate even at this level. Blood pressures that are markedly elevated (e.g., systolic >180 mm Hg or diastolic >110 mm Hg) or those associated with evidence of existing end-organ damage may require immediate pharmacologic intervention. In general, whether pharmacologic intervention is initiated, a nonpharmacologic approach is the foundation of any management strategy.[1]

Nonpharmacologic Therapeutic Approaches

Information concerning dietary modifications, exercise, weight reduction, the role of cations, and the possible role of relaxation and stress management techniques for reducing blood pressure have opened the door for greater acceptance of multiple nonpharmacologic approaches to the treatment of hypertension. The 1988 report of the Joint National Committee (JNC) on the Detection, Evaluation, and Treatment of High Blood Pressure recommended that "nonpharmacological approaches be used both as definitive intervention and as an adjunct for pharmacological therapy and should be considered for all antihypertensive therapy."

Several studies have shown positive correlation of increased blood pressure with alcohol consumption of more than 2 ounces/day.[3] Although smoking has not been shown to cause sustained hypertension, it is associated with increased cardiovascular, pulmonary, and hypertension risks, and therefore should be eliminated.[4]

Weight reduction has a strong correlation with decreased blood pressure in obese individuals. Stamler et al[5] reported that a 10-pound weight loss maintained over a 4-year period allowed 50% of participants previously on pharmacologic management to remain normotensive and free of medication.

Sodium restriction has been a mainstay of hypertension control, as a 100-mEq drop in daily intake can result in a 2- to 9-mm Hg decline in systolic blood pressure in salt-sensitive individuals. This goal is one of the easiest for a patient to accomplish, as moderate restriction can be accomplished by eliminating table salt for cooking, avoiding salty foods, and using a salt substitute.[6]

Regular aerobic exercise not only assists with weight reduction but also appears to lower diastolic blood pressure. Cade and associates[7] reported a decline from 117 to 97 mm Hg diastolic blood pressure after 3 months of daily walking or running for 2 miles. This effect appeared to be independent of weight loss, and some benefit persisted even if the patient became sedentary.

Vegetarian diets high in polyunsaturated fats, potassium, and fiber result in lower blood pressures than diets high in saturated fats. Dietary fat control also contributes to the reduction of cholesterol and coronary artery disease risk.[8] The role of cations such as potassium, magnesium, and calcium in lowering blood pressure has now been investigated. High potassium intake (>80 mEq/day) may result in a modest decline in blood pressure while offering a natriuretic and cardioprotective effect. These effects are more pronounced in hypokalemic individuals.[9] Magnesium and calcium supplementation of more than 300 mg/day and 800 mg/day, respectively, have been shown to lower the relative risk of developing hypertension in a large cohort of women. The impact of individual supplementation is less clear, and the role of these substances is still controversial.[10]

Stress management and relaxation techniques over a 4-year period have been shown to reduce systolic blood pressure 10 to 15 mm Hg and diastolic blood pressure 5 to 10 mm Hg. However, these results are variable and are largely dependent on the instructor–patient relationship.[11]

The effects of nonpharmacologic approaches can be additive and certainly are beneficial even if the patient requires drug therapy. Stamler and associates[12] documented that reducing weight and lowering salt and alcohol intake allowed 39% of patients previously on therapy to remain normotensive without medication over a 4-year period. In the mildly hypertensive individual, these lifestyle modifications should be tried for at least 6 months before initiating pharmacologic therapy.

Pharmacologic Therapy

The decision to initiate drug therapy requires consideration of individual patient characteristics, such as age, race, sex, family history, cardiovascular risk factors, concomitant disease states, compliance, and ability to purchase the prescribed therapeutic agent. Pharmacologic therapy is recommended when the systolic blood pressure is higher than 160 mm Hg and the diastolic blood pressure remains higher than 100 mm Hg. Treatment of stage 2 and 3 hypertension (systolic pressure >160 and diastolic pressure >100 mm Hg) has reduced cardiovascular morbidity and mortality dramatically since the 1960s. The incidence of stroke, congestive heart failure, and left ventricular hypertrophy has also decreased among treated stage 1 hypertensives, and therapy is recommended if patients have one or more cardiovascular risk factors and have not controlled their blood pressure after 6 months of lifestyle modification.

The ideal antihypertensive agent would improve quality of life, reduce coronary heart disease risk factors, maintain normal hemodynamic profiles, reduce left ventricular hypertrophy, have a positive impact on concomitant disease states, and reduce end-organ damage while effectively lowering blood pressure on a convenient dosing regimen at minimal cost to the patient. This "magic bullet" has yet to be synthesized, although several of the newer antihypertensive classes offer the possibility of many of these positive outcomes.

The selection of an appropriate antihypertensive agent may be based on the current recommendations of the JNC on the Detection, Evaluation, and Treatment of High Blood Pressure or individualized to the specific medical, social, psychological, and economic situation of each patient.[1] The previous stepped-care approach has been modified by the JNC into an algorithm that permits an individualized approach to the patient (Fig. 75.1). Many clinicians have moved away from the stepped-care philosophy toward a monotherapy approach, which maximizes the dose of one drug before substituting or adding another. Combination therapy with lower doses of several agents may also be utilized to minimize adverse effects. Therapeutic choices must be based on a sound understanding of the mechanism of action, pharmacokinetics, adverse effect profile, and cost of available agents.

Major Antihypertensive Classes

ACE Inhibitors

Angiotensin-converting enzyme (ACE) inhibitors (Table 75.3) block the conversion of angiotensin I to angiotensin II, resulting in decreased aldosterone production with subsequent increased sodium and water excretion. Renin and potassium levels are usually increased as a result of this medication. The hemodynamic response includes decreased peripheral resistance, increased renal blood flow, and minimal changes in cardiac output and glomerular filtration rate. There is little change in insulin and glucose levels or in the lipid fractions. The adverse effects of

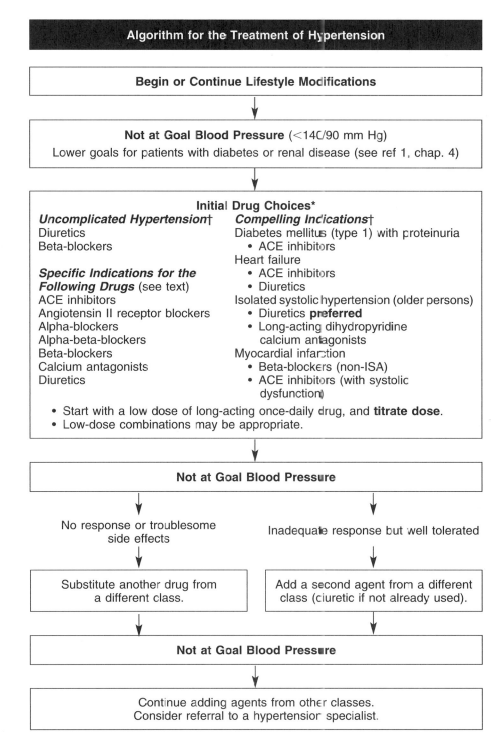

Algorithm for the Treatment of Hypertension

Begin or Continue Lifestyle Modifications

↓

Not at Goal Blood Pressure (<140/90 mm Hg)
Lower goals for patients with diabetes or renal disease (see ref 1, chap. 4)

↓

Initial Drug Choices*

Uncomplicated Hypertension†   *Compelling Indications†*
Diuretics   Diabetes mellitus (type 1) with proteinuria
Beta-blockers   • ACE inhibitors
                                  Heart failure
Specific Indications for the   • ACE inhibitors
Following Drugs (see text)   • Diuretics
ACE inhibitors   Isolated systolic hypertension (older persons)
Angiotensin II receptor blockers • Diuretics **preferred**
Alpha-blockers   • Long-acting dihydropyridine
Alpha-beta-blockers   calcium antagonists
Beta-blockers   Myocardial infarction
Calcium antagonists   • Beta-blockers (non-ISA)
Diuretics   • ACE inhibitors (with systolic
                                    dysfunction)

• Start with a low dose of long-acting once-daily drug, and **titrate dose.**
• Low-dose combinations may be appropriate.

↓

Not at Goal Blood Pressure

↓   ↓

No response or troublesome   Inadequate response but well tolerated
side effects

↓   ↓

Substitute another drug from   Add a second agent from a different
a different class.   class (diuretic if not already used).

↓   ↓

Not at Goal Blood Pressure

↓

Continue adding agents from other classes.
Consider referral to a hypertension specialist.

*Unless contraindicated. ACE indicates angiotensin-converting enzyme; ISA, intrinsic sympathomimetic activity.
†Based on randomized controlled trials (see ref. 1, chaps. 3 and 4).

Fig. 75.1. Algorithm for the treatment of hypertension. (From National Institutes of Health.[1])

ACE inhibitors include cough (1–30%), headache, dizziness, first-dose syncope in salt- or volume-depleted patients, acute renal failure in patients with renal artery stenosis, angioedema (0.1–0.2%), and teratogenic effects in the human fetus. Thus, ACE inhibitors should not be used during the second and third trimesters of pregnancy. Captopril (Capoten) has a higher incidence of rash, dysgeusia, neutropenia, and proteinuria than the others due to a sulfhydryl group in the ring structure.[13]

The ACE inhibitors are good first-line agents for patients with diabetes, congestive heart failure, peripheral vascular

Table 75.3. **Antihypertensive Drugs**

Drug class	Available doses (mg)	Usual dose/schedule (mg/day)	Half-life (hours)	Peak (hours)	Pregnancy class
ACE inhibitors					
Benazepril (Lotensin)	5, 10, 20, 40	10–40 qd	10	2–4	C (1st trimester) D (2nd and 3rd trimester)
Captopril (Capoten)	12.5, 25, 50, 100	25–50 bid–tid	2	1–2	C (1st trimester) D (2nd and 3rd trimester)
Enalapril (Vasotec)	2.5, 5, 10, 20	5–40 qd	11	4	C (1st trimester) D (2nd and 3rd trimester)
Fosinopril (Monopril)	10, 20	10–40 qd	12	2–6	C (1st trimester) D (2nd and 3rd trimester)
Lisinopril (Prinivil, Zestril)	2.5, 5, 10, 20, 40	10–40 qd	12	6	C (1st trimester) D (2nd and 3rd trimester)
Moexipril (Univasc)	7.5, 15	7.5–30 qd	2–10	1.5	C (1st trimester) D (2nd and 3rd trimester)
Quinapril (Accupril)	5, 10, 20, 40	10–80 qd	2	2–4	C (1st trimester) D (2nd and 3rd trimester)
Perindopril (Aceon)	2, 4, 8,	4–8qd	3–10	3–7	C (1st trimester) D (2nd and 3rd trimester)
Ramipril (Altace)	1.25, 2.5, 5, 10	2.5–20 qd	2	3–6	C (1st trimester) D (2nd and 3rd trimester)
Trandolapril (Mavik)	1, 2, 4	2–4 mg qd	10	4–10	C (1st trimester) D (2nd and 3rd trimester)
Beta-Blockers				*Selectivity*	
Atenolol (Tenormin)	25, 50, 100	50–100 qd	9	B_1	C
Acebutolol (Sectral)	200, 400	400–800 qd	4	B_1, ISA	B
Betaxolol (Kerlone)	10, 20	10–20 qd	22	B_1	C
Bisoprolol (Zebeta)	5, 10	5–20 qd	11	B_1	C
Carteolol (Cartrol)	2.5, 5	2.5–10 qd	6	B_1, B_2, ISA	C
Labetalol (Normodyne)	100, 200, 300	100–400 bid	6	B_1, B_2, α	C
Nadolol (Corgard)	20, 40, 80, 120, 160	40–80 qd	24	B_1, B_2	C
Metoprolol (Lopressor)	50, 100	100–450 qd	3	B_1	C
Penbutolol (Levatol)	20	20–80 qd	5	B_1, B_2, ISA	C
Pindolol (Visken)	5, 10	10–30 qd	4	B_1, B_2, ISA	B
Propranolol (Inderal)	60, 80, 120, 160, SR;	80–160 SR qd	10	B_1, B_2	C
	10, 20, 40, 60, 80, 90	20–120 bid	4	B_1, B_2	C
Timolol (Blocadren)	5, 10, 20	10–30 bid	4	B_1, B_2	C
Calcium entry antagonists					
Amlodipine (Norvasc)	2.5, 5, 10	2.5–10		6–12	C
Diltiazem (Cardizem)	SR 60, 90, 120	SR 60–120 bid		6–11	C
	CD 120, 180, 240, 300	CD 180–360 qd	6	12	
	30, 60, 90, 120,	30–90 qid		2–3	
(Dilacor XR)	120, 180, 240	120–360 qd	4	4–6	C
Felodipine (Plendil)	SR 2.5, 5, 10	5–20 qd	16	2–5	C
Isradipine (DynaCirc)	2.5, 5	2.5–5 bid	8	1.5	C
Nicardipine	SR 30, 45, 60	SR 30–60 bid			
(Cardene)	20, 30	20–40 tid	4	0.5–2	C
Nifedipine (Adalat Procardia)	SR 10, 20, 30, 60, 90	30–120 qd	5	0.5–6	C
Nisoldipine (Sular)	10, 20, 30, 40	20–40 qd	10	6–12	C
Verapamil (Calan, Covera, Isoptin, Verelan)	SR 120, 180, 240 40, 80, 120	240–480 qd	7	1–2	C
α_1-blockers					
Doxazosin (Cardura)	1, 2, 4, 8	1–16 mg qd	22	2–3	B
Prazosin (Minipress)	1, 2, 5	1–5 bid–tid	3	3	C
Terazosin (Hytrin)	1, 2, 5, 10	1–10 qd	12	1–2	C
Central α_2-agonists					
Clonidine (Catapres)	0.1, 0.2, 0.3	0.2–1.2 qd	16	3–5	C
	TTS 1, 2, 3	1 patch weekly	19	2–3 days	
Guanabenz (Wytensin)	4, 8	4–8 bid	6	2–4	C
Guanfacine (Tenex)	1, 2	1–3 qd	17	3	B
Methyldopa (Aldomet)	125, 250, 500	250–500 tid–qid	2	2–4	B

(Continued on next page)

Table 75.3. Antihypertensive Drugs (Continued)

Drug class	Available doses (mg)	Usual dose/ schedule (mg/day)	Half-life (hours)	Peak (hours)	Pregnancy class
Vasodilators					
Hydralazine (Apresoline)	10, 25, 50, 100	10–50 qid	7	0.5–2	C
Minoxidil (Loniten)	2.5, 10	10–40 qd	4	2–3	C
$\alpha\beta$-Blockers					
Carvedilol (Coreg)	6.25, 12.5, 25	6.25–12.5 bid	7	3–4	C
Labetalol (Normodyne)	100, 200, 300	100 mg–400 bid	6	2–4	C
Selected thiazide diuretics					
Chlorothiazide (Diuril)	250–500	500–2000 qd	6–12	4	
Hydrochlorothiazide (HydroDIURIL)	25, 50, 100	25–50 qd	6–12	4–6	
Chlorthalidone (Hygroton)	25, 50, 100	25–100 qd	24–72	2–6	
Indapamide (Lozol)	1.25, 2.5	2.5–5 qd	36	2	B
Metolazone (Zaroxolyn)	0.5, 2.5, 5, 10	2.5–5 qd	12–24	2.6	B
Loop diuretics					
Bumetanide (Bumex)	0.5, 1, 2	0.5–2 qd	4–6	1–2,	C
Furosemide (Lasix)	20, 40, 80	20–40 qd–bid	6–8	1–2	C
Potassium-sparing diuretics					
Amiloride (Midamor)	5	5–20 qd	24	6–10	B
Spironolactone (Aldactone)	25, 50, 100	25–100 qd	48–72	48–72	D
Triamterene (Dyrenium)	50, 100	100 bid	12–16	6–8	B
Angiotensin receptor antagonists					
Eprosartan (Teveten)	400, 600	400–800 qd	5–9	3–6	C (1st trimester) D (2nd and 3rd trimester)
Irbesartan (Avapro)	75, 150, 300	150–300 qd	11–15	3–6	C (1st trimester) D (2nd and 3rd trimester)
Losartan (Cozaar)	25, 50	25–100 qd	2–9	1–4	C (1st trimester) D (2nd and 3rd trimester)
Telmisartan (Micardis)	20, 40, 80	20–80 qd	24	0.5–1	C (1st trimester) D (2nd and 3rd trimester)
Valsartan (Diovan)	80, 160	80–320 qd	6	2–4	C (1st trimester) D (2nd and 3rd trimester)

ISA = Intrinsic sympathomimetic activity; D = positive evidence of human fetal risk; C = fetal risk documented in animals; B = low fetal risk; SR = slow release; CD = controlled delivery.

disease, elevated lipids, and renal insufficiency. This class is effective in all races and ages, although black patients respond better with the addition of a diuretic.[14,15]

Angiotensin Receptor Antagonists

Angiotensin receptor antagonists, a newer class of antihypertensive agents, binds to the angiotensin II receptors, resulting in blockade of the vasoconstrictor and aldosterone-secreting effects of angiotensin II. In addition, bradykinin production is not stimulated. The first agent available in the United States was losartan (Cozaar). The physiologic effects of losartan include a rise in plasma renin and angiotensin II levels and a decrease in aldosterone production. There is no significant change in plasma potassium levels and no effect on glomeru-

lar filtration rate, renal plasma flow, heart rate, triglycerides, total cholesterol, high-density lipoprotein (HDL) cholesterol, or glucose. Losartan use does produce a small uricosuric effect with lowering of plasma uric acid levels.

These agents are effective antihypertensives in adults and the elderly. Blood pressure–lowering effects are not as significant in black patients. Adverse effects include muscle pain, dizziness, cough, insomnia, and nasal congestion. As with ACE inhibitors, angiotensin receptor antagonists should not be used during the second and third trimesters of pregnancy.

At this time the role of angiotensin receptor antagonists is not completely defined. Further study of the hemodynamic effects in large populations is needed to determine the role in cardiac patients. These agents are an alternative antihypertensive agent for patients experiencing adverse effects from ACE inhibitors.

Calcium Entry Antagonists

Calcium entry antagonists (CEAs) inhibit the movement of calcium across cell membranes in myocardial and smooth muscles. This action dilates coronary arteries, and additional peripheral arteriole dilation reduces total peripheral resistance, resulting in decreased blood pressure. Although the mechanism of action for lowering blood pressure is similar for these agents, structural differences result in varying effects on cardiac conduction and adverse effect profiles. Verapamil (Calan, Covera, Isoptin, Verelan) and diltiazem (Cardizem, Dilacor, Tiazac) slow atrioventricular (AV) node conduction and prolong the effective refractory period in the AV node. Cardiac output is increased by nifedipine (Procardia), nicardipine (Cardene), isradipine (DynaCirc), and felodipine (Plendil).

The calcium entry antagonists are contraindicated in patients with heart block, cardiogenic shock, or acute myocardial infarction. Common adverse effects include peripheral edema, dizziness, headache, asthenia, nausea, constipation, flushing, and tachycardia. Calcium entry antagonists have no significant impact on lipid profiles or glucose metabolism.[1]

These agents are effective at all ages and in all races. They are good choices for patients with diabetes, angina, migraine, chronic obstructive pulmonary disease (COPD)/asthma, peripheral vascular disease, renal insufficiency, and supraventricular arrhythmias.[14,15]

Diuretics

Thiazide, loop, and potassium-sparing diuretics have been the mainstay of antihypertensive therapy since the 1960s. They remain as first-line agents in the JNC VI approach, although the ACE inhibitors and calcium entry antagonists are rapidly replacing diuretics as monotherapy for hypertension.

Thiazide diuretics increase renal excretion of sodium and chloride at the distal segment of the renal tubule, resulting in decreased plasma volume, cardiac output, and renal blood flow and increased renin activity. Potassium excretion is increased, and calcium and uric acid elimination is decreased.[13] Thiazides adversely affect lipid metabolism by increasing the total cholesterol level 6% to 10% and the low-density lipoprotein (LDL) cholesterol 6% to 20%, and by causing a possible 15% to 20% rise in triglycerides.[15] Plasma glucose levels increase secondary to a decrease in insulin secretion. Clinical adverse effects include nausea, vomiting, diarrhea, dizziness, headache, fatigue, muscle cramps, gout attacks, and impotence. Thiazides are inexpensive choices for initial therapy, but caution must be exercised in patients with preexisting cardiac dysfunction, lipid abnormalities, diabetes mellitus, and gout. The lowest effective dose is recommended to minimize these potential adverse effects. Suggested daily doses are hydrochlorothiazide (HydroDIURIL) 25 mg, chlorthalidone (Hygroton) 25 mg, and indapamide (Lozol) 2.5 mg daily. Indapamide is unique among thiazides in that it has minimal effects on glucose, lipids, and uric acid. Thiazides are good choices for volume/salt-dependent, low-renin hypertensives. Thiazides improve blood pressure control when added to ACE inhibitors, beta-blockers, vasodilators, and alpha-blockers.

The loop diuretics—furosemide (Lasix), torsemide (Demadex), and bumetanide (Bumex)—inhibit sodium and chloride reabsorption in the proximal and distal tubules and the loop of Henle. These diuretics are effective in patients with decreased renal function. The primary adverse effects include ototoxicity with high doses in patients with severe renal disease and in combination with an aminoglycoside, photosensitivity, excess potassium loss, increased serum uric acid, decreased calcium levels, and impaired glucose metabolism. Patients may experience nausea, vomiting, diarrhea, headache, blurred vision, tinnitus, muscle cramps, fatigue, or weakness. Furosemide and bumetanide are utilized in patients with compromised renal function or congestive heart failure (CHF) and as adjuncts to volume-retaining agents such as hydralazine (Apresoline) and minoxidil (Loniten).

The potassium-sparing diuretics spironolactone (Aldactone), triamterene (Dyrenium), and amiloride (Midamor) are useful for preventing potassium wastage from thiazide and loop diuretics. Spironolactone competitively inhibits the uptake of aldosterone at the receptor site in the distal tubule, thereby reducing aldosterone effects. It is used for treatment of primary aldosteronism, CHF, cirrhosis with ascites, hypertension, and hirsutism. Triamterene is used in combination with hydrochlorothiazide as Dyazide or Maxzide and effectively prevents potassium loss. Amiloride inhibits potassium excretion at the collecting duct. Adverse reactions associated with spironolactone include gynecomastia, nausea, vomiting, diarrhea, muscle cramps, lethargy, and hyperkalemia. Triamterene and amiloride have adverse effects similar to those seen with the thiazide diuretics.[13-15]

Antiadrenergic Agents

Beta-Blockers

β-adrenergic blocking agents compete with β-agonists for B_1 receptors in cardiac muscles and B_2 receptors in the bronchial and vascular musculature, inhibiting the dilator, inotropic, and chronotropic effects of β-adrenergic stimulation. Clinical responses to β-adrenergic blockade include decreased heart rate, cardiac output, blood pressure, renin production, and bronchiolar constriction; there is also an initial increase in total peripheral resistance, which returns to normal with chronic use.

Beta-blockers are contraindicated for sinus bradycardia, second- or third-degree heart block, cardiogenic shock, cardiac failure, and severe COPD/asthma. The adverse effect profile of beta-blocking agents is partially dependent on their receptor selectivity (Table 75.3). Acebutolol (Sectral), penbutolol (Levatol), carteolol (Cartrol), and pindolol (Visken) have intrinsic sympathomimetic activity (ISA), resulting in less effect on cardiac output and lipid profiles. Beta-blockers without ISA slow the heart rate, decrease cardiac output, increase peripheral vascular resistance, and cause bronchospasm. Common adverse effects include fatigue, impotence, depression, shortness of breath, cold extremities, cough, drowsiness, and dizziness. The more lipid-soluble agents, such as propranolol and metoprolol, have a higher incidence of central nervous system (CNS) effects. In diabetic patients beta-blockers may mask the usual symptoms of hypoglycemia, such as tremor, tachycardia, and hunger.[13] Increased triglycerides

(30%) and decreased HDL cholesterol (1–20%) occur with non-ISA agents.[15] Beta-blockers are effective agents in the young and white populations. Black patients may not respond as well to monotherapy because of their lower renin levels. Beta-blockers are good choices for patients with supraventricular tachycardia, high cardiac output, angina, recent myocardial infarction, migraine, and glaucoma. Caution should be exercised in those with diabetes, CHF, peripheral vascular disease, COPD/asthma, and an elevated lipid profile.[14]

Central Acting Drugs

Methyldopa (Aldomet), clonidine (Catapres), guanfacine (Tenex), and guanabenz (Wytensin) are central α_2-agonists. These agents decrease dopamine and norepinephrine production in the brain, resulting in a decrease in sympathetic nervous activity throughout the body. Blood pressure declines with the decrease in peripheral resistance. Methyldopa exhibits a unique adverse effect profile as it induces autoimmune disorders, such as those with positive Coombs' and antinuclear antibody (ANA) tests, hemolytic anemia, and hepatic necrosis. The other agents produce sedation, dry mouth, and dizziness. Abrupt clonidine withdrawal may result in rebound hypertension. These drugs are good choices for patients with asthma, diabetes, high cholesterol, and peripheral vascular disease.

Peripheral Acting Drugs

Guanadrel (Hylorel), reserpine (Serpasil), and guanethidine (Ismelin) are peripheral antiadrenergic agents. Their mechanism of action is at the storage granule level of norepinephrine release. They are infrequently chosen because of their significant side effects, which include profound hypotension, sedation, depression, and impotence.

α_1-Blockers

α_1-Receptor blockers have an affinity for the α_1-receptor on vascular smooth muscles, thereby blocking the uptake of catecholamines by smooth muscle cells. This action results in peripheral vasodilation. The currently available agents are prazosin (Minipress), terazosin (Hytrin), and doxazosin (Cardura). There is a marked reduction in blood pressure with the first dose of these drugs. It is recommended that they be started with 1 mg at bedtime and titrate slowly upward over 2 to 4 weeks. When adding a second antihypertensive the α-blocker dose should be decreased and titrated upward again. Often a diuretic is added to α_1-blocker therapy to reduce sodium and water retention. The primary adverse effects of these three drugs are dizziness, sedation, nasal congestion, headache, and postural effects. They do not significantly affect lipids, glucose, electrolytes, or exercise tolerance. α_1-Blockers are good choices for young active adults and patients with diabetes, renal insufficiency, CHF, peripheral vascular disease, COPD/asthma, or elevated lipids.

The Antihypertensive and Lipid Lowering Treatment to Prevent Heart Attack Trial (ALLHAT) was initiated in 1994 to evaluate the impact of various classes of antihypertensives on outcomes. In early 2000 the doxazosin treatment arm was discontinued because a twofold higher incidence of CHF was noted compared to those on chlorthalidone.[16]

Vasodilators

The two direct vasodilators, hydralazine (Apresoline) and minoxidil (Loniten), dilate peripheral arterioles, resulting in a significant fall in blood pressure. A sympathetic reflex increase in heart rate, renin and catecholamine release, and venous constriction occur. The renal response includes sodium and water retention. The patient often experiences tachycardia, flushing, and headache. Addition of a diuretic and a beta-blocker relieves the major adverse effects of the vasodilators. Hydralazine may cause a lupus-like reaction with fever, rash, and joint pain. Chronic use of minoxidil often results in hirsutism with increased facial and arm hair. These drugs are third- or fourth-line agents because of their adverse side-effect profile.[13–15]

Quality-of-Life Issues

The need for lifestyle changes and probable drug therapy increases the possibility that the patient's quality of life will be altered. The adverse physical, mental, and metabolic effects of antihypertensive therapy results in significant nonadherence to prescribed regimens. In 1982 Jachuck and associates[17] investigated the effect of medications on their patients by asking them, their closest relatives, and their physicians a series of questions concerning their quality of life since starting the blood pressure medications. The physicians and patients thought there was either no change or improvement, whereas 99% of the relatives thought the patients were worse. They cited side effects such as memory loss, irritability, decreased libido, hypochondria, and decreased energy as major problems.[17] Other studies during the 1980s confirm that nonselective beta-blockers, diuretics, and methyldopa compromised quality of life to a far greater extent than ACE inhibitors or calcium entry antagonists.[17–19] Further research in this area is necessary to assist the physician in determining the optimum strategy for blood pressure control to improve adherence and quality of life.

Antihypertensive Selection

It is important to consider the patient's lifestyle, economic status, belief systems, and concerns about treatment when selecting an antihypertensive agent. Therapy should be initiated with one drug in small doses to minimize adverse effects. It is important to educate the patient about the long-term benefits of therapy, including the decreased incidence of stroke and renal and cardiac disease. Adequate follow-up visits are scheduled to assess adherence and adverse effects. During these visits the patient is asked to describe the mental, physical, and emotional changes that have occurred as a result of therapy. If adverse effects are bothersome, consider an alternative selection from a different drug class and attempt to maintain monotherapy. If a second drug is needed, agents can be combined that improve efficacy without significantly altering the adverse-effect profile (e.g., adding a diuretic to an ACE inhibitor).

There are some special considerations when prescribing medications. Concomitant disease states must be considered and drugs selected that either improve or at least maintain the current clinical condition. Hypertension is a major risk factor for thrombotic and hemorrhagic strokes; smoking, CHF, diabetes, and coronary artery disease increase the risk. Patients with coronary artery disease may benefit from a calcium entry antagonist or beta-blocker with ISA to decrease anginal pain while resulting in minimal changes in lipid profiles. CHF and hypertension respond well to ACE inhibitors and diuretic therapy. Diabetes may be adversely affected by thiazide diuretics and beta-blockers. ACE inhibitors, calcium entry antagonists, and central α_2-agonists are appropriate choices.

Patients with severe renal disease are most effectively treated with loop diuretics, whereas ACE inhibitors and CEAs may decrease proteinuria and slow the progress of renal failure. As renal function declines, ACE inhibitors must be used with some caution as increased potassium and decreased renal perfusion may occur. A few agents such as methyldopa, clonidine, atenolol, nadolol, and captopril need dosage reduction in the presence of renal failure (see Chapter 97).

Asthma and COPD patients may be effectively treated with calcium entry antagonists, central α_2-agonists, and α_1-blockers. Beta-blockers and possibly diuretics should be avoided because they might exacerbate bronchospasm.

The elderly are of special concern when selecting an antihypertensive. They have decreased receptor sensitivity, changing baroreceptor response, atherosclerosis, decreased myocardial function, declining total body water, decreased renal function, and memory loss. Blood pressure should be lowered cautiously using smaller than normal doses that are slowly titrated upward. Calcium entry antagonists, ACE inhibitors, and diuretics are possible choices for the elderly. Beta-blockers are effective in the elderly especially in conjunction with diuretics. Larger doses may result in declining mental function, depression, fatigue, and impotence. α_1-Blockers and central α_2-agonists may be used with caution. First-dose syncope and sedation are the major concerns (see Chapter 24).

Black patients may not respond as well to ACE inhibitors or beta-blockers as other races, perhaps due in part to low renin, salt/volume-dependent hypertension. Thiazide diuretics may adversely affect diabetes, gout, and lipids. Calcium entry antagonists, α_1-blockers, central α_2-agonists, and ACE inhibitors are possible choices.

Young women with hyperdynamic hypertension may respond best to a beta-blocker to slow the heart rate and relieve symptoms of stress. An active young man would be better served with an ACE inhibitor, calcium entry antagonist, or alpha-blocker, as beta-blockers and diuretics may cause impotence and exercise intolerance.[14]

Severe Hypertension and Emergencies

Patients with a diastolic blood pressure (DBP) over 115 mm Hg must be treated upon diagnosis. The blood pressure should be lowered in 5- to 10-mm Hg increments with a goal of lowering it to less than 100 mm Hg after several weeks of therapy. Often more than one drug must be used initially to control the blood pressure. A hypertensive emergency exists if the DBP is over 130 mm Hg and evidence of end-organ damage exists, such as retinal hemorrhage, encephalopathy, pulmonary edema, myocardial infarction, or unstable angina. Drugs available for treatment in this situation include sodium nitroprusside, nitroglycerin, hydralazine, phentolamine, labetalol, and methyldopa. Patients must be hospitalized for appropriate monitoring. Hypertensive urgency exists when the DBP is over 115 mm Hg without evidence of end-organ damage. Oral agents such as clonidine, captopril, and minoxidil may be used to lower the DBP 10 to 15 mm Hg over several hours.[1] Nifedipine should not be used in this situation as many serious adverse events have been reported including severe hypotension, acute myocardial infarction, and death.[20]

Conclusion

Pharmacologic management of hypertension challenges the physician to understand the patient's social, psychological, and economic status in order to select an antihypertensive regimen that effectively lowers the blood pressure, alleviates concomitant disease states, and allows easy adherence to the regimen. Continual assessment of therapy is necessary to determine the effectiveness of the regimen, adverse side effects, and the patient's quality-of-life issues.

Acknowledgment

The assistance of Janet Pick-Whitsitt, Pharm. D., with Table 75.3 is gratefully acknowledged.

References

1. National Institutes of Health. Sixth Report of the Joint National Committee on Detection, Evaluation, and Treatment of High Blood Pressure. National High Blood Pressure Education. NIH publication no. 98-4080. Bethesda: National Heart, Lung and Blood Institute, 1997.
2. Haynes RB, Sackett DL, Taylor DW, et al. Increased absenteeism from work after detection and labeling of hypertensive patients. N Engl J Med 1978;297:741–4.
3. Gordon T, Doyle JT. Alcohol consumption and its relationship to smoking, weight, blood pressure, and blood lipids. Arch Intern Med 1986;146:262–5.
4. Pooling Project Research Group. Relationship of blood pressure, serum cholesterol, smoking habit, relative weight and ECG abnormalities to incidence of major coronary events. J Chronic Dis 1978;31:201–6.
5. Stamler J, Farinaro E, Majonnier LM, et al. Prevention and control of hypertension by nutritional-hygienic means. JAMA 1980;243:1819–23.
6. Rose G, Stamler J. The Intersalt Study: background, methods and main results: Intersalt Cooperative Research Group. J Hum Hypertens 1989;3:283–8.
7. Cade R, Mars D, Wagemaker H, et al. Effect of aerobic exercise training on patients with systemic arterial hypertension. Am J Med 1984;77:785–90.

8. Margetts BM, Beilin LJ, Armstrong BK. A randomized control trial of a vegetarian diet in the treatment of mild hypertension. Clin Exp Pharmacol Physiol 1985;12:263–5.

9. Kaplan NM. Non-drug treatment of hypertension. Ann Intern Med 1985;102:359–73.

10. Witteman JC, Willett WC, Stampfer MJ, et al. A prospective study of nutritional factors and hypertension among US women. Circulation 1989;80:1320–7.

11. Patel C, Marmot MG. Stress management, blood pressure and quality of life. J Hypertens 1987;5(suppl 1):521–8.

12. Stamler R, Stamler J, Grimm R, et al. Nutritional therapy for high blood pressure. JAMA 1987;257:1484–91.

13. American Hospital Formulary Service Drug Information. Bethesda: American Society of Hospital Pharmacists, 2001.

14. Kaplan NM. Clinical hypertension, 7th ed. Baltimore: Williams & Wilkins, 1998.

15. Houston MC. New insights and new approaches for the treatment of essential hypertension: selection of therapy based on coronary heart disease, risk factor analysis, hemodynamic pro-files, quality of life and subsets of hypertension. Am Heart J 1989;117:911–51.

16. ALLHAT Collaborative Research Group. Major cardiovascular events in hypertensive patients randomized to doxazosin vs. chlorthalidone: the antihypertensive and lipid-lowering treatment to prevent heart attack trial (ALLHAT) JAMA 1999; 283(15):1967–75.

17. Jachuck SJ, Brierly H, Jachuck S, et al. The effect of hypotensive drugs on quality of life. J R Coll Gen Pract 1982;32:103–5.

18. Croog SH, Levine S, Testa MA, et al. The effects of antihypertensive therapy on the quality of life. N Engl J Med 1986; 314:1657–64.

19. Steiner SS, Friedhoff AJ, Wilson BL, et al. Antihypertensive therapy and quality of life: a comparison of atenolol, captopril, enalapril and propranolol. J Hum Hypertens 1990;4:217–25.

20. Grossman E, Messerli FH, Grodzicki T. Should a moratorium be placed on sublingual nifedipine capsules given for hypertensive emergencies and pseudoemergencies? JAMA 1996; 276(16):1328–31.

76
Ischemic Heart Disease

Jim Nuovo

Cardiovascular disease remains the most significant cause of morbidity and mortality in the United States. In 1998 approximately 1.3 million Americans experienced a myocardial infarction (MI) and 700,000 of them died.[1] It is estimated that 12.4 million Americans are alive today with a history of MI, angina, or both. The financial impact of this disease is enormous. The cost estimate for cardiovascular disease in 1998 was over $110 billion. It is important for all primary care providers to implement screening and preventive care programs to reduce the burden of cardiovascular disease. Because of the high morbidity and mortality it is also important to recognize the early manifestations of this disease.

Unfortunately, in up to 20% of patients the first manifestation of ischemic heart disease (IHD) is sudden cardiac arrest.[2] Most deaths from IHD occur outside the hospital and within 2 hours of the onset of symptoms. Since the 1960s a great deal of effort has been directed toward the practice of cardiopulmonary resuscitation and emergency cardiac care. These efforts have been directed toward minimizing the number of cardiac deaths. Recently revised evidence-based guidelines present a summary of the collaborative effort of the American Heart Association and the International Liaison Committee on Resuscitation.[2] Furthermore, there has been a substantial undertaking to identify and treat individuals with significant cardiovascular risk factors with the goal of lowering morbidity and mortality (see Chapter 7). This effort has been successful as noted by the decline in death rates from myocardial ischemia and its complications. This chapter discusses three issues, relevant to the family physician, regarding IHD: the evaluation of patients with chest pain, the diagnosis and management of angina pectoris, and the diagnosis and management of MI.

Chest Pain

Chest pain is one of the common reasons for patients visiting primary care physicians.[3] The major diagnostic considerations for chest pain are listed in Table 76.1. Of the diagnostic considerations, which are the most commonly seen by family physicians? A Family Practice Research Network investigated this issue. Over 1 year the Michigan Research Network (MIRNET) prospectively collected information on 399 patients with episodes of chest pain. The most common diagnostic findings were (1) musculoskeletal pain (20.4%); (2) reflux esophagitis (13.4%); (3) costochondritis (13.1%); and (4) angina pectoris (10.3%).[4] The highest priority is generally given to distinguishing cardiac from noncardiac chest pain. Of the many diseases listed, the most common differential diagnostic considerations are of esophageal and psychiatric etiologies.

Noncardiac Chest Pain

Noncardiac chest pain remains a complex diagnosis and management problem. Studies have demonstrated that 10% to 30% of patients with chest pain who undergo coronary arteriography have no arterial abnormalities.[5,6] Follow-up studies of these patients have shown that the risk of subsequent myocardial infarction is low.[7,8] Fifty to seventy-five percent of these patients have persistent complaints of chest pain and disability.[9,10] The most common noncardiac problems in the differential are esophageal disorders, hyperventilation, panic attacks, and anxiety disorders (see Chapters 31 and 87).

Esophageal Chest Pain

Of the patients who have undergone coronary arteriography and have been found to have normal coronary arteries, as many as 50% have demonstrable esophageal abnormalities.[11] Richter et al[12] critically reviewed 117 articles on recurring chest pain of esophageal origin to clarify issues related to this disease. They paid specific attention to the following controversial issues: potential mechanisms of esophageal pain, differentiation of cardiac and esophageal causes, evaluation of esophageal motility disorders, use of esophageal tests for evaluating noncardiac chest pain, usefulness of techniques for prolonged monitoring of intraesophageal pressure and pH, and

Table 76.1. **Common Causes of Chronic and Recurrent Chest Pain**

Cardiac causes
  Hypertrophic cardiomyopathy
  Ischemic heart disease
  Mitral valve prolapse
  Pericarditis
Chest wall problems
  Costochondritis
  Myofascial syndrome
Gastrointestinal causes
  Esophageal motility disorders
  Gastroesophageal reflux
Neurologic causes
  Radiculopathy
  Zoster (postherpetic neuralgia)
Psychiatric causes
  Anxiety
  Depression
  Hyperventilation
  Panic disorder

the relation of psychological abnormalities to esophageal motility disorders. They concluded that (1) specific mechanisms that produce chest pain are not well understood; (2) esophageal chest pain has usually been attributed to the stimulation of chemoreceptors (acid and bile) or mechanoreceptors (spasm and distention); and (3) studies done to confirm direct associations between these factors and pain have not been consistent in their findings.

It appears that the triggers for esophageal chest pain are multifactorial and often idiosyncratic to the individual. Differentiating cardiac from esophageal disease can be frustrating. As many as 50% of patients with coronary disease have esophageal disease.[13] There are many esophageal disorders that produce pain mimicking myocardial ischemia. Areskog et al[14] have shown that esophageal abnormalities are common in patients who are admitted to a coronary care unit and are later found to have no evidence of cardiac disease. The clinical history frequently does not differentiate between cardiac and esophageal chest pain, although features may be helpful in this process. Features suggesting esophageal origin include pain that continues for hours, pain that interrupts sleep or is meal-related, pain relieved by antacids, or the presence of other esophageal symptoms (heartburn, dysphagia, regurgitation). Conversely, it is well documented that gastroesophageal reflux may be triggered by heavy exercise and may produce exertional chest pain mimicking angina even during treadmill testing.

Tests that can be done to determine the presence of esophageal disease include esophageal motility testing, continuous ambulatory esophageal pH monitoring, and provocative testing (e.g., acid perfusion and balloon distension).[15] Although findings from these tests have produced a better understanding of the pathologic conditions leading to the development of chest pain with esophageal disorders, there is no consensus as to the usefulness of these tests for the specific patient with chest pain. As noted by Pope,[16] "What is needed is a simple and safe provocative esophageal ma-

neuver to turn on chest pain that possesses a high degree of sensitivity."

There is clearly an interaction between psychological abnormalities and esophageal disorders. Patients with esophageal disorders have been shown to have significantly higher levels of anxiety, somatization, and depression.[17] It is not clear if there is a cause-and-effect relation. Given the aforementioned difficulties in the diagnosis of esophageal chest pain, the differentiation of this pain from cardiac disease, and the close relation between cardiac, esophageal, and psychiatric disease, it is wise to maintain a consistent approach to the evaluation of these patients. Richter et al[12] developed a stepwise approach for patients with recurring chest pain. They recommended exclusion of cardiac disease, with the subsequent evaluation to rule out structural abnormalities of the upper gastrointestinal (GI) tract (barium swallow, upper GI series, and endoscopy). Also recommended is a trial of antireflux therapy for 1 to 2 months. In those patients who fail to respond, specialized testing may then be appropriate (esophageal motility, 24-hour pH monitoring, provocative testing, and psychological evaluation).[15]

Psychiatric Illness

There has long been a connection between psychiatric disorders and noncardiac chest pain. Katon et al[18] reported the results of an evaluation of 74 patients with chest pain and no history of organic heart disease. Each patient underwent a structured psychiatric interview immediately after coronary arteriography. Patients with chest pain and negative coronary arteriograms were significantly younger, more likely to be female, more apt to have a higher number of autonomic symptoms (tachycardia, dyspnea, dizziness, paresthesias) associated with chest pain, and more likely to describe atypical chest pain. These patients also had significantly higher scores on indices of anxiety and depression that met *Diagnostic and Statistical Manual of Mental Disorders*, 3rd edition (DSM-III) criteria for panic disorder, major depression, and phobias.

The strong association between anxiety and depression disorders in patients with noncardiac chest pain has been observed in many other studies. Specific medical therapy directed at anxiety and depression may help some of these patients. Cannon et al[19] reported a study on a group of patients with chest pain despite normal coronary angiograms. Imipramine was shown to improve their symptoms. Patients who were given 50 mg nightly had a statistically significant reduction (52%) in episodes of chest pain.

Cardiac Chest Pain: Angina Pectoris

Angina is not simply one type of pain; it is a constellation of symptoms related to cardiac ischemia. The description of angina may fit several patterns:

1. *Classic angina.* Classic angina presents as an ill-defined pressure, heaviness (feeling like a weight), or squeezing sensation brought on by exertion and relieved by rest. The pain is most often substernal and left-sided. It may radiate to the jaw, interscapular area, or down the arm. Angina usually begins gradually and lasts only a few minutes.

2. *Atypical angina.* Similar symptoms are experienced but with the absence of one or more of the criteria for classic angina. For example, the pain may not be consistently related to exertion or relieved by rest. Conversely, the pain may have an atypical character (sharp, stabbing), but the precipitating factors are clearly anginal.

3. *Anginal equivalent.* The sensation of dyspnea is the sole or major manifestation.

4. *Variant (Prinzmetal's) angina.* This angina occurs at rest and may manifest in stereotyped patterns, such as nocturnal symptoms or symptoms that appear only after exercise. It is thought to be caused by coronary artery spasm. Its symptoms often occur periodically, with characteristic pain-free intervals, and are associated with typical electrocardiographic (ECG) changes, most commonly ST segment elevation.

5. *Syndrome X (microvascular angina).* Some patients with the clinical diagnosis of coronary artery disease have no evidence of obstructive atherosclerosis. Several reports investigating this population have found a subset with metabolic evidence for ischemia (myocardial lactate during induced myocardial stress as evidence for ischemia). The term *syndrome X* has been proposed.[20] It has been suggested that some of these patients have microvascular angina.

It is important for clinicians to recognize the factors that may confound the clinical diagnosis of angina pectoris: (1) The severity of pain is not necessarily proportional to the seriousness of the underlying illness. (2) The physical examination is not generally helpful for differentiating cardiac from noncardiac disease. A normal examination cannot be counted on to rule out significant cardiac disease. (3) The ECG is normal in more than 50% of patients with IHD. A normal ECG cannot be used to rule out significant cardiac disease. (4) Denial is a significant component in the presentation of chest pain caused by MI. (5) Some of the diseases common in the differential diagnosis of chest pain may present concurrently. Major depressive disorder and panic disorder are known to be prevalent in patients with esophageal disorders. Colgan et al[21] reported that of 63 patients with chest pain and normal angiograms 32 (51%) had evidence of an esophageal disorder, and 19 of the 32 (59%) had a current psychiatric disorder (anxiety or depression). Patients with concurrent disorders are particularly challenging to the clinician sorting out the cause of the chest pain.

Clinical Tools Used to Distinguish Cardiac from Noncardiac Chest Pain

Despite the difficulties noted above, there are important clinical tools that can be used to distinguish cardiac from noncardiac chest pain.

History

Despite the cited difficulties, the history is key to distinguishing cardiac from noncardiac etiologies of chest pain. Noncardiac chest pain is often fleeting, brief, sharp, or stabbing. The

Table 76.2. **Pretest Likelihood of Significant Ischemic Heart Disease (IHD) Based on Symptoms**

Age (years)	Likelihood of IHD, M/F (%)		
	Nonanginal	Atypical angina	Typical angina
30–39	5.0/0.8	22/4	69/26
40–49	14/3	46/13	87/55
50–59	21/8	59/32	92/79
60–69	28/18	67/54	94/90

Source: Diamond and Forrester[22] Copyright© 1979 Massachusetts Medical Society. Reprinted with permission. All rights reserved.

pain may be reproduced by palpating the chest wall. The duration of pain is also important. Symptoms that last many hours or days are not likely to be anginal. A great deal of work has been done to assess the probability of IHD in a given patient based on the clinical presentation. In 1979 Diamond and Forrester[22] presented such an approach. Using data from the clinical presentation correlated with autopsy and angiographic information, they presented a pretest likelihood of coronary artery disease in symptomatic patients according to age, sex, and type of chest pain (nonanginal, atypical angina, or typical angina). Several observations can be made from this chart (Table 76.2): Men have a substantially greater risk than women for any given type of chest pain and at any given age. A middle-aged man with atypical chest pain is at high risk for having significant coronary artery disease. Young women (ages 30–40 years) with classic angina have a relatively low risk of having significant coronary artery disease.

Diagnostic Testing

After establishing a pretest probability of IHD, there are a variety of tests available to help establish an accurate diagnosis. Although many tests are now firmly established in clinical practice, none is particularly suited to wide-scale, cost-effective application because each has limitations concerning sensitivity and specificity.

Exercise Tolerance Testing. In 1997 the American College of Cardiology and the American Heart Association Task Force on Assessment of Cardiovascular Procedures set guidelines for exercise treadmill testing (ETT).[23] For patients with symptoms suggestive of coronary artery disease there are five basic indications for undertaking exercise stress testing: (1) as a diagnostic test for patients with suspected IHD, (2) to assist in identifying those patients with documented IHD who are potentially at high risk due to advanced coronary disease or left ventricular dysfunction, (3) to evaluate patients after coronary artery bypass surgery, (4) to quantify a patient's functional capacity or response to therapy, and (5) to follow the natural course of the disease at appropriate intervals. The purpose of ETT for the patient with chest pain is to help establish whether the pain is indeed due to IHD.

Although there are many exercise protocols available, the protocols proposed by Bruce in 1956 remain appropriate. A review of the ETT for family physicians has been published.[24,25] In the standard ETT (Bruce protocol) the patient is asked to exercise for 3-minute intervals on a motorized treadmill device while being monitored for the following: heart rate and blood pressure response to exercise, symptoms during the test, ECG response (specifically ST segment displacement), dysrhythmias, and exercise capacity. Contraindications to ETT include unstable angina, MI, rapid atrial or ventricular dysrhythmias, poorly controlled congestive heart failure (CHF), severe aortic stenosis, myocarditis, recent significant illness, and an uncooperative patient. A significant (positive) test includes an ST segment depression of 1.0 mm below the baseline. Many factors influence the results of an ETT and can lead to false-positive or false-negative findings. Factors leading to false-positive results include (1) the use of medications such as digoxin, estrogens, and diuretics; and (2) conditions such as mitral valve prolapse, cardiomyopathy, and hyperventilation. Factors leading to false-negative results include (1) the use of medications such as nitrates, beta-blockers, calcium channel blockers; and (2) conditions such as a prior MI or a submaximal effort.[26] The sensitivity of the ETT has been estimated to range from 56% to 81% and the specificity from 72% to 96%.[26] The key point is that given the vagaries of the ETT for diagnosing IHD (generally low sensitivity and specificity) a patient with a high pretest likelihood of IHD (e.g., a 50-year-old man with typical angina) still has a high probability of having significant disease even in the face of a normal (negative) test. Furthermore, a patient with a low probability of IHD (e.g., a 40-year-old woman with atypical chest pain) still has a low chance of significant disease even if the test is positive.[22] The optimal use of diagnostic testing is for those patients with moderate pretest probabilities (e.g., a 40- to 50-year-old man with atypical pain).

In addition to the diagnostic implications of an ETT, there are prognostic implications. The following are considered to be parameters associated with poor prognosis or increased disease severity: failure to complete stage 2 of a Bruce protocol, failure to achieve a heart rate over 120 bpm (off beta-blockers), onset of ST segment depression at a heart rate of less than 120 bpm, ST segment depression over 2.0 mm, ST segment depression lasting more than 6 minutes into recovery, ST segment depression in multiple leads, poor systolic blood pressure response to exercise, ST segment elevation, angina with exercise, and exercise-induced ventricular tachycardia.[26]

Radionuclide Perfusion Imaging. There are patients in whom the standard ETT is not a useful diagnostic tool and in whom a radionuclide procedure would be more appropriate. Patients with baseline ECG abnormalities due to digitalis or left ventricular hypertrophy with strain or those with bundle branch block (especially left bundle branch block) cannot have proper evaluation of the ST segment for characteristic ischemic changes. In these patients a radionuclide stress test is appropriate. The principle behind radionuclide testing is as follows: Myocardial thallium 201 chloride uptake is proportional to the coronary blood flow. A myocardial segment supplied by a stenotic coronary artery receives less flow relative to normal tissue, causing a thallium perfusion defect. Thallium washout is also slower in stenotic areas. With perfusion imaging, both stress and rest images are compared for perfusion. As a general rule, a defect is visible on thallium imaging if there is 50% or greater stenosis in a coronary artery. In the standard exercise thallium test, repeat imaging is performed 3 to 4 hours after completion of the ETT. Some investigators advocate 24-hour imaging in patients with perfusion defects to look for delayed reversibility.

For patients unable to exercise, thallium imaging can be performed using dipyridamole (Persantine) as a coronary vasodilator. Adenosine may also be used. Its advantages over dipyridamole include an ultrashort half-life (less than 10 seconds) and better coronary vasodilation. Two technetium radiopharmaceuticals [technetium sestamibi (Cardiolyte) and technetium teboroxime (Cardiotec)] have been approved for myocardial perfusion imaging. These agents may eventually replace thallium because of more favorable imaging characteristics.[27]

Compared to the standard ETT, the thallium 201 ETT has the advantage of increased sensitivity (80–87%) and specificity (85–90%).[27] Dipyridamole, adenosine, and technetium perfusion testing has a sensitivity ranging from 70% to 95% and specificity from 60% to 100%. Unfortunately, the cost of these procedures is more than five times as great as a standard ETT ($1000–$1400 versus $175–$250).[25]

Stress Echocardiography. Ischemic heart disease can be detected with stress echocardiography. During stress-induced myocardial ischemia, the affected ventricular walls become hypokinetic. Studies suggest that physical exercise and dobutamine may be the preferable means of provoking ischemia in patients undergoing stress echocardiography.[28,29] Preliminary data suggest a higher sensitivity and specificity than for the standard ETT and increased usefulness for predicting subsequent myocardial events; however, the primary utility of this test appears to be for detection of ischemia in patients who are unable to exercise adequately. Similar values for sensitivity and specificity between stress echocardiography and perfusion imaging have been reported. Stress echocardiography may be particularly valuable in patients who have a questionable defect on perfusion imaging.

The advantages and disadvantages of each of these diagnostic tests for IHD, as well as gender-specific issues, are presented in a summary by Redberg.[30]

Response to Nitroglycerin. Another approach employs clinical information to determine the probability of coronary artery disease based on response to treatment. One such study involved the use of sublingual nitroglycerin to determine the likelihood of disease. Horwitz et al[31] evaluated the usefulness of nitroglycerin as a diagnostic aid for IHD. They found a sensitivity of 76% and a specificity of 80% in 70 patients with chest pain of anginal type. It was concluded that 90% of patients with recurrent, angina-like chest pain who exhibit a prompt response to nitroglycerin (within 3 minutes) have IHD; however, a delayed or absent response paradoxically indicates either an absence of IHD or unusually severe disease. Therefore failure to respond to nitroglycerin should not be used to exclude the diagnosis of IHD.

Angina Pectoris

Once the diagnosis of angina is established, there are several important management considerations for this disease. The first is related to disease prognosis, the second to drug therapy, and the third to further investigative tests and invasive therapeutic interventions. Comprehensive management guidelines were prepared in 1999 by the American College of Cardiology and American Heart Association Task Force.[32]

Prognosis

Three major factors determine the prognosis of patients with angina pectoris: the amount of viable but jeopardized left ventricular myocardium, the percentage of irreversibly scarred myocardium, and the severity of underlying coronary atherosclerosis. A number of studies were reported before invasive therapies were available that assess the prognosis of patients with stable angina. Most of them appeared between 1952 and 1973 and reported an annual mortality of 4%. Since cardiac catheterization has come into general use, the prognosis has been modified and is based on the number of diseased vessels. Currently, the annual mortality rates for patients with one-vessel disease, two-vessel disease, three-vessel disease, and left main coronary artery disease (CAD) are 1.5%, 3.5%, 6.0%, and 8.0% to 10.0%, respectively.[33]

Exercise tolerance testing has been used to establish the prognosis in patients with symptomatic IHD. The exercise test parameters associated with a poor outcome have been described above.[26]

When does angina signal severe coronary disease? Pryor et al[34] developed a nomogram based on a point scoring system to help answer this question. They based the nomogram on the following factors: type of chest pain (typical, atypical, nonanginal), sex, selective cardiovascular risk factors (hypertension, smoking, hyperlipidemia, diabetes mellitus), anginal duration (months), and the presence of carotid bruits. By applying the nomogram for the individual patient one can determine the probability of severe disease (i.e., 75% narrowing of the left main coronary artery or three-vessel disease).

Drug Therapy

In patients with stable exertional angina who do not have severe disease, the goal of therapy is to abolish or reduce anginal attacks and myocardial ischemia and to promote a normal lifestyle. For the relief of angina, the treatment strategy is to lower myocardial oxygen demand and increase coronary blood flow to the ischemic regions.

Patients are screened for the presence of significant cardiovascular risk factors and are advised to modify any that are present. Three classes of antianginal drugs are commonly used: nitrates, beta-blockers, and calcium channel blockers. Each reduces myocardial oxygen demand and may improve blood flow to the ischemic regions. The mechanisms by which these agents reduce myocardial oxygen demand or increase coronary blood flow to ischemic areas differ from one class of drug to another. No greater efficacy in relieving chest pain or decreasing exercise-induced ischemia has been shown for one or another group of drugs.

Nitrates

Nitrates are potent venous and arterial dilators. At low doses venous dilation predominates, and at higher doses arterial dilation occurs as well. Nitrates decrease myocardial oxygen demand in the following ways: Decreased venous return reduces left ventricular end-diastolic volume and ventricular wall stress. Increased arterial compliance and cardiac output lowers systolic blood pressure and decreases peripheral resistance (afterload). It also enhances myocardial oxygen supply by preventing closure of stenotic coronary arteries during exercise, dilating epicardial coronary arteries, and decreasing left ventricular end-diastolic pressure, thereby enhancing subendocardial blood flow and inhibiting coronary artery spasm. Nitrates are inexpensive and have a well documented safety record. Both short- and long-acting nitrates are available. Short-acting preparations are used for relief of an established attack, whereas long-acting nitrates are used for prevention. The most significant concern about the long-acting nitrates is tolerance. Most studies have shown that tolerance develops rapidly when long-acting nitrates are given for anginal prophylaxis.[34]

With nitroglycerin patches tolerance can develop within 24 hours, and further therapy can lead to complete loss of the antianginal effect.[35] Various dosing strategies with oral and transdermal formulations have been used to overcome the development of nitroglycerin tolerance. Patch-free intervals of 10 to 12 hours are commonly used to retain the antianginal effectiveness. For oral administration, nitroglycerin isosorbide dinitrate three times daily at 7 A.M., noon, and 5 P.M. appears to prevent the development of tolerance. Because of the concern for intervals during which patients remain unprotected, it is common to add another antianginal agent to the nitroglycerin regimen. Other problems with nitroglycerin include the fact that 10% of patients do not respond and 10% have associated intolerable headaches that may necessitate discontinuation.[35]

Beta-Blockers

The antianginal effect of beta-blockers is well established.[36] These agents improve exercise tolerance and reduce myocardial ischemia. The effect produces a reduction in myocardial oxygen demand through a reduction in heart rate and contractility. Many beta-blockers are available. They may be divided into those that are nonselective (β_1 and β_2) (i.e., propranolol, timolol, nadolol), those that are β_1 selective (i.e., atenolol, metoprolol, acebutolol), and those that are nonselective and produce vasodilatory effects through the ability to block α_1-receptors and dilate blood vessels directly (i.e., labetalol). All beta-blockers, irrespective of their selective properties, are equally effective in patients with angina.[36]

Some 20% of patients do not respond to beta-blockers. Those who do not respond are more likely to have severe IHD. Furthermore, some patients do not tolerate the adverse side effects, such as fatigue, depression, dyspnea, and cold extremities. Other concerns include a small but significant aggravation of hyperlipidemia and precipitation of CHF and bronchospasm in susceptible individuals. Generally, beta-blockers are dose-adjusted to achieve a heart rate of 50 to 60 bpm. Patients should be cautioned to not stop beta-blockers abruptly, thereby avoiding a rebound phenomenon.

Calcium Channel Blockers

Calcium channel blockers are a diverse group of compounds, all of which impede calcium ion influx into the myocardium and smooth muscle cells. These agents relieve myocardial ischemia by reducing myocardial oxygen demand secondary to decreased afterload and myocardial contractility. In addition, they dilate coronary arteries. There are three classes of calcium channel blockers: papaverine derivatives (verapamil), dihydropyridines (nifedipine, nicardipine), and benzothiazepines (diltiazem). Each of the drugs in the three classes has different effects on the atrioventricular (AV) node, heart rate, coronary vasodilation, diastolic relaxation, cardiac contractility, systemic blood pressure, and afterload. All three classes are effective for the management of patients with stable angina.[37] Most studies have shown them to have effects equal to those of beta-blockers. Calcium channel blockers may be preferred in patients with obstructive airway disease, hypertension, peripheral vascular disease, or supraventricular tachycardia. In general, they are well tolerated. The most troublesome side effects include constipation, edema, headache, and aggravation of congestive heart failure.

Concern has developed that short-acting calcium channel blockers may be associated with an increased risk of MI. There has been evidence of a 58% to 70% increase in risk of MI compared to that in patients on beta-blockers or diuretics. The phenomenon has been noted to be dose-related. At present the National Heart, Lung, and Blood Institute has issued a statement recommending caution with the use of short-acting calcium channel blockers.[38]

Combination Therapy

It is important to maximize therapy with any one class of antianginal drug before considering it a failed trial. If monotherapy fails, it is appropriate to add another agent. Generally beta-blockers and nitrates or calcium channel blockers and nitrates complement each other. Calcium channel blockers and beta-blockers can be used together. Combination therapy may be more effective than either agent alone. It is important to be cautious, as some combinations produce deleterious effects. For example, verapamil and beta-blockers may produce extreme bradycardia or heart block.

Aspirin

Aspirin is effective for primary and secondary prevention of MI, presumably by inhibiting thrombosis. Although there is controversy as to the ideal therapeutic dose, low-dose therapy (81–325 mg) is generally recommended.[39] Alternative antiplatelet regimens to aspirin include ticlopidine and clopidogrel. A 1994 review found no evidence that any antiplatelet regimen was more effective than medium-dose aspirin alone in the prevention of vascular events.[40] Another review of randomized trials comparing either ticlopidine or clopidogrel with aspirin found several trials showing a small additional benefit of these two drugs over aspirin in reducing the odds of a vascular event.[41]

Invasive Testing

Cardiac catheterization is not routinely recommended for initial management of patients with stable angina. Patients who warrant such an evaluation are those who exhibit evidence of severe myocardial ischemia on noninvasive testing or who have symptoms refractory to antianginal medications. In patients who undergo catheterization, the most important determinant of survival is left ventricular function followed by the number of diseased vessels. Patients with left main artery disease or three-vessel disease with diminished left ventricular function are candidates for a coronary artery bypass graft procedure. Others (those with one- or two-vessel disease) are managed medically or considered for percutaneous transluminal coronary angioplasty (PTCA).

Unstable Angina Pectoris

Unstable angina manifests clinically either as an abrupt onset of ischemic symptoms at rest or as an intensification or change in the pattern of ischemic symptoms in a patient with a history of IHD. This intensification may be manifested by an increase in the frequency, severity, and duration of symptoms as well as an increasing ease of provocation (symptoms at rest or with minimal effort). Recurrence of ischemic symptoms soon after an MI (usually within 4 weeks) is also considered a sign of unstable angina. Unstable angina is generally diagnosed on clinical grounds alone. Because of the episodic nature of ischemia in unstable angina, however, transient ECG abnormalities (ST segment depression or elevation or T wave abnormalities, i.e., inversion, flattening, or peaking) may not be documented in 50% to 70% of patients with the clinical diagnosis of unstable angina. In studies in which prolonged Holter monitoring was used during the in-hospital phase of unstable angina, transient ischemic ST segment deviations have been described in 60% to 70% of cases, more than 70% of them being clinically unsuspected or silent.[42]

Prognosis

The prognosis of patients with unstable angina is not as good as those with chronic stable angina. Mortality is increased in those who fail to respond to initial therapy, who have severe left ventricular dysfunction, and who have multivessel CAD (particularly left main artery disease).

Management Strategy

An important development in the management of unstable angina was the 1994 report of the Agency for Health Care Policy and Research.[43] This report includes clinical practice guidelines that are based on a consensus panel of experts. The guidelines allow physicians to consider outpatient management for a select subgroup of patients with unstable angina, specifically those who are thought to be at low risk for MI. According to the report, in the initial management physicians should use the information in Table 76.3 to determine whether a particular patient has high, intermediate, or low likelihood

Table 76.3. **Likelihood of Significant Coronary Artery Disease (CAD) in Patients with Symptoms Suggesting Unstable Angina**

High likelihood (any of the listed features)	Intermediate likelihood (absence of high-likelihood features and any of the listed features)	Low likelihood (absence of high- or intermediate-likelihood features but may have the listed features)
Known history of CAD	Definite angina: men <60, women <70	Chest pain, probably not angina
Definite angina: men ≥60 women ≥70	Probable angina: men >60 or women >70	One risk factor but not diabetes
Hemodynamic changes or ECG changes with pain	Probably not angina in diabetics or in nondiabetics with ≥two other risk factors[a]	T wave flat or inverted <1 mm in leads with dominant R waves
Variant angina	Extracardiac vascular disease	Normal ECG
ST increase or decrease ≥1 mm	ST depression 0.05 to 1.00 mm	
Marked symmetric T wave inversion in multiple precordial leads	T wave inversion ≥1 mm in leads with dominant R waves	

Source: Braunwald et al.[43]

[a]CAD risk factors include diabetes, smoking, hypertension, and elevated cholesterol.

of having significant CAD. For example, the patient with low likelihood might be nondiabetic, have atypical chest pain, be younger (<60 years for men, <70 years for women), and have a normal ECG. The next step is to determine the level of risk for MI. The information in Table 76.4 allows a similar stratification of risk. For example, a low-risk patient is one with a history of angina that is now provoked at a lower threshold but not at rest, and the ECG is normal or unchanged. Low-risk patients may be treated with aspirin, nitroglycerin, beta-blockers, or a combination. Follow-up should be no later than 72 hours. High- or moderate-risk patients should be admitted for intensive medical management. Intensive medical management includes consideration of aspirin, heparin, nitrates, beta-blockers, calcium channel blockers (if the patient is already on adequate doses of nitrates and beta-blockers or unable to tolerate them), and morphine sulfate.

Once patients are stable, they should be considered for non-invasive exercise testing to further define the prognosis and direct the treatment plan. Low-risk patients can be managed medically. Those at intermediate risk should be considered for additional testing (either a cardiac catheterization, radionuclide stress test, or echocardiographic stress test). Those at high risk should be referred for cardiac catheterization.[43]

Since the publication of the 1994 report, efforts have been directed at the use of markers of cardiac injury, i.e., cardiac troponins (troponin T and troponin I). Their detection, even at low levels, is highly sensitive and specific for injury. Troponin elevation in patients otherwise considered to have unstable angina identifies a subset of patients requiring more aggressive intervention. Hamm and Braunwald[44] have proposed a risk-stratification algorithm that incorporates troponin testing.

Table 76.4. **Short-Term Risk of Death or Nonfatal Myocardial Infarction in Patients with Symptoms Suggesting Unstable Angina**

High risk (at least one of the listed features must be present)	Intermediate risk (no high-risk feature but must have any of the listed features)	Low risk (no high- or intermediate-risk feature but may have any of the listed features)
Prolonged ongoing (>20 min) rest pain	Rest angina now resolved but not low likelihood of CAD	Increased angina frequency, severity, or duration
Pulmonary edema	Rest angina (>20 min or relieved with rest or nitroglycerin)	Angina provoked at a lower threshold
Angina with new or worsening mitral regurgitation murmurs	Angina with dynamic T wave changes	New-onset angina within 2 weeks to 2 months
Rest angina with dynamic ST changes ≥1 mm	Normal or unchanged ECG	Nocturnal angina
Angina with S_3 or rales	New onset of CCSC III or IV angina during past 2 weeks but not low likelihood of CAD	
Angina with hypotension	Q waves or ST depression ≥1 mm in multiple leads	
Age >65 years		

Source: Braunwald et al.[43]

CCSC = Canadian Cardiovascular Study Class.

Antiplatelet Therapy

Antiplatelet therapy is an important addition for patients with unstable angina. A number of studies have demonstrated that a common cause of crescendo angina is platelet aggregation and thrombus formation on the surface of an ulcerated plaque. In the Veterans Administration Cooperative Study, men with unstable angina who received aspirin (325 mg/day) had a 50% reduction in subsequent death from MI.[45] As noted previously, ticlopidine and clopidogrel are alternative antiplatelet regimens to aspirin.

Percutaneous Transluminal Coronary Angioplasty

There has been a marked increase in the use of angioplasty over the past 20 years. The American College of Cardiology and the American Heart Association Task Force have published guidelines for the selection of patients for coronary angioplasty.[46] Among patients with unstable angina, PTCA is recommended for those who do not show an adequate response to medical treatment (continued chest pain or evidence of ongoing ischemia during ECG monitoring) or who are intolerant of medical therapy because of uncontrollable side effects.

The long-term outcome after successful angioplasty has been reported to be excellent even when compared with patients undergoing bypass surgery.[47] Further research is important in the areas of long-term outcome for multiple lesions, extensive disease, and avoidance of complications. Technologies such as stents, laser angioplasty, and atherectomy await further evaluation.

Coronary Artery Bypass Graft

Large randomized trials have shown that surgical revascularization is more effective than medical therapy for relieving angina and improving exercise tolerance for at least several years. Development of atherosclerosis in the coronary artery bypass graft resulting in angina generally occurs within 5 to 10 years. However, patients with internal mammary artery grafts have substantially fewer problems with graft occlusion (90% patency rate at 10 years). Improved survival with surgical versus medical therapy is seen only in the subset of patients with severe CAD or left ventricular dysfunction.[48]

Silent Ischemia

Many investigations have established that most ischemic episodes in patients with stable angina are not accompanied by chest pain (silent ischemia). What remains unclear is the precise nature of events that accompany ischemic events that do or do not produce pain. Patients with predominantly silent ischemia may be hyposensitive to pain in general; denial may play a role, or they may experience pain but attribute the symptoms to a less significant event. It is well documented that personality-related, emotional, and social factors can modulate the perception of pain. It is not surprising that the symptoms among cardiac patients with the same degree of disease vary greatly. Personality inventory studies have shown that patients with reproducible angina have higher scores on indices of nervousness and excitability than do those who are free of symptoms. Many studies have shown that stress of various types can influence the frequency and duration of ischemic episodes in patients with angina.[49]

Silent ischemia is prevalent. Seventy percent of ischemic episodes in patients with IHD are estimated to be asymptomatic. Among patients with stable angina who undergo 24-hour Holter monitoring, 40% to 72% of the episodes are painless. Among patients with unstable angina, more than half manifest painless ST segment depression.

In 1988 Cohn[50] proposed classifying silent ischemia into three clinical types to help clarify the prevalence, detection, prognosis, and management of this syndrome. Type 1 includes persons with ischemia who are asymptomatic, never having had any signs or symptoms of cardiovascular disease. Type 2 includes persons who are asymptomatic after an MI but still show painless ischemia. Type 3 includes patients with both angina and silent ischemia. From Cohn's data 2.5% to 10.0% of middle-aged men have type 1 silent ischemia. Among middle-aged men known to have CAD, 18% have type 2 and 40% have type 3.

Methods of Detection

Certain tests can be used to assess the presence of silent ischemia: ETT, ambulatory ECG for ST segment changes (Holter monitor), radionuclide tests including thallium scintigraphy and gated pooled [multiple gated acquisition (MUGA)] scan, and stress echocardiography. Of these tests, the most commonly considered are ETT and Holter monitoring.

For Holter monitoring, when ST segment changes that meet strict criteria are seen in a patient with known IHD, it is generally accepted that they represent episodes of myocardial ischemia. Ischemic criteria include at least 1.0 mm of horizontal or down-sloping ST segment depression that lasts for at least 1 minute and is separated from other discrete episodes by at least 1 minute of a normal baseline. The methodology has limitations, including difficulty reading ST segment changes in patients with an abnormal baseline (left ventricular hypertrophy with strain) or in those with a left bundle branch block.

It is not thought at this time that any of the methods to detect silent ischemia are useful for screening for the presence of IHD in apparently healthy populations. Although this subject remains controversial, it may be wise to screen those patients at high risk (i.e., diabetics or patients with two or more cardiac risk factors).

Prognostic Implications

The presence of frequent, prolonged ischemic episodes despite medical therapy in patients with stable and unstable angina has been associated with a poor prognosis. Using Cohn's classification system, those patients with type 2 silent ischemia have the worst prognosis, especially those with left ventricular dysfunction and three-vessel disease. Exercise tests done 2 to 3 weeks after an MI have shown an adverse 1-year prognosis associated with silent ischemia.[50] It is unclear whether those with type 3 have a worse prognosis.

Management

Antiischemic medical and revascularization therapies have been shown to reduce asymptomatic ischemia. It is prudent to consider patients with persistent asymptomatic ischemia to be at higher risk for subsequent events and therefore to warrant more aggressive therapy. Patients with type 1 are advised to modify risk factors and avoid activities known to produce ischemia. Those with strongly positive tests can be considered for angiography. For patients with types 2 or 3, treatment with beta-blockers for a cardioprotective effect should be considered. It remains unresolved whether asymptomatic ischemia has a causal relation with subsequent MI and cardiac death or is merely a marker of high risk.[51]

Myocardial Infarction

Clinical Presentation

The classic initial manifestations of an acute MI include prolonged substernal chest pain with dyspnea, diaphoresis, and nausea. The pain may be described as a crushing, pressing, constricting, vise-like, or heavy sensation. There may be radiation of the pain to one or both shoulders and arms or to the neck, jaw, or interscapular area. Only a few patients have this classic overall picture. Although 80% of patients with an acute MI have chest pain at the time of initial examination, only 20% describe it as crushing, constricting, or vise-like.[52] The pain may also be described atypically, such as sharp or stabbing, or it can involve atypical areas such as the epigastrium or the back of the neck. "Atypical" presentations are common in the elderly.

Pathy[53] found that the initial manifestations of an acute MI were more likely to include symptoms such as sudden dyspnea, acute confusion, cerebrovascular events (e.g., stroke or syncope), acute CHF, vomiting, and palpitations. There is strong evidence that a substantial proportion of MIs are asymptomatic. In an update of the Framingham Study, Kannel and Abbott[54] reported that 28% of infarcts were discovered only through the appearance of new ECG changes (Q waves or loss of R waves) observed on a routine biennial study. These infarctions had been previously unrecognized by both patient and physician.

Physical Examination

For the patient with an "uncomplicated MI" there are few physical examination findings. The main purpose of the examination is to assess the patient for evidence of complications from the MI and to establish a baseline for future comparisons. Signs of severe left ventricular dysfunction include hypotension, peripheral vasoconstriction, tachycardia, pulmonary rales, an S_3, and elevated jugular venous pressure (see Chapter 79). Preexisting murmurs should be verified. A new systolic murmur can result from a number of causes: papillary muscle dysfunction, mitral regurgitation as a result of ventricular dilatation, ventricular septal rupture, and acute severe mitral regurgitation due to papillary muscle rupture.

Electrocardiography

The classic ECG changes of acute ischemia are peaked, hyperacute T waves, T wave flattening or inversion with or without ST segment depression, horizontal ST segment depression, and ST segment elevation. Changes associated with an infarction are (1) the fresh appearance of Q waves or the increased prominence of preexisting ones; (2) ST segment elevations; and (3) T wave inversions. It is important to recognize that with acute MI the ECG may be entirely normal or contain only "soft" ECG evidence of infarction.

In the past infarcts were classified as transmural or subendocardial, depending of the presence of Q waves. This terminology has now been replaced by the terms *Q-wave* and *non–Q-wave* MI. This distinction has more clinical relevance, as several studies have indicated differences in etiology and outcome. The key differences between these two groups are as follows: (1) Q-wave infarctions account for 60% to 70% of all infarcts and non–Q-wave infarctions for 30% to 40%. (2) ST segment elevation is present in 80% of Q-wave infarctions and 40% of non–Q-wave infarctions. (3) The peak creatine kinase tends to be higher in Q-wave infarctions. (4) Postinfarction ischemia and early reinfarction are more common with non–Q-wave infarctions. (5) In-hospital mortality is greater with Q-wave infarctions (20% versus 8% for non–Q-wave infarctions). In general, it is thought that the non–Q-wave infarction is a more unstable condition because of the higher risk of reinfarction and ischemia.

Laboratory Findings

Elevation of the creatine kinase muscle and brain subunits (CK-MB) isoenzyme is essential for the diagnosis of acute MI. In general, acute elevations of this enzyme are accounted for by myocardial necrosis. Detectable CK-MB from noncardiac causes is rare except during trauma or surgery. The peak level appearance of CK-MB is expected within 12 to 24 hours after the onset of symptoms; normalization is expected in 2 to 3 days. Therefore patients should have a CK-MB level determined on admission and every 8 to 12 hours thereafter (repeated twice). Reliance on a single CK assay in an emergency room setting to rule out MI is not sensitive and should be discouraged. Cardiac troponins (T and I) are newer markers for cardiac injury. The troponins first become detectable after the first few hours following the onset of myocardial necrosis, and they peak after 12 to 24 hours. Normalization of troponin T levels requires 5 to 14 days; troponin I levels requires 5 to 10 days.[55]

Management Guidelines

Comprehensive management guidelines were prepared in 1999 by the American College of Cardiology and American Heart Association Task Force.[46] The main priority for patients with an acute MI is relief of pain. The frequent clinical observation of rapid, complete relief of pain after early reperfusion with thrombolytic therapy has made it clear that the pain of an acute MI is due to continuing ischemia of living jeopardized myocardium rather than to the effects of completed myocardial necrosis.

Effective analgesia should be administered at the time of diagnosis. Analgesia can be achieved by the use of sublingual nitroglycerin or intravenous morphine (or both). Sublingual nitroglycerin is given immediately unless the systolic blood pressure is less than 90 mm Hg. If the systolic blood pressure is under 90 mm Hg, nitroglycerin may be used after intravenous access has been obtained. Long-acting oral nitrate preparations are avoided for management of early acute MI. Sublingual or transdermal nitroglycerin can be used, but intravenous infusion of nitroglycerin allows more precise control. The intravenous dose can be titrated by frequently measuring blood pressure and heart rate. Morphine sulfate is also highly effective for the relief of pain associated with an acute MI. In addition to its analgesic properties, morphine exerts favorable hemodynamic effects by increasing venous capacitance and reducing systemic vascular resistance. The result is to decrease myocardial oxygen demand. As with nitroglycerin, hypotension may occur. The hypotension may be treated with intravenous fluids or leg elevation.

Oxygen

Supplemental oxygen is given to all patients with an acute MI. Hypoxemia in a patient with an uncomplicated infarction is usually caused by ventilation-perfusion abnormalities. When oxygen is used it is administered by nasal cannula or mask at a rate of 4 to 10 L/min. In patients with chronic obstructive pulmonary disease it may be wise to use lower flow rates (see Chapter 83).

Thrombolytic Therapy

In addition to relieving pain and managing ischemia, thrombolytic therapy must be considered. Thrombosis has a major role in the development of an acute MI. Approximately 66% of patients with MIs have ST segment elevation, making it likely that the process is caused by an occlusive clot. The goal of thrombolytic therapy is reperfusion with a minimum of side effects. The most commonly used thrombolytic agents are streptokinase, anisoylated plasminogen streptokinase activator complex (APSAC), recombinant tissue-type plasminogen activator (rt-PA), urokinase, and pro-urokinase.

Early administration of thrombolytic therapy, within 6 to 12 hours from the onset of symptoms, has been associated with a reduction in mortality. Indications for thrombolytic therapy include typical chest pain >30 minutes but <12 hours that is unrelieved by nitroglycerin, and ST segment elevation in more than two contiguous leads (>1 mm in limb leads or >2 mm in chest leads) or ST segment depression in only V_1 and V_2 or a new left bundle branch block. Relative contraindications for thrombolytic therapy include history of stroke, active bleeding, blood pressure >180 mm Hg systolic, major surgery/trauma in the last 3 to 6 months, recent noncompressible vascular puncture, and possible intracranial event/unclear mental status.[56] Wright and colleagues[56] present a summary of the major thrombolytic trials. Advances in this therapeutic modality during the past 5 years include new third-generation fibrinolytic agents and various strategies to enhance administration and efficacy of these agents. A number of ongoing trials are attempting to determine whether the combination of fibrinolytic therapy with low molecular weight heparin enhances coronary reperfusion and reduces mortality and late reocclusion. Also presented is a dose and cost summary of the available fibrinolytic agents.[56]

Complications (Mechanical)

The most common complications of an acute MI are mechanical and electrical. Mechanical complications include those that are quickly reversible and those that are clearly life-threatening. Reversible causes of hypotension include hypovolemia, vasovagal reaction, overzealous therapy with antianginal or antiarrhythmic drugs, and brady- and tachyarrhythmias. Other, more serious etiologies include primary left ventricular failure, cardiac tamponade, rupture of the ventricular septum, acute papillary muscle dysfunction, and mitral regurgitation (see Chapter 80).

Killip and Kimball[57] developed a classification of patients with acute MI.

Class 1: Patients with uncomplicated infarction without evidence of heart failure as judged by the absence of rales and an S_3.

Class 2: Patients with mild to moderate heart failure as evidenced by pulmonary rales in the lower half of the lung fields and an S_3.

Class 3: Patients with severe left ventricular failure and pulmonary edema.

Class 4: Patients with cardiogenic shock, defined as systolic blood pressure less than 90 mm Hg with oliguria and other evidence of poor peripheral perfusion.

Cardiogenic shock has emerged as the most common cause of in-hospital mortality of patients with an acute MI. Despite advances in medical therapy, cardiogenic shock has a dismal prognosis (80–90% mortality). The management of patients with cardiogenic shock includes adequate oxygenation, reduction in myocardial oxygen demands, protection of ischemic myocardium, and circulatory support (see Chapter 80). The potential for myocardial salvage with emergency reperfusion should be considered in all cases.

Complications (Electrical)

The past 30 years has seen major developments in the recognition and treatment of arrhythmias (see Chapter 77). The most common include the brady- and tachyarrhythmias, AV conduction disturbances, and ventricular arrhythmias. Organized treatment protocols have been developed for each of these dysrhythmias.[58]

Post-MI Evaluation

Recommendations for pre- and postdischarge evaluations of patients with an acute MI have been outlined by the American College of Cardiologists, the American Heart Association, and the American College of Physicians.[46] They include recommendations for testing exercise tolerance and strategies to determine those who would benefit from medical or surgical intervention. These recommendations include a submaximal ETT at 6 to 10 days and at 3 weeks to determine functional capacity.

Rehabilitation

The goal of cardiac rehabilitation includes maintenance of a desirable level of physical, social, and psychological functioning after the onset of cardiovascular illness.[59] Specific goals of rehabilitation include risk stratification, limitation of adverse psychological and emotional consequences of cardiovascular disease, modification of risk factors, alleviation of symptoms, and improved function. Risk stratification is accomplished by exercise tolerance testing. Additionally, high-risk patients include those with CHF, silent ischemia, and ventricular dysrhythmias. All patients should undergo an evaluation to reduce risk factors (smoking, hyperlipidemia, and hypertension) (see Chapters 7 and 8). Risk modification of these factors has been associated with significant reduction in subsequent cardiac events. Enrollment in a cardiac rehabilitation program with particular emphasis on exercise has been shown to reduce cardiovascular mortality.[60]

References

1. 2001 Heart and Stroke Statistical Update. American Heart Association. *http://www.americanheart.org.*
2. Guidelines 2000 for cardiopulmonary resuscitation and emergency cardiovascular care. An international consensus on science. The American Heart Association in Collaboration with the International Liaison Committee on Resuscitation. *http://www.americanheart.org/ECC/index.html.*
3. Fulp SR, Richter JE. Esophageal chest pain. Am Fam Physician 1989;40:101–16.
4. Klinkman MS, Stevens D, Gorenflo DW. Episodes of care for chest pain: a preliminary report from MIRNET. J Fam Pract 1994;38:345–52.
5. Kemp HG, Vokonas PS, Cohn PF, Gorlin R. The anginal syndrome associated with normal coronary arteriograms: report of a six-year experience. Am J Med 1973;54:735–42.
6. Marchandise B, Bourrassa MG, Chairman BR, Lesperance J. Angiographic evaluation of the natural history of normal coronary arteries and mild coronary atherosclerosis. Am J Cardiol 1978;41:216–20.
7. Proudfit WL, Bruschke AVG, Sones FM. Clinical course of patients with normal or slightly or moderately abnormal coronary arteriograms: 10-year follow-up of 521 patients. Circulation 1980;62:712–17.
8. Kemp HG, Kronmal RA, Vlietstra RE, Frye RL. Seven year survival of patients with normal or near normal coronary arteriograms: a CASS registry study. J Am Coll Cardiol 1986;7:479–83.
9. Ockene IS, Shay MJ, Alpert JS, Weiner BH, Dalen JE. Unexplained chest pain in patients with normal coronary arteriograms: a follow-up study of functional status. N Engl J Med 1980;303:1249–52.
10. Lavey EB, Winkle RA. Continuing disability of patients with chest pain and normal coronary arteriograms. J Chronic Dis 1979;32:191–6.
11. Davies HA, Jones DB, Rhodes J. Esophageal angina as the cause of chest pain. JAMA 1982;248:2274–8.
12. Richter JE, Bradley LA, Castell DO. Esophageal chest pain current controversies in pathogenesis, diagnosis and therapy. Ann Intern Med 1989;110:66–78.
13. Schofield PM, Bennett DH, Whorwell PJ, et al. Exertional gastro-oesophageal reflux: a mechanism for symptoms in patient with angina pectoris and normal coronary angiograms. BMJ 1987;294:1459–61.
14. Areskog M, Tibbling L, Wranne B. Noninfarction in coronary care unit patients. Acta Med Scand 1981;209:51–7.
15. Glade MJ. Continuous ambulatory esophageal pH monitoring in the evaluation of patients with gastrointestinal reflux: Diagnostic and therapeutic technology assessment (DATTA). JAMA 1995;274:662–8.
16. Pope CE. Chest pain: heart? gullet? both? neither? [editorial]. JAMA 1992;248:2315.
17. Clouse RE, Lustman PJ. Psychiatric illness and contraction abnormalities of the esophagus. N Engl J Med 1983;309:1337–42.
18. Katon W, Hall ML, Russo J, et al. Chest pain: relationship of psychiatric illness to coronary arteriographic results. Am J Med 1988;84:1–9.
19. Cannon RO, Quyyumi AA, Mincemoyer R, Stine AM, Gracely RH, Smith WB. Imipramine in patients with chest pain despite normal coronary angiograms. N Engl J Med 1994;330:1411–17.
20. Cannon RO. Angina pectoris with normal coronary angiograms. Cardiol Clin 1991;9:157–66.
21. Colgan SM, Schofield PJ, Whorwell DH, Bennett DH, Brook NH, Jones PE. Angina-like chest pain: a joint medical and psychiatric investigation. Postgrad Med J 1988;64:743–6.
22. Diamond GA, Forrester JS. Analysis of probability as an aid in the clinical diagnosis of coronary-artery disease. N Engl J Med 1979;300:1350–8.
23. ACC/AHA guidelines for exercise testing: a report of the American College of Cardiology/American Heart Association Task Force on Practice Guidelines (Committee on Exercise Testing). J Am Coll Cardiol 1997;30:260–311.
24. Evans CH, Karunaratne HB. Exercise stress testing for the family physician. Part 1. Performing the test. Am Fam Physician 1992;45:121–32.
25. Evans CH, Karunaratne HB. Exercise stress testing for the family physician. Part 2. Am Fam Physician 1992;45:679–88.
26. Ellestad MH. Stress testing: principles and practice, 4th ed. Philadelphia: FA Davis, 1995.
27. Botvinick EH. Stress imaging: current clinical options for the diagnosis, localization, and evaluation of coronary artery disease. Med Clin North Am 1995;79:1025–61.
28. Afridi I, Quinones MA, Zoghbi WA, Cheirif J. Dobutamine stress echocardiography: sensitivity, specificity, and predictive value for future cardiac events. Am Heart J 1994;127:1510–15.
29. Beleslin BD, Ostojic M, Stepanovic J, et al. Stress echocardiography in the detection of myocardial ischemia: head-to-head comparison of exercise, dobutamine, and dipyridamole tests. Circulation 1994;90:1168–76.
30. Redberg RF. Diagnostic testing for coronary artery disease in women and gender differences in referral for revascularization. Cardiol Clin 1998;16:67–77.
31. Horwitz LD, Herman MV, Gorlin R. Clinical response to nitroglycerin as a diagnostic test for coronary artery disease. Am J Cardiol 1972;29:149–53.
32. 1999 update: ACC/AHA guidelines for the management of patients with chronic stable angina. A report of the American College of Cardiology/American Heart Association Task Force on Practice Guidelines (Committee on Management of chronic stable angina). J Am Coll Cardiol 1999;33:2092–197.
33. Hilton TC, Chaitman BR. The prognosis in stable and unstable angina. Cardiol Clin 1991;9:27–39.
34. Pryor DB, Shaw L, Harrell FE, et al. Estimating the likelihood of severe coronary artery disease. Am J Med 1991;90:553–62.

35. Bomber JW, Detullio PL. Oral nitrate preparations: an update. Am Fam Physician 1995;52:2331–6.
36. Howard PA, Ellerbeck EF. Optimizing beta-blocker use after myocardial infarction. Am Fam Physician 2000;62:1853–60.
37. Opie LH. Calcium channel antagonists. Part II. Use and comparative properties of prototypical calcium antagonists in ischemic heart disease, including recommendations based on analysis of 45 trials. Rev Cardiovasc Drug Ther 1987;1:4461–75.
38. Psaty BM, Heckbert ER, Koepsell TD, et al. The risk of myocardial infarction associated with antihypertensive drug therapies. JAMA 1995;274:670–5.
39. Hennekens CH, Buring JE. Aspirin in the primary prevention of cardiovascular disease. Cardiol Clin 1994;12:443–50.
40. Antiplatelet Trialists' Collaboration. Collaborative overview of randomized trials of antiplatelet therapy—I. Prevention of death, myocardial infarction, and stroke by prolonged antiplatelet therapy in various categories of patients. BMJ 1994;308:81–106.
41. Hankey GJ, Sudlow CLM, Dunbabin DW. Thienopyridine derivatives (ticlopidine, clopidogrel) versus aspirin for preventing stroke and other serious vascular events in high vascular risk patients. In: The Cochrane Library, issue 1. Oxford: Cochrane Library, 2000.
42. Shah PK. Pathophysiology of unstable angina. Cardiol Clin 1991;9:11–26.
43. Braunwald E, Mark DB, Jones RH, et al. Diagnosing and managing unstable angina: quick reference guide for clinicians, number 10. AHCPR publication no. 94-0603. Rockville, MD: US Department of Health and Human Services, Public Health Service, Agency for Health Care Policy and Research and National Heart, Lung, and Blood Institute, 1994.
44. Hamm CW, Braunwald E. A classification of unstable angina revisited. Circulation 2000;102:118–22.
45. Lewis HD, Davis JW, Archibald DG, et al. Protective effects of aspirin against acute myocardial infarction and death in men with unstable angina: results of a Veterans Administration cooperative study. N Engl J Med 1983;309:396–403.
46. 1999 update: ACC/AHA guidelines for the management of patients with acute myocardial infarction. A report of the American College of Cardiology/American Heart Association Task Force on Practice Guidelines (Committee of Management of Acute Myocardial Infarction). J Am Coll Cardiol 1999;34:890–911.
47. Faxon DP. Percutaneous coronary angioplasty in stable and unstable angina. Cardiol Clin 1991;9:99–113.
48. Sherman DL, Ryan TJ. Coronary angioplasty versus bypass grafting: cost-benefit considerations. Med Clin North Am 1995;79:1085–95.
49. Barsky AJ, Hochstrasser B, Coles A, et al. Silent myocardial ischemia is the person or the event silent? JAMA 1990;264:1132–5.
50. Cohn PF. Silent myocardial ischemia. Ann Intern Med 1988;109:312–17.
51. Gottlieb SO. Asymptomatic or silent myocardial ischemia in angina pectoris: pathophysiology and clinical implications. Cardiol Clin 1991;9:49–61.
52. Lavie CJ, Gersh BJ. Acute myocardial infarction: initial manifestations, management, and prognosis. Mayo Clin Proc 1990;65:531–48.
53. Pathy MS. Clinical presentation of myocardial infarction in the elderly Br Heart J 1967;29:190–9.
54. Kannel WB, Abbott RD. Incidence and prognosis of unrecognized myocardial infarction: an update on the Framingham study. N Engl J Med 1984;311:1144–7.
55. Mair J Morandell D, Genser N. Equivalent early sensitivities of myoglobin, creatine kinase MB mass, creatine kinase isoform ratios, and cardiac troponins I and T for acute myocardial infarction. Clin Chem 1995;41:1266–72.
56. Wright RS, Kopecky SL, Reeder GS. Update on intravenous fibrinolytic therapy for acute myocardial infarction. Mayo Clin Proc 2000;75:1185–92.
57. Killip T, Kimball JT. Treatment of myocardial infarction in a coronary care unit: a two-year experience with 250 patients. Am J Cardiol 1967;20:457–61.
58. Guidelines 2000 for cardiopulmonary resuscitation and emergency cardiovascular care. International consensus on science. Circulation 2000;102:1–384.
59. Squires RW, Gau GT, Miller TD, Allison TG, Lavie CJ. Cardiovascular rehabilitation: status 1990. Mayo Clin Proc 1990;65:731–55.
60. O'Connor GT, Buring JE, Yusuf S, et al. An overview of randomized trials of rehabilitation with exercise after myocardial infarction. Circulation 1989;80:234–44.

77
Cardiac Arrhythmias

Michael S. Klinkman

Cardiac arrhythmias are frequently seen in routine primary care practice, and "palpitations" or patient concerns about "skipped heartbeats" are among the most common presenting complaints in primary care. However, in this area the linkage between symptom and disease is tenuous: symptomatic patients often do not have significant cardiac arrhythmias, whereas many clinically significant arrhythmias are detected in asymptomatic patients. This creates a difficult balancing act for the primary care clinician, whose job it is to effectively uncover treatable disease while avoiding unnecessary health care utilization or specialty consultation.

Although diagnosis and treatment are rapidly moving from the office to the electrophysiology laboratory, many cardiac arrhythmias can still be diagnosed and managed within the primary care setting. This chapter focuses on identification and outpatient management of these common arrhythmias and includes a primer of relevant physiology and pharmacology. Because of the specialized and complex nature of cardiac electrophysiology in children, discussion is limited to the adult and older adolescent patient. The goals of this chapter are threefold: to assist family physicians in the diagnosis of common arrhythmias, to provide basic management advice for conditions treatable in the office, and to point to conditions for which more specialized diagnostic testing and referral are indicated.

Basic Electrophysiology of the Heart

All cardiac cells share the ability to automatically contract (automaticity) at an inherent rate (rhythmicity). Myocardial cells contract when a transmembrane action potential (AP) develops. Fully polarized cells have a transmembrane electrical potential (TEP) of -90 mV. After stimulation by an electrical impulse, the membrane allows a slow inward leak of sodium ions. When the TEP has been reduced to a critical level of -60 mV, a "fast" sodium ion channel opens momentarily to actively transport ions across the membrane and depolarize the cell (phase 0 of the AP of the cell). Following depolarization the sodium channel closes, and a complex exchange of sodium, potassium, and calcium ions occurs during phases 1 and 2 of the AP. During phase 3 potassium ions are pumped out of the cell, the TEP returns to slightly below baseline, and the cell cannot contract (absolute refractory period). During phase 4 potassium moves in and sodium out of the cell through specific ion channels, and a strong electrical stimulus can cause depolarization and contraction (relative refractory period). The cell is now ready for its next beat in response to an impulse. If no electrical impulse occurs, the slow inward transport of positive ions eventually results in spontaneous depolarization and contraction at a rate specific to the type of cell (e.g., 40 per minute for ventricular myocardial cells). The protein structures of the ion channels are controlled by several recently identified genes on chromosomes 3, 4, 7, 11, and 21.[1]

Normal cardiac rhythm depends on the automaticity and conductivity of the specialized group of cells that compose the conduction system, and the receptivity of individual myocardial cells to impulses conducted over the system. The sinoatrial (SA) node, located high in the left atrium, controls the normal heart rate. Cells in the SA node spontaneously "fire" (transmit electrical impulses) at regular intervals owing to increased membrane permeability to sodium and calcium. The AP is transmitted as an electrical impulse from the SA node through the atria to the atrioventricular (AV) node, then through the His system and bundle branches to the Purkinje fibers in the ventricle, then to ventricular myocardial cells. This cell-to-cell communication is controlled by connexins, specialized proteins functioning in the gap junction between cardiac cells. A slight delay occurs at the AV node, which has a pattern of automaticity similar to that of the SA node. Cells in the two nodes also have an absolute and relative refractory period, which is an important factor in the genesis of reentrant arrhythmias.

General Causes of Arrhythmias

The identification of several mutations in the genes that encode the protein structures of sodium and potassium ion channels[1-3] has revolutionized our understanding of arrhythmias. It is increasingly clear that mutations in any of the genes responsible for ion channel, connexin, or myosin protein structure can either directly cause arrhythmias or predispose individuals to an arrhythmia under any of the circumstances described below. We are entering the era of "molecular epidemiology," in which genotyping and variable gene expression will be important parts of diagnosis and treatment.

Anything that can influence cardiac automaticity or conductivity can cause an arrhythmia (Table 77.1) in a susceptible heart. Autonomic nervous system input can greatly influence both automaticity and conductivity. Sympathetic input through the stellate ganglion stimulates cardiac β_1-receptors and increases automaticity and conductivity, and parasympathetic input through the vagus nerve stimulates muscarinic receptors and inhibits β_1-receptors, decreasing automaticity and conductivity. The presence of stressful external events or circumstances commonly stimulates sympathetic activity and can cause arrhythmias, whereas some mental health conditions (e.g., anxiety, panic attacks, panic disorder) are also associated with increased sympathetic activity. The central nervous system (CNS) can also alter baseline sympathetic and parasympathetic tone and predispose to arrhythmias. Local or mechanical factors can influence conductivity and automaticity through the autonomic nervous system. For example, pressure on the neck can stimulate the carotid sinus and increase parasympathetic output, and placing an extremity or the face in ice water can greatly stimulate parasympathetic activity.

Anatomic alterations in the conduction system may also cause arrhythmias. Accessory or alternate pathways for the conduction of cardiac impulses can be present from birth or develop over time. Under certain circumstances these pathways can provide a bypass tract that replaces the normal sinus node–generated rhythm with a reentrant rhythm. This process is believed to cause most supraventricular arrhythmias.

Alterations in extracellular electrolyte concentrations, particularly potassium, calcium, magnesium, and sodium, can alter automaticity and conductivity by affecting TEP generation and recovery. Extracellular oxygen content can greatly influence cardiac rhythm; low oxygen tension can decrease conductivity and contractility of myocardial cells and promote arrhythmia, as seen with myocardial infarction (MI), cardiac ischemia, and some cases of congestive heart failure (CHF). Decreased extracellular pH, often seen with MI or cardiac ischemia, can cause similar decreases in conductivity and result in arrhythmia. Endocrine mediators can also have direct or indirect effects on cardiac rhythm. Increased amounts of circulating catecholamines or thyroid hormone can increase contractility and automaticity through the sympathetic nervous system and by direct effect on myocardial cells, whereas decreases in circulating thyroid hormone or corticosteroid concentrations can decrease contractility and automaticity.

Ingested substances can also have profound effects on cardiac rhythm. Caffeine and other sympathomimetic substances can increase conductivity, whereas CNS depressants such as alcohol have the opposite effect. Illicit drugs such as amphetamines and cocaine have strong, well-known stimulatory effects on cardiac rhythm, but other street drugs can also precipitate arrhythmias. A multitude of prescription and nonprescription drugs have been associated with cardiac rhythm disturbances. Cardiac medications (e.g., digoxin and all classes of antiarrhythmics) and tricyclic antidepressants are perhaps the best known groups of medications with proarrhythmic effects, but combinations of medications (astemizole and ketoconazole) and some over-the-counter medications (pseudoephedrine) can also affect conductivity and automaticity.

Localized damage to cardiac muscle, such as the destruction of myocardial and conduction system cells seen with MI or damage from surgery to repair congenital anomalies, can result in decreased conductivity and contractility and create reentrant circuits.

Finally, senescence of cardiac conduction system cells and myocardial cells may affect automaticity and conductivity in elderly individuals. This phenomenon can occur directly, through fibrotic degradation in the conduction system, or indirectly, through the increased susceptibility of cardiac cells to the agents mentioned above.

Table 77.1. **General Causes of Arrhythmias**

Autonomic nervous system input
  Sympathetic input through stellate ganglion
  Parasympathetic input through vagus nerve
Autonomic response to stressful external factors
Autonomic response to mental health conditions (e.g., anxiety disorder)
Autonomic response to physical factors (e.g., carotid sinus pressure)
Anatomic alterations in the conduction system (bypass tracts)
Alterations in extracellular electrolyte concentrations
Alterations in circulating endocrine mediators (e.g., thyroid hormone)
Decreased tissue oxygenation
Decreased extracellular pH
Destruction of or damage to myocardial cells
Endocrine mediators (e.g., thyroid hormone)
Genetic mutations
Ingested substances
  Stimulants (e.g., caffeine) and sympathomimetics
  Depressants (e.g., alcohol)
  Prescription drugs
  Illicit drugs
Senescence in cardiac conduction system or myocardial cells

Approach to the Diagnosis of Cardiac Arrhythmias

The initial step in managing arrhythmias in the primary care setting is to determine if the patient is hemodynamically stable. Unstable patients require immediate management and may benefit from transfer to an emergency or inpatient facility. Stable patients can be evaluated in the office using a stepwise approach (Table 77.2). Although the diagnosis of specific cardiac arrhythmia rests on the presence of specific electrocardiographic (ECG) or electrophysiologic (EP) study

Table 77.2. **Diagnostic Approach for Patients with Arrhythmias**

Determine whether patient is hemodynamically stable and triage appropriately
Obtain clinical history
   Circumstances surrounding onset of symptoms, duration of symptoms
   Brief review of systems
   Complete substance use and diet history
   Past medical history
   Brief mental health screen
Perform physical examination as directed by history
   Search for evidence of medical conditions associated with arrhythmias
   Cardiac auscultation
Obtain electrocardiogram (ECG)
Consider other laboratory tests (serum chemistries and electrolytes) as directed by history
Options for additional diagnostic studies
   Graded exercise test (GXT, "stress test")
   24- or 48-hour ambulatory ECG monitoring
   Long-term, continuous-loop, event monitoring
   Echocardiography
   Electrophysiologic (EP) study
   Cardiac catheterization

findings, valuable clues regarding the clinical significance and cause of the arrhythmia can be obtained by a careful clinical history and physical examination.

History

Patients may present with nonspecific symptoms suggestive of cardiac arrhythmia, such as palpitations, sensation of a racing heart, dizziness, or sudden fatigue. In these circumstances four key questions help determine the clinical significance of the symptoms and sometimes point to likely cause(s):

1. *When did the symptom(s) start?* After starting a new medication? A long time ago? Yesterday?
2. *What sets it off?* Exertion? Emotional stress? Ingestion of a meal or certain foods such as coffee? Taking a dose of medication? Lying down or sudden position change? A tight shirt collar or tie?
3. *How long does it last?* Moments? Or does it go on for hours or days?
4. *What else happens?* Chest pain? Dyspnea? Orthopnea? Nausea? Tingling in the hands or around the mouth?

Clinicians who discover arrhythmias in asymptomatic patients may get little help from patients' answers to these questions. However, a complete drug history, including prescription, non-prescription, and illicit drug use, should be obtained for all patients, as well as a smoking, alcohol, and brief dietary history. A brief review of systems should also be completed, focusing on symptoms of cardiac or endocrine conditions. Reviewing the patient's medical history for the presence of conditions associated with arrhythmia may reveal a likely cause. Finally, screening for mental health problems such as anxiety, panic, or depression provides valuable clues in some cases.

Physical Examination

The physical examination should look for evidence of medical conditions associated with arrhythmias. For example, sudden weight gain, the presence of bibasilar rales on pulmonary examination, ankle edema, and an audible S_3 on cardiac auscultation may indicate the presence of congestive heart failure, whereas moist skin, the presence of a fine tremor, hypertension, and lid lag suggest the hyperthyroid stage of Graves' disease. Cardiac auscultation alone can point to specific arrhythmias, as an irregularly irregular rhythm almost always signifies atrial fibrillation.

Electrocardiogram

The ECG is necessary to establish a specific diagnosis and may be the point at which evaluation of arrhythmia begins for asymptomatic patients. Lead II is the best single lead for evaluation of cardiac rhythm in most patients, as the P and QRS electrical vectors in patients without axis deviation are most positive in this lead. A long rhythm strip is often valuable for evaluating arrhythmias, particularly in the case of AV conduction defects. Although an increasing number of primary care offices use ECG equipment that prints out a computerized diagnostic assessment on the tracing, these algorithm-based diagnoses are often incomplete or inaccurate. Clinicians are urged to read and interpret the ECG themselves, paying particular attention to P wave appearance, intervals (PR, PP, and QT) and the relation between the P wave and QRS complex. Several reference books are available to assist clinicians in ECG interpretation.

Other Diagnostic Studies

Depending on the type of arrhythmia and its clinical presentation, additional diagnostic evaluation may be helpful. Simple graded exercise testing (GXT) can sometimes reproduce arrhythmia patterns in patients with exercise-induced symptoms. If the clinical history is suspicious for arrhythmia but the physical examination and ECG do not confirm its presence, 24- or 48-hour continuous ambulatory ECG monitoring (Holter monitoring) or long-term, continuous-loop, event recorder monitoring may be performed to capture occasional periods of cardiac arrhythmia.[4] However, studies have shown that rhythm abnormalities noted in the monitor tracing often have little temporal correspondence with patient symptoms as recorded in a symptom diary,[5,6] and the clinical significance of this pattern of results is not clear. Echocardiography, particularly transesophageal echocardiography (TEE), can also be useful to look for structural changes that may predispose to arrhythmias or affect management decisions, such as an enlarged left atrium or left atrial appendage in patients with atrial fibrillation.[7–9] Electrophysiologic studies are a powerful diagnostic tool, although they require the patient to undergo cardiac catheterization. Programmed electrical stimulation of specific areas of the conduction system or cardiac tissue via catheter can uncover ectopic pacemakers, find accessory or bypass tracts responsible for reentry arrhythmias, and in combination with radiofrequency ablation (RFA) eliminate the cause of many arrhythmias.[10–14] Although most family physicians do not perform these tests, it is important that they know the appropriate indications for each test and how to interpret test results.

Approach to Therapy for Cardiac Arrhythmias

Many cardiac arrhythmias are of little clinical significance and do not require therapy other than careful discussion with the patient and reassurance. For other arrhythmias, clinicians should begin by searching for and treating any reversible underlying causes or medical conditions. If the arrhythmia persists, four types of treatment are available: drug therapy, cardioversion, radiofrequency or surgical ablation, and implantable devices (pacemakers and defibrillators).

Correction of Underlying Problems

Medication use or ingestions (e.g., caffeine) are the most commonly seen reversible causes of arrhythmias, and changing or discontinuing medications or discontinuing use of caffeine or other substances may eliminate the problem. Correction of electrolyte imbalances can also eliminate arrhythmias. In patients with CHF or ischemic heart disease and arrhythmia, effective therapy for the underlying condition may improve tissue oxygen delivery and local pH and result in return to sinus rhythm. Clinicians should look for and correct all potentially reversible causes before initiating drug or ablative therapy.

Drug Therapy

Antiarrhythmic drugs have been assigned to classes based on their mode of action. Table 77.3 lists examples of drugs in each of the Vaughan-Williams classes.[15] Class I agents act on the sodium ion channel, with slight differences between IA, IB, and IC agents in specific actions. Randomized controlled trials of drug therapy for ventricular arrhythmia have shown no improvement in survival, and in some cases excess mortality, in patients using class I antiarrhythmics. Use of these agents is declining,[16–19] although there may be a role for class IC agents propafenone and flecainide in supraventricular arrhythmias.[19–21] The use of class II drugs (beta-blockers) has been shown to have a beneficial effect on survival in post-MI patients, presumably due to suppression of lethal ventricular arrhythmia. They are also useful as adjunctive treatment to implantable cardiac defibrillators (ICDs), as an alternative to RFA for AV nodal reentrant tachyarrhythmias, and to control rate in atrial fibrillation.[13,19,22] Class III drugs prolong the AP by increasing refractoriness. Amiodarone has emerged as an effective agent for both ventricular and supraventricular arrhythmias.[23,24] Dofetilide and ibutilide have also shown promise in recent clinical trials, while sotalol (a combined class II and III agent) appears to be less effective than other class III agents.[19,25–27] Class IV agents (calcium channel blockers) are effective for many supraventricular arrhythmias.[19,28]

The major drawback to the use of any of these agents is their potential for inducing complex arrhythmias (proarrhythmic effect).[19,29,30] The best known example is the emer-

gence of torsades de pointes arrhythmia in patients with prolonged QT intervals treated with class I antiarrhythmics,[31] but all antiarrhythmic drugs have proarrhythmic potential and their use must be carefully monitored.

Cardioversion

Urgent or emergent direct current (DC) cardioversion is most commonly used in hemodynamically unstable patients with atrial or ventricular arrhythmias, but elective cardioversion can be an effective treatment for selected supraventricular arrhythmias. It has been successfully employed either before or after medication to convert atrial fibrillation or flutter to sinus rhythm,[14] and it has a place in the nonpharmacologic management of other supraventricular tachyarrhythmias.[32] Microcurrent catheter-based cardioversion is currently being studied.

Ablative Therapy

The ablative approach rests on identification and localization of an aberrant conduction pathway responsible for the arrhythmia, usually through an EP study. Ablation is clearly effective in treating supraventricular tachyarrhythmias. Physical interruption of aberrant pathways via sharp surgical dissection during open-heart surgical procedures became common during the 1980s; the maze procedure (named for the procedure that creates a pattern that looks like a maze and traps the reentrant circuit) and its variants are the best example of this approach.[33,34] More recently, cryoablation and RFA techniques have become the nonpharmacologic treatment of choice for selected supraventricular tachyarrhythmias.[10–12] In RFA, application of radiofrequency energy to a portion of the aberrant pathway produces thermal injury and a permanent refractory state in the tissue, preventing any further aberrant conduction. High success rates have been reported for RFA in most settings,[10–12] and it may prove to be the most cost-effective approach to management of many supraventricular tachyarrhythmias.[35–37] RFA also has a growing role in treatment of monomorphic ventricular tachycardia refractory to drug therapy.[10]

Pacemakers and Defibrillators

Implantable cardiac pacemakers have been available for many years and provide effective therapy for many bradyarrhythmias and other conduction disturbances. Although pacemakers have been developed for use in supraventricular tachyarrhythmias, they are infrequently used.[38] Implantable cardiac defibrillators have evolved rapidly in size, sophistication, and ease of insertion over the past decade. Recent clinical trials have confirmed their superior effectiveness as compared to drug therapy in reducing mortality in survivors of cardiac arrest and patients at high risk for sudden cardiac death (SCD).[39–42] ICDs are now considered the treatment of choice for secondary prevention of SCD, and an emerging standard for primary prevention of SCD in high-risk patients, despite the absence of good data on their relative cost-effectiveness.[43]

Automatic external defibrillators (AEDs) combine computerized detection of ventricular fibrillation with low-energy

Table 77.3. Dosing, Indications, and Contraindications for Common Antiarrhythmic Drugs Listed by Vaughan-Williams Class

Name	Dosing	Indications	Contraindications • clinical notes
Class IA			
Disopyramide		VT	CHF (relative); 2nd- or 3rd-degree AV block prolonged QT interval
Norpace	100–200 mg po q6–8h		• Proarrhythmic effects
Norpace CR	200–400 mg po q12h		
Procainamide		Primary: VT	CHF relative; complete heart block
Pronestyl	375–500 mg q3–4h	Secondary: VT, AT in	• Drug-induced lupus
Pronestyl SR	500–1000 mg q6–8h	WPW syndrome	• Blood dyscrasias
Procan SR	500–750 mg q6–8h		• Proarrhythmic effects
Quinidine		VT	2nd- or 3rd-degree AV block prolonged QT interval
Quinidine sulfate	200–300 mg q6–8h		• Proarrhythmic effects
Quinidex Extentabs	300–600 mg q8–12h		
Quinaglute	324–648 mg q8–12°		
Class IB			
Lidocaine	IV: 1 mg/kg bolus followed by 1–4 mg/min infusion	VT, VF	• CNS side effects
Mexiletine		Primary: VT	2nd- or 3rd-degree AV block
Mexitil	150–300 mg po q8–12h	Secondary: SVT in WPW syndrome	• ?Hepatic toxicity • CNS side effects • Proarrhythmic effects
Tocainide		VT	2nd- or 3rd-degree AV block
Tonocard	400–600 mg po q8h		• Blood dyscrasias • Pulmonary fibrosis • Proarrhythmic effects
Class IC			
Flecainide	IV: 2 mg/kg over 5–10 min	Primary: VT	CHF (relative) 2nd- or 3rd-degree AV block; bifascicular block
Tambocor	50–200 mg po q12h	Secondary: SVT, paroxysmal AF, atrial flutter	• Proarrhythmic effects
Propafenone		Primary: VT	CHF; 2nd- or 3rd-degree AV block; severe asthma
Rythmol	150–300 mg po q8h	Secondary: SVT in WPW syndrome	• Proarrhythmic effects
Moricizine		Primary: VT	Cardiogenic shock; 2nd-3rd-degree AV block; bifascicular block
Ethmozine	200–300 mg po q8h	Secondary: SVT	• Proarrhythmic effects
Class II (beta-blockers)			
Propranolol		AT; sinus tachycardia; SVT; VT prophylaxis; SVT in WPW syndrome; VPB post-MI	CHF; severe asthma; severe bradycardia; 2nd- or 3rd-degree AV block
Inderal	20–80 mg po q6h		
Inderal LA	20–160 mg po q12h		
Acebutolol		Same as propranolol	CHF; severe bradycardia; 2nd- or 3rd-degree AV block
Sectral	200–600 mg po BID		
Atenolol		Same as propranolol	CHF; severe bradycardia; 2nd- or 3rd-degree AV block
Tenormin	50–100 mg po q12h		
Bisoprolol		Same as propranolol	CHF; severe asthma; severe bradycardia; 2nd- or 3rd-degree AV block
Zebeta	2.5–20 mg po qd		
Esmolol	IV: 0.5 mg/kg bolus, 0.05 to 0.2 mg/min infusion	SVT; VT; AF	CHF; severe asthma; severe bradycardia; 2nd- or 3rd-degree AV block
Brevibloc			
Labetalol	IV: 1–2 mg/kg bolus, 0.5–2 mg/min infusion	SVT	CHF (relative); severe asthma; severe bradycardia; 2nd- or 3rd-degree AV
Normodyne	100–400 mg po q8–12h	Same as propranolol	
Trandate	100–400 mg po q8–12h		
Metoprolol	IV: 2.5–5.0 mg over 2 min, up to 15 mg total	SVT	CHF; severe bradycardia; 2nd- or 3rd-degree AV block
Toprol XL	50–200 mg po qd	Same as propranolol	
Lopressor	50–100 mg po q8–12h		

(Continues on next page)

Table 77.3. Continued

Name	Dosing	Indications	Contraindications • clinical notes
Nadolol Corgard	40–240 mg po qd	Same as propranolol	CHF; severe asthma; severe bradycardia; 2nd- or 3rd-degree AV block
Timolol Blocadren	10–20 mg po q12h	Same as propranolol	CHF; severe asthma; severe COPD; severe bradycardia; 2nd- or 3rd-degree AV block
Pindolol Visken	2.5–30 mg po q12h	Same as propranolol	CHF; severe asthma; severe bradycardia; 2nd- or 3rd-degree AV block
Class III			
Amiodarone Cordarone	IV: 5 mg/kg over 10–15 min bolus, then 0.5–1 mg/min 800–1600 mg po qd or q12h for 1–2 weeks (loading dose); 200–400 mg po qd (maintenance)	Primary: VT; VF prophylaxis Secondary: AF; VPB post-MI	Severe bradycardia; 2nd- or 3rd-degree AV block (unless pacemaker capability) • proarrhythmic effects • pulmonary toxicity • hepatic toxicity • corneal deposits • thyroid abnormalities
Sotalol Betapace	IV: 1–1.5 mg/kg over 10 min 80–160 mg po q12h	VT; VF prophylaxis	CHF; severe asthma; severe bradycardia; 2nd- 3rd-degree AV block; prolonged QT interval • Proarrhythmic effects
Ibutilide Corvert	IV: 1–2 mg over 10 min	AF (termination); SVT	• Proarrhythmic effects
Dofetilide Tikosyn	125–500 mg po q12h	AF	Prolonged QT interval; renal impairment; use with verapamil, cimetidine, trimethoprim or ketoconazole
Class IV (calcium channel blockers)			
Diltiazem Cardizem Cardizem Cardizem SR	IV: 0.25 mg/kg bolus followed by 10–15 mg/hr infusion 30–90 mg po q6h 60–180 mg po q12h	AT; sinus tachycardia; SVT; AF; atrial flutter	Sick sinus syndrome severe bradycardia; 2nd- or 3rd-degree AV block
Verapamil Isoptin Isoptin Isoptin SR Calan Calan SR	IV: 5–10 mg over 2 min, repeat in 30 min if needed 80–120 mg q6–8h 180–480 mg po q12h to qd 80–120 mg q6–8h 180–180 mg po q12h to qd	AT; sinus tachycardia; SVT; AF; atrial flutter	Sick sinus syndrome; severe bradycardia; 2nd- or 3rd-degree AV block; concomitant use of IV and IV beta-blockers; AF in WPW
Miscellaneous			
Adenosine Adenocard	IV: 6 mg over 1–2 sec, may repeat bolus twice with 12 mg over 1–2 min if needed	SVT; SVT in WPW syndrome	Sick sinus syndrome; AV block 2nd or 3rd-degree • may cause dyspnea, chest pain, flushing
Digoxin Lanoxin	IV: 0.5 mg bolus followed by 0.1–0.3 mg q4–6h Loading dose: 0.5–0.75 mg po followed by 0.125–0.25 mg q6h 0.125–0.25 mg po qd	AF; atrial flutter; AT	VF • proarrhythmic effects

AF = atrial fibrillation; AT = (paroxysmal) atrial tachycardia; CHF = congestive heart failure; CNS = central nervous system; COPD = chronic obstructive pulmonary disease; MI = myocardial infarction; SVT = supraventricular tachycardia; VPB = ventricular premature beat; VT = ventricular tachycardia; WPW syndrome = Wolff-Parkinson-White syndrome.

Note: VPBs are not included in list of indications, as treatment is generally not indicated for VPBs.

biphasic waveform defibrillation.[44] They have also evolved rapidly over the past decade in size, cost, and ease of use, and have emerged as a central part of new emergency and "public access" defibrillation protocols employed by first-response emergency personnel.[44–46]

Specific Cardiac Arrhythmias: Diagnosis and Management

This section describes the salient clinical features and management options for the most common cardiac arrhythmias, including sample ECG tracings where appropriate. Table 77.4 lists arrhythmias by class in the order addressed in the text, and Table 77.5 lists treatments of choice and alternative treatments for specific arrhythmias.

Sinus Bradycardia

Sinus bradycardia consists of normally conducted cardiac impulses originating in the sinus node at a rate less than 60 beats per minute (bpm). It occurs in individuals at a high level of athletic conditioning, as a result of vagal hyperactivity or pain, and during sleep. It can be a symptom of hypothyroidism and is often associated with medication use (e.g., narcotic analgesics, calcium channel antagonists, beta-blockers, digoxin, quinidine, procainamide). It can also occur in the setting of an inferior wall MI. It can present significant problems when it appears in elderly patients, if it is the result of sinus node disease or fibrosis, or if it is associated with an acute inferior wall MI.

The clinical history may vary from no symptoms to fatigue, dizziness, syncope or near-syncope, or chest pain (if associated with MI). Clinicians should look for signs or symptoms

Table 77.4. **Common Cardiac Arrhythmias**

Supraventricular arrhythmias—slow to moderate rate
  Sinus bradycardia
  Sinus pause/sinus arrest
  Atrial premature beats (premature atrial complexes)
Supraventricular tachyarrhythmias
  Sinus tachycardia
  Atrial tachycardia
  Multifocal atrial tachycardia
  AV nodal reentrant tachycardias (paroxysmal
    supraventricular tachycardia)
  AV reciprocating tachycardias ("preexcitation" syndromes)
  Atrial fibrillation
  Atrial flutter
Other atrioventricular conduction abnormalities
  1st-degree AV block
  2nd-degree AV block, Mobitz type I (Wenckebach block)
  2nd-degree AV block, Mobitz type II
  3rd-degree AV block
Ventricular arrhythmias
  Ventricular premature beats (premature ventricular
    complexes)
  Ventricular tachycardia—nonsustained and sustained
  Ventricular fibrillation

AV = atrioventricular.

of hypothyroidism, CHF, and MI. The ECG appears normal except for a slow heart rate. No other tests are necessary, unless an associated medical condition is suspected.

Treatment is not necessary unless the patient is symptomatic or is at high risk for complications related to slow heart rate (e.g., an elderly patient at risk for falls). In general, treat an underlying cause first whenever possible: if associated with medication use, discontinue the offending medication; if due to hypothyroidism, begin treatment with thyroid hormone. Patients who do not have a likely cause or who do not respond to treatment may require pacemaker insertion. Emergent treatment for unstable patients can be initiated in the office with atropine until definitive care can be arranged.

Sinus Pause/Sinus Arrest

As its name suggests, sinus pause/sinus arrest consists of an unexpected pause in an otherwise normal pattern of cardiac impulses. The sinus node does not fire, and a pause of up to several seconds may occur followed by resumption of a regular rhythm or emergence of a nodal or idioventricular "escape" rhythm. It commonly occurs in individuals during deep sleep, but when frequent and associated with escape rhythms it may also indicate a fibrotic and malfunctioning SA node, sick sinus syndrome, or medication effect (digoxin, quinidine, calcium channel blocker, or beta-blocker overdosing).

The condition may be asymptomatic or associated with recurrent dizziness, near-syncope, or syncope, and resumption of cardiac impulses may be perceived by the patient as palpitations. The ECG shows normal sinus rhythm with a sudden pause during which P waves are absent, followed either by resumption of P waves and normal sinus rhythm or appearance of a junctional or ventricular QRS complex. With sick sinus syndrome, other types of arrhythmia or conduction disturbance are seen as well.

Treatment is not always necessary, but in light of the potential for significant symptoms and the possibility of significant underlying cardiac disease, referral for cardiac evaluation is warranted. If symptomatic patients do not respond to correction of known underlying causes, cardiac pacemaker insertion may be necessary. Emergent office-based treatment for full sinus arrest consists of intravenous atropine or isoproterenol until definitive care can be arranged.

Premature Atrial Complexes

The terms *premature atrial complexes* (PACs) and *atrial premature beats* (APBs) are both used, and they represent the same phenomenon. Cardiac impulses are initiated in one or more ectopic atrial foci but are otherwise conducted as for a normal beat. They often occur in individuals with a normal heart and can be precipitated by anxiety, fatigue, ingestion of a number of substances (alcohol, tobacco, caffeine, sympathomimetic drugs), and possibly sleep deprivation. They can also occur in the presence of atrial enlargement, CHF, myocardial ischemia and infarction, pericarditis, or as a response to hypoxia, elevated local pH, or electrolyte imbalance.

The APBs are usually asymptomatic, but patients may present with palpitations. Physical examination is nonspecific, ex-

Table 77.5. **Treatment of Choice and Alternative Treatments for Common Cardiac Arrhythmias**

Arrhythmia	Treatment(s) of choice	Alternative treatment
Sinus bradycardia	Atropine (emergent) Pacemaker	Isoproterenol
Sinus pause/arrest	Atropine (emergent) Pacemaker	
Atrial premature beats, junctional premature beats	Treatment often not necessary	Beta-blockers, verapamil
Sinus tachycardia	Beta-blockers	Verapamil
Atrial tachycardia	Beta-blockers RFA (curative)	Verapamil
Multifocal atrial tachycardia	IV verapamil (conversion) Beta-blockers, verapamil	RFA of AV node plus pacemaker
AV nodal reentrant tachycardias (SVT) and AV reciprocating tachycardias ("preexcitation")	IV adenosine (conversion) IV verapamil (conversion) Carotid sinus pressure, vagal maneuvers (conversion) Beta-blockers (prophylaxis) Calcium channel blockers (prophylaxis) RFA (curative)	IV esmolol (conversion) DC cardioversion Pacemaker Class IC antiarrhythmics (prophylaxis) Class III antiarrhythmics (prophylaxis) Digoxin (conversion and prophylaxis; use with caution)
Atrial fibrillation	DC cardioversion Amiodarone Beta-blockers Calcium-channel blockers Digoxin Aspirin, coumadin (CVA prevention)	Class I antiarrhythmics Class III antiarrhythmics RFA of ectopic focus (if present) RFA of AV node plus pacemaker Surgical ablation (Cox maze procedure)
Atrial flutter	DC cardioversion Rapid atrial pacing (conversion) Beta-blockers Calcium channel blockers RFA of reentrant circuit (curative)	Ibutilide (conversion) Class IA antiarrhythmics RFA of AV node plus pacemaker
1st-degree AV block and 2nd-degree (Mobitz type I)	Treatment often not necessary	Pacemaker (symptomatic Mobitz type I)
2nd-degree (Mobitz type II) and 3rd-degree AV block	Pacemaker	
Ventricular premature beats	Treatment often not necessary	Beta-blockers Amiodarone
Ventricular tachycardia, nonsustained	With no heart disease: no treatment necessary With heart disease and VT on EP study: implantable cardiac defibrillator With heart disease and no VT on EP study: treat heart disease (see text)	With heart disease: amiodarone EP study with RFA of ectopic focus
Ventricular tachycardia, sustained	ACLS protocol, transfer for definitive care Postevent: implantable cardiac defibrillator	
Ventricular fibrillation	ACLS protocol, automatic external defibrillator, transfer for definitive care Postevent: implantable cardiac defibrillator	

ACLS = advanced cardiac life support; AV = atrioventricular; CVA = cerebrovascular accident; EP = electrophysiologic; RFA = radiofrequency ablation; VT = ventricular tachycardia.

cept for signs of underlying conditions. On ECG (Fig. 77.1a), the amplitudes and axes of ectopic P waves differ from that seen in sinus rhythm, as a different part of the atrium is depolarizing. The PR interval of the APB is usually prolonged, as conduction between the ectopic focus to the AV node is slowed. A prolonged PP interval is often seen between the APB and a subsequent normal beat. The QRS complex appears normal, unless aberrant conduction bypassing the AV node or ventricular conduction disturbance is also present.

APBs may occur in patterns such as bigeminy or trigeminy, in couplets, or as short runs.

Treatment is directed at correcting the underlying cause but is otherwise not necessary. In patients with an unacceptable level of symptoms, verapamil or beta-blockers can be used to suppress APBs with relatively mild side effects. However, clinicians should carefully consider the risk/benefit ratio of drug therapy for this benign condition before initiating drug therapy.

Figure 1a: Premature atrial complexes (atrial premature beats) [beats #3,6,9]

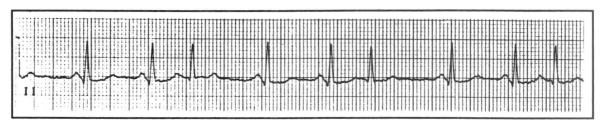

Figure 1b: Sinus tachycardia

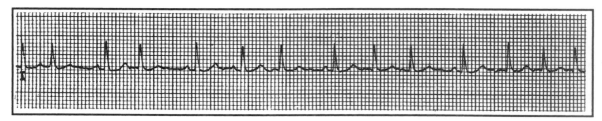

Figure 1c: Multifocal atrial tachycardia

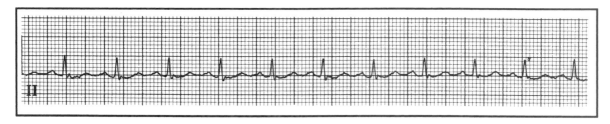

Figure 1d: Supraventricular tachycardia

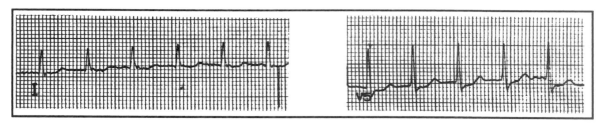

Figure 1e: AV reciprocating tachycardias ("preexcitation" syndromes)
[example: Wolff-Parkinson-White syndrome]

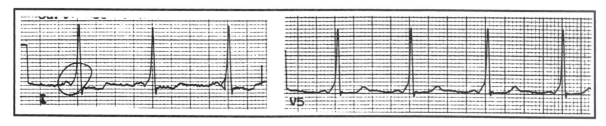

Fig. 77.1. Selected supraventricular arrhythmias: sample electrocardiogram (ECG) tracings. ECG leads from which tracings were obtained are listed in the lower left corner. See text for discussion of specific ECG features of each arrhythmia.

Supraventricular Tachyarrhythmias

Increased experience with EP studies and our growing knowledge of molecular genetics have combined to fundamentally change our understanding of the supraventricular tachyarrhythmias (SVTs). SVTs include all tachyarrhythmias that originate above the bifurcation of the bundle of His, and are present in roughly 1% of the United States population.[13] Terminology in this area is evolving and confusing. A practical way to stratify SVTs is by involvement of the AV node: AV-node–*dependent* arrhythmias are more responsive to medications or procedures that slow or block conduction at the AV node than are *independent* arrhythmias that bypass the node. Reentry is now believed to be the underlying mechanism of most SVTs, with a smaller proportion caused by abnormal automaticity or triggered activity without a bypass tract.

Sinus Tachycardia

Sinus tachycardia consists of normally conducted cardiac impulses originating in the sinus node at a rate of over 100 bpm. It may be asymptomatic or symptomatic, often described by patients as "palpitations" or a "racing heart." This rhythm is an appropriate response to the need for increased cardiac output and can be a normal finding in distressed or exercising individuals. However, its occurrence at rest is not normal and should lead to a search for an underlying cause. Possible causes include hyperthyroidism, fever, anemia, hypoxia, CHF, hypovolemia, anxiety, caffeine or other stimulants, illicit drug ingestion, and medication use (common nonprescription medications such as cold preparations with sympathomimetic effects, as well as tricyclic antidepressants, prazosin, and theophylline). In some cases a reentrant process at the SA node may be the cause.

Symptoms are generally nonspecific, although in patients with underlying ischemic heart disease sinus tachycardia can precipitate acute ischemia. The ECG (Fig. 77.1b) is normal except for the rate; all waves and complexes have normal morphology. Evaluation depends on the likelihood of significant underlying illness.

Treatment is directed at the underlying cause. Treatment with rate-lowering drugs is indicated only for relief of hemodynamically significant symptoms (syncope, near-syncope, ischemia) when no underlying cause can be found.

Atrial Tachycardia

Atrial tachycardia (also known as automatic or paroxysmal atrial tachycardia) might be considered a variant of sinus tachycardia, in which an ectopic atrial pacemaker or an intraatrial reentry mechanism initiates a rapid regular rhythm using the normal conduction system. The heart rate may vary from 100 to 300 bpm, depending on whether AV block is present. Atrial tachycardia with AV block is strongly associated with digoxin intoxication; otherwise, it has many of the same precipitating factors as sinus tachycardia. It can be distinguished from sinus tachycardia by the appearance of abnormal P waves or by retrograde or nonconducted P waves when some degree of AV block is present.

Treatment depends on the cause. If symptoms are significant, treatment with rate-lowering drugs may be indicated.

Referral to a cardiologist for an EP study may allow identification and ablation of a causative intraatrial reentry tract.

Multifocal Atrial Tachycardia

Multifocal atrial tachycardia (MAT) is characterized by the appearance of multiple ectopic atrial foci, with a rapid and slightly irregular rhythm the result of transmission of these multiple foci through the AV node. It is usually associated with respiratory failure due to chronic pulmonary disease, although it is also seen with chronic heart disease and with the use of thioxanthene drugs. Hypoxia and hypokalemia have been hypothesized as the major causative mechanisms.[47]

The arrhythmia itself rarely causes symptoms, but the underlying condition is usually all too clear. Because the pulse is often irregularly irregular, MAT can be mistaken for atrial fibrillation on clinical examination. The ECG (Fig. 77.1c) shows an atrial rate over 100 bpm with at least three distinct P wave morphologies. The PP, PR, and RR intervals are irregular due to the varying conduction pathways, and some P waves are not conducted. If the ectopic P waves are of low amplitude, the ECG can also resemble that seen with atrial fibrillation.

Treatment is directed at correcting the presumed metabolic abnormalities. Administration of supplemental oxygen for pulmonary failure or treatment of associated CHF may alleviate hypoxia. Intravenous bolus administration of verapamil has been shown to convert MAT to sinus rhythm, and oral verapamil or beta-blockers can slow the ventricular rate. However, these medications are often poorly tolerated in MAT patients with severe cardiac or pulmonary disease, and drug therapy is usually reserved for patients who develop ischemia or hemodynamic instability. Patients refractory to drug therapy may benefit from AV nodal ablation followed by pacemaker insertion.[13,12]

AV Nodal Reentrant Tachycardias

Many clinicians recognize AV nodal reentrant tachycardia (AVNRT) by the commonly used term *paroxysmal supraventricular tachycardia* (PSVT). It consists of a regular and rapid rhythm, usually between 140 and 220 bpm, caused by a reentry mechanism dependent on a dual conduction pathway within the AV node. Regular beats are transmitted through the node along a "fast" pathway. A premature atrial beat initiates the arrhythmia; it is blocked from antegrade passage through the fast pathway during its refractory period but transmitted antegrade through a "slow" pathway in the node. This impulse is then transmitted both antegrade to the ventricles and retrograde through the fast pathway (now nonrefractory) back to the slow pathway, where the process is repeated. This arrhythmia is often seen in young, healthy individuals with otherwise normal hearts, but it may occur with myocarditis, cardiac ischemia, chronic obstructive pulmonary disease (COPD), or other conditions potentially affecting AV nodal function.

Many patients are asymptomatic during episodes. Young patients may note only palpitations but may also have associated weakness, dizziness, or mild dyspnea; they are usually hemodynamically stable during an episode. Older patients, particularly those with underlying cardiac or pulmonary disease, may develop angina, CHF, or cerebrovascular insufficiency during episodes; syncope is rarely reported. Cardiac auscultation reveals a regular, rapid rhythm. The ECG (Fig. 77.1d) shows a regular rhythm with normal QRS complexes (unless aberrant ventricular conduction is also present), but P waves are abnormal owing to retrograde conduction. In many cases of AVNRT, P waves are absent as atria depolarize at the same time as the ventricles. In other cases, a slight difference in depolarization timing creates slurs in the normal QRS due to atrial activity.

Treatment depends in large part on the level of symptoms and the patient's hemodynamic stability. Unstable patients require emergent conversion by DC cardioversion or intravenous bolus administration of adenosine, verapamil, or esmolol. Intravenous adenosine is currently the treatment of choice in many centers, as it terminates SVT in more than 90% of cases.[48] Other class I antiarrhythmics may produce conversion to sinus rhythm at high rates, but their high risk/benefit ratios essentially preclude their use in this setting. Rapid digitalization has been used for urgent conversion in the past with high success rates, but it does not result in immediate correction and may predispose to the development of other arrhythmias.[13] Nonpharmacologic techniques such as carotid sinus massage, Valsalva maneuver, or other vagal maneuvers such as facial ice bag application or ice bucket immersion prolong AV node refractory periods and can produce conversion to sinus rhythm in selected situations.

Once converted to sinus rhythm, several drugs are effective in preventing recurrence, including oral verapamil, diltiazem, beta-blockers, and digoxin. Because digoxin appears to exert its effect indirectly through the vagus nerve, exercise may lead to recurrence of SVT in patients treated with this drug. Class IC and class III agents have shown some success in preventing recurrence of SVT but in general are less desirable because of their high incidence of side effects.

Asymptomatic SVT in young, healthy patients generally does not require treatment. Infrequent symptomatic episodes may be treated with the nonpharmacologic techniques described above as well as by preventive pharmacotherapy. Some patients may be able to administer self-treatment at the onset of SVT, using either the Valsalva maneuver or a single dose of medication (oral propranolol or verapamil or sublingual verapamil).

Nonpharmacologic therapeutic interventions aimed at eliminating the reentrant pathway have developed rapidly in recent years. RFA has been widely and successfully employed and may be the most cost-effective approach to therapy for patients with breakthrough SVT while on medication.[36]

AV Reciprocating Tachycardias

Atrioventricular reciprocating tachycardias (AVRTs), also known as "preexcitation" syndromes or accessory pathway arrhythmias, are characterized by a regular, rapid rhythm, usually between 140 and 220 bpm. They are caused by an anatomically distinct accessory pathway that conducts in retrograde fashion from ventricle to atrium, establishing a reentry circuit between the AV node and the pathway that causes paroxysmal bursts of supraventricular tachycardia. The reentry can be either orthodromic (antegrade transmission to the ventricles through the normal pathway for a normal QRS complex during tachycardia, retrograde transmission to the atria through the accessory pathway) or antidromic (antegrade transmission to the ventricles through the accessory pathway, which may alter the QRS). It is technically more correct to say that preexcitation syndromes cause AVRTs, as tachycardia is the intermittently occurring consequence of the presence of the pathway. The two best known examples of AVRT are the Wolff-Parkinson-White (WPW) and Lown-Ganong-Levine (LGL) syndromes.

This condition is often seen in young adults with otherwise normal hearts, but it is also associated with hypertrophic cardiomyopathy, several congenital cardiac anomalies, and possibly mitral valve prolapse. Patients have the same range of symptoms as seen with other types of SVT. Unlike most AVNRTs, preexcitation syndromes can be diagnosed between episodes by their ECG appearance. The classic ECG appearance of WPW between episodes of tachycardia is a short PR interval (<0.12 second) and a widened QRS complex with a slurred up-sloping initial component called the delta wave (Fig. 77.1e). With orthodromic conduction, episodes of tachycardia will have an ECG appearance indistinguishable from other types of SVT; however, delta waves can be seen during tachycardia in antidromic conduction, and if large can cause a widened QRS complex easily mistaken for ventricular tachycardia. LGL syndrome is less unique in its ECG appearance, consisting of a short PR interval (<0.12 second) and a normal QRS, leading some experts to question whether it simply represents a short but otherwise normal atrial conduction process in patients with AVNRT from other causes.

Treatment follows the same general principles as for SVT. Digoxin should be used with caution, as it may cause emergence of other arrhythmias, and verapamil may cause heart rate acceleration rather than conversion in those with WPW syndrome. Surgical ablation of the accessory pathway has largely given way to RFA as the curative therapy of choice.[10,13]

Atrial Fibrillation

Atrial fibrillation (AF) is the most common sustained supraventricular arrhythmia and is primarily a disease of elderly patients, by one estimate currently affecting over 2.3 million U.S. adults, including 4% of adults over 60 years of age and 9% of those over 80.[49] It represents a major cause of morbidity and mortality in the United States, particularly due to its association with embolic stroke. A tremendous research effort has been targeted to determine its mechanism and optimal management. It now appears that AF represents a chaotic form of intraatrial reentry involving multiple circuits generating 350 to 700 wavelets per minute with variable conduction through the atrium and the rest of the conduction system. In some patients, an ectopic focus in or near the pulmonary veins has been identified as the source of the reentrant activity.[50] Over time, these reentrant circuits alter the electrical milieu to promote maintenance of the arrhythmia in a process called electrical remodeling, leading to the new aphorism that "AF begets AF."[51] Although a few cases may occur in elderly patients with otherwise normal hearts ("lone AF"), it is most commonly seen in patients with increased atrial mass, valvular heart disease, and other types of chronic cardiac or pulmonary disease. In patients with underlying cardiac or pulmonary disease, any of the general causes of arrhythmias listed in Table 77.1 can precipitate AF.

Atrial fibrillation can present as either a sustained or intermittent arrhythmia. Symptoms may or may not be present and range from palpitations to dizziness to exacerbation of associated chronic conditions; in the elderly, syncope and falls may occur as a consequence of poor perfusion. Cardiac auscultation reveals an irregularly irregular rhythm, a first heart sound of variable intensity, often a variable pulse, and other clinical findings consistent with underlying disease(s). The ECG (Fig. 77.2a,b) is characterized by an irregular, wavy baseline representing chaotic atrial depolarization, the absence of P waves, and irregularly appearing QRS complexes. A ventricular rate of more than 100 bpm is labeled a "rapid" ventricular response, between 60 and 100 bpm a "moderate" response, and less than 60 bpm a "slow" response. Slow ventricular rates suggest AV nodal disease, hypothyroidism, or the presence of drugs that increase AV node refractory time (digoxin, beta-blockers, calcium channel blockers, and possibly class I antiarrhythmics).

Figure 2a: Atrial fibrillation with slow ventricular response

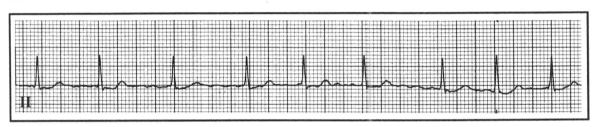

Figure 2b: Atrial fibrillation with rapid ventricular response

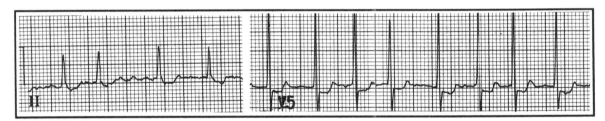

Figure 2c: Atrial flutter

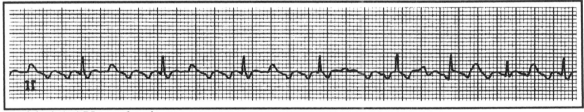

with 4:1 AV conduction

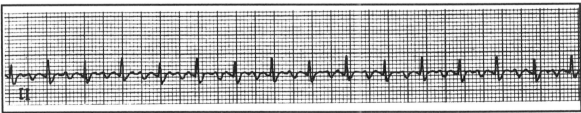

with 2:1 AV conduction

Fig. 77.2. Atrial fibrillation and flutter. Sample ECG tracings for atrial fibrillation with slow and rapid ventricular response and atrial flutter. ECG leads from which tracings were obtained are listed in the lower left corner.

A detailed discussion of the management of atrial fibrillation is beyond the scope of this chapter, but important management principles for common clinical situations can be described. If AF precipitates acute CHF, hypotension, syncope, cerebral hypoperfusion, or angina at rest, or if patients are otherwise hemodynamically unstable, urgent treatment (usually in the hospital or emergency department setting) is required. This situation is most likely to occur with AF with a rapid ventricular response. Because a significant proportion of unstable AF patients may have had an acute MI, clinicians should carefully consider this possibility when evaluating the patient. Cardioversion can be attempted in the emergency or inpatient setting for unstable patients, but caution is needed to minimize the risk of embolism at the time of conversion. When time allows, drug therapy can be initiated with digoxin, beta-blockers, verapamil, or diltiazem to help control the ventricular rate and increase the likelihood of successful cardioversion.

In the clinically stable patient with newly diagnosed AF, the duration of the episode and the presence of underlying cardiac disease are the main factors determining treatment. In patients with good cardiac function, spontaneous conversion to sinus rhythm (SR) within 24 hours of onset is common.[52] In patients with known duration of AF less than 48 hours and no significant cardiac disease, active treatment is also likely to result in conversion to SR; after acute anticoagulation, either DC cardioversion or medication (IV ibutilide or oral propafenone, flecainide, or quinidine) has shown good success in terminating AF.[50] For patients with over 48 hours or unknown duration of AF or with underlying cardiac disease, TEE can be used to guide therapy. If TEE shows no evidence of atrial thrombus or stasis, heparinization and DC cardioversion followed by 4 weeks of anticoagulation with warfarin has been shown to be safe and effective in restoring SR in the short term.[8] If thrombus or stasis is present on TEE, 3 weeks of therapeutic anticoagulation with warfarin, followed by DC cardioversion and at least 4 more weeks of anticoagulation, is the current recommendation.

The long-term success of cardioversion depends primarily on the patient's age, duration of AF, underlying disease, and left atrial diameter, but in most patients AF recurs after cardioversion.[50,53] Despite the theoretical appeal of maintenance drug therapy to prevent recurrence, its role is controversial. Clinical trials have shown both improved success in maintaining SR and excess mortality from proarrhythmic side effects.[17,54,55] Amiodarone appears to offer the best combination of effectiveness and safety in this role, although 12-month recurrence rates are still high.[55] Some experts recommend DC cardioversion alone for a first AF episode, with cardioversion followed by amiodarone for a first relapse.[56] For patients with an ectopic focus near the pulmonary veins, RFA to eliminate the focus offers a potential cure for AF, but preliminary reports have yielded inconsistent results.[56,57] RFA of the AV node followed by permanent pacemaker insertion may be necessary in symptomatic patients refractory to other treatment.

Paroxysmal AF can be considered a special case of symptomatic recurrent AF, and results of clinical trials of drug therapy mirror those for maintenance drug therapy. Several drugs, including propafenone, flecainide, and sotalol, increase the length of time between paroxysms but do not abolish them, and may predispose to proarrhythmia.[19,50]

In general, management of persistent or recurrent AF should not focus on restoring and maintaining sinus rhythm but on maximizing ventricular function and reducing the risk of stroke, which approaches 6% per year in AF patients.[58] Three types of antiarrhythmic drug can be used to block AV node conduction, slow a rapid ventricular rate, and improve ventricular function: digoxin, beta-blockers, and calcium channel blockers. Digoxin has been used extensively in elderly patients because of its effectiveness in enhancing left ventricular contractility, but it may be less effective in controlling the rate than either of the other two medications. Digoxin and atenolol have been used in combination with some success.[56] Unfortunately, beta-blockers and calcium channel blockers (particularly verapamil) may precipitate or worsen CHF.

Reducing the risk of stroke is the major goal of treatment of AF. The results of several clinical trials of stroke prevention in AF support the use of warfarin in most clinical circumstances.[59–63] Pooled analysis of clinical trial data highlights several risk factors for stroke: mitral stenosis, hypertension (treated or untreated), previous transient ischemic attack or stroke, CHF, left ventricular dysfunction, and age over 75 years.[63–65] Unless contraindicated, warfarin is recommended for all patients with one or more risk factors, with either warfarin or aspirin recommended for those between 65 and 75 years of age with no risk factors. Aspirin is recommended for those under 65 with no additional risk factors, but there is little data on the effectiveness of aspirin in this group. Aspirin is indicated for those unable to use warfarin, although its effectiveness is unknown. The risk of hemorrhagic complications from warfarin can be minimized by dosing adjustment to maintain an international normalized ratio (INR) between 2.0 and 3.0.[65]

Atrial Flutter

Atrial flutter is virtually always caused by a reentry circuit in the right atrium, which creates a wavefront of depolarization most often moving in a counterclockwise direction across the atria ("typical," "common," or "counterclockwise" atrial flutter), but occasionally traveling clockwise ("atypical," "uncommon," "rare," or "clockwise" flutter). It is associated with underlying cardiac disease such as myocarditis, myocardial infarction, coronary artery disease, or acute ischemia. The underlying atrial rate is approximately 300 bpm (250–350 bpm, although it can be higher), with the ventricular rate dependent on the degree of AV block present. If an AV bypass tract is present, 1:1 conduction occurs for a ventricular rate of about 300 bpm, and conduction through a healthy AV node results in a 2:1 block and ventricular rate of about 150 bpm. A higher degree of block (3:1 or 4:1) may occur with a diseased or fibrotic AV node, resulting in a ventricular rate of 70 to 100 bpm.

Patients may be asymptomatic, or symptoms may resemble those seen with SVT or atrial fibrillation. Physical examination most often reveals a rapid heart rate, and hypotension or CHF may be seen if ventricular filling is low due to the rapid rate. Pulses may be variable and irregular if variable AV block is present. On ECG (Fig. 77.2c), the atrial rate is regular, usually between 250 and 350 bpm, and has a wave-like or sawtooth pattern ("flutter waves") seen best in leads II, III, and aVF. If 1:1 conduction occurs, these waves are hidden by QRS complexes; they may still be difficult to appreciate with a 2:1 block but can be seen more easily with a 3:1 or greater block. If atrial flutter is suspected in the setting of rapid ventricular rates, vagal maneuvers such as carotid sinus massage or an intravenous bolus of adenosine may increase the AV block and reveal the sawtooth pattern.

Atrial flutter is considered an unstable rhythm, and its termination is indicated whenever possible. If the ventricular rate is rapid, the patient is hemodynamically unstable, or underlying disease such as angina or CHF is exacerbated, immediate DC cardioversion under controlled circumstances is indicated. In patients with severe underlying cardiac disease or on potentially arrhythmogenic medications such as digoxin, rapid atrial pacing in a cardiac laboratory setting may be a safer alternative for conversion to sinus rhythm. For more stable patients, reversible underlying conditions or precipitating factors can be corrected before conversion is attempted. Cardioversion is successful in restoring sinus rhythm in more than 95% of cases.[14] Although DC cardioversion and atrial pacing have been considered the preferred treatments, medical cardioversion with ibutilide is emerging as an acceptable alternative.[66] Class IA, IC, or III antiarrhythmics can be effective as pretreatment before DC cardioversion or atrial pacing to increase the likelihood of sustaining sinus rhythm. Beta-blockers, calcium channel blockers, or digoxin may slow a rapid ventricular rate but are not considered effective for conversion to sinus rhythm.

Drug therapy has been shown to be of limited effectiveness in preventing recurrent atrial flutter.[14] In the absence of underlying heart disease, class IC agents flecainide and propafenone may be effective in reducing the number of recurrences, but class IA and IC agents have been associated with serious side effects in patients with underlying heart disease. With improved atrial mapping techniques, RFA of the reentrant circuit has emerged as an effective and potentially curative treatment option; in patients with highly symptomatic atrial flutter unresponsive to other treatments, RFA of the AV junction followed by permanent pacemaker insertion should be considered.[14] The association between stroke and atrial flutter is unclear at present, with conflicting reports regarding risk of stroke after conversion to SR and with drug therapy. Current opinion supports the use of warfarin for cardioversion, but no standard has emerged for long-term anticoagulation.

Other AV Conduction Abnormalities

Conduction disturbances in the AV node–His–Purkinje pathway are a relatively common occurrence, ranging from asymptomatic first-degree AV block to potentially lethal third-degree AV block. A full description of the pathophysiology and electrophysiology of AV block is beyond the scope of this chapter, so a summary of the most common types follows.

First-degree block (Fig. 77.3a) is commonly caused by increased vagal tone or as a drug side effect (digoxin). It is characterized by a prolonged PR interval of more than 0.2 second with an otherwise normal ECG. Unless it is accompanied by significant bradycardia, treatment is not necessary.

There are two varieties of second-degree AV block. Mobitz type I (Wenckebach block) (Fig. 77.3b) is often transient, occurring after cardiac surgery, during an acute MI, or with digoxin toxicity. It is characterized by a constant PP interval, progressive prolongation of the PR interval, and shortening of the RR interval followed by complete block of an atrial impulse and a dropped beat. This rhythm may be perceived on cardiac auscultation as grouped beats followed by a missed beat in a regular pattern. Treatment is generally not necessary. If significant bradycardia and hypoperfusion occur, a cardiac pacemaker may be needed. Mobitz type II block (Fig. 77.3c) is associated with damage to the His–Purkinje system, often due to organic heart disease. Its ECG appearance is as a dropped beat after a normal P wave with otherwise constant PR intervals. It is often associated with intraventricular conduction delays and a slightly wide or atypical QRS complex. This pattern is usually not transient, as it is associated with damage to the conduction system, and is likely to progress to complete heart block. Treatment with a cardiac pacemaker is usually indicated.[67]

Third-degree AV block (complete heart block) (Fig. 77.3d) indicates complete absence of AV conduction. It is usually caused by serious organic heart disease. P waves are present but not conducted, and QRS complexes are usually atypical and widened, reflecting their junctional or ventricular origin. The ventricular rate is most often the idioventricular "escape" frequency of 30 to 40 bpm, but faster heart rates or episodes of asystole can occur. Treatment with a cardiac pacemaker is necessary.

Ventricular Arrhythmias

Most ventricular arrhythmias (VAs) arise from a reentry mechanism involving ventricular myocardium or the portion of the cardiac conduction pathway located below the AV node.[68] Predisposing factors include ischemic or valvular heart disease, structural congenital anomalies, cardiomyopathy, CHF, genetic mutations in ion channel proteins (the cause of congenital long QT syndrome), and autonomic hypersensitivity. Their clinical importance lies in their association with SCD, which accounts for over 350,000 deaths in the U.S. annually.[69] In patients without underlying cardiac disease, the risk of SCD is low and treatment necessary only in special circumstances ["complex" VA such as ventricular tachycardia (VT) or frequent multifocal ventricular premature beats]. However, the risk of SCD in VA is much higher in the presence of underlying cardiac disease, particularly CHF, cardiomyopathy, or in the post-MI setting. The emergence of the ICD as an effective preventive intervention has reduced drug therapy to a secondary and supportive role in treatment of VA. Because most VAs occur outside of the hospital setting, major efforts are now being made to integrate AEDs into out-of-hospital resuscitation protocols.

In general, in the routine office setting family physicians should diagnose this arrhythmia based on ECG, Holter mon-

Figure 3a: First-degree atrioventricular block

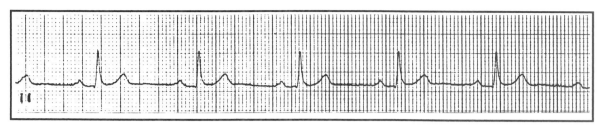

Figure 3b: Second-degree atrioventricular block, Mobitz type I ("Wenckebach"block)

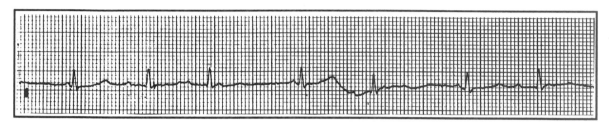

Figure 3c: Second-degree atrioventricular block, Mobitz type II

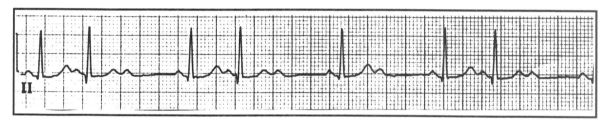

Figure 3d: Third-degree atrioventricular block

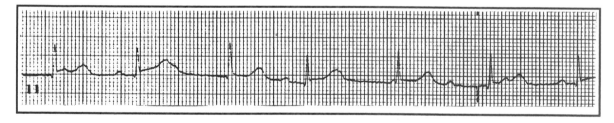

Fig. 77.3. Selected atrioventricular (AV) conduction abnormalities: sample ECG tracings. ECG leads from which tracings were obtained are listed in the lower left corner. Note the progressive prolongation of the PR interval prior to the missed beat in Mobitz type I block (b), the fixed PR interval prior to the missed beat in Mobitz type II block (c), and complete dissociation of atrial and ventricular depolarization in third-degree block (d). See text for discussion of specific ECG features of each arrhythmia.

itoring, or cardiac event monitoring, and search for evidence of underlying cardiac disease or reversible precipitating factors before deciding on therapy. Drug therapy should be initiated with caution and only when clearly indicated.

Ventricular Premature Beats

Ventricular premature beats (VPBs) are the single most common cardiac arrhythmia and perhaps the most overtreated of all cardiac conditions. They are usually the result of reentry in ventricular myocardium or the terminal portion of the Purkinje system; one to several reentry circuits can be present in an individual. They commonly occur in the absence of underlying heart disease and are precipitated by anxiety, emotional stress, exercise, caffeine and other sympathomimetics, electrolyte or acid–base abnormalities, alcohol, and many medications. They also occur in patients with underlying heart disease and in the setting of acute ischemia or MI, acute infection, CHF, chronic ischemia, cardiomyopathy, and some forms of valvular or structural heart disease, including mitral valve prolapse.

The VPBs are most often asymptomatic and are found on routine auscultation or an ECG obtained for other reasons.

Patients with frequent VPBs may report palpitations, dizziness, or weakness. On physical examination, VPBs are noted as an early beat with a following compensatory pause. The ECG (Fig. 77.4a) shows baseline sinus rhythm with the VPB seen as an early QRS, which is wide (>0.12 second), notched, and slurred, and not preceded by a P wave. The T wave is often opposite in direction from the QRS due to aberrant repolarization. A P wave following the QRS or embedded in the

Figure 4a: Ventricular premature beats (premature ventricular complexes)

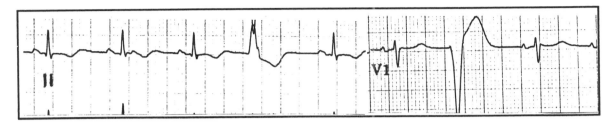

Figure 4b: Nonsustained ventricular tachycardia

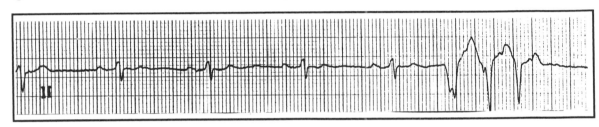

Figure 4c: Sustained ventricular tachycardia

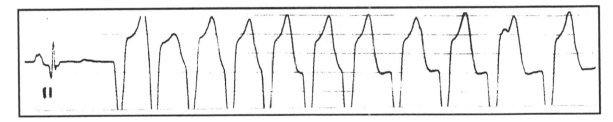

Figure 4d: Ventricular fibrillation

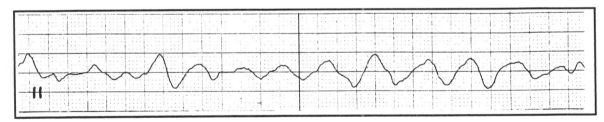

Figure 4e: Torsades de pointes (at initiation)

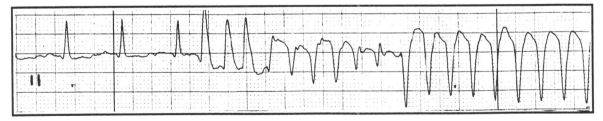

Fig. 77.4. Selected ventricular arrhythmias: sample ECG tracings. ECG leads from which tracings were obtained are listed in the lower left corner. See text for discussion of specific ECG features of each arrhythmia

T wave may be seen, the result of retrograde conduction. The SA node is generally not depolarized by the VPB, creating a "compensatory pause" following the early beat; one sinus beat is suppressed due to a refractory myocardium and conduction system, but the regular SA node pacing is maintained. VPBs can be unifocal or multifocal (the result of more than one reentrant focus), and can occur in patterns such as trigeminy (once every three beats), bigeminy, or couplets (two in a row).

The Lown classification, formerly used to grade the risk of various types of VPB, has largely been replaced by the following treatment "rules." In patients without heart disease, VPBs are not associated with an increased risk of sudden death or other coronary events and generally should not be treated. In the presence of severe symptoms, a careful discussion of risks and benefits of therapy with patients should take place prior to initiating drug therapy. Beta-blockers are the first choice for therapy under most circumstances. The use of class I agents in patients with VPBs has been repeatedly shown to increase the risk of sudden death or coronary events, and these agents should be avoided.[18,19,22] In the post-MI setting, treatment with beta-blockers and angiotensin-converting enzyme inhibitors (ACEIs), preferably in combination, has been shown to have a beneficial effect regarding mortality.[70] Low-dose amiodarone may be helpful in patients who cannot use beta-blockers or ACEIs. Calcium channel blockers are not effective and should not be used. Some experts now recommend that post-MI patients with VPBs undergo EP study so that patients at high risk for SCD (those with inducible VT) can receive an ICD.[71]

Ventricular Tachycardia

Ventricular tachycardia (VT) is defined as the presence of three or more consecutive VPBs; it is further divided into non-sustained VT (NSVT), lasting less than 30 seconds, and sustained, lasting more than 30 seconds. It may be monomorphic (one site of origin) or polymorphic (two or more sites of origin). Monomorphic VT may occur in healthy individuals during exercise, with vagal stimulation, or with excitement or fright, and may be caused by any number of drugs or other substances, notably class I antiarrhythmics, tricyclic antidepressants, and phenothiazines. Polymorphic VT (torsades de pointes being the most familiar example) is associated with congenital long QT syndrome and organophosphate poisoning, and it can be precipitated by electrolyte abnormalities, digoxin, most antiarrhythmic and tricyclic medications, and medication combinations such astemizole and itraconazole. Either type of VT is commonly seen in the setting of acute MI and other serious heart disease.

Nonsustained VT is often asymptomatic but may produce palpitations, weakness, and presyncope; sustained VT is rarely asymptomatic and presents with symptoms ranging from palpitations to sudden death. On auscultation the heart rate may be slightly irregular, with the pulse ranging from 100 to 300 bpm. Other clinical findings vary, as cardiac perfusion changes from beat to beat. With monomorphic VT, the ECG shows a single QRS morphology with the QRS duration more than 0.12 second and the T wave polarity opposite to the QRS polarity. Atrial activity is usually not discernible.

Polymorphic VT (Fig. 77.4b) shows several QRS morphologies. Torsades de pointes (Fig. 77.4e) is characterized by alternation of QRS polarity or amplitude (or both) in repeated cycles of 5 to 20 beats.

Most experts do not recommend treatment for NSVT in the absence of underlying heart disease, as there appears to be no increased risk of SCD. If underlying heart disease is present, a careful search to identify those at high risk for SCD is indicated. Various tests have been studied alone or in combination, including echocardiography, Holter monitoring, enhanced ECG-based methods (QT interval dispersion, T-wave alternans, heart rate variability, and signal-averaged ECG), baroreflex sensitivity, and inducibility of VT on EP study, but no standard protocol has yet emerged. Many experts now recommend that patients with underlying heart disease and NSVT undergo an EP study, with the presence of inducible VT identifying high-risk patients who will benefit from ICD placement.[71] The major role for drug therapy is in treatment of underlying cardiac disease: beta-blockers and ACE inhibitors reduce mortality post-MI and in CHF, but it is not clear whether they reduce the rate of SCD. Although amiodarone has been shown to reduce mortality in patients at high risk for SCD,[72] clinical trials directly comparing ICD placement to amiodarone have confirmed the superior effectiveness of ICDs.[73,74] EP studies paired with RFA offer potentially curative therapy for reentrant NSVT and are currently under study.

Sustained VT (Fig. 77.4c) requires emergent treatment guided by current advanced cardiac life support (ACLS) protocols, followed by transfer to an appropriate facility for definitive care.

Ventricular Fibrillation

Ventricular fibrillation (VF) is a state of chaotic ventricular activity caused by the random firing of multiple ectopic foci, probably due to a complex reentry mechanism.[75] It may result from degeneration of VT and most often occurs in the setting of an acute MI. The arrhythmia results in random, ineffective activity in the ventricles, preventing effective blood circulation. Death occurs within minutes if effective resuscitation is not initiated. The ECG (Fig. 77.4d) shows erratic oscillations without any recognizable complexes; an amplitude of more than 1 mm is termed "coarse" VF and is considered to be more amenable to defibrillation than "fine" VF.

Treatment should begin immediately with cardiopulmonary resuscitation efforts as outlined in Basic Life Support (BLS) and ACLS protocols, including the use of AEDs as soon as possible.[44] Transfer to the hospital for definitive care should occur as soon as possible. Patients who survive VF are candidates for ICD placement.

Conclusion

Although diagnostic and treatment options for patients with cardiac arrhythmias are growing rapidly, successful management still rests on a careful and thorough clinical approach to this problem. Family physicians should be able to (1) correctly diagnose common specific arrhythmias, (2) search for and treat underlying or predisposing conditions, (3) determine whether specific treatment is indicated and initiate therapy where possible, and (4) effectively work with consultants when specialized diagnostic or therapeutic approaches are required.

References

1. Priori SG, Barhanin J, Hauer RN, et al. Genetic and molecular basis of cardiac arrhythmias: impact on clinical management parts I and II. Circulation 1999;99:518–28.
2. Bennett PB, Yazawa K, Makita N, George AL Jr. Molecular mechanism for an inherited cardiac arrhythmia. Nature 1995;376:683–5.
3. Splawski I, Timothy KW, Vincent GM, Atkinson DL, Keating MT. Molecular basis of the long-QT syndrome associated with deafness. N Engl J Med 1997;336:1562–7.
4. Zimetbaum PJ, Josephson ME. The evolving role of ambulatory arrhythmia monitoring in general clinical practice. Ann Intern Med 1999;130:848–56.
5. Graboys T. Appropriate indications for ambulatory electrocardiographic monitoring. Cardiol Clin 1992;10:551–4.
6. Weitz HH, Weinstock PJ. Approach to the patient with palpitations. Med Clin North Am 1995;79:449–56.
7. Thamilarasan M, Klein AL. Transesophageal echocardiography (TEE) in atrial fibrillation. Cardiol Clin 2000;18:819–31.
8. Klein AL, Grimm RA, Murray RD, et al. Use of transesophageal echocardiography to guide cardioversion in patients with atrial fibrillation. N Engl J Med 2001;344:1411–20.
9. Grimm RA. Transesophageal echocardiography-guided cardioversion of atrial fibrillation. Echocardiography 2000;17:383–92.
10. Morady F. Radio-frequency ablation as treatment for cardiac arrhythmias. N Engl J Med 1999;340:534–44.
11. Jais P, Shah DC, Haissaguerre M, Hocini M, Peng JT, Clementy J. Catheter ablation for atrial fibrillation. Annu Rev Med 2000; 51:431–41.
12. Grubb NR, Furniss S. Science, medicine, and the future: radiofrequency ablation for atrial fibrillation. BMJ 2001;322:777–80.
13. Chauhan VS, Krahn AD, Klein GJ, Skanes AC, Yee R. Supraventricular tachycardia. Med Clin North Am 2001;85:193–223.
14. Waldo AL, Mackall JA, Biblo LA. Mechanisms and medical management of patients with atrial flutter. Cardiol Clin 1997; 15:661–76.
15. Vaughan—Williams EM. A classification of antiarrhythmic actions reassessed after a decade of new drugs. J Clin Pharmacol 1984;24:129–47.
16. Morganroth J, Goin JE. Quinidine-related mortality in the short-to-medium-term treatment of ventricular arrhythmias. A meta-analysis. Circulation 1991;84:1977–83.
17. Echt DS, Liebson PR, Mitchell LB, et al. Mortality and morbidity in patients receiving encainide, flecainide, or placebo. The Cardiac Arrhythmia Suppression Trial. N Engl J Med 1991;324: 781–8.
18. Epstein AE, Bigger JT Jr, Wyse DG, Romhilt DW, Reynolds-Haertle RA, Hallstrom AP. Events in the Cardiac Arrhythmia Suppression Trial (CAST): mortality in the entire population enrolled. J Am Coll Cardiol 1991;18:14–9.
19. Chaudhry GM, Haffajee CI. Antiarrhythmic agents and proarrhythmia. Crit Care Med 2000;28:N158–64.
20. Boriani G, Biffi M, Capucci A, et al. Oral propafenone to convert recent-onset atrial fibrillation in patients with and without underlying heart disease. A randomized, controlled trial. Ann Intern Med 1997;126:621–5.
21. Chimienti M, Cullen MT, Casadei G. Flecainide and Propa-

22. fenone Italian Study Group. Safety of long-term flecainide and propafenone in the management of symptomatic paroxysmal atrial fibrillation. Am J Cardiol 1996;77:66A–71A.
22. Teo KK, Yusuf S, Furberg CD. Effects of prophylactic antiarrhythmic drug therapy in acute myocardial infarction. An overview of results from randomized controlled trials. JAMA 1993; 270:1589–95.
23. Sim I, McDonald KM, Lavori PW, Norbutas CM, Hlatky MA. Quantitative overview of randomized trials of amiodarone to prevent sudden cardiac death. Circulation 1997;96:2823–9.
24. Peuhkurinen K, Niemela M, Ylitalo A, Linnaluoto M, Lilja M, Juvonen J. Effectiveness of amiodarone as a single oral dose for recent-onset atrial fibrillation. Am J Cardiol 2000;85:462–5.
25. Mason JW. A comparison of seven antiarrhythmic drugs in patients with ventricular tachyarrhythmias. Electrophysiologic Study versus Electrocardiographic Monitoring Investigators. N Engl J Med 1993;329:452–8.
26. Miller MR, McNamara RL, Segal JB, et al. Efficacy of agents for pharmacologic conversion of atrial fibrillation and subsequent maintenance of sinus rhythm: a meta-analysis of clinical trials. J Fam Pract 2000;49:1033–46.
27. Falk RH, Pollak A, Singh SN, et al. Intravenous dofetilide: a class III antiarrhythmic agent, for the termination of sustained atrial fibrillation or flutter. J Am Coll Cardiol 1997;340:385–90.
28. Vukmir RB. Cardiac arrhythmia therapy. Am J Emerg Med 1995;13:459–70.
29. Kerin NZ, Somberg J. Proarrhythmia: definition, risk factors, causes, treatment, and controversies. Am Heart J 1994;128:575–85.
30. Naccarelli GV, Wolbrette DL, Luck JC. Proarrhythmia. Med Clin North Am 2001;85:503–26.
31. Faber TS, Zehender M, Just H. Drug-induced torsade de pointes: incidence, management and prevention. Drug Safety 1994;11: 463–76.
32. Trohman RG, Parrillo JE. Direct current cardioversion: indications, techniques, and recent advances. Crit Care Med 2000;28: N170–3.
33. Cox JL, Ferguson TB. Cardiac arrhythmia surgery. Curr Probl Surg 1989;26:193–278.
34. Schaff HV, Dearani JA, Daly RC, Orszulak TA, Danielson GK. Cox-Maze procedure for atrial fibrillation: the Mayo Clinic experience. Semin Thorac Cardiovasc Surg 2000;12:30–7.
35. Hogenhuis W, Stevens SK, Wang P, et al. Cost-effectiveness of radio-frequency ablation compared with other strategies in Wolff-Parkinson-White syndrome. Circulation 1993;88(5 pt 2): II:437–46.
36. Kalbfleisch SJ, Calkins H, Langberg JJ, et al. Comparison of the cost of radiofrequency catheter modification of the atrioventricular node and medical therapy for drug-refractory atrioventricular node reentrant tachycardia. J Am Coll Cardiol 1992;19:1583–7.
37. Fitzpatrick AP, Kourouyan HD, Siu A, et al. Quality of life and outcomes after radiofrequency His-bundle catheter ablation and permanent pacemaker implantation: impact of treatment in paroxysmal and established atrial fibrillation. Am Heart J 1996; 131:499–507.
38. Gregoratos G, Cheitlin MD, Conill A, et al. ACC/AHA guidelines for implantation of cardiac pacemakers and antiarrhythmia devices: a report of the American College of Cardiology/American Heart Association Task Force on Practice Guidelines (Committee on Pacemaker Implantation). J Am Coll Cardiol 1998;31: 1175–209.
39. The Antiarrhythmics versus Implantable Defibrillators (AVID) Investigators. A comparison of antiarrhythmic-drug therapy with implantable defibrillators in patients resuscitated from near-fatal ventricular arrhythmias. N Engl J Med 1997;337:1576–83.
40. Connolly SJ, Gent M, Roberts RS, et al. Canadian implantable

defibrillator study (CIDS): a randomized trial of the implantable cardioverter defibrillator against amiodarone. Circulation 2000; 101:1297–302.

41. Buxton AE, Lee KL, Fisher JD, Josephson ME, Prystowsky EN, Hafley G. A randomized study of the prevention of sudden death in patients with coronary artery disease. Multicenter Unsustained Tachycardia Trial Investigators. N Engl J Med 1999;341: 1882–90.

42. Gollob MH, Seger JJ. Current status of the implantable cardioverter-defibrillator. Chest 2001;119:1210–21.

43. O'Brien BJ, Yee R. Chapter 10: Current evidence on the cost effectiveness of the implantable cardioverter defibrillator. Can J Cardiol 2000;16(suppl C):45C–7C.

44. Atkins DL, Bossaert LL, Hazinski MF, et al. Automated external defibrillation /public access defibrillation. Ann Emerg Med 2001;37:S60–S67.

45. White RD, Hankins DG, Bugliosi TF, et al. Seven years' experience with early defibrillation by police and paramedics in an emergency medical services system. Resuscitation 1998;39: 145–51.

46. Stiell IG, Wells GA, Field BJ, et al. Improved out-of-hospital cardiac arrest survival through the inexpensive optimization of an existing defibrillation program: OPALS Study Phase II. JAMA 1999;281:1175–81.

47. Schwartz M, Rodman D, Lowenstein SR. Recognition and treatment of multifocal atrial tachycardia: a critical review. J Emerg Med 1994;12:353–60.

48. Camm AJ, Garratt AJ. Adenosine and supraventricular tachycardia. N Engl J Med 1991;32:1621–7.

49. Go AS, Hylek EM, Phillips KA, et al. Prevalence of diagnosed atrial fibrillation in adults: national implications for rhythm management and stroke prevention: the Anticoagulation and Risk Factors in Atrial Fibrillation (ATRIA) Study. JAMA 2001;285: 2370–5.

50. Falk RH. Atrial fibrillation. N Engl J Med 2001;344:1067–78.

51. Nattel S, Li D, Yue L. Basic mechanisms of atrial fibrillation— very new insights into very old ideas. Annu Rev Physiol 2000; 62:51–77.

52. Danias PG, Caulfield TA, Weigner MJ, Silverman DI, Manning WJ. Likelihood of spontaneous conversion of atrial fibrillation to sinus rhythm. J Am Coll Cardiol 1998;31:588–92.

53. Carlsson J, Neuzner J, Rosenberg YD. Therapy of atrial fibrillation: rhythm control versus rate control. Pacing Clin Electrophysiol 2000;23:891–903.

54. Dries DL, Exner DV, Gersh BJ, Domanski MJ, Waclawiw MA, Stevenson LW. Atrial fibrillation is associated with an increased risk for mortality and heart failure progression in patients with asymptomatic and symptomatic left ventricular systolic dysfunction: a retrospective analysis of the SOLVD trials. J Am Coll Cardiol 1998;32:695–703.

55. Roy D, Talajic M, Dorian P, et al. Amiodarone to prevent recurrence of atrial fibrillation: Canadian Trial of Atrial Fibrillation Investigators. N Engl J Med 2000;342:913–20.

56. Carlson MD. How to manage atrial fibrillation: an update on recent clinical trials. Cardiol Rev 2001;9:60–9.

57. Haissaguerre M, Jais P, Shah DC, et al. Electrophysiological end point for catheter ablation of atrial fibrillation initiated from multiple pulmonary venous foci. Circulation 2000;101:1409–17.

58. Wolf PA, Abbott R, Savage D. Atrial fibrillation as an independent risk factor for stroke: the Framingham Study. Stroke 1991;22:983–8.

59. Petersen P, Boysen G, Godtfredson J, Andersen E, Andersen B. Placebo-controlled, randomized trial of warfarin and aspirin for prevention of thromboembolic complications in chronic atrial fibrillation: the Copenhagen AFASAK study. Lancet 1989;1:175–9.

60. Connolly SJ, Laupacis A, Gent M, Roberts RS, Cairns JA, Joyner C. Canadian Atrial Fibrillation Anticoagulation (CAFA) study. J Am Coll Cardiol 1991;18:349–55.

61. Ezekowitz MD, Bridges SL, James KE, et al. Warfarin in the prevention of stroke associated with nonrheumatic atrial fibrillation. Veterans Affairs Stroke Prevention in Nonrheumatic Atrial Fibrillation Investigators. N Engl J Med 1992;327:1406–12.

62. Boston Area Anticoagualation Trial for Atrial Fibrillation Investigators. The effect of low-dose warfarin on the risk of stroke in patients with nonrheumatic atrial fibrillation. N Engl J Med 1990;323:1505–11.

63. Blackshear JL, Baker VS, Rubino F, et al. Adjusted-dose warfarin versus low-intensity, fixed-dose warfarin plus aspirin for high-risk patients with atrial fibrillation: Stroke Prevention in Atrial Fibrillation III randomized clinical trial. Lancet 1996;348:633–8.

64. Atrial Fibrillation Investigators. Risk factors for stroke and efficacy of antithrombotic therapy in atrial fibrillation: analysis of pooled data from five randomized controlled trials. Arch Intern Med 1994;154:1449–57.

65. Segal JB, McNamara RL, Miller MR, et al. Anticoagulants or antiplatelet therapy for non-rheumatic atrial fibrillation and flutter (Cochrane Review). In: The Cochrane Library, issue 1. Oxford: Update Software, 2001.

66. Stambler BS, Wood MA, Ellenbogen KA, Perry KT, Wakefield LK, VanderLugt JT. Efficacy and safety of repeated intravenous doses of ibutilide for rapid conversion of atrial flutter or fibrillation. Ibutilide Repeat Dose Study Investigators. Circulation 1996;94:1613–21.

67. Barold SS, Hayes DL. Second-degree atrioventricular block: a reappraisal. Mayo Clin Proc 2001;76:44–57.

68. Alpert MA, Mukerji V, Bikkina M, Concannon MD, Hashimi MW. Pathogenesis, recognition, and management of common cardiac arrhythmias. Part I: ventricular premature beats and tachyarrhythmias. South Med J 1995;88:1–21.

69. Myerburg RJ, Kessler KM, Castellanos A. Sudden cardiac death. Structure, function, and time-dependence of risk. Circulation 1992;85:I2–10.

70. Burkart F, Pfisterer M, Kiowski W, Follath F, Burckhardt D. Effect of antiarrhythmic therapy on mortality in survivors of myocardial infarction with asymptomatic complex ventricular arrhythmias: Basel Antiarrhythmic Study of Infarct Survival (BASIS). J Am Coll Cardiol 1990;16:1711–8.

71. Windhagen-Mahnert B, Kadish AH. Application of noninvasive and invasive tests for risk assessment in patients with ventricular arrhythmias. Cardiol Clin 2000;18:243–63.

72. Investigators of Amiodarone Trial Meta-Analyses. Effect of prophylactic amiodarone on mortality after acute myocardial infarction and in congestive heart failure: meta-analysis of individual data from 6500 patients from randomized trials. Lancet 1997;350:1417–24.

73. Moss AJ, Hall WJ, Cannon DS, et al. Improved survival with an implanted defibrillator in patients with coronary disease at high risk for ventricular arrhythmia. Multicenter Automatic Defibrillator Implantation Trial Investigators. N Engl J Med 1996; 335:1933–40.

74. Zipes DP, Wyse DG, Friedman PL, et al. A comparison of antiarrhythmic drug therapy with implanatable defibrillators in patients resuscitated from near-fatal ventricular arrhythmias. N Engl J Med 1997;337:1576–83.

75. Jalife J. Ventricular fibrillation: mechanisms of initiation and maintenance. Annu Rev Physiol 2000;62:25–50.

78
Valvular Heart Disease

Eric Walsh

Introduction

Timely and appropriate diagnosis and treatment of valvular heart disease is an important skill for family physicians. Excessive consultation and diagnostic testing of patients who present with murmurs creates unnecessary anxiety and cost. Yet the failure to make a timely diagnosis of valvular heart disease, or to refer when appropriate, can lead to irreversible cardiac damage, decreased functional status, and even death. In making the diagnosis of valvular heart disease, it is important to know the clinical maneuvers that can help refine the bedside diagnosis of murmurs. It is useful to know when third and fourth heart sounds (S_3 and S_4) are abnormal, and how to distinguish innocent and physiologic murmurs from murmurs caused by valvular heart disease.

Third Heart Sound

An S_3 is considered normal in patients under 30 who have no other signs of heart disease. An S_3 heard in patients between ages 30 and 40 is suspicious. In this age group, conditions such as thyrotoxicosis, pregnancy, anxiety, and postexercise states can cause an S_3 not associated with heart disease.

An S_3 heard past age 40 should be considered a likely sign of heart disease. It can be caused by three types of cardiac disease: ventricular diastolic overload, ventricular dysfunction, and constrictive pericarditis. Ventricular diastolic overload is most commonly caused by mitral regurgitation or aortic insufficiency. The S_3 heard with these states of ventricular diastolic overload is almost invariably associated with a murmur. An S_3 not associated with a ventricular diastolic overload state suggests global ventricular dysfunction. Diastolic overload over long periods of time can lead to ventricular dysfunction, which is the most serious and irreversible cause of the S_3. Other nonvalvular problems, such as chronic ischemia can also lead to global dysfunction and an S_3. Pericardial dis-

ease can cause an S_3. In the case of pericardial disease, it is the sudden deceleration of ventricular relaxation and filling caused by the pericardial pathology that creates the S_3.

Fourth Heart Sound

There is debate about whether an S_4 can be considered normal in the geriatric population, where there is some physiologic loss of ventricular compliance; but as a general rule, an audible S_4 should be considered pathologic. In contrast to an S_3, which gets louder as ventricular compliance decreases, the S_4 becomes softer as the underlying ventricular dysfunction progresses. The underlying cardiac pathology leading to the production of an S_4 is similar to the factors causing an S_3, with two important additions: whereas an S_3 is not heard with hypertrophic cardiomyopathy or left ventricular hypertrophy (LVH) caused by hypertension, an S_4 is common with these conditions.

Innocent and Physiologic Murmurs

Between 90% and 95% of murmurs identified by family physicians are innocent or physiologic murmurs. Innocent murmurs are those present in patients with no cardiac pathology. Murmurs are physiologic when there is an identifiable cause but the heart is normal. Examples of physiologic murmurs include the murmurs heard with anemia, thyrotoxicosis, the increased blood volume of normal pregnancy, and the high output state caused by fever.

Characteristics

Murmurs can be appreciated in 50% to 60% of healthy children, depending on the listening conditions and the cooperation of the child.[1] Soft murmurs can be heard in 30% to 40%

of healthy adults.[1] Innocent murmurs are usually best heard along the left sternal border, between the second and the fourth intercostal spaces. Innocent murmurs are always systolic and are rarely louder than grade 2/6. In young patients innocent murmurs are evanescent and usually do not radiate to the carotid area. In older patients it can be more difficult to distinguish pathologic from innocent murmurs. The decreased compliance of the large arteries associated with aging can cause an innocent murmur to be heard in the neck. There are several associated findings that make the diagnosis of an innocent or physiologic murmur less likely. These findings include the presence of more than one sound at S_1, abnormal splitting of S_2, a loud or soft S_1, or a hyperdynamic or sustained ventricular impulse.

Physical Maneuvers

There are a number of simple bedside maneuvers useful for diagnosing an innocent versus a pathologic murmur. These maneuvers increase or decrease preload and increase afterload. The presence of extrasystolic beats, which change the hemodynamics, can affect the quality of murmurs in ways that aid the diagnosis.

Increased Afterload

The best method to increase afterload is the handgrip maneuver. The physician instructs the patient to squeeze the examiner's hand as hard as possible, and the physician returns the pressure. The handgrip should decrease outflow murmurs, including innocent murmurs, physiologic murmurs, and pathologic aortic outflow murmurs.

Decreased Preload

Decreased preload is created by the Valsalva maneuver or by sudden sitting or standing. Both of these mechanisms cause decreased venous return to the heart. Decreased preload diminishes murmurs that are increased by blood volume, including innocent murmurs, physiologic murmurs, outflow murmurs, and mitral and tricuspid regurgitation. The murmurs of mitral valve prolapse and hypertrophic cardiomyopathy should become louder with a decreased preload.

Increased Preload

Two simple maneuvers can increase preload. The first is lifting the patient's legs while the patient is in the supine position. The second is asking the patient to squat. Increased preload should dilate, to some extent, the left ventricle and thereby decrease the murmurs caused by mitral valve prolapse and hypertrophic cardiomyopathy. The effect of increased preload on other murmurs is variable, but most outflow murmurs become louder with this maneuver.

Ectopic Beats

A premature ventricular beat creates a diagnostic opportunity. If the murmur is an aortic stenosis murmur, it becomes louder after an extrasystolic beat because of the increased pressure gradient across the stenotic valve. The prolonged diastole does not affect most flow murmurs or the murmur caused by mitral regurgitation.

Valvular Heart Disease

Incidence

An important clinical issue is the incidence in the general population of heart murmurs caused by heart disease. If a heart murmur is heard, what is the likelihood that it is caused by heart disease? The incidence of valvular heart disease in the general population is difficult to determine. Murmurs and the pathology that causes them can resolve spontaneously. The loud childhood murmur of a ventricular septal defect can disappear when the defect closes spontaneously. Murmurs can disappear as the pathology worsens; for example, a mitral regurgitant murmur can disappear as the left atrial pressure rises and left ventricular failure occurs. Murmurs that are not pathologic can become so later in life. A bicuspid aortic valve can produce a murmur without a significant gradient early in life, but as valvular calcification develops, significant aortic stenosis can appear. Lastly, the incidence of valvular heart disease depends on the methods by which it is sought: the findings on clinical examination, echocardiography, and autopsy differ.

Good raw data regarding the incidence of valvular heart disease in the general (male) population were obtained in World War I, during which time 2.5 million young men from their late teens to about 30 years old were examined by army doctors.[2] A total of 85,143 men (3.4%) were classified on clinical grounds as having valvular heart disease; 73.4% were diagnosed as having mitral regurgitation, and the remaining 26.6% were about evenly distributed between mitral stenosis, aortic stenosis, and aortic regurgitation, with a small number having right-sided valvular heart disease and nonvalvular heart murmurs such as patent ductus arteriosus (PDA) or ventricular septal defect (VSD). Since World War I the incidence of rheumatic heart disease has declined, making mitral stenosis, which is almost solely caused by rheumatic disease, much rarer.

The use of echocardiography and autopsy increases estimates of the frequency of valvular heart disease. A survey of 18,132 autopsies showed that 6.3% of patients at autopsy had valvular heart disease, 49% involving the mitral valve, 42% the aortic valve, 9% the tricuspid valve, and 0.3% the pulmonic valve.[3] A study of patients over 65 years old found that aortic stenosis was present in 2% overall, with a twofold increase in incidence for each 10 years of life.[4] In 1999, the Framingham Heart Study reported a series of 3,589 color Doppler echocardiograms done on participants between 26 and 83 years old in that ongoing study. The study reported on valvular incompetence, but not valve stenosis.

Using this sophisticated technology, the incidence of valvular incompetence was much higher than previously reported: mitral regurgitation was found in 19.1%, and aortic regurgitation in 10.8%. But when "trivial" and "mild" valvular incompetence are excluded from the analysis, the incidence of "moderate" or "severe" valvular incompetence is reported as 1.9% for the mitral valve, and 0.69% for the aortic valve.[5] Interestingly, a decreased body mass index (BMI) was associated with an increased risk for mitral but not aortic incompetence. A report from the Strong Heart Study, which evaluated echocardiographic data from 3,486 Native Americans, found mitral regurgitation in 21.0% of participants, although regurgitation was moderately severe in only 0.3% and severe in only 0.2%.[6] This study also confirmed the association of lower BMI, as well as female gender, older age, and higher blood pressure with mitral regurgitation.[6]

More recently, the use of anorectic drugs for weight loss, specifically dexfenfluramine, has been associated with an increased risk of the development of valvular regurgitation, most commonly mitral, but also tricuspid and aortic regurgitation (odds ratio 3.1; 95% confidence interval 1.34–7.13).[7] There is reassuring evidence that clinical auscultation is an adequate method of screening for valvular lesions associated with dexfenfluramine, and that discontinuing the drug probably halts progression of the valvular lesions.[7,8]

Mitral Valve Regurgitation

Etiology

There are a large number of causes of mitral regurgitation. Degenerative lesions include the myxomatous change of mitral valve prolapse and the congenital abnormalities of Marfan syndrome, Ehlers-Danlos syndrome, and others. Degenerative changes also include mitral annulus calcification. Inflammatory and infective causes of mitral regurgitation include endocarditis, rheumatic fever, lupus, and scleroderma (see Chapters 82 and 113). Ischemia is one of the most important causes of mitral regurgitation. Mitral regurgitation in the setting of ischemia is due to dysfunction of the papillary muscles and/or remodeling of the ventricle. There is a statistically significant association of mitral regurgitation with increasing age, hypertension, and a lower BMI.[5]

Symptoms

Mitral regurgitation may progress for decades without causing symptoms. Symptoms usually occur insidiously. The first symptom is usually fatigue because of decreased cardiac output. Later dyspnea, orthopnea, and paroxysmal nocturnal dyspnea occur as the left atrial pressure and pulmonary vascular pressure rise. The causes of rapid progression of symptoms with mitral regurgitation include the onset of atrial fibrillation and severe papillary muscle dysfunction or rupture.

Physical Findings

The pulse associated with mitral regurgitation is collapsing in nature. The apical impulse is hyperkinetic and becomes laterally displaced and more diffuse as the disease progresses. The heart sounds are unremarkable. It is unusual to hear an S_4, and the presence of an S_3 indicates advanced disease. The murmur of mitral regurgitation is a holosystolic murmur. It is described as plateau in intensity and blowing in quality. Throughout most of the natural history of mitral regurgitation, the murmur starts at S_1 and ends at S_2. As left atrial pressure and pulmonary pressure rise, the murmur may end before S_2. The murmur of mitral regurgitation becomes softer during the late stages of the disease.

Increasing afterload should increase the intensity of the murmur. Decreasing preload should make the murmur softer, and increasing preload usually makes little or no difference

in the murmur. When there is a premature beat and a compensatory pause, the murmur of mitral regurgitation does not change appreciably in the postextrasystolic beat.

Natural History, Complications, Medical Therapy, and Timing of Surgery

As Stapleton[2] suggested, "mitral incompetence is the most benign of left heart valvular lesions. . . . Patients may do well on medical therapy for years after the onset of symptoms." Medical therapy consists of afterload reduction with angiotensin-converting enzyme (ACE) inhibiting agents. As left ventricular function declines, digoxin and diuretics may be added. Atrial fibrillation is a late occurrence and requires rate control. Atrial fibrillation usually denotes marked atrial enlargement, and electrical cardioversion is rarely successful on a long-term basis. The timing of surgery is more controversial for mitral regurgitation than for other valvular heart disease because of the relatively slow course of progression in most cases. Clear indications for valve replacement include left ventricular (LV) failure caused by mitral regurgitation, hemodynamic decompensation with decreased cardiac output (even with normal ejection fraction) at rest or with exercise, and rapid (more than 2 cm per year as measured by echocardiography or chest radiography) increase in ventricular size.[9] More recently, criteria for early replacement of the mitral valve in patients selected as high risk based on low LV ejection fraction (>45%) or low right ventricular (RV) ejection fraction (>30%) have been proposed.[10] Mitral regurgitation that is secondary to ischemia carries a worse prognosis, and mitral valve replacement should be considered earlier than in nonischemic mitral regurgitation. Decisions about valve replacement at the time of coronary artery bypass graft (CABG) surgery should be made on grounds of the severity of heart failure symptoms and LV function, and the clinical severity of regurgitation. Often this is best assessed by intraoperative transesophageal echocardiography (TEE).[11] Mitral regurgitation as a result of myocardial infarction (MI) worsens prognosis independently of other variables, including age and ventricular function. Patients with mitral regurgitation secondary to an MI had a 5-year total mortality of 62% ± 5% vs. total mortality in the control group with MI but no mitral regurgitation of 39% ± 6%. The 5-year cardiac mortality in the group with post-MI mitral regurgitation was 50% ± 6% vs. 30% ± 5% mortality in the control group (both $p < .001$).[11]

Mitral Valve Prolapse

Mitral valve prolapse warrants special mention for a number of reasons. While mitral valve prolapse was previously thought to be common, recent evidence indicates a prevalence of about 2%.[12] There are several unique aspects to the history and physical examination in patients with mitral valve prolapse, and treatment modalities differ in some ways from other causes of mitral regurgitation. In addition, some clinicians have postulated the existence of a mitral valve prolapse syndrome,[13] which involves diffuse autonomic and connective tissue pathology.

Mitral valve prolapse is caused by a combination of factors. There is an abnormality of the connective tissue in the mitral valve, which leads to myxomatous degeneration of the valve and the chordae. Excessive or redundant mitral valve tissue is present and there is often an increased orifice size. Lastly, the length, position, or physiologic function of the papillary muscle and chordae apparatus is abnormal.

Symptoms and Physical Findings

The symptoms of mitral valve prolapse that relate to mitral regurgitation are the same as those seen with other causes of mitral regurgitation. Until recently, it had been reported that palpitations, caused by ventricular ectopy or exaggerated awareness of the heartbeat, and atypical chest pain were more common in patients with mitral valve prolapse. A recent study of mitral valve prolapse, using the Framingham database, has called that association into question.[12]

The mitral valve prolapse syndrome has been defined as mitral valve prolapse associated with increased autonomic tone. Studies have shown increased catecholamine levels and changes in diurnal variation of catecholamine levels in some patients with mitral valve prolapse. In addition, these patients have abnormalities of β-adrenergic receptors and evidence of decreased intravascular volume.[2] Patients with this syndrome may complain of anxiety and show signs of increased adrenergic tone, such as unexplained elevations of the resting pulse. On physical examination S_1 and S_2 are normal, and S_3 and S_4 are usually not present.

Mitral valve prolapse is different from other causes of mitral regurgitation because of the presence of a high-pitched mid-systolic click and the fact that the murmur is not holosystolic. The murmur is mid- to late systolic, follows the click, and often ends before S_2. The findings in mitral valve prolapse are inconstant. There may be no click or murmur one day, but the next day these findings are obvious. An increase in afterload or preload makes the click and murmur occur later, and a decrease in preload makes the click earlier and the murmur louder. The click and murmur of mitral valve prolapse should occur later and may be softer during the beat following the compensatory pause after a premature beat.

Controversies, Complications, Treatment, and Natural History

It is reasonable to wonder when mitral valve prolapse is a disease and when it is a normal variant. Population based studies[12] indicate a low incidence and a benign prognosis. Studies of patients who present with end stage mitral valve regurgitation demonstrate a subgroup of patients with mitral valve prolapse who have serious progressive disease.[14,15] How much workup should be done if an isolated click is heard? What about a click with a murmur? Answering these questions is difficult, particularly when one notes that auscultation may be normal one day and a loud regurgitant murmur may be present the next. The best evidence suggests that the pathology of mitral valve prolapse relates to the degree of mitral regurgitation.[14–16] Risk factors associated with serious mitral valve prolapse requiring valve replacement include increasing age, male sex, increased BMI, and hypertension.

When the severity of mitral valve regurgitation is defined, the medical treatment is the same as for other causes of mitral regurgitation. The adrenergic symptoms, atypical chest pain, and palpitations associated with mitral valve prolapse often respond to beta-blockers.

Mitral Stenosis

Etiology

Mitral stenosis has a single cause: rheumatic heart disease. Although only 50% of patients with mitral stenosis can recall an episode of rheumatic fever, the surgical pathology of stenotic mitral valves virtually always reveals the changes associated with rheumatic heart disease. Congenital mitral stenosis is exceedingly rare.[16] Symptoms can occur as early as 3 years after the episode of rheumatic fever, but most commonly 15 to 25 years elapse between the episode of rheumatic fever and the detection of mitral stenosis. As would be expected, findings and symptoms typically begin during the third to fifth decade of life. The incidence of mitral stenosis has been declining for the last 50 years along with the decline in rheumatic fever.

Symptoms

Symptoms associated with mitral stenosis are directly related to the mitral valve area.[16] With a valve area of more than 2.5 cm^2, assuming a sinus rhythm, no symptoms are present. With a valve area of 1.4 to 2.5 cm^2, there is minimal dyspnea with exertion. With a valve area of 1.0 to 1.3 cm^2, dyspnea on exertion is severe, and orthopnea and paroxysmal nocturnal dyspnea can occur. At valve areas of less than 1 cm^2, resting dyspnea, severe pulmonary edema, and disability occur. The onset of atrial fibrillation, common with advanced mitral stenosis, causes a sudden worsening of symptoms, often frank congestive heart failure (CHF). Pregnancy, infection, and surgery can also cause CHF. Other symptoms associated with mitral stenosis include hemoptysis, which may be the presenting symptom, and frequent bronchitis and wheezing, caused by hyperemia of the bronchi due to increased pulmonary vascular pressure.

Physical Findings and Diagnosis

There are many characteristic physical findings with mitral stenosis, but they are subtle and often overlooked. Ventricular underfilling can cause the carotid pulses to be brisk and brief. The cardiac apex is in the normal location, and the point of maximal impulse (PMI) is small and nonsustained. In fact, the presence of a sustained PMI rules out isolated mitral stenosis. Fine pulmonary crackles may be present, but signs of right heart failure or peripheral edema are typically a sign of end-stage disease.

S_1 is loud with mitral stenosis; in fact, an accentuated S_1, particularly in the setting of atrial fibrillation, should alert the clinician to the possibility of mitral stenosis. As the disease progresses and mitral mobility decreases, S_1 may become softer, but by that time symptoms are usually advanced, and the diagnosis should be obvious. S_2 is either normal or has a loud P2, which can be heard at the apex. S_3 and S_4 are rare because of normal ventricular size, compliance, and slowed diastolic filling.

One of the characteristic heart sounds of mitral stenosis is the opening snap, which occurs after S_2, and is sharper and higher pitched than an S_3. Patients with mitral stenosis usually have a diastolic murmur that is soft, low-pitched (a rumble), and occurs during mid- to late diastole. If the rhythm is sinus, there is presystolic accentuation of the murmur with atrial contraction. Maneuvers that increase or decrease afterload or preload have little effect on the murmur of mitral stenosis.

Natural History, Complications, Medical Therapy, and Timing of Surgery

Mitral stenosis has a more rapid progression and a higher case-fatality rate than mitral regurgitation. Among patients with mild symptoms, 58% are dead in 10 years without surgery; and 85% of patients with mild to moderate symptoms are dead in 10 years without surgery.[16] Rare cases of mitral stenosis remain clinically stable for years, but progression is the rule.

Medical therapy for mitral stenosis is aimed at reducing complications and does not affect the progression of the disease. Diuretics are used to treat pulmonary edema, but digoxin or afterload reduction do not work for this problem. Rate control for atrial fibrillation is essential, and ventricular rates of 50 to 60 beats per minute (bpm) should be the goal of treatment. Digoxin or beta-blockers can be used for rate control. With the onset of atrial fibrillation, electrical cardioversion is attempted and anticoagulation considered, especially if atrial fibrillation persists or recurs.

The assessment of thrombotic risk is an important issue in the diagnosis and treatment of mitral stenosis. Studies have suggested that thrombotic risk is increased with mitral stenosis even with sinus rhythm[17] and with selected echocardiographic findings in atrial fibrillation.[18] Coronary artery disease is rare in the setting of mitral stenosis.

When mitral stenosis is diagnosed, even if symptoms are not present, a workup is initiated to determine left atrial size, valve area, and the atrio-ventricular (AV) pressure gradient. Usually, an echocardiogram is sufficient for this purpose. When moderate symptoms are present or with symptoms such as paroxysmal nocturnal dyspnea or hemoptysis, which suggest significantly elevated pressures, the patient should be referred for surgery. Mitral valve commissurotomy is preferred to mitral valve replacement if possible, although the final decision usually cannot be made until the time of surgery.[18]

Aortic Insufficiency

Etiology

There are multiple etiologies for aortic insufficiency. In an age of a declining incidence of syphilis and rheumatic heart disease, the most common cause is a structural abnormality of the aorta, such as an abnormal valve or aneurysm. In addition to syphilis and rheumatic fever, aortic insufficiency can be caused by subacute bacterial endocarditis, rheumatoid arthritis, ankylosing spondylitis, Reiter's disease, and lupus erythematosus (see Chapters 82 and 113). Congenital connective tissue diseases such as Marfan and Ehlers-Danlos syndromes can cause aortic insufficiency, as can severe hypertension.

Symptoms

Patients with aortic insufficiency remain asymptomatic for decades. Early on, patients may complain of palpitations or awareness of heartbeat and mild orthostatic light-headedness. When more severe symptoms occur, they typically begin with fatigue, followed by dyspnea and orthopnea. Later, patients experience angina due to decreased coronary artery flow secondary to the low diastolic pressure in the aorta.

Physical Findings

Patients with aortic insufficiency are often described as flushed and sweaty. Their skin is warm, and until the late stages of the disease they look healthy. Blood pressure can be normal in aortic insufficiency. With severe regurgitation, there is a wide pulse pressure, and the width of the pulse pressure correlates with the severity of the disease until the left ventricle starts to fail. The fourth Korotkoff sound, muffling, is a more valid indicator of diastolic pressure than the fifth sound, which can sometimes be heard down to 0 mm Hg. The peripheral pulses are bounding and collapsing in nature. The first heart sound is soft with aortic insufficiency. Although S_2 is normal, the aortic component may be lost, so S_2 can sound single. Because of elevated diastolic pressure before the atrial contraction, S_4 is rare until the ventricle is markedly dilated and failing, but an S_3 is common.

The murmur of aortic insufficiency is a high-pitched, soft, blowing diastolic murmur heard best with the diaphragm. It is most audible along the left sternal border with the patient leaning forward and holding expiration. The murmur is sometimes heard at the apex, where it is a lower-pitched rumble (the Austin–Flint murmur) that can be confused with the murmur of mitral stenosis. Because of the greatly elevated stroke volume seen with aortic insufficiency, an outflow murmur mimicking aortic stenosis is common and may be the only murmur appreciated initially. Although one would expect that increasing afterload by the handgrip maneuver would increase the diastolic murmur of aortic insufficiency, it is not always the case. Transient arterial occlusion with two blood pressure cuffs inflated above systolic pressure on the upper extremities often increases the intensity of the murmur. The related outflow murmur usually diminishes with increased afterload. The diastolic murmur does not change appreciably with other maneuvers or after extrasystolic beats.

Natural History, Complications, Medical Therapy, and Timing of Surgery

Stapleton[2] evaluated cases of aortic insufficiency treated medically and noted that among low-risk patients [normal blood pressure, normal electrocardiogram (ECG), no cardiomegaly] 96% were alive 15 years after diagnosis. Among high-risk patients who had two or three ECG abnormalities, cardiomegaly, and an abnormal pulse, 70% were alive at 15 years. Medical therapy consists of providing the kind of follow-up that ensures the appropriate timing of surgical intervention if it becomes necessary. Even before the onset of symptoms, afterload reduction with ACE inhibitors can be done. As symptoms progress, surgery should be strongly considered.

A number of parameters are used as indicators for surgical

intervention in patients with asymptomatic or minimally symptomatic aortic insufficiency, but the best combination of these parameters is still a matter of debate. Surgery should be considered if the pulse pressure is more than 100 mm Hg, if there is LVH or ST-T wave abnormalities on the ECG, or if the chest radiograph reveals cardiomegaly, particularly if the cardiothoracic ratio is more than 60%.

Echocardiographic criteria for surgical consultation include an end-diastolic LV diameter of more than 70 mm or an end-systolic diameter of more than 50 mm. An ejection fraction of 40% or less is also an indication for surgical consultation. A decline in ejection fraction during exercise has been shown to identify a cohort of patients at high risk for complications in whom surgery should be considered earlier.[19,20] Because of the embolic and anticoagulation risks of prosthetic aortic valves, the goal of timing surgery is to wait as long as possible, without subjecting the patient to an irreversible loss of LV function.

Aortic Stenosis[21,22]

Etiology

After mitral regurgitation, aortic stenosis is the second most common cause of valvular heart disease in the general population. Male sex predominates by about a 2:1 ratio. Most cases of aortic stenosis are caused by one of three factors: a bicuspid aortic valve, rheumatic fever, or degenerative changes associated with aging (aortic sclerosis). A bicuspid aortic valve is present in 1% to 2% of all births, but it is not known what proportion of these patients progress to having hemodynamically significant aortic stenosis. Isolated cases present with severe symptoms during the teenage years, childhood, or even infancy. Rheumatic fever as a cause of aortic stenosis is declining, whereas age-related aortic stenosis is increasing with increasing life expectancy. An echocardiographic study of patients over 65 found aortic sclerosis in 26% and aortic stenosis in 2%. Risk factors for aortic stenosis include older age, male gender, current smoking, history of hypertension, and elevated low-density lipoprotein and total cholesterol.[4] The risk factors for coronary artery disease are also risk factors for more rapidly progressive aortic stenosis,[21,22] so the index of suspicion for the presence of aortic stenosis or its more rapid progression should be heightened in patients with risk factors for coronary artery disease.

Symptoms

When symptoms due to aortic stenosis develop, they are serious and life-threatening, and the disease is advanced. Angina due to increased LV mass, oxygen consumption, and wall tension can occur even with normal coronary arteries. Medically treated angina due to aortic stenosis is associated with a 5-year life expectancy. Syncope is a frequent presenting symptom of aortic stenosis. Without surgery life expectancy after syncope is 3 years. CHF is also a presenting symptom of aortic stenosis and if not treated surgically carries a 2-year life expectancy. Sudden death is the first symptom of aortic stenosis in 15% of patients with the disease. It is rare for aortic stenosis to present with less serious symptoms.

Physical Findings

Patients with aortic stenosis have normal or low blood pressure. In patients under age 60 an elevated systolic pressure (above 160 to 170 mm Hg) makes severe aortic stenosis unlikely, whereas in elderly patients with diffuse loss of arterial compliance an elevated systolic pressure can be found with moderate to moderately severe aortic stenosis. Low systolic blood pressure and a narrow pulse pressure are ominous signs. Early in the course of aortic stenosis a short, high-pitched opening sound may be heard in the second right intercostal space and may radiate to the neck. As the valvular disease progresses, the opening sound disappears.

The carotid pulse provides the best clue to the presence and severity of aortic stenosis. Called *parvus et tardus* (weak and slow), the carotid pulse rises slowly and often with a shudder. The changes in the carotid pulse are often correlated to the severity of the valvular gradient and the severity of the disease. The cardiac apex is diffuse and often displaced laterally. The PMI is forceful and prolonged. S_1 is usually normal with aortic stenosis. With advanced disease S_2 can be paradoxically split due to prolonged left ventricular systole. An S_3 is rare, but S_4 is common.

The murmur of aortic stenosis is best heard at the second right intercostal space and often radiates to the neck. It is coarse and usually loud. It is described as a crescendo-decrescendo murmur or a diamond-shaped murmur; the later the peak of the crescendo, the more severe is the gradient. The closer to S_2 the murmur ends, the more severe is the disease. The murmur of aortic stenosis is decreased by increased afterload and by decreased preload. The murmur becomes louder with increased preload. The marked accentuation of the murmur after a postextrasystolic beat is one of the most important clues to the presence of aortic stenosis. The physical findings most correlated with severity of disease are a late carotid upstroke; low amplitude of the carotid upstroke; louder, late peaking murmur; and a single second heart sound.[23]

Natural History, Complications, Medical Therapy, and Timing of Surgery

The natural history of aortic stenosis is variable, and the disease can present with clinical symptoms during childhood or during the ninth decade. Once aortic stenosis has been detected, it should be considered a progressive lesion. Presymptomatic medical management should ensure that the rate of progression is well defined. The development of LVH or strain on the ECG and increased cardiac size on the chest radiograph should be followed at least yearly and more often if clinical concern warrants. Serial echocardiography is useful for assessing outflow gradient and LV wall thickness, as the development of a thickened left ventricle can precede the cardiac enlargement seen by radiography.

During the asymptomatic phase of the disease, no medical intervention is indicated. Once symptoms occur, surgery should be considered quickly. Surgery may be considered before symptoms develop if there is ventricular enlargement, segmental wall motion abnormalities suggesting ischemia, severe ECG changes, or frequent ectopy, which might place the patient at risk for sudden death. It has been argued that elderly (older than 75) asymptomatic patients with aortic stenosis who are in sinus rhythm, without bundle branch block and without atrial enlargement, can be followed clinically, no matter what the echocardiographic findings are.[24]

If CHF develops, the use of ACE inhibitors is controversial. Other treatments for complications, pending surgery, consist of accepted medical regimens: digoxin and diuretics for heart failure, cardioversion and chemical stabilization with quinidine for atrial fibrillation (rate control with digoxin or a beta-blocker if cardioversion fails), and nitrates and beta-blockers or calcium channel blockers for angina pectoris.

Hypertrophic Cardiomyopathy

Hypertrophic cardiomyopathy, also known as idiopathic hypertrophic subaortic stenosis (IHSS) and hypertrophic obstructive cardiomyopathy (HOCM), is a hereditary condition causing a murmur that originates in the area below the aortic valve. The murmur is created by thickening of the myocardium with disproportionate septal thickening and subsequent narrowing of the outflow tract. The Venturi effect in the area of subaortic narrowing can cause movement of the anterior mitral valve toward the outflow tract, further worsening the obstruction. The ventricle in patients with hypertrophic cardiomyopathy is hyperkinetic, and systolic emptying of the ventricle is rapid and nearly complete. There is also abnormal relaxation and markedly decreased compliance of the ventricle that causes severe diastolic abnormalities.

The characteristics of this murmur are similar to those of the murmur of aortic stenosis with some key differences. With subaortic stenosis a brisk carotid upstroke is maintained, even in the face of a severe gradient. Contrary to the murmur of aortic stenosis, the murmur of subaortic stenosis becomes softer with increased preload or after a compensatory pause[18] and is louder with decreased preload. Like aortic stenosis, the murmur is softer with increased afterload. The gradient increases with decreased ventricular filling and with lowered systemic resistance. This point is particularly important for athletes, because after exercise both of these conditions are present. Although subvalvular aortic stenosis is an uncommon condition, it causes a disproportionate percentage of unexpected sudden deaths in healthy young people, usually immediately after exercise. Beta-blockers are the medical treatment of choice, but surgery to thin the septum is often necessary.

Right-Sided Heart Murmurs

Right-sided heart murmurs are far less common than left-sided murmurs. The pressures sustained by the valves are lower, which means that valvular dysfunction is less likely to occur. Right-sided murmurs have many of the same characteristics as murmurs involving the analogous left-sided valves with some key differences.

Left-sided murmurs involving the mitral valve cause pulmonary congestion, whereas similar right-sided murmurs involving the tricuspid valve cause central venous congestion and peripheral edema. Whereas left-sided murmurs typically stay the same or diminish slightly with inspiration, right-sided

heart murmurs usually become noticeably louder. Increasing afterload by handgrip does not affect right-sided murmurs, nor does the compensatory pause after an extrasystolic beat. Changes in preload, however, affect right-sided murmurs in the same way they affect murmurs originating from the left side of the heart. Lastly, there is no tricuspid analogy to mitral valve prolapse.

Congenital Heart Disease

Murmurs During Infancy

Murmurs are an uncommon finding during infancy. A murmur in an infant should be considered an important finding. A murmur heard during the first 24 hours of life carries a 1 in 12 chance of being caused by congenital heart disease. The most common cause of pathologic murmurs in this age group is patent ductus, which normally resolves spontaneously by 8 weeks of age. A murmur heard at 6 months of age has a one in seven chance of being caused by congenital heart disease, and a murmur heard at 1 year has a 1 in 50 chance of representing congenital heart disease. Table 78.1 lists the frequencies of various types of congenital heart diseases based on a number of epidemiological studies.[25–30]

There are four general findings on physical examination and office laboratory testing that should alert the family physician to pursue the possibility of congenital heart disease in an infant: (1) failure to thrive; (2) abnormal oxygenation, with normal defined as an oxygen saturation of more than 95% in room air (oxygen saturation should not consistently decrease with feeding); (3) signs of CHF, including tachycardia, tachypnea, poor feeding, and sweating; and (4) signs of syndromes (e.g., Down syndrome) or other congenital anomalies.

Maternal risk factors for congenital heart disease in the infant include smoking and gestational diabetes.[31,32] A weak protective effect has been demonstrated for periconceptional multivitamin use (defined as starting at least 3 months before pregnancy and continuing at least 3 months into pregnancy)[33] (see Chapters 10 and 11).

Table 78.1. **Frequency of Congenital Heart Disease (CHD)**

Condition	Percent
Ventricular septal defect (VSD)	32
Pulmonic stenosis	9
Patent ductus arteriosus (PDA)	8
Atrial septal defect (ASD)	7
Coarctation of aorta	7
Aortic stenosis	4
Tetralogy of Fallot	4
Atrioventricular septal defect	4
Hypoplastic left heart	3
D-transposition of vessels	3
Hypoplastic right heart	2
Truncus arteriosus	2
Double outlet right ventricle	1
Single ventricle	1
All other types of CHD	13

Table 78.2. **Recurrence Risk of Congenital Heart Disease**

Defect	Siblings (%)	Offspring (%)
Ventricular septal defect (VSD)	6	4
Atrial septal defect (ASD)	3	4–10
Atrioventricular (AV) septal defect	2	5–10
Patent ductus arteriosus (PDA)	2.5	3
Valvular aortic stenosis	3	5–10
Valvular pulmonic stenosis	2	6
Coarctation of aorta	2	3
D-transposition of arteries	2	5
Tetralogy of Fallot	2	4
Hypoplastic left heart	1–2	5
Hypoplastic right heart	1	5
Anomalous pulmonary vein	3	5
Truncus arteriosis	8	8
Double outlet ventricle	2	4
Atrial isomerism	5	1
Single ventricle	3	5
Ebstein's malformation	1	5

The risk of recurrence of congenital heart disease in siblings and offspring is summarized in Table 78.2.

Ventricular Septal Defect (VSD)

Because VSD is the most common murmur caused by a congenital heart defect, it is important to review its presentation. Newborns and children with a VSD present with a holosystolic murmur similar to the murmur of mitral regurgitation. Murmurs caused by VSDs are typically louder and coarser than the murmur of mitral regurgitation. A VSD is heard best at the left sternal border, and the murmur is often associated with a thrill. About 24% of VSDs close spontaneously by 18 months and 75% by 10 years of age. Those that do not close can cause irreversible pulmonary hypertension, cardiac disability, and early death. If the family physician suspects a VSD, early diagnosis, referral, and close follow-up are critical. Frequent examinations for respiratory status, feeding, and weight gain are mandatory. Any signs of failure to thrive or of RV volume or pressure overload require workup for possible surgical intervention.

Murmurs During Pregnancy

A large percentage of pregnant women develop murmurs because of an increased plasma and blood volume (see Chapter 12). Studies have shown that most murmurs during pregnancy are benign, and investigations such as echocardiography add little or no benefit to the outcomes of most pregnancies. That is no reason for complacency, however, because certain types of valvular heart disease are likely to become much more se-

rious during pregnancy, even to the point where they threaten the life of the mother or fetus. Pregnant women with known valvular heart disease or in whom there is a diastolic murmur, pansystolic murmur, loud murmur (grade 3 or more), or symptoms of cardiovascular disease must be evaluated for valvular heart disease.

Mitral stenosis, which may be clinically silent prior to conception, can become an important problem during pregnancy. Maternal morbidity and mortality are significantly increased owing to pulmonary edema caused by increased intravascular volume. The fetus suffers from poor growth, and there is increased fetal loss. Mitral regurgitation, on the other hand, is usually well tolerated during pregnancy.

Aortic regurgitation is also well tolerated during pregnancy, except when it is secondary to Marfan syndrome. Increased blood volume can cause dilatation and dissection or rupture of the aortic root. Pregnancy should be avoided in women with Marfan syndrome. Aortic stenosis, although rare in women of childbearing age, causes significant problems during pregnancy. Maternal mortality rates of up to 17% have been reported, and because of sudden depletion of intravascular volume, mortality rates of up to 40% after termination of pregnancy have been reported.[2] Subvalvular aortic stenosis, seen with hypertrophic cardiomyopathy, causes increased maternal morbidity during pregnancy, especially at delivery, when blood loss can worsen outflow obstruction. Any cause of severe left-to-right shunt or pulmonary hypertension creates a contraindication to pregnancy.

Murmurs in the Athlete[34–36]

One of the most important aspects of the physical examination of the athlete is to identify the rare patient in whom risk of sudden death can be avoided. In patients older than 40 years, the most likely cause of sudden death during sports participation is coronary artery disease (see Chapter 76). In the young athlete the most common causes of sudden death are hypertrophic cardiomyopathy,[1,36] and possibly mitral valve prolapse.[34] A 1998 study looked at all sudden deaths in athletes and nonathletes ages 35 or younger in a defined geographical area in Italy with population of 4.4 million people older than 17. This study included 33,735 people who had been screened during that time. The causes of sudden death that would have presented with a murmur, all defined by autopsy, are listed in Table 78.3.[35]

The physical findings associated with these problems are covered elsewhere in this chapter. Because hypertrophic cardiomyopathy is a congenital disease, a history of unexplained syncope and a family history of sudden death are key pieces of information. The finding of arrhythmias, a history of syn-

Table 78.3. **Valvular Causes of Sudden Death in 33,735 Athletic Screenings**

Cause of death	Athletes $n = 49$ (%)	Nonathletes $n = 220$ (%)	Total $n = 269$ (%)
Mitral valve prolapse	5 (10.2%)	21 (9.5%)	26 (9.7%)
Hypertrophic cardiomyopathy	1 (2.0%)	16 (7.3%)	17 (6.3%)

cope, or a family history of sudden death should prompt the family physician to further work up a patient with mitral valve prolapse before sanctioning exercise. Aortic stenosis and other congenital heart conditions associated with pulmonary hypertension are also potential causes of sudden death in young athletes. Current recommendations from the American College of Sports Medicine and the American College of Cardiology for participation in sports by patients with all types of congenital heart disease are found in the Bethesda conference of 1994.[36]

References

1. Harvey WP. Cardiac pearls. Dis Month 1994;40:41–113.
2. Stapleton JF. Natural history of chronic valvular disease. Cardiovasc Clin 1986;16:105–47.
3. Rose AG. Etiology of acquired valvular heart disease in adults. A survey of 18,132 autopsies and 100 consecutive valve replacement operations. Arch Pathol Lab Med 1986;110:385–8.
4. Stewart BF, Siscovick D, Lind BK, et al. Clinical factors associated with aortic valve disease. Cardiovascular health study. J Am Coll Cardiol 1997;29:630–4.
5. Singh JP, Evans JC, Levy D. et al. Prevalence and clinical determinants of mitral, tricuspid and aortic regurgitation (the Framingham Heart Study). Am J Cardiol 1999;83:897–902.
6. Jones EC, Devereux RB, Roman MJ et al. Prevalence and correlates of mitral regurgitation in a population based sample (the Strong Heart Study). Am J Cardiol 2001;87:298–304.
7. Roldan CA, Gill EA, Shivley BK. Prevalence and diagnostic value of precordial murmurs for valvular regurgitation in obese patients treated with dexfenfluramine. Am J Cardiol 2000;86:535–9.
8. Weissman NJ, Panza JA, Tighe JF, Gwynne JT. Natural history of valvular regurgitation 1 year after discontinuation of dexfenfluramine therapy. A randomized double-blind, placebo-controlled trial. Ann Intern Med 2001;134:267–73.
9. Saenz A, Hopkins CB, Humphries JO. Valvular heart disease. In: Chung EK, ed. Quick reference to cardiovascular diseases. Baltimore: Williams & Wilkins, 1987;71–92.
10. Wencker D, Borer JS. Hochreiter C, et al. Preoperative predictors of late postoperative outcome among patients with nonischemic mitral regurgitation with "high risk" descriptors and comparison with non-operated patients. Cardiology 2000;93:37–42.
11. Grigioni F, Enriques-Sarano M, Zehr KJ, et al. Ischemic mitral regurgitation: long term outcome and prognostic implications with quantitative Doppler assessment. Circulation 2001;103:1759–64.
12. Freed LO, Levy D, Levine RA, et al. Prevalence and clinical outcome of mitral valve prolapse. N Engl J Med 1999;339:1–7.
13. Fontana ME, Sparks EA, Harsios B, Wooley CF. Mitral valve prolapse and the mitral valve prolapse syndrome. Curr Probl Cardiol 1991;16:315–68.
14. Singh RG, Cappucci R, Kramer-Fox R, et al. Severe mitral regurgitation due to mitral valve prolapse: risk factors for development, progression and need for mitral valve surgery. Am J Cardiol 2000;85:193–8.
15. Kolibash AJ, Kilman JW, Bush CA, et al. Evidence of progression from mild to severe mitral regurgitation in mitral valve prolapse. Am J Cardiol 1986;58:762–7.
16. Fukuda M, Oki T, Iuchi A, et al. Predisposing factors for severe mitral regurgitation in idiopathic mitral valve prolapse. Am J Cardiol 1995;76:503–7.
17. Cheng-Wen C, Sing-Kai L, Yu-Shien K, et al. Predictors of sys-

temic embolism in patients with mitral stenosis: a prospective study. Ann Intern Med 1998;128:885–9.
18. Gonzalez-Torreciella E, Garcia-Fernandez MA, Perez-David E, et al. Predictors of left atrial contrast and thrombi in patients with mitral stenosis and atrial fibrillation. Am J Cardiol 2000;86:529–34.
19. Lindsay J, Silverman A, Van Voorhees LB, Nolan NG. Prognostic implications of left ventricular function during exercise in patients with aortic regurgitation. Angiology 1987;38:386–92.
20. Wahi S, Haluska B, Pasquet A, et al. Exercise echocardiography predicts development of left ventricular dysfunction in medically and surgically treated patients with asymptomatic severe aortic regurgitation. Heart 2000;84:606–14.
21. Palta S, Pai AM, Gill KS, Pai RG. New insights into the progression of aortic stenosis: implications for secondary prevention. Circulation 2000;101:2497–502.
22. Nassimiha D, Aronow WS, Ahn C, Goldman ME. Association of coronary risk factors with progression of aortic valvular stenosis in older persons. Am J Cardiol 2001;87:1313–4.
23. Munt B, Legget ME, Kraft CD et al. Physical examination in valvular aortic stenosis: correlation with stenosis severity and prediction of clinical outcome. Am Heart J 1999;137:298–306.
24. Pierri H, Nussbacher A, Decourt LV, et al. Clinical predictors of prognosis in severe aortic stenosis in unoperated patients > or = to 75 years of age. Am J Cardiol 2000;86:801–4.
25. Samanek N, Voriskova M. Congenital heart disease among 815,569 children born between 1980–1990 and their 15-year survival: a prospective Bohemia survival study. Pediatr Cardiol 1999;20:411–7.
26. Ainsworth S, Wyllie JP, Wren C. Prevalence and significance of cardiac murmurs in neonates. Arch Dis Child (Fetal Neonatal Ed) 1999;80:F43–5.
27. Bosi G Scorrano M, Tosato G, et al. The Italian Multicentric Study on Epidemiology of Congenital Heart Disease: first step of the analysis. Working Party of the Italian Society of Pediatric Cardiology. Cardiol Young 1999;9:291–9.
28. Wren C, Richmond S, Donaldson L. Presentation of congenital heart disease in infancy: implications for routine examination. Arch Dis Child (Fetal Neonatal Ed) 1999;80:F49–53.
29. Meberg A, Otterstad JE, Froland G, et al. Early clinical screening of neonates for congenital heart defects: the cases we miss. Cardiol Young 1999;9:169–74.
30. Samanek M. Congenital heart malformations: prevalence, severity, survival, and quality of life. Cardiol Young 2000;10:179–85.
31. Kallen K. Maternal smoking and congenital heart defects. Eur J Epidemiol 1999;15:731–7.
32. Aberg A, Westbom L, Kallen B. Congenital malformations among infants whose mothers had gestational diabetes or preexisting diabetes. Early Hum Dev 2001;61:85–95.
33. Botto LD, Mulinare J, Erickson JD. Occurrence of congenital heart defects in relation to maternal multivitamin use. Am J Epidemiol 2000;151:878–84.
34. Maron BJ, Thompson PD, Puffer JC, et al. Cardiovascular preparticipation screening of competitive athletes: a statement for health professionals from the sudden death committee (clinical cardiology) and congenital heart defects committee (cardiovascular disease in the young), American Heart Association. Circulation 1996;94:850–6.
35. Corrado D, Basso C. Schiavon M, Thiene G. Screening for hypertrophic cardiomyopathy in your athletes. N Engl J Med 1998;339:364–5.
36. Graham TP, Bricker JT, James FW, Strong WB. 26th Bethesda Conference: recommendations for determining eligibility for competition in athletes with cardiovascular abnormalities. Task Force 1: congenital heart disease. Med Sci Sports Exerc 1994;26:S46–53.

79
Heart Failure

William A. Norcross and Denise D. Hermann

Heart failure (HF) is defined as the inability of the heart to generate a cardiac output sufficient to meet the metabolic needs of body tissues at rest or with activity. This definition is sufficiently broad to include systolic and diastolic failure, high-output failure, and cor pulmonale. The adjective "congestive" is appropriate only when there are symptoms or signs of systemic or pulmonary fluid volume overload, typically related to sodium and water retention secondary to activation of the neurohumoral axis (renin-angiotensin-aldosterone system and arginine-vasopressin system) with HF.

Heart failure affects 4.9 million people in the United States and is the only major cardiovascular disorder with increasing incidence and prevalence. Two factors thought to contribute to this phenomenon are increases in average life expectancy and medical advances that have diminished morbidity and mortality from most cardiovascular disorders. The diagnosis of HF accounts for annual health care costs in the United States of more than $18 billion, half of which, it is estimated, could be saved by improvements in outpatient management. Despite modern therapies, however, the morbidity and mortality associated with HF remain high, averaging 10% mortality at 1 year and 50% at 5 years.[1]

The causes of HF are listed in Table 79.1. Coronary artery disease is presently the most common etiology and represents the etiology of HF in nearly 70% of patients with systolic dysfunction in the United States. Idiopathic dilated cardiomyopathy, valvular heart disease, and hypertensive cardiomyopathy are also common (see Chapters 75, 78, and 82).

Diastolic (lusitropic) failure occurs when the left ventricle becomes stiff and noncompliant and elevated left ventricular filling pressures develop. Systolic function is generally preserved, and therefore the ejection fraction remains normal to slightly reduced. The cardiac output is preserved at the expense of increased diastolic filling pressure, and is diminished in the setting of hypovolemia and/or excessive systemic afterload. Diastolic failure most commonly results from an-

tecedent hypertension or coronary artery disease. Although the prevalence of chronic diastolic HF in a primary care setting is unknown, studies from tertiary care centers suggest that up to 40% of patients with HF may have primarily diastolic dysfunction.[2] It is important to recognize diastolic dysfunction because certain treatments for systolic dysfunction (diuretics, digoxin) may worsen the patient's hemodynamic profile or clinical condition.

High-output HF is uncommonly encountered in a primary care practice. It is important to recognize because the conditions that cause it (Table 79.1) are often responsive to treatment.

Acute Heart Failure/Cardiogenic Pulmonary Edema

Diagnosis

Although severe acute heart failure (AHF) can manifest in a patient with mild to moderate chronic symptoms, for the purposes of this section the patient with new onset of severe symptoms is described. Air hunger, dyspnea, and anxiety are the most notable symptoms. Classically, the patient expectorates pink, frothy sputum, occasionally blood-streaked due to pulmonary edema and rapid alveolar filling from either pressure or volume overload or both. Physical findings include tachypnea with use of accessory muscles, tachycardia, engorged neck veins, rales, and wheezing (cardiac asthma). The extremities are pale and cool, and peripheral cyanosis may be present. The chest roentgenogram typically shows cardiomegaly (although the heart size and shape may be normal in the setting of acute myocardial infarction, hypertensive crisis, or acute valvular emergency), pulmonary vascular redistribution, Kerley B lines, and perihilar infiltrates with a classic "bat wing" appearance and pleural effusions may be noted (right-sided or bilateral effusions are the rule).

Table 79.1. Causes of Heart Failure

Most common
Coronary artery disease
  Diastolic dysfunction
  Systolic dysfunction
Hypertensive cardiomyopathy
  Diastolic dysfunction
  Systolic dysfunction (late)

Common
  Idiopathic cardiomyopathy
  Alcoholic cardiomyopathy
  Hypertrophic cardiomyopathy
  Diabetic cardiomyopathy
  Valvular heart disease
  Cor pulmonale (right heart failure only)
    Chronic lung disease
    Pulmonary embolic disease
    Primary/secondary pulmonary hypertension

Uncommon
  Infectious cardiomyopathy (viral, bacterial, fungal, parasitic)
  Doxorubicin-induced cardiomyopathy
  Bleomycin-induced cardiomyopathy
  Constrictive pericarditis
  Restrictive cardiomyopathy
    Amyloidosis
    Hemochromatosis
    Sarcoidosis
  Collagen vascular disease-induced cardiomyopathy
  High-output failure
    Anemia
    Arteriovenous shunt
    Paget's disease of bone
    Thyrotoxicosis
  Thiamine deficiency (beriberi) cardiomyopathy
  Radiation-induced cardiomyopathy
  Cardiomyopathy of pregnancy
  Uremic cardiomyopathy
  Endocardial fibroelastosis

Initial diagnostic testing must include an electrocardiogram (ECG) to rapidly exclude acute myocardial infarction (MI) or a significant arrhythmia, blood chemistries, a complete blood count (CBC), arterial blood gases, and any other tests indicated by the clinical history and examination. Early bedside echocardiography may be helpful, especially for diagnosing acute valvular cardiac disease, helping to differentiate cardiac from noncardiac pulmonary edema, and defining left ventricular (LV) function as preserved or impaired. Severely ill patients (e.g., those with hypotension, oliguria, diminished mentation (cardiogenic shock), or failure to rapidly respond to therapy) require central hemodynamic monitoring by placing an indwelling pulmonary artery catheter (e.g., Swan-Ganz catheter).

Treatment

Acute HF is a medical emergency. Unless severely hypotensive, the patient is placed in a seated position to assist venous pooling and diminish preload. In the absence of chronic obstructive pulmonary disease (COPD) with retention of carbon dioxide, high-flow 100% oxygen is delivered by way of a tight-fitting mask to maintain peripheral oxygen saturation

above 94%. Vascular access is established and cardiac monitoring instituted. Rotating tourniquets and phlebotomy are rarely utilized in the modern era, as they have been replaced by aggressive pharmacologic therapy. An acute MI with signs of HF or shock should prompt a rapid evaluation by a cardiologist for percutaneous transluminal coronary angioplasty (PTCA) or administration of thrombolytic agents.

First-Line Agents

Furosemide is generally a first-line agent if the patient is not severely hypotensive. When given intravenously it acts initially as a venodilator and subsequently as a diuretic. The patient is given twice the customary daily oral dose intravenously. If the patient does not take a diuretic, the furosemide dose is 0.5 to 1.0 mg/kg IV slow push. (Rapid, large doses of intravenous furosemide have been associated with permanent ototoxicity.)

Morphine has long had a role in the treatment of cardiogenic pulmonary edema but must be used with caution. It is a potent venodilator and also reduces anxiety. On the other hand, it can cause or worsen hypotension and may mask symptoms and signs that are important for the clinician to observe when sequentially assessing patients with a suspected acute coronary syndrome. The starting dose is 2 to 4 mg IV; subsequent doses can be titrated according to the patient's response. Nitroglycerin, a potent venodilator, may also be considered a first-line drug, especially in patients with concomitant chest pain or ischemia. Because of the peripheral vasoconstriction associated with AHF, topical nitroglycerin is avoided. Nitroglycerin 0.3 mg sublingually or a similar dose of the oral spray may be used and repeated depending on the patient's response. Care is taken to avoid symptomatic hypotension, especially in patients with diastolic HF, those in whom right ventricular infarction is suspected, and those with an acute coronary syndrome.

Second-Line and Third-Line Agents

The choice of a second-line agent depends on the patient's clinical parameters. It is reasonable to use the guidelines of the American Heart Association adopted from the recommendations made at the International Guidelines Conference on Cardiopulmonary Resuscitation (CPR) and Emergency Cardiac Care (ECC).[3] If systolic blood pressure is below 70 mm Hg, consider norepinephrine 0.5 to 30.0 μg/min IV. If the systolic blood pressure is between 70 and 100 mm Hg, and there are symptoms or signs of shock, consider using dopamine in a range of 2.5 to 15.0 μg/kg/min IV. If the systolic blood pressure is between 70 and 100 mm Hg, and there are no symptoms or signs of shock, use dobutamine 2 to 20 μg/min IV. If the systolic blood pressure is above 100 mm Hg and the patient is not significantly hypertensive, consider nitroglycerin 10 to 20 μg/min IV. If the diastolic blood pressure is above 110 mm Hg, consider nitroglycerin at a starting dose of 10 to 20 μg/min IV and titrate to the desired or optimal effect, or use nitroprusside 0.1 to 5.0 μg/kg/min IV.

By the time third-line agents are required, and possibly before, it is presumed that such a patient would be admitted to a coronary care unit (CCU) and a cardiologist consulted. In patients who do not respond promptly to initial treatment, right heart catheterization (e.g., Swan-Ganz catheter) is desirable to rule out noncardiogenic pulmonary edema and to guide subsequent therapy. Along with drug therapy, it is also reasonable to consider the institution of positive end-expiratory pressure (PEEP), continuous positive airway pressure (CPAP), or intubation with ventilatory support. Third-line agents include amrinone, milrinone, and aminophylline. Other interventions that may be appropriate, depending on the clinical situation, include intraaortic balloon counterpulsation and various surgical procedures such as coronary artery bypass grafting (CABG), valve replacement, and even cardiac transplantation.

Chronic Heart Failure

Clinical Manifestations

The New York Heart Association (NYHA) classification system is widely used to grade heart failure according to symptoms. Unfortunately, it lacks objectivity. NYHA class I patients have no limitation of physical activity. Class II patients are comfortable at rest, but "ordinary" physical activity results in symptoms (e.g., fatigue, dyspnea). Class III patients are comfortable at rest but have symptoms with low levels of activity. Class IV patients experience symptoms at rest. Classes II and III are often difficult to distinguish. Maintaining a frame of reference to the normal activities of an age- and sex-matched normal individual is helpful.

Risk factors for chronic heart failure include aging, coronary heart disease, diabetes, hypertension, and obesity. Unlike the classic presentation of severe AHF, chronic heart failure can be of slow and insidious onset. Patients at risk for the development of heart failure should be screened for symptoms of *f*atigue, *a*ctivity intolerance, *c*ongestive symptoms, *e*dema, and *s*hortness of breath (FACES). Several studies have convincingly demonstrated that the symptoms, signs, and radiographic findings classically associated with chronic HF have poor positive and negative predictive values.[4] Moreover, left ventricular dysfunction can be asymptomatic or symptoms with exercise can be rationalized and attributed to poor physical conditioning or to aging. Although the individual

symptoms and signs of HF are often unreliable, diagnostic accuracy is improved directly with the number of symptoms and signs observed and the acuity of the presentation.

The symptoms and signs of chronic HF are shown in Table 79.2. It is critical to note that symptoms cannot distinguish systolic from diastolic ventricular dysfunction. It is helpful therapeutically to distinguish signs of low cardiac output from congestion (left, right, or biventricular volume overload). The former respond favorably to inotropic agents and vasodilators and the latter to diuretics and vasodilators. In the patient with predominant diastolic ventricular dysfunction, dyspnea on exertion may be the primary symptom. In such patients signs often include hypertension and a prominent S_4. The echocardiogram typically shows normal ventricular dimensions and preserved systolic function; Doppler interrogation of mitral valve inflow and pulmonary vein flow demonstrate diastolic filling abnormalities. Left atrial enlargement and left ventricular hypertrophy (LVH) are common. LVH without systemic hypertension (HTN) warrants an evaluation for infiltrative or primary myocardial disease. In the patient with isolated right ventricular (RV) failure, the most likely etiology is primary or secondary pulmonary disease. RV dysplasia and pericardial constriction may be considered as well, but are uncommon.

Diagnosis

Chronic HF is a clinical syndrome whose diagnosis should be confirmed by further evaluation. All patients with symptoms or signs consistent with HF should undergo an assessment of LV function. Specifically, the ejection fraction should be measured by echocardiography or radionuclide ventriculography. These tests also help distinguish systolic from diastolic dysfunction. After confirming the diagnosis, the next step is to determine the etiology of chronic HF. If there are significant risk factors for coronary artery disease (CAD) or if CAD is otherwise suspected, noninvasive testing or direct coronary angiography should be considered (see Chapter 76). Although it is tempting to treat HF patients empirically based on clinical grounds alone, we strongly recommend the use of a confirmatory test for two reasons: (1) the delivery of a diagnosis with such a grave prognosis (50% mortality at 5 years) mandates precision, and reversible or treatable factors must not be over-

Table 79.2. **Symptoms and Signs of Chronic Heart Failure**

Parameter	Low cardiac output	"Left-heart" congestion (pressure or volume overload, or both)	"Right-heart" or biventricular congestion (pressure or volume overload, or both)
Symptoms	Fatigue, anorexia, poor energy, malaise, decreased exercise capacity, weight loss, weakness, impaired concentration or memory	Dyspnea (rest or exertion), orthopnea, paroxysmal nocturnal dyspnea, cough, nocturia	RUQ or epigastric pain or fullness, abdominal bloating, nausea or anorexia, ankle/leg swelling, weight gain
Signs	Resting tachycardia, S_3, low carotid pulse volume, cool or vasoconstricted extremities, cachexia, reduced urine output, altered mentation	Cardiomegaly, abnormal apical impuse, S_3, tachypnea, rales, loud P_2	Jugular distension, hepatomegaly, hepatojugular reflux, pleural effusions or ascites, dependent edema, RV gallop or lift, loud P_2

RUQ = right upper quadrant; RV = right ventricular.

looked; and (2) useless or inappropriate therapies may be dangerous to the patient and are expensive in their own right.

One study demonstrated the ECG to be a useful screening tool for HF.[5] Of 96 patients with impaired LV systolic function, as determined by two-dimensional, M-mode, and Doppler echocardiography, 90 had major ECG abnormalities (atrial fibrillation, LVH, prior MI, bundle branch block, or left axis deviation) and none had a completely normal ECG. Using major ECG abnormalities as a marker in this study gives a sensitivity of 94% for systolic HF. If these data are borne out by other, similar studies, the ECG may become a useful test when deciding which patients may benefit from assessment of the ejection fraction (EF). Unfortunately, a high sensitivity for major ECG abnormalities has not been demonstrated for diastolic dysfunction, RV failure, or high-output failure. For instance, the sensitivity and specificity of the ECG for detecting LVH vary widely with the grading criteria employed.

Radionuclide ventriculography and echocardiography with Doppler are appropriate tools for the evaluation of the EF. Compared to the EF as measured by cineangiography, the correlation of radionuclide ventriculography ($r = 0.88$) is slightly better than that of echocardiography ($r = 0.78$).[6] However, most clinicians prefer echocardiography with Doppler sonography because of its added ability to quantitate chamber size and detect LVH and valvular dysfunction. The advantages and disadvantages of the two tests are compared in Table 79.3.

Because HF is often asymptomatic or minimally symptomatic, and because early treatment has been documented to diminish mortality and ameliorate the progression of the disease, it would be desirable to have a simple, inexpensive, accurate test for the diagnosis of HF. Natriuretic peptide assays hold promise for this purpose. Natriuretic peptides are secreted in high levels in systolic HF secondary to atrial and ventricular wall stress. Their properties include natriuresis, vasodilation, and inhibition of the renin-angiotensin-aldosterone axis. The data to date suggest brain natriuretic peptide (BNP, a 32 amino acid peptide originally named because it was thought to be a neurotransmitter in pig brain, but now known to be secreted by the cardiac ventricle) and N-terminal proBNP (NT-proBNP, the circulating amino terminal portion of the BNP prohormone) correlate best with the diagnosis of systolic heart failure. Test characteristics for BNP

show sensitivities of 77% to 97%, specificities of 73% to 87%, and positive predictive values of 16% to 70%.[7] For NT-proBNP sensitivities range from 82% to 94%, specificities from 55% to 69%, and positive predictive values from 50% to 58%.[7] As expected, the test characteristics for both tests depend on the assay utilized and the pretest likelihood of HF in the study population (there is improved accuracy in populations at high risk for systolic HF.) These assays have not been well studied in diastolic HF or high-output HF. There is currently no national consensus as to the best test or specific assay to use, but the technology is promising. Such a test may be used in cases where the diagnosis remains uncertain after conventional diagnostic testing has been performed. The assay may be particularly helpful in the emergency department or outpatient clinic.

Once the clinical syndrome of HF is diagnosed, the etiology can often be ascertained by way of a careful history and physical examination, ECG, chest radiography, chemistry panel, thyroid-stimulating hormone (TSH) assay, CBC, and echocardiography. Some would argue the case for serum iron, iron-binding capacity, and ferritin assays to evaluate for the presence of hemochromatosis.

Alcoholic cardiomyopathy, thought to play a role in 20% to 30% of patients with "idiopathic" cardiomyopathy, is probably more commonly encountered than we realize. A sensitive exploration of the issue is necessary for all patients (see Chapter 59). Also, alcoholic cardiomyopathy seems to correlate well with the presence of the skeletal myopathy of alcoholism[8]; therefore, a careful neurologic examination is important. Similarly, a history of cocaine or amphetamine abuse, which may result in premature large or small vessel CAD and infarct, may be difficult to elicit.

Prognosis

Despite medical and surgical advances in the treatment of HF, the prognosis generally remains grim. Overall mortality for HF optimally treated with angiotensin-converting enzyme (ACE) inhibitors, digoxin, and diuretics is about 10% annually, with a 5-year mortality of 50%. Approximately 30% to 50% of these deaths are sudden. Data from the Framingham study suggest that this 5-year mortality has not changed appreciably since the 1930s. African Americans have about a

---

Table 79.3. **Echocardiography Versus Radionuclide Ventriculography for Evaluating Left Ventricular Performance**

Test	Advantages	Disadvantages
Echocardiography	Permits concomitant assessment of valvular disease, LV hypertrophy, and LA size Less expensive than radionuclide ventriculography in most cases Able to detect pericardial effusion and ventricular thrombus	Difficult to perform in patients with lung disease Usually only semiquantitative estimate of EF provided Technically inadequate in up to 18% of patients under optimal circumstances
Radionuclide ventriculography	More precise and reliable measurement of EF Better assessment of RV function	Requires venipuncture and radiation exposure Limited assessment of valvular heart disease and LV hypertrophy

Source: Konstam et al.[1]

LV = left ventricular; LA = left atrial; EF = ejection fraction; RV = right ventricular.

Table 79.4. **Prognostic Factors for Chronic Heart Failure**

Etiology of Ventricular Dysfunction
  Predominant systolic impairment
  Ischemic heart disease
  Idiopathic, hypertensive, or valvular heart disease
  Other
    Myocarditis: infectious, autoimmune, giant cell
    Hypertrophic cardiomyopathy
    Toxin-related cardiomyopathy (e.g., alcohol,
      anthracyclines)
    Infiltrative diseases (e.g., amyloid, hemochromatosis)
Patient demographics
  Race
  Gender
  Age
Comorbidities
  Diabetes, systemic or pulmonary hypertension, sleep apnea,
    renal or hepatic dysfunction
Easily measured variables
  Symptoms—NYHA classification, specific activity scale
  Ejection fraction in left and right ventricles
  Exercise capacity: VO_2 max, 6-minute walk distance
  Hemodynamics
  Serum sodium
  Thyroid function
  Arrhythmias/ECG (antiarrhythmic therapy)
  Doppler echocardiography (mitral inflow pattern)
  LV size, volumes, shape, and mass
Other markers; research tools
  Neurohormones: plasma norepinephrine, renin activity,
    aldosterone, atrial natriuretic factor
  Markers of autonomic dysfunction (heart rate variability)
  Signal-averaged ECG
  Endomyocardial biopsy

NYHA = New York Heart Association.

1.5-fold higher risk of mortality from HF than whites. The following variables have been found to be independent predictors of a poor prognosis in HF: severely depressed ejection fraction (<30%); LV size and morphology (globular is worse); functional class (NYHA class IV: 30–50% mortality at 1 year); concomitant RV failure or pulmonary hypertension; increased cardiothoracic ratio on chest roentgenogram; older age; reduced exercise capacity; hyponatremia; atrial and ventricular arrhythmias; and neuroendocrine activation [elevated levels of norepinephrine, angiotensin II, aldosterone, atrial natriuretic factor, tumor necrosis factor-α (TNF-α) and other cytokines] (Table 79.4). TNF-α is responsible for inducing "cardiac cachexia," a chronic muscle wasting syndrome seen frequently in advanced heart failure, cancer, and AIDS. At present, the treatment is directed at the underlying disease, although a clinical trial evaluating the effect of a TNF receptor blocker (etanercept) on prognosis in chronic HF is under way, with results expected in 2002.

Management Principles
Patient Counseling

The establishment of a caring, open, compassionate relationship with the patient and the family is necessary for effective treatment of HF. The clinician should not hesitate to enlist the help of dietitians, pharmacists, nurse educators, and com-munity groups. Home health care resources can be especially helpful. It is believed that better patient education and compliance improve morbidity and mortality statistics and save billions of dollars in health care expenditures.

General Counseling

The patient and family should be informed of the pathophysiology of HF, including an explanation of the symptoms observed, the rationale for complying with treatment recommendations, and, if known or suspected, the cause of the HF. The patient and family are told what symptoms or signs suggest a deteriorating course and what to do in the event such symptoms develop. All treatments are explained carefully, and the patient's responsibilities in treatment are reinforced. When family members are involved in the treatment plan, their responsibilities are also clearly delineated. The patient and family should be referred to appropriate support groups and community organizations (e.g., American Heart Association).

Patients should weigh themselves daily and record the results. Because a few pounds may be important, it is important to standardize the method of weighing. It is recommended that the patient be weighed in the morning after awakening, after urinating, but before eating. Although the significance of change in weight is related to "baseline" body mass, a change of 3 to 5 pounds is generally sufficient to merit a call to the primary care provider. Well-educated and compliant patients and their families may adjust the diuretic dosage at home based on daily weights. However, frequent adjustments in diuretic dosage require more frequent monitoring of electrolytes, especially potassium and magnesium.

Every effort is made to get smoking patients to stop. There are few things, if any, more dangerous to patients with HF. Community organizations [American Heart Association (AHA), American Cancer Society (ACS), American Lung Association (ALA)] may be helpful in this regard. HF patients are prime targets for pulmonary infections and therefore should receive appropriate immunizations against influenza and pneumococcus (see Chapter 7).

Sharing the prognosis with the patient and family is a difficult but necessary task of the primary care provider. It is made more difficult by the imprecision inherent in such a process, particularly when the underlying etiology may be unknown or other conditions affect the patient's health. Still, patients and their families deserve this information so they may plan their lives accordingly. Patients should be advised to create advance directives.

Activity/Exercise

Regular moderate, symptom-limited aerobic exercise may be safely recommended to all patients with stable NYHA class I to III HF; it may improve functional capacity and quality of life and diminish symptoms. Concerns about sexual activity must be fully explored, as patients are unlikely to initiate conversation on this matter. Patients with stable NYHA class I to III HF may engage safely in sexual activity, although practices may have to be altered to accommodate patients with diminished exercise tolerance. Although no specific training or cardiac rehabilitation program can be routinely recommended, such programs may be of benefit to certain patients, particularly those with concerns about exercising and those with concomitant CAD. An observed maximal stress test is often useful to objectively document exercise capacity and provide the patient with reassurance that the resulting exercise prescription (roughly to 60% of maximum) is safe.

Diet

All patients should be placed on a 3-g sodium diet, which is palatable, inexpensive, and achievable for most patients. Patients with continued congestive symptoms or fluid retention on high doses of diuretics may require a 2-g or even 1-g sodium diet, though these are much less palatable and compliance is more difficult to obtain. Low-fat diets must be considered with caution, as many patients with HF are elderly and subject to malnutrition. A vitamin supplement may be reasonable, especially if the patient is at risk for loss of water-soluble vitamins because of diuretics. Alcohol, an agent known to be cardiotoxic and capable of acutely depressing myocardial contractility and causing arrhythmias, should be avoided altogether. If the patient is unwilling to stop, ingestion of more than one drink (total of 1 ounce of alcohol) daily should be strongly discouraged. Because of the critical importance of diet in the successful management of HF, it is recommended that the patient and spouse be referred to a health care professional, such as a dietitian for counseling. Nonsteroidal antiinflammatory drugs, both prescription and over the counter (OTC), should be avoided because of the high risk of renal injury (especially in diabetics and those with underlying renal insufficiency) and decompensation of HF.

Compliance with Treatment

Compliance is the cornerstone of treatment of HF. Excellent compliance with the treatment plan should result in improved quality of life, alleviation of symptoms, lower mortality, decreased emergency room visits and hospitalizations, and much lower cost of care. Research shows that patients are noncompliant because of one or more of the following factors: (1) failure to understand the treatment plan, (2) disbelief that the treatment plan can be effective, (3) forgetfulness, and (4) constraints upon following the treatment plan (e.g., financial). During the period following diagnosis, frequent office visits are necessary to titrate medications, reinforce teaching and treatment, and assess side effects.

Patients should know their drug regimen, including drug name, dosage, and method of taking it. Patients should bring all their drugs, including OTC drugs, to the office visit with the primary care provider immediately after hospitalizations, changes in the regimen, and at intervals throughout the year. Patients should also have a written record of their current drug regimen at home and on their person. Home health services or family support may be necessary for patients with memory problems or other intellectual deficits, as well as for those who are blind or frail or have other major physical limitations. A home care evaluation by knowledgeable staff often yields clues to pitfalls to therapy in refractory patients. Compliance has been shown to improve when the patient and family are involved in the development of the treatment plan, feel fully informed about all aspects of the treatment, and experience open, helpful communication with all members of the treatment team.

A nurse-directed, multidisciplinary outpatient intervention in elderly patients with HF has been shown to produce a significant reduction in hospitalizations, improved quality-of-life scores, and savings in health care costs of $460 per patient over 90 days compared to that for patients assigned to conventional care.[9] The intervention consists of intensive education about HF, dietary instruction by a dietitian, analysis and simplification of the drug regimen, and intensive follow-up through home care services and visits and calls from study team members.

Drugs

Vasodilators

Angiotensin-converting enzyme inhibitors (ACEIs) are the cornerstone of the pharmacologic management of systolic HF, and contemporary therapy of systolic HF mandates an ACEI unless contraindicated. Although the reason that ACEIs are more effective than other vasodilators in reducing HF mortality is not fully known, the Survival and Ventricular Enlargement Trial (SAVE),[10] Cooperative North Scandinavian Enalapril Survival Study (CONSENSUS),[11] Vasodilator-Heart Failure Trial-II (V-HeFT II),[12] and Studies of Left Ventricular Dysfunction (SOLVD)[13] trials demonstrated an approximate 20% reduction in mortality compared to placebo. ACEIs reduce afterload, improve neurohumoral abnormalities, improve symptoms and quality of life, and decrease hospitalizations. In the prevention arm of the SOLVD trials, it was further demonstrated that ACEIs delayed the onset of symptoms of HF and first hospitalization for HF in patients with clinically silent LV dysfunction.

The ACEIs are generally well tolerated. Side effects are infrequent and include rash, angioedema, cough, hypotension, hyperkalemia, and impaired renal function. Some of these side effects may be avoided by using specific angiotensin II receptor blockers (ARBs, e.g., losartan). The Evaluation of Losartan in the Elderly-2 (ELITE-2) trial[14] directly compared the use of ACEIs and ARBs on mortality in chronic heart failure in elderly patients with systolic LV dysfunction and found no significant difference. Because of the study population profile, extrapolation of these data to all subsets of patients is not advised. With the exception of patients who develop angioedema or allergic rash, ACEIs remain preferred therapy. Studies of the combined use of both ACEIs and ARBs in systolic HF are now ongoing. Preliminary results are of concern because of an increase in mortality when ACEIs and ARBs are used in combination with beta-blockers (discussed below). It is premature to recommend the combined use of ACEIs and ARBs at present.

Although a survival benefit in regard to HF has been demonstrated in clinical trials of ACEIs, it has not been translated into a survival benefit for the general HF population, largely because these drugs are underused or underdosed by primary care physicians, generally because of unfounded concerns about excessive blood pressure reduction. In the SOLVD trial, systolic blood pressure decreased by only 5 mm Hg, on average, and diastolic blood pressure by 4 mm Hg. Even in the CONSENSUS trial, which enrolled patients with NYHA class IV HF, only 5.5% of patients treated with enalapril were withdrawn because of symptomatic hypotension.

Therefore, all patients with HF should be offered a trial of ACEIs, except those with specific contraindications: (1) a history of allergy or intolerance to ACEIs; (2) a serum potassium level higher than 5.5 mEq/L that cannot be reduced by conventional means; or (3) symptomatic hypotension, even without ACEI treatment. Caution and careful monitoring are used for patients with systolic blood pressures less than 90 mm Hg and patients with a creatinine level above 3.0 mg/dL or a creatinine clearance less than 30 mL/min. Half the usual dosage of ACEI is given to patients with renal insufficiency, and renal function must be monitored frequently.

In stable patients who are not at high risk for symptomatic hypotension, ACEIs may be started as for the treatment of hypertension, with the dosage titrated upward every 2 to 4 weeks to a target dose equivalent to those used in the large-scale clinical trials of ACEIs for HF. Examples of target doses are captopril 50 mg tid and enalapril 10 mg bid. All ACEIs are believed to be equally effective for the treatment of HF, and a corresponding dosage of any other ACEI may be used.

Patients at high risk for symptomatic hypotension should be treated with a low dose of a short-acting ACEI (e.g., captopril 6.25 mg). It is reasonable to consider hospitalizing patients at especially high risk for hypotension, though most patients can be safely monitored in the outpatient setting. If the first dose is tolerated, the patient may be started on captopril 6.25 to 12.5 mg tid. If this dose is tolerated, the patient may be switched to an ACEI with qd or bid dosing intervals and slowly titrated up to the target dose. Patients with renal insufficiency or high risk for hypotension should initially be seen at least weekly and the serum creatinine and potassium levels monitored carefully. In the event of worsening renal function (increased serum creatinine of 0.5 mg/dL or more), hyperkalemia (5.5 mEq/L or higher), or symptomatic hypotension, the patient is reevaluated and the regimen modified. Excessive diuretic administration is a common reason for ACEI intolerance.

Beta-Blockers

Beta-blocker therapy should be added to standard therapy in all patients with NYHA class II or III systolic HF. There are insufficient data to make firm recommendations regarding the efficacy and risk/benefit ratio of treatment of patients with NYHA class I or IV HF with beta-blockers. There is strong evidence to support a mortality benefit and reduced hospitalizations with the use of carvedilol,[15] bisoprolol,[16] and metoprolol CR/XL[17] in patients with NYHA class II or III systolic HF. Unlike ACEIs and ARBs, beta-blockers do not exhibit a "class effect," so that the administration of such agents to patients with HF should be limited to the agents studied in clinical trials. Studies comparing the agents mentioned above are ongoing, but at presently convincing data do not support the use of one drug over another. Regardless of the choice of agent, similar recommendations can be made for the addition of beta-blockers to standard therapy. First, patients should be carefully assessed for clinical stability. Patients with worsening edema, dyspnea, or other manifestations of decompen-

sating HF should be stabilized and should be stable for at least 1 week before beta-blockers are started. The dosage of beta-blockers should be individualized and patients must be closely monitored. Beta-blockers should be started at low dose and titrated upward no more frequently than every 2 weeks. When increasing the dosage, it is wise to give the new dose in the office and to observe the patient for at least 1 hour afterward for symptoms of dizziness or light-headedness or marked changes in vital signs. Patients who do manifest worsening HF should first have their other drugs (diuretics, ACEIs, etc.) adjusted to try to compensate, or the dose of beta-blocker decreased or discontinued. With careful management, most patients can tolerate beta-blocker therapy, even those whose HF may transiently decompensate while titrating therapy. The starting dose of carvedilol (Coreg) is 3.125 mg orally twice daily. If tolerated, the dose can be doubled every 2 weeks to a maximum of 25 mg twice daily for patients weighing less than 85 kg and 50 mg twice daily for those weighing 85 kg or more. The starting dose of metoprolol CR/XL is 25 mg orally daily for patients with NYHA class II and 12.5 mg daily for those with NYHA Class III. The dose is titrated upward every 2 weeks to a target dose of 200 mg daily. The starting dose of bisoprolol is 1.25 mg orally daily titrated upward in a similar manner to a maximum dose of 10 mg daily.

For patients unable to take ACEIs or ARBs, the currently accepted alternate regimen, for which a mortality benefit has been demonstrated at 1 and 3 years,[18] is the combination of hydralazine and isosorbide dinitrate. However, compared to ACEIs, this combination has a worse side-effect profile, and in clinical trials 18% to 33% of patients discontinued one or both agents. Headaches, palpitations, nasal congestion, and hypotension are the most common side effects. The two agents are started concurrently and slowly titrated upward. Isosorbide dinitrate is started at a dose of 10 mg tid and titrated to 40 mg tid. Hydralazine is started at a dose of 10 to 25 mg tid and titrated to 75 mg tid. The drugs are then titrated upward incrementally and no sooner than weekly. In the V-HeFT II trial,[12] which compared the hydralazine–isosorbide dinitrate regimen to enalapril in patients with HF, the average total daily doses were hydralazine 200 mg and isosorbide dinitrate 100 mg. It is unknown if lower dosages would be effective.

Digoxin

A number of studies have found digoxin to improve symptoms and functional status in patients with systolic HF[19]; yet two centuries after its first use in HF by Withering, its effect on mortality has only recently been determined. The National Heart, Lung and Blood Institute: Digitalis Investigation Group (NHLBI-DIG) study found no overall mortality benefit attributable to digoxin in systolic HF; however, a morbidity benefit was observed in that over an average follow-up period of 37 months there were 6% fewer hospitalizations for HF in the digoxin-treated group.[20] It is clear, also, that digoxin withdrawal precipitates clinical worsening and increases hospitalizations.[19]

Even among cardiologists there is debate about when to initiate digoxin in the clinical course of patients with systolic HF. Some clinicians routinely prescribe digoxin for all patients with LV systolic dysfunction (EF <40%). Others institute digoxin only if symptoms and functional status are not satisfactorily improved by ACEIs, beta-blockers, and diuretics. Most agree that digoxin should be prescribed for patients with severe HF and in HF patients with concurrent atrial fibrillation and a rapid ventricular response. The primary mechanism of action of digoxin for symptom alleviation in HF may not be its mild positive inotropic action but rather its vagotonic effects, which antagonize the sympathetic nervous system activation during HF.

Prior to instituting digoxin, the patient's serum electrolytes, blood urea nitrogen (BUN), and creatinine must be tested and a recent ECG reviewed. For stable patients in the outpatient setting, digoxin is started orally and loading doses are almost never required. In younger patients with normal renal function, a dose of 0.25 mg once daily may be prescribed. In elderly, small, or hypothyroid patients, start with 0.125 mg daily. For patients with renal insufficiency, consult one of the widely available nomograms to determine the digoxin dose. When digoxin levels have achieved steady state (approximately 1 week for patients with normal renal function and 3 weeks for those with renal insufficiency), determine the serum digoxin level and repeat the serum BUN, creatinine, and electrolytes. Also obtain and review the ECG.

After steady state has been reached and the patient is stable on a dose of digoxin that results in serum levels within the therapeutic range, it is usually not helpful to determine digoxin levels regularly. Many clinicians recommend checking the digoxin level annually, and it must be obtained if the patient (1) develops symptoms or signs of digoxin toxicity (nausea, mental status change, visual disturbance, ectopy); (2) suffers deterioration of cardiac status; (3) suffers deterioration of renal status; or (4) is prescribed a drug known to interact with digoxin (verapamil, quinidine, amiodarone, antibiotics, and anticholinergic agents).

Diuretics

Diuretic therapy is used only in patients with HF who demonstrate symptoms or signs of fluid volume overload ("congestive" heart failure). Diuretics improve the clinical status of patients with CHF by promoting renal excretion of sodium and water, but they also activate the renin-angiotensin-aldosterone axis, potentiate the hypotensive effect of ACEIs, and may decrease cardiac output, especially in patients with diastolic dysfunction. While diuretics should not be used routinely in all patients with HF, most patients will require them during their clinical course.

Thiazide diuretics may be useful for mild CHF, but they are ineffective when the glomerular filtration rate (GFR) falls below 30 mL/min. Patients with moderate to severe CHF, a GFR less than 30 mL/min, or marked fluid volume overload should be given a loop diuretic such as furosemide, orally or intravenously, depending on the acuity of the clinical situation. Average oral starting doses of furosemide range from 10 to 40 mg. (Initial, target, and suggested maximal doses for most of the drugs commonly used in HF can be found in Table 79.5.)

Most patients respond to a single daily morning dose of diuretic. If a larger dose of diuretic is needed, increasing the morning dose rather than splitting the dose generally achieves a better diuresis. An alternative to increasing the dose of diuretic, especially when it has superseded the target dose, is to add a diuretic from a different class (e.g., addition of triamterene to the regimen of a patient taking furosemide).

Metolazone is a diuretic commonly reserved for patients with severe or refractory HF because of its potency. It must be used with great caution. A typical starting dose of metolazone is 2.5 mg once daily. The major side effects are similar to those of other diuretic agents: volume depletion, hypotension, hypokalemia, and hypomagnesemia. The combination of furosemide and metolazone is exceptionally potent and necessitates frequent monitoring of fluid status and serum electrolytes. Although there are no set rules for following serum potassium and magnesium levels, it seems reasonable to check levels when starting or changing the regimen of diuretics and ACEIs. Stable patients on diuretics should have the serum potassium measured every 3 to 6 months, but this suggestion is clearly a guideline and should not supplant clinical judgment. It must also be recalled that potassium is a predominantly intracellular cation, and that serum levels do not often accurately reflect intracellular stores. Therefore, clinicians should consider potassium supplementation in patients whose serum potassium falls below 4 mEq/dL. Potassium supplementation is undertaken with great caution in patients with renal insufficiency (including the elderly with a "normal" BUN and creatinine) and those on ACEIs or potassium-conserving diuretics. High-dose diuretic regimens also may cause excessive renal excretion of magnesium and calcium. It may be necessary to replace these nutrients as well.

The Randomized Aldactone Evaluation Study (RALES) Trial[21] demonstrated a mortality benefit in patients in NYHA class III or IV from spironolactone 25 mg orally daily. The study has not been duplicated and its results can be applied only to patients with moderate to severe systolic HF. Although little hyperkalemia was seen in the study, clinicians must be particularly concerned about this risk in general practice because the drug will generally be added to a regimen that already contains potassium-conserving drugs in patients with renal hypoperfusion. Candidates for spironolactone therapy should have NYHA class III or VI systolic HF, be normokalemic and have a creatinine less than 2.5 mg/dL. Strong consideration should be given to discontinuing supplemental potassium when spironolactone is added to the regimen. The serum potassium and sodium should be checked at weekly intervals until stable, frequently thereafter, and at any time there is a change in regimen or clinical status.

Anticoagulants

Although some clinicians have suggested the use of warfarin routinely in patients with HF, there is insufficient evidence to support such a recommendation at this time. As 60% to 75% of HF populations have concomitant CAD, antiplatelet therapy may be strongly indicated and empiric use of warfarin increases bleeding risk. HF patients with primary valvular disease, atrial fibrillation, pulmonary embolism or other systemic embolic event, or an LV thrombus should be anticoagulated to an international normalization ratio (INR) in the range of 2.0 to 3.0.

Table 79.5. **Drugs Commonly Used for Chronic Heart Failure**

Drug	Initial dose (mg)	Target dose (mg)	Recommended maximum dose (mg)	Average wholesale price (AWP) for 100 tablets at average or target dose (generic used, when available)
Thiazide diuretics				
Hydrochlorothiazide	25 qd	As needed	50 qd	$7.74
Chlorthalidone	25 qd	As needed	50 qd	$18.40
Loop diuretics				
Furosemide	10–40 qd	As needed	240 bid	$14.30
Bumetanide	0.5–1.0 qd	As needed	10 qd	$75.18
Ethacrynic acid	50 qd	As needed	200 bid	$53.24
Thiazide-related diuretic				
Metolazone	2.5 (test dose)	As needed	10 qd	$93.18
Potassium-sparing diuretic				
Spironolactone	25 qd	As needed	100 bid	$45.94
Triamterene	50 qd	As needed	100 bid	$87.12
Amiloride	5 qd	As needed	40 qd	$47.57
ACE inhibitors				
Enalapril	2.5 bid	10 bid	20 bid	$107.22
Captopril	6.25–12.5 tid	50 tid	100 tid	$131.46
Lisinopril	5 qd	20 qd	40 qd	$108.29
Quinapril	5 bid	20 bid	20 bid	$95.99
Benazepril	10 qd	20 qd	40 qd	$90.01
Ramipril	2.5 qd	10 qd	20 qd	$131.45
Fosinopril	10 qd	20 qd	40 qd	$87.74
Beta blockers				
Bisoprolol	1.25 qd	10 qd		$131.10
Carvedilol	3.125 bid	25 bid		$163.21
Metoprolol succinate	12.5 qd	200 qd		$80.10

Source: Adapted from Konstam et al.[1]

Pacemaker Therapy of Systolic Heart Failure

Increasingly it is becoming recognized that systolic heart failure is characterized by conduction system abnormalities and rhythm disturbances in addition to the well-known problems with myocardial contractility and neurohumoral imbalances. In some HF patients, conduction disturbances diminish cardiac output through reduced diastolic filling, abnormal wall motion and prolonged regurgitation through the mitral and tricuspid valves. Some studies have shown benefit from biventricular pacing in patients with significantly widened QRS complex on quality of life scores, exercise tolerance, and improvement in NYHA functional class.[22] At present, application of this therapy should be individualized. Ongoing studies will define the risks and benefits of this treatment, characterize the survival benefit, and identify those patients most likely to be helped by it.

Drug Management of Diastolic Heart Failure

Although some causes of diastolic dysfunction are irreversible (e.g., myocardial fibrosis), potentially reversible conditions are found in many patients. Therapies that reduce arterial blood pressure, diminish myocardial ischemia, and promote regression of LVH may reverse some of the diastolic abnormalities. Supraventricular arrhythmias are common and

poorly tolerated, as tachycardia reduces LV filling time and further increases diastolic pressures.

Because of LV stiffness, patients with diastolic HF are sensitive to changes in LV end-diastolic volume. Diuretics are almost always necessary for congestive symptoms, but overly aggressive diuresis may reduce stroke volume and cardiac output. With hypertrophic cardiomyopathy (HCM), even a mild positive inotrope such as digoxin can worsen outflow tract obstruction. Beta-blockers and calcium channel blockers promote myocardial relaxation and are usually considered first-line agents for the treatment of diastolic HF. ACEIs have not been extensively studied for diastolic HF. However, because tissue-based ACE activity is upregulated in LVH secondary to pressure overload and because it, in turn, leads to reductions in LV relaxation, it is tempting to speculate that ACEIs may have a salutary effect on diastolic function at the level of the myocardium.[23]

Revascularization

Despite the widespread use of CABG and PTCA, few data exist on the efficacy of aggressive treatment of asymptomatic coronary arterial lesions in patients with HF; moreover, there are no randomized, controlled clinical trials that have evaluated outcomes of any procedure in patients with systolic LV dysfunction, other than transplantation for end-stage heart failure. Several cohort studies evaluating the effect of CABG have shown a survival benefit from CABG in patients with clinically symptomatic HF or severe systolic dysfunction and severe or activity-limiting angina.[24–26] Neither CABG nor PTCA has been proved to improve survival in HF patients without angina. Nonetheless, because of the high prevalence of CAD in patients with HF, the suspected high prevalence of "silent" ischemia in this population, and our increasing understanding of "hibernating" myocardium (nonfunctioning or hypofunctioning heart wall that is underperfused but viable), it is conceivable that detection and revascularization of stenotic coronary arteries may improve prognosis via the prevention of future MIs and the diminishing mortality due to HF (see Chapter 76).

Because of the uncertainty surrounding this issue and the high stakes involved, the Heart Failure Guideline Panel of the Agency for Health Care Policy and Research (AHCPR) has developed an algorithm to help patients and providers deal with this clinical situation.[1] These guidelines were devised in 1994, and updated recommendations are expected in 2001–2002 from the combined American College of Cardiology/American Heart Association Task Force and the Heart Failure Society of America. PTCA has not been shown to improve survival in patients with HF of any type, so CABG is considered the procedure of choice. The clinician and patient, though, must also use judgment when choosing a revascularization procedure. A patient may not be a candidate for revascularization if CABG or PTCA is not an acceptable procedure to the patient, anatomic or technical factors (e.g., prior chest irradiation, severe distal disease) jeopardize the likelihood of a successful result, severe comorbid diseases exist, or the ejection fraction is low (<20%).

Once a patient has been determined to be a candidate for revascularization, the HF guideline panel recommended that HF patients be categorized and offered evaluation and treatment as follows:

1. Heart failure patients with severe or activity-limiting angina, frequent episodes of pulmonary edema, or angina decubitus should be advised to undergo coronary arteriography as the first diagnostic modality, to be followed by CABG, if operable lesions are found (see Chapter 76). This group of patients is at greatest risk, has the highest likelihood of having treatable CAD, and is likely to receive the greatest benefit from revascularization.
2. Heart failure patients with mild angina or a history of MI should be advised to undergo a noninvasive test for myocardial ischemia as the first diagnostic modality. Appropriate tests include exercise or pharmacologic stress myocardial perfusion scintigraphy (e.g., thallium scanning), exercise or pharmacologic stress (dobutamine) echocardiography, or stress radionuclide angiocardiography. Patients with evidence of ischemic myocardium should be advised to undergo coronary angiography with revascularization to follow if operable lesions are discovered.
3. Heart failure patients without angina or a history of any manifestation of CAD are, along with their physicians, in a

quandary. There are no data to support routine evaluation of this group for myocardial ischemia. The patient and physician should discuss this issue thoroughly and consider the presence of risk factors that make CAD likely or those that explain the patient's HF (e.g., alcoholism) by way of another etiology. If the patient and physician agree that it would be appropriate to screen for myocardial ischemia, the evaluation should begin with one of the noninvasive tests.

Patient Monitoring

Office Visit

The family physician inquires about changes in chronic symptoms or the development of new symptoms. Special attention is given to inquiring about dyspnea or fatigue on exertion, orthopnea, edema, and paroxysmal nocturnal dyspnea. At selected intervals the physician reviews all of the areas covered in the section on patient counseling, especially activity and functional ability, diet, medication regimen, and mental health issues. Patients should bring a record of daily weights to the office visit, and, if requested by the physician, all of their medications (prescription and OTC). Evidence of snoring, episodes of apnea or hypopnea, or other signs of sleep disturbance is sought from the patient and sleep partner.

In a study of 42 patients with stable, "optimally treated" HF, 45% were found to have a moderate to severe degree of sleep-disordered breathing, often associated with prolonged and severe hypoxemia.[27] Patients in whom sleep apnea-hypopnea is suspected are referred to a sleep disorder specialist.

The physical examination includes weight, vital signs, and assessment for edema, rales, or findings suggestive of pleural effusion, jugular venous distention, hepatomegaly, and hepatojugular reflux. A careful cardiac examination is performed with attention to changes in heart rate, cardiac impulse, murmurs and gallops, and especially a third heart sound (S_3). The use of the echocardiogram or any other noninvasive or invasive testing for the purposes of routinely monitoring a patient with HF is not recommended.

All of the data obtained from the history and physical examination at the time of the office visit are carefully considered and used to make appropriate changes, when necessary, in the patient's therapeutic regimen. It is believed that this careful outpatient clinical assessment and subsequent adjustment of therapy is critical for improving quality of life, decreasing mortality, maintaining functional status, and decreasing the frequency of hospital admissions for HF patients.

Exacerbations

Although HF patients and their physicians are disappointed and sometimes alarmed when an episode of clinical deterioration occurs, the occasion can also be used for education that may prevent future decompensations. The physician must search for intercurrent or comorbid diseases that may have caused the deterioration (e.g., thyroid disease, anemia, infection, sleep apnea, arrhythmias, MI, pulmonary embolism, cardiac valvular disease, renal insufficiency, hepatic dysfunction, diabetes, uncontrolled hypertension). The physician must also search for etiologies related to patient noncompliance (e.g., not taking medications or following diet, alcohol or illicit drug abuse) or iatrogenic or OTC drugs that either conserve sodium (nonsteroidal antiinflammatory drugs) or have negative cardiac inotropic effects (e.g., diltiazem, verapamil, beta-blockers, quinidine, disopyramide). Episodes of clinical deterioration in HF patients should not be accepted as part of the natural history of HF. Rather, a careful, thoughtful search for the etiology is almost always fruitful and provides important information that can be used to educate patient and physician alike and prevent future incidents of decompensation.

Prevention of HF

Primary Prevention

Family physicians practicing good preventive medicine and health promotion are already preventing HF (see Chapters 7 and 8). Hypertension and CAD are the two most commonly encountered antecedents of HF, and aggressive detection and treatment of hypertension and other treatable risk factors for CAD (smoking, dyslipidemia, obesity, inactivity, diabetes) can do much to prevent HF. Additionally, physicians must counsel their patients to drink alcohol in moderation (≤ 2 oz daily) or not at all and to abstain completely from the use of cocaine and other illicit drugs.

Some have made a strong case for routine screening for hemochromatosis,[28] but this recommendation has not been met with widespread enthusiasm. The issue is not addressed by the U.S. Preventive Services Task Force in the second edition of the *Guide to Clinical Preventive Services*.

Secondary Prevention

All patients found to have an EF of less than 40% should be treated with a "target dose" of an ACEI, unless contraindications exist. All patients who suffer a nonfatal MI (except those with small, uncomplicated, non–Q-wave inferior MIs and who have not previously had an MI) should have their EF measured noninvasively prior to discharge and within 6 to 12 months thereafter. If an ACEI was not initiated during peri-infarction management, all those with an EF of less than 40% should be treated with target doses of an ACEI.

Future Therapy for Heart Failure

The morbidity and mortality related to the diagnosis of heart failure averages 10% annually despite treatment with ACE inhibitors. It approaches 40% to 50% annually for the most symptomatic patients. Surgical procedures such as cardiomyoplasty, implantation of ventricular assist devices, and cardiac transplantation are viable options for a few such patients. Pharmaceutical agents with additive survival benefit have been sought with great interest. Despite exhibiting great promise in early trials, a number of agents have been demonstrated to be ineffective or actually increase the mortality rate compared to placebo. The latter group includes oral milrinone, flosequinan, and vesnarinone, suggesting that chronic inotropic stimulation is disadvantageous in heart failure.

Refractory Chronic Heart Failure and the Heart Failure Specialist

Primary care providers should consider referral to a heart failure specialist or cardiologist to assist in case management when patients remain symptomatic (NYHA class III or IV) despite (or are intolerant of) "standard therapy." There are other specific indications for referral: when the presence or severity of heart failure is uncertain; patients with two or more hospitalizations or emergency room visits for heart failure within 6 months; patients with suspected acute myocarditis; heart failure with moderate to severe aortic or mitral regurgitation; patients with evidence of myocardial ischemia or potentially reversible myocardial dysfunction; and consideration of clinical trial participation.

Patients in whom cardiac transplantation might be considered during the next 1 or 2 years should be referred early, as serial assessment is invaluable to the transplant team for determining the tempo of disease progression. An "elective" transplant evaluation and the concomitant educational process typically is conducted over several weeks. Once the patient has been listed for transplantation, the wait for an appropriate donor organ may exceed 10 to 14 months, depending on the patient's blood type, body habitus, and other conditions. Urgent transplantation places the patient at increased risk of morbidity from renal or hepatic damage, a prolonged hospitalization and recovery phase, or death while awaiting surgery. Valuable relationships with members of the transplant team are also more difficult to develop in emergent situations.

References

1. Konstam M, Dracup K, Baker D, et al. Heart failure: evaluation and care of patients with left-ventricular systolic dysfunction. Clinical practice guideline no. 11. AHCPR publication no. 94-0612. Rockville, MD: Agency for Health Care Policy and Research, Public Health Service, U.S. Department of Health and Human Services, 1994.
2. Bonow RO, Udelson JE. Left ventricular diastolic dysfunction as a cause of congestive heart failure. Ann Intern Med 1992;117:502–10.
3. International Guidelines on CPR and ECC. Circulation 2000;102(suppl):1–384.
4. Chakko CS, Woska D, Martinez H, et al. Clinical, radiographic, and hemodynamic correlations in chronic congestive heart failure: conflicting results may lead to inappropriate care. Am J Med 1991;90:353–9.
5. Davie AP, Francis CM, Love MP, et al. Value of the electrocardiogram in identifying heart failure due to left ventricular systolic dysfunction. BMJ 1996;312:222–6.
6. Folland ED, Parisi AF, Moynihan PF, et al. Assessment of left-ventricular ejection fraction and volumes by real-time, two-dimensional echocardiography: a comparison of cineangiographic and radionuclide techniques. Circulation 1979;60:760–6.
7. Talwar S, Downie PF, Ng LL, et al. Towards a blood test for heart failure: the potential use of circulating natriuretic peptides. Br J Clin Pharmacol 2000;50:15–20.
8. Urbano-Marquez A, Estruch R, Navarro-Lopez F, et al. The effects of alcoholism on skeletal and cardiac muscle. N Engl J Med 1989;320:409–15.
9. Rich MW, Beckham V, Wittenberg C, et al. A multidisciplinary

intervention to prevent the readmission of elderly patients with congestive heart failure. N Engl J Med 1995;333:1190–5.

10. Pfeffer MA, Braunwald E, Moyé LA, et al. Effect of captopril on mortality and morbidity in patients with left-ventricular dysfunction after myocardial infarction: results of the survival and ventricular enlargement trial. N Engl J Med 1992;327:669–77.

11. CONSENSUS Trial Study Group. Effects of enalapril on mortality in severe congestive heart failure. N Engl J Med 1987; 316:1429–35.

12. Cohn JN, Johnson G, Ziesche S, et al. A comparison of enalapril with hydralazine-isosorbide dinitrate in the treatment of chronic congestive heart failure. N Engl J Med 1991;325:303–10.

13. SOLVD Investigators. Effect of enalapril on mortality and the development of heart failure in asymptomatic patients with reduced left-ventricular ejection fractions. N Engl J Med 1992; 327:685–91.

14. Pitt B, Poole-Wilson PA, Segal R, et al. Effect of losartan compared with captopril on mortality in patients with symptomatic heart failure: randomized trial—the Losartan Heart Failure Survival Study ELITE II. Lancet 2000;355:1582–87.

15. Packer M, Bristow MR, Cohn JN, et al. The effect of carvedilol on morbidity and mortality in patients with chronic heart failure. N Engl J Med 1996;334:1349–55.

16. CIBIS-II Investigators and Committees. The Cardiac Insufficiency Bisoprolol Study II: a randomised trial. Lancet 1999;353: 9–13.

17. Hjalmarson A, Goldstein S, Fagerberg B, et al. Effects of controlled-release metoprolol on total mortality, hospitalizations, and well-being in patients with heart failure. JAMA 2000;283: 1295–302.

18. Cohn JN, Archibald DG, Ziesche S, et al. Effect of vasodilator therapy on mortality in chronic congestive heart failure: results of a Veteran's Administration Cooperative Study. N Engl J Med 1986;314:1547–52.

19. Packer M, Gheorghiade M, Young D, et al. Withdrawal of digoxin from patients with chronic heart failure treated with angiotensin-converting-enzyme inhibitors. N Engl J Med 1993;329:1–7.

20. The Digitalis Investigation Group. The effect of digoxin on mortality and morbidity in patients with heart failure. N Engl J Med 1997;336:525–33.

21. Pitt B, Zannad F, Remme WJ, et al. The effect of spironolactone on morbidity and mortality in patients with severe heart failure. N Engl J Med 1999;341:709–17.

22. Bryce M, Spielman SR, Greenspan AM, et al. Evolving indications for permanent pacemakers. Ann Intern Med 2001;134: 1130–41.

23. Katz AM. The cardiomyopathy of overload: an unnatural growth response in the hypertrophied heart. Ann Intern Med 1994;121: 363–71

24. Bounous EP, Mark DB, Pollock BG, et al. Surgical survival benefits for coronary disease patients with left-ventricular dysfunction. Circulation 1988;78(suppl I):151–7.

25. Coronary Artery Surgery Study (CASS) Principal Investigators and Associates. Coronary artery surgery study: a randomized trial of coronary artery bypass surgery: survival data. Circulation 1983;68:939–50.

26. Califf RM, Harrell FE Jr, Lee KL, et al. The evolution of medical and surgical therapy for coronary artery disease: a 15-year perspective. JAMA 1989;261:2077–86.

27. Javaheri S, Parker TJ, Wexler L, et al. Occult sleep-disordered breathing in stable congestive heart failure. Ann Intern Med 1995;122:487–92.

28. Edwards CQ, Kushner JP. Screening for hemochromatosis. N Engl J Med 1993;328:1616–20.

80
Cardiovascular Emergencies

William J. Hueston and A. Kesh Hebbar

Cardiac disease accounts for the largest proportion of deaths in the United States. Many patients with underlying cardiac problems present to family physicians with conditions that can lead to death if not properly evaluated and treated. This chapter examines several cardiac emergencies that may be encountered by patients in a primary care practice.

Syncope

Syncope refers to transient loss of consciousness with loss of motor tone. Near-syncope generally refers to patients who lose some motor activity and have a decreased level of consciousness, but do not completely pass out. These conditions are frightening to patients and their family and usually result in patients' seeking care immediately. In one series, syncope-related problems accounted for 3% of all emergency department visits and 6% of all general medical hospital admissions.

Syncope can be the symptom of many different conditions including multiple noncardiac conditions. However, syncope associated with cardiac problems carries a much higher risk of subsequent death than when caused by other noncardiac diseases. In a prospective study of patients identified with syncope, it was found that patients whose syncope was linked to a cardiac cause had a 1-year mortality of 30% compared to 12% when a neurologic diagnosis was made and 6% with syncope from unknown causes.[1] For this reason, the identification of a cardiac problem contributing to syncope is important.

The causes of syncope can be divided into three broad categories: cardiac, neurologic, and other. A list of causes of syncope is shown in Table 80.1.[1,2] This chapter focuses on cardiac causes of syncope and cardiac medications that can result in syncope.

Pathophysiology and Differential Diagnosis

The symptom of syncope usually develops as a result of transient decreases in oxygen delivery to the neurologic centers that control consciousness. Any cardiac, circulatory, or neurologic condition that reduces perfusion to this area of the brain can cause syncope. In a prospective trial of 204 patients presenting with syncope in the early 1980s, Kapoor and colleagues[1] were able to classify 26% as having cardiac problems and another 26% with noncardiac conditions that caused their symptoms. In the remaining 48%, no cause could be found despite extensive investigation.[2]

Cardiac Syncope

Cardiac causes of syncope lead to a reduction in cardiac output that results in decreased perfusion of the brain. This includes cardiac dysrhythmias, cardiac ischemia, and obstruction to cardiac outflow.

The most common cause of transient reductions in cardiac outflow is an acute dysrhythmia. Of the types of rhythm disturbances, nonsustained ventricular tachycardia is the most common dysrhythmia associated with syncope. Since ventricular tachycardia can occur in association with ischemia, patients may have reduced cardiac output preceding the onset of the rhythm disturbance. The other dysrhythmia frequently resulting in syncope is sick sinus syndrome (tachycardia-bradycardia syndrome). In this instance either the tachycardic phase or the bradycardic phase can result in transitory decreases in cardiac output.

Ischemia also should be considered in the patient presenting with syncope (also see Chapter 76). The ischemic event can result in myocardial infarction or can be transient such as that occurring with aortic stenosis. Both of these possibilities should be entertained especially when the syncope is associated with exercise in a patient with risk factors for valvular or atherosclerotic disease. In younger patients, another potential for ischemic-related syncope is hypertrophic cardiomyopathy. Young individuals with exercise-induced syncope should be carefully evaluated for the possibility of hypertrophic cardiomyopathy before being allowed to participate in sports or other exertional activities.

Table 80.1. **Causes of Syncope**

Cardiac syncope
Dysrhythmias
  Ventricular tachycardia
  Supraventricular tachycardia
  Sick-sinus syndrome
  Sinus pause
  Complete heart block
Cardiac ischemia
  Myocardial infarction
  Aortic stenosis
  Hypertrophic cardiomyopathy
Obstruction of inflow/outflow
  Pulmonary embolism
  Aortic dissection
  Atrial myxoma
  Pericardial tamponade

Neurogenic syncope
Vasovagal syncope
Vascular obstruction
  Subclavian steal syndrome
  Vertebral-basilar transient ischemic attacks
Carotid hypersensitivity
Autonomic neuropathies

Other
Idiopathic orthostatic hypotension
Hypovolemia
Medications
Hyperventilation
Psychiatric syncope/conversion reaction

Obstructive cardiac conditions resulting in syncope are uncommon. The most common obstructive cause of syncope is pulmonary embolism. Another emergent cause of syncope that obstructs cardiac filling is cardiac tamponade. In addition, rare cardiac abnormalities can cause syncope. These include atrial myxomas that may obstruct blood flow through the mitral valve, cardiac tumors that can obstruct valvular flow, and thoracic aortic dissection, which can obstruct blood flow to the cerebral vessels. Finally, cardiac tamponade can restrict cardiac filling and result in decreased cardiac output.

Other Causes of Syncope

A variety of neurologic conditions can cause syncopes. These include posterior circulation transient ischemic attacks, vasopressor/vasovagal syncope, and carotid hypersensitivity. Additionally, seizures can mimic syncope. If the syncopal episode is witnessed, tonic-clonic motor activity can indicate an underlying seizure disorder. If the episode is not witnessed, a generalized seizure should remain in the differential diagnosis until a cause is found.

Other nonneurologic conditions to consider that can be associated with syncope include decreased intravascular fluids that occur with hemorrhage or profound dehydration. In addition, psychiatric conditions also should be considered, especially when the syncope tends to occur in dramatic fashion and always in the presence of onlookers. Psychiatric problems such as hyperventilation also can cause the loss of consciousness.

Some common associated findings with each disorder are shown in Table 80.2.[3]

Table 80.2. **Associated History and Physical Examination Findings for Common Causes of Syncope**

Cause	Onset	Other history	Physical exam
Dysrhythmia	Quick, little warning	Higher risk with CAD; family history of hypertrophic cardiomyopathy	Murmur of aortic stenosis; irregular rhythm or rate disturbance
Ischemic heart disease	With exertion	Risk factors for CAD; previous angina	No specific findings
Aortic stenosis	With exercise	Recurrent syncope; rheumatic heart disease	Systolic murmur
Hypertrophic cardiomyopathy	With exercise	Family history of sudden death	Murmur accentuated by Valsalva maneuver
Seizure disorder	May have aura	History of seizures; drug use that reduces seizure threshold; alcohol or other drug withdrawal	Postictal state; loss of bladder or bowel continence
Vertebrobasilar transient ischemic attack	Sudden onset	Risk factors for vascular disease	May find carotid bruits; usually no specific findings
Subclavian steal syndrome	Onset with exercise using left arm	Recurrent syncope with exercise; higher incidence in women	Decreased pulse and blood pressure in left arm
Orthostatic syncope	Usually gradual onset with episodes of near-syncope	Usually progressive in nature; associated with drugs that can cause orthostasis (alpha-blockers, tricyclic antidepressants); associated with diabetes mellitus	Orthostatic drop in blood pressure with rising; with autonomic neuropathy (associated with diabetes) see drop in blood pressure without an accompanying rise in pulse
Psychogenic syncope	Dramatic event	Occurs in times of stress; patient rarely injured in fall	No specific cardiac or neurologic findings

CAD = coronary artery disease.

Evaluation

The most important aspects of the evaluation are the history, physical examination, and electrocardiogram testing. These three techniques have been found to yield the diagnosis in about 50% of cases of syncope.[4]

History

As part of a comprehensive history of the event and general health of the patient, several areas should be emphasized. The occurrence of prodromal symptoms and what these symptoms were like may be useful in suggesting a potential cause for the syncope. Generally, neurologic or neurovascular events occur with little warning. Vasovagal syncope often produces a prodrome that includes flushing, sweating, nausea, and anxiety. Some cardiac dysrhythmias are associated with palpitations, but many, such as ventricular tachycardia, may occur without warning; thus, palpitations can be a specific indicator of a cardiac source, but is not very sensitive.

The specific circumstances surrounding the syncope also should be determined. As indicated earlier, events that occur when the neck is turned or compressed or associated with micturition, cough, or straining may indicate carotid hypersensitivity. Orthostatic hypotension occurs with standing or other sudden position changes. Subclavian steal is associated with upper extremity use.

The occurrence of syncope with exertion is worrisome and raises the possibility of ischemic heart disease from either fixed vessel obstruction or aortic stenosis. Younger patients with syncope or near-syncope during athletic activities should be evaluated for hypertrophic cardiomyopathy.

Past medical history is important to assess the presence and risk factors for atherosclerotic disease. In addition, a number of drugs are associated with syncope (Table 80.3), so a complete medication history is essential.[1,2] A family history of syncope, sudden death (especially at a young age, as frequently occurs in hypertrophic cardiomyopathy), and other illnesses might suggest specific conditions.

In addition, information from an onlooker about what happened during the event may be useful. In particular, the presence of tonic-clonic motor activity may differentiate seizure activity from syncope. Furthermore, information about how the individual fell and his or her activity while "passed out" can be useful in identifying patients with psychiatric syncope.

Physical Examination

A careful physical examination can help confirm some of the conditions suspected from the history. Assessment of the blood pressure in both arms while lying, sitting, and standing with simultaneous measure of the pulse is very useful. Blood pressure testing can reveal orthostasis (with or without pulse increases) and may detect differences in left and right arm blood pressures suggestive of subclavian steal.

Attention to the carotid arteries should include listening for bruits and palpating the pulse. In addition, gentle carotid massage can be useful in assessing for carotid hypersensitivity. Carotid pressure should be avoided if bruits are present to reduce the risk of causing a cerebrovascular embolism with massage. In addition, in patients with a high likelihood for

Table 80.3. Drugs Associated with Syncope

Vasodilating agents
  Nitrates
  Calcium channel blockers
  ACE inhibitors
  Minoxidil (topical and systemic)
  Alpha-blocking agents
Psychoactive drugs
  Tricyclic antidepressants
  Phenothiazines
  MAO inhibitors
Drugs lengthening the QT interval
  Type I (quinidine, procainamide, disopyramide, flecainide, encainide)
  Sotalol
  Amiodarone
Diuretics
Others
  Alcohol
  Cocaine
  Digitalis
  Vincristine and other neuropathic drugs
  Marijuana

ACE = angiotensin-converting enzyme; MAO = monoamine oxidase.
Source: Kapoor,[2] with permission.

carotid hypersensitivity, intravenous access may be warranted to treat the resulting sinus pause or third-degree atrioventricular (AV) block (also see Chapter 77).

The cardiac examination is important as well. Determination of the resting heart rate and any rhythm disturbances can be signs of a rate problem. The presence of murmurs may signal aortic stenosis or other valvular heart disease (see Chapter 78). The emergence of a murmur or accentuation of a soft aortic murmur while the patient does a Valsalva maneuver and the physician listens over the aortic outflow tract may indicate hypertrophic cardiomyopathy. A pericardial rub can indicate restrictive pericarditis.

Other Testing

Evaluation of the patient with syncope can be performed on an outpatient basis if the patient has not suffered any injury from the fall, has not had recurrent episodes, and is at low risk for ischemic cardiac events or malignant dysrhythmias. This description would most often apply to young healthy individuals for whom this is an isolated, brief episode with full recovery and no injury. Young healthy patients with clear antecedents to the event that suggest a clear cause, such as vasovagal syncope, may require no additional workup for a single event.

Initial evaluation of the patient with syncope should include an electrocardiogram (ECG) to establish the cardiac rhythm and assess for signs of cardiac injury or syncope. If the history is suggestive of a cardiac rhythm disturbance and the initial ECG is normal, further evaluation with a Holter monitor is indicated. If patients experience multiple near-syncope episodes, consideration may be given to an event recorder rather than Holter monitoring, especially if the events are not frequent and are likely to be missed over the 24- or 48-hour period that the Holter monitor is in place.[5]

Patients at risk for ischemic events should have cardiac enzymes determined to rule out myocardial infarction. For patients with syncope related to exertion, further evaluation for ischemia is warranted with a cardiac stress test.

An echocardiogram may be useful in patients with a rub or murmur. Echocardiography will allow for visualization of the valves, and Doppler flow can estimate whether significant pressure gradients exist across the heart valves. Additionally, the echocardiogram may detect areas of previous myocardial injury or hypertrophy, and it evaluates the pericardium.

Routine brain imaging is not likely to be useful in patients without carotid bruits, no other neurologic symptoms, and a normal neurologic examination. Without evidence of motor activity during the event, electroencephalograms are not likely to be helpful.[6]

For patients in whom the previous evaluation has been unrevealing, two additional types of evaluations may be indicated. In patients with suspected or known cardiac disease or whose history is suggestive of a cardiac dysrhythmia, further evaluation with electrophysiologic (EPS) testing may be indicated. In several studies of patients with cardiac disease and unexplained syncope, EPS testing uncovered a presumptive cause for the syncope in 18% to 75% of cases.[3] Treatment of syncope in these cases resulted in a cessation of symptoms in 75% to 85% of patients. In contrast, in patients without cardiac disease, response to treatment ranges from 12% to 20% suggesting that EPS abnormalities uncovered in these individuals were not causing the symptoms.

Patients in whom a vagally mediated mechanism is suspected can be evaluated using the head-up tilt test. The tilt test involves positioning of the tilt table at a 60- to 80-degree angle for 10 to 60 minutes supplemented with the infusion of isoproterenol. A recurrence of symptoms in this circumstance is usually indicative of vasovagal syncope. The tilt test is most useful in patients with recurrent symptoms but no evidence of suspected cardiac disease in whom other evaluations have been unfruitful.

In some patients, psychiatric evaluation is indicated. Psychiatric problems can be uncovered in as many as 25% of patients who have recurrent syncope.[4] Patients at higher risk for psychiatric disorders include those in whom syncope is also witnessed and is dramatic, who have had five or more episodes in 1 year, and have other suspected underlying psychiatric disorders.

Management

Because syncope is a symptom, appropriate management includes identifying the underlying cause and providing effective therapy.

The most important types of syncope to treat are those associated with dysrhythmias and with ischemic heart disease. Once a cardiac problem has been established as the cause of the syncopal episodes, further evaluation with EPS testing and evaluation for underlying ischemic heart disease may be warranted. Control of potential malignant dysrhythmias such as ventricular tachycardia or supraventricular tachycardias with ischemia are essential to prevent sudden death.

A second important aspect in managing syncope is to avoid drugs that can exacerbate orthostasis or contribute to depressed sinus or AV nodal function. Patients who are currently taking these medications should be offered trials of alternatives that may not cause as much orthostatic hypotension. Patients who are prone to orthostasis should be advised to remain well hydrated and avoid situations where they may lose excessive fluids without adequate replacement, such as long hikes in hot, dry environments. Wearing elastic hose to prevent venous pooling and intermittently contracting the leg muscles to promote venous return also may be helpful.[7]

Syncope in Children and Adolescents

Syncope also is a common symptom in children and adolescents. Some studies estimate that up to 20% of all children or adolescents will have at least one fainting episode before reaching adulthood.[8] The challenge for the physician is to differentiate when these episodes are due to benign causes such as breath-holding or hyperventilation and when they signal more serious problems.

In one small study of pediatric patients presenting to an emergency department with syncope, over half of all patients with syncope had a vasovagal attack.[9] In all patients except the 9% in which the cause remained unknown, a benign reason was identified for the attack.

While syncope from serious illness is uncommon in children, there are some warning signs of cardiac disease that should prompt a more thorough investigation[8] (Table 80.4). These include syncope that occurs when the patient is lying down or with no forewarning, syncope provoked by exercise, episodes accompanied by chest pain or palpitations, and loss of consciousness for more than 5 minutes. In addition, children or adolescents who have a family history of cardiomyopathies, sudden death, or aortic stenosis should be evaluated more extensively.

Cardiogenic Shock

Traditional classification of shock states has been based on broad but discrete hemodynamic defects. These categories include hypovolemic shock (e.g., hemorrhage, gastroenteritis), obstructive shock (acute pulmonary embolism), distributive shock (anaphylactic and septic shock), and cardiogenic shock. Survival from shock states is dependent on the initial resuscitative efforts to establish tissue perfusion and reverse the underlying etiologic process. Table 80.5 lists the major hemodynamic patterns seen in each of these shock states.

Table 80.4. **Factors Associated with Cardiac-Induced Syncope in Children**

Attack when recumbent
Little or no prodrome preceding attack
Attack associated with exercise
Unconsciousness lasting more than 5 minutes
History of cardiac disease in family member
History of sudden death in family member

Table 80.5. **Classification of Types of Shock**

Type of shock	CI	SVR	PVR	PaOP
Cardiogenic shock, e.g., AMI	↓	↑	N	↑
Hypovolemic shock	↓	↑	N	↓
Distributive shock, e.g., septic shock	↑		N	N–↓
Obstructive shock, e.g. pulmonary embolism	↓	↑–N	↑	N–↓

AMI = acute myocardial infarction; CI = cardiac index; SVR = systemic vascular resistance; PVR = pulmonary vascular resistance; PaOP = pulmonary artery occlusion pressure; N = normal; ↑ = increased; ↓ = decreased.

The most frequent cause of cardiogenic shock is acute myocardial infarction (AMI). Anterior MI is by far the most common type of infarction precipitating cardiogenic shock. In the case of an acute anterior wall MI, left anterior descending artery occlusion is usually detected. Lateral wall MIs are not often associated with cardiogenic shock. Inferior MI alone infrequently causes shock.

In the past cardiogenic shock was reported to occur in up to 15% to 20% of individuals with AMI, but with the advent of thrombolytic therapy the incidence has decreased to about 7%.[10,11] The majority of patients do not present initially in shock but develop this state during hospitalization and usually it is due to an infarct extension. The differential diagnosis of cardiogenic shock is summarized in Table 80.6.

Pathophysiology

Obstruction of coronary blood flow produces myocardial ischemia. Ischemia causes myocardial wall dysfunction, which is reversible if blood flow is reestablished. During these brief episodes of wall dysfunction, pulmonary edema may develop. However, wall motion abnormalities abate with restoration of blood flow, so heart failure usually responds to the usual aggressive management.

In acute MI, ischemia is not relieved. This results in cell necrosis. Loss of myocardial muscle results in irreversible impairment in myocardial contractility and ventricular performance. The resulting decline in cardiac output reduces arterial blood pressure and coronary perfusion pressure. This in turn leads to further cardiac ischemia and extension of the necrosis.

Cardiogenic shock often involves multivessel disease with substantial amount of myocardial damage. At autopsy more than two thirds of patients with cardiogenic shock demonstrated stenosis of 75% or more of luminal diameter of all

Table 80.6. **Differential Diagnosis of Cardiogenic Shock**

Acute myocardial infarction
Septal wall rupture
Dilated cardiomyopathy
Myocarditis
Pericardial tamponade
Right ventricular failure
Arrhythmias

three major coronary vessels and exhibited necrosis of at least 40% of the left ventricle.[12,13]

Diagnosis

The criteria for the diagnosis of cardiogenic shock include evidence of myocardial wall motion abnormalities combined with (1) hypotension with systolic blood pressure less than 90 mm Hg for at least 30 minutes and the need for vasopressors; (2) clinical evidence of end-organ dysfunction, e.g., cool clammy skin, altered mental status, oliguria (less than 20 mL/h); or (3) confirmatory hemodynamic features, i.e., pulmonary capillary wedge pressure (PCWP) >15 mm Hg and cardiac index <2.2 L/min/m^2.

In evaluating patients with cardiogenic shock, it is important to exclude mechanical complications (e.g., septal rupture, papillary muscle rupture, right ventricular infarction) because they may need urgent operative intervention. These complications can be detected quickly by echocardiography or angiography.

Management

When cardiac shock occurs, immediate resuscitative measures should be undertaken. Oxygenation should be optimized with obtaining a PaO$_2$ over 60 mm Hg as the goal. Noninvasive ventilation with bilevel positive airway pressure (BiPAP) or intubation and mechanical ventilation may be needed to achieve appropriate oxygenation. Fluid management should be carefully titrated to maintain filling pressure of the left ventricle but avoiding fluid overload. The hematocrit should be maintained at or greater than 30% to improve oxygen delivery to the myocardium.

Vasopressors and inotropic therapy are usually used in the management of cardiogenic shock, but should be considered as supportive and not curative. Supportive therapy without attempts to attain reperfusion does not appear to improve prognosis.

Vasoconstricting agents useful in the management of cardiogenic shock include dopamine, dobutamine and norepinephrine. Dopamine can be used at doses ranging between 5 and 20 μg/kg/min. Low doses help in renal and splanchnic blood flow by vasodilation (2–3 μg/kg/min). At doses of 4 to 6 μg/kg/min dopamine increases cardiac contractility and at higher doses (>10 μg/kg/min) increases blood pressure by activation of peripheral α-receptors. Dobutamine is a powerful inotropic agent and also reduces afterload by peripheral vasodilation. The dose of dobutamine is titrated for effect. The usual starting dose is 2 to 5 μg/kg/min and can be increased to 20 μg/kg/min. Norepinephrine also has α- and β-adrenergic activity and a potent vasoconstricting agent. Among these agents, dopamine is usually preferred because of the multiple effects that can be obtained simply by altering the infusion rate.

Intraaortic balloon pump counterpulsation (IABP) is another option to assist ventricular function and usually is performed on patients who do not respond to medical therapy. The balloon is inserted percutaneously via a femoral catheter and floated to the proximal aorta. The balloon then fills during diastole and deflates during systole. The function of the balloon is controlled electronically and is synchronized with the cardiac cycle. IABP is not a permanent solution, but allows for patient transfer to another facility and gives physicians time to initiate revascularization procedures to reverse ischemia. IABP has consistently been shown to lower in-hospital mortality.[14]

The key to treatment is obtaining revascularization of the threatened myocardium so that myocardial wall function is improved. This can be achieved either surgically or, for patients who present early in the process of an infarction, through clot lysis using a thrombolytic agent. Patients receiving either thrombolytic therapy or IABP have lower mortality rates than those not receiving these therapies. Combining the two approaches appears to confer even greater benefit than either alone.[15]

Even with aggressive management, outcomes for cardiogenic shock are poor. The randomized international SHOCK trial (*sh*ould we emergently revascularize *o*ccluded *c*oronaries for cardiogenic sho*ck*) assessed the effects on 30-day mortality of a direct invasive strategy (emergency early revascularization) compared with initial medical stabilization (including thrombolysis and IABP).[16] Overall, the trial enrolled 302 patients and showed no significant difference in the 30-day mortality for patients treated with early intervention compared to those who were treated with initial medical stabilization. However, when the trial looked at the subset of patients under the age of 75, early revascularization did show significant benefits. In this group, early revascularization was calculated to save 13 lives per 100 patients under age 75.

Sudden Cardiac Death (SCD)

According to the most widely used estimates, between 300,000 and 400,000 people die of sudden cardiac death in the United States every year.[17] Two age-related peaks occur: between 5 and 6 months of age and between 45 and 75 years of age.

In adults, coronary heart disease is by far the structural basis for at least 80% of SCD. Consequently, those at highest risk for coronary heart disease, such as men, are at higher risk for SCD. Additionally, poor cardiac function is a risk factor for SCD. In fact, an ejection fraction equal to or less than 30% is the single most powerful predictor for sudden cardiac death.[18]

It is important to have an understanding of the other causes of sudden cardiac death because recognizing them may be lifesaving. Table 80.7 reviews the causes of SCD.

Sudden Cardiac Death in Infants, Children, and Adolescents

An estimated 5,000 to 7,000 children die suddenly in the United States annually; this does not include the 5,000 to 7,000 deaths from sudden infant death syndrome (SIDS).[19] Those at highest risk are patients with congenital heart disease who have structural abnormalities that cannot be fully corrected. The development of severe pulmonary hypertension (Eisenmenger syndrome) confers the highest risk. A history of early or sudden unexplained death in other family members should raise the index of suspicion for congenital diseases that increase the risk of SCD such as hypertrophic

Table 80.7. **Causes of Sudden Cardiac Death**

Coronary artery abnormalities
    Coronary atherosclerosis
    Congenital abnormalities of coronary arteries
    Coronary arteritis
Hypertrophy
    Left ventricular hypertrophy with coronary artery disease
    Hypertensive heart disease
    Valvular heart disease
    Hypertrophic cardiomyopathy (HCM)
    Primary or secondary pulmonary hypertension
Myocardial disease
    Ischemic cardiomyopathy
    Alcoholic cardiomyopathy
    Postpartum cardiomyopathy
    Acute myocarditis
Congenital heart disease
Electrical abnormalities
    Fibrosis of conduction system
    Prolonged QT syndrome
    Drug effect
Miscellaneous
    Acute cardiac tamponade
    Massive pulmonary embolism
    Dissecting aneurysm of aorta
    Sudden infant death syndrome (SIDS)

cardiomyopathy, long QT syndrome, congenital coronary abnormalities, and Marfan syndrome. In children with family members with these disorders, symptoms of chest pain, palpitations, exertional dizziness or syncope may need to be investigated thoroughly before a benign cause is assigned for the symptoms.

In contrast to adults, coronary artery disease is rare in childhood and is usually associated with other disorders such as lipid abnormalities or infectious diseases like Kawasaki syndrome. Kawasaki syndrome is the most common cause of acquired coronary artery disease in infants and young children (see Chapter 18). SCD occurs in 1% to 2% of patients with untreated Kawasaki syndrome.

Unfortunately for most patients, SCD may be the presenting symptom in many cases, and the underlying condition(s) may be discovered only at the time of autopsy. Although SCD is relatively uncommon, its psychosocial impact is devastating.

Sudden infant death syndrome is defined as sudden death of an apparently healthy infant whose death remains unexplained even after autopsy. Risk factors for SIDS are prematurity, infants of teenage mothers, and exposure to tobacco and cocaine. Apnea is considered to be the main etiology but occlusive lesions of the cardiac conduction tissue arteries have been demonstrated in some children.[20] An observational study by Schwartz et al[21] suggested that abnormal prolongation of QT interval may be the cause of SIDS.

Sudden Death in Young and Middle-Aged Athletes

The incidence of sudden cardiac death in athletes is low and the cause varies with the age of the population studied. In young competitive athletes hypertrophic cardiomyopathy

(HCM) is the most frequent cause followed by aberrant coronary arteries. For individuals older than 35 years, coronary artery atherosclerosis is by far the most common cause of sudden cardiac death. These individuals tend to start running at an older age and usually have a strong family history of heart disease or have other recognized risk factors.

Some studies estimate that up to 50% of sudden death in young athletes are due to HCM.[22] Some of the older terms used to describe the condition were *idiopathic hypertrophic subaortic stenosis* (IHSS), *hypertrophic obstructive cardiomyopathy* (HOCM), and *muscular subaortic stenosis*. The characteristic physiologic abnormality is diastolic dysfunction and increased left end-diastolic pressure, which results in pulmonary congestion and dyspnea.

HCM is an autosomal-dominant disease and is identified most often in adults in their 30s and 40s. The majority of the patients are asymptomatic. If patients do experience problems, the most common complaint is dyspnea. Other less common symptoms include angina, fatigue, dizziness on exertion, presyncope, and syncope. On physical examination of patients with HCM the apical impulse is often displaced laterally and forceful. A systolic murmur is sometimes present that resembles aortic stenosis but usually does not radiate to the neck vessels and increases in intensity with Valsalva maneuver and standing. The ECG is usually abnormal in symptomatic patients with evidence of left ventricular hypertrophy (LVH) and ST segment and T wave abnormalities. Prominent Q waves in leads II and III, AVF, and sometimes in the precordial leads can also be seen. Echocardiogram shows the characteristic features of the hypertrophied septum, outflow tract obstruction, and diastolic dysfunction. Screening asymptomatic athletes with echocardiogram is not cost-effective because of the low prevalence of the disease.

The mechanisms of sudden death in HCM include tachyarrhythmias or ischemia from small vessel disease.[23] Beta-blockers remain the mainstay of medical therapy, and dual-chamber pacemakers and surgery are options for the high-risk patient.[24,25]

Causes of sudden death in athletes are summarized in Table 80.8.

Sudden Death in Dilated Cardiomyopathy and Heart Failure

Patients with coronary heart disease are living longer with the aggressive therapeutic interventions over the last two decades. However, while people live longer the proportion of patients with stable heart failure who die suddenly has

Table 80.8. Causes of Sudden Cardiac Death in Athletes

Coronary atherosclerosis
Hypertrophic cardiomyopathy
Idiopathic left ventricular hypertrophy
Right ventricular hypertrophy
Coronary artery anomalies
Long QT syndrome
Myocarditis

Table 80.9. Potential Problems Associated with an Implantable Cardiac Defibrillator (ICD)

Potential problems with insertion or maintenance
  Frequent shocks
  Infection or hematoma at time of insertion
  Pacing malfunction
  Lead dislodgment
Special precautions for patients with ICD
  Procedures needing electrocautery
  Magnetic resonance imaging (MRI) is contraindicated
  ICD may continue to function after death (need to disconnect)

increased.[26] The primary mechanism of death appears to be due to an acute arrhythmia. In particular, a high incidence of ventricular arrhythmias has been observed during follow-up of patients with aortic valve surgery, multiple valve surgery or cardiomegaly.[27]

For patients who have experienced an acute arrhythmia or who are found to be at high risk for sudden cardiac death, an implantable cardiac defibrillator (ICD) may be lifesaving. ICDs are multiprogrammable devices capable of delivering high-energy defibrillation shocks, antitachycardia pacing, and pacing for bradyarrhythmias. The unit runs on a battery that has a charge capacity that varies from 5 to 9 years.

Two recent major trials have shown convincingly that ICD is superior to antiarrhythmic drugs in certain situations. The Antiarrhythmics Versus Implantable Defibrillators (AVID) trial showed significantly better survival rate over a 3-year

Table 80.10. Algorithm for Recent Cardiopulmonary Resuscitation (CPR) Protocols

Primary ABCD survey
(airway, breathing, circulation, defibrillate)
↓
Assess rhythm after first three shocks
↓
If persistent or recurrent ventricular fibrillation/tachycardia
↓
Secondary ABCD survey
Place airway device, confirm breathing, establish circulation by inserting intravenous line, and differential diagnosis for reversible causes
↓
1 mg epinephrine intravenously and repeat every 3–5 min
or
40 units of vasopressin intravenous, one time dose
↓
Resume attempt to defibrillate
↓
Consider antiarrhythmics
Amiodarone for persistent or recurrent ventricular fibrillation/tachycardia
Lidocaine for persistent of recurrent ventricular fibrillation/tachycardia
Magnesium for hypomagnesemic patient
Procainamide
↓
Resume attempts to defibrillate

Table 80.11. **Some Medications Useful in CPR**

Medication	Indication	Adult dose
Amiodarone	VF or pulseless V-tach	300 mg initial followed by 150 mg repeated doses
	Stable V-tach	150 mg over 10 min followed by 1 mg/min infusion for 6 hours, then 0.5 mg/min
	Supraventricular tachycardia	Same as stable V-tach
Atropine	Bradycardia	0.5–1.0 mg IV every 3–5 minutes
	Asystole	1 mg IV repeated every 3–5 minutes
Epinephrine	VF or pulseless V-tach	1 mg IV repeated every 3–5 minutes
	Pulseless electrical activity	As above
	Asystole	As above
	Bradycardia unresponsive to atropine	1–10 μg/min IV titrated to heart rate
Lidocaine	VF or pulseless V-tach	1–1.5 mg/kg IV may repeat in 3–5 minutes
Vasopressin	VF or pulseless V-tach	40 units single dose

V-tach = ventricular tachycardia; VF = ventricular fibrillation.
Source: Adapted with permission from Eisenberg and Mengert.[35] Copyright© 2001 Massachusetts Medical Society. All rights reserved.

follow-up in patients who had survived a near-fatal ventricular fibrillation or had sustained ventricular tachycardia.[28] The Multicenter Automatic Defibrillator Implantation Trial (MADIT) included patients with low ejection fraction and episodes of unsustained ventricular tachycardia, and compared ICD with no therapy.[29] The trial was terminated prematurely because of a marked survival benefit with ICDs. After ICD placement, routine visits at 3- to 6-month intervals are arranged for pacing malfunction and battery failure. Some of the emergencies for patients with ICD are highlighted in Table 80.9.

In patients with an ICD, antibiotic prophylaxis is not recommended for procedures that may induce bacteremia.[30] However, an ICD should be disabled during electrocautery use. An ICD constitutes a strong contraindication to magnetic resonance imaging (MRI). ICD system infection is an uncommon problem but will need removal of the system and IV antibiotics to eradicate infection.[31]

ICDs may have to be inactivated in terminally ill patients when frequent arrhythmias triggers ICD shocks. Consent to inactivate the ICD should be specifically obtained even in a patient with a do-not-resuscitate order.[32] In a patient who is pacemaker dependent, inactivating the ICD bradycardia pacing is not recommended as this may be mistakenly interpreted as physician-assisted suicide. Careful counseling and an informed consent should be in place before deactivating ICD devices.

Cardiopulmonary Resuscitation

More than 200,000 people in the United States die suddenly each year from coronary artery disease before they reach the hospital. An estimated 500,000 patients also will experience a cardiac arrest during their hospitalization.[33] Cardiopulmonary resuscitation (CPR) was designed to intervene in these circumstances and restore a normal cardiac rhythm so that the underlying disease can be addressed and normal health restored.

CPR is guided by protocols approved by the American Heart Association. These protocols are reviewed and updated periodically. The last review was completed in 2000. The published Guidelines 2000 for CPR and Emergency Cardiovascular Care[34] is the first attempt to base recommendation on evidence and make them adaptable to the resources available in different countries.

The fundamentals of CPR have remained the same for the past several decades and continue to include four basic sequential steps: (1) the call for help, (2) chest compression and mouth-to-mouth resuscitation, (3) rapid defibrillation, and (4) medical management of specific cardiac arrhythmias. An algorithm for progressing through CPR is shown in Table 80.10. The prognosis for patients with pulseless electrical activity and asystole is very poor. Potentially treatable conditions should be addressed first. The failure to identify a treatable condition signals poor likelihood to respond to resuscitation efforts.

Common rhythm disturbances encountered in cardiac arrest include ventricular fibrillation, pulseless ventricular tachycardia, pulseless electrical activity, and asystole. Medications useful in cardiac resuscitation are listed in Table 80.11.[35]

Two changes in the CPR protocols should be highlighted. First is the addition of vasopressin for use in patients with shock-resistance ventricular fibrillation. There are no data on the performance of vasopressin in cardiac arrest, but the consensus conference adopting current recommendations believed that this drug would be more effective than epinephrine in shock-resistant ventricular fibrillation. Second is the addition of amiodarone as the antiarrhythmic of choice for most ventricular arrhythmias. The substitution of amiodarone for other antiarrhythmics is based on evidence from the Amiodarone for Resuscitation After Out-of-Hospital Cardiac Arrest Due to Ventricular Fibrillation (ARREST) trial. In this study, patients who received amiodarone had improved survival in shock-resistant ventricular fibrillation. No other antiarrhythmics, including lidocaine, has demonstrated any effectiveness in this situation.

A number of controversies persist in the use of CPR. These include issues such as when CPR should be terminated for patients who are not responding, and when CPR is not appropriate. These issues require further clarification and at the present time are left to the best judgment of the clinician caring for the patient and to the family.

References

1. Kapoor WN, Karpf M, Wieland S, et al. A prospective evaluation and follow-up of patients with syncope. N Engl J Med 1983; 309;197–204.
2. Kapoor WN. Evaluation and management of the patient with syncope. JAMA 1992;268:2553–60.
3. Manolis AS, Linzer M, Salem D, Estes NAM. Syncope: current diagnostic evaluation and management. Ann Intern Med 1990; 112:850–63.
4. Linzer M, Yang EH, Estes M, et al. Diagnosing syncope: part 1: value of history, physical examination, and electrocardiography. Ann Intern Med 1997;126:989–96.
5. Linzer M, Prystowsky EN, Brunetti LL, et al. Recurrent syncope of unknown origin diagnosed by ambulatory continuous loop ECG recording. Am Heart J 1988;116:1632–4.
6. Davis TL, Freeman FR. Electroencephalography should not be routine in the evaluation of syncope in adults. Arch Intern Med 1990;150;2027–9.
7. Willis J. Syncope. Pediatr Rev 2000;21:201–3.
8. Braden DS, Games CH. The diagnosis and management of syncope in children and adolescents. Pediatr Ann 1997;26:422–6.
9. Lerman-Sagie T, Lerman P, Mukamel M, Blieden L, Mimouni M. A prospective evaluation of pediatric patients with syncope. Clin Pediatr 1994;33:66–70.
10. Scheidt S, Ascheim R, Killip T. Shock after acute myocardial infarction: a clinical and hemodynamic profile. Am J Cardiol 1970;26:556.
11. Califf RM, Bengston JR. Cardiogenic shock. N Engl J Med 1994;330:1724.
12. Wackers FJ, Lie KI, Becker AE, et al. Coronary artery disease in patients dying from cardiogenic shock or congestive heart failure in the setting of acute myocardial infarction. Br Heart J 1976;38:906.
13. Page DL, Caulfield JB, Kastor JA, et al. Myocardial changes associated with cardiogenic shock. N Engl J Med 1971;285:133.
14. Waksman R, Weiss AT, Gotsman MS, Hasin Y. Intraaortic counterpulsation improves survival in cardiogenic shock complicating acute myocardial infarction. Eur Health J 1993;14: 1–74.
15. Sanborn TA, Sleeper LA, Bates ER, et al, for the SHOCK Investigators. Impact of thrombolysis, aortic counterpulsation, and their combination in cardiogenic shock: a report from the SHOCK Trial registry. J Am Coll Cardiol 2000;36:1123–9.
16. Hochman JS, Sleeper LA, Godfrey E, et al, for the SHOCK Investigators. Should we emergently revascularize occluded coronaries for cardiogenic shock? An international randomized trial of emergency PTCA/CABG-Trial design. Am Heart J 1999;137: 313–21.
17. Myerburg RJ, Kessler KM, Castellanos A. Sudden cardiac death: epidemiology, transient risk, and intervention assessment. Ann Intern Med 1993;119:1187.
18. Bigger JT, Fleiss JL, Kleiger R, et al. The relationships among ventricular arrhythmias, left ventricular dysfunction and mortality in the 2 years after myocardial infarction. Circulation 1984;69:250.
19. Driscoll DJ, Edwards WD. Sudden unexpected death in children and adolescents. J Am Coll Cardiol 1985;5:118B–21B.
20. Anderson KR, Hill RW. Occlusive lesions of the cardiac conduction tissue arteries in sudden infant death syndrome. Pediatrics 1982;69:50.
21. Schwartz PJ, Stramba-Badiale M, Segantini A, et al. Prolongation of the QT interval and the sudden infant death syndrome. N Engl J Med 1998;338:1709–14.
22. Maron BJ, Epstein SE, Roberts WC. Causes of sudden death in competitive athletes. J Am Coll Cardiol 1986;7:240.
23. Maron BJ, Roberts WC, McAllister HA, et al. Sudden death in young athletes. Circulation 1980;62:218–29.
24. Fananapazir L, Cannon RO III, Tripodi D, et al. Impact of dual chamber permanent pacing in patients with obstructive hypertrophic cardiomyopathy with symptoms refractory to verapamil and beta adrenergic blocker therapy. Circulation 1992;85:2149.
25. Robbins RC, Stinson EB. Long term results of left ventricular myotomy and myectomy for obstructive hypertrophic cardiomyopathy. J Thorac Cardiovasc Surg 1996;111:586.
26. Packer M. Sudden unexpected death in patients with congestive heart failure: a second frontier. Circulation 1985;72:681.
27. Konishi Y, Matsuda K, Nishiwaki N, et al. Ventricular arrhythmias late after aortic and/or mitral valve replacement. Jpn Circ J 1985;49:576.
28. The Antiarrhythmics Versus Implantable Defibrillators (AVID) Investigators. A comparison of antiarrhythmic drug therapy with implantable defibrillators in patients resuscitated from near fatal ventricular arrhythmias. N Engl J Med 1997;337:1569–75.
29. Moss AJ, Hall WJ, Cannon DS, et al. Improved survival with an implanted defibrillator in patients with coronary disease at high risk for ventricular arrhythmia. N Engl J Med 1996;335: 1933–40.
30. Dajani AS, Taubert KA, Wilson W, et al. Prevention of bacterial endocarditis. Recommendations by the American Heart Association. JAMA 1997;277:1794.
31. O'Nunain S, Perez I, Roelke M, et al. The treatment of patients with infected implantable cardioverter defibrillator systems. J Thorac Cardiovasc Surg 1997;133:121–9.
32. Braun TC, Hagen NA, Hatfield RE et al. Cardiac pacemakers and implantable defibrillators in terminal care. J Pain Symptom Manag 1999;18:126–131.
33. Ballew KA, Philbrick JT. Causes of variation in reported in-hospital CPR survival: a critical review. Resuscitation 1995;30:203–15.
34. Guidelines 2000 for cardiopulmonary resuscitation and emergency cardiovascular care: international consensus on science. Circulation 2000;102(suppl 1):1–138.
35. Eisenberg MS, Mengert TJ. Cardiac resuscitation. N Engl J Med 2001;344:1304–13.

81
Venous Thromboembolism

Glenn S. Rodriguez and Thomas M. Schwartz

Venous thromboembolism causes substantial disability and death. The incidence of deep venous thrombosis (DVT) is about 1 per 1000 person years. The most serious and potentially preventable complication, pulmonary embolus, kills an estimated 50,000 Americans each year.[1] Venous stasis secondary to chronic valvular incompetence, often a consequence of venous thrombosis, causes varying degrees of pain, edema, and ulceration. The changing demographic patterns, particularly the aging of society, are increasing the risk of venous thromboembolism and the importance of prevention. Recent identification of inherited defects causing thrombosis (inherited thrombophilias) allows improved prevention through identification of individuals at high risk. The knowledge and tools for effective prevention and treatment are available but currently underused.[2] Early identification, office-based diagnostic tests, safer treatments, and targeted education programs for physicians may offer the chance to reduce the incidence of venous thromboembolism and associated morbidity.

Pathophysiology

Virchow hypothesized three factors that predispose a person to venous thrombosis: a hypercoagulable state, injury to the vascular intima, and venous stasis. A century of research has verified this hypothesis. DVT is now understood to be a multifactorial disorder, involving a combination of genetic risk factors and acquired conditions.[3] Known genetic causes are present in 25% of unselected DVT cases and 63% of familial cases.[4] This percentage will probably increase as research identifies more genetic causes. Some conditions that predispose to thrombosis have both genetic and acquired components. Examples are elevated levels of factor VIII[5] and high plasma homocysteine levels. Stasis is the most common precipitating factor. Vascular injury is often the result of surgery or trauma.

A hypercoagulable state results from a disruption of the normal balance between the procoagulant system and the anticoagulant system. The natural anticoagulant system works to confine a beneficial thrombosis to the site of injury and prevent propagation. Major components of this system include antithrombin III, protein C, and protein S. Protein C is activated to the enzyme APC, which functions as a natural anticoagulant by inactivating procoagulant factors Va and VIIIa in the presence of protein S. Antithrombin III directly inhibits thrombin.

Modern molecular genetics is rapidly elucidating the prothrombotic mutations that contribute to hypercoagulable states. The anticoagulant system is impaired by the factor V Leiden mutation, and by deficiencies of proteins C and S and antithrombin. Raised plasma levels of prothrombin 20210A and factor VIII increase risk by accelerating the procoagulant system.

Epidemiology

Reliable incidence data for DVT are not available. Autopsy series show that DVT is often present when not clinically suspected, so hospital discharge diagnosis and death certificate data underestimate the true prevalence. Declining autopsy rates in the United States compound the problem. The best incidence data are from Malmö General Hospital in Sweden, which has maintained an autopsy rate greater than 75% since 1957. The incidence of DVT and fatal pulmonary embolism has been remarkably stable at 35%, representing 9% of all hospital deaths.[6] The Worcester DVT study, a regional survey of hospital discharge diagnoses, reported a diagnosis of DVT in 0.9% of all hospital discharges. The incidence rate increased exponentially with age, rising by a factor of approximately 200 between ages 20 and 80 years.[7] Studies using screening techniques to evaluate hospitalized patients identified surgery of the pelvis or lower extremity and anes-

Table 81.1. **Prevalence of Risk Factors for Thrombosis**

Factor	General population[a]	Patients with thrombosis (%)
Genetic		
Factor V Leiden mutation (APC resistance)	~1 in 20	~20[b]
Prothrombin 20210A	~1 in 50	~6
Protein C deficiency	~1 in 300	~3
Protein S deficiency	~1 in 300	~1–2
Antithrombin deficiency	~1 in 3000	~1
Mixed (genetic and acquired components)		
High concentration factor VIII	1 in 10	25
Hyperhomocystinemia	1 in 20	10

[a]Varies significantly in different ethnic populations.

[b]Up to 60% in pregnant patients with deep venous thrombosis (DVT).

thesia lasting more than 30 minutes as the highest risk events (see Chapter 57). More patients hospitalized for medical reasons experience an episode of DVT than did surgical patients because of the greater number of total admissions.

Table 81.1 lists the prevalence of risk factors for venous thrombosis.[3] The most common inherited thrombophilia is APC resistance caused by a point mutation producing an abnormal protein known as factor V Leiden. It is present in 5% of Caucasian Americans but has a much lower prevalence in other ethnic groups.[8,9] Women with the factor V Leiden mutation are at increased risk for DVT when taking oral contraceptives. The lifetime risk for DVT in factor V Leiden heterozygotes is approximately 10% and for homozygotes is >80%. Direct molecular genetic testing for the R506Q mutation in the factor V gene is available. Genetic testing can distinguish homozygotes and is the definitive test. The American College of Medical Genetics recommendations for who should be tested for factor V Leiden are listed in Table 81.2.[10] General population screening is not recommended.

Clinical Approach

A logical set of principles are basic to the structure of the clinical approach:

1. Venous thrombosis is common. Thrombosis results when an individual with an inherited predisposition to thrombo-

Table 81.2. **American College of Medical Genetics (ACMG) Guidelines for Factor V Leiden Testing**

Testing is recommended for individuals who have:
  Any venous thrombosis and are <50 years of age
  Venous thrombosis in unusual sites
  Recurrent venous thrombosis at any age
  Venous thrombosis and a strong family history of thrombotic disease
  Venous thrombosis during pregnancy or in women taking oral contraceptives
  Relatives with venous thrombosis who are under age 50

sis suffers venous stasis or vascular injury. Testing to identify the causes of thrombophilia is important.

2. The location of the thrombus is important. The primary source (90%) of pulmonary emboli is the deep veins of the proximal lower extremities. Thrombi limited to the calf pose limited risk (<5%) of pulmonary embolism, but extension to proximal veins occurs.[11] This point is critical to the diagnostic approach outlined in this chapter.

3. Pulmonary embolism is not an independent disease but a complication of DVT. Pulmonary embolism is discussed in Chapter 86.

4. Pulmonary embolism kills quickly; 75% to 90% of those affected die within the first few hours. With limited opportunity for effective diagnosis and treatment, identification of high-risk individuals and primary prevention of DVT is the goal.

Prevention

The key to prevention of thromboembolism is physician recognition of patients at risk, vigorous use of effective treatment, and prophylactic regimens. Selection of appropriate treatments to prevent DVT is imperative whenever a hypercoagulable state is identified or when venous stasis or vascular injury is likely. The 1986 National Institutes of Health (NIH) Consensus Conference outlined such a strategy, and it has been updated.[12] Prophylactic regimens to prevent DVT are discussed in Chapter 57.

Clinical Risk Stratification

Evaluation of the patient with suspected DVT begins with a thorough history and physical examination. DVT occurs predominantly in patients with clinical risk factors. The limita-

Table 81.3. **Clinical Risk Factors and Physical Findings Associated with Deep Venous Thrombosis (DVT)**

Risk factors	Physical findings
Active malignancy	Localized tenderness along distribution of deep veins
Recently bedridden	Unilateral pitting edema
Recent paralysis/paresis	Thigh or calf swelling >3 cm compared to the asymptomatic limb
Recent limb immobilization	Dilated superficial (nonvaricose) veins in symptomatic limb only
Trauma	Erythema in symptomatic limb only
Hospital or nursing home confinement	
Pregnancy/puerperium	
Strong family history of DVT	

tions of physical examination to identify DVT are well known, but physical findings are useful when present. Table 81.3[13,16] lists clinical risk factors and findings that are associated with DVT. Formal clinical risk scoring systems have been developed to stratify patients with suspected first DVT into low, moderate and high-risk groups. Risk stratification then helps guide evaluation as described below, especially the need for follow-up evaluation if initial studies are negative.[13–16]

Diagnostic Tests

D-Dimer Assay

D-dimer, a degradation product of cross-linked fibrin, is released into the blood during fibrinolysis. D-dimer testing is highly sensitive, but has poor specificity in the diagnosis of DVT because many conditions can lead to elevated serum D-dimer levels.[17] It has been studied as an adjunctive test to help rule out DVT. There are several types of D-dimer assays currently available for clinical use, including enzyme-linked immunosorbent assay (ELISA), latex agglutination, and whole blood agglutination. ELISA testing is very accurate, but the conventional test takes at least several hours and may not be practical for clinical use. Several rapid ELISAs that can be run in less than an hour are now available and have sensitivity that is roughly equivalent to standard ELISA.[18] Latex agglutination assays are inexpensive and rapid, but lack sufficient sensitivity to be useful as screening tests.[19] Whole blood agglutination assays have several advantages. They require only a drop of blood, rather than plasma, and provide results in as little as 2 minutes. Their sensitivity is reported to be similar to that of ELISA.[20] Two studies suggest that DVT can be reliably ruled out in low-risk patients using formal risk stratification in whom whole blood agglutination assay D-dimer testing is negative.[15,16]

Ultrasonography/Duplex Scanning

Real-time compression ultrasonography has been demonstrated to be a reliable technique for noninvasive evaluation of proximal venous thrombosis.[21,22] With this technique the veins under evaluation are visualized and the ability to compress the vein with probe pressure measured. The technique is accurate for thrombi above the knee, with sensitivity and specificity reported to be more than 90% in most series. It is less useful for diagnosing thrombi below the knee. Real-time ultrasonography is widely available, but the reliability of the results may vary with the expertise of the technologist performing the study. Duplex scanning combines real-time ultrasonography with a pulsed Doppler study to diagnose DVT.[23] The reported sensitivity and specificity of this test ranges from 85% to 95%. It also is of limited value for diagnosing calf thrombi.

Duplex scanning should not be confused with a Doppler study. Doppler evaluation of the lower extremity requires only a small hand-held unit and does not use B-mode ultrasonography. It detects only venous occlusion, so significant mural thrombi may be missed. The test has poor sensitivity and no role as a definitive diagnostic test.

Contrast Venography

Contrast venography has long been considered the standard by which all other diagnostic tests for DVT are measured. Performed according to defined techniques, it is highly accurate and has the advantage of reliably diagnosing thrombosis below the knee.[24] Risks include phlebitis, contrast allergy, local extravasation of dye, and discomfort. The overall complication rate is 4%, and the risk of major complications due to a contrast reaction is 1%. Its main use currently is in the evaluation of high-risk patients with a negative compression ultrasound or for diagnosis of recurrent DVT.

Other Diagnostic Tests

Impedance plethysmography and radiofibrinogen scanning are other tests that have been used in the past for diagnosis of DVT. Because of the wide availability of compression ultrasonography, these tests are now rarely used.

Diagnostic Approach

Many diagnostic strategies for the evaluation of DVT have been proposed,[25] and the preferred strategy will likely change over time. Based on current data we propose the diagnostic approach outlined in Figure 81.1. Using this approach, the evaluation of the patient with suspected DVT should begin with clinical risk stratification. Existing formal scoring systems that allow rapid stratification of patients as low, moderate, or high risk have been clinically validated.[13,16] Moderate- and high-risk patients should promptly undergo compression ultrasound or duplex scanning. A negative study in these patients should be followed by either venography or repeat ultrasound within 1 week. Patients with low clinical risk may undergo D-dimer testing or immediate ultrasound. If D-dimer or ultrasound is negative, then further evaluation is not required. Patients with a positive D-dimer should have ultrasound. Patients with a positive ultrasound or venogram should be treated with anticoagulation.

Treatment

The diagnosis of proximal DVT requires prompt institution of anticoagulation with heparin or low molecular weight heparin. The traditional approach is intravenous administration of unfractionated heparin. Standard heparin is a heterogeneous mixture of polysaccharide chains ranging in molecular weight from about 3,000 to 30,000. It acts by binding to plasma antithrombin III and inactivating thrombin and factor Xa. These enzymes are protected by fibrin, so higher doses are required to stop extension of a thrombus than to prevent its initial formation. Heparin does not directly prevent embolism or promote thrombus dissolution.

Heparin therapy is usually administered intravenously with an initial 80 U/kg bolus followed by continuous infusion of 18 U/kg/h.[26] The goal of therapy is to maintain the partial thromboplastin time (PTT) at 1.5 to 2.0 times the control value. Optimal timing of PTT measurements has yet to be firmly established. The American College of Chest Physicians

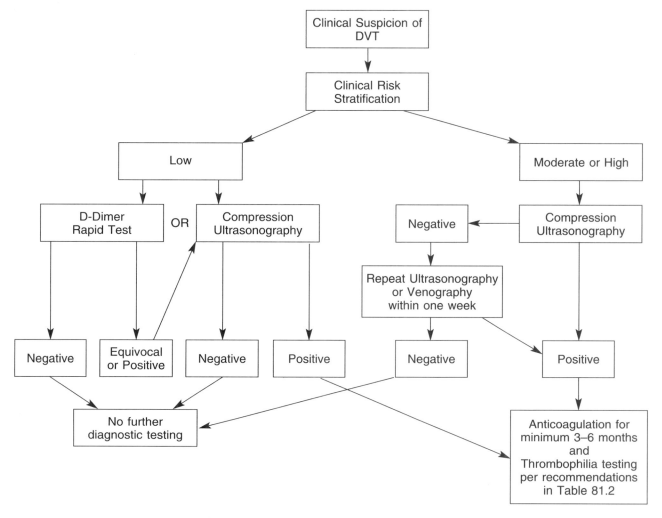

Fig. 81.1. Diagnostic approach to the patient with suspected lower extremity deep venous thrombosis (DVT).

(ACCP) recommends treating with heparin for 4 to 5 days, until warfarin therapy increases the international normalized ratio (INR) to the 2.0 to 3.0 range. The INR is a worldwide system used to standardize prothrombin times among laboratories.

The major complications of heparin therapy include hemorrhage, thrombocytopenia, osteoporosis, and anaphylaxis. The risk of hemorrhage increases with age, significant coexistent illness, and the presence of known bleeding sites. Platelet count should be checked daily to monitor for thrombocytopenia during heparin therapy. The effects of heparin can be terminated by intravenous injection of protamine sulfate.

Low molecular weight heparins (LMWHs) are fragments of standard heparin with mean molecular weights of 4000 to 6000. There are three LMWHs available in the United States: dalteparin, enoxaparin, and tinzaparin. LMWHs are theoretically superior to unfractionated heparin because of greater anticoagulant specificity (primary action on factor Xa), a more predictable anticoagulant response, fewer complications, and a longer plasma half-life.[27] Many studies have evaluated specific LMWHs for the treatment of DVT, and a meta-analysis concluded that LMWHs administered subcutaneously in fixed doses, adjusted for body weight, and without laboratory monitoring are more effective and safer than adjusted-dose standard heparin.[28] A Cochrane Database systematic review found LMWH to be at least as effective as heparin in preventing recurrent thromboembolism with lower risk of hemorrhage and lower overall mortality.[29] Although LMWHs are more expensive on a per-unit basis, they may lower the total cost of treatment per episode of DVT. LMWH should be continued for 4 to 5 days until the patient is therapeutic on warfarin with an INR of 2.0 to 3.0.[26]

Two studies have compared the safety and efficacy of subcutaneous LMWH administered at home with intravenous heparin in the hospital.[30,31] These studies demonstrated equivalent safety and efficacy. However, 30% to 60% of potentially eligible patients were excluded from the studies because of additional risk factors. A more recent study compared treatment of DVT with LMWH in hospital for 10 days vs. starting therapy at home.[32] There was no significant difference in outcome between the two groups; however, total costs for the home treatment group were 56% less than the costs for the hospital treat-

Table 81.4. **Relative and Absolute Contraindications to Home Treatment of DVT**

Concurrent pulmonary embolism
Active bleeding or high clinical risk for bleeding
    Familial bleeding disorder
    Thrombocytopenia
    Severe liver disease
Hemodynamic instability
Limited cardiopulmonary reserve
Significant renal insufficiency
Pregnancy
Severe leg pain and swelling
Uncertain compliance or follow-up

ment group. Home-based treatment of DVT with LMWH is becoming more common. Effective protocols for home therapy with LMWH involve a multidisciplinary approach including the physician, pharmacy, and home health nurse. Contraindications to home treatment are listed in Table 81.4.[33]

After treatment with heparin or LMWH, anticoagulation is continued with warfarin. Warfarin should be started concurrently with heparin or LMWH. The duration of warfarin therapy is controversial.[34] The ACCP guideline gives the following recommendations regarding duration of anticoagulation: 3 to 6 months for DVT associated with transient known risk (e.g., surgery), >6 months for idiopathic DVT, and lifelong therapy for recurrent DVT or if associated with a persistent risk factor.[26] The dosage of warfarin is adjusted to maintain a prothrombin time approximately 1.5 times control or an INR of 2.0 to 3.0.[26]

Anticoagulation therapy carries substantial risk of hemorrhage. Warfarin has a narrow therapeutic ratio and is a major cause of preventable adverse drug reactions. Current recommendations suggest daily measurement of the prothrombin time during initiation of warfarin therapy. Once the INR is in the therapeutic range for two consecutive measurements, weekly monitoring is acceptable. The measurement interval can be extended to 2 to 4 weeks for patients on long-term anticoagulation with stable prothrombin times.[26,33] Optimal management of anticoagulation therapy requires a coordinated program of patient education, drug–drug and drug–food interaction detection, systematic adjustment of warfarin dosage based on prothrombin times, fail-safe systems to communicate the recommendations to patients, and implementation of a patient registry. Organized anticoagulation clinics are cost-effective and demonstrate superior outcomes.[35]

Thrombolytic therapy for DVT has been investigated because it theoretically could prevent postphlebitic syndrome by lysing the clot. It may be appropriate for selected patients with massive iliofemoral DVT. Unfortunately, studies of this therapy have shown a significant increase in major hemorrhage and it is not generally recommended for uncomplicated DVT.[33,36]

References

1. Silverstein MD, Heit JA, Mohr DN, Petterson TM, O'Fallon WM, Melton LJ. Trends in the incidence of deep vein thrombosis and pulmonary embolism: a 25-year population-based cohort study. Arch Intern Med 1998;158:585–93.
2. Anderson FA, Wheeler HB, Goldberg RJ, et al. Physician practices in the prevention of venous thromboembolism. Ann Intern Med 1991;115:591–5.
3. Rosendaal FR. Venous thrombosis: prevalence and interaction of risk factors. Haemostasis 1999;29(suppl S1):1–9.
4. Heijboer H, Brandjes DPM, Buller HR, Sturk A, ten Cate JW. Deficiencies of coagulation-inhibiting and fibrinolytic proteins in outpatients with deep-vein thrombosis. N Engl J Med 1990;323:1512–16.
5. Kyrle P, Minar E, Hirschl M, et al. High plasma levels of factor VIII and the risk of recurrent venous thromboembolism. N Engl J Med 2000;343:457–62.
6. Lindblad B, Sernby NH, Bergqvist D. Incidence of venous thromboembolism verified by necropsy over 30 years. BMJ 1991;302:709–11.
7. Anderson FA, Wheeler HB, Goldberg RJ, et al. A population-based perspective of the hospital incidence and case-fatality rates of deep vein thrombosis and pulmonary embolism. Arch Intern Med 1991;1512:933–8.
8. Ridker PM, Miletich UP, Hennekens CH, Buring JE. Ethnic distribution of factor V Leiden in 4047 men and women: implications for venous thromboembolism screening. JAMA 1997;227:1305–7.
9. Gregg JP, Yamane A, Grody WW. The prevalence of the factor V Leiden mutation in four distinct American ethnic populations. Am J Med Genet 1997;73:334–6.
10. Grody W, Griffen J, Taylor A, Korf B, Heit J. American college of medical genetics consensus statement on factor V Leiden mutation testing. Genet Med 2001;3(2)139–48.
11. Philbrick JT, Becker DM. Calf deep venous thrombosis: a wolf in sheep's clothing? Arch Intern Med 1988;148:2131–8.
12. Clagett GP, Anderson FA, Heit J, et al. Prevention of venous thromboembolism. Chest 1995;108:321S–34S.
13. Wells PS, Anderson DR, Bormanis J, et al. Value of assessment of pretest probability of deep-vein thrombosis in clinical management. Lancet 1997;350:1795–8.
14. Miron MJ, Perrier A, Bounameaux H. Clinical assessment of suspected deep vein thrombosis: comparison between a score and empirical assessment. J Intern Med 2000;247(2):249–54.
15. Kearon C, Ginsberg JS, Douketis J, et al. Management of suspected deep venous thrombosis in outpatients by using clinical assessment and D-dimer testing. Ann Intern Med 2001;135:108–11.
16. Lennox AF, Delis KT, Serunkuma S, et al. Combination of a clinical risk assessment score and rapid whole blood D-dimer testing in the diagnosis of deep vein thrombosis in symptomatic patients. J Vasc Surg 1999;30:794–804.
17. Brill-Edwards B, Lee A. D-dimer testing in the diagnosis of acute venous thromboembolism. Thromb Haemost 1999;82(2):688–94.
18. Lee AY, Ginsberg JS. Laboratory diagnosis of venous thromboembolism. Baillieres Clin Haematol 1998;11:1–18.
19. Becker DM, Philbrick JT, Bachhuber TL, Humphries JE. D-dimer testing and acute venous thromboembolism. A shortcut to accurate diagnosis? Arch Intern Med 1996;156:939–46.
20. Wells PS, Brill-Edwards P, Stevens P, et al. A novel and rapid whole-blood assay for D-dimer in patients with clinically suspected deep vein thrombosis. Circulation 1995;91:2184–7.
21. Perrier A, Desmarais S, Miron M, et al. Non-invasive diagnosis of venous thromboembolism in outpatients. Lancet 1999;353:190–5.
22. Cogo A, Lensing A, Koopman M, et al. Compression ultrasonography for diagnostic management of patients with clinically suspected deep vein thrombosis: prospective cohort study. BMJ 1998;316:17–20.
23. Langsfeld M, Hershey FB, Thorpe L, et al. Duplex B-mode im-

aging for the diagnosis of deep venous thrombosis. Arch Surg 1987;122:587–91.

24. Hull R, Hirsh J, Sackett DL, et al. Clinical validity of a negative venogram in patients with clinically suspected venous thrombosis. Circulation 1981;64:622–5.

25. Kearon C, Julian J, Math M, Newman T, Ginsberg J. Noninvasive diagnosis for deep venous thrombosis. Ann Intern Med 1998;128:663–77.

26. Hirsch J, Dalen J, Guyatt G. The sixth (2000) ACCP guideline for antithrombotic therapy for prevention and treatment of thrombosis. Chest 2001;119(suppl 1):1S–2S.

27. Schafer AI. Low-molecular-weight heparin—an opportunity for home treatment of venous thrombosis. N Engl J Med 1996;334:724–5.

28. Lensing AW, Prins MH, Davidson BL, et al. Treatment of deep venous thrombosis with low-molecular-weight heparins. Arch Intern Med 1995;155:601–7.

29. Schraibman IG, Milne AA, Royle EM. Home versus in-patient treatment for deep vein thrombosis. Cochrane Database of Systematic Reviews 2001;issue 2.

30. Levin M, Gent M, Hirsh J, et al. A comparison of low-molecular-weight heparin administered primarily at home with un-fractionated heparin administered in the hospital for proximal deep-vein thrombosis. N Engl J Med 1996;334:677–81.

31. Koopman MMW, Prandoni P, Piovella F, et al. Treatment of venous thrombosis with intravenous unfractionated heparin administered in the hospital as compared with subcutaneous low-molecular-weight heparin administered at home. N Engl J Med 1996;334:682–7.

32. Boccalon H, Elias A, Chale J-J, Cadene A, Gabriel S. Clinical outcome and cost of hospital vs. home treatment of proximal deep vein thrombosis with a low-molecular-weight heparin. Arch Intern Med 2000;160:1769–73.

33. Yacovella T, Alter M. Anticoagulation for venous thromboembolism. Postgrad Med 2000;108:43–54.

34. Hutten BA, Prins MH. Duration of treatment with vitamin K antagonists in symptomatic venous thromboembolism. Cochrane Database of Systematic Reviews 2001;issue 2.

35. Asell JE. The value of an anticoagulation management service. In: Managing oral anticoagulation therapy. Gaithersburg, MD: Aspen, 2000;1–6.

36. Sanson B-J, Buller H. Is there a role for thrombolytic therapy in venous thromboembolism? Haemostasis 1999;29(suppl 1):81–3.

82
Selected Disorders of the Cardiovascular System

David E. Anisman

Pericarditis

Pericarditis may be divided into two types—acute and constrictive. Acute pericarditis (AP), which is an inflammatory condition of the membranes lining the heart, affects men more frequently than women, and is seen with increasing frequency with advancing age. While AP is diagnosed in less than 1% of hospital admissions, it has an estimated prevalence of 2% to 6% in the general population, underscoring the frequency with which it is either clinically not apparent or not considered in the differential diagnosis.[1] The most common etiologies are idiopathic, viral (which may actually account for most idiopathic cases), and in association with cardiac ischemia (Table 82.1). Indeed, the chest pain associated with AP may make it difficult to distinguish from acute myocardial ischemia. Constrictive pericarditis (CP), formerly known as Pick's disease, is characterized by a thickened, adherent, and fibrous pericardium that impairs diastolic filling, leading to the gradual onset of symptoms consistent with systemic venous congestion, such as congestive heart failure (CHF). It is a postinflammatory sequela of many of the same etiologies as AP, but the clinician should always maintain a high suspicion for tuberculosis, which is still the leading cause of CP in developing countries.[2]

Presentation and Diagnosis

Acute pericarditis may be heralded by a viral prodrome, and classically presents with a triad of chest pain, pericardial friction rub, and characteristic electrocardiographic (ECG) changes. The chest pain is usually rather abrupt in onset, retrosternal in location, and made worse with recumbency, deep inspiration, and swallowing. It is often eased by sitting up and leaning forward. The pain may radiate to the trapezius ridge, or may mimic the pain of acute myocardial ischemia with radiation into the left arm. Respiratory symptoms are generally the result of secondary pleural irritation rather than a primary effect of AP on cardiac function. The pathognomonic pericardial friction rub is classically described as triphasic (atrial systole, ventricular systole, and diastole), with the ventricular systolic component most readily and most often heard. The rub is scratchy or "Velcro-like" and best heard with the patient sitting upright and leaning forward, with respirations interrupted, and by placing the diaphragm over the left lower sternal border and cardiac apex. Confusion with murmurs can be avoided by recognizing that the rub does not radiate or vary in either loudness or timing with maneuvers that typically are used for murmur identification.

The four classic stages of ECG changes in AP are summarized in Table 82.2; not all phases need be present to confirm the diagnosis. Because PR segment depression may coexist with ST segment elevation, it is crucial to use the TP segment as a baseline.[3] Acute pericarditis may be differentiated from acute myocardial infarction (AMI) by the diffuseness of ST changes, the absence of Q waves, and the characteristically concave up-sloping morphology of the ST segment. Benign early repolarization (BER) also may present with diffusely elevated ST segments, but use of the ST/T ratio (Fig. 82.1) is helpful in making the distinction.

Because of the wide variety of presenting signs and symptoms, CP is difficult to diagnose solely on history and physical examination.[2] Symptoms of right-sided CHF, such as abdominal distention, peripheral edema, and anorexia reflect impaired diastolic filling and chronically depressed cardiac output. Left-sided CHF symptoms such as dyspnea and orthopnea also occur, but are less frequent.[4] Common examination findings include Kussmaul's sign (jugular venous pressure *increasing* with inspiration), ascites, cachexia, hepatomegaly, and a pericardial knock (an early diastolic sound heard best with the diaphragm and increased with squatting). Though rarely normal, the ECG findings are nonspecific, revealing generalized low voltage, T-wave inversions, conduc-

Table 82.1. Etiologies of Pericarditis

Infectious
  Bacterial: pneumococcus, staphylococcus, *Neisseria meningitidis*, streptococcus, mycoplasma, tuberculosis, *Haemophilus influenzae*, rickettsia
  Viral: coxsackie, echovirus, adenovirus, influenza, varicella-zoster, HIV
  Fungal: histoplasmosis, aspergillosis, blastomycosis, coccidioidomycosis
Trauma: blunt chest trauma, post-thoracic surgery
Medications: procainamide, phenytoin, isoniazid, penicillin, heparin, warfarin, cromolyn sodium, methysergide
Cardiac: AMI, Dressler's syndrome, endocarditis, aortic dissection
Radiation therapy
Neoplastic: breast, bronchogenic lung, lymphoma, leukemia
Uremia: poorly controlled or while on hemodialysis
Autoimmune: systemic lupus erythematosus, rheumatoid arthritis, inflammatory bowel, acute rheumatic fever, scleroderma, polyarteritis nodosa, dermatomyositis
Other: sarcoidosis, amyloidosis

AMI = acute myocardial infarction.

tion delays, and atrial dysrhythmias (especially atrial fibrillation).[4,5] When the presentation suggests constrictive or restrictive pathophysiology, a chest x-ray showing pericardial calcification argues for CP over other etiologies. Better still, magnetic resonance imaging (MRI) and computed tomography (CT) are the preferred methods for identifying the pericardial thickening of CP. Echocardiography is often helpful in evaluating ventricular function and documenting the impaired diastolic filling characteristic of CP. Cardiac catheterization is the gold standard for resolving the diagnostic dilemmas via demonstration of equalized diastolic pressures between atria and ventricles.

Differential Diagnosis

Differential considerations for AP include AMI, pulmonary embolism, aortic dissection, cardiac contusion, mediastinitis, esophageal spasm, esophagitis, and pneumonia. A thorough history, examination, ECG analysis, and selected diagnostic testing and imaging will usually address these concerns, but the distinction between AP and AMI may remain difficult, complicating subsequent therapy. Constrictive pericarditis must be differentiated from tamponade, restrictive cardiomyopathy, intraabdominal malignancy, and hepatic cirrhosis. Liver function

tests in CP patients are typical for passive congestion (elevated alkaline phosphatase and γ-glutamyl transpeptidase), while cirrhotic patients show diminished albumen and increased prothrombin times. Echocardiogram, CT, and MRI are also helpful in making these distinctions. Where confusion between constrictive and restrictive etiologies persists, catheterization with endomyocardial biopsy is indicated.[1,5]

Intervention

Initial management of AP focuses on treating the underlying cause, if possible. Purulent pericarditis requiring IV antibiotics must be documented by pericardiocentesis and is a medical emergency, with mortality rates of up to 77%.[6] Clinicians should monitor AP for pericardial effusion and the development of cardiac tamponade, requiring emergent pericardiocentesis. Analgesia for AP is critical, and is best achieved with nonsteroidal antiinflammatory drugs (NSAIDs) such as aspirin (650 mg po q4h) or indomethacin (25 to 50 mg po q6h). Intravenous ketorolac (30 mg IM or IV q6h) is also effective. Since the high doses of corticosteroids needed for pain control have both immune and adrenal suppressive effects, it is prudent to withhold them for at least 48 hours to determine if NSAIDs will be effective for symptom management. When the patient is pain free for 5 to 7 days, all antiinflammatory agents should be tapered. Recurrent pericarditis is treated by reinstituting high-dose NSAIDs, followed by tapering these agents over several months. Colchicine has also been used with some success. Even though the presence of AP is a relative contraindication to administration of thrombolytics, the incidence of post-AMI AP can be decreased by the appropriate use of thrombolytic therapy for the AMI, since decreasing the size of the AMI will decrease the likelihood for development of AP.

The progressive nature of CP demands referral to a cardiovascular surgeon for all symptomatic patients, since the earlier stage at which pericardiectomy is performed, the better the outcome. Improvement is usually dramatic and sustained. Temporizing measures include the use of diuretics. Rate-slowing drugs should be used with caution, if at all, since maintaining an adequate cardiac output in CP is often rate-dependent.

Prevention

The most common etiologies of AP do not lend themselves to effective preventive efforts, and prevention of CP is usu-

Table 82.2. Electrocardiographic Findings for the Four Stages of Acute Myopericarditis

Stage	Duration	Electrocardiographic finding
I	Days–2 weeks	Diffuse PR segment depression (I, II, III, aVL, V2–6) (with reciprocal PR segment elevation in aVR, V1) Diffuse ST segment elevation (I, II, III, aVL, V2–6) (with reciprocal ST segment depression in aVR, V1)
II	1–3 weeks	ST segment normalization T wave flattening with decreased amplitude
III	3–several weeks	T wave inversion
IV	Several weeks	Normalization and return to baseline ECG

Source: Chan et al,[3] with permission.

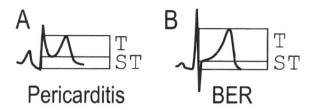

Pericarditis BER

Fig. 82.1. This PR segment–ST segment discordant ratio may also help in discriminating between the ST segment elevation resulting from benign early repolarization (BER) and acute myopericarditis. It is objectively assessed by comparing the heights of the ST segment and T wave in lead V6: the ST segment/T wave magnitude ratio. Using the PR segment as the baseline for the ST segment and the J point as the beginning of the T wave, the heights are measured with calculation of the ratio. If the ratio is 0.25 or greater, pericarditis is the likely diagnosis; with results less than 0.25, one should consider BER. (From Chan et al,[3] with permission.)

ally dependent on prevention of AP. Focusing efforts on preventable etiologies, such as coronary artery disease (CAD), malignancy, management of uremic conditions, and judicious use of certain medications are most likely to be productive measures.

Myocarditis

Occurring most commonly in 20- to 50-year-old men, myocarditis is the inflammation of cardiac myocytes and associated structures (vascular, interstitium, and pericardium). Viral infection in general, and Coxsackie B virus in particular, is the most common cause in North America (Table 82.3). Myocyte damage during the first 3 days appears to be due to a direct viral effect, which is terminated by antibody-mediated viral clearance. A persistent T-cell–mediated response in a subset of patients seems to underlie the evolution of abnormal ventricular architecture and the eventual development of dilated cardiomyopathy (DCM).[7,8] While most cases of myocarditis are asymptomatic and resolve spontaneously, one third of patients have residual cardiac abnormalities ranging from subtle ECG changes to CHF, which may be acute and life-threatening. The more mild cases generally respond well to conventional CHF management, whereas the more severe cases may require mechanical ventricular assist devices or even transplant. Cases of sudden death have been reported, presumably secondary to ventricular dysrhythmia.

Presentation and Diagnosis

Symptomatic patients often note a nonspecific flu-like prodrome, occasionally accompanied by palpitations. One third note chest pain that may mimic ischemia, and a small number present with symptoms of CHF. Examination may reveal tachycardia, a muffled first heart sound, or a murmur of tricuspid or mitral regurgitation. Severe cases will have findings consistent with CHF. Electrocardiogram commonly re-

veals a sinus tachycardia with nonspecific ST and T wave changes (often superimposed on those of pericarditis). Conduction delays are not uncommon, and intraventricular delays often denote more serious myocardial damage and a worse prognosis. White blood count is elevated in a quarter of patients, and the erythrocyte sedimentation rate (ESR) is increased in up to 60%. Serology is rarely clinically useful. Echocardiography may show increased left ventricular (LV) wall thickness similar to that seen in other forms of cardiomyopathy, and is very important in identifying ventricular wall motion abnormalities, detecting ventricular thrombus, and measuring LV ejection fraction (LVEF). A near-normal baseline LVEF is currently the best predictor of a good outcome; findings on light microscopy from biopsy specimens have not correlated well with prognosis.[9,10]

Myocardial biopsy is most useful if performed within the first 3 to 4 days when the diagnostic yield is highest. Even then, however, it is uncommon that biopsy findings will significantly change management decisions. Some authorities consider biopsy to be the gold standard in the diagnosis of myocarditis and recommend it in all cases of ventricular dysfunction where the cause is unclear.[11] Others question this recommendation, noting the low yield of biopsy due to the patchy nature of inflammatory infiltrates, and the difficulty with which current pathologic criteria are employed.[9]

Differential Diagnosis

Several serious cardiac conditions must be differentiated from myocarditis. These include AMI, CHF due to other causes (e.g., ischemia, hypertension), dysrhythmias, and pericarditis. Complicating the evaluation is the fact that all of these conditions may coexist with myocarditis.

Intervention

If an infectious agent is identified, appropriate therapy should be instituted immediately. Most patients with mild to moder-

Table 82.3. **Etiologies of Myocarditis**

Infectious
  Bacterial: clostridia, diphtheria, gonococcus, haemophilus, legionella, meningococcus, mycobacteria, mycoplasma, salmonella, staphylococcus, streptococcus (especially pneumococcus)
  Spirochetes: borrelia, leptospira, syphilis
  Fungal: actinomyces, aspergillus, candida, coccidioides, histoplasma
  Protozoal: toxoplasma, trypanosoma
  Rickettsia: Q fever, Rocky Mountain spotted fever, scrub typhus, typhus
  Viral: adenovirus, Coxsackie, cytomegalovirus, Epstein-Barr, hepatitis, herpes simplex, HIV, influenza A and B, rabies, respiratory syncytial virus, varicella zoster
Medications: hydrochlorothiazide, lithium, penicillins, sulfamethoxazole/trimethoprim, tetracycline
Physical agents: radiation therapy
Autoimmune: rheumatoid arthritis, systemic lupus erythematosus
Other: giant cell myocarditis, hypersensitivity reactions, Kawasaki disease, peripartum myocarditis, rheumatic fever, sarcoidosis

ate symptoms require supportive measures specific to their presentation. Bed rest is critical to limit continued damage to the myocardium. Treatment of the systemic symptoms typical of viral infection with analgesics and antipyretics is indicated, but NSAIDs should be avoided in the first 2 weeks due to the potential for myocardial cell damage. Conventional treatment with digoxin, diuretics, nitrates, and angiotensin-converting enzyme inhibitors (ACEIs; especially when ejection fraction is less than 40%) is appropriate when CHF is present.[7,11] Temporary cardiac pacing is indicated in cases of third-degree or symptomatic second-degree type II atrioventricular block. Anticoagulation may be warranted for ventricular thrombus or to prevent development of thrombus in the presence of atrial fibrillation. Cardiac transplantation is used only as a last ditch effort, often after intraaortic balloon pump or LV assist device have failed. Antiviral therapies such as interferon-α and polyclonal immunoglobulin (Ig) are rarely useful, since they are only of benefit when started before or during viral infection.[12] Alpha-, beta-, and calcium channel blocking drugs may be of benefit due to their vasodilating properties, but as yet remain investigational.[12] Steroids and other immunosuppressive agents have not been found to produce a significant benefit in clinical outcomes. In fact, they may be harmful in the acute phase of viral myocarditis, possibly due to decreased antibody-mediated clearance of virus. Their use is suggested only in biopsy-proven cases after other treatments have failed, and prior to transplant.[7,9,12] One exception is in the treatment of autoimmune causes such as giant cell myocarditis or systemic lupus, where it is the treatment of choice. Future therapies may include immunomodulating agents if such can be found to target T cells only.[8]

Prevention

The majority of viruses that constitute the most common causes of myocarditis are not amenable to effective prevention measures. Less common causes such as sexually transmitted diseases are preventable through counseling on risk-limiting behavioral mechanisms. Others causes such as pneumococcus, influenza, hepatitis, and diphtheria may be prevented through immunization, though the risk of myocarditis in the general population does not warrant a change in current immunization strategy.

Endocarditis

Infectious endocarditis (IE) is an infection of the endocardial surface mainly due to bacteria, but rarely may be caused by fungi and protozoa. The interaction between the infecting organisms and the host's immune response gives rise to the classic though not universally found lesion of IE: the valvular vegetation. These vegetations may interfere with valvular function leading to CHF, and may embolize to produce a wide variety of focal and systemic signs and symptoms. Acute bacterial endocarditis (ABE) is a subset of IE in which the clinical course may become fulminant in as little as 3 to 5 days, tends to be caused by more virulent organisms such as *Staphylococcus aureus*, and generally affects patients with previ-

ously normal valves, intravenous drug users (IVDUs), and those with prosthetic valves. Because of its aggressive course, the complications of ABE tend to be severe. In contrast, subacute bacterial endocarditis (SBE) is more gradually progressive, often taking weeks to months before being diagnosed. The subacute form of IE is caused by less virulent organisms (e.g., *Streptococcus viridans*), has severe complications less often than ABE, and primarily affects patients with abnormal valvular architecture, either congenital or prosthetic. The overall incidence of IE in the United States is estimated at between 1.6 and 6.0 cases per 100,000 population, with a slight male predominance and a median age of 50 years.[13] This demographic is changing due to the decreased prevalence of rheumatic heart disease, advances in the surgical management of children with congenital cardiac disease, and a steady rise in intravenous drug abuse. As a result, children and IVDUs make up an increasing proportion of those with IE. Untreated, IE is almost uniformly fatal. Therefore, if IE is suspected, aggressive evaluation and treatment, to include early surgery in some cases, is essential. Such a strategy has decreased mortality rates to as low as 40% in non-addicts with *S. aureus* ABE and 0% to 10% in IVDUs.[14]

Effective management of IE relies on targeting treatment to specific organisms. Gram-positive bacteria are the most common cause of IE, with over 80% of cases due to staphylococcal and streptococcal species.[13,14] Gram-negative bacteria account for 10% to 20% of cases, with *Pseudomonas* occurring primarily in IVDUs and those with prosthetic valve endocarditis (PVE), and the HACEK group (*Haemophilus* species, *Actinobacillus actinomycetemcomitans*, *Cardiobacterium hominis*, *Eikenella corrodens*, and *Kingella kingae*) occurring most commonly in native valve, non-IVDUs. While IE is rare in children overall, those with congenital cardiac disease most often have *S. viridans* or *S. aureus* as causative agents.[15] More than half of IE in IVDUs is due to *S. aureus*, but gram-negative bacteria, especially *Pseudomonas*, and fungi are common as well. In addition, IVDUs have a very high incidence of right-sided valvular involvement, especially the tricuspid valve. Prosthetic valve endocarditis is most often due to *S. viridans*, *S. aureus*, and *Staphylococcus epidermidis*, as well as *Pseudomonas* and other gram-negative bacilli. As a general rule, a normal vaginal delivery poses little increased risk of IE. However, bacteremia during delivery carries an increased risk of enterococcal, group B streptococcal, and *S. aureus* IE.[13] Nosocomial IE is most commonly due to staphylococcal species, enterococci, fungi, and *Pseudomonas*, and is seen in patients with burns, extended intensive care unit stays, and placement of intravascular and intracardiac devices or urinary catheters.

Presentation and Diagnosis

Though the primary lesion in IE is in the heart itself, many of its presenting signs and symptoms reflect the systemic nature of the disease. Fever, myalgias, fatigue, headache, and abdominal pain are common in all types of IE, but are more severe and persistent in ABE. Findings consistent with CHF develop in up to 60% of all cases of IE, and are often a poor prognostic sign as CHF carries a mortality of up to 80% and

Table 82.4. Criteria for Diagnosis of Infective Endocarditis

Definite infective endocarditis
  Pathologic criteria
    Microorganisms: demonstrated by culture or histology in
    a vegetation, *or* in a vegetation that has embolized, *or*
    in an intracardiac abscess, *or*
    Pathologic lesions: vegetation or intracardiac abscess
    present, confirmed by histology showing active
    endocarditis
  Clinical criteria, using specific definitions listed in Table 82.5
    2 major criteria, *or*
    1 major and 3 minor criteria, *or*
    5 minor criteria
Possible infective endocarditis
  Findings consistent with infective endocarditis that fall short
  of "definite," but not "rejected"
Rejected
  Firm alternate diagnosis for manifestations of endocarditis,
  or
  Resolution of manifestations of endocarditis, with antibiotic
  therapy for 4 days or less, *or*
  No pathologic evidence of infective endocarditis at surgery
  or autopsy, after antibiotic therapy for 4 days or less

Source: Durack et al,[17] with permission.

is the most common cause of death in all types of IE.[16] Vegetations can embolize to almost any location, causing distant infection or infarction; such embolization occurs in about 12% to 40% of patients with SBE and 40% to 60% of patients with ABE.[13] Right-sided embolic events may lead to specific complaints of chest pain, cough, and hemoptysis. Left-sided embolic events can present as mental status changes, stroke, myocardial infarction, splenic infarction, and renal abscess. Up to 90% of patients with *Streptococcus pneumoniae* ABE have an associated meningitis. Other complications of IE include osteomyelitis, septic arthritis, and mycotic aneurysms.

With the exception of Janeway lesions, which are found most commonly with ABE, few physical findings are highly specific for IE. Nonetheless, Roth spots, Osler's nodes, petechiae, splinter hemorrhages, and splenomegaly occur in up to 25% of cases of IE, and when more than one occur together it is strongly suggestive of the diagnosis. Cardiac murmurs in IE are most often regurgitant, but frequently are not present on initial evaluation. While a change in a preexisting murmur is of uncertain significance, a new aortic regurgitant murmur in association with fever is strongly associated with IE.[13] Laboratory evaluation is frequently of less value in making the early diagnosis of IE than are the history and examination, but usually shows granulocytosis, especially in ABE. In SBE, anemia, a positive rheumatoid factor, elevated Veneral Disease Research Laboratory (VDRL) titers, and circulating immune complexes are common. Other laboratory findings and imaging may reflect other complications as mentioned above. Electrocardiogram may reveal conduction abnormalities, indicating the extension of an aortic valve infection to a valve-ring abscess, which carries a worse prognosis.[13]

In 1994, with the goal of increasing the proportion of def-

Table 82.5. Definitions of Terminology Used in the Diagnostic Criteria of Infective Endocarditis

Major criteria
  Positive blood culture for infective endocarditis
    Typical microorganism for infective endocarditis from two separate blood cultures
      Viridans streptococci,[a] *Streptococcus bovis*, HACEK group, *or*
      Community-acquired *Staphylococcus aureus* or enterococci, in the absence of a primary focus, *or*
    Persistently positive blood culture, defined as recovery of a microorganism consistent with infective endocarditis from
      Blood cultures drawn more than 12 hours apart, *or*
      All of three or a majority of four or more separate blood cultures, with first and last drawn at least 1 hour apart
  Evidence of endocardial involvement
    Positive echocardiogram for infective endocarditis
      Oscillating intracardiac mass, on valve or supporting structures, *or* in the path of regurgitant jets, *or* on implanted
      material, in the absence of an alternative anatomic explanation, *or*
      Abscess, *or*
      New partial dehiscence of prosthetic valve, *or*
    New valvular regurgitation (increase or change in preexisting murmur not sufficient)
Minor criteria
  Predisposition: predisposing heart condition or intravenous drug use
  Fever: ≥38.0°C (100.4°F)
  Vascular phenomena: major arterial emboli, septic pulmonary infarcts, mycotic aneurysm, intracranial hemorrhage,
    conjunctival hemorrhages, Janeway lesions
  Immunologic phenomena: glomerulonephritis, Osler's nodes, Roth spots, rheumatoid factor
  Microbiologic evidence: positive blood culture but not meeting major criterion as noted previously[b] *or* serologic evidence
    of active infection with organism consistent with infective endocarditis
  Echocardiogram: consistent with infective endocarditis but not meeting major criterion as noted previously

HACEK = *Haemophilus* spp., *Actinobacillus actinomycetemcomitans*, *Cardiobacterium hominis*, *Eikenella* spp., and *Kingella kingae*.

[a]Including nutritional variant strains.

[b]Excluding single positive cultures for coagulase-negative staphylococci and organisms that do not cause endocarditis.

Source: Durack et al,[17] with permission.

inite diagnoses of IE correctly identified, Durack and colleagues[17] proposed a revised set of diagnostic criteria patterned after the Jones criteria for rheumatoid arthritis. Under these so-called Duke criteria, the diagnosis of definite IE is arrived at either through one of two pathologic criteria or through one of several combinations of major and minor clinical criteria (Table 82.4). The clinical criteria emphasize two main areas: positive blood cultures and evidence of endocardial involvement (Table 82.5). The latter clinical criterion takes advantage of both transthoracic (TTE) and transesophageal (TEE) echocardiography as safe yet highly sensitive means for identifying endocardial lesions.[16] It is recommended that TTE be the initial study of choice for most patients. However, where TTE is negative and clinical suspicion remains high, or in cases involving a prosthetic valve, possible abscess, or valve perforation, TEE is preferable, as it has higher sensitivity in such cases. In spite of a negative predictive value of 80%, a negative TEE should be repeated frequently in high-risk patients.[16] The Duke criteria have been extensively studied and found to have sensitivity ranging from 75% to 100% while maintaining excellent specificity (92–99%) and a negative predictive value of at least 92%.[17–20] These criteria have also been validated for both the adult and pediatric populations, as well as special groups such as those with PVE.[21–23] However, since an adequate amount of clinical data must be collected before the Duke criteria can be applied, early empiric therapy should not be delayed if IE is suspected. In this regard, the criteria are best used to assist in sculpting medical therapy and determining a need for surgical intervention.

Differential Diagnosis

Virtually any systemic infection should be considered in the differential diagnosis of IE. These include, but are not limited to, pneumonia, meningitis, pericarditis, abscess, osteomyelitis, tuberculosis, and pyelonephritis. Noninfectious etiologies to be considered include stroke, myocardial infarction, rheumatic fever, vasculitis, malignancy, and fever of unknown origin.

Intervention

Because bacteria in valvular vegetations are relatively protected from host immune defenses, antibiotics chosen to treat IE must be bactericidal, and regimens for their administration must be aggressive and of adequate duration to completely eradicate the organism and prevent relapse (Tables 82.6 to 82.9).[24,25] Repeat blood cultures should be negative within 48 hours of beginning antibiotic therapy, especially for staphylococcal infection. Cultures should also be repeated at 4 and 8 weeks after completion of antibiotic therapy. If positive, those with native valve IE should receive a repeat course of antibiotics; those with PVE or resistant enterococcus should receive both repeat antibiotics and possible surgical intervention.[25] Careful attention should be given to identifying and treating complications. CHF in particular must be treated aggressively, since there is a dramatic worsening of prognosis as CHF becomes more severe.[26] Therapy of CHF should be initiated with conventional medications (ACEIs and diuretics), but the timing of surgical intervention should be given particular emphasis. To that end, early surgical, infectious disease, and cardiology consultations are warranted for all patients with suspected IE.

In general, surgery should not be delayed because of active IE. Indications for surgical intervention include CHF that is progressive despite appropriate antibiotic and medical management, periannular or myocardial abscess, valvular obstruction, persistent bacteremia despite appropriate antibi-

Table 82.6. **Treatment Regimens for Viridans Streptococci[a] Bacterial Endocarditis**

Penicillin susceptibility	Antibiotics	Duration
High (MIC ≤0.1 μg per mL)	Aqueous penicillin, 12 to 18 million U day *or*	4 weeks
	Ceftriaxone, 2 g daily *or*	4 weeks
	Penicillin, 12 to 18 million U per day, plus gentamicin, 1 mg per kg every 8 hours[b]	2 weeks
Moderate (MIC >0.1, <0.5 μg per mL)	Penicillin, 18 million U per day *plus*	4 weeks
	Gentamicin, 1 mg per kg every 8 hours[b]	2 weeks
Low (MIC ≥0.5 μg per mL)	Penicillin, 18 million U per day, plus gentamicin, 1 mg per kg every 8 hours[b]	4 to 6 weeks
In patients with penicillin allergy		
MIC <0.5 μg per mL	Vancomycin, 15 mg per kg every 12 hours[b]	4 weeks
MIC ≥0.5 μg per mL	Vancomycin, 15 mg per kg every 12 hours,[b] plus gentamicin, 1 mg per kg every 8 hours[b]	4 to 6 weeks

MIC = minimal inhibitory concentration.

[a]These regimens also apply to treatment of endocarditis caused by *Streptococcus bovis.*

[b]Dosages need to be adjusted based on renal function.

Source: Giessel et al,[24] as adapted from Wilson et al.[2] with permission.

Table 82.7. **Treatment Regimens for Enterococcal Bacterial Endocarditis**

Penicillin-allergic patient	Penicillin-susceptible organism	Antibiotics	Duration
No	Yes	Penicillin, 18 to 30 million U per day, plus gentamicin, 1 mg per kg every 8 hours[b] or	4 to 6 weeks[a]
		Ampicillin, 12 g per day, plus gentamicin, 1 mg per kg every 8 hours[b]	4 to 6 weeks
No	No	Vancomycin, 15 mg per kg every 12 hours,[b] plus gentamicin, 1 mg per kg every 8 hours[b]	4 to 6 weeks
Yes	No or yes	Vancomycin, 15 mg per kg every 12 hours,[b] plus gentamicin, 1 mg per kg every 8 hours[b]	4 to 6 weeks

[a]Six-week course of therapy for endocarditis involving a prosthetic valve or when symptoms have been present for longer than 3 months.

[b]Dosages need to be adjusted based on renal function.

From Giessel et al,[24] as adapted from Wilson et al,[25] with permission.

otics, dehiscence of a prosthetic valve, fungal infection, conduction delay or heart block, enlarging vegetations, and recurrent emboli.[13,14,26]

Once the diagnosis of IE is suspected, antibiotic therapy should be instituted without delay. Until culture results and sensitivities are available to guide antibiotic selection, choice of empiric therapy should primarily rely on whether the clinical scenario is acute or subacute.[13] Other factors to be considered include nosocomial vs. community-acquired infection, presence of prosthetic material, and intravenous drug use. In the acute setting, nafcillin (2.0 g IV q4h) plus ampicillin (2.0 g IV q4h) plus gentamicin (1.5 mg/kg IV q8h) should be used; vancomycin (1.0 g IV q12h) should replace nafcillin when methacillin-resistant *S. aureus* is a concern. For SBE, ampicillin (2.0 g IV q4h) plus gentamicin (1.5 mg/kg IV q8h) is indicated.

Table 82.8. **Treatment Regimens for Staphylococcal Bacterial Endocarditis**

Penicillin-allergic patient	Methicillin-susceptible organism	Involved valve	Antibiotics	Duration
No	Yes	Native	Nafcillin, 2 g every 4 hours,[a] or oxacillin, 2 g every 4 hours plus	4–6 weeks
			(Optional) Gentamicin, 1 mg per kg every 8 hours[a]	3–5 days
Yes[b]	Yes	Native	Cefazolin, 2 g every 8 hours[a] plus	4–6 weeks
			(Optional) Gentamicin, 1 mg per kg every 8 hours[a]	3–5 days
Yes[c] No or yes	No or yes No	Native Native	Vancomycin, 15 mg per kg every 12 hours[a]	4–6 weeks
No	Yes	Prosthetic	Nafcillin, 2 g every 4 hours,[a] or oxacillin, 2 g every 4 hours plus	≥6 weeks
			Rifampin, 300 mg every 8 hours plus	≥6 weeks
			Gentamicin, 1 mg per kg every 8 hours[a]	2 weeks
No Yes[c]	No No or yes	Prosthetic Prosthetic	Vancomycin, 15 mg per kg every 12 hours[a] plus	≥6 weeks
			Rifampin, 300 mg every 8 hours plus	≥6 weeks
			Gentamicin, 1 mg per kg every 8 hours[a]	2 weeks
Yes	No	Prosthetic	Cefazolin, 2 g every 8 hours[a] plus	≥6 weeks
			Rifampin, 300 mg every 8 hours plus	≥6 weeks
			Gentamicin, 1 mg per kg every 8 hours[a]	2 weeks

[a]Dosages need to be adjusted based on renal function.

[b]History of allergy that does not involve immediate-type hypersensitivity.

[c]History of immediate-type hypersensitivity.

Source: Giessel et al,[24] as adapted from Wilson et al,[25] with permission.

Table 82.9. **Treatment Regimens for Bacterial Endocarditis caused by HACEK Organisms**

Antibiotic	Dosage and route	Duration
Ceftriaxone[a]	2 g once daily IV or IM	4 weeks
Ampicillin[a]	12 g per day IV, either continuously or in 6 equally divided doses	4 weeks
plus		
Gentamicin[b]	1 mg per kg IM or IV every 8 hours	4 weeks

HACEK = *Haemophilus* spp., *Actinobacillus actinomycetemcomitans*, *Cardiobacterium hominis*, *Eikenella* spp., and *Kingella kingae*.

[a]Experience in treating HACEK organisms with other than β-lactam antibiotics is limited; for patients unable to tolerate β-lactam antibiotics, consult an infectious disease specialist.

[b]Dosages need to be adjusted based on renal function.

Source: Wilson et al,[25] with permission.

Prevention

Prevention of IE in those with abnormal valvular architecture is covered in detail in Chapter 57. In those with normal valves, prevention is mainly an issue of education on the avoidance of IV drug use.

Cardiomyopathies

In 1995, the World Health Organization's classification of cardiomyopathies (CMs) recognized two main groupings.[27] The *functional* CMs describe anatomic and hemodynamic changes, and include dilated, hypertrophic, and restrictive forms, as well as the less common arrhythmogenic right ventricular CM. The *specific* CMs describe particular etiologies, and include ischemic, hypertensive, valvular, inflammatory, metabolic, general system disease, muscular dystrophies, neuromuscular disorders, toxic reactions, and peripartal. The specific CMs generally have the clinical features of one or more functional types. Indeed, many CMs previously labeled idiopathic are now known to be primary disorders of the myocardium caused by well-defined genetic mutations. In general, the clinician first recognizes a particular functional type of CM, and then proceeds to search for a specific etiology, since treatment of an underlying cause may arrest the cardiomyopathic process. Management of all the CMs should include early consultation with a cardiologist well versed in the pertinent and complex issues surrounding diagnosis and treatment.

Most CMs present with some manifestations of CHF, and so have two primary underlying pathogenic mechanisms: activation of the renin-angiotensin system and of the adrenergic nervous system. As a result, treatment with ACEIs and beta-blocking agents are often a mainstay of treatment. Diuretics are used for volume overload states, with digoxin as a second- or third-line agent for symptom control. Anticoagulation is indicated for a history of embolic phenomena and the dysrhythmias that might predispose to them, or significantly depressed LVEF.

Dilated Cardiomyopathy

Dilated cardiomyopathy (DCM) is characterized by an increase in LV diastolic and systolic volumes with an associated reduction in LVEF, and is the leading cause of CHF. The idiopathic form is the most common subtype, demonstrating

myocyte hypertrophy and interstitial fibrosis on histology, and may be due to chronic myocarditis, either viral or autoimmune. Etiologies of DCM include primary genetic abnormalities (which are often autosomal dominant, making family history very important), toxic (including alcohol induced), and drug related (e.g., anthracyclines, cocaine). It may also be secondary to systemic conditions such as myocardial ischemia, hypertension, and valvular abnormalities.[28]

Patients with DCM often present with generalized symptoms of fatigue and dyspnea worsening over months to years; sudden death and embolic phenomena are less common. Physical examination reveals pulmonary and, less often, systemic venous congestion. When atrial fibrillation occurs, the presentation is often one of acute decompensation. Screening laboratory tests include ESR; creatinine kinase (to screen for inherited muscular dystrophies); renal, liver, and thyroid function studies; iron studies (to identify hemochromatosis); and, if the presentation is acute, viral serologies. The ECG may be normal, but often shows T wave changes, septal Q waves, atrioventricular conduction abnormalities, and bundle branch blocks. Sinus tachycardia and supraventricular dysrhythmias are common, and nonsustained ventricular tachycardia occurs in 20% to 30%.[28] Echocardiogram is essential to demonstrate the diagnostic criteria of ejection fraction <0.45, fractional shortening <25%, and LV end diastolic volume >112%. If diastolic dysfunction is demonstrated, endomyocardial biopsy should be performed to rule out infiltrative disease.

Treatment follows the basic precepts for CHF, with several notable caveats. In DCM secondary to hypertension or valvular disease, afterload reduction is best achieved by adding hydralazine or nitrates to the standard CHF regimen. Recent studies have suggested that the combination of angiotensin II receptor antagonists with ACEIs may be more effective than either agent alone.[29] In patients with New York Heart Association class IV failure and an LVEF <35%, adding 25 mg of spironolactone to the standard CHF regimen has been shown to decrease overall mortality by 30%.[30] Transplantation may be the only option for select, severely symptomatic patients, especially those with idiopathic DCM.

Hypertrophic Cardiomyopathy

Hypertrophic cardiomyopathy (HCM) is defined as increased LV wall thickness, either symmetric or asymmetric, and either global or regional, with overall normal (or slightly reduced)

LV chamber size. Twenty-five percent of patients with HCM have dynamic outflow tract obstruction due to ventricular septal hypertrophy and anterior displacement of the papillary muscles, with associated abnormal mitral valve formation.[31,32] This obstruction may be a cause of sudden death, and is increased by activities that increase myocardial contractility (e.g., strenuous exercise), or by maneuvers or agents that decrease venous return (e.g., Valsalva, diuretics). Conversely, obstruction is decreased by agents that decrease myocardial contractility (e.g., beta-blockers) or by maneuvers that increase venous return (e.g., squatting). The risk for sudden death is highest in children and young adults, and may be the initial presentation. Possible risk factors for sudden death include recurrent syncope, prior cardiac arrest, sustained ventricular tachycardia, massive LV hypertrophy, and a family history of sudden death from HCM.[32] Hypertrophic CM is a primary, heterogeneous disease of the sarcomere, with autosomal dominant inheritance demonstrated most commonly.[32,33]

In addition to the common CHF symptoms such as fatigue, dyspnea, and orthopnea, patients with HCM often complain of palpitations (due to atrial fibrillation caused by left atrial enlargement), presyncope, and syncope. Since most HCM is nonobstructive, auscultation generally reveals no murmur. Patients with outflow tract obstruction often demonstrate a 3–4/6 systolic murmur heard over both the left sternal border (due to outflow obstruction) and the axilla (due to mitral regurgitation). An S$_4$ is often heard due to increased filling from the enlarged atria. Pulmonary congestion is rare except with severe outflow obstruction or end-stage HCM (when systolic and diastolic dysfunction become manifest), or with atrial fibrillation. The ECG usually reveals a wide array of nonspecific changes including LV hypertrophy, ST changes, T wave inversion, left atrial enlargement, and Q waves. The chest radiograph is often normal or suggestive of atrial enlargement. As with DCM, echocardiogram with Doppler studies is essential, with the transesophageal approach useful to define subtle mitral valve abnormalities. Nuclear angiography and MRI may yield additional information on myocardial dysfunction.

There is no consensus on the utility of prophylactic treatment of asymptomatic patients with HCM, but avoiding strenuous exercise is critical for all patients, as is antibiotic prophylaxis for SBE.[31] For symptomatic patients with obstruction, beta-blocking agents are essential to decrease outflow obstruction by increasing diastolic filling time and decreasing filling pressures. Other negative inotropic agents may be used to similar effect, but the vasodilating properties of many calcium antagonists (especially verapamil) may counter this effect, leading to decreased filling, increased obstruction, and sudden death. Oral disopyramide at 600 to 800 mg per day is the drug of choice according to some authors.[32] In symptomatic patients with obstruction who have failed medical management, dual-chamber pacing has been shown to be effective.[33] Restoration and maintenance of sinus rhythm in patients with atrial fibrillation is usually achieved with either sotalol or amiodarone. In end-stage HCM, systolic and diastolic dysfunction may necessitate the use of standard CHF drug regimens, with particularly cautious use of digitalis and diuretics. Myectomy and valve replacement are often effective at resolving obstruction, but the relief may be temporary, due to surgically induced dysrhythmias and progression of the underlying primary myopathic process.

Restrictive Cardiomyopathy

Diastolic dysfunction is the hallmark of restrictive cardiomyopathy (RCM); LV size and shape, and systolic function are either normal or nearly so. The least common of all functional cardiomyopathies, restrictive pathophysiology may be seen in both HCM and hypertensive CM. Other etiologies include infiltrative diseases such as hemochromatosis and amyloid (the most common systemic cause of RCM), scleroderma, carcinoid, sarcoidosis, radiation therapy, and anthracycline use. Idiopathic RCM also occurs and may be an autosomal-dominant condition associated with skeletal myopathies.[34]

The pathophysiology is characterized by decreased cardiac output, increased jugular venous pressure, and pulmonary congestion. Biatrial enlargement accounts for frequent thromboembolic events, a presenting symptom in up to one third of patients with RCM.[34] Both right- and left-sided CHF symptoms are common presenting scenarios. Examination reveals increased jugular venous pulse and decreased pulse pressure. An S$_3$ due to abrupt cessation of early rapid filling is common. The ECG is invariably abnormal, showing left bundle branch blocks more commonly than right, decreased voltage (especially in amyloidosis), and a wide variety of dysrhythmias (particularly in the infiltrative diseases). Chest radiograph reveals evidence of pulmonary and venous hypertension and congestion. Echocardiogram is essential to rule out other causes of the patient's symptoms, and to assess filling rates and pressures. CT and MRI are often very helpful in distinguishing RCM from its most important differential consideration—constrictive pericarditis. Cardiac catheterization is critical to define hemodynamic parameters and to perform endomyocardial biopsy. If the distinction between RCM and constrictive pericarditis remains unclear, exploratory surgery and empiric pericardectomy are often attempted.

Treatment with diuretics is indicated for congestive symptoms, but caution must be exercised to avoid decreasing preload to the extent that cardiac output is compromised further. Because of its proarrhythmic effects, digitalis should be avoided if systolic function is normal; amiodarone is preferred for maintenance of sinus rhythm. For clinically significant conduction abnormalities that are refractory to medical therapy, pacemaker implantation is indicated. As a last resort, transplantation may be considered in idiopathic RCM, but has a poor prognosis in amyloidosis and sarcoidosis, as these diseases tend to recur in the transplanted heart.[34]

Prevention

Because so many instances of CM are secondary to treatable causes, early and appropriately aggressive prevention and treatment of hypertension, CAD, and alcohol and illicit drug abuse, as well as optimizing control of the host of metabolic conditions that may predispose to CM, form the mainstay of preventive strategy. While little can be done to prevent the types of CM having a primarily genetic etiology, it is imperative to perform careful screening of all first-degree relatives with a thorough history, physical examination, and echocardiogram.

Pulmonary Hypertension

Pulmonary hypertension (PH) is a rare disease with a universally fatal outcome if untreated. It is defined by a mean pulmonary artery (PA) pressure >25 mm Hg at rest and >30 mm Hg during exercise.[35] The incidence of primary pulmonary hypertension (PPH) is one to two cases per million population, with a female predominance (1.7:1), a mean age at diagnosis in the mid-30s, and a median survival of 2 years after diagnosis; the 5-year survival is less than 40%. It has been shown that 6% to 10% of PPH is familial, with autosomal-dominant inheritance and incomplete penetrance.[36] Many common congenital cardiac defects as well as a long list of acquired conditions may also lead to the development of PH. The final common pathway for all causes of PH is right ventricular failure (RVF). With recent advances in the characterization and management of PH, early diagnosis is imperative since starting therapy before pulmonary vasculature has lost its responsiveness increases the likelihood of therapeutic success.

All etiologies of PH are felt to have one or more underlying pathophysiologic mechanisms: vascular injury (PA plexogenic arteriopathy of PPH), an alteration in the balance of vasodilatation and vasoconstriction normally controlled by local vascular factors, and thrombotic changes in the pulmonary vasculature. Numerous secondary etiologies of PH have been identified. Atrial and ventriculoseptal defects (ASD and VSD) and patent ductus arteriosus lead to a hyperkinetic state with increased flow to the right heart. Pulmonary venous hypertension may be caused by mitral stenosis, pulmonary obstruction (tumor, pulmonary embolism, sickle cell disease), or LV failure. If detected early, hyperkinetic states and pulmonary venous hypertension are often reversible, as is the pulmonary arterial hypertension that results. Pulmonary hypertension secondary to other causes is often less reversible, and these causes include parenchymal lung disease, obstructive sleep apnea, chest wall deformities and neuromuscular disorders that impair the mechanics of ventilation, CREST syndrome (calcinosis, Raynaud's phenomenon, esophageal dysmotility, sclerodactyly, and telangiectasias), pulmonary vasculidities (Raynaud's, dermatomyositis, rheumatoid arthritis, systemic lupus erythematosus), hepatic cirrhosis with portal hypertension, and human immunodeficiency virus (HIV) disease. Conditions less strongly associated with PH include hypothyroidism and the use of appetite suppressants.

Presentation and Diagnosis

Because the presentation can be so nonspecific, the physician's challenge is to be aware of the risk factors for PH and to have an appropriate index of suspicion. The goal of the evaluation and early consultation is to identify an underlying cause and to define the extent of pulmonary vascular pathology and RV dysfunction. The most common presenting symptoms include dyspnea (initially only with exertion), angina due to RV ischemia, and syncope or near-syncope due to reduced cardiac output. Examination may reveal increased jugular venous distention, RV heave, and a prominent P_2. Significant RVF may be evidenced by an S_4, peripheral edema, hepatomegaly, and ascites. With more severe PH one may appreciate an S_3, the holosystolic murmur of tricuspid regurgitation, or the early diastolic murmur of pulmonic regurgitation (the Graham Steell murmur). Chest radiograph may show increased hilar structures and enlarged RV and right atrium. Electrocardiogram usually reveals a normal sinus rhythm, right chamber enlargement, and a strain pattern. Transthoracic echocardiogram with Doppler is the screening method of choice,[37] allowing measurement of RV systolic pressures and morphologic abnormalities, LV function, valvular assessment, and identification of intracardiac shunts.

Definitive diagnosis requires right heart catheterization and measurement of PA pressures. Specific studies that are useful for the evaluation of specific causes of PH include TEE for selected intracardiac abnormalities; polysomnography for obstructive sleep apnea; pulmonary function testing for parenchymal lung disease; serologic tests for connective tissue disorders (e.g., lupus anticoagulant, anticardiolipin and antinuclear antibodies); platelet count and liver functions for cirrhosis and portal hypertension; HIV screening; hemoglobin electrophoresis for sickle cell disease; serum coagulation tests; and ventilation-perfusion scan and possibly CT for chronic pulmonary emboli (PE). If chronic PE is suspected, pulmonary angiography is indicated.

Differential Diagnosis

Coronary artery disease and cardiomyopathies leading to RV dysfunction may account for the presenting symptoms and signs of PH. This broad diagnostic overlap often results in nearly a 2-year delay in diagnosing PH.[36]

Intervention

Due to the invasive means necessary to diagnose and treat PH, early consultation is a must to determine the feasibility and timing of surgical therapies for potentially reversible causes (e.g., ASD, VSD, mitral stenosis). General measures to be recommended include supplemental oxygen on airplanes, and avoiding high altitudes, pregnancy (a hemodynamically high flow state), and oral contraceptive drugs (due to clotting risk).[35] Supplemental oxygen is otherwise only useful for documented hypoxemia, which is usually found only with exertion, though patients with parenchymal lung disease may need it at rest. Digoxin may be used for overt RV failure, but other agents commonly used for LV failure (e.g., beta-blockers and ACEIs) are contraindicated due to their tendency to depress RV function. Diuretics should be used only for signs of systemic congestion, and then with extreme caution as RV function is preload dependent. Anticoagulation is associated with increased survival times, and warfarin is indicated to achieve an international normalized ratio of 2.0. Approximately one third of patients respond to vasodilating agents with a decrease in PA pressures and resistance, and can be placed on oral dihydropyridine calcium antagonists. However, empiric trials of these agents should never be undertaken, since nonresponders may decompensate precipitously. Responder status is best determined during right heart catheterization with the administration of potent, short-acting IV vasodilators while monitoring PA pressure and resistance. Those who do not respond may benefit from epoprostenol, a prostacyclin administered continuously via a Hickman catheter. Originally used as a temporizing measure while awaiting organ donation, epoprostenol allowed many such patients to avoid the need for transplant altogether. In addition to its vasodilating action, it is believed that epoprostenol's antiplatelet and vascular remodeling effects may underlie its success.

Except for repairing the underlying defects mentioned earlier, surgical interventions are generally options of last resort. Pulmonary thromboendarterectomy is indicated in severe PH caused by a clot that is proximal enough in the pulmonary vascular tree to be amenable to removal. Atrial septostomy, which creates a right to left shunt, thereby unloading the RV and increasing cardiac output, may be used in patients with recurrent syncope or RV failure when medical therapy has failed, and generally only as a bridge to transplant. Single or bilateral lung, and heart–bilateral lung transplant yields up to a 44% 5-year survival without recurrence of PH, though bronchiolitis obliterans is common.[37]

Prevention

Early repair of anatomic defects causing either a hyperkinetic state or pulmonary venous hypertension is paramount. Efforts to prevent or effectively manage parenchymal lung disease are also important. All first-degree relatives of patients with either PPH or a congenital cardiac anomaly should be screened with TTE at the time of diagnosis of the index case.

Peripheral Vascular Disease

While the prevalence of peripheral vascular disease (PVD) in the general population is 30%, only 5% have symptoms of claudication.[38] Coronary artery disease and stroke occur 2 to 4 times more often in symptomatic patients with PVD than in those without symptoms, and 2 to 3 times more often in patients with asymptomatic PVD compared to those without PVD. In addition, 70% to 80% of patients with symptomatic PVD are stable over 5 to 10 years. Amputation rates range from 0.8% to 1.0% per year, and are higher in smokers and diabetics. Therefore, the primary importance in diagnosing PVD lies in its role in identifying patients at risk for CAD morbidity and mortality.

Atherosclerosis is the most common cause of PVD, just as it is for CAD and stroke. Risk factors for PVD parallel those for CAD and include smoking, diabetes, hypertension, hyperlipidemia, age over 50 years, male gender, obesity, and postmenopausal status. Putative risk factors whose link to PVD is less well established include homocystinemia, elevated fibrinogen and uric acid levels, and chlamydia infection.[39]

Presentation and Diagnosis

The cardinal symptom of PVD is claudication, although patients may also present with complaints of poorly healing ul-

cerations. Numbness, paresthesias, and rest pain are often associated with severely compromised circulation. Aortoiliac disease is heralded by low back and buttock pain, and when accompanied by impotence is termed Leriche's syndrome. Thigh pain indicates iliac or common femoral artery disease, whereas foot pain is usually due to infrapopliteal disease. Calf pain is most commonly caused by superficial femoral arterial disease, but may be the result of occlusion at any level above this. However, since 83% of PVD patients are asymptomatic, findings on physical examination may be the only clinical clue to the presence of disease. Significant signs include diminished pulses and increased capillary refill time; atrophic changes such as muscle wasting, changes in skin color, and hair loss; and decreased warmth and dependent rubor. A bruit found with a decreased pulse indicates a hemodynamically significant obstruction, but does not quantify its severity. Evaluation of collateral circulation carries important treatment implications and is performed by placing the patient in the supine position and elevating the limb to 45 degrees; pallor in the distal extremity indicates inadequate collateral circulation.

The key diagnostic study is the ankle-brachial index (ABI), normally 1.0 to 1.1. An ABI <0.8 indicates significant PVD, and <0.5 indicates multilevel disease. In either case, further imaging is indicated with either duplex ultrasound and Doppler color flow (which localizes diseased segments and grades lesion severity) or MR angiography (especially good for evaluation of arterial dissection and wall morphology). Where noninvasive techniques are inadequate and surgery is indicated, fluoroscopic angiography is the test of choice.

Differential Diagnosis

The most common differential considerations include neurogenic claudication due to either disk disease, spinal stenosis, or osteophytic changes, and shin splints (in younger persons). Less common causes are Buerger's disease (thromboangiitis obliterans) and congenital anatomic abnormalities such as popliteal artery entrapment.

Intervention

As smokers with PVD have a tenfold risk of amputation, tobacco cessation is essential. Other nonspecific interventions include diets low in cholesterol and fat and high in fruits and vegetables, keeping the feet warm and dry and nails trimmed, and inspecting the feet daily and reporting any trauma to the physician immediately. Graded exercise programs improve exercise tolerance in up to 30% of patients. Pharmacologic measures to decrease blood pressure and serum lipid levels are also indicated, with similar end points to those for treating CAD. Aspirin (75–325 mg po qd) with or without dipyridamole (150–400 mg po qd) has been shown to decrease CAD and stroke risk, and is indicated for PVD as well. Ticlopidine (250 mg po bid with meals) and clopidogrel (75 mg po qd) have both been shown to be effective in decreasing the incidence of vascular morbidity in general, and ticlopidine has also been shown to improve symptoms and objective measures of PVD. However, ticlopidine is associated with significant adverse hematologic effects which may limit its utility.[40] Pentoxifylline (400 mg po tid) offers no consistently significant clinical benefit, but may be considered in severely impaired patients for whom even small symptomatic improvements would be meaningful. Vasodilator and anticoagulant therapy have not been shown to be useful in chronic PVD. Surgical consultation is indicated for occupation or lifestyle limiting symptoms where nonsurgical therapy has failed or for signs or symptoms of ischemia at rest.

References

1. Lorell BH. Pericardial diseases. In: Braunwald E, ed. Heart disease: a textbook of cardiovascular medicine, 5th ed. Philadelphia: WB Saunders, 1997;1478–505.
2. Myers RBH, Spodick DH. Constrictive pericarditis: clinical and pathophysiologic characteristics. Am Heart J 1999;138(2): 219–32.
3. Chan TC, Brady WJ, Pollack M. Electrocardiographic manifestations: acute myopericarditis. J Emerg Med 1999;17(5):865–72.
4. Vaitkus PT, LeWinter MM. Pericardial disease. In: Bone RC, Alpert JS, eds. Current practice of medicine. Philadelphia: Churchill Livingstone, 1996;II:21.1–8.
5. Osterberg L, Vagelos R, Atwood JE. Case presentation and review: constrictive pericarditis. West J Med 1998;169(4):232–9.
6. Sagrista-Sauleda J, Barrabes JA, Permanyer-Miralda G, Soler-Soler J. Purulent pericarditis: review of a 20-year experience in a general hospital. J Am Coll Cardiol 1993;22:1661–5.
7. Caforio ALP, McKenna WJ. Recognition and optimum management of myocarditis. Drugs 1996;52(4):515–25.
8. Kawai C. From myocarditis to cardiomyopathy: mechanisms of inflammation and cell death. Circulation 1999;99(8):1091–100.
9. Pisani B, Taylor DO, Mason JW. Inflammatory myocardial diseases and cardiomyopathies. Am J Med 1997;102(5):459–69.
10. Mendes LA, Picard MH, Dec GW, Hartz VL, Palacios IF, Davidoff R. Ventricular remodeling in active myocarditis. Am Heart J 1999;138(2):303–8.
11. Parrillo JE. Myocarditis: How should we treat in 1998? J Heart Lung Transplant 1998;17(10):941–4.
12. Rezkalla SH, Raikar S, Kloner RA. Treatment of viral myocarditis with focus on captopril. Am J Cardiol 1996;77(8):634–7.
13. Durack DT. Infective endocarditis. In: Alexander RW, Schlant RC, Fuster V, eds. Hurst's the heart, arteries and veins, 9th edition. New York: McGraw-Hill, 1997;2205–39.
14. Cunha BA, Gill MV, Lazar JM. Acute infective endocarditis: diagnostic and therapeutic approach. Infect Dis Clin North Am 1996;10(4):811–34.
15. Brook MM. Pediatric bacterial endocarditis: treatment and prophylaxis. Pediatr Clin North Am 1999;46(2):275–87.
16. Kemp WE, Citrin B, Byrd BF. Echocardiography in infective endocarditis. South Med J 1999;92(8):744–54.
17. Durack DT, Lukes AS, Bright DK. New criteria for diagnosis of infective endocarditis: utilization of specific echocardiographic findings. Am J Med 1994;96(3):200–9.
18. Cecchi E, Parrini I, Chinaglia A, et al. New diagnostic criteria for infective endocarditis: a study of sensitivity and specificity. Eur Heart J 1997;18(7):1149–56.
19. Hoen B, Beguinot I, Rabaud C, et al. The Duke criteria for diagnosing infective endocarditis are specific: analysis of 100 patients with acute fever or fever of unknown origin. Clin Infect Dis 1996;23(2):298–302.
20. Dodds GA, Sexton DJ, Durack DT, Bashore TM, Corey GR, Kisslo J. Negative predictive value of the Duke criteria for infective endocarditis. Am J Cardiol 1996;77(5):403–7.
21. Stockheim JA, Chadwick EG, Kessler S, et al. Are the Duke criteria superior to the Beth Israel criteria for the diagnosis of infective endocarditis in children? Clin Infect Dis 1998;27(6): 1451–6.
22. Del Pont JM, De Cicco LT, Vartalitis C, et al. Infective endocarditis in children: clinical analyses and evaluation of two diagnostic criteria. Pediatr Infect Dis J 1995;14(12):1079–86.
23. Nettles RE, McCarty DE, Corey GR, Li J, Sexton DJ. An evaluation of the Duke criteria in 25 pathologically confirmed cases of prosthetic valve endocarditis. Clin Infect Dis 1997;25(6): 1401–3.
24. Giessel BE, Koenig CJ, Blake RL. Management of bacterial endocarditis. Am Fam Physician 2000;61(6):1725–32.
25. Wilson WR, Karchmer AW, Dajani AS, et al. Antibiotic treatment of adults with infective endocarditis due to streptococci, enterococci, staphylococci, and HACEK microorganisms. JAMA 1995;274(21):1706–13.
26. Moon MR, Stinson EB, Miller DC. Surgical treatment of endocarditis. Prog Cardiovasc Dis 1997;40(3):239–64.
27. Richardson P, McKenna W, Bristow M, et al. Report of the 1995 World Health Organization/International Society and Federation of Cardiology Task Force on the definition and classification of cardiomyopathies. Circulation 1996;93(5):841–2.
28. Elliott P. Diagnosis and management of dilated cardiomyopathy. Heart 2000;84(1):106–12.
29. McKelvie RS, Yusuf S, Pericak D, et al. Comparison of candesartan, enalapril and their combination in congestive cardiac failure. Randomized evaluation of strategies for left ventricular dysfunction (RESOLVD) pilot study. Circulation 1999;100(10): 1056–64.
30. Pitt B, Zannad F, Remme WJ, et al. The effect of spironolactone on morbidity and mortality in patients with severe heart failure. N Engl J Med 1999;341(10):709–17.
31. Louie EK, Edwards LC III. Hypertrophic cardiomyopathy. Prog Cardiovasc Dis 1994;36(4):275–308.
32. Wigle ED, Rakowski H, Kimball BP, Williams WG. Hypertrophic cardiomyopathy: clinical spectrum and treatment. Circulation 1995;92(7):1680–92.
33. Maron BJ. Hypertrophic cardiomyopathy. In: Alexander RW, Schlant RC, Fuster V, eds. Hurst's the heart, arteries and veins, 9th edition. New York: McGraw-Hill, 1997;2057–74.
34. Kushwaha SS, Fallon JT, Fuster V. Restrictive cardiomyopathy. N Engl J Med 1997;336(4):267–76.
35. Barst RJ. Recent advances in the treatment of pediatric pulmonary artery hypertension. Pediatr Clin North Am 1999;46(2): 331–45.
36. Peacock AJ. Primary pulmonary hypertension. Thorax 1999;54: 1107–18.
37. Krowka MJ. Pulmonary hypertension: diagnostics and therapeutics. Mayo Clinic Proc 2000;75:625–30.
38. Fowkes FGR. Epidemiology of peripheral vascular disease. Atherosclerosis 1997;131(suppl):29–31.
39. Powers KB, Vacek JL, Lee S. Noninvasive approaches to peripheral vascular disease: what's new in evaluation and treatment? Postgrad Med 1999;106(3):52–64.
40. Jackson MR, Clagett GP. Antithrombotic therapy in peripheral arterial occlusive disease. Chest 1998;114(5 suppl):666S–82S.

83

Obstructive Airway Disease

Howard N. Weinberg

Obstructive airway disease includes two entities that share many common characteristics, asthma and chronic obstructive pulmonary disease (COPD). Chronic cough, a prominent symptom of both ailments, is also discussed in this chapter.

Background

Asthma

Asthma is a disorder of the pulmonary airways characterized by reversible obstruction, inflammation, and hyperresponsiveness.[1] Approximately 9 million to 12 million Americans are affected by this disease, with an annual mortality of 4000 to 5000.[2] Initial onset can be at any age, in either sex, and in every race. The severity of this illness is difficult to predict; some victims suffer a rapidly worsening course, whereas others appear to "outgrow" the disease.

The bronchospasm and inflammation may be triggered by allergens, infection, and psychophysiologic stressors. Allergens include inhaled substances such as molds, pollens, dust, animal danders, industrial pollutants, tobacco smoke, smoke from wood stoves, and cosmetics. Oral inducers may be food preservatives containing sulfiting agents and medications, especially aspirin and β-adrenergic antagonists (including selective agents and topical preparations).

Respiratory infections, particularly viral, are also major stimulators.[3] Occasionally a virus, such as the respiratory syncytial virus, induces bronchospasm in nearly all patients. Some patients have attacks only with infections.

Psychological factors certainly play a role in inducing asthma episodes. These triggers may be difficult to recognize and may manifest as part of a panic attack, as fear of the disease itself, or as a symptom of abuse. Panic attacks can also be confused with and misdiagnosed as asthma (see Chapter 31).

Chronic Obstructive Pulmonary Disease (COPD)

Chronic obstructive pulmonary disease is characterized by abnormal expiratory flow that does not change significantly over time. This delineation was intended to exclude asthma as well as specific upper airway diseases such as cancers and conditions affecting the lower airways such as bronchiectasis, sarcoidosis, and cystic fibrosis.[4] Traditionally included in this category has been chronic bronchitis and emphysema. In some patients, however, the overlap with asthma is so strong that a significant distinction cannot be made. Indeed, the term COPD was developed in recognition of the tremendous overlap between asthma, chronic bronchitis, and emphysema.

Chronic bronchitis is defined as a cough that occurs at least 3 months a year for 2 consecutive years and involves excess mucous secretion in the large airways. A malady of adults, chronic bronchitis affects about 20% of men and is primarily caused by smoking. Unfortunately, the incidence in women is increasing as the percentage of women smokers increases. Other contributing factors include air pollution, occupational exposures, and infection.[5]

Emphysema is defined as a permanent enlargement of distal air spaces with destruction of the acinar walls without fibrosis. This entity can be further subdivided into centriacinar, panacinar, and distal acinar types.[6] Like chronic bronchitis, this illness is found primarily in smokers. There is, however, a rare type of congenital emphysema and also a genetic syndrome associated with the lack of α_1-antitrypsin.

Chronic Cough

Although cough is an essential component of the presentation of both COPD and asthma, there are many other entities that can cause chronic coughing. The four most common causes are postnasal drip syndrome, COPD, asthma, and gastroesophageal reflux.[7] Other causes include acute and chronic infection, other lung diseases (embolism, cancer), aspiration, psychogenic factors, and cardiac failure. Cough can also result from medications, such as angiotensin-converting enzyme (ACE) inhibitors. Also, a significant number of patients have two or more causes for cough.

Clinical Presentation

Asthma

The classic symptoms of asthma are cough, dyspnea, and wheezing. The wheezing may be audible or require auscultation. Infrequently, a patient may be so "tight" that wheezing is detected only after initial therapy. The patient might be resting comfortably or be in extreme respiratory distress. At such times there may be accessory muscle movement (subcostal, intercostal, or supraclavicular), nasal flaring (particularly in children), cyanosis, or altered mental status. Auscultation often reveals rhonchi, wheezing, and a reversal of the normal 2:1 inspiratory/expiratory ratio. An increase in respiratory rate, independent of fever, is also a cardinal sign.

Sometimes, especially in children, the only presentation of asthma is a chronic night cough. Another symptom complex includes wheezing and shortness of breath that occurs following exercise. This entity is known as exercise-induced asthma (EIA) or bronchospasm (EIB). Many Olympic-caliber athletes have EIB.

COPD

The typical picture of COPD is prominent cough, dyspnea, and often wheezing. In severe situations tachypnea, accessory muscle movement, breathing through pursed lips, cyanosis, and agitation are present. Long-standing disease may be indicated by a pronounced barrel chest (i.e., an increase in the anterior-to-posterior dimension). Copious sputum production may also be noted. Chest auscultation may reveal wheezes, rales, or rhonchi in varying intensity, or it can be normal. Heart sounds might be distant, or a gallop indicative of secondary heart disease may be detected. Examination of the extremities might reveal cyanosis of the nailbeds or clubbing of the fingers.

Cough

Clinical presentation of cough is self-explanatory: the patient is coughing. It is important to note whether the cough is dry or productive of sputum (thick, thin, purulent, bloody). The time of day or night often provides a clue to the extensive differential diagnosis as can evidence of allergy such as rhinitis, allergic shiners, or a transverse nose crease (the allergic salute). Of particular note are symptoms related to gastro-esophageal reflux (e.g., heartburn, water brash, or increased belching). Finally, these patients may present with the signs and symptoms of a multitude of underlying diseases.

Diagnosis

Asthma and COPD

The diagnosis of asthma or COPD should be fairly evident after the history and physical examinations are completed. Laboratory and radiographic data by themselves usually cannot establish the diagnosis of either disorder but may provide confirmatory information and assist in the assessment of severity.

Pulmonary Function Tests

Although extensive pulmonary testing may be indicated in the occasional patient, the most useful information is obtained from evaluating the forced expiratory volume in 1 second (FEV_1), the forced vital capacity (FVC), the FEV_1/FVC ratio, and the peak expiratory flow rate (PEFR). Obstructive disease is indicated by a reduced FEV_1 in the presence of a normal FVC, which also causes a reduction in the FEV_1/FVC ratio. Restrictive diseases (pure emphysema), on the other hand, show a normal FEV_1, a decreased FVC, and an increased FEV_1/FVC ratio.

With asthma a useful test is to observe the change in FEV_1 following treatment with a bronchodilator. An increase of 15% is indicative of reversible airway disease.[4] Three stimulators—exercise, histamine, methacholine—may be used for provocative testing. A decrease in FEV_1 of 20% is considered positive. The PEFR may be obtained using a peak flowmeter and can be measured in the office or at home. It provides a quick, objective indication of the severity of an episode and can serve as a signal to start certain treatments. It is also a measure of the response to therapeutic intervention. It is highly recommended that patients be provided with peak flowmeters and instructed about how to use them. These devices must be demonstrated and practiced. Many patients have trouble mastering the technique. To be fully effective, this device must be used when patients are feeling well in order to define a personal "best" for later comparison. With COPD the spirometric abnormalities may be a mixture of obstructive and restrictive diseases. In asymptomatic patients, especially smokers, abnormal results can serve as an indicator of early illness and, it is hoped, as a stimulus to quit smoking. In symptomatic patients, these measurements can serve as a sign of progression. Finally, the FEV_1 or PEFR may be used to evaluate the asthmatic component in the COPD patient.

Arterial Blood Gases

Evaluation of the severity of disease may be assisted by the measurement of arterial blood gases (ABGs). Severe hypoxemia in the asthmatic or hypercapnia in the chronic lung patient might serve as an important factor in the decision to hospitalize a patient. Most outpatients do not need ABG measurements.

Other Laboratory Tests

Useful tests in ill patients include measurement of blood leukocytes as a sign of acute infection, and hematocrit as indicative of an additional reason for hypoxemia if it is low or as a sign of long-standing hypoxemia if polycythemia is noted. Sputum evaluation is useful for identifying the pathogen in an acute infection.

Chest Radiography

It is not necessary to obtain a chest radiograph on every patient with asthma or COPD. A radiograph may be useful in the undiagnosed patient with chronic cough and may help to identify complications in patients with obstructive disease. These problems might include pneumonia, pneumothorax, pneumomediastinum, or subcutaneous emphysema. In the newly discovered asthmatic (especially children) radiography should be done if foreign body aspiration is suspected. The chest radiograph of the COPD patient may be normal; show a mild increase in lung markings; demonstrate the hyperlucency, overinflation, and bullae often seen with emphysema; or show an enlarged heart or the pulmonary congestion seen with heart failure. On occasion, a chest film holds the key to differentiating congestive heart failure with wheezing (cardiac asthma) from asthma (see Chapter 79). Other radiologic procedures, such as lung scans, computed tomography (CT) scans, and angiography have a role only in the management of complications.

Chronic Cough

The diagnosis and workup of chronic cough is often difficult, time-consuming, and expensive. Irwin and associates[7] presented a schema for evaluating previously undiagnosed patients. Their suggestions, in decreasing order of usefulness, include the history, physical examination, pulmonary function tests, methacholine challenge, upper gastrointestinal radiology, measurement of esophageal pH, sinus and chest radiography, and bronchoscopy. Following this approach a diagnosis is possible in 99% of patients.

Management

The management of asthma and COPD is best viewed from a standpoint of both disease complexes. It includes avoidance, immunotherapy, exercise, drug treatment, and psychosocial support (Fig. 83.1).

Avoidance

The lifestyle of the patient with pulmonary problems may be drastically affected by environmental factors: climate, outdoor air pollution, and indoor air pollution.

Climate

Both asthmatic and COPD sufferers may be affected by changes in wind velocity, humidity, and temperature. Low wind velocity allows accumulation of allergens; high humidity leads to an increase in pollen-producing plants and molds; and sudden temperature drops cause a fall in airway conduction.[8] Barometric pressure changes are also associated with exacerbations of asthma and COPD. Extremes in climatic

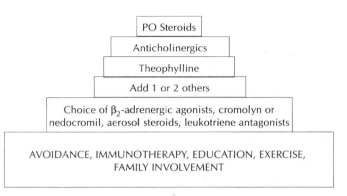

Asthma Maintenance

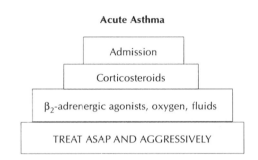

Acute Asthma

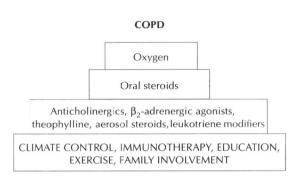

COPD

Fig. 83.1. Recommended step treatment plan for asthma and chronic obstructive pulmonary disease (COPD). ASAP = as soon as possible.

events, such as prolonged heat waves or air inversions, often result in increased mortality among COPD patients. Although patients cannot avoid climatic changes, they can stay inside on particularly bad days and can minimize the effects by using filtered air-conditioning and heating systems maintained at fairly constant temperature year round.

Outdoor Air Pollution

Potential allergens include man-made (e.g., smoke and chemical fumes) and natural substances (e.g., pollens, dusts, and molds). Although difficult to avoid, some factors can be minimized by controlling the type of grass, ornamental shrubs, and flowering vegetation around the home.

Indoor Air Pollution

Fortunately, indoor allergens are much more readily controlled. It is of paramount importance to eliminate tobacco smoke. Other potential irritants include building materials, cleaning agents, air fresheners, pest control chemicals, decorative plants, dried flowers, cockroachs, scented candles, and cosmetics. The bedroom is a critical room to allergy-proof. Attention is directed to pillows, mattresses, carpets, drapes, blankets, shelf ornaments, and stuffed animals (especially in the bed). Wood stoves and kerosene heaters have been shown to aggravate respiratory problems. Sometimes families must give up their pets. This entire aspect of avoidance must be stressed to all patients and may obviate the need for further treatment.

Education of patients is essential regarding all aspects of management. Excellent material is available from the National Asthma Education Program.[9]

Immunotherapy

Desensitization

If avoidance fails, allergic patients should be tried on antihistamines and nasal sprays and considered for allergy desensitization.[10]

Immunization

Influenza and pneumococcal vaccines should be given to all patients with significant respiratory illness. Influenza vaccine is administered yearly about 2 to 3 months prior to anticipated outbreaks. October and November are the prime times to immunize in the United States. If a patient misses the vaccine, consideration should be given to prophylaxis with antiviral medications. Pneumococcal vaccine should be supplemented with booster injections once after 5 years, although this recommendation may change.

Exercise

Aerobic exercise is important for both asthmatics and COPD patients. Proper and consistent exercise at least three times a week can lead to improved tolerance and endurance and an increase in the feeling of wellness.[11] Consider ordering pulmonary rehabilitation.

Drug Treatment

The choice of medication for these illnesses has greatly expanded since the 1980s and is presently continuing to undergo rapid changes in philosophy. It is especially true for asthma, where emphasis has shifted from treating just bronchospasm to treating inflammation as well.[1] Unfortunately, those who suffer with COPD have not experienced as great a revolution in drug treatment.

β_2-Adrenergic Agonists

The β_2-adrenergic agonist class of medication (beta-2s) is now the first step for treating bronchospasm. Available as liquids, short- and long-acting tablets, metered-dose inhalers (MDIs), dry powder inhalers, nebulizable solutions, and injectables, these agents have many potential uses. Available in the United States are albuterol (Proventil, Ventolin), bitolterol (Tornalate), metaproterenol (Alupent, Metaprel), pirbuterol (Maxair), terbutaline (Brethaire, Brethine), and salmeterol (Serevent) (Table 83.1).

The choice of preparation depends on the patient's age and the acuteness of the situation. MDIs and nebulizers have an almost instantaneous onset of action, and sustained-released tablets offer assistance with nocturnal symptoms. Oral forms have their greatest use in young children. It is rarely necessary to use both the oral and inhalation route at the same time, a situation that leads to increased toxicity with little gain in benefit.

Beta-2s are the treatment of choice for episodic or mild asthmatics and for EIB. Once the need is established for continual usage, as for moderate and severe asthmatics, some authorities use these agents as first-line treatment whereas others reserve their use for rescue efforts, preferring to use antiinflammatory drugs first. Certainly, every patient with significant obstructive disease should always have this medication on hand.

The newest member of this class, salmeterol, is unique in its 12-hour action. It is indicated for maintenance and nocturnal symptoms of both asthma and COPD. Shorter-acting agents may still be used between doses if rescue is needed, although tolerance may become a problem.[12]

In the near future, dry-powder forms of MDIs should be available. It is hoped this advance will reduce the problems associated with propellant gases and also be more compatible with the environment.

For the treatment of acute situations, beta-2s are the agents of choice. They can be administered by nebulizer (and repeated at 60- to 90-minute intervals if needed[13]) or by MDI using an InspirEase at the rate of one inhalation per minute for 5 minutes. The use of these agents has supplanted the need for older agents such as ephedrine, isoproterenol, and epinephrine. Even in the emergency situation, beta-2s have been found to be equally effective with significantly less toxicity when compared to subcutaneous epinephrine.[14]

Some patients experience great trouble utilizing an MDI. Proper technique must be taught and observed. For those too young or who cannot master the MDI, the following spacer devices are available: InspirEase, Inhal-aid, Paper tube, and Aerochamber.[15] Home-made alternatives are the inside of a paper towel roll or a small paper lunch bag. Any of these devices should work with all inhalers.

In the COPD patient these drugs have less application but are still valuable when bronchospasm is present. Pulse and blood pressure should be monitored.

Corticosteroids

The use of steroids for asthma has received considerable impetus in recent years. Traditionally thought to be too strong for chronic use, the advent of MDI preparations has minimized side effects and pushed corticosteroids to the forefront. In addition, recognition of the importance of inflammation in the pathophysiology of asthma has made many authorities advocate corticosteroids as first-line treatment.[16] Unfortunately,

Table 83.1. **Recommended Dosages for Theophylline, β_2-Adrenergic Agonists and Corticosteroids**

Medication	Age group (years)	Route	Usual dosage
Theophylline	<1	po	Varies
	1–9	po	24 mg/kg/day
	9–12	po	20 mg/kg/day
	12–16	po	18 mg/kg/day
	>16, smoker	po	18 mg/kg/day
	>16, nonsmoker	po	13 mg/kg/day
Albuterol	>2	po	0.1 mg/kg/tid–qid, max 2 mg tid
	>2	MDI	1–2 inhal q4h
	>12	Nebulizer	2.5 mg q4h
Bitolterol	>12	MDI	2 inhal q4h or 3 inhal q6h
Metaproterenol	<6	po	1.3–2.6 mg/kg/day tid–qid
	>6	po	10–20 mg tid/qid
	>2	MDI	1–2 inhal q4h
	>12	Nebulizer	0.2–0.3 ml q4h
Pirbuterol	>12	MDI	1–2 inhal q4h
Salmeterol	>12	MDI	2 inhal q12h
Terbutaline	>12	po	1.25–5.00 mg tid
	>12	MDI	2 inhal q4h
Beclomethasone	>6	MDI	2–4 inhal bid/qid, max 20/day
Budesonide	>6	MDI	1–2 inhal bid, max 8/day
Flunisolide	>6	MDI	2 inhal bid, max 8/day
Fluticasone	>6	MDI	Three different strengths
Triamcinolone	>6	MDI	1–2 inhal tid/qid, max 16/day
Prednisone	1–12	po	1–2 mg/kg/day, taper 5–10 days
	>12	po	40–80 mg/day, taper 5–10 days

Source: Data are from the Physicians' Desk Reference.[17]

MDI = Multiple-dose inhaler; inhal = inhalations.

the probably unfounded fear of the effect of steroids on growth and adrenal function has caused a reluctance to utilize this medication. For the moderate to severe asthmatic, for the unstable patient, and during an acute crisis, however, there should be no hesitancy to use steroids.

Aerosol preparations include beclomethasone (Beclovent, Vanceril), budesonide (Pulmicort), flunisolide (AeroBid), fluticasone (Flovent), and triamcinolone (Azmacort). The effect of these medications may not be fully seen for up to 4 to 8 weeks and are therefore not effective for the acute attack. They also do not protect against adrenal insufficiency. Oral medication must be tapered when switching to an aerosol (Table 83.1).[17]

A new product combining fluticasone and salmeterol (Advair) in three dosage strengths was released in April 2001. Initial reports show significant advantages over either medication used alone.[18] Oral steroids, usually in the form of prednisone, are essential for use during the acute exacerbation or for the severe, chronic patient with asthma or COPD. When used early during an episode, steroids may prevent a relapse[19] or the need for hospitalization. Some physicians prescribe oral steroids to any patient needing treatment in an emergency setting. Patients with long-standing disease often develop recognizable patterns of deterioration, such as with acute upper respiratory infections. These patients can be instructed to use steroids early to prevent exacerbations. Dosage varies with age and weight. For chronic treatment, every-other-day administration is preferred, whereas multiple daily dosing may be most effective in the acute situation.

Corticosteroids are also available for intravenous use, which is indicated whenever hospitalization is being considered. Unfortunately, there is no definitive proof as to the effectiveness of intravenous steroids for preventing hospitalization. In addition, their onset of action is at least 4 hours.

Cromolyn and Nedocromil

Primarily used as prophylactic agents for asthma, cromolyn and nedocromil are antiinflammatory and, due to their almost complete lack of side effects, represent a significant therapeutic advantage. Unfortunately, not all patients respond to them.

Cromolyn (Intal) is available for MDI or nebulizer. Its onset of action can be as long as 1 to 2 months. Dosage is two inhalations qid; tapering to less frequent dosage can be attempted. Once it is begun, this medication should be used throughout an acute episode so as not to lose the prophylaxis. Along with beta-2s and inhaled steroids, cromolyn is useful for EIB.

Nedocromil (Tilade) is the newer of the two agents, and its safety is comparable to that of cromolyn. Dosage recommendations are also similar. In addition, nedocromil may be effective in preventing the cough caused by ACE inhibitors.

Leukotriene Modifiers

This is a new class of medications consisting of three agents: montelukast (Singulair), 10 mg in the evening, 4 or 5 mg for children; zafirlukast (Accolate), 20 mg bid avoiding food, 10 mg in children; and zileuton (Zyflo), rarely used due to qid dosing and the need to monitor liver enzymes. The first two products are occasionally also of benefit in COPD.[20]

Theophylline

Long the cornerstone of asthma treatment, theophylline is no longer the initial drug of choice. A bronchodilator, theophylline is best utilized for patients needing more than one maintenance drug and for those with pronounced nocturnal symptoms. It is also worth a trial in COPD patients.

There are various formulations of theophylline: liquid, capsule, tablet, slow-release products, and the intravenous form. Most patients require several days of continuous usage to reach maximal effectiveness. Once a steady state is reached, it is best to maintain the same brand, as bioavailability may vary from product to product. Smokers and children tend to need higher doses due to rapid metabolism. Significant interactions are possible with erythromycins, fluoroquinolones, cimetidine, phenytoin, and oral contraceptives. Also, dosages need to be closely monitored in patients with liver failure or congestive heart failure. Serum theophylline levels are recommended for all the above situations and in difficult patients where fine-tuning is needed. The serum therapeutic level has been changed from 10 to 20 μg/mL to 5 to 15 μg/mL.[21] Older preparations that contain subtherapeutic doses of theophylline, Marax and Tedral, are no longer considered appropriate therapy (Table 83.1).

Children require close monitoring. As they grow, their dosage requires constant readjustment. Theophylline has come under scrutiny with regard to potential interference with school performance, but no significant effect has been established.

In the acute situation (office or emergency room) theophylline (as aminophylline) is no longer considered appropriate for intravenous usage as it does not represent a therapeutic advantage but does significantly increase toxicity.[22] It may be useful, however, in hospitalized patients.

Anticholinergics

The current choice of anticholinergic drug is ipratropium (Atrovent) for MDI or nebulizer. For COPD, because of fewer side effects, ipratropium may well be the preferred bronchodilator. The usual dosage is two inhalations qid, but this dosage can be exceeded in COPD patients.[21] For asthma, use ipratropium if other treatment is not effective. Several studies combining nebulized ipratropium with a β_2-agonist have produced unclear results when used in severe asthma.[23]

Calcium Channel Blockers

Calcium channel blockers have been suggested to have a mild bronchodilatory effect, but it has not been clinically demonstrated. They are, however, effective for the treatment of hypertension in obstructive disease, especially compared to beta-blockers and ACE inhibitors.

Antibiotics

For acute bacterial infections in patients with asthma and COPD, antibiotics are essential. There has been debate concerning when to treat the COPD-afflicted patient. The use of broad-spectrum antibiotics appears to be indicated when COPD sufferers have at least two of the following three symptoms: an increase in dyspnea, an increase in sputum production, and an increase in sputum purulence.[24]

Mucolytics and Expectorants

The value of mucolytics and expectorants has not been demonstrated in objective studies.

Oxygen

Except in the acute situation, oxygen should be reserved for chronic patients who are in distress when breathing room air. With COPD patients who retain high levels of carbon dioxide, the only functioning respiratory drive may be related to hypoxia. It is therefore critical to adjust the oxygen to a level where the hypoxic drive is not lost.

Pregnancy and Breast-Feeding

Pregnancy is complicated by asthma about 1% of the time, with a potentially large risk to the fetus if hypoxia develops. The use of theophylline, beta-2s, cromolyn, Singulair, Accolate, and steroids is generally considered safe.[20] Some antibiotics and decongestants, live virus vaccines, and iodides must be avoided.

For lactating mothers the same medications considered safe during pregnancy are acceptable. Breast-feeding should be strongly encouraged, as studies suggest it delays the onset of allergies and asthma in the infant.[1,19]

Psychosocial Support

Psychosocial support is a critical component in any management plan and is addressed later in the chapter.

Prevention

Asthma and COPD are at opposite extremes when it comes to treatment and prevention. Whereas there are several fine alternatives for asthma treatment, management of COPD is at best symptomatic. On the other hand, asthma is essentially unpreventable, whereas COPD should not exist.

Smoking cessation is the key to relegating COPD to medical history. Except for a rare genetic or occupational case (which should also be preventable with good industrial hygiene), most COPD is directly related to smoking. The United States is moving in the direction of encouraging nonsmokers' rights, but unfortunately children have ready access to tobacco products and are still starting to smoke in large numbers. Physicians therefore must remind every smoker at every appointment to begin the process of cessation.

Control of smoking is also key to decreasing the morbidity of asthma. Even side-stream smoke has been shown to result in more attacks, more complications, and more frequent need for emergency services. It is critical that the parents of asthmatic children never smoke in the house or car. Prevention of death has always been a priority within the medical profession. It is certainly appropriate for asthma and COPD.

Asthma is usually viewed as a nonfatal disease, but it does carry the potential for death. Most studies show that preventable deaths and hospitalizations have been the result of delayed treatment due primarily to two factors: the patient's or family's inability to recognize the severity of an attack, and the physician's poor assessment of the severity of an attack.[25,26] Suggestions for prevention include frequent use of peak flowmeters as an objective guide to severity, establishing effective maintenance therapy, and emphasizing patient and family education. Education is aimed at recognizing an attack, knowing what measures to take at home, and learning to call for help early. The material provided in the national education program is superb and should be made available to all patients.[9]

On the other hand, COPD is a highly fatal disease, the fourth leading cause of mortality in the United States and still increasing.[27] Although little can be done to reverse this disease, good management of the environment, appropriate medication, and smoking cessation aid in improving the quality of life for the affected individual. Extremely severe cases may be considered for lung volume reduction surgery or transplantation.[11]

Family and Community Issues

Family support is an essential factor in the successful treatment of chronic lung disease. This point is especially true for children and the debilitated, who might be unable to care for themselves.

Asthma

Patient and family attitudes are critical in the patient's acceptance of this disease. Several factors have been identified with regard to poor patient attitude: the unpredictable nature of asthma leading to a feeling of "beyond my control"; a feeling of stigmatization; a false perception that asthma is psychogenic and therefore "in my head"; a tendency to deny the disease; and the fear elicited by an experience of being unable to breathe.[28] These attitudes may handicap all attempts at treatment and should be addressed via thorough patient and family education.

Also important is the tendency for families to label their asthmatics as ill. It is best to view the patient as a person with asthma and not as an asthmatic person. All activities should be continued, especially sports and physical education. It is far better to use an MDI and run than to sit on the sidelines and watch.

COPD

Emotional difficulties are common in COPD sufferers. The dyspnea and fatigue of this disease often leads to depression and fear. Quality of life may be reduced in all areas, including social, sexual, vocational, and recreational activities, leading to further loss of self-esteem and isolation.[29] Patients should be encouraged to do as much as possible for themselves and must be given every opportunity to participate in the usual family and community events, even if a wheelchair and oxygen are needed. When the illness becomes terminal, patients should be counseled to keep control of their own lives by participating in the decisions of how and where to die. They can be encouraged to make living wills or execute powers of attorney. If appropriate, patients should be allowed to die at home, and physicians should be willing to make house calls. This measure improves the final quality of life by affording the patient the comfort of dying in a familiar setting, surrounded by family and friends.

References

1. Guidelines for the diagnosis and management of asthma. National Asthma Education Program, expert panel report 2. NIH publ. no. 97-4051. Bethesda: National Heart, Lung and Blood Institute, 1997.
2. Shuttari MF. Asthma: diagnosis and management. Am Fam Physician 1995;52:2225–35.
3. Johnston SL, Pattemore PK, Sanderson G, et al. Community study of role of viral infections in exacerbations of asthma in 9–11 year old children. BMJ 1995;310:1225–9.
4. American Thoracic Society. Standards for the diagnosis and care of patients with chronic obstructive pulmonary disease (COPD) and asthma. Am Rev Respir Dis 1987;136:225–44.
5. Ingram RH. Chronic bronchitis, emphysema, and airways obstruction. In: Harrison's principles of internal medicine, 15th ed. New York: McGraw-Hill, 2001;1456-63, 1491–99.
6. Snider GL, Kleinerman J, Thurlbeck WM, Bengali ZH. The definition of emphysema: report of a National Heart, Lung and Blood Institute, Division of Lung Diseases workshop. Am Rev Respir Dis 1985;132:182–5.
7. Irwin RS, Curley FJ, French CL. Chronic cough, the spectrum and frequency of causes, key components of the diagnostic evaluation, and outcome of specific therapy. Am Rev Respir Dis 1990;141:640–7.
8. Kemp JP, Metzer EO. Getting control of the allergic child's environment. Pediatr Ann 1989;18:801–8.
9. Teach your patients about asthma: a clinician's guide. NIH publ. no. 92-2737. Washington, DC: National Institutes of Health, 1992.
10. Abramson MJ, Puy RM, Weiner JM. Is allergen immunotherapy effective in asthma? A meta-analysis of randomized controlled trials. Am J Respir Crit Care Med 1995;151:969–74.
11. Ries AL, Kupferberg DH, What's new in COPD the latest treatment options. J Respir Dis 2000;21:304–20.
12. Anderson CJ, Bardana EJ. Asthma in the elderly: interactions to be wary of. J Respir Dis 1995;16:965–76.
13. Fanta CH, Israel E, Sheffer AL. Managing—and preventing—severe asthma attacks. J Respir Dis 1992;13:94–108.
14. Becker AB, Nelson NA, Simons FER. Inhaled salbutamol (albuterol) vs. injected epinephrine in the treatment of acute asthma in children. J Pediatr 1983;102:465–9.
15. Plaut TF. Holding chambers for aerosol drugs. Pediatr Ann 1989;18:824–6.
16. Szefler SJ. A comparison of aerosol glucocorticoids in the treatment of chronic bronchial asthma. Pediatr Asthma Allergy Immunol 1991;5:227–35.
17. Physicians' desk reference, 55th ed. Oradell, NJ: Medical Economics, 2001.

18. Kavura M. Salmeterol and fluticasone propionate combined in a new powder inhalation device for the treatment of asthma: a randomized, double-blind, placebo controlled trial. J Allergy Clin Immunol 2000;105:1108–16.

19. Chapman KR, Verbeck PR, White JG, Rebeeck AS. Effect of a short course of prednisone in the prevalence of early relapse after the emergency room treatment of acute asthma. N Engl J Med 1991;324:788–94.

20. The Medical Letter on Drugs and Therapeutics 2000(6 March); 42:19–24.

21. Gross NJ. COPD management: achieving bronchodilatation. J Respir Dis 1996;17:183–95.

22. Seigel D, Sheppard D, Gelb A, Weinberg PF. Aminophylline increases the toxicity but not the efficacy of an inhaled beta-adrenergic agonist in the treatment of acute exacerbations of asthma. Am Rev Respir Dis 1985;132:283–6.

23. Herner SJ, Seaton TL, Mertens MK. Combined ipratropium and

β2 adrenergic receptor agonist in acute asthma. J Am Board Fam Pract 2000;13:1:55–65.

24. Anthonisen NR, Manfreda J, Warren CPW, Hershfield EJ, Harding GKM, Nelson NA. Antibiotic therapy in exacerbation of COPD. Ann Intern Med 1987;106:196–204.

25. Morray B, Redding G. Factors associated with prolonged hospitalization of children with asthma. Arch Pediatr Adolesc Med 1995;149:276–9.

26. Strunk RC. Death caused by asthma: minimizing the risks. J Respir Dis 1989;10:21–36.

27. Fraser KL, Chapman KR. Chronic obstructive pulmonary disease, prevention, early detection, and aggressive treatment can make a difference. Postgrad Med 2000;108:103–16.

28. Dirks JF. Patient attitude as a factor in asthma management. Pract Cardiol 1986;12(1):84–98.

29. Dowell AR. Quality of life: how important is managing COPD? J Respir Dis 1991;12:1057–72.

84
Pulmonary Infections

Jonathan E. Rodnick and James K. Gude

Pneumonia

Pneumonia is a parenchymal lung infection that usually presents with fever and cough and is diagnosed by a new infiltrate on a chest radiograph. Community-acquired pneumonia (CAP) is any pneumonia that is acquired outside of the hospital setting.

A family physician with 2000 patients would see, on average, 25 to 30 patients with CAP per year, and four to five of these would likely need hospitalization. There are an estimated 4 million cases of pneumonia yearly in the United States with 600,000 hospitalizations. The mortality rate averages 14% of hospitalized patients.[1] With 75,000 deaths yearly, pneumonia is the sixth leading cause of death in the U.S.

Etiology

Given the fact that a specific etiology cannot be identified in 40% to 50% of patients, a probable order of frequency of etiologies of CAP is that 20% to 60% are caused by *Streptococcus pneumoniae* (pneumococcus); 5% to 20% by *Mycoplasma pneumoniae*; 5% to 15% by *Chlamydia pneumoniae*; 2% to 10% by *Haemophilus influenzae*; 2% to 5% by *Legionella* sp.; 1% to 5% by *Staphylococcus aureus*; 1% to 3% by gram-negative bacilli; 3% by miscellaneous causes including *Moraxella catarrhalis* and *Chlamydia psittaci*; and 3% to 6% by aspiration.[2,3] The frequency differs by age. In the elderly the *Chlamydia* and *Mycoplasma* percentages decrease (although they still are seen), whereas *S. pneumoniae* increases in importance.

In influenza epidemics, *S. aureus* is a more frequent cause. With trauma, alcoholic intoxication, coma, and strokes, anaerobic and gram-negative pneumonias are more common. Healthy individuals' lungs do not become colonized by gram-negative bacteria. With underlying chronic obstructive pulmonary disease, *H. influenza* and *M. catarrhalis* are more often encountered as causes of CAP.

Clinical Presentation

One study found that the presenting symptoms of CAP include cough in 88%, dyspnea in 71%, sputum production in 69%, chest pain in 64%, hemoptysis in 17%, and confusion in 17%.[4] An upper respiratory infection precedes pneumonia only about one third of the time. Confusion is a common presenting symptom in older patients, the majority of whom have no fever.

The initial signs of community-acquired pneumonia are nonspecific. Abdominal pain may mimic appendicitis or cholecystitis with inflammation of the diaphragmatic pleura. Abnormal vital signs—tachypnea, tachycardia, and/or fever—increase the likelihood of pneumonia. A chest exam with careful auscultation and percussion has moderate usefulness. The most helpful examinations are percussion dullness and listening with the stethoscope for crepitations/crackles with the patient in the upright sitting position (highest sensitivity) and in the lateral decubitus position (highest specificity).[5] If the chest examination is entirely clear, pneumonia is unlikely. Many of the classic signs such as percussion dullness, tracheal breath sounds, egophony, and pectoriloquy are encountered as the pneumonia progresses, so that they are not initially helpful, but they assist in following the course of the pneumonia. It takes about 1 month for a classic pneumococcal pneumonia to resolve on physical exam, but the chest x-ray resolution takes longer. Persisting abnormal crepitations may indicate bronchiectasis or a persisting organized pneumonia, and persisting dullness with absent breath sounds may indicate pleural thickening or empyema.

Diagnosis

The presenting chest x-rays can be helpful in characterizing community-acquired pneumonias into the classic typical and atypical types. However, the descriptions are not absolute and not all presentations or chest x-rays fall into one or the other category. Table 84.1 differentiates typical pneumonias (which are usually due to *S. pneumoniae, H. pneumoniae,* and *Legionella* spp.) from the atypical (which are due more often to viral, *Mycoplasma,* or *Chlamydia* causes).

The typical pneumonias tend to start abruptly with rigor, chills, and fever, and have localized roentgenographic findings, whereas the atypical pneumonias are gradual in onset without marked toxicity and have diffuse x-ray involvement, often in excess of physical findings. The mortality of the typical pneumonias exceeds that of the atypical.

With CAP proven by an abnormal chest film or thought highly likely despite a negative chest film (an uncommon occurrence except with *Pneumocystis carinii* pneumonia or in those with severe dehydration or neutropenia), a sputum Gram stain with culture and sensitivity if there is a productive cough, two blood cultures, a complete blood count, chemistry panel, a measurement of oxygenation, and an HIV test are recommended. The Gram stain of the sputum should be scanned for areas where there are more than 25 neutrophils per high-powered field and less than 10 squamous cells. If this is found, the predominant Gram-stained species should be noted. If it is Gram-positive, lancet-shaped diplococci, *S. pneumoniae* is likely. For pneumococcal pneumonia, the positive predictive value of the Gram stain is 80% to 90%. However, the sensitivity is low. If it is void of organisms, viral, *Mycoplasma,* or *Chlamydia* causes are more likely. If gram-negative small rods are seen, *H. influenzae* is the likely cause. The Gram stain, if adequate, helps with the initial selection of antibiotics. The use of the Gram stain is debated, but it is immediate and at times very informative. The sputum culture is less informative initially but is recommended as it may reveal drug-resistant *S. pneumoniae.* For definitive cultures only blood cultures, transtracheal aspirates, pleural effusion sampling, or direct needle aspirates of the involved lung give trustworthy results of the infecting organism behind the pneumonia. But these samplings are often difficult to do and take 1 or more days for culture results.

A white blood cell count greater than 15,000/mm^3 favors a typical pneumonia, whereas less than 15,000 indicates a likely atypical infection. A high percent of band forms, especially if greater than 20%, is more suggestive of typical pneumonia The chemistry panel is valuable in detecting hyponatremia, azotemia, metabolic acidosis, and hyperglycemia. Blood cultures are recommended for all hospitalized patients. Bacteremia is most common in pneumococcal pneumonia.

The chest films may show pleural effusions, which can be from congestive failure, inflammatory reaction, or empyema. Air fluid levels can be seen in lung abscesses. It takes clinical judgment to decide when to perform a thoracentesis, when to place a chest tube, when to perform bronchoscopy, and when to place a Swan-Ganz catheter for hemodynamic monitoring. As a guideline, if the effusion is less than 2 cm on a lateral decubitus film, if the patient is not toxic, and if the patient responds to initial antibiotic therapy, no thoracentesis is needed. If an empyema is diagnosed by putrid odor, by Gram stain, or by culture, a chest tube is mandatory. With major mucus plugging or overwhelming bronchorrhea, bronchoscopy may help. When adult respiratory distress syndrome and congestive heart failure cannot be distinguished, a Swan-Ganz pulmonary artery catheter is needed for therapeutic decisions.

A follow-up chest film is important, and most pneumonias have cleared by 3 months. If the patient is a smoker and if the pneumonia does not clear, there is up to a 50% chance of having an underlying obstructive lung cancer. If there is not complete resolution in a smoker, an investigation is warranted, usually with a chest computed tomography (CT) scan and/or bronchoscopy.

Mycoplasma and *Chlamydia* are grown with great difficulty, so culture is not an option in most settings. They are usually diagnosed after the fact with paired complement fixation titers showing at least a fourfold titer rise in specimens drawn 3 to 4 weeks apart. However, cold agglutinins are suggestive of *Mycoplasma* if the titer is high. Other one-time serologies that can be suggestive of infection are a single com-

Table 84.1. **Characteristic Findings of Community-Acquired Pneumonia**

Characteristic	Typical pneumonia	Atypical pneumonia
Onset	Often sudden	Usually gradual
Myalgia/headache/photophobia	Not prominent	Often prominent
Rigors	Common	Rare
Toxicity	Marked	Mild to moderate
Cough	Productive, purulent, or bloody sputum	Nonproductive paroxysms or only scant mucoid sputum
Pleuritic pain	Common	Rare
Fever	>38.9°C (>102°F)	<38.9°C (<102°F)
Physical findings	Percussion dullness with signs of lung consolidation	Often minimal
Roentgenographic findings	Localized; findings correlate well with physical examination	Involvement in excess of findings on physical examination
Leukocyte count	>15,000/mm^3	<15,000/mm^3
Pathogen	Bacteria, including *Legionella*	*Mycoplasma pneumoniae, Chlamydia pneumoniae,* viruses

plement fixation titer for *Mycoplasma* pneumonia >1:64 and for *Chlamydia*, an immunofluorescence assay showing an immunoglobulin M (IgM) titer of >1:16.[6] A nasal wash specimen, if available, may be tested for rapid viral detection assays. It is almost as good as culture, and results are available in hours. If influenza A virus is suspected, a culture should also be requested. Other diagnostic tests, when clinically indicated, include induced sputa for *P. carinii* and a skin test and sputum smear and culture for tuberculosis.

Management

The art of medicine is using the clinical presentation, chest x-rays, physical examination, lab tests, and current epidemiology in the community to select appropriate antibiotic therapy. Table 84.2 lists the factors associated with increased mortality in patients with CAP, and these factors should be used as a guide to decide whether the patient should be admitted.[7] About 20% of patients with community-acquired pneumonias require admission to the hospital. Both typical and atypical pneumonias can be treated as an outpatient if no comorbidity factors are present. Table 84.3 reviews the causative organisms and recommended antibiotics based on the presence or absence of comorbid factors. Most pneumonias in otherwise healthy individuals younger than age 65 and with no comorbid factors can be treated with an oral macrolide or doxycycline or a fluoroquinolone (preferentially those with anti-pneumococcal activity such as moxifloxacin, gatifloxacin, or levofloxacin). Table 84.4 reviews the typical dosage schedule for the antibiotics mentioned in Table 84.3. For patients older than 65 or those with significant comorbid factors, one of the following regimens is recommended: an oral antipneumococcal fluoroquinolone *or* a macrolide or doxycycline *plus*

Table 84.2. **Factors Associated with Increased Mortality from Pneumonia**

Age >65
Male sex
Nursing home resident
Underlying conditions, such as alcoholism, neurologic disease, COPD, congestive heart failure, diabetes, postsplenectomy, cancer, malnutrition, chronic liver or renal disease, HIV infection, or other immunodeficiency
Confusion
Fever (temperature >38.3°C or 101°F)
Tachycardia (pulse >125/min)
Tachypnea (respiratory rate >30/min)
Hypotension (diastolic <60 mm Hg or systolic <90 mm Hg)
Arterial pH <7.35
Hypoxemia (O_2 saturation <90% or PaO_2 <60 mm Hg)
Hypercapnia ($PaCO_2$ >45 mm Hg)
Hyponatremia (sodium <130 mEq/L)
Anemia (hematocrit <30% or hemoglobin <9 g/dL)
Leukopenia (<4000 WBC/mm³)
Pronounced leukocytosis (>30,000 WBC/mm³)
Elevated serum creatinine level
Bacteremia
Bilateral or multilobe densities or large pleural effusion on chest film
Suspicion of staphylococcal or gram-negative infection

an oral second-generation cephalosporin, such as cefuroxime, or amoxicillin/clavulanate. Those situations where patients are unable to hold down oral medicines, or are not able to be hospitalized despite indications, IM or IV ceftriaxone may be used for one to two doses followed by oral cefpodoxime *plus* a macrolide or doxycycline.

If there are factors associated with increased mortality, admission to the hospital and treatment with a combined regimen of a parenteral second- or third-generation cephalosporin (cefuroxime or ceftriaxone) and a parenteral macrolide is recommended. If there are allergies to these antibiotic selections or if there is a high community prevalence of *S. pneumoniae* resistance to penicillin [usually defined as minimum inhibitory concentration (MIC) values ≥4 mg/dL], a parenteral antipneumococcal fluoroquinolone (used alone) is recommended. For those who are sick enough to be admitted to the intensive care unit (ICU), penicillin-resistant *S. pneumoniae* (PRSP), gram-negative bacteria, *Legionella* spp., *S. aureus*, and occasionally *Pseudomonas aeruginosa* need to be covered. Additional antibiotics to be considered for treating PRSP in this setting include not only the antipneumococcal fluoroquinolones, but also vancomycin and clindamycin. The choice of antibiotics is outlined in Table 84.3. It is not known how long antibiotic therapy should be continued. Bacterial pneumonia is usually treated for 7 to 14 days (the longer period for those with comorbidities), and atypical pneumonia for 14 days. For inpatients on parenteral therapy, the switch to oral therapy is usually done when the patient is afebrile for 24 to 48 hours, the white cell count is decreasing, and the patient has a functioning gastrointestinal tract.

Prevention and Family Issues

Yearly influenza vaccine is recommended for all adults older than 50 and all others with chronic disease or impaired immune systems as well as all medical personnel. Influenza epidemics occur yearly and are associated with excess pneumonias and deaths. The influenza pandemic of 1918 caused over 20 million deaths. Another pandemic is probable, but when? No other respiratory virus produces morbidity and mortality like the influenza virus. Both influenza A and B are associated with significant illnesses, but influenza A is associated with more virulence and antigenic heterogeneity. Influenza vaccination protects 70% to 90% of young adults if the vaccine viruses match the infecting community viruses. The elderly have a lesser degree of protection, probably around 60%. With influenza outbreaks in institutions, vaccination and the prophylactic use of amantadine or rimantadine for influenza A, or topical zanamivir or oseltamivir for either influenza A or B for 2 weeks (until the vaccine becomes effective), limits the spread of influenza. These agents are also used to treat influenza pneumonia. It is important to remember that hand washing—for medical personnel, friends, and family members—can reduce the spread of respiratory viruses.

Pneumococcal vaccination (23 strains) is recommended for persons older than 65 years, for younger patients with chronic conditions, and for medical personnel who might be exposed

Table 84.3. Guidelines for Empiric Antimicrobial Therapy of Adults with Community-Acquired Pneumonia

Outpatient pneumonia		Inpatient pneumonia	
Patients age ≤65 and no comorbidities	Patients age >65 and/or comorbidities	Non-ICU care	Patients requiring ICU care
Common etiologies *Streptococcus pneumoniae* *Mycoplasma pneumoniae* Respiratory viruses *Chlamydia pneumoniae* *Haemophilus influenzae* Miscellaneous (*Legionella*, *Mycobacterium tuberculosis*)	**Common etiologies** *Streptococcus pneumoniae* *Mycoplasma pneumoniae* *Chlamydia pneumoniae* Respiratory viruses *Haemophilus influenzae* Miscellaneous (*Legionella*, aerobic gram-negative bacilli, *Moraxella*)	**Common etiologies** *Streptococcus pneumoniae* *Haemophilus influenzae* Aerobic gram-negative bacilli *Legionella* species *Staphylococcus aureus* *Chlamydia pneumoniae* Respiratory viruses Miscellaneous (*Mycoplasma pneumoniae*, *Moraxella*) Polymicrobial (including anaerobic bacteria)	**Common etiologies** *Streptococcus pneumoniae* *Legionella* species Aerobic gram-negative bacilli *Mycoplasma pneumoniae* Respiratory viruses *Staphylococcus aureus* *Hemophilus influenzae* therapy
Therapy choices Macrolide (erythromycin, clarithromycin, azithromycin) or doxycycline or fluoroquinolone (moxifloxacin, gatifloxacin, levofloxacin) if allergy to above, or frequent penicillin-resistant *S. pneumoniae* (PRSP) in community	**Therapy choices** A fluoroquinolone (moxifloxacin, gatifloxacin, or levofloxacin) *OR* a macrolide (erythromycin, clarithromycin or azithromycin) *plus* amoxicillin/clavulanate or 2nd-generation cephalosporin (cefuroxime). Use a fluoroquinolone of frequent PRSP in community	**Therapy choices** Parenteral 2nd- or 3rd-generation cephalosporin (cefuroxime or cefuroxime *plus* macrolide (erythromycin, clarithromycin, azithromycin) or fluoroquinolone (moxifloxacin, gatifloxacin, levofloxacin) if allergy to above or frequent PRSP in community	**Therapy choices** Piperacillin-tazobactam or 3rd-generation cephalosporin with anti-*Pseudomonas* activity (ceftazidime or imipenem) or, ciprofloxacin and macrolide (azithromycin); if penicillin-resistant *S. pneumoniae* is suspect, add vancomycin, moxifloxacin, gatifloxacin, levofloxacin, or clindamycin; if *Pseudomonas* is suspected, add a second coverage with an aminoglycoside, such as gentamicin or tobramycin
	A parenteral option is ceftriaxone for 1–2 doses, followed by oral cefpodoxime *plus* a macrolide or doxycycline.		

Source: Based on refs. 2, 3, 8–11.

Table 84.4. Antibiotics: Names and Doses

Names	Dose
Amoxicillin (Polymox)	500 mg to 1.0 g po every 8 hours
Amoxicillin/clavulanate (Augmentin)	500 to 875 mg twice daily
Azithromycin (Zithromax)	500 mg po on day 1 followed by 250 mg po daily for 4 more days, or 500 mg IV daily
Cefpodoxime (Vantin)	100 to 200 mg po twice daily
Ceftazidime (Fortaz)	1 g IV every 8 hours
Cefuroxime (Ceftin, Zinacef)	500 mg po every 12 hours or 750 to 1500 mg IV every 8 hours
Ciprofloxacin (Cipro)	500 mg po twice daily or 400 mg IV every 12 hours
Clarithromycin (Biaxin)	500 mg twice daily
Clindamycin (Cleocin)	600 or 900 mg IV every 8 hours
Doxycycline (Vibramycin, Doryx, Vibra-Tabs, Monodox)	100 mg po or IV every 12 hours
Erythromycin (numerous preparations)	250 to 500 mg po every 6 hours, or 500 mg IV every 6 hours
Gatifloxacin (Tequin)	400 mg po or IV daily
Gentamicin (Garamycin)	3 mg/kg/day in equally divided doses every 8 hours
Imipenem/cilastatin sodium (Primaxin)	500 mg every 6 hours
Levofloxacin (Levaquin)	400 mg po or IV daily
Moxifloxacin (Avelox)	400 mg po or IV daily
Penicillin	500 mg po every 6 hours for 7 to 10 days, or 1 g IV every 6 hours
Piperacillin-tazobactam (Zosyn)	3.375 g IV every 6 hours
Tobramycin (Nebcin, Tobramycin Sulfate)	3 mg/kg/day in equally divided doses every 8 hours
Vancomycin (Vancocin)	1 g every 12 hours

to PRSP. The vaccine should be given to all splenectomy patients. In high-risk individuals, it should be repeated every 7 years. It reduces the chances of pneumonococcal pneumonia by 60% to 80%. Hemophilus B vaccine is indicated for children and for those with immunodeficiency at high risk, as it decreases the incidence of *H. influenzae* respiratory infections.[12] Patients who smoke cigarettes should strongly be encouraged to quit. An episode of pneumonia may be a moti-

vating factor that will move someone from contemplation to action.

Atypical Pneumonias: *Mycoplasma* and *Chlamydia*

The main causes of the atypical pneumonias are *Mycoplasma pneumoniae*, *Chlamydia pneumoniae*, *Chlamydia trachomatis*, *Chlamydia psittaci*, *Coxiella burnetii* or Q-fever, influenza A and B, respiratory syncytial virus (RSV), parainfluenza virus, rhinovirus, and many other viruses. In children and young adults, these atypical causes of pneumonia are more common than typical bacterial causes.[13,14]

M. pneumoniae infections are caused by one of a class of bacterial L-forms, which are the smallest free-living organisms. Infection is endemic in humans, and epidemics occur every 3 to 7 years. Infection is thought to be transmitted by droplets coughed by an infected person.

Diagnosis of *Mycoplasma*

M. pneumoniae usually produces a tracheobronchitis with an incubation of 2 to 4 weeks. It is manifested by a dry cough following an upper respiratory infection characterized by sore throat, malaise, fever, chills, and headache. The cough is particularly severe at night, and can last over a month. Maculopapular rashes and diarrhea may occur, and occasionally a bullous myringitis is diagnostic. Dyspnea and chest pain are unusual. Uncommon extrapulmonary complications include hepatitis, pericarditis, hemolysis, erythema multiformis, aseptic meningitis, transverse myelitis, and Guillain-Barré syndrome. On physical examination one usually hears only scattered crepitations. Signs of consolidation are unusual. The chest x-ray shows segmental infiltrates that are usually unilateral but occasionally bilateral. Pleural effusions are unusual. It may take months for the infiltrates to resolve. The white blood cell count is usually normal, and there can be false-positive immunologic tests, such as rheumatoid factor and syphilis serologic tests. The bacterial L-forms are difficult to culture. Serologic tests were reviewed above (see Diagnosis under Pneumonia).

Diagnosis of *Chlamydia*

The bacterial genus *Chlamydia* contains three species that infect humans: *C. trachomatis*, *C. psittaci*, and *C. pneumoniae*. *C. trachomatis* causes infant inclusion conjunctivitis and pneumonia. *C. psittaci* is contracted from infected birds, usually imported, and presents as an abrupt onset febrile illness. The cough can diminish within hours of starting treatment. *C. pneumoniae* is usually a mild, atypical pneumonia with initial upper respiratory symptoms of sore throat and hoarseness. The headache can be impressive. Wheezing often occurs. The chest infiltrates are not specific, tending to be unilateral more than bilateral, patchy, or dense. Serologic tests were reviewed above. Infection can occur without seroconversion, and this failure of immunity may explain why these pneumonias can be recurrent.

Management

Treatment (see Table 84.3) for both *Mycoplasma* and *Chlamydia* spp. is with a macrolide, doxycycline, or a fluoroquinolone for at least 2 weeks to prevent relapse.

Legionnaire's Disease

Legionnaire's disease was named after an outbreak of a new pneumonia in Philadelphia at an American Legion convention in 1976. Thirty species and serotypes have been recognized; the most common agent is *Legionella pneumophila*. Middle-aged and elderly men are most commonly affected. Risk factors include immunosuppression, cigarette smoking, chronic obstructive pulmonary disease (COPD), diabetes mellitus, and chronic cardiac or renal disease. *Legionella* bacteria are found in water, and institutional water systems (cooling towers, showers, nebulizers) are important sources of infections.

Diagnosis

This typical pneumonia presents with abrupt-onset fevers, rigors, myalgias, and headache. Hemoptysis, pleurisy, diarrhea, and confusion occur. Chest x-rays show patchy infiltrates progressing to involve contiguous lobes. Pleural effusions are common. Hyponatremia is often seen. The Gram stain usually does not show this weakly gram-negative organism. A *Legionella* antigen in the urine can be detected in about 70% of the patients. A fourfold rise in the IgG titer by immunofluorescence assay supports the diagnosis.

Management

Treatment is usually with azithromycin, or one of the fluoroquinolones such as levofloxacin, gatifloxacin, or moxifloxacin for 10 to 21 days. Rifampin is sometimes added.[15] Mortality from Legionnaire's disease is 5% to 20% and can be 50% in the immunocompromised. If suspected, hospitalization is recommended. Patient isolation is not needed, but infection control or the health department should be notified to investigate the source.

Pneumocystis carinii Pneumonia

Pneumocystis carinii pneumonia is the most common life-threatening disease for the patient infected with HIV (also see Chapter 42). When the CD4 count is <200, the stage is set for this pneumonia. It typically presents with over a month of progressive breathlessness including a nonproductive cough, fever, and malaise. On physical exam there are nonspecific diffuse crepitations or crackles. The chest film can be normal, but it usually shows a diffuse ground-glass appearance indicative of an interstitial and alveolar process. Effusions and hilar adenopathy are unusual. There is usually lymphopenia with a total lymphocyte count of <1,000/mL and hypoxemia. A carbon monoxide diffusion capacity is characteristically low (<80% of predicted). The organism is found in induced sputa about 60% of the time and bronchoalveolar lavage over 95% of the time. An algorithm for diagnosis is presented in Figure 84.1.

Management

Trimethoprim-sulfamethoxazole (TMP-SMX) is the treatment of choice. It can be given orally or intravenously. The dose is based on 15 mg/kg/day of the TMP component.[16] Side effects are common, occurring in over 50% of patients including skin rashes (Stevens-Johnson syndrome), neutropenia, hepatitis, hyponatremia, and drug fever. Treatment should continue for 21 days. There are many alternatives for treatment. Three frequently used are intravenous pentamidine (3 mg/kg/day), oral dapsone (100 mg/day) plus TMP (15 mg/kg/day), or IV clindamycin (600 mg q6h) plus oral primaquine (3 mg/day).[17] Glucose-6-phosphate deficiency should be checked before starting dapsone or primaquine. Corticosteroids are indicated if hypoxemia ($PaO_2 < 70$ mm Hg) is present. Prednisone is started at 80 mg and tapered over 2 weeks.

Prevention and Family Issues

If the CD4 T cell count is <200, *Pneumocystis* prophylaxis with TMP/SMX-DS one tablet daily is cost-effective. Alternatives include dapsone 100 mg/day or twice weekly or inhaled pentamidine 300 mg every 4 weeks. Without prophylaxis, up to 80% of patients with a low CD4 count will develop pneumocystic pneumonia. With new antiretroviral regimens, if the CD4 count rises above 200, prophylaxis can be discontinued.

Histoplasmosis

Histoplasmosis is caused by a fungus found in moist soil throughout the temperate zones of the world (in the United States it occurs especially in the Ohio and Mississippi River Valleys). Growth of the fungus is enhanced by bird droppings. Humans inhale mycelial fragments, which then convert to a yeast phase in the lung, followed by hematogenous dissemination to other organs, including lumph nodes, liver, and spleen. Subsequent calcifications are then seen, which can have a characteristic concentric or target pattern.

Clinical Manifestations

The primary infection is often asymptomatic in healthy individuals. Flu-like symptoms (fever, malaise, cough) may develop and patients may become dyspneic and hypoxic. If there is a heavy inoculum of spores, pleuritic pain, dyspnea, and hypoxia may develop. Symptoms generally run a course of days to several weeks. Occasionally, rheumatologic syndromes (arthralgia, erythema nodosum) are present and may mimic sarcoidosis. Chronic cavitary histoplasmosis can develop, especially in those with underlying chronic lung disease. Disseminated histoplasmosis usually reflects a defective immune system (most commonly due to HIV). Fever, weight loss, anemia, hepatosplenomegaly, and gastrointestinal (GI) ulceration are common, but pulmonary manifestations are not.

Diagnosis

Diagnosis is based on clinical suspicion, characteristic radiographics, positive sputum or tissue stains or cultures, and/or serologic tests. With chronic cavitary or disseminated histo-

Fig. 84.1. Workup of those suspected of having *Pneumocystis carinii* pneumonia (PCP).

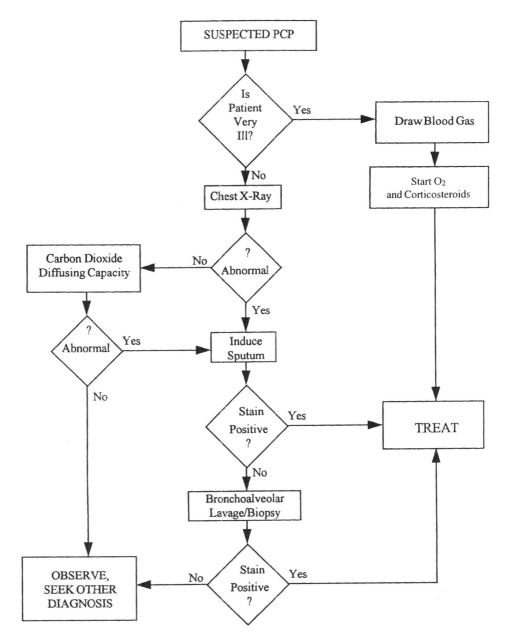

plasmosis, a sputum or tissue stain or culture is the best way to make the definitive diagnosis. Complement-fixation (CF) tests can be used for diagnosis, but are not specific. A titer of 1:32 or more or a fourfold rise provides presumptive evidence of acute infection. It is important to remember that CF titers rise in response to the skin test antigen, which is one of the reasons the skin test is not used as a diagnostic aid.

With primary disease, the chest radiographs frequently show a bilateral patchy lower lobe pneumonia, hilar adenopathy, and rarely a small pleural effusion.

Nodular residua can remain that may resemble a metastatic neoplasm or "buckshot" calcification.

Management

In a normal host, no treatment is usually needed for those with acute symptoms of less than 1 month's duration. Patients who have symptoms for more than 1 month, who have chronic and progressive pulmonary histoplasmosis, or who have disseminated histoplasmosis (most of whom are immunosuppressed) need to be treated. Itraconazole 200 or 400 mg/day is the treatment of choice for chronic pulmonary disease in the immunocompetent host. Oral ketaconazole or fluconazole are alternatives. In those who are immunocompromised or who are sick enough to be hospitalized, amphotericin B is recommended as initial treatment, followed by an oral azole. Long-term maintenance therapy is necessary to prevent relapse.[18]

Coccidioidomycosis

Coccidioides, a fungus, is found in the soil of the semiarid Southwest. Dust storms, outdoor recreation, and new construction are associated with an increased risk of infection.

There are an estimated 100,000 primary infections per year in the U.S. resulting from inhaling the arthrospore.

Clinical Manifestations

The primary infection is usually asymptomatic, although up to 40% have symptoms of acute "valley fever" with cough, low-grade fever, and often arthralgias or erythema nodosum. A few infected persons (0.5% to 1.0%) develop progressive pulmonary or disseminated disease (common sites are the meninges, bones and joints, and soft tissues). People of African or Filipino descent, pregnant women, infants, and the immunosuppressed are at greatest risk.

Diagnosis

The main difficulty is failure to consider the diagnosis. The chest radiograph of the primary infection is nonspecific with transient infiltrates and occasionally hilar adenopathy or pleural effusions. Multiple nodules or thin-walled cavities develop in 5% to 10% of those infected. Sputum smears and cultures are sometimes positive, but not always, in those with abnormal chest radiographs. Serologic testing can also be helpful. Seventy-five percent of people with primary infections develop IgM acute-phase antibodies. IgG CF antibodies develop later and are a marker (>1:16) for disseminated extrapulmonary disease. Changes in the antibody titer are useful for monitoring the course of the disease. Culture is diagnostic, but many labs are reluctant to do it because of the possibility of aerosolizing spores and causing iatrogenic disease.

Therapy

Over 95% of patients recover without therapy. Most authorities do not recommend treating asymptomatic patients with no risk factors, even those with a solitary nodule or a pulmonary cavity. Those with symptomatic cavities, fibrocavitary pneumonia, or disseminated extrapulmonary infection such be treated long-term with oral azole antifungals such as itraconazole, 200 mg a day, or fluconazole 400 to 800 mg a day for at least 1 year. Those with immunosuppression and diffuse pneumonia or widespread dissemination may require intravenous amphotericin B. Duration of therapy ranges from months to years.[19,20]

Tuberculosis

Tuberculosis (TB) is an enormous worldwide problem. Over one third of the world's population is infected. An estimated 8 million new cases of active disease occur each year and TB causes an estimated 2 or 3 million deaths yearly.[21] Tuberculosis incidence in the United States decreased steadily from 80/100,000 in 1930 to about 10/100,000 in 1985, but then rose in concert with the HIV epidemic and increased immigration. Fortunately, since 1992 the incidence has decreased again and is now about 6.5/100,000. The incidence of TB is disproportionately higher in African Americans and Hispanics. The homeless and immigrants from countries where TB is more prevalent (Mexico, the Philippines, Vietnam, China,

India, and Haiti) are especially vulnerable. In the United States it is estimated that 15 million persons are infected with *Mycobacterium tuberculosis* (i.e., are skin test-positive).

Tuberculosis is caused by a small bacterium with a thick lipid wall, making it particularly resistant to destruction by either macrophages or drugs. It multiplies slowly and can lay dormant for long periods. The infection usually starts by inhaling droplets from an infected person's cough to the periphery of the lung, where they cause a local inflammatory reaction. There is usually some hematogenous spread: kidneys, liver, and bone are the most common organs seeded. Clinical disease rarely occurs at this stage, although occasionally foci irritate or rupture into the pleura causing a pleural effusion.

After this initial asymptomatic infection, individuals are thought to have a latent infection and are left only with a positive skin test and sometimes a parenchymal lung calcification (Ghon lesion), which can be associated with calcified hilar lymph nodes (Ranke complex).

Between 70% and 90% of active TB is reactivation, that is, a breakdown of these latent foci years later. Why it happens is poorly understood. Risk factors for active TB include recent weight loss (associated with malnutrition or alcoholism), poorly controlled diabetes, and immunosuppression (from steroids, AIDS, or cancer). HIV has been called the most potent activator of TB ever detected. Persons infected with both HIV and TB have a 100 times greater risk of developing active TB compared to persons who have been infected with TB but are not HIV positive (also see Chapter 42).

Of those newly infected with bacilli (i.e., skin test converters), it is estimated that about 3% to 5% develop active TB within the first year after exposure. The risk is higher in infants and adolescents and those with immunodeficiency. Of all those with positive skin tests, no risk factors, a normal chest radiograph, and who are thought not to be recent converters, approximately 1 of 2000 persons develop active TB each year. Over a lifetime, most people whose skin tests convert run about a 3% to 5% chance of developing the disease initially and another 3% to 5% chance of developing TB over the rest of their lives.

Clinical Presentation

Active pulmonary tuberculosis usually presents with a progressively severe cough, productive of mucopurulent sputum. Hemoptysis is not common, but when present can be massive. Malaise, low-grade fever, and weight loss are often present. Dyspnea and chest pain is uncommon. The physical examination may demonstrate crepitations, decreased breath sounds, or percussion dullness due to pleural effusion.

Extrapulmonary TB can involve any system and is seen in up to 15% of patients with active disease and over 50% of those with immunodeficiency and tuberculosis. Extrapulmonary disease can affect lymph nodes (including hilar adenopathy), bone marrow, liver, kidneys, meninges, pericardium, and the GI tract.

Diagnosis

The chest radiograph in patients with active TB most frequently shows a fibronodular upper lobe infiltrate. Cavities

Table 84.5. **Dosage Recommendations for the Initial Treatment of Tuberculosis in Adults**

Drug	Daily dose (mg/kg)	Twice-weekly dose (mg/kg)	Thrice-weekly dose (mg/kg)
Isoniazid	5 Max 300 mg	15 Max 900 mg	15 Max 900 mg
Rifampin	10 Max 600 mg	10 Max 600 mg	10 Max 600 mg
Pyrazinamide	15–30 Max 2.0 g	50–70 Max 4.0 g	50–70 Max 3.0 g
Ethambutol	15–25 Max 2.5 g	50	25–30

may form, and hilar adenopathy, pleural effusion, or upper lobe volume loss may be present. The definitive diagnosis of active disease is based on a smear and culture of the sputum or other infected material. Smears may be done using a Ziehl-Neelsen or an acid-fast technique, causing the organisms to appear red ("red snappers"), but more frequently a fluorescence technique is used. Rapid culture techniques and identification using nucleic acid probes have decreased the time required for laboratory identification to less than 2 weeks. All initial isolates should be tested for drug sensitivity.

Patients whose smears are positive should be in respiratory isolation. After 2 to 3 weeks of therapy, most patients (even those who remain smear-positive) are thought to be noninfectious. Follow-up monthly sputum cultures are used to monitor compliance and resistance. Cultures should be negative after 2 to 3 months of therapy. HIV testing should be performed on all patients with newly diagnosed TB.

Management

The increased incidence of TB has been accompanied by an increase in drug resistance. Up to 10% of TB isolates are isoniazid [isonicotinic acid hydrazide (INH)] resistant and 1% to 2% are resistant to multiple drugs. Because using one drug to treat active disease often results in resistant organisms, rather than a cure, the current adult recommended antituberculosis therapy for active disease is INH 300 mg qd, rifampin (RIF) 600 mg qd, and pyrazinamide (PZA) 15 to 30 mg/kg/day and ethambutol (EMB) 15 to 25 mg/kg/day for the first 2 months. Then INH and RIF (daily or twice weekly) are continued for a total of 6 months of therapy.[22] The drugs are best given together; there is no need for split dosages. See Table 84.5 for dosages of common antituberculosis medications and Table 84.6 for common medication side effects.

TB in immunocompromised patients should be treated for 9 to 12 months with two drugs to which the organism is sensitive. Occasionally, intramuscular streptomycin is used in those with drug resistance, the noncompliant patient, or those whose visual acuity cannot be monitored (monitoring is necessary for ethambutol). Secondary oral agents, including ethionamide, cycloserine, and *p*-aminosalicylic sodium are used in patients with multiple drug resistance.

To ensure compliance, directly observed therapy (DOT) is often used by health departments—a health care worker gives patients their medication and watches them swallow it. DOT using a twice-weekly regimen can be substituted for daily therapy after the first 2 weeks of therapy. An alternative is

giving three times weekly DOT therapy with all four drugs for 6 months. All patients should be monitored with monthly physician visits to obtain sputum smears and cultures and liver function tests as well as to check for other adverse drug reactions. Treatment completion rates on DOT exceed 90%.[23]

If a patient remains symptomatic or has a positive culture after the initial 2 months of a three- or four-drug regimen, noncompliance or drug resistance is likely. These patients should be referred to a TB specialist or health department clinic. To prevent the development of drug resistance, never add one drug at a time to a failing regimen. DOT is strongly recommended for those who are HIV positive, have a history of drug or alcohol abuse, have a history of previous TB treatment, the homeless, or those with a major psychiatric or cognitive disorders. Because of drug interactions, the use of rifampin is difficult in HIV-positive patients who are on antiretroviral therapy. Consultation is recommended. In these patients rifabutin is sometimes substituted for rifampin.

Prevention and Family Issues

The TB skin test is one of the oldest diagnostic tests still in use today, having been initially developed by Koch more than 100

Table 84.6. **Antibiotics for Tuberculosis**

Drug	Common side effects
Isoniazid	Hepatotoxicity (see test)—monitor lever functions Peripheral neuropathy—use vitamin B₆ 25 mg qd Increases phenytoin level May decrease efficacy of hypoglycemics (?) CNS reactions
Rifampin	Colors urine, stool, saliva, and sweat orange Accelerates metabolism of certain drugs: oral contraceptives, statins, Coumadin, methadone, steroids Thrombocytopenia Hepatotoxicity Febrile reactions
Ethambutol	Optic neuritis (rare at dose of 15 mg/kg) Loss of red-green perception Skin rash
Pyrazinamide	Hepatotoxicity Hyperuricemia GI disturbance Arthralgias

years ago. The Mantoux test is recommended using 0.1 mL [5 tuberculin units (5TU)] of purified protein derivative (PPD) injected subcutaneously, with the result (induration, not erythema) read in 48 to 72 hours. Tests read after 72 hours underestimate the true size of induration. Multiple-puncture tests are not recommended.

A positive reaction indicates latent infection from past exposure (at least 2 to 3 months ago). Unfortunately, the test often can be negative in the elderly and immunosuppressed (up to 60% of patients with AIDS and TB have a false-negative test). All patients with a positive test should have a chest radiograph to rule out active disease. The skin test usually remains positive for years, but waning occurs with age. Repeated skin testings enhances reactivity (the booster phenomenon). Bacille Calmette-Guérin (BCG) vaccination, often given in underdeveloped countries, may cause a positive skin test for many years.

Tuberculin skin testing is indicated in anyone who has HIV infection, has a possible exposure to anyone with active TB, is an immigrant from a country with a high prevalence of TB, has symptoms or a chest radiograph compatible with TB, or who is a resident or worker in hospitals, nursing homes, mental institutions, or jails.[24] Routine skin testing of children at low risk for TB is not necessary. Children who reside in high-prevalence areas should be considered for skin testing at 4 to 6 years of age and again at 11 to 16 years. The key to prevention of TB in children is good contact investigation of patients with active disease. Anergy skin testing is not recommended in those who are skin test negative, but in whom tuberculosis is still suspected.[25]

There is at least 80% efficacy in preventing future active disease with INH treatment in those who are skin test positive. The definition of a positive skin test is different for different groups. A cut point of ≥5 mm induration is recommended in those who are immunosuppressed, are household members or close contacts of a newly diagnosed patient, or who have an abnormal chest radiograph consistent with old TB (more than calcified nodes or pleural thickening). A cut point of ≥10 mm is recommended for those who have a high likelihood of being infected, but do not have the above risk factors. This group includes persons from countries with a high prevalence of TB, IV drug users, homeless individuals, nursing home residents, or those with diabetes, renal failure, on corticosteroids, or who have had a significant weight loss. A cut point of ≥15 mm is sometimes recommended for healthy persons with none of the above risks who are in low-prevalence populations.[24] The predictive value of a positive test is this group is low. Persons who have positive results need to have active TB ruled out with a chest film.

In those with stable or negative films, the preferred treatment regimen is INH (5 mg/kg or 300 mg max) daily for 9 months, although 6 months is acceptable in those at lower risk. Twice weekly therapy with DOT is indicated if there is a concern with adherence. An alternative is RIF and PZA daily for 2 months in those who can't take INH. Treatment is usually delayed until the postpartum period when pregnant women are found to be skin test positive. There are no longer age criteria for chemoproplylaxis.[26]

The most common concern about INH is drug-induced hepatitis. The overall incidence is about 1%, although it is age-related. In persons under age 20, hepatitis is rare, whereas in those over age 35 it occurs in about 0.2%.[27] Prodromal symptoms, such as tiredness and anorexia, may occur weeks to months before clinical toxicity. Seventy percent of hepatitis occurs during the first 3 months of therapy. The best way to follow patients on INH is regularly (monthly) to ask about prodromal symptoms of hepatitis, such as fatigue.

Monitoring liver transaminases in those over age 35, heavy drinkers, and those with other liver disease is reasonable. Up to 20% may show mild, asymptomatic rise in liver enzymes (less than five times normal). In those individuals, INH does not need to be discontinued, but they should be followed more closely.

The BCG vaccination is used in many countries where TB is prevalent. Its efficacy is probably about 50%, but the consensus is that its efficacy is greater for preventing extrapulmonary disease (e.g., TB meningitis) in children. BCG vaccination usually leaves a keloid or scar where given (often on the left shoulder). In the United States the BCG vaccination is rarely indicated.[28] If BCG was given more than 5 years previously, it should not be considered as a cause of a positive skin test.

Mycobacterium Avium Complex

Mycobacterium avium intracellulare complex (MAC) disease is seen as a late-stage infection in AIDS patients. Its risk is inversely correlated with the CD4 lymphocyte count. The organism is found in soil and water; it is not thought to be transmitted human to human. Before AIDS, MAC disease was uncommon, and seen primarily in older patients with COPD or prior tuberculosis.

The symptoms of MAC infection in AIDS patients are nonspecific: fever, anorexia, weight loss, fatigue, diarrhea, and abdominal pain; pulmonary symptoms are uncommon. Blood cultures are frequently positive. The organism is also found in the sputum and stool and in tissue biopsies. When found on a sputum smear, treatment for active tuberculosis should be initiated until the culture results are known. Treatment for MAC decreases symptoms and possibly increases survival. Because of resistance, multiple drugs are used. The current regimen is clarithromycin (500 mg bid) plus ethambutol (15 mg/kg/day). Rifabutin (300 mg qd) is often added.[17] Duration of treatment is indefinite, unless the CD4 count is above 100 for at least 6 months and the patient is asymptomatic. Current data suggest that twice daily clarithromycin or weekly azithromycin will help prevent MAC disease in those with CD4 counts of less than 50 cells/mm³. Prophylaxis may be stopped when CD4 counts are greater than 100 for 6 months. In those who are HIV negative and who develop chronic pulmonary MAC, the usual drug regimen is triple therapy with the above drugs. This is continued 12 months beyond culture negativity (usually about 18 months total).

References

1. Fine MJ, Smith MA, Carson CA, et al. Prognosis and outcomes of patients with community-acquired pneumonia: a meta-analysis. JAMA 1996;275:134–41.

2. Bernstein JM. Treatment of community-acquired pneumonia—IDSA guidelines. Chest 1999;115:95–135.

3. American Thoracic Society. Guidelines for the initial empiric therapy of community-acquired pneumonia. Am J Respir Crit Care Med 2001;163:1730–54.

4. British Thoracic Society Research Committee. Community-acquired pneumonia in adults in British hospitals in 1982–1983; a survey of aetiology, mortality, prognostic factors and outcomes. Q J Med 1987;62:195–220.

5. Wipt JE, Lipsky BA, Hirschmann JV, et al. Diagnosing pneumonia by physical examination. Arch Intern Med 1999;159:1082–7.

6. Skerrett SJ. Diagnostic testing for community-acquired pneumonia. Clin Chest Med 1999;20:531–48.

7. Fine MJ, Auble TE, Yealy DM, et al. A prediction rule to identify low risk patients with community-acquired pneumonia. N Engl J Med 1997;336:243–50.

8. Bartlett JG, Breiman RF, Mandel LA, et al. Community-acquired pneumonia in adults: guidelines for management. Clin Infect Dis 1998;26:811–38.

9. Marrie TJ, Lau CY, Wheeler SL, et al. A controlled trial of a critical pathway for treatment of community-acquired pneumonia. JAMA 2000;283:749–55.

10. Heffelfinger, JD, Dowell SF, Jorgensen, JH, et al. Management of community-acquired pneumonia in the era of pneumococcal resistance. Arch Intern Med 2000;160:1399–408.

11. Mandell LA. Antibiotic therapy for community-acquired pneumonia. Clin Chest Med 1999;20:589–98.

12. Steinhoff MC, Auerbach BS, Nelson MD, et al. Antibody responses to *Haemophilus influenzae* type B vaccines in men with human immunodeficiency virus infection. N Engl J Med 1991;325:1837–42.

13. Fang GD, Fine M, Orloff J, et al. New and emerging etiologies for community-acquired pneumonia with implications for therapy; a prospective multicenter study of 359 cases. Medicine 1990;69:307–16.

14. Block S, Hedrick J, Hammerschlag MR, et al. Mycoplasmal pneumoniae and Chlamydia pneumoniae in pediatric community-acquired pneumonia: comparative efficacy and safety of clarithromycin vs. erythromycin ethylsuccinate. Pediatr J Infect Dis 1995;14:471–7.

15. Bartlett JG, Dowell SF, Mandell LA, File TM Jr, Musher DM, Fine MJ. Practice guidelines for the management of community-acquired pneumonia. Clin Infect Dis 2000;31:347–82.

16. Schliep TC, Yarrish RL. Pneumocystis carinii pneumonia. Semin Respir Infect 1999;14:333–43.

17. Goldschmidt RH, Dong BJ. Treatment of AIDS and HIV-related conditions: 2000. J Am Board Fam Pract 2000;13:274–98.

18. Wheat J, Sarosi G, McKinsey D, et al. Practice guidelines for the management of patients with histoplasmosis. Clin Infect Dis 2000;30:688–95.

19. Stevens D. Coccidioidomycosis. N Engl J Med 1995;16:1077–82.

20. Galgiani JN, Ampel NM, Catanzaro A, Johnson RH, Stevens DA, Williams PL. Practice guideline for the treatment of coccidioidomycosis. Infectious Diseases Society of America. Clin Infect Dis 2000;30:658–61.

21. Dye C, Scheele S, Dolin P, Pathania V, Raviglione MC, for the WHO Global Surveillance and Monitoring Project. JAMA 1999;282:677–86.

22. American Thoracic Society. Treatment of tuberculosis and tuberculosis infection in adults and children. Am J Respir Crit Care Med 1994;149:1359–74.

23. Chaulk CP, Kazandjian VA, for the Public Health Tuberculosis Guidelines Panel. JAMA 1998;279:943–8.

24. American Thoracic Society. Targeted tuberculin testing and treatment of latent tuberculosis infection. MMWR 2000;49(RR-6):1–51.

25. Slovis BS, Plitman JD, Haas DW. The case against anergy testing as a routine adjunct to tuberculin skin testing. JAMA 2000;283:2003–7.

26. Salpeter SR, Sanders GD, Salpeter EE, Owens DK. Monitored isoniazid prophylaxis for low-risk tuberculin reactors older than 35 years of age: a risk benefit and cost-effectiveness analysis. Ann Intern Med 1997;127:1051–61.

27. Nolan CM, Goldberg SV, Buskin SE. Hepatotoxity associated with isoniazid preventive therapy: a 7-year survey from a public health tuberculosis clinic. JAMA 1999;281:1014–8.

28. Centers for Disease Control. The role of BCG in the prevention and control of tuberculosis in the United States. MMWR 1996;45(RR-4):1–18.

85
Lung Cancer

Michael E. Clark and Daniel K. Onion

Lung cancer is now the leading cause of cancer mortality in both men and women in the United States. It has long been the leading cause of cancer death in men, but in 1987 lung cancer surpassed breast cancer to become the leading cause of cancer death in women. In the United States 87% of lung cancer is caused by cigarette smoking.[1] In 2000 it is estimated that there will have been 164,100 new cases of lung cancer and 156,900 deaths, accounting for 28% of all cancer deaths. The National Cancer Institute has calculated the lifetime risk of being diagnosed with lung cancer to be 7.82% in males and 5.66% in females with the highest risk seen among black males (8.58%). The risk of dying from lung cancer is 7.62% for men and 4.77% in women.[1]

The gap between men and women with lung cancer is expected to continue to narrow. Lung cancer rates among women have increased by more than 500% since 1950.[2] In the early 1900s cigarette smoking prevalence in women was only 6%. This prevalence increased steadily until the 1960s when it peaked at 34.2%. While mortality from lung cancer in men has plateaued or even decreased slightly, it is estimated that lung cancer mortality in women will continue to increase over the next 10 years as the population of women with the highest smoking prevalence ages. In addition, while smoking prevalence in both sexes has declined, the rate of decline has been greater in men than in women.

Prevention/Early Detection

Prevention is generally divided into three categories. Primary prevention involves those measures that are intended to prevent a disease from occurring (also see Chapter 7). Secondary prevention is aimed at identifying and treating disease in asymptomatic individuals. Tertiary prevention encompasses the treatment of patients with clinically apparent disease and will be covered later in this chapter.

Primary Prevention

Lung cancer lends itself well to primary prevention. Given that the vast majority of lung cancer is smoking related, it is a very preventable disease. In addition to cigarette smoking, there are several other exposures that increase risk of lung cancer, and are largely preventable.

Tobacco

Smoking remains the leading cause of preventable death in the United States, killing an estimated 419,000 people per year.[3] Cigarette smoke contains many known carcinogens. Nicotine is not carcinogenic but is responsible for the highly addictive nature of cigarettes. There is a linear relationship between the number cigarettes smoked per day and the risk of lung cancer.[4] Smoking prevalence in the United States decreased significantly during the 1970s and 1980s. However, the decline has plateaued over the last decade. Even more concerning is the fact that cigarette smoking is on the increase among high school students.[5] The long-term consequences of increased smoking prevalence in young Americans could be great. The benefits of smoking cessation are enormous, and newer options with improved efficacy make this one of the more effective interventions for a family physician. This subject is covered in detail in Chapter 8.

Occupational and Environmental Exposure

In the United States, approximately 10% of lung cancer is occupationally related. Asbestos exposure has long been associated with lung cancer. As many as 24% of the deaths in workers exposed to high levels of asbestos are due to lung cancer. Cigarette smoking increases the carcinogenicity of asbestos tenfold.[6] Mesothelioma is a neoplasm that is essentially unheard of in the absence of asbestos exposure. However the incidence is approximately 8% in asbestos workers. Silica, like asbestos, does not directly cause damage to DNA.

Rather it causes a chronic inflammatory state with an increased production of reactive oxygen species, which in turn produce mutations. Arsenic, nickel, polyaromatic hydrocarbons, and chromium compounds are all considered to be carcinogenic to the lung. Radon was first linked to lung cancer in miners exposed to very high levels of the gas. Radon at lower levels is ubiquitous in the air and water of most homes. The relationship between radon exposure and lung cancer appears to be linear; however, a reasonably safe level of radon has yet to be established.[7,8]

Nutrition

There is evidence that diets rich in fruits and vegetables decrease the risk of cigarette smoke–induced lung cancer.[9] Higher levels of antioxidants in this diet may play a role in this protective effect. Reactive oxygen species seem to be involved in the carcinogenicity of cigarette smoke and many other causative agents of lung cancer.[6,9] But it has been difficult to prove a direct link between antioxidants and prevention of lung cancer. In fact both clinical and animal studies have shown an increased incidence of lung cancer with β-carotene supplementation.[9,10]

Genetics

Cigarette smoking is well established as a cause of lung cancer; however, most smokers never develop lung cancer, suggesting that other factors are important. Several studies have shown a significant increase in the risk of mortality from lung cancer in first-degree relatives of patients with the disease.[11] The relative risk is 2 to 2.5 times the risk for controls. Many of the carcinogenic compounds in cigarette smoke including polycyclic aromatic hydrocarbons and nitrosamines must be activated by cytochrome P-450 prior to binding to DNA. Specific mutations in the P-450 genes have been associated with an increased susceptibility to the carcinogenic effects of smoking. Other enzymes such as glutathione transferase conjugate carcinogenic compounds, making them inactive. Deficiencies in these enzymes also increase lung cancer.

Carcinogenesis in the lung is believed to be a multistep process. After exposure to a carcinogen, cells within the lung will progress from normal to hyperplastic, to dysplastic, and finally to carcinoma. Along the way different oncogenes are expressed at each stage. Oncogene products act as growth factors and regulatory proteins within normal cells, but an increased production of these proteins is associated with tumor formation. Many oncogenes have been associated with lung cancer and the degree of their expression seems to play a major role in the proliferation of the tumor. K-*ras* mutations have been shown to decrease the latent phase in bronchogenic carcinoma. Overproduction of the C-*erb*-B2 gene product is associated with an increased likelihood of distant metastases, shortened survival, and resistance to chemotherapy.[12] Tumor suppressor genes also play an important role in the development of lung cancer. Mutations in the *p53* tumor suppressor gene are the most common abnormality seen in human tumors. A normal *p53* gene introduced into cell lines with active oncogenes will suppress tumor formation, whereas mutant *p53* genes increase tumorigenicity of normal cells.[13]

Secondary Prevention

The most recent recommendation of the U.S. Preventive Services Task Force is that routine screening of asymptomatic patients for lung cancer using chest x-ray or sputum cytology is not recommended ("D" recommendation).[14] Intuitively it seems that there would be a benefit to screening for lung cancer. As the leading cause of cancer death in the United States the burden of disease is great. There is also evidence that early detection improves 5-year survival.[15] Unfortunately, four large randomized controlled studies in the 1980s revealed no effect on disease-specific mortality. This discrepancy between the improved survival without a decrease in disease specific mortality is believed to be secondary to lead time or overdiagnosis bias.

Recently interest in lung cancer screening has intensified. New screening tests offer the potential to diagnose high-risk individuals at an earlier stage of their disease. Low-dose computed tomography (CT) scans are able to detect much smaller nodules (5 mm or less) than standard chest radiograghs.[16–18] Positron emission tomography (PET) and single photon emission computed tomography (SPECT) scanning are also being touted for their ability to detect lung cancer at an earlier stage.[19] Theoretically these modalities may have merit over more traditional imaging since they measure biologic function, not just anatomy. Lastly, there is increasing interest in the use of genetic assays to aid in the early diagnosis and screening of lung cancer. The addition of screens for genetic mutations (K-*ras*, *p53*, etc.) to sputum cytology or bronchoalveolar lavage may significantly increase the sensitivity of these tests.[20,21] Despite the promise of new technology, several concerns raised by previous studies will have to be resolved before widespread screening for lung cancer is indicated. The first concern is that it is not clear that the prognosis for a 5-mm nodule is better than the prognosis for a 30-mm nodule.[15] The next concern has to do with overdiagnosis bias. There is some evidence from the initial randomized studies that improved survival was due to the detection of small clinically insignificant tumors. Lastly, once effectiveness of screening is determined, cost would need to be evaluated.

Classification of Lung Cancer

Histologically, lung cancer is divided into three groups (Table 85.1). Small cell carcinoma accounts for 15% to 25%, non–small cell lung cancer 70% to 80%, and miscellaneous types ~5%. These three groups are then further subdivided. Small cell lung carcinoma (SCLC) consists of (1) oat cell carcinoma, (2) intermediate cell type, and (3) combined oat cell carcinoma. Non–small cell lung cancer (NSCLC) consists of (1) squamous cell carcinoma, (2) adenocarcinoma, and (3) large cell carcinoma. The miscellaneous types include carcinoid tumor, adenosquamous carcinoma, bronchial gland carcinoma, and other less common tumors.[22] Adenocarcinoma is the most common form of lung cancer in the United States. Squamous cell carcinoma is the most closely correlated with smoking history, while bronchoalveolar carcinoma does not appear to be related to tobacco exposure. The histology of the

Table 85.1. **Histologic Classification of Lung Cancer**

Small cell lung cancer (SCLC)
    Oat cell carcinoma
    Intermediate cell type
    Combined oat cell carcinoma
Non–small cell lung cancer (NSCLC)
    Squamous cell carcinoma
        Epidermoid carcinoma
        Spindle cell carcinoma
    Adenocarcinoma
        Acinar
        Papillary carcinoma
        Solid carcinoma with mucous secretion
        Bronchioloalveolar carcinoma
    Large cell carcinoma
        Giant cell carcinoma
        Clear cell carcinoma
Miscellaneous tumors
    Adenosquamous carcinoma
    Carcinoid tumors
    Bronchial gland carcinoma

tumor plays an important role in prognosis and treatment. Bronchoalveolar carcinoma has the best prognosis, with a 30% to 35% 5-year survival. The only hope for cure with most lung cancers is with early detection and surgical treatment. However, small cell carcinoma metastasizes at a very early stage and therefore does poorly with surgical treatment. Survival with small cell carcinoma is low; however, if caught at an early stage, there is chance for cure with chemotherapy and radiation.

Diagnosis and Staging

Clinical Presentation

The initial presentation of patients with lung cancer is largely dependent on the location of the tumor. Since most lung cancers are endobronchial in origin, cough is the most common presenting complaint. Hemoptysis and dyspnea are other early symptoms. Frequently, tumors in asymptomatic patients are detected on routine chest x-ray. Sputum production is usually not excessive in most lung cancers, except bronchioloalveolar carcinoma, which does produce profuse watery sputum. Peripheral tumors frequently are asymptomatic until they metastasize or invade the chest wall. Later symptoms include fatigue, weight loss, anorexia, pleuritic shoulder pain, pleurisy, and fever (usually from postobstructive pneumonia). Clinically patients may have unilateral wheezing or stridor, pneumonia, or a pleural effusion on lung exam. Clubbing is seen in almost one third of patients, more commonly in women than men.

There are several syndromes associated with lung cancers that may produce other signs and symptoms. Horner's syndrome and Pancoast syndrome are both caused by apical tumors invading local nerves. The two may coexist or occur separately. Horner's syndrome consists of ptosis, miosis, enophthalmos, and ipsilateral facial anhidrosis. Pancoast syndrome is caused by invasion of the brachial plexus and usu-

ally the first rib, leading to pain, numbness, and weakness in the affected arm. Enlarging metastatic lesions in the vertebral body can cause spinal cord compression; distal weakness and pain are the primary symptoms; steroids and irradiation are sometimes beneficial. Carcinomatous meningitis may also produce focal neurologic deficits as individual nerve roots are involved.

Tumors can spread locally to invade the esophagus, causing obstruction or fistulas, or the pericardium, producing cardiac tamponade. Large mediastinal tumors or those with significant lymphatic invasion may obstruct venous drainage, producing the superior vena cava syndrome. These patients may have jugular venous distention, orthopnea, dyspnea, facial edema, edema of the upper extremity and chest, and central nervous system (CNS) symptoms. Most cases of superior vena cava syndrome are due to lung cancer. Treatment is radiation therapy to the affected area.

Paraneoplastic syndromes, systemic effects that are not caused directly by local growth or metastasis of the primary tumor, are common with lung cancer. Hypertrophic pulmonary osteoarthropathy is seen in NSCLC. It is responsible for clubbing and can affect distal portions of other long bones. Eaton-Lambert syndrome is a myasthenia-like syndrome associated with small cell carcinoma which produces proximal muscle weakness. Electromyography (EMG) differentiates Eaton-Lambert from myasthenia gravis. SCLC also can cause the syndrome of inappropriate secretion of antidiuretic hormone (SIADH) producing hyponatremia and Cushing's syndrome secondary to increased production of adrenocorticotropic hormone (ACTH). Squamous cell carcinoma may produce a parathyroid hormone–like substance, which leads to hypercalcemia. Squamous cell carcinoma may also cause disseminated intravascular coagulopathy (DIC).

Diagnostic Approach

In patients with a history suspicious for lung cancer, a chest x-ray is generally obtained. If a lung nodule is found, the x-ray should be compared to previous radiographs. A nodule that has not changed in size over a 2-year period does not require further workup, because it is very unlikely to be malignant. A CT scan of the chest and upper abdomen is the first step in the evaluation of a suspicious lesion. This will allow for better clarification of the nodule and more sensitive detection of adenopathy or mediastinal involvement. Unfortunately, chest CT alone has a 79% sensitivity for detecting mediastinal lymph nodes and a sensitivity of only 62% for detecting mediastinal and chest wall invasion.[22] Positron emission tomography (PET) increases the sensitivity (89–93%) and specificity (94–100%) of noninvasive staging of lung cancer significantly.[23] The PET scan uses fluorine-18–labeled D-glucose, which is injected into the patient. Malignant nodules have a high uptake of the labeled glucose and will show up as hot spots on the scan. More widespread availability of PET scanning may improve the accuracy of preoperative staging, and prevent inappropriate surgery. PET scans are also being used to monitor response to therapy.

Tissue Diagnosis

Sputum cytology is the safest and least expensive source of tissue. However, more invasive methods are usually used because they offer a higher likelihood of getting an adequate sample. In a patient with central lesion and hemoptysis, sputum cytology may be very useful. Flexible bronchoscopy is very effective in the presence of a centrally located lesion, with a diagnostic yield of 70% to 90%. Bronchoscopy is much less useful for peripheral lesions. Transthoracic needle biopsy (TNB) is the procedure of choice for diagnosing peripheral nodules. The diagnostic yield of this procedure is very dependent on the size of the nodule. For large lesions the yield is greater than 90%, but for lesions smaller than 2 cm the yield is 15%.[24] A negative transthoracic biopsy does not exclude cancer. Between 20% and 30% of patients with negative TNB had malignant lesions.[24] Endoscopic ultrasonography with fine-needle aspiration is currently being used to biopsy lymph nodes in the posterior mediastinum, aortopulmonary window, and subcarinal region. This test seems to have a high sensitivity and specificity and is becoming more widely used. Thoracentesis is a safe and easy procedure that can be done on most patients with effusions. Cytology is positive in ~65% of patients with malignancy.

Mediastinoscopy is the method of choice for biopsy of paratracheal and hilar nodes. This procedure is also very sensitive and safe, with a complication rate of ~2%. Thoracoscopy is used only when staging cannot be completed by less invasive methods.

Staging Non–Small Cell Lung Cancer

The initial decision in the staging process for NSCLC is to determine whether the tumor is resectable for cure. NSCLC is staged based on the T, N, M system (Tables 85.2 and Table 85.3). Stage I and stage II patients who do not have a surgical contraindication benefit from resection of the tumor. Prior to attempting cure, every attempt should be made to confirm that the patient is appropriately staged. Invasion into the mediastinum might preclude surgery, but, as stated previously, CT scan is neither sensitive nor specific for mediastinal involvement. PET scan may eventually be helpful with this problem. Similar concerns arise with the poor specificity of CT scan to detect malignant nodes. Mediastinal or subcarinal metastases would also preclude surgery; however, it is not unusual for 2- to 3-cm nodes to be disease free. Therefore, current recommendations are to biopsy all nodes greater than 1 cm prior to thoracotomy.[24] Malignant pleural effusions are also a contraindication to surgery. Since 65% of pleural ef-

Table 85.3 **Staging of Lung Cancer**

Stage	TNM subsets
0	Tis N0 M0
IA	T1 N0 M0
IB	T2 N0 M0
IIA	T1 N1 M0
IIB	T2 N1 M0
	T3 N0 M0
IIIA	T3 N1 M0
	T1–3 N2 M0
IIIB	T4 N0–2 M0
	Any T N3 M0
IV	Any T Any N M1

Source: Adapted from Mountain CF. Revisions in the international system for staging lung cancer. Chest 1997;111:1710–17, with permission.

Table 85.2. **TNM Classification of Lung Cancer**

Primary tumor (T)

Tx	Tumor that cannot be assessed, or malignant cells in sputum or bronchial washings but not visualized by imaging or bronchoscopy
Tis	Carcinoma in situ
T0	No evidence of primary tumor
T1	Tumor ≤3 cm, in a lobar bronchus or distal airways, and surrounded by lung or visceral pleura
T2	Tumor that is either >3 cm; involving the main bronchus (≥2 cm of the carina); invading the visceral pleura; or with atelectasis or obstructive pneumonitis that extends to the hilar region but does not involve the entire lung
T3	Tumor of any size that invades: chest wall (including superior sulcus tumors), diaphragm, mediastinal pleura; parietal pericardium; or tumor in the main bronchus <2 cm from, but not involving, the carina; or associated atelectasis or obstructive pneumonitis of the entire lung
T4	Tumor of any size that invades: mediastinum, heart, great vessels, trachea, esophagus, vertebral body, carina; or presence of malignant/pericardial effusion; or satellite tumor nodule within ipsilateral primary-tumor lobe of the lung

Lymph Nodes (N)

Nx	Regional lymph nodes cannot be assessed
N0	No regional lymph nodes metastasis
N1	Metastasis to ipsilateral peribronchial or ipsilateral hilar lymph nodes, and intrapulmonary nodes by direct extension
N2	Metastasis to ipsilateral mediastinal or subcarinal lymph nodes
N3	Metastasis to contralateral mediastinal, contralateral hilar, scalene, or supraclavicular lymph nodes

Distant metastasis (M)

Mx	Distant metastasis cannot be assessed
M0	No distant metastasis
M1	Distant metastasis present

Source: Adapted from Mountain CF. Revisions in the international system for staging lung cancer. Chest 1997;111:1710–7, with permission.

fusions in lung cancer patients contain malignant cells, thoracentesis should be done on all pleural effusions prior to surgery. Finally, any distant metastasis makes a patient stage IV. The search for distant metastases should be focused. All patients should have a complete history and physical, complete blood count (CBC), complete metabolic panel, and chest CT extending to the adrenal glands. A CT scan of the head need only be done if the patient has CNS symptoms (seizure or headache) or has signs of diffuse metastasis such as profound weight loss or anemia. Unless the patient has known metastases, elevated alkaline phosphatase levels, bone pain, or elevated calcium should be evaluated with a bone scan. In the presence of metastases, these abnormalities can be assumed to be from bony metastases.

Staging Small Cell Lung Cancer

More than 70% of SCLC is metastatic at diagnosis. Because of this SCLC is divided into two stages, limited and extensive. Limited-stage SCLC is disease that can be confined to one radiation field. This includes tumors confined to one hemithorax. Limited-stage SCLC may have ipsilateral hilar or supraclavicular nodes, or ipsilateral or contralateral mediastinal nodes. All other SCLC is extensive stage. The search for metastases in SCLC should be systematic. All patients should get a complete history and physical, CBC, and complete metabolic panel. Abnormalities on any of these tests should help focus further workup. Once a patient meets criteria for extensive disease, there is no need for further workup since it will not influence staging. Tests that can be considered are cranial CT scan, bone scan, abdominal CT scan, and bone marrow biopsies. In completely asymptomatic patients, cranial CT scan may be the place to start since 15% of patients will have a positive scan.

Treatment

Non–Small Cell Carcinoma

Prognosis and treatment of NSCLC are dependent on staging. While survival for many other cancers has improved greatly over the last 25 years with improved treatment and supportive care, lung cancer survival has remained at 10% to 14%.[1] Recently there has been some renewed optimism regarding treatment for NSCLC. The advent of multimodality treatment for advanced disease, new chemotherapeutic agents, and the potential for gene therapy are all promising.

Early-stage lung cancer has a reasonable prognosis. Published 5-year survival for stage IA disease is 67% to 80%.[25] Treatment for stage I and stage II disease is surgical. Several studies in the 1980s confirmed that survival was higher and recurrence rate was much lower with lobectomy compared to limited resection of the tumor. Even with appropriate surgical treatment, the local recurrence rate for early-stage NSCLC is high (36–75% for stage I and 49–82% for stage II). Many studies have evaluated the role of adjuvant therapy in early-stage disease. The use of adjuvant chemotherapy in stage I and II disease is controversial. Several studies have shown a

significant improvement in 5-year survival with postoperative chemotherapy; however, others have shown an increased risk of death. The discrepancy in these studies may be due to the chemotherapeutic agents used. Trials are currently under way using newer agents, which it is hoped will clarify the situation. Meta-analysis of nine randomized control trials on the use of postoperative radiation therapy (RT) clearly showed that patients who received RT after surgery had a worse survival rate than those who received only surgery. Combined adjuvant chemo-radiotherapy has not yet been shown to prolong survival. Since adjuvant chemotherapy and radiation therapy have not shown significant benefit, recent studies have evaluated neoadjuvant (preoperative) chemotherapy in early-stage disease (stage I and II). Two separate trials have shown a significant improvement in survival.[25,26]

Treatment and prognosis for stage III NSCLC is dependent on the clinical presentation. Patients with stage IIIA disease are actually a very diverse group. Those with incidental N2 disease (not evident by clinical staging and found on mediastinal node dissection) actually have a fair survival rate (24–34%) with surgery alone. Patients with minimal N2 disease are considered to be potentially resectable, but they do poorly with surgery alone. Those who have bulky N2 disease with nodes that are visible on chest x-ray are considered to be nonresectable. Three small randomized studies have found significant improvement in survival of stage IIIA patients given neoadjuvant chemotherapy; one study showed no improvement.[24] Preliminary studies on the use of chemoradiotherapy preoperatively for stage IIIA suggest some potential benefit of combined therapy.[25] Traditionally the treatment of nonresectable stage IIIA and stage IIIB disease was radiotherapy alone. Survival rates were very poor (3–5%). Currently these patients receive chemotherapy followed by radiation, or concurrent chemotherapy and radiation therapy, which produces a modest survival benefit.

A large portion (40%) of patients present with advanced disease. These patients have metastasis, locally invasive disease, or malignant pleural effusions. Radiotherapy alone yields an average survival of 9 to 10 months. A combination of radiotherapy and newer chemotherapeutic agents (paclitaxel/carboplatin, gemcitabine/cisplatin, or vinorelbine/cisplatin) improves both 1- and 3-year survival.[26,27] More importantly, two recent studies showed that patients with advanced disease who received chemotherapy had an improved quality of life as compared to patients receiving best supportive care.[25]

Treatment of Small Cell Lung Cancer

SCLC is a very aggressive disease. One third of patients present with limited-stage disease and two thirds present with extensive disease. Most patients respond well to chemotherapy initially (65–85% response rate); however, 5-year survival remains extremely poor at 5%.[28] Several new chemotherapy regimens have been evaluated over the last decade. Paclitaxel, gemcitabine, vinorelbine, topotecan, and irinotecan have all been used with variable effectiveness. These new drugs in combination with radiotherapy have been shown to increase response rate and frequency of complete remission. The small size of most trials has made it difficult to prove survival benefit.

Molecular Biology and Lung Cancer Treatment

Improved understanding of the biochemistry and molecular biology of lung cancer has led to novel approaches to treatment. Lung cancers have a tendency to early metastasis. Matrix metalloproteinases (MMPs) are enzymes produced by tumor cells that destroy basement membranes in normal cells, leading to metastasis. MMP inhibitors are currently being used in phase III trials in patients with complete remission following induction chemotherapy.[28] Angiogenesis is the formation of new blood vessels, and is believed to be an important step in metastasis. Antivascular endothelial growth factor antibodies and thalidomide, which also inhibits angiogenesis, are both in clinical trials. A *p53* tumor suppressor gene mutation is the most common mutation seen in lung cancer. In vitro studies have shown replacement of the mutant gene with wild-type *p53* inhibits lung tumor growth.[29] Systemic delivery of gene therapy has proven difficult, but local injection of normal *p53* into a metastatic lesion did produce some tumor regression. Other tumor suppressor genes are also being investigated. Overproduction of oncogenes is frequently associated with both SCLC and NSCLC. The *myc* oncogenes are associated with SCLC. In vitro *myc* genes can be inhibited by transfection with mutant *myc* genes and therefore prevent cell proliferation. The *ras* oncogene is associated with poor prognosis in adenocarcinoma. Several drugs that are known to inhibit *ras* activation are now in clinical trials.

References

1. Trends in lung cancer morbidity and morality. Available at *www.lungusa.org.*
2. Tanoue L. Cigarette smoking and women's respiratory health. Clin Chest Med 2000;21:47–65.
3. Nair A, Brandt E. Effects of smoking on health care costs. J Okla State Med Assoc 2000;93:245–52.
4. Vineis P, Kogevinas M, Simonato L, Brennan P, Boffetta P. Leveling-off of the risk of lung and bladder cancer in heavy smokers: an analysis based on multicentric case-control studies and a metabolic interpretation. Mutat Res 2001;463:103–10.
5. Kumra V, Markoff B. Who's smoking now? The epidemiology of tobacco use in the United States and abroad. Clin Chest Med 2000;21:1–9.
6. Ding M, Shi X, Castranova V, Vallyathan V. Predisposing factors in occupational lung cancer: inorganic minerals and chromium. J Environ Pathol Toxicol Oncol 2000;19:129–38.
7. Samet JM, Eradze GR. Radon and lung cancer risk: taking stock at the millennium. Environ Health Perspect 2000;108(suppl 4):635–41.
8. Gustavsson P, Jakobsson R, Nyberg F, Pershagen G, Jarup L, Scheele P. Occupational exposure and lung cancer risk: a population-based case-referent study in Sweden. Am J Epidemiol 2000;152:32–40.
9. Traber M, van der Vliet A, Reznick A, Cross C. Tobacco-related diseases—is there a role for antioxidant micronutrient supplementation. Clin Chest Med 2000;21:173–87.
10. Alpha-Tocopherol, Beta Carotene Cancer Prevention Study Group. The effect of vitamin E and beta carotene on the incidence of lung cancer and other cancers in male smokers. N Engl J Med 1994;330:1029–35.
11. Christiani D. Smoking and the molecular epidemiology of lung cancer. Clin Chest Med 2000;21:87–93.
12. Toloza E, Roth J, Swisher S. Molecular events in bronchogenic carcinoma and their implications for therapy. Semin Surg Oncol 2000;18:91–9.
13. Walker C, Robertson LJ, Myskow MW, et al. p 53 expression in normal and dysplastic bronchial epithelium and in lung carcinomas. Br J Cancer 1994;70:297–303.
14. Guide to clinical preventive services, 2nd ed. Report of U.S. Preventive Service Task Force. Baltimore: Williams & Wilkins 1996;135–52.
15. Patz E, Goodman P, Bepler G. Screening for lung cancer. Curr Concepts MA Med Soc 2000;343:1627–33.
16. Miettinen O. Screening for lung cancer. Radiol Clin North Am 2000;38:479–86.
17. Henschke C, Yankelevitz D. CT screening for lung cancer. Radiol Clin North Am 2000;38:487–94.
18. Porter J, Spiro S. Detection of early lung cancer: early lung cancer action project: overall design and findings from baseline screening. Thorax 2000;55(suppl 1):S56–S62.
19. Goldsmith S, Kostakoglu L. Nuclear medicine imaging of lung cancer. Radiol Clin North Am 2000;38:511–25.
20. Gruidl M, Shaw Wright G. Potential biomarkers for the early detection of lung cancer. J Thorac Imag 2000;15:13–20.
21. Minamoto T, Mai M, Ronai Z. K-ras mutation: early detection in molecular diagnosis and risk assessment of colorectal, pancreas, and lung cancers—a review. Cancer Detect Prevent; 2000;24:1–12.
22. Mountain C. The evolution of the surgical treatment of lung cancer. Chest Surg Clin North Am 2000;10:83–104.
23. Park B, Louie O, Altorki N. Staging and the surgical management of lung cancer. Radiol Clin North Am 2000;38:545–61.
24. Hyer J, Silvestri G. Diagnosis and staging of lung cancer. Clin Chest Med 2000;21:95–106.
25. Reif M, Socinski M, Rivera M. Evidence-based medicine in the treatment of non-small-cell lung cancer. Clin Chest Med 2000;21:107–17.
26. Rosell R, Felip E. Role of multimodality treatment for lung cancer. Semin Surg Oncol 2000:18:143–51.
27. Johnson D. Locally advanced, unresectable non-small cell lung cancer. Chest 2000;117:123S–6S.
28. Kelly K. New chemotherapy agents for small cell lung cancer. Chest 2000;117:156S–62S.
29. Bunn P, Soriano A, Johnson G, Heasley L. Biology and molecular biology come of age. Chest 2000;117:163S–8S.

86
Selected Disorders of the Respiratory System

*George C. Coleman, Richard H. Hoffman, Michael R. Lustig,
John G. King, and David W. Marsland*

Respiratory Failure

Normal respiration results in uptake of oxygen and elimination of carbon dioxide, and is a process involving both the movement of gases and the circulation of blood. Respiratory failure results from any condition that severely affects the lungs' ability to maintain arterial oxygenation, with or without adequate carbon dioxide elimination. Respiratory failure can occur as an acute or chronic condition, and can be divided into two main categories: a failure of gas exchange manifested primarily by hypoxemia, and a failure of ventilation whose primary consequence is hypercapnia. Because ventilatory failure ultimately leads to a failure of gas exchange, respiratory failure may present clinically as severe hypoxemia or as severe hypercapnia with hypoxemia.

Hypoxic respiratory failure exists when arterial oxygen tension is severely reduced (PaO_2 <60 mm Hg) and cannot be corrected by increasing inspired oxygen concentration beyond 50% (FIO_2 >0.5). Reductions in arterial oxygen tension below 60% coincide with the beginning of a steep descent of the oxygen-hemoglobin dissociation curve. This leaves minimal reserve for tissue oxygenation, and patients are usually symptomatic. Patients may complain of headache, anxiety, somnolence, or altered mental status, including confusion and seizures. Physical findings of mild hypoxemia include tachycardia, tachypnea, diaphoresis, and hypertension. As hypoxemia progresses, cyanosis and ultimately bradycardia and hypotension develop.

Acute hypercapnic respiratory failure is defined as a partial carbon dioxide pressure ($PaCO_2$) exceeding 50 mm Hg associated with respiratory acidosis. This excludes patients with chronic hypercapnia in whom renal compensation has nearly normalized the pH. The development of symptoms depends on both the degree of hypercapnia and the rate at which the $PaCO_2$ increases. Acute elevations in $PaCO_2$ to 80 to 90 mm Hg may produce neurologic symptoms including confusion, headaches, and sometimes convulsions progressing to coma.

Physical findings may include tremor, slurred speech, agitation, and asterixis. Complications may include arrhythmias, hyperkalemia, and gastrointestinal bleeding.

Diagnosis of acute respiratory failure should be considered in any patient presenting with these symptoms and signs, and is confirmed if hypoxemia with or without hypercapnia is found by arterial blood gases. The many underlying causes can be grouped into two categories by chest radiograph: conditions causing diffuse or patchy infiltrates [acute respiratory distress syndrome (ARDS), pneumonia, cardiogenic pulmonary edema, severe atelectasis, pulmonary contusion, alveolar hemorrhage, progressive interstitial lung disease, and aspiration] and conditions with a clear film [acute exacerbation of chronic obstructive pulmonary disease (COPD), asthma, neuromuscular disease or central nervous system (CNS)-mediated respiratory depression such as drug overdose].[1] The most important causes of arterial hypoxemia include alveolar hypoventilation and ventilation-perfusion mismatching.

In addition to treating the underlying illness, therapy focuses on restoring adequate arterial oxygen. This requires a patent airway and oxygen supplementation. With nasal cannulae and loose-fitting masks, oxygenation steadily increases with flow rates up to 6 L/min. However, because an FIO_2 greater than 0.5 can seldom be maintained with any open delivery system, treatment generally requires an intensive care unit setting with a non-rebreathing mask or endotracheal intubation. In cases of acute respiratory failure, noninvasive positive-pressure ventilation with a face mask has been shown to be as effective in improving gas exchange as ventilation via endotracheal intubation. When endotracheal intubation can be avoided, the development of ventilator-associated pneumonia is unlikely.[2] Mechanical ventilation can be cycled based on volume or pressure. Volume-cycled ventilation can be divided into two types: assisted/controlled, which allows for greater patient rest, and synchronized intermittent, which gives better coordination between patient and ventilator and allows some exercising of respiratory muscles. Pressure-support ventilation requires the patient initiate every breath. Initial mechanical ventilator settings include a tidal volume between 8 and 10 mL/kg body weight, at 11 to 14 breaths per minute, and are adjusted based on serial determinations of arterial blood gases. Positive end expiratory pressure (PEEP) may be added to further improve oxygenation. Complications of mechanical ventilation include both pulmonary and nonpulmonary types. Pulmonary complications include pneumonia,[3] sinusitis, alveolar overdistention, and atelectasis. Nonpulmonary complications include thromboembolic disorders,[4] gastrointestinal bleeding, pressure ulcers, acute renal failure, and neuromuscular weakness.[5]

Acute Respiratory Distress Syndrome

Acute respiratory distress syndrome is a severe pulmonary injury occurring in medical or surgical patients. It has a mortality of 40% to 50% and can be caused by direct or indirect lung injury with pneumonia, severe trauma, sepsis, and aspiration being the most common causes. In these conditions, the alveolar-capillary barrier is damaged either on the alveolar epithelial or the microvascular endothelium side, and this allows the leakage of protein-rich fluid into the alveolar or interstitial spaces. An inflammatory reaction can last for weeks and may result in fibrosis of the alveoli if the patient survives. The criteria for ARDS are acute onset, bilateral chest infiltrates on chest x-ray, pulmonary wedge pressure under 18, and a PaO_2/FIO_2 ratio equal to or less than 200.[6] The diagnosis of ARDS should be considered in any patient with one of the known causes who develops dyspnea and tachypnea with severe hypoxia and lung infiltrates. Noteworthy is the fact that unlike the edema of congestive heart failure that clears with diuretics, the edema of acute lung injury fails to clear.

Treatment requires mechanical ventilation in an intensive care setting that maintains adequate oxygen delivery but yet does not cause additional damage, search for treatable causes such as infection, and nutritional support. Considerations in mechanical ventilation include lower tidal volumes that improve mortality possibly by reducing further lung injury and decreasing inflammatory mediator release,[7] and optimal PEEP levels to recruit atelectatic, undamaged alveoli while avoiding high peak transalveolar pressures to prevent barotrauma. Acceptance of some hypercapnia (which can be treated with infusion of intravenous sodium bicarbonate) may allow lower alveolar pressures.[8] Studies of glucocorticoids and inhaled nitric oxide and other vasodilators do not show improved outcomes. Ongoing studies of patient positioning and surfactant may reveal other methods of optimizing outcomes.[1]

Pulmonary Embolism

Pulmonary embolism is a frequent cause of morbidity and mortality but remains difficult to diagnose despite new diagnostic methods. It is thought that annually there are 150,000 deaths in the United States due to pulmonary embolism.[9]

Risk factors include inherited and acquired disorders. Common inherited risk factors include mutations in the factor V gene (factor V Leiden), the prothrombin (factor II) gene, and the methylenetetrahydrofolate reductase gene, resulting in hypercoagulability by increasing production or reducing neutralization of thrombin. Less common inherited disorders include deficiencies of proteins C and S, the anticoagulant proteins. Patients with these disorders may present in early adulthood with thromboembolic events. Acquired risk factors include orthopedic and pelvic surgery, spinal and neurologic trauma, malignancy, nephrotic syndrome, estrogens, pregnancy and the puerperium, antiphospholipid antibodies, and hyperhomocystinemia (of genetic or acquired etiology).[10]

Most pulmonary emboli originate from the deep veins of the thigh and pelvis. Thrombi usually develop from vein bifurcations or valve cusps; they may also arise in the calf but rarely embolize. Deep vein thrombosis may arise in the upper extremity, with most cases seen in patients with central venous catheters, although spontaneous deep vein thrombosis of the upper extremity does occur.[11,12] Right atrial thrombus during atrial fibrillation is also a potential source.

Diagnosis

Deep vein thrombosis is difficult to diagnose. Patients may have a completely normal exam and have a clot. Clinical findings may include unilateral leg edema, venous distention, leg pain, tenderness, and cyanosis. However, these symptoms are very nonspecific and make objective testing to confirm the diagnosis mandatory especially in light of the potential complications of treatment. Ultrasonography, impedence plethysmography, and ascending venography may be used to evaluate the venous system of the lower extremity. Venography can evaluate the entire venous system, whereas the other two methods can evaluate only the proximal system. Strategies to diagnose deep vein thrombosis and pulmonary embolism may also include use of the plasma D-dimer level, a fibrin degradation product.[13] The D-dimer [enzyme-linked immunosorbent assay (ELISA)] is a sensitive test for thromboembolism, and a negative test is good evidence against these disorders; however, the D-dimer is frequently elevated in hospitalized patients limiting its usefulness in those patients most likely to develop thromboembolic disease.[14] The D-dimer can also be normal in angiographically confirmed pulmonary embolism.[15]

Pulmonary embolism has a similarly variable clinical picture. Emboli may occur silently[16] or present with symptoms mimicking other cardiopulmonary disorders. Pulmonary embolism should be considered when the diagnoses of pneumonia, congestive heart failure, myocardial infarction, and asthma are made.

Signs and symptoms of pulmonary emboli are nonspecific, and no finding or combination of findings is diagnostic. In addition, the clinical picture can vary depending on the size, location, and number of emboli. Symptoms can vary from transient dyspnea with small emboli to sudden severe shortness of breath, chest pain, and syncope with massive emboli. The most common symptoms are dyspnea, pleuritic pain, apprehension, and cough. Hemoptysis occurs in about one third of patients. The most common signs are tachypnea, rales, increased P_2 heart sound, tachycardia, and fever. Only one third of patients have clinically evident lower extremity phlebitis.

Patient evaluation includes chest x-ray, electrocardiogram, arterial blood gases, and D-dimer. These tests help identify disorders with similar symptoms. The chest x-ray is usually abnormal but nonspecific, showing, for instance, pleural effusion, infiltrate, atelectasis, or elevation of the hemidiaphragm. The electrocardiogram (ECG) is also often abnormal and nonspecific. Atrial arrhythmias (sinus tachycardia, atrial fibrillation), ST segment and T wave changes and QRS changes are often found.[16–18] Most patients with pulmonary embolism are hypoxic and have an increased alveolar-arterial oxygen gradient, although pulmonary emboli have been shown to occur in patients with a Pao_2 of more than 90 mm Hg and a normal alveolar-arterial oxygen gradient. Age- and disease-related changes in normal arterial blood gases further limit their usefulness for diagnosing pulmonary embolism.[19]

Because of the unreliability of the clinical diagnosis of pulmonary embolism, objective testing must be undertaken to either exclude or confirm the diagnosis in at-risk patients. Over the past decade, the ventilation-perfusion (VQ) scan has been a key test. A normal scan excludes the diagnosis of pulmonary embolism, and a high-probability scan (based on the size and number of unmatched perfusion defects) is correlated with a 98% chance of angiographically confirmed pulmonary embolism. Unfortunately, many scans are read as intermediate or low probability, results still associated with a significant percentage of emboli (40% and 15%, respectively).[20] Venous ultrasound of the proximal veins of the legs can be used in patients suspected of having pulmonary embolism when the patient has a nondiagnostic VQ scan. A deep vein thrombosis is found in 5% to 10% of these patients, but if the test is normal, pulmonary embolism is still not excluded.[21] Traditionally, those patients in whom the diagnosis has not been excluded have been evaluated by pulmonary angiography.

Additional methods may be used in patient evaluation that may augment or replace VQ scans and angiography. Alveolar dead-space (alveoli ventilated but not perfused to allow gas exchange) is increased in pulmonary embolism. A volumetric capnogram can measure multiple respiratory parameters and combined with a blood-gas measurement of $Paco_2$ can give a determination of alveolar dead-space. Normal dead-space measurement when combined with a normal D-dimer excludes pulmonary embolism with the same sensitivity as a normal VQ scan.[22,23]

Helical, or spiral, computed tomography (CT) is rapidly emerging as the imaging study of choice for various steps along the path toward establishing a diagnosis of pulmonary embolus. It may be used to confirm pulmonary embolism or evaluate those patients with nondiagnostic VQ scans.[24] When compared to VQ scans, spiral CT has been shown to have better sensitivity and greater interobserver agreement, i.e., greater consistency of interpretation among radiologists.[25] Unlike a VQ scan, it also provides images of the lung parenchyma, mediastinum, and thoracic wall, and thus may reveal the presence of an alternative cause of the presenting symptoms such as pneumonia, interstitial lung disease, or cardiovascular disease.[26] Spiral CT findings also correspond closely to pulmonary

angiography, with a sensitivity and specificity for emboli to main through segmental arteries of 94%.[27] Further, it may be more readily available than conventional pulmonary angiography because it does not require a fully staffed cardiac catheterization laboratory. Spiral CT may be more cost-effective than conventional pulmonary angiography.[28] Nonetheless, angiography remains the gold standard and can be used whenever the evaluation has failed to yield definitive results.

Prevention and Treatment

Occurrence of thromboembolic disease is very predictable for many clinical conditions and preventative strategies that reduce that risk are well documented (also see Chapter 81). For instance, deep vein thrombosis occurs in as many as 64% of total knee replacement patients without prophylaxis. With oral anticoagulant prophylaxis, the DVT rate was 46%, and with low molecular weight heparin, the rate was 31.5%, a risk reduction of over 50%. Prophylaxis should also be undertaken in patients undergoing surgery for hip replacement, hip fracture repair, open urologic surgery, gynecologic malignancy surgeries, and general surgery depending on age and the type of procedure. Trauma patients, especially spinal cord injury patients, benefit from preventive strategies. Medical patients with conditions such as myocardial infarction, stroke, and malignancy are also candidates for prophylaxis. Prevention can be accomplished with oral coumadin, low-dose heparin, or low molecular weight heparin. Prevention should be withheld in patients having spinal puncture or epidural anesthesia due to the risk of perispinal hematoma and in patients at particularly high risk of hemorrhage.[29]

There are several options for the treatment of deep vein thrombosis and pulmonary embolism. Low molecular weight heparin or intravenous unfractionated heparin should be given for 5 days, and if ongoing treatment with warfarin is planned, this should overlap the heparin treatment for 4 to 5 days. Longer courses of heparin are recommended for patients with massive emboli or severe iliofemoral thrombosis. Warfarin therapy should achieve a prothrombin time in an international normalized ratio (INR) range of 2.0 to 3.0, and treatment should extend for 3 months in patients with reversible risk factors. Treatment for 6 months is recommended for patients with idiopathic thromboembolism. The role of thrombolytic therapy in thromboembolism is unclear; patients with hemodynamic compromise and massive emboli are possible candidates. Inferior vena cava filters are used in patients with recurrent emboli despite appropriate anticoagulation and in patients in whom anticoagulation is contraindicated.[30] Patients treated with heparin should be observed for thrombocytopenia which is immune mediated and can be accompanied by venous and arterial thrombi.[31] Warfarin interacts with multiple medications and should be avoided in pregnancy. Agents that can cause gastrointestinal bleeding should be avoided.

Pulmonary Hypertension[32–37]

Pulmonary hypertension is characterized by a fixed elevation in mean pulmonary-artery pressure above 25 mm Hg at rest, or more than 30 mm Hg during exercise.[32] Traditionally pulmonary hypertension was classified as either "primary," which is exceedingly rare, or "secondary," which includes numerous diverse etiologies. In 1998, the World Health Organization (WHO) sponsored a symposium on primary pulmonary hypertension. From this meeting came a new classification system that divides the causes into categories, based on common aspects of etiology and treatment.

Classification

The WHO classification system divides pulmonary hypertension into five categories: (1) associated with disorders of the respiratory system and/or hypoxia, (2) due to chronic thrombotic or embolic disease, (3) due to pulmonary venous hypertension, (4) due to pulmonary arterial hypertension, and (5) due to disorders directly affecting the pulmonary vasculature. Underlying causes within each category are listed in Table 86.1.[37]

Evaluation

Dyspnea on exertion and fatigue are the primary symptoms of pulmonary hypertension. As the disease progresses, chest pain, dizziness, cough, hemoptysis, and syncope may develop. A thorough review of systems should be done searching for symptoms suggestive of associated and underlying conditions (Table 86.1). Specific inquiry regarding prior use of anorexic agents is also important. Physical findings arise from compensatory changes in the right ventricle. The most frequent finding is an increase in the intensity of the second heart sound, with P_2 being louder than A_2 in the pulmonic listening area (left upper sternal border). Later, a prominent right ventricular impulse develops and may progress to a right ventricular heave. Murmurs of pulmonic insufficiency or tricuspid regurgitation may also develop. Neck vein distention and lower extremity edema are signs of advanced disease.

When pulmonary hypertension is considered, the most useful diagnostic study is the transthoracic echocardiogram, specifying a search for pulmonary hypertension as a reason for the study. Doppler estimation of pulmonary artery pressure is necessary to identify pulmonary hypertension and is not included in routine echocardiograms at all centers. Mean pressures of 26 to 35 mm Hg are considered mild, 36 to 45 mm Hg are moderate, and over 45 mm Hg is considered severe pulmonary hypertension.[33] Other studies should then be done to look for secondary factors and associated conditions. Evidence of congenital heart disease and the status of the heart valves and septum can also be determined by the echocardiogram. A chest radiograph and pulmonary function studies, including lung volumes, diffusion capacity, and spirometry, may point to emphysema or pulmonary fibrosis. In overweight patients with loud snoring or hypersomnolence, a sleep study is done to evaluate for obstructive sleep apnea. Possible thromboembolic disease should be evaluated as discussed in the previous section. Lastly, blood tests are ordered based on suspicion of underlying diseases and may include a complete blood count (CBC), sedimentation rate, antinuclear antibody (ANA), cardiolipin antibody, hepatic function studies, HIV antibody, and thyroid studies.[34]

Table 86.1 Diagnostic Classification of Pulmonary Hypertension

1. Pulmonary arterial hypertension
   1.1. Primary pulmonary hypertension
      1.1.1. Sporadic
      1.1.2. Familial
   1.2. Related to:
      1.2.1. Collagen vascular disease
      1.2.2. Congenital systemic-to-pulmonary shunts
      1.2.3. Portal hypertension
      1.2.4. HIV infection
      1.2.5. Drugs/toxins
         1.2.5.1. Anorexigens
         1.2.5.2. Other
      1.2.6. Persistent pulmonary hypertension of the newborn
      1.2.7. Other
2. Pulmonary venous hypertension
   2.1. Left-sided atrial or ventricular heart disease
   2.2. Left-sided valvular heart disease
   2.3. Extrinsic compression of central pulmonary veins
      2.3.1. Fibrosing mediastinitis
      2.3.2. Adenopathy/tumors
   2.4. Pulmonary veno-occlusive disease
   2.5. Other
3. Pulmonary hypertension associated with disorders of the respiratory system and/or hypoxemia
   3.1. Chronic obstructive pulmonary disease
   3.2. Interstitial lung disease
   3.3. Sleep disordered breathing
   3.4. Alveolar hypoventilation disorders
   3.5. Chronic exposure to high altitude
   3.6. Neonatal lung disease
   3.7. Alveolar-capillary dysplasia
   3.8. Other
4. Pulmonary hypertension due to chronic thrombotic and/or embolic disease
   4.1. Thromboembolic obstruction of proximal pulmonary arteries
   4.2. Obstruction of distal pulmonary arteries
      4.2.1. Pulmonary embolism (thrombus, tumor, ova and/or parasites, foreign material)
      4.2.2. In-situ thrombosis
      4.2.3. Sickle cell disease
5. Pulmonary hypertension due to disorders directly affecting the pulmonary vasculature
   5.1. Inflammatory
      5.1.1. Schistosomiasis
      5.1.2. Sarcoidosis
      5.1.3. Other
   5.2. Pulmonary capillary hemangiomatosis

At this point, if pulmonary arterial hypertension is suspected, cardiology consultation and right-heart catheterization are indicated to confirm the diagnosis, determine the prognosis, and decide on the therapy.

A 6-minute walk test is very useful for establishing a baseline to follow response to therapy. This involves exercise oxymetry during a timed 6-minute walk. Functional classification of patients with pulmonary hypertension follows the New York Heart Association (NYHA) scheme for congestive heart failure.

Table 86.2. **Treatment of Underlying Conditions Associated with Pulmonary Hypertension**

Category	Treatment goal	Interventions
Disorders of the respiratory system and/or hypoxemia	Maximize pulmonary function and normalize oxygenation	Long term oxygen Steroids Bronchodilators Nocturnal CPAP
Pulmonary venous disease	Reduce left atrial pressure to decrease PAP	Afterload reduction Diuretics
Chronic thromboembolic disease	Restore luminal patency and reduce vascular resistance	Lifelong anticoagulation Vena caval filter Thromboendarterectomy
Pulmonary arterial disease related to infection, inflammatory conditions, toxins	Reduce vascular resistance, endothelial and smooth muscle dysfunction	Vasodilators Disease modifying antiinflammatory agents Antiinfectious agents Avoiding toxin or causative drugs (anorexics)
Primary pulmonary hypertension	Reduce vascular resistance, endothelial and smooth muscle dysfunction	Vasodilator therapy

CPAP = continuous positive airway pressure; PAP = positive airway pressure.

Treatment

Treatment begins with therapy targeted to any underlying factors identified, and are listed in Table 86.2. Current treatment strategies use vasodilators to reduce right ventricular overload. Indications for vasodilator therapy are based on right heart catheterization findings and results of a vasodilator trial, often performed at the time of catheterization. Agents that have been useful include calcium channel blockers for class I and II patients and vasodilatory prostaglandins, such as epoprostenol for class III and IV patients. While shown to prolong life in severe cases, these agents are quite expensive and difficult to administer, requiring continuous intravenous infusion.[35] Drugs under investigation include inhaled nitric oxide and inhaled prostacyclin analogues.[36,37]

Pneumothorax

A pneumothorax is defined as the presence of gas within the pleural space. This gas may enter through the chest wall and parietal pleura, as occurs in trauma. It may originate from gas-filled gastrointestinal structures such as a ruptured esophagus or bowel with subsequent escape of gas across the diaphragm from a pneumoperitoneum. Most often the gas originates in the lung with leakage following alveolar or tracheobronchial injury or through the visceral pleura due to focal pulmonary processes.[38] Examples of the latter process include bronchogenic carcinoma, rheumatoid lung nodules, thoracic endometriosis, and pulmonary infarcts, which cause localized damage to lung tissue leading to pneumothorax.[39] In the same way, tuberculosis and more recently *Pneumocystis carinii* pneumonia have been found to cause pneumothorax.[40] Traditional classification schemes identify three types, spontaneous, traumatic, and tension.

Spontaneous Pneumothorax

Primary spontaneous pneumothorax occurs suddenly in healthy individuals and may be the result of a ruptured subpleural bleb.

The incidence is 4.3 cases per 100,000 patient-years, and peaks in persons between 20 and 30 years of age. The likelihood is five times higher for men than women, and is more common among taller individuals. An increased incidence of spontaneous pneumothorax has been found among smokers. There appears to be a higher risk in some families. In some cases patients have been identified with an anomalous bronchial tree anatomy suggesting a congenital predisposition.[41] Secondary spontaneous pneumothorax is also seen in patients with underlying lung disease such as COPD, tuberculosis, sarcoidosis, and cancer.

The most common symptoms include sudden onset of chest pain and dyspnea. The chest pain may be dramatic and severe, localized over the area of pneumothorax and sometimes radiating to the ipsilateral shoulder. Small leaks in healthy individuals may cause only moderate degrees of pain. It is not unusual for patients to recall prior episodes of similar pain, milder in degree and briefer in duration for which they did not seek care. The dyspnea experienced can also vary in intensity, being more severe in patients with underlying lung disease and in those with large leaks. Physical examination usually reveals normal vital signs except for a mild tachycardia. Chest percussion reveals a more resonant note than usual over the affected side. The hyperresonance of a pneumothorax is best found by percussing over the mid-clavicle with the patient sitting or standing.[42] Breath sounds are absent or decreased on the affected side. Arterial blood gases may reveal hypoxia. Patients with secondary spontaneous pneumothorax usually have more severe symptoms due to diminished baseline pulmonary function. Healthy individuals who have a small pneumothorax may present with mild symptoms and subtle physical findings.[43] The chest roentgenogram is diagnostic, showing a lucent area of pleural space devoid of the normal vascular markings that divide the edge of the lung from the chest wall.[44] While it is difficult to estimate the size of the pneumothorax by chest x-ray, a 1-inch lucent rim corresponds approximately to a 30% collapse of the lung. In patients too ill to remain upright, a supine chest x-ray will show lucency in the costophrenic sulcus rather than the apex.

Treatment options depend on the size of the pneumothorax and the severity of symptoms. Small pneumothoraces involving less than 15% of the hemithorax may resolve without therapy, provided no additional leakage occurs. Complete resolution is expected in 10 days. Supplemental oxygen can facilitate resolution by increasing the pressure gradient of nitrogen from the pleural space into the capillaries. Mildly symptomatic patients will often respond to needle aspiration.[45] A large pneumothorax or a patient with severe symptoms requires removal of the air by insertion of a large-bore chest tube that allows for reexpansion of the lung.

Recurrence rates for both types of spontaneous pneumothorax are high, ranging from 20% to 50%, and the choice of treatment does not appear to affect these recurrence rates. Smoking cessation can reduce the risk of recurrence.[46] Surgical or chemical pleurodesis is considered after two ipsilateral spontaneous pneumothoraces or when a 5- to 7-day course of chest tube therapy fails to result in lung reexpansion.[43]

Traumatic Pneumothorax

A traumatic pneumothorax can result from penetrating or nonpenetrating chest trauma as well as from such invasive procedures as bronchoscopy, thoracentesis, central line placement, mechanical ventilation, and cardiopulmonary resuscitation. Most traumatic pneumothoraces seen in hospitals today are iatrogenic due to numerous invasive procedures. Symptoms, physical examination, and radiologic findings are similar to those of spontaneous pneumothorax. Treatment depends on size of the pneumothorax and symptoms; however, traumatic pneumothoraces resulting from direct trauma require tube thoracostomy, as a hemothorax is often present.[43,44]

Tension Pneumothorax

A tension pneumothorax can result from either a spontaneous or a traumatic pneumothorax and is a life-threatening emergency. Tension develops as air freely enters the pleural space during inspiration but is unable to escape during expiration. The result of this one-way valve is further lung collapse, with shifting of the trachea and mediastinum away from the pneumothorax. Patients with a tension pneumothorax are in acute respiratory distress and have dilated neck veins, tracheal deviation, and absence of breath sounds on the affected side. They are in danger of impending cardiovascular collapse unless prompt treatment ensues. Immediate insertion of a large-bore needle (16 gauge) into the affected pleural cavity at the second intercostal space releases the trapped air, relieves the

pressure, and results in rapid improvement in cardiac output and blood pressure. Following this emergent procedure, a chest roentgenogram can be performed and a chest tube inserted to prevent recurrence.[43,44]

Pleural Effusion

Pleural effusion is defined as an accumulation of fluid in the pleural space that occurs as a result of a disparity between fluid formation and resorption. While not a disease in itself, pleural effusions may be a result of more than 50 disease processes. Six diseases—congestive heart failure (CHF), cirrhosis with ascites, pleuropulmonary infections, malignancy, pulmonary embolism, and pancreatitis—account for more than 90% of all cases. By using the history, physical findings, and thoracentesis to sample and analyze the pleural fluid, the physician can establish the etiology in approximately 75% of cases.[47]

Evaluation

Patients with pleural effusions may be asymptomatic. When symptoms are present, they are the result of pleural inflammation or mechanical effects of the fluid volume. The most common presenting complaints include pleuritic chest pain, dyspnea, nonproductive cough, and fever. Occasionally pain may be referred to the abdomen or ipsilateral shoulder. Physical examination of the chest characteristically reveals decreased breath sounds over the area of the effusion. Tactile fremitus, dullness to percussion, and a pleural friction rub are sometimes found over the area of the effusion.

The posteroanterior (PA) and lateral chest roentgenogram is the most informative initial diagnostic study when a pleural effusion is suspected. Effusions that blunt the costophrenic angle represent more than 100 mL of fluid. When 500 mL of fluid is present, chest x-rays correctly reveal the presence of an effusion in virtually all cases.[48] If uncertainty exists, ultrasound can accurately identify effusions over 100 mL in size. Lateral decubitus views are necessary to confirm that the effusion is not loculated.[49]

Once the presence of a pleural effusion is confirmed, the etiology should be sought. This is best done through analysis of pleural fluid obtained by thoracentesis. The fluid should first be categorized as either a transudate or exudate based on analysis of several simple laboratory tests outlined in Table 86.3. Other laboratory studies may aid in the diagnosis, including cytology, glucose, Gram stain, bacterial and fungal

Table 86.3. **Pleural Fluid Characteristics**

Characteristic	Transudate	Exudate
Pleural fluid protein/serum protein ratio	<0.5	>0.5
Pleural fluid LDH/serum LDH ratio	<0.6	>0.6
Pleural fluid LDH	<Two-thirds of upper limit of normal serum LDH	>Two-thirds of upper limit of normal serum LDH
pH	>7.40	<7.40
WBC count	Usually <1000/μL	Usually >1000/μL

LDH = lactate dehydrogenase; WBC = white blood cell.

cultures, acid-fast bacillus (AFB) stain, amylase, rheumatoid factor, and lipid studies. However, these tests should be performed based on the nature of the fluid and the clinical presentation.[50]

Etiology

Congestive heart failure is the most common cause of a transudative effusion, and is usually bilateral. The failing left ventricle leads to increased pulmonary capillary pressure that forces fluid into the interstitium. The failing right ventricle contributes to an effusion by elevating capillary hydrostatic force in the parietal pleura, thus diminishing reabsorption. Signs and symptoms of heart failure are also present, and the diagnosis is usually straightforward, based upon the total clinical picture. Hepatic cirrhosis is associated with a transudative right-sided effusion in 5% to 10% of cases where ascites is present. Pancreatitis and subphrenic abscesses can also produce right-sided effusions. While these typically begin as transudates, they usually convert to exudative effusions. Nephrotic syndrome and hypoalbuminemia produce transudates as a part of a generalized process of increased interstitial edema. Pulmonary embolus is accompanied by effusion in 50% of cases. Typically small and localized to the area of pleuritic chest pain, the embolus may be transudate, resulting from localized interstitial edema or bloody exudates due to infarction.

Exudates result from injury, inflammation, or infiltrative disease processes affecting the pleura. They may also develop due to lymphatic obstruction. Exudative effusions are often due to neoplasms, most commonly bronchogenic, breast metastases, and mesotheliomas. While most acute bacterial pneumonias do not lead to effusions, a parapneumonic effusion is seen in 5% of cases of pneumococcal pneumonia. Viral and mycoplasma pneumonia may also cause effusions. Tuberculosis should always be considered in the workup (also see Chapter 84). Tuberculous pleural fluid usually shows a low glucose and a predominance of lymphocytes. Unfortunately, organisms are rarely found on acid-fast stain, and cultures are positive in only 25% of cases. It is of note that pleural tuberculosis can be diagnosed using adenosine deaminase as a pleural fluid marker.[51]

Other less frequent causes of exudates include collagen vascular disease such as systemic lupus and rheumatoid arthritis and intraabdominal pathology as mentioned above.[52]

Management

Treatment of a pleural effusion should be directed at the underlying disease process. Appropriate antibiotic therapy usually results in resolution of a parapneumonic pleural effusion, although some effusions require chest tube drainage. Pleurodesis is used for management of recurrent malignant effusions and for transudative effusions that do not respond to maximal medical treatment.

Many pleural effusions reflect chronic disease, thereby requiring family education and physician support. Hospice care may be beneficial for the terminal patient and his or her family. Some infectious diseases such as tuberculosis require that the family physician screen and treat family members.

Interstitial Lung Disease

The interstitial lung diseases (ILDs) are a group of heterogeneous disorders that are classified together because of similar clinical, pathologic, physiologic, and roentgenographic findings.[53] In the United States the prevalence of ILD is estimated to be 20 to 40 per 100,000 population.

Interstitial lung diseases have common histologic findings, including derangement of the alveolar structures in the lung with inflammation (alveolitis) and fibrosis of the alveolar walls, air spaces, and pulmonary capillaries. The initiating agent is unknown in most cases but is thought to be precipitated by a toxin or antigen, which leads to alveolitis and fibrosis. These changes result in decreased lung compliance and volumes as well as limitation in transfer of oxygen from air to blood.

More than 150 ILDs have been identified and are classified by etiology. Sixty-five percent of them have an unknown etiology. A smaller group is responsible for the vast majority of clinical cases. Table 86.4 is an abbreviated list of the more commonly seen ILDs.

The predominant clinical symptoms are cough and breathlessness. Typically, patients exhibit insidious exertional breathlessness, dry cough, fatigue, and malaise. Less frequent complaints include chest pain, hemoptysis, fever, anorexia, and weight loss. Detailed history is the most useful diagnostic tool and should include questions about the duration and progression of symptoms, presence of fever or other constitutional symptoms, a comprehensive occupational history, a review of medications, and symptoms of or exposure to HIV. Physical examination may reveal bibasilar dry, Velcro-like rales, clubbing, and cyanosis. The exam may be normal.

Chest roentgenography may reveal a diffuse interstitial, alveolar, or mixed pattern in the lung fields that often progresses to a honeycomb pattern. A normal chest film is present in 10% of patients despite significant clinical disease. Arterial blood gases (ABGs) may be normal or show a mild hypoxemia that worsens with exercise. Hypercarbia is rare, and hypocarbia may be present. Most laboratory studies are

Table 86.4. **Some Common Interstitial Lung Diseases**

Known etiology	Unknown etiology
Inhaled inorganic dusts	Sarcoidosis
Silicosis	Collagen vascular disorders
Asbestosis	Systemic lupus erythematosus
Coal workers'	Rheumatoid arthritis
pneumoconiosis	Idiopathic pulmonary fibrosis
Berylliosis	Eosinophilic pneumonitis
Hypersensitivity	Histiocytosis X
pneumonitis	Pulmonary hemorrhage syndrome
Farmer's lung	
Drug-induced	
Cytotoxic drugs	
Nitrofurantoin	
Amiodarone	
Gold	
Penicillamine	
Radiation pneumonitis	

normal except for an often elevated erythrocyte sedimentation rate. Pulmonary function tests demonstrate a restrictive pattern with reduced vital capacity, carbon monoxide diffusing capacity of the lungs (DL_{co}), and total lung volume as well as a normal or above normal forced expiratory volume in first second/forced vital capacity ratio (FEV_1/FVC).

High-resolution CT may be helpful in evaluating diffuse interstitial lung disease, and attempts have been made to correlate findings with specific diagnoses.[54] More invasive diagnostic measures can be utilized when clinical indications such as atypical or progressive symptoms, extrapulmonary involvement, the absence of a plausible clinical diagnosis, consideration of toxic therapies, and assessment of disease activities exist. Transbronchial biopsy and bronchoalveolar lavage, and thoracoscopic lung biopsy are often utilized in these cases.[55]

The goal of the treatment in ILD is to suppress the alveolitis and prevent further lung damage. Untreated, most ILDs progress to end-stage lung disease with cor pulmonale and death due to respiratory failure. The mainstay of treatment for ILDs of unknown etiology is corticosteroids to decrease the inflammation. Immunosuppressive and cytotoxic agents have also been used. Bronchodilators and oxygen therapy are often useful during the later stages of the disease. With known ILDs, initial treatment begins with identification and removal of the causative agent, followed by corticosteroids if the inflammation fails to resolve.

All patients with ILD are susceptible to bacterial lung infections and must be monitored closely. Smoking cessation and avoidance of bystander smoke should be encouraged.

Pulmonary Sarcoidosis

Sarcoidosis is a multisystem granulomatous disease of unknown etiology that affects all races and age groups, but most commonly affects black women of ages 20 to 40 years. Pulmonary involvement is by far the most frequent clinical problem, and is responsible for the bulk of the morbidity and mortality. Granulomas form in the alveoli, bronchi, and pulmonary vessels, leading to derangement of pulmonary function.[55] The etiology remains unknown.

The most frequent symptoms are dyspnea and cough. Patients may present initially with nonpulmonary symptoms such as fever, arthralgias, malaise, and erythema nodosum. However, patients with sarcoidosis are frequently asymptomatic and are identified on the basis of abnormalities on a chest roentgenogram performed for other reasons. The most common radiographic findings are bilateral hilar lymphadenopathy (stage I) and diffuse infiltrates (stage II). Ninety percent or more of patients will have some abnormality on the chest x-ray. DL_{co} and vital capacity are generally adversely effected.

It is important to distinguish pulmonary sarcoidosis from other granulomatous diseases and other infiltrative lung diseases that may have identical clinical presentation. High-resolution CT scan can reveal a number of abnormalities. Bronchoscopy with transbronchial lung biopsy is the preferred diagnostic modality for documenting the presence of noncaseating granulomas. Serum angiotensin-converting enzyme levels are elevated in 75% of patients and may aid in diag-

nosis.[57] The course of sarcoidosis is variable, with some patients experiencing resolution of all symptoms, and others having slowly progressive disease. Corticosteroids are quite effective at relieving symptoms but have not been shown to modify the overall course of the disease. For this reason, treatment with corticosteroids is usually reserved for patients with worsening symptoms or organ-threatening pulmonary or extrapulmonary disease. The usual treatment of symptomatic sarcoidosis is prednisone 40 to 60 mg/day with slow tapering of the dose over several months. The patient may then be maintained on lower doses as required; a typical dose might be 10 to 20 mg every day or every other day for as long as a year. For patients who cannot tolerate steroids, alternative regimens may include immunosuppressive, cytotoxic, and antimalarial drugs. Unfortunately, as many as two thirds of patients will relapse after termination of treatment.

Atelectasis[58-70]

Atelectasis, or lung collapse, can be subsegmental or lobar, and these types are defined by their clinical findings and x-ray appearance.

Subsegmental (plate-like) atelectasis can be asymptomatic, or present with cough, sputum production, fever, dyspnea, tachypnea, and end-inspiratory crackles. X-rays show linear densities in the lower lung fields. In the postoperative setting other pulmonary complications such as pulmonary embolus, aspiration, pneumonia, and bronchospasm should be considered, especially if associated with pleuritic chest pain, hemoptysis, hypoxia, hypoventilation, or fever. Early postoperative fever does not correlate well with atelectasis.[58,59]

Risk factors include abdominal or chest surgery (23% abdominal, 8–29% laparoscopic cholecystectomy, 54–100% in coronary artery bypass), inadequate preoperative education, chronic lung disease (FEV_1 less than 1.5 L), smoking, obesity, cardiac disease, age over 55, recent respiratory infection, muscle weakness, excessive secretions, inadequate postoperative pain relief (rates decrease with patient controlled[66] and epidural anesthesia[67]), and sickle cell crisis. In the perioperative period, pre- and postoperative deep breathing and coughing and postoperative postural drainage have been shown to reduce atelectasis by more than half.[60,66] Early ambulation and voluntary deep-breathing exercises (sustained maximum inspiration with incentive spirometry—10 deep breaths with a 3- to 5-second inspiratory hold every 1 to 2 waking hours) reduce pulmonary morbidity. At the preoperative physical, the family physician must explain the importance of these maneuvers to the patient and enlist family members in compliance supervision. Smoking cessation counseling at least 2 months prior to elective procedures should be offered.

Lobar atelectasis produces dullness to percussion, with decreased vocal fremitus and breath sounds over the affected lobe. X-ray findings can be difficult to interpret,[69] but may show elevation of the hemidiaphragm, displacement of fissures and hilum, and shift of the mediastinum toward the collapsed lobe with homogeneous consolidation of the affected lobe. Lobar atelectasis in infants most often involves the right upper lobe. Children are more likely to collapse the left lower or right middle lobe. Most of these are postpneumonic and usually clear in a few weeks to 3 months. Other considerations in the differential diagnosis of lobar collapse in children are foreign body aspiration (more commonly causes hyperinflation, 40% have atelectasis), congenital malformations of the bronchial skeleton, external compression from vascular or other structures, and chronic inflammation. Recurrent collapse is common in asthma and cystic fibrosis. In adults malignancies and asthma are common.[70] Atelectasis should be considered when there is worsening oxygenation on mechanical ventilation.

Treatment of lobar collapse requires attention to diagnosis and management of underlying disease. Chest percussion and postural drainage with assistance of respiratory therapists or family members can be beneficial. Bronchoscopy is helpful for foreign body removal, persistent collapse not responsive to conservative measures, definitive diagnosis, and direct laser treatment of obstructive lesions.

Other forms of atelectasis are the patchy atelectasis of infectious pneumonia in toddlers, which usually clears with treatment. Rounded atelectasis is an uncommon peripheral pseudotumor, 87% of which are related to asbestos exposure.[61] Widespread diffuse atelectasis due to inadequate surfactant occurs in the premature infant with respiratory distress syndrome or from the lung injury of vapor or smoke inhalation.

Hyperventilation

Hyperventilation is symptomatic hypocapnea (lowering of arterial Pco_2) most commonly caused by mild to moderate asthma, anxiety, and drug or alcohol abuse. Other etiologies include CNS lesions, metabolic acidosis, hormone replacement therapy, heart failure, pulmonary embolus, acclimatization to high altitude, heat illness, exercise, pregnancy, and chronic pain. Symptoms include dypnea at rest or with minimal exertion, air hunger or inability to take a deep breath, paresthesias (circumoral or acral), chest tightness, and dizziness. Signs may be absent, but prominent upper thoracic movement, lack of costal expansion, decreased diaphragmatic breathing, and sighs and gasps may be noted. Voluntary breath-holding time is often abnormally short (<10 seconds). Symptoms associated with the hyperventilation provocation test do not correlate with hypocapnea.[71] Panic attacks can be provoked by breathing higher concentrations of CO_2.[72] A focused psychiatric interview should be performed to evaluate the possibility of an underlying panic disorder.

Underlying conditions should be treated. With anxiety-related hyperventilation, explanation and reassurance are important. Controlled diaphragmatic breathing and relaxation training[63,64] can be taught to the patient by the family physician and behavioral therapist. Associated anxiety disorders may require behavioral or medical treatment.

Bronchiectasis

Bronchiectasis is the irreversible widening of small airways. Often a significant lung injury such as pneumonia (bacterial, tuberculosis, pertussis) or foreign body aspiration precedes

symptoms by 10 to 20 years. Cystic fibrosis, *Helicobacter pylori* colonization, *Mycobacterium avium-intracellulare*, bronchopulmonary aspergillosis, immotile cilia syndrome, α_1-antitrypsin deficiency, hypogammaglobulinemia, rheumatoid arthritis, Sjögren's syndrome, and Kartagener's syndrome are other predisposing diseases.

Bronchiectasis presents with chronic productive cough (purulent, noncopious, non–foul smelling, and often worse after lying down). Other findings are dyspnea, recurrent fever, pleurisy, hemoptysis, and sputum production with upper respiratory infections. Common signs are crackles, squeaks, rhonchi, and wheezing.[65] Lung sounds may vary with cough and posture or be localized and persistent. Different from other chronic lung disease is its occurrence in nonsmokers, predominance in women (70%), and chest x-ray abnormalities (91%) that show patchy chronic or recurrent infiltrates, or dilated and thickened airways (parallel lines, ring shadows in cross section) sometimes with air-fluid levels. If doubt remains, high-resolution CT is diagnostic.

Management includes pneumococcal and influenza vaccination, and treatment of any underlying disease such as gamma globulin replacement in hypogammaglobulinemia. Chest physiotherapy three to four times daily appears to be beneficial but has not been proven effective.[73] Oral antibiotics are used to treat exacerbations[74] (amoxicillin, tetracycline, or trimethoprim-sulfamethoxazole as the first line to cover *Haemophilus influenzae* and *Streptococcus pneumoniae*) and oral or aerosolized forms are used as prophylaxis. Aerosolized bronchodilators[75] (β_2-agonists and anticholinergics) and antiinflammatory agents are helpful in some patients. Other therapeutic considerations include arterial embolization for life-threatening hemoptysis, and surgery for those who have failed conservative therapy, or have localized disease. Aerosolized recombinant human rh DNase is effective for cystic fibrosis but not idiopathic bronchiectasis.[76]

References

1. Greene KE, Peters JI. Pathophysiology of acute respiratory failure. Clin Chest Med 1994;15(1):1–12.
2. Antonelli M, Conti G, Bufi M. A comparison of noninvasive positive pressure ventilation and conventional mechanical ventilation in patients with acute respiratory failure. N Engl J Med 1998;339(7):429–35.
3. Cook DJ, Kollef MH. Risk factors for an ICU-acquired pneumonia. JAMA 1998;279(20):1605–6.
4. Hirsch DR, Ingenito EP, Goldhaber SZ. Prevalence of deep venous thrombophlebitis among patients in medical intensive care. JAMA 1995;274(4):335–7.
5. Chad DA, Lacomis D. Critically ill patients with newly acquired weakness: the clinicopathological spectrum. Ann Neurol 1994;35(3):257–9.
6. Ware LB, Matthay MA. The acute respiratory distress syndrome. N Engl J Med 2000;342:1334–49.
7. The acute respiratory distress syndrome network. Ventilation with lower tidal volumes as compared with traditional tidal volumes for acute lung injury and the acute respiratory distress syndrome. N Engl J Med 2000;342:1301–8.
8. Marini JJ, Wright LA. Acute respiratory failure. In: Baum GL,

Crapo JD, Celli BR, Karlinsky JB. Textbook of Pulmonary Disease, 6th ed. Philadelphia, Lippincott-Raven, 1997.

9. Baum GL, Crapo JD, Celli BR, Karlinsky JB. Textbook of pulmonary medicine, 6th ed. Philadelphia: Lippincott-Raven, 1998.

10. Seligsohn U, Lubetsky A. Genetic susceptibility to venous thrombosis. N Engl J Med 2001;344(16):1222–31.

11. Horattas MC, Wright DJ, Fenton AH, et al. Changing concepts of deep vein thrombosis of the upper extremity—report of a series and review of the literature. Surgery 1988;104:561–7.

12. Monreal M, Lafox E, Ruiz J, Valls R, Alastrue A. Upper extremity deep vein thrombosis and pulmonary embolism. Chest 1991;99:280–3.

13. Perrier A, Desmarais S, Miron MJ, et al. Non-invasive diagnosis of venous thromboembolism in outpatients. Lancet 1999;353: 190–5.

14. Raimondi P, Bongard O, Moerloose P, et al. D-dimer plasma concentration in various clinical conditions: implications for the use of this test in the diagnostic approach of venous thromboembolism. Thromb Res 1993;69:125–30.

15. Kutinsky I, Blakley S, Roche V. Normal D-dimer levels in patients with pulmonary embolism. Arch Intern Med 1999;159: 1569–72.

16. Nielson HK, Husted SE, Drussell LR, Fasting H, Charles P, Hansen HH. Silent pulmonary embolism in patients with deep vein thrombosis. J Intern Med 1994;235(5):457–61.

17. Bell WG, Simon TL, DeMets DL. The clinical features of submassive and massive pulmonary emboli. Am J Med 1977;62: 355–60.

18. Fulkerson WJ, Coleman RE, Raven VE, Saltman HA. Diagnosis of pulmonary embolism. Arch Intern Med 1976;146:961–7.

19. Overton DT, Bocka JJ. The alveolar-arterial oxygen gradient in patients with documented pulmonary embolism. Arch Intern Med 1988;45:1617–19.

20. PIOPED Investigators. Value of the ventilation/perfusion scan in acute pulmonary embolism: results of the prospective investigation of the pulmonary embolism diagnosis(PIOPED). JAMA 1990;263:2753–9.

21. Kearon C, Ginsberg JS, Hirsh J. The role of venous ultrasonography in the diagnosis of suspected deep vein thrombosis and pulmonary embolism. Ann Intern Med 1998;129:1044–9.

22. Kline JA, Israel EG, Michelson EA, et al. Diagnostic accuracy of a bedside D-dimer assay and alveolar dead-space measurement for rapid exclusion of pulmonary embolism. JAMA 2001;285(6):761–8.

23. Kline JA, Johns KL, Colucciello SA, Israel EG. New diagnostic tests for pulmonary embolism. Ann Emerg Med 2000;35(2):168–80.

24. Ost D, Rozenshtein A, Saffran L, Snider A. The negative predictive value of spiral computed tomography for the diagnosis of pulmonary embolism in patients with nondiagnostic ventilation-perfusion scans. Am J Med 2001;110:6–21.

25. Mayo JR, Remy-Jardin M, Muller NL, et al. Pulmonary embolism: prospective comparison of spiral CT with ventilation-perfusion scintigraphy. Radiology 1997;205(2):447–52.

26. Kim KI, Muller NL, Mayo JR. Clinically suspected pulmonary embolism: utility of spiral CT. Radiology 1999;210:693–7.

27. ACCP Consensus Committee on Pulmonary Embolism. Opinions regarding the diagnosis and management of venous thromboembolic disease. Chest 1998;113:499–504.

28. Remy-Jardin M, Remy J. Spiral CT angiography of the pulmonary circulation. Radiology 1999;212:615–36.

29. Geerts WH, Heit JA, Clagett GP, et al. Prevention of venous thromboembolism. Chest 2001;119(1)(suppl):133–75.

30. Hyers TM, Agnelli G, Hull RD, et al. Antithrombotic therapy for venous thromboembolic disease. Chest 2001;119(1)(suppl): 176–93.

31. Hirsh J, Warkentin TE, Shaughnessy SG, et al. Heparin and low-molecular-weight heparin. Chest 2001;119(1)(suppl):64–94.

32. Rich S, Dantzker DR, Ayres SM, et al. Primary pulmonary hypertension: a national prospective study. Ann Intern Med 1987;107:216–23.

33. Russo-Magno PM, Hill N. New approaches to pulmonary hypertension. Hosp Pract 2001;36(3):29.

34. Gaine S. Pulmonary hypertension. JAMA 2000;284(24):3160–8.

35. Barst RJ, Rubin LJ, McGoon MD, Caldwell EJ, Long WA, Levy PS. Survival in primary pulmonary hypertension with long-term continuous intravenous prostacyclin. Ann Intern Med 1994;121: 409–15.

36. Hoeper MM, Olschewski H, Ghofrani HA, et al. A comparison of the acute hemodynamic effects of inhaled nitric oxide and aerosolized iloprost in primary pulmonary hypertension. J Am Coll Cardiol 2000;35:176–82.

37. Rich S. Executive Summary of the World Symposium on PPH, 1998. http://www.who.int/ncd/cvd/pph.html#Diagnosis, accessed May 2, 2001.

38. Schramel FM, Postmus PE, Vanderschueren RG. Current aspects of spontaneous pneumothorax. Eur Respir J 1997;10(6):1372–9.

39. Joseph J, Sahn SA. Thoracic endometriosis syndrome: new observations from an analysis of 110 cases. Am J Med 1996;100(2): 164–70

40. Metersky ML, Colt HG, Olson LK, et al. AIDS-related spontaneous pneumothorax: risk factors and treatment. Chest 1995; 108(4):946–51.

41. Bense L, Lewander R, Ekund G, et al. Bilateral bronchial anomaly: a pathogenetic factor in spontaneous pneumothorax. Am Rev Respir Dis 1992;146(2):513–61.

42. Orriols R. A new physical sign in pneumothorax. Ann Intern Med 1987;107(2):255.

43. Jenkinson SG. Pneumothorax. Clin Chest Med 1985;6(1):153–61.

44. Weinberger SE. Principles of pulmonary medicine, 2nd ed. Philadelphia: WB Saunders, 1992.

45. Andrivet P, Djedaini K, Teboul JL, et al. Spontaneous pneumothorax: comparison of thoracic drainage vs immediate or delayed needle aspiration. Chest 1995;108(2):335–9.

46. Sadikot RT, Greene T, Meadows K, et al. Recurrence of primary spontaneous pneumothorax. Thorax 1997;52(9):805–9.

47. Jay SJ. Diagnostic procedures for pleural disease. Clin Chest Med 1985;6(1):33–48.

48. Bartter T, Akers SM, Pratter MR. The evaluation of pleural effusion. Chest 1994;106:1209–14.

49. Henschke CI, Davis SD, Remeno PM, Yankelevitz DF. The pathogenesis, radiologic evaluation, and therapy of pleural effusions. Radiol Clin North Am 1989;27:1241–55.

50. Peterman TA, Speicher CE. Evaluating pleural effusions: a two-stage laboratory approach. JAMA 1984;252:1051–3.

51. Feinsilver SH, Houston MC, Sahn SA. Fast-track effusion care. Patient Care 1992;26(3):92–133.

52. Sahn SA. State-of-the-art: the pleura. Am Rev Respir Dis 1988; 138:184–234.

53. Schwarz MI, King TE Jr. Interstitial lung disease, 2nd ed. Philadelphia: Mosby-Year Book, 1993.

54. Wells A. Clinical usefulness of high resolution computed tomography in cryptogenic fibrosing alveolitis. Thorax 1998;53:1080.

55. Thurlbeck WM, Miller RR, Muller NL, et al. Diffuse diseases of the lung. A team approach. Philadelphia: BC Decker, 1991.

56. Newman LS, Rose CD, Maier LA. Sarcoidosis. N Engl J Med 1997;45:234.

57. Studdy PR, Bird R. Serum angiotensin converting enzyme in sarcoidosis—its value in present clinical practice. Ann Clin Biochem 1989;26:13.

58. Massard G, Wihlm JM. Postoperative atelectasis. Chest Surg Clin North Am 1998;8(3):503–28, viii.

59. Dept. of Anesthesia, St. Vincent Medical Center, Toledo, OH. Lack of association between atelectasis and fever. Chest 1995; 107(1):81–4.

60. Thoren L. Postoperative pulmonary complications and their prevention by means of physiotherapy. Acta Chir Scand 1954; 107–93.

61. Hillerdal G. Rounded atelectasis. Clinical experience with 74 patients. Chest 1989;95(4):836–41.

62. Howell JBL. Behavioral breathlessness. Thorax 1990;45:287–92.

63. Garssen B, Rijken H. Clinical aspects and treatment of the hyperventilation syndrome. Behav Psychother 1986;14:46–68.

64. Hegel MT, Abel GG, Etscheidt M, Cohen-Cole S, Wilmer CI. Behavioral treatment of angina like chest pain in patients with hyperventilation syndrome. J Behav Ther Exp Psychiatry 1989; 20(1):31–9.

65. Nicotra MB, Rivera M, Dale AM. Clinical, pathophysiologic, and microbiologic characterization of bronchiectasis in an aging cohort. Chest 1995;108:955–61.

66. Gust R, Pecher S, Gust A, Hoffmann V, Bohrer H, Martin E. Effect of patient-controlled analgesia on pulmonary complications after coronary artery bypass grafting. Crit Care Med 1999; 27(10):2218–23.

67. Ballantyne JC, Carr DB, deFerranti S, et al. The comparative effects of postoperative analgesic therapies on pulmonary outcome: cumulative meta-analyses of randomized, controlled trials. Anesth Analg 1998;86(3):598–612.

68. Chumillas S, Ponce JL, Delgado F, Viciano V, Mateu M. Prevention of postoperative pulmonary complications through respiratory rehabilitation: a controlled clinical study. Arch Phys Med Rehabil 1998;79(1):5–9.

69. Ashizawa K, Hayashi K, Aso N, Minami K. Lobar atelectasis: diagnostic pitfalls on chest radiography. Br J Radiol 2001; 74(877):89–97.

70. Greene R. Acute lobar collapse: adults and infants differ in important ways. Crit Care Med 1999;27(8):1677–9.

71. Hornsveld HK, Garssen B, Dop MJ, van Spiegel PI, de Haes JC. Double-blind placebo-controlled study of the hyperventilation provocation test and the validity of the hyperventilation syndrome. Lancet 1996; July 20;348(9021):154–8.

72. Battaglia M, Bertella S, Ogliari A, Bellodi L, Smeraldi E. Modulation by muscarinic antagonists of the response to carbon dioxide challenge in panic disorder. Arch Gen Psychiatry 2001; 58(2):114–9.

73. Jones A, Rowe BH. Bronchopulmonary hygiene physical therapy in bronchiectasis and chronic obstructive pulmonary disease: a systematic review. Heart Lung 2000;29(2):125–35.

74. Mysliwiec V, Pina JS. Bronchiectasis: the "other" obstructive lung disease. Postgrad Med 1999;106(1):123–6, 128–31.

75. Hassan JA, Saadiah S, Roslan H, Zainudin BM. Bronchodilator response to inhaled beta-2 agonist and anticholinergic drugs in patients with bronchiectasis. Respirology 1999;4(4):423–6.

76. O'Donnell AE, Barker AF, Ilowite JS, Fick RB. Treatment of idiopathic bronchiectasis with aerosolized recombinant human DNase I. rhDNase study group. Chest 1998;113(5):1329–34.

87

Gastritis, Esophagitis, and Peptic Ulcer Disease

Alan M. Adelman and Peter R. Lewis

Dyspepsia/Epigastric Pain

Gastritis, esophagitis, and peptic ulcer disease present commonly with epigastric pain, or dyspepsia. Dyspepsia refers to upper abdominal pain or discomfort and may be associated with fullness, belching, bloating, heartburn, food intolerance, nausea, or vomiting. Dyspepsia is a common problem. Despite discoveries about the cause and treatment of peptic ulcer disease, dyspepsia remains a challenging problem to evaluate and treat.

Epidemiology

Dyspepsia is a common problem, with an annual incidence of 1% to 2% in the general population and a prevalence that may reach 20% to 40%. The four major causes of dyspepsia are nonulcer dyspepsia (NUD), peptic ulcer disease (PUD), gastroesophageal reflux disease (GERD), and gastritis. NUD, PUD, GERD, and gastritis account for more than 90% of all causes of dyspepsia. Other, less common causes of dyspepsia are cholelithiasis, irritable bowel disease, esophageal or gastric cancer, pancreatitis, pancreatic cancer, Zollinger-Ellison syndrome, and abdominal angina (see Chapters 89, 90, and 93). Patients who seek medical attention for dyspepsia are more likely to be concerned about the seriousness of the symptom, worried about cancer or heart disease, and experiencing more stress than individuals who do not seek medical attention for dyspepsia.

Presentation

No single symptom is helpful for distinguishing between the causes of dyspepsia, but some patient characteristics are predictive of serious disease. For example, as single symptoms, nocturnal pain, relief of pain by antacids, worsening of pain by food, anorexia, nausea, and food intolerance are not helpful for distinguishing the causes of dyspepsia. Patients older than 45 years or with alarm symptoms (i.e., weight loss, dysphagia, persistent vomiting, gastrointestinal bleeding, hematemesis, melena) are more likely to have serious underlying disorder. With the possible exceptions of peptic ulcer disease and duodenitis, there was no association of clinical value between endoscopic findings and dyspeptic symptoms. It is important to inquire about the use of nonsteroidal antiinflammatory drugs (NSAIDs), as their use is a frequent cause of peptic ulcer disease. To summarize, symptoms are not useful for differentiating the causes of dyspepsia.

General Approach

Individuals with evidence of complications of PUD (e.g., gastric outlet obstruction or bleeding) or systemic disease (e.g., weight loss, anemia) should be promptly evaluated. Because age is the strongest predictor of finding "organic" disease on endoscopy, individuals over the age of 45 years should be thoroughly evaluated. For the remaining patients there are three commonly used strategies for the evaluation and management of dyspeptic symptoms: (1) empiric therapy; (2) evaluation, usually with endoscopy, for a specific cause of the dyspeptic symptoms; and (3) test for *Helicobacter pylori* and treat if positive (test and treat).

Empiric treatment for dyspepsia consists of standard antiacid therapy (Table 87.1). Histamine-2 receptor antagonists (H_2RA) are available over-the-counter. If an H_2RA or proton pump inhibitor (PPI) fails to relieve symptoms, further workup should be undertaken. A recent review showed that PPIs, while more costly, are more effective than other antiacid agents in relieving symptoms.[1]

The second approach to the patient with dyspepsia is thorough evaluation for a specific cause of the dyspeptic symptoms. When available, upper endoscopy is the preferred procedure. Although an upper gastrointestinal (UGI) series is less

Table 87.1. **Usual Daily Dosage of Antiacid Medications**

Generic (brand) name	Usual daily dosage	Average wholesale price (AWP)[a] ($)[b]
Antacids (Maalox, Mylanta)	15–30 mL 0.5 hour and 2 hours after meals and at bedtime	30–60
Histamine-2 receptor antagonists		
Cimetidine (Tagamet)	800 mg hs	62
Famotidine (Pepcid)	20 mg bid	104
Nizatidine (Axid)	150 mg bid	94
Ranitidine (Zantac)	150 mg bid	89
Sucralfate	1 qid	88
Proton pump inhibitors		
Omeprazole (Prilosec)	20–40 mg qd	125–178
Lansoprazole (Prevacid)	15–30 mg qd	114–116
Rabeprazole (Aciphex)	20 mg qd	114
Esomeprazole (Nexium)	20–40 mg qd	120
Pantoprazole (Protonix)	40 mg qd	90

[a]Source for AWP: Red Book. Montvale, NJ: Medical Economics Company, Inc. Accessed Internet version at *http://physician.pdr.net/physician/static.htm?path=controlled/searchredbook.htm* on July 11, 2001. Where multiple generic equivalents are available, the least expensive AWP is listed.

[b]Amount rounded to the nearest dollar.

expensive and may be more readily available, it has a false-negative rate that exceeds 18% in some studies and a false-positive rate of 13% to 35%. In addition, the UGI series is poor for diagnosing GERD and gastritis, two of the most common causes of dyspepsia. A negative UGI does not rule out disease, and if indicated, further evaluation with upper endoscopy should be pursued. Although more expensive, upper endoscopy has lower false-positive and false-negative rates, biopsies can be undertaken, and testing for *H. pylori* can be performed.

The third common approach to the evaluation of patients with dyspepsia is to test for *H. pylori* and treat if positive. (For further information on the evaluation and treatment of *H. pylori*, on Peptic Ulcer Disease, below.) This approach is favored by recently published American and Canadian guidelines.[2,3] Several decision analyses also support this approach.[4,5] And finally, several reviews[6,7] and clinical trials also favor the test-and-treat approach for the patient with dyspepsia.[8–11]

The eradication of *H. pylori* in patients with NUD (with negative endoscopy) is controversial. A meta-analysis by Moayyedi et al[12] showed a small but statistically significant benefit to eradication, while a more recent meta-analysis by Laine et al[13] showed no benefit.

Gastroesophageal Reflux Disease

Gastroesophageal reflux disease (GERD) is a common problem. About 10% of the general population report heartburn daily and 15% to 40% experience it monthly. Lifetime estimates of GERD symptoms in the general population may be greater than 50%.[14] The incidence of GERD increases during pregnancy and with obesity and tobacco use. Several factors may lead to GERD including hiatal hernia, incompetence of the lower esophageal sphincter (LES), inappropriate LES relaxation, impaired esophageal peristalsis and acid clearance, impaired gastric emptying, and repeated vomiting. Exposure to excessive acid or pepsin can lead to damage of the esophageal mucosa, resulting in inflammation and ultimately scarring and stricture formation. Medications (e.g., theophylline, calcium channel blockers, and β-adrenergic agonists), foods (e.g., caffeine and chocolate), and alcohol may lower LES pressure and lead to GERD. Medications such as alendronate (Fosamax) may cause local irritation of the esophagus. GERD may occur as an isolated entity or as part of a systemic disorder such as scleroderma. GERD is a risk factor for esophageal adenocarcinoma, one of the fastest growing cancers in the United States.

Presentation

The most reliable symptom of GERD is heartburn, a retrosternal burning sensation that may radiate from the epigastrium to the throat. Patients may also complain of pyrosis or water brash, the regurgitation of bitter-tasting material into the mouth. Belching is frequently described. Symptoms may be worse after eating, bending over, or lying down. Nocturnal symptoms may awaken the patient. GERD can cause respiratory problems including laryngitis, chronic cough, aspiration pneumonia, and wheezing. Atypical chest pain can also be caused by GERD (see Chapter 76). Finally, patients may complain of hoarseness, a globus sensation, odynophagia (pain with swallowing), or dysphagia.

Diagnosis

A young patient with no evidence of systemic illness requires no further workup and can be treated empirically. Older patients, particularly those with the complaint of odynophagia or dysphagia, require evaluation to rule out tumor or stricture. Upper endoscopy is the evaluation of choice. Ambulatory 24-hour pH monitoring is the most sensitive test for demonstrating reflux if endoscopy is negative. A barium swallow study or esophageal manometry may be necessary if a motility disorder is suspected, as endoscopy is often normal in patients with this problem.

Management

GERD is treated by both nonpharmacologic and pharmacologic means.[15,16] It is important to note that whereas patients with mild disease may respond to nonpharmacologic treatment, patients with moderate to severe symptoms or recurrent disease must continue to observe lifestyle changes while drug therapy is added or intensified.

All patients with GERD should be advised to reduce weight (if over their ideal body weight), avoid large meals (especially several hours before going to sleep), refrain from lying down after meals, and refrain from wearing tight clothing around the waist. Patients who experience nocturnal symptoms often find relief by putting the head of the bed on blocks 4 to 6 inches in height. Sleeping on more pillows or on a wedge may be less effective because of nocturnal movements. Because nicotine lowers LES pressure, smoking cessation is recommended. Medications and foods that can lower LES pressure as well as alcohol should be avoided.

Patients who do not respond to lifestyle and medication changes alone are treated with pharmacologic agents. The pharmacologic treatment of GERD can be approached as a stepwise process. For mild, intermittent symptoms, antacids or over-the-counter H2RAs can be used. For persistent or severe symptoms, prescription-strength H2RAs or PPIs are the mainstay of treatment, although other agents are available. H2RAs can be tried first and, if ineffective, PPIs can be substituted. Once a patient's symptoms are controlled, a trial of decreasing the dose of medication (e.g., from twice daily to once daily) or switching from the more expensive PPIs to less expensive H2RAs may be warranted.

H2RAs suppress acid secretion by competing with histamine, thereby blocking its effect on parietal cells of the stomach. H2RAs are effective, but both daytime and nocturnal acid production must be inhibited; therefore, twice-daily dosing is recommended rather than just nocturnal dosing. If symptoms are controlled for 6 to 8 weeks, just nocturnal dosing to control symptoms can be tried. For severe or refractory GERD, doubling the standard dose of H2RAs may be effective. Combining H2RAs with a prokinetic agent may be better than using either agent alone.

PPIs irreversibly block the final step in parietal cell acid secretion and are the most potent antisecretory agents available. In more severe GERD, PPIs are more efficacious than H2RAs for symptom control including extraesophageal manifestations, esophageal healing, and reducing the risk of stricture formation and recurrence.[17] PPIs are less effective when taken on an as-needed basis. They are effective when dosed daily before breakfast, although some patients may require twice daily (before meals) dosing to achieve symptom control and/or esophageal healing. PPIs are the treatment of choice for erosive esophagitis. Side effects (chiefly headache and diarrhea) resulting in medication discontinuation are rare. As is true for H2RAs, different PPIs, while having different pharmacokinetic properties at equivalent doses, are roughly comparable in terms of clinical efficacy. Patients unresponsive to one H2RA or PPI may be responsive to another agent within the same medication class. Rarely, patients unresponsive to PPIs may respond to H2RAs.

Prokinetic agents can increase esophageal contraction amplitude, increase LES pressure, and accelerate gastric emptying, three of the most significant motility problems in the pathogenesis of GERD. Metoclopramide, the only prokinetic drug available, is a dopamine antagonist that can cause extrapyramidal symptoms and, rarely, tardive dyskinesia. It is considered a second-line agent for GERD.

Sucralfate has also been shown to be efficacious for mild to moderate GERD. Sucralfate is a sulfated disaccharide that appears to protect against acid by local effects on the mucosa.

For the minority of patients with GERD who require maintenance medication, periodic examination, coupled with efforts to try to reduce medication, is warranted. A concern in patients with chronic GERD is Barrett's esophagus. Barrett's esophagus is metaplasia of the cells of the distal esophagus and is considered a precancerous lesion. The risk of development of adenocarcinoma of the esophagus may be as high as 2%. Unfortunately, neither aggressive medical therapy nor surgical therapy for GERD has been shown to alter the progression between Barrett's esophagus and esophageal adenocarcinoma.[18] There is uncertainty as to the efficacy and optimal frequency of endoscopic surveillance of patients with Barrett's esophagus. When dysplasia, the stage between metaplasia and adenocarcinoma, is identified, the recommended frequency of surveillance with esophagogastroduodenoscopy (EGD) and repeat biopsy varies, depending on the severity of dysplasia.

Individuals who are intolerant or unresponsive to optimal medical therapy are suitable operative candidates. Other indications for surgery are young age, nonadherence to medical therapy, or complications of GERD, such as recurrent esophageal strictures or bleeding. Surgical approaches to GERD attempt to create a more functional LES, limiting the potential for pathologic reflux of gastric contents. Although a VA Cooperative Trial comparing medical to surgical therapy reported improved results for the surgical cohort, a 10-year follow-up to this study showed no difference between the groups in terms of patient satisfaction, symptoms, and complications, including cancer.[19] Of note, 62% of the surgery group reported regular use of antireflux medications. Laparoscopic procedures provide effective treatment without the morbidity of open procedures. A case series of patients treated with laparoscopic surgery reported rare postoperative medication use.[20]

Peptic Ulcer Disease

Most peptic ulcers are caused by either *H. pylori* or NSAIDs. Although infection with *H. pylori* appears to be common, most individuals with *H. pylori* do not develop ulcers. Peptic ulcers may involve any portion of the UGI tract, but ulcers are most often found in the stomach and duodenum. Duodenal ulcers are approximately three times as common as gastric ulcers. About 10% of the population suffers from duodenal ulcers at some time in their lives. In the past, PUD was marked by periods of healing and recurrence. Successful treatment of ulcers associated with *H. pylori* infection greatly diminishes recurrences.

Presentation

Epigastric pain is the most common presenting problem of both duodenal and gastric ulcer disease. The pain may be described as gnawing, burning, boring, aching, or severe hunger pains. Patients with duodenal ulcers typically experience pain within a few hours after meals and complete or partial relief of pain with ingestion of food or antacids. Pain in gastric ulcer patients is more variable; pain may worsen with eating. Both duodenal and gastric ulcers may occur and recur in the absence of pain. Pain is variable among patients with both kinds of ulceration and correlates poorly with ulcer healing. Physical examination usually reveals epigastric tenderness midway between the xiphoid and umbilicus, but maximal tenderness is sometimes to the right of midline. Other findings may include a succussion splash due to a mixture of air and fluid in the stomach when gastric outlet obstruction results from an ulcer in the duodenum or pyloric channel or abdominal rigidity is apparent in the presence of perforation.

Diagnosis

There are two ways that PUD may be diagnosed. First, an ulcer may be diagnosed by either radiographic studies or endoscopy. Although duodenal and gastric ulcers can be diagnosed by UGI studies, when available, upper endoscopy is the investigation of first choice. Gastric ulcers more than 3 cm in diameter or without radiating mucosal folds are more likely to be malignant. In addition to the indications listed earlier in the chapter, endoscopy should be considered in patients with negative radiographic studies, those with a history of deformed duodenal bulbs (thus making radiographic examination difficult), and in patients with GI bleeding. If an ulcer is diagnosed endoscopically, a rapid *Campylobacter*-like organism urease test (CLOtest) is a quick, sensitive test for determining the presence of *H. pylori*. False positives are uncommon, and false negatives occur in approximately 10% of cases. The presence of *H. pylori* can also be determined histologically and by culture. Culture with drug sensitivities is important when drug resistance is suspected.

In the second approach, test and treat, a patient is tested for *H. pylori* and if positive, antibiotic therapy can be initiated without documenting an ulcer. There are several ways that *H. pylori* infection can be documented. Both qualitative (sensitivity 71%, specificity 88%) and quantitative [enzyme-linked immunosorbent assay (ELISA): sensitivity 85%, specificity 79%] serology tests are available. The stool antigen test is more accurate than serology tests (sensitivity 92%, specificity 88%). Urea breath test, using a carbon isotope (^{13}C or ^{14}C), is the most accurate noninvasive test (sensitivity 95%, specificity 96%).[21] The use of proton pump inhibitors, bismuth preparations, and antibiotics can suppress *H. pylori* and lead to false-negative results.

Most patients, especially those who are asymptomatic posttreatment, do not require documentation of eradication of *H. pylori*. If one wishes to test for cure, a urea breath test (4 weeks after therapy) or stool antigen test can be performed. A falling ELISA titer (1, 3, and 6 months after therapy) may also be used to document eradication. If a repeat endoscopy is performed, a CLOtest may be used.

Treatment

All patients with PUD who smoke should be advised to stop. Smoking can delay the rate of healing of ulcers. If PUD is associated with the use of an NSAID, the NSAID should be discontinued and traditional antiulcer therapy begun with either an H₂RA or PPI. If the NSAID cannot be stopped, then a PPI or misoprostol should be started. For patients who test positive for *H. pylori*, antibiotic treatment should be given. A number of drug regimens have been shown to be effective (Table 87.2).[22] If not part of the antibiotic regimen, a H₂RA or PPI should be added to hasten pain relief. Patients with *H. pylori*–negative ulcers are treated with traditional antiacid agents alone for 4 to 6 weeks. There is no evidence that the use of two or more antiacid agents (e.g., sucralfate and an H₂RA) offers any advantage over the use of a single antiacid agent.

There are a number of problems with the current antibiotic regimens. First, compliance may be a problem because of cost, duration of therapy, and side effects. GI side effects can occur with metronidazole, amoxicillin, and clarithromycin. There is a trade-off between better compliance with the shorter duration of therapy and better eradication rate with longer duration of therapy. A second problem is the emergence of antibiotic resistance against both metronidazole and clarithromycin, which favors the use of triple-drug regimens.

All H₂RAs effectively heal ulcers in equipotent doses (Table 87.1). About 75% to 90% of ulcers are healed after 4 to 6 weeks of therapy. The PPIs heal ulcers more quickly than H₂RAs, but healing rates at 6 weeks are not significantly improved over those with H₂RAs. PPIs should be considered for patients with severe symptoms, gastric ulcers, a potential for complications, or with refractory disease. Healing rates with sucralfate (Carafate) are comparable to those with H₂RAs. There are no significant side effects.

Table 87.2. **Treatment for Eradication of *Helicobacter pylori*-Associated Peptic Ulcer Disease**[a22]

Therapies with proton pump inhibitor (PPI)[b]
  PPI + metronidazole 250 mg qid + clarithromycin 500 mg bid–tid
  PPI + amoxicillin 1000 mg bid or 500 mg qid + clarithromycin 500 mg bid–tid[c]
  PPI + bismuth subsalicylate 2 tablets qid + metronidazole 250 mg qid + tetracycline hydrochloride 500 mg qid
Other
  Bismuth subsalicylate 2 tablets qid + metronidazole 250 mg qid + tetracycline hydrochloride 500 mg qid[d]

[a]All regimens are given for 14 days.
[b]Continue PPI for total of 28 days
[c]Lansoprazole/clarithromycin/amoxicillin available as Prevpac.
[d]Available as Helidac; in addition, give H₂-receptor blocker for 28 days.

Prostaglandins protect the gastric mucosa, possibly by enhancing mucosal blood flow. Misoprostol, a prostaglandin E_1 analogue, can be used to prevent ulcers due to NSAIDs. Misoprostol also heals ulcers at approximately the same rate as H_2RAs, but severe diarrhea may limit patient compliance. Stimulation of uterine contractions and induction of abortions are the most serious side effects of misoprostol.

Dietary therapy is now limited to the elimination of foods that exacerbate symptoms and the avoidance of alcohol and coffee (with or without caffeine) because alcohol and coffee increase gastric acid secretion.

Refractory Ulcers and Maintenance Therapy

Most duodenal ulcers heal within 4 to 8 weeks of the start of therapy. After 12 weeks of therapy, 90% to 95% of ulcers are healed. Higher doses of H_2RAs (e.g., ranitidine 600–1200 mg/day) or PPIs may be used to heal refractory ulcers. Gastric ulcers heal more slowly than duodenal ulcers, but 90% are healed after 12 weeks of therapy. PPIs are the drug of choice for gastric ulcers.

Individuals with persistent or recurrent symptoms after therapy should be reevaluated. Compliance with previous recommendations and a search for NSAID use should be reviewed. Endoscopy should be performed to document healing. Drug resistance may be a factor in persistence of ulcers secondary to *H. pylori*. Gastric cancer should be excluded by biopsy if a gastric ulcer remains unhealed (see Gastric Cancer, below). Zollinger-Ellison syndrome is also considered in the case of refractory ulcers.

In patients successfully treated for *H. pylori* or who have discontinued the use of NSAIDs, maintenance treatment with H_2RAs or PPIs should not be needed. Patients with ulcers in the absence of *H. pylori*, complicated PUD (e.g., bleeding or perforation), a history of refractory ulceration, age greater than 60 years, or a deformed duodenum are candidates for at least 1 year of maintenance therapy with H_2RAs or PPIs.

Gastritis/Gastropathy

Gastritis represents a group of entities characterized by histologic evidence of inflammation. Gastropathy is characterized by the absence of histologic evidence of inflammation of the gastric mucosa. Both gastritis and gastropathy may be either acute or chronic. It may be difficult to distinguish the two entities by clinical, radiographic, and visual endoscopic examinations. Gastritis and gastropathy may occur simultaneously and/or overlap with conditions such as GERD or PUD, or may be a manifestation of less common conditions such as Crohn's or celiac disease or sarcoidosis.

Acute gastritis may be due to infections (mainly *H. pylori*; less commonly viral, fungal, mycobacterial, or parasitic causes), autoimmune conditions (e.g., pernicious anemia), and chronic acid suppression. Histologic variants of uncertain cause include lymphocytic and eosinophilic gastritis. Gastropathy is commonly due to medications [e.g., NSAIDs including aspirin and cyclooxygenase-2 (COX-2) inhibitors, bisphosphonates, potassium, and iron], alcohol, refluxed bile,

ischemia ("stress," as is seen in patients with shock, sepsis, trauma, or burns), or vascular congestion (as in portal hypertension or congestive heart failure).

Chronic gastritis may be preceded by episodes of symptomatic acute gastritis (e.g. *H. pylori*) or present without prior warning, with dyspepsia and constitutional symptoms. *H. pylori* is the most common cause of chronic gastritis, this effect may be accentuated in patients receiving chronic PPI therapy. Pernicious anemia may be associated with chronic gastritis.

Taken together these conditions range in presentation from asymptomatic to life threatening. Of particular interest to the clinician are acute and chronic erosive changes that may be complicated by symptomatic anemia or frank hemorrhage (presenting with melena or hematemesis—see Upper Gastrointestinal Bleed, below) and chronic atrophic changes that may progress to gastric cancer. Treatment consists of managing the underlying disease and removing gastric irritants.

Upper Gastrointestinal Bleed

Upper gastrointestinal bleed is defined as GI blood loss above the ligament of Treitz. If the bleeding is clinically evident, it may present in one of three ways. Hematemesis may be bright red or coffee-grounds–appearing material and usually means active bleeding. Melena signifies that the blood has transited through the GI tract, causing digestion of blood. Melena may also be caused by lower GI bleeding. And finally, although uncommon, an UGI bleed may present as hematochezia if bleeding is brisk. If subacute or chronic, the UGI bleed may be discovered during the workup of iron-deficiency anemia or hemoccult positive stools.

Causes

The four most common causes of UGI bleeding are peptic ulceration, gastritis/gastropathy, esophageal varices, and esophagogastric mucosal tear (Mallory-Weiss syndrome). The causes of gastritis/gastropathy are described above. Bleeding due to varices is usually abrupt and massive. Varices may be due to alcohol cirrhosis or any other cause of portal hypertension such as portal vein thrombosis. Mallory-Weiss syndrome classically presents with retching followed by hematemesis. Other causes of UGI bleeding include gastric carcinoma, lymphoma, polyps, and diverticula.

Diagnosis and Management

The diagnosis and management of the patient with UGI bleeding depends on the site and extent of bleeding. Vomitus and stool should be tested to confirm the presence of blood. Initial management for all patients includes assessment of vital signs including orthostatic changes. Patients with significant blood loss should be typed and matched for blood replacement and large-bore intravenous lines placed for fluid and blood replacement.

A nasogastric tube should be placed and the aspirate tested for blood. Absence of blood may mean that the bleeding has ceased. If the aspirate consists of red blood or coffee-grounds material, the stomach is lavaged with saline.

Once the patient is hemodynamically stable, upper endoscopy can be performed. Rapid upper endoscopy upon presentation of patients in stable condition may hasten diagnosis and limit hospitalization.[23] Endoscopy may not reveal an obvious source of bleeding in cases of resolved blood loss due to Mallory-Weiss tears or vascular malformations, or distal duodenal lesions. Massive hemorrhage from varices can make endoscopy useless. The other more common causes will be readily apparent. If the patient continues to bleed and a source has not been identified, a tagged red blood cell scan or angiography may be used to identify the source of bleeding. Upper endoscopy can be therapeutic as well as diagnostic. Sclerotherapy or ligation of esophageal varices can be performed through the endoscope. A variety of endoscopic treatments are available for bleeding peptic ulcers including thermal coagulation, injection therapy with alcohol or epinephrine, and endoclips.

When bleeding is refractory to medical and endoscopically administered therapies, interventional radiological (e.g., embolization or transjugular intrahepatic portasystemic shunt, TIPS) or surgical (resection or shunting) interventions should be considered.

There are two additional therapies for bleeding varices. Peripherally administered somatostatin or balloon tamponade are effective alternative treatments for bleeding varices.

Prevention of GI bleeding is more effective than treatment. Treatment of *H. pylori*–positive PUD or maintenance therapy for *H. pylori*–negative PUD may decrease subsequent bleeding episodes. Nonselective beta-blockers (propranolol or nadolol) can prevent and reduce the mortality rate associated with GI bleeding in patients with cirrhosis and varices.

Gastric Cancer

While the incidence of distal gastric cancer has declined significantly in the United States since the 1930s, there has been an increase of proximal stomach cancers. African-American males have a higher incidence of gastric adenocarcinoma. Individuals moving from Japan to the United States lower their risk of gastric cancer, suggesting that dietary and environmental factors play roles in the pathogenesis of this disorder. Additional risk factors include gastric polyps, Barrett's esophagus, subtotal gastric resection, and chronic gastritis. Ninety percent of the gastric cancers are adenocarcinomas; lymphomas (the stomach is the most common extranodal site of lymphoma) and leiomyosarcomas comprise the remainder.

Early gastric cancers are usually asymptomatic. As the cancer grows, patients may complain of anorexia or early satiety, vague discomfort, or steady pain. Weight loss, nausea and vomiting, and dysphagia (more common with proximal cancers) may also be present. Rarely, paraneoplastic manifestations occur. The physical examination is usually normal in patients with early disease, but a palpable abdominal mass or supraclavicular nodes, enlarged liver, or ascites may be present with advanced or metastatic disease. Patients with gastric cancer may present with GI bleeding, overt or otherwise occult, although this represents a minority of presentations.

Upper gastrointestinal (UGI) x-ray studies can usually detect gastric cancer. In younger patients (<45 years) without alarming symptoms, UGI is adequate to diagnose a benign gastric ulcer. These patients should be followed radiographically to ensure healing of the ulcer. Benign gastric ulcers should heal within 6 to 12 weeks. If an ulcer is suspicious in appearance, alarming symptoms are present, or the patient is >45 years of age, EGD with biopsy is the preferred procedure. If the initial biopsies are benign, then endoscopy should be repeated at 12 weeks to ensure that the ulcer has healed completely.

While surgical treatment is the only definite chance for a cure, unfortunately only one third of patients present early enough to achieve a surgical cure. Despite advanced surgical treatments 5-year survival rates remain low. Postoperative (adjuvant) chemotherapy with or without radiation for patients undergoing tumor resection may be recommended.

References

1. Delaney BC, Innes MA, Deeks J, et al. Initial management strategies for dyspepsia. The Cochrane Library, Oxford, England: Updated February 23, 2000.
2. American Gastroenterological Association. American Gastroenterological Assoication medical position statement: evaluation of dyspepsia. Gastroenterology 1998;114:579–81.
3. Hunt RH, Fallone CA, Thomson ABR, Canadian *Helicobacter Pylori* Study Group. Canadian *Helicobacter Pylori* Consensus Conference update: infection in adults. Can J Gastroenterol 1999;13:213–17.
4. Fendrick AM, Chernow ME, Hirth RA, Bloom BS. Alternative management strategies for patients with suspected peptic ulcer disease. Ann Intern Med 1995;123:260–8.
5. Ebell MH, Warbasse L, Brenner C. Evaluation of the dyspeptic patient: a cost-utility study. J Fam Pract 1997;44:545–55.
6. Smucny J. Evaluation of the patient with dyspepsia. J Fam Pract 2001;50:538–43.
7. Ofman JJ, Rabeneck L. The effectiveness of endoscopy in the management of dyspepsia: a qualitative systematic review. Am J Med 1999;106:335–46.
8. Lassen AT, Pedersen FM, Bytzer P, de Muckadell OBS. *Helicobacter pylori* test-and-eradicate versus prompt endoscopy for management of dyspeptic patients: a randomized trial. Lancet 2000;356:455–60.
9. Jones R, Tait C, Sladen G, Weston-Backer J. A trial of test-and-treat strategy for *Helicobacter pylori*-positive dyspeptic patients in general practice. Int J Clin Pract 1999;53:413–16.
10. Heaney A, Collins JSA, Watson RGP, McFarland RJ, Bamford KB, Tham TCK. A prospective randomised trial of a "test ant treat" policy versus endoscopy based management in young *Helicobacter pylori* positive patients with ulcer-like dyspepsia, referred to a hospital clinic. Gut 1999;45:186–90.
11. Delaney BC, Wilson S, Roalfe A, et al. Randomised controlled trial of *Helicobacter pylori* testing and endoscopy for dyspepsia in primary care. BMJ 2001;322:1–5.
12. Moayyedi P, Soo S, Deeks J, et al, on behalf of the Dyspepsia Review Group. Systematic review and economic evaluation of *Helicobacter pylori* eradication treatment for non-ulcer dyspepsia. BMJ 2000;321:659–64.
13. Laine L, Schoenfeld P, Fennerty MB. Therapy for *Helicobacter pylori* in patients with nonulcer dyspepsia: a meta-analysis of randomized, controlled trials. Ann Intern Med 2001;134:361–9.

14. Locke GR 3rd, Talley NJ, Fett SL, Zinsmeister AR, Melton LJ 3rd. Prevalence and clinical spectrum of gastroesophageal reflux; a population-based study in Olinsted County, Minnesota. Gastroenterology 1997;112:1448–56.
15. DeVault KR, Castell DO. Updated guidelines for the diagnosis and treatment of gastroesophageal reflux disease. The Practice Parameters Committee of the American College of Gastroenterology. Am J Gastroenterol 1999;94:1434–42.
16. Scott M, Gelhot AR. Gastroesophageal reflux disease: diagnosis and management. Am Fam Physician 1999;59:1161–9.
17. Chiba N, DeGara CJ, Wilkinson JM, Hunt RH. Speed of healing and symptoms of relief in grade II to IV gastroesophageal reflux disease: a meta-analysis. Gastroenterology 1997;112:1798–810.
18. Kahrilas PJ. Management of GERD: medical versus surgical. Semin Gastrointest Dis 2001;12:3–15.
19. Spechler SJ, Lee E. Ahnen D, et al. Long-term outcome of medical and surgical therapies for gastroesophageal reflux disease: follow-up of a randomized controlled trial. JAMA 2001;285:2331–8.
20. Peters JH, DeMeester TR, Crookes P, et al. The treatment of gastroesophageal reflux disease with laparoscopic Nissen fundoplication: prospective evaluation of 100 patients with "typical" symptoms. Ann Surg 1998;228:40–50.
21. Vairea D, Vakil N. Blood, urine, stool, breath, money, and Helicobacter pylori. Gut 2001;48:287–9.
22. Howden CW, Hunt RH. Guidelines for the management of Helicobacter pylori infection. Am J Gastroenterol 1998;93:2330–8.
23. Lee JG, Turnipseed S, Romano PS, et al. Endoscopy-based triage significantly reduces hospitalization rates and costs of treating upper GI bleeding: a randomized controlled trial. Gastrointest Endosc 1999;50:755–61.

88
Diseases of the Large and Small Bowel

David M. James

Infectious Diarrhea Syndromes

After upper respiratory tract infections, acute gastroenteritis is the second most common illness in the United States. Most cases are brief and self-limited, however, the attack rate is estimated at 1.5 to 1.9 attacks per person per year, and is ultimately responsible for 10,000 deaths per year nationally.[1] Viral organisms are the most common cause of infectious diarrhea; however, bacterial pathogens including *Shigella,* nontyphoidal *Salmonella, Escherichia coli, Campylobacter jejuni,* and *Yersinia* account for the most severe episodes. Protozoal gastroenteritis caused by *Entamoeba histolytica* and *Giardia lamblia* is common in travelers, and may produce intermittent symptoms (also see Chapter 9).

Socioeconomic conditions and living conditions play a distinct role in the attack rate of enteric infection. Contaminated water sources, undercooked foods (especially meats), institutionalization, and inadequate sanitation are major risk factors for enteric infection.

Clinical Approach to the Patient with Acute Diarrhea

A complete history and physical examination should be conducted to address the following issues:

1. Does the diarrhea originate in the large or small intestine? Small-bowel pathology is usually associated with frequent, large-volume stools described as watery and related to eating. Large-bowel diarrhea is usually more frequent, with smaller stool volumes (1–2 L/day) and may be associated with tenesmus and bloody stools.
2. Are there other contacts with similar illness? Viral diarrhea commonly presents in clusters of affected patients; this is especially true of infections contacted in day-care centers, schools, or health care institutions.
3. Has there been recent travel? Possible causes could include enterotoxigenic *E. coli,* or the protozoa *E. histolytica* and *G. lamblia.*
4. Has there been consumption of undercooked poultry or hamburger meat? This might suggest *Salmonella* or enterohemorrhagic *E. coli.*
5. Has there been any antibiotic use within the previous 6 weeks, suggesting a postantibiotic colitis with *Clostridium difficile* overgrowth?
6. Are there any other predisposing medical conditions for diarrhea, especially diabetes, HIV disease, or bowel surgery?

If the illness is prolonged, consider the following diagnostic investigations:

1. Stool examination for fecal leukocytes (bacterial infection), culture and sensitivity, ova and parasites, and *C. difficile* toxin.
2. In cases that are culture-negative, a nonprepped flexible sigmoidoscopy or colonoscopy may be indicated for seriously ill patients.
3. If no colon pathology is identified, consider an esophagogastroduodenoscopy (EGD) with small-bowel biopsies.

Viral Infections

Viral enteric infection is responsible for the majority of gastrointestinal complaints seen in the office or emergency department. Patients may present with one or more symptoms of diarrhea, nausea, fever, abdominal pain or cramping, headache, and general malaise. Causative viral agents include echoviruses, reoviruses (especially Norwalk virus), and adenoviruses. In the majority of patients, however, the specific viral agent remains unidentified.[2]

Physical examination of the patient may reveal hyperactive bowel sounds, and mild lower abdominal discomfort with palpation. If history and physical examination are insufficient to make a diagnosis, obtain a complete blood count (CBC) and a stool sample. The CBC should reveal a normal white blood cell count with a slight lymphocytosis. Stool examination reveals an excess of water without pus or blood.

Treatment includes fluid replacement, either orally or parenterally. Outpatient therapy should restrict solid food and dairy products for 24 to 48 hours, while encouraging oral rehydration with an appropriate electrolyte/glucose solution [Pedialyte, Gastrolyte, or other World Health Organization (WHO)-approved oral rehydration solution]. Stool cultures may be obtained to exclude other etiologies. In most patients, the diarrhea typically subsides by 3 to 5 days. The diet may be advanced as tolerated. If vomiting is severe, hospital admission for parenteral fluid rehydration is warranted, especially in the very young or elderly patient.

Bacterial Infections

Bacterial enteric infections are associated with the gastrointestinal symptoms of diarrhea, vomiting, and abdominal discomfort. The symptoms result as a direct effect of bacterial toxin on the intestinal wall stimulating secretion of water into the intestinal lumen, or by the actual invasion of bacteria into the intestinal wall.

Escherichia coli

This bacterium may cause diarrhea by either of the previously mentioned mechanisms. At least five forms of gastroenteritis may result, including enteropathogenic, enterotoxigenic, enteroinvasive, enterohemorrhagic, and enteroadherent types. Diagnosis is often difficult, because E. coli is found commonly in the stool as normal flora. The enterotoxigenic type of gastritis is associated with travel (traveler's diarrhea), while enterohemorrhagic gastritis may be associated with undercooked poultry or hamburger meat. Most cases of coliform gastroenteritis are brief and the symptoms of fever, diarrhea, and abdominal cramps are self-limited. However, the enterohemorrhagic variety may produce severe illness with bloody diarrhea and possibly hepatorenal failure in very young patients or the elderly.[1]

In patients with significant symptoms and suspected invasive disease, a Gram or Wright stain of the stool reveals numerous polymorphonuclear leukocytes and erythrocytes. Stool cultures should be obtained to exclude other bacterial agents. Treatment is supportive, providing fluid supplementation and antispasmodic agents. Chronic cases of E. coli enteritis may require antibiotic therapy for resolution (ciprofloxacin 250–500 mg po bid is a reasonable choice).

Salmonella

Five distinct clinical syndromes are associated with Salmonella infections: (1) gastroenteritis (about 75% of infections); (2) bacteremia with and without gastrointestinal involvement (10% of cases); (3) typhoidal "enteric" fever (8% of cases); (4) localized infections in bones, joints, and meninges (5%); and (5), a symptomatic carrier gallbladder state.

Salmonella enteritidis, serotype typhimurium, produces a typical case of mild gastroenteritis with headache, nausea, vomiting, diarrhea, and fever lasting for 2 to 4 days. Solid food restriction, antispasmodic agents, and fluid and electrolyte repletion are effective treatment. Other serotypes may produce a more severe illness lasting up to 3 weeks, occasionally accompanied by bacteremia. Stool examination in these cases will reveal fecal leukocytes, and culture is required to identify the organism. Antibiotics are generally not required in patients with mild illness who are not bacteremic, as the drugs will only prolong the carrier state. Patients with more severe illness or documented bacteremia may require hospitalization for IV fluid therapy, and treatment with ciprofloxacin 400 mg IV q12h, or 500 mg po q12h for 10 days, or trimethoprim-sulfamethoxazole (TMP-SMX) one DS tablet bid for 14 days.[3]

Campylobacter jejuni

Campylobacter jejuni is probably the most common cause of inflammatory diarrhea in developed countries. Infection may vary from an asymptomatic case to severe enterocolitis. A typical episode begins with fever and malaise, followed within 24 hours by nausea, vomiting, diarrhea, and abdominal pain. The diarrhea is profuse, and contains blood and leukocytes. Infection is usually self-limited, and lasts less than 1 week. Reservoirs of infection include contaminated water, milk, meat, and poultry; also implicated are domestic pets, especially cats and dogs. Diagnosis may not be obvious from history and physical examination, thus stool culture is mandatory for accurate diagnosis.[4] Treatment includes fluid repletion, and in severe cases, antibiotic treatment with ciprofloxacin 500 mg po bid for 7 days, or TMP-SMX one DS tablet bid for 7 days.

Yersinia

Yersinia enterocolitica is responsible for a spectrum of illness, ranging from simple gastroenteritis to invasive ileitis and colitis. In older children and adults, Yersinia infections may cause a mesenteric adenitis, with symptoms mimicking acute appendicitis. Diarrhea is a fairly constant feature, with fever and abdominal cramping generally accompanying the diarrhea. Duration of illness ranges from 14 to 46 days. Interestingly, Yersinia infection may cause radiographic findings similar to those seen with Crohn's colitis, including bowel wall nodularity, mucosal thickening, and aphthous ulceration. The illness is usually self-limited, and antibiotics are often not necessary.[5]

Shigella

Shigella organisms may cause a severe, invasive diarrhea (dysentery), especially in infants and the elderly. The diarrhea is frequent, bloody, and mucoid, due to the invasion of the colonic epithelium by the organism. The clinical course is biphasic, beginning with watery diarrhea, malaise, and fever; this is followed by tenesmus and frank dysentery within 24 hours. Children seem to have milder infections, lasting 1 to 3 days; symptoms in adults persist for 7 days. In severe cases, symptoms may last 2 to 4 weeks. The stool will contain pus and blood, and a stool culture is mandatory for accurate diagnosis. Therapy involves fluid and salt repletion, as well as antibiotics (ciprofloxacin 500 mg po bid, or TMP-SMX one DS tablet bid; either drug is used for a 2-week course).

Protozoal Gastroenteritis

The most common causes of protozoal gastroenteritis in the United States are *E. histolytica* and *G. lamblia*. Amebiasis may produce either an intermittent diarrheal syndrome, or a severe, fulminating illness with a presentation similar to that of inflammatory bowel disease. Giardiasis produces a more chronic diarrheal illness often accompanied by epigastric distress due to the duodenal infestation with parasites. Travel history is critical to the diagnosis. Amebiasis is common in travelers to the tropics, while giardiasis is endemic to certain Western nations, especially Russia. Other important clues to a giardiasis history are day-care participation, camping, and immunocompromise (i.e., HIV). Amebiasis may produce occult blood in the stool, with a proctoscopic examination showing an erythematous, friable rectal mucosa.[2] Definitive diagnosis is made by examination of fresh stool, with identification of cysts or trophozoites. Amebiasis is treated with metronidazole 750 mg po tid for 10 days, followed by iodoquinol 650 mg po tid for 3 weeks. Giardiasis may be treated with metronidazole 250 mg po tid for 5 days, or quinacrine 100 mg po tid for 5 days.

Antibiotic-Associated Enterocolitis

Also known as pseudomembranous colitis, the diarrheal symptoms are mediated by a toxin produced by an overgrowth of *C. difficile,* an organism commonly inhabiting the bowel. Typically, this illness develops subsequent to, or concurrently with, exposure to potentially any antibiotic. Diarrhea in these cases is typically profuse and watery, but is bloody in 5% of cases. Proctosigmoidoscopy reveals multiple discrete yellow plaques, which on biopsy reveal the features of a pseudomembrane.[1,6] Diagnosis is most reliably made by identification of *C. difficile* toxin in the stool. Treatment includes metronidazole 500 mg po bid for 10 days, with a toxin-binding resin such as cholestyramine 4 g qid for 5 days, alternatively, vancomycin 125 mg po qid for 10 days may be used.

Malabsorption

Malabsorption syndrome refers to the inability to absorb or digest one or more nutrients. The segment of involved intestine specifies the extent of the malabsorption. Patients with malabsorption will complain of diarrhea characterized by large, loose, foul-smelling stools with associated weight loss.

Pathophysiology

The small bowel is involved in the absorption of nutrients. Fats, iron, calcium, and folic acids are absorbed in the proximal small bowel. Pathologic processes that disrupt intraluminal or mucosal absorption in this region of the small bowel (e.g., Whipple's disease, pancreatic failure, celiac sprue, eosinophilic gastroenteritis) may result in fat malabsorption, osteopenia, and microcytic anemia. The ileum is involved in the absorption of bile acids and vitamin B_{12}. Disorders of this region of the small bowel, such as Crohn's disease or lymphoma, or surgical resection of this area, may result in diarrhea, weight loss, and macrocytic anemia.

Clinical Approach to the Patient with Malabsorption

It is prudent to begin with a complete history and physical examination. Document any travel history.

To provide qualitative evidence of malabsorption, perform a Sudan stain for fecal fat. This is done by heating on a glass slide a small amount of the patient's stool, acetic acid, and saline, followed by application of Sudan stain. In the presence of malabsorption, a large number of fat droplets will be present.

To provide a quantitative determination of stool fat, obtain a 72-hour collection of stool from the patient while the patient is following a diet containing 100 g of fat daily. Stool fat in excess of 7 g per 24 hours indicates fat malabsorption.

To check the integrity of the small intestinal mucosal, perform a D-xylose test. D-xylose is a 5-carbon pentose sugar that is absorbed across the intact intestinal mucosal. A 25-g dose is given orally, followed by a 5-hour urine collection, and a 2-hour postingestion serum level. A normal individual will secrete more than 5 g of D-xylose in the urine, and have D-xylose present in the serum sample. If an abnormally low level of D-xylose is found in the urine or serum, endoscopy of the small intestine with mucosal biopsies and aspiration for cultures should be performed to exclude mucosal disease or bacterial overgrowth. If the D-xylose test is normal, consider a pancreatic cause for the malabsorption.[6,7]

Treatment of malabsorption is directed at the underlying cause.

Irritable Bowel Syndrome

Irritable bowel syndrome (IBS) is one of the most common gastrointestinal problems encountered in family practice. Patients with IBS may have some or all of the symptoms of abdominal pain, distention, altered bowel habit, urgency, flatus, and a sense of incomplete evacuation. Synonymous terms include spastic colon, mucous colitis, and irritable colon. Patients with IBS have abnormal intestinal motility of the entire gut. IBS has no underlying anatomic abnormality or inflammatory component; however, patients with IBS tend to have some element of secondary psychiatric morbidity, with anxiety, depression, and somatization being common. IBS is typically found in young or middle-aged adults, with a 2:1 female-to-male ratio.[8]

Clinical Presentation

The hallmark of IBS is abdominal pain associated with defecation. Usually, symptoms begin in adolescence or early adulthood. Diagnostic criteria for supporting the diagnosis of IBS include a history of abdominal pain for 12 weeks (not necessarily consecutive) or more within the preceding 12 months which is relieved by defecation, and/or associated with a change in frequency of stool, and/or associated with a change in stool form. The frequency of stool is usually more than three bowel motions daily or less than three motions weekly. Mucus passed with stool, and a feeling of incomplete evacuation is also associated strongly with IBS.

Clinical Approach to the Patient with Suspected IBS

The extent of investigation depends on how closely the history and patient physical examination fits the characteristic features of IBS. Typically, the physical examination is normal in IBS, apart from possible lower quadrant abdominal tenderness or palpable bowel loops. Features on history and physical that argue against IBS include a steady downhill course, significant weight loss, nocturnal symptoms, onset after age 60, cachexia, or abdominal mass. As a general rule, obtain a CBC, serum albumin (to rule out malabsorption), erythrocyte sedimentation rate (ESR), stool culture, and stool for ova and parasites. Colonoscopy is indicated for those patients over age 40, especially if symptoms are of recent onset, or if there is a family history of bowel malignancy[6,8] (see Chapter 92).

Be aware of four conditions that mimic IBS. Giardiasis resembles IBS in every way. The clue to diagnosis is demographics (travel, day care, camping, immunocompromised patients), stool examination for ova and parasites, and possible small bowel aspirate and/or biopsy. Crohn's disease may cause IBS-like symptoms in young people; endoscopy and/or small bowel enema is helpful in sorting out these patients who may present with significant postprandial pain.

Lactose intolerance should be considered if symptoms appear after consumption of dairy products. Microscopic colitis is a condition found in middle-aged women with watery diarrhea and abdominal pain. Endoscopy in these patients reveals a normal-appearing mucosa; however, mucosal biopsy shows inflammation.

Management

Treatment must be individualized and directed toward reduction of symptoms and reduction of secondary anxiety. After an appropriate workup, reassurance that there is no underlying physical pathology is very helpful. Dietary restrictions are probably unnecessary, except in cases of lactose intolerance. The mainstays of treatment are bulking agents (Metamucil, Citrucel, FiberCon) taken once or twice a day with sufficient fluids to produce one or two bowel motions daily. These agents tend to reduce diarrhea, alleviate constipation, and reduce the cramping sensation as well. Loperamide (Imodium) may be effective in reducing urgency and fecal soiling in patients with persisting diarrhea. Antispasmodics (hyoscyamine sulfate or dicyclomine) may be helpful in conjunction with bulking agents. Tricyclic antidepressants may be considered when there is a coexisting affective disorder.

Diverticular Disease

Diverticulosis of the colon results from herniation of the mucosal and submucosal layers through the muscularis layer. This often occurs at points where nutrient arteries penetrate the muscularis. The incidence of diverticulosis in Western populations increases with age, and is observed to include roughly 65% of individuals by age 85. Diverticulitis is the inflammatory complication of diverticulum, and is seen in 20% of patients with diverticulosis.[9] The risk of diverticulitis increases with the number and distribution of diverticula.

Clinical Presentation

Colonic diverticula are generally asymptomatic, and found incidentally on barium enema or lower GI endoscopy. They are most commonly found on the left side of the colon. Inflammation of diverticula is usually due to mechanical obstruction by a fecalith, or some other nondigestible remnant, such as a seed or popcorn kernel. The obstruction increases the susceptibility of the thin-walled diverticular sac to invasion by colonic bacteria. This in turn leads to microperforation of the sac wall with localized inflammation (peridiverticulitis), localized peridiverticular abscess formation, or, in some cases, wider inflammation with pericolonic abscess formation. Generally, only one diverticulum in the sigmoid colon is involved, and the peridiverticulitis remains localized and heals with a residual area of pericolonic fibrosis. Repeated attacks of diverticulitis may lead to segmental narrowing and even colonic obstruction.

Diverticulitis with a large perforation may lead to a pericolonic abscess, which can extend along the bowel wall or rupture into adjacent organs, creating fistulas between the colon and the vagina, urethra, bladder, or overlying abdominal wall. Rarely, free perforation of a diverticulum may occur and present with frank peritonitis.

Patients generally present for medical care with complaints of variable severity. Left lower quadrant pain is a common theme, although pain may also be located in the right lower quadrant (cecal diverticulitis; also think of appendicitis). Signs of peritoneal irritation, fever, leukocytosis, and possibly a palpable mass may also be present in advanced cases.

Diagnosis

A patient history, physical examination, and an awareness of the disease provide a starting point for diagnosis. For an acute episode, include a CBC, and a computed tomography (CT) scan of the abdomen and pelvis with oral contrast for delineation of the areas of inflamed bowel and to rule out abscess formation or free air. Plain abdominal radiographs are less helpful, but they are useful to demonstrate any concomitant bowel obstruction or free air under the diaphragm.

In nonacute cases, flexible sigmoidoscopy, colonoscopy, or air-contrast barium enema will reveal the disease, as well as helping to rule out other disorders such as inflammatory bowel disease or colonic carcinoma. Keep in mind that a common cause of colonic bleeding is from a ruptured diverticulum. The right colon is the source of 70% of these bleeds, which are usually bright red and copious. Luckily, they are often self-limiting. Evaluation of these bleeds will require endoscopy and occasionally angiography.

Treatment

Asymptomatic patients require no specific treatment apart from general advice to increase dietary fiber intake. Patients with only mild tenderness, no fever, and no leukocytosis may be managed as outpatients, with increased fiber, increased fluids, and oral antibiotics (ciprofloxacin 500 mg po bid plus metronidazole 500 mg po bid; or TMP-SMX DS tablets bid plus metronidazole; or clindamycin 300 mg po tid). Acutely ill patients should be managed in the hospital with intravenous fluids, bowel rest, and intravenous antibiotics (ampicillin-sulbactam 1.5 g IV q6h, or clindamycin 300 mg IV q8h, or ciprofloxacin 500 mg IV bid plus metronidazole 500 mg IV q8h are a few acceptable regimens). A surgical consultation is prudent.

Inflammatory Bowel Disease

Inflammatory bowel disease (IBD) includes at least two forms of idiopathic intestinal inflammation: ulcerative colitis (UC), and Crohn's disease (also known as regional ileitis). In the absence of any other identifiable cause of colon inflammation (radiation, infection, or ischemia), both UC and Crohn's may be defined empirically by their typical clinical, laboratory, endoscopic, and pathologic features.

The incidence of UC and Crohn's disease varies between 5 and 10 per 100,000. Both disorders occur equally in men and women, with spikes of peak incidence between ages 15 and 30, and then again between ages 55 and 65.[10]

Clinical Presentation

Crohn's Disease

Crohn's disease produces a transmural inflammation of the alimentary tract anywhere along its length, with ulceration of the mucosa and formation of granulomas, abscesses, and fistulas. The inflammation may be segmental, with relatively normal tissue interposed between involved areas ("skip lesions"). Involvement of the terminal ileum and colon is common. Symptoms commonly encountered include diarrhea, fever, colicky abdominal pain, and weight loss. Pain is often located in the right lower quadrant, and may be associated with a palpable mass due to chronic inflammation. With colonic involvement, the diarrhea is bloody. Perianal disease may also occur, with formation of fissures, fistulas, sinus tracts, or abscesses to other organ structures in the abdomen. Extraintestinal manifestations of Crohn's disease include seronegative arthropathy, uveitis, erythema nodosum, spondyloarthritis, pericholangitis, and chronic dermatoses.[11]

Ulcerative Colitis

In contrast to Crohn's disease, UC produces a nontransmural inflammation of the mucosa and superficial submucosa, typically of the rectum and distal colon. Inflammation may occur proximally, extending into the right colon. Major symptoms include abdominal pain, fever, rectal bleeding, diarrhea, and tenesmus. The severity of symptoms correlates with the intensity of inflammation and the extent of bowel involved.[12]

Diagnosis

Diagnosis of IBD requires a careful history, a general physical examination of the patient, and appropriate radiologic and endoscopic examinations. Stool samples are generally heme positive, with microscopic examination also revealing neutrophils and eosinophils. Colitis caused by bacterial pathogens as *Salmonella, Shigella, Campylobacter, C. difficile,* or protozoans (amebiasis) may mimic IBD; obtain a stool culture for these as part of the workup.

Radiologic studies include plain films, contrast studies, and CT scanning. In the presence of severe UC, plain films may reveal irregularity of the colonic mucosa due to edema of the bowel wall. Plain films may also reveal the hugely dilated lengths of bowel, which define toxic megacolon, a serious complication of UC. Barium enema is contraindicated if the colon is dilated in UC, but in Crohn's, air contrast enemas will reveal the extent of colonic disease, and the presence of fistulas, submucosal edema, and pseudodiverticula formation. Upper GI barium studies with small bowel follow-through are useful for diagnosis of small bowel disease. CT scanning with oral contrast is also useful to delineate the extent of disease in UC and Crohn's, especially in an ill patient. In a patient with an acute abdomen, CT scanning may reveal associated IBD pathology, including abscesses, fistulas, mesenteric edema/streaking, free fluid, and bowel wall thickening.

Endoscopy plays a central role in the diagnosis of IBD. Proctosigmoidoscopy is easily and quickly performed in the nonprepped bowel for initial evaluation of colitis. Early signs of UC include hyperemia and edema of the mucosa; with more advanced inflammation, the mucosa is friable, granular, erythematous, and superficially ulcerated without "skip areas." Colonoscopy is contraindicated in the presence of severe inflammation, and should be reserved for follow-up when the disease is quiescent. Colonoscopy also is able to obtain tissue biopsies for pathologic study to differentiate between UC and Crohn's, and to provide a tissue diagnosis of associated masses or strictures found within the colon. A complete colonoscopy will allow evaluation of the terminal ileum by intubation of the ileocecal valve. Upper GI endoscopy may assist in the assessment of upper GI symptoms in a patient with known Crohn's disease. Repeated colonoscopies are unnecessary to follow the severity of inflammation in Crohn's disease, as there is poor correlation of the endoscopic appearance with clinical remission.

Complications

Toxic megacolon is a serious complication of UC. The colon is massively dilated (greater than 10 cm in diameter), and the patient is often gravely ill. The condition may be precipitated by a barium enema (or the bowel preparation) in the presence of severe colitis, potassium depletion, antidiarrheal medications, or narcotic pain relievers. Colonic cancer may occur in patients with long-standing UC (10 years or more), and the risk rises to between 0.5% and 1% annually after 15 years. Periodic colonoscopy is recommended for surveillance. Crohn's disease is not as strongly associated with bowel or colonic cancer, although Crohn's sufferers have a somewhat higher risk than the general population.[13]

Crohn's disease may be complicated by fistula formation between the bowel and other organs, including the vagina, bladder, urethra, prostate, and skin. Other extraintestinal manifestations may be present, including spondyloarthropathy of the spine and sacroiliac joints, oligoarthropathies involving the large joints of the arms and legs, and inflammatory conditions of the eye (anterior uveitis) and skin (erythema nodosum). A severe skin complication is pyoderma gangrenosum. Hepatic involvement includes gallstone formation and sclerosing cholangitis. Renal involvement includes formation of calcium oxalate stones, and hydronephrosis due to the ureteric obstruction from an ileal mass.

Management

Medical management of UC and Crohn's disease share common themes. Sulfasalazine (1000 mg po tid–qid) is effective in inducing remission in mild to moderate UC, ileocolitis, and Crohn's colitis. It will reduce the frequency and severity of UC, but does not maintain remission of Crohn's disease. It is safe in pregnancy and lactation. Adverse effects are encountered in 25% of patients using sulfasalazine, and include anorexia, rash, headache, fever, aplastic anemia, leukemia, hepatotoxicity, and hemolytic anemia. Patients unable to tolerate sulfasalazine may alternatively use mesalamine.

Mesalamine is the 5-aminosalicylate moiety of sulfasalazine. It is available in topical and oral forms. Enemas and suppositories (Rowasa) are beneficial for active distal colitis, including active disease unresponsive to topical steroids. The tablet form (Asacol, Dipentum, and Pentasa) is useful for maintenance of remission of UC and Crohn's disease, and may reduce recurrence following surgery for cure of ileitis and ileocolitis.

Corticosteroids are useful for patients with active moderate to severe UC, active small or large bowel Crohn's, or for extraintestinal manifestations of Crohn's (eye, skin, joints). Severely ill patients will require parenteral methylprednisolone (60–125 mg IV q6–12h), while more stable patients may receive oral prednisone or dexamethasone. Corticosteroids are not effective in maintaining remission of disease, or preventing postoperative recurrence. They may be used safely in pregnancy to control IBD. Keep in mind the side effects of long-term administration. Steroid enemas, foams, and suppositories are useful for controlling IBD confined to the rectum.[14]

Immunosuppressive agents such as 6-mercaptopurine, azathioprine, and cyclosporine are reserved for the management of chronic active disease, refractory disease, and complications of Crohn's such as fistulas and perianal disease. The immunosuppressives, despite having the advantage of saving the patient from large doses of corticosteroids, are nephrotoxic, and should be avoided in pregnancy.

Antibiotics useful in IBD include metronidazole and ciprofloxacin. In patients with active colonic Crohn's disease, metronidazole 250 mg po tid is as effective as sulfasalazine in obtaining disease control. Metronidazole and ciprofloxacin (500 mg po bid) are both useful in healing active perianal disease, and as adjunctive therapy (with surgical drainage) in treatment of abscesses.[14]

Surgery to remove the entire rectum and colon is curative for UC. Colectomy is also required in fulminant cases of toxic megacolon. In Crohn's, disease recurrence is the rule; surgery should be reserved for patients with fistulas, bowel obstruction, abscess formation, perforation, or bleeding. Rarely should medically refractory disease be operated upon. Percutaneous abscess drainage and endoscopic balloon dilatation may be useful alternatives to surgery in selected patients. Efforts should be sought to avoid multiple bowel resections because of the risk of producing short-bowel syndrome. Involving a surgical consultant early on during the management of patients hospitalized with IBD is prudent.

References

1. Geurrant RL, Bobak DA. Bacterial and protozoal gastroenteritis. N Engl J Med 1991;325:327–40.
2. Jenkins J, Braen GR. Manual of emergency medicine, 4th ed. Philadelphia: Lippincott Williams & Wilkins, 2000;243–9.
3. Glynn JR, Hornick RB, Levine MM. Infecting dose and severity of typhoid: analysis of volume data and examination of the influence of the definition of illness. Epidemiol Infect 1995;115:23–6.
4. Blaser MJ, Reller LB. *Campylobacter* enteritis. N Engl J Med 1981;305:1444–7.
5. Cover TL, Aber RC. *Yersinia enterocolitica.* N Engl J Med 1989;321:16–20.
6. Yamada T, Alper D, eds. Textbook of gastroenterology, 2nd ed. Philadelphia: Lippincott, 1995.
7. Olsen WA. A pathophysiologic approach to the diagnosis of malabsorption. Am J Med 1987;67:1007–18.
8. Kandel G. Irritable bowel syndrome. Can J Diagn 2000;12(12):72–83.
9. Thompson WG, Patel DG. Clinical picture of diverticular disease of the colon. Clin Gastroenterol 1986;15:903–10.
10. Kirsner JB, Shorter RG, eds. Inflammatory bowel disease, 4th ed. Philadelphia: Lea & Febiger, 1995.
11. Colombel JF, Grandbastien B, Gower-Rousseau C. Clinical characteristics of Crohn's disease. Gastroenterology 1996;111:604–20.
12. Gionchetti P, Campieri M. Medical treatment of ulcerative colitis. Curr Opin Gastroenterol 1996;12:352–65.
13. Provencale D. Prophylactic colectomy or surveillance for chronic ulcerative colitis. Gastroenterology 1995;109:111–8.
14. Hanauer SB. Drug therapy: inflammatory bowel disease. N Engl J Med 1996;334:841–5.

89
Diseases of the Pancreas

Michael R. Spieker

Diseases of the pancreas cause significant morbidity and mortality in Western countries. In addition to caring for the acutely ill patient, family physicians can more successfully care for patients with pancreatic diseases by effective intervention in the patient's lifestyle and family issues. Such interventions may disrupt a pattern of chronic alcohol abuse and provide supportive care for the family of the patient.

Acute Pancreatitis

Background

Acute pancreatitis is a locally intense inflammation of the pancreas with variable involvement of other regional tissues or remote organ systems. It accounts for over 100,000 admissions and over 2000 deaths annually in the United States. Most cases of acute pancreatitis are mild and can be managed by close observation and supportive care without relying on sophisticated medical interventions. However, 25% of cases are severe and may require complex monitoring or surgical intervention.

Pancreatitis develops when trypsinogen is activated to trypsin by an inciting event. Trypsin subsequently activates other pancreatic enzymes including chymotrypsin, elastase, carboxypeptidase, and phospholipase A that cause local and systemic manifestations ranging from local pain to the systemic inflammatory response syndrome (SIRS). Overt sepsis and infected pancreatic necrosis have mortality rates over 50%.

Causes

Cholelithiasis and chronic excessive alcohol use are the leading causes of acute pancreatitis and account for 80% of the cases in the United States. Gallstone pancreatitis predominantly affects women (6:1), while alcohol-induced pancreatitis affects men more often (3:1). Pancreatitis can develop after an alcoholic binge, but it usually occurs in patients who have been drinking alcohol excessively for 7 to 10 years. About 10% of cases are idiopathic, but recent studies of these cases demonstrate microlithiasis as the probable cause in a significant proportion. Other less common causes of acute pancreatitis include medications (nonsteroidal antiinflammatories, oral contraceptives, tetracyclines, sulfonamides, didanosine, thiazide diuretics, furosemide, and propofol); metabolic conditions (familial hyperlipidemia, hyperparathyroidism, hypercalcemia); infections (mumps, cytomegalovirus, hepatitis A, B, and C, coxsackievirus, and tuberculosis); and pancreatic ductal obstruction due to a tumor mass. The incidence of acute pancreatitis is much higher in patients with acquired immunodeficiency syndrome (AIDS) (see Chapter 42). In children, trauma is the most common cause of pancreatitis and should raise suspicions of child abuse (see Chapter 27).

Diagnosis

Acute pancreatitis causes patients to have relatively sudden onset of midepigastric pain, nausea, and vomiting. Pain may vary from mild to intense, and patients describe it as an inescapable, constant, boring pain that often radiates to the right upper quadrant or back. Intensity of the pain does not correlate with severity of pancreatic inflammation or necrosis.

Patients with acute pancreatitis appear acutely ill with protracted vomiting and are unable to find a position to ease the relentless abdominal pain. A low-grade temperature may be present, although this does not necessarily indicate an infectious process. The abdomen is exquisitely tender in the midepigastrium and may exhibit diffuse tenderness throughout the abdomen due to peritoneal irritation. Bowel sounds are diminished or completely absent if an ileus is present. Patients often present with signs of hypovolemia and occasionally present in frank shock due to protracted vomiting and shifting of fluid into the third space. Periumbilical ecchymoses

Table 89.1. **Criteria for Assessment of Acute Pancreatitis**

Ranson's criteria for alcoholic pancreatitis	
At admission	During initial 48 hours
Age >55 years	Hct falls >10%
WBC >16,000 per mm^3	BUN rise >5 mg/dL
Glucose >200 mg/dL	Arterial PO_2 <60 mm Hg
LDH >350 IU/L	Serum Ca^{2+} <8.0 mg/dL
AST >250 U/L	Base deficit >4 mEq/L
	Estimated fluid sequestration >6 L

Mortality <1% with 0–2 signs; 15% with 3–4 signs; 40% with 5–6 signs; 100% with 7 or more signs.

Modified Glasgow criteria: within 48 hours of hospitalization
Age >55 years
WBC >15,000 per mm^3
Glucose >180 mg/dL
BUN >45 mg/dL
LDH >600 U/L
Ca^{2+} <8.0 mg/dL
Albumin <3.2 g/dL
Arterial PO_2 <60 mm Hg

Mortality or surgical intervention 6% with 0–2 signs; 40% with 3 or more signs.

AST = aspartate aminotransferase; BUN = blood urea nitrogen; LDH = lactate dehydrogenase; WBC = white blood count.

(Cullen's sign) or flank ecchymoses (Grey Turner sign) are uncommon, but when present serve as evidence of hemorrhagic necrosis of the pancreas.

Abnormal laboratory findings in acute pancreatitis include elevated serum amylase and lipase. Although very sensitive, the serum amylase is not specific for pancreatitis. Mild elevations up to three times normal can be seen in asymptomatic alcoholics. Because amylase rises rapidly in acute pancreatitis and clears in 2 to 3 days the elevation may be missed in patients who delay seeking treatment. Serum lipase is less sensitive but more specific for pancreatitis, and it has a longer half-life than amylase. Urine amylase determinations and amylase clearance to creatinine clearance ratios provide minimal additional useful diagnostic information. The white blood cell count may be elevated to 25,000/μL in patients with acute pancreatitis, even in the absence of a bacterial infection, and the hematocrit may be elevated due to hemoconcentration. Electrolyte abnormalities are common due to vomiting; hyperglycemia may be present secondary to glucagon secretion and decreased insulin production. Serum albumin and calcium may be low. Liver function tests are elevated in patients with obstructive causes of pancreatitis with aspartate aminotransferase/alanine aminotransferase (AST/ALT) levels >150 IU/L having a specificity of >95% for gallstone pancreatitis.[1]

Plain films of the abdomen are generally nonspecific, but are important to exclude other causes of abdominal pathology such as a ruptured viscus. Ultrasound is the most sensitive study to evaluate pancreatitis caused by biliary tract obstruction, but its utility for evaluating the pancreas itself is in identifying abscesses and pseudocysts. Up to 30% of patients with mild disease have a normal contrast-enhanced computed tomography (CT) scan of the pancreas. Early CT scanning is justified when the clinical diagnosis is in doubt; when the patent has severe abdominal symptoms, leukocytosis, or fever; when the patient fails to improve with medical management over 48 to 72 hours; or when the patient has three or more of Ranson's risk factors (Table 89.1) for severe acute pancreatitis.[2] Dynamic contrast-enhanced CT scanning has a 92% positive predictive value for pancreatic necrosis.[3] The distinction between pancreatic abscess and infected necrosis is critical because pancreatic necrosis has double the mortality rate and requires a markedly different therapeutic approach from that for pancreatic abscess. Endoscopic retrograde cholangiopancreatography (ERCP) should be considered to rule out gallbladder microlithiasis in patients who have been completely evaluated and in whom a definitive cause of pancreatitis has not been found.[4]

Management

Patients who develop severe disease require more intensive care, have higher rates of morbidity and mortality, and are not easily identified by their initial clinical presentation.[5] In 1992, members of the International Symposium of Acute Pancreatitis defined severe acute pancreatitis as pancreatitis with evidence of organ failure (shock, pulmonary insufficiency, renal failure or gastrointestinal bleeding) and/or local complications such as pancreatic necrosis, abscess, or pseudocyst.[6] Several grading systems (Tables 89.1 and 89.2) help to objectively quantify the severity of disease and stratify the prognosis for the patient with acute pancreatitis.[2,7-8] While all the grading systems have a relatively low sensitivity of predicting a severe attack, the Acute Physiology and Chronic Health Evaluation (APACHE) II illness grading system may provide the most useful estimate of the severity of the illness.[8] The Ranson[2] and Glasgow[7] criteria, by their nature, delay characterizing the severity of pancreatitis, while APACHE II can be applied at any time during the hospitalization and used sequentially to monitor the progress of treatment. The mean score for patients with uncomplicated outcomes was 6.29 compared to 9.35 and 14.2 for those with complicated and fatal outcomes, respectively.

Therapy for acute pancreatitis has advanced little beyond supportive care.[9] Fortunately, three fourths of patients have mild disease and respond quickly to diminished oral intake, generous intravenous fluid hydration, and parenteral analgesia. Patients may require several liters of fluid to replace losses from protracted vomiting and fluid shifts. Nasogastric tubes do not relieve pain or shorten hospital stays, although they may afford symptomatic relief in patients with severe vomiting or ileus. Other therapies have been evaluated and have been found to be of no additional benefit in mild disease. Cimetidine, calcitonin, somatostatin, glucagon, and enzyme inhibitors have not decreased the severity of the disease or mortality rates.[10] Total parenteral nutrition (TPN) has been similarly found to be ineffective in shortening the hospital course, but it still plays an important role for patients who develop complications and require prolonged bowel rest. Enteral nutrition delivered distal to the ligament of Treitz may offer advantages over TPN and decrease septic complications.[11]

Patients with severe pancreatitis, infected pancreatic necrosis, or systemic complications require invasive monitoring of

Table 89.2. **Acute Physiology and Chronic Health Evaluation (APACHE II) Criteria**

Physiologic variable	High abnormal range				0	Low abnormal range			
	+4	+3	+2	+1		+1	+2	+3	+4
Temp, rectal (°C)	≥41	39–40.9		38.5–38.9	36–38.4	34–35.9	32–33.9	30–31.9	≤29.9
Mean arterial pressure (mm Hg)	≥160	130–159	110–129		70–109		50–69		≤49
Heart rate	≥180	140–179	110–139		70–109		55–69	40–54	≤39
Respiratory rate	≥50	35–49		25–34	12–24	10–11	6–9		≤5
Oxygenation F$_i$O$_2$ >0.5 record A$_{aDO_2}$	≥500	350–499	200–349		<200				
F$_i$O$_2$ <0.5 record PaO$_2$					PO_2>70	PO_2 61–70		PO_2 55–60	PO_2<55
Arterial pH	≥7.7	7.6–7.69		7.5–7.59	7.33–7.49		7.25–7.32	7.15–7.24	<7.15
Serum Na$^+$ (mmol/L)	≥180	160–179	155–159	150–154	130–149		120–129	111–119	≤110
Serum K$^+$ (mmol/L)	≥7	6–6.9		5.5–5.9	3.5–5.4	3–3.4	2.5–2.9		<2.5
Serum Cr (mg/dL) double score for acute renal failure	≥3.5	2–3.4	1.5–1.9		0.6–1.4		<0.6		
Hematocrit (%)	≥60		50–59.9	46–49.9	30–45.9		20–29.9		<20
White blood count (×10^3/mm^3)	≥40		20–39.9	15–19.9	3–14.9		1–2.9		<1
Glasgow Coma Scale (GCS): Score – 15 actual GCS									
Acute physiology score (APS) (sum of the 12 variables)									
Serum HCO$_3$ (venous-mmol/L); use if no ABGs	≥52	41–51.9		32–40.9	22–31.9		18–21.9	15–17.9	<15

APACHE II score is given by the sum of the acute physiology score (APS), the age points, and the chronic health points

Age points: Age 45, zero; 45–54, 2 points; 55–64, 3 points; 65–74, 5 points; and ≥75, 6 points.

Chronic health points are assigned if the patient has a history of severe organ system insufficiency or is immunocompromised as follows: nonoperative or emergency postoperative patients, 5 points; elective postoperative patients, 2 points. Organ insufficiency or immunocompromised state must have been evident before hospital admissions must conform to the following criteria: liver, biopsy-proven cirrhosis and documented portal hypertension, episodes of past UGI bleeds attributed to portal hypertension, or prior episodes of hepatic failure/encephalopathy/coma; cardiovascular, NYHA class IV; respiratory, chronic restrictive, obstructive or vascular disease resulting in severe exercise restriction; renal, receiving chronic dialysis; immunocompromised, received therapy that suppresses resistance to infection.

A$_{aDO_2}$ = alveolar-arterial oxygen difference; PaO$_2$ = arterial partial pressure of oxygen; F$_i$O$_2$ = fraction of inspired oxygen; ABGs = arterial blood gases; NYHA = New York Heart Association; UGI = upper gastrointestinal.

cardiovascular, pulmonary, and renal systems, as well as observation for sepsis, abscess formation, and pseudocysts. Surgical intervention is indicated for evidence of abscess formation or infected pancreatic tissue. The role of the surgeon in patients with severe necrotizing pancreatitis without evidence of infection is less clear. Imipenem and cefuroxime have shown preliminary success in reducing septic complications from pancreatitis, but mortality may be reduced only in specific subsets.[12–14]

Future Directions

New diagnostic tests and therapeutic strategies may favorably impact the morbidity and mortality associated with pancreatitis. Though not yet clinically applicable, tests that measure C-reactive protein, trypsinogen activation peptides, and leukocyte elastase have shown promise in determining the severity of the disease. Selective decontamination of the gut with antibiotics has not proven to reduce mortality in a randomized clinical trial.[15] Though not conclusively demonstrated, immediate endoscopic removal of gallstones may prove to be more effective than surgery,[16] intraarterial infusion of antibiotics or protease inhibitors has shown promise,[17] and long-term peritoneal dialysis (7 days) may improve outcomes. Therapies directed at the active molecules of the SIRS response such as platelet-activating factor (PAF) offer hope in reducing multiple organ failure.[18] However, these treatments have not been evaluated by large controlled studies.

Chronic Pancreatitis

Background

Chronic pancreatitis is a progressive inflammation of the pancreas manifested by recurrent abdominal pain and a progressive loss of both exocrine and endocrine pancreatic function. Prevalence rates of 3.5 to 4 per 100,000 probably underestimate the true incidence of the disease since many patients are asymptomatic, while others with undiagnosed abdominal pain may have chronic pancreatitis. Mortality rates as high as 50% have been reported 25 years after diagnosis. Patients with chronic pancreatitis are at higher risk for pancreatic cancer.

Pancreatic acinar cells hypersecrete protein that precipitates to form intraductal plugs that result in obstruction of the ducts and activation of pancreatic enzymes. Intraductal stones form if the precipitate includes calcium carbonate. Elevated ductal pressures may contribute to the development of the disease.

Causes

Heavy, prolonged alcohol use is associated with 70% to 90% of chronic pancreatitis in Western countries.[19] Most investigators believe that acute pancreatitis does not lead to chronic pancreatitis unless complications such as pseudocysts or ductal strictures occur. Up to 30% of cases have no discernible cause and are deemed idiopathic. Obstructing lesions of the pancreatic duct (pseudocysts, tumors, or posttraumatic strictures), tropical pancreatitis, intraductal stones, hypoparathyroidism, and cystic fibrosis are unusual causes of the disease.

Patients with chronic pancreatitis are more likely to have mutations in the gene associated with cystic fibrosis.[20] Smoking increases the risk of chronic pancreatitis tenfold.

Diagnosis

Most patients with chronic pancreatitis have a long history of heavy alcohol use (greater than 150 mL/day), and chronic, recurrent episodes of abdominal pain associated with nausea and vomiting. However, up to 20% of patients are asymptomatic. Diabetes and malabsorption are relatively nonspecific and late findings. Physical examination often reflects the usual sequelae of long-term alcohol use, including ruddy complexion, spider nevi, gynecomastia, and hepatomegaly. Serum amylase, lipase, and electrolytes are most often normal. The white blood cell count is normal. Liver function abnormalities are found in chronic alcohol users. Pancreatic calcifications are pathognomonic for chronic pancreatitis and can be identified in plain abdominal radiographs in 30% of cases. Ultrasound and CT are moderately sensitive and specific for making the diagnosis while the roles for magnetic resonance imaging and endoscopic ultrasonography are not yet well defined. ERCP remains the gold standard imaging procedure, but it is infrequently used to make the diagnosis due to its invasive nature. Pancreatic function tests may be useful in diagnosing patients with normal laboratory and imaging findings.

Management

Alcohol avoidance is the cornerstone to managing chronic pancreatitis. Patients with chronic pancreatitis who consume even small amounts of alcohol ($<$50 mL/day) have more frequent severe pain, calcifications, and complications.[21] Larger intakes reduce the time to pancreatic calcification and death. Patients who fail to respond to noninvasive management of alcohol abstinence, analgesics, and nerve blocks may benefit from internal surgical drainage procedures or ductal stent placement if there is evidence of large duct obstruction. Low-fat diets and oral administration of bicarbonate and pancreatic enzymes may help reduce fat malabsorption and diarrhea but offer no apparent pain control benefit.[22–23] Persistent or large pseudocysts require surgical intervention. Pancreatic resection may improve long-term pain.[24,25]

Pancreatic Cancer

Background

Pancreatic cancer is the fourth and fifth most common cause of cancer-related death in males and females, respectively. The incidence rate of 9/100,000 has remained steady since 1973. Data indicate clear evidence of increased risk with smoking; however, no data support any direct effect from alcohol intake or specific occupational exposures. Risk of pancreatic cancer increases by 2% per decade in patients with chronic pancreatitis, and dietary nitrosamines from smoked foods have also been implicated as a risk factor. Long-standing diabetes doubles the risk of pancreatic cancer.[26] Five-year survival rates are dismal; however, in the past decade the rates have increased from 1% to 3% in whites and from 3% to 5% in blacks. Advances in the area of genetic markers have not yet significantly impacted morbidity and mortality rates because of the inability to detect the tumor while it is still potentially curable.

Clinical Manifestations

Clinical features of pancreatic cancer are initially vague and nonspecific and frequently contribute to a delay in diagnosis. Jaundice is the most common physical finding; however, weight loss, epigastric pain, or incapacitating back pain may be the presenting complaint. Glucose intolerance develops 6 to 12 months prior to the diagnosis in 10% to 15% of patients. The clinical constellation of glucose intolerance, vague gastrointestinal symptoms, and weight loss in a patient under the age of 60 with no family history of diabetes mellitus should alert the clinician to the possibility of pancreatic cancer. A palpable gallbladder (Courvoisier's sign) in the absence of cholangitis, while present in only 25% of patients, suggests a malignant obstruction of the common bile duct until proven otherwise. Distant metastases, ascites, cervical adenopathy, and a periumbilical mass may also be noted on physical examination.

Diagnosis and Staging

Although the spectrum of malignant pancreatic neoplasms includes islet cell tumors, cystadenocarcinomas, and other rare neoplasms, adenocarcinoma of ductal origin represents about 90% of pancreatic carcinomas. The cancer occurs in the head of the pancreas in 70% of patients, in the pancreatic body in 20%, and in the tail in 10%.

No single laboratory test is diagnostic. In clinical practice, tumor-associated antigen CA 19-9 has been found to be the most useful in diagnosis, but elevated liver enzymes, coagulopathy, and anemia are common. Sensitivities of carbohydrate antigen CA 19-9, carcinoembryonic antigen (CEA), and CA-125 for identifying pancreatic carcinomas are 71%, 62%, and 27%, respectively.[27] Most investigators believe that these tumor markers are unreliable for diagnosing pancreatic cancer.

Ultrasound, plain film abdominal radiographs, and upper gastrointestinal series are not sensitive as diagnostic tests. CT is the diagnostic procedure of choice for the jaundiced patient with a suspected malignancy because of its relative diagnostic accuracy, availability, and cost. State-of-the art spiral CT may obviate the routine use of staging laparoscopy.[28] Magnetic resonance imaging has no advantage over CT. ERCP remains the most sensitive diagnostic test and is the gold standard for delineating the exact site of obstruction. Advances with endoscopic ultrasound make it the most sensitive imaging test to date in detecting small lesions.[29]

The TNM (tumor, nodes, metastases) system for staging pancreatic cancer represents the most important factor for determining resectability and prognosis. Preoperative endoscopic or percutaneous biopsy is required to confirm the diagnosis before appropriate palliative chemotherapy or radiation therapy can be initiated. Laparoscopy is being evaluated as an additional staging modality.

Management

Pancreatic resection provides the only opportunity for cure. However, patients should carefully consider outcomes before undergoing surgical exploration. Ninety percent of patients with all types of pancreatic cancer have tumors that are unresectable at the time of diagnosis and overall 5-year survival is poor. Pancreaticoduodenectomy (Whipple procedure) is the procedure of choice for ductal adenocarcinoma of the pancreatic head. Despite sophisticated preoperative staging methods, 60% to 70% of patients with apparently resectable adenocarcinoma of the pancreatic head have metastatic or locally invasive disease precluding resection at laparotomy. Total pancreatectomy has been proposed; however, no appreciable survival benefit has been shown. Obstructive jaundice, duodenal obstruction, and back pain often require palliative operative intervention or endoscopically placed drainage stents. Of single-agent chemotherapies, only fluorouracil (5-FU) has demonstrated a response rate greater than 20%. Combination therapy with radiation and 5-FU increases survival, but the median survival for patients with unresectable cancers is only 12 months. Pancreatic cancer recurs locally, with incapacitating constant back pain a disabling sign of disease progression.

Future Directions

If available, spiral CT allows for very rapid three-dimensional evaluation of small pancreatic tumors and accurate assessment of resectability relative to the amount of vascular encasement with tumor mass. Circulating polypeptides such as peptide islet amyloid polypeptide (IAPP) produced by the beta cells of the pancreas, and gene abnormalities, especially those associated with cystic fibrosis remain fertile grounds for research attempts to identify useful diagnostic tools.[30–31]

Therapeutic trials with the endogenous gastrointestinal hormone, peptide YY, demonstrate reduced cancer cell growth if given prior to traditional 5-FU chemotherapy, and gemcitabine, a nucleoside analogue that exhibits antitumor activity, decreased pain intensity, increased survival, and increased time to progressive disease in a phase II trial.[32] In another small phase II study interferon-α as adjuvant chemotherapy to 5-FU and radiotherapy significantly improved survival.[33]

Until tools for early diagnosis are widely available, the role of the primary care physician is to provide aggressive palliation of the constant back pain pancreatic cancer patients suffer and to maintain dialogue with the patient and family, especially with regard to hospice care. Prevention of this devastating disease through modification of diet, smoking, and alcohol intake should be the family physician's most important goal.

References

1. Tenner S, Bubner H, Steinberg W. Predicting gallstone pancreatitis with laboratory parameters: a meta-analysis. Am J Gastroenterol 1994;89:1863–6.
2. Ranson JHC, Rifkind KM, Roese DF, Fink SD, Eng K, Spencer FC. Prognostic signs and the role of operative management in acute pancreatitis. Surg Gynecol Obstet 1974;139:69–81.
3. Stanten R, Frey CF. Comprehensive management of acute

necrotizing pancreatitis and pancreatic abscess. Arch Surg 1990; 125:1269–75.

4. Venu RP, Geemen JE, Howgan W, Stone J, Johnson GK, Soergel K. Idiopathic recurrent pancreatitis: an approach to diagnosis and treatment. Dig Dis Sci 1989;34:56–60.

5. vanSonnenberg E, Stabile BE, Varney RR, Christensen RR. Percutaneous drainage of infected and non-infected pseudocysts. Radiology 1989;170:757–62.

6. Bradley EL. A clinically based classification system for acute pancreatitis. Summary of the international symposium on acute pancreatitis. Arch Surg 1993;128:586–90.

7. Blamey SL, Imrie CW, O'Neill J, Gilmour WH, Carter DC. Prognostic factors in acute pancreatitis. Gut 1984;25:1340–6.

8. Wilson C, Heath DI, Imrie CW. Prediction of outcome in acute pancreatitis: a comparative study of APACHE II, clinical assessment and multiple factor scoring systems. Br J Surg 1990; 77:1260–4.

9. Steinberg WM, Tenner S. Acute pancreatitis. N Engl J Med 1994;330:1198–210.

10. Andriulli A, Leandro G, Clemente R, et al. Meta-analysis of somatostatin octreotide and gabexate mesilate in the therapy of acute pancreatitis. Aliment Pharmacol Ther 1998;12:237–45.

11. Al-Omran M, Wilke D. Enteral versus parenteral nutrition for acute panreatitis. In: The Cochrane Library: Update Software, Issue 1. Cambridge: Oxford, 2001.

12. Pederzoli P, Bassi C, Vesentini S, Campedelli A. A randomized multicenter clinical trial of antibiotic prophylaxis of septic complications in acute necrotizing pancreatitis with imipenem. Surg Gynecol Obstet 1993;176:480–93.

13. Golub R, Siddiqi F, Pohl D. Role of antibiotic in acute pancreatitis: a meta-analysis. J Gastrointest Surg 1998;2:496–503.

14. Kramer KM, Levy H. Prophylactic antibiotics for severe acute pancreatitis: the beginning of an era. Pharmacotherapy 1999;19: 592–602.

15. Luiten EJT, Hop WCJ, Lange JF, et al. Controlled clinical trial of selective decontamination for the treatment of severe acute pancreatitis. Ann Surg 1995;222:57–65.

16. Neoptolemos JP, Carr-Locke DL. Controlled trial of urgent endoscopic retrograde cholangiopancreatography and endoscopic sphincterotomy versus conservative treatment for acute pancreatitis due to gallstones. Lancet 1988;2:979–83.

17. Schmid SW, Uhl W, Friess H, Malfertheiner P, Buchler MW. The role of infection in acute pancreatitis. Gut 1999;45:311–16.

18. Kingsnorth AN, Galloway SW, Formella LJ. Randomized, double-blind phase II trial of lexipafant, a platelet activating factor antagonist in human pancreatitis. Br J Surg 1995;82:1414–20.

19. Worning H. Chronic pancreatitis: pathogenesis, natural history and conservative treatment. Clin Gastroenterol 1984;13:871–94.

20. Sharer N, Schwarz M, Malone G, et al. Mutations of the cystic fibrosis gene in patients with chronic pancreatitis. N Engl J Med 1998;339:645–52.

21. Lankisch MR, Imoto M, Layer P, DiMagno EP. The effect of small amounts of alcohol on the clinical course of chronic pancreatitis. Mayo Clin Proc 2001;76:242–51.

22. Lankisch PG, Lohr-Happe A, Otto J, Creutzfeldt W. Natural course in chronic pancreatitis: pain, exocrine and endocrine pancreatic insufficiency and prognosis of the disease. Digestion 1993;54:148–55.

23. Brown A, Hughes M, Tenner S, Banks PA. Does pancreatic enzyme supplementation reduce pain in patients with chronic pancreatitis: a meta-analysis. Am J Gastroenterol 1997;92:2032–5.

24. Berney T, Rudisuhli T, Oberholzer J. Caulfield A, Morel P. Long-term metabolic results after pancreatic resection for severe chronic pancreatitis. Arch Surg 2000;135:1106–11.

25. Sakorafas GH, Farnell MB, Nagorney DM, Sarr MG, Rowland CM. Pancreatoduodenectomy for chronic pancreatitis: long-term results in 105 patients. Arch Surg 2000;135:517–23.

26. Everhart J, Wright D. Diabetes mellitus as a risk factor for pancreatic cancer: a meta-analysis. JAMA 1995;273:1605–9.

27. Murr M, Sarr M. Pancreatic cancer. CA J Clin Cancer 1994; 44:304–18.

28. Pisters PW, Lee JE, Vanthey JN, Charnsangavej C, Evans DB. Laparoscopy in the staging of pancreatic cancer. Br J Surg 2001;88:325–37.

29. Midwinter MJ, Beveridge CJ, Wilsdon JB, Bennett MK, Baudouin CJ, Charnley RM. Correlation between spiral computed tomography, endoscopic ultrasonography and findings at operation in pancreatic and ampullary tumors. Br J Surg 1999;86: 189–93.

30. Urrutia R, DiMagno E. Genetic markers: the key to early diagnosis and improved survival in pancreatic cancer? Gastroenterology 1996;110:306–10.

31. Tada M, Ohashi M. Analysis of K-ras gene mutation in hyperplastic duct cells of the pancreas without pancreatic disease. Gastroenterology 1996;110:227–31.

32. Carmichael J, Fink U, Russell RC, et al. Phase II study of gemcitabine in patients with advanced pancreatic cancer. Br J Cancer 1996;73:101–5.

33. Nukui Y, Picozzi VJ, Traverso LW. Interferon based adjuvant chemoradiation therapy improves survival after pancreaticoduodenectomy for pancreatic adenocarcinoma. Am J Surg 2000; 179:367–71.

90
Diseases of the Liver

Dan E. Brewer

Clinical Presentation

Signs and Symptoms

Diseases of the liver can have a wide spectrum of clinical presentations from asymptomatic chronic hepatitis that is found only as the result of screening to fulminant hepatitis progressing rapidly to complete liver failure. The classic symptoms of acute hepatitis are nausea, fatigue, anorexia, pruritus, and jaundice. Patients who develop chronic hepatitis usually have an asymptomatic phase that lasts for many years. As the disease progresses, they may develop fatigue, myalgias, and nonspecific abdominal pain. Chronic hepatitis may progress to cirrhosis and/or hepatocellular carcinoma.

History

The history obtained by the physician should focus on the time course of the illness and carefully search for any possible exposures to viral hepatitis. Sexual exposures and exposure to blood products may lead to hepatitis B or C, and food- or water-borne exposures may lead to hepatitis A. Alcohol intake should always be explored. Family history, travel history, occupational exposures, and a careful drug history are also important.

A relatively abrupt onset of nausea, anorexia, and aversion to smoking followed by the development of jaundice suggests a viral hepatitis. A more gradual development of jaundice associated with pruritus suggests obstruction of the biliary tree (cholestasis). If these obstructive symptoms are accompanied by acute or intermittent episodes of pain, gallstones are the most common cause. If the patient has signs of cholestasis but no pain, cancer of the head of the pancreas must be considered, especially if weight loss is also present. Painful jaundice associated with fever suggests acute cholangitis.

Physical Examination

The physical examination of a patient with suspected liver disease should include special attention to the skin, abdomen, and neurology. Jaundice is an abnormal yellow tint to the skin and sclera that is the result of elevations of bilirubin. Palmar erythema, spider angiomas, and bruising may be present on the skin exam.

Liver size and character should be assessed by palpation and percussion. In acute hepatitis, the liver may be enlarged and tender. Alcoholic disease or other causes of fatty infiltration may cause enlargement without tenderness. In cirrhosis, the liver is often small and nodular to palpation and may be accompanied by splenomegaly. Murphy's sign (tenderness to palpation over the gallbladder) usually indicates cholelithiasis.[1] The abdominal examination may show evidence of ascites. The most reliable signs on examination for ascites are "shifting dullness," a palpable fluid wave and bulging flanks in the recumbent position.[2] Ascites is often accompanied by peripheral edema of the lower extremities. In advanced cirrhosis with severe portal hypertension, there may be superficial dilation of veins surrounding the umbilicus ("caput medusae").

In severe cases of liver disease, there may be neurologic and psychiatric manifestations. The classic peripheral finding of asterixis is characterized by a "flapping" tremor of the hands and can be elicited by having the patient hold the arms straight with full extension of the wrists. Hepatic encephalopathy presents with typical manifestations of organic delirium: clouded consciousness, disrupted sleep/arousal cycles, and visual hallucinations.

Laboratory Evaluation

Liver function tests (LFTs) provide indirect evidence of hepatobiliary disease but must always be interpreted in the context of the clinical scenario. Abnormal test results occur in as many as one third of asymptomatic patients screened with multiple test panels, but the incidence of clinically significant unsuspected liver disease is approximately 1%.[3] Aspartate aminotransferase (AST, formerly SGOT) and alanine aminotransferase (ALT, formerly SGPT) are the most commonly used hepatocellular enzymes or transaminases on standard laboratory panels. They are released into the blood when hepatocellular membranes are damaged. AST is found in significant concentrations in many organs of the body, while ALT is more specific to the liver. The pattern of AST and ALT elevations may be a clue to the underlying disease state. In general, alcoholic liver disease has an AST/ALT ratio of 2:1 or greater. Acute viral hepatitis usually has higher ALT levels than AST.

γ-Glutamyltransferase (GGT) is another transaminase that is used on many multiphasic laboratory panels. It may be elevated with minimal hepatocellular damage or with acute alcohol intake without evidence of any histologic damage. Clinically, therefore, it is used mostly to identify the source of elevated alkaline phosphatase levels rather than as a stand-alone test of hepatocellular damage. An increased GGT in the presence of an increased alkaline phosphatase indicates that the alkaline phosphatase is of hepatic origin.

Alkaline phosphatase (AP) is a family of enzymes that are found in liver, bone, placenta, intestine, and kidney. More than 80% of circulating alkaline phosphatase is from the liver and bone. In the liver AP is synthesized by bile epithelial cells, and its synthesis is increased in response to obstruction of the bile duct.[4] For this reason, an elevated AP of liver origin often indicates cholestasis. Liver AP can also rise in infiltrative diseases such as amyloidosis. There are many causes

of elevated AP levels other than primary liver diseases. Adolescents and pregnant women have elevated levels. Levels can also be increased in hyperthyroidism, cardiac failure, trauma, lymphoma, and metastatic cancers. Alkaline phosphatase should only be evaluated in the fasting state.

Bilirubin is a breakdown product of hemoglobin that is actively secreted into the bile ducts by hepatocytes after being conjugated to increase its solubility in water. It may be elevated in either hepatocellular damage or cholestatic disease. Normally 70% of the bilirubin in circulation is unconjugated ("indirect"). An elevation of the unconjugated fraction suggests hemolysis or Gilbert's syndrome. If more than 50% of the bilirubin is conjugated ("direct"), then primary liver disease is more likely to be the cause. The serum conjugated bilirubin does not usually rise until at least one half of the liver's excretory capacity has been disrupted.[4] It is very unusual for extrahepatic obstruction to cause the bilirubin level to rise above 15 mg/dL.

Serum albumin and the prothrombin time (PT) are commonly available blood tests that demonstrate the ability of the liver to produce proteins. Abnormalities of the PT may occur fairly quickly, whereas a low albumin level usually indicates that liver disease has been present for 3 weeks or longer.

When investigating LFT abnormalities, any single abnormal liver test should be confirmed with a second test. For example, an elevated alkaline phosphatase should be followed by a GGT, and an elevated AST should be confirmed with an ALT. The clinician should always search for potential offending drugs, occupational exposures, or other ingestions that may cause reversible LFT abnormalities (Table 90.1). Once a general category of liver disease is suspected, more specific laboratory evaluation may include viral serologies,

Table 90.1. **Common Liver Function Tests**

Test	Abnormality	Common causes	Comments
AST	Hepatocellular damage	Viral hepatitis Toxic/drug reactions Alcoholic disease	AST:ALT >2 suggests alcoholic disease, value rarely greater than 500
ALT	Hepatocellular damage	Viral hepatitis Toxic/drug reactions Alcoholic disease	ALT > AST in acute viral hepatitis, values often in the 1000s
GGT	Hepatocellular damage	Same as above	Use only to confirm that AP is of liver origin; too sensitive to be used alone for diagnosis
AP	Obstruction/infiltration	Cholelithiasis Cholangitis Cancer of pancreas Amyloid	Nonhepatic causes of elevation include bone disease, pregnancy, childhood, nonfasting state
Bilirubin	Hepatocellular, obstructive, or biochemical	Any liver disease	Isolated elevations in Gilbert's disease and hemolysis
Prothrombin time	Biochemical dysfunction	Any process that creates widespread hepatocellular dysfunction	Can be prolonged with dietary deficiency or malabsorption of vitamin K
Albumin	Biochemical dysfunction	Any process that creates widespread hepatocellular dysfunction	Requires 3 weeks of hepatic dysfunction; may also be reduced in acute inflammation, malnutrition or acute illness

ALT = alanine aminotransferase; AP = alkaline phosphatase; AST = aspartate aminotransferase; GGT = γ-glutamyltransferase.

Table 90.2. **Less Common Causes of Chronic Liver Disease and Cirrhosis**

Disorder	Laboratory test	Treatment
Hemochromatosis	Transferrin saturation, ferritin, marrow biopsy	Phlebotomy
Wilson's disease	Ceruloplasmin, serum copper	D-penicillamine
Primary biliary cirrhosis	Antimitochondrial antibody	Ursodiol
Autoimmune hepatitis	Antinuclear antibody, anti–smooth muscle antibody	Immunosuppression
α_1-antitrypsin (A1A) deficiency	A1A activity	α_1-proteinase inhibitor

and tests for hemochromatosis, Wilson's disease, α-antitrypsin deficiency, or autoimmune hepatitis[5] (Table 90.2).

If anatomic imaging is needed, an ultrasound of the liver, gallbladder, and bile ducts is usually the initial study. Computed tomography (CT), magnetic resonance imaging (MRI), and radionuclide studies are usually second-line tests in evaluating liver disease. Liver biopsy is occasionally required for diagnosis and/or management of chronic hepatitis, but it is rare for biopsy to be required in acute hepatitis.

Viral Hepatitis

Viral hepatitis classically presents with a prodrome of generalized fatigue, anorexia, and myalgia prior to the onset of jaundice. Symptoms then progress to nausea, vomiting, and abdominal pain. Other features may include headache, fever, and arthralgias. It is clear from serologic evidence, however, that many people are exposed to viral hepatitis but have only a nonspecific illness or are totally asymptomatic. Certain hepatitis viruses (hepatitis B, C, and D viruses) may cause a chronic illness that can progress to cirrhosis, hepatocellular carcinoma, and liver failure. Any patient with a chronic hepatitis is more likely to progress to these more severe outcomes if there is a second insult to the liver such as ongoing alcohol abuse or acquired immunodeficiency syndrome (AIDS).

Hepatitis A

Hepatitis A virus (HAV) is an RNA enterovirus that is highly contagious and is spread directly or indirectly by the fecal-oral route. It causes an acute, self-limited hepatitis and has no known chronic state.[6] Severe hepatitis from HAV occurs rarely and is more common in the elderly and in patients with underlying chronic hepatitis or cirrhosis from another cause. The average incubation period for the virus is approximately 30 days, and peak viral shedding in the stool occurs prior to the onset of clinical jaundice.

Contamination of food or water with HAV can create epidemics of acute hepatitis. Outbreaks have also been described in day-care and institutional settings. Several parts of the world are endemic for HAV, and travelers from the United States are advised to either be immunized or take immune globulin prior to visiting these areas (current recommendations can be found at the Web site *www.cdc.gov/travel*).[7] The antigenic composition of HAV is remarkably similar throughout the world, which explains the excellent effectiveness of the hepatitis A vaccine.[8]

The diagnosis of acute HAV depends on identification of the immunoglobulin M (IgM)-specific anti-HAV antibody.

This is usually present in the serum by the time jaundice is clinically apparent and is cleared within 4 to 6 months. The immunoglobulin G (IgG) antibody to HAV that subsequently appears persists throughout the patient's lifetime and confers immunity. Treatment of hepatitis A is supportive, and hospitalization is usually necessary only if significant dehydration occurs due to protracted vomiting.

Hepatitis B

Hepatitis B virus (HBV) is a DNA virus that is spread directly through sexual contact, blood exposure, or vertical transmission in the perinatal period. There is both an acute HBV illness and a chronic disease state.[6] Groups at high risk for hepatitis B include intravenous drug users, patients with multiple sexual partners, and patients and staff in institutions for the mentally impaired or prisons. Health care workers are also at increased risk through exposure to infected body fluids.

The incubation of HBV is 4 to 6 weeks, and the prodromal symptoms tend to be more prolonged than in HAV infection. Acute fulminant hepatitis occurs to a small percentage of patients with acute hepatitis B infection, and 5% to 10% of patients develop an acute serum sickness with fever, rash, and arthralgias. Ten percent of patients with acute HBV infection have a relapse of symptoms 2 to 6 months after the original symptoms, but this relapse is usually less severe than the original infection.

The diagnosis of acute hepatitis B infection is made by identification of hepatitis B surface antigen (HBsAg) in the serum. It usually appears before the onset of jaundice and is present for up to 6 months after the acute infection. If the HBsAg persists in the serum beyond 6 months, the patient is considered to have a chronic hepatitis B infection. The disappearance of the HBsAg and the appearance of the hepatitis B surface antibody (HBsAb or anti-HBs) indicate that the patient has cleared the infection and has developed immunity. Anti-HBs will also be found in most patients who have received the hepatitis B vaccine series.

Hepatitis B core antibody (HBcAb or anti-HBc) indicates exposure to the HBV. This antibody first appears during the acute infection and persists for many years or for life. The presence of the anti-HBc does not imply that the HBV has been cleared—chronic carriers will have anti-HBc. Occasionally, anti-HBc is the only identifiable serologic marker found in a patient who has acute HBV infection. This occurs in the "window" between the disappearance of the HBsAg and the appearance of an adequate titer of anti-HBs Figures 90.1 and 90.2 and Table 90.3 provide more detail on the interpretation of HBV serology.

Patients with chronic HBV infection may have an "e" anti-

Fig. 90.1. Typical time course of hepatitis B serology with recovery. (*Source: www.CDC.gov/ NCIDOD/diseases/hepatitis.*)

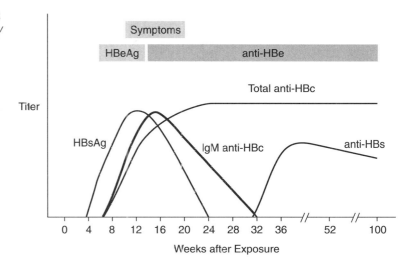

gen (HBeAg, which is not the same as hepatitis E virus) in their serum. The e antigen is a marker for active viral replication, and its presence indicates that the patient is at higher risk for progression to cirrhosis and indicates a higher likelihood of infecting another person if exposure to blood or body fluids occurs.

There is no specific treatment for acute HBV infection other than supportive care. About 5% to 10% of adults, 20% of children, and 90% of neonates and infants who are infected with HBV will go on to chronic infection. Chronic infection leads to cirrhosis in approximately 20% to 30% of patients, and a small percentage of these will go on to hepatocellular carcinoma.

Patients with chronic HBV infection should be evaluated for antiviral therapy to reduce their chance of progressing to cirrhosis and/or hepatocellular carcinoma. The most effective regimen currently in use is a combination of interferon-α and lamivudine.[9] Those patients who develop end-stage liver disease may require liver transplantation.

Hepatitis C

Hepatitis C virus (HCV) is an RNA virus that is transmitted by blood products and by perinatal vertical transmission. Sex-

ual transmissions have been documented but are less common. This virus is responsible for the majority of cases that were previously called "non-A, non-B posttransfusion hepatitis."[6] In comparison to hepatitis B, the acute phase is more likely to be asymptomatic or mild, but patients who acquire HCV are much more likely to develop a chronic hepatitis.[10] Eighty to eighty-five percent of patients infected with HCV develop chronic hepatitis and 20% of these develop cirrhosis (Fig. 90.3).[11]

Although the blood supply in the United States is now quite safe with respect to transmission of HCV,[11] anyone who received a transfusion, organ transplant, or cryoprecipitate prior to 1992 is at risk of having chronic HCV infection and should be screened.[12]

Hepatitis C is diagnosed by demonstrating antibody to HCV in the blood. The initial screening test is usually an enzyme-linked immunoassay (EIA), and a recombinant immunoblot assay (RIBA) is used for confirmation if there is any concern about the initial test being falsely positive.[13]

A quantitative or qualitative RNA viral load test can be done to demonstrate viral particles in the bloodstream. The qualitative test is as much as ten times more sensitive than

Fig. 90.2. Typical time course of hepatitis B serology with chronic infection. (*Source: www. CDC.gov/NCIDOD/diseases/hepatitis.*)

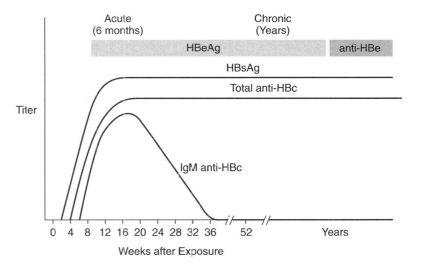

Table 90.3. **Interpretation of the Hepatitis B Panel**

Tests	Results	Interpretation
HBsAg	Negative	Susceptible
Anti-HBc	Negative	
Anti-HBs	Negative	
HBsAg	Negative	Immune due to
Anti-HBc	Negative	vaccination
Anti-HBs	Positive with	
	≥10 mIU/mL[a]	
HBsAg	Negative	Immune due to
Anti-HBc	Positive	natural infection
Anti-HBs	Positive	
HBsAg	Positive	Acutely infected
Anti-HBc	Positive	
IgM anti-HBc	Positive	
Anti-HBs	Negative	
HBsAg	Positive	Chronically infected
Anti-HBc	Positive	
IgM anti-HBc	Negative	
Anti-HBs	Negative	
HBsAg	Negative	Four interpretations
Anti-HBc	Positive	possible[b]
Anti-HBs	Negative	

[a]Postvaccination testing, when it is recommended, should be performed 1–2 months following dose #3.

[b]1. May be recovering from acute HBV infection.

2. May be distantly immune and the test is not sensitive enough to detect a very low level of anti-HBs in serum.

3. May be susceptible with a false-positive anti-HBc.

4. May be chronically infected and have an undetectable level of HBsAg present in the serum.

Source: Immunization Action Coalition publication "Needle Tips," available at *www.immunize.org.*

the quantitative test.[14] Unlike the viral load testing of human immunodeficiency virus (HIV) infection, the quantitative level of RNA copies in HCV does not correlate with the current severity or predict the future progression of disease. The test is useful, however, in following treatment protocols for the patient with HCV. A patient who has a high viral load prior to beginning antiviral treatment has a poorer likelihood of responding to treatment. If a patient receives antiviral therapy and the viral load has not decreased significantly after 3 to 4 months of treatment, the patient's HCV is considered to be nonresponsive to the regimen.[13]

HCV can be separated into several major genotypes and at least 50 different subtypes. This genotypic variability is one of the factors that has made development of a vaccine against HCV difficult.[14] The various genotypes have different levels of responsiveness to current antiviral therapies. Genotype 1 is the most common genotype in the United States, making up approximately 70% of cases. Genotype 1 is the most resistant to current therapies.

One important task for family physicians caring for patients with HCV infection is to decide whether referral for liver biopsy and consideration of treatment is needed. Because treatment decisions are based on the amount of inflammation on the liver biopsy and LFTs are an inconsistent marker for this inflammation, the majority of patients diagnosed with HCV will need to have a liver biopsy. On the other hand, liver biopsy should only be done if it will make a difference in management strategy, so anyone who has a contraindication to treatment should not have a biopsy. Recommendations of the National Institutes of Health (NIH) consensus panel for treatment are listed in Table 90.4.

One of the most controversial topics in the management of HCV has been whether to biopsy a patient who has normal LFTs. A patient with any elevation of LFTs should be considered for treatment because the level of elevation does not correlate with the inflammation found on biopsy. A patient who has normal LFTs at one point in time may have intermittent elevations that are the result of hepatic inflammation. With this in mind, some authorities have stated that every patient who does not have a contraindication to biopsy or treatment should have a liver biopsy. Patients with persistently normal LFTs, however, have a benign course and are very unlikely to progress to cirrhosis of the liver.[15] The NIH consensus conference on hepatitis C that met in 1997 recom-

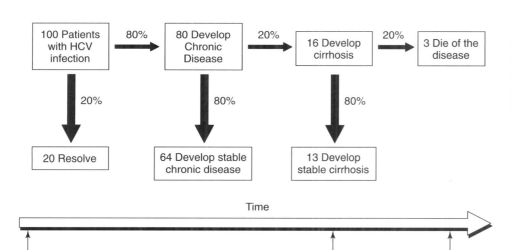

Fig. 90.3. The natural history of HCV infection—the "80/20 rule." These percentages are approximate and vary with population studied and coexistent illnesses.

Table 90.4. **Indications and Contraindications to Treatment of Hepatitis C: Who Should Be Treated for Chronic Hepatitis C?**

Persons recommended for treatment
Treatment is recommended for patients with chronic hepatitis C who are at greatest risk for progression to cirrhosis, as characterized by
Persistently elevated ALT levels;
Detectable HCV RNA; and
A liver biopsy indicating either portal or bridging fibrosis or at least moderate degrees of inflammation and necrosis.

Persons for whom treatment is unclear
Included are
Patients with compensated cirrhosis (without jaundice, ascites, variceal hemorrhage or encephalopathy);
Patients with persistent ALT elevations, but with less severe histologic changes. (In these patients, progression to cirrhosis is likely to be slow, if at all; therefore, observation and serial measurements of ALT and liver biopsy every 3–5 years is an acceptable alternative to treatment with interferon); and
Patients aged <18 years or >60 years.

Persons for whom treatment is not recommended
Included are
Patients with persistently normal ALT values;
Patients with advanced cirrhosis who might be at risk for decompensation with therapy;
Patients who are currently drinking excessive amounts of alcohol or who are injecting illegal drugs; and
Persons with major depressive illness, cytopenias, hyperthyroidism, renal transplantation, evidence of autoimmune disease, or who are pregnant.

Source: Centers for Disease Control and Prevention. Recommendations for prevention and control of hepatitis C virus infection and HCV-related chronic disease. MMWR 1998;47(RR-19):1–54.

mended against treating patients with HCV infection and persistently normal transaminase levels even though most such patients have some evidence of inflammation on liver biopsy.[13] This recommendation may change in the future if more effective and less toxic antiviral regimens are found.

Most patients being treated for HCV infection currently receive a combination of interferon and ribavirin for 6 to 12 months. A new form of interferon known as pegylated interferon has improved overall response rates to therapy and allows once-weekly dosing. Treatment of HCV infection is an area of active research, and treatment regimens are likely to change rapidly in the next several years.

Other Viral Agents

Hepatitis D and E are far less common than the viral hepatitides described above. Hepatitis D (formerly called delta hepatitis) occurs only as a co-infection with hepatitis B but frequently causes a much more severe acute illness than HBV alone. Fulminant hepatitis and death are more common with hepatitis D than the other viral hepatitides. Hepatitis E is similar to hepatitis A in that it is transmitted enterically and is generally a self-limited illness. Hepatitis G has recently been described and has been found in about 1% of American blood donors. Its clinical significance is uncertain at this time. Epstein-Barr virus, cytomegalovirus, and other herpesviruses can also cause an acute hepatitis.

Human Immunodeficiency Virus

Although the human immunodeficiency virus (HIV) does not commonly cause a primary viral hepatitis, it is important in the natural history and treatment of patients with chronic hepatitis due to other viruses. Co-infection of HIV with both HBV and HCV is common, especially among intravenous drug abusers. Patients with co-infection are more likely to have progression of their chronic hepatitis. They are more likely to have a suboptimal response to antiviral therapies aimed at HCV and often have their treatment complicated by medication interactions and direct liver toxicity of their antiretroviral therapy. Any patient discovered to have chronic HBV or HCV infection should have serologic testing for HIV (also see Chapter 42).

Prevention of Viral Hepatitis

Preventive measures for hepatitis A include rigorous hand washing, particularly among food handlers and day-care workers, and proper sanitation and wastewater disposal. Patients who believe they have been recently exposed to HAV should receive immune globulin within 2 weeks of the exposure at a dose of 0.02 mg/kg intramuscularly. Anyone who anticipates a future exposure (such as foreign travel to an endemic region) should be vaccinated. The vaccine provides protection against HAV within 4 weeks of the initial dose. The complete vaccination series, which provides extended immunity, includes a second vaccination 6 months after the first.[7]

Because of the increased risk of severe hepatitis, patients with chronic hepatitis or cirrhosis should receive hepatitis A vaccine. The vaccine and/or immune globulin are also given under the direction of public health authorities in specific outbreaks of HAV.

Prevention of hepatitis B and C involves proper blood bank screening procedures, universal blood exposure precautions for health care workers, avoidance of multiple sexual contacts and the sharing of intravenous needles, surveillance of pregnant women, and immunization.[16,17]

All pregnant women should be screened for the presence of HBsAg early in pregnancy, and this should be repeated if the patient is at risk of acquiring the infection during the preg-

Table 90.5. **Doses of Hepatitis A and B Vaccines**

Recommended dosages and schedules of hepatitis A vaccines					
Vaccine	Age group	Dose	Volume	# Doses	Schedule
Havrix	2–18 years	720 El.U.	0.5 mL	2	0, 6–12 months
(GlaxoSmithKline)	19 years and older	1440 El.U.	1.0 mL	2	0, 6–12 months
Vaqta	2–18 years	25 U	0.5 mL	2	0, 6–18 months
(Merck & Co.)	19 years and older	50 U	1.0 mL	2	0, 6–12 months

El.U. = Elisa units; U = units.

Recommended dosages of hepatitis B vaccines[a]				
Vaccine brand	Age group	Dose	Volume	# Doses
Engerix-B	0–19 years	10 μg	0.5 mL	3
(GlaxoSmithKline)	20 years and older	20 μg	1.0 mL	3
Recombivax HB	0–19 years	5 μg	0.5 mL	3
(Merck & Co.)	11–15 years	10 μg	1.0 mL	2
	20 years and older	10 μg	1.0 mL	3

[a]The schedule for hepatitis B vaccination is flexible and varies. Consult the ACIP statement on hepatitis B (11/91), AAP's *2000 Red Book*, or the package insert for details.

Note: For adult dialysis patients, the Engerix-B dose required is 40 μg/2.0 mL (use the adult 20 μg/mL formulation) on a schedule of 0, 1, 2, and 6 months. For Recombivax HB, a special formulation for dialysis patients is available. The dose is 40 μg/1.0 mL and it is given on a schedule of 0, 1, and 6 months.

Source: CDC.[17] Immunization Action Coalition publication, "Needle Tips," available at *www.immunize.org.*

nancy. Infants born to mothers with HBsAg should receive hepatitis B immune globulin (HBIG) and their first HBV vaccine within the first 12 hours of life.[17]

When HBV vaccine was first available, a strategy of immunizing high-risk individuals was begun. This was very successful in reaching health care workers, patients with hemophilia, and those on dialysis, but was unsuccessful in reaching intravenous drug users, prostitutes, and others at risk on the basis of lifestyle. Because of this, universal infant hepatitis B vaccination is now standard in the United States. Catch-up vaccination schedules for adolescents and adults who are not yet immunized but are at risk for HBV are available as well. Anyone who is not immune to HBV but becomes exposed should receive HBIG and begin a primary immunization series. Table 90.5 lists the dosing of vaccines for HAV and HBV.

Alcoholic Hepatitis

Alcohol and its metabolites are toxic to hepatocytes and can cause both acute hepatitis and chronic liver disease. Acute alcoholic hepatitis is clinically very similar to the acute viral hepatitis described in the previous section with the exception that there is usually no fever or viral prodrome. The AST/ALT ratio is usually 2:1 or greater in alcoholic injury and the GGT is usually at least twice normal.[5] With abstinence from alcohol and supportive care, the acute liver injury may be totally reversible. Patients with alcoholic liver disease are often malnourished and require nutritional supplementation, especially thiamine and folate. Markers for poor prognosis include abnormal coagulation studies, azotemia, bilirubin level >15 mg/dL, and encephalopathy.[18]

Alcohol is the most common cause of chronic liver disease, cirrhosis, and hepatocellular carcinoma in the United States and is often a cofactor in patients with chronic liver disease

from other causes. Patients with cirrhosis from any cause who continue to abuse alcohol have a much worse prognosis with increased risk of progression to end-stage liver disease and hepatocellular carcinoma.

Toxic Hepatic Injury

Many drugs have the potential to cause acute liver injury. Many more can cause transient hepatocellular enzyme elevations that are of uncertain clinical significance.[5] One of the most frequent causes of toxic hepatic injury is acute or chronic overdose of acetaminophen. Other common medications that may cause liver injury include sulfonamides, estrogens, isoniazid, nitrofurantoin, amiodarone, methotrexate, allopurinol, valproic acid, and any of the hepatic hydroxymethylglutaryl coenzyme A (HMG CoA) reductase inhibitors.[19] Other toxic exposures, including industrial exposure to carbon tetrachloride and vitamin A overdose, may also cause serious liver disease (see Table 90.6 for a more complete list).

Other Causes of Chronic Liver Disease

Although a significant majority of chronic liver disease in the United States is caused by alcohol and viral agents, physicians must also consider some of the other potential causes.[5] Table 90.2 lists several of the less common causes of liver disease that may require investigation.

Hemochromatosis is particularly important because of its relative frequency, its subtle clinical presentation, and the need for early diagnosis and treatment. Patients with hemochromatosis have an inherited propensity to absorb excess iron leading to high levels of iron stored in the body. Hereditary hemochromatosis (HH) is an autosomal-recessive dis-

Table 90.6. **Substances That Are Reported to Cause Liver Damage**

Class	Examples
Nonsteroidal antiinflammatory agents	Ibuprofen, naproxen, ketoprofen, rofecoxib, celecoxib, others
Pain relievers	Acetaminophen
HMG CoA reductase inhibitors	Atorvastatin, lovastatin, simvastatin, others
Niacin	
Fibric acid derivatives	Gemfibrozil, fenofibrate
Thiazolidinediones	Pioglitazone, rosiglitazone
Sulfonylureas	Glipizide
Anticonvulsants	Carbamazepine, phenytoin, valproic acid
Cholinesterase inhibitors	Tacrine
Antibiotics	Sulfonamides, nitrofurantoin, ciprofloxacin, synthetic penicillins, isoniazid
Antifungals	Ketoconazole, fluconazole, amphotericin
Antivirals	Dideoxyinosine (ddI), zidovudine (AZT)
Protease inhibitors	Ritonavir, indinavir
Hormones	Estrogens, tamoxifen
Antirheumatic agents	Methotrexate
Cardiovascular agents	Amiodarone, methyldopa
Nutritional supplements	Chaparral, comfrey, germander, pennyroyal, ephedra, ji bu huan, gentian, senna, shark cartilage, scutellaria ("skullcap"), alchemilla ("lady's mantle"), valerian, high-dose vitamin A
Substances of abuse	Cocaine, phencyclidine ("angel dust"), glues and solvents, MDMA ("ecstasy"), anabolic steroids

This list includes many substances that are known to cause liver damage but is not a comprehensive list of all known toxins.

ease with an estimated gene frequency of 8% in the North American population and a clinical prevalence of 4 to 6 per 1000 in primary care populations.[20] Clinical manifestations of hemochromatosis occur earlier and more frequently in men because iron loss through menstruation, pregnancy, and breast-feeding are partially protective for women. HH causes a wide array of symptoms in many systems of the body including sexual impotence with testicular atrophy, a "bronzing" hyperpigmentation of the skin, arthropathy, type II diabetes mellitus, hyperlipidemia, and heart failure. In the liver, hemosiderin deposition leads to cirrhosis.[21]

The diagnosis of HH is made on the basis of abnormal iron studies. A transferrin saturation of greater than 45% is the most commonly recommended screening test. Any patient with an elevated transferrin saturation should have a repeat fasting transferrin saturation and a serum ferritin level. A fasting transferrin saturation of greater than 55% along with a serum ferritin of greater than 200 μg/L in women or greater than 300 μg/L in men is highly suggestive of HH. Liver biopsy will show increased iron stores in the liver and is usually recommended to make a definitive diagnosis. Prognosis for patients who are identified early and undergo therapeutic phlebotomy is excellent. When a patient is identified with HH, family members should be screened with either iron studies or genotyping since early treatment with phlebotomy is beneficial.

Cirrhosis of the Liver

Cirrhosis is the common end stage of a number of chronic liver diseases. The clinical features of cirrhosis are the result of liver scarring with subsequent portal hypertension and abnormal protein production. Esophageal varices, ascites, and splenomegaly may be caused by portal hypertension. Hypoalbuminemia, low levels of vitamin K–dependent clotting factors, thrombocytopenia, and anemia may also occur. Hyponatremia is a common finding in patients with cirrhosis and may be complicated by diuretics and sodium restriction. If the cirrhosis progresses, death is usually the result of gastrointestinal bleeding (from portal hypertension and coagulopathy), hepatorenal syndrome, encephalopathy, or bacterial peritonitis.

Effective therapy of the underlying cause of the cirrhosis can arrest progression of liver injury in many cases and may permit substantial clinical improvement.[22] Management of cirrhosis is supportive with particular attention to maintaining abstinence from alcohol and giving nutritional support. Patients with cirrhosis are often malnourished for many reasons. Thus, protein restriction is no longer routinely recommended, even in patients with encephalopathy. Most patients need routine supplementation of thiamine, folate, calcium, and a multivitamin. They should generally avoid iron supplementation.

Sodium restriction (88 mmol/day or 2000 mg/day) as well as diuretics may be beneficial for patients with symptomatic ascites. Fluid restriction is not usually necessary, and the hyponatremia commonly seen in cirrhotic ascites seldom needs treatment. An agent active at the distal tubule, such as spironolactone (Aldactone) is usually the first diuretic used. In severe cases, loop diuretics such as furosemide (Lasix) may need to be added.[23]

Patients who are at risk for or have had an episode of bacterial peritonitis should be on daily prophylactic antibiotics to prevent recurrence. Regimens that have been studied include ciprofloxacin (Cipro) 750 mg once weekly, trimethoprim-sulfamethoxazole (Septra, Bactrim) one double-strength tablet 5 days/week, and norfloxacin (Noroxin) 400 mg daily.[24]

Patients who are at moderate risk for variceal hemorrhage

should receive a nonselective beta-blocker such as propranolol (Inderal) or nadolol (Corgard) to reduce this risk. Those at high risk (especially those with a previous bleeding episode) should have banding or sclerotherapy of the varices.

Patients with encephalopathy should have potential underlying causes (particularly infection) investigated and treated appropriately. In addition, they should receive oral lactulose in doses adjusted to produce several loose stools daily. Metronidazole (Flagyl) is now favored over neomycin sulfate for long-term suppression of intestinal bacterial flora because of the ototoxicity and nephrotoxicity of the neomycin. Metronidazole should not be used in the face of active alcohol consumption.[23]

Liver Transplantation

Patients with advanced cirrhosis of the liver may be candidates for liver transplantation. One- and five-year survival rates at established transplantation centers are typically 90% and 80% or better. Contraindications to transplantation include active alcoholism or substance abuse, seropositivity for HIV, and severe cardiac or pulmonary disease. Most transplantation centers require a minimum of 6 months of abstinence from alcohol before placing a patient on the waiting list for transplantation. The greatest barrier to transplantation remains a shortage of transplantable organs. Each year the number of eligible transplant recipients exceeds the supply of available organs by a factor of 5 to 10.[25]

Hepatocellular Carcinoma

Metastatic tumors are by far the most common cancers found in the liver, with colon cancer being the most common primary source (see Chapter 92). Most cases of primary hepatocellular carcinoma (HCC) arise in patients who have chronic liver damage. Surveillance studies suggest an annual rate of HCC of 1% to 4% in patients with established cirrhosis. The average time from the onset of hepatitis to the development of HCC is 30 years. Worldwide, hepatitis B is the most common cause, while alcoholic liver disease and hepatitis C are the most common causes in North America. A larger percentage of patients with chronic liver disease from HCV go on to HCC than those infected with HBV. Patients who are co-infected with HCV and HIV are at particular risk to progress to hepatocellular carcinoma. There is no effective chemotherapy for HCC, and recurrence after resection is common.

Many authorities recommend screening for the development of HCC in patients with cirrhosis with serum α-fetoprotein (AFP) testing and serial imaging studies. This strategy has not been adequately evaluated in randomized trials, and there is no evidence that it reduces mortality.[26]

Summary

The evaluation of abnormal liver function tests and management of patients with alcoholic and viral hepatitis are the most common liver problems encountered by family physicians. Although the incidence of new infections with HCV and HBV have diminished significantly with better blood banking procedures and HBV vaccination, there is still a large cohort of patients who have chronic hepatitis from previous infection. These patients will continue to need medical care as they develop complications of their hepatitis during the next several decades. Further prevention of new cases requires aggressive vaccination strategies, public health measures, and education to reduce the spread of hepatitis through intravenous drug use and sexual transmission.

Screening and intervention strategies for alcoholism and other substance abuse are discussed in Chapter 59. Alcoholism is encountered in almost every conceivable setting of family practice, and all family physicians should be familiar with this illness.

References

1. Naylor CD. Physical examination of the liver. JAMA 1994;271:1859–65.
2. Williams JW, Simel DL. Does this patient have ascites? JAMA 1992;267:2645–8.
3. Kamath PS. Clinical approach to the patient with abnormal liver test results. Mayo Clin Proc 1996;71:1089–95.
4. Johnston DE. Special considerations in interpreting liver function tests. Am Fam Physician 1999;59:2223–30.
5. Pratt DS. Kaplan MM. Evaluation of abnormal liver-enzyme results in asymptomatic patients. N Engl J Med 2000;342:1266–71.
6. Hepatitis, 2001. Available at *www.cdc.gov/ncidod/disease/hepatitis.htm.*
7. Prevention of hepatitis A through active or passive immunization: recommendations of the advisory committee on immunization practices (ACIP). MMWR 1999;48:1–37.
8. Keeffe EB, Iwarson S, McMahon BJ, et al. Safety and immunogenicity of hepatitis A vaccine in patients with chronic liver disease. Hepatology 1998;27:881–6.
9. Terrault NA. Combined interferon and lamivudine therapy: is this the treatment of choice for patients with chronic hepatitis B virus infection? Hepatology 2000;32:675–7.
10. Hoofnagle JH. Hepatitis C: The clinical spectrum of disease. Hepatology 1997;26(suppl 1):15S–20S.
11. Seeff LB. Natural history of hepatitis C. Hepatology 1997; 26(suppl 1):21S–28S.
12. Recommendations for prevention and control of hepatitis C virus (HCV) infection and HCV-related chronic disease. MMWR 1998; 47:1–39.
13. National Institutes of Health consensus development conference panel statement: management of hepatitis C. Hepatology 1997; 26(suppl 1):1S–10S.
14. Larson AM, Carithers RL. Hepatitis C in clinical practice. J Intern Med 2001;249:111–20.
15. Marcellin P, Levy S, Erlinger S. Therapy of hepatitis C: patients with normal aminotransferase levels. Hepatology 1997;26(suppl 1):133S–6S.
16. Update: recommendations to prevent hepatitis B virus transmission—United States. JAMA 1995;274:603–4.
17. CDC. Hepatitis B virus: a comprehensive strategy for eliminating transmission in the United States through universal childhood vaccination: recommendations of the ACIP. MMWR 1991;40:1–19.
18. Lieber CS. Medical disorders of alcoholism. N Engl J Med 1995; 333:1058–65.

19. Lewis JH. Drug-induced liver disease. Med Clin North Am 2000;84:1275–311.
20. Phatak PD, Sham RL, Raubertas RF, et al. Prevalence of hereditary hemochromatosis in 16,031 primary care patients. Ann Intern Med 1998;129:954–61.
21. Hemochromatosis management working group. Management of hemochromatosis. Ann Intern Med 1998;129:932–9.
22. Habib A, Bond WM, Heuman DM. Long-term management of cirrhosis. Postgrad Med 2001;109:101–8.
23. Runyon BA. Management of adult patients with ascites caused by cirrhosis. Hepatology 1998;27:264–72.
24. Rimola A, Garcia-Tsao G, Navasa M, Piddock LJ, Planas R, Bernard B. Diagnosis, treatment and prophylaxis of spontaneous bacterial peritonitis: a consensus document. J Hepatol 2000;32: 142–53.
25. United network for organ sharing, 2001. Available at *www.unos.org*.
26. Collier J, Sherman M. Screening for hepatocellular carcinoma. Hepatology 1998;27:273–8.

91
Diseases of the Rectum and Anus

Thomas J. Zuber

Anorectal disorders represent some of the most common, yet poorly understood conditions in primary care. Any discussion of these conditions requires a thorough understanding of the anorectal anatomy (Figs. 91.1 and 91.2). The anal canal spans 2 to 3 cm from the lower border of the anal crypts at the dentate line to the anal verge (external skin).[1] The anal canal is lined with a specialized squamous epithelium called anoderm.[1] Sensory innervation from the external skin extends upward to the dentate line. Most patients have no sensation above the dentate line and are exquisitely sensitive below it.

Internal and external hemorrhoids are discussed here in detail, as patients often attribute all anorectal complaints to "hemorrhoids." Other conditions that are reviewed include anal fissures, abscesses, fistulas, incontinence, rectal prolapse, pruritus ani, infectious proctitis, hidradenitis suppurativa, condyloma acuminatum, and anal carcinoma.

Hemorrhoids

It is estimated that 50% to 75% of United States adults suffer at some time from hemorrhoids.[2,3] Hemorrhoids are distended vascular cushions that line the anal canal.[4-7] Internal hemorrhoids are composed, in part, of the dilated terminal tributaries of the superior and middle rectal veins, appearing above the dentate line.[2] External hemorrhoids are composed of the dilated tributaries of the inferior rectal vein, appearing below the dentate line[2] (Fig. 91.1). Mixed hemorrhoids are composed of both internal and external hemorrhoids.

The anal cushions are composed of arterioles and venules,[6,7] so describing internal hemorrhoids as simple "varicose veins" is inaccurate. The submucosal anchoring and connective tissue structure inside an anal cushion can become worn by chronic straining or from trauma from passing inspissated stool.[3] Ablative treatments for internal hemorrhoids attempt to re-create connective tissue anchoring by scarring the mucosa to the underlying tissues.[3]

The entire anal canal must be thoroughly investigated before initiating treatment for hemorrhoids. Patients can be examined in the knee-chest position, but most practitioners prefer the Sims' or left lateral decubitus position. The slotted Ives anoscope (Redfield Corporation, Montvale, NJ) provides excellent visualization of a full anal cushion or hemorrhoids above and below the dentate line. Once the pathology is identified, patients can be offered appropriate treatment interventions for their stage or severity of disease (Table 91.1).

Hemorrhoids tend to be a recurring problem.[5] Lifestyle changes are important to limit the need for repeated treatments and should be recommended for all patients.[4] The initial use of stool softeners and the long-term use of stool bulking agents can reduce straining and trauma to the anal canal.[4,5,8-10] Patients should be encouraged to drink six full glasses of water a day and consume at least five servings of fresh fruits and fresh vegetables daily.[9] Prolonged sitting should be avoided, and patients should be educated not to delay toileting once the rectum fills.

Internal Hemorrhoids

Most patients with internal hemorrhoids present with painless rectal bleeding. Internal hemorrhoids generally develop at the fixed positions of the anal cushions within the anal canal[2,4,5,8] (Fig. 91.2). Several new ablative techniques offer effective, less expensive treatments (Table 91.1). Patients with severe bleeding, persistent prolapse, or failure to respond to conservative modalities may require surgical intervention.[5]

The rubber band ligation technique effectively strangulates the internal hemorrhoid.[1,3] A small rubber band is loaded onto a hollow applicator, the hemorrhoid is pulled inside the applicator, and the rubber band is released to the base of the hemorrhoid.[1,5,8] The hemorrhoid sloughs off during the following 1 to 2 weeks.[3] Moderate pain can follow this procedure, as can the rare but significant complication of pelvic sepsis.[8,11] Any patient with pelvic pain, fever, and inability

Fig. 91.1. Anorectal anatomy and hemorrhoids.

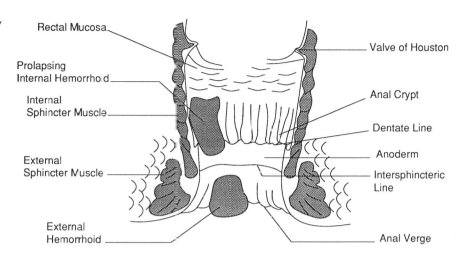

to urinate following rubber band ligation must be immediately evaluated for this potentially fatal complication.[11]

Infrared photocoagulation is an easily performed office treatment for internal hemorrhoids.[3] A 15-volt tungsten-halogen lamp provides a controlled energy emission at the tip of the instrument.[3] The energy causes tissue destruction up to 3 mm in depth, and subsequent scar formation tethers the hemorrhoidal vessels to the underlying tissues and reduces blood flow into the hemorrhoid.[3] Multiple timed pulses lasting 1.0 to 1.5 seconds are administered at the upper (proximal) portion of the internal hemorrhoid.

Infrared treatments have been described as a "painless" intervention by some authors.[3] Most patients experience a mild

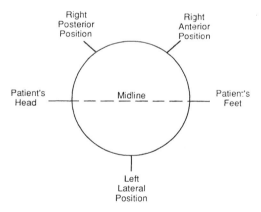

Fig. 91.2. When examining a patient who is lying in the left lateral decubitus (Sims') position, the patient's head is to the left and the feet are to the right. The midline of the canal is parallel to the floor. The circle represents the dentate line. The three anal cushions (and locations for the development of internal hemorrhoids) generally are located at the 10 o'clock position (right posterior), 2 o'clock position (right anterior), and 6 o'clock position (left lateral). This type of circular drawing can be included in the patient's chart when evaluating hemorrhoids, with pathology drawn inside (above the dentate line) or outside the circle to document disease location and severity.

burning sensation,[10] but the treatment is performed without anesthesia and is well tolerated. Pelvic sepsis has not been noted following infrared treatment.

Bipolar diathermy and galvanic destruction are two methods of electrosurgical destruction of internal hemorrhoids.[3] Both treatments appear to be effective and safe, and each can be used for higher grade (grade 3 or 4) hemorrhoids. The galvanic destruction technique requires at least 10 minutes of treatment time, compared to a few seconds for infrared or bipolar diathermy treatments.

Some therapies for internal hemorrhoids have been largely discontinued. Sclerotherapy has significant risks, including mucosal sloughing, thrombosis, abscess formation, and bacteremia.[5] Cryotherapy has a high cure rate but produces tremendous watery discharge and can result in sphincter muscle damage and anal stenosis.[3,5] Surgical excision is occasionally required, but other destructive modalities can be employed first. Laser hemorrhoidectomy is expensive and is associated with slower healing rates than standard surgical excision.[12]

External Hemorrhoids

Uncomplicated, nonthrombosed external hemorrhoids rarely require surgical intervention.[5] Novice examiners may mistake external tags for a true external hemorrhoid.[2] A tag results from a prior hemorrhoid that has thrombosed, scarred, and effectively lost its blood supply.[2] Rarely tags cause itching or interfere with hygiene, but they generally are left untreated.

Thrombosed external hemorrhoids can cause extreme pain and disability and are common in pregnant patients and young adults.[13] Patients present with a tender perianal mass, and the bluish blood clot often can be seen through the skin. If the patient presents with the thrombosed hemorrhoid during the first few days or if it ruptures, excision of the thrombosed hemorrhoid is indicated.[5,8] Simple incision and drainage of the clot frequently results in spontaneous reclosure of the skin, rethrombosis, and recurrent pain in 24 hours.[5,8]

Excision of a thrombosed external hemorrhoid can be facilitated by adequate exposure created by an assistant retracting the buttocks laterally.[5] Lidocaine (1–2%) can be ad-

Table 91.1. **Grading and Treatment Recommendations for Internal Hemorrhoids**

Grade	Appearance	Treatment options
I	Excessive bulging above the mucosal surface without prolapse	Conservative management with fiber, stool bulking agents, dietary vegetables
II	Prolapse with defecation and spontaneous reduction	Dietary management Infrared coagulation Electrosurgical ablation Rubber band ligation
III	Prolapse that requires manual reduction	Infrared coagulation Electrosurgical ablation Rubber band ligation Surgical or laser hemorrhoidectomy
IV	Prolapse that cannot be reduced manually	Surgical hemorrhoidectomy Laser hemorrhoidectomy Electrosurgical ablation

ministered above and around the hemorrhoid. An elliptical excision is performed, removing overlying skin and the entire clot.[1,5,14] Electrocautery can be employed for hemostasis, and the wound can be left open or closed with a running subcuticular absorbable suture.

Thrombosed hemorrhoids that have been present for more than 48 to 72 hours generally are best treated conservatively.[5,14,15] After 3 days time, the pain produced by surgical intervention frequently is greater than the pain that occurs with spontaneous resolution. The mass usually reduces slowly over the next few weeks.[5]

Nonhemorrhoidal Anorectal Diseases

Anal Fissure

A fissure is a crack or tear in the anal mucosa, usually produced by the passage of hard stool.[16,17] The lesion classically is associated with bleeding and intense pain at defecation.[16,17] Patients often complain of a sharp, cutting, or tearing sensation. Nearly half of the patients present with the complaint of hemorrhoids.[16]

Anal fissures most commonly appear in the midline of the anal canal, with 90% in the posterior midline.[8,16,17] Fissures outside the midline can be associated with other disease states such as Crohn's disease, tuberculosis, or syphilis.[8] A search for associated pathology should be initiated whenever a fissure is found outside the midline (see Chapters 41 and 88).

Because fissures develop in the heavily innervated anoderm, the pain of a fissure often is out of proportion to the lesion's size.[9] They can be diagnosed from the history, digital examination, and anoscopy. When examining for fissures, the sphincter muscle spasm can be overcome by gentle but persistent lateral separation of the edges of the anal orifice using traction of the gloved fingers to the side of the anus.[17]

Once discovered, many fissures heal over a few weeks time with rigorous efforts to soften the stools.[8,16] Stool softeners, increased fluid intake, sitz baths, and stool bulking agents may be helpful.[8,9,16] Lidocaine 2% jelly may assist with pain when applied to the tissues just prior to a bowel movement.

Unhealed fissures can give rise to chronic, intermittent, or continuous symptoms.[16] Recurrent tearing of the anoderm with the passage of each stool can result in a chronic fissure. The anal crypt immediately above the chronic fissure (at the dentate line) can become swollen and edematous, resulting in a hypertrophied anal papilla or polyp.[16,17] Distal to the fissure (at the anal verge) may be a larger sentinel skin tag or sentinel pile.[17] This swelling on the outer edge of the anal canal can serve as a marker for a fissure immediately above.[16,17]

The internal anal sphincter muscle may develop spasm from the presence of the overlying fissure. Over time the fissure may deepen, and the spastic muscle becomes fibrotic and contracted.[17] Conservative measures often fail once the muscle becomes fibrosed. Topical nitroglycerin ointment can reduce sphincter muscle contraction while the fissure is healing.[18–20] Early studies used 0.2% ointment; commercially available products in the United States (2% nitroglycerin ointment) generally should be diluted.[19,20] The ointment sometimes produces headaches and syncope in young patients. Botulinum toxin 20 units injected in two divided doses into the anal sphincter on both sides of the canal appears even more effective.[21,22]

Surgery for anal fissures usually is limited to patients who have persisting fissures unresponsive to conservative measures. Lateral internal sphincterotomy, which releases the contracted muscle, is the most widely recommended intervention.[16,17] This surgery is performed by inserting a thin cataract or no. 11 blade through the perianal skin between the external and internal sphincter muscles. The blade is teased toward a gloved finger in the rectum, dividing the fibrotic internal sphincter. The blade should not cut all the way through to the mucosa.[17] Incontinence occasionally results from the procedure, limiting the use of surgery for fissures.

Anorectal Abscess

An anorectal abscess results from cellulitis or infection of the glands and crypts at the dentate line.[8,17,23] Both aerobic and anaerobic bacteria may be noted within an anorectal abscess.[17] Some reports suggest a higher incidence of the abscesses among men. Anorectal abscesses usually are obvious, producing diffuse swelling, erythema, and pain around the anus. Most abscesses are aggravated by sitting, coughing, sneezing, and defecating.[17] Anterior abscesses in women are occasionally confused with Bartholin's abscesses (see Chapter 102).

Anorectal abscesses are classified according to their location. A common classification system divides them into perianal, ischiorectal, submuous (or high intermuscular), and pelvirectal.[8,17,23] Perianal abscesses represent half of all anorectal abscesses[8] and appear as ovoid swellings in close proximity to the anus. Fluctuance may be noted on the perianal skin, and spontaneous drainage of a perianal abscess commonly occurs.

Ischiorectal abscesses produce a more diffuse, brawny swelling of the entire perianal region.[17] Digital examination may reveal a bulging in the anal canal. High intermuscular abscesses can be difficult to diagnose. They can produce a chronic aching that is relieved once the abscess bursts and drains pus into the rectum.[17]

Anorectal abscesses should be surgically drained upon discovery.[8,17,23] Perianal abscesses can be drained by a cruciate incision (in the shape of a plus sign) made as close as possible to the anal verge.[8] Direct compression of the tissues expresses the pus, and an iodoform gauze drain can be placed within the abscess cavity for 24 hours or replaced for longer treatment periods. Antibiotics should not be used in place of surgical drainage, and their use after drainage is debated.

Anal Fistula

An anal fistula is a chronic granulating tract connecting two epithelial-lined surfaces.[8,17] Simple fistulas usually have a single external skin opening and a single internal opening in the anal canal or rectal mucosa. More complicated fistulas can have a complex course and multiple external openings. The wall of the tract is lined with a thick, tough layer of fibrous tissue.[17]

Anal fistulas most commonly develop following pyogenic abscesses.[8,17] Small crypt abscesses along the dentate line may serve as a reservoir for repeated infection from enteric bacteria.[17] Three fourths of all fistulas are low anal or low intersphincteric fistulas.[17] Low intersphincteric fistulas extend upward from the skin between the external and internal sphincter muscles and then dive through the internal sphincter to the dentate line.

Anal fistulas are predominantly found in middle-aged men.[17] Patients frequently give the history that they had a prior abscess that burst, producing a chronic intermittent discharge.[17] Anal fistulas generally are painless, but when associated with inflammatory bowel disease patients may complain of additional bowel symptoms (see Chapter 88). When examining a patient with a fistula, inquiry should be made about changes in bowel habits, passage of mucus and blood, abdominal pain, and weight loss.

The anal skin can exhibit a single or multiple fistular openings. An opening may be situated on the summit of a pink or red nodule of granulation tissue, and palpation of the perianal skin may express pus through the opening. Gentle injection of a dye solution or the use of a probe can identify the course of a fistula tract. Probing in the office setting is discouraged, as it may result in pseudotracts and distortion of the anatomy.[8] Any patient identified with a fistula should be referred for definitive surgical care.[8]

Many surgical and ablative procedures have been devised for fistulas. Most authors recommend opening the fistula tract,

with healing accomplished by wound granulation or by performing primary closure.[17] Setons made of silk or rubber bands can be threaded through the fistula and tightened sequentially, producing necrosis of the overlying tissues and externalization of the fibrous tract.[17]

Anal Incontinence

Anal incontinence is loss of control of flatus and feces.[17,24] There are many causes for anal incontinence, some of which appear in Table 91.2. Young patients with incontinence may suffer from congenital anorectal deformities, secondary megacolon from chronic constipation, or trauma to the anal sphincter apparatus.[17,24] Ulcerative colitis can produce anorectal abscesses that destroy the sphincter musculature (see Chapter 88). Mass lesions such as carcinoma, rectal prolapse, or large hemorrhoids also can produce mechanical interference in canal closure and subsequent incontinence.[17]

Functional fecal incontinence is defined as recurrent uncontrolled passage of fecal material in a person without evidence of neurologic or structural etiologies.[25] The new definition suggests that an individual must be at least 4 years of age, and that the incontinence can be associated with either diarrhea or constipation in an individual with a normal anal sphincter structure.[25] The new definition for functional disease includes the 25% of patients with diarrhea-predominant irritable bowel syndrome who experience incontinence.[25]

Older women are particularly at risk for incontinence due to progressive denervation of the pelvic floor musculature from prior birth-related injury.[24] The aging process can produce decreasing resting sphincter pressures, increased colonic transit time, and decreased sensitivity to rectal distention in both genders. Debilitated elderly patients or those with dementia are particularly prone to incontinence. Efforts should be made to establish a routine of daily stooling, fiber, and stool bulking agents to limit soiling by the elderly (see Chapter 24).

Incontinence frequently is associated with fecal impaction

Table 91.2. **Some Causes of Anal Incontinence**

Congenital abnormalities (before and after surgery), such as ectopic anus
Neurologic conditions such as tabes dorsalis, spina bifida, cerebral vascular accident, dementia
Birth-related neurologic damage to the pelvic floor musculature resulting from compression injury by the head at delivery
Trauma
    Accidental impalement into the anorectal tissues
    Obstetric tears
    Operative trauma (fistula, hemorrhoids)
    Rectal surgery such as internal sphincterotomy, fistulectomy
Secondary megacolon due to chronic constipation
Rectal prolapse
Large prolapsing third- or fourth-degree hemorrhoids
Ulcerative colitis with perirectal abscesses
Carcinoma of the anal canal
Amebic dysentery
Impaction of feces
Old age and general debility
Rectovaginal fistula
Radiation enteritis
Diarrheal states

in the elderly.[17] Fecal impaction occurs when a large, firm, immovable mass of stool develops in the rectum owing to incomplete evacuation of stool.[26] Fecal impaction can be managed by breaking up the mass with a gentle gloved finger or instrument and removing the inspissated stool.[17,26]

Rectal Prolapse

Complete rectal prolapse, or procidentia, is the abnormal descent of all layers of the rectal wall with or without protrusion through the anus.[27] Partial rectal prolapse, or prolapse of only the rectal mucosa, is most frequently encountered in children between the ages of 1 and 5, and in the elderly. Partial prolapse is believed to be caused by an abnormality in the attachment of the mucosa to the submucosal layer. Straining may produce both partial and complete prolapse. Partial prolapse creates a protruding mass with radiating furrows (like the spokes on a wheel) and associated hemorrhoids.[27] True procidentia (full-thickness rectal prolapse) creates circular furrows.[26]

The initial treatment of partial prolapse is removal of contributing factors such as colon polyps, diarrhea, constipation, or laxative use. In infants the prolapse should be manually reduced following each defecation, with gauze placed over the anus, and the buttocks then taped together.[27] As the child grows older, the partial prolapse often decreases in size and frequency until it subsides altogether. If additional intervention is necessary, injection sclerotherapy, rubber band ligation, or surgical hemorrhoidectomy may be beneficial.

In adults, complete rectal prolapse is more common in older women. Multiparity and obstetrical trauma to the anal sphincter may predispose to this increase in women. The majority of adults present with the protruding rectal tissue, although bleeding, mucous discharge, and pain may be reported. The treatment for procidentia (complete prolapse) is surgical. There are many operations used for this condition, and all can result in some degree of incontinence. About 40% of the elderly who undergo abdominal proctopexy do not regain continence.[27]

Pruritus Ani

Pruritus ani is the symptom complex consisting of intense itching and burning discomfort of the perianal skin.[28] The itching and subsequent scratching can lead to skin breakdown, maceration, weeping, and superinfection. Itching is most common after a bowel movement or just before falling asleep. Multiple causes exist for pruritus ani, and attempts should be made to identify the specific cause and institute specific treatment[16,28–30] (Table 91.3). Patients with pruritus ani are generally healthy, vigorous men (4:1 male/female ratio) aged 20 to 50 years.[16,28]

A complete skin examination with focus on the mouth, scalp, and nails may provide evidence for a coexisting dermatologic condition (see Chapter 115). The perianal tissues should be closely inspected for primary perianal pathology. Pinworms and *Candida* infections are the most common infections associated with pruritus ani.[30] Unfortunately, in most patients there is no demonstrable cause.[16]

Table 91.3. **Conditions Associated with Pruritus Ani**

Systemic illness
  Diabetes mellitus
  Hyperbilirubinemia
  Leukemia
  Aplastic anemia
  Thyroid disease
Mechanical factors
  Chronic diarrhea
  Chronic constipation
  Anal incontinence
  Soaps, deodorants, perfumes
  Hemorrhoids producing leakage
  Prolapsed hemorrhoids
  Alcohol-based anal wipes
  Rectal prolapse
  Anal papilloma
  Anal fissure
  Anal fistula
Skin sensitivity from foods
  Tomatoes
  Caffeinated beverages
  Beer
  Citrus products
  Milk products
Medications
  Colchicine
  Quinidine
Dermatologic conditions
  Psoriasis
  Seborrheic dermatitis
  Intertrigo
  Neurodermatitis
  Bowen's disease
  Atopic dermatitis
  Lichen planus
  Lichen sclerosis
  Contact dermatitis
Infections
  Erythrasma (*Corynebacterium*)
  Intertrigo (*Candida*)
  Herpes simplex virus
  Human papillomavirus
  Pinworms (*Enterobius*)
  Scabies
  Local bacterial abscess
  Gonorrhea
  Syphilis

Patients should be educated about proper perineal hygiene. Soaps and talcum powders should be avoided, and patients should use white, undyed, unscented toilet tissue to limit allergic skin reactions. Excessive anal wiping is discouraged as it may produce skin lichenification.[30] Loosely fitting, dry cotton undergarments should be worn. Men who sweat excessively during the day can be encouraged to change their underwear at midday to limit moisture on the skin.

Pruritus ani can be difficult to treat. An empiric trial of a combination steroid and antifungal cream often is recommended but may not be successful.[29] Limited symptomatic relief may be gained from the use of antihistamines.[29] Additional treatment recommendations appear in Table 91.4. Dermatologic referral can be considered for refractory cases.

Table 91.4. **Treatment Guidelines for Patients with Pruritus Ani**

Cleanse perianal tissues following defecation with water
Avoid applying soaps or vigorous scrubbing to tissues
Dry tissues with patting of cotton towel or hair dryer
Apply a thin cotton pledget dusted with unscented cornstarch
   between bowel movements
Consume high-fiber diet to regulate bowel movements
Eliminate foods that promote itching such as tomatoes,
   chocolate, nuts, citrus fruits, colas, coffee, tea, beer
Avoid topical medications as they create irritation
Use 1% hydrocortisone cream sparingly for itching
Systemic antihistamines may relieve itching at bedtime

Infectious Proctitis

Proctitis describes an inflammation limited to the distal 10 cm of the rectum.[31–35] Infectious proctitis usually is caused by sexually transmitted diseases such as *Neisseria gonorrhoeae* and *Chlamydia trachomatis.*[23] Proctitis is considered when patients complain of rectal discomfort, tenesmus, rectal discharge, and constipation.[23] The anorectal mucosa may appear red and friable, and a mucopurulent discharge often is noted (see Chapter 41).

Gonorrheal proctitis is most common in homosexual men. Rectal gonorrhea in women usually results in spread from the genital tract, although 6% of women with rectal involvement are culture-negative from the cervix.[23] The majority of infected individuals are asymptomatic.[25,36,37] The ability to express pus from the anal crypts is highly suggestive of gonorrhea.[37] Nearly one half of rectal swabs may be falsely negative for gonorrhea, and empiric treatment is warranted when a high suspicion for the disease exists. Intramuscular ceftriaxone has replaced procaine penicillin G as the recommended treatment due to increasing penicillinase-producing *N. gonorrhoeae*[23,31] (see Chapter 41). Reculturing is recommended in 1 to 2 months, as treatment failure rates may be as high as 35%.[23]

Chlamydia trachomatis is recovered in 15% of asymptomatic homosexual men.[23] Because of the high rate of coexisting disease, all persons with gonorrhea should be treated for presumed *Chlamydia* infection (Table 91.5). Lymphogranuloma venereum (LGV), also caused by *C. trachomatis* serovars, can produce proctocolitis, inguinal adenopathy, and fistulas.[31] The sigmoidoscopic appearance with LGV is usually more severe, whereas *Chlamydia* proctitis usually produces a nonspecific erythema of the mucosa.

Viral infections can cause proctitis. Herpes simplex virus may produce vesicles, ulcers, itching, fever, sacral paresthesias, urinary retention, and impotence.[23] The anoscopic findings include erythema, diffuse ulcerations, and occasional pustules. Acyclovir can be used to shorten the clinical course or decrease shedding (400 mg five times daily for 10 days) or used daily (400 mg twice a day) to prevent recurrences.[32]

Syphilis proctitis generally produces multiple painless chancres in the perianal or anal area. Inguinal adenopathy may be present, and ulcers may be painful if secondarily infected.[23] Darkfield examination of scrapings or serologic testing can be used to document the infection. Follow-up serology is recommended 3 and 6 months following treatment.

Hidradenitis Suppurativa

Hidradenitis suppurativa is a chronic, inflammatory disease of the apocrine sweat glands of the skin.[17] Hidradenitis can develop in the perianal tissues, and often the skin changes are mistaken for perianal fistulas. Hidradenitis develops after puberty and is more common in individuals with oily skin. The patient may develop firm nodules that can coalesce into bands or plaques. Induration, drainage, and tenderness commonly are seen. Surgical treatment includes complete excision of the affected skin in single or multiple stages.[17]

Condyloma Acuminatum

Anal condyloma are caused by the human papillomavirus (HPV), usually types 6 and 11.[33] Anal warts appear to be most common in young men, especially those engaging in anal intercourse.[31] Women with anal warts often have coexisting warts on the cervix and labia. Smoking and alterations in immune system function [poor nutrition, human immunodeficiency virus (HIV) disease, severe allergies] may predispose to HPV infection (see Chapter 116).

Anal warts often are multiple and extend from the anal skin into the anal canal. Anoscopy is always indicated to evaluate the extent of disease.[34] Most patients exhibit only slight symptoms, such as irritation, moisture on the tissues, and occasional bleeding with defecation. Malignant degeneration of the underlying tissues can occur, especially in patients with HIV disease.[35] The goal of therapy is amelioration of signs and symptoms—not the eradication of HPV.[31]

The presence of anogenital warts in children incites high emotional response, and management is controversial.[34] While up to half of these children have been sexually abused,

Table 91.5. **Commonly Recommended Treatments for Infectious Proctitis**

Causative organism	Treatment
Neisseria gonorrhoeae[a]	Ceftriaxone 250 mg IM (single dose)
Chlamydia trachomatis	Doxycycline 100 mg po two times daily for 7 days
Herpes simplex virus	Acyclovir 800–1600 mg/day po for 10 days
Syphilis (*Treponema pallidum*)	Benzathine penicillin G 2.4 million units IM
Entamoeba histolytica	Metronidazole 750 mg po three times daily for 10 days
Shigella species	Trimethoprim-sulfamethoxazole DS po two times daily for 7 days
Campylobacter jejuni	Erythromycin 500 mg po four times daily for 7 days

[a]Consider empiric treatment with doxycycline because of the high rate of concomitant infection with *Chlamydia trachomatis.*

many acquire the infection by vertical transmission at birth. Assessment by a multidisciplinary team with set procedures for the consideration of abuse is appropriate.[34]

Multiple therapies exist for anogenital condylomas.[31,33] Podophyllin (25% concentration, applied for 5 to 10 minutes) and bichloracetic acid are topical agents applied weekly to destroy the warts.[32] Bichloracetic acid can be used in the anal canal,[32] an important consideration as up to 70% of homosexual men with external warts will have lesions up to the dentate line.[34] Both treatments can produce significant local skin irritation. Cryotherapy also is an effective destructive treatment but often is painful when applied to the perianal tissues.

Scissors excision following local anesthesia, and electrosurgical excision and destruction are effective techniques for removing condyloma.[32] The smoke plume generated at electrosurgery carries HPV particles, and an appropriate smoke evacuator should be used to protect both the patient and health care providers. Intralesional recombinant interferon-α is approved for treatment of condyloma (1 million units injected into each lesion three times a week on alternate days for 3 weeks).[32] Historically, application of topical 5-fluorouracil (5-FU) cream has been used to eliminate perianal warts. The potential for severe local skin effects has all but eliminated use of 5-FU cream.

Anal Carcinoma

Five types of malignant epithelial growths may develop in the anal region. Adenocarcinomas are the most common malignancies in the region, and most descend from the rectum above.[17] Between 2% and 6% of all anal cancers are squamous cell carcinomas.[17] Squamous cell carcinomas of the anal canal, historically aggressive tumors, are treated with irradiation, chemotherapy, and abdominopelvic resection.[17] Malignant melanomas, basal cell carcinomas, and primary adenocarcinomas of the anal canal are encountered much less commonly (see Chapter 117).

References

1. Pemberton JH. Anatomy and physiology of the anus and rectum. In: Zuidema GD, ed. Shackelford's surgery of the alimentary tract, 3rd ed. Philadelphia: WB Saunders, 1991;242–74.
2. Leibach JR, Cerda JJ. Hemorrhoids: modern treatment methods. Hosp Med 1991;27:53–68.
3. Dennison AR, Wherry DC, Morris DL. Hemorrhoids: nonoperative management. Surg Clin North Am 1988;68:1401–9.
4. Smith LE. Anal hemorrhoids. Neth J Med 1990;37:S22–32.
5. Schussman LC, Lutz LJ. Outpatient management of hemorrhoids. Prim Care 1986;13:527–41.
6. Medich DS, Fazio VW. Hemorrhoids, anal fissure, and carcinoma of the colon, rectum, and anus during pregnancy. Surg Clin North Am 1995;75:77–88.
7. Thomson WHF. The nature of haemorrhoids. Br J Surg 1975;62:542–52.
8. Stahl TJ. Office management of common anorectal problems. Postgrad Med 1992;92:141–51.
9. Zuber TJ. Anorectal disease and hemorrhoids. In: Taylor RB, ed. Manual of family practice. Boston: Little, Brown, 1997;381–4.
10. Ferguson EF. Alternatives in the treatment of hemorrhoidal disease. South Med J 1988;81:606–10.
11. Russel TR, Donohue JH. Hemorrhoidal banding: a warning. Dis Colon Rectum 1985;28:291–3.
12. Senagore A, Mazier WP, Luchtefeld MA, MacKeigan JM, Wengert T. Treatment of advanced hemorrhoidal disease: a prospective, randomized comparison of cold scalpel vs. contact Nd:YAG laser. Dis Colon Rectum 1993;36:1042–9.
13. Friend WG. External hemorrhoids. Med Times 1988;116:108–9.
14. Buls JG. Excision of thrombosed external hemorrhoids. Hosp Med 1994;30:39–42.
15. Grosz CR. A surgical treatment of thrombosed external hemorrhoids. Dis Colon Rectum 1990;33:249–50.
16. Mazier WP. Hemorrhoids, fissures, and pruritus ani. Surg Clin North Am 1994;74:1277–92.
17. Goligher J, Duthie H, Nixon H. Surgery of the anus rectum and colon, 5th ed. London: Baillière, 1984.
18. Gorfine SR. Treatment of benign anal disease with topical nitroglycerin. Dis Colon Rectum 1995;38:453–7.
19. Madoff RD. Pharmacologic therapy for anal fissure [editorial]. N Engl J Med 1998;338:257–9.
20. Carapeti EA, Kamm MA, McDonald PJ, Chadwick SJD, Melville D, Phillips RKS. Randomized controlled trial shows that glyceryl trinitrate heals anal fissures, higher doses are not more effective, and there is a high recurrence rate. Gut 1999;44:727–30.
21. Brisinda G, Maria G, Bentivoglio AR, Cassetta E, Gui D, Albanese A. A comparison of injections of botulinum toxin and topical nitroglycerin ointment for the treatment of chronic anal fissure. N Engl J Med 1999;341:65–9.
22. Minguez M, Melo F, Espi A, et al. Therapeutic effects of different doses of botulinum toxin in chronic anal fissure. Dis Colon Rectum 1999;42:1016–21.
23. Bassford T. Treatment of common anorectal disorders. Am Fam Physician 1992;45:1787–94.
24. Toglia MR. Anal incontinence: an underrecognized, undertreated problem. Female Patient 1996;21:17–30.
25. Whitehead WE, Wald A, Diamant NE, Enck P, Pemberton JH, Rao SS. Functional disorders of the anus and rectum. Gut 1999;45(suppl II):II55–9.
26. Knight AL. Fecal impaction. In: Rakel RE, ed. Saunders manual of medical practice. Philadelphia: WB Saunders, 1996;259–60.
27. Abcarian H. Prolapse and procidentia. In: Zuidema GD, ed. Shackelford's surgery of the alimentary tract, 3rd ed. Philadelphia: WB Saunders, 1991;331–48.
28. Dailey TH. Pruritus ani. In: Zuidema GD, ed. Shackelford's surgery of the alimentary tract, 3rd ed. Philadelphia: WB Saunders, 1991;281–5.
29. Zellis S, Pincus SH. Pruritus ani and vulvae. In: Rakel RE, ed. Conn's current therapy 1996. Philadelphia: WB Saunders, 1996;815–6.
30. Aucoin EJ. Pruritus ani: practical therapy for persistent itching. Postgrad Med 1987;82:76–80.
31. Centers for Disease Control and Prevention. 1993 Sexually transmitted diseases treatment guidelines. MMWR 1993;42 (RR-14):1–102.
32. Modesto VL, Gottesman L. Sexually transmitted diseases and anal manifestations of AIDS. Surg Clin North Am 1994;74:1433–64.
33. Bonnez W, Reichman RC. Papillomaviruses. In: Mandell GL, Bennett JE, Dolin R, eds. Mandell, Douglas and Bennett's principles and practices of infectious diseases, 4th ed. New York: Churchill Livingstone, 1995;1387–400.
34. Von Krogh G, Gross G. Anogenital warts. Clin Dermatol 1997;15:355–68.
35. Palefsky JM. Anal cancer and its precursors: an HIV-related disease. Hosp Physician 1993;Jan:35–42.
36. Toglia MR. Pathophysiology of anorectal dysfunction. Obstet Gynecol Clin North Am 1998;25:771–81.
37. Janicke DM, Pundt MR. Anorectal disorders. Emerg Med Clin North Am 1996;14:757–88.

92
Colorectal Cancer

Gregory L. Brotzman and Russell G. Robertson

Colorectal cancer (CRC) continues to be one of the predominant cancers in the Western world, surpassed only by lung cancer in mortality rates. It is estimated that 135,400 new cases of colorectal cancer will be diagnosed in 2001 and that 56,700 people will die from the disease during the same period.[1] Despite advances in early detection, screening, and treatment, these mortality figures have remained relatively constant. The fiscal implications of CRC management are staggering, with approximately $6.5 billion spent on CRC-related care in the United States annually.[2] There are emerging differences in racial mortality rates, with African Americans having the highest mortality rates (50.7 per 100,000 people) compared to Caucasians (43.6 per 100,000 people). American Indians have the lowest incidence (16.3 per 100,000 people). Colorectal cancer affects men and women equally.[1]

Advancing age remains the single greatest risk factor favoring the development of CRC. Therefore, the costs of managing colorectal cancer are likely to increase as the population ages. Today Americans have a 5% chance of developing this cancer during their lifetime.[3] Certain risk factors substantially increase an individual's chances of developing CRC: inflammatory bowel disease, colonic adenomas, a family history of CRC, and a high-fat/low-fiber diet.[4] Although the etiology of CRC is not completely understood, environmental, genetic, and dietary factors are believed to be responsible for 85% to 90% of all cases.[5]

There is cause for some optimism, however, as the advent of colonic endoscopy, our improved understanding of the adenoma-carcinoma continuum, and elegant cellular and molecular biologic techniques have made CRC now one of the best models for translating research into useful clinical practice. Improvements in fiberoptic technology and sound screening protocols have made elimination of CRC as a major cause of death a theoretic possibility.[6–8] Efforts continue toward the development of more effective strategies aimed at early diagnosis and prevention.[5]

Presentation

Variability in the signs and symptoms of CRC poses a significant challenge to the physician (Table 92.1). CRC may be asymptomatic, with the diagnosis being made by a CRC screening examination or serendipitously while evaluating the patient for an unrelated illness. For symptomatic CRC the signs and symptoms vary depending on the location of the lesion. Right-sided tumors present most commonly with anemia, abdominal pain, weight loss, or a change in bowel habits. If the lesion is left-sided, the most common presenting findings are change in bowel habits, rectal blood loss, and abdominal pain.[9,10]

Right-sided colon tumors rarely produce changes in bowel habits but are more likely to be the source of chronic occult bleeding that can lead to symptoms consistent with iron deficiency anemia (fatigue, dizziness, palpitations). When a postmenopausal woman or adult man develops such symptoms in the absence of an obvious cause, CRC should be suspected. Pain in the lower abdomen is an occasional symptom of tumors located in the transverse or left colon. These patients are more likely to notice a change in bowel habits, as either diarrhea or constipation can occur owing to a constricting lumen. The stool may be dark or maroon-colored, and passage may be associated with bloody mucus. Weight loss and fever are occasionally reported as well but seldom as the sole presenting symptom.[3] The first signs of colon cancer may be produced by metastatic disease. Colon cancer metastasizes to the liver and lung, whereas rectal cancer metastasizes primarily to the lung and bone.[11] An otherwise asymptomatic patient may have pruritus and jaundice due to liver involvement. Ascites, enlarged ovaries, and scattered deposits in the lungs may also result from the otherwise undetected presence of CRC.

Obstruction and perforation are the conditions most often associated with the acute presentation of CRC. Obstruction

Table 92.1. **Common Signs and Symptoms of Colorectal Cancer**

Anemia
Abdominal pain
Weight loss
Change in bowel habits
Rectal blood loss
Heme-positive stools

Table 92.2. **Known or Suspected Risk Factors for the Development of Colorectal Cancer**

Polyps
Family member with polyps
Obesity
High-fat diet
Low-fiber diet
Smoking and alcohol
Environmental factors
Inflammatory bowel disease
Family cancer syndrome
Familial polyposis syndrome

of the large bowel is highly suggestive of cancer, particularly in older patients. Complete obstruction occurs in up to half of patients, depending on the location of the tumor. Long-term survival rates are poorer for patients who have obstruction at the time of diagnosis. Perforation is a surgical emergency and may precipitate complications such as peritonitis and abscess formation.[3,11]

Risk Factors

Polyps

Polyps are a risk factor for CRC, particularly if they are adenomatous in type (Table 92.2). Siblings and parents of patients with adenomatous colorectal polyps have a 1.78 relative risk for developing CRC. The age at the time of polyp diagnosis is an important prognostic factor for the risk of cancer development. Siblings of patients with adenomatous polyps diagnosed before age 60 have a 2.59 relative risk for developing CRC.[12] Polyp size and histology are directly related to the risk of CRC, with villous polyps larger than 2 cm having a 50% greater chance of containing cancer than smaller or nonvillous polyps.[3,13]

There is concern that a small distal colorectal polyp, whether adenomatous or hyperplastic, is a proximal neoplasm marker. In study of 366 patients without a history of CRC or polyps, Pennazio et al[14] demonstrated that 34% of patients with distal small colorectal polyps also had proximal polyps noted on colonoscopic examination. These proximal lesions might have been missed had colonoscopy not been performed.[14]

Familial Adenomatous Polyposis

Familial adenomatous polyposis is an autosomal-dominant disease, with an occurrence rate of 1:7000 to 1:10,000 individuals. The colon is virtually completely lined with polyps. Approximately 50% to 75% of these patients develop CRC by age 35 if colectomy is not performed.[15] Diagnosis is by genetic testing of family members.

Dietary Factors

Dietary fat increases bowel transit time and increases the concentration of fecal bile acids, such as cholic and deoxycholic acid. These bile acids act as potential carcinogens on the colonic mucosa.[11] In contrast to fat, fiber decreases bowel transit time and therefore exposure of the bowel to these carcinogens.[3] Fiber, particularly wheat fiber, has been reported

to have a protective effect against the development of CRC. A randomized study of high-dose wheat bran fiber and calcium supplementation reported reduced colonic levels of total and secondary fecal bile acids compared to controls. It is postulated that because bile acids may be carcinogenic, reduction of their concentrations in the colon may be the mechanism by which a high-fiber diet reduces the risk of developing CRC.[16] However, a recent long-term study of 61,463 Swedish women (average 9.6 years of follow-up) revealed no decrease in the risk of colorectal cancer with high consumption of cereal fiber. The study did find that those women who had very low intake of fruits and vegetables had a much higher risk of developing colorectal cancer. [17]

A diet rich in carbohydrates, fruits, and fiber may bestow a strong protective effect from adenoma development, whereas ingestion of a high-fat diet increase the risk of CRC development more than twice that of control groups.[4] Dietary factors also play a role in the development of CRC in individuals who consume alcohol. Men who eat a diet low in folate and methionine accompanied by substantial consumption of alcohol (more than two drinks per day) have a 3.3 relative risk for development of colon cancer compared to individuals who drink less than two drinks a day and who have a balanced diet.[18]

Environmental Factors

Environmental influences exert a definite influence on the development of CRC. Industrialized countries are at a relatively increased risk compared to less developed countries or countries that traditionally had high-fiber/low-fat diets. This point is exemplified by the fact that persons from a low-risk country who migrate to the United States over time develop CRC rates similar to those among native U.S. citizens.[3,19] This increased rate of CRC is probably directly related to dietary changes that accompany migration (i.e., changing from a high-fiber/low-fat diet to a low fiber/high fat diet).

Smoking and Alcohol

Cigarette smoking and alcohol consumption have been reported to increase the relative risk of an individual to develop colonic adenomas and CRC. The relative risk of developing small adenomas is 3.6 for smokers with more than a 20-pack-a-year history. Alcohol consumption (especially when beer is the alcohol being consumed) increases the risk of developing

CRC two- to threefold over baseline.[20] Alcohol consumption and tobacco use are independently related to the risk of developing large colorectal adenomas[21] (also see Chapter 7).

Family History of Cancer

Although frequently neglected, a family medical history is an integral component of CRC risk detection.[6,22] Cancer family syndrome, an autosomal-dominant disorder, incurs a 33% risk that a patient will develop cancer by the age of 50. Common cancers in these individuals include multiple adenocarcinomas of the colon (especially the proximal colon) or endometrium. Patients who have other types of cancer are at a relative increased risk of developing CRC. If a patient has a first-degree relative with CRC, the patient is at a two- to fourfold increased risk of developing CRC him- or herself.[3,12]

Inflammatory Bowel Disease

There is a substantial increased risk of CRC in patients with ulcerative colitis, with the risk being inversely proportional to the age of onset of the colitis and directly proportional to the extent of colonic involvement.[23] Twenty-five percent of patients with ulcerative colitis develop CRC after 25 years of disease.[18] Crohn's disease is also associated with the development of CRC but to lesser degree than ulcerative colitis. Patients with Crohn's disease may have a 4- to 20-fold increased risk of developing CRC compared to the general population, but this association is less clear-cut than for ulcerative colitis.[18,24]

Incidence and Location

The incidence of CRC increases with age and is highest during the eighth decade of life.[11] Colorectal cancer has shown a gradual shift in location from left-sided to right-sided tumors over the past several decades.[25] Rosato and Marks[26] compared the distribution of CRC from 1939 to 1957 to that for a group of patients from 1970 to 1977. Percentages of cancers based on location for 1939 to 1957 and 1970 to 1977, respectively, have shifted as follows: rectum colon 51% versus 32%, sigmoid colon 13% versus 31%, descending colon 20% versus 5%, transverse colon 4% versus 13%, and ascending colon 12% versus 16%. In a prospective study, Tedesco et al.[27] evaluated 642 patients and found that 66% of polyps and cancers were located within 60 cm of the anus, and that 5% of polyps and 28% of cancers were located within the first 25 cm. Knowledge of this shift from predominantly left-sided to right-sided tumors is an important consideration when discussing diagnostic studies.

Anatomy and Pathogenesis

The colon runs from the cecum to the rectum. Lymphatic drainage occurs in both a segmental and a circumferential fashion. This segmented drainage pattern explains why CRCs may appear as a localized, apple-core-type lesion.[3] Histologically, normal colonic columnar epithelium is proliferative only in the lower two thirds of the glandular crypts. The upper one third and surface cells are normally nonproliferative.[3] When exposed to carcinogens, mutational activation of oncogenes and the inactivation of tumor suppresser genes occur. At least four or five mutations are required to produce a malignant tumor. Cumulative mutations are responsible for the biologic properties of the tumor.[28]

Exposure of normal colonic epithelium to carcinogens leads to the movement of proliferative cells from the basal two thirds of the crypts to the surface cell layer. These cells replicate but do not exfoliate, leading to increasing numbers of cells and eventual polyp formation. Polyps can be sessile (broad-based) or pedunculated (on a stalk), with the polyp's histology being hyperplastic or neoplastic. If neoplastic, polyps are classified as adenomatous (tubular), villous (finger-like), or mixed (intermediate). Adenomatous polyps, if left untreated, may become progressively more dysplastic and eventually develop into carcinoma in situ or invasive CRC.[3]

Diagnosis and Screening for Colorectal Cancer

Colorectal cancer is common and readily treated in many cases, making it an ideal cancer to try to prevent using screening strategies. Because almost all colorectal cancers arise from adenomatous polyps, one might conclude that the vast majority of deaths from CRC would be preventable if screening tests were used to their maximum benefit.[29] Yet, in general, less than 50% of persons for whom screening is recommended have been screened.[30] In 1997, a large population-based study of 52,754 persons age 50 or older assessed whether people had had fecal occult blood testing (FOBT) and/or sigmoidoscopy within the recommended 1 or 5 year intervals, respectively.[31] Only 19.8% said they had FOBT within the prior year and 30.4% had sigmoidoscopy. In that light, it is incumbent on the medical profession and those concerned with the public's health to better identify the barriers to screening so that its maximum benefit can be achieved.

There are a variety of methods available for the diagnosis of CRC, each having its own associated controversy. In addition, there are several currently accepted screening guidelines being employed for the purpose of detecting CRC in otherwise asymptomatic patients with no additional risk factors. Although similarities exist, new information regarding the utility of endoscopic and radiographic techniques may change significantly those established recommendations.

Beginning at age 50, the U. S. Preventive Services Task Force recommends annual FOBT and flexible sigmoidoscopy (periodicity unspecified).[7] The American Cancer Society recommends one of five screening options[32]:

- Yearly FOBT
- Flexible sigmoidoscopy every 5 years
- Yearly FOBT plus flexible sigmoidoscopy every 5 years
- Double contrast barium enema every 5 years
- Colonoscopy every 10 years

Digital Rectal Examination

Digital rectal examination has traditionally aided in the diagnosis of many rectal cancers.[8] Today, however, the proximal shift in the distribution of CRCs makes a greater number of lesions undetectable with digital rectal examination alone. As digital rectal examination at best can reach only the most distal 5 to 7 cm of the rectum, its diagnostic virtue lies only in its simplicity and low cost but in no way should be considered a substitute for a more thorough examination.[7]

Fecal Occult Blood Testing

Fecal occult blood testing continues to be the subject of significant study. Its allure remains its relatively low cost, the potential for mass screening, and most importantly the detection of asymptomatic cancers. Most currently available guaiac tests rely on a peroxidase-like reaction to the heme component of blood. Despite the flaws associated with FOBT, including failure to detect 75% of adenomas and 30% to 50% of colorectal carcinomas in association with an overall false-negative rate of 40%, most reports on their use emphasize that a relatively high percentage of the cancers detected are early-stage lesions.[33,34] The 33% reduction in mortality observed in individuals who underwent annual FOBT screening in the Minnesota Colon Cancer Control Study strongly supports FOBT as a useful diagnostic approach.[31] Dietary precautions prior to collection of the FOBT can decrease the likelihood of false positives. Patients should be instructed to avoid aspirin and nonsteroidal antiinflammatory drugs (NSAIDs) for 1 week prior to collection of specimens, and red meat and vitamin C for 3 days prior.[35] Current recommendations are for obtaining a total of six samples (two from each of three specimens).

Barium Enema

The air contrast barium enema (ACBE) has proved to be a valuable study for the diagnosis of CRC. Its advantages include its sensitivity for the detection of small polyps, its detection rate for rectal lesions, and its efficacy in diagnosing early inflammatory bowel disease as well as relatively low cost and lower complication rates when compared with colonoscopy.[6] Disadvantages of ACBE are the need for more patient cooperation and the radiation exposure compared to that incurred with colonoscopy. ACBE can still be of significant value to physicians with limited access to colonoscopy.[36]

Flexible Sigmoidoscopy

Sigmoidoscopy in asymptomatic persons appears to be a highly sensitive method for early detection of both cancer and adenomatous polyps of the distal colon and rectum. In trained hands, a 60-cm flexible sigmoidoscope can reach the descending colon and detect two to three times more neoplasms than the rigid sigmoidoscope.[6] Sigmoidoscopy has a relatively low cost, requires no sedation, is sensitive, specific, safe, easy to perform, and is a useful means of reducing both the incidence of cancer and its associated mortality.[37] However, the value of flexible sigmoidoscopy has recently been questioned due to its inability to detect lesions in the proximal colon.

Two studies demonstrated that sigmoidoscopic screening will fail to detect a substantial proportion of asymptomatic CRCs or polyps associated with a high risk of cancer.[38,39]

Overview of Flexible Sigmoidoscopy Technique

After informed consent is obtained, the patient is placed in the left lateral supine position after bowel preparation with two Fleet-type enemas. Perform a digital exam, and then insert the lubricated tip of a flexible 60- to 70-cm sigmoidoscope into the rectum about 10 cm. The scope is held with the left hand and the fingers of the left hand will operate the scope levers, allowing it to turn various directions. The shaft is advanced with the right hand. The goal is to insert the scope maximally, with examination for pathology occurring primarily during withdrawal of the scope. Air needs to be insufflated to expand the bowel cavity, but too much air will lead to cramping and spasm, making the examination more difficult. Do not advance if there is resistance or if there is a "red out" where the scope is in direct contact with the bowel wall. If the bowel appears not to move as you advance the scope, the scope is likely "telescoping," and will cause discomfort to the patient. The scope should be retracted until the bowel moves away from the field of view. The scope can then be advanced again to allow for a fuller length of the bowel to be examined. Another way to maximize the length of bowel examined is by torquing of the scope about 30 degrees against a mucosal fold and retracting about 5 cm. This technique will allow the bowel to bunch up on the scope, permitting a longer section of the bowel to be examined. After maximal insertion or if patient is not able to tolerate any further advancement, begin to slowly withdraw the scope. Note any diverticula, masses, or other abnormalities and document your findings. Biopsy can be performed through a biopsy port on the scope. Avoid biopsy of vascular areas and be sure all bleeding is stopped after the biopsy before completing your examination.[40]

Colonoscopy

Examination of the entire colon by colonoscopy remains the gold standard for visualization, biopsy, and when possible removal of colonic neoplasms.[6] Colonoscopy is an expensive procedure involving sedation and has a higher complication rate than other diagnostic modalities. In some reports, just over 17% of colonoscopies failed to reach the cecum.[41] In a recent Veterans Administration (VA) study, 3121 asymptomatic men with a mean age of 62.9 years underwent a screening colonoscopic examination; 37.5% had one or more neoplastic lesions detected, with invasive cancer diagnosed in 1% of the patients. In this study, 52% of the 128 patients with advanced proximal colon lesions had no distal adenomas that a sigmoidoscopy would detect.[38] The authors also found that hyperplastic polyps had an odds ratio of 1.5 for advanced proximal disease.

The selection of a particular screening technique poses several challenges to the family physician. The gold standard for screening is currently colonoscopy due to the definitive nature of the procedure's complete visualization of the large intestine. However, the procedure is associated with risks of perforation, anesthetic complications, and patient discomfort. The high cost of colonoscopy can be a deterrent either to the individual or payer if not a covered benefit for the purpose of screening the low-risk asymptomatic patient. In the most capable hands, a flexible sigmoidoscope will reach only the first part of the descending colon, missing lesions of the right and transverse colon that may be present in asymptomatic patients. The Minnesota Study documents the effectiveness of FOBT as a screening technique with its inherent limitations. Computed tomography (CT)-guided colonography, also known as virtual colonoscopy, holds a great deal of promise as a noninvasive approach to screening that eliminates several of the risks of colonoscopy.[42] While promising, CT-guided colonography costs have yet to be delineated, it has yet to be proven an effective substitute for colonoscopy, and it also lacks the capability for biopsy afforded during endoscopic colonoscopy.

The challenge for the family physician is selecting the method most appropriate for our patients that may be determined by cost, availability of technology, and the ability of a patient to tolerate a procedure. There are courses available to teach colonoscopy with biopsy to nongastroenterologists. Following such training, a preceptorship is needed to develop both technical and diagnostic expertise in colonoscopy. The key issue is having sufficient volume in one's practice to maintain the acquired skill and a supportive environment (staff and facilities) to maximize patient care and minimize the risk of complications.

Colorectal Cancer Classification Systems

The two most common classification systems are the Dukes and TNM (tumor/node/metastasis) systems. The original Dukes system was developed for classification of rectal cancers. Dukes A describes a rectal tumor that has not penetrated the wall and has no nodal involvement. Dukes B involves a penetrating cancer through the rectal wall but with no nodal involvement. Dukes C indicates lymph node involvement. The Dukes system was modified by Kirklin in 1949, extending the classification to include colon cancers. Turnbull in 1967 added Dukes D to describe metastases to distant organs. The Dukes classification fails to take into account the number of involved nodes and clinical factors, but it is still the single best predictor of survival.[43]

The TNM system is based on the anatomic extent of the cancer. T stands for the extent of the primary tumor, N for the condition of the regional lymph nodes, and M for the presence or absence of distant metastases at the time of diagnosis.[44] The National Cancer Institute recently convened an expert panel to develop guidelines for colon and rectal surgery. As a result of this meeting, the panel recommended using the TNM system for tumor staging based on a review of the best available evidence.[45]

Treatment

Approximately 85% of patients with CRC can have a curative operation to remove the involved colon and mesentery. Patients need a preoperative colonoscopy and CT of the abdomen to rule out liver metastases.[23] Any colonic or rectal polyps are removed.[9] Resections that save the sphincter in patients with rectal cancer assist in reducing the number of abdominoperineal excisions necessary.[44] 5-Fluorouracil (5-FU) is a cytostatic drug that inhibits DNA synthesis in cancer cells. The postoperative use of 5-FU along with levamisole, an immunomodulator drug, improves postoperative cure rates.[46] Levamisole is believed to antagonize the effect of 5-FU on RNA synthesis, potentially reducing the toxicity associated with 5-FU administration. Similarly, improved cure rates are noted when leucovorin, a folic acid derivative, is used along with 5-FU.[47] Because the prognosis is poor for advanced-stage CRC, these patients should be enrolled in clinical trials to possibly improve their prognosis and associated survival.[48]

Prognosis

Increased age may be associated with a shorter survival time. Women have a better prognosis than men in general. The CRC prognosis worsens when moving from the right to the left side of the colon.[1,44] Histologic grading and operative findings are important prognostic factors for CRC. Nodal involvement is an essential component of both the Dukes and the TNM staging systems. Poorly differentiated histology is associated with a poorer prognosis compared to well-differentiated histology.[11] The 5-year survival rate is most favorable for CRC of the descending colon and rectum. The overall 5-year survival figures after surgery for CRC Dukes A is 70% to 83%, Dukes B 48% to 62%, and Dukes C 22% to 33%.[44]

Prevention

Prevention of colon cancer remains a theoretic possibility and ought to be pursued, especially for patients whose family histories place them at high risk. Identifying genetic predisposition, dietary modifications, cessation of alcohol and tobacco use, and chemoprevention represent the spectrum of preventive modalities. None of these has proved to be completely effective for preventing CRC. The role of genetic predisposition in CRC is most prominent for patients with familial polyposis, inflammatory bowel disease, a family history of colon cancer, and a family history of adenomatous polyps.[3] The first two categories require aggressive and regular surveillance to identify the development and removal of early adenomas up to and including total colectomy. Siblings and parents of patients with adenomatous polyps are at an increased risk for CRC, particularly when the adenoma is diagnosed before the age of 60 or, in the case of siblings, when a parent has CRC.[12] Some recommend screening with colonoscopy or ACBE the first-degree relatives of patients with adenomatous polyps diagnosed before age 60.[12] The American Cancer Society recommends colonoscopy or ACBE every 3 to 5 years starting at age 35 to 40 for patients with a first-degree relative having CRC with an age of onset of 55 or less. Screening should be earlier for patients with familial polyposis syndrome, a family history of nonpolyposis CRC, or inflammatory bowel disease. If patient has colorectal adenomas, they should be removed. When an adenoma is found on flexible sigmoidoscopy, colonoscopy must be done to detect and remove all polyps.[14] Most patients with history of adenomas require colonoscopy every 3 to 5 years. Individualized evaluation is necessary for the aged and for patients with a malignant adenoma, multiple adenomas, or a sessile adenoma.[21,49] Genetic testing is available for patients at risk for familial adenomatous polyposis (FAP). A patient with a negative genetic test has essentially zero risk for FAP, whereas a patient with a positive genetic result has a 100% likelihood of developing FAP.[15]

Chemoprevention has shown significant signs of promise. Recent observations suggest that aspirin and other NSAIDs, supplemental folate and calcium, and postmenopausal hormone replacement therapy (estrogen) have a chemopreventive benefit.[50] Although encouraging, the value of chemoprevention has not yet been substantiated through more extensive study and should not replace standard screening techniques or risk-reducing lifestyle changes.

References

1. Greenlee RT, Hill-Harmon MB, Murray T, Thun M. Cancer statistics, 2001. CA Cancer J Clin 2001;51:15–36.
2. Schrag D. Weeks J. Costs and cost-effectiveness of colorectal cancer prevention and therapy. Semin Oncol 1999;26:561–8.
3. Fry R, Fleshman J, Kodner I. Cancer of colon and rectum. Clin Symp 1989;41:2–32.
4. Sandler R, Lyles C, Peipins L, et al. Diet and risk of colorectal adenomas: macronutrients, cholesterol, and fiber. J Natl Cancer Inst 1993;85:884–91.
5. Vargas P, Alberts D. Primary prevention of colorectal cancer through dietary modification. Cancer 1992;70:1229–35.
6. Toribara N, Sleisenger M. Screening for colorectal cancer. N Engl J Med 1995;332:861–7.
7. U.S. Preventive Services Task Force. Guide to clinical preventative services, 2nd ed. Baltimore: Williams & Wilkins, 1996.
8. Bard J. Colorectal cancer update. Prevention, screening, treatment & surveillance for high risk groups. Med Clin North Am 2000;84:1163–79.
9. Wayne M, Cath A, Pamies R. Colorectal cancer: a practical review for the primary care physician. Arch Fam Med 1995;4:357–66.
10. Lieberman D, Smith F. Screening asymptomatic subjects for colon malignancy with colonoscopy. Am J Gastroenterol 1991;86:946–51.
11. Sinnige H, Mulder N. Colorectal carcinoma: an update. Neth J Med 1991;38:217–28.
12. Winawer S, Zauber A, Gerdes H, et al. Risk of colorectal cancer in the families of patients with adenomatous polyps. N Engl J Med 1996;334:82–7.
13. Stryker S, Wolff B, Culp C, et al. Natural history of untreated colonic polyps. Gastroenterology 1987;93:1009–13.
14. Pennazio M, Arrigoni A, Risio M, Spandre M, Rossini F. Small rectosigmoid polyps as markers of proximal neoplasms. Dis Colon Rectum 1993;36:1121–5.
15. Peterson G, Boyd P. Gene tests and counseling for colorectal cancer risk: lessons from familial polyposis. J Natl Cancer Inst 1995;17:67–71.
16. Alberts D, Ritenbaugh C, Story J, et al. Randomized, double-blinded, placebo-controlled study of effect of wheat bran fiber and calcium on fecal bile acids in patients with resected adenomatous colon polyps. J Natl Cancer Inst 1995;88:81–92.
17. Terry P, Giovannucci E, Michels K, et al. Fruit, vegetables, dietary fiber, and risk of colorectal cancer. J Natl Cancer Inst 2001;93:525–33.
18. Giovannucci E, Rimm E, Ascherio A, Stampfer M, Colditz G, Willett W. Alcohol, low-methionine-low-folate diets, and risk of colon cancer in men. J Natl Cancer Inst 1995;87:265–73.
19. Levin K, Dozois R. Epidemiology of large bowel cancer. World J Surg 1991;15:562–7.
20. Kune G, Vitetta L. Alcohol consumption and the etiology of colorectal cancer: a review of the scientific evidence from 1957 to 1991. Nutr Cancer 1992;18:97–111.
21. Martinez M, McPherson S, Annegers J, Levin B. Cigarette smoking and alcohol consumption as risk factors for colorectal adenomatous polyps. J Natl Cancer Inst 1995;87:274–9.
22. Levin B, Murphy G. Revision in American Cancer Society recommendations for the early detection of colorectal cancer. CA Cancer J Clin 1992;42:296–9.
23. DeCosse J, Tsioulias G, Jacobson J. Colorectal cancer: detection, treatment and rehabilitation. CA Cancer J Clin 1994;44:27–42.
24. Bachwich D, Lichtenstein G, Traber P. Cancer in inflammatory bowel disease. Med Clin North Am 1994;78:1399–412.
25. Axtell L, Chiazze L. Changing relative frequency of cancers of the colon and rectum in the United States. Cancer 1966;19:750–4.
26. Rosato F, Marks G. Changing site distribution patterns of colorectal cancer at Thomas Jefferson University Hospital. Dis Colon Rectum 1981;24:93–5.
27. Tedesco F, Wayne J, Avella J, Villalobos M. Diagnostic implications of the spatial distribution of colonic mass lesions (polyps and cancers): a prospective colonoscopic study. Gastroenterol Endosc 1980;26:95–7.
28. Cho K, Vogelstein B. Genetic alterations in the adenoma–carcinoma sequence. Cancer 1992;70:1727–31.
29. Winawer SJ, Zauber AG, Ho MN, et al. Prevention of colorectal cancer by colonoscopic polypectomy. N Engl J Med 1993;329:1977–83.
30. Tomeo CA, Colditz GA, Willet WC, et al. Harvard report on cancer prevention: vol. 3: prevention of colon cancer in the United States. Cancer Causes Control 1999;10:167–80.
31. Screening for colorectal cancer—United States, 1997. MMWR 1999;48:116–21.
32. Smith R, von Eschenback A, Wender R, Levin B, Byers T, et al. American Cancer Society guidelines for the early detection of cancer: update of early detection guidelines for prostate, colorectal, and endometrial cancers and Update 2001: testing for early lung cancer detection. CA Cancer J Clin 2001;51:38–75.
33. Simon J. Occult blood screening for colorectal carcinoma: a critical review. Gastroenterology 1985;88:820–37.
34. Van Dam J, Bond J, Sivak M. Fecal occult blood screening for colorectal cancer. Arch Intern Med 1995;155:2389–402.
35. Mandel J, Bond J, Church T, et al. Reducing mortality from colorectal cancer by screening for fecal occult blood. N Engl J Med 1993;328:1365–71.
36. Freedman S. The role of barium enema in detecting colorectal disease: a radiologist's perspective. Postgrad Med 1992;92:245–51.
37. Selby J, Friedman G, Quesenberry C, Weiss N. A case-control study of screening sigmoidoscopy and mortality from colorectal cancer. N Engl J Med 1992;326:653–7.
38. Lieberman D, Weiss D, Bond J, Ahnen D, Garewal H, Chejfec G. Use of colonoscopy to screen asymptomatic adults for colorectal cancer. N Engl J Med 2000;343:162–8.
39. Imperiale TF, Wagner DR, Lin CY, et al. Risk of advanced proximal neoplasms in asymptomatic adults according to the distal colorectal findings. N Engl J Med 2000;343:169–74.
40. Varma J, Pfenninger J. Flexible sigmoidoscopy. In: Pfenninger

J, Fowler G, eds. Procedures for primary care physicians. St. Louis: Mosby, 1994;907–27.

41. Barthel J, Hinojosa T, Shah N. Colonoscope length and procedure efficiency. J Clin Gastroenterol 1995;21:30–2.

42. Johnson CD, Dachman AH. CT colonography: the next colon screening examination? Radiology 2000;216(2):331–41.

43. Deans G, Parks T, Rowlands B, Spence R. Prognostic factors in colorectal cancer. Br J Surg 1992;79:608–13.

44. Kronborg O. Staging and surgery for colorectal cancer. Eur J Cancer 1993;29A:575–83.

45. Nelson H, Petrelli N, Carlin A, et al. Guidelines 2000 for colon and rectal surgery. J Natl Cancer Inst 2001;93:583–96.

46. Abdalla E, Blair E, Jones R, Sue-Ling H, Johnston D. Mechanism of synergy of levamisole and fluorouracil: induction of human leukocyte antigen class I in colorectal cancer cell line. J Natl Cancer Inst 1995;87:489–96.

47. Connell MJ, Mailliard JA, Kahn MJ, et al. Controlled trial of fluorouracil and low-dose leucovorin given for 6 months as postoperative adjuvant therapy for colon cancer. J Clin Oncol 1997; 15:246.

48. Verschraegen C, Pazdur R. Medical management of colorectal carcinomas. Tumor 1994;80:1–11.

49. Winawer S, St. John D, Bond J, et al. Prevention of colorectal cancer: guidelines based on new data. WHO Bull OMS 1995;73:7–10.

50. Janne P, Mayer J. Chemoprevention of colorectal cancer. N Engl J Med 2000;342:1960–8.

93
Surgical Problems of the Digestive System

E. Chris Vincent and Mike Purdon

Advances in the field of general surgery over the last decade have sparked a revolution in the care of patients with digestive diseases. Pressure from third-party payers to reduce hospital costs without sacrificing quality as well as the adaptation of the video-laparoscope for routine cholecystectomy ushered in an era of "minimally invasive" surgery. Improvements in diagnostic tools such as ultrasonography and computer-assisted tomography contributed to the change. Nevertheless, the principles of general surgery remain unchanged. Careful preoperative patient preparation, meticulous surgical technique, and prevention of postoperative complications remain as important as ever.

Abdominal Pain

Abdominal pain can be one of the most perplexing and potentially serious patient complaints evaluated by the family physician. Even symptoms that are less remarkable, such as anorexia, nausea, and minor gastrointestinal bleeding may indicate severe underlying pathology. Family physicians should carefully evaluate abdominal symptoms to ensure timely diagnosis and to determine if surgical or other treatment is necessary.

Etiology

Abdominal pain can result from myriad intra- and extraperitoneal diseases (Table 93.1). In studies done in Great Britain in the late 1980s, 16% of all patients admitted for abdominal pain had acute appendicitis and 13% had intestinal obstruction. A urologic cause for the abdominal pain was found in 8%. No etiology was found in 35% of patients; thus for many years nonspecific abdominal pain (NSAP) was thought to be the most frequent cause of hospital admissions for abdominal pain.[1,2] A more recent study, however, suggests that the astute practitioner can make a definitive diagnosis in most patients admitted for NSAP.[3]

Evaluation

History

There are three types of gastrointestinal pain: visceral, deep somatic, and referred. Visceral pain arises from tension in the walls of hollow viscera or from capsular stretching of a solid organ. It is a diffuse, poorly localized pain, often associated with autonomic symptoms such as sweating, bradycardia, and nausea. Somatic pain arises from the abdominal wall, especially the parietal peritoneum. It is sharp and easily localized. Referred pain is usually superficial and often a considerable distance from the diseased organ.

Important features of the pain are its character (colicky, burning, boring, knife-like) and its duration. In general, pain that lasts more than 6 hours is caused by conditions of surgical importance. Pain that awakens the patient is usually an indicator of disease. Vomiting can be due to absorbed toxins or occur as a result of peritoneal irritation or obstruction. It is a nonspecific finding, but its timing can be a helpful clue. It appears early with ureteral and biliary colic as well as intestinal obstruction but late with acute appendicitis.[4]

Physical Examination

The careful abdominal examination provides necessary information for deciding if the patient has a "surgical abdomen," especially if it is repeated every 2 to 3 hours by the same person as the pain evolves. The most gentle portions of the examination—inspection and auscultation—should be done first. A "scaphoid" abdomen does not mean that it is "unremarkable," only that it is sunken-in under the effects of gravity. An abdomen should appear symmetric or nearly so. If the patient is writhing, one should suspect ureteral or biliary colic. Restricted motion suggests peritonitis. Auscultation of the ab-

Table 93.1. Causes of Abdominal Pain

Gastrointestinal and intraperitoneal causes

Inflammatory factors:
  Peritonitis: bacterial, chemical, perforated hollow viscus,
    ruptured ovarian cyst
  Inflamed hollow viscus: appendix, gallbladder, peptic ulcer,
    colitis, diverticulitis, Meckel's diverticulitis,
    gastroenteritis, Crohn's disease, ulcerative colitis
  Solid organ: hepatitis, pancreatitis
  Other: lymphadenitis, pelvic abscess or infection
Obstruction: intestinal, biliary
Solid organ distention: acute hepatomegaly or splenomegaly
Pelvic organs: ovarian cyst distention, ovarian torsion, ectopic
  pregnancy, endometriosis
Intraperitoneal bleeding: ruptured liver, spleen, or hollow
  viscus; ruptured aortic aneurysm; ruptured ectopic
  pregnancy; perforated ulcer
Ischemia: bowel, omental
Trauma
Metabolic: lactase deficiency
Functional: irritable bowel syndrome, biliary dyskinesia

Extraperitoneal causes

Abdominal wall: trauma, hematoma, abscess, hernia
Cardiopulmonary: pneumonia, myocardial infarction,
  empyema, pulmonary embolism
Hematologic: leukemia, sickle cell disease
Neurologic: herpes zoster, spinal cord tumor, spinal
  osteomyelitis
Genitourinary: prostatitis, seminal vesiculitis, epididymitis,
  urinary calculi, tumor, infection
Metabolic: uremia, porphyria, diabetes, addisonian crisis
Musculoskeletal: spinal cord disorders
Drugs, toxins, heavy metals
Factitious and psychogenic

domen is a low-yield procedure, but it may help diagnose small-bowel obstruction if the examiner happens to listen during a period of rushes and tinkles.[4]

Abdominal palpation, feeling for localized areas of muscle rigidity (guarding), can help diagnose peritonitis. Absent guarding, however, does not exclude underlying pathology. Palpation and percussion of the right upper quadrant (RUQ) is essential for assessing the liver and gallbladder. Murphy's sign—pain in the RUQ upon palpation with deep inspiration—has a sensitivity of only 27%; therefore, its absence does not rule out gallbladder disease.[5]

Additional Testing

For most acute abdominal conditions, urinalysis, and a complete blood count (CBC) are helpful. Urinalysis helps to evaluate for infection, diabetes, porphyria, and nephrolithiasis. Anemia may be noted with chronic or subacute blood loss; leukocytosis may indicate infection. Additional tests may include measurement of serum amylase, lipase, transaminase, pregnancy test, glucose, and electrolytes. Stool may be easily checked for gross or occult blood. Other initial tests may include electrocardiography (ECG), chest radiography, diagnostic peritoneal lavage, culdocentesis, and special imaging studies such as computed tomography (CT) or ultrasonography (US). Plain film abdominal radiographs are rarely diagnostic

unless the patient has an intestinal obstruction, perforated viscera, or renal stone.[6] In the less acute situation, upper or lower endoscopy may play a role. Laparoscopy or laparotomy may be a part of the initial diagnosis and management; prompt surgical consultation should be considered.

Preparing the Patient for Surgery

Preoperative Testing

Evaluation of a patient about to undergo an abdominal operation depends on the severity of the illness, the presence of concomitant medical problems, and the surgical urgency. Abnormal laboratory values are often found in acutely ill patients who require emergent procedures. These patients should have, as a minimum, a CBC, serum electrolyte analysis, glucose, creatinine or blood urea nitrogen (BUN), ECG, and chest radiograph (also see Chapter 57). Indiscriminate laboratory testing of all healthy patients prior to elective surgery is not recommended. Instead, the clinician should perform a review of systems and physical examination looking for unsuspected cardiac, pulmonary, renal, and hematologic diseases. Selective "routine" testing can then be performed based on indications (Table 93.2).[7-9]

Fluid Therapy

Except for the most emergent abdominal problems, fluid imbalances should be corrected before surgery. These disorders usually involve volume depletion due to fluid loss or "third-spacing" and serum electrolyte abnormalities. It is important to ensure adequate urine output before potassium supplements are given.

Diabetic Control

Minor and elective surgical procedures require little alteration in the insulin or oral hypoglycemic medication dose. Most gastrointestinal surgery is stressful enough to alter the patient's metabolic status. A common practice is to begin an intravenous infusion of 5% dextrose solution on the day of surgery and administer one half to two thirds of the usual insulin dose subcutaneously. For prolonged operations on ill or septic patients, intravenous insulin and glucose infusions are often used, with careful intraoperative and postoperative glucose monitoring. For patients who do not eat for the first few days after surgery, modifications of their usual insulin doses are required. In general, frequent blood glucose monitoring and continuous intravenous insulin and glucose infusions are recommended.[10]

Laparoscopic Surgery

Since the early 1900s, surgeons have used a laparoscope to perform intraabdominal operations through small incisions. It was not until the late 1980s, when video-camera technology allowed visualization of the viscera by more than one person, that cholecystectomy via the laparoscope became possible. Since that time there has been such rapid acceptance of the

Table 93.2. **Indications for Selective Preoperative Testing Prior to Elective Surgery**

Test	Indication
Urinalysis	Renal disease
	Diabetes
	Recent genitourinary infection
Complete blood count	Anticipated blood loss (major surgery)
	Renal disease
	Hematologic disorder
	Malignancy or chemotherapy use
Coagulation studies	Anticoagulation therapy
	Personal or family history of bleeding disorder
	Hepatic disease
Electrolytes	Hypertension
	Renal disease
	Diabetes
	Adrenal or thyroid disease
	Malignancy or chemotherapy use
Blood urea nitrogen/creatinine	Age >60 years
	Hypertension
	Renal disease
	Diabetes
Serum glucose	Age >45 years
	Hypertension
	Renal disease
	Diabetes
	Obesity (consider)
Pregnancy test	Women of childbearing age with uncertain status based on menstrual history
Electrocardiogram	Age >40 years
	Hypertension
	Renal disease
	Diabetes
	Symptoms of coronary artery disease
Chest radiography and pulmonary function testing	Age >60 years
	Smoking history
	Pulmonary disease, symptoms, or findings
	Symptoms of coronary artery disease
	Upper abdominal surgery

Source: Adapted from Litaker,[7] King,[8] and McPherson.[9]

technique that most gallbladders are now removed with laparoscopic assistance.

The advantages of laparoscopic surgery include fewer wound infections, less blood loss, shorter hospital stays, and earlier ambulation and return to work. Most patients leave the hospital on the first postoperative day and are back to work within 2 weeks. Disadvantages include increased cost and the carbon dioxide (CO_2) pneumoperitoneum that must be created to visualize abdominal organs.[11]

Complications that are unique to the laparoscopic approach include perforation of visceral or vascular structures by a trocar or needle and harmful effects of the CO_2 pneumoperitoneum such as hypercarbia, decreased cardiac output, pneumothorax, and gas embolism. Inadvertent injuries to nerves, vessels, and viscera may go unrecognized owing to the lack

of depth perception compounded by the restricted movement and lack of sense of touch that is inherent in laparoscopic instruments.[11] Absolute contraindications to laparoscopic surgery are similar to those for "open" procedures. Relative contraindications include previous abdominal surgery, suspected adhesions, morbid obesity, severe chronic obstructive pulmonary disease (COPD), and pregnancy.[12]

Abdominal Trauma

Trauma is the leading cause of death in children and adults up to age 44 years and kills more Americans age 1 to 34 years than all other diseases. Approximately 60 million people are injured annually, accounting for approximately one in six hospital admissions. The total cost of injury in the United States is estimated at approximately $200 billion per year and these costs continue to increase.[13]

Clinical Presentation

Patients with blunt abdominal trauma can pose difficult diagnostic challenges. Nearly 50% of patients have no complaints or external signs of abdominal injury on admission.[14] Initial attention should address the ABCs of resuscitation: airway, breathing, and circulation. Laboratory analysis may include an initial urinalysis and CBC followed by serial hematocrits. Additional adjunctive tests are often required because physical examination is frequently nonspecific and patients may look well initially but then worsen.

Diagnostic peritoneal lavage (DPL) has been used increasingly since its introduction in 1965. After placement of a nasogastric tube and urinary catheter, an infraumbilical catheter is introduced by open or closed (Seldinger) technique. Immediate aspiration of 5 to 10 mL of blood constitutes a positive test, terminating the procedure. Otherwise, 1 L of a balanced salt solution is instilled and then siphoned out. This fluid is examined for red (RBCs) and white (WBCs) blood cells, amylase, bacteria, and bile. The presence of lavage fluid in a chest tube or urinary catheter is also noted. This technique has been shown in case series to be sensitive and specific for detecting intraabdominal bleeding.[15] It is especially useful in patients with altered sensorium, multiple trauma, or unexplained hypotension. It does not identify the source of bleeding and cannot detect retroperitoneal injuries. DPL may also miss subcapsular hematomas that have not ruptured into the peritoneum. Relative contraindications include pregnancy, previous major abdominal surgery, and bleeding disorders. The advantages are that it is an inexpensive, sensitive test that can be rapidly performed in the emergency department, avoiding treatment delay. It has been criticized as overly sensitive as bleeding detected can provoke laparotomy for liver and spleen injuries that may be better managed nonoperatively. Also, complications may arise in as many as 5% of patients.[15]

Helical CT is readily available in many hospitals and is the imaging procedure of choice in hemodynamically stable patients. CT is especially useful for evaluating liver and spleen injuries, which account for 40% and 20%, respectively, of abdominal organ injuries after blunt trauma.[16] It also detects retroperitoneal bleeding missed by DPL and fractures of the ribs, spine, and pelvis. CT may be more limited in patients with penetrating abdominal injuries due to uncertain sensitivity for the detection of hollow viscus injury and is not reliable in patients with diaphragmatic injury.[15] In penetrating flank and back wounds, CT scanning with triple contrast has an accuracy rate of 97% to 100% and is appropriate in the evaluation of patients with suspected retroperitoneal injury.[17]

Helical CT technology has improved sensitivity for pancreatic trauma but subtle injuries may be missed.[16] Other disadvantages of CT include its high cost, the time needed for the test, the requirement for hemodynamic stability, and the expertise necessary to interpret the study. Ultrasonography has been used extensively in Europe and Japan to determine the extent of abdominal injuries. The advantages are that it can be rapidly done at the bedside with minimal preparation and can be easily used for serial examinations. US does not require contrast agents and can elucidate abnormalities above the diaphragm, such as pericardial tamponade. US has been shown to be comparable with DPL and CT for the detection of hemoperitoneum and superior to both because of its rapidity, noninvasiveness, portability, and low cost.[18] US is helpful for evaluating solid organs (liver, spleen, kidney), although CT is more sensitive. US is somewhat operator dependent, and injuries that do not result in hemoperitoneum may be missed on initial scanning.[15]

Other adjunctive studies to consider include radiography, diatrizoate meglumine and diatrizoate sodium (Gastrografin, MD-Gastroview) duodenography, intravenous pyelography, cystography, and urethrography. Laparoscopy is expensive, invasive, and rarely helpful in blunt trauma, but may be the best method for evaluating diaphragmatic injuries after penetrating thoracoabdominal injuries.[13]

Penetrating abdominal trauma is usually due to gunshot and knife wounds. As with blunt trauma, the first priority is to stabilize the patient. Diagnostic tests such as CT and US should not delay urgent laparotomy in patients with obvious signs of abdominal visceral injury, overt peritonitis, or abdominal distention and hypotension. DPL may be useful in detecting diaphragmatic injuries and for determining penetration of gunshot wounds.[17]

Management

Family physicians should initiate management with volume replacement, baseline laboratory testing, typing and crossmatching blood, and bladder catheterization (when not contraindicated). With penetrating trauma an initial preoperative dose of antibiotic such as ampicillin/sulbactam or cefoxitin is appropriate. Although blunt abdominal trauma does not always obligate laparotomy, surgical consultation is advisable.

Appendicitis

Despite the steady decrease in the incidence of and mortality from appendicitis, it remains a prevalent problem.[19–21] The lifetime incidence of appendicitis is approximately 7%. The disease is rare in infants and the elderly but is common during ado-

lescence.[1,21,22] The etiology is usually idiopathic or associated with a fecalith. Rarely, appendicitis is secondary to foreign bodies, parasitic worms, or tumors (Kaposi's sarcoma).[23,24]

Clinical Presentation

The diagnosis of appendicitis remains a challenge. "Typical" appendicitis begins as a dull, periumbilical, or epigastric pain accompanied by anorexia and nausea. Within a few hours the pain becomes sharper, more intense, and localized to the right lower quadrant (RLQ). Physical examination reveals a low-grade fever, rebound tenderness, and muscle guarding. A positive psoas sign (increased pain with passive right hip extension) raises the likelihood of appendicitis. A review of the symptoms and signs of acute appendicitis found that the diagnosis should be questioned if one of the following is found: (1) absence of RLQ pain; (2) absence of pain migration to the RLQ; (3) presence of a previous episode of similar pain; or (4) lack of RLQ tenderness, rigidity, or guarding.[25] Signs with little diagnostic value included rectal tenderness, Rovsing's sign [pain in the RLQ when pressure is applied to the lower left quadrant (LLQ)], and bowel sound changes.[19,25,25]

One-third of all patients are "atypical" resulting in an incorrect or delayed diagnosis. A patient whose appendix is retrocecal or below the pelvic brim may complain of flank or back pain and diffuse abdominal tenderness. In this situation a positive psoas sign may signal appendicitis.[27] The diagnosis in children, the elderly, and reproductive-age females is frequently missed, and perforations are more common. Children with limited verbal skills may have a loss of appetite, unusual irritability, and a tendency to be quiet and lie down; vomiting is common and may precede pain.[28] Elderly patients may note only nonspecific symptoms such as indigestion and abdominal distention without localizing pain or tenderness.[26] Women with appendicitis are frequently misdiagnosed with pelvic inflammatory disease, gastroenteritis, or urinary tract infections (UTI).[29] Pregnancy presents a special challenge: a gravid uterus displaces the appendix superiorly and at term the pregnant woman with appendicitis may complain of RUQ pain. Because of abdominal muscle laxity she may not demonstrate rigidity or guarding.[19]

There are no blood tests that confirm or exclude the diagnosis, although a leukocytosis with a left shift (elevated bands) is often seen. For this reason, diagnostic imaging has become popular, especially in young children, the elderly (over age 60), women of reproductive age, and those with an "atypical" presentation.[30] Plain film radiography is not diagnostic but may help to rule out other conditions. Barium enema may show a nonfilling appendix but is not used for the acute presentation, largely because of advances in US and CT technology.[19,31]

Graded-compression US is readily available, inexpensive, and safe. Because US does not use ionizing radiation and can assist in diagnosing acute gynecologic conditions, it is the preferred imaging study for children and reproductive-age women. The diagnostic accuracy of US in patients with appendicitis is high; in research studies the positive (PPV) and negative (NPV) predictive values are 91% to 94% and 89% to 97%, respectively.[31] In actual practice, the real PPV and

NPV of US may be lower than 90% to 95% because US is very operator dependent. Also, the PPV for US in patients with perforated appendicitis is much lower than 90% because the diagnostic sign, a noncompressible appendix, is present in only 38% to 55% of patients. CT, though expensive, is more accurate than US for diagnosing appendicitis. The PPV and NPV are 92% to 98% and 95% to 100%, respectively.[31] Additionally, complications such as perforation or abscess formation are better demonstrated with CT than with US. Because of this CT is rapidly becoming the imaging procedure of choice for most patients in whom the diagnosis is not clear.[19,31] Other advantages of CT imaging in patients with suspected appendicitis include a reduction in the false-negative (i.e., unnecessary) appendectomy rate and potential overall cost savings.[32,33]

Several conditions may mimic appendicitis. Pelvic inflammatory disease accounts for 35% to 45% of the negative laparotomies for presumed appendicitis. Others include terminal ileitis, pyelonephritis, diverticulitis, ureteral calculus, pancreatitis, and subphrenic abscess. Mesenteric adenitis, a self-limited condition, may also masquerade as appendicitis.[27]

Management

Surgical removal of the appendix via a McBurney or transverse muscle-splitting incision is the standard definitive treatment. Laparoscopic removal is also possible, although most studies fail to demonstrate an advantage over the traditional "open" technique. Women of childbearing age are an exception, as they may benefit from laparoscopic diagnosis and possibly treatment of a gynecologic disease, accounting for their symptoms.[22,30] Elderly patients who initially present several days into the course of their illness and who are improving may be managed without surgery.[19]

The routine use of prophylactic antibiotics in patients with uncomplicated appendicitis is controversial; however, most authors recommend them. All patients with complicated, gangrenous, or perforated appendicitis should receive intravenous antibiotics for 7 to 10 days or until clinical improvement. Appendicitis-related infections are polymicrobial; therefore, the antibiotics used should have both aerobic and anaerobic activity. Effective antibiotic regimens include (1) single-agent therapy with a second- or third-generation cephalosporin, and (2) metronidazole in combination with a β-lactamase inhibitor, a cephalosporin, or an aminoglycoside. Wound irrigation with topical antibiotics and delayed wound closure may be beneficial. If a periappendiceal abscess is present, it should be drained and the appendix removed after recovery.[19,22]

Complications, Morbidity, and Mortality

Wound infection is the most frequent complication of appendicitis. Other problems include urinary retention, intestinal obstruction, abscess formation, UTI, pneumonia, intestinal fistula, and infertility. A perforated appendix increases the complication rate threefold. Mortality is only 0.03% for simple appendicitis but increases to 0.2% with perforation. As expected, very young, elderly, immunosuppressed, and "atypical" patients suffer higher mortality rates.[19,22]

Cholecystitis and Cholelithiasis

The prevalence of gallstones in adults in Western industrialized nations averages 10% to 15%. It is lower (5%) in Asians and Africans and higher (up to 70%) in Native Americans. Women are two times as likely as men to develop gallstones. Incidence increases with age; 25% of persons over age 65 and 50% over age 75 have cholelithiasis. A family history of cholelithiasis and a diet rich in carbohydrates and fats are additional risk factors for gallstone formation.[34–36]

Clinical Presentation

Patients with acute cholecystitis usually complain of a rapid onset of severe, cramping RUQ abdominal pain with associated low-grade fever, nausea, and vomiting. Physical findings may include RUQ or epigastric tenderness, guarding, and Murphy's sign. The gallbladder may be palpable in up to 20% of patients.[37,38] Patients with chronic cholecystitis have a more indolent course. Fever is uncommon, and abdominal pain, nausea, and vomiting are less severe. Episodes are shorter in duration and recurrent.

Ninety to 95% of patients with cholecystitis have gallstones; however, abdominal pain in patients with gallstones may not be due to cholecystitis. Typical biliary colic is a steady, RUQ, or epigastric pain that lasts 1 to 5 hours and may be associated with nausea and vomiting. It commonly occurs at night, usually around the same time. Postprandial pain, dyspepsia, bloating, flatulence, and fatty food intolerance are not specific for gallstone related pain. Physicians who encounter patients with these symptoms should consider other diagnoses.[37,39]

Laboratory findings of acute cholecystitis include a leukocytosis of 12,000 to 15,000 cells/mm^3 and mild increases in the serum transaminase, amylase, and alkaline phosphatase levels. In the absence of common bile duct stones, the total serum bilirubin is usually less than 4 mg/dL.[37,38] Patients with chronic cholecystitis rarely have abnormal laboratory values.

Abdominal radiographs seldom help diagnose cholecystitis but may exclude other conditions. US is 95% sensitive and specific for diagnosing gallstones and has largely supplanted oral cholecystography (OCG). CT imaging may identify gallstones when the US cannot because of overlying fat or bowel gas. Radionucleotide cholescintigraphy with hepato-iminodiacetic acid (HIDA scan) is the test of choice in patients without gallstones and patients who have an atypical presentation. Nonvisualization of the gallbladder in spite of normal visualization of the liver and bile ducts is 90% to 95% sensitive and specific for acute cholecystitis. It accurately proves cystic duct obstruction and can be used despite high serum bilirubin levels. The major disadvantage is the high false-positive rate in the patient who is fasting, alcoholic, or receiving parenteral alimentation.[37,38]

Management

Moderately ill patients with suspected cholecystitis are hospitalized for intravenous fluid replacement and diagnostic evaluation. Intravenous antibiotics, although controversial, are usually recommended. Cholecystectomy should be performed within 24 to 72 hours in most patients with acute cholecystitis, as complications are more likely with delayed surgery. Patients with peritonitis or whose condition deteriorates should have immediate surgery.[37,38,40]

Laparoscopic cholecystectomy is the procedure of choice for uncomplicated acute and chronic cholecystitis. Patients with pancreatitis, peritonitis, sepsis, coagulopathy, gallbladder cancer, or cholecystoenteric fistulas are usually best managed by open cholecystectomy. Male gender, advanced age, and a history of multiple prior painful attacks are additional factors favoring an open operation. US evidence of a stone more than 20 mm, gallbladder wall thickness more than 4 mm, or common bile duct (CBD) diameter more than 6 mm also increases the likelihood of converting to an open procedure. Cholecystostomy (percutaneous gallbladder drainage and stone removal) remains an option for patients who are poor surgical candidates.[37,41]

Medical management may be considered for patients with chronic cholecystitis who are poor operative candidates or who decline surgery. Options include oral bile acids (ursodiol), direct contact with methyl tert-butyl ether (MTBE), or extracorporeal shock wave lithotripsy (ESWL). Optimal stones for dissolution by ursodiol or MTBE are radiolucent, less than 10 mm in diameter, and "float" when viewed by US or OCG. The gallbladder must be functioning, as noted by OCG or HIDA scan. Because of these restrictions, only 30% of patients with chronic cholecystitis are candidates for dissolution treatment. Complete dissolution rates average 30% to 90%, depending on the size of stones. Gallstones recur within 5 years in 50% of successfully treated patients, although maintenance therapy with ursodiol reduces this recurrence rate to 25%.[37,42] Experience with ESWL is limited; in optimal patients, the efficacy is 70% to 90%. Disadvantages include restricted applicability and availability, the need for concomitant oral dissolution therapy, a high incidence of biliary colic, and a stone recurrence rate similar to those for other nonsurgical methods.[34,37]

Most persons with asymptomatic or "silent" stones discovered incidentally by US can be managed expectantly, as only 1% to 2% become symptomatic each year.[34,37] Cholecystectomy should be considered in patients with a calcified ("porcelain") gallbladder or who undergo laparotomy for an unrelated condition. Diabetes is not an indication for elective cholecystectomy, although diabetics with symptomatic stones should be treated promptly.[38,41,43]

Complications, Morbidity, and Mortality

In patients with cholelithiasis, 10% to 15% of those younger than age 60 and 30% to 95% older than age 60 have CBD stones. History and physical examination may be unremarkable, but usually patients with CBD stones present with some variation of Charcot's triad (jaundice, RUQ pain, and fever). Serum liver tests [direct bilirubin, alkaline phosphatase, and γ-glutamyltranspeptidase (GGT)] are usually elevated. A dilated CBD on US suggests choledocholithiasis; however, this finding is seen in only 50% of patients.

For three decades endoscopic retrograde cholangiopancreatography (ERCP) has been the "gold standard" for diagnos-

ing CBD stones. Advantages include a high sensitivity and specificity (up to 95%) with comparable success rates for stone removal. Disadvantages include a small but significant risk of complication (usually pancreatitis) and availability (mainly limited by operator skill). Magnetic resonance cholangiography (MRC), helical CT cholangiography (HCTC), and endoscopic US (EUS) are newer additions to the list of noninvasive tests. All are highly sensitive and specific (80–100%) and are comparably safe. None is therapeutic, however, and they may not be as widely available as ERCP.[37,44,45]

If found, CBD stones should usually be removed due to a high complication rate.[34,37] The technique depends on operator availability and experience. Preoperative ERCP with endoscopic sphincterotomy is more than 90% successful in expert hands. Intraoperative cholangiography should be seriously considered in most young and all elderly patients who have not had preoperative ERCP, MRC, HCTC, or EUS. Most CBD stones discovered at surgery should be removed either via laparoscopic exploration, conversion to an "open" procedure, or postoperative ERCP.[37,41]

Gallbladder perforation occurs in 3% to 12% of patients with acute cholecystitis. Diabetics, elderly, and immunocompromised patients or patients with systemic vascular disease are at higher risk for perforation. Elderly or diabetic patients are also more likely to develop emphysematous cholecystitis, a rare but serious condition with a 15% mortality. Patients with large (usually >2 cm diameter) stones who have cholecystenteric fistulas may develop intestinal obstruction ("gallstone ileus") if the stone passes via fistula into bowel.[37,38]

Mortality from cholecystectomy is only 0.2%. Most deaths occur in elderly or critically ill patients. Injury to the bile ducts is slightly more common with laparoscopic compared to open cholecystectomy.[40,41]

Inguinal Hernia

Inguinal hernias are defined on the basis of their anatomic relation to the inferior epigastric vessels. Direct inguinal hernias lie medial to the inferior epigastrics in Hesselbach's triangle; indirect hernias appear lateral to the vessels and protrude through the internal inguinal ring. The fundamental problem is a defect in the endoabdominal fascia, allowing the peritoneum, and in some cases viscera, to bulge. Predisposing factors are listed in Table 93.3.[46,47]

Several classification systems have been developed for the purpose of communication and comparison of repair results. Most systems are based on the size and location of the defect. Unfortunately, no single classification system is universally accepted.[46,48]

Clinical Presentation

In children inguinal hernias are usually present at birth or shortly thereafter. The onset in adults is often insidious, although rapid onset is possible and is almost invariably associated with unusual straining or exertion. Patients may feel little or no discomfort, complaining only of a protrusion in the groin with coughing or lifting that subsides when the pa-

Table 93.3. **Factors Predisposing to Inguinal Hernias**

Factor	Cause
Increased intraabdominal pressure	Lifting, coughing, sneezing, straining, obesity, chronic obstructive pulmonary disease, ascites, prostatic hypertrophy, pregnancy
Weak or attenuated abdominal muscles and fascia	Advanced age, poor physical fitness, chronic illness, weight loss
Patent processus vaginalis or dilated inguinal ring[a]	Congenital
Denervation of musculature of internal ring[a]	Injury to nerve during appendectomy or other abdominal surgery

[a]Indirect hernias only.

Source: Adapted from Eubanks[46] and Abrahamson.[47]

tient is resting supine.[49] When present, the pain of an inguinal hernia is usually described as a soreness or burning. Examination reveals a dynamic mass that increases in size and turgor with the Valsalva maneuver, coughing, or standing; it resolves when the patient relaxes or lies down.

Radiography and laboratory tests are seldom used to confirm the diagnosis. It has been taught that patients over age 45 should be evaluated for malignant ascites or a partial bowel obstruction due to colon cancer.[49] Research, however, has failed to show an association between inguinal hernias and colon cancer.[50]

Management

Repair of a reducible inguinal hernia is rarely emergent. Many small, asymptomatic, direct hernias can be treated conservatively with a hernia belt or truss. A truss will not cure a hernia but may help identify patients with hernias but atypical symptoms; those who gain relief from the truss may benefit from surgery. Surgical repair is usually indicated for all indirect hernias, especially in the elderly, because the morbidity and mortality risk of incarceration or strangulation is much higher than the risks associated with surgery.[46,49,51]

The "traditional" reinforcement of the posterior wall of the inguinal canal and high ligation of the sac was first described by Bassini in 1884. Since that time, many repair techniques have been developed, and no particular operation has emerged as the gold standard. The Shouldice procedure has a low recurrence rate but requires extensive dissection. Lichtenstein's group reported excellent results using prosthetic mesh in a "tension-free" hernioplasty.[46,52]

Laparoscopic hernia repair has emerged as an alternative to the "traditional" operations. Several techniques have been tried, and many studies comparing various laparoscopic to open procedures have been done. Disadvantages of the laparoscopic hernioplasty include increased direct costs and the need for prosthetic mesh as well as general anesthesia. Advantages include less postoperative pain and more rapid return to work. Although the issue of "open" versus "minimally invasive" repair remains controversial, the laparoscopic approach may be better suited for patients with bilateral or recurrent hernias.[46,53–56]

Complications, Morbidity, and Mortality

Recurrence is the most frequent complication of inguinal hernia repair, with failure rates averaging 10%. Faulty technique, rather than type of repair, may be the cause of most failures.

Exceptions include the Shouldice procedure and repairs that employ a prosthetic mesh; their reported failure rates are usually less than 5%. Minor complications of hernia repair include hemorrhage, wound infection, and injury to the bowel, bladder, testicles, vas deferens, and nerves. The mortality from elective hernia repair is negligible.[46,53,57]

Bowel Obstruction

Bowel obstruction may be classified as mechanical or neurogenic (ileus). Table 93.4 lists some of the causes of obstruction by age group. The three leading causes of obstruction are adhesions (60%), hernias (20%), and neoplasms (10%).[58] Most obstructions occur in the small bowel. In complete obstructions, up to 42% have strangulation of the blood supply.[59] Delay in diagnosis increases patient pain, total duration of hospital stay, the need for intensive care, and mortality.[60]

Clinical Presentation

A history of constipation, previous abdominal surgery, age over 50, and distention are important historical clues.[60] Crampy pain typically occurs in paroxysms every 4 to 5 minutes.[58] Patients with a high small bowel obstruction (SBO) have early vomiting and little distention. Symptoms develop rapidly, and patients may pass stool or flatus. The symptoms of low SBO progress more slowly. Vomiting occurs later, is less profuse, and may be feculent. Colonic obstruction causes early constipation and marked abdominal distention but little vomiting.[58]

Physical examination may reveal shock, dehydration, tachycardia, or fever, especially if there is a high SBO or if there has been strangulation or perforation. Early, bowel sounds are hyperactive but become hypoactive if treatment is delayed or there is peritonitis. Tenderness may be absent in early cases but is invariably present later on. The physician should palpate the hernial orifices and perform a rectal examination. Discovery of a mass suggests strangulation or neoplasm. Scars from previous abdominal surgery imply obstruction due to adhesions.

The symptoms and signs of neurogenic bowel obstruction are variable.[59] In general, however, the onset of symptoms is gradual, and physical findings moderate. Ileus may occur postlaparotomy, or as a result of electrolyte derangements, drugs, intraabdominal inflammation, retroperitoneal hemorrhage or inflammation, intestinal ischemia, thoracic processes,

Table 93.4. **Causes of Bowel Obstruction**

Age	Mechanical	Neurogenic/paralytic
All ages	Cystic fibrosis Intussusception (more common in infants) Malrotation Strangulated hernia Volvulus (more common in elderly)	Familial visceral myopathy or neuropathy Nonfamilial visceral myopathy or neuropathy Medications (opiates, psychotropics, antiparkinsonian) Metabolic (hypokalemia, uremia, hypothyroid) Postoperative Peritonitis Retroperitoneal syndrome
Neonates/infants	Congenital atresia Imperforate anus Meconium ileus	Hirschsprung's disease
Adults	Adhesions Bezoars Carcinoma Crohn's disease Gallstones Parasites Pregnancy Radiation injury	Collagen vascular disease Diabetes
Elderly	Same as adults; also diverticulitis	

or sepsis.[59] Laboratory studies are usually nonspecific, although a CBC, serum electrolyte assays, urea nitrogen, and creatinine should be measured.[59] Leukocytosis suggests strangulation, but it is not always present. If the patient has been vomiting, electrolytes are frequently abnormal and should be corrected prior to surgery.

Traditionally, plain films have been used to confirm the presence or absence of SBO, but sensitivity ranges from 40% to 70%.[61] The distribution of air in the bowel is the most important finding. In patients with high complete SBO there is little air in the bowel. More distal SBO produces a "stepladder" pattern of air-fluid levels within bowel loops. With distal colon blockage, gas shadows are located peripherally. Haustral folds can be distinguished from valvulae conniventes (small bowel folds); the former are deeper, more irregular, and do not traverse the gut.

Up to 40% of patients with bowel obstruction have normal radiographs.[61] Computed tomography may be useful in patients with intestinal obstruction who have a suspicious clinical presentation and normal abdominal radiographs. If there is a history of abdominal cancer, CT may show peritoneal carcinomatosis or evidence of solid organ metastases, localizing the point of obstruction. Adhesions may be inferred in areas of transition from dilated to nondilated bowel without apparent cause but are often a diagnosis of exclusion. CT is also able to detect early signs of strangulation or volvulus with high accuracy.[61] If the diagnosis is uncertain, a barium or water-soluble contrast study may be useful. The choice of agent is controversial. The risk of barium impaction proximal to the obstruction is probably small; nevertheless, it should not be used if perforation is suspected. Diatrizoate is thought to be safer, but mucosal detail is often lacking, and the hyperosmolar effect may produce intravascular volume depletion and electrolyte imbalance. Recurring or low-grade obstruction is best defined by barium studies such as enteroclysis. Disadvantages include the need for nasoenteric intubation, slow transit time through a fluid-filled hypotonic small bowel, and the need for specialized radiologic technique and interpretation.[58] All patients suspected of having colonic obstruction (in the absence of peritonitis) should undergo proctosigmoidoscopy. Although colonoscopy may be useful in patients with partial colonic obstruction, it has little role in the initial evaluation of patients with complete colonic obstruction. The insufflation of air, or even carbon dioxide, through the endoscope into the obstructed bowel may exacerbate colonic distention and precipitate perforation.[59]

Management

Surgery is the treatment of choice for most bowel obstructions. All patients should be allowed nothing by mouth and be given intravenous fluids. Some surgeons recommend broad-spectrum antibiotics because of the risk of bacterial translocation across the bowel wall.[58] Decompression of the upper gut may reduce the discomfort of distention and lessen the risk of aspiration.[59] The role of long intestinal tubes is controversial, as they have been associated with more complications. In patients with neurogenic obstruction, treatment is entirely supportive and correction of the underlying condition may relieve the blockage.[58] Surgery may be avoided in patients with partial intestinal blockage due to adhesions if they improve with nasogastric suction. Patients treated conservatively must have serial examinations and radiographs. The optimal length of a nonoperative trial of therapy is controversial, ranging from 12 to 120 hours.[62] Complete SBO necessitates early laparotomy.

Complications, Morbidity, and Mortality

Surgical complications include inadvertent enterotomy, recurrent obstruction, wound infection, intraabdominal abscesses, respiratory failure, atelectasis, pneumonia, electrolyte imbalance, urinary tract infection, and renal failure. In one series the morbidity was 30%. The mortality rate continues to drop and is now less than 10%. Old age, comorbidity, nonviable strangulation, and a treatment delay of more than 24 hours all increased the death rate. Age older than 75 years and comorbidity increased the risk of death four to five times compared with younger and healthy patients.[63]

Prevention

Many agents have been tested with the hope of reducing abdominal adhesions due to surgery. To date, none is recommended. Careful handling of the abdominal viscera at the time of surgery, avoidance of excessive suturing or peritoneal closure, the exclusion of foreign materials from the peritoneal cavity, and placement of the omentum between the gut and abdominal wall when closing may prevent adhesion formation.[58]

References

1. Irvin TT. Abdominal pain: a surgical audit of 1190 emergency admissions. Br J Surg 1989;76:1121–5.
2. Hawthorn IE. Abdominal pain as a cause of acute admission to hospital. J R Coll Surg Edinb 1992;37:389–93.
3. Decadt B, Sussman L, Lewis MPN, et al. Randomized clinical trial of early laparoscopy in the management of acute non-specific abdominal pain. Br J Surg 1999;86:1383–6.
4. Jones RS. Acute abdomen. In Townsend CM, ed. Sabiston textbook of surgery, 16th ed. St. Louis: WB Saunders, 2001;802–15.
5. Gunn A, Keddie N. Some clinical observations on patients with gallstones. Lancet 1972;2:239–41.
6. Anyanwu AC, Moalypour SM. Are abdominal radiographs still overutilized in the assessment of acute abdominal pain? A district general hospital audit. J R Coll Surg Edinb 1998;43:267–70.
7. Litaker D. Preoperative screening. Med Clin North Am 1999;83:1565–81.
8. King MS. Preoperative evaluation. Am Fam Physician 2000;62:387–96.
9. McPherson DS. Preoperative laboratory testing: should any tests be "routine" before surgery? Med Clin North Am 1993;77:289–309.
10. Hoogwerf BJ. Perioperative management of diabetes mellitus: striving for metabolic balance. Cleve Clin J Med 1992;59:447–9.
11. Chekan EG, Pappas TN. Minimally invasive surgery. In: Townsend CM, ed. Sabiston textbook of surgery, 16th ed. St. Louis: WB Saunders, 2001;292–310.
12. Curet MJ. Special problems in laparoscopic surgery. Previous abdominal surgery, obesity, and pregnancy. Surg Clin North Am 2000;80:1093–110.
13. Hoyt DB, Coimbra R, Winchell RJ. Management of acute trauma. In Townsend CM, ed. Sabiston textbook of surgery, 16th ed. St. Louis: WB Saunders, 2001;311–45.
14. Chiquito PE. Blunt abdominal injuries. Diagnostic peritoneal lavage, ultrasonography and computed tomography scanning. Injury 1996;27:117–24.
15. Amoroso TA. Evaluation of the patient with blunt abdominal trauma: an evidence based approach. Emerg Med Clin North Am 1999;17:63–75.
16. Novelline RA, Rhea JT, Bell T. Helical CT of abdominal trauma. Radiol Clin North Am 1999;37:591–612.
17. Ferrada R, Birolini D. New concepts in the management of patients with penetrating abdominal wounds. Surg Clin North Am 1999;79:1331–56.
18. McKenny KL. Ultrasound of blunt abdominal trauma. Radiol Clin North Am 1999;37:879–93.
19. Lally KP, Cox CS, Andrassy RJ. Appendix. In Townsend CM, ed. Sabiston textbook of surgery, 16th ed. Philadelphia: WB Saunders, 2001;917–28.
20. Williams NM, Jackson D, Everson NW, et al. Is the incidence of acute appendicitis really falling? Ann R Coll Surg Eng 1998;80:122–4.
21. Addiss DG, Shaffer N, Fowler BS, et al. The epidemiology of appendicitis and appendectomy in the United States. Am J Epidemiol 1990;132:910–25.
22. Hale DA. Appendectomy: a contemporary appraisal. Ann Surg 1997;225:252–61.
23. Green SM, Schmidt SP, Rothrock SG. Delayed appendicitis from an ingested foreign body. Am J Emerg Med 1994;12:53–6.
24. Ravalli S, Vincent RA, Beaton HL. Acute appendicitis secondary to Kaposi's sarcoma in the acquired immunodeficiency syndrome. NY State J Med 1991;91:383–4.
25. Wagner JM, McKinney WP, Carpenter JL. Does this patient have appendicitis? JAMA 1996;276:1589–94.
26. Kraemer M, Franke C, Ohmann C, et al. Acute appendicitis in late adulthood: incidence, presentation, and outcome. Results of a prospective multicenter acute abdominal pain study and a review of the literature. Langenbecks Arch Surg 2000;385:470–81.
27. Hardin DM Jr. Acute appendicitis: review and update. Am Fam Physician 1999;60:2027–34.
28. Rothrock SG, Pagane J. Acute appendicitis in children: emergency department diagnosis and management. Ann Emerg Med 2000;36:39–51.
29. Rothrock SG, Green SM, Dobson M, et al. Misdiagnosis of appendicitis in nonpregnant women of childbearing age. J Emerg Med 1995;13:1–8.
30. Wilcox RT, Traverso LW. Have the evaluation and treatment of acute appendicitis changed with new technology? Surg Clin North Am 1997;77:1355–70.
31. Birnbaum BA, Wilson SR. Appendicitis at the millennium. Radiology 2000;215:337–48.
32. Schuler JG, Shortsleeve MJ, Goldenson RS, et al. Is there a role for abdominal computed tomographic scans in appendicitis? Arch Surg 1998;133:373–6.
33. Rao PM, Rhea JT, Novelline RA, et al. Effect of computed tomography of the appendix on treatment of patients and use of hospital resources. N Engl J Med 1998;338:141–6.
34. Hermann RE. The spectrum of biliary stone disease. Am J Surg 1989;158:171–3.
35. Kratzer W, Mason RA, Kachele V. Prevalence of gallstones in sonographic surveys worldwide. J Clin Ultrasound 1999;27:1–7.
36. Caroli-Bosc FX, Deveau C, Peten E, et al. Cholelithiasis and dietary risk factors: an epidemiologic investigation in Vidauban, Southeast France. Dig Dis Sci 1998;43:2131–7.
37. Ahmed A, Cheung RC, Keeffe EB. Management of gallstones and their complications. Am Fam Physician 2000;61:1673–80.
38. Sharp KW. Acute cholecystitis. Surg Clin North Am 1988;68:269–79.
39. Rigas B, Torosis J, McDougall CJ, et al. The circadian rhythm of biliary colic. J Clin Gastroenterol 1990;12:409–14.
40. Lo CM, Liu CL, Fan ST, et al. Prospective randomized study of early versus delayed laparoscopic cholecystectomy for acute cholecystitis. Ann Surg 1998;227:461–7.
41. Strasberg SM. Laparoscopic biliary surgery. Gastroenterol Clin North Am 1999;28:117–32.
42. Rubin RA, Kowalski TE, Khandelwal M, et al. Ursodiol for hepatobiliary disorders. Ann Intern Med 1994;121:207–18.
43. Aucott JN, Cooper GS, Bloom AD, et al. Management of gallstones in diabetic patients. Arch Intern Med 1993;153:1053–8.
44. Soto JA. Bile duct stones: diagnosis with MR cholangiography and helical CT. Semin Ultrasound CT MR 1999;20:304–16.
45. Polkowski M, Palucki J, Regula J, et al. Helical computed to-

mographic cholangiography versus endosonography for suspected bile duct stones: a prospective blinded study in non-jaundiced patients. Gut 1999;45:744–9.

46. Eubanks SW. Hernias. In Townsend CM, ed. Sabiston textbook of surgery, 16th ed. Philadelphia: WB Saunders 2001; 783–801.

47. Abrahamson J. Etiology and pathophysiology of primary and recurrent groin hernia formation. Surg Clin North Am 1998;78: 953–72.

48. Rutkow IM, Robbins AW. Classification systems and groin hernias. Surg Clin North Am 1998;78:1117–27.

49. Berliner SD. When is surgery necessary for a groin hernia? Postgrad Med 1990;87:149–52.

50. Wheeler WE, Wilson SL, Kurucz J, et al. Flexible sigmoidoscopy screening for asymptomatic colorectal disease in patients with and without inguinal hernia. South Med J 1991;84:876–8.

51. Schumpelick V, Treutner KH. Inguinal hernia repair in adults. Lancet 1994;344:375–9.

52. Kurzer M. The Lichtenstein repair. Surg Clin North Am 1998; 78:1025–46.

53. Schumpelick V, Treutner KH. Inguinal hernia repair in adults. Lancet 1994;344:375–9.

54. Crawford DL, Phillips EH. Laparoscopic repair and groin hernia surgery. Surg Clin North Am 1998;78:1047–62.

55. Collaboration EH. Laparoscopic compared with open methods of groin hernia repair: systematic review of randomized controlled trials. Br J Surg 2000;87:860–7.

56. Lucas SW, Arregui ME. Minimally invasive surgery for inguinal hernia. World J Surg 1999;23:350–5.

57. Bendavid R. Complications of groin hernia surgery. Surg Clin North Am 1998;78:1089–103.

58. Evers BM. Small bowel. In: Townsend CM, ed. Sabiston textbook of surgery, 16th ed. Philadelphia: WB Saunders 2001;873–916.

59. Turnage RH, Bergen PC. Intestinal obstruction and ileus. In: Feldman M, ed. Sleisinger and Fordtran's gastrointestinal and liver disease, 6th ed. Philadelphia: WB Saunders 1998;1799–808.

60. Bohner H, Yang Q, Franke C, et al. Simple data from history and physical examination help to exclude bowel obstruction and to avoid radiographic studies in patients with acute abdominal pain. Eur J Surg 1998;164:777–84.

61. Daneshmand S. The utility and reliability of computed tomography scan in the diagnosis of small bowel obstruction. Am Surg 1999;65:922–6.

62. Miller G, Boman J, Shrier I, et al. Natural history of patients with adhesive small bowel obstruction. Br J Surg 2000;87:1240–7.

63. Fevang BT. Complications and death after surgical treatment of small bowel obstruction: a 35-year institutional experience. Ann Surg 2000;231:529–37.

94
Selected Disorders of the Digestive System and Nutrition

Robert L. Buckley

Ischemic Bowel Diseases

Acute Arterial Disease

Vascular diseases affecting the colon can occur acutely or chronically and often mimic other conditions, such as bacterial gastroenteritis and inflammatory bowel disease, making diagnosis difficult. While these conditions most often are seen in the sixth decade of life and beyond, they can occur in younger patients with hypercoagulable states, with medications that increase coagulation, and with recreational drug use. The ischemic injury can involve the full thickness of the bowel or more superficial levels. The small intestine and right colon are perfused by the superior mesenteric artery (SMA), and the inferior mesenteric artery (IMA) supplies the left colon and most of the rectosigmoid. Watershed areas in the vascular supply to the bowel may be particularly susceptible to ischemic injury. When the colon is involved, the patient is said to have ischemic colitis, although this does not imply etiology. Ischemic colitis may involve multiple conditions that may result in acute, subacute, or chronic injury that may be superficial or transmural. Approximately half of all patients with mesenteric ischemia present with ischemic colitis, most commonly associated with generalized arteriosclerosis.[1,2]

Clinical Presentation

Mesenteric arteriopathy may present acutely, subacutely, or chronically. The mesenteric vessels can become occluded from emboli, thrombi, or vasospasm. The most common presenting symptom is abdominal pain. In patients with SMA occlusion, the pain is often severe and out of proportion to the physical examination, localized or diffuse, colicky or constant. Patients with ischemic colitis commonly have pain localized to the left lower quadrant that may be mild in intensity and associated with an urge to defecate. Gastrointestinal bleeding is common with occlusion of the SMA or IMA. The patient may have a prior history of unexplained weight loss or postprandial pain and complain of nausea, vomiting, or diarrhea. Thirty percent of elderly patients with SMA involvement present with mental status changes. Signs of SMA occlusion include fever, tachycardia, abdominal distention, rigidity, and rebound tenderness. On examination the patient's bowel sounds are frequently hypoactive. Patients may have unexplained abdominal distention in both acute SMA occlusion involving the small intestine and ischemic colitis. Patients with acute occlusion of the SMA may present with hypotension.[2] Approximately 20% of patients with ischemic colitis go on to develop chronic colitis with stricture, continued diarrhea that may be bloody, and weight loss.[1]

Diagnosis

The diagnosis of mesenteric arteriopathy requires a high level of suspicion in an elderly patient or in a patient with a hypercoagulable state. Laboratory studies are nonspecific. Patients may have leukocytosis, metabolic acidosis, hyperamylasemia, elevated alkaline phosphatase, and hemoconcentration in proportion to the extent of bowel involvement. Stools may be positive for occult blood or show frank bleeding. Plain films of the abdomen can be normal or show gas-filled loops of bowel with thickened folds and air-fluid levels. Late x-ray findings include thumb printing, aperistaltic loops, and pneumoperitoneum. Computed tomography (CT) of the abdomen may suggest other possible etiologies for the symptoms and signs such as mesenteric vein thrombosis, but can be nondiagnostic for arterial disease. Doppler ultrasound is diagnostic in 28% of cases. Colonoscopy can be used to rule out other etiologies of the patient's symptoms and can confirm the diagnosis of ischemic colitis. Angiography allows identification of vascular lesions and allows planning for surgical intervention.[2]

Management

Supportive therapy for patients with acute superior mesenteric arteriopathies includes fluid management to correct electrolyte abnormalities and restore blood pressure. Decompression with the use of a nasogastric tube and/or rectal tube may improve circulation to the affected bowel. Broad-spectrum antibiotics should be started to treat sepsis. Intraarterial vasodilators such as selective infusion of papaverine at 30 to 60 mg per hour can be used while preparing for surgical intervention in occlusive disease of the SMA. The patient on papaverine should be monitored for worsening abdominal pain or hypotension. In patients with nonocclusive disease, the papaverine may be continued for 24 hours and the arteriogram repeated.[2]

Patients with ischemic colitis may be initially treated medically if they do not show signs of peritonitis. Patients are put at bowel rest and IV fluids are given. Patients with signs of significant malnourishment, or with a prolonged course, are candidates for hyperalimentation. Broad-spectrum antibiotics may be indicated to reduce colonic injury and treat sepsis. Patients usually rapidly improve within 24 hours on medical management. Patients who show signs of worsening pain, with laboratory findings such as leukocytosis and metabolic acidosis, or peritoneal signs are candidates for surgical intervention.[1] Patients should be evaluated for the etiology of the ischemic bowel disease including cardiac evaluation for embolic events and for other evidence of vascular disease.

Prevention and Family and Community Issues

Patients with risk factors for arterial disease should take all possible steps to reduce their risk by treating their hypertension, normalizing cholesterol, and avoiding tobacco products and recreational drugs such as cocaine. Patients with a family history of hypercoagulable states should be cautious in the use of medications that may enhance coagulation. Patients with significant atherosclerotic vascular disease should be warned to report unexplained abdominal pain. Patients who have had an episode of ischemic bowel are at risk for vascular disease elsewhere and should be warned about the risks of heart disease as well as other vascular problems.

Chronic Mesenteric Ischemia

Chronic mesenteric ischemia can occur at any age, although the mean age of presentation is 58.[3] The majority of these patients are smokers.

Clinical Presentation

The classic presentation of chronic mesenteric ischemia is periumbilical or epigastric abdominal pain 20 to 30 minutes after a meal. The pain lasts 1 to 3 hours.[4] Patients may also present with weight loss as the primary complaint, since they may decrease oral intake to avoid the abdominal pain. Patients may complain of nausea, vomiting, diarrhea, or constipation. On examination, patients may have an abdominal bruit and show signs of malnutrition. The abdominal examination typically does not localize the pain, and peritoneal findings are usually absent.

Diagnosis

Computed tomography (CT) of the abdomen is usually not diagnostic but may help rule out other etiologies for the symp-

toms. Colonoscopy and esophagoduodenoscopy are often normal; however, biopsy may reveal manifestations of ischemia. Duplex ultrasound can be diagnostic, showing decreased flow. Intestinal pH readings have been used to help make the diagnosis, with a drop in pH noted at the onset of pain after eating a test meal. Angiography allows confirmation of the diagnosis and planning for surgical therapy.[3]

Treatment

The treatment of chronic mesenteric ischemia remains surgical. Long-acting nitrates may provide symptomatic improvement. Nutritional abnormalities should be corrected; however, the patient may not be able to tolerate nutritional supplements due to exacerbation of the abdominal pain. Surgery is indicated to correct high-grade lesions or those lesions associated with symptoms.[1] Patients should also be evaluated for other vascular problems including coronary artery disease.

Prevention and Family and Community Issues

Risk factors for arteriosclerosis should be minimized to the degree possible. Patients should be encouraged to avoid or stop the use of tobacco products. Hypertension, hypercholesterolemia, and diabetes should be controlled to the degree possible. Patients should be warned about the increased risk of other vascular problems including coronary artery disease.

Acute Superior Mesenteric Venous Thrombosis

Superior mesenteric venous (SMV) thrombosis is an uncommon condition that occurs most often in patients of ages 40 to 60. These patients most often have an identifiable hypercoagulable state. SMV thrombosis may lead to congestion of the involved intestine with resulting infarction.

Clinical Presentation

The clinical course and presenting symptoms of SMV thrombosis are usually more subtle than SMA occlusion. The patient most often presents with worsening abdominal pain of more than a day's duration and may be associated with gastrointestinal bleeding. Patients can complain of anorexia, nausea, vomiting, or diarrhea. On examination, the findings will vary with the severity of the condition and the patient may have a normal abdominal examination or show signs of peritonitis. Patients may have fever, tachycardia, and hypotension.

Diagnosis

Laboratory abnormalities are nonspecific and include leukocytosis, hyperamylasemia, and metabolic acidosis. Plain films of the abdomen show only nonspecific changes, most often an ileus pattern. CT scans of the abdomen are frequently diagnostic in this condition. Ultrasound is often less useful due to overlying bowel gas. Ateriography can be useful where arterial disease cannot be ruled out based on the results of the other studies. Endoscopy can be used to help rule out other etiologies for the patient's symptoms.

Treatment

Intravenous (IV) fluids are given to replace fluid losses and to correct electrolyte imbalances. Heparin is used to prevent propagation of the thrombus if the patient does not have acute gastrointestinal bleeding. Once adequately anticoagulated, the patient is then treated with warfarin to maintain an international normalized ratio (INR) between 2 and 3. Patients who show progression in their signs or symptoms with medical management and those with findings of peritonitis on presentation may require surgical intervention followed by continued anticoagulation.[2]

Prevention and Family and Community Issues

Patients with hypercoagulable states are at risk for SMV thrombosis and should be cautious in the use of drugs such as birth control pills that may enhance coagulation. They may benefit from carrying a medical identification bracelet and should inform all treating physicians of their condition. Patients who have had one episode of thrombosis are at much greater risk of another episode, particularly within the first month. Patients may need lifelong anticoagulation.[5]

Food Allergies

Food allergy is an immunologic reaction to a dietary product. About 0.3% to 7.5% of the general population and up to 33% of children with atopic dermatitis have food allergies.[6,7] Nonimmunologic adverse reactions to food, such as Chinese restaurant syndrome, scromboid fish poisoning, and lactose intolerance, must be differentiated from food allergies.

Clinical Presentation

Patients with food allergies present with abdominal pain, rhinitis, diarrhea, vomiting, exacerbation of asthma, angioedema, urticaria, or atopic dermatitis. Oral symptoms include pruritus and swelling of the lips, tongue, and palate. Deaths have been reported from anaphylaxis. Food allergens are predominately water-soluble glycoproteins 10,000 to 60,000 daltons.[8] In adults the most common food allergies are to fish, shellfish, tree nuts, and peanuts, and in children to eggs, peanuts, milk, soy, and wheat.[9]

Diagnosis

Symptoms may occur rapidly after ingestion of the allergen or be delayed up to 24 hours. The history should include the timing of symptoms and a family history of atopic disease (see Chapter 36). A symptom and food diary may be helpful. A modified elimination diet may be used when anaphylaxis has not occurred. Skin prick and radioallergosorbent testing (RAST) for food allergens can be done, but the accuracy is limited by the variability in commercially supplied extracts and the instability of some of the antigens.[10] A positive skin test does not conclusively prove the presence of a food allergy; however, a negative test does make an immunoglobulin (IgE)-mediated food allergy unlikely.[8] Definitive diagnosis of food allergies requires demonstrating that removal of the offending food eliminates the allergic symptoms and that these symptoms recur with reintroduction of the food.

Management

The only effective management of food allergies is avoidance. Infants with cow's milk allergy can be managed with a formula containing casein hydrolysate (i.e., Alimentum, Nutramigen, Progestimil). Soy protein–based formulas are avoided in these infants, as approximately 20% of infants with cow's milk allergy are allergic to soy protein.[7]

The H_1-antihistamines are useful for controlling the rhinitis and urticaria caused by food allergies. Caution must be taken when administering egg-derived vaccines to patients with severe allergies to eggs or chicken.

Prevention and Family and Community Issues

Breast-feeding is encouraged, particularly for infants who have a family history of atopic disease. For high-risk infants, a casein hydrolysate formula is used if a supplement is needed. Children with a strong family history of atopic disease should not be given eggs, peanuts, or cow's milk before the age of 3.[8,9] Family members preparing meals are taught to read food labels so as to avoid "hidden" foods. Patients and their family members can learn more about reading labels and other food allergy information on the Food Allergy Network Web page (*http://www.foodallergy.org*). Under some circumstances, 1 to 2 years of complete avoidance of an allergen may result in the loss of sensitivity; however, patients and their families should be cautioned that this is unlikely to occur with allergies to peanuts, tree nuts, fish, or shellfish.[8]

Lactose Intolerance

Lactose is the primary sugar of mammalian milk and is present in many prepared foods and medications. The ability to digest lactose varies with age and race. In the United States it is estimated that 22% of Caucasians, 65% of African Americans, and almost 100% of Vietnamese are lactose malabsorbers.[11–13]

Clinical Presentation

Patients with lactose intolerance may have no symptoms or may present with abdominal bloating, cramping abdominal pain, flatulence, and watery diarrhea. Symptoms may be intermittent and depend on the amount of lactose ingested, the speed of gastric emptying, and the bacterial flora of the colon.

Diagnosis

The clinical diagnosis of lactose intolerance is difficult, as symptoms can be intermittent in nature and patients may not be aware that foods they have ingested contain lactose. In addition to milk products, lactose can be found in commercially baked bread, doughnuts, cereals, breakfast drinks, salad dressing, cake mixes, and as a filler in over-the-counter and prescription drugs.[11] Variations in the speed of gastric emptying may cause differences in tolerance of lactose, making elimination diets and rechallenges difficult to interpret. The symptom complex has significant overlap with irritable bowel, further complicating the diagnosis.[14] The diagnosis of lactose intolerance can be supported by evaluating the stool for a pH less than 5.8 and reducing substances, and by the breath hydrogen test.[11]

Management

Patients with lactase deficiency may still be able to tolerate lactose in reduced amounts. Foods high in fat or fiber slow gastric emptying and delivery of lactose to the intestine, allowing more complete digestion.[11] Prehydrolyzed milk is available commercially. Lactase produced from the yeast *Kluyveromyces lactis* and from the fungus *Aspergillus oryzae* (Lactaid, Lactrase, Dairy Ease) is available and may be added to milk products or taken prior to consuming lactose-containing foods.[11] Patients on a lactose-reduced diet may require an oral calcium supplement.

Family and Community Issues

Populations at high risk for lactose intolerance should be targeted for dietary education. School lunch programs must take into account these differences when planning and preparing meals.

Bacterial Food Poisoning

Food poisoning and food-borne illnesses are a significant cause of morbidity and mortality. *Campylobacter, Salmonella, Shigella, Escherichia coli*, and *Staphylococcus* are the most common bacterial pathogens implicated in the United States (Table 94.1).[15] Bacterial food poisoning may result from ingestion of the bacteria, as with *Salmonella, Shigella, Campylobacter*, and *E. coli* or from ingestion of toxins produced by the bacteria as in staphylococcal food poisoning.

Campylobacter infections have become the most common cause of bacterial gastroenteritis in the United States. Outbreaks occur most often in the spring and fall and have been associated with contaminated water, unpasteurized milk, and contaminated beef and poultry.[16]

Staphylococcal food poisoning accounts for 7.8% of reported cases of food poisoning in the United States.[17] Symptoms are caused by ingestion of extracellular toxins produced by the staphylococcus (usually *Staphylococcus aureus*). Foods with a low water content, such as ham and cured meats, are most often implicated. *Salmonella enteriditis* and *Salmonella typhimurium* are the most common species seen in *Salmonella* food poisoning and are found in both wild and domestic animals. Chicken and eggs are most frequently implicated in cases of *Salmonella* food poisoning.[16,18]

Shigella outbreaks in the United States have been associated with contaminated water and foods such as lettuce, tofu, and shellfish.[19–21] Ingested organisms colonize the small bowel and then invade the colonic mucosa, where they replicate intracellularly, producing a severe inflammatory response and superficial ulceration. Cytotoxins are produced that may inhibit fluid absorption.[22]

Pathogenic strains of *E. coli*, usually from contaminated water, are the most common cause of traveler's diarrhea[23] (see Chapter 9). Four pathologic presentations of *E. coli* food poisoning have been recognized: enteropathic, enteroinvasive, enterotoxigenic, and enterohemorrhagic. Enteropathic *E. coli* is unusual in developed countries but is a common cause of infant diarrhea in the Third World. Enteroinvasive *E. coli* invades the mucosal epithelium and replicates intracellularly, leading to areas of ulceration of the mucosa. Enterotoxigenic *E. coli* is most commonly seen in persons traveling to tropical areas. In the United States outbreaks have been associated with contaminated water in a national park.[23] Food-borne en-

Table 94.1. **Bacterial Food Poisoning**

Pathogen	Symptoms	Food	Diagnosis	Treatment
Campylobacter	Watery or bloody diarrhea, headache, abdominal pain	Poultry, beef, contaminated milk, water	Culture stool, characteristic motion on smear, leukocytes on stool smear	Symptomatic; macrolides, doxycycline
Staphylococcus	Nausea, vomiting, watery diarrhea	Meats	Clinical symptoms	Symptomatic
Salmonella	Diarrhea, abdominal pain, low-grade fever, enteric fever, prolonged fever, shaking chills	Poultry, eggs, meats, water	Stool cultures, blood cultures, clinical presentation	Symptomatic; for severe cases: quinolones, ceftriaxone, trimethoprim-sulfamethoxazole
Shigella	Watery or bloody diarrhea, abdominal cramps, rectal urgency	Water, shellfish, lettuce and other fecal-contaminated foods	Stool cultures, blood cultures, in stool smear, hemorrhagic ulcerations on proctosigmoidoscopy	Symptomatic; trimethoprim-sulfamethoxazole, quinolones
Escherichia coli	Watery or bloody diarrhea, abdominal pain, hemolytic-uremic syndrome	Water, ground beef	Stool culture, leukocytes on smear, may see hemorrhagic ulceration on proctosigmoidoscopy	Symptomatic for *E.coli* O157:H7; doxycycline, quinolones, bismuth subsalicylate for travelers diarrhea

terohemorrhagic *E. coli* is most commonly caused by the serotype O157:H7 and is now the leading cause of hemolytic-uremic syndrome in the U.S. with a 2% to 5% mortality (see Chapter 21). Outbreaks in the U.S. have been most associated with the ingestion of undercooked ground beef, lettuce, unpasteurized cider, milk, and contaminated water.[16,24] *E. coli* O157:H7 is the most common infectious cause of grossly bloody diarrhea in the United States.[25]

Clinical Presentation

Campylobacter infection has an incubation period of 2 to 7 days. Patients present with watery diarrhea that frequently becomes bloody, headache, chills, sweats, anorexia, lethargy, and severe abdominal pain. The illness usually resolves in less than 1 week. Relapses may occur, which can be confused with ulcerative colitis or Crohn's disease. Extracolonic manifestations include reactive arthritis and the Guillain-Barré syndrome with up to 36% of patients with Guillian-Barré syndrome having positive serology to *Campylobacter*.[16,26,27]

Patients with staphylococcal food poisoning present with nausea, vomiting, watery diarrhea, and abdominal pain 2 to 6 hours after ingestion. The symptoms last 1 to 3 days.

Salmonella infections may present in two distinct ways: enteritis or enteric fever. *Salmonella* enteritis is manifested by diarrhea, abdominal pain, low-grade fever, chills, nausea, vomiting, headache, and generalized malaise beginning 5 to 72 hours after ingestion of contaminated food and lasting 2 to 5 days. Complications of *Salmonella* enteritis include septicemia, pericarditis, neurologic and muscular disorders, arteritis, and malabsorption. *Salmonella* enteric fever is most frequently caused by *Salmonella typhi* and *Salmonella paratyphi* types A, B, and C with an incubation period of 7 to 28 days. Patients present with generalized malaise, headache, high fever, body aches, weakness, abdominal pain, nausea, vomiting, coughing, shaking chills, and anorexia. Fever may last several weeks. Stools may remain positive for up to 3 months, although carrier states are more common in women and the elderly, particularly after antibiotic treatment, and may last for years.[18]

The incubation period for *Shigella* is 36 to 72 hours. Patients present with watery or bloody diarrhea, fever, cramps, tenesmus, rectal urgency, and abdominal pain. Extracolonic manifestations include lethargy, headache, arthritis, and seizures.[28] Hemolytic-uremic syndrome has been reported in patients with shigellosis.

Patients infected with enterotoxigenic strains of *E. coli* present with fever and watery or bloody diarrhea lasting 3 to 6 days. Enteroinvasive strains cause diarrhea that may be bloody. Patients with enterohemorrhagic *E. coli* present with fever, chills, emesis, abdominal cramps, and bloody diarrhea. Symptoms last approximately 7 days. Signs of the hemolytic-uremic syndrome may develop 5 to 9 days after the onset of diarrhea and are more commonly seen in young children.[29]

Diagnosis

The diagnosis of bacterial food poisoning is made predominantly on clinical grounds. Stools may be bloody or positive for leukocytes in infections due to *Campylobacter, Shigella,*

and *E. coli*. Sigmoidoscopy may show areas of hemorrhage or ulceration, particularly with infections due to *Shigella* and *E. coli*. Cultures of stool are diagnostic except for staphylococcal food poisoning. Blood or urine cultures can be positive in patients with *Shigella* and *Salmonella* infections. Staphylococcal toxin can be detected in food using an immunoassay.

Management

Treatment of bacterial food poisoning is usually symptomatic only. Antibiotic therapy is indicated for severe disease. When antibiotic therapy is warranted, erythromycin and the newer macrolides are the antibiotics of choice for the treatment of *Campylobacter*. Alternative treatments include doxycycline, tetracycline, and the quinolones.[30,31]

Antibiotics are used only in severe cases of *Salmonella* infection because of concerns about induction of a carrier state. In adults the quinolones (Cipro, Floxin) may be the drugs of choice. Other alternative treatments in adults include ceftriaxone (Rocephin), trimethoprim-sulfamethoxazole (TMP-SMX) (Bactrim, Septra), and ampicillin for susceptible strains. In children, intravenous ceftriaxone, cefotaxime, chloramphenicol, ampicillin, or TMP-SMX may be used depending on sensitivity patterns.[31]

Drug-resistant *Shigella* is becoming increasingly more common. The quinolones should be considered for use in adults. TMP-SMX remains the drug of choice in children. Alternative drugs include azithromycin, ampicillin, and ceftriaxone based on sensitivities.[31]

Treatment of *E. coli* food poisoning consists of fluid and electrolyte replacement. Results of studies on the use of antibiotics are conflicting. One study showed prolongation of diarrhea and an increased risk of hemolytic-uremic syndrome in patients with enterohemorrhagic *E. coli* treated with TMP-SMX.[29] Doxycycline and the quinolones are effective against *E. coli*. Bismuth subsulfate (Pepto-Bismol) has been shown to be effective as a prophylactic agent for travelers' diarrhea, as have the quinolones.[32]

Family and Community Issues

Foods may become cross-contaminated with *Campylobacter*, *Salmonella, E. coli*, or *Shigella* when food preparers do not wash their hands between handling uncooked and cooked foods. Foods must be adequately cooked and promptly refrigerated if not served immediately. Raw milk and undercooked eggs should be avoided. In tropical areas flies may contaminate food with *Shigella* if it is not properly protected.[33] Person-to-person transmission of *E. coli* O157:H7 has been reported after initial food-borne illness, and so careful hand washing is important when there has been a case in the family.[25]

Food Poisonings Associated with Neurologic Disorders

A number of food ingestions cause neurologic symptoms that require prompt diagnosis and treatment, including botulism, ciguatera, paralytic shellfish poisoning, and amnestic shellfish poisoning. These syndromes are caused by toxins produced by the action of bacteria on food, in the case of botulism, or by the accumulation of toxin from the food chain, as in ciguatera, paralytic shellfish poisoning, and amnestic shellfish poisoning.

Botulism is caused by toxins produced by *Clostridium botulinum* under anaerobic conditions. In the U.S. it is most often caused by serotypes A, B, and E. Serotypes A and B are most often encountered in improperly canned, smoked, or fermented foods. Serotype E is most commonly encountered in association with seafood. Infant botulism has an incidence of 100 cases per year in the U.S., and is most often associated with honey ingestion.[34,35]

Ciguatera poisoning is caused by heat-stable, tasteless toxins produced by a dinoflagellate that accumulates in the food chain of reef fish. Due to jet travel and refrigerated shipment of fish, the problem is now seen worldwide. The larger carnivorous species, such as snapper, amberjack, grouper, barracuda, mullet, mackerel, and jackfish are most often implicated with ciguatera.

Paralytic shellfish poisoning is caused by ingestion of mollusks that concentrate toxins produced by a dinoflagellate. Most cases occur during the summer months in New England and on the Pacific Coast in the United States. Amnestic shellfish poisoning is caused by domoic acid, which accumulates in shellfish from microalgae in their food chain.[36,37]

Clinical Presentation

Botulism commonly occurs after an incubation period of 12 to 72 hours. Initial symptoms include diplopia, dysarthria, dysphagia, descending motor weakness, and paralysis. Mental status changes and sensory disturbances are not usually seen. Infants most frequently present with poor feeding, altered cry, hypotonia, and a poor suck reflex.[34,35]

Symptoms of ciguatera usually occur 2 to 12 hours after ingestion of contaminated fish. Initially the patient has nausea, vomiting, abdominal cramps, and watery diarrhea. The gastrointestinal symptoms generally resolve over 1 to 2 days. The hallmarks of the disorder are the neurologic symptoms, which may appear early in the course or be delayed by several days after other symptoms have resolved. Patients experience a reversal of hot and cold sensation, paresthesias of the lips and digits, weakness, and myalgias. Patients may have a sensation that their teeth are loose and have vertigo, hypersalivation, visual disturbances, and ataxia. Less common symptoms and findings include hypotension, cardiac conduction abnormalities, coma, respiratory failure, and shock. Improvement occurs spontaneously, although residual symptoms may last for weeks or even months.[38]

Patients with paralytic shellfish poisoning can develop symptoms within 30 minutes to 3 hours of ingestion. Initial symptoms include paresthesias of the mouth and extremities, headache, vertigo, a floating sensation, and, less frequently, gastrointestinal symptoms. The patient progresses to ataxia, cranial nerve dysfunction, and paralysis. The mortality rate is 1% to 12%, predominantly due to respiratory failure. Spontaneous recovery begins within 18 hours with those surviving 24 hours having a good prognosis. Symptoms usually resolve within 3 days.[37] Patients with amnestic shellfish poisoning develop symptoms 15 minutes to 38 hours after ingestion of toxic mussels. Initial symptoms include vomiting, diarrhea, and abdominal cramps. Neurologic symptoms develop, including headache, short-term memory loss, and confusion. Patients may experience severe bronchorrhea requiring intubation and may progress to coma. Deaths have resulted from the poisoning. Patients who recover may have prolonged symptoms and learning disorders.[36]

Diagnosis

Descending paralysis and a normal spinal fluid analysis help differentiate botulism from Guillain-Barré syndrome. The lack of sensory symptoms and the longer time of onset of botulism differentiates it from ciguatera and paralytic shellfish poisoning. The marine intoxications are diagnosed predominantly on clinical grounds. Samples of food can be analyzed for botulism toxin. Duodenal aspirates and stools can be cultured for *Clostridium*. The patient's serum can be tested for botulism toxin using a mouse assay.[35,39]

Management

Treatment of botulism is initiated on clinical grounds while awaiting laboratory confirmation.[35] If ingestion has been recent, attempts are made to remove unabsorbed toxin. Early use of botulism antitoxin may reduce the severity of the symptoms. Penicillin given parenterally may prevent germination of any ingested spores and further toxin production. Vital capacities should be followed, and ventilatory support may be required if it falls to below one-third the predicted value or below 1 L in adults.[40]

Ciguatera is treated with symptomatic support, with spontaneous resolution of symptoms in 1 to 4 weeks. Hypovolemia may require treatment with IV fluids to correct the fluid and electrolyte abnormalities. Patients with severe symptoms including those with coma may respond to an infusion of 20% mannitol, 1 g/kg over 30 minutes, after hypovolemia has been corrected.[36,38] Amitriptyline can be used to treat the paresthesias. A high-protein, high-carbohydrate diet has been advocated for the first 6 months after an episode of ciguatera. Fish, nuts, and alcohol should be avoided.[38]

Treatment of amnestic shellfish poisoning is predominantly supportive. With paralytic shellfish poisoning, gastric lavage with 2% sodium bicarbonate may be useful, as the toxin is labile in a basic pH.[36,37]

Family and Community Issues

People who do home canning should take particular care in the preparation of foods. Home-canned foods should be heated at 80°C for 5 minutes. Public health officials and those in the military must be alert to the potential use of botulism toxin as a biologic weapon.[39] Patients who have had an episode of ciguatera should be advised to avoid reexposure to the toxin and should avoid eating reef-dwelling fish if possible. Male patients with ciguatera and their partners should be warned that the toxin can be concentrated in semen and passed to sexual partners during intercourse.[38] In parts of the United States and Canada there is a quarantine on shellfish harvesting at times when concentrations of dinoflagellates are highest (most often in the spring and summer months in the United States), and shellfish are monitored for toxin concentrations.[36,37]

References

1. Cappell M. Gastrointestinal disorders and systemic disease, part II: intestinal (mesenteric) vasculopathy II ischemic colitis and chronic mesenteric ischemia. Gastroenterol Clin North Am 1998;27(4):827–60.
2. Cappell MS. Gastrointestinal disorders and systemic disease, part II: intestinal (mesenteric) vasculopathy I acute superior mesenteric arteriopathy and venopathy. Gastroenterol Clin North Am 1998;27(4):783–825.
3. Moawad J, Gewertz B. Chronic mesenteric ischemia clinical presentation and diagnosis. Surg Clin North Am 1997;77(2):357–69.
4. Stanton P, Hollier P, Seidel T, Rosenthal D, Clark M, Lamis P. Chronic intestinal ischemia: diagnosis and therapy. J Vasc Surg 1986;4:338–44.
5. Rhee R, Gloviczki P. Mesenteric ischemia mesenteric venous thrombosis. Surg Clin North Am 1997;77(2):327–38.
6. Bernhisel-Broadbent J. Food allergy: current knowledge and future directions diagnosis and management of food hypersensitivity. Immunol Allergy Clin North Am 1999;19(3):463–77.
7. Schreiber RA, Walker WA. Food allergy: facts and fiction. Mayo Clin Proc 1989;64:1381–91.
8. Burks AW. Pediatric allergy and immunology childhood food allergy. Immunol Allergy Clin North Am 1999;19(2):397–407.
9. Sampson HA. Food allergy. J Allergy Clin Immunol 1989;84:1062–7.
10. Bahna SL. Diagnostic tests for food allergy. Clin Rev Allergy 1988;6:259–84.
11. Saavedra JM, Perman JA. Current concepts in lactose malabsorption and intolerance. Annu Rev Nutr 1989;9:475–502.
12. Montes RG, Perman JA. Lactose intolerance: pinpointing the source of nonspecific gastrointestinal symptoms. Postgrad Med 1991;89:175–84.
13. Rings EHHM, Grand RJ, Buller HA. Lactose intolerance and lactase deficiency in children. Curr Opin Pediatr 1994;6:562–7.
14. Shaw A, Davies G. Lactose intolerance problems in diagnosis and treatment. J Clin Gastroenterol 1999;28(3):208–16.
15. Karras DJ. CDU Update incidence of foodborne illness: preliminary data from the Foodborne Diseases Active Surveillance Network (FoodNet). Ann Emerg Med 2000;35(1):92–3.
16. Slutsker L, Altekruse S, Swerdlow D. Emerging infectious diseases: foodborne diseases emerging pathogens and trends. Infect Dis Clin North Am 1998;12(1):199–216.
17. Tranter HS. Foodborne illness: foodborne staphylococcal illness. Lancet 1990;336:1044–6.
18. Baird-Parker AC. Foodborne illness: foodborne salmonellosis. Lancet 1990;336:1231–5.
19. Davis H, Taylor JF, Perdue JN, et al. A shigellosis outbreak traced to commercially distributed shredded lettuce. Am J Epidemiol 1988;128:1312–21.
20. Lee LA, Ostroff SM, McGee HB, et al. An outbreak of shigellosis at an outdoor music festival. Am J Epidemiol 1991;133:608–15.
21. Reeve G, Martin DL, Pappas J, Thompson RE, Greene KD. An outbreak of shigellosis associated with the consumption of raw oysters. N Engl J Med 1989;321:224–7.
22. Hale TL. Genetic basis of virulence in Shigella species. Microbiol Rev 1991;55:206–24.
23. Doyle MP. Foodborne illness: pathogenic Escherichia coli, Yersinia enterocolitica, and Vibrio parahaemolyticus. Lancet 1990;336:1111–5.
24. Bell BP, Goldoft M, Griffin PM, et al. A multistate outbreak of Escherichia coli O157:H7-associated bloody diarrhea and hemolytic uremic syndrome from hamburgers: the Washington experience. JAMA 1994;272:1349–53.
25. Berkelman RL. Emerging infectious diseases in the United States, 1993. J Infect Dis 1994;170:272–7.
26. Blaser MJ, Reller LB. Campylobacter enteritis. N Engl J Med 1981;305:1444–52.
27. Callegaro L, Jack DB, Samson JC. Campylobacter infections, Guillain-Barré syndrome, and parenteral gangliosides. Lancet 1991;337:789–94.
28. Lahat E, Katz Y, Bistritzer T, Eshel G, Aladjem M. Recurrent seizures in children with Shigella-associated convulsions. Am Neurol Assoc 1990;28:393–5.
29. Pavia AT, Nichols CR, Green DP, et al. Hemolytic-uremic syndrome during an outbreak of Escherichia coli O157:H7 infections in institutions for mentally retarded persons: clinical and epidemiologic observations. J Pediatr 1990;116:544–51.
30. DuPont HL. Practice guidelines: guidelines on acute infectious diarrhea in adults. Am J Gastroenterol 1997;92(11):1962–75.
31. The choice of antimicrobial drugs. Med Lett Drugs Ther 1999;41(1064):95–104.
32. Advice for travelers. Med Lett Drugs Ther 1999;41(1051):39–42.
33. Dupont HB, Levine MM, Hornick RB, Formal SB. Inoculum size in shigellosis and implications for expected mode of transmission. J Infect Dis 1989;159:1126–8.
34. Muensterer O, Cheng T. Infant botulism. Pediatr Rev 2000;21(12):427.
35. Shapiro R, Hatheway C, Swerdlow D. Botulism in the United States: a clinical and epidemiologic review. Ann Intern Med 1998;129(3):221–8.
36. Underman AE, Leedom JM. Fish and shellfish poisoning. Curr Clin Top Infect Dis 1993;13:203–25.
37. Mines D, Stahmer S, Shepherd S. Travel-related emergencies: poisonings food, fish, shellfish. Emerg Med Clin North Am 1997;15(1):157–77.
38. Beadle A. Ciguatera fish poisoning. Milit Med 1997;162(5):319–22.
39. Arnon S, Schechter R, Inglesby T, et al.: Botulism toxin as a biologic weapon, medical and public health management. JAMA 2001;285(8):1059–70.
40. Shneerson JM. Botulism: a potentially common problem [editorial]. Thorax 1989;44:901–2.

95
Urinary Tract Infections

Boyd L. Bailey, Jr.

Urinary tract infection (UTI) is a cause of significant discomfort, acute and long-term morbidity, and loss of productivity, resulting in over 7 million office visits with an estimated 1 million episodes annually of UTI-related illness requiring hospitalizations.[1] Among children, 1 in 20 girls and 1 in 50 boys have a UTI each year.[2]

Four major risk groups[3] for community-acquired UTIs have been identified: school-age girls, young women in their sexually active years (including pregnancy), males with prostate obstruction, and the elderly. This chapter discusses important clinical issues in the following categories: UTI in children, UTI in pregnancy, acute uncomplicated lower UTI in young women, recurrent infection in women, acute uncomplicated pyelonephritis in young women, complicated UTIs, UTIs in young men, catheter-associated UTIs, asymptomatic bacteriuria without a catheter, chronic UTI in the elderly, UTIs with spinal cord injuries, and fungal UTIs. The primary aim of UTI diagnosis and management is the prevention of long-term complications of progressive events that affect later-life morbidity or mortality.

UTIs in Children

For boys and girls the incidence of symptomatic infection during the first 6 months of life is similar, but after 6 months to a year it falls off rapidly for boys. Among girls, the first-year incidence is more evenly distributed through the year. During the first 3 months, boys are infected more often, presumably related to the uncircumcised susceptibility.[2] In neonates the prevalence is threefold higher among premature infants.[4] For girls the incidence steadily rises with a small transient increase at preschool time and then remains level until sexual activity becomes a factor. Asymptomatic bacteriuria is absent in boys until later in adult life when obstructive problems occur. In girls asymptomatic bacteriuria is present early in infancy and remains fairly constant until the late teens.[1]

The primary host-related factors that lead to the development of UTI include infancy, female sex, abnormal defense mechanisms, the presence of urinary tract abnormalities, sexual activity, and instrumentation.[4] In children without urinary tract abnormalities, periurethral bacterial colonization, for unclear reasons, is a risk factor for UTI.[5] Voiding dysfunction (urgency, frequency, dysuria, hesitancy, dribbling of urine, and overt incontinence) can be recognized with an eye toward modification.[6]

Escherichia coli accounts for as much as 80% of cases of UTI.[2,4] In neonates and complicated cases, *Proteus mirabilis* (mainly in boys), *Klebsiella pneumoniae*, *Pseudomonas aeruginosa*, Enterobacter species, *Staphylococcus aureus* (mainly in older children), *Streptococcus viridans*, enterococci, and *Candida albicans* are to be considered.[4]

Diagnosis
Urinalysis and Culture

In any febrile infant or child the differential diagnosis should include UTI. Screening by urinalysis for pyuria and bacteriuria is not adequately sensitive to allow UTI to be ruled out without a culture.[4,7] In a properly collected specimen (urethral catheterization or suprapubic aspiration in infants), a presumptive diagnosis can be made with the presence of any bacteria and five leukocytes per high-power field (hpf).[8]

Imaging Evaluation

Imaging tests should be conducted after the first episode of UTI in girls younger than 5 years, boys of any age, older sexually inactive girls with recurrent UTI, and any child with pyelonephritis.[8] Debate continues about the best radiologic approach for evaluating of UTI.[7,9] The issue centers around the role of radionuclide scans, and how these methods may replace or be used in conjunction with traditional ultrasonography (US), voiding cystourethrography (VCUG), intravenous pyelography (IVP), and spiral computer-assisted tomography (CT).

Radionuclide cystography, a method using scintigraphic imaging, gives accurate information similar to that of contrast based VCUG, with the possible advantage of significantly less radiation exposure.[10] The scintigraphic study using 99m-technetium dimercaptosuccinic acid (DMSA) has become a leading choice for gauging renal function and identifying renal cortical defects. The DMSA scan is quickly becoming a gold standard for diagnosis of acute pyelonephritis. When applied at 6 to 12 months after cortical defects have first developed, the DMSA scan may be the best test for renal scarring. US has the obvious advantage of being a noninvasive test that is strong at ruling out obstruction. IVP gives comprehensive structural information, and is very good for detecting kidney stones, but transient swelling during infection weakens the predictive capability of the test. The spiral CT is becoming the first choice for the presence of obstructive stone disease. VCUG gives comprehensive lower tract information and allows grading the severity of reflux.[7]

An imaging strategy can be summarized this way. Use renal/bladder US to look for obstruction; use a DMSA scan to identify cortical defects and assess differential function; use a VCUG to detect bladder anomalies, neurogenic defects, residual urine, and urethral abnormalities such as posterior valves, urethral strictures, and the presence of vesicoureteral reflux; and use spiral CT to determine the presence of stones.[7]

Management

Early diagnosis and prompt treatment of UTI in infants and young children are crucial. With vesicoureteral reflux, or other urinary tract abnormalities, immediate treatment reduces the risk of renal scarring. In the history, inquire about the defecation pattern and preceding use of antibiotics such as amoxicillin or a cephalosporin. Physical examination should include a rectal examination to detect a large fecal reservoir.[6]

Symptomatic neonates should be treated for 7 to 10 days with a parenteral combination of ampicillin and gentamicin. Young infants with UTI, children with clinical evidence of acute pyelonephritis, and children with upper tract infection associated with urologic abnormalities or surgical procedures can be treated with a combination of an aminoglycoside and ampicillin, or an aminoglycoside and a cephalosporin.[4] Duration of therapy remains unsettled. For complicated infection, 7 to 14 days has been arbitrarily recommended; for uncomplicated infection, 3 to 5 days has shown adequacy.[7]

For uncomplicated UTI, oral agents may include amoxicillin, ampicillin, sulfisoxazole acetyl, trimethoprim-sulfamethoxazole, nitrofurantoin, or cephalosporins for a duration of 5 to 10 days.[7] Antibiotic treatment of asymptomatic bacteriuria in children is controversial based on certain issues: there is limited evidence that renal damage is prevented or loss of function reduced; replacement of a low-virulence organism with a more virulent one may occur; and the child may experience unknown long-term side effects of antibiotics.[4] A reasonable approach with asymptomatic bacteriuria is to treat children younger than 5 years or those who have urinary tract structural abnormalities.

UTIs During Pregnancy

Pregnant women with UTIs are at greater risk of delivering infants with low birth weight, premature infants, preterm infants with low birth weight, and infants small for gestational age. In addition, the likelihood is greater for premature labor, hypertension/preeclampsia, anemia, and amnionitis. There is strong evidence that UTI causes low birth weight through premature delivery rather than growth retardation[11] (see Chapter 12).

The risk of pyelonephritis from antepartum bacteriuria may be as high as 30%. Identification and eradication reduces this risk to less than 5%. Antepartum bacteriuria has an estimated prevalence of 2% to 12%, with an increasing relation to age, parity, and lower socioeconomic status.[12]

An optimal time for screening all pregnancies has been suggested to be around 16 weeks (see Chapter 11). Although often the first prenatal visit is before 16 weeks, a practical approach to screening is to obtain a culture at this first visit. If negative, no further cultures are necessary unless there is a history of prior UTI, or the patient becomes symptomatic. If the screening culture result is 10^5 colony-forming units (CFU)/mL or higher, the test should be repeated to improve on the specificity of a single culture. If the repeat culture is positive, treatment for asymptomatic bacteriuria follows.[12]

As in nonpregnant females, E. coli is the most common cause of UTI during pregnancy, accounting for more than 80% of isolates. Other organisms include Enterobacter species, Klebsiella species, Proteus species, enterococci, and Staphylococcus saprophyticus.

The first concern regarding treatment during pregnancy is the safety of antibiotics. Considered reasonably safe are penicillins, cephalosporins, and methenamine. Cautious use can be considered with sulfonamides [allergic reaction, kernicterus, glucose-6-phosphate dehydrogenase (G6PD) deficiency], aminoglycosides (eighth nerve and renal toxicity), nitrofurantoin (neuropathy, G6PD deficiency), clindamycin (allergic reaction, pseudomembranous colitis), and erythromycin estolate (cholestatic hepatitis).[12,13]

For asymptomatic bacteriuria, a regimen of 3 to 7 days is used with antibiotics chosen with safety in mind. There is little support for single-dose therapy, although for a pregnant female with a history of recurrent UTIs, or who develops a UTI early in pregnancy, a single postcoital prophylactic dose may be considered. Appropriate postcoital single oral doses are either cephalexin 250 mg or nitrofurantoin 50 mg.[14] Pyelonephritis is managed the same as with nonpregnant females.[12]

Acute Uncomplicated Lower UTI In Young Women

The risk for UTI is increased by sexual intercourse, delayed postcoital voiding (although controversial[15]), diaphragm and spermicidal gel, and a history of recurrent UTIs.[16] One of three types of infection can account for these infections: acute cystitis, acute urethritis, or vaginitis.[17]

Cystitis pathogens include E. coli, S. saprophyticus, Proteus species, or Klebsiella species. Symptoms are abrupt in onset, severe, and usually multiple; they include dysuria, increased frequency, and urgency. Suprapubic pain and tenderness and sometimes low back pain also occur. Pyuria is usually present and occasionally hematuria.

Urethritis pathogens include *Chlamydia trachomatis*, *N. gonorrhoeae*, and herpes simplex virus. Symptoms are more likely to be gradual in onset and mild (including dysuria and possibly vaginal discharge and bleeding from a concomitant cervicitis), and include lower abdominal pain. Suspicion is raised if the patient has a new sexual partner or evidence of cervicitis on examination. Pyuria is usually present.

Vaginitis pathogens include *Candida* species and *Trichomonas vaginalis*. Symptoms include vaginal discharge or odor, pruritus, dyspareunia, and external dysuria without increased frequency or urgency. Pyuria and hematuria are rarely present (see Chapter 102).

With no complicating clinical factors, reasonable empiric treatment for presumed cystitis, prior to organism identification, is a 3-day regimen of any of the following: oral trimethoprim-sulfamethoxazole (TMP-SMX), trimethoprim, norfloxacin, ciprofloxacin, ofloxacin, lomefloxacin, or enoxacin (Table 95.1). With the complicating factors of diabetes, symptoms for more than 7 days, recent UTI, use of a diaphragm, or age over 65 years, a 7-day regimen can be considered using these same antibiotics.[17]

For cystitis during pregnancy, consider a 7-day regimen that includes oral amoxicillin, macrocrystalline nitrofurantoin, cefpodoxime proxetil, or TMP-SMX. Avoid using fluoroquinolones in pregnant women, and use gentamicin cautiously because of fetal eighth nerve threat. TMP-SMX has not been approved for use during pregnancy but is widely used. Once the causative organisms have been identified, the antibiotics can be modified.[17]

Recurrent Infections (Cystitis) in Women

Recurrent cystitis can be termed relapse or reinfection. Relapse is defined as a recurrence within 2 weeks of completing therapy for the same pathogen. Reinfection is defined as a recurrence more than 2 weeks after completing therapy for a different species or strain. For relapse, efforts should be made to rule out a urologic abnormality and to treat for an extended time, such as 2 to 6 weeks. For reinfection, the following strategy is useful: If a spermicide and diaphragm are being used, changing the contraceptive method is recom-

Table 95.1. **Antibiotic Regimens for Adult Cystitis, Pyelonephritis, and Prophylaxis**

Antibiotic	Oral (cystitis)	Oral (pyelonephritis and complicated UTIs)	Parenteral	Daily prophylaxis	Single-dose postcoital
Amoxicillin	250 mg every 8 h	500 mg every 8 h			
Ampicillin			1 g every 6 h		
Trimethoprim	100 mg every 12 h			100 mg every 24 h	
Trimethoprim-sulfamethoxazole	160 plus 800 mg every 12 h	160 plus 800 mg every 12 h	160 plus 800 mg every 12 h	40 plus 200 mg every 24 h	40 plus 200 mg
Norfloxacin	400 mg every 12 h	400 mg every 12 h		200 mg every 24 h	
Ciprofloxacin	250 mg every 12 h	500 mg every 12 h	200 to 400 mg every 12 h		
Ofloxacin	200 mg every 12 h	200 mg followed by 300 mg every 12 h			
Lomefloxacin	400 mg every day	400 mg every day			
Enoxacin	400 mg every 12 h	400 mg every 12 h			
Macrocrystalline nitrofurantoin	100 mg four times a day			100 mg every 24 h	50 to 100 mg
Cephalexin				250 mg every 24 h	250 mg
Cefpodoxime proxetil	100 mg every 12 h	200 mg every 12 h			
Cefixime	400 mg every day	400 mg every day			
Ceftriaxone			1 to 2 g every day		
Gentamicin			1 mg/kg of body weight every 8 h, or 3 to 5 mg/kg every 24 h		
Imipenem-cilastatin			250 to 500 mg every 6 to 8 h		
Ampicillin-sulbactam			1.5 g every 6 h		
Ticarcillin-clavulanate			3.2 g every 6 to 8 h		
Piperacillin-tazobactam			3.375 g every 6 to 8 h		
Aztreonam			1 g every 8 to 12 h		

Sources: Data sources include Pfau and Sacks,[14] Stamm and Hooten,[17] and Johnson.[18]

mended. For two or fewer incidents of UTI per year, physician- or patient-initiated therapy can be started, based on symptoms, using either single-dose or 3-day therapy. For three or more UTIs per year, the relation to coitus must be considered. If the UTI is not related to coitus, a low-dose antibiotic, daily or three times weekly, is recommended. This regimen is commonly continued for 3 to 6 months.[15,17] If the recurrent UTIs are related to coitus, a single low-dose postcoital treatment may be preferable (Table 95.1).

Usually not attributable to predisposing anatomic defects, recurrent UTIs in women most likely are related to an underlying biologic predisposition or to behavior promoting UTI.[18]

Although perineal cleansing methods are partially protective, oral antimicrobial therapy is probably most effective. It can be accomplished as chronic prophylaxis, postcoital prophylaxis, or intermittent self-administered therapy.

Acute Uncomplicated Pyelonephritis in Young Women

Uncomplicated pyelonephritis exhibits findings suggestive of upper tract tissue penetration and inflammation, such as fever and flank pain. Underlying factors that impede the response to natural host responses are minimized. The infecting organism should be highly susceptible to most antibiotics.

Characteristic pathogens in acute uncomplicated pyelonephritis in young women include *E. coli, Proteus mirabilis, K. pneumoniae*, and *S. saprophyticus*. Outpatient management is reasonable for mild to moderate illness without nausea and vomiting. A 10- to 14-day regimen of the following is appropriate: oral TMP-SMX, norfloxacin, ciprofloxacin, ofloxacin, lomefloxacin, or enoxacin (Table 95.1). For severe illness or possible urosepsis requiring hospitalization, the following regimen can be followed: parenteral TMP-SMX, ceftriaxone, ciprofloxacin, gentamicin (with or without ampicillin), or ampicillin-sulbactam until afebrile then oral TMP-SMX, norfloxacin, ciprofloxacin, ofloxacin, lomefloxacin, or enoxacin (Table 95.1) to complete a 14-day course of therapy.[17]

During pregnancy hospitalization is the optimal course with the following suggested regimen: parenteral ceftriaxone, gentamicin (with or without ampicillin), aztreonam, ampicillin-sulbactam, or TMP-SMX until afebrile, then oral amoxicillin, amoxicillin-clavulanate, a cephalosporin, or TMP-SMX to complete a 14-day course of therapy.[17]

Complicated UTIs

Clinically, a complicated UTI may present in the same way as an uncomplicated one. A complicated infection occurs in urinary tracts that have a functional, metabolic, or anatomic derangement predisposing to a more difficult infectious process including more resistant organisms.

Characteristic organisms present in complicated urinary tract infections include *E. coli, Proteus* species, *Klebsiella* species, *Pseudomonas* species, *Serratia* species, enterococci, and staphylococci. Outpatient management is reasonable for mild to moderate illness without nausea or vomiting. The best

oral antibiotic course, administered for 10 to 14 days, is norfloxacin, ciprofloxacin, ofloxacin, lomefloxacin, or enoxacin. TMP-SMX, amoxicillin, or cefpodoxime proxetil could also be used. For severe illness or possible urosepsis, hospitalization is necessary with treatment by parenteral ampicillin and gentamicin, ciprofloxacin, ofloxacin, ceftriaxone, aztreonam, ticarcillin-clavulanate, piperacillin-tazobactam, or imipenem-cilastatin until afebrile, then oral TMP-SMX, norfloxacin, ciprofloxacin, ofloxacin, lomefloxacin, or enoxacin for a total of 14 to 21 days.[17]

UTIs in Younger Men

Without underlying structural urologic abnormalities, risk factors for UTIs in young men include homosexuality, lack of circumcision,[19] and a sex partner colonized with uropathogens.[17]

Management of symptomatic cystitis without obvious complicating factors requires a urine culture to establish the pathogen. This step establishes sensitivity and helps define relapse or reinfection in the event of recurrence. Once the culture is obtained, a 7-day course of TMP-SMX, trimethoprim, or a fluoroquinolone is initiated.

The traditional approach of undertaking a thorough post-UTI evaluation to rule out a urologic abnormality has been disputed.[20,21] If pursued in young men who have responded to treatment, the chance of finding a urinary tract defect is low.[18]

Catheter-Associated UTIs

Mortality from UTIs is increased threefold in hospitalized patients with an indwelling catheter. Catheterization is associated with a 5% to 10% incidence of UTI per day of catheterization. A 3-day presence of an indwelling catheter has been identified as a risk factor for UTI. Catheter-associated UTI (CAUTI) is the most common acquired infection in long-term-care facilities. Complications include catheter obstruction, fever, stones, pyelonephritis, chronic interstitial nephritis, bacteremia, renal failure, and death. In the intensive care setting, 95% of nosocomial UTIs are CAUTI.[22]

With short-term catheterization, *E. coli* is the most common organism, followed by *Pseudomonas aeruginosa, K. pneumoniae, Proteus mirabilis, Serratia marcescens, Citrobacter* spp., *Staphylococcus epidermidis*, and enterococci.[23] With long-term catheterization, significant infection may be due to the ordinarily nonuropathogenic *Providencia stuartii* or *Morganella morganii*. Yeast may become an isolated pathogen when antibiotics are in use.[22,23]

Treatment revolves around three modes of action: prevention, antimicrobials for acquired asymptomatic bacteriuria and symptomatic lower UTI, and antimicrobials for a symptomatic (complicated) upper UTI. Prevention focuses on avoiding catheterization if possible. If catheterization is a mandatory, minimize the duration and use a closed drainage system. Short-term use of silver alloy catheters in hospitalized patients reduces the incidence of symptomatic UTI and bacteremia, and is likely to result in cost savings.[24] For short-term catheterization of 3 to 14 days, daily prophylactic norfloxacin, ciprofloxacin, or amoxicillin has shown benefit.[18] For acquired asymptomatic bacteriuria and symptomatic lower UTI after short-term catheter use, a single-dose of TMP-SMX (320–1600 mg) has been shown to be as effective as a 10-day course.[25]

Asymptomatic Bacteriuria in Patients Without a Catheter

With the exception of pregnancy and prior to urologic surgery, screening for asymptomatic bacteriuria has no apparent value. Even among the elderly where there may be an association between asymptomatic bacteriuria and mortality, a causal link has not been demonstrated.[17]

Chronic UTIs in the Elderly

Among males the incidence of bacteriuria essentially disappears after infancy and reappears during later adulthood as obstructive elements come into play. With aging, both symptomatic infection and asymptomatic bacteriuria occur. The incidence of UTI in both sexes steadily rises with age during the elderly years.[1] The place of residence helps predict incidence. For those over age 65, estimates of incidence are as follows: (1) at home—women 20%, men 10%; (2) in nursing homes—women 25%, men 20%. In hospitals the incidence is high for both sexes.[26] The elderly behave in a dynamic fashion, with high turnover of those with bacteriuria and those with a UTI.[26]

Many factors come into play for elderly men and women that balance the incidence of UTI: lack of estrogen in women, and prostatic secretion in men,[27] and bacterial adhesion factors in both sexes[26] (see Chapter 24).

Whereas *E. coli* and *S. saprophyticus* are the most common cause of UTI in young adults, some significant shifts in causative organism occur with the elderly. For nursing homes, *E. coli* remains the most common causative organism, and *Enterococcus* organisms have become the second most common. For the most part, *S. saprophyticus* does not occur in this setting. *E. coli* drops in frequency for women, and gram-positive organisms can dominate among men.[28] This shift to non–*E. coli* organisms can easily be attributed to an increased rate of hospitalization of the elderly.[26]

A debatable issue that has become somewhat clearer is that asymptomatic bacteriuria does not seem to influence mortality in elderly women.[29] Previous studies have pointed in both directions,[30] with some clearly showing increased functional disability even if an effect on mortality is not clear.[31]

Basically, a lower UTI presents with dysuria, urgency, and frequency. An upper UTI may present with clear signs of fever, chills, and flank pain with tenderness. In a fair percentage of cases, possibly 20%, these signs and symptoms can be absent or obscured by a presentation that might include fever, altered mental status (confusion) with variable gastrointestinal symptoms and signs (nausea and vomiting, abdominal tenderness), apathy, incontinence, and even respiratory symptoms.[26] Alternatively, not all nonspecific "mental status" changes can be at-

tributed to a UTI, and focusing on antibiotic therapy alone is inappropriate.[27] A difficult question is whether bacteriuria is really asymptomatic in the elderly.[32]

Laboratory screening is a little more direct in men than women, but does not, unfortunately, substitute for a culture in the elderly, as it can in younger people.

The management of UTIs in the elderly was addressed in specific areas of this chapter (see Recurrent Infections (Cystitis) in Women, Complicated UTIs, and Catheter-Associated UTIs, above). In the elderly, antibiotics in general require minimal dose adjustment. Consider total body weight and renal function. Duration of treatment is similar to that in other age groups.[24] Antibiotic choices are shown in Table 95.1. Regular use of cranberry juice (300 mL/day) appears to reduce both bacteriuria and pyuria, and leads to fewer symptomatic infections and less antibiotic use.[33]

UTI in Spinal Cord Injuries

Special considerations for increased risk of UTI with spinal cord injuries include bladder overdistention, vesicoureteral reflux, high-pressure voiding, large postvoid residuals, stones in the urinary tract, and outlet obstruction.[34]

Management of infection risks focuses primarily on proper drainage of the bladder. A turning point that occurred during the 1960s was the understanding of the value of intermittent catheterization in reducing the risk of significant bacteriuria.[35] Development of bacteriuria is certain with an indwelling catheter and suprapubic catheter. Although not fully understood, bacteriuria and the incidence of symptomatic UTIs are reduced by intermittent catheterization. In addition, intermittent catheterization performed by the affected person is preferable to having it done by a caregiver.[34] There are many variations in the technique of intermittent catheterization. The critical predictor for improved outcome is intermittent catheterization rather than having an indwelling catheter.

Diagnostic signs and symptoms are poorly sensitive and specific.[34] Estimation of pyuria is generally considered the best indication of UTI.

Fungal UTIs

Fungal UTI is most commonly caused by *Candida*, and occasionally by *Cryptococcus neoformans*, *Aspergillus* species, and the endemic mycoses. Clinical clues are CAUTI, obstructed urinary tracts, especially in diabetics, and immunosuppressive therapy. Antibiotics, and none are exempt, can play a role in the emergence of candiduria upon use or immediately following.

For asymptomatic colonization with *Candida* (except following renal transplant, and in whom urologic instrumentation or surgery is planned), no specific antifungal therapy is required.

Candida cystitis is best treated with amphotericin B bladder instillation (50 μg/mL), systemic therapy (single-dose intravenous 0.3 mg/kg), or fluconazole 200 mg po for 14 days.

Ascending pyelonephritis and *Candida* urosepsis require

Table 95.2. **Diagnostic Information on Common Urine Screening Tests, Individually and in Various Combinations**[a]

Screening test	Sensitivity	Specificity	Positive likelihood ratio	Negative likelihood ratio
Nitrite (present or absent)	0.5	0.95	10.00	0.53
Bacteria				
Unstained, spun (2+ on scale of 4+)	0.75	0.8	3.75	0.31
Gram stain, unspun (1/hpf)	0.8	0.85	5.33	0.24
Microscopic pyuria				
Spun (5 WBCs/hpf)	0.6	0.85	4.00	0.47
Unspun (50 WBC/mm³)	0.65	0.9	6.50	0.39
WBCs + bacteria				
Standard spun[b]	0.66	0.99	66.00	0.34
Enhanced unspun[c]	0.85	0.98	42.50	0.15
Leukocyte esterase (present or absent)	0.2	0.95	4.00	0.84
Leukocyte esterase + nitrite	0.5	0.98	25.00	0.51
Methylene blue	0.6	0.98	30.00	0.41
Uriscreen	0.9	0.9	9.00	0.11
Bac-T-screen	0.9	0.7	3.00	0.14
Chemstrip LN	0.9	0.7	3.00	0.14

[a]Values have been taken from several sources,[39–41] rounded by the author, and represent reasonable numbers to use in clinical practice.

[b]5 WBCs/hpf + any bacteria in spun urinalysis.

[c]10 WBCs/mm³ + any bacteria by Gram stain.

hpf = high-power field; WBC = white blood cell count.

systemic antifungal therapy with IV amphotericin B at 0.6 mg/kg/day, duration depending on severity but in general involving a total dose of 2 g. An alternative is fluconazole at 5 to 10 mg/kg/day (IV or po).[36]

Laboratory Guides and Interpretation

The organisms that cause UTIs are few in number, but there are growing pressures for more efficient and timely screening measures to determine the likelihood of a UTI. Ideal screening for a UTI would involve a highly sensitive test that confidently excludes the disease, thereby eliminating the need to proceed to more costly follow-up tests of culturing and antibiotic sensitivity. The ideal screening test would be highly specific for detecting or identifying the disease for which empiric treatment has been initiated while uropathogen identity and antimicrobial sensitivity are pending. Unfortunately, the ideal screening test does not exist.

Pyuria

From a practical standpoint, pyuria represents readily measurable evidence of host injury. The most accurate method, or gold standard, of defining significant pyuria is the leukocyte excretion rate. There is evidence that the significant rate is 400,000 white blood cells (WBC)/hour.[37] This measurement is cumbersome—hence the popularity of quicker, simpler, but less accurate screening tests. They include microscopic examination of unspun urine in a counting chamber (WBC/mm³), spun urine under a coverslip (WBC/hpf), and leukocyte esterase.[38] In general, the WBC/hpf is approximately

11% of the WBC/cubic mm³.[39] Diagnostic information related to these tests is displayed in Table 95.2.[38–46]

Bacteriuria

A UTI can be defined as the presence of significant numbers of pathogenic bacteria in appropriately collected urine.[38]

Table 95.3. **Suggested Culture Colony Count Thresholds for Significant Bacteriuria**

Various clinical settings	Significant bacteriuria (CFU/mL)
Infants and children	
Voided	≥10³
Catheter	≥10³
Suprapubic aspirate (SPA)	≥10³
External collection devices	≥10⁴
Adult	
Midstream, clean-catch	
Female	
Asymptomatic	≥10⁵
Symptomatic	≥10²
Male	≥10³
In-and-out (straight) catheterization	≥10²
Chronic indwelling catheter	≥10²
Indwelling catheter or SPA in spinal injuries	Any detectable colony count
External collection devices	≥10⁵
Condom collection device in spinal injuries	≥10⁴

Sources: Data are from Cardenas and Hooton[34] and Eisenstadt and Washington.[46]

Urine culture is considered the gold standard for defining significant bacteriuria. All other tests are simply screening devices chosen to balance immediate, simple results with accuracy. The most common tests are direct microscopy and the dipstick (nitrite and leukocyte esterase). Many methods have been used with variable accuracy.[45] Commonly used screening tests with approximated diagnostic information are shown in Table 95.2.

Urine Culture

It is important to realize that even though the culture is universally used as a gold standard for significant bacteriuria in UTIs against which other tests are measured, it is not the perfect test and falls short of being 100% sensitive and specific. Bacterial culture methods include, in order of decreasing predictive accuracy, the quantitative culture (pour plate method), semiquantitative culture (surface streak procedure), and miniaturized culture (filter paper, roll tube, and dipslide methods). The colony count that represents significant bacteriuria varies with factors that include age, sex, anatomic location of the infection, and symptoms. Although the urine culture is considered the gold standard for defining significant bacteriuria, the level of significance is not uniform across the clinical spectrum of disease. Colony counts of what can currently be considered as significant bacteriuria for infection are shown in Table 95.3.[34,46]

References

1. Warren JW. Clinical presentations and epidemiology of urinary tract infections. In: Mobley LT, Warren JW, eds. Urinary tract infections: molecular pathogenesis and clinical management. Washington, DC: ASM Press, 1996;3–28.
2. Stull TL, LiPuma JJ. Epidemiology and natural history of urinary infections in children. Med Clin North Am 1991;75(2):287–98.
3. Stamm WE, Hooton TM, Johnson JR, et al. Urinary tract infections: from pathogenesis to treatment. J Infect Dis 1989;159(3):400–6.
4. Zelikovic I, Adelman RD, Nancarrow PA. Urinary tract infections in children. An update. West J Med 1992;157(5):554–61.
5. Shortliffe LM. The management of urinary tract infections in children without urinary tract abnormalities. Urol Clin North Am 1995;22(1):67–73.
6. Hellerstein S. Urinary tract infections in children: Why they occur and how to prevent them. Am Fam Physician 1998;57(10):2440–6.
7. Linshaw MA. Controversies in childhood urinary tract infections. World J Urol 1999;17(6):383–95.
8. Carmack MA, Arvin AM. Urinary tract infections—navigating complex currents [editorial]. West J Med 1992;157(5):587–8.
9. Hellerstein S. Evolving concepts in the evaluation of the child with a urinary tract infection [editorial comment]. J Pediatr 1994;124(4):589–92.
10. Conway JJ, Cohn RA. Evolving role of nuclear medicine for the diagnosis and management of urinary tract infection [editorial comment]. J Pediatr 1994;124(1):87–90.
11. Schieve LA, Handler A, Hershow R, et al. Urinary tract infection during pregnancy: its association with maternal morbidity and perinatal outcome. Am J Public Health 1994;84(3):405–10.
12. Zinner SH. Management of urinary tract infections in pregnancy: a review with comments on single dose therapy. Infection 1992;20(suppl 4):S280.
13. Chow AW, Jewesson PJ. Use and safety of antimicrobial agents during pregnancy. West J Med 1987;146:761–4.
14. Pfau A, Sacks TG. Effective prophylaxis for recurrent urinary tract infections during pregnancy. Clin Infect Dis 1992;14:810.
15. Madersbacher S, Thalhammer F, Marberger M. Pathogenesis and management of recurrent urinary tract infection in women. Curr Opin Urol 2000;10(1):29–33.
16. Hooton TM, Hillier S, Johnson C, et al. Escherichia coli bacteriuria and contraceptive method. JAMA 1991;265(1):64–9.
17. Stamm WE, Hooton TM. Management of urinary tract infections in adults. N Engl J Med 1993;329:1328.
18. Johnson JR. Treatment and prevention of urinary tract infections. In: Mobley LT, Warren JW, eds. Urinary tract infections: molecular pathogenesis and clinical management. Washington, DC: ASM Press, 1996;95–118.
19. Spach DH, Stapleton AE, Stamm WE. Lack of circumcision increases the risk of urinary tract infection in young men. JAMA 1992;267:679.
20. Krieger JN, Ross SO, Simonsen JM. Urinary tract infections in healthy university men. J Urol 1993;149(5):1046–8.
21. Pfau A. Re: urinary tract infections in healthy university men [letter]. J Urol 1994;151(3):705–6.
22. Burrows LL, Khoury AE. Issues surrounding the prevention and management of device-related infections. World J Urol 1999;17(6):402–9.
23. Warren JW. The catheter and urinary tract infection. Med Clin North Am 1991;75:481–95.
24. Saint S, Veenstra DL, Sullivan SD, Chenoweth C, Fendrick AM. The potential clinical and economic benefits of silver alloy urinary catheters in preventing urinary tract infection. Arch Intern Med 2000;160(17):2670–5.
25. Harding GKM, Nicolle LE, Ronald AR, et al. How long should catheter-acquired urinary infection in women be treated? A randomized controlled study. Ann Intern Med 1991;114:713.
26. Baldassarre JS, Kaye D. Special problems in urinary tract infection in the elderly. Med Clin North Am 1991;75(2):375–90.
27. Nicolle LE. Urinary tract infections in long-term care facilities. Infect Control Hosp Epidemiol 1993;14(4):220–5.
28. Lipsky BA, Ireton RC, Gihn SD, et al. Diagnosis of bacteriuria in men specimen collection and culture interpretation. J Infect Dis 1987;155:847–54.
29. Abrutyn E, Mossey J, Berlin JA, et al. Does asymptomatic bacteriuria predict mortality and does antimicrobial treatment reduce mortality in elderly ambulatory women? Ann Intern Med 1994;120(10):827–33.
30. Nordenstam GR, Brandberg CA, Oden AS, et al. Bacteriuria and mortality in an elderly population. N Engl J Med 1986;314:1152–6.
31. Nicolle LE, Henderson E, Bjornson J, et al. The association of bacteriuria with resident characteristics and survival in elderly institutionalized men. Ann Intern Med 1987;106:682–6.
32. Hamilton-Miller JMT. Issues in urinary tract infections in the elderly. World J Urol 1999;17:396–401.
33. Avorn J, Monane M, Gurwitz JH, et al. Reduction of bacteriuria and pyuria after ingestion of cranberry juice. JAMA 1994;271(10):751–4.
34. Cardenas DD, Hooton TM. Urinary tract infection in persons with spinal cord injury. Arch Phys Med Rehabil 1995;76(3):272–80.
35. Ronald AR, Pattullo ALS. The natural history of urinary tract infection in adults. Med Clin North Am 1991;75(2):299–312.
36. Sobel JD, Vazquez JA. Fungal infections of the urinary tract. World J Urol 1999;17(6):410–4.
37. Stamm WE. Measurement of pyuria and its relation to bacteriuria. Am J Med 1983;75(1B):53–8.
38. Pappas PG. Laboratory in the diagnosis and management of urinary tract infections. Med Clin North Am 1991;75(2):313–26.

39. Alwall N. Pyuria: deposit in high-power microscopic field—wbc/hpf—versus wbc/mm^3 in counting chamber. Acta Med Scand 1973;194:537–40.

40. Bailey BL. Urinalysis predictive of urine culture results. J Fam Pract 1995;40(1):45–50.

41. Hoberman A, Wald ER, Penchansky L, Reynolds EA, Young S. Enhanced urinalysis as a screening test for urinary tract infection. Pediatrics 1993;91(6):1196–9.

42. Bachman JW, Heise RH, Naessens JM, Timmerman MG. A study of various tests to detect asymptomatic urinary tract infections in an obstetric population. JAMA 1993;270(16):1971–4.

43. Lockhart GR, Lewander WJ, Cimini DM, Josephson SL, Linakis JG. Use of urinary gram stain for detection of urinary tract infection in infants. Ann Emerg Med 1995;25(1):31–5.

44. Carroll KC, Hale DC, Von Boerum DH, et al. Laboratory evaluation of urinary tract infections in an ambulatory clinic. Am J Clin Pathol 1994;101(1):100–3.

45. Jenkins RD, Fenn JP, Matsen JM. Review of urine microscopy for bacteriuria. JAMA 1986;255(24):3397–403.

46. Eisenstadt J, Washington JA. Diagnostic microbiology for bacteria and yeasts causing urinary tract infections. In: Mobley LT, Warren JW, eds. Urinary tract infections: molecular pathogenesis and clinical management. Washington, DC: ASM Press, 1996;29–68.

96

Fluid, Electrolyte, and Acid-Base Disorders

Joseph Hobbs

Fluid, electrolyte, and acid-base disorders are frequently associated with problems encountered in family medicine. Rapid detection and treatment of these disorders are important, as they affect the quantity and quality of vital organ profusion. These disorders are seen in all age groups and various clinical settings; but the very young, the very old, and those with chronic diseases are particularly vulnerable to serious complications because of inadequate or immature mechanisms of compensation, correction, and prevention.[1,2]

Differential Diagnosis

Fluid, electrolyte, and acid-base disorders are likely to occur in patients with problems that can cause alterations in total body and/or the effective circulating volume. These disorders are often detected initially from the results of routinely performed electrolyte panels and other biochemical profiles before clinical manifestations are apparent. These disorders frequently result in abnormalities in the measurement of plasma concentrations of sodium, potassium, bicarbonate, chloride, glucose, blood urea nitrogen (BUN), and creatinine. Suspected acid-base abnormalities should be further evaluated by measuring the arterial plasma partial pressure of CO_2 (i.e., Pco_2) and pH. Less frequent abnormalities of magnesium, calcium, and phosphate concentration may be present as primary disorders (e.g., parathyroid disorders) or as a consequence of more common disorders (e.g., chronic renal disease). Renal conservation or loss of electrolytes and water can be determined by measuring the urinary concentrations of sodium, potassium, chloride, magnesium, phosphate, and hydrogen and urine osmolality.[3,4] Differential diagnoses of common plasma and urine electrolyte abnormalities are as follows.

Hyponatremia ($[Na^+]$ <135 mEq/L) and **hypoosmolality** (i.e., plasma osmolality <275 mOsm/kg) indicate excess water content relative to sodium caused by renal retention of ingested water [e.g., hypovolemic-induced antidiuretic hormone (ADH) release, syndrome of inappropriate secretion of ADH (SIADH)], excess water ingestion greater than renal free water clearance, or both. Hyponatremia occurs without hypoosmolality (i.e., pseudohyponatremia) in the presence of hyperproteinemia and hyperlipidemia. Hyponatremia with hyperosmolality occurs as a result of hyperglycemia (Fig. 96.1; see Table 96.1, below). **Hypernatremia** ($[Na^+]$ >145 mEq/L) and **hyperosmolality** (i.e., plasma osmolality >290 mOsm/kg) reflect a water deficit relative to sodium caused by excess water loss, decreased water intake, decreased water retention (e.g., lack of ADH effect), or excess intake of sodium salts (Fig. 96.2; see Tables 96.2 and 96.3).

Hypokalemia ($[K^+]$ <3.5 mEq/L) results when there is excessive total body potassium losses or intracellular sequestration (e.g., alkalosis) of potassium. **Hyperkalemia** ($[K^+]$ >5.5 mEq/L) occurs when there is excess intake, decreased excretion, or intracellular extrusion (e.g., acidosis) of potassium.[3]

Hypobicarbonatemia (i.e., $[HCO_3^-]$ <24 mEq/L: Primary event in metabolic acidosis or the compensatory event in respiratory alkalosis (see Table 96.6).

Hyperbicarbonatemia ($[HCO_3^-]$ >28 mEq/L) is the primary event in metabolic alkalosis or the compensatory event in respiratory acidosis (see Table 96.6). $[HCO_3^-]$ does not fall as much as $[Na^+]$ and $[Cl^-]$ in hypoosmolar states because of renal regeneration of HCO_3^-.

Hypochloremia ($[Cl^-]$ <98 mEq/L) occurs in metabolic alkalosis or as a part of the metabolic compensation in respiratory acidosis. **Hyperchloremia** ($[Cl^-]$ >106 mEq/L) occurs in normal anion gap metabolic acidosis or as a part of the metabolic compensation in respiratory alkalosis. Chloride concentration can be altered by the H_2O content relative to sodium, such that excess water causing hyponatremia can cause hypochloremia, and water deficits leading to hypernatremia can cause hyperchloremia. Plasma chloride concentration changes caused by os-

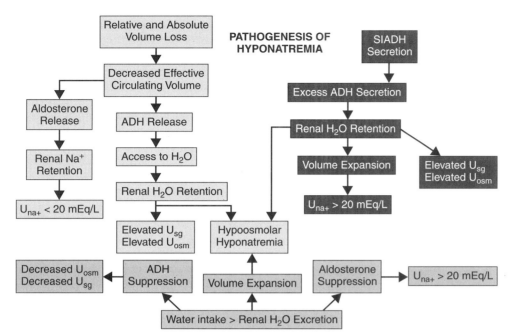

Fig. 96.1. Pathogenesis of hyponatremia. U_{Na} = urine sodium concentration; U_{osm} = urine osmolality; U_{sg} = urine specific gravity; ADH = antidiuretic hormone; SIADH = syndrome of inappropriate ADH secretion.

molality changes are directly proportional to changes in plasma sodium concentration. Bromism can falsely elevate Cl^-.

The **anion gap** ($[Na^+] + [K^+] - [HCO_3^-] + [Cl^-] = 16 \pm 4$ mEq/L), when elevated, suggests the increased presence of unmeasured anions of fixed endogenous acids or unmeasured anions caused by the addition of exogenous acids, which cause metabolic acidosis. The anion gap, when decreased, suggests increased unmeasured cations (e.g., increased cationic proteins of plasma cell dyscrasia, lithium intoxication, and rarely severe hypercalcemia and hypermagnesemia usually occurring concurrently), decreased unmeasured anions (e.g., hypoalbuminemia and severe hypoosmo-

lality), and errors in measurements of $[Na^+]$, $[C^-]$, and $[HCO_3^-]$ in severe hypernatremia.

Elevated arterial plasma Pco_2 (Pco_2 >44 mm Hg) is the primary event in respiratory acidosis or the compensatory event in metabolic alkalosis. **Decreased arterial plasma Pco_2** (Pco_2 <36 mm Hg) is the primary event in respiratory alkalosis or the compensatory event in metabolic acidosis.

Decreased arterial plasma pH (pH <7.38) is caused by metabolic acidosis, respiratory acidosis, or a combination of these two events with other primary acid-base disturbances where acidosis predominates. **Elevated arterial plasma pH** (pH >7.42) is caused by metabolic alkalosis, respiratory al-

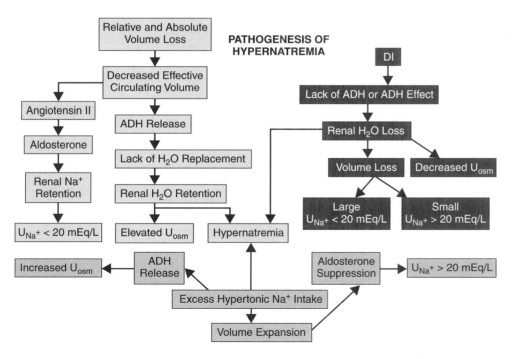

Fig. 96.2. Pathogenesis of hypernatremia. DI = diabetes insipidus. (See Fig. 96.1 for other abbreviations.)

kalosis, or a combination of these two events with other acid-base disturbances where alkalosis predominates. A normal systemic pH could exist with abnormal values of P_{CO_2} and $[HCO_3^-]$, which is the reason the quantitate relation of the three acid-base parameters, via rules of expected compensation for primary acid-base disorders, must be determined to identify specific disorders.

Elevated BUN concentration [BUN] (>20 mg/dL) suggests the presence of prerenal azotemia, intrinsic renal disease, postrenal disease, excessive cellular catabolism, or gastrointestinal tract bleeding. **Low [BUN]** (<10 mg/dL) occurs with protein deficiency and hemodilution.

Plasma creatinine concentration ([PCr]) varies directly with muscle mass and renal function. High [PCr] (>1.4 mg/dL) is associated with renal dysfunction or massive muscle destruction (i.e., rhabdomyolysis). Low [PCr] occurs in the debilitated elderly and in other settings where there is decreased skeletal muscle mass. The creatinine clearance (C_{Cr}) approximates the glomerular filtration rate and is a clinical estimation of renal function. C_{Cr} declines 1 ml/min/year in those over age 40, and is different in men and women. The renal creatinine clearance can be estimated using [PCr] such that

$$C_{CR} \cong \frac{(140 - age) \times lean\ body\ weight\ (Kg)}{PCr \times 72}$$

for males, and these results multiplied by 0.85 for females. Renal creatinine clearance can also be obtained using a 24-hour urine collection and calculating

$$C_{Cr} = \frac{Ucr\ (mg/dL) \times volume\ (mL/min)}{PCr}$$

Normal C_{Cr} is 120 ± 25 mL/min for men and 95 ± 20 ml/min for women. Low C_{Cr} implies declining intrinsic renal function. High C_{Cr} suggests the presence of hyperfiltration associated with early glomerular damage. Diabetic ketoacidosis can decrease the renal clearance of creatinine leading to an elevated [PCr].

Hyperglycemia (glucose >110 mg/dL fasting) is caused by insulin deficiency or resistance and is associated with volume depletion and hyperosmolality. **Hypoglycemia** (glucose <60 mg) can be caused by insulin excess, reduced carbohydrate consumption, or both.

Hypomagnesemia (Mg^{2+} <1.5 mEq/L) associated with urinary magnesium (U_{mg}) conservation (U_{mg} <10 mg/day) can be caused by decreased magnesium intake (e.g., protein–calorie malnutrition), decreased magnesium absorption, and extrarenal magnesium loss. Hypomagnesemia associated with urinary magnesium excretion (U_{mg} >10 mg/day) can be caused by excessive renal magnesium loss (e.g., diuretic use, hypokalemia, hypercalciuria, hypervolemia, and hyperthyroidism). Hypomagnesemia is also caused by chronic magnesium wasting and treatment-induced intracellular magnesium redistribution (e.g., diabetic ketoacidosis and alcoholism).

Hypermagnesemia (Mg^{2+} >2.5 mEq/L) results when magnesium intake exceeds renal excretion (U_{mg} >20 mg/day) and when there is decreased renal excretion (U_{mg} <20 mg/day) caused by excessive renal magnesium tubular reabsorption (e.g., hyperparathyroidism, hypovolemia, hypocalcemia, and hypothyroidism) and decreased glomerular filtration rate (GFR) (e.g., acute and chronic renal failure and hypovolemia).[5,6]

Hypocalcemia (Ca^{2+} <8.5 mg/dL or ionized Ca^{2+} <4.1 mg/dL) associated with normal or subnormal parathyroid hormone (PTH) is caused by PTH-deficient hypoparathyroidism and severe hypomagnesemia. Hypocalcemia associated with elevated PTH is caused by chronic renal failure, vitamin D deficiency, malabsorption, drug-induced microsomal enzyme induction (e.g., mithramycin and phenytoin), osteomalacia, and causes of severe acute hyperphosphatemia such as acute pancreatitis, hepatic failure, and other causes of massive tissue necrosis. **Hypercalcemia** (total $[Ca^{2+}]$ >10.5 mg/dL or ionized $[Ca^{2-}]$ >5.1 mg/dL) associated with elevated PTH is caused by primary hyperparathyroidism (i.e., excessive production of PTH) and severe secondary hyperparathyroidism of chronic renal failure. Hypercalcemia associated with normal PTH is caused by vitamin D excess, sarcoidosis, hyperthyroidism, increased bone calcium release (e.g., immobilization and bony metastasis), extracellular fluid depletion, thiazides, or milk-alkali syndrome. Because calcium is bound to albumin, changes in plasma albumin levels alter total Ca^{2+}. Ionized Ca^{2+} must be measured to validate nonbound (i.e., free) plasma calcium levels.[6,7]

Hypophosphatemia (plasma phosphorus <2.5 mg/dL) is caused by increased phosphate renal excretion (i.e., U_{po4} >100 mg/24 hr) in diabetic ketoacidosis, hypokalemia, and phosphate deficiency (U_{po4} <100 mg/24 hr) in hypoparathyroidism and decreased phosphate intake (e.g., alcoholism, vitamin D deficiency, and use of phosphate binders), as well as intracellular phosphate shifts (U_{po4} <100 mg/24 hr) in metabolic and respiratory alkalosis. **Hyperphosphatemia** (phosphorus >4.8 mg/dL) associated with U_{po4} >1500 mg/24 hr is caused by increased release of phosphates into the extracellular fluid by cell lysis (e.g., rhabdomyolysis) and initial anionic redistribution of metabolic acidosis (e.g., diabetic ketoacidosis and lactic acidosis). Hyperphosphatemia associated with U_{po4} <1500 mg/24 hr is caused by decreased renal phosphate excretion (e.g., volume depletion, acute and chronic renal failure, and hyperparathyroidism).[6–9]

Urine osmolality (U_{osm}) and **Urine specific gravity** (U_{sg}) reflect the renal dilutional capacity (U_{osm} less than that of plasma or 350 mOsm/kg to U_{osm} <100 mOsm/kg; or urine specific gravity 1.010–1.000) or renal concentrating capacity (U_{osm} greater than that of plasma or 350 mOsm/kg; and specific gravity >1.010).[4,10] Urine osmolality of 200 mOsm/kg indicates the presence of ADH in euvolemic and normal plasma osmolar states. However, urine osmolality must be compared to serum osmolality to assess appropriateness of renal water concentration and dilution.

Urine sodium concentration (U_{Na}) reflects renal sodium conservation capacity (U_{Na} <20 mEq/L) in hypovolemia and renal hypoperfusion, and prerenal azotemia) or appropriate renal sodium excretion (U_{Na} >20 mEq/L) in euvolemia based on sodium intake. Urinary sodium conservation capacity is disrupted with diuretics, osmotic diuresis, and sodium-losing nephropathies. With hypovolemia, U_{Na} <20 mEq/L suggests an extrarenal source of volume loss; U_{Na} >40 mEq/L suggests that renal sodium loss is contributing to the hypovolemia. Fractional excretion of sodium ($FeNa^+$) is the ratio of the amount of filtered sodium to the amount of sodium excreted. $FeNa^+$ <1% suggests renal failure caused by prerenal factors; $FeNa^+$ >2% suggests acute tubular necrosis or postrenal factors.[4,10–12] Urinary potassium concentration (U_K) reflects renal potassium conservation capacity (U_K <25 mEq/L) in extracellular and total body hypokalemia caused by extrarenal factors or appropriate renal potassium excretion (U_K >25 mEq/L) based on potassium intake in normal potassium states. U_K >25 mEq/L also occurs in extracellular hypokalemia as a result of diuretic use and osmotic diuresis and in extracellular hyperkalemia with total body potassium depletion caused by acidosis. Urinary potassium excretion also occurs with metabolic alkalosis caused by chloride deficiency (e.g., vomiting), increased distal tubular sodium reabsorption (e.g., vomiting or mineralocorticoid excess), or both.[4,10]

Urine magnesium concentration (U_{Mg}) reveals urinary magnesium conservation (U_{Mg} <10 mg/day) and excretion (U_{Mg} >10 mg/day). Hypermagnesemia (U_{Mg} >10 mg/day) suggests renal magnesium loss; hypomagnesemia (U_{Mg} <10 mg/day) suggests extrarenal magnesium loss.[13]

Urinary pH reflects the degree of urinary acid fixation and varies in response to acid base disorders. Low urine pH (i.e., pH <5.5) occurs as a result of metabolic acidosis or metabolic alkalosis caused by volume contraction. High urine pH (i.e., pH >6.5) occurs during the recovery from metabolic alkalosis, chronic hypercapnia, milk-alkali syndrome, and urinary tract infection with urease-producing organisms.[10]

Volume Depletion

Volume depletion is caused by actual volume losses through the gastrointestinal (GI) tract, kidneys, and skin, or relative volume losses caused by redistribution of fluids (e.g., the "third spacing" of pancreatitis and edema formation caused by decreased plasma oncotic pressure), loss of perfusion pressures (e.g., cardiogenic shock), or loss of vascular compliance (e.g., septic shock). Both absolute and relative volume depletion causes decreased "effective circulating volume" (ECV), which is sensed by cardiac and arterial baroreceptors as a fall in mean arterial pressure. The common central response to decreased ECV includes norepinephrine-induced increased heart rate, cardiac contractility, and peripheral arterial vasoconstriction, all of which cause a relative increase in the perfusion effectiveness of the remaining circulating volume. Central volume receptors cause the production of renin, which is degraded to angiotensin II, also a potent vasoconstrictor. Angiotensin II is converted to aldosterone, which causes renal sodium retention at accelerated rates to reduce the net quantity of volume loss from the depleted vascular bed. Volume depletion-induced se-

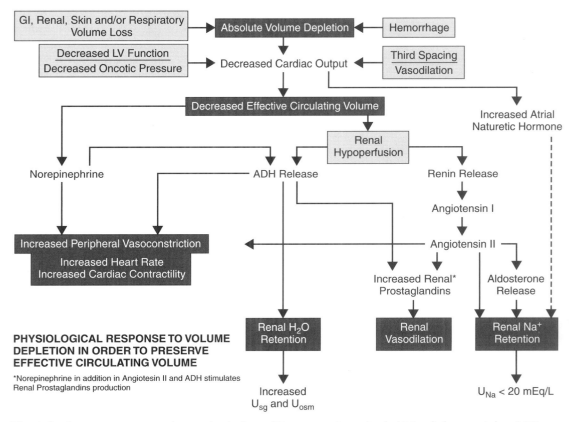

Fig. 96.3. Physiologic response to volume depletion. GI = gastrointestinal; LV = left ventricle; ACE = angiotensin-converting enzyme. (See Fig. 96.1 for other abbreviations.)

cretion of ADH also causes vasoconstriction and decreased renal water clearance in an attempt to restore the ECV. The hypoosmolality-induced inhibition to ADH secretion can be overridden by the more potent stimulus to ADH secretion, volume depletion (Fig. 96.3).[14] Each of these physiologic vasoconstrictors promotes cardiac and cerebral blood flow at the expense of less vital organs.

Volume depletion results in decreased renal blood flow, which causes the release of intrarenal prostaglandins with vasodilating properties. These prostaglandins blunt the hypovolemia-induced vasoconstriction in the renal vasculature, thereby disproportionally preserving renal blood flow and glomerular filtration. This renoprotective response can be diminished by the use of nonsteroidal antiinflammatory drugs (NSAIDs) and angiotensin-converting enzyme (ACE) inhibitors.[15–17]

Volume depletion may cause palpitations, postural dizziness, and light-headedness, especially when moving from a recumbent to an erect position. Volume depletion can exacerbate hypoperfusion caused by vascular disease and produce organ-specific or local symptoms such as angina in coronary heart disease and the abdominal pain of the ischemic bowel in mesenteric atherosclerosis. Severe volume depletion can lead to multisystem failure, circulatory collapse, and death. The amount of fluid intake and loss estimated by the patient may indicate the severity of the volume depletion, but this information is difficult to obtain from children and patients with chronic or acute cognitive deficits. Edema and weight gain may occur when decreased ECV is accompanied by excessive renal sodium and water conservation (e.g., congestive heart failure, cirrhosis, and nephrosis) and the addition of volume disproportionately added to the interstitial fluid space because of increased hydrostatic pressure, decreased plasma oncotic pressure, or loss of vascular integrity.

Although the clinical presentation of volume depletion is obvious in its most severe and acute forms, its earlier presence and chronic forms are associated with more subtle findings (e.g., general malaise, weakness, anorexia, and mental status changes). Volume depletion may cause resting tachycardia, excessive postural pulse and blood pressure changes [systolic blood pressure drops of >15 mm Hg and an increase in pulse rate of >20 beats per minute (bpm) from supine to sitting positions], and hypotension.

Volume loss caused by sepsis may be associated with hyperthermia, hypothermia, or hyperventilation. Internal jugular venous pressures may be low except when decreased ECV is caused by heart failure and resulting venous hypertension. Decreased effective circulating volume caused by absolute volume loss causes decreased skin turgor, whereas decreased ECV caused by left ventricular dysfunction, decreased oncotic pressures, and loss of vascular integrity may be associated with edema formation. Documentation of weight loss could further support the presence of absolute volume loss, and weight gain may reflect the compensatory sodium retention seen in the edematous states caused by a decreased ECV.

With volume depletion the urine specific gravity and urine osmolality are high (i.e., >1.015 and >350 mOsm/kg, respectively) as a result of ADH-induced renal water conservation, and the urine sodium concentration is less than 20 mEq/L, reflecting renal sodium conservation in the absence of intrinsic renal disease, diuretic use, or osmotic diuresis. Volume losses that occur with the ingestion or administration of hypotonic fluids have the potential to result in hyponatremia (e.g., mild volume depletion in an infant with diarrhea receiving an oral hypotonic electrolyte solution). Volume depletion without adequate access to free water can result in hypernatremia (e.g., a febrile patient with dementia).[18] The alteration in acid-base balance depends on the source of volume loss (e.g., metabolic acidosis caused by diarrhea and metabolic alkalosis caused by vomiting). Significant quantities of potassium can be lost with most sources of volume depletion. When volume depletion is severe, renal potassium excretion can be compromised in normal and abnormal kidneys, thereby increasing the potential that potassium repletion could lead to hyperkalemia without careful monitoring.[15,16]

Blood urea nitrogen is retained in volume-depleted states such that the normal 10:1 BUN/creatinine ratio is elevated (e.g., to >20:1) because of renal hypoperfusion, resulting in prerenal azotemia and non-intrinsic or functional acute renal failure. Elevation of BUN and maintenance of a BUN/creatinine ratio of 10:1 in the presence of volume depletion may be indicative of protein starvation or acute renal failure caused by postrenal obstruction [e.g., benign prostatic hypertrophy (BPH), carcinoma, stones, blood clots, papillary necrosis] or intrinsic renal disease caused by hypotension-induced renal ischemia causing acute tubular necrosis (ATN). The fractional excretion of sodium is less than 1% with prerenal causes of acute renal failure caused by decreased ECV not associated with intrinsic renal dysfunction (e.g., Na^+-losing nephropathies and diuretic use) and more than 2% in ATN. The urine sediment in volume depletion and prerenal azotemia is acellular, but with ATN caused by acute or severe hypotensive states the urine sediment could contain renal tubular epithelial cells and casts.[14] With prerenal causes of acute renal failure the renal urinary concentration capacity to osmolalities of more than 350 mOsm/kg is preserved, but this ability to concentrate urine may be lost in patients with ATN. A similar disturbance is seen with urinary Na^+ conservation such that prerenal causes of acute renal failure results in a U_{Na} of <20 mEq/L and a U_{Na} of >40 mEq/L in those with ATN.[19]

Volume depletion is treated by incremental restoration of the ECV using oral electrolyte solutions in mild volume depletion, the infusion of isotonic fluid in more severe settings, and the cessation of volume loss. Volume repletion must also include the replacement of daily obligate fluid losses. The rate of volume repletion depends on the severity of the volume depletion and associated complications. Volume repletion must proceed with caution in patients who have left ventricular dysfunction and the age-related decrease in cardiac function seen in the elderly. In febrile and other states of increased physiologic stress, estimation of the insensible losses becomes difficult and is a frequent cause of insufficient volume repletion. Daily weighing reveals the net result of volume repletion, persistent volume losses, and the potentially unmeasurable insensible losses. Restoration of ECV results in the loss of abnormal postural blood pressure and pulse changes, urinary excretion of sodium (i.e., urinary sodium >20 mEq/L), and restoration of body weight.[16]

Once the volume status has been restored, treatment can be directed to restoring electrolyte loss (e.g., potassium) and normal osmolality by providing free water in hypernatremic states. If hyponatremia occurs as a result of volume depletion–induced ADH secretion, restoration of the circulating volume would result in a water diuresis (i.e., dilute urine) and normalization of plasma osmolality.[14] If acute volume loss is caused by significant blood loss, transfusion with whole blood plus isotonic fluid infusion may be necessary. If effective circulating volume depletion is caused by left ventricular dysfunction, efforts to increase cardiac contractility and decrease cardiac afterload may be used to increase the ECV. Increased hepatic protein production and decreased renal protein losses can restore oncotic pressures and the ECV in patients with nephrosis or cirrhosis. Removal of any drug and the treatment of any infectious disease that causes inappropriate peripheral vasodilatation must also be pursued.

Volume Excess

Volume excess, or hypervolemia, can be caused by decreased ECV, which results in renal sodium and water conservation and edema formation (e.g., hypoalbuminemia and left ventricular dysfunction). Volume excess can also be caused by chronic renal failure, mineralocorticoid excess, and infusion of sodium and water at rates exceeding renal excretion, ultimately resulting in total body hypervolemia and increased ECV. Significant volume retention can occur in local areas because of chronic venous or lymphatic obstruction with no alteration of the ECV (Table 96.1).[20]

Total body volume excess caused by decreased ECV and edema formation may cause symptoms of vital organ hypoperfusion (e.g., syncope, unstable angina). Weight gain may reflect the quantity of the volume retention. Evidence of edema may be found in the lower extremities in an ambulatory patient but may be more evident in the presacral area in a recumbent patient. Depending on the etiology of volume excess, physical findings of congestive heart failure (CHF), hepatic cirrhosis, and nephrosis might be present. Edema and hypertension may be associated with renal failure or mineralocorticoid excess.

Edematous states caused by decreased ECV result in U_{Na} and U_{osm} consistent with those of absolute volume depletion except when there is intrinsic renal disease, osmotic diuresis, or diuretic use. Hypervolemia associated with increase ECV causes urinary sodium wasting ($U_{Na} > 20$ mEq/L) and no excessive water retention (assuming normal osmolality). Hypoalbuminemia suggests cirrhosis, nephrosis, or a protein-losing enteropathy as a potential cause of volume excess. Hypokalemia and hypertension are associated with volume excess caused by mineralocorticoid excess.

Treatment of volume excess caused by decreased ECV involves increasing the cardiac output (e.g., afterload reduction and increasing the force of cardiac contraction) and restoring intravascular oncotic forces in patients with cirrhosis and hypoalbuminemia. Removal of some edema by diuretics may be required, especially if the retained fluid compromises venti-

Table 96.1. Causes of Hyponatremia

Decreased effective circulating volume, inducing aldosterone-mediated sodium retention, angiotensin II vasoconstriction, and ADH vasoconstriction and renal water retention (decreased plasma osmolality; $U_{Na}^+ < 20$ mEq/L; $U_{osm} > 350$ mOsm/kg)
Edematous states
   Congestive heart failure
   Hypoalbuminemia
      Cirrhosis
      Nephrosis
      Protein malnutrition and protein-losing enteropathies
   Nonsteroidal antiinflammatory drugs
   Chronic use of vasodilating drugs
   Severe hypokalemia
   Decreased vascular integrity (e.g., sepsis, anaphylaxis)
   Third-space sequestration
      Bowel obstruction, pancreatitis, peritonitis, ascites
      Massive tissue injury (e.g., crush injuries and burns), venous obstruction
Hypovolemic states
   GI volume losses (e.g., diarrhea, vomiting)
   Skin volume losses
   Renal loss (urine sodium >40 mEq/L)
      Osmotic
      Diuretics
         Thiazides (most common)
         Loop diuretics (least common and variable urine osmolality)
      Adrenal insufficiency
      Na^+-losing nephropathies (variable urine osmolality)
      Cerebral salt wasting

Inappropriate secretion of ADH, causing renal water retention and volume excess (decreased plasma osmolality; $U_{Na}^+ > 20$ mEq/L; $U_{osm} > 200$ mOsm/kg even with H_2O loading)
SIADH
Severe pain and/or stress

Excess water intake ($U_{Na}^+ > 20$ mEq/L, $U_{osm} < 100$ mOsm/kg)
   Primary polydipsia
   Renal failure
   Hypothyroidism

Hyponatremia not caused by H_2O excess
   Normal plasma osmolality (e.g., hyperproteinemia, hyperlipidemia)
   Elevated plasma osmolality (e.g., hyperglycemia, mannitol infusion)

Reset osmolality (e.g., cirrhosis and chronic decreased ECV)

ADH = antidiuretic hormone; GI = gastrointestinal; SIADH = syndrome of inappropriate secretion of ADH; ECV = effective circulating volume.

lation (e.g., pulmonary edema and tense ascites). Third-space fluids should be removed with caution, as removal of large amounts causes rapid reaccumulations extracted from the circulating volume, resulting in hypotension. Third-space fluid cannot be rapidly removed with diuretics, as the vascular interface with the general circulation is small, and aggressive diuresis increases the risk of hypotension and vascular collapse. Aggressive therapeutic diuresis, when required, should be pursued only when there is peripheral edema, which can serve as an internal source of volume repletion in the event that overdiuresis and hypotension inadvertently occur. With states of aldosterone excess (hepatic cirrhosis with ascites), an aldosterone antagonist (i.e., spironolactone) is used to decrease sodium reabsorption and edema formation, and, if possible, the source of the hyperaldosteronism is removed. With renal failure, diuresis with potent loop diuretics may be required to remove excess volume and any factor that can acutely decrease existing compromised renal function (e.g., infection, volume depletion, use of nephrotoxic agents). Overzealous diuresis must be avoided in patients with end-stage congestive cardiomyopathy, where a certain amount of venous hypertension may be required to maintain a cardiac output consistent with survival. Treatment with diuretics is associated with many complications, the most significant of which are hypokalemia, hypovolemia, metabolic alkalosis (i.e., thiazides and loop diuretics), metabolic acidosis (carbonic anhydrase inhibitors and the distal tubular diuretics amiloride, triamterene, and spironolactone), hypomagnesemia, and worsening glucose tolerance (especially thiazides).

Hyponatremia

Hyponatremia is caused by (1) excessive addition of water to body fluids because of volume depletion–induced secretion of ADH, (2) SIADH, and (3) addition of water at rates that exceed renal water clearance capability. Hyponatremia may also occur in settings where osmolality is normal (i.e., pseudo-hyponatremia caused by severe hyperlipidemia and hyper-proteinemia)[21–24] and in others where the osmolality is elevated (e.g., hyperglycemia)[25] (Table 96.1, Fig. 96.1). Volume depletion–induced hyponatremia occurs when consumption of free water is used as the primary source of volume repletion, resulting in retention of the ingested water because of the nonosmotic (i.e., hypovolemia-induced vasoconstriction) presence of ADH.[26–29] Diuretic-induced volume depletion and hyponatremia are most often caused by thiazide diuretics because these drugs do not impair the renal concentrating mechanism, as is the case with medullary loop diuretics.[29–33] Hyponatremia can also occur with the edematous states of CHF, cirrhosis, and nephrosis caused by decreased ECV for similar reasons.[34] SIADH occurs when excess ADH is secreted in the absence of volume or osmotic stimuli, resulting in water excess and hyponatremia [e.g., ADH-secreting tumors, central nervous system (CNS) disorders, and pulmonary disease] (Table 96.2). There are rare occasions where patients with CNS disease will develop hyponatremia not caused by SIADH, but by CNS factors that induce renal salt wasting and hypovolemia. Adrenal insufficiency causes hyponatremia by both volume and nonvolume stimulation of ADH secretion.[35] The ingestion of large quantities of water (i.e., 10–15 L in 24 hours)[34] at rates exceeding renal water excretion, leading to hyponatremia, can be accomplished at times without the polydipsia being apparent to casual observers (i.e., primary polydipsia). Patients with renal dysfunction, however, may develop hyponatremia with much less ingested water because of an associated decreased renal water clearance capability (Table 96.2, Fig. 96.1).[34,36]

The symptoms associated with hyponatremia depend on the

Table 96.2. Causes of Syndrome of Inappropriate Antidiuretic Hormone Secretion

Central nervous system disorders causing increased hypothalamic production of antidiuretic hormone
  Infections (e.g., meningitis, HIV infection)
  Vascular problems (e.g., subdural hemorrhage)
  Primary and metastatic cancers
  Psychosis
  Postpituitary surgery
  Hypothalamic infiltrative disease (e.g., sarcoidosis)
  Others (e.g., Guillain-Barré syndrome)

Pharmacologic agents
  Stimulants of hypothalamic antidiuretic hormone secretion
    Haloperidol
    Amitriptyline
    Thioridazine
    Thiothixene
    Carbamazepine
    Fluoxetine and sertraline[50–52]
    Monoamine oxidase inhibitors[53]
    Others (e.g., bromocriptine mesylate)
  Potentiators of antidiuretic hormone effect
    Chlorpropamide
    Tolbutamide
    Carbamazepine
  Exogenous antidiuretic hormone preparations
    Vasopressin
    Oxytocin

Pulmonary disorders causing increased antidiuretic hormone production
  Pneumonias
  Tuberculosis
  Acute respiratory failure
  Others (e.g., asthma, pneumothorax)

Ectopic production of antidiuretic hormone (e.g., bronchogenic carcinoma, oat cell carcinoma of the lung, pancreatic carcinoma)

Pancreatic carcinoma

Prolactinoma

Others
  Postoperative patient
  Severe nausea

Source: Rose BD. Hypoosmolal states—hyponatremia. In: Rose BD, Post TW. Clinical physiology of acid-base and electrolyte disorders. Part three: physiologic approach to acid-base and electrolyte disorders, 5th ed. New York: McGraw-Hill, Health Professions Division, 2001;696–745, with permission.

factors causing excessive water retention. Excessive water ingestion suggests the presence of primary polydipsia, especially in those with chronic renal disease or unstable psychiatric disorders. Symptoms caused directly by hypoosmolality are mostly neurologic and are directly related to the degree and acuteness with which hyponatremia develops. Slowly developing hyponatremia may remain asymptomatic at lower levels of plasma sodium concentration (compared to rapidly developing hyponatremia) because of the adaptive potential of brain cells to hypoosmolality.[37] Problems such as weakness, nausea, vomiting, confusion, irritability, postural dizziness, syncope, and falls are common; focal neurologic problems such as seizures and coma are less common.[38]

Hyponatremia caused by absolute volume depletion is associated with findings that suggest decreased ECV (e.g., weight loss), whereas the edematous causes of hyponatremia are associated with findings characteristic of CHF, nephrosis, cirrhosis, and severe renal insufficiency (e.g., weight gain and edema formation). Weight gain without evidence of edema or volume depletion is consistent with SIADH and primary polydipsia.

The presence of hyponatremia and hypoosmolality is confirmed by low measured and calculated plasma osmolality. Plasma osmolality (P_{osm}) is the total osmolality of the solutes in the plasma and can be calculated as

$$P_{osm} = 2[Na^+] + \frac{[glucose]}{18} + \frac{[BUN]}{2.8}$$

Because BUN freely diffuses across cell membranes, it does not hold water in extracellular spaces; therefore, the effective P_{osm} is two times $[Na^+]$ plus $[glucose]/18$, or 270 to 280 mOsm/kg. In those with hyponatremia and hypoosmolality, the plasma $[Cl^-]$ is decreased proportionally, assuming an absence of underlying acid-base disorders. Moreover, the $[HCO_3^-]$ does not decrease as much as $[Na^+]$ and $[Cl^-]$ because of HCO_3^- renal regeneration. Therefore, a proportional $[HCO_3^-]$ decrease to $[Na^+]$ or $[Cl^-]$ would indicate the presence of an acid-base disorder in true hypoosmolar states. Hyponatremia with normal plasma osmolality suggests the presence of severe hyperlipidemia and hyperproteinemia (i.e., pseudohyponatremia). Hyponatremia and high osmolality are caused by hyperglycemia (plasma sodium concentration decreased by 1 mEq/L for every 62-mg increase in glucose concentration above normal) and mannitol infusion. The calculated plasma osmolality (two times $[Na^+]$ plus $[glucose]/18$ plus $[BUN]$ should approximate the measured plasma osmolality. However, the measured plasma osmolality value can be increased by the presence of ethanol, methanol, ethylene glycol, and increased amounts of BUN, but because these substances freely diffuse across cellular membranes they do not affect the distribution of water, and the plasma sodium concentration remains unchanged.

Hyponatremia caused by renal water retention secondary to volume depletion, or SIADH, results in a high urine specific gravity and high urine osmolality. The urine sodium concentration is less than 20 mEq/L with hyponatremia caused by volume depletion (except with intrinsic renal disease, diuretic use, and osmotic diuresis). Urinary sodium concentration is more than 20 mEq/L with hyponatremia secondary to SIADH because of water-induced total body volume expansion. With hyponatremia caused by primary polydipsia, urine specific gravity and osmolality are low, and there is mild renal salt wasting.[39] Plasma osmolality <270 mOsm/L totally suppresses ADH secretion, resulting in a urine osmolality no greater than 60 mOsm/kg.

Treatment of hyponatremia and hypoosmolality caused by true volume depletion is isotonic volume repletion via the oral or intravenous route; only in severe cases of hyponatremia (neurologic symptoms or plasma $[Na^+]$ less than 110 mEq/L) caused by hypovolemia is water restriction or infusion of hypertonic saline (or both) required. Once the ECV has been restored, a water diuresis ensues, and the plasma osmolality normalizes. With hyponatremia and hypoosmolality occurring in edematous states, restoring the ECV by enhancing ventricular dysfunction in patients with CHF and increasing oncotic pressures in those with nephrosis and cirrhosis is the primary focus of therapy. For hyponatremia caused by SIADH or primary polydipsia and in patients with severe renal failure, water restriction is the main modality used to restore normal plasma osmolality. Efforts are made to remove, if possible, the source of SIADH secretion and to treat the underlying psychopathology that caused excessive ingestion of water by those with primary polydipsia. With symptomatic SIADH that causes significant hypoosmolality, it becomes necessary to treat the hypotonic state acutely with hypertonic saline infusion in a hospital setting. For patients who are asymptomatic, the plasma sodium concentration should be increased at a rate of 0.5 mEq/L/hr until a level of 120 mEq/L is reached. More rapid correction of hyponatremia may be required for those patients who have severe neurologic symptoms (1.0–1.5 mEq/L/hr for the first 10 mEq/L elevation in the plasma sodium concentration). These attempts to avoid correction too rapidly of hyponatremia decrease the occurrence of infrequent but potentially devastating central pontine demyelinization.[40–49]

Hypernatremia

Hypernatremia and hyperosmolality are caused by increased insensible, renal, and GI hypotonic fluid loss at rates exceeding hypotonic fluid intake. Chronic ingestion of hypotonic fluids at rates less than obligate daily insensible loss can also lead to hypernatremia and hyperosmolality, especially in patients with debilitating disease or hypothalamic disorders that result in a decreased thirst response to hypernatremia and those with immature (i.e., infants) or impaired (e.g., chronic renal failure) renal concentrating mechanisms. Hypernatremia can result from pure water loss through skin (e.g., fever), through the respiratory tract (e.g., hyperventilation), and in the presence of nephrogenic and central diabetes insipidus when there is a reduction in secretion or action of ADH.[50–56] The hypernatremic state can also be caused by excess addition of sodium salts to body fluid compartments (Table 96.3).[57]

The symptoms associated with hypernatremia are related directly to the rate and severity of the water loss or solute gain. The symptoms occur because of the extracellular hyperosmolality and resultant volume loss of cells, especially those of the CNS.[37] Early symptoms may be nonspecific and include weakness and irritability; later seizures and other alterations of consciousness may occur. Symptoms associated with volume depletion could be present if hypernatremia is caused by pure water or hypotonic fluid losses. The presence of polyuria suggests a renal loss of pure water (e.g., diabetes insipidus), osmotic diuresis (e.g., glycosuria), or sodium-induced diuresis caused by diuretics when there is no access to water or hypotonic fluid replacement. Hypernatremia caused by the addition of sodium salts is associated with shortness of breath and swelling (signs of ECV expansion). The physical findings of hypernatremia are those related to vol-

Table 96.3. **Causes of Hypernatremia**

Volume depletion caused by water losses exceeding
  sodium losses and/or inadequate water access (increased
  plasma osmolality; U_{osm} >600 mOsm/kg; U_{Na} <20 mEq/L)[a]
  Renal hypotonic volume losses (U_{Na} >20 mEq/L, U_{osm}
    <plasma osmolality)
    Osmotic diuresis
    Diuretics
  Gastrointestinal hypotonic volume loss
  Skin hypotonic volume loss
  Respiratory hypotonic volume loss

Volume expansion with sodium salts (increased plasma
  osmolality; U_{Na} >20 mEq/L; U_{osm} >600 mOsm/kg)[a]

Pure water loss (increased plasma osmolality;
  U_{osm} >600 mOsm/kg; U_{Na} <20 mEq/L)[a]
  Respiratory infections, tachypnea
  Increase sweating, fever
  Diabetes insipidus (U_{osm} <300 mOsm/kg and
    U_{Na} >20 mEq/L when polyuria is present)

[a]Assuming absence of salt-losing nephropathy, diuretic use, or osmotic diuresis.

ume depletion (i.e., pure water and hypotonic volume loss) and those of volume expansion (i.e., addition of Na⁺ salts), such as edema, weight gain, systemic hypertension, venous hypertension, S_3 gallop, and pulmonary edema.

Hypernatremia, or hyperosmolality, is confirmed by plasma osmolality values greater than 300 mOsm/kg. Plasma hyperosmolality and hyperglycemia may present with hyponatremia, normonatremia, or hypernatremia because of the net osmotic movement of intracellular water into the ECV. Hypernatremia caused by volume loss from nonrenal sources and inadequate hypotonic volume replacement results in a urine sodium concentration of less than 20 mEq/L and high urine osmolality (e.g., >600 mOsm/kg) unless intrinsic renal disease or drugs impair renal sodium and water conservation. Hypernatremia caused by renal volume losses and inadequate hypotonic volume replacement is associated with a urine sodium concentration greater than 20 mEq/L and a urine osmolality that may be less than 350 mOsm/kg. When hypernatremia is caused by the addition of sodium salts, the urine osmolality is usually more than 350 mOsm/kg and the urine sodium concentration more than 20 mEq/L. Significant hypernatremia without maximum concentrated urine (i.e., 800–1200 mOsm/kg) suggests diabetes insipidus, intrinsic renal disease, osmotic diuresis, or diuretic use.[14,55,58]

Hypernatremia caused by hypotonic volume loss that results in a decreased ECV must initially be treated by restoring the circulating volume with isotonic saline until signs of hypovolemia have been removed. The isotonic saline infusion may also contribute to the lowering of the plasma osmolality because it is hypotonic to patients with hyperosmolality. Once the ECV has been restored, hypotonic fluids can be administered to provide free water in order to decrease plasma osmolality. Correction of asymptomatic hyperosmolality must proceed slowly (i.e., [Na⁺] reduction of 0.5 mEq/L/hr) to avoid cerebral edema and resultant neurologic dysfunction (e.g., seizures). Pure water losses from the skin and kidneys is replaced with hypotonic solutions [e.g., half or quarter

normal saline or dextrose 5% in water (D_5W) depending on concurrent Na⁺ losses].[2,59] Hypernatremia caused by the addition of Na⁺ salts is treated with D_5W and diuretics. Hypernatremia caused by hypodipsia and lack of access to water or a hypotonic solution is treated by removing the obstacles to hypotonic fluid ingestion.[60] Because older persons have a decreased thirst response to rising plasma osmolality, hypotonic fluid administration in settings such as fever and pneumonia should be anticipatory to prevent the development of hypernatremia, assuming that significant volume deficits have not occurred. Hypokalemia in the presence of hypernatremia must be treated not only because of its potential dangerous cardiac effects but also because hypokalemia may exacerbate urinary concentrating deficiency.

Treatment of central diabetes insipidus is the administration of ADH preparation acutely (e.g., aqueous vasopressin) and chronically (e.g., vasopressin in oil and vasopressin nasal sprays). Nephrogenic diabetes insipidus is treated only if the polyuria makes daily routines difficult to manage or the rate of water ingestion is less than renal water loss. Nephrogenic diabetes insipidus can be treated with hydrochlorothiazide and a low-sodium diet. NSAIDs have likewise been helpful in these settings. NSAIDs and hydrochlorothiazide can also be used effectively to treat central diabetes insipidus.

Hyperglycemia

The impact of glucose at normal levels of osmolality is no greater than an additional 3.3 to 5.7 mOsm/L. However, in states where extracellular glucose is elevated, severalfold, the impact on fluid and electrolyte balance is substantial. Excessive hyperglycemia obligates large amounts of additional water to extracellular spaces by osmotic-induced intracellular water loss (i.e., cellular dehydration). This glucose-induced increase in extracellular water dilutes plasma sodium such that there is a 1 mEq/L decrease in plasma sodium concentration for every 62 mg/dL increase in serum glucose concentration.[61] If this dilutional effect of hyperglycemia, which should affect all extracellular anions, does not occur, substantial water losses (greater than sodium) are present. Hyperglycemia creates an osmotic diuresis that causes loss of salt and water, which, if substantial and not repleted, leads to total body volume depletion. Volume depletion causes decreased renal perfusion, which decreases renal excretion of excessive glucose, thus adding to the degree of hyperglycemia. This hyperglycemic diuresis also promotes urinary potassium losses as well. In diabetic ketoacidosis the insulin levels are lower causing not only gluconeogenesis but ketogenesis as well. Common to both disorders is hyperosmolality caused by hyperglycemia and volume and potassium depletion.

Treatment is aimed at restoring effective circulating volume, using isotonic saline until hemodynamic stability has been attained. Volume repletion will decrease plasma glucose levels substantially and glomerular filtration rate is increased. In hyperosmolar hyperglycemic nonketotic syndrome, if insulin is required, blood glucose lowering is usually accomplished with small amounts. In diabetic ketoacidosis (DKA), larger and continuous doses of insulin are absolutely required not only to reduce glucose levels, but also to halt ketogenesis. In both these disorders, the rate of glucose hyperglycemia is suddenly exposed to a decrease in plasma osmolality caused by insulin-induced lowering of glucose levels. A plasma glucose level of 300 mg/dL but no lower is the aim of therapy in these hyperosmolar states to avoid cerebral edema. This can be accomplished by change to dextrose sodium and water IV infusion and decreasing the amount of administered insulin.

Hypotonic fluid repletion to restore water loss can be started once hemodynamic stability has been attained. Potassium deficits that are substantial in both disorders must be repleted to enhance cellular glucose uptake, restore renal concentrating capacity, and avoid cardiac dysrhythmias. Insulin's promotion of cellular glucose uptake requires potassium, and in hyperglycemia, caused by the endogenous lack of insulin, the use of exogenous insulin may exacerbate plasma hypokalemia.

Hyperglycemia is caused by two states of insulin deficiency. Hyperosmolar hyperglycemic nonketotic syndrome generally has enough insulin, albeit low, to prevent lipolysis. However, the insulin levels are too low to provide adequate cellular glucose uptake that stimulates gluconeogenesis, which adds to the accumulating hyperglycemia[62] (also see Chapter 120).

Hypokalemia

Hypokalemia, the most frequent electrolyte abnormality seen in family medicine, is usually caused by the use of medullary and cortical loop diuretics (e.g., furosemide and hydrochlorothiazide). Plasma hypokalemia, reflecting potassium loss from all body fluid compartments (i.e., total body potassium depletion), can occur as a result of excessive urinary, GI, and skin potassium losses. Renal potassium losses (i.e., U_K >25 mEq/L) leading to total body hypokalemia can result from diuretic use, polyuria, sodium-losing nephropathies, primary mineralocorticoid excess, vomiting, and hypomagnesemia. Medullary and cortical loop diuretics and sodium-losing nephropathies cause excessive kaliuresis because of increased flow to the distal renal tubule. Vomiting results in small amounts of K^+ loss in gastric fluid, but initially large K^+ losses are caused by chloride depletion, increased distal tubule reabsorption of Na^+ and urinary K^+ excretion, and HCO_3^- retention. Hypokalemia caused by chloride deficits (e.g., vomiting) and primary and secondary mineralocorticoid excesses are usually associated with metabolic alkalosis. Diabetic ketoacidosis and renal tubular acidosis are associated with increased urinary K^+ loss and total body K^+ depletion, which may be masked by an acidosis-induced increase in $[K^+]$. The $[K^+]$ falls with the treatment of acidemic states.

If hypokalemia occurs with high U_K without obvious causes (e.g., diuretic use, vomiting, or polyuria), a renin assay is required, especially if the patient has hypertension. If renin levels are high or normal, continued diuretic use, renovascular hypertension, sodium-losing nephropathies, and Cushing's disease must be considered as possible causes. If the renin levels are low, the aldosterone level should be measured. High aldosterone levels with hypokalemia suggest primary hyperaldosteronism, and low aldosterone levels suggest an extrinsic source of excess mineralocorticoid activity (i.e., licorice ingestion).

Total body potassium depletion and hypokalemia can also result from inadequate intake (e.g., clay ingestion and starvation) to replete daily losses. Hypokalemia with normal total body potassium is seen when potassium is shifted between fluid compartments as a result of respiratory and metabolic alkalosis, an acute increase in erythropoiesis (i.e., treatment of severe megaloblastic anemias), increased insulin activity, delirium tremens, and hypothermia. Total body hypokalemia can occur without evidence of plasma hypokalemia (e.g., acidemia and states of sodium excess) (Table 96.4).[63,64]

Generalized weakness is the most common symptom associated with hypokalemia. Other symptoms include polyuria, polydipsia, anorexia, nausea, vomiting, constipation, palpitations, muscle cramps, and muscle tenderness (e.g., hypokalemia-induced rhabdomyolysis). Hypokalemia also increases the sensitivity of cardiac muscle to the cardiotoxic effects of digitalis, which may include syncope, dizziness, palpitations, and symptoms of worsening CHF and angina.

Signs associated with hypokalemia include objective evidence of proximal muscle weakness disorders of cardiac per-

Table 96.4. **Causes of Hypokalemia**

Renal K⁺ loss (U_K >25 mEq/L)
Diuretics,, current use
Vomiting and nasogastric tube drainage
Magnesium depletion
Mineralocorticoid excess (e.g., primary and secondary hyperaldosteronism, Cushing's disease, licorice ingestion, hyperreninism, Bartter syndrome)
Diabetic ketoacidosis
Renal tubular acidosis
Ureterosigmoidostomy
Polyuria
Osmotic diuresis
Correction of chronic hypercapnia

Extrarenal loss (U_K <25 mEq/L)
Diarrhea
Excess sweating
Intestinal fistulas
Rectal villous adenoma
Geophagia
Laxative abuse
Chloride-losing diarrhea

Intracellular K⁺ sequestration
Metabolic and respiratory alkalosis (Tables 96.1 and 96.2)
Excess insulin
Treatment of megaloblastic anemias
β-adrenergic agonist
Hypothermia
Catecholamine excess
Hypokalemic periodic paralysis

Pseudohypokalemia
Prolonged standing of collected blood with extremely high WBC count
Blood specimen collected immediately after insulin administration

Total body K⁺ depletion with plasma eukalemia
Diabetic ketoacidosis
Renal tubular acidosis

Decreased K⁺ intake
Starvation

formance, rate and rhythm, and ileus. Measurements of the plasma potassium concentration can confirm the presence of true hypokalemia unless there is a redistribution of potassium because of alkalemia (0.4 mEq/L decrease in $[K^+]$ for every 0.1 increase in plasma pH) and other causes of intracellular potassium sequestration. Sampling error can mask true hypokalemia when there is significant hemolysis during blood collection. When blood samples from patients with extremely high white blood cell (WBC) counts (e.g., leukemia) are permitted to stand for long periods, K^+ is sequestered intracellularly, thereby reducing $[K^+]$ secretion (i.e., pseudohypokalemia).

Hypokalemia occurring with a urine potassium concentration of less than 25 mEq/L is consistent with a nonrenal route of potassium loss (e.g., skin and lower GI tract). Hypokalemia with a urine potassium concentration higher than 25 mEq/L is consistent with renal potassium loss (e.g., diuretics, hypomagnesemia, polyuria, or mineralocorticoid excess) as a contributing cause to the potassium deficit.[10] Pseudohypokalemia can occur when a blood sample containing a significantly elevated number of WBCs is permitted to stand and the cells take up the available extracellular potassium. Hypokalemia may diminish renal concentration and acidification capacity. Severe hypokalemia causes skeletal muscle dysfunction and increases the potential of muscle injury (i.e., rhabdomyolysis) under certain stresses revealed by the presence of myoglobinuria. Electrocardiographic (ECG) changes associated with hypokalemia include decreased magnitude of T waves, U wave formation, ST segment depression, and cardiac dysrhythmias that occur because of the increased myocardial tissue automaticity and prolonged ventricular repolarization, thereby permitting reentrant pathways to develop.

Treatment of hypokalemia includes increased dietary intake of potassium-rich foods (e.g., fruits and vegetables), the administration of potassium chloride, and stopping the renal, GI, and skin losses of potassium.

Potassium chloride can be given orally as an elixir, an effervescent liquid, or a slow-release preparation in amounts necessary to correct hypokalemia. Hypokalemia resistant to replacement therapy in diuretic-induced hypokalemia suggests the potential presence of magnesium deficiency, which must be corrected to maximize the effectiveness of potassium repletion. Slow oral repletion (i.e., 60 mEq of potassium per liter per day) is sufficient for mild nonsymptomatic hypokalemia (i.e., 3.5–3.0 mEq/L). If a large amount of potassium is required, the intravenous route for repletion is used adding KCl to glucose free IV fluids. KCl in concentrations greater than 60 mEq/L through peripheral veins is inadvisable because of the potential for resultant local pain and venous sclerosis. With severe symptomatic hypokalemia (i.e., <2.5 mEq/L) accompanied by life-threatening symptoms, potassium repletion can proceed more rapidly, usually not exceeding 10 to 20 mEq/hr. In all cases of potassium repletion, the impact of a given amount of potassium must be monitored by frequent plasma potassium measurements.[65] Distal diuretics in combination with medullary loop and cortical diuretics may decrease kaluresis, thereby decreasing the potential for developing hypokalemia. These potassium-sparing diuretics may be helpful for treating the hypokalemia associated with primary hyperaldosteronism.

Hyperkalemia

Hyperkalemia results when potassium is added to the ECV at rates exceeding renal, skin, and GI potassium excretion. This increased extracellular potassium content can represent an absolute increase in total body potassium or shifts of potassium from intracellular to extracellular sites. A total body potassium increase occurs with increased potassium intake and decreased potassium excretion due to volume depletion, renal dysfunction including hypoaldosteronism, or both. Drugs capable of causing hypoaldosteronism and hyperkalemia include distal tubular diuretics (e.g., spironolactone, amiloride, and triamterene), ACE inhibitors, and NSAIDs.[66] Shifting of intracellular potassium to extracellular fluid spaces occurs with metabolic acidosis (0.2–1.7 mEq/L increase in $[K^+]$ for every 0.1 decrease in pH), cellular destruction, digitalis intoxication, excessive physical exercise, insulin deficiency and hyperglycemia, hyperkalemic periodic paralysis, β-adrenergic blockage, and spurious elevations of potassium. Spurious elevations, or pseudohyperkalemia, can be caused by hemolysis of red blood cells as a result of collection or storage, release of K^+ during coagulation of blood samples with increased WBCs (e.g., WBCs $>100,000/mm^3$ in leukemia) or increased platelets (i.e., $>1,000,000/mm^3$), and sampling blood from an ischemic extremity (Table 96.5).[64,67]

Symptoms associated with hyperkalemia include muscle weakness, paresthesia, and in severe cases paralysis. ECG manifestations include peaked T waves, flattening of the P waves, increased PR interval, increased QRS duration, shortened QT interval, and sine wave development with resultant ventricular fibrillation and asystole.

Once hyperkalemia has been confirmed, treatment must be

Table 96.5. **Causes of Hyperkalemia**

Increased K^+ intake

Decreased K^+ excretion
  Acute and chronic renal failure
  Decreased effective circulating volume
  Hypoaldosteronism
    K^+-sparing diuretics (e.g., Aldactone, amiloride, triamterene)
    Hyporenin hypoaldosteronism in mild renal disease
    NSAIDs
    ACE inhibitors
    Adrenal insufficiency

Intracellular K^+ extrusion
  Metabolic and respiratory acidosis
  Tissue injury (e.g., crush)
  Insulin deficiency in diabetic ketoacidosis; hyperosmolality
  Drugs (e.g., β-adrenergic blockers, digitalis intoxication, succinylcholine, and arginine HCl)
  Excessive exercise
  Hyperkalemic periodic paralysis

Pseudohyperkalemia
  Thrombocytosis
  Leukocytosis
  Hemolysis of blood sample
  Blood collection from ischemic extremity

ACE = angiotensin-converting enzyme; NSAID = nonsteroidal antiinflammatory drug.

aimed at decreasing the addition of potassium and promoting potassium removal from the ECV. The latter can be accomplished by enhancing potassium cellular entry using insulin and glucose. With severe symptomatic hyperkalemia, removal of an excessive amount of potassium from the total body water using polystyrene sulfurate, diuretics, and dialysis (for patients with renal dysfunction) may be required. If metabolic acidosis is present, decreasing fixed acid production and retention as well as the use of $NaHCO_3$ reverses the movement of potassium out of cells. If hyperkalemia is associated with life-threatening dysrhythmias, calcium as calcium gluconate can be used to increase the threshold of myocardial tissue excitability induced by hyperkalemia, thereby reducing the chances of serious cardiac events.

Hypobicarbonatemia

Decreased concentration of bicarbonate can occur as a result of the primary event in metabolic acidosis or the compensatory event in respiratory alkalosis. Bicarbonate is lowered on an equivalent mEq/L basis to the increase in the anion gap in large anion gap acidosis. A large anion gap with normal, or increased plasma $[HCO_3^-]$ also represents the presence of a large anion gap metabolic acidosis albeit mix with other acid base disturbances. Decreased plasma $[HCO_3^-]$ without a maximally acidified urine indicates an intrinsic or extrinsic problem with renal acidification. Hypobicarbonatemia caused by respiratory alkalosis is usually not less than 12 mEq/L.

Metabolic Acidosis

Metabolic acidosis is a primary reduction in plasma bicarbonate concentration leading to hypobicarbonatemia, which stimulates compensatory hyperventilation and hypocapnia (i.e., decreased P_{CO_2}). In metabolic acidosis, the compensatory hyperventilation decreases the P_{CO_2} 1.2 mm Hg for each 1.0 mEq/L decrease in the plasma bicarbonate concentration. The limit of compensatory hyperventilation in metabolic acidosis is 10 mm Hg and may be more difficult to reach and maintain in the acute processes (e.g., DKA) when compared to chronic processes (e.g., chronic renal failure). If the rate of the P_{CO_2} decrease is less or more than predicted, a mixed acid-base disturbance consisting of metabolic acidosis and respiratory acidosis or respiratory alkalosis, respectively, is present.[18,68–70] The hypobicarbonatemia is caused by GI bicarbonate loss (e.g., diarrhea), renal bicarbonate loss (e.g., renal tubular acidosis), or bicarbonate titration with fixed endogenous acids (e.g., ketoacids) and exogenous acids (e.g., salicylate intoxication). Metabolic acidosis caused by pure bicarbonate loss is characterized by hyperchloremia and a normal anion gap. However, when metabolic acidosis is caused by the addition (e.g., methanol ingestion), retention (e.g., renal failure),[71] or excess production (e.g., lactic acidosis) of fixed acids that titrate bicarbonate, acidic anions remaining in extracellular body fluids cause expansion of the anion gap and a normal chloride concentration.[72–74] Metabolic acidosis causes extracellular hyperkalemia due to cellular buffering of hydrogen ions (failure of acidosis-induced hyperkalemia suggests total body potassium depletion), but because significant

volume loss is a frequent complication (e.g., DKA), total body hypokalemia must always be expected (chronic renal failure and hypoaldosteronism may be an exception) (Table 96.6).[64] The ingestion of acid toxins (e.g., paraldehyde, methanol, ethylene glycol, and salicylates) is associated not only with the distinct acid metabolite but also lactic acid as vascular collapse ensues (Table 96.6).

Symptoms suggestive of the origin of metabolic acidosis include those associated with the ingestion of acid toxins (e.g., tinnitus of salicylate intoxication, acute loss of visual acuity of methanol ingestion and mental status changes, and flank pain of ethylene glycol ingestion), an infection in a patient with insulin-dependent diabetes mellitus (IDDM), or a history of a prolonged hypotensive episode (e.g., lactic acidosis). Patients with acute metabolic acidosis may show obvious tachypnea, but with chronic states the rapid rate of respiration may be replaced with an increased depth of respiration. Findings associated with volume depletion ranging from postural hypotension to shock may also be present. Mental status may vary from confusion to coma depending on the quantity and acuteness of the fixed acid load, the adequacy of the circulating volume, and the severity of the acidemia. A funduscopic examination could reveal the retinal edema of methanol intoxication. Hyperkalemia induced by metabolic acidosis might be present early, but this process promotes urinary potassium wasting and total body potassium depletion. Cardiac rhythm disturbances and skeletal muscle weakness could therefore be a part of the presenting findings. If ingestions are suspected, measure plasma salicylate levels and assay for ethylene glycol, calculate the osmolal gap (i.e., difference between measured and calculated plasma osmolalities) to detect methanol and ethylene glycol ingestions, and examine the urinary sediment to detect oxalate crystals of ethylene glycol. If arterial blood gases and other electrolytes confirm metabolic acidosis, assess the adequacy of urinary acidification (less than maximal acidic urine suggests renal tubular acidosis).

Therapy for metabolic acidosis is initially directed at restoration of the systemic pH to levels that do not compromise cardiac function or predispose to cardiac dysrhythmias. These levels differ depending on the etiology of the acidosis; in general, however, safe systemic pH exists at 7.2 for most acidic ingestions and states where the source of bicarbonate loss cannot be immediately stopped. Severe forms of metabolic acidosis therefore require administration of sodium bicarbonate in amounts necessary to restore the pH to this safe level (and only to this level), with care taken to avoid volume excess and posttreatment metabolic alkalosis by overaggressive alkali therapy.

If the metabolic acidosis is severe enough to warrant alkali therapy, the $[HCO_3^-]$ required to give the desired pH can be determined by solving the following expression of the bicarbonate/P_{CO_2} buffer system to avoid overcorrection and posttreatment metabolic alkalosis.

$$\text{Desired pH} = [H^+] = \frac{24 \times \text{existing } P_{CO_2}}{[HCO_3^-]}$$

$[H^+]$ is estimated in nanoequivalents per liter (i.e., nanoEq/L) rather than pH units. A pH of 7.4 = 40 nanoEq/L, and for every pH unit increase there is a 0.8 reduction in $[H^+]$ (e.g., pH 7.50 = 0.8 × 40 = 32 nanoEq/L). For every pH unit de-

Table 96.6. **Causes of Hypobicarbonatemia**[a]

Metabolic acidosis (i.e., decreased pH, decreased [HCO_3^-][b] and decreased P_{CO_2}[c])
  Hyperchloremia, normal anion gap
    Bicarbonate loss (hypokalemia and urine pH <5.5)
      GI tract bicarbonate loss (e.g., diarrhea, ureterosigmoidostomy, fistulas, tube drainage, and cholestyramine chloride ingestion)
      Renal bicarbonate loss (e.g., type II renal tubular acidosis with viable urine pH depending on HCO_3^- loading and acute recovery from chronic hypocapnia, carbonic anhydrase inhibitors)
      Renal bicarbonate production failure (e.g., type I renal tubular acidosis with urine pH >5.5 and type IV renal tubular acidosis)
      HCl addition (e.g., NH_3Cl and some hyperalimentation fluids)
    Hypoaldosteronism (hyperkalemia, submaximal urinary acidification)
      Primary adrenal insufficiency
      Hyporeninemic hypoaldosteronism (e.g., during early chronic renal failure, acute renal failure interstitial nephritis angiotensin-converting enzyme inhibition, and nonsteroidal antiinflammatory drug use)
      Aldosterone resistance (e.g., spironolactone, amiloride, triamterene)
      Intestinal nephritis
      Early renal failure
      Acute renal failure
    Initial recovery from organic acidosis (variable [K^+] and urine pH)
  Normochloremia, large anion gap (urine pH <5.5)
    Excessive production of endogenously generated organic acids
      Diabetic ketoacidosis (i.e., excessive β-hydroxybutyrate and acetoacetate)
      Starvation ketosis (as above)
      Alcoholic ketosis (as above)
      Lactic acidosis (excessive lactate)
      Muscle necrosis (as above)
    Decreased excretion of endogenous acid metabolites
      Renal failure
    Ingestion of exogenous agents causing organic acidosis
      Methanol (formaldehyde, formic acid, and lactic acid accumulation)
      Ethylene glycol (glycolic and oxalic acid accumulation)
      Paraldehyde (formic and lactic acid accumulation)
      Salicylates (salicylic acid, ketones, and lactate accumulation)

Respiratory alkalosis (i.e., increased pH, decreased [HCO_3^-][c] and decreased P_{CO_2}[b])
  Increased CNS stimulation
    Physiologic and psychogenic hyperventilation
    CNS disease (e.g., infectious, trauma, infarct, bleeding, tumors, heat stroke)
    Pregnancy
    Progesterone-producing tumors
    Hepatic encephalopathy
    Methylxanthines, nicotine, salicylates
    Sepsis
  Hypoxia
    High altitude
    Anemia, severe
    Pulmonary embolus, pulmonary edema, pneumothorax
    Carbon monoxide poisoning
    Mechanical overventilation

[a]Hypobicarbonatemia = decreased [HCO_3^-].

[b]Primary acid-base event.

[c]Secondary or compensatory acid-base event.

crease there is a 1.25 increase in the [H^+] (e.g., pH 7.2 = $1.25 \times 1.25 \times 40 = 63$ nanoEq/L). Most acid-base maps provide the [H+] equivalent for pH values. Because the respiratory hyperventilation present with metabolic acidosis remains stable for hours, small increments in the [HCO_3^-] may return a severely acidemic state to a less dangerous systemic pH of about 7.2.

Volume repletion is essential to restore circulatory hemodynamics, which prevents volume depletion–induced lactic acidosis and ensures the appropriate distribution of any infused alkali or other intravenously administered therapeutic agents (i.e.,

insulin). The source of the acidosis must be removed (urinary alkalinization for salicylate intoxication) and halted (insulin administration to patients with DKA), and the ECV restored. However, when the source of the acidosis produces an organic anion (ketoacids and lactate) that can be metabolized into bicarbonate, much lower pH levels (i.e., 6.9–7.0) may be accepted before the use of any alkali, especially with DKA, where the source of the acidosis can be stopped with volume repletion and insulin infusion. Even then the problems associated with alkali use (e.g., volume overload and hypokalemia) must be weighed against any anticipated beneficial effect—the subject of much controversy.[75–78] Treatment of organic acidosis with volume repletion results in the metabolism of organic acid ions, converting a large anion gap acidosis into a normal anion gap acidosis (hyperchloremia) during the later stages of acid-base normalization.[5,79] Potassium depletion must be anticipated with most forms of metabolic acidosis as a consequence of the primary process, which involves intracellular shifts of potassium, thus increasing plasma [K$^+$], which leads to increased kaluresis. Potassium losses associated with volume depletion caused by osmotic diuresis and gastric fluid losses and vomiting must also be corrected. Treatment can further exacerbate extracellular hypokalemia when acidosis is corrected or ECV is restored, or with insulin use.[18,64,70,80–85]

Respiratory Alkalosis

Respiratory alkalosis is a primary reduction in the PCO_2 (i.e., hypocapnia), which stimulates a compensatory cellular and renal reduction in bicarbonate concentration. With primary acute and chronic respiratory alkalosis, the compensatory bicarbonate loss occurs at a rate of 2.0 mEq/L, or 5.0 mEq/L for every 10 mm Hg decrease in the PCO_2. The limits of these metabolic compensations in acute and chronic respiratory alkalosis are 18 and 12 mEq/L, respectively. If the rate of compensatory bicarbonate loss is less or more than predicted, a mixed acid-base disturbance is present consisting of respiratory alkalosis and metabolic alkalosis and metabolic acidosis, respectively. Respiratory alkalosis is caused by hypoxia (e.g., pulmonary embolus), psychogenic and physiologic (e.g., pregnancy) hyperventilation, and abnormal stimulation of the CNS respiratory center (e.g., fever, gram-negative sepsis, salicylate intoxication, hepatic encephalopathy, cerebrovascular accidents, and CNS tumors and inflammatory processes) (Table 96.6).[86–88]

Acute hypocapnia may be associated with circumoral and digital paresthesias, light-headedness, carpopedal spasm, and tetany. The associated hyperventilation is obvious, as it is mostly rate-driven. With chronic hypocapnia the respiratory rate may be normal, and the depth of respiration may predominate as the mechanism of PCO_2 removal. Treatment is directed to the underlying cause.

Hyperbicarbonatemia

Increased concentration of [HCO$_3$$^-$] is caused by the primary event in metabolic alkalosis and the compensatory event in respiratory acidosis. The bicarbonate concentration increase should be proportional to the decrease in plasma chloride concentration. If these relationships do not exist, then one must consider the presence of mixed acid-base disturbances.

Metabolic Alkalosis

Metabolic alkalosis is a primary increase in plasma bicarbonate concentration (i.e., hyperbicarbonatemia) that causes a compensatory reduction in ventilation and relative hypercapnia (i.e., increased PCO_2). With primary metabolic alkalosis the compensatory hypoventilation occurs at a rate of 0.7 mm Hg increase in the PCO_2 for every 1.0 mEq/L increase in the bicarbonate concentration. The limit of this compensatory

hypoventilation is 55 mm Hg because of hypoxia-induced ventilation. If the rate of PCO_2 increase is less or more than predicted, a mixed acid-base disturbance consisting of metabolic alkalosis and respiratory alkalosis or acidosis is present. Hypochloremia occurs as a consequence of primary loss (e.g., vomiting) or from displacement caused by hyperbicarbonatemia. Hypokalemia caused by actual loss and intracellular sequestration is also caused by metabolic alkalosis. The hyperbicarbonatemia is caused by the retention and generation (e.g., diuretic overuse) of excess bicarbonate, intake of excess bicarbonate at rates exceeding renal bicarbonate excretion (e.g., milk-alkali syndrome), and hydrogen loss (e.g., vomit-

Table 96.7. Causes of Hyperbicarbonatemia[a]

Metabolic alkalosis (i.e., increased [HCO$_3$$^-$][b] increased P$CO_2$, increased pH)
  Hypovolemia and chloride depletion (i.e., hypochloremia, hypokalemia: urine Na$^+$ <10 mEq/L, Cl$^-$ <10 mEq/L, pH <6, K$^+$ <10 mEq/L
    Vomiting
    Postdiuretic use
    Congenital chloride diarrhea
    Bartter syndrome
    Acute correction of hypercapnia in hypovolemia
  Hypervolemia (i.e., hypochloremia, hypokalemia; urine Na$^+$ >10 mEq/L, Cl$^-$ >10 mEq/L, pH <6.0)
    Mineralocorticoid excess
    Renal artery stenosis
    Primary aldosteronism
    Adrenal hyperplasia
  Excessive alkali (hypochloremia, hypokalemia; urine Na$^+$ >10 mEq/L, Cl$^-$ >10 mEq/L, pH >7.0)
    Excessive exogenous alkali (e.g., absorbable antacids, milk-alkali syndrome, excessive infusion of NaHCO$_3$)
    Excessive endogenous alkali (e.g., NaHCO$_3$)
    Acute correction of chronic hypercapnia in euvolemia
    Metabolism of β-hydroxybutyrate, acetoacetate, lactate, and citrate
  Severe hypokalemia
  Hypercalcemia (e.g., primary hyperparathyroidism)
Respiratory acidosis (i.e., lactate, increased PCO_2,[b] increased [HCO$_3$$^-$]
  Suppression of CNS respiratory center
    Drugs (e.g., sedatives
    Oxygen-induced acute PCO_2 retention in chronic obstructive pulmonary disease (COPD)
    Sleep apnea
  Disorders of respiratory muscles
  Obstructed airway
    Extrinsic foreign body
    Aspiration
    Laryngeal edema or spasm
    Bronchospasm
  Disturbances of gas exchange across alveolar membrane
    Pulmonary edema
    Adult respiratory distress syndrome
    Diffuse pneumonia
    COPD
  Loss of ventilatory volume
    Pneumothorax
    Hemothorax
    Pleural effusions

[a]Hyperbicarbonatemia = increased [HCO$_3$$^-$].
[b]Primary acid-base event.

ing) (Table 96.7). Metabolic alkalosis caused by volume depletion is characterized by a urinary chloride concentration of less than 10 mEq/L (i.e., saline-responsive), whereas metabolic alkalosis due to a primary increase in distal renal tubule activity (e.g., mineralocorticoid excess) and increased alkali ingestion is characterized by a urinary chloride concentration higher than 10 mEq/L (i.e., saline-resistant). Paradoxically, the urinary pH is usually acidic except when the disorder is caused by excessive alkali ingestion.[89–91]

Signs and symptoms associated with metabolic alkalosis are those of volume depletion and hypokalemia in saline-responsive states, and hypokalemia and volume excess (e.g., edema and hypertension) in saline-resistant states. Treatment of saline-responsive metabolic alkalosis requires volume repletion with isotonic normal saline, which inhibits the volume depletion–induced retention of bicarbonate, resulting in an alkaline diuresis. With saline-resistant metabolic alkalosis, the source of the excess alkali ingestion must be removed or inhibited. Potassium deficits must also be repleted using potassium chloride.[91]

Respiratory Acidosis

Respiratory acidosis is a primary increase in the P_{CO_2} (i.e., hypercapnia), which stimulates compensatory cellular and renal retention of bicarbonate. With primary acute and chronic respiratory acidosis, the compensatory bicarbonate retention occurs at a rate of 1.0 mEq/L or 4.0 mEq/L for every 10 mm Hg increase in the P_{CO_2}. The limits of the metabolic compensations during acute and chronic respiratory acidosis are 30 and 45 mEq/L, respectively. If the rate of compensatory bicarbonate retention is less or more than predicted, a mixed acid-base disturbance consisting of respiratory acidosis and metabolic acidosis or alkalosis is present. Respiratory acidosis is caused by CNS respiratory center inhibition (e.g., sedatives), disorders of the respiratory and chest wall muscles (e.g., Guillain-Barré syndrome), obstruction to ventilation (e.g., sleep apnea), and pulmonary perfusion and diffusion dysfunction (e.g., severe diffuse pneumonias) (Table 96.7).[87]

Symptoms of respiratory acidosis include shortness of breath and the mental status changes associated with progressive acute and chronic hypercapnia. The treatment of respiratory acidosis is directed to the primary cause to increase the effectiveness of ventilation and pulmonary gas exchange.[92]

Mixed Acid-Base Disturbances

The presence of a mixed acid-base disturbance is usually detected when a primary acid-base event fails to demonstrate the expected compensation. This failure of compensation can predict the presence of a respiratory and metabolic acid-base event occurring concurrently but does not predict the presence of mixed metabolic events or mixed respiratory events. Acid-base maps have similar diagnostic limitations. The mixture of more than two events can be determined by other laboratory evidence but is best detected when historical evaluations suggest multiple acid-base events. Although laboratory data may be the first evidence of acid-base disturbances, utilization of these tools to predict primary and mixed acid-base disturbances must be related with clinical data to ensure that the information is appropriately interpreted (Table 96.8).

Table 96.8. **Common Mixed Acid-Base Disturbances**

Disorder	Examples
Predicted by rules of compensation	
Metabolic acidosis and respiratory alkalosis (partial pressure of carbon dioxide reduction greater than predicted for metabolic acidosis)	Chronic renal failure and septicemia
Metabolic alkalosis and respiratory acidosis (partial pressure of carbon dioxide reduction less than predicted for metabolic acidosis)	Lactic acidosis and chronic obstructive pulmonary disease
Metabolic and respiratory alkalosis (partial pressure of carbon dioxide elevation less than predicted for metabolic alkalosis)	Diuretic overuse and psychogenic hyperventilation
Metabolic alkalosis and respiratory acidosis (partial pressure of carbon dioxide elevation greater than predicted for metabolic alkalosis)	Vomiting and adult respiratory distress syndrome
Not predicted by rules of compensation	
Hyperchloremia and large anion gap metabolic acidosis (nonequivalent changes in chloride and bicarbonate concentrations and an elevated anion gap)	Diarrhea and chronic renal disease
Metabolic alkalosis and large anion gap acidosis (nonequivalent changes in chloride bicarbonate concentrations and an elevated anion gap)	Vomiting and chronic renal failure
Acute and chronic respiratory alkalosis ($[HCO_3^-]$ reduction greater than predicted for acute respiratory alkalosis and less than predicted for chronic respiratory alkalosis)	Septicemia and psychogenic hyperventilation
Acute and chronic respiratory acidosis ($[HCO_3^-]$ elevation greater than predicted for acute respiratory acidosis and less than predicted for chronic respiratory acidosis)	Acute respiratory failure and COPD
Chronic respiratory acidosis and acute respiratory alkalosis ($[HCO_3^-]$ elevation or reduction inconsistent with expected P_{CO_2} elevation or reduction for either of these disorders, respectively)	COPD and pulmonary embolus
Metabolic alkalosis and nonanion gap metabolic acidosis (difficult to recognize because $[Cl^-]$ and $[HCO_3^-]$ changes depend on which disorder predominates; if each disorder is of equal magnitude, then $[Cl^-]$, $[HCO_3^-]$, P_{CO_2}, and pH are normal)	Chronic diuretic overuse and diarrhea

COPD = chronic obstructive pulmonary disease.

The presence of a mixed acid-base disturbance is best detected by anticipating its presence in clinical settings, although some laboratory findings can be helpful. The compensation in acid-base disturbances minimizes changes in systemic pH but never totally corrects the pH (the possible exception is chronic hypocapnia in persons living at high altitudes). Therefore, the presence of a normal pH with normal $[HCO_3^-]$ and P_{CO_2} indicates the presence of a mixed acid-base disturbance. Likewise, with primary acid-base disturbances the compensatory event is in the same direction as the primary event; therefore, acid-base disturbances where the compensatory event and the primary event are in opposite directions also indicate the presence of a mixed acid-base disturbance. A large anion gap metabolic acidosis occurring concurrently with a hyperchloremia metabolic acidosis (e.g., a patient with diabetic ketoacidosis and diarrhea) is detected when the anion gap does not account for the amount of $[HCO_3^-]$ concentration reduction. An example of this mixed disturbance is a sign of recovery during the appropriate treatment of DKA as β-hydroxybutyrate and acetoacetate (ketone bodies) are hepatically converted to $[HCO_3^-]$, resulting in a transition from the original large anion gap metabolic acidosis to a hyperchloremia metabolic acidosis with less severe systemic pH reductions. The presence of a large anion gap, regardless of the systemic pH, indicates the presence of metabolic acidosis. For example, a patient with plasma metabolic alkalosis caused by diuretic use may have a $[HCO_3^-]$ of 36 mEq/L, and if the hypovolemia becomes severe enough lactic acidosis may ensue. However, an 8 mEq/L drop in $[HCO_3^-]$ caused by titration of lactic acid would result in a $[HCO_3^-]$ of 28 mEq/L, essentially no change in $[Cl^-]$, and an appropriate P_{CO_2} response with the pH still slightly alkalemic. This process can be detected early based on the concurrent increase in the anion gap as $[HCO_3^-]$ is consumed in the titration with lactic acid and elevated plasma lactic acid—if the potential for this disorder had been anticipated clinically.[68,69,72,93]

The limits of compensation are important factors to consider especially when suspecting respiratory acidosis in a patient with metabolic alkalosis. Although the compensation for metabolic alkalosis is P_{CO_2} retention, P_{CO_2} values higher than 55 mm Hg do not occur because the resulting hypoxia stimulates ventilation. Therefore, in patients with metabolic alkalosis and a P_{CO_2} higher than 55 mm Hg, primary impairment of ventilation causing respiratory acidosis must also be present. Because the limits of compensation in chronic respiratory alkalosis is a $[HCO_3^-]$ of 14 mEq/L, $[HCO_3^-]$ less than that implies the additional presence of metabolic acidosis. Likewise, the limits of compensation for chronic respiratory acidosis is renal HCO_3^- retention to 45 mEq/L, and higher $[HCO_3^-]$ concentrations imply the additional presence of metabolic alkalosis.[94] Because chronic renal disease in its end stages results in a $[HCO_3^-]$ of 12 to 14 mEq/L, greater $[HCO_3^-]$ reductions would suggest additional causes of metabolic acidosis (e.g., vomiting).

Mixtures of acute and chronic respiratory acidosis as well as acute and chronic respiratory alkalosis can be detected using the rules of compensation for primary acid-base disorders and by plotting P_{CO_2} and $[HCO_3^-]$ on acid-base maps. Points that define mixtures of acute and chronic respiratory alkalosis or respiratory acidosis may also be consistent with a mixture of acute respiratory and metabolic alkalosis or acute respiratory acidosis and metabolic alkalosis. Mixtures of respiratory acidosis and respiratory alkalosis pose special problems. The more profound event may alter the P_{CO_2} enough to leave the respiratory-induced metabolic compensation unopposed for hours to days (e.g., a patient with chronic obstructive pulmonary disease who is mechanically hyperventilated, thereby decreasing the P_{CO_2} and leaving the P_{CO_2}-induced $[HCO_3^-]$ elevation until renal $[HCO_3^-]$ excretion occurs over the following hours to days).

References

1. Hobbs J. Acid-base disorders. Postgrad Med 1988;83(suppl 2):91–8.
2. Beck LH. The aging kidney. Defending a delicate balance of fluid and electrolytes. Geriatrics 2000 Apr;55(4):26–8, 31-2.
3. Hobbs J. Acid-base, fluid and electrolyte disorders. In: Rakel RE, editor. Textbook of family practice, 4th ed. Philadelphia: WB Saunders, 1990.
4. Kamel KS, Ethier JH, Richardson RMA, et al. Urine electrolytes and osmolality: when and how to use them. Am J Nephrol 1990; 10:89.
5. Oh MS, Carroll HJ, Goldstein DA, Fein IA. Hyperchloremic acidosis during the recovery phase of diabetic ketosis. Ann Intern Med 1978;89:925–30.
6. Healey DM, Jacobson EJ. Acid-base and electrolyte disorders. In: Common medical diagnosis and an algorithmic approach, 2nd ed. Philadelphia: WB Saunders, 1996;80–104.
7. Kumar R. Calcium disorders. In: Kokko JP, Tannen RL, eds. Fluid and electrolytes, 3rd ed. Philadelphia: WB Saunders, 1996; 391–419.
8. Alperin RJ, Saxton CR, Seldin DW. Clinical interpretation of laboratory values. In: Kokko JP, Tannen RL, eds. Fluids and electrolytes, 3rd ed. Philadelphia: WB Saunders, 1996;391–419.
9. Dennis VW. Phosphate disorders. In: Kokko JP, Tannen RL, eds. Fluid and electrolytes, 3rd ed. Philadelphia: WB Saunders, 1996;359–90.
10. Rose BD. Meaning and application of urine chemistries. In: Rose BD, ed. Clinical physiology of acid-base and electrolyte disorders, 5th ed. New York: McGraw-Hill, 2001;404–14.
11. Musch W, Thimpont J, Vandervelde D, Verhaeverbeke I, Berghmans T, Decaux G. Combined fractional excretion of sodium and urea better predicts response to saline in hyponatremia than do usual clinical and biochemical parameters. Am J Med 1995; 99(suppl 4):348–55.
12. Steiner RW. Interpreting the fractional excretion of sodium. Am J Med 1984;77:699.
13. Rude RK. Magnesium disorders. In Kokko JP, Tannen RL, eds. Fluid and electrolytes, 3rd ed. Philadelphia: WB Saunders, 1996; 421–45.
14. Briggs JP, Singh IIJ, Sawaya BE, Schnermann J. Disorders of salt balance. In: Kokko JP, Tannen RL, eds. Fluids and electrolytes, 3rd ed. Philadelphia: WB Saunders, 1996;3–62.
15. Rose BD. Regulation of the effective circulating volume. In: Rose BD, ed. Clinical physiology of acid-base and electrolyte disturbances, 5th ed. New York: McGraw-Hill, 2001;258–84.
16. Rose BD. Hypovolemic states. In: Rose BD, ed. Clinical physiology of acid-base and electrolyte disturbances, 5th ed. New York: McGraw-Hill, 2001;415–46.
17. Brady HR, Brenner BM. Acute renal failure. In: Isselbacher KJ, Braunwalde E, et al, eds. Harrison's principles of internal medicine, 13th ed. New York: McGraw-Hill, 1996;1265–74.
18. Narins RG, Jones ER, Stom MC, et al. Diagnostic strategies in

disorders of fluid, electrolyte and acid-base homeostasis. Am J Med 1982;72:496–504.

19. Hays SR. Ischemic acute renal failure. Am J Med Sci 1992; 304(suppl 2):93–108.

20. Rose BD. Edematous states. In: Rose BD, ed. Clinical physiology of acid-base and electrolytes disorders, 5th ed. New York: McGraw-Hill, 2001;478–534.

21. Albrink MJ, Hald PM, Man EB, Peters JP. The displacement of plasma water by the lipids of hyperlipemic plasma: a new method for the rapid determination of plasma water. J Clin Invest 1955;34:1481.

22. Tarail R, Buchwald KW, Holland JF, Selawry OS. Misleading reductions of plasma sodium and chloride: association with hyperproteinemia in patients with multiple myeloma. Proc Soc Exp Biol Med 1962;110:145.

23. Worth HGJ. Plasma sodium concentration: bearer of false prophecies? BMJ 1983;287:567.

24. Vaswani SK, Sprague R. Pseudohyponatremia in multiple myeloma. South Med J 1993;86(suppl 2):251–2.

25. Katz M. Hyperglycemia-induced hyponatremia: calculation of expected plasma sodium depression. N Engl J Med 1973;289: 843–4.

26. Keating JP, Schears GJ, Dodge PR. Oral water intoxication in infants: an American epidemic. Am J Dis Child 1991;145:985–90.

27. Wattad A, Chiang ML, Hill LL. Hyponatremia in hospitalized children. Clin Pediatr (Phila) 1992;31(suppl 3):153–7.

28. Kleinfeld M, Casimir M, Borra S. Hyponatremia as observed in a chronic disease facility. J Am Geriatr Soc 1979;27:156–61.

29. Ashouri OS. Severe diuretic-induced hyponatremia in the elderly. Arch Intern Med 1986;146:1355.

30. Anderson OK, Gudbrandsson T, Jamerson K. Metabolic adverse effects of thiazide diuretics: the importance of normokalemia. J Intern Med Suppl 1991;735:89–96.

31. Friedman E, Shadel M, Halkin H, Farfel Z. Thiazide induced hyponatremia: reproducibility by single dose rechallenge and an analysis of pathogenesis. Ann Intern Med 1989;110:24–30.

32. Ayus JC. Diuretic-induced hyponatremia. Arch Intern Med 1986;146:1295–6.

33. Sonnenblick M, Algur N, Rosin A. Thiazide induced hyponatremia and vasopressin release. Ann Intern Med 1989;110:751.

34. Rose BD. Hypoosmolal states-hyponatremia. In: Rose BD, ed. Clinical physiology of acid-base and electrolytes disorders, 5th ed. New York: McGraw-Hill, 2001;696–745.

35. Harrigan MR. Cerebral salt wasting syndrome. Crit Care Clin 2001 Jan;17(1):125–38.

36. Oh MS, Carroll HJ. Disorders of sodium metabolism: hypernatremia and hyponatremia. Crit Care Med 1992;20:94–103.

37. Trachtman H, Futterweit S, Hammer E, Siegel TW, Oates P. The role of polyols in cerebral cell volume regulation in hypernatremic and hyponatremic states. Life Sci 1991;49:677–88.

38. Disorders of water and salt metabolism. In: Porush JG, Faugert PF, eds. Renal disease in the aged. Boston: Little, Brown, 1991. pg 15–33.

39. Mulloy AL, Caruana RJ. Hyponatremic emergencies. Med Clin North Am 1995;79(suppl 1):155–68.

40. Mickel HS, Oliver CN, Starke-Reed PE. Protein oxidation and myelinolysis occur in brain following rapid correction of hyponatremia. Biochem Biophys Res Commun 1990;172:92–7.

41. Norenberg MD. Treatment of hyponatremia: the case for a more conservative approach. In: Narins RG, ed. Controversies in nephrology and hypertension. New York: Churchill-Livingstone, 1984. pg. 379–391.

42. Ayus JC, Krothapalli RK, Arieff AL. Changing concepts in treatment of severe symptomatic hyponatremia: rapid correction and possible relation to central pontine myelinolysis. Am J Med 1985;78:897–902.

43. Sterns RH, Riggs JE, Schochet SS Jr. Osmotic demyelination

syndrome following correction of hyponatremia. N Engl J Med 1986;314:1535.

44. Narins RG. Therapy of hyponatremia: does haste make waste? N Engl J Med 1986;314:1573.

45. Vieweg WV. Treatment strategies in the polydipsia-hyponatremia syndrome. J Clin Psychiatry 1994;55(suppl 4): 154–60

46. Karp BI, Laureno R. Pontine and extra pontine myelinolysis: a neurologic disorder following rapid correction of hyponatremia. Medicine (Baltimore) 1993;72(suppl 6):359–73.

47. Harris CP, Townsend JJ, Baringer JR. Symptomatic hyponatremia: can myelinolysis be prevented by treatment? J Neurol Neurosurg Psychiatry 1993;56(suppl 6):626–32.

48. Pirzada NA, Ali II. Central pontine myelinolysis. Mayo Clin Proc 2001 May;76(5):559–62.

49. Gross P, Reimann D, Henschkowski J, Damian M. Treatment of severe hyponatremia: conventional and novel aspects. J Am Soc Nephrol 2001 Feb;12 Suppl 17:S10–4.

50. Jackson C, Carson W, Markowitz J, Mintzer J. SIADH associated with fluoxetine and sertraline therapy. Am J Psychiatry 152:809, 1995.

51. ten Holt WL, van Iperen CE, Schrijver G, et al. Severe hyponatremia during therapy with fluoxetine. Arch Intern Med 156:681, 1996.

52. Liu BA, Mittmann N, Knowles SR, et al. Hyponatremia and the syndrome of inappropriate secretion of antidiuretic hormone associated with the use of selective serotonin reuptake inhibitors: A review of spontaneous reports. Can Med Assoc J 155:519, 1996.

53. Peterson JC, Pollack RW, Mahoney JJ, Fuller RJ. Inappropriate antidiuretic hormone secondary to a monoamine oxidase inhibitor. JAMA 239:1422, 1978.

54. Snyder NA, Feigal DW, Arieff AL. Hypernatremia in elderly patients: a heterogeneous, morbid and iatrogenic entity. Ann Intern Med 1987;107:309–19.

55. Rose BD. Hyperosmolal states—hypernatremia. In: Rose BD, ed. Clinical physiology of acid-base and electrolytes disorders, 5th ed. New York: McGraw-Hill, 2001;746–93.

56. Phillips PA, Rolls BJ, Ledingham GG, et al. Reduced thirst after water deprivation in healthy elderly men. N Engl J Med 1984;311:753–9.

57. Moder RG, Hurley DL. Fatal hypernatremia from exogenous salt intake: report of a case and review of the literature. Mayo Clin Proc 1990;65:1587–94.

58. Sterns RH, Spital A. Disorders of water balance. In: Kokko JP, Tannen RL, eds. Fluids and electrolytes, 2nd ed. Philadelphia: WB Saunders, 1990;139–94.

59. Park YJ, Kim YC, Kim MO, Ruy JH, Han SW, Kim HJ. Successful treatment in the patient with serum sodium level greater than 200 mEq/L. J Korean Med Sci 200 Dec;15(6):701-3.

60. Amirlak I, Dawson K. Hypernatremia in early infancy. Ann Trop Paediatr 2000 Sep;20(3):173-7; discussion 177-8.

61. Katz MA. Hyperglycemia-induced hyponatremia—calculation of expected serum sodium depression. New England Journal of Medicine 1973;289:843-844.

62. Liamis G, Gianoutsos, C, Elisaf MS. Hyperosmolar nonketotic syndrome with hypernatremia: how can we monitor treatment? Diabetes Metab 2000 Nov;26(5):403-5.

63. Disorders of potassium metabolism. In: Porush JG, Faugert PF, eds. Renal disease in the aged. Boston: Little, Brown, 1991.

64. Adrogue HJ, Madias NE. Changes in plasma potassium concentration during acute acid-base disturbances. Am J Med 1981;71:456.

65. Paltiel O, Salakhov E, Ronen I, Berg D, Israeli A. Management of severe hypokalemia in hospitalized patients: a study of quality of care based on computerized databases. Arch Intern Med 2001 Apr 23;161(8):1089-95.

66. Schepkens H, Vanholder R, Billiouw JM, Lameire N. Life-threatening hyperkalemia during combined therapy with angiotensin-converting enzyme inhibitors and spironolactorne: an analysis of 25 cases. Am J Med 2001 Apr 15;110(6):438-41.

67. Tannen RL. Potassium disorders. In: Kokko JP, Tannen RL, eds. Fluids and electrolytes, 3rd ed. Philadelphia: WB Saunders, 1996;111–99.

68. Narins RG, Emmett M. Simple and mixed acid-base disorders: a practical approach. Medicine (Baltimore) 1980;59:161–87.

69. Rose BD. Introduction to simple and mixed acid-base disorders. In: Rose BD, ed. Clinical physiology of acid-base and electrolytes disorders, 5th ed. New York: McGraw-Hill, 2001;535–50.

70. Rose BD. Metabolic acidosis. In: Rose BD, ed. Clinical physiology of acid-base and electrolytes disorders, 5th ed. New York: McGraw-Hill, 2001;578–646.

71. Prough DS. Physiologic acid-base and electrolyte changes in acute and chronic renal failure patients. Anesthesiol Clin North America 2000 Dec;18(4):809-33, ix.

72. Oster JR, Perez GO, Materson BJ. Use of the anion gap in clinical medicine. South Med J 1988;81:225–37.

73. Emmett M, Narins RG. Clinical use of the anion gap. Medicine (Baltimore) 1977;56:38.

74. Gabow PA, Kaehny WD, Fennessey PV, et al. Diagnostic importance of an increased anion gap. N Engl J Med 1980;303:854.

75. Stackpoole PW. Lactic acidosis: the case against bicarbonate therapy. Ann Intern Med 1986;105:276–9.

76. Narins RG, Cohen JJ. Bicarbonate therapy for organic acidosis: the case for its continued use. Ann Intern Med 1987;106:615–18.

77. Cooper JD, Walley KR, Wiggs BR, Russell JA. Bicarbonate does not improve hemodynamics in critically ill patients who have lactic acidosis. Ann Intern Med 1990;112:492–8.

78. Okuda Y, Adrogue HJ, Field JB, Nohara H, Yamashita K. Counterproductive effects of sodium bicarbonate in diabetic ketoacidosis. J Clin Endocrinol Metab 1996;81(suppl 1):314–20.

79. Oh MS, Carroll HJ, Uribarri J. Mechanisms of normochloremic and hyperchloremia acidosis in diabetic ketoacidosis. Nephron 1990;54:1–6.

80. Foster DW, McGarry JD. The metabolic derangements and treatment of diabetic ketoacidosis. N Engl J Med 1983;309:159–65.

81. Kitabchi AE, Wall BM. Diabetic ketoacidosis. Med Clin North Am 1995;79(suppl 1):9–37.

82. Lipsky MS. Management of diabetic ketoacidosis. Am Fam Physician 1994;49(suppl 7):1607–12.

83. Kitabchi AE. Diabetic ketoacidosis. Med Clin North Am 1995;79(suppl 1):9–37.

84. Fish LH. Diabetic ketoacidosis: treatment strategies to avoid complications. Postgrad Med 1994;96(suppl 3):75–8,81,85.

85. Lipsky MS. Management of diabetic ketoacidosis. Am Fam Physician 1994;49:1607–12.

86. Giebisch GE, Berger L, Pitts RF. The extrarenal response to acute acid-base disturbances of respiratory origin. J Clin Invest 1955;34:231–5.

87. Rose BD. Respiratory alkalosis. In: Rose BD, ed. Clinical physiology of acid-base and electrolytes disorders, 5th ed. New York: McGraw-Hill, 2001;673–81.

88. Masotti L, Ceccarelli E, Cappelli R, Barabesi L, Forconi S. Arterial blood gas analysis and alveolar-arterial oxygen gradien in diagnosis and prognosis of elderly patients with suspected pulmonary embolism. J Gerontol A Biol Sci Med Sci 2000 Dec;55(12)M761-4.

89. Rose BD. Metabolic alkalosis. In: Rose BD, ed. Clinical physiology of acid-base and electrolytes disorders, 5th ed. New York: McGraw-Hill, 2001;551–77.

90. Jacobson HR, Seldin DW. On the generation, maintenance, and correction of metabolic alkalosis. Am J Physiol 1983;245:F425.

91. Amundson DE, Diamant J. Severe metabolic alkalosis. South Med J 1994;87(suppl 2):275–7.

92. Rose BD. Respiratory acidosis. In: Rose BD, editor. Clinical physiology of acidbase and electrolytes disorders. 5th ed. New York: McGraw-Hill, 2001:647-72.

93. Paulson WD, Gadallah MF. Diagnosis of mixed acid-base disorders in diabetic ketoacidosis. Am J Med Sci 1993;306(suppl 5):295–300.

94. Bia M, Thier SO. Mixed acid-base disturbance: a clinical approach. Med Clin North Am 1981;65:347.

97
Diseases of the Kidney

Joseph E. Ross

The incidence of end-stage renal disease (ESRD) continues to rise.[1] Complications of renal failure are numerous. New strategies that prevent or cause remission/regression of renal disease are needed. Modification of risk factors associated with the development and progression of renal disease are essential. These include hyperglycemic control, treatment of hypertension, control of hyperlipidemia, discontinuance of smoking, and correction of proteinuria.[2]

Acute Renal Failure

Despite advances in the treatment of acute renal failure (ARF), the overall mortality rate has improved little since the 1960s. ARF itself, regardless of other illnesses, increases the risk of severe complications and mortality. ARF complicates 5% of hospital and 30% of intensive care unit (ICU) admissions. Acute mortality approaches 50%; of those who survive ARF, 50% have persistent deterioration of renal function.[3]

Emphasis needs to shift to the prevention of ARF and delaying its progression to chronic renal failure. Risk factors that predispose to ARF include advanced age, preexisting renal disease, coexisting cardiovascular disease, inadequate fluid replacement (medical, trauma, and surgical patients), delayed treatment of sepsis, and lack of recognition of nephrotoxic drugs.

ARF is characterized by a sudden and rapid decline in renal function. ARF is classified as prerenal, intrinsic renal, or postrenal (Table 97.1). Prerenal failure is rapidly reversible. It is primarily caused by renal hypoperfusion, nonsteroidal antiinflammatory drugs (NSAIDs), and angiotensin-converting enzyme (ACE) inhibitors. Intrinsic renal disease most commonly presents in the form of acute tubular necrosis (ATN) and acute interstitial nephritis (AIN). ATN is caused by ischemia, toxins, and glomerulonephritis. AIN is primarily caused by nephrotoxic drugs. Postrenal failure is due to bladder outlet or ureteral obstruction.

Evaluation

The initial presentation of ARF is decreased urine output. Clinical manifestations vary, but nausea, weakness, and fatigue are most common. Initial evaluation includes a urinalysis to evaluate urine pH, specific gravity, proteinuria, hematuria, or pyuria. Red blood cell casts are seen with glomerulonephritis, white blood cell casts with pyelonephritis, and epithelial cells and granular casts with ischemic damage. Transient urinary eosinophilia occurs in 80% of AIN. Serum chemistries include electrolytes, blood urea nitrogen (BUN), and creatinine for baseline and to monitor progression of ARF. The glomerular filtration rate (GFR) can be decreased by 50% before a change in creatinine is observed. Twenty-four-hour urine collections for creatinine clearance and protein may be necessary. Creatinine clearance is reduced by half for each doubling of the serum creatinine. The serum BUN/creatinine ratio, the urine/serum creatinine ratio, and fractional excretion of urinary sodium are not helpful for determining the origin of ARF.

Renal ultrasonography can determine kidney size and evaluate the collecting system. Small kidneys reflect chronic renal disease. Hydronephrosis is seen with obstructive nephropathy. Renal biopsy may be indicated in patients with nephrotic syndrome, hematuria, or casts suggestive of glomerular disease, as the biopsy may guide therapy and provide prognostic information. If ARF continues or worsens, serum calcium, magnesium, phosphate, uric acid, and protein levels should also be followed.

Treatment

Prerenal ARF

The treatment goal is to improve urine output. Hemodynamic monitoring with central venous pressure (CVP) or Swan-Ganz system may be necessary. Normal saline (500–1000 mL over 30–60 minutes) may help improve renal perfusion. In the case

Table 97.1. **Etiology of Acute Renal Failure**

Prerenal (55–60%)
Intravascular volume depletion
  Dehydration
  Blood loss
  Over-diuresis
  Sepsis
  Burns
Hypotension
Severe congestive heart failure
Drugs
  Alpha-blockers
  ACE inhibitors
  NSAIDs
Liver failure

Intrinsic renal (35–40%)
Ischemic acute tubular necrosis
  Septic shock
  Hypotension
  Major surgery
Nephrotoxins
  Contrast dye
  Toxins (NSAIDs, aminoglycosides, sulfonamides, acyclovir,
    heavy metals, organic solvents)
  Myoglobinuria/hemoglobinuria
  Crystal deposition (hyperuricosuria)
Vascular injury
  Hypertension
  Diabetes mellitus
  Vasculitis
  Thrombotic thrombocytopenic purpura
  Hemolytic uremic syndrome
  Eclampsia
  Embolic (cholesterol plaques, status post–renal stent
    placement)
Glomerulonephritis (see Table 97.5)
Interstitial disease
  Drugs (β-lactam antibiotics, NSAIDs)
  Infectious (pyelonephritis, tuberculosis)
  Systemic (sarcoidosis, multiple myeloma)
  Allergic

Postrenal (less than 5%)
Ureteral obstruction
  Stone
  Clot
  Neoplasm
  External compression
  Stricture
Bladder outlet obstruction
  Benign prostatic hypertrophy
  Prostate neoplasms
  Clot
  Plugged Foley catheter
  Neurogenic bladder
  Anticholinergic drugs

ACE = angiotensin-converting enzyme; NSAID = nonsteroidal antiinflammatory drug.

of recent surgery or trauma, transfusion should be considered. Diuretic therapy may include use of furosemide (Lasix) 80 to 360 mg IV, doubling dosages every 30 minutes until active urine output is obtained. Alternative loop diuretics [ethacrynic acid (Edecrin) 50 to 200 mg IV] may be employed. Metola-zone (Zaroxolyn) 5 to 10 mg PO may induce diuresis if it is not obtained with other diuretics. If these measures are ineffective, osmotic diuretics (solutions of 20% mannitol by continuous intravenous infusion at rates of 10 to 20 mL/hr) may be used. They may not become effective for 6 to 12 hours and should be discontinued if there is no effect after 12 hours. Low-dose dopamine (2–3 μg/kg/min) may be tried, but if no improvement in renal function is noted over 6 to 12 hours, discontinue therapy.

Intrinsic Renal ARF

Contrast agents cause the creatinine level to peak within 72 hours and then slowly recover over 7 to 14 days if appropriate therapy is instituted. It may be prevented by hydration with intravenous fluids 24 hours prior to and after the contrast procedures or using mannitol 25 g in 1 L of 5% dextrose (D5) 0.45 normal saline at a rate of 100 to 150 mL/hr IV beginning 4 hours prior to the procedure and continuing for 2 to 4 hours after the contrast procedure is done. Aminoglycoside-induced ARF is more prevalent with increasing patient age, volume depletion, more than 5 days of use, large doses, preexisting liver disease, and preexisting renal insufficiency. Correcting preexisting volume depletion and monitoring the appropriate drug levels are necessary for prevention. NSAID-induced AIN can be minimized by the judicious use of NSAIDs in the elderly and in the presence of preexisting renal insufficiency. NSAID-induced AIN is more common with the use of ibuprofen, naproxen, and fenoprofen. Acute glomerulonephritis (GN) rarely occurs in the hospital setting.

Postrenal ARF

Obstruction of the bladder can be diagnosed and treated by bladder catheterization. Renal ultrasonography can exclude ureteral obstruction.

Management of Complications

Volume depletion decreases renal perfusion and worsens ARF. Measuring daily patient weights, fluid intake and output measurements, and frequent electrolyte BUN and creatinine levels are necessary. Once ARF stabilizes, fluid replacement should be equal to insensible losses (500 mL/day) plus urinary or other drainage losses (Table 97.2).

Dietary restrictions include sodium, potassium, phosphorus, protein, and magnesium. Total caloric intake of 35 to 50 kcal/kg/day should be maintained with most calories provided by carbohydrates (100 g/day).

Hypertension is exacerbated by fluid overload. The use of antihypertensive agents that do not decrease renal blood flow (non-dihydropyridine calcium channel blockers, cardioselective beta-blockers, and central acting agents) can be considered. Metabolic acidosis control is aided by restriction of dietary protein. Treatment is not required until serum bicarbonate levels are less than 16 mEq/L. Mild elevations of uric acid frequently occur. Hyperphosphatemia can usually be controlled by restriction of dietary phosphate. Hypocalcemia can be corrected with oral calcium carbonate or intravenous calcium gluconate. Anemia is common, caused by increased red blood cell (RBC) loss and decreased RBC production.

Table 97.2. **Management of Complications of Acute Renal Failure**

Complication	Treatment
Fluid overload	Salt restriction of 2–4 g/day of NaCl Limit replacement to insensible losses plus urine output and drainage losses Diuretics as needed (furosemide, ethacrynic acid, metolazone) Ultrafiltration or dialysis
Diet restrictions	Protein 0.6 g/kg/day, potassium intake less than 40 mEq/day, phosphorus intake less than 800 mg/day No magnesium containing compounds
Hypertension	Restriction of free water intake Correction of volume overload Antihypertensive agents
Hyperphosphatemia	Restriction of dietary phosphate intake Aluminum hydroxide 15 to 30 mL tid and once the phosphate level is normal, calcium carbonate 500 to 1000 mg tid/qid
Hypocalcemia	Calcium carbonate (as above) unless symptomatic, then calcium gluconate 10 to 20 mL of 10% solution
Hyperuricemia	Allopurinol 100 mg/day if uric acid level greater than 15 mg/dL
Metabolic acidosis	Restriction of dietary protein if bicarbonate level greater than 16 mEq/L Sodium bicarbonate 325 to 650 mg tid po if less than 16 mEq/dL If acidosis is severe (pH less than 7.2), IV sodium bicarbonate
Hyponatremia	Fluid restriction
Hyperkalemia	Mild (less than 5.5 mEq/L): potassium dietary restriction, elimination of potassium supplements and potassium sparing diuretics Moderate (5.5 to 6.5 mEq/L): administration of potassium binding resins, sodium polystyrene (Kayexalate) 15 to 30 g every 4 hours with sorbitol 50 to 100 mL in 20% solution (by mouth or as retention enema) Severe (greater than 6.5 mEq/1): 10 units of regular insulin plus 50 mL of 50% dextrose solution, plus one ampule of sodium bicarbonate intravenous Also consider calcium gluconate 10 mL of a 10% solution IV
Drugs	Drug dosage needs to be adjusted for degree of renal impairment
Infection	Therapy directed at infectious process Avoid potentially nephrotoxic agents
Anemia	Rule out GI bleed Transfusion Erythropoietin if long-term therapy
Hypermagnesemia	Discontinue magnesium antacids

Drug dosages must be adjusted for the degree of renal failure. Platelet dysfunction may occur secondary to the uremia and present as gastrointestinal (GI) bleeding. Infection is common and should be treated aggressively if it occurs.

Dialysis is reserved for (1) treatment of symptoms of uremia (pericarditis, seizures, or encephalopathy); (2) management of volume overload; (3) hyperkalemia; and (4) acidosis refractory to conservative therapy. Dialysis does not appear to hasten recovery from ARF. Peritoneal or hemodialysis use must be individualized. Ultrafiltration of plasma without dialysis can be used to treat intractable volume overload. Slow, continuous hemofiltration is an alternative if conventional dialysis is not tolerated or peritoneal dialysis cannot be done.

Chronic Renal Failure

The etiology of chronic renal failure (CRF) is an important determinant for progression to ESRD. CRF is typically asymptomatic until late in its course. In 1998 more than 390,000 patients were treated for ESRD in the United States. In excess of $15 billion is spent annually for ESRD therapy. The dialysis 1-year survival is 80% and 5-year survival is 29%.[1]

Diabetes mellitus is the most common cause of CRF and accounts for more than one third of all ESRD. Other common causes include hypertension (21%), glomerulonephritis (11%), and polycystic kidney disease (5%).[4] The peak incidence of ESRD is between ages 65 and 74, and patients over age 75 have the largest rate of growth of ESRD. The incidence of ESRD in blacks and Native Americans is greater than that in the white population.[3]

Prevention

Glomerulosclerosis is the common histologic change that leads to renal failure in diabetes and hypertension. Matrix injury is associated with overproduction of plasminogen activator inhibitor, angiotensin, and transforming growth factor-β.[5] These lead to the development of proteinuria. The magnitude of proteinuria is a strong independent predictor of

Table 97.3. **Regression/Remission Strategies in Renal Disease**

Dietary
   Protein—low-protein diet 0.6 g/kg/day
   Cholesterol—diet/drugs (statins, niacin, fibrates)
   Homocystinemia—folic acid 1 mg/day

Diabetes mellitus
   Maintain HbA_{1c} less than 7%
   Urine for microalbuminuria yearly
   Blood pressure less than 130/85; if proteinuria less than
     125/75

Proteinuria
   ACE inhibitor/combination with ARB

Hypertension
   ACE inhibitor/ARB
   Nondihydropyridine agents
   Cardioselective beta-blockers
   Diuretics (low dose) if fluid retention

ACE = angiotensin-converting enzyme; ARB = angiotensin receptor blocker; HbA_{1c} = adult hemoglobin component 1c.

progression of renal disease. ACE inhibitors and angiotensin receptor blockers (ARBs) decrease these levels. ACE inhibitors and ARBs also improve existing glomerular damage by reducing intraglomerular capillary pressure by decreasing efferent arteriolar tone, which reduces basement membrane remodeling and protein leakage. This effect is independent of their hypertensive effects. Hypertension initiates and potentiates glomerulosclerosis changes by increasing arterial pressure, which causes increased glomerular pressure. This results in remodeling, protein leaks, fibrosis, and nephron loss. Hypertension also accelerates arteriosclerosis in preglomerular arterioles and increases glomerular capillary pressure. Hypertension arises from and accelerates diabetic nephropathy; 70% of patients with non–insulin-dependent diabetes mellitus (NIDDM), and greater than 50% of insulin-dependent diabetics mellitus (IDDM) have hypertension.[6]

A model strategy for the remission of renal disease is shown in Table 97.3: (1) low-protein diet of 0.6 g/kg/body weight per day; (2) tight diabetic control including maintenance of adult hemoglobin component HbA_{1c} levels less than 7%; (3) maximized dose of ACE inhibitor possibly in conjunction with ARB to control blood pressure and proteinuria; and (4) optimum control of other renal and cardiac risk factors.[7] Optimum blood pressure in diabetes without proteinuria should be less than 130/85 mm Hg. If coexisting hypertension or proteinuria is present, desired blood pressure should be less than 125/75.

Yearly screening for microalbuminuria in hypertensives and diabetics is recommended. Microalbuminuria is seen in 20% to 30% of patients with hypertension. Institution of ACE inhibitors with or without ARB medications is indicated should proteinuria arise. Nondihydropyridine calcium channel blockers (verapamil/diltiazem/amlodipine) can also be used. Dihydropyridine calcium blockers are not recommended as they dilate afferent arterioles and paradoxically increase glomerular pressure if systemic blood pressure is not adequately reduced. Thiazide diuretics for fluid overload or fluid retention are used if creatinine clearance is greater than 30 mL per minute. Loop diuretics are necessary if creatinine clearance falls to lower levels. Nonselective beta-blockers can reduce renal blood flow secondary to decreased cardiac output (except nadolol/labetalol/carvedilol/metoprolol).

ACE inhibitors are safe until creatinine levels reach 3 mg/dL. Renal function should be monitored the first few weeks after institution of therapy, as a 20% to 25% rise in creatinine is not unexpected and usually plateaus within a few weeks. Continued rise may be secondary to concomitant diuretic use or renal vascular disease, which should be evaluated. Combinations of ACE inhibitors and ARBs appear to have additive antiproteinuric effects in short-term studies.[4]

Control of other renal and cardiovascular risk factors include smoking cessation, weight reduction, regular exercise, reduction of cholesterol, reduction of homocysteine levels, and daily aspirin in diabetics.

Treatment

A common cause of deterioration in CRF is volume depletion. Patients should be slightly volume-expanded, as evidenced by trace peripheral edema. States causing depressed cardiac output must be addressed and drugs that exacerbate CRF avoided (Table 97.4).

Dietary modifications include protein restriction when the creatinine clearance is less than 25 mL/min. Potassium, sodium, fluid, and magnesium restrictions apply. Hyperphosphatemia therapy is directed at maintaining phosphorus levels at 4.5 to 6.0 mg/dL. Aluminum may accumulate in patients with CRF and cause osteomalacia and encephalopathy. Calcium carbonate can be used once serum phosphate levels are less than 7.0 mg/dL. Vitamin D analogues such as calcitriol may be necessary to maintain serum calcium between 8.5 and 11.0 mg/dL. Parathyroidectomy may be required to control severe secondary hyperparathyroidism due to hyperphosphatemia.

When the GFR becomes less than 10 mL/min, metabolic

Table 97.4. **Treatment of Chronic Renal Failure**

Fluids	Oral fluids should be limited to daily urine output plus insensible losses (500 cc)
Diet	No-added-salt diet (8 g of sodium chloride per day)
	Protein restriction of 0.6 g/kg/day when GFR less than 25 mL/min
	No magnesium antacids or supplements
Calories	35–50 kcal/kg/day
Potassium	Less than 40 mEq/day when GFR less than 25 mL/min
Phosphate and calcium	Dietary phosphorus restriction 800–1000 mg/day when GFR less than 50 mL/min
	Limit aluminum hydroxide antacids
	Calcium carbonate for maintenance
	Calcitriol 0.25 to 1.0 μg po qd
	Parathyroidectomy
Hypertension	See ARF (Table 97.2)
Metabolic acidosis	See ARF (Table 97.2)
	May need diuretic to compensate for additional sodium from bicarbonate
Anemia	Recombinant human erythropoietin
	Supplemental oral iron and folate

ARF = acute renal failure; GFR = glomerular filtration rate.

abnormalities can often no longer be controlled conservatively, and dialysis or renal transplant is considered. Indications for dialysis are similar to those in ARF. The frequency, duration, and type of dialysis are based on the patient's metabolic, nutritional, and volume needs.

Anemia is a common complication of chronic renal failure. Erythropoietin (80 to 100 units kg/week, subcutaneous in two to three doses per week) therapy can be instituted when hemoglobin is less than 10 g/dL and causes other than chronic renal failure have been eliminated. Iron supplementation of 200 mg per day and folic acid 1 mg per day is recommended before starting erythropoietin. Hemoglobin is monitored every 1 to 2 weeks until a hemoglobin level of 12 g/dL is obtained and is stable; then hemoglobin is monitored every 4 weeks.[8] Blood pressure may initially increase and require adjustment or institution of antihypertensive therapy.

Renal transplantation survival rates are improving with advances in the donor–recipient selection progress, immunosuppressive drug regimens, surgical techniques, and methods for treating transplant graft rejection. Patients with nephropathy secondary to IDDM do better long term with renal transplantation than dialysis. Acquired polycystic kidney disease, which worsens in ESRD, is improved by renal transplantation.

The care of renal transplant patients is becoming an increasingly shared responsibility of family practitioners and transplant specialists. Almost 75% of transplant recipients now live longer than 10 years after surgery. Their risk for hypertension, hyperlipidemia, coronary artery disease, and malignancy is higher than in nontransplant patients.[9,10]

Ninety percent of transplant patients have hypertension prior to the transplant and 50% need ongoing therapy. The risk of graft failure increases as blood pressure rises. Target blood pressure is 130/85 without proteinuria and 125/75 with proteinuria. Cardiovascular disease is now the number one cause of mortality after the first year. Elevated lipids are exacerbated due to steroid and cyclosporine use in transplant patients. The target low-density lipoprotein (LDL) level should be less than 100 and may be treated with hepatic hydroxymethylglutaryl coenzyme A (HMG CoA) inhibitors. The incidence of diabetes is 40%. Diabetic control is worsened by steroid use, which impairs insulin production and cyclosporine, which decreases secretion. There is a 20% increase in bone loss in the first 6 to 12 months after transplant, making the transplant patient a high risk for osteoporosis. Malignancies of the skin and lip are higher than in the general population and incidence increases over time. Non-Hodgkin's lymphoma is higher than expected in the first year after transplant. Transplant recipients need to be watched for opportunistic infections secondary to immunosuppression. Close observation for interactions with transplant medications and prescription drugs is important.

Glomerulonephritis

Deposition of immune complexes and reduction of serum complement occurs with most forms of glomerulonephritis. Manifestations include (1) asymptomatic proteinuria; (2) asymptomatic hematuria; (3) nephritic syndrome; (4) nephrotic syndrome; (5) hypertension; (6) rapidly progressive

ARF; and (7) ESRD. Glomerulonephritis presents with a nephritic/nephrotic syndrome. Nephritic syndrome is characterized by the sudden onset of hematuria often with RBC casts, proteinuria, increasing azotemia, and salt and water retention. This situation causes edema, periorbital or peripheral (or both), and hypertension. As the amount of proteinuria increases, the nephritic syndrome develops into a nephrotic syndrome. The nephrotic syndrome is characterized by increased proteinuria (>3.5 g/day), hypoproteinemia, peripheral edema, and hyperlipidemia. Early treatment offers a higher likelihood for preservation and improvement in renal function. Early referral for a renal biopsy is essential to detect treatable causes (Table 97.5).[11,12]

Table 97.5. Secondary Causes of Glomerulonephritis

Minimal change glomerulonephritis
  Drugs (NSAIDs, lithium, interferon, ampicillin)
  Hodgkin's
  Infectious (viral, parasitic)
  Allergies (food, dust, pollen, contact, bee stings)

Membranous glomerulonephritis
  Drugs (gold, penicillamine, captopril, mercury)
  Neoplasms (melanoma, carcinoma)
  Infectious causes (hepatitis B/C, malaria, syphilis)
  Systemic lupus erythematosus

Focal segmental glomerulonephritis
  IV drug use
  HIV
  Neoplasm
  Lithium
  Obesity
  Sickle cell disease
  Connective tissue disease

IgA nephropathy
  Hepatic cirrhosis
  Celiac disease
  Seronegative arthropathies
  Toxoplasmosis
  HIV
  Henoch-Schönlein purpura

Diffuse proliferative glomerulonephritis
  Post-streptococcal
  Viral
  Parasitic

Membranoproliferative glomerulonephritis
  Cryoglobinuria
  Neoplasm (lymphoma, leukemia)
  Infectious causes (hepatitis B/C, endocarditis,
    schistosomiasis, malaria, infected shunt)
  Rheumatologic (SLE, sarcoid, scleroderma)

Rapidly progressive (crescentic) glomerulonephritis
  Antiglomerular basement membrane disease (Goodpasture's)
  Pauci-immune complex (Wegener's vasculitis)
  Henoch-Schönlein purpura
  Rheumatologic disease (SLE)
  Infectious causes (endocarditis, postinfectious
    glomerulonephritis)
  Neoplasm (lymphoma, leukemia)
  Drugs (hydralazine, penicillamine)

HIV = human immunodeficiency virus; IgA = immunoglobulin A; NSAID = nonsteroidal antiinflammatory drug; SLE = systemic lupus erythematosus.

Nephritic/nephrotic patients should follow a no-added-salt, normal-protein diet. Diuretic therapy can control peripheral edema. Overdiuresis must be avoided as it may aggravate renal failure. ACE inhibitors may reduce proteinuria considerably and aid in hypertensive control. NSAIDs may also reduce proteinuria. NSAID and ACE inhibitor use must be monitored as both can also cause a decline in GFR. Severely nephrotic patients may need antithrombotic and antiinfective prophylaxis. Hypercholesterolemia is controlled by diet and medication.

Minimal Change Glomerulonephritis

Minimal change disease is responsible for 70% to 90% of nephrotic syndromes in children under 10 years old, 50% in older children, and 10% to 15% in adults.[10] Its onset is usually sudden. Renal function remains normal as do complement levels. Biopsy is recommended (1) if clinical features suggest an alternative diagnosis; (2) onset occurs before 1 one year of age or after 6 years of age; or (3) there is an inadequate response to treatment. Children are initially treated with prednisone for 8 to 12 weeks. More than 90% respond within 8 weeks of therapy, but the risk of relapse is less when therapy is extended to 12 weeks. Adults treated with steroids initially respond more slowly, and 25% fail to respond within 3 to 4 months. Adults tend to relapse less often than children. Alternative second-line agents include cyclophosphamide, chlorambucil, and cyclosporine.

Membranous Glomerulonephritis

Membranous nephropathy is the commonest cause (40%) of primary glomerulonephritis-induced nephrotic syndrome in adults. One third of patients have spontaneous remission, one third have partial remission and remain stable, and one third develop progressive renal failure. Treatment with steroids and cytotoxic drugs has been shown to increase the likelihood of remission and improve preservation of renal function when severe proteinuria is present.

Focal Segmental Glomerulonephritis

Focal segmental glomerulonephritis causes up to 15% of cases of nephrotic syndrome. Up to 40% of patients respond to steroids with complete remission. Cyclophosphamide and cyclosporine are unlikely to be of benefit if there is no initial response to prednisone.

Immunoglobulin A Nephropathy

Immunoglobulin A (IgA) nephropathy is the commonest form of glomerulonephritis. Typically it presents as recurrent episodes of macroscopic hematuria 5 to 10 days after an upper respiratory infection; 10% to 20% develop renal insufficiency over time. Rapid deterioration occurs in some patients, resulting in ESRD. There is no specific treatment currently recommended. Steroids are sometimes employed if minimal change disease is also present. Cyclophosphamide, dipyridamole, warfarin, and fish oil have all been tried with little long-term benefit.[10]

Diffuse Proliferative Glomerulonephritis

Diffuse proliferative glomerulonephritis is often called poststreptococcal glomerulonephritis. Patients present with nephritic syndrome 1 to 3 weeks after a streptococcal infection. It more commonly occurs after a respiratory infection than a skin infection except in endemic outbreaks. The disease rarely progresses to nephrotic syndrome. Recovery occurs in 7 to 14 days with supportive care. Specific treatment directed against the immunologic underlying process is not indicated.

Membranoproliferative Glomerulonephritis

Two types of membranoproliferative glomerulonephritis exist based on immune deposits. Type I is the most common. Spontaneous remission rates of up to one third are seen, while one third develop renal insufficiency, and one third develop ESRD. Type II disease is rare. Steroids, cytotoxic drugs, anticoagulants, antiplatelet drugs, and cyclosporine have been tried for both types with limited success.

Rapidly Progressive (Crescentic) Glomerulonephritis

Clinical features are variable depending on the underlying cause of the glomerulonephritis. A rapidly progressive form is seen with antiglomerular basement membrane disease. Untreated patients die rapidly from pulmonary hemorrhage (Goodpasture's) or renal failure. Pauci-immune glomerulonephritis is the result of small-vessel vasculitis. Crescentic glomerulonephritis secondary to systemic lupus erythematosus can lead to rapidly progressive renal failure.

Cystic Kidney Disease: Inherited and Acquired

Solitary cysts of the kidney are commonly found on routine screening for other medical problems. They are usually unilateral but can be bilateral. The cyst growth is slow and does not cause progression or development of renal failure. No active treatment is necessary.

Autosomal-Dominant Polycystic Kidney Disease

Autosomal-dominant polycystic kidney disease (ADPKD) occurs in 1:1000 individuals, affecting 500,000 Americans; it is present in approximately 10% of patients with ESRD. It is the most common hereditary disease—20 times more common than Huntington's chorea, 15 times more common that cystic fibrosis, and 10 times more common than sickle cell disease. Mutation of a gene on chromosome 16 causes 90% of ADPKD cases. Renal cysts occur in the renal tubules. As the cysts enlarge they disconnect from the tubule and become isolated cysts. Only 1% to 2% of the nephrons are involved in the cystic process. Factors associated with rapid progression of renal failure in ADPKD include (1) onset at childhood; (2) male gender; (3) coexistent hypertension; (4) urinary tract infection; (5) black race; and (6) sickle cell disease.

The gene carrying ADPKD can also be detected in family

members. ADPKD can be diagnosed in utero by amniocentesis and chorionic villous sampling. Medical and ethical considerations must be weighed when counseling potentially affected family members.

Complications

Renal complications occur by the fourth or fifth decade: flank pain (60%), hematuria (35%), proteinuria (33%), hypertension (30% of children, 60% of adults), and renal calculi (20%).

Pain can be secondary to enlargement of the cyst, hemorrhage into a cyst, renal stone formation, or infection. NSAIDs are avoided as they may aggravate renal failure. Treatment consists of conservative management with pain medication. Percutaneous cyst decompression or open cyst reduction surgery is sometimes required in severe cases.

Hematuria is secondary to cyst rupture, urinary tract infection, or coexisting renal cancer. If severe, the hematuria can affect renal function. Initial treatment consists of hydration and bed rest. If hematuria is persistent, further investigation is warranted to rule out renal carcinoma.

Hypertension in those with ADPKD is associated with increased renin levels. Treatment with ACE inhibitors is recommended. Calcium channel blockers (nondihydropyridine group) are also effective. Diuretics are used cautiously as they may cause electrolyte imbalance and elevated uric acid levels.

Proteinuria is usually not in the nephrotic range. The degree of proteinuria is not indicative of the degree of cystic involvement. When urinary tract infections occur, bacteriuria is often not present, as many cysts are disconnected from the tubule. Treatment with an antibiotic that penetrates the cyst wall is needed [trimethoprim-sulfamethoxazole (TMP-SMX), quinolones, chloramphenicol, erythromycin, tetracyclines, or metronidazole]. Kidney stones are primarily calcium oxalate or uric acid. Stones are difficult to diagnose within cysts, and at times computed tomographic (CT) scanning is needed. Treatment for kidney stones in ADPKD is the same as if no cystic disease existed. Renal cell cancers are no more common with polycystic kidney disease than in the general population.

Extrarenal Manifestations

ADPKD is a systemic disease. In addition to renal cysts, cysts develop in the liver, pancreas, spleen, seminal vesicles, ovaries, and central nervous system (CNS). Extrarenal cysts increase with age. The incidence of hepatic cysts at age 20 to 29 is 10%, whereas it is 75% at age 60 or older. Massive hepatic cysts are primarily seen in women. The number of hepatic cysts increases with ESRD development.

Other extrarenal manifestations include mitral valve prolapse (26%) with palpitations and atypical chest pain, aortic valve disease that often needs surgical valve replacement, and increased incidence of berry aneurysms of the brain, and colonic diverticula (80%) that have a higher likelihood for perforation than in the normal population.

Autosomal-Recessive Polycystic Kidney Disease

Autosomal-recessive polycystic kidney disease (ARPKD) has an incidence of 1:10,000 to 1:40,000. The chromosomal gene location is unknown. Patients develop massive cystic kidneys with renal failure presenting at birth. Extrarenal cysts do not develop as in ADPKD, but hepatic fibrosis and portal hypertension are severe. There is no specific therapy for ARPKD. Dialysis for newborns and infants is necessary. Kidneys are often removed owing to respiratory compromise.

Acquired Polycystic Kidney Disease

Acquired polycystic kidney disease is present in more than 35% of patients on dialysis. The development of bilateral renal cysts often precedes ESRD. These patients have no history of hereditary cystic kidney disease.

Cyst formation increases with the duration of ESRD. Cyst regression occurs with renal transplantation and restoration of normal renal function. The incidence of adenocarcinoma of the kidney is increased in acquired polycystic kidney disease.

Renal Cancers

Renal Adenocarcinoma

Renal cell carcinoma is twice as common in men than in women, and most commonly occurs between the ages of 50 and 70 years. Several factors increase one's risk for developing renal cell carcinoma: (1) smoking doubles the risk; (2) work exposure to asbestos; (3) cadmium exposure (battery, paint, and welding workers); (4) overweight; (5) high-fat diet; (6) dialysis patients who develop kidney cysts; (7) history of tuberous sclerosis; and (8) family history of renal carcinoma.

Cure rates for renal adenocarcinoma (hypernephroma, renal cell carcinoma), which accounts for 85% of renal cancers, are related to the stage of the tumor. Cure is possible when the tumor is localized to the kidney and the immediate surrounding tissue. Even when regional lymph node and blood vessels are involved, significant cure rates can be achieved. Distant metastatic disease signals a poor prognosis.

Surgical resection is the mainstay of treatment. Even with disseminated disease, debulking the tumor improves the clinical course. Systemic chemotherapy is of only limited effectiveness. Abnormal liver function tests may be secondary to a paraneoplastic syndrome and not necessarily imply metastatic disease. CT scanning is the preferred scanning tool for evaluating tumor size and the extent of any metastatic disease.

Transitional Cell Carcinoma

Transitional cell carcinoma, accounting for 15% of renal cancers, is curable in 90% of cases if it is superficial and confined to the renal pelvis or ureter. With unconfined tumors, which become deeply invasive, cure rates drop to 10% to 15%. Tumors that penetrate the ureteral wall or are metastatic are not curable. Lymph node dissection does not seem to improve outcome. Although ureteroscopy and pyeloscopy can be used to biopsy the tumor, total excision of the ureter, bladder cuff, pelvis, and kidney is recommended. Treatment of extensive disease is not aided by irradiation or chemotherapy, and enrollment in a clinical trial is recommended. The incidence of opposite-side transitional cell carcinoma is 3% to 4%. The incidence of bladder cancer after surgery is 30% to 50%.

Bladder Carcinoma

Bladder cancer is the sixth most common cancer in the United States. It is two-and-one-half times more likely in men than women, and two times more likely in whites than in African Americans. The incidence increases with age and 80% of new cases are diagnosed older than 50 years of age. Risk factors include (1) tobacco use, (2) obesity, (3) occupational exposure to asbestos or coke ovens in steel plants, (4) pelvic radiation therapy, (5) dialysis patients, and (6) familial history of bladder cancer.

Hematuria is the first symptom 85% of the time; 90% of bladder carcinomas are transitional cell carcinomas, 6% to 8% are squamous cell carcinomas, and 2% are adenocarcinomas. Superficial cancer treatment is achieved by transurethral resection with or without intravesical chemotherapy. For deeply invasive tumors or for patients with regional distal metastasis, segmental or radical cystectomy often combined with radiation and chemotherapy is necessary.

Wilms' Tumor

Wilms' tumors account for almost all renal neoplasms during childhood. The median age at diagnosis is 3 years. Five hundred new cases are diagnosed yearly. The tumor is usually found by discovering an asymptomatic abdominal mass that is generally unilateral. Hypertension is present in 60% of cases. State-of-the-art therapy requires the combined efforts of the family physician, surgeon, oncologist, and radiation oncologist and it necessitates referral to an appropriate treatment center.[13]

Wilms' tumor is curable with more than 90% 4-year survivorship.[12] The prognosis depends on the stage, histopathologic features of the tumor, the patient's age, and tumor size. Anaplastic and sarcomatous histologic patterns are associated with a worse prognosis and an increased incidence of relapse and death. Therapy consists primarily of surgery, followed by chemotherapy and in some patients irradiation.

References

1. U.S. Renal Data System. USRDS 2000 annual data report. Bethesda, MD: National Institute of Diabetes and Digestive and Kidney Diseases, National Institutes of Health (NIH), DHHS, 2000. Available at *www.usrds.org*.
2. Bakris GL. Preserving renal function in adults with hypertension and diseases: a consensus approach. Am J Kidney Dis 2000; 36:646–61.
3. Agrawd M, Swartz R. Acute renal failure. Am Fam Physician 2000;61:2077–88.
4. Schmitz PG. Progressive renal insufficiency. Postgrad Med 2000;108:145–54.
5. Wali RK, Weir MR. Slowing the progression of chronic glomerulosclerosis. Res Staff Physician 2000;46:16–38.
6. Ritz ER, Orth SR. Nephropathy in patients with type 2 diabetes mellitus N Engl J Med 1999;341:1127–33.
7. Brenner, BM. Multimodal therapy in remission/regression of renal disease. In: Proceedings from the symposium at the 8th annual clinical nephrology meetings. CMF Monograph, Comprehensive Medical Communications, Inc., 2000;3–4.
8. Schmidt RJ, Besgrab A. When to treat the anemia of chronic renal insufficiency. Fam Pract Recert 2001;23:38–44.
9. Kolpak S, Mehler P. Medical issues in treating renal transplant patients. Hosp Pract 2001;June:50–56.
10. Peddi VR, First MR. Primary care of patients with renal transplants Med Clin North Am 1997;81:767–84.
11. Falk, RJ. Primary glomerular disease. In: Brenner BM, ed. The kidney, 6th ed. Philadelphia: WB Saunders, 2000;1268–77.
12. Jennette JC, Falk RJ. Diagnosis and management of glomerular diseases. Med Clin North Am 1997;81:653–77.
13. Neville HL, Ritchey ML. Wilms tumor: overview of National Wilms Tumor Study Group results. Urol Clin North Am 2000; 27:435–42.

98
Diseases of the Prostate

Paul T. Cullen

Prostatitis

Prostatitis is the most common urological diagnosis in men under age 50.[1] Up to 35% of men report at least one symptom of prostatitis and 10% have symptoms consistent with chronic prostatitis. Prostatitis is an important consideration in a man with perineal pain and voiding problems.

The National Institutes of Health (NIH) classification system separates prostatitis into four categories: acute bacterial, chronic bacterial, and the chronic pelvic pain syndrome (CPPS) with and without inflammation.[2] The symptoms of prostatitis are similar except for acute bacterial prostatitis, which is accompanied by fever, systemic symptoms, and a tender prostate. Perineal, suprapubic, or genital pain accompanied by irritative and obstructive voiding symptoms are typical features of one of the chronic prostatitis syndromes. The findings on digital examination of the prostate are inconsistent and nonspecific.[3]

Microscopic examination of the expressed prostatic secretions (EPSs) and urine following prostatic massage and a urine culture are useful in the evaluation of a man with suspected chronic prostatitis. EPSs are obtained by compressing the prostate with the examining finger from its lateral edges toward the median sulcus. The secretions are collected in a sterile specimen container. Microscopic examination of the initial urine voided after prostatic massage is an alternative to the EPS. The presence of 10 or more white blood cells per high power field (WBCs/hpf) in the EPS or postmassage urine is consistent with bacterial prostatitis or CPPS with inflammation.[4] Significant bacterial growth of more than 10^5 organisms in the urine is present in either acute or chronic bacterial prostatitis. The absence of WBCs and a negative urine culture indicates noninflammatory CPPS. A simplified classification and treatment of prostatitis is described in Table 98.1.

CPPS (Nonbacterial Prostatitis)

In as many as 90% of patients, chronic prostatitis does not have a proven bacterial etiology. The diagnosis of chronic pelvic pain syndrome is primarily based on symptoms. Although two categories of CPPS are recognized based on the presence of inflammatory cells, the clinical value of this distinction is often unclear. A wide variety of causes have been postulated, including infection, sexual activity, autoimmune disorders, prostatic cysts and calculi, and activation of inflammatory cytokines. Up to 50 % of patients with CPPS have features of depression or somatization. There is no scientific evidence of the benefit of any specific type of treatment.[5] Empiric treatment with antibiotics for 2 to 4 weeks is often recommended if inflammatory cells are present. Symptomatic treatment with nonsteroidal antiinflammatory drugs, sitz baths, prostatic massage, and frequent ejaculation is used for control of discomfort. α-Adrenergic blockers can be used if obstuctive voiding symptoms are present.

Bacterial Prostatitis

Chronic bacterial prostatitis should be suspected in any man with recurrent urinary infection.[6] It is often accompanied by vague pain and voiding dysfunction. Aerobic gram-negative rods are the most common causative bacteria. Four weeks of fluoroquinolone antibiotic therapy is recommended. Patients who experience frequent relapses may benefit from longer courses of therapy or daily suppressive antibiotics.

Acute bacterial prostatitis is uncommon in the office setting. It may be misdiagnosed as pyelonephritis. Typical symptoms include the sudden onset of fever, chills, dysuria, perineal pain, frequency, urgency, and slowing of the urinary stream. Prostatic edema may result in acute urinary retention. The prostate gland is boggy and tender on examination. The prostate should not be vigorously massaged because of the risk of bacteremia. Pyuria and bacteriuria are present, and gram-negative bacilli are

Table 98.1. **Evaluation and Management of Prostatitis**

Type of prostatitis	EPS/postmassage U/A (WBC/hpf)	Urine/EPS culture	Treatment
Chronic pelvic pain syndrome without inflammation	<10	Negative	Non-steroidal antiinflammatory drugs Alpha-blockers if obstructive voiding symptoms present Treat anxiety/depression if present Sitz baths Avoid spicy food, caffeine, alcohol
Chronic pelvic pain syndrome with inflammation	>10	Negative	2-week course of doxycycline or erythromycin Alpha-blockers if obstructive voiding symptoms present Sitz baths Avoid spicy food, caffeine, alcohol
Chronic bacterial	>10	Positive	1-month course of quinolone antibiotic Watch for relapse
Acute bacterial	>10	Positive	2–4 week course of quinolone antibiotic Hospitalize if "toxic"

EPS = expressed prostatic secretion; U/A = urinalysis.

present in the urine culture. The severely ill patient should be hospitalized and treated with intravenous antibiotics.

Because the symptoms and findings in the prostatitis syndromes are not specific, it is important to consider other urologic problems that may masquerade as prostatitis. If symptoms persist and a cause for the patient's complaint remains elusive, a complete urologic evaluation to exclude other pathology should be performed.

Benign Prostatic Hyperplasia

Benign prostatic hyperplasia (BPH) is the most common benign tumor in men. BPH appears microscopically in 50% of men by age 60 and in 90% of men who live to age 85. By age 80 about 25% of men are symptomatic with BPH. Aging and androgens are required for the development of BPH. Progressive BPH may lead to acute urinary retention, chronic renal failure, urinary tract infection, and bladder stones.

Clinical Presentation

The symptoms attributed to BPH result from mechanical obstruction of urine outflow with a dynamic component dependent on smooth muscle tone in the prostate and bladder neck and secondary irritative uninhibited bladder contractions. *Lower urinary tract symptoms* (LUTS) is the term used to describe these complaints. The severity of LUTS does not correlate well with the severity of prostatic enlargement. Since symptoms are not directly correlated with prostate size, *benign prostatic obstruction* (BPO) is a more accurate term for this syndrome. Prostatitis, urinary tract infection, neoplasms of the bladder or prostate, and neurogenic bladder are other common problems that may present with similar symptoms.

The patient with BPH usually seeks treatment because the symptoms are affecting his quality of life. A self-administered scoring system, the American Urological Association (AUA) Symptom Scoring Index (Table 98.2), has been developed and has proved to have validity and reliability for measuring BPH symptoms and the response to treatment. The index be should

be used to initially quantify the patient's symptoms and then to monitor the response to therapy. The total symptom score is classified into three categories: mild (0–7), moderate (8–18), or severe (19–35).[7]

The initial history should review other causes of outflow obstruction, such as urethral stricture, and neurologic disorders (diabetes, stroke, Parkinson's disease) that can impair bladder function and produce similar symptoms. Asking about hematuria and previous urinary tract problems is indicated. A review of medications that diminish bladder contractility (anticholinergics) or increase outflow resistance (sympathomimetics) is necessary.

A digital rectal examination (DRE) can be used to estimate the size of the prostate gland, but there is little correlation with the degree of obstructive symptoms. With BPH the prostate is firm and often symmetrically enlarged. Areas of significant induration, nodularity, or asymmetry are investigated for the possibility of prostate cancer.

Initial studies include a urinalysis and a serum creatinine assay. Renal ultrasonography should be obtained in patients with BPH if there is a history of urinary tract surgery, an elevated serum creatinine level, hematuria, urinary tract infection (UTI), or renal stones. Measuring the postvoid residual urine is optional and not well correlated with signs and symptoms of prostatism. The serum prostate-specific antigen (PSA) level is not uniformly recommended for evaluating BPH. There are no data to indicate men with symptoms of BPH are at increased risk for prostate cancer.[8] A PSA level can be obtained to screen for prostate cancer, but elevations between 4 and 10 ng/mL will be the result of BPH in up to 75% of patients (see Screening for Prostate Cancer, below).

Treatment

In most patients the primary goal of treatment is relief of the lower urinary tract symptoms that result from BPH. To accurately evaluate the effectiveness of therapy, it is important to initially quantify the severity of the patient's complaints by using the AUA symptom scoring index. Longitudinal stud-

Table 98.2. **American Urological Association (AUA) Symptom Index**

Questions (All refer to over the past month)	Not at all	Less than 1 time in 5	Less than half the time	About half of the time	More than half of the time	Almost always
1. How often have you had the sensation of not completely emptying your bladder after you finished urinating?	0	1	2	3	4	5
2. How often have you had to urinate less than 2 hours after you finished urinating?	0	1	2	3	4	5
3. How often have you found you stopped and started again several times when you urinated?	0	1	2	3	4	5
4. How often have you found it difficult to postpone urination?	0	1	2	3	4	5
5. How often have you had a weak urinary stream?	0	1	2	3	4	5
6. How often have you had to push or strain to begin urination?	0	1	2	3	4	5
7. How often do you get up at night from the time you go to bed from the time you get up in the morning?	0	1	2	3	4	5

Sum of 7 circled numbers: _____

Symptom score (sum):
  0–7 = mild prostatism
  8–18 = moderate prostatism
  19–35 = severe prostatism.

Source: Barry et al,[7] with permission.

ies of untreated patients with symptomatic BPH have demonstrated a significant variation in the severity of symptoms, with periods of improvement and worsening.

For patients with a symptom score in the mild range (0–7), the most appropriate course is to monitor the patient and provide no active treatment. For a symptom score in the moderate to severe range, active treatment of BPH is a strong consideration. It is appropriate to exercise "watchful waiting" for some patients with moderate symptoms. Medications that alleviate the symptoms of BPH should be prescribed for patients whose symptoms are severe enough to warrant treatment. Transurethral resection of the prostate (TURP) is the traditional treatment for BPH not responding to medical therapy.

α-Adrenergic Antagonists

The α-adrenergic antagonist drugs block the receptors of the bladder neck and prostatic urethra, decreasing smooth muscle tone and diminishing the dynamic component of outflow resistance. Alpha-blockers may also provide long-term benefits by accelerating programmed cell death in prostate tissue. Representative alpha-blockers used to treat BPH include terazosin (Hytrin), doxazosin (Cardura), and tamsulosin (Flomax). Alpha-blockers reduce symptom scores by 50% to 60% and provide long-term control of the symptoms of BPH. The response is seen within weeks (Table 98.3), and there is a dose-dependent relation to symptom improvement with terazosin and doxazosin. A titration dosage schedule is recommended when using these alpha-blockers. A first-dose hypotensive response complicated by syncope can occur with terazosin and can be avoided if the first dose is taken at bedtime. Weakness, dizziness, and postural hypotension are common side effects of alpha-blocker therapy and result in discontinuation in about 10% of men. The antihypertensive effect is much greater in hypertensive than normotensive men. The

Table 98.3. **Medications for Benign Prostatic Hypertrophy**

Medication	Selective alpha-blocker (tamulosin)	Alpha blockers (terazosin, doxazosin)	Saw palmetto	Finasteride
Onset of action	Days to weeks	Days to weeks	Weeks to a few months	Months
Side effects	Minimal, ejaculatory dysfunction (5%)	Dizziness, orthostasis (10%), ?CHF	Headache, dyspepsia	Minimal, decreased libido, impotence
Efficacy	50% decrease in symptoms	50% decrease in symptoms	Varies, up to 20%	20% decrease in symptoms
Dosing schedule	No titration, two dosages	Titration required	320 mg of lipophyllic extract daily	Single dose
Cost	$500/yr	$360–$400/yr	$360/yr	$750/yr
Effect on PSA	None	None	None	Reduces by 50%

CHF = congestive heart failure; PSA = prostatic specific antigen.

mean decrease in systolic blood pressure is 18 mm Hg in hypertensive patients, but a drop of only 4 mm Hg occurs in normotensive men. Tamsulosin does not require a titration schedule and has a lower frequency of orthostasis, although ejaculatory dysfunction has been reported. A maximal therapeutic effect for a given dosage of alpha-blocker is seen in 4 to 6 weeks. A degree of concern may be warranted about nonselective alpha-blockers because of an increase in cardiovascular events observed in patients treated with terazosin for hypertension during the Antihypertensive and Lipid Lowering Trial to Prevent Heart Attack (ALLHAT).[9]

Androgen Deprivation Therapy

Benign prostatic hypertrophy does not develop in the absence of androgens. The removal of androgens decreases the size of the prostate and diminishes the mechanical component of obstructive symptoms. Testosterone, the most potent endogenous androgen, requires conversion to its active form dihydrotestosterone by an intracellular enzyme 5α-reductase. Finasteride (Proscar), an inhibitor of this enzyme, is approved for treatment of BPH. Finasteride is given as a 5-mg dose once daily. It is effective in about 40% of patients, reducing their symptoms scores by 20%. It is most effective in patients with significantly enlarged prostate glands. Finasteride must be taken for 3 to 6 months to produce a significant effect. Its few side effects include a decrease in libido, ejaculatory dysfunction, and impotence (5%). Finasteride is useful for long-term management, and the symptom alleviation it produces has been shown to persist for a minimum of 4 years. There is no evidence of an increased benefit from the addition of finasteride to alpha-blockers alone.[10]

Phytotherapy

Nonprescription therapy using herbal therapy derived from the saw palmetto berry (*Sernoa repens*) is one of the most widely used treatments for BPH (also see Chapter 128). Saw palmetto may decrease dihydrotestosterone concentration in the prostate. Although a meta-analysis of 18 randomized trials found it more effective than placebo, many of the studies were of short duration and insufficient quality.[11] Inconsistency in the preparation and bioavailability of herbal therapies complicates the determination of an effective dose. Saw palmetto has relatively few side effects. An extract of the African plum tree bark (Prostata) is also available, although there are few quality studies to support its effectiveness.

Invasive Therapies

The most effective treatment for the relief of the symptoms of BPH is TURP, with 80% of treated patients reporting "good" resolution of symptoms.[12] There is a 0.2% operative mortality and common complications include thrombophlebitis, retrograde ejaculation, urinary infection, impotence, and incontinence. The indications for surgical intervention in BPH include progressive symptoms with failure of medical therapy, urinary retention, renal failure from obstructive uropathy, recurrent UTIs, persistent hematuria, bladder calculi, and large bladder diverticuli.

Transurethral incision of the prostate gland is an effective alternative to TURP if the prostate is moderate in size. It can be done under local anesthesia, is associated with less blood loss, and does not result in retrograde ejaculation.

Additional less invasive options include microwave heating, electrovaporization, and laser prostatectomy. Although these procedures are often performed in the outpatient setting and are associated with a low rate of complications, they may be somewhat less effective than TURP.

Prostate Cancer

Adenocarcinoma of the prostate gland is the most common noncutaneous neoplasm in men. Every year approximately 200,000 new cases are identified in the United States. Prostate cancer kills about 32,000 men yearly and is second only to lung cancer as a cause of cancer deaths in men. The number of men dying from prostate cancer in the U.S. began to decrease slightly in 1995. The disease is more common and often more aggressive in African-American men. In relation to total deaths from all cancers, prostate cancer is responsible for 6% of cancer deaths in whites and 9% in African Americans. A positive family history of prostate cancer in a first-degree relative is the most important risk factor for prostate cancer.[13] Only about 25% of men who develop clinically recognized prostate cancer die from it; 30% to 40% of men over age 50 have clinically silent prostate cancer that never results in any health consequences. About 40% of deaths from prostate cancer occur in men ages 80 or older.

Screening for Prostate Cancer

The American Cancer Society and the American Urological Association recommend screening with an annual digital rectal exam beginning at age 40. These groups also recommend an annual serum PSA level beginning at age 40 to 45 for African-American men or men who have a family history of prostate cancer, and for all men starting at age 50. The American Academy of Family Physicians and American College of Physicians recommend the physician discuss the risks and benefits of screening and decide based on individual patient preference. In 1996, the U.S. Preventative Services Task Force recommended against screening and it is likely their position will not change until 2004, when evidence from randomized controlled trials on the benefit of screening becomes available.

The presence of a hard nodule, significant asymmetry, or an area of induration on DRE is suspicious for cancer. PSA is an enzyme produced by epithelial cells of the prostate that hydrolyzes the ejaculate and has a function in male fertility. The PSA level can be elevated in BPH, prostatitis, prostate cancer, prostate trauma, prostate surgery, and after an ejaculation. "Routine" DRE does not raise the PSA significantly. The normal PSA level is less than 4 ng/mL. Approximately 20% of men with prostate cancer have a PSA level of 2 to 4.[14] Prostate cancer is rare (<1%) if the PSA is less than 2. Reducing the lower limit of PSA to 2.5 ng/mL would to improve the sensitivity of the test. The improvement in sensitivity would be offset by a large increase in false-positive test results requiring additional diagnostic tests and producing substantial patient anxiety. Levels between 4 and 10 ng/mL may be the result of benign or malignant disease, but only 25% of those in this range will have cancer. As the level rises above 10 ng/mL the probability of cancer increases to 50% or greater. A PSA value above 50 ng/mL is highly suggestive of metastatic disease. In addition to the absolute level of PSA, age-specific normal levels, the rate of increase of PSA, and the ratio of free PSA to total PSA have been used to improve the predictive value; however, there is no conclusive evidence to suggest that these techniques be used routinely.[15] A PSA level that increases by 0.75 ng/mL/year or more may indicate a developing malignancy. If patients are being treated with finasteride, the normal value for PSA should be reduced by 50%.

Cancers detected by PSA screening are equivalent in malignant grade to those diagnosed clinically.[16] Radical prostatectomy or radiation therapy are options for treating cancer that is confined to the prostate, but more than 10 years is required before an increase in survival is evident. The argument for screening is based on the concept that surgery or radiotherapy produces a survival benefit for confined asymptomatic cancer that is likely to become clinically significant before the patient dies from another cause. This situation is most likely in young patients who harbor silent high-grade tumors. It is difficult to justify screening a man who is not expected to live at least 10 years. For healthy men under age 70 and extremely healthy and vigorous men over age 70, individual factors should be weighed in the decision to recommend screening. African Americans and men with a family history of prostate cancer are at greater risk for cancer, and screening these groups should confer a larger benefit. The patient must be informed that abnormal findings detected will lead to urologic consultation, biopsy, and the possibility of surgery. For patients who are offered screening, the DRE and PSA are complementary and should both be performed. Significant abnormalities of DRE or PSA should be referred to a urologist for further evaluation. Until 2004, when the results of randomized prospective trials become available, controversy about the benefit of prostate cancer screening will continue.

Diagnosis and Staging

The prognosis for prostate cancer depends on the histologic grade of the tumor, the PSA level, and whether it is confined within the prostate gland. Once the tumor penetrates the capsule and involves adjacent tissues or lymph nodes, eradication is unlikely. The Gleason system is most commonly used to grade the tumor histology. It has a range of scores between 2 and 10; scores of 2 to 4 indicate well-differentiated (low-grade), 5 to 7 moderately differentiated, and 8 to 10 poorly differentiated (high-grade) malignancies. Either the TMN or the Whitmore Jewett (W-J) staging system is used to estimate anatomically the size and extent of spread of the tumor. TMN stage T3 or W-J stage C and D cancers extend beyond the capsule of the prostate and usually cannot be completely removed. It is common for the stage to be more advanced at surgical resection than the original estimate. The diagnosis of

cancer is confirmed by needle biopsy using transrectal ultrasonography of the prostate to direct the sampling of six anatomic zones (sextant) and any suspicious areas. PSA level, chest radiograph, radionuclide bone scan, and computed tomography (CT) scanning may be used to estimate the stage before planning treatment.

Treatment

A primary consideration when choosing the method of treatment for prostate cancer is the likelihood of the tumor shortening the patient's life or producing significant symptoms. At present there are no definitive randomized trials directly comparing the effectiveness of various treatments for localized prostate cancer. In the absence of compelling evidence, the decision to select surgical or radiation therapy is often influenced by the specialty of the treating physician.

If the cancer is localized to the prostate, treatment should prevent future spread while maintaining bladder, bowel, and sexual functions. If the patient has a low-grade confined tumor (Gleason 2–5) and his expected life span is less than 10 years, "watchful waiting" is a reasonable approach. This strategy may not be appropriate for men under age 65, as their cancer is more likely to become symptomatic. Moderate and poorly differentiated tumors (Gleason 6 to 10) are more likely to become clinically significant. If the patient's expected life span is more than 10 years, radical prostatectomy and radiation therapy are effective treatments in confined prostate cancer.[17] Radical prostatectomy has a 0.4% mortality rate, and 30% to 70% of patients maintain sexual functioning. Urinary incontinence develops in 5% to 30% of patients after surgery. After successful surgery the PSA level should remain undetectable. Traditional external beam radiation therapy, three-dimensional (3D) conformational treatment planning with highly focused beam therapy, and the implantation of radioactive seeds into the prostate (brachytherapy) are options for the patient who is unwilling to undergo surgery. Acute complications of traditional irradiation include proctitis, cystitis, urinary retention, and scrotal edema in 30% to 50% of patients. Chronic proctitis, diarrhea, and cystitis occur in a small percentage given radiation therapy, but 50% are impotent at 7 years following treatment; 3-D conformational radiation therapy and brachytherapy have a lower rate of side effects than standard external beam therapy.

Radiation therapy is preferred if complete surgical removal of the tumor is unlikely. A Gleason score of 7 or higher, a PSA level greater than 20, or evidence the tumor has penetrated the prostate capsule (stage T3) is an indication for primary radiation therapy.[18]

For men who present with prostate cancer that has already metastasized to lymph nodes or other sites, palliative therapy is all that can be offered. Prostate cancer spreads locally to the seminal vesicles and base of the bladder. The obturator and hypogastric lymph nodes are often involved. Common sites of osteoblastic bony metastases are the spine, pelvis, ribs, sternum, and skull. The lung, liver, and adrenal gland are sites of visceral metastases. Prostate cancer is influenced by androgens, and about 85% of patients have an objective response to androgen removal. Hormonal therapy delays the progression of cancer and provides local control for patients with advanced local disease or high-grade tumors confined to the prostate. Androgen removal is also beneficial if the PSA level is steadily rising, or when nodal or distant metastases are present. Treatment options include orchiectomy, gonadotropin-releasing hormone agonists (leuprolide/Lupron, goserelin/Zoladex), agents that interfere with androgen binding to cellular receptors (flutamide/Eulexin, bicalutamide/Casodex), and adrenal steroid inhibitors (ketoconazole, aminogluthetimide). A common combination often referred to as total androgen blockade combines a gonadotropin-releasing hormone agonist and an androgen receptor blocker.[19] Eventually prostate cancer becomes androgen insensitive, and may paradoxically respond for a short time to discontinuing androgen blockade. Chemotherapy has very limited benefit for disease that has become resistant to hormone therapy. Local irradiation can achieve temporary control with symptoms of soft tissue or bony metastases.

References

1. Collins M, Stafford R, O'Leary M, Barry M. How common is prostatitis? A national survey of physician visits. J Urol 1998; 159:1224–8.
2. Krieger JN, Nyberg LJ, Nickel JC. NIH consensus definition and classification of prostatitis. JAMA 1999;282:236–7.
3. Nickel CJ. Prostatitis syndromes: an update for urologic practice. Can J Urol 2000;7:1091–7.
4. Ludwig M, Schroeder-Printxen I, Lüdecke G, Weidner W. Comparison of expressed prostatic secretions with urine after prostatic massage—a means to diagnose chronic prostatitis/inflammatory chronic pelvic pain syndrome. Urology 2000;55: 175–7.
5. Collins M, MacDonald R, Wilt T. Diagnosis and treatment of chronic abacterial prostatitis: a systematic review. Ann Intern Med 2000;133:367–81.
6. Lipsky B. Prostatitis and urinary tract infection in men: what's new; what's true? Am J Med 1999;106:327–34.
7. Barry M, Fowler FJ, O'Leary MP, et al. The American Urological Association symptom index for benign prostatic hyperplasia. J Urol 1992;148:1549.
8. Young J, Muscatello DJ, Ward JE. Are men with lower urinary tract symptoms at increased risk of prostate cancer? A systematic review and critique of the available evidence. Br J Urol 2000;85:1037–48.
9. ALLHAT officers and coordinators for the ALLHAT Collaborative Research Group. Major cardiovascular events in hypertensive patients randomized to doxazosin vs chlorthalidone. JAMA 2000;283:1967–75.
10. Roehrborn C. Is there a place for combination medical therapy? Curr Opin Urol 2001;11:17–25.
11. Ceullar D, Kyprianou N. Future concepts in the medical therapy of benign prostatic hyperplasia. Curr Opin Urol 2001;11: 27–33.
12. Chow RD. Benign prostatic hyperplasis. Patient evaluation and relief of obstructive symptoms. Geriatrics 2001;56:33–8.
13. Barry M. Prostate specific antigen testing for early diagnosis of prostate cancer. N Engl J Med 2001;344:1373–7.
14. Babaian R, Johnston D, Naccarato W, Ayala A, Bhadkamkar V, Fritsche A. The incidence of prostate cancer in a screening population with a serum prostate specific antigen between 2.5 and 4.0 ng/ml: relation to biopsy strategy. J Urol 2001;165:757–60.
15. Hoffman RM, Clanon DL, Littenberg B, Frank JJ, Peirce JC. Using the free to total inconsistency in the preparation and bioavailability of herbal therapies complicate the determination of an effective dose prostate-specific antigen ratio to detect prostate cancer in men with nonspecific elevations of prostate-specific antigen levels. J Gen Intern Med 2000;15:739–48.
16. Gilliland FD, Gleason DF, Hunt WC, Stone N, Harlan LC, Key C. Trends in Gleason score for prostate cancer diagnosed between 1983 and 1993. J Urol 2001;165:846–50.
17. Scher H Isaacs J, Zelefsky M, Scardino P. Prostate cancer. In: Abeloff M, Armitage J, Lichter A, Niederhuber J, ed. New York, Edinborough, London, Madrid, Melbourne, San Francisco, Tokyo Churchill Livingstone Clinical oncology, 2nd ed. 2000 p. 1842.
18. Horwitz E, Hanks G. External beam radiation therapy for prostate cancer. CA Cancer J Clin 2000;50:349–75.
19. Labrie F. Screening and hormonal therapy of localized prostate cancer shows major benefits of survival. Cancer J Sci Am 2000; suppl 2:S182–7 Vol 6.

99
Surgery of the Male Genital System

John P. Fogarty

Acute Scrotal Pain

Acute scrotal pain and swelling is a common presentation in boys and young men. While there are several causes, it is critical to rule out testicular torsion early because the likelihood of salvage of the torsed testicle diminishes with time. Testicular torsion represents a surgical emergency and the family physician must quickly exclude this condition.[1] Common conditions to be considered causing acute scrotal pain include torsion of a testicular appendage, epididymitis, trauma, hernia, hydrocele, and varicocele.[2]

A careful history and physical examination will usually narrow the differential diagnosis of the acute scrotum. Torsion occurs rarely in the neonatal period, and when it does occur, it is usually in association with an inguinal hernia. It most commonly occurs in young men below age 25, with 85% between the ages of 12 and 18.[3] Torsion of the testicular appendage tends to occur earlier, usually between the age of 7 and 12.[4] Torsion is typically associated with pain of sudden onset, with nausea, vomiting, and swelling of the ipsilateral scrotum.[5] A history of trauma does not exclude torsion.

The most difficult clinical distinction is between acute torsion and epididymo-orchitis. Distinction is important, since one may be treated medically while the other needs immediate surgical intervention. Epididymitis typically occurs in sexually active men below the age of 35, with or without fever and pyuria, or in older men with prostate disease. It is likely to have a gradual onset over several days as opposed to torsion, which usually presents abruptly with severe pain.

On physical examination, the patient with torsion appears in moderate to severe pain and the inguinal area should be inspected for presence of hernias, swelling, or edema. The scrotum should be assessed for discrepancies in size, swelling, or erythema of the two sides. Unilateral swelling without erythema suggests the diagnosis of hernia or hydrocele. A high-riding testis with an abnormal (transverse lie) position suggests

torsion. For both torsion and epididymitis, the affected hemiscrotum will typically demonstrate significant erythema and swelling after 24 hours. With torsion, there is usually an absent cremasteric reflex, elicited by stroking the inner aspect of the thigh and observing the scrotal response. For both conditions, loss of testicular landmarks occurs late in the clinical course.

Next the examiner should palpate the testicle. With epididymitis, the tenderness and swelling should be posterolateral to the testis and the testis itself is usually not tender. Tenderness limited to the upper pole of the epididymis suggests torsion of the testicular appendage and may be accompanied by a "blue dot" sign, a visible and palpable hard tender nodule.[1,4] In early torsion, the entire testis is swollen and tender and is usually larger than the unaffected side. If relief is elicited with elevation of the scrotum, the diagnosis of epididymitis is more likely (Prehn's sign). If torsion is suspected, manual derotation of the testis away from the midline can be attempted. Prompt relief confirms the diagnosis and the patient should be referred for orchiopexy as soon as possible. In equivocal cases, surgical consultation and possible exploration are indicated.[4]

Color Doppler imaging has become the most common diagnostic study in the initial evaluation of the acute scrotum to differentiate between those cases requiring surgical exploration and those that can be observed or treated medically. It has the advantages of ease of use and avoids the time delay of nuclear medicine scanning. Color Doppler is able to reliably image acute epididymitis and in cases where there is evidence of diminished or absent blood flow to the testis, prompt surgical intervention and exploration is mandatory.[1,2,4]

Testicular Cancer

While testicular cancer accounts for only about 1% of all cancers in males, it is the most common cancer between ages 15 and 35 years.[6,7] Risk factors associated with testicular cancer include white race, a history of cryptorchidism, testicular atrophy, and family history.[8] Testicular cancer occurs four to five times more frequently in whites than in blacks, and 10% of males diagnosed with testicular cancer give a positive history of recent trauma. It is thought that this trauma does not cause the cancer, but may help bring the cancer to the attention of the patient and physician.[9] There is no association between the incidence of testicular cancer and vasectomy, occupational or environmental exposures, or viral illness.

The largest proportion of testicular cancers are of germ cell origin, and are further subdivided into seminomas and nonseminomas. Nonseminomatous tumors include yolk sac, embryonal cell, teratomas, and choriocarcinomas, and surgical therapy or chemotherapy is the usual approach. Seminomatous tumors comprise 40% of germ cell tumors and are usually extremely radiosensitive.

The most typical presentation in the patient later found to have testicular cancer is the discovery of a painless hard lump in the testicle. Delay in both presentation by the patient and diagnosis by the physician is common, with delays reported between 4 and 18 months.[10,11] In addition to the painless lump, the patient may also present with diffuse swelling or hardness in the scrotum or with signs of distant metastases to bone or the lungs. Any patient presenting with a testicular mass should have an ultrasound of the scrotum and any intratesticular mass should be considered cancer until proven otherwise. The staging workup of the new diagnosis of testicular cancer includes serum markers [β-subunit of human chorionic gonadotropin (HCG), α-fetoprotein (AFP), and lactate dehydrogenase (LDH)], chest x-ray, and computed tomographic (CT) scan of the abdomen.[12]

Treatment will depend on the cell type and the staging of the tumor. Testicular cancer is a highly curable neoplasm with an overall survival rate exceeding 95%.[13] While testicular cancer has a low incidence and excellent cure rate, more is needed in prevention and screening by increasing awareness of this condition in high-risk groups and encouraging young males to perform self-examination.

Erectile Dysfunction

Erectile dysfunction is defined as the inability to achieve and maintain penile erection sufficient to perform satisfactory sexual activity. A very common problem, it affects 20 to 30 million men in the United States and is present in approximately 30% of men 40 to 70 years of age.[14,15] The incidence increases with advancing age. This disorder can be characterized as organic, psychogenic, or mixed. Organic causes comprise over 70% and are associated with many chronic medical conditions, including peripheral vascular disease, diabetes, hypertension, and liver or kidney dysfunction. Queries about smoking and alcohol use along with a detailed medication history may elicit common causes. A history of surgery or trauma to the pelvis region may also be contributory. Psychogenic causes usually involve partner relationship issues, anxiety, or depression. A careful history, including medications and alcohol use, and a medical examination, along with targeted

laboratory studies, are usually sufficient to categorize erectile dysfunction.[16]

Therapy for erectile dysfunction includes medications, vacuum devices, penile therapies, or surgical implants. Psychogenic causes may require individual or couples counseling for resolution. Sildenafil (Viagra) therapy has a very favorable response rate for both psychogenic and organic causes, but should be used with caution in patients with known coronary disease or patients using nitrate medication. Primary care physicians will frequently encounter patients with this complaint and should be able to manage the majority with advice, counseling, medications, and support.

Newborn Circumcision

Routine newborn circumcision remains controversial. Despite efforts by organized medicine to provide accurate and unbiased information for parents, precise information about risks and benefits of the procedure and potential harm is not easy to present in an informed consent process.[17] Some favor the procedure to reduce medical problems, including sexually transmitted disease and urinary tract infection, while others view circumcision as unnecessary and disfiguring.[18] Circumcision is probably performed as much for religious and cultural indications as medical ones, but data demonstrate that it has a low incidence of complications and provides modest medical benefits.[17] The use of routine anesthesia for this procedure is becoming more common, particularly among younger physicians.[19]

Anesthesia for this procedure includes dorsal penile nerve block (injecting approximately 1 mL of 1% plain lidocaine over the dorsum of the penis at the 10 and 2 o'clock positions), ring block (0.8 mL of plain lidocaine injected in a band or ring around the penis, halfway along the shaft), or topical anesthetic [lidocaine 2.5%, prilocaine 2.5% (EMLA) cream applied around the distal half of the penis and allowed to remain for 10 minutes]. One study demonstrated that the ring block is the most effective, with the topical anesthetic least effective.[18]

Techniques used are named for the instruments for circumcision and include the Hollister-Stier Plastibell, Mogan clamp, and Gomco clamp.[20] The techniques are not reviewed here, as residents are likely to learn one or all three in their obstetrics rotations and later with their own continuity patients. Complications are infrequent, with an incidence of 0.2%, and include local bleeding, infection, adhesions, penile trauma, and poor cosmetic result.

Phimosis/Paraphimosis

Phimosis and paraphimosis occur only in uncircumcised or partially circumcised males. Paraphimosis refers to the condition in which the foreskin, once pulled back behind the glans penis, cannot be returned to its original position. It represents a surgical emergency because if left untreated it can have severe consequences.[21] Phimosis refers to a nonemergent condition in which the foreskin cannot be completely pulled back or retracted.

Paraphimosis most often occurs in medical settings after penile examination or urethral catheterization where the practitioner fails to return the retracted foreskin after the procedure. As the foreskin remains behind the corona, it may swell, forming a tight constricting band. This ring may subsequently impair the flow of blood or lymphatic fluid to and from the glans and the prepuce. If left untreated, this continued swelling could compromise blood flow and result in gangrene and autoamputation of the glans.

Patients with paraphimosis typically present with penile pain with or without obstructive voiding symptoms. The glans appears enlarged and congested with a collar of swollen foreskin around the base. A tight band is usually apparent behind the head of the penis. There may be a history of recent penile manipulation, instrumentation, or self-retraction of the uncircumcised foreskin. Examination should focus on the presence of the foreskin, color of the glans, the degree of constriction, and turgor of the prepuce.

Treatment should focus on reducing the condition as quickly as possible, to reduce the penile edema and replace the foreskin to its original position. An attempt at immediate reduction at diagnosis is appropriate since further delay increases swelling, symptoms, and risk of complications. If unsuccessful or too painful, anesthesia may be necessary. Topical anesthetics, including ice, 2% lidocaine gel, or 2.5% lidocaine and 2.5% prilocaine (EMLA cream) applied for several minutes may help before manipulation. A penile nerve block similar to those used in newborn circumcision may be necessary. After satisfactory anesthesia and ice application to decrease swelling, gentle pressure with the thumbs on the glans and fingers wrapped around the prepuce is attempted to reduce the trapped foreskin. If unsuccessful, it may be necessary to cut an emergency dorsal slit, similar to the initial slit in a circumcision procedure, to release the constricting band. Regardless of method of reduction, the patient should have a follow-up circumcision to prevent future episodes.

Phimosis typically occurs secondary to repeated infection and scarring and may lead to painful erections along with difficulties with proper hygiene. Initial mild episodes may be treated with antibiotic ointments or topical steroids. The best treatment for recurrent episodes is circumcision.

Vasectomy

Vasectomy is a common procedure performed in family practice offices and is the safest, simplest, and least expensive method of permanent birth control.[22] It has a slightly higher rate of minor complications over tubal ligation, but tubal failures can result in ectopic pregnancy, while vasectomy results can be checked at any time using sperm counts.[23] Ideally the patient and his partner should be seen together for evaluation and counseling before vasectomy. The history should include information about the patient's marital status, present number of children, and motivation for the procedure. Consent for the procedure should emphasize the permanence of the procedure despite the potential for reversal. Patients should understand that if further children are desired, other forms of contraception would be more appropriate, or the patient could

consider a sperm bank as an option. The physician should fully explain the risks and benefits of the procedure and perform a full examination of the scrotum, testes, and inguinal areas. Contraindications for vasectomy include a history of a bleeding disorder, including present anticoagulation therapy, and local infection. Aspirin should be avoided within 1 to 2 weeks of the procedure and other platelet inhibitors or anticoagulants should be withheld for 3 to 4 days.

The patient should prepare for the procedure by clipping the local hair rather than shaving to avoid postoperative infection and to shower and fully cleanse the genital area on the day of surgery. He should not eat for at least 2 hours prior to the procedure. The patient is instructed to bring a clean athletic supporter to wear after the procedure until recovery is complete. Some clinicians will prescribe a short-acting hypnotic, such as lorazepam 1 mg, 30 minutes to 1 hour prior to the procedure to help with relaxation.

Techniques and procedures vary considerably, but the "no-scalpel" method appears to provide the least postoperative discomfort and bleeding.[24,25] The results are highly dependent on the skill of the surgeon. The typical vasectomy tray is a minor surgery set with either a No. 15 blade or the no-scalpel instruments. The approach is either midline along the median raphe of the scrotum or bilateral with two separate entry points. Patient size and ease of isolation of the vas on each side may influence the preferred approach. Each vas may be located and isolated using the three-point method in which the vas is elevated with the thumb and forefinger above the scrotum and the middle finger beneath (Fig. 99.1). Anesthesia with 1% or 2% lidocaine without epinephrine is used to anesthetize the skin and is then extended to the cord structures around the vas, using 3 to 5 mL on each side. To grasp and isolate the vas deferens, operators will commonly use the no-scalpel clamp, small Allis forceps, or small towel clips.

When adequate anesthesia is obtained, the vas deferens is held in place with a towel clip or the no-scalpel fixation clamp

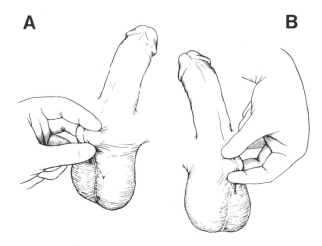

A   B

Fig. 99.1. Three-finger method for stabilizing the vas for a standard vasectomy. (Courtesy of the Association for Voluntary Surgical Contraception and David Rosenzweig. © 1991 American Urological Association Inc., with permission.)

and the surgeon releases the three-finger grip. With the clamp held parallel to the skin and tenting the vas tense against the skin, a scalpel or sharp dissecting forceps is used to pierce the scrotal skin and separate the layers down to the vas deferens. At this point a small hemostat or the sharp dissecting forceps may be used to separate the vas from its surrounding tissue. With the no-scalpel technique, the sharp tine of the forceps is used to skewer the vas and deliver it through the wound. The fixation clamp or towel clip is used to grasp the isolated vas, the forceps is introduced below the clamp, and with gentle pressure the vas is separated from its sheath for at least a 1-cm length.

The vas deferens is then incised and a small portion is removed. The prostatic end is typically cauterized using a small battery-powered cautery and is then allowed to retract within the sheath, which is then closed with an absorbable suture. The testicular end is usually left outside the sheath to prevent revascularization. Studies suggest that there is less postoperative congestion and discomfort if this end is left open. The entry site, if entered via the sharp dissecting instrument, may not need any suturing or the skin can be closed with one or several absorbable sutures. A small amount of antibiotic ointment may be applied and a gauze pad placed for both protection and pressure on the area.

After the procedure, postoperative care instructions include application of intermittent ice packs to the scrotum for eight to 12 hours, bed rest, and scrotal support for 48 hours and avoidance of any heavy lifting for at least 1 week. Sexual activity may be resumed when the patient feels well but he should remember that he is not sterile until at least 15 to 20 ejaculations after the procedure. A semen analysis should be performed at 6 to 8 weeks after the procedure and if no sperm are seen, birth control methods may be discontinued.

Potential complications of vasectomy include bleeding or hematoma (1–4%), incisional infection (2–6%), sperm granuloma (15–40%), and congestive epididymitis (0.4–6%).[22,24,25] Bleeding, the largest concern for both patient and physician, usually can be prevented through good surgical technique and careful patient instructions. Most hematomas can be controlled initially with ice packs and then with heat after the hematoma has organized. They rarely require surgical evacuation. Infections occur in less than 2% to 6% of procedures and most commonly are superficial wound infections, which are easily treated with suture removal and topical antibiotics.[26]

The Undescended Testicle

Cryptorchidism, or undescended testicle, is most commonly diagnosed as part of the routine newborn examination or during well-child care. The rationale for treatment of this fairly common condition is to prevent the adverse sequelae, including decreased fertility, testicular torsion, inguinal hernia, and neoplasms of the testicle.[27] While it is well documented that men with a history of undescended testicle have an increased incidence of testicular cancer, this risk is probably not as great as once thought, and while greater than the normal population, is in the range of 1:1000 to 1:2500 of males with this history.[28]

Most undescended testicles are present at birth and this condition is much more common in premature infants. Up to one third of premature males are born with an undescended testicle, while only 3% to 5% of term infants are affected.[29] By 3 months of age the incidence is reduced to 0.8% and does not change thereafter. Approximately 20% of infants who present with cryptorchidism have at least one nonpalpable testicle. Through surgical exploration, about one half of nonpalpable testicles are found to be intraabdominal, while the rest represent either absent or atrophic testicles.

Undescended testicles may either be "true" undescended testicles (including intraabdominal or anywhere along the normal anatomic path) or retractile, which are not truly undescended and require no therapy. The physical exam should include a general survey for syndromes that may be associated with cryptorchidism, including Prader-Willi, Kallmann's syndrome, or Laurence-Moon-Biedl. The genitalia should be examined carefully for hypospadias or ambiguity, signs that may point to gonadal dysgenesis or true hermaphroditism. The exam should be performed with the two-hand technique, one hand starts at the hip and sweeps along the inguinal canal, while the other palpates the scrotum. The retractile testicle will easily be moved into the scrotum, but may again retract, while the undescended testicle may be felt along the path. Urologic consultation may be required to distinguish the retractile from undescended testicle. If both testicles are nonpalpable, this may suggest a workup for congenital adrenal hyperplasia, including ultrasound and hormonal evaluations.

For the normal infant boy with a unilateral palpable undescended or nonpalpable testicle, referral to urology at 6 months is indicated. Treatment may involve hormonal manipulation with human chorionic gonadotropin or surgery, using laparoscopy or open exploratory surgery.[27]

References

1. Galejs LE, Kass EJ. Diagnosis and treatment of the acute scrotum. Am Fam Physician 1999;59:817–24.
2. Blaivas M, Batts M, Lambert M. Ultrasonographic diagnosis of testicular torsion by emergency physicians. Am J Emerg Med 2000;18:198–200.
3. Tumeh SS, Benson CV, Richie JP. Acute diseases of the scrotum. Semin Ultrasound CT MRI 1991;2:115–30.
4. Sidhu PS. Clinical and imaging features of testicular torsion: role of ultrasound. Clin Radiol 1999;54:343–52.
5. Rabinowitz R, Hulburt WC. Acute scrotal swelling. Urol Clin North Am 1995;22:101–5.
6. Kincade S. Testicular cancer. Am Fam Physician 1999;59: 2539–44.
7. Devesa SS, Blot WJ, Stone BJ, Miller BA, Tarone RE, Fraumeni JF. Recent cancer trends in thte United States. J Am Cancer Inst 1995;87:175–82.
8. Nicholson PW, Harland SJ. Inheritance and testicular cancer. Br Cancer J 1995;71:421–6.
9. Bosl GJ, Motzer RJ. Testicular germ-cell cancer. N Engl J Med 1997;337:242–53.
10. Diekmann KP, Becker T, Bauer HW. Testicular tumors: presentation and role of diagnostic delay. Urol Int 1987;42:241–7.
11. Moul JW, Paulson DF, Dodge RK, Walther PJ. Delay in diagnosis and survival of testicular cancer: impact of effective therapy and changes during 18 years. J Urol 1990;143:520–3.

12. Rowland RG, Foster RS, Donahue JP. Scrotum and testis. In: Adult and pediatric urology, Gillenwater JY, Howards SS, Grayhack JT, Duckett JW, ed., 3rd ed. St. Louis: Mosby, 1996;1917–49.

13. Einhorn LH Testicular cancer. In: Follow-up of Cancer: a handbook for physicians, Fischer DS, ed. 4th ed. Philadelphia: Lippincott, 1995;68–73.

14. Burnett AL. Erectile dysfunction: a practical approach for primary care. Geriatrics 1998;53:34–48.

15. Lawliss C, Cree J. Oral medications in the management of erectile dysfunction. J Am Board Family Pract 1998;11:307–14.

16. Epperly TD, Moore KE. Health issues in men: Part I. Common genitourinary disorders. Am Fam Physician 2000;61:3657–64.

17. Christakis DA, Harvey E, Zerr DM, Feudtner C, Wright JA, Connell FA. A trade-off analysis of routine newborn circumcision. Pediatrics 2000;105:246–9.

18. Lander J, Brady-Fryer B, Metcalfe JB, Nazarali S, Muttitt S. Comparison of ring block, dorsal penile nerve block, and topical anesthesia in neonatal circumcision. JAMA 1997;278:2157–62.

19. Stang HJ, Snellman LW. Circumcision practice patterns in the United States. Pediatrics 1998;101:E5.

20. Peleg D, Steiner A. The Gomco circumcision: common problems and solutions. Am Fam Physician 1998;58:891–8.

21. Choe JM. Paraphimosis: current treatment options. Am Fam Physician 2000;62:2623–26.

22. Clenney TL, Higgins JC. Vasectomy techniques. Am Fam Physician 1999;60:137–46.

23. Greek G. Vasectomy. Procedures in primary care. Postgrad Med 2000;108:173–9.

24. Bass R, Abdouch I, Halm D. et al. Office surgery. Monograph, edition no. 232, Home Study Self-Assessment Program. Kansas City, MO: American Academy of Family Physicians, September 1998.

25. Stockton MD, Davis LE, Bolton KM. No-scalpel vasectomy: a technique for family physicians. Am Fam Physician 1992;46:1153–64.

26. Raspa RF. Complications of vasectomy. Am Fam Physician 1993;48:1264–8.

27. Docimo SG, Silver RI, Cromie W. The undescended testicle: diagnosis and management. Am Fam Physician 2000;62:2037–44.

28. Pinczowski D, McLaughlin JK, Lackgren G, Adami HO, Perrson I. Occurrence of testicular cancer in patients operated on for cryptorchidism and inguinal hernia. J Urol 1991;146:1291–4.

29. Scorer CG, Farrington GH. Congenital deformities of the testis and epididymis. New York: Appleton-Century-Crofts, 1971.

100
Selected Disorders of the Genitourinary System

Evan A. Ashkin and David K. Ornstein

This chapter discusses genitourinary system disorders not addressed in prior chapters. There are three main topic areas covered: scrotal mass, including testicular and nontesticular scrotal pathology; urothelial tumors (bladder cancer); and urolithiasis.

Scrotal Mass

Some genitourinary (GU) disorders present as a scrotal mass and are commonly seen by family physicians for initial evaluation and management. These nontesticular masses include hydrocele, varicocele, indirect hernia, spermatocele and epididymitis, and testicular masses such as testicular cancer.

Nontesticular Masses

Hydrocele and Indirect Inguinal Hernia

In infants, hydroceles and indirect inguinal hernias are caused by incomplete obliteration of the processus vaginalis. This results in a collection of peritoneal fluid between the parietal and visceral layers of the tunica vaginalis surrounding the testicle. In a communicating hydrocele fluid freely flows between the peritoneal cavity and the tunica vaginalis. In a noncommunicating hydrocele there is obliteration of the processus vaginalis at some point between the peritoneal cavity and the tunic vaginalis. Hydroceles occur more frequently on the right and are often bilateral.[1]

Pediatric hernias are present in 10 to 20 per 1000 live births. Risk factors include prematurity and low birth weight. Eighty percent to 94% of newborns have a patent processus vaginalis; most close spontaneously by 1 to 2 years of age.[2] Sudden presentation in an adult of a noncommunicating hydrocele may be secondary to torsion, neoplasm, injury, or infection.

Hydroceles and indirect inguinal hernias usually present as a painless swelling in the groin or scrotum. On physical examination scrotal palpation shows a smooth mass ascending up the spermatic cord toward the external inguinal ring. With an upright position or Valsalva maneuver, hernia and noncommunicating hydrocele, as well as varicocele, will increase in size. Hydroceles are translucent by transillumination.

In the pediatric age group inguinal hernia or communicating hydrocele are indications for surgery. In infants noncommunicating hydroceles often spontaneously close by 1 to 2 years of age and should not be repaired until that time. Adult hydroceles require no treatment unless they are uncomfortable. Repair is the same for both hydrocele and inguinal hernia, being a high ligation of the patent processus vaginalis.

Varicocele

Dilated veins in the pampiniform plexus cause a varicocele. The majority are left sided resulting from higher pressures on the left compared to the right, as the left testicular vein drains into the renal vein, whereas the right drains into the vena cava. Varicoceles are present in 20% of men and occur in 30% of men being evaluated for infertility.[3] Repair is indicated for infertility and in adolescent boys if testicular growth arrest occurs. If onset in an adult is sudden for left-sided varicocele, consider renal tumor; if on the right, consider obstruction of the vena cava.

Physical examination reveals the classic "bag of worms" posterior and superior to the testicle. In adolescent boys evaluation of testicular size is important to determine the need for surgical correction. Sonography, a comparative orchidometer, or punched out elliptical rings can be used to determine size. A volume difference between the testicles of greater than 2 cm^3 is the minimal requirement for surgical repair.

Spermatocele and Epididymal Cyst

A spermatocele or epididymal cyst presents as a painless mass superior and posterior to the testicle and is completely separate from the testicle. It represents cysts of the rete testes, epididymis, or ductuli efferentes. It requires surgical removal only if enlarged and symptomatic.

Epididymitis

Epididymitis may cause a painful swelling of the testicle and is a common cause of a painful testicle in postpubertal males. Presentation is usually of increasing testicular pain and discomfort and can be accompanied by urethral discharge. On exam the epididymis is enlarged and may be indistinguishable from the testicle. The swelling is tender and may be indurated.

In prepubertal boys and men 35 years and older, bacterial urinary tract infection (UTI) is a common cause, probably secondary to prostatic reflux. In postpubertal boys and men younger than 35 years old, *Neisseria gonorrhoeae* and *Chlamydia trachomatis* are more common causes.

Treatment should be directed at the most likely cause. For suspected UTI, ciprofloxacin (Cipro) 500 mg orally twice daily for 10 to 14 days is usually adequate. In prepubertal boys an evaluation of the GU system to include urinary system sonography and a voiding cystourethrogram should be done.[4] When a sexually transmitted disease (STD) is suspected, adequate treatment can be provided with a single dose of ceftriaxone (Rocephin) 250 mg given intramuscularly (IM) to cover gonorrhea, and doxycycline (Vibramycin) 100 mg orally twice daily for 10 days to cover *Chlamydia*. No further workup is needed but one should offer STD prevention counseling as well as testing for syphilis and human immunodeficiency virus (HIV), and encourage the patient to contact sexual partners for treatment (see Chapter 41).

Testicular Masses

Testicular Torsion

Testicular torsion or torsion of the testicular appendages present as a painful testicle that is often enlarged or demonstrates a mass. These topics are covered in Chapter 99.

Acute Orchitis

Acute orchitis presents with sudden onset of testicular pain and high fever, and may be associated with nausea and vomiting. On exam the testicle is tender, enlarged, and may be indurated. Urinalysis may demonstrate proteinuria or hematuria.

Pyogenic bacteria and viral infections are the most common causes. Mumps orchitis occurs in 20% to 35% of cases of mumps parotitis and presents 3 to 4 days after onset of parotid symptoms.[3] Management of acute orchitis includes bed rest, scrotal support, ice, and analgesics. If a bacterial cause is suspected, appropriate antibiotics should be initiated. Spermatogenesis may be permanently diminished but infertility is rare, as only 15% of cases are bilateral.

Testicular Cancer

Epidemiology and Risk Factors

Although relatively infrequent, testicular cancer is the most common solid tumor among men between the ages of 20 and 34 years old. It is estimated that there will be 7200 new testicular cancers cases diagnosed in 2001 in the United States.[5] The most important risk factor for testicular cancer is cryptorchidism. Cryptorchidism increases testicular cancer risk 3- to 14-fold, and it has been estimated that 10% of testicular cancer patients have a history of cryptorchidism. Early orchidopexy (before 1 year of age) may reduce, but does not eliminate, this increased risk.

Pathology

Germ cell tumors account for more than 90% of all testes tumors, the majority of which are classified as pure seminomas or nonseminomas. Most nonseminomatous germ cell tumors are composed of a combination of the following histologic patterns: embryonal carcinoma, teratoma, teratocarcinoma, and choriocarcinoma.

The most common non–germ cell testicular tumors are Sertoli and Leydig cell tumors. The majority of these tumors are benign. Leydig cell tumors can present with sequelae of increased androgen production such as precocious puberty in boys and virilization in girls.

Diagnosis and Evaluation

All intratesticular masses should be considered a malignancy until proven otherwise. Patients with testicular masses should have a scrotal sonogram to confirm the presence of a solid intratesticular mass and to evaluate the contralateral testicle. For the most part, patients with intratesticular masses should undergo radical orchiectomy through an inguinal approach. There is no role for needle biopsy, and testicular masses should not be removed by a transscrotal approach. Prior to orchiectomy, patients should be evaluated with serum tumor markers, α-fetoprotein (AFP), and human chorionic gonadotropin (β-HCG). More than 90% of patients with nonseminomatous germ cell tumors have either an elevated AFP, β-HCG, or both. In contrast only 10% of seminomas are associated with an elevated β-HCG. AFP is never produced by pure seminomas, so patients with elevated an AFP should be treated as through they have nonseminomatous tumors.

Germs cell tumors spread sequentially to the retroperitoneal lymph nodes and then to other distant sites. Patients with a diagnosis of a germ cell neoplasm should be staged with an abdominal computed tomography (CT) scan and chest radiographs. Other serum markers such as lactate dehydrogenase (LDH) can provide useful prognostic information as well.

Treatment

The development of cis-platinum–based chemotherapy for testicular cancer has made cure possible in most cases. Today, treatment decisions are based on maximizing chance for cure while reducing treatment-related morbidities. The primary treatment for all testicular tumors is radical orchiectomy. Subsequent treatment depends on histology and clinical stage.

Seminoma is very sensitive to radiation, and effective doses can be delivered with minimal morbidity. Therefore, even though only 15% of patients with clinical stage I seminoma have micrometastatic lymph node involvement, it is recommended that most of these patients receive a low dose of adjuvant radiation to the retroperitoneum. Patients with lymph node metastasis <5 cm in diameter are also treated with radiation. Patients with bulky adenopathy ≥ 5 cm or distant disease, are treated with three to four courses of cis-platinum–based chemotherapy.

Nonseminomas are less sensitive to radiation than seminomas but respond very well to cis-platinum–based chemotherapy. Treatment options for stage I nonseminomas include retroperitoneal lymph node dissection (RPLND), surveillance, or primary chemotherapy.

Treatment recommendations are based on histologic features of the primary tumor as well as patient's desires to avoid treatment-related side effects. Approximately 30% of patients with clinical stage I disease have micrometastatic lymph node involvement, but the presence of more than 50% embryonal elements or lymphovascular invasion increases this risk to greater than 50%.[6] Although RPLND is a major surgical procedure, it can now be performed with minimal morbidity. Development of "template" dissection techniques preserves the sympathetic chain so that the patient's seminal emission and antegrade ejaculation will be retained.[7] Patients with pathologic stage II disease following RPLND are usually treated with two cycles of platinum-based chemotherapy. Observation protocols can achieve cure rates similar to that of RPLND but require intensive follow-up with serum markers, chest x-ray (CXR), and abdominal CT scan every 2 to 4 months for 2 years and yearly for an additional 3 years.[8] Another potential disadvantage of surveillance is that patients who develop recurrences require three to four rather than two cycles of chemotherapy. The addition of a third and fourth cycle increases morbidity substantially. Although excellent cure rates can also be achieved with primary chemotherapy, long-term morbidity has yet to be determined.

All patients with stage II or higher non-seminomas should be treated with three to four cycles of cis-platinum–based chemotherapy. Patients with persistently elevated tumor markers following orchiectomy are presumed to have residual metastatic disease and should be treated with chemotherapy. Those with residual retroperitoneal masses larger than 3 cm usually undergo a postchemotherapy RPLND.

Urothelial Tumors (Bladder Cancer)

Epidemiology and Risk Factors

It is estimated that in 2001, 54,300 people (39,200 men and 15,100 women) will be diagnosed with, and 12,400 people (8300 men and 4100 women) will die from, bladder cancer in the U.S.[5] Bladder cancer is the fourth most common noncutaneous malignancy among men in the U.S., representing 4% of all male cancer cases. Among women, bladder cancer is the eighth most common cancer and accounts for 2% of all cases diagnosed. The incidence of bladder cancer increases with age in men and women. The median age at the time of diagnosis is 69 years for men and 71 years for women.[9]

The most significant risk factor for bladder cancer is cigarette smoking. It has been estimated that cigarette smoking accounts for approximately 60% of all bladder cancer cases,[10]

and increases bladder cancer risk by 2.5-fold.[11,12] Occupational exposures can also be important risk factors for bladder cancer; aniline and other chemical dyes, combustion gases from coal, and heavy metals have all been implicated.[13] Consumption of large quantities of phenacetin-containing analgesics can lead to bladder cancer development as long as 25 years from the time of exposure. Although some have suggested that coffee and artificial sweeteners may increase bladder cancer risk, this has never been shown in a case-controlled epidemiologic study. Patients treated with cyclophosphamide (Cytoxan) have up to a ninefold increased risk, with a latency period of 6 to 13 years after the exposure.[14] Studies have shown that administration of 2-mercaptoethanesulfonic acid (Mesna) can reduce the carcinogenic properties of cyclophosphamide. Pelvic irradiation can also increase bladder cancer risk by as much as twofold.[15]

Pathology

The vast majority of bladder cancers diagnosed in the U.S. are transitional cell carcinomas. These tumors can manifest in a variety of growth patterns including papillary, sessile, nodular, and flat. Histologic grading is primarily based on the degree of anaplasia of the tumor cells. Multiple grading schemes have been used; most commonly tumors are grouped into three grades—low, moderate, and high. There is a strong correlation between tumor grade and stage, such that low-grade transitional cell carcinoma is most commonly superficial and high-grade tumors most commonly invasive. Histologic grade is also a strong predictor of tumor aggressiveness and the risk of disease progression with low-grade tumors is 10% compared to 50% for high-grade tumors. There is a strong correlation between histologic grade and stage. Carcinoma in situ (CIS) is characterized microscopically by cellular atypia confined to the urothelium. This premalignant lesion is the precursor lesion to a high-grade invasive bladder cancer and its presence in association with noninvasive tumor portends a poor prognosis.

Squamous cell carcinoma accounts for 3% to 7% of bladder cancers in the U.S.[9] and 80% in Egypt. Chronic infection with *Schistosomiasis haematobium* is the cause of most Egyptian bladder cancers. In nonendemic regions such as the U.S., squamous cell carcinoma of the bladder is most commonly the result of chronic irritation from long-term (many years) indwelling Foley catheter, chronic infections, or bladder diverticulum. Adenocarcinoma of the bladder is rare, accounting for fewer than 2% of all bladder cancers. Most commonly adenocarcinoma of the bladder develops from an urachal remnant or in patients who were born with bladder exstrophy.

Location

The vast majority of urothelial malignancies occur in the bladder. Upper tract (ureters and collecting system) tumors occur in 2% to 3% of patients with bladder tumors, while 30% to 75% of upper tract tumors have associated bladder tumors. Bilateral involvement occurs in 2% to 5% of all patients with upper tract transitional cell carcinomas.

Diagnosis and Staging

Hematuria is the most common presenting sign or symptom of bladder cancer. Other less common signs include urinary frequency, irritability, and dysuria. Although the vast majority of bladder cancers are associated with microscopic hematuria, the hematuria frequently is intermittent and a negative urinalysis does not exclude bladder cancer. All patients with hematuria should be evaluated with a urine cytology, cystoscopy, and intravenous urogram. Those with gross hematuria should be further evaluated with a renal sonogram or CT.

Cystoscopy is the primary diagnostic tool for bladder cancer, and the cystoscopic appearance of a tumor can usually provide significant diagnostic and prognostic clues regarding the grade and stage of the tumor. Low-grade superficial tumors appear as delicate fronds, while high-grade invasive tumors appear like a solid mass, usually with areas of necrosis. A transurethral resection is performed to confirm the diagnosis and to determine the tumor stage. The primary goal of staging is to determine if the cancer is superficial or invasive. Superficial tumors (Ta) are confined to the mucosal layer of the bladder while invasive tumors extend into the muscle (T2) or perivesicle fat (T3). Tumors extending into the submucosa or lamina propria (T1) are technically considered noninvasive, but since these tumors are likely to progress to "muscle invasive" disease these patients must be followed more closely than those with Ta tumors. Furthermore, since transurethral resection can frequently understage patients, particularly those with high-grade tumors, it is critical to biopsy an adequate sample of bladder muscle to reliably exclude the presence of muscle-invasive disease. Frequently patients with high-grade T1 disease are treated as if they had muscle-invasive disease.

CT examination of the abdomen and pelvis should be obtained in patients with muscle-invasive bladder cancer (T2 or higher) and/or high-grade disease to evaluate the perivesicle soft tissue, pelvic and retroperitoneal lymph nodes, as well as the liver and adrenal glands. CT scans are relatively unreliable in determining depth of tumor invasion and may fail to detect lymph node metastasis in up to 40% of patients with them.

Intravenous urograms or retrograde ureteropyelograms should be obtained in all patients with bladder cancer to exclude the presence of an upper tract transitional cell carcinoma.

Treatment

Superficial Disease

The majority of patients with superficial tumors can be effectively treated with transurethral resection alone. Patients with recurrent or multifocal superficial transitional cell carcinoma as well as those with CIS should receive adjuvant intravesical therapy. Bacille Calmette-Guérin (BCG) is the most effective and most commonly used form of intravesical immunotherapy.[16,17] A standard course of BCG consists of six weekly instillations. For those patients who fail a single course of BCG, a second course can be administered safely and effectively. Overall, BCG reduces tumor recurrences rates from around 50% to 20%. Among patients with CIS, BCG induces durable complete responses in 50% to 70% of cases. Some studies have shown that BCG may reduce progression rates and improve long-term survival among bladder cancer patients, but other studies have not. Intravesical chemotherapy can also be effective in reducing recurrences rates and the most commonly used agent is mitomycin C.

Invasive Disease

The standard treatment for muscle-invasive bladder cancer is radical cystoprostatectomy (removal of bladder, prostate, and seminal vesicles) for men and anterior exenteration (removal of bladder, uterus, ovaries, and cuff of vagina) in women. The recurrence rate after radical cystectomy is dependent on pathologic stage, but the overall 10-year recurrence free survival in contemporary series is 66%.[18,19] The early complication rate and perioperative mortality after cystectomy is 28% and 3%, respectively.[19] Partial cystectomy is rarely performed because of the high risk for local recurrence. Bladder salvage protocols that involve "aggressive" transurethral resection, external beam radiation, and chemotherapy have been evaluated, but to date long-term results are less favorable than for radical cystectomy.[20]

Urinary reconstruction following cystectomy is an important component in the management of patients with invasive bladder cancer. An ileal conduit is a small segment of ileum that is brought up to the abdominal wall as a stoma and allowed to drain freely into an appliance. Recently continent urinary diversions have become popular and there are a wide variety of types that use either small or large bowel or a combination of both. Continent cutaneous diversions involve creation of a catheterizable stoma on the abdominal wall. Orthotopic diversions in which the reservoir is connected directly to the native urethra provide the best opportunity to dramatically lessen the impact of cystectomy on quality of life. These diversions can be performed successfully in men and women. Radical cystectomy can be accomplished with preservation of the neurovascular bundles in men and the vagina in women. Thus normal urinary and sexual function can be retained despite curative therapy for invasive bladder cancer. The most common long-term complication from all types of urinary diversions is ureteroenteric anastomotic strictures, so patients must be followed closely for the development of hydronephrosis and/or deterioration of renal function. Patients with continent diversions can develop hyperchloremic metabolic acidosis and vitamin B_{12} deficiency.

Urolithiasis

Urolithiasis is a common problem that family physicians manage and need to distinguish from other causes of abdominal and flank pain. Conditions that may be similar to or mimic renal colic include cholecystitis, dissecting abdominal aortic aneurysm, appendicitis, diverticulitis, colitis, ovarian pathology, testicular pathology, ectopic pregnancy, hernia, constipation, and ureteral tumors.

Epidemiology

Lifetime risk of developing urolithiasis is approximately 12% in white males.[21] In the U.S. urolithiasis is twice as prevalent in the southeast.[22] It is two to three times more common in males than females, and affects Caucasians more than Asians and blacks. Incidence peaks between 30 and 50 years old and recurrence rates are as high as 40% to 75% over 25 years. Frequency of different stone types varies greatly with the population studied. In the U.S. calcium stones are by far the most common, with calcium oxalate stones accounting for 36% to 76%, and calcium phosphate stones accounting for 6% to 20%. Less common are mixed type, magnesium ammonium phosphate (struvite), uric acid, and least common cystine stones.[22]

Etiology

Diseases such as primary hyperparathyroidism, type 1 renal tubular acidosis (RTA), Crohn's disease, primary hyperoxaluria, and cystinuria are associated with recurrent urolithiasis but account for less than 5% of patients with stone disease. An etiology for urolithiasis can be determined 97% of the time after an appropriate workup. Etiologies of urolithiasis are listed in Table 100.1. Metabolic abnormalities account for the majority of disease. Sixty percent of calcium stone disease is caused by idiopathic hypercalciuria. Hyperuricosuria, followed by hypocitraturia and hyperoxaluria, are the next most common metabolic abnormalities causing disease. Medications that may also play a role in stone disease include indinavir (Crixivan), acetazolamide (Diamox), and triamterene (Dyrenium).

Presentation

Urolithiasis causes pain when a stone partially or completely obstructs the collecting system or ureter. Distal ureteral stones may be associated with dysuria, frequency, and penile or labial pain. Classically the patient presents with severe, colicky, unilateral flank or lower abdominal pain. The pain may radiate to the groin, scrotum, or labia, and be associated with nausea and vomiting. Fever is present when associated with UTI.

Evaluation

A thorough history including present symptoms, medical history (gouty diathesis, bowel disease), medications (prescriptions, over the counter, and supplements), diet, and family history of stone disease or related illnesses is necessary. Phys-

Table 100.1. **Etiologies of Urolithiasis**

Idiopathic hypercalciuria (absorptive types I and II)
Renal hypercalciuria
Unclassified hypercalciuria
Cystinuria
Primary hyperparathyroidism
Hyperuricosuria
Gouty diathesis
Infection lithiasis
Renal tubular acidosis type 1
Hypocitraturia
Hypomagnesuria
Hyperoxaluria

ical exam should focus on the flank, abdomen, groin, and genitals, and pay careful attention to other possible diagnoses. Urinalysis with urinary pH and microscopic examination for crystals should be done and urine culture obtained to evaluate for coexistent infection. Diagnostic imaging is the next step in evaluation. Where available, unenhanced helical CT is the test of choice with reported sensitivity of 95% to 100% and specificity of 94% to 96% in diagnosing urolithiasis. Advantages of this imaging technique include avoidance of intravenous contrast, short duration (approximately 5 minutes to perform), ability to visualize all stone types, localization of stone within the ureter, identification of secondary signs of obstruction when a stone has recently passed, and ability to diagnose other abdominal and pelvic pathology when urolithiasis is not present.[23] Using Hounsfield density helical CT allows one to differentiate uric acid, cystine, and calcium-containing stones from one another, and to subtype calcium stones.

Plain radiography has numerous limitations in the initial workup of urolithiasis. Only calcium containing stones are radiopaque and calcifications seen on plain radiograph may or may not be associated with the urinary system. Sensitivities as low as 59% have been reported for plain radiography in detecting urolithiasis.

Intravenous urography (IVU) has been the standard for the diagnosis of urolithiasis and when unenhanced helical CT is unavailable remains the imaging study of choice. IVU can usually detect ureteral obstruction based on dilation of the collecting system or ureter, a delayed nephrogram or delayed excretion of contrast. IVU is limited in that signs of obstruction may not appear acutely, radiolucent stones cannot be visualized, and many other causes of abdominal pain cannot be evaluated. Intravenous contrast is necessary when performing an IVU and can cause postcontrast nephropathy and numerous systemic reactions. Ultrasound can play a role in visualizing dilation of the collecting system but has poor sensitivity for detecting stones in the ureter.

Approach to Management

Once a diagnosis of acute urolithiasis has been established, management is directed by the location and size of the stone as well as complicating factors such as urosepsis or renal failure. Immediate urologic consultation is recommended in the setting of urolithiasis with urosepsis, anuria, or renal failure, as well as with refractory pain and overall poor medical status. Patients with urosepsis require immediate drainage by percutaneous nephrostomy or retrograde ureteral stent insertion. In the absence of the conditions stated above, stone size determines the next step. Ureteral stones with a width of ≤5 mm can be managed conservatively and when 4 mm or less will spontaneously pass in 80% of patients. Patients with ureteral stones >5 mm in width require urologic consultation as rates of spontaneous passage are only 35% and fall to 25% when stones are 7 mm in width.

Patients with stones <5 mm in width may be selected for conservative management. Adequate analgesia and maintaining urine volumes greater than 2 L a day are essential. Patients should be instructed to strain their urine and bring in any stones for analysis and should follow up immediately for symptoms of urosepsis. Stone passage may be monitored with weekly plain radiographs, and a urologic referral made if stones are not passed within 4 to 6 weeks.

Analgesia

Adequate control of pain often requires a combination of nonsteroidal antiinflammatory drugs (NSAIDs) and narcotics. Commonly used NSAIDs include ketorolac (Toradol) 10 mg orally every 4 to 6 hours, diclofenac (Voltaren) 50 mg orally every 8 hours, ibuprofen (Motrin, Advil) 800 mg orally every 8 hours, aspirin 650 mg orally every 4 hours, and indomethacin (Indocin) 50 mg orally every 8 hours. NSAIDs must be held for 3 days prior to extracorporeal shock-wave lithotripsy (ESWL) because of antiplatelet effects and risk of bleeding and aspirin should be held for 7 days prior to ESWL. The newer cyclooxygenase-2 inhibitors may also be effective for analgesia with less antiplatelet effects. Narcotics used for breakthrough pain include meperidine (Demerol) 50 mg orally every 3 to 4 hours as needed, hydrocodone 10 mg with acetaminophen 500 mg (Lortab 10/500) orally every 4 to 6 hours as needed, oxycodone 5 mg with acetaminophen 325 mg (Percocet 5/325) orally every 4 to 6 hours as needed, and codeine 30 mg with acetaminophen 300 mg (Tylenol with codeine No. 3) orally every 4 to 6 hours as needed. An antiemetic such as promethazine (Phenergan) 25 mg orally every 4 to 6 hours may also be helpful.

Urologists have a number of different modalities available for stone removal or destruction, when such intervention is needed. Stone location and size will determine the optimal procedure. ESWL is a minimally invasive procedure effective for calculi <1 cm in the ureter and <2 cm in the kidney. Basket retrieval through a cystoscope or ureteroscope is indicated for lower ureteral stones not amenable to ESWL. Larger stones may be treated with percutaneous nephrolithotomy alone or in combination with ESWL. Staghorn renal calculi should always be treated because of their high complication rates. Asymptomatic renal stones do not require treatment but become symptomatic in 50% of patients over 5 years.

Metabolic Evaluation

All patients with stone disease should have a basic workup to identify underlying metabolic or environmental factors causing stone formation. A more extensive workup is recommended for patients with recurrent stone disease and initial stone disease with risk factors (family history of stones, gout, nephrocalcinosis, bowel disease, concomitant UTI).[24]

Pak and Resnick[24] suggest a four-step evaluation process for a thorough workup and a one-step minimum evaluation for all patients. Minimal evaluation should include urinalysis with urine culture, stone analysis when possible, and serum calcium, phosphorus, uric acid, creatinine, and electrolytes. When stone analysis confirms a cystine stone, cystinuria is diagnosed. Struvite stones are diagnostic of infection lithiasis. Uric acid stones indicate hyperuricosuria or a condition associated with low pH such as gout or chronic diarrhea. Cal-

cium phosphate stones are seen with primary hyperparathyroidism, RTA, and sodium alkali therapy. Calcium oxalate stones, which are the most common, are seen in numerous conditions and of less help in confirming a diagnosis. Primary hyperparathyroidism will show elevated serum calcium and low phosphate. RTA is associated with hypokalemia and metabolic alkalosis. Gouty diathesis is often associated with elevated serum uric acid.

Step two, when indicated, includes a 24-hour urine collection for a stone risk profile (commercially available) on a patient's customary diet. The stone risk profile includes urine calcium, oxalate, uric acid, citrate, pH, total volume, sodium, sulfate, phosphorus, magnesium, and urinary saturation of calcium oxalate, brushite, monosodium urate, and uric acid.

Step three involves dietary modifications based on the results of step two and an increase of fluid intake to maintain a urine volume of >2 L a day. After 1 week the stone risk profile is repeated. Dietary modifications include a sodium restriction of 200 mEq daily for all patients. If urinary oxalate is >45 mg per day, patients should avoid tea, spinach and dark roughage, chocolate, and nuts, and take no more than 500 mg of vitamin C daily. When urinary calcium is >250 mg per day, a moderate calcium restriction is recommended. Protein intake should be limited if uric acid levels are >700 mg per day or if sulfate levels are >30 mmol per day. When urinary pH, citrate or potassium are low, patients should be instructed to increase intake of potassium-rich citrus fruits like grapefruit, orange, and cranberry.

In step four the two completed stone profiles are compared, and if abnormalities are corrected by dietary modification and increased hydration, then environmental changes are recommended. If abnormalities persist, then patients are determined to be metabolic, and appropriate treatment is initiated.

Treatment

All patients are recommended to drink a minimum of 2 L of fluid a day, eat a diet high in potassium-rich citrus fruits, and to restrict intake of protein, oxalate, and sodium.

Hypercalciuria

Patients with hypercalciuria (>250 mg per day) associated with hypercalcemia should be evaluated for primary hyperparathyroidism. When hypercalciuria is seen with excess urinary sodium, dietary restriction of sodium 100 mEq per day is recommended. Absorptive hypercalciuria or renal hypercalciuria are the probable causes when the above-mentioned conditions are not present. Both can be treated with thiazides such as trichlormethiazide (Metahydrin) 4 mg daily with potassium citrate 20 mEq twice daily. Doses of potassium citrate may be adjusted based on follow-up serum potassium and urinary citrate levels.

Hyperoxaluria

Hyperoxaluria (>45 mg per day), if not secondary to excess intake of oxalate, is seen with inflammatory bowel disease, small bowel resection, and intestinal malabsorption of fat. Dietary restriction of oxalate is the main form of treatment.

Hypocitraturia

Mild to moderate hypocitraturia (100–320 mg per day) is usually secondary to high intake of animal proteins and is best treated with dietary restriction and potassium citrate 20 mEq twice daily. Severe hypocitraturia (<100 mg per day) is seen with chronic diarrhea and complete distal RTA. Correction of the diarrhea should be attempted and potassium citrate 20 to 40 mEq twice daily may be given.

Hyperuricosuria

Hyperuricosuria (>700 mg per day) without elevated serum uric acid is found with excess intake of purines from animal protein. Along with dietary modification, allopurinol (Zyloprim) 300 mg daily and potassium citrate may be useful in preventing further stones. Elevated serum uric acid with hyperuricosuria and low urinary pH is found in patients with gouty diathesis. Allopurinol 300 mg daily, along with potassium citrate if urinary pH is low, are recommended (also see Chapter 123).

Prevention of Urolithiasis

By taking a thorough history that includes medical conditions, diet, and family history, physicians can identify patients at risk for urolithiasis. These patients should be advised to maximize fluid intake; avoid dehydration; moderate sodium, protein, and oxalate intake. These patients warrant special attention when placed on medications that are known to increase their risk for stone disease.

References

1. Kapur P, Caty MG, Glick PL. Pediatric hernias and hydroceles. Pediatr Clin North Am 1998;45:773–89.
2. Skoog SJ. Benign and malignant pediatric scrotal masses. Pediatr Clin North Am 1997;44:1229–49.
3. Junnila J, Lassen P. Testicular masses. Am Fam Physician 1998; 57:685–92.
4. Galejs LE, Kass EJ. Diagnosis and treatment of the acute scrotum. Am Fam Physician 1999;59:817–24.
5. Greenlee RT, Hill-Harmon MB, Murray T, Thun M. Cancer statistics 2001. CA 2001;51:15–36.
6. Levin HS. Prognostic features of primary and metastatic testis germ-cell tumors. Urol Clin North Am 1993;20:39–53.
7. Foster RS, Donohue JP. Retroperitoneal lymph node dissection for the management of clinical stage I nonseminoma. J Urol 2000;163:1788–92.
8. Lowe BA. Surveillance versus lymphadenectomy in stage I nonseminomatous germ-cell tumors. Urol Clin North Am 1993;20: 75–83.
9. Lynch CF, Cohen MB. Urinary system. Cancer 1995;75:316–9.
10. Brennan P, Bogillot O, Cordier S, et al. Cigarette smoking and bladder cancer in men: a pooled analysis of case controlled studies. Int J Cancer 2000;15:289–94.
11. Cohen SM, Shirai T, Steineck G. Epidemiology and etiology of premalignant urothelial changes. Scand J Urol Nephrol 2000; 205:105–15.
12. Chiu BC, Lynch CF, Cerhan JR, Cantor KP. Cigarette smoking and risk of bladder, pancreas, kidney, and colorectal cancers in Iowa. Ann Epidemiol 2001;11:28–37.
13. Sadetzki S, Densal D, Blumstein T, Novikov I, Modan B. Selected risk factors for transitional cell bladder cancer. Med Oncol 2000;17:179–82.
14. Vlaovic P, Jewett MA. Cyclophosphamide-induced bladder cancer. Can J Urol 1999;6:745–8.
15. Sella A, Dexeus FH, Chong C, Ro JY, Logothetis CJ. Radiation therapy-associated invasive bladder tumors. Urology 1989; 33:185–8.
16. Catalona WJ, Ratliff TL. Bacillus Calmette-Guerin and superficial bladder cancer: clinical experience and mechanisms of action. Surg Ann 1990;22:263–7.
17. Malkowicz SB. Intravesical therapy for superficial bladder cancer. Semin Urol Oncol 2000;18(4):280–8.
18. Stein JP, Lieskovsky G, Cote R, Groshen S, Feng AC, Boyd S. Radical cystectomy in the treatment of invasive bladder cancer: long-term results in 1,054 patients. J Clin Oncol 2001;19: 666–75.
19. Dalbagni G, Genega E, Hashibe M, et al. Cystectomy for bladder cancer: a contemporary series. J Urol 2001;165:1111–6.
20. Dunst J, Rodel C, Zietman A, Schrott KM, Sauer R, Shipley WU. Bladder preservation in muscle-invasive bladder cancer by conservative surgery and radiochemotherapy. Semin Surg Oncol 2001;20:24–32.
21. Portis AJ, Sundaram CP. Diagnosis and initial management of kidney stones. Am Fam Physician 2001;63:1329–38.
22. Saklayen MG. Medical management of nephrolithiasis. Med Clin North Am 1997;81:785–99.
23. Smith RC, Levine J, Rosenfeld AT. Helical CT of urinary tract stones. Radiol Clin North Am 1999;37:911–52.
24. Pak CY, Resnick MI. Medical therapy and new approaches to management of urolithiasis. Urol Clin North Am 2000;27: 243–53.

101

Family Planning and Contraception

Grant M. Greenberg and Barbara S. Apgar

Hormonal Contraception

Oral Contraceptives Pills (Combined Dose)

The suppression of follicle-stimulating hormone (FSH) by oral contraceptive pills (OCPs) is caused by the negative feedback of ethinyl estradiol (EE) on the pituitary. Implantation is inhibited by altered development of the endometrium, rendering it less favorable for implantation. Cervical mucus also thickens, making it more difficult for sperm penetration. The first year failure rate for typical users is 3%. Smoking may impair the effectiveness of OCPs through an antiestrogenic effect, and escape ovulation could occur.[1]

Over 1 million unintended pregnancies are related to OCP use, misuse, or discontinuation. Depending on the population, discontinuation rates may be high by the end of the first year especially if abnormal bleeding is present. Smokers who use OCPs with 20 to 30 μg of EE report spotting or bleeding at a significantly higher rate than nonsmokers.[2] Therefore, smokers may be more likely to discontinue OCPs and incur higher rates of unintended pregnancy.

Since OCPs were first marketed, the amounts of estrogen and progesterone have been significantly reduced. This is important because adverse reactions are dose-related. The amount of estrogen most commonly administered is 30 to 35 μg of EE daily. The ultralow-dose OCPs containing $\leq$20 μg of EE were introduced to address the continuing concern that the dose of estrogen is related to the risk of myocardial infarction (MI), stroke, and venous thromboembolism (VTE). The decrease in cardiovascular risk has to be balanced with an acceptable efficacy rate. In a study of 1708 women taking a low-dose OCP (100 μg levonorgestrel, 20 μg EE), 18 pregnancies occurred during 26,554 cycles, of which six were due to subject noncompliance.[3] Results of this study provided evidence that reducing the estrogen and progestin dose did not compromise contraceptive efficacy. The overall safety profile of the ultralow-dose regimens is similar to OCPs containing 35 μg of EE. The ultralow-dose OCPs also provide menstrual cycle control equivalent to that obtained with triphasic combinations and a 75% higher EE dose.[4]

Cancer

Concern about cancer remains a significant reason why women fear taking OCPs. Protection of OCPs against some gynecologic cancers is largely unknown by the public. The conclusion of an analysis of 54 epidemiologic studies is that there is no overall association between breast cancer and OCP use.[5] Age of user, duration of use, dosage, and family history were not found to be associated with breast cancer risk. A 40% decrease in the incidence of epithelial ovarian cancer in OCP users has been observed.[6] Results suggest that 5 years of OCP use by nulliparous women can reduce their ovarian cancer risk to that of parous women who never used OCPs. Women who used OCPs for at least 12 months have an age-adjusted relative risk of endometrial cancer of 0.6.[7] Significant controversy exists about the association, if any, of OCPs with cervical cancer. Much of the early data were confounded because of the failure to control for the presence of human papillomavirus. OCPs may increase the risk of adenocarcinomas of the cervix more than squamous disease.[8]

Cardiovascular Disease and OCPs

Women who smoke and use OCPs have the highest risk of death from cardiovascular (CV) disease.[9] The risk of death attributable to smoking among young women not using OCPs is approximately 16 times higher than the risk attributable to OCP use in nonsmokers. From these data, it is recommended that women older than 35 should not use OCPs if they smoke. Even heavy smokers who use low-dose OCPs carry the same risk as those using higher-dose OCPs. The low-dose OCPs do not reduce the risk in heavy smokers, and the current warning on OCP package inserts is still appropriate.

Many of the current recommendations are based on studies of older higher dose OCPs and in women with significant risk factors for CV disease. Current use of low-dose OCPs appears to be unrelated to an increased risk of MI among non-smokers and even light smokers, but users who smoke heavily are at greatly increased risk.[10] In a pooled analysis of women aged 18 to 44 with incident MI who had no prior history of ischemic heart disease or CV disease, there was no evidence of an increased risk of MI associated with use of low-dose OCPs.[11] In the one study that found a five-fold increased risk of MI associated with current OCP use, the increased risk probably reflected the more frequent use of OCPs by women with CV risk factors who had undergone less screening such as routine blood pressure evaluations.[12] In the pooled analysis data, there was no evidence of interaction between current OCP use and cigarette smoking, in contrast with earlier studies performed with higher-dose OCPs. The discrepancy between the results of the World Health Organization (WHO) study and the pooled U.S. studies may reflect unmeasured hypertension among smokers in the WHO study.

There is an increased risk of VTE among OCP users.[13] In 1995, three case-control studies linked the use of OCPs containing desogestrel or gestodene with an increased risk of nonfatal VTE compared to those containing levonorgestrel. This represented an increase of 10 to 15 cases of VTE in nonusers of OCPs to 20 to 30 cases per 100,000 in women using these formulations. A fourth study evaluated 12 OCP formulations and demonstrated no risk differences of VTE among the various OCPs including those containing gestodene and desogestrel. The minor changes in levels of the natural anticoagulant proteins sometimes observed with OCP use may be insufficient to trigger thrombosis unless an inherited clotting defect exists. In summary, OCPs containing the third-generation progestins appear to produce minor effects on coagulation and present a relatively low thrombotic risk to non-smokers with no clotting defects.

The risk of developing deep vein thrombosis (VT) appears to be greatest in the first 6 months and the first year of OCP use.[13] Women who developed VT in the early periods of use were more often thrombophilic, which increased the risk 19-fold in the first 6 months. Women with inherited clotting defects who used OCPs more often and sooner developed VTs. However, the inherited clotting defects explain only part of the effect. When women continue to use OCPs, their risk of developing VT does not disappear and is also present in those who have no inherited defect.

The American College of Medical Genetics recommends factor V Leiden testing in women with recurrent VT or VT in unusual sites and those with VT during pregnancy or while using OCPs.[14] Testing for prothrombin 20210A and plasma homocysteine levels should also be included. Mutations in the prothrombin gene and the factor V gene are associated with cerebral thrombosis.[15] The use of OCPs is strongly and independently associated with cerebral-vein thrombosis. The presence of the prothrombin gene mutation and OCP use increases the risk of cerebral-vein thrombosis by a factor of 20. It is recommended that carriers of the prothrombin gene mutation who have had an episode of thrombosis discontinue

Table 101.1. Noncontraceptive Benefits of Oral Contraceptive Pills (OCPs)

Decreased rate of hospitalization for pelvic inflammatory disease
Decreased rate of fibrocystic breasts and fibroadenomas
Decreased rate of functional ovarian cysts
Decreased rate of dysfunctional uterine bleeding and anemia
Increased bone mass density in patients with amenorrhea
Protection against uterine and ovarian cancer

OCPs. Asymptomatic carriers should be counseled about alternative methods of contraception.

A meta-analysis was performed on 16 studies evaluating the association between ischemic stroke and OCP use.[16] Eleven studies showed a significant association between current OCP use and ischemic stroke risk. The risk persisted for low-estrogen preparations in population-based studies that controlled for smoking and hypertension, suggesting that current OCP use is a risk factor for ischemic stroke. The analysis also indicated that the ischemic stroke risk of OCP use is independent of smoking, hypertension, migraine history, and age. Based on these data, an OCP user's annual stroke risk would be expected to increase from 4.4 to 8.5 per 100,000 cases. This increased risk must be balanced with the known health benefits of OCP use (Table 101.1).

Combination Injectable Contraceptive Agents

The once-a-month injectable contraceptive agent containing a progestin and an estrogen provides a safe contraceptive option and an alternative for women who wish to use injectable formulations that cause less disruption of normal bleeding patterns. The Food and Drug Administration (FDA)-approved medroxyprogesterone acetate (MPA) /estradiol cypionate (E2C) combination (Lunelle-Pharmacia and Upjohn) contains 25 mg of MPA and 5 mg of E2C suspended in 0.5 mL of an aqueous solution that is administered within the first 5 days after the onset of menses. Repeat injections are administered every 28 days. E2C is a long-acting ester of estradiol that delays the hormonal degradation and produces more regular withdrawal bleeding. Because this preparation contains only 25 mg of MPA, it is cleared more rapidly from the circulation allowing faster return to fertility than depomedroxyprogesterone acetate (DMPA).

The efficacy of this combination results from the inhibition of follicle maturation, ovulation, and formation of the corpus luteum. The failure rate has been reported as 0.1 pregnancies per 100 woman years. More than 1150 women from 13 countries received MPA/E2C in a WHO-sponsored study, with 731 women completing the 12-month trial.[17] Two pregnancies were reported. Efficacy rates are unaffected if the injection is administered within 5 days before or after the 28-day period. The first postpartum injection should be administered within 4 to 6 weeks after delivery. If switching from OCPs, the first injection of MPA/E2C can be given during the active pills or within 7 days of the last active pill. If switching from DMPA, the first injection should be administered within 13 weeks of the last DMPA injection. Patient acceptability is high, with 84% of users reporting a favorable opinion of the method. Fertility rates after discontinuing

MPA/E2C are comparable to those achieved following discontinuation of OCPs.

MPA/E2C is associated with a significantly lower incidence of ovarian follicular development compared to an OCP containing 20 μg ethinyl estradiol and 0.1 mg levonorgestrel.[18] Withdrawal bleeding occurs within 10 to 20 days after injection. After discontinuation of the injections, ovulation typically resumes in about 60 to 90 days. More than two thirds of women have regular cycles, and discontinuation due to bleeding-related problems occurred half as often as with DMPA. For women with DMPA-induced amenorrhea, switching to MPA/E2C resulted in monthly withdrawal bleeding in 82% of the women after 6 months of use.[19]

Progestational Agents

Progestin-only pills (POPs) are less effective than OCPs, with failure rates varying from 1.1 to 9.6 pregnancies per 100 women in the first year of use.[20] The POPs show high efficacy for lactating women and do not decrease milk production, as OCPs do. However, there are very few studies on the effects of POPS on lactation when administered prior to the sixth postpartum week. Since progesterone withdrawal is the likely stimulus that initiates lactation, it appears that progesterone levels should decline to baseline before POPs are started. Therefore, use of POPs should be delayed for at least 3 days after delivery. To be effective, POPs must be taken at exactly the same time each day.

Depomedroxyprogesterone Acetate (DMPA)

The injectable contraceptive agent, DMPA or Depo-Provera, has a typical failure rate of 1 per 100 woman years.[20] One of the reasons for the high efficacy rate is that each 150-mg injection provides 3 months of protection followed by a 4- to 6-week grace period before the next injection. Amenorrhea, secondary to endometrial atrophy, occurs in over 90% of women who use DMPA for more than 2 years.[21] Use of DMPA does not result in irreversible suppression of ovulation, but patients need to clearly understand that there may be a delay in return to fertility. It has also been demonstrated that DMPA produces a systemic hypoestrogenic state. DMPA can be safely initiated immediately postpartum with the first injection given within 5 days of delivery

The amenorrhea produced by DMPA was a frequently cited reason for continuation of the method by adolescents. Adolescents using DMPA also have lower incidence of repeat pregnancy at 12 months postpartum than those using OCPs. However, 93% of adolescents using DMPA reported that side effects including weight gain, nausea, and irregular menstrual cycles were the reason for discontinuation of contraception.[22] There appears to be an association between depressive symptoms and DMPA use that seems to subside on discontinuation.[23] Given all side-effect profiles, women who were told to return to the clinic if side effects occurred were 2.7 times more likely to continue using DMPA than women who did not receive that advice.[24] As for any contraceptive method, health care providers play an important role in ensuring the highest possible continuation rates for DMPA.

The reported loss of bone density with use of DMPA is concerning, but because of methodologic flaws in the research (variation in age of subjects, duration of use, use of other medication, and cigarette smoking) it is difficult to extract meaningful data. It is well established, however, that a decrease in ovarian function and a consequent reduction in estrogen secretion cause an increase in bone turnover that results in a decrease in bone density. Therefore, it is suggested that the suppression of ovulation and the reduction in estrogen production by DMPA could be the principal mechanism by which users exhibit a lower bone density than nonusers. In a cross-sectional study of 200 DMPA users, the bone density was significantly lower in DMPA users whether they were smokers or not.[25] The impact of DMPA on bone density might be greatest in adolescents and women with very long-term use and in heavy smokers. At the present time, no specific change in recommendations is warranted. However, clinicians need to make cautious recommendations for DMPA use in adolescents who may be at particular risk for bone loss, such as those who have hypoestrogenic amenorrhea.

Subdermal Contraceptive Implants

Subdermal contraceptive implants (Norplant) are inserted directly under the skin and provide effectiveness for 5 years. Studies have shown a pregnancy rate of 0.6/100 woman years after 1 year and a cumulative rate of 1.5/100 woman years at 5 years.[26] Users with heavier body weight experience higher pregnancy rates. For continuing implant users, annual pregnancy rates <1.0/100 in years 6 and 7, together with low cumulative pregnancy rates, demonstrate that contraceptive implants remain highly effective for 7 years. Levonorgestrel is released from each of the capsules at a steady rate. The primary mechanism of action is suppression of ovulation, although not as much as seen in DMPA users. This may be due to sporadic surges and withdrawals of estradiol, which contribute to abnormal bleeding patterns. Duration of use of the Norplant device does not affect the future pregnancy rate, and discontinuation results in normal fertility.

Despite the fact that 50% of women experience 8 or more days of continuous bleeding during the first 6 months of use, acceptability is high as indicated by a 1-year continuation rate of 93.7% of those reporting excessive bleeding.[27] It appears that the rate of menstrual disturbances peaks at 73% after 3 months and consistently decreases to 20% after 5 years.[28] If the endometrium is especially atrophic, more irregular bleeding can be expected. Levonorgestrel, EE, and ibuprofen were administered to women experiencing 8 or more consecutive days of bleeding or spotting during a 2-week period.[28] Each of the active drugs decreased the bleeding and spotting per treatment interval better than placebo. The duration rather than the frequency of bleeding was the most significantly reduced.

A new single 4-cm-rod contraceptive implant (Implanon) containing 58 mg of etonogestrel (3-keto desogestrel) is being studied for use in the U.S. Initially, 67 μg etonogestrel is released daily. A major advantage is that it can be placed with a large-bore needle so that an incision is unnecessary. Implanon was inserted in a mean time of 0.61 minutes compared with a Norplant insertion requiring 3.9 minutes.[29] Typically, implant removal through an incision appears to be fast and uncomplicated. Women exposed to Implanon for 644 women-years experienced no pregnancies during the 2-year study period.

Implanon is associated with acceptable bleeding patterns, although bleeding irregularities are the primary reason for discontinuation during the first 2 years of use.[30] Compared with Norplant users, women with Implanon experienced fewer irregular bleeding episodes and a higher rate of amenorrhea. Bone mineral density does not appear to decrease during use.

Intrauterine Contraceptive Devices

The intrauterine contraceptive device (IUCD) has not increased in popularity despite testimony to its effectiveness and safety. The reticence partially stems from media coverage of problems with the Dalkon Shield, which was associated with pelvic inflammatory disease (PID) due to multifilamented strings that are no longer used in IUCDs. The decision to discontinue marketing most IUCDs was based on an economic decision rather than a medical one.

There has been false belief that the mode of action of the IUCD is as an abortifacient. Research has demonstrated that the IUCD exerts its effects by interfering with the reproductive process before fertilization occurs. The rate of recovery of eggs from tubal flushings in women with and without IUCDs at known intervals after the midcycle peak of luteinizing hormone (LH) demonstrated that no fertilized eggs were recovered from the uterine cavities of any IUCD users.[31] It has been postulated that the copper IUCD stimulates a foreign-body inflammatory response that may cause toxicity to both the spermatocytes and oocytes. A 98.7% increase in the numbers of inflammatory cells in endometrial washings 18 weeks after insertion of an IUCD has been demonstrated.[32] The progesterone IUCDs produce a less pronounced foreign-body response.

Currently there are three types of IUCD marketed in the United States: the TCU 380A (ParaGard), a progesterone-releasing IUCD (Progestasert), and the most recent levonorgestrel releasing IUCD (Mirena). The Mirena IUCD releases 20 mcg per day of levonorgestrel and can remain in place for up to 5 years. It has a similar side effect and efficacy profile to Progestasert. Older IUCDs such as the copper T and Lippes loop, even though they are not marketed currently, are FDA-approved and need not be removed prematurely unless the patients develop problems associated with their use.

The T-shaped IUCD was developed to conform to the shape of the uterine cavity when it is tightly contracted, thereby minimizing distortion of the uterine wall. Adding copper wire around the stem increases the effectiveness. The ParaGard has copper wrapped around each of the horizontal arms and around the stem and retains its effectiveness for at least 10 years. The Progestasert releases 65 mcg of progesterone daily, which is sufficient to prevent pregnancy but not enough to cause an increase in serum progesterone. Because the progesterone in the device is depleted after 18 months, the Progestasert must be replaced annually. The Progestasert may reduce the amount of cramping and uterine blood flow, but there are no data available from randomized controlled trials to support this indication. However, good evidence is available for the use of the levonorgestrel releasing IUCD (Mirena) as an effective and well-tolerated treatment for menorrhagia.[33]

Optimal candidates for IUCDs are women who have had at least one child, are in a mutually monogamous relationship, are at low risk for sexually transmitted disease, and do not desire permanent sterilization. Nulliparity is not an absolute contraindication. The presence of sexually transmitted disease carries the highest probability of complications. The clinician should be thoroughly familiar with the manufacturer's package insert information. The patient and clinician must both sign the informed consent. The IUCD may be inserted anytime during the menstrual cycle if the patient is not pregnant. Concern about PID and uterine perforation has limited this procedure in the past, but available evidence implies safety and efficacy despite package labeling to the contrary.[34] Approximately 2% of women spontaneously expel the IUCD during the first year.

Patients who are not candidates for an IUCD include those who have an acute pelvic infection or a history of PID, have had previous surgery that might predispose to ectopic pregnancy, have uterine anomalies resulting in distortion of the uterine cavity, or who have known or suspected genital carcinoma. Specific contraindications to the ParaGard include Wilson's disease and allergy to copper. Neither device should be inserted in a uterus that sounds less than 6.5 cm from the external os. Although use of the IUCD in women with type II or non–insulin-dependent diabetes mellitus is not recommended in the current product labeling for the ParaGard, more recent studies do not support this recommendation. Users of Progestin IUCDs have a markedly higher ratio of ectopic to normal pregnancies, varying inversely with dose. Copper and nonmedicated IUCDs have age-specific ectopic pregnancy rates six times those of controls.

An association between PID and IUCD use has been well documented. The mechanism appears to be direct spread of microorganisms to the fallopian tubes. However, it appears that the risk of PID has been overestimated by methodologic errors in earlier case-controlled studies. In fact, recent meta-analyses have supported previous assertions that IUCD-associated PID occurs more frequently in women with preexisting genital infection, but there is no increased risk in uninfected women.[35] The actual risk of PID may be quite low even in the presence of sexually transmitted diseases (STDs).[36] The risk of PID after insertion of an IUCD falls to baseline by 5 months after insertion. PID acquired more than 4 months after insertion appears to be due to acquisition of a new STD. The administration of prophylactic antibiotics at the time of insertion may not influence the rate of PID in low-risk populations.[37]

Actinomycotic PID is associated with IUCD use. *Actinomyces* species identified on a Papanicolaou (Pap) smear of an IUD user should be investigated, although the relation between a Pap smear positive for *Actinomyces* and the eventual development of pelvic actinomycosis is unclear. There is no evidence of the need to treat the asymptomatic patient with *Actinomyces* on Pap smear with antibiotics. Removing the IUCD and repeating the cytology in 2 months to verify clearance of the organism should allow the patient to have the IUCD reinserted at that time. Symptomatic patients should be treated with parenteral antibiotics and have the IUD removed.

Although menorrhagia is associated with copper IUD use, women appear to tolerate an increased menstrual blood loss without developing anemia. Prostaglandin synthetase inhibitors administered during menstruation have been shown to decrease the blood loss significantly.

A uterine length of more than 7.0 cm and good insertion technique are associated with a decreased risk of removal due to bleeding and pain. Perforation rates are reported to occur in 1/1000 IUCD insertions and are generally related to the force exerted during insertion. If the IUCD cannot be located inside the uterus, an ultrasound study is performed. Any IUCD located outside the uterus is electively removed by laparoscopy. Severe peritoneal reactions can occur if an abdominal IUCD is not removed. If the IUCD is found to be located in the uterus but no string is visible, a cylindrical brush used for obtaining a Pap smear can be used to extract the IUCD string.[38]

The incidence of spontaneous abortion in a patient who conceives with an IUCD in place is about 55%, about three times greater than controls. If the IUCD is removed, the incidence decreases to 29%. When compared to hormonal methods of contraception, short-term users of IUCDs show a quicker return to fertility after discontinuation of the method. However, long-term IUCD use (greater than 6 years) appears to be associated with fertility impairment, especially in nulliparous women.[39]

Barrier Contraceptives

Diaphragm

The contraceptive diaphragm is a dome-shaped rubber cup attached to a flexible rim. The rim enables the dome to make a tight seal with the vaginal wall to provide a barrier to sperm and infectious agents. The diaphragm also prevents cervical mucus from neutralizing vaginal acidity, so the vaginal environment remains hostile to the sperm. The diaphragm is inserted in the vagina before intercourse so the posterior rim rests behind the cervix in the posterior fornix and the anterior rim fits snugly behind the symphysis pubis. Spermicidal jelly, placed into the dome and around the rim before insertion, helps create a seal between the diaphragm rim and the vaginal wall.

Diaphragms are manufactured in four shapes to accommodate the anatomic variance of the female pelvis. They differ in the construction of the diaphragm rim. The *arcing spring* diaphragm has a strong rim and spring. This diaphragm arcs when folded and makes insertion easy. The arcing diaphragm can be worn by most patients, even those with a cystocele, rectocele, or laxity of the muscle tone. The *coil spring* diaphragm has a strong rim and spring. This diaphragm folds

flat for insertion and can be used with a plastic introducer. Most patients who have average muscle tone and pubic arch can wear the coil spring. The *flat spring* diaphragm has a thin delicate rim and strength. A woman with strong muscular support may be able to wear this diaphragm easier than the flex or coil rim. It folds flat for insertion and may be used with an introducer. The *wide seal* diaphragm has a flap of soft rubber attached to the inner edge of the rim that creates a tight seal with the vaginal wall. The rubber flap also helps keep the spermicide inside the diaphragm. This diaphragm is not available by prescription and is available only from the manufacturer.

Diaphragms must be properly fitted to be effective. Diaphragms that are too big or too small are not effective in preventing pregnancy. A change in size may be needed after pregnancy or with the gain or loss of significant weight. A wide discrepancy exists among reported failure rates of 1.0 to 19.4 per 100 woman-years.[40] The risk of failure is approximately doubled when the user is younger than 30 or has intercourse four or more times per week. Despite women being motivated and properly instructed, it has been demonstrated that the pregnancy rate is higher during the first year with continuation rates at 12 months of only 35%.

Diaphragm type and duration of use may affect the risk of urinary tract infections (UTIs). Too large a diaphragm may increase the risk by encouraging incomplete or infrequent urination. The longer the diaphragm is worn beyond the recommended time, the greater is the risk of residual urine. Toxic shock syndrome has been reported when the diaphragm is worn longer than 36 hours.

Condoms

The condom is the oldest form of barrier contraception and is gaining in popularity because of its safety and protection from STDs. The greatest increase in condom purchases occurred in 1987 after the U.S. Surgeon General's report on acquired immunodeficiency syndrome (AIDS) was released. When used properly and consistently, the effectiveness of the condom is better than 97% alone or 99% with use of vaginal contraception.[40] The ability of the condom wall to maintain its integrity throughout intercourse is critical to its effectiveness. It has been demonstrated that condom breakage occurs in approximately 1 of 100 acts of intercourse. Factors associated with breakage included vaginal intercourse and minimal foreplay, and breakage also occurred prior to ejaculation. Data from a longitudinal study indicate that when condoms are consistently used during heterosexual intercourse when one partner is human immunodeficiency virus (HIV)-positive and the other is seronegative, transmission of HIV is effectively prevented.[41] However, inconsistent use of condoms resulted in a seroconversion rate of 12.7% after 24 months of exposure.

The female condom is a polyurethane pouch that lines the vagina and covers the cervix and vulva by the application of flexible rings at each end. Theoretically it is an effective barrier contraceptive, but the typical 6-month failure rate has been reported to be as high as 15% to 26%. The female condom was marketed with little supporting data on its effectiveness as a barrier contraceptive. The FDA has required that product labeling state that the male condom is the method of choice for preventing STDs.

Spermicides

Spermicides are used in conjunction with other forms of contraception, namely the diaphragm and condom. Spermicides are rarely used as single contraceptive agents despite the fact that they are simple to use and readily available. Spermicidal agents consist of two components: (1) an inert base (foam, cream, jelly, suppository, tablet) that ensures dispersion and holds the spermicidal agent in the vagina; and (2) the spermicidal agent, usually nonoxynol-9. Nonoxynol-9–containing spermicides are generally considered to have minimal side effects. If used perfectly, the initial-year failure rate among perfect users is 3%, but the initial-year failure rate among typical users is about 21%.[40] Consistent use is the most important factor in preventing pregnancy. Nonoxynol-9 may protect against transmission of both gonorrhea and chlamydial infections, especially when condoms are used consistently.

Surgical Contraception

Tubal Ligation

Sterilization remains the most common method of family planning by married women. Almost 50% of female sterilization procedures occur while women are hospitalized for another surgery or childbirth. A "posttubal sterilization syndrome" that includes alterations of menstrual flow, exacerbation of premenstrual symptoms, and pelvic pain has been reported after tubal ligation.[42] The early literature was flawed and did not take into account that many women undergoing tubal ligations had recently discontinued OCPs or IUCDs and that they might have been returning to menstrual patterns that existed prior to use of their current contraceptive method.

Vasectomy

Vasectomy remains a safe, effective, but often overlooked method of contraception. Performed as an outpatient procedure, it has a very low complication rate. Concerns about associations with prostate and testicular cancer in vasectomized men are unfounded, with the weight of recent evidence suggesting no increased risk.[43] Most men achieve azoospermia within 4 months of the procedure, with long-term sterility greater than 99%.[44]

Natural Family Planning

Natural family planning methods may be useful for those who wish to avoid hormonal, barrier, and surgical methods of contraception. The basis for these methods involves abstinence from intercourse during periods of fertility, and requires either recognition or detection of ovulation and the assumption that ovulation occurs only once during the same menstrual cycle. Methods of ovulation detection may incorporate charting cervical mucus changes (the ovulation method), a combination of mucus charting, symptom identification, and confirmation of a rise in basal body temperature to confirm postovulatory infertility (the symptothermal method), and more recently urinary testing for luteinizing hormone levels.

The Creighton Model Natural Family Planning System is a standardized system of teaching couples how to perform the method accurately. Proponents of the natural family planning model cite the absence of side effects of artificial methods of contraception, the benefits of increased communication between partners, and the opportunity to explore aspects of the sexual relationship other than intercourse. Pregnancy rates with this method can be as low as 0.14/100 couples.[45] This method is not opposed by any religious organization, but does require motivated couples, careful education, and close follow-up to optimize efficacy. The lactation-amenorrhea method is useful only for women who are less than 6 months postpartum and are exclusively breast-feeding.[46] It is based on the idea that the elevated prolactin levels that occur with consistent breast-feeding inhibit ovulation. The standard days method involves periodic abstinence from days 8 to 19 of each menstrual cycle and requires regular menstrual cycles between 26 and 32 days in length.

It is difficult to determine the effectiveness of the natural family planning methods. Reported pregnancy rates can vary anywhere between 2% and 30%. A number of reasons account for the wide variability in the data. The classification of pregnancies that occurred while a specific method was used was not consistent and the same method of ovulation prediction was not used. Use-effectiveness could have been taken to mean method failures or desired pregnancy results.

Postcoital (Emergency) Contraception

Postcoital contraception, also known as emergency contraception or the "morning-after pill," has been found to reduce the rates of unwanted pregnancy after unprotected intercourse associated with contraceptive failure (e.g., breakage of a condom). The original method, the Yuzpe regimen, involves the use of combined OCPs to provide 100 μg EE and 0.5 mg of levonorgestrel in two doses 12 hours apart within 72 hours of unprotected intercourse. The first dose is taken as soon as possible after the unprotected intercourse so the term "morning-after pill," if not clarified, may be misunderstood by the patient. Most studies have recommended treatment within 72 hours to increase efficacy. However, use up to 5 days after unprotected intercourse provides significant contraceptive benefit, and later presentation for emergency contraception should not prohibit its use.[47] When used properly, emergency contraception can reduce the risk of unintended pregnancy by at least 74%.

The primary mode of action of the morning-after pill does not appear to be ovulation suppression, the production of a luteolytic effect, tubal transport modification, or an embryotoxic effect. It appears that the mechanism of action is modification of the nidation site, making it unsuitable for implantation. However, because of the variability in research

Table 101.2. **Emergency Contraception Options**

Pill brand	Pills per dose	EE per dose (μg)	Levonorgestrel per dose (mg)
Alesse	5 pink	100	0.50
Levlen	4 light-orange	120	0.60
Levlite	5 pink	100	0.50
Levora	4 white	120	0.60
Lo/Ovral	4 white	120	0.60
Nordette	4 light-orange	120	0.60
Ovral	2 white	100	0.50
Ovrette	20 yellow	0	0.75
Plan B	1 white	0	0.75
Preven	2 blue	100	0.50
Tri-Levlen	4 yellow	120	0.50
Triphasil	4 yellow	120	0.50
Trivora	4 pink	120	0.50

All regimens involve two doses, 12 hours apart.
EE = ethinyl estradiol.

designs, it is difficult to draw firm conclusions. It has been suggested that the depression of progesterone-associated endometrial protein by high-dose ethinyl-norgestrel administration could affect the immunosuppressive capability of the gestational endometrium and enhance rejection of the implanting fetus.

The only World Health Organization contraindication to use of postcoital contraception is pregnancy, while FDA contraindications include known coronary artery disease, clotting disorders, and history of thromboembolic disease. However, side effects related to the high dose of estrogens are common, such as nausea, vomiting, dizziness, and fatigue. Providing an antiemetic agent such as meclizine 50 mg 1 hour prior to each dose has been shown to effectively relieve some of the gastrointestinal symptoms. If vomiting occurs within a short time of pill ingestion, consideration should be given to readministering the regimen. The use of a progestin-only method (levonorgestrel 0.75 mg in two doses 12 hours apart) has been found to have lower rates of side effects with comparable efficacy.[48] Whichever regimen is selected, a consistent method of contraception should be utilized until the next menstrual period. The menstrual period following use of the emergency contraception may be abnormal. If menses fails to occur within 3 weeks after emergency contraception, a pregnancy test should be obtained. Multiple regimens are known to be effective (Table 101.2)

References

1. Vessey MP, Villard-Mackintosh L, Jacobs HS. Anti-estrogenic effect of cigarette smoking [letter]. N Engl J Med 1987;317:769.
2. Rosenberg MJ, Waugh MS, Long S. Unintended pregnancies and use, misuse and discontinuation of oral contraceptives. J Reprod Med 1995;40:355–60.
3. Archer DF, Maheux R, DelConte A, et al. Efficacy and safety of a low-dose monophasic combination oral contraceptive containing 100 μg levonorgestrel and 20 μg ethinyl estradiol (Alesse). Am J Obstet Gynecol 1999;181:s39–s44.
4. Reisman H, Martin D, Gast MJ. A multicenter randomized comparison of cycle control and laboratory findings with oral contraceptive agents containing 100 μg levonorgestrel with 20 μg ethinyl estradiol or triphasic norethindrone with ethinyl estradiol Am J Obstet Gynecol 1999;181:s45–s52.
5. Collaborative Group on Hormonal Factors in Breast Cancer. Breast cancer and hormonal contraceptives: collaborative re-analysis of individual data on 53,297 women with breast cancer and 100,239 women without breast cancer from 54 epidemiologic studies. Lancet 1996;347:1713–27.
6. Gross TP, Schlesselman JJ. The estimated effect of oral contraceptive use on the cumulative risk of epithelial ovarian cancer. Obstet Gynecol 1994;83:419–24.
7. The Cancer and Steroid Hormone Study of the Centers for Disease Control and the National Institute of Child Health and Human Development. Combination oral contraceptive use and the risk of endometrial cancer. JAMA 1987;257(6):796–800.
8. Thomas DB, Ray RM. Oral contraceptives and invasive adenocarcinomas and adenosquamous carcinomas of the uterine cervix. The WHO Collaborative Study of Neoplasia and Steroid Contraceptives. Am J Epidemiol 1996;144:281–9.
9. Schwingle PJ, Ory HW, Visness CM. Estimates of the risk of cardiovascular death attributable to low-dose oral contraceptives in the United States. Am J Obstet Gynecol 1999;180:241–9.
10. Rosenberg L, Palmer JR, Rao RS, Shapiro S. Low-dose oral contraceptive use and the risk of myocardial infarction. Arch Intern Med 2001;161:1065–70.
11. Sidney S, Siscovick DS, Petitti DB, et al. Myocardial infarction and use of low-dose oral contraceptives. A pooled analysis of 2 US studies. Circulation 1998;98:1058–63.
12. WHO Collaborative Study of Cardiovascular Disease and Steroid Hormone Contraception. Acute myocardial infarction and combined oral contraceptives: results of an international multicentre case-control study. Lancet 1997;349:1201–9.
13. Bloemenkamp KW, Rosendaal FR, Helmerhorst FH, Vandenbroucke JP. Higher risk of venous thrombosis during early use of oral contraceptives in women with inherited clotting defects. Arch Intern Med 2000;160:49–52.
14. American College of Medical Genetics. New guidelines for factor V Leiden testing. Genet Med 2001;3:139–48.
15. Martinelli E, Sacchi E, Landi G, et al. High risk of cerebral-vein thrombosis in carriers of a prothrombin gene mutation and in users of oral contraceptives. N Engl J Med 1998;1793–7.
16. Gillum LA, Mamidipudi SK, Johnston SC. Ischemic stroke risk with oral contraceptives. A meta-analysis. JAMA 2000;284:72–8.
17. WHO Task Force on Long-Acting Systemic Agents for Fertility Regulation, Special Programme of Research, Development and Research Training on Human Reproduction. A multicentered phase III comparative study of two hormonal contraceptive preparations given once-a-month by intramuscular injection. I: comparative efficacy and side effects. Contraception 1988;37:1–20.
18. Jain JK, Ota F, Mishell DR. Comparison of ovarian follicular activity during treatment with a monthly injectable contraceptive and a low-dose oral contraceptive. Contraception 2000;61:195–8.
19. Piya-Anant M, Koetsawang S, Patrasupapong N, et al. Effectiveness of Cyclofem in the treatment of depot medroxyprogesterone acetate induced amenorrhea. Contraception 1998;57:23–8.
20. Trussel J, Kost K. Contraceptive failure in the United States: a critical review of the literature. Stud Fam Plann 1987;18:237–83.
21. Mishell DR. Pharmacokinetics of depot medroxyprogesterone acetate contraception. J Reprod Med 1996;41(suppl):381–90.
22. O'Dell CM, Forke CM. Polaneczky MM, et al. Depot medroxyprogesterone acetate or oral contraception in postpartum adolescents. Obstet Gynecol 1998;91:609–14.
23. Civic D, Scholes D, Ichikawa L, et al. Depressive symptoms in

users and non-users of depot medroxyprogesterone acetate. Contraception 2000;61:385–90.

24. Hubacher D, Goco N, Gonzalez B, Taylor D. Factors affecting continuation rates of DMPA. Contraception 1999;60:345–51.

25. Cundy T, Cornish J, Roberts H, Elder H, Reid IR. Spinal bone density in women using depot medroxyprogesterone contraception. Obstet Gynecol 1998;92:569–73.

26. Su-Juan G, Ming-Kun M, Ling-De Z, et al. A 5-year evaluation of Norplant contraceptive implants in China. Obstet Gynecol 1994;83:673–8.

27. van Amerongen D. Removal rates of subdermal levonorgestrel implants. J Reprod Med 1994;39:873–6.

28. Diaz S, Croxatto NB, Pavez M, et al. Clinical assessment of treatments for prolonged bleeding in users of Norplant implants. Contraception 1990;42:97–109.

29. Zheng SR, Zheng HM, Qian SZ, Sang GW, Kaper RF. A randomized, multicenter study comparing the efficacy and bleeding pattern of a single-rod (Implanon) and a six-capsule (Norplant) hormonal contraceptive implant. Contraception 1999;60: 1–8.

30. Croxatto HB, Urbancsek J, Massai R, Bennink C, van Beek A. A multicentre efficacy and safety study of the single contraceptive implant, Implanon. Hum Reprod 1999;14:976–81.

31. Alvarez F, Brache V, Fernandez E, et al. New insights on the mode of action of intrauterine contraceptive devices in women. Fertil Steril 1988;49:768–73.

32. Moyer DL, Mishell DR. Reactions of human endometrium to the intrauterine foreign body. Am J Obstet Gynecol 1971;111: 66–79.

33. Lethaby AE, Cooke I, Reese M. Progesterone/progestogen releasing intrauterine systems versus either placebo or any other medication for heavy menstrual bleeding. Cochrane Database Systematic Reviews 2000;issue 2.

34. Grimes D, Schulz K, Stanwood N. Immediate post-abortal insertion of intrauterine devices. Cochrane Database Systematic Reviews 2000;issue 2.

35. Grimes DA. Intrauterine device and upper genital tract infection. Lancet 2000;356:1013–19.

36. Shelton JD. Risk of clinical pelvic inflammatory disease attrib-utable to an intrauterine device. Lancet 2001;357:443–6.

37. Grimes DA, Schulz KF. Prophylactic antibiotics for intrauterine device insertion: a meta-analysis of the randomized trials. Contraception 1999;60:57–63.

38. Ben-Rafael Z, Binder D. A new procedure for removal of a "lost" intrauterine device. Obstet Gynecol 1996;87:785–6.

39. Doll H, Vessey M, Painter R. Return of fertility in nulliparous women after discontinuation of the intrauterine device: comparison with women discontinuing other methods of contraception. Br J Obstet Gynaecol 2001;108:304–14.

40. Craig S, Hepburn S. The effectiveness of barrier methods with and without spermicide. Contraception 1982;26:347–59.

41. DeVincenzi I for the European Study Group on Heterosexual Transmission of HIV. A longitudinal study of human immunodeficiency virus transmission by heterosexual partners. N Engl J Med 1994;31:341–6.

42. Shain RN, Miller WB, Mitchell GW, et al. Menstrual pattern change 1 year after sterilization: results of a controlled, prospective study. Fertil Steril 1989;52:192–203.

43. Schwingle PJ, Guess HA. Safety and effectiveness of vasectomy. Fertil Steril 2000;73:923–36.

44. Haldar N, Cranston D, Turner E, MacKenzie I, Guillebaud J. How reliable is a vasectomy? Long-term follow-up of vasectomized men. Lancet 2000;356:43–4.

45. Howard MP, Stanford JB. Pregnancy probabilities during use of the Creighton model fertility care system. Arch Fam Med 1999; 8:391–402.

46. Tommaselli GA, Guida M, Palomba S, Barbato M, Nappi C. Using complete breastfeeding and lactational amenorrhea as birth spacing methods. Contraception 2000;61:253–7.

47. Rodrigues I, Grou F, Joly J. Effectiveness of emergency contraceptive pills between 72 and 120 hours after unprotected sexual intercourse. Am J Obstet Gynecol 2001;184:531–7.

48. Task Force on Postovulatory Methods of Fertility Regulation. Randomized controlled trial of levonorgestrel versus the Yuzpe regimen of combined oral contraceptives for emergency contraception. Lancet 1998;352:428–33.

102
Vulvovaginitis and Cervicitis

Mary Willard

Although modern medical practice has often relegated vaginal symptoms to the realm of the specialist gynecologist, the range of symptoms and diagnoses covered under this category with the concomitant preventive health and risk management issues is ideally suited to the expertise of the family physician. Excellence in the diagnosis and management of these diseases is the standard of care and can be achieved with a minimal investment of equipment, time (a 1-minute slide examination), and cost to the patient. Patients with vaginal complaints account for an estimated 10% of office visits each year,[1] and many more may be inaccurately diagnosed by phone. This chapter reviews the systematic approach to the evaluation and treatment of vaginal diseases as well as issues of particular interest to family physicians.

Diagnostic Assessment

It is critical for the family physician to remember that few complaints are more annoying to the female patient than vaginal itching and discharge. Tolerance of low-grade symptomatology is the norm for some patients until a flare turns the problem into a midnight emergency. Although the history and physical examination are helpful, only appropriate testing can make the diagnosis.

Laboratory Equipment and Technique

The equipment needed for accurate diagnosis of vaginal complaints is simple: saline in small containers, nonsterile cotton-tipped applicators, slides, coverslips, a good microscope with 10× and 40× capacity (i.e., low- and high-dry power), 10% potassium hydroxide solution (KOH) preparation, diagnostic tests for *Chlamydia* and gonococci, and a small magnifying lens. Vaginal fluid should be examined as soon as possible after the fluid is obtained, as *Trichomonas vaginalis* is fragile and may die quickly.

The technique of examining vaginal fluid is straightforward. After inserting the vaginal speculum, a plain cotton-tipped applicator is swept into the vaginal fluid, withdrawn (preferably with a "clump" of discharge), and placed immediately into a small container with only 1 mL of saline. Small pediatric red-topped tubes containing saline can be kept in all rooms where pelvic examinations may be performed so they are immediately available. For maximal results, the smallest amount of saline and the largest sample of vaginal fluid should be used. Once the sample of vaginal fluid is obtained, cervical cultures can be prepared if necessary, the pelvic examination completed, and the saline examined.

The vaginal fluid in saline is examined microscopically using gloves as per universal precautions. Take the cotton applicator from the tube and place a drop of fluid on two slides, one for the saline examination and one for a KOH preparation. If a diagnosis of yeast is being entertained, it is critical to try to get a "clump" of the discharge onto the designated KOH slide. A drop of a 10% KOH solution (made by mixing 90 mL distilled water with 10 g KOH) is dropped on it and immediately smelled for a fishy odor, which may be an indicator of bacterial vaginosis. If further evaluation for hyphae is to be done, place a coverslip and allow the slide to sit until the saline slide is examined. The KOH destroys some of the vaginal epithelial and white blood cells (WBCs), leaving only hyphae for inspection.

Next examine the saline slide with coverslip under low power. Search for motion of cells, sheets of epithelial cells compatible with denuding of mucosa, or "clue cells." The latter are vaginal epithelial cells "studded" with bacteria that adhere for unknown reasons. These epithelial cells look dense and tend to glitter when the focus is varied. Although clue cells are present normally in up to 10% of the field, a preponderance of them, especially when combined with a fishy odor on the KOH preparation, supports the diagnosis of bacterial vaginosis.[2]

Once the examination under low power is completed, it is appropriate to scan the field under high-dry power to check for *T. vaginalis* and to better examine the epithelial cells. Trichomonads appear as motile triangular cells, somewhat larger than WBCs, with long moving tails. Because many bacteria are part of the normal vaginal ecosystem and are nonpathogenic,[3] Gram stains and routine cultures are not first-line tests for diagnosing vaginal diseases. If the high-power field has more than 10 WBCs, consider the possibility of an upper genital tract infection.

If an examination for yeast is necessary, place the KOH preparation under the microscope. Hyphae and spores are best seen on this specimen by focusing under low power to find a "clumped" area and then going immediately to high-dry power and focusing on the edges of the clump. The clumped material usually represents epithelial cells and hyphae tissue not desiccated by the KOH preparation; the edge of the clump is the best place to identify the hyphae. Certainly if the history so warrants and the cervical os reveals discharge from above, appropriate tests for *Chlamydia*, gonococci, or both are performed.

When analyzing vaginal complaints, few tests other than those noted above are needed except in specific circumstances or in refractory cases (which are discussed in relevant sections). One area of controversy is the role of vaginal pH tests. Because the premenopausal vaginal ecosystem keeps the pH under 4.5, assessment of change might be of some value. Although sensitive, this test is not specific and can be influenced greatly by fluids from the cervix, by semen, or by douching. It has, therefore, limited application in the office. There is also investigation into the use of monoclonal antibodies and DNA analysis. Unfortunately, none of these tests is of sufficient reliability to replace the simple slide evaluations.

History

As with any clinical problem, the history is a critical clue to diagnosis and must be obtained methodically from each patient. The ambiguous nature of the problem, however, means that the diagnosis cannot be made solely on historical clues, such as a "cheesy" discharge. Most women can, with minimal clarification by the physician, reveal a clear history of their complaint. Because there is individual variation in the amount and character of the vaginal discharge that is "normal," the family physician role is to help patients distinguish a change from that pattern. Ask about skin lesions, internal or external itching, odor, dyspareunia, and the use (and frequency) of douching, new soaps, or deodorant sprays. Always inquire about previous similar episodes, but ask how these diagnoses were made, especially in the patient treated over the phone. Many patients who state that they "always get yeast infections" have never had an accurate diagnosis made, and any vaginal cream has the potential of calming an inflamed mucosa (thereby diminishing the symptoms until the next flare).

One of the most commonly missed presentations of vaginitis is the complaint of dysuria (see Chapter 95). Treating all patients with dysuria as cystitis results in the inevitable phone call 48 to 72 hours later from a patient who is no better. Because women with vulvitis complain of pain externally with urination, clarification of the type of dysuria at the initial encounter assists in determining which patients require additional evaluation for vaginitis.

It is essential that the family physician obtain a complete sexual history from these patients and assess them for risk of sexually transmitted diseases (see Chapter 41). If the patient is sexually active, the physician should inquire about any new spermicidal agents or condoms, symptom complaints from a partner(s), a new sexual partner, and sexual practices. Moreover, the patient should be educated about sexual practices that minimize risk of disease.

Physical Examination

Although the pelvic examination can be tailored by the history, patients with vaginal complaints must be evaluated systematically. The external genitalia are thoroughly assessed for clues using a hand-held magnifying lens if necessary. The urethra, labia, and vulvae are completely checked for ulcerations, warts, tears, cysts, abscesses, erythema, and edema. Additionally, the vaginal mucosa itself must be inspected for color, lesions, and edema. Normal vaginal mucosa is pink with moist folds. A fiery red or weepy mucosa is a sign of inflammation. Any plaque-type lesions are scraped for adherence to vaginal mucosa, a sign of possible candidiasis.

As part of the complete evaluation, observe the cervical os for pus as a cause of discharge. Using a large cotton swab (e.g., one used for proctoscopic examinations), clean the cervix of all discharge, and observe the os for a short time, usually 10 seconds. If purulent fluid appears at the os opening from above, it is an indicator of upper pelvic infection for which *Chlamydia* and gonococci must be tested. At this point, a bimanual examination should also be performed to assess adnexal tenderness or masses.

Clinical Presentation

It is impossible, given the constraints of space, to discuss all possible forms of vaginitis or other vaginal diseases. Instead, the focus here is on the more common etiologies and important vaginal skin diseases that may masquerade as "itch." This approach assists in clarifying most vaginal complaints.

Traditional medical training clearly defined the classic presentations for vaginitis. Unfortunately, this "eyeball" method correctly diagnoses only one third of the cases,[4] making thorough clinical evaluation necessary (Fig. 102.1). Nevertheless, an appreciation of the textbook presentations is necessary when teasing apart the significant historical details given by the patient. It is equally important to realize the change in epidemiology of vaginitis since the 1970s. The most common cause of vaginitis is now bacterial vaginosis, followed by mycotic diseases (e.g., *Candida* sp.), and then trichomoniasis.[5] Whatever the reason for this shift, knowledge of the probabilities is useful.

Contact and Chemical Dermatitides

Contact and chemical dermatitides are much overlooked diagnoses for the patient with vulvitis. Any topical agent used

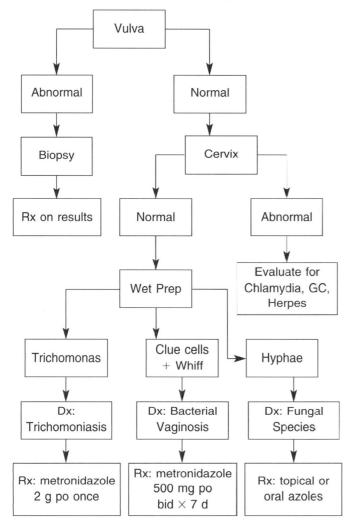

Fig. 102.1. Diagnostic algorithm for vaginal symptoms. Dx = diagnosis; GC = gonococcus; Rx = treatment.

in the genital area (including nonoxynol-9 and rubber in condoms) can be an allergen. A reddened, swollen vulva or a vaginal mucosa exuding a clear exudate characterizes this problem. Equally important is the patient who has been douching repeatedly and with increasing frequency. This practice sets up a denuding phenomenon that inflames and strips the mucosa. The appropriate treatment for this category of inflammation is to discontinue the product and consider using a short-term course of topical external steroids for symptomatic relief.[6]

Mycotic Diseases

Although the incidence is rising,[5] contrary to popular belief among patients and physicians, true fungal infections probably account for approximately one third of all vaginal infections. The textbook presentation is a patient complaining of a vaginal itch and cheesy exudate, with white plaques adherent to the vaginal wall and a KOH preparation showing multiple hyphae. The diagnosis should not be made unless hyphae are seen on the slide. Because as many as 20% of asymptomatic women have positive cultures,[7] it is obvious that culture methods are too sensitive and should be reserved for refractory cases,[8] frequent relapses, or when yeast is suspected clinically but the KOH preparation is negative. In this case, suspect *Candida glabrata*, which may present with vaginal burning and, as a spore former, can be diagnosed only on Gram stain. This infection is often refractory to the standard duration of treatment and may require protracted therapy.[6]

Yeast infections typified by *Candida albicans* have been erroneously ascribed to many causes. For example, yeast infections probably do not occur any more frequently in diabetic women but may be more difficult to eradicate.[6] Therefore, consider diabetes in the patient with chronic infections, not frequent ones. There is also little proved association between yeast infection and use of birth control pills.[9] For frequent relapses, consider treating the sexual partner(s) to achieve full eradication and changing the patient's diet, as high calories and crude fiber have been associated with susceptibility to infection.[10] Remember, too, that women with human immunodeficiency virus (HIV) disease may manifest persistent or diffuse candidiasis as a presenting symptom (see Chapter 42).

Treatment is straightforward and consists of either topical azole applications or an oral one-time dose of fluconazole (Diflucan).[11] To date, no data prove oral routes to be superior and they are associated with side effects such as headache, drug reactions, and gastrointestinal (GI) toxicity.[11] Additionally, there is no proved superiority of one drug over another or of creams over tablets, although general data show the azoles to be slightly more efficacious than nystatin.[12] Use of a cream allows external and internal application and may be more soothing acutely. Most of these are now available in over-the-counter (OTC) formulations that have similar costs to prescription items. Physician and patient preferences dictate the specific drug and route, and there is no risk associated with treatment during pregnancy. Truly refractory cases may require longer treatment courses, and the patient with frequent relapses may benefit from oral ketoconazole (Nizoral) 100 mg/day or oral fluconazole (Diflucan) 150 mg every week or month except during pregnancy.[12,13]

Trichomoniasis

The syndrome caused by *T. vaginalis* may cause severe itching or pain often accompanied by frequency of urination because of concomitant cystitis from the organism. On examination the vulva and the vaginal mucosa is fiery red with cervical petechiae ("strawberry cervix"). The typical discharge is yellow-green and bubbly in nature, but any range of color and texture may be seen, making slide examination critical. As noted above, the diagnosis is made by finding motile trichomonads on the saline smear. Because of the low positive predictive value of *Trichomonas* reported on Papanicolaou smears,[7] all of these results should be confirmed by a wet preparation before therapy is initiated. Although the culture methodology for *T. vaginalis* may have better sensitivity and specificity in theory, there is still debate over the ideal medium and methods, so the technique is not useful.

The drug of choice in therapy is metronidazole (Flagyl), with the best response noted after a 2-g single dose.[13] An alternative regimen of 500 mg bid for 7 days is best used for refractory cases only, as it produces no higher an initial cure than the one-time dose. Metronidazole has a significant Antabuse-type reaction, so patients must be cautioned to use no alcohol, including cough medicine, during the treatment. As a sexually transmitted disease, it is critically important for the patient's sexual partner(s) to be treated concurrently to prevent reinfection, and although there are some resistant cases, resistance is not an all-or-none phenomenon. Rather, resistance may range from mild (where treatment is effective) to severe, necessitating a treatment dose of 2.5 g/day in divided doses for 7 to 10 days.[14] At this time, no other medication available in the United States provides better therapeutic results.

Trichomoniasis during pregnancy is difficult to treat. Although the literature is scant, oral metronidazole may be teratogenic during the first trimester and is therefore contraindicated until the second trimester and reserved for severe infections only. Both intravaginal clotrimazole and clindamycin may be effective in controlling the symptoms during the first trimester, although they may not produce eradication.[6,13]

Bacterial Vaginosis

Formerly known as *Gardnerella* or nonspecific vaginitis, bacterial vaginosis has been credited with as many as 50% of all diagnoses of vaginitis.[15] It represents an overgrowth in the vagina of anaerobic organisms classically known as *Gardnerella vaginalis* and now noted to be multiple organisms. It produces no vulvar symptoms, no change in vaginal mucosa, little itching, and no pain, unless the discharge is so profuse the vulvae are simply macerated. Because its course is usually indolent, it does not cause an acute change in symptoms. The patient may note only a slight change in normal discharge and an odor that may be more pronounced after intercourse. Patients are frequently inured to the symptoms until treatment is finished and the discharge gone. There may not be an odor immediately on examination, but KOH releases the amines in the epithelial cells and produces the classic fishy odor that is diagnostic when clue cells are present. Because *Gardnerella* bacteria may be a normal inhabitant of the vagina, culture of the organism for a diagnosis has poor specificity and so has not been recommended.[7]

Treatment for this syndrome is metronidazole 500 mg po bid for 7 days or metronidazole gel 0.75% 5 g intravaginally bid for 5 days (Fig. 102.1).[13] Alternatively, clindamycin 2% vaginal cream can be used for 7 days. Unfortunately, the one-time dose used to treat trichomoniasis is insufficient for bacterial vaginosis. For refractory cases or as an alternate, oral clindamycin 300 mg bid for 7 days can be used.[13]

Because some association has been noted between bacterial vaginosis and premature rupture of membranes or postpartum endometriosis, therapy should be considered during pregnancy.[16] The recommended drug during pregnancy is a 2% clindamycin vaginal cream at night for 7 days or oral metronidazole 250 mg tid for 7 days[16] (see above).

At this time, the role of sexual transmission of this disorder is unclear. Studies can be found to support either opinion, and partner therapy has not produced an improved cure rate, at least at conventional dosage.[16] Equally unclear is the role of treatment in the asymptomatic patient, but it may be considered in someone undergoing vaginal surgery because of a potential role in pelvic inflammation.[16]

Atrophic Vaginitis

A common cause of vaginal symptoms in the postmenopausal woman, atrophic vaginitis should be considered concomitantly with the evaluation for other etiologies. Lack of estrogen produces thin vaginal epithelium and cells deficient in the acids that provide the premenopausal woman with a balanced vaginal ecosystem. Therefore, the mucosa easily denudes and becomes traumatized. Thus presenting symptoms may include lack of vaginal lubrication with coitus, pruritus, and dyspareunia, with or without discharge (see Chapter 104).

On examination the vaginal folds are flattened, and the mucosa is pale pink and shows lack of lubrication. The cervix is usually atrophic and frequently friable, and the wet preparation is negative. Hormone replacement therapy is the treatment of choice, but vaginal estrogen creams used nightly can provide short-term relief.[17] The patient must be reminded that a vaginal discharge may recur as the cells mature back to a premenopausal pattern.

Sexually Transmitted Diseases

Several sexually transmitted diseases (STDs) that present with predominantly vaginal symptoms are discussed more fully in Chapter 41.

Chlamydia *Infection*

As an STD, *Chlamydia* infection is discussed Chapter 41. Even though *Chlamydia* does not produce vaginitis (except in adolescents), it does cause mucopurulent cervicitis. On examination, the cervix may be eroded and present a mucopurulent discharge that when wiped quickly re-forms at the os. When this condition is seen, the alert clinician performs appropriate tests, examining wet preparations for concomitant vaginal infections, as patients with one STD are at high risk of having more.

Once a diagnosis of *Chlamydia* is suspected, empiric treatment is warranted, especially in a high-risk patient (defined as sexually active, nonmonogamous, and young). The standard treatment is doxycycline (Vibramycin) 100 mg po bid for 7 days or azithromycin (Zithromax) 1 g po once.[13] If the patient is allergic to tetracycline (rare) or pregnancy is suspected, an appropriate alternative is erythromycin 500 mg po qid for 7 days. Partners should be treated aggressively, but a test of patient cure is considered unnecessary.

Herpesvirus *Infection*

Especially in the case of recurrences, patients with herpesvirus infection may present only with symptoms of external burning and minimal liquid discharge. Without ulcerations externally or on the cervix, this diagnosis should not be entertained unless there is a known history of a positive culture (see Chapter 41).

Human Papillomavirus Infection

Current trends indicate that most human papillomavirus (HPV) disease presents as warts either externally or internally. Therefore, HPV is unlikely to be a cause of any symptoms unless the growth is large enough to cause an exudative process. Because HPV is associated with cervical dysplasia, a Papanicolaou smear must be examined regularly. No form of treatment has proved to be superior or to eradicate the virus. Topical podophyllin externally and cryotherapy internally remain standard options. Both podofilox (0.5% solution) and an immunomodulating agent, Aldara (imiquimod), are available by prescription for patient home use.[13] Neither is superior to office treatment, but both offer the advantage of patient home use. A self-administered regimen of 5% imiquimod cream applied externally overnight three times a week for 16 weeks will produce no more toxicity than podophyllin and may be the best initial choice.[18]

Leukorrhea Secondary to Birth Control Pills

On some occasions, the only cause of leukorrhea is an eroded cervix secondary to the use of birth control pills (see Chapter 101). The hormones in birth control pills cause more endocervix to be exposed to the environment of the vagina, producing irritation and weeping of the mucosa. It is usually asymptomatic. If a patient is having symptoms, this diagnosis is excluded.

Vulvar Diseases

It is critical to remember that many skin diseases manifest with vaginal symptoms. Most, such as seborrheic dermatitis, psoriasis, tinea, and pediculosis, have unique characteristics that are obvious. Without these unique characteristics, diagnosis and appropriate therapy may best be achieved by performance of a simple punch biopsy or referral to dermatology. Patients must be told that the treatment effect may take months to realize. In addition, any pigmented lesion should be biopsied and the patient referred if indicated by biopsy results.

Vestibulitis

With vestibulitis there is variable redness and edema of the vestibular glands, frequently with a lesion. The number of glands involved can range from 1 to 100, and the symptoms are vulvar pain with dyspareunia. The etiology is still hotly debated, but probably HPV is involved. Treatment results are best with vestibular resection or intralesional interferon, but no therapy is 100% effective.[19]

Lichen Sclerosis

Lichen sclerosis is a hyperplastic condition with a white lesion seen predominantly in women over age 50. There is a typical "keyhole" pattern on both sides of the vulva. The lesion may eventually cover the entire vulva with adhesion and eventual obliteration of the labia minora to the majora. Treatment is a topical testosterone ointment (30 mL of testosterone in oil with 120 g petrolatum) twice a day for 4 to 6 months and then one or two times a week for life.[17] If the patient cannot tolerate the side effects, alternative therapy of progesterone cream can be used. There is a high recurrence rate, even with surgery or laser, so dramatic treatment is best avoided.

Lichen Simplex Chronicus

Caused by chronic itching or irritation, lichen simplex chronicus is a thick, scaly condition with localized vulvar lesions without adhesions. Treatment is symptomatic with topical steroids for 1 to 2 months. Because the only recurrences are seen in patients treated by surgery, this intervention is no longer acceptable.[20]

Lichen Planus

Lichen planus may involve mucous membranes in other organ systems (see Chapter 118). There is vulvar burning, leukorrhea, and redness of the inner labia. Patients may have violaceous papules externally and small, lacy, gray, reticular patterns on the inner labia. Without these identifying marks, this lesion may appear similar to that of atrophic vaginitis; it should be entertained as a diagnosis whenever therapy for atrophic vaginitis fails. Treatment is topical with either a potent fluorinated steroid or a medium potency steroid under occlusion.[20] The patient must be reminded that this condition flares and remits over long periods.

When the Tests Are Negative

A dilemma ensues when, despite the best efforts of the clinician, the examination and tests reveal no reason for the patient's symptoms. In such cases, the clinician should review the history, the adequacy of specimen collection, the performance of the laboratory tests, and the possibility of *Chlamydia*, and should obtain any history previously overlooked and consider the diagnosis of an acid-base change in the vaginal environment known as cytolytic vaginosis. Although not easily diagnosed, this entity is caused by an overgrowth of acidophilic Döderlein's lactobacilli, producing an increase in enzymes that degrade intracellular glycogen to lactic acid and causing massive desquamation and cytolysis and a watery discharge. Because the luteal phase epithelial cells are richer in lactic acid, this syndrome may be cyclic in nature. The hallmark for diagnosis is epithelial cells that have a moth-eaten appearance, often called pseudo-clue cells, and a few WBCs on the wet preparation. In addition, because this process is driven by an acidic environment, the symptoms worsen with douching using conventional acidic agents. Instead, these patients can be treated with a douching mixture of sodium bicarbonate and water (1–2 tablespoons in 500 mL water) used three times a week while symptomatic.[4]

If the workup was adequate, the clinician should resist the urge to perform "shotgun" or even empiric treatment, as such treatment perpetuates old myths, and instead be supportive and understanding of the symptoms and encourage the patient to be checked for subsequent recurrences.

Special Considerations for the Family Physician

Much of the success of therapy depends on the unique relationship between the family physician and the patient.

Compliance

The trusting relationship between the patient and the family physician enhances compliance with often distasteful regimens. The patient is encouraged to finish the full course of therapy despite symptom resolution, and when the therapy demands partner compliance, the patient must be instructed to abstain from intercourse until therapy is completed. Role-playing this partner discussion with the patient may help allay anxiety. Choose the shortest regimen possible and make sure the patient understands side effects (including local irritation), route of usage, and use of medication during menses. Negotiate with the patient the best time to begin treatment and inform her of the possibility of recurrence or treatment failure. In addition, it is critical to assess the patients' attribution of disease in this condition. Clarity about sexual transmission is important; if possible, use printed information for the patient to read and give to her partner(s).

Issues of self-support and control of symptoms can be critical to compliance as well. These points can be reinforced through good patient education. Sources of self-help for the patient can be found in women's health literature such as *Our Bodies, Our Selves* or its revision.[21] These references may provide the patient with more detailed information on hygiene, as well as alternative remedies. The physician, however, should first read the relevant sections to be sure that the information is consonant with good care and to explain areas of disagreement. (For example, there is scant scientific evidence for the use of intravaginal yogurt.) Some patients work best with a combination of conventional medical therapy and time-honored suggestions.

Recurrent or Persistent Vaginitis

Nothing is more frustrating to the patient or physician than recurrence (defined as symptoms recurring after a 1-month disease-free interval) or persistence of symptoms. In this situation the physician should start over with the history, emphasizing compliance with previous therapy and focusing attention on details of diet, clothing, and irritants. Question the patient about high dairy intake, increased simple sugars, use of new deodorant tampons or pads, or other topical agents such as perfumes or home remedies. Explore the relation to tight clothing, exercise gear, the use of dildos or vibrators, and the use of hot tubs or pools.

The examination and basic tests should be repeated, but if the history reveals no further clues, culture the cervix for *Chlamydia* and the vaginal vault for bacteria and *Candida* and perform any necessary vulvar biopsies. In the diabetic patient the blood glucose must be controlled concomitantly while re-instituting therapy.

Results of the tests dictate therapy. Persistent *Candida* or *Trichomonas* infection may need prolonged (*Candida*) or increased (*Trichomonas*) therapy. Consider treating according to the results of the bacterial culture using an antibiotic[6] targeted to the dominant organism.

If tests are negative, provide support and sympathy, educate the patient about good hygiene and sexual behaviors that minimize risk, and proscribe anything that might exacerbate symptoms. Encourage the patient to return to be examined when symptoms recur.

Management of the HIV-Positive Patient

Other than the fact that patients who are HIV-seropositive may have problems with HPV, treatment of vaginal disorders follows the same recommendations as for nonpositive patients. Although refractory candidiasis may be a clue for the physician to check a patient for HIV status, a normal vaginal infection should not be of concern.[22]

Role of Colposcopy

The role of colposcopy is not well defined regarding vaginal symptoms. It may be a useful tool in the future, but its current usage is in the evaluation of an abnormal Papanicolaou smear or cervix. Therefore, use it in a patient with persistent cervicitis only to screen for abnormal areas to biopsy. Additionally, conventional wisdom dictates that patients with HPV undergo colposcopy to detect a precancerous state of the cervix.

Prevention of Vaginitis

When an STD has caused the vaginitis, the family physician must educate the patient about the difference between a disease that can arise de novo and then be propagated between partners and one acquired from someone else. Patients are understandably concerned about where they got the disease, but the clinician can help focus the patient on treatment, give basic relevant information, and plan a subsequent visit to continue pursuing their concerns. Clarity about sexual transmission is important, as the patient may also need to be concerned about hepatitis and HIV risk. Acquisition of an STD is certainly threatening to partners who thought of themselves as mutually monogamous, and relationship issues are frequently topics for subsequent visits.

In addition to concerns about sexual transmission, the physician should educate the patient about the causative or associative factors found to be significant in the history. Use of local irritants, clothing, and other offending behaviors must be discouraged. Above all, encouraging the patient to come in for evaluation of subsequent infections is critical, as the etiology may differ from the current one.

References

1. Paavonen J, Stamm WE. Lower genital tract infections in women. Infect Dis Clin North Am 1987;1179–98.
2. Bump RC, Zuspan FP, Buesching WJ, Ayers LW, Stephens T. The prevalence, six-month persistence and predictive values of laboratory indicators of bacterial vaginosis (nonspecific vaginitis). Am J Obstet Gynecol 1984;150:917–23.
3. Faro S. Bacterial vaginitis. Obstet Gynecol 1991;34:582–6.
4. Cibley LJ, Cibley LJ. Cytolytic vaginosis. Am J Obstet Gynecol 1991;165:1245–8.
5. Kent HL. Epidemiology of vaginitis. Am J Obstet Gynecol 1991;165:1168–76.
6. Horowitz BJ, Mardh PA, eds. Vaginitis and vaginosis. New York: Wiley Liss, 1991.
7. Eschenbach DA, Hiller SL. Advances in diagnostic testing for vaginitis and cervicitis. J Reprod Med 1989;34(suppl 18):555–64.
8. Horowitz BJ. Mycotic vulvovaginitis: a broad overview. Am J Obstet Gynecol 1991;165:1188–92.
9. Roy S. Vulvovaginitis: causes and therapies: nonbarrier contraceptives and vaginitis and vaginosis. Am J Obstet Gynecol 1991;165:1240–4.
10. Reed B, Slatery M, French T. Diet and vaginitis. J Fam Pract 1989;29:509–15.
11. Drugs for vulvovaginal candidiasis. Med Lett Drugs Ther 2001;43:3,4.
12. Watson MC, Grimshaw JM, Bond CM, et al. Oral versus intravaginal imidazole and triazole anti-fungal treatment of uncomplicated vulvovaginal candidiasis. Cochrane Review. The Cochrane Library 2001;1.
13. Drugs for sexually transmitted infections. Med Lett Drugs Ther 1999;41:85–90.
14. Forna F, Gulmezoglu AM. Interventions for treating trichomoniasis in women. Cochrane Review. The Cochrane Library 2001;1.
15. Eschenbach DA, Hiller S, Critchlow C, Stevens C, DeRowen T, Holmes KK. Diagnosis and clinical manifestations of bacterial vaginosis. Am J Obstet Gynecol 1988;158:819–23.
16. Joesoef MR, Schmid GP, Hillier SL. Bacterial vaginosis: review of treatment options and potential clinical indications for therapy. CID 1999;28(suppl 1):S57–S65.
17. Byyny RL, Speroff L. A clinical guide for the care of older women. Baltimore: Williams & Wilkins, 1990.
18. Gall SA. Female genital warts: global trends and treatments. Infect Dis Obstet Gynecol 2001;9(3):149–54.
19. McKay M, Frankman O, Horovitz BJ, Lecart C, Micheletti L, Ridley C. Vulvar vestibulitis and vestibular papillomatoses: report of the ISSVD committee on vulvodynia. J Reprod Med 1991;36:413–5.
20. McKay M. Vulvar dermatoses. Clin Obstet Gynecol 1991;34:614–29.
21. Boston Women's Health Book Collective. The new our bodies, ourselves. New York: Simon & Schuster, 1992.
22. Hammill HA, Murtagh CP. Gynecologic care of the human immunodeficiency virus-positive woman. Clin Obstet Gynecol 1991;34:599–604.

103
Menstrual Disorders

Peggy R. Cyr and Ann K. Skelton

Menstrual Cycle

Women experiencing menstrual difficulties frequently call upon family physicians. The disorders range from a failure to menstruate to excessive menstrual bleeding. Menstrual disorders stem from multiple etiologies, spanning the breadth of many disciplines including genetics, metabolism, endocrinology, gynecology, and psychology. Menstrual disorders are best addressed through a comprehensive primary care approach.

Normal Physiology and Patterns

Regulation of the menstrual cycle is a product of complex, delicate interactions among hormones of the hypothalamus, pituitary, and ovaries. The hypothalamus secretes gonadotropin-releasing hormone (GnRH) in a pulsatile manner. The pituitary secretes luteinizing hormone (LH) and follicle-stimulating hormone (FSH), which act primarily on the theca and granulosa cells of the ovary respectively. With FSH and estradiol stimulation, a dominant follicle develops and releases an egg. Estradiol has a negative feedback effect on FSH, resulting in decreased stimulation of the several other less mature follicles that develop monthly. FSH also stimulates the development of LH receptors in the ovarian granulosa cells. When the concentration of estradiol reaches a threshold level for a specific duration, the LH surge occurs. The LH surge triggers ovulation and formation of the corpus luteum. The corpus luteum produces estrogen and progesterone, which have a negative feedback result on GnRH and FSH, eventually leading to decreased levels of estrogen and progesterone and corpus luteum involution if pregnancy has not taken place. In the absence of pregnancy, menstruation occurs and FSH levels increase to prepare for the next cycle.[1]

The follicular phase of the menstrual cycle, under control primarily of FSH, results in ovulation and usually lasts 10 to 14 days. During this phase, the endometrium proliferates under estrogen stimulation, and progesterone receptors are synthesized on endometrial epithelial cells. The luteal phase of the menstrual cycle refers to the period after the LH surge stimulates ovulation. The corpus luteum produces progesterone, which causes endometrial glandular secretory changes and changes in the endometrial stroma. The luteal phase consistently lasts 14 days after the mid-cycle LH surge. In the absence of pregnancy, the regression of the corpus luteum and drop in progesterone result in endometrial sloughing. Figure 103.1 is a graphic illustration of the interaction of key hormones during the menstrual cycle.

Normal menstrual cycle intervals are 21 to 45 days from the first day of one cycle to the first day of next, with bleeding lasting 3 to 7 days. Average blood loss is 30 to 40 mL per cycle. The average age of menarche in the United States is 12 years, and menopause is 52.

Disorders of Menstruation

The following terminology describes the key features of menstrual history and disorders of menstruation:

Amenorrhea: absence of menstrual periods

Menarche: onset of first menses

Menometrorrhagia: menses at irregular intervals with varying amounts of blood loss

Menopause: cessation of menses for 6 months, not due to pregnancy

Menorrhagia: loss of more than 80 mL of blood during a menstrual cycle or menstrual duration of more than 7 days

Metrorrhagia: bleeding between menstrual cycles

Oligomenorrhea: menstrual cycles of 36 days or more

Polymenorrhea: menstrual cycles shorter than 21 days

Primary amenorrhea: lack of menarche by age 14 in girls without development of secondary sexual characteristics or by age 16 in those with secondary sexual characteristics

Fig. 103.1. Hormonal changes through the menstrual cycle.

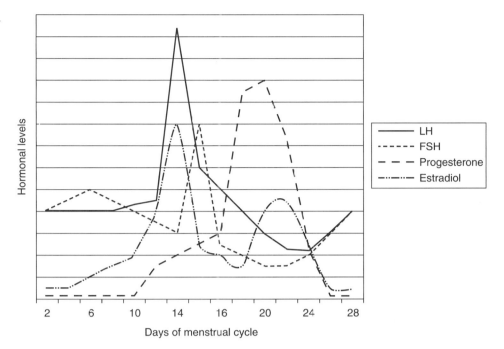

Secondary amenorrhea: absence of menses for six consecutive cycles in a previously menstruating woman, or for 12 months in a woman with oligomenorrhea

General Approach

Any woman presenting with a menstrual disorder should have a thorough and pertinent history and physical examination.

Table 103.1. **Elements of History Taking for Menstrual Disorders**

Menstrual history	Age of menarche
	Usual menstrual pattern (cycle length, duration, flow)
	First day of last menstrual period
	Moliminal symptoms (breast tenderness, mittelschmerz)
	Dysmenorrhea
Gynecologic and sexual history	Use of contraception
	Pregnancies, deliveries, complications
	GYN procedures (e.g., D&C)
	Pelvic pain
Family history	Age of onset of menarche and menopause in sister(s) and mother
	Similar menstrual dysfunction in others
	Congenital syndromes or anomalies
	Endocrine disorders
General medical history	Changes in weight
	Emotional stressors
	Signs of excessive exercise (e.g., stress fractures)
	Sexually transmitted diseases
	Medications
	Previous chemotherapy or radiation
	Other endocrine or metabolic disorders
	Disordered eating

The key components of the history are a family history, a menstrual and reproductive history, and a general medical history including medications used, and nutritional, exercise, and emotional assessments. Details are listed in Table 103.1.

The focus of the physical exam is to look for abnormal genital anatomy such as an imperforate hymen or enlarged fibroid uterus. Additional areas of attention during the physical exam are listed in Table 103.2. The pertinent areas include looking for signs of androgen excess, estrogen deficiency, or an endocrinopathy.

Primary Amenorrhea

Congenital anomalies are the main cause of primary amenorrhea. These include imperforate hymen or a vaginal septum that will be detected on exam and can be treated surgically. Congential absence of the uterus and vagina can occur. An andro-

Table 103.2. **Elements of Physical Exam for Menstrual Disorders**

Skin	Acne, alopecia, hirsutism, abdominal striae
Neurologic	Visual field deficit
Neck	Thyroid nodules or enlargement
Breasts	Tanner stage, galactorrhea
Abdomen	Adrenal mass
External genitalia and vagina	Imperforate hymen, vaginal septum, atrophic vaginal mucosa, scant cervical mucus, enlarged clitoris
Cervix	Friability, inflammation, polyps, duplication
Uterus and ovaries	Enlargement of uterus or ovaries

gen insensitivity syndrome leads to a 46,XY female who has no uterus or tubes and a blind vaginal pouch. Testes are found within the abdomen or inguinal hernias and require surgical removal due to the risk of malignant transformation. Women with Turner's syndrome (45,XO) never menstruate because the ovaries are not developed. Patients with congential anomalies require specialty consultation. Women with primary amenorrhea and normal sexual development should undergo the same evaluation as patients with secondary amenorrhea (also see Chapter 16).

Secondary Amenorrhea

The most common etiology of secondary amenorrhea is pregnancy. Secondary amenorrhea is seen commonly in endurance athletes and anorexic patients. Each etiology will be discussed below under the workup of amenorrhea, presented in a stepwise fashion.

Workup for Amenorrhea

The production of menstrual flow requires an integrated hypothalamic-pituitary-ovarian axis, a hormonally responsive uterus, and an intact outflow tract. The most important task in the diagnostic evaluation of amenorrhea is to identify the malfunctioning element (Table 103.3).

First Step

Check a urine pregnancy test. Pregnancy is the most common cause of secondary amenorrhea and may be a cause of primary amenorrhea in a young woman who is sexually active around the onset of menarche.

Second Step

Check serum levels of thyroid-stimulating hormone (TSH) and prolactin. Hyperprolactinemia and hypothyroidism can be the cause of amenorrhea.

Amenorrhea Secondary to Elevated Prolactin Level. About one third of women with no obvious cause of amenorrhea will have an elevated prolactin level.[2] Hyperprolactinemia is most commonly the result of a pituitary microadenoma (<10 mm in diameter), which in and of itself should not affect pituitary function. A plain x-ray with a cone-down view of the sella turcica will detect the presence of a large tumor. If the cone-down view is abnormal, the prolactin level is >100 ng/mL, and the patient has headaches or visual disturbances, then magnetic resonance imaging (MRI) of the brain is indicated. Elevated prolactin levels inhibit the pulsatile release of GnRH from the hypothalamus, which ultimately inhibits estrogen production and leads to amenorrhea. Dopamine agonist therapy (bromocriptine) is reserved for prolactin-secreting tumors with rapid growth or large tumors, and for patients who want to become pregnant or who have intolerable galactorrhea. Surgery is for tumors unresponsive to medical therapy. Microadenomas can be managed by checking yearly serum prolactin and brain MRI every 2 to 3 years.

Three main types of medications can also elevate prolactin levels, resulting in amenorrhea: antipsychotics; antidepressants, both tricyclic and monoamine oxidase inhibitors (MAOIs); and antihypertensive agents, including calcium channel blockers and methyldopa. Stopping these agents will generally result in a quick return to menstruation.

Amenorrhea Secondary to Hypothyroidism. Thyroid failure is associated with elevated prolactin levels since hypothalamically released thyrotropin-releasing hormone also stimulates prolactin production. There may also be a direct effect of hypothyroidism on the feedback control of LH, FSH, and estradiol on the hypothalamus and pituitary.[3] Treatment of hypothyroidism results in prompt return of ovulatory cycles and menses ensue.

Of note, galactorrhea is present in only one third of women with increased prolactin levels, and one third of women with galactorrhea have normal menses.[4]

Table 103.3. **Workup for Amenorrhea**

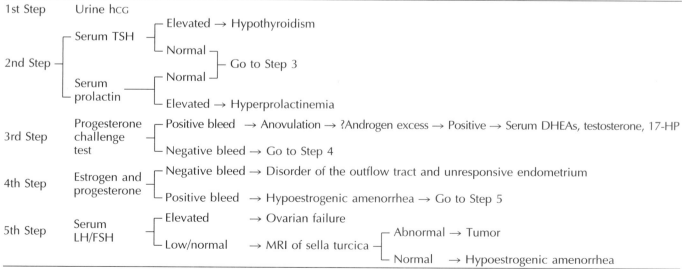

DHEA = dehydroepiandrosterone; FSH = follicle-stimulating hormone; hCG = human chorionic gonadotropin; 17-HP = 17-hydroxyprogesterone; LH = luteinizing hormone; TSH = thyroid-stimulating hormone.

Third Step

Perform a progesterone challenge test. This test evaluates the functional endogenous estrogen status and competence of the outflow tract. The standard regimen is 10 mg of medroxyprogesterone orally, daily for 10 days. Any bleeding within 2 to 10 days after stopping the progesterone is a positive sign indicating the presence of anovulation.

Amenorrhea Secondary to Anovulation. These women will have withdrawal bleeding after taking the progesterone challenge test. This type of amenorrhea is frequently associated with high androgen levels as seen in polycystic ovarian syndrome, and, in rare cases, adrenal tumors or adrenal enzyme deficiencies, which cause elevated progesterone levels. Hyperandrogenic chronic anovulation is present in 37% of amenorrheic women and 90% of infertile women with oligomenorrhea.[5]

If high androgen levels are suspected on physical exam, additional tests include serum testosterone, dehydroepiandrosterone sulfate (DHEAS), and serum 17-hydroxyprogesterone (17-HP). Serum testosterone >200 mg/dL indicates an androgen-secreting tumor. Serum DHEAS >7000 ng/dL indicates an adrenal tumor. Serum 17-HP between 200 and 800 ng/dL indicates possible adrenal hyperplasia, which can be further evaluated by an adrenocorticotropic hormone (ACTH) stimulation test. Serum 17-HP >800 ng/dL indicates 21-hydroxylase deficiency.[6]

A negative progesterone withdrawal test indicates one of three possibilities:

1. A disorder of the outflow tract.
2. A nonreactive endometrium.
3. Inadequate estrogen stimulation of the endometrium.

When there is no withdrawal bleed, proceed to the fourth step.

Fourth Step

Prescribe a 1-month regimen of estrogen and progesterone. Two possible regimens are oral contraceptives or 1.25 mg of conjugated equine estrogen on days 1 to 21 and 10 mg medroxyprogesterone acetate on days 17 to 21. A positive withdrawal bleed with use of estrogen and progesterone confirms an unobstructed outflow tract and a responsive endometrium.

Amenorrhea Secondary to Disorders of the Outflow Tract. Most of the disorders of the outflow tract are congenital in origin and are outlined in the section under primary amenorrhea. Asherman's syndrome is an acquired form of amenorrhea in which intrauterine adhesions prevent endometrial stimulation by estrogen and/or block the outflow of menstrual blood. The adhesions may form after vigorous curettement of the postabortion or postpartum endometrium or scarring by endometritis. Diagnosis is made by a hysterosalpingogram or hysteroscopy, and the syndrome may be treated surgically by lysis of adhesions. Tuberculosis can also cause intrauterine lesions that can block the outflow of menstrual blood.

Amenorrhea Secondary to Unresponsive Endometrium. The endometrium will not respond to progesterone withdrawal in rare circumstances of high levels of androgens such as seen in adrenal tumors, polycystic ovarian syndrome, or adrenal enzyme deficiency. These situations should be expected when there are signs of androgen excess.

Amenorrhea Secondary to Inadequate Stimulation of the Endometrium. These patients will have menstrual bleeding with the administration of estrogen and progesterone. This type of amenorrhea is referred to as hypoestrogenic amenorrhea. Proceed to the fifth step.

Fifth Step

Measure serum levels of the gonadotropins: LH and FSH. The serum gonadotropins LH and FSH can be elevated, normal, or low. Elevated levels are termed hypergonadotropic amenorrhea, normal levels are called normogonadotropic amenorrhea, and low levels indicate hypogonadotropic amenorrhea.

Hypergonadotropic Amenorrhea—Elevated LH/FSH. The primary cause of amenorrhea associated with elevated LH/FSH is ovarian failure. Ovarian failure is termed premature if a woman is less than 40 years of age. A karyotype should be obtained in these women to check for 45,XO (Turner's syndrome), 46,XY (pure gonadal dysgenesis), and 46,XX in idiopathic premature ovarian failure.

Twenty to forty percent of cases of premature ovarian failure are associated with autoimmune disorders.[7] A workup for autoimmune diseases is recommended. Adrenal failure can follow ovarian failure and should be monitored with periodic morning cortisol levels.

Chemotherapeutic agents can also cause ovarian failure by direct ovarian toxicity. This effect may be reversible.

Hormonal therapy with estrogen and progesterone should be strongly considered in all patients with ovarian failure. Due to the low estrogen state, there is an increased risk of osteoporosis and a concern of increased cardiovascular risk.[8] Oral contraceptives and calcium and vitamin D supplementation are recommended.

Normo- or Hypogonadotropic Amenorrhea—Normal or Low LH/FSH. If the FSH and LH are normal or low in this low estrogen state, it indicates pituitary or hypothalamic dysfunction. Tumors of the hypothalamus (craniopharyngiomas) or tumors of the pituitary (adenomas) or ischemic necrosis of the pituitary as seen in obstetrical shock (Sheehan's syndrome) all can cause this type of amenorrhea. A MRI of the brain is the most sensitive imaging study of the pituitary in these conditions.[9] If the MRI is negative, a defect in the pulsatile release of GnRH from the hypothalamus is the probable cause. This is a diagnosis of exclusion and is commonly associated with emotional stress (acute or chronic), nutritional deficiencies as seen in anorexia nervosa, and excessive strenuous physical exercise.

If contraception is desired, oral contraception pills (OCPs) are recommended. If pregnancy is desired, referral to an infertility specialist is indicated for either pulsatile GnRH in hypothalamic failure or menotropins in the case of pituitary failure. This low-estrogen state requires estrogen, calcium, and vitamin D supplementation as well.

Additional Medications Causing Amenorrhea. Amenorrhea is a common side effect of oral contraceptives, Depo-Provera, or Norplant. Rule out pregnancy and reassure the patient. Digitalis and marijuana can also cause amenorrhea through estrogen-like effects.

Female Athlete Triad

The female athlete triad, one feature of which is amenorrhea, warrants special note because of its common presentation to primary care physicians and because of its potential consequences. Osteoporosis and disordered eating are the other two aspects of the triad. In this syndrome, vigorous athletic training and weight changes produce hypothalamic dysfunction and primary or secondary amenorrhea. The associated low estrogen levels may produce osteoporosis, which is especially devastating if it occurs in adolescence when bone density should be peaking. Osteoporosis increases the risk of stress fractures and other fractures in athletes. The disordered eating associated with the female athlete triad may not meet the strict definitions of anorexia nervosa or bulimia but is prevalent among female athletes. Since amenorrhea or a fracture is often the presenting complaint of women with this triad, physicians should review exercise and eating habits for those presenting with amenorrhea or fractures. Evaluation, as outlined above for primary or secondary amenorrhea, should take place for those young women who have missed three menstrual periods. If no other cause is found, treatment of the eating disorder, through counseling, nutritional advice, and, in some cases, serotonin reuptake inhibitors, and a change in exercise patterns will usually result in resumption of menses. Important adjuncts in treatment of the female athlete triad include screening for osteoporosis and preventive measures including intake of calcium and vitamin D, and hormone replacement with oral contraceptives or regimens similar to those used in postmenopausal women (also see Chapter 51).

Polycystic Ovarian Syndrome

Polycystic ovarian syndrome (PCOS) is a common disorder with varying features, including menstrual disorders. A 1990 National Institutes of Health consensus lists the following definite criteria of the syndrome: hyperandrogenism with clinical features, menstrual dysfunction, and the exclusion of congenital adrenal hyperplasia. Probable criteria included insulin resistance, perimenarchal onset, and elevation in the LH/FSH ratio and ultrasonographic evidence of polycystic ovaries.[10]

The common feature in all patients with PCOS is anovulation. Menstrual manifestations of anovulation in PCOS range from amenorrhea to oligomenorrhea to metrorrhagia. The usual hypothalamic, pituitary, and ovarian interactions are disrupted.

LH levels and its patterns of pulsatile release are characteristically abnormal in women with PCOS and result in production of androgens by the thecal cells of the ovary. The obesity often associated with the syndrome decreases the levels of sex binding hormone, increasing the circulating levels of testosterone and estrogens. Usual feedback mechanisms are disrupted by chronic stimulation of hormones, and the delicate balance needed to produce ovulation is upset. Ovulation may occur from time to time in women with PCOS, and contraception should be discussed.

In addition to the virilization associated with chronic anovulation and high levels of circulating androgens and estrogens, potential consequences of PCOS include infertility, an increased risk of endometrial cancer, and possibly breast cancer. The insulin resistance, hyperinsulinemia, and hyperandrogenism associated with the syndrome increase the risk of diabetes and heart disease.

The amenorrhea, oligomenorrhea, or metrorrhagia resulting from PCOS should be fully evaluated to rule out other causes. Although a characteristic elevation in the LH/FSH ratio, similar to that seen at midcycle, is common, most patients are diagnosed on a clinical basis after ruling out other abnormalities. Most often, the menstrual irregularities begin at menarche, and are associated with clinical features of hyperandrogenism and obesity.

Treatment of PCOS is aimed at achieving pregnancy if desired, preventing cancers, treating associated hirsutism, alopecia or acne, and preventing type II diabetes and coronary artery disease. Weight reduction alone may lead to resumption of ovulation, pregnancy for those who desire it and significant reduction in metabolic and cardiac consequences of PCOS. For those who desire conception, ovulation induction can help achieve pregnancy. Interrupting the chronic estrogen and androgen stimulus can help prevent endometrial cancer, and patients who do not desire conception may be treated with oral contraceptives or cyclic progesterone. Hirsutism and alopecia may respond to oral contraceptives or spironolactone, which may need to be used for at least 6 months before noting improvement. Screening for diabetes with fasting or random glucose tests is recommended, especially in obese patients (see Chapter 120). The effect of exercise and weight reduction on increasing insulin sensitivity should be stressed with patients. Finally, monitoring lipid profiles can help identify and treat women with "male pattern" lipid profiles. Because progesterone characteristically increases levels of LDL, oral contraceptives may be a better choice than progesterone for treatment of women with PCOS who have abnormal lipid profiles.

Irregular Vaginal Bleeding

Irregular vaginal bleeding is another common menstrual disorder seen by primary care physicians. If careful evaluation for anatomic problems, systemic illness, and medication influences do not yield a cause, the bleeding is termed "dysfunctional uterine bleeding." Table 103.4 lists the most common conditions to be considered in the differential diagnosis of irregular vaginal bleeding.

Evaluation of Irregular Vaginal Bleeding

Evaluation begins with the history and physical exam. The patient's age may point toward the anovulation common around menarche before the full maturation of the hypothalamic-pitu-

Table 103.4. **Causes of Irregular Vaginal Bleeding**

Anatomic	Anovulation	Coagulopathy	Other
Fibroids	Hypo- or hyperthyroidism	Von Willebrand's disease	Pregnancy and its complications,
Polyps: cervical	Hyperprolactinemia	Leukemia	including postpartum conditions
or endometrial	PCOS	Cirrhosis/liver failure	Medications: hormones,
Adenomyosis	Cushing's syndrome	Use of anticoagulants,	phenothiazines, antidepressants,
Endometriosis	Addison's syndrome	aspirin, NSAIDs	anticholinergics, morphine,
Endometrial	Ovarian/adrenal tumors with	Thrombocytopenia	anticoagulants, steroids
hyperplasia or	hyperandrogenism		Infections: cervicitis, endometritis,
cancer	Menarche		PID
Cervical cancer	Menopause		IUD use
Sarcoma	Obesity		
	Hypothalamic anovulation		

IUD = intrauterine device; NSAID = nonsteroidal antiinflammatory drug; PCOS = polycystic ovary syndrome; PID = pelvic inflammatory disease.

itary-ovarian axis, or toward anovulatory cycles close to menopause. Other historical features listed in Table 103.1 will help guide the evaluation toward etiologies including infection, tumors, endocrinopathies, and coagulopathies. Presence of risk factors for endometrial cancer, including hypertension, diabetes, family history, obesity, early menarche, or late menopause, should heighten concern for cancer.

The general appearance of a patient with irregular vaginal bleeding may direct the physician toward PCOS or the female athlete triad as causes for the irregularity. Table 103.2 lists pertinent physical findings that may indicate other disorders.

Just as for amenorrhea, the laboratory evaluation for women with irregular bleeding begins with a pregnancy test. Pregnancy-related conditions are very common and some, such as ectopic pregnancy, are life threatening. Since examination is not very sensitive in diagnosis of thyroid conditions or hyperprolactinemia, a TSH and prolactin level should be included early in the evaluation for most women. An evaluation for anemia with a hemoglobin or hematocrit should be done if there is any indication of excessive blood loss. If the history or examination points toward a coagulopathy, a complete blood count, protime, partial thromboplastin time, and bleeding time will help in determining the diagnosis. Young patients may present with heavy or irregular vaginal bleeding as a first sign of coagulation disorder, so these studies are especially important in younger women. Cultures of the cervix are helpful in those women whose history or physical examination suggests infection as an etiology. A pelvic ultrasound may confirm or reveal fibroids as a cause of heavy and sometimes irregular bleeding, and an endometrial lining thickness of less than 5 mm helps to reassure that irregular vaginal bleeding is not due to endometrial hyperplasia or cancer. A meta-analysis found that a vaginal ultrasound with an endometrial lining of greater than 5 mm was 96% sensitive for cancer of the endometrium and 92% sensitive for endometrial disease of any kind, including cancer, polyps, or hyperplasia.[11] However, any patient over age 35 with irregular vaginal bleeding must have an endometrial biopsy or dilation and curettage (D&C) to rule out hyperplasia or cancer. The endometrial biopsy is 100% sensitive for endometrial cancer when compared to hysteroscopy and guided biopsy.[12] If no other cause is found, hysteroscopy can sometimes identify

uterine polyps or adenomyosis (ectopic endometrial tissue within the myometrium) and can help direct sites for biopsy.

Treatment of Irregular Vaginal Bleeding

Treatment is aimed at the primary etiology if one can be found. If a cause cannot be found, the bleeding is termed dysfunctional uterine bleeding (DUB). Treatment of DUB is outlined below.

Dysfunctional Uterine Bleeding

Dysfunctional uterine bleeding may be ovulatory (15%) or anovulatory (85%). The presence of moliminal symptoms such as breast tenderness, cramping, and bloating points toward ovulation. Ovulatory dysfunctional bleeding is usually due to progesterone withdrawal and is more regular than anovulatory DUB. The treatment of DUB focuses on two aspects: control of bleeding and prevention of endometrial hyperplasia. Treatment may be medical or surgical and depends on the presence or absence of ovulation, degree of symptoms, desirability of pregnancy, and the patient's preferences.

Acute menorrhagia with hemodynamic compromise is treated with estrogens, intravenously over 24 hours. If there is no change, a D&C is performed.

For those patients who do not want to conceive, the polymenorrhea, oligomenorrhea, menorrhagia, or metrorrhagia of dysfunctional uterine bleeding often can be controlled hormonally. Oral contraceptives usually result in regular, lighter menses and help prevent endometrial hyperplasia. Using a combination oral contraceptive three times a day for a week can help stop heavy anovulatory bleeding, as long as other pathologies have been ruled out. From there, the patient can transition to the usual daily oral contraceptive pill if she is younger than 35 or up until menopause in nonsmokers without contraindications. Progesterone, given either as depomedroxyprogesterone or orally as medroxyprogesterone acetate, will change bleeding patterns and protect against hyperplasia as well. With depomedroxyprogesterone, 70% of women will have scant or no bleeding, 20% will have fairly regular bleeding patterns, and 10% will continue to have irregular vaginal bleeding. An alternative delivery system for progesterones is the progesterone containing intrauterine contraceptive device (IUD), which also decreases menstrual blood flow.

Nonsteroidal antiinflammatory drugs (NSAIDs) can decrease blood loss in women with menorrhagia by 25%, and often decrease dysmenorrhea as well. Their effect on blood loss is a result of their antiprostaglandin nature, which increases the thromboxane to prostacyclin ratio, resulting in vasoconstriction and platelet aggregation.[13]

Danazol is a synthetic androgen, which acts as an antiestrogen to inhibit ovulation and LH and FSH production. The result is amenorrhea. It produces a high incidence of androgenic side effects, which often lead to its discontinuation.

GnRH analogues decrease estrogen production, resulting in amenorrhea or decreased flow. Side effects include menopausal symptoms and decrease in bone density. Its expense and side-effect profile prevent its long-term use, but it may be useful for women who desire future fertility but have failed other treatments. "Add-back" estrogen and progesterone can help decrease the incidence of osteoporosis associated with GnRH analogue use.

Surgical approaches include D&C, which is a temporizing measure that stops heavy bleeding but does not change the underlying process. Endometrial ablation by a variety of means is done with hysteroscopic visualization and results in amenorrhea or light periods. It should never be undertaken without first ruling out endometrial atypia, hyperplasia, and cancer. Hysterectomy clearly represents a definitive treatment for dysfunctional vaginal bleeding, but is associated with complications and is not recommended as first-line treatment.

Dysmenorrhea

Dysmenorrhea is defined as cramping pain in the lower abdomen occurring at the onset of menses. Dysmenorrhea is commonly divided into two main categories:

Primary dysmenorrhea, when there is no discernible pelvic pathology
Secondary dysmenorrhea, which is due to pelvic pathology such as endometriosis.

Primary dysmenorrhea is a diagnosis of exclusion. A thorough history and physical will help determine if there is any pelvic pathology. Table 103.5 will help to differentiate primary from secondary dysmenorrhea.

Primary Dysmenorrhea

Primary dysmenorrhea is the most common menstrual disorder in women.[14] Women with dysmenorrhea often experience sharp, intermittent spasms of pain, usually centered in the suprapubic area. Pain may radiate to the back of the legs or the low back. Systemic symptoms of nausea, vomiting, diarrhea, fatigue, fever, headache, or light-headedness are fairly common. Pain usually starts within hours of onset of menses and peaks within the first 1 to 2 days.

There are some theories that smoking, obesity, and alcohol consumption are related to more dysmenorrhea, but these remain controversial. The etiology of primary dysmenorrhea is not precisely understood, but most symptoms can be explained by the action of uterine prostaglandins, particularly PGF_2. This prostaglandin is released as the endometrium sloughs, causing uterine contractions.

Treatment of Primary Dysmenorrhea

NSAIDs are the first choice for treatment. NSAIDs work through prostaglandin synthetase inhibition.[15] Prostaglandins are felt to be responsible for the uterine contractions and the systemic symptoms mentioned such as nausea and diarrhea. If one particular NSAID is not effective, try one from another class.

Oral contraceptives are second-line therapy unless a woman is also seeking contraception, then they would become first-line therapy. Oral contraceptives are 90% effective in improving primary dysmenorrhea[16] and work by reducing menstrual blood volume and suppressing ovulation. It may take up to 3 months for the oral contraceptives to become effective. Norplant and Depo-provera are also effective since these methods often induce amenorrhea.

For the 10% of patients who do not respond to NSAIDs and/or oral contraceptives, a wide range of alternative therapies have been proven effective, including transcutaneous electrical nerve stimulation (TENS), acupuncture, omega-3 fatty acids, transdermal nitroglycerin, thiamine, and magnesium supplements.[17]

Secondary Dysmenorrhea

The onset of secondary dysmenorrhea generally occurs after age 25. The pelvic pathology can be divided into uterine causes and extrauterine causes. The uterine causes are adenomyosis,

Table 103.5. **Differentiating Primary from Secondary Dysmenorrhea**

Historical points	Primary dysmenorrhea	Secondary dysmenorrhea
Onset	Adolescence, within first 3 years of menarche	First one or two cycles after menarche (congenital outflow obstruction) or after age 25
Menstrual flow	Normal	Heavy and/or irregular
Pain with intercourse	No	Yes
Infertility	No	Yes
History of PID	No	Maybe
Pelvic exam	Normal	Abnormal, bulky uterus; nodular uterosacral ligaments
Response to NSAID/OCP	Good	Little or no response

OCP = oral contraceptive pill.

pelvic inflammatory disease, cervical stenosis, polyps, fibroids, and IUDs. The extrauterine causes are endometriosis; inflammation and scarring (adhesions); functional ovarian cysts; benign or malignant tumors of the ovary, bowel, or bladder; and inflammatory bowel disease.[18] Some of these disorders can be determined by a careful pelvic exam. The two most important diagnostic steps are a pelvic ultrasound, including an intravaginal probe component, and laparoscopy.

Treatment of Secondary Dysmenorrhea

Treatment should focus on the underlying condition. For patients with a mass lesion or enlarged uterus on exam or ultrasound referral to a gynecologic specialist is indicated. For adenomyosis, gynecologic consultation is warranted. If a woman has an IUD, dysmenorrhea may be an indication for removal.

Although endometriosis (ectopic functioning endometrial tissue located in such places as the ovaries, uterosacral ligaments, cul de sac, and peritoneum) can be suspected on exam, it must be confirmed by laparoscopy. Endometriosis is a common cause of secondary dysmenorrhea. In fact, approximately 24% of women who complain of pelvic pain are subsequently found to have endometriosis.[19] This condition is often associated with infertility. If pain relief is the goal, medical options include oral contraceptives, danazol, progestational agents, and GnRH agonists. If pain is severe or infertility is an issue, laparoscopic surgical excision and ablation of lesions is indicated. If pain is intractable and childbearing is not a factor, hysterectomy and oopherectomy are indicated.

References

1. Speroff L, Glass RH, Kase NG, eds. Clinical gynecologic endocrinology and infertility. 6th ed. Philadelphia: Lippincott Williams & Wilkins, 1999;201–10.
2. Schlechte J, Sherman B, Halmi N, et al. Prolactin-secreting pituitary tumors in amenorrheic women: a comprehensive study. Endocr Rev 1980;1:295–308.
3. McIver B, Romanski SA, Nippoldt TB. Concise review for primary-care physicians: evaluation and management of amenorrhea. Mayo Clin Proc 1997;72:1164.
4. Speroff L, Glass RH, Kase NG. Clinical gynecologic endocrinology and infertility. 6th ed. Philadelphia: Lippincott Williams & Wilkins, 1999;421–8.
5. Hull MG. Epidemiology of infertility and polycystic ovarian disease: endocrinological and demographic studies. Gynecol Endocrinol 1987;1:235–45.
6. Kiningham RB, Apgar BS, Schwenk TL. Evaluation of amenorrhea. Am Fam Physician 1996;53:1192.
7. Alper MM, Garner PR. Premature ovarian failure: its relationship to autoimmune disease. Obstet Gynecol 1985;66:27–30.
8. Barrett-Connor E, Bush TL. Estrogen and coronary heart disease in women. JAMA 1991;265:1861–7.
9. Davajan V, Kletzky OA. Secondary amenorrhea without galactorrhea or androgen excess. In: Mishell DR Jr, Davajan V, Lobo RA, eds. Infertility, contraception and reproductive endocrinology, 3rd ed. Boston: Blackwell Scientific, 1991;372–95.
10. Gordon CM. Menstrual disorders in adolescents. Pediatr Clin North Am 1999;46(3):520.
11. Smith-Bindman R, et al. Endometrial ultrasound to exclude endometrial abnormalities. JAMA 1998;280:1510–17.
12. Van Den Bosch T, Vandendael A, Van Schoubroeck D, Wrantz PAB, Lombard CJ. Combining vaginal ultrasonography and office endometrial sampling in the diagnosis of endometrial disease in postmenopausal women. Obstet Gynecol 1995;85(3):349–52.
13. Chen BH, Giudice LC. Dysfunctional uterine bleeding. West J Med 1998;169(5):280–4.
14. Jamieson DJ, Steege JF. The prevalence of dysmenorrhea, dyspareunia, pelvic pain, and irritable bowel syndrome in primary care practices. Obstet Gynecol 1996;87:55–8.
15. Dawood MY. Nonsteroidal anti-inflammatory drugs and changing attitudes toward dysmenorrhea. Am J Med 1988;84:23–9.
16. Dawood MY. Dysmenorrhea. Clin Obstet Gynecol 1990;33:168–78.
17. Coco AS. Primary dysmenorrhea. Am Fam Physician 1999;60:489–96.
18. Smith RP. Gynecology in primary care. Baltimore: Williams & Wilkins, 1997;389–404.
19. Eskenazi B, Warner M. Epidemiology of endometriosis. Obstet Gynecol Clin North Am 1997;24:235–58.

104
Menopause

Pepi Granat

The defining feature of menopause, ovarian failure, has a variable effect among women. Tailoring treatment to each woman's circumstance is crucial to menopause management. Not all changes are unwelcome. Many women are happy to be free of possible pregnancy, menstrual bleeding, dysmenorrhea, and/or fibroids. Many report midlife as their happiest and most productive period.

Lack of estrogen is thought to produce most of menopause's unwanted changes when they occur. Androgen depletion also may play a role.[1] Artificial or premature menopause may occur due to surgery, radiation, or disease. Table 104.1 lists conventional terms describing menopause.[2] Emerging research on estrogen's actions, especially at the molecular level, clarifies its central importance, yet uncertainties can produce fluctuating practice options, especially when studies conflict with clinical experience and patient preference.

Not all women lack estrogen after menopause. Adrenal androstenedione can be converted in fat stroma to estrogen especially, but not exclusively, in obese women who are then exposed to unopposed endogenous estrogen, with risk of endometrial hyperplasia and cancer.

Choosing from a plethora of products for estrogen or hormone replacement therapy (ERT or HRT) and coordinating with treatment of chronic and acute diseases of aging require judgment. Since patients' adherence to prescribed regimens is historically poor,[3] physicians must create uniquely suitable methods of shared decision making and patient education. The physician's knowledge base, experience, personal preference, and enthusiasm are key, since women adhere better to regimens presented convincingly.[4,5]

Effects of Estrogen Deficiency

Urogenital Atrophy

Vaginal dryness, soreness, bleeding, urinary infections, dysuria, and dyspareunia can occur.[6] As sexual activity declines, the vagina can constrict, making intercourse or even pelvic examination impossible. Function is restored with estrogen therapy, systemically or locally. Since healthy functioning contributes to well-being,[7] prevention of genital atrophy warrants emphasis in decision making.[8]

Breast Cancer

Although women have a 1 in 28 chance of dying of breast cancer and a 1 in 5 chance of dying of coronary heart disease (CHD), they fear breast cancer much more than heart disease. Estrogen may promote a lower grade of breast cancer of low virulence with good outcome.[9] Mortality in women who develop breast cancer while on estrogen is lower than if breast cancer develops off hormones.[10]

Oral Health; Ear, Nose, and Throat

Estrogen repletion yields less periodontitis and tooth loss.[11] The voice and laryngeal mucosa are also affected.[12] Women singers and speakers have lowered vocal range due to a net androgenic effect, unless estrogen is replaced.

Skin and Hair Changes

Adrenal production of androgens usually yields predominance of androgenic effect, leading to loss of scalp hair and growth of facial and body hair. Skin becomes thin and loses collagen.

Weight Change

Menopause itself causes weight gain, an effect mistakenly attributed to hormones.[13] Progestogens may retain fluid and cause bloating. In a 12-year prospective study of body mass in 290,827 women,[14] lean and heavy women showed significant benefit from ERT/HRT, with lean women benefiting most.

Cardiovascular Disease

Menopause is a risk factor for CHD[15] (also see Chapter 76). Studies consistently report from one half to one third the amount of CHD in women taking estrogen. More than 30 observational studies reveal a pooled estimate of a relative risk of CHD of 0.65 [95% confidence interval (CI) 0.59–

Table 104.1. **Menopause Glossary**

Menopause	End of menstruation, after 12 months of amenorrhea without obvious other cause, or after damage or removal of ovaries; median age 51 years
Perimenopause	Period of time up to 6 years before and 1 year after menopause
Induced menopause	Cessation of menses after surgery, radiation, or other damage to both ovaries
Premature menopause	Menopause before age 40
Postmenopause	All years after menopause and perimenopause
Confirmation of menopause	By signs, history, and symptoms; may use FSH (30–40 mIU/mL on more than one measurement)

FSH = follicle-stimulating hormone

0.71) for ever-users vs. never-users of estrogen. Despite the association, biases could account for some of the effect. Various biases identified are surveillance bias, healthy-user bias, compliance bias and healthy-survivor bias.[16] Prospective, randomized, double-blind studies of primary prevention are in progress and not completed yet, but observational studies, meta-analyses, animal and in vitro studies, and biologic plausibility uphold opinions that estrogens lessen lipid accretion in arteries. Protection against future events in women with existing heart disease (secondary prevention) has been challenged by recent studies.[17] There is evidence of beneficial effects for at-risk subsets such as women with small dense low-density lipoprotein (LDL) or elevated lipoprotein a [Lp(a)] levels,[18] as well as caution for subsets with certain prothrombotic factors.[19]

Bone

Estrogen favorably affects fracture rate and builds bone. For women whose bone density is inadequate, whether taking ERT/HRT or not, bisphosphonates (etidronate, alendronate, or risedronate) can be added or started. An abnormal peripheral screening bone density should trigger more precise dual-energy x-ray absorptiometry (DEXA) scanning (also see Chapter 122). Adequate calcium (1500 mg) and vitamin D (400 U) is imperative, but without estrogen, bone resorption occurs. Beneficial effects begin whenever ERT/HRT is started after menopause and are lost when stopped, dissipating after 5 years. Progestogens may enhance antiresorptive effects of estrogen but are insignificant alone.[20]

Treatment Options

General Approach to Hormonal Treatments

Hot flashes (or flushes) cause women to seek relief. Instability of estrogen levels produces the hot flush. Although phytoestrogens (isoflavones, lignans, etc.) give some relief,[21] estrogen is predictably efficacious and safe.[22]

Apart from using high-dose estrogen for heavy uterine bleeding, estrogens may be marketed in the United States for three indications: alleviation of hot flushes, prevention of osteoporosis, and treatment of symptomatic urogenital atrophy. When drugs are used "off-label," it is important to document informed consent and shared choice. Such discussions should be revisited often. Contraindications are undiagnosed genital bleeding, pregnancy, known or suspected breast cancer, and active thrombophlebitis. Other contraindications are relative.

The physician's caring approach to inevitable family and life changes cements the relationship, encouraging patient compliance. It helps immensely to elicit a woman's opinion and prior experience with ERT/HRT or oral contraceptives (OCs). Communication by visit, fax, telephone, or e-mail should occur a few weeks after starting a regimen. Women should be seen at least yearly for blood pressure, weight check, and symptom review, with breast, pelvic exam, and Papanicolaou smear, along with mammogram, fecal occult blood, and total assessment for nongynecologic problems, especially surveillance and treatment of ongoing medical conditions as appropriate for age.[23]

Assessment of Estrogen Status

Cycle lengths may shorten early in perimenopause and lengthen later. Heavy bleeding can occur. Unusual bleeding patterns (frequent, heavy, or with clots) may require ultrasound or endometrial biopsy (see Chapter 103). Perimenopause in nonsmokers can be treated with low-dose OCs. HRT will not prevent pregnancy. A follicle-stimulating hormone (FSH) level just before starting a new pill pack can help confirm menopausal status. The switch to HRT can be made after age 51 or 52.

Hormonal blood levels in perimenopause and postmenopause are not always useful, unless estradiol measurement is very low (<20 pg/mL), since wide fluctuations occur. Moreover, serum levels may not reflect target tissue activity. Estradiol levels before menopause are 50 to 500 pg/mL. After menopause they are 5 to 25 pg/mL. Replacement therapy usually yields levels of 40 to 100 pg/mL.[22] FSH levels over 30 or 40 mIU usually indicate menopause. Estrogen status is estimated by symptoms, physical exam of vaginal mucosa, bleeding pattern, and maturation index (microscopical examination for parabasal, intermediate, or superficial epithelial cells of vagina).

Treatment is guided by circumstance and likelihood of adherence. When the uterus is present, progestogen or other endometrial protection must be undertaken.

Treatment, Expectations, and Tolerance

Approach to Options

A usual dose of estrogen (0.625 mg conjugated estrogen or 1 to 2 mg estradiol) plus a progestogen (2.5 mg of medroxyprogesterone or 100 mg of natural micronized progesterone) daily is a starting point for most women. Irregular bleeding can be expected up to 6 to 9 months. Some women prefer a monthly cycle with expected bleeding, which entails giving a progestogen cyclically. If any bleeding would provoke nonadherence, a very low dose regimen of estrogen/progestogen should be chosen. A thin, white, or Asian woman whose mother had osteoporosis might accept transient or cyclical bleeding and tolerate side effects in the hope of preventing bone loss. Fearful or skeptical women should start low, possibly with estrogen alone. Progestogens can be added in 1 to 3 months. Tolerable treatment plans are possible in almost all cases.

Which Estrogen? Estrogen Substitutes? What about SERMs?

Conjugated equine estrogens have a history of 60 years of use. Multiple studies showing benefits of estrogen have been done mostly with this product in the United States. Estradiol has been used more in Europe. Synthetic conjugated equine estrogen mimics natural equine estrogen and comes from plants. It is approved by the Food and Drug Administration (FDA) for hot flashes but not for osteoporosis prevention or treatment. Most of the estrogen in conjugated estrogens is in the form of estrone (E1), which converts to estradiol (E2) mainly in the mucosa of the intestine and in other cells. The circulating hormone that acts at a cellular level is estradiol, which is made by the ovary. Estrone is a reservoir of estrogen in the body, constantly converting between E1 and E2. Estradiol, not conjugated estrogens or estrone, can be applied transdermally, avoiding first-pass hepatic effects on coagulation factors, but also blunting beneficial effects on lipids, especially high-density lipoprotein (HDL). Conjugated estrogens are available in vaginal cream form, are absorbed, and can cause endometrial hyperplasia or cancer, as can even the weak estrogen, estriol, when taken orally, but not when in a vaginal cream. Table 104.2 lists various estrogen products available.

Selective estrogen receptor modulators (SERMs) have variable pro- and antiestrogen actions either alone or in combination with estrogen with or without progestogen. They may become more useful as more evidence accumulates. The finding that tamoxifen exerts proestrogenic effects on bone in the early 1990s led to the understanding that there are two types of estrogen receptors (ERs) in nuclei of target cells, ERα and ERβ.[24,25] Future research may allow tailoring tissue effects using designed molecules to enhance estrogen's many desirable actions while blocking its problematic ones.

Currently, tamoxifen is indicated as adjuvant treatment for breast cancer, and possibly breast cancer prevention in lower doses in high-risk women. Some physicians are using tamoxifen along with estrogen/progesterone regimens after breast cancer. Raloxifene is indicated for osteoporosis prevention but does not have as strong antiresorptive actions as estrogen or bisphosphonates. It will cause, not prevent, hot flushes.

Another product under study is tibolone, a tissue-specific steroid with beneficial effects on vasomotor symptoms, bone, brain, and lipids. It has inhibitory effects on endometrium and breast.[26] It also has androgenic properties.[27]

The Progestogen Problem

Many of the side effects of HRT come from progestogens. Different preparations can be tried to find a tolerable one. Tables 104.3 and 104.4 list combined estrogen/progestogen products and progestogen only products, respectively. Micronized natural progesterone has less dampening effect on some of estrogen's advantageous actions.[28] The progestogen can be given monthly, as was usual in the past, rather than daily. Duration counts more than dose for reducing the risk of endometrial hyperplasia. The dose should be 5 to 10 mg of medroxyprogesterone or 200 mg of natural micronized progesterone or 2.5 to 5 mg of norethindrone acetate daily for a minimum of 12 days monthly, along with the estrogen of choice. The woman should be reassured she may have a period, but this does not mean return of pregnancy potential. Women can take progestogens every 3 to 6 months, but they should be advised their protection from endometrial hyper-

Table 104.2. **Estrogen Products Approved by the Food and Drug Administration**

Estrogen type	Oral	Transdermal	Vaginal	Comment
Conjugated equine estrogens	Premarin		Premarin cream	Derived from pregnant mare's urine
Synthetic conjugated estrogens	Cenestin			Derived from plant material
Esterified estrogens	Estratab, Menest			Plant-derived
Estropipate (piperazine estrone sulphate)	Ortho-Est, Ogen		Ogen cream	Plant-derived
Micronized 17β-estradiol	Estrace	Matrix: Alora, Esclim, Climara, Vivelle, Vivelle-Dot Reservoir: Estraderm	Estrace vaginal cream Estring vaginal ring	
Estradiol hemihydrate			Vagifem vaginal tablet	
Dienestrol			Ortho Dienestrol vaginal cream	Synthetic
Ethinyl estradiol	Estinyl			Synthetic
Chlorotrianisene	TACE			Estrogenic and antiestrogenic properties

Table 104.3. **Estrogen Plus Progesterone Regimens: FDA-Approved Products**

Oral: continuous estrogen/cyclic progesterone	Conjugated equine estrogens (CEEs) and medroxyprogesterone acetate (MPA)	Premphase
Oral: continuous combined (estrogen and progesterone)	CEE and MPA Ethinyl estradiol and norethindrone acetate 17-β estradiol and norethindrone acetate	Prempro Femhrt Activella
Oral: continuous estrogen/intermittent progesterone	17-β estradiol and norgestimate	Ortho-Prefest
Dermal patch: continuous estrogen/cyclic progesterone	17-β estradiol and norethindrone acetate	CombiPatch
Dermal patch: continuous combined (estrogen and progesterone)	17-β estradiol and norethindrone acetate	CombiPatch

plasia is lessened slightly. Women can be offered yearly endometrial biopsy, or yearly ultrasound followed by biopsy if endometrial lining is thickened.

Global Health and Adherence to Prescribed Regimens

General, nonhormonal measures for good health are foremost. All women should cooperate with physicians to achieve smoking cessation; eat favorable food choices; perform aerobic and strengthening exercise; take calcium and vitamin D using supplements if diet or sunlight is inadequate; be screened for degenerative diseases and cancer; pay attention to safety issues such as using seatbelts and bicycle helmets, and domestic violence prevention; and enhance their spiritual, social, and emotional health.

The facts about estrogen and ERT/HRT are a work in progress. Women's adherence to (compliance with) ERT/HRT is 22% to 30%.[2,29,30] If physicians recommend it based on data and experience, they must convey enthusiasm in order to improve these adherence rates.[3] Academic research and physicians' opinions can be upstaged by commercial agendas. Popular stores and magazines scorn the "medicalization" of menopause, promoting untested products. Pharmaceutical campaigns cast doubt about hormones in order to market substitutes.

An estrogen-deficient woman who commits to ERT/HRT appears to be healthier and longer-lived than one who omits it. Several objective decision analyses support this view, based on available evidence. One study using a Markov model concluded that most women would benefit from ERT/HRT, not just in quality of life, but also in length of life, with a gain of at least 6 months.[31] A few women with no cardiac or fracture risk but with high breast-cancer risk may show reduced life expectancy. Another study, which also used Markov model computer analysis, showed high benefit in all groups with no reduction in life expectancy.[32] Even in a worst-case scenario, the benefit of estrogen was maintained, although to a lesser degree. These and other authors[33] conclude that their analyses support broader use of ERT/HRT.

Subsequent data showing lower breast cancer mortality in estrogen users, although the incidence may have been higher, could reveal yet more benefit if factored into these decision analyses. Conversely, current data revealing more secondary cardiac events in the first year on HRT could skew these analyses toward less benefit.[17]

One recent randomized study calls these conclusions into question.[34] This was an 8-year NIH study in healthy women, one arm of which compared conjugated equine estrogens plus MPA with placebo, found a slight increase (26%, 38 vs 30 per 10,000 woman-years) in invasive breast cancer, which almost reached nominal significance. For this slight increase, which exceeded the preset limit, the study had to be stopped after 5.2 years because preset criteria for globally significant benefit versus harm were met. There was no increase in total mortality. The study confirmed much of what is known about estrogen's benefits and risks, and is the first to show reduction in fractures on estrogen plus MPA. It failed to show a reduction in coronary heart disease, yielding a relative hazard risk of 1.29. There was a 37% decrease in colon cancer. In all, there were 19 excess events per 10,000 woman-years. The conclusion of

Table 104.4. **Progestogen Products in Use**

Progestogen type	Oral tablet or pill	IUD/implant/injectable	Vaginal gel	Product
Progestin	Medroxyprogesterone acetate Norethindrone Norethindrone acetate Norgestrel Levonorgestrel	Depo-Provera Injection Norplant, subdermal Mirena, IUD		Cycrin, Provera Micronor, Nor-QD Aygestin Nordette
	Megestrol			Megace
Progesterone	Progesterone USP (in peanut oil) Progesterone	Progestasert IUD	 Crinone	Prometrium

Types of progestogens: progestogen = any substance with progestogenic activity in the body; progesterone = natural progesterone as found in the body; progestin = synthetic progesterone.

the authors was that estrogen plus MPA should not be used or continued primarily for prevention of chronic diseases, but rather for known indications. The estrogen-only arm of the study (in hysterectomized women) has not to date shown the same effects and is scheduled to end in 2005. Despite the discordance of incidence and mortality of breast cancer in many studies (slight increase in incidence, but significant decrease in mortality on estrogen)[35] some women and physicians may be less willing to trade possible breast cancer risk for cardioprotection until definitive studies, possibly at onset of menopause, provide data that supports inferences from observational and cohort studies, animal studies, and biochemical mechanisms, that ERT/HRT may be cardioprotective.

More research, new products, and future analyses will present fresh challenges. Physicians' and women's belief systems are key. High-quality data are difficult to obtain and interpret. Reports and studies must be coupled with clinical experience and patient preference to tailor treatment choices always to the individual woman. Menopause management must take into account how beliefs are formed and changed. The physician is one of the more accurate and stronger forces influencing women's choices.

References

1. Randolph JF, Dennerstein L. Female androgen deficiency syndrome: a hard look at a sexy issue. Medscape Women's Health 2001;6(2).
2. North American Menopause Society (NAMS). *www.menopause.org*.
3. Ravnikar VA. Compliance with hormone replacement therapy: are women receiving the full impact of hormone replacement therapy preventative health benefits? Women's Health Issues 1992;2:75–82.
4. Granat P. Persuasive education for physician and patient. Abstract, Women's Health and Research: multidisciplinary models for excellence. Gainesville, FL: University of Florida (Gainesville), 1997;37.
5. Hill DA, Weiss NS, LaCroix AZ. Adherence to postmenopausal hormone therapy during the year after the initial prescription: a population-based study. Am J Obstet Gynecol 2000;182:270–6.
6. Cardozo L, Bachmann G, McClish D, et al. Meta-analysis of estrogen therapy in the management of urogenital atrophy in postmenopausal women: second report of the Hormones and Urogenital Therapy Committee. Obstet Gynecol 1998;92:722–7.
7. Leiblum SR. Redefining female sexual response. Contemp Obstet/Gynecol 2000;45(11):120–126.
8. Freedman M. Sexuality in post-menopausal women. Menopausal Med 2000;8(4):1–5.
9. Gapstur SM, Morrow M, Sellars TA. Hormone replacement therapy and risk of breast cancer with a favorable histology: results of the Iowa Women's Health Study. JAMA 1999;281:2091–7.
10. Bergkvist L, Adami HO, Persson I, Bergstrom R, Krusemo UB. Prognosis after breast cancer diagnosis in women exposed to estrogen and estrogen-progestogen replacement therapy. Am J Epidemiol 1989;130:221–8.
11. Krall EA, Dawson-Hughes B, Hannan MT, Wilson PW, Kiel DP. Postmenopausal estrogen replacement and tooth retention. Am J Med 1997;102:536–42.
12. Abitbol J, Abitbol P, Abitbol BJ. Sex hormones and the female voice. Voice 1999;13(3):424–46.
13. Chmouliovsky L, Habicht F, James RW, Lehmann T, Cam-
pana A, Golay A. Beneficial effect of hormone replacement therapy on weight loss in obese menopausal women. Maturitas 1999;32(3):147–53.
14. Rodriguez C, Calle EE, Patel AV, et al. Effect of body mass on the association between estrogen replacement therapy and mortality among elderly US women. Am J Epidemiol 2001;153(2):145–52.
15. Gohlke-Barwolf C. Coronary artery disease—is menopause a risk factor? Basic Res Cardiol 2000;95(suppl 1):I77–83.
16. Sturgeon SR, Schairer C, Brinton LA, Pearson T, Hoover RN. Evidence of a healthy estrogen user survivor effect. Epidemiology 1995;6:227–31.
17. Hulley S, Grady D, Bush T, et al. Randomized trial of estrogen plus progestin for secondary prevention of coronary heart disease in postmenopausal women. JAMA 1998;280:605–13.
18. Shlipak MG, Simon JA, Vittinghoff E, et al. Estrogen and progestin, lipoprotein(a), and the risk of recurrent coronary heart disease events after menopause. JAMA 2000;283(14):1845–52.
19. Psaty BM, Smith NL, Lemaitre RN, et al. Hormone replacement therapy, prothrombotic mutations, and the risk of incident nonfatal myocardial infarction in postmenopausal women JAMA 2001;285:906–13.
20. Alkhom D, Vokes T. Treatment of postmenopausal osteoporosis. JAMA 2001;285:1215–8.
21. Potter SM. Soy protein and isoflavones: their effects on blood lipids and bone density in postmenopausal women. Am J Clin Nutr 1998;68(suppl):1375s–9s.
22. Speroff L, Glass RH, Kase NG. Postmenopausal hormone therapy. In: Clinical gynecologic endocrinology and infertility, 6th ed. Philadelphia: Lippincott Williams and Wilkins, 1999;725–67.
23. U.S. Preventive Services Task Force. Guide to clinical preventive services: report of the U.S. Preventive Services Task Force, 2nd ed. Washington, DC: US Preventive Services Task Force, 1996.
24. Love RR, Mazes RB, Barden HS, et al. Effect of tamoxifen on bone mineral density in post-menopausal women with breast cancer. N Engl J Med 1992;326:852–6.
25. Foegh ML, Ramwell PW. Cardiovascular effects of estrogen: implications of the discovery of the estrogen receptor subtype beta. Curr Opin Nephrol Hypertens 1998;7(1):83–9.
26. Kloosterboer HJ. Tibolone: a steroid with a tissue-specific mode of action. J Steroid Biochem Mol Biol 2001;76(1–5):231–8.
27. Morley JE. Androgens and aging. Maturitas 2001;38(1):61–71.
28. The Writing Group for the PEPI Trial. Effects of estrogen or estrogen/progestin regimens on heart disease risk factors in postmenopausal women. The Postmenopausal Estrogen/Progestin Interventions (PEPI) Trial. JAMA 1995;273:199–208.
29. Udoff L, Langenberg P, Adashi EY. Combined continuous hormone replacement therapy: a critical review. Obstet Gynecol 1995;86:306–16.
30. Hammond CB. Women's concerns with hormone replacement therapy—compliance issues. Fertil/Steril 1994;62(suppl 2):157S–60S.
31. Col NF. Patient-specific decisions about hormone replacement therapy in postmenopausal women. JAMA 1997;277(14):1140–7.
32. Zubialde JP, Lawler F, Clemenson N. Estimated gains in life expectancy with use of postmenopausal estrogen therapy: a decision analysis. J Fam Pract 1993;36:271–80.
33. Gorsky RD, Koplan JP, Peterson HB, Thacker SB. Relative risks and benefits of long-term estrogen replacement therapy: a decision analysis. Obstet Gynecol 1994;83:161–6.
34. Writing Group for the Women's Health Initiative Investigators. Risks and benefits of estrogen plus progestin in healthy postmenopausal women. Principle results from the women's health initiative randomized control trial. JAMA 2002;288:321–33.
35. Bush TL, Whiteman M, Flaws JA. Hormone replacement therapy and breast cancer: a qualitative review. Obstet Gynecol 2001 Sep;98(3):498–508.

Tumors of the Female Reproductive Organs

Kathi D. Clement and Ronald L. Malm

Common tumors of the female reproductive system include leiomyomas and cervical, endometrial, and ovarian carcinomas.

Leiomyomas

Leiomyoma or fibroid is one of the most frequently encountered disorders of the female genital tract; most are asymptomatic benign findings on a routine pelvic examination. Until recently, diagnosis and treatment for symptomatic leiomyomas was hysterectomy. Diagnostic studies now include pelvic ultrasonography, computed tomography (CT) scan, hysteroscopy, and rarely magnetic resonance imaging (MRI). Treatment may include hysteroscopic procedures such as endometrial ablation for bleeding or hysteroscopic myomectomy, laparoscopic myomectomy, gonadotropin-releasing hormone to reduce the size of the fibroid and induce amenorrhea, and hysterectomy.

Signs and Symptoms

Most leiomyomas are asymptomatic and noted as a pelvic mass at the time of a routine gynecologic examination. The most common type is intramural or subserous (Fig. 105.1). The etiology of leiomyomas is unknown, but there is clear evidence of estrogen dependence because fibroids invariably shrink after menopause. If estrogen therapy is instituted with menopause, leiomyomas may not decrease in size—this occurs with transdermal estrogen, rather than with oral conjugated estrogen.[1] The growth usually appears between ages 30 and 40. The prevalence increases among black women.

Symptoms include abnormal bleeding, pelvic pressure, lower abdominal mass, and less commonly pelvic pain and vaginal discharge. Rarely, symptoms occur because of pressure on the ureters or rectum. Patients with foul discharge, pain, and heavy bleeding may have an infected prolapsing submucous fibroid. Other painful tumors include leiomyomas that enlarge so rapidly avascular degeneration occurs; these lesions occur more frequently during pregnancy.

Differential Diagnosis

Evaluation of a pelvic mass is designed to rule out an ovarian tumor or uterine sarcoma. Noninvasive methods include transvaginal ultrasonography as an initial diagnostic tool, with CT and MRI to further delineate the mass.[2] Hysteroscopy, although invasive, may provide both diagnosis and treatment via dissection of some submucous fibroids and destruction of the endometrium by endometrial ablation.[3] Finally, hysterectomy is the definitive diagnostic and treatment method.

Abnormal bleeding from a myomatous uterus requires further evaluation. Several etiologies for this condition are endometrial hyperplasia or malignancy, distortion of the endometrial cavity by the fibroid, disturbance of the pituitary-ovarian axis, and anovulatory bleeding. The workup may include endometrial biopsy or curettage, hysteroscopy, hysterosalpingography, timed endometrial biopsies, ultrasonography, and serial plasma progesterone assays.

Complications

Major complications of leiomyomas can occur during pregnancy (see Chapter 13). The fibroid can grow so rapidly that avascular necrosis results. Also, with incomplete abortions in the myomatous uterus, placental fragments can become infected, hemorrhage can occur, and curetting may become not only difficult but also dangerous. Other complications include abnormal labor patterns, malpresentations, infertility, and chronic abortion. Bleeding myomas may lead to anemia.

Management

The key to management is the control of symptoms once a benign diagnosis is established. Considerations include the

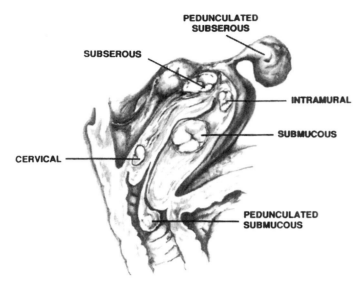

Fig. 105.1. Most common types of leiomyomas: intramural or subserous.

patient's age, fertility status, and reliability; other medical problems that might influence surgical status; and the effect of the tumor on surrounding tissue. If fertility is a factor and there are major symptoms, a reasonable approach is myomectomy. Although a leiomyoma can recur, this situation occurs less frequently with women who have had a child after myomectomy.[4] A gonadotropin-releasing hormone (GnRH) agonist, leuprolide (Lupron), can reduce fibroid size and symptoms.[5-7] A single, daily dose of leuprolide acetate results in an initial increase of luteinizing hormone (LH) and follicle-stimulating hormone (FSH).[8] This action leads to a transient increase in estrone and estradiol in premenopausal women. Continuous daily doses decrease the LH and FSH levels in all patients. In premenopausal women estrogens are reduced to postmenopausal levels. After therapy, the fibroid may enlarge, but symptoms do not necessarily recur. Long-term, continuous therapy (2 years or more) increases bone loss because of the induced hypoestrogenic state.[9,10] In some cases, leuprolide has become an adjunct to presurgical therapy for reducing fibroid size, so laparoscopic myomectomy or vaginal hysterectomy can be done.[11]

Cervical Carcinoma

Epidemiology and Etiology

The cervical cancer death rate in the United States has decreased 63% over a 30-year span (1960–1990) but has increased in recent years in women under 50. Yet 65,000 cases of cervical cancer in situ, 12,900 cases of invasive cervical carcinoma, and 4400 deaths were expected in 2001.[12] Despite decreasing rates of invasive cervical cancer, preinvasive lesions of the cervix remain a leading cause of morbidity in young women. Invasive cervical cancer is the third most common gynecologic malignancy and one of the leading causes of cancer death in women. Human papillomavirus (HPV) has been implicated as a sexually transmitted etiology for cervical dysplasia and carcinoma, as certain strains of the HPV virus have oncogenic potential[13] (see Chapter 102).

Major risk factors for cervical carcinoma include a present or past history of an abnormal Papanicolaou (Pap) smear; multiple sexual partners; early age at first intercourse[14]; being African American, Hispanic, or Native American[15]; history of genital warts or other sexually transmitted diseases[16,17]; smoking[18,19]; using oral contraceptives (especially the high-dose estrogen pills used during the 1960s and 1970s)[20]; an immunocompromised state; a partner with genital warts; a sexual partner who has had intercourse with a female who developed cervical cancer; and being a woman whose mother had taken diethylstilbestrol during her pregnancy.[21]

Screening

Not a diagnostic tool but, rather, a screening method, the Pap smear remains the first step when evaluating for cervical carcinoma. Some of the inadequacies of the screening process are Pap smear false negatives (5–56%), failure to identify high-risk patients, inaccurate or incomplete laboratory reports, poor patient compliance, and inadequate follow-up by the physician.[22] Because the Pap smear contains cells from only a small area, cancerous or precancerous lesions can be missed if the abnormality is small, deep in the canal, or an advanced invasive lesion where infection and necrotic tissue obscure the true cytology; consequently the smear is reported as squamous atypia and inflammation.

Because cervical intraepithelial neoplasia (CIN) arises within the transformation zone, an adequate sample must contain columnar epithelium from the endocervix, immature metaplastic cells, or both. Adequate sampling becomes more difficult when the transformation zone is less accessible, such as with premenarcheal, pregnant, postmenopausal, or postcervical irradiation patients.[23] Today, sampling tools for cervical cytology include cytobrush, broom brush, and/or plastic spatula. An alternative to the conventional Pap smear is liquid-based mono-layer cytology, which increases the sensitivity in detecting both high- and low-grade lesions. This one-brush technique provides better cellular adequacy, increased detection of squamous intraepithelial lesions (SILs), and can also be used for HPV typing.[24-26] It is costlier, two to four times more expensive than the Pap smear. Cervicography, which incorporates a photograph of the cervix stained with acetic acid that is sent to a diagnostic center where trained colposcopists review it, is no longer thought to be an adjunct for cytologic screening.[27]

Terminology on the Pap report is a description of the cytology. The Bethesda System provides a standard terminology for Pap smear reports. The new Bethesda System 2001 simplifies the Pap smear report (Table 105.1). Epithelial abnormalities are Bethesda-classified as squamous or glandular. According to current Bethesda guidelines, patients with atypical squamous cells of undetermined significance (ASC-US) should have repeat Pap smears at 6-month intervals for 2 years plus; if the smear suggests inflammation, studies to rule out cervical and vaginal infection should be done. The atypical

Table 105.1. **Bethesda System 2001**

Specimen type: Indicate conventional smear (Pap smear) vs. liquid based vs. other

Specimen adequacy
 Satisfactory for evaluation (describe presence or absence of endocervical/transformation zone component and any other quality limiting factors)
 Unsatisfactory for evaluation (specify reason)
  Specimen rejected (specify reason)
  Specimen processed and examined, but unsatisfactory for evaluation of epithelial abnormality because of (specify reason)

General categorization (optional)
 Negative for intraepithelial lesion or malignancy
 Epithelial cell abnormality: see interpretation/result (specify squamous or glandular as appropriate)
 Other: see interpretation/result

Automated review
If case examined by automated device, specify device and result

Ancillary testing
Provide a brief description of the test methods and report the results so that it is easily understood

Interpretations/result
 Negative for intraepithelial lesion or malignancy
  Organisms
   Trichomonas vaginalis
   Fungal organisms morphologically consistent with *Candida* spp.
   Shift in vaginal flora suggestive of bacterial vaginosis
   Bacteria morphologically consistent with *Actinomyces* spp.
   Cellular changes associated with herpes simplex virus
  Other nonneoplastic findings (optional to report; not inclusive)

Reactive cellular changes associated with
 Inflammation (includes typical repair)
 Radiation
 Intrauterine contraceptive device (IUD)
Glandular cells status posthysterectomy
Atrophy
Other
 Endometrial cells (in a woman ≥40 years of age)
Epithelial cell abnormalities
 Squamous cell
  Atypical squamous cells
   Of undetermined significance (ASC-US)
   Cannot exclude HSIL (ASC-H)
  Low-grade squamous intraepithelial lesion (LSIL) encompassing: HPV/mild dysplasia/CIN 1
  High-grade squamous intraepithelial lesion (HSIL) encompassing: moderate and severe dysplasia, CIS/CIN 2 and CIN 3
   With features suspicious for invasion (if invasion is suspected)
  Squamous cell carcinoma
 Glandular cell
  Atypical
   Endocervical cells
   Endometrial cells
   Glandular cells
  Atypical glandular/endocervical cells, favor neoplastic
  Endocervical adenocarcinoma in situ
  Adenocarcinoma
   Endocervical
   Endometrial
   Extrauterine
   Not otherwise specified (NOS)
Other Malignant Neoplasms

glandular cell report represents a dilemma, as adenocarcinoma in situ often lies beyond the limits of colposcopy and has no colposcopic appearance. In addition, 37% to 50% of patients with an atypical glandular cell report may have a histologic diagnosis of dysplasia or cancer.[28] These women should undergo colposcopy and endocervical curettage, and they may also need cone biopsy.[29] Other cytologic terms found within the Bethesda System that may require clarification include low- and high-grade squamous intraepithelial lesions (LGSILs and HGSILs). LGSIL encompasses mild dysplasia, HPV, and/or cervical intraepithelial neoplasm 1 (CIN 1), and HGSIL indicates moderate to severe dysplasia, CIN 2 or 3.

Diagnosis

An abnormal Pap smear, high-risk history, or suspicious lesions of the cervix, vulva, or vagina necessitate further evaluation by colposcopy and colposcopically directed biopsies (Fig. 105.2). During colposcopy, which magnifies the area, abnormalities indicating probable cervical neoplasia can be noted and biopsied. Abnormalities include epithelium that turns white with acetic acid, leukoplakia, gross lesions, or abnormal vascular patterns including punctation (pinpoint ves-

sels) and mosaicism (abnormal pattern of vessels). Biopsies during pregnancy can be omitted if microinvasion or invasive carcinoma is not suspected.[30] The entire squamocolumnar junction must be visualized, and an endocervical curettage (ECC) is performed, except during pregnancy, to rule in or out endocervical canal/transformation zone involvement. Finally, the cytology, colposcopic impression, and histology of the biopsies should correspond. If they do not, further evaluation and biopsies are done, as the histology may not yet reflect the true biologic potential.[31] If the biopsies reveal preinvasive disease and the ECC is negative, cryotherapy, a loop electrosurgical excision procedure (LEEP), or laser therapy is indicated, with a follow-up Pap smear in 3 to 4 months. Although cryotherapy has been proved to be not only cost-effective but also most effective for CIN 1 or 2, there are some restrictive criteria. For instance, no more than the proximal 5 mm of the canal can be involved, the lesion must be covered by the cryoprobe, and lesions that are large and encompass more than two quadrants of the cervix should be treated by LEEP or laser ablation. LEEP is an electrosurgical excision that is exceptionally fast, technically simple, and utilized more frequently than laser ablation, as it is more cost-effective and an office procedure. LEEP (or laser ablation) is preferred for

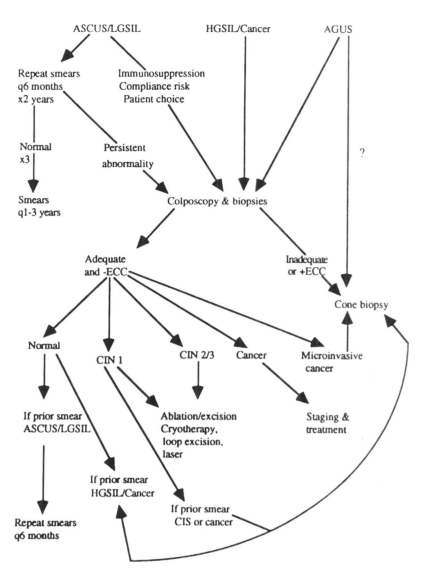

Fig. 105.2. Evaluation process of an abnormal Papanicolaou smear, high-risk history, or suspicious lesions of the cervix, vulva, or vagina. ASCUS = atypical cells of undetermined significance; LGSIL = low-grade squamous intraepithelial lesion; HGSIL = high-grade squamous intraepithelial lesion; AGUS = atypical glandular cells of undetermined significance; ECC = endocervical curettage; CIN = cervical intraepithelial neoplasia; CIS = carcinoma in situ.

large lesions, high-grade (CIN 3) lesions, or lesions that extend into the canal. Contraindications for cervical LEEP include lesions suggestive of invasion, any situation where thermal artifact could preclude diagnosis, and pregnancy.[32,33]

Conization is used for cases with a positive ECC, discordance between cytology and histology, unsatisfactory colposcopy results, or the need to distinguish between microinvasion and true invasive carcinoma. The cervical cone should include the external cervical os, a part of the portio vaginalis, and a portion of the endocervical canal. If the invasion is more than 3 mm, one proceeds with a staging evaluation.[34]

To help with clinical staging, cystoscopy, flexible sigmoidoscopy, intravenous urography, chest radiography, CT, MRI, and bone scans may be warranted.[35] A lymphangiogram detects changes in the internal architecture of nodes contained within a metastatic deposit. When the node is completely replaced by tumor, the node no longer opacifies, and the lymphatic channel may or may not be obstructed. Thus these two markers of metastasis could be read as falsely negative. These nodes can be discerned by CT and MRI. MRI is more accurate than CT for assessing the thickness of cervical stromal invasion.[36] Accurate staging is essential to determine the mode of therapy.[37]

Cervical cancer spreads locally into the uterine corpus and vagina. Involvement of the uterine corpus increases the incidence of distant metastasis and worsens prognosis.[37] Usually, bladder and rectal involvement is rare without extensive disease. After extensive local involvement, hematogenous spread occurs with metastases to the lung (26.5%), liver (16%), bone (14%), and bowel (8%).[38] Lymphatic dissemination usually involves the pelvic lymph nodes, followed by the paraaortic lymph nodes, and finally the scalene nodes.

Treatment

In the past cure of cervical cancer included simple amputation of the cervix, but now surgical procedures for the cancer focus on hysterectomy and lymphadenectomy. The role of radical hysterectomy and pelvic lymphadenectomy has increased as more patients present with early-stage cervical carcinoma. From 1983 to 1991 more than 54% of white women and 39% of black women with cervical carcinoma were diagnosed with localized disease.[39] Considerations for radiation therapy rather than surgery include morbid obesity, significant health problems that would compromise surgical recovery, and tumor bulk. Recent phase III trials of advanced cancer populations or women with early-stage disease but poor prognostic factors (metastatic disease with pelvic lymph node involvement, parametrial disease, or positive surgical margins) show improved survival for cisplatin-based therapy given concurrently with radiation therapy.[39] Surgery usually conserves one or both ovaries, thereby preventing most of the effects of estrogen deprivation and sexual dysfunction. The latter is especially important, as the effects of radiotherapy on the vagina include shortening, fibrosis, and atrophy. Ovarian ablation may occur, and there is an 8% chance of developing genitourinary or gastrointestinal fistulas.[40] Although most cervical cancers are radiosensitive and radiation therapy is standard for advanced cancers, radical hysterectomy is preferable in the young, healthy woman with early lesions (stage IIA or less), as this form of treatment leaves a woman's tissue in a better state of preservation.

Endometrial Hyperplasia and Cancer

Epidemiology and Etiology

Endometrial cancer is the most common pelvic malignancy in American women today. The average woman has a 1% chance of developing endometrial cancer during her lifetime. It is estimated that in 2001 there will be 38,300 new cases of endometrial cancer and 6600 deaths.[41] The incidence of endometrial cancer remained fairly constant from the 1940s to 1960s at 23.9 cases per 100,000 women.[41] The incidence then increased significantly from 1960 to 1975, attributed to more frequent use of exogenous estrogen[42] (see Chapter 104). After 18 months of unopposed estrogen use, women had a 30% incidence of endometrial hyperplasia. Fifteen years of unopposed estrogen use resulted in a seven times greater chance for the development of endometrial cancer compared with women who did not use estrogen.[43] Estrogens promote endometrial cell reproduction and may accelerate changes that lead to neoplasia in the endometrium.[44] In the past, endometrial hyperplasia (EH) was thought to be a precursor of endometrial carcinoma. The International Society of Gynecologic Pathologists have classified EH into categories of simple and complex, with most simple EH regressing spontaneously or with progestin suppressive therapy.[45] The complex hyperplasia with atypia is a precursor of endometrial carcinoma.

Risk Factors

Although the literature is not in complete agreement on all risk factors associated with the development of endometrial cancer, each bears review and attention.[46] Data suggest that a significant number of women without any predisposition for endometrial cancer based on these risk factors will develop the disease.[47] Most of these risk factors are somehow related to estrogen, whether exogenous or endogenous. Age seems to be the only constant indicator for endometrial carcinoma.[47]

1. Age: Patients in their mid-fifties frequently have more aggressive cancers and higher mortality rates (75%).[47] However, any woman can develop endometrial hyperplasia and

carcinoma. The significance of age is most likely related to the onset of menopause or recent postmenopause.[48] Women in their sixties and seventies have the highest incidence of the cancer; on the other hand, fewer than 5% of women develop the disease before age 40.[49]

2. Obesity: Numerous studies have associated obesity with an increased incidence of endometrial cancer.[50–53] Large concentrations of fat in the upper body (android obesity) put women at greater risk for developing endometrial cancer.[54] Many women who are not obese do develop endometrial hyperplasia and carcinoma, so obesity is not necessarily a causal factor for the disease.

3. Previous breast cancer: Research has identified an association between breast cancer and the risk of developing endometrial carcinoma (see Chapter 107). This association represents a modest increase in risk, but the increasing number of women presenting with breast cancer represents a potential increase in endometrial cancer.[55] Women who are overweight (80 kg or more) and have a history of breast cancer are at even greater risk for developing endometrial carcinoma.[56] Women receiving tamoxifen therapy for breast cancer may also be at increased risk.[57]

4. Nulliparity: Research associates nulliparity with increased risk of endometrial cancer, but it is not necessarily a causal factor for the disease. Parous women have a 30% lower risk of endometrial cancer than nulliparous women. Risk decreases as the mother's age at the last pregnancy increases.[58]

5. Late onset of menopause: Women who enter menopause after 52 years of age are at increased risk for endometrial cancer when compared with women who have finished menopause by 49 years[59] (see Chapter 104).

Diagnosis

Clinical presentation includes abnormal bleeding in about 80% of patients. This bleeding may be premenstrual, intermenstrual, or postmenstrual. Bleeding in premenopausal women is usually described as excessive flow at the time of menstruation. Women over age 80 with postmenopausal bleeding account for 50% to 60% of the cases of diagnosed endometrial carcinoma. Approximately 10% of patients also have lower-abdominal cramping as well as bleeding. Women who experience menstrual irregularities and are over age 40 should undergo endometrial sampling to rule out malignancy. Those women who are extremely anxious or who present with stenosis or large leiomyomas should not be tested in the office.[60]

Sampling techniques include the following:

1. Papanicolaou smear: Whereas this technique is excellent for cervical cancers, it is ineffective when screening for endometrial cancer and should not be used.

2. Dilation and curettage (D&C): This technique has a 90% accuracy rate, but it is costly, painful, and may result in infection, perforation, and hemorrhage.[61]

3. Aspiration curettage: This technique has an 80% to 90% accuracy rate; adequate samples are usually obtained, and it is cost-effective. Problems associated with the technique include pain in the event of myometrium adherence and

the physician's lack of experience. Negative findings should never be considered definitive.[61]

4. Endometrial biopsy: This technique has an accuracy of 90% to 95%,[62,63] and usually causes less cramping than other techniques.

5. Pelvic ultrasonography: Ultrasonography is proving to be a useful tool for diagnosing endometrial carcinomas.[64–66] The thickness of the endometrium can be measured relatively easily, and the endometrial–myometrial junction has a distinct halo-like appearance. Measurements of less than 4 mm are reassuring but alone are not diagnostic.[67] Ultrasonography may be able to detect benign causes of abnormal bleeding, such as submucous myomas or polyps.

6. Hysteroscopy: Although used more frequently for evaluation of recurrent miscarriage, infertility due to endometrial abnormalities, or removal of an impacted intrauterine contraceptive device (IUD), hysteroscopically directed biopsies may be more accurate than D&C.[68]

Treatment

Management options for endometrial hyperplasia and carcinoma range from periodic sampling of the endometrial cavity in the case of simple hyperplasia to hysterectomy for atypical hyperplasia. The most successful treatments for endometrial carcinoma typically include surgery and irradiation; radiation therapy and surgery combined tend to be more successful than surgery alone.[69] Progesterone has been used in women unable to tolerate surgery and irradiation. Posttreatment follow-up includes physical examination, vaginal cytology, and a serum CA-125 assay, all performed at 6-month intervals for 3 years.[70]

Ovarian Cancer

Epidemiology and Etiology

Although few women develop ovarian cancer, it is the fourth most common cause of female cancer death. The American Cancer Society estimates that 23,400 new cases of ovarian cancer will be diagnosed in 2001 and 13,900 women will die from this disease.[41] Although ovarian cancer ranks second in incidence among gynecologic cancers, it causes more deaths than any other cancer of the female reproductive tract. From 1973 to 1991, the relative 5-year survival for all stages of the disease increased from 36% to only 42%.[71] Since the early 1980s any decrease in overall mortality of patients with ovarian cancer may be directly attributed to the excellent survival of the 1400 patients diagnosed annually with germ-line tumors, due to widespread curability of these relatively rare tumors. Epithelial ovarian cancer is the most common lethal malignancy of the female genital tract. Because 70% of women present with advanced-stage disease (stage III or IV), the prognosis of ovarian cancer is generally poor. At best, this group has a 15% to 20% chance of 5-year survival despite aggressive treatment. With early diagnosis and treatment, the relative survival rate jumps to 90%, but early diagnosis is rare.[71]

The etiology of ovarian cancer is unknown, although hereditary, environmental, dietary, reproductive, endocrine, and viral factors may be associated with it.[72] Although a positive family history of ovarian cancer increases a woman's risk 20-fold, 95% of women with ovarian cancer have no family history for it.[73] Familial ovarian cancer is thought to be inherited in an autosomal-dominant pattern with variable penetrance. First-degree relatives (i.e., mother, sister, daughter) who share one-half of a patient's genes have as high as a 50% chance of developing the disease. This propensity contrasts with the 1.4% (1/70) for women with a negative family history for ovarian cancer.[74]

Pregnancy and the use of oral contraceptives may protect against the development of ovarian cancer.[72] However, recent research suggests that oral contraceptives may not be protective in women who carry the BRCA1 or BRCA2 gene mutation.[75] Conversely, nulliparity or low parity and the lack of oral contraceptive use are considered risk factors for ovarian cancer. The model developed by Pike[73] suggests that 5 years of combination-type oral contraceptive use may decrease the lifelong risk of ovarian cancer by approximately 50%. Other possible risk factors include a history of breast, endometrial, or colon cancer; viruses including rubella and mumps; noncontraceptive estrogens; blood group A; and being Caucasian or from an industrialized nation.[76]

Screening Tests

Ovarian cancer is often "silent," showing no obvious signs or symptoms until late in its development. The changes in management by surgery, chemotherapy, and radiotherapy have done little to improve survival rates.[75] Consequently, more emphasis on early screening may solve the problem (see Chapter 7). Young et al[77] suggested that if cancer is detected when it is confined to the capsule of the ovary, the outcome following surgery may be improved. Although pelvic examination is an important part of the gynecologic examination, small ovarian lesions are often missed. Bourne et al[76] noted that little success has been achieved using culdocentesis or radioimmunoscintigraphy for early screening. Consequently, the development of a screening test has focused on changes in tumor-related antigens in the peripheral circulation and pelvis and transvaginal ultrasonography.

A glycoprotein tumor-associated antigen, CA-125 has been investigated as a clinically useful marker. The serum level of CA-125 is more than 35 U/mL in about 80% of women with epithelial ovarian cancer.[74] However, only 50% of women with stage I disease have an elevated CA-125.[74] There may be marked elevations of CA-125 with benign ovarian tumors, salpingitis, endometriosis, benign gastrointestinal disorders such as cirrhosis or pancreatitis, and other malignancies including pancreatic, liver, gastric, lung, colorectal, and even breast carcinoma.[78] Consequently, the specificity is not adequate to fulfill true screening criteria. CA-125 is also useful for following the patient's response to therapy.[79]

Campbell et al[80] proposed screening for ovarian cancer with ultrasonography (US). The newer use of transvaginal US leads to improved image quality, which may lead to increased detection of ovarian abnormalities.[75] Evaluation of any US abnormality should include a repeat scan to avoid removal of ovaries that are only undergoing transient physiologic changes.

Advances in Treatment

Currently, treating patients with advanced ovarian cancer consists of surgery followed by systemic chemotherapy with a platinum-containing regimen.[80] Because the success rate is limited, several modalities are being investigated, and new treatments are clearly needed.[81] Throughout most of its course, ovarian cancer remains within the confines of the abdominal cavity. Consequently, intraperitoneal administration of cytotoxic agents has many theoretic advantages over systemic administration.

Efforts to develop biologic agents that circumvent the usual resistance patterns in tumors partially treated with chemotherapy are under way.[82] Monoclonal antibody conjugates can be used for tumor localization and delivery of cytotoxic substances to tumor cells. Interferons have been used both systemically and intraperitoneally. Other biologic agents, such as interleukin-2, tumor necrosis factor, and lymphokine-activated killer cells, are currently undergoing clinical trials. Likewise, the use of some compounds in photodynamic therapy is being investigated.

Conclusion

Information contained in this chapter leads to an obvious conclusion: We must emphasize prevention and early detection in the office setting to decrease mortality. Prevention includes teaching patients the early warning signs of various reproductive problems, continuing to read the literature for developments in screening and treatment techniques, and knowing that, despite best efforts, many of these cancers are missed.

References

1. Sener AB, Seckin NC, Ozman S, et al. The effects of hormone replacement therapy on uterine fibroids in postmenopausal women. Fertil Steril 1996;65:354–7.
2. Weinreb JC, Barkoff ND, Megibow A, et al. The value of MR imaging in distinguishing leiomyomas from other solid pelvic masses when sonography is indeterminate. AJR 1990;154:295–9.
3. American College of Obstetricians and Gynecologists. Surgical alternatives to hysterectomy in the management of leiomyomas ACOG practice bulletin 16. Washington, DC: ACOG, May 2000; 1–10.
4. Candiani GB, Fedele L, Parazzini F, et al. Risk of recurrence after myomectomy. Br J Obstet Gynaecol 1991;98:385–9.
5. Friedman AJ, Hoffman DI, Comite F, et al. Treatment of leiomyomata uteri with leuprolide acetate depot: a double blind, placebo-controlled, multicenter study: the leuprolide study group. Obstet Gynecol 1991;77:720–5.
6. Stovall TG, Ling FW, Henry LC, et al. A randomized trial evaluation: leuprolide acetate before hysterectomy as treatment for leiomyomas. Am J Obstet Gynecol 1991;164:1420–3.
7. Pace JN, Miller JL, Rose LI. GnRH agonists: gonadorelin, leuprolide, and nafarelin. Am Fam Physician 1991;44:1777–82.
8. Physicians' desk reference, 55th ed. Montvale, NJ: Medical Economics, 2001;3176.
9. Friedman AF, Lobel SM, Rein MS, et al. Efficacy and safety considerations in women with uterine leiomyomas treated with gonadotrophin-releasing hormone agonists: the estrogen threshold hypothesis. Am J Obstet Gynecol 1990;163:1114–9.
10. Barbieri RL. Gonadotrophin-releasing hormone agonists and es-

11. Zullo F, Pellicano M, De Stefano R, et al. A prospective randomized study to evaluate leuprolide acetate treatment before laparoscopic myomectomy: efficacy and ultrasonographic predictors. Am J Obstet Gynecol 1998;178:108–12.
12. Greenlee R, Hill-Harmon M, Murray T, et al. Cancer statistics 2001. CA Cancer J Clin 2001;51(1):15–36.
13. Lungu O, Sun XW, Felix J, et al. Relationship of human papillomavirus type to grade of cervical intraepithelial neoplasia. JAMA 1992;267:2493–6.
14. Brinton LA, Frammeni JF. Epidemiology of uterine cervical cancer. J Chronic Dis 1986;39:1051–68.
15. Centers for Disease Control. Black-white differences in cervical cancer mortality: United States, 1980–1987. MMWR 1990; 39:245–8.
16. Moscicki A, Palefsky JM, Gonzales J, et al. The association between human papillomavirus, deoxyribonucleic acid status, and the results of cytologic rescreening tests in young, sexually active women. Am J Obstet Gynecol 1991;165:67–71.
17. Carmichael JA, Maskens PD. Cervical dysplasia and human papillomavirus. Am J Obstet Gynecol 1989;160:916–8.
18. Slattery ML, Robison LM, Schuman KL, et al. Cigarette smoking and exposure to passive smoke are risk factors for cervical cancer. JAMA 1989;261:1593–8.
19. Brinton LA, Schairer C, Haenszel W, et al. Cigarette smoking and invasive cervical cancer. JAMA 1986;255:3265–9.
20. Brinton LA, Juggin GR, Lehman HF, et al. Long-term use of oral contraceptives and risk of invasive cervical cancer. Int J Cancer 1986;38:339–44.
21. Devesa SS, Young JL, Brinton LA, et al. Recent trends in cervix uteri cancer. CA Cancer J Clin 1989;64:2184–90.
22. Boring CC, Squires TS, Tong T. Cancer statistics: 1992. CA Cancer J Clin 1992;42:13–38.
23. Nelson JH, Averette HE, Richart RM. Cervical intraepithelial neoplasia (dysplasia and carcinoma in situ) and early invasive cervical carcinoma. CA Cancer J Clin 1989;39:157–78.
24. Bishop JW, Bigner SH, Colgan JJ. Multicenter masked evaluation of AutoCyte PREP thin layers with matched conventional smears including initial biopsy results. Acta Cytol 1998;42: 189–97
25. Lee KR, Ashfaq R, Birdsong GG, et al. Comparison of conventional Papanicolaou smears and a fluid-based thin-layer system for cervical cancer screening. Obstet Gynecol 1997;90:278–84.
26. Sherman ME, Schiffman MH, Lorincz AT, et al. Cervical specimens collected in liquid buffer are suitable for both cytologic screening and ancillary human papillomavirus testing. Cancer 1997;81(2):89–97.
27. Baldauf JJ, Dreyfus M, Ritter J, et al. Cervicography. Does it improve cervical cancer screening? Acta Cytol 1997;41: 295–301.
28. Kaferle JF, Malouin JM. Evaluation and management of the AGUS Papanicolaou smear. Am Fam Physician 2001;63:2239–44.
29. Kurman RJ, Henson DE, Herbst AL, et al. Interim guideline for management of abnormal cervical cytology. JAMA 1994;271: 1866.
30. Benedet JL, Selke PA, Nickerson KG. Colposcopic evaluation of abnormal Papanicolaou smears in pregnancy. Am J Obstet Gynecol 1987;157:932–7.
31. Stafl A, Mattingly RF. Angiogenesis of cervical neoplasia. Am J Obstet Gynecol 1975;121:845–51.
32. Wright TC, Gagnon S, Ferenczy AF, et al. Excising CIN lesions by loop electrosurgical procedure. Contemp Obstet Gynecol 1991;35:57–73.
33. Wright TC, Gagnon MD, Richart RM, et al. Treatment of cervical intraepithelial neoplasia using the loop electrosurgical excision procedure. Obstet Gynecol 1992;79:173–8.

34. Stringer CA. When the Pap is positive: confirming the diagnosis, verifying extent of disease. Prim Care Cancer 1989;9:15–18.

35. Cervix uteri. In: American Joint Committee on Cancer: AJCC cancer staging manual, 5th ed. Philadelphia: Lippincott-Raven, 1997;189–94.

36. Kim SH, Chol BI, Lee HP, et al. Uterine cervical carcinoma: comparison of CT and MR findings. Radiology 1990;175:45–51.

37. Perez CA, Zivnuska F, Askin F, Kumar B, Camel HM, Powers WE. Prognostic significance of endometrial extension from primary carcinoma of the uterine cervix. CA Cancer J Clin 1975;35:1493–504.

38. Lifshitz S, Buchsbaum HJ. The spread of cervical carcinoma. In: Sciarra J, ed. Gynecology and obstetrics. Philadelphia: Lippincott, 1999;7(4):1–3.

39. Morris M, Eifel PJ, Lu J, et al. Pelvic radiation with concurrent chemotherapy compared with pelvic and para-aortic radiation for high-risk cervical cancer. N Engl J Med 1999;340:1137–43.

40. Van Nagell JR, Parker JC, Maruyama Y, Utley J, Luckett P. Bladder or rectal injury following radiation therapy for cervical cancer. Am J Obstet Gynecol 1974;119:727–32.

41. American Cancer Society. Cancer facts and figures 2001. Atlanta, GA: American Cancer Society, 2001.

42. Fu YS, Gambone JC, Berek JS. Pathophysiology and management of endometrial hyperplasia and carcinoma. West J Med 1990;153:50–61.

43. Whitehead M, Fraser D. Controversies concerning the safety of estrogen replacement therapy. Am J Obstet Gynecol 1987;156:1313–22.

44. Gal D. Endometrial hyperplasia: diagnosis and management. In: Sciarra J, ed. Gynecology and obstetrics. Philadelphia: Lippincott, 1999;(4)13:1–11.

45. Silverberg SG. Hyperplasia and carcinoma of the endometrium. Semin Diagn Pathol 1988;5:135.

46. Gursberg SB, Chen SY, Cohen CJ. Endometrial cancer: factors influencing the choice of treatment. Gynecol Oncol 1974;2:308–13.

47. Ferenczy A. Methods for detecting endometrial carcinoma and its precursors. In: Buchsbaum HJ, Sciarra J, eds. Gynecology and obstetrics. New York: Harper & Row, 1982;4:1–8.

48. Gilman CJ. Management of early-stage endometrial carcinoma. Am Fam Physician 1987;35:103–12.

49. Gallup DG, Stock RJ. Adenocarcinoma of the endometrium in women 40 years of age or younger. Obstet Gynecol 1984;64:417–20.

50. Damon A. Host factors in cancer of the breast and uterine cervix. J Natl Cancer Inst 1960;24:483–516.

51. Wynder EL, Escher GC, Mantel N. An epidemiologic investigation of cancer of the endometrium. Cancer 1966;19:489–520.

52. Dunn LJ, Bradbury JT. Endocrine factors in endometrial carcinoma: a preliminary report. Am J Obstet Gynecol 1967;97:465–71.

53. Hershcopf RJ, Bradlow HL. Obesity, diet, endogenous estrogens, and the risk of hormone-sensitive cancer. Am J Clin Nutr 1987;45:283–9.

54. Schapira DV, Jumar NB, Lyman GH, Cavanagh D, Roberts WS, LaPolla J. Upper-body fat distribution and endometrial cancer risk. JAMA 1991;226:1808–11.

55. Lucas WE. The epidemiology of endometrial cancer. In: Sciarra J, ed. Gynecology and obstetrics. Philadelphia: Lippincott, 1990;7–10.

56. Staszewski J. Breast cancer and body build. Prev Med 1977;6:410–5.

57. Fisher B, Constantino JP, Redmond CK, et al. Endometrial cancer in tamoxifen-treated breast cancer patients: findings from the National Surgical Adjuvant Breast and Bowel Project (NSABP) B-14. J Natl Cancer Inst 1994;86:527.

58. Parazini F, La Vecchia C, Negri E, Fedele L, Balotta F. Reproductive factors and risk of endometrial cancer. Am J Obstet Gynecol 1991;164:522–7.

59. Elwood JM, Cole P, Rothman KJ, Kaplan SD. Epidemiology of endometrial cancer. J Natl Cancer Inst 1977;59:1055–60.

60. Koonings PP, Grimes DA. Endometrial sampling techniques for the office. Am Fam Physician 1989;40:207–10.

61. Lacey CG. Premalignant and malignant disorders of the uterine corpus. In: Pernoll MI, ed. Current obstetrics and gynecologic diagnosis and treatment. Norwalk, CT: Appleton & Lange, 1998; 937–52.

62. American College of Obstetricians and Gynecologists. Carcinoma of the endometrium. Technical bulletin no. 162. Washington, DC: ACOG, 1991.

63. Canavan TP, Doshi NR. Endometrial cancer. Am Fam Physician 1999;59:3069–76.

64. Nasri MN. The role of vaginal scan in measurement of endometrial thickness in postmenopausal women. Br J Obstet Gynaecol 1991;98:470.

65. Ascher SM, Frost AR, Garra BS, Potkul R, Zeman RK. Endometrial ultrasound of the uterus: correlation with histopathology. J Ultrasound Med 1992;11:1159.

66. Volksen M, Dietrich M, Osmers R, Kuhn W. Early diagnosis of carcinomas of the endometrium via transvaginal sonography. J Ultrasound Med 1992;11:1155.

67. Varner RE, Sparks JM, Cameron CD, et al. Transvaginal sonography of the endometerium in postmenopausal women. Obstet Gynecol 1991;78:195.

68. Loffer FD. Hysteroscopy with selective endometrial sampling compared with D and C for abnormal uterine bleeding: the value of a negative hysteroscopic view. Obstet Gynecol 1989;73:16.

69. Boronow RC. Advances in diagnosis, staging, and management of cervical and endometrial cancer, stages 1 and II. Cancer 1990;65(suppl 3):648–59.

70. Berchuck A. Post-treatment surveillance of patients with early-stage endometrial cancer. Gynecol Oncol 1995;59:20–4.

71. Oram DH, Jacobs IJ, Brady JL, Prys-Davies A. Early diagnosis of ovarian cancer. Br J Hosp Med 1990;44:320–4.

72. Piver MS, Baker TR, Piedmonte M, Sandecki AM. Epidemiology and etiology of ovarian cancer. Semin Oncol 1991;18:177–85.

73. Pike MC. Age-related factors in cancers of the breast, ovary, and endometrium. J Chronic Dis 1987;40(suppl 2):59S–69S.

74. Partridge EE, Barnes MN. Epithelial ovarian cancer: prevention, diagnosis, and treatment. CA Cancer J Clin 1999;49:297–320.

75. Modan B, Hartge P, Hirsh-Yechezkel G, et al. Parity, oral contraceptives and the risk of ovarian cancer among carriers and noncarriers of a BRCA1 or BRCA2 mutation. N Engl J Med 2001;345:235–40.

76. Bourne T, Reynolds K, Campbell S. Ovarian cancer. Eur J Cancer 1991;27:655–9.

77. Young RC, Walton LA, Ellenberg SS, et al. Adjuvant therapy in stage I and stage II epithelial ovarian cancer: results of two prospective randomized trials. N Engl J Med 1990;322:1021–7.

78. Bast RC, Jacobs I. The CA-125 tumor associated antigen: a review of the literature. Hum Reprod 1989;4:1.

79. Friedlander ML, Dembo AJ. Prognostic factors in ovarian cancer. Semin Oncol 1991;18:205–12.

80. Campbell S, Goessens L, Goswamy R, Whitehead MI. Real-time ultrasonography for determination of ovarian morphology and volume: a possible new screening test for ovarian cancer? Lancet 1982;1:425–6.

81. Averette HE, Donato DM. Ovarian carcinoma. Cancer 1990;65(suppl 3):703–8.

82. Omura GA, Brady MF, Homesley HD, et al. Long-term follow-up and prognostic factor analysis in advanced ovarian carcinoma: the gynecologic oncology group experience. J Clin Oncol 1991;9:1138–50.

106
Benign Breast Conditions and Disease

Kathryn M. Andolsek and Joyce A. Copeland

Benign breast conditions and diseases are commonly encountered in primary care. Primary health care providers must be able to:

Elicit an accurate history

Perform an accurate examination of the breasts

Differentiate between benign and medically significant complaints or findings

Utilize available office procedures for evaluation of breast lesions

Reassure patients with benign disorders

Manage common symptoms

Counsel patients regarding preventive strategies and risk factors for breast cancer

Apply appropriate screening modalities for breast cancer

Educate patients regarding the value and management of breast-feeding.

Anatomy and Physiology

The breast is composed of 6 to 20 lobes and contains glandular, ductal, fibrous, and fatty tissue. More lobes are present in the outer quadrants, especially the upper outer quadrants; therefore, many breast conditions (among them, breast cancer) occur more frequently in these regions. Each lobe contains several lobules within which are ducts that join to form one of the 6 to 10 major ducts emerging at the areola. Six to 10 pinhole openings are present on the areola, each draining a single lobe. Accessory breast tissue frequently occurs along the embryonic milk line. The normal breast changes in size and texture throughout the menstrual cycle. During the premenstrual phase, acinar cells increase in number and size, the ductal lumen widens, and breast size and turgor increase. These changes reverse during the postmenstrual phase. Patients frequently have many questions about breast development throughout the life cycle.

Hypertrophy of breast tissue, noted in many newborns, is a result of stimulation by maternal hormones and usually spontaneously regresses. Breast bud development (thelarche) generally is the first sign of puberty in girls, occurring at an average age of 11 years. Thelarche is considered premature if it occurs earlier than 8 years of age. Thelarche has been occurring in younger girls. Some experts attribute it to a higher percentage of body fat or environmental exposure to estrogen-like substances. Premature thelarche without other signs of pubertal development or accelerated growth is usually benign and requires no treatment after medical evaluation has excluded true precocious puberty, estrogen-producing tumors, ovarian cysts, or exogenous estrogen exposure.[1]

Assessment of a Woman with Breast Complaints

History

A woman with breast complaints requires a review of her age; menstrual and reproductive history; family history of breast disease and cancer; use of hormonal agents, as well as other drugs (prescribed, over the counter, recreational, and herbal); and if pertinent, prior breast-feeding experience, personal cancer history, and previous breast surgery. Most patients present with breast complaints that involve a mass, pain, or discharge. Specific details of the history as outlined in Table 106.1 help the clinician differentiate between benign and malignant conditions.

Physical Examination

Examination of the breast should be performed in a well-lighted room. Facilitate privacy by draping portions of the breast not being examined. Consider having a chaperone present during the examination. The examination includes inspec-

Table 106.1. **History Taking Pertinent for a Patient with Breast Complaints**

Menstrual/reproductive history
  Menarche: age at onset
  Menopause: symptoms, chronologic relation to breast cancer (when applicable)
  Parity: age of first term pregnancy; nulliparity
  Pregnancy: current pregnancy status
  Contraception or hormonal therapy
  Breast-feeding: has patient breast-fed?
Socioeconomic status
Age
Cancer history
  Breast, ovarian, endometrial, colon
Family history
  Breast, ovarian, endometrial, colon cancer, prostate
  Relationship to patient
  Chronologic relation of breast cancer to menopause
Self-breast examination (SBE)
  Does the patient perform SBE?
  How did she learn the procedure?
  How often does she perform the examination?
History of breast surgery
  Document when surgery was performed any reasons; include results for any biopsies.
Previous biopsy
Symptoms/mass
  Onset
  Setting of symptoms/mass
  Change in symptoms/mass over time
  Relation of symptoms/mass to menstrual cycle
  History of similar symptoms
  Presence of discharge: color, location on nipple, spontaneous or expressed, recent breast-feeding or pregnancy, medications, history of the symptom, visual changes
Pain: caffeine intake, hormonal therapy, contraception
Presence of a mass: circumstances of discovery

tion and palpation. Inspection is initiated with the woman seated, arms at her side. The breasts are assessed for symmetry, alterations in contour, or significant differences in sizes of the breasts. Slight differences are common; however, visible retractions are not normal and require further evaluation. Changes can be detected earlier if the patient is asked to tense the pectoralis muscle while raising her hands above her head and placing her hands on her hips. Extreme differences in size and symmetry are uncommon, and only rarely are there endocrinologic or pathologic abnormalities in women with large pendulous breasts (macromastia). Deviations from normal skin color and contour should be noted. Characteristics that may be associated with malignancy include dimpling, edema, and thickening of the skin with enlarged pores (*peau d'orange*), crusting or scaling, or retraction of the nipple. Nipples should be evaluated for inversion, rashes, discharge, or ulceration. Inverted nipples are a normal variation as long as the nipple is not fixed and is capable of eversion. Accessory nipples occur in approximately 1% of women. The clinician should note the color and characteristics of any nipple discharge.

Palpation should be performed with the patient in the seated and supine positions. In the supine position the examination

is enhanced by having the patient extend her arm, flex her elbow, and rest her hand under her head on the ipsilateral side. Palpation is accomplished by compressing the breast tissue gently with the pads of the middle three fingers. Palpation is best accomplished when the fingers move in contiguous circles with consecutively smaller concentric circles from the periphery to the center. A gradual increase in the degree of pressure of exertion helps to explore the entire depth of the breast. All four quadrants of the breast must be examined systematically to ensure coverage of the entire breast. The tail of the breast, which extends toward the axilla, must be included in the process. Palpation of the nipple includes gently squeezing the region to determine if a discharge can be elicited. Any discomfort the patient feels during the examination should be noted.

Patients presenting with a mass should be asked to identify the location. Careful palpation of this region includes compression of the overlying skin to detect fixation and consistency. Findings may be recorded as descriptive text or by an illustration in the medical record.

Palpation is completed by examination of the axillary, supraclavicular, and infraclavicular regions to determine if lymphadenopathy is present. The evaluation of the axilla is best accomplished with the patient seated, the examiner supporting the arm on the side being examined. The anterior border, posterior border, chest wall, and inner portion of the arm are included. Documentation of physical findings is outlined in Table 106.2.

Common Conditions and Diseases

Mastodynia/Mastalgia

Benign breast pain is a common presenting complaint occurring at some point in 41% to 69% of women. It is most commonly unilateral but may be bilateral; in two thirds of women

Table 106.2. **Documentation of Objective Findings Relating to the Breast**

Mass
  Consistency: soft, firm, hard
  Mobility: fixed, mobile
  Margins: well circumscribed/smooth, irregular
  Skin changes: color, ulcerations, crusting, *peau d'orange*
  Size: centimeters
  Location: quadrant

Nipple discharge
  Nipple description: crusting, inversion, ulcerations
  Character: color, bleeding
  Location of discharge
  Unilateral or bilateral
  Number of ducts involved
  Occult bleeding
  Cytology (limited usefulness)

Node
  Axillary
  Supraclavicular
  Infraclavicular

Table 106.3. **Therapeutic Modalities for Fibrocystic Breasts**

Modality	Comments
Clothing	
Well-padded support brassiere	
Loose-fitting clothing	
Analgesics	
Acetaminophen	Topical NSAIDs available in other countries
NSAIDs	Not been demonstrated efficacious in controlled studies
Ice packs	
Weight reduction	Possibly useful for women body mass index >27
Dietary changes	Inconsistent findings of efficacy
Restrict caffeine and other methylxanthines	4–6 month trial needed; 1 small RCT suggests benefit from low fat high carbohydrate diet
Thiamine	50–100 mg/day ; no RCTs support its use
Vitamin E	400–600 IU/day; no RCTs support its use
Evening primrose oil	1500–3000 mg/day
Cis-linoleic acid	Insufficient evidence of efficacy
Diuretics	Spironolactone 25 mg qd to qid
	5/6 RCTs support its use
Hormonal regulation	Low-estrogen, high-progesterone oral contraceptive pill
	Medroxyprogesterone 5–10 mg 10 days prior to menses
	Progesterone cream massage daily for week prior to menses
	4–6 month trial; no consistent improvement in controlled studies
Danazol	200–600 mg po qd until desired effect; then 50–100 mg qd maintenance for 4–6 months
	Luteal phase danazol: 200 mg per day during luteal phase demonstrates comparable efficacy with fewer adverse effects
	Only FDA-approved medication for this indication
Tamoxifen	10–20 mg/day for 3–4 months; or for day 15–25 of monthly menstrual cycle
Bromocriptine	1.25 mg hs to 2.5 mg bid; in general should be avoided due to potential for severe adverse reactions; 2 RCTs suggest limited benefit
Luteinizing hormone releasing agents	Significant adverse effects
	Possible adverse effects on bone metabolism
Calcium supplementation	Mixed results in studies, possibly effective

NSAID = nonsteroidal antiinflammatory drug; RCT = randomized clinical trial.

the pain is cyclical; in one third it is noncyclic. Women with cyclical pain may have fibrocystic condition; however, not all women with fibrocystic breast condition, an extremely common finding, have painful breasts.[2] Table 106.3 presents commonly recommended interventions and their potential adverse effects. Almost half of women can expect resolution of their symptoms.[3]

Fibrocystic Changes and Conditions

Fibrocystic breast condition is the most common benign condition of the breast. It is so prevalent as to be considered part of the natural history of the breast, not a disease. Fibrocystic complex has been defined as a condition in which mastalgia and breast tenderness are associated with palpable lumps. Prevalence increases with age and is most common in women 35 to 45 years of age. The condition is rare in postmenopausal women. Mastodynia, the most frequent symptom associated with fibrocystic breasts, is thought to be due to breast swelling. The pain is usually located in the denser upper outer quadrant of the breasts and is usually bilateral. It characteristically begins just prior to menses and diminishes when menses begins. Patients may perceive increased breast size during this period. Family history of this condition is common. Physical examination reveals the presence of cysts,

ranging in size from 1 mm to many centimeters. The cysts are irregular, easily movable bilateral lumps or areas of local tenderness without a discrete mass; compression causes tenderness. Resolution of cysts following the menstrual cycle supports the diagnosis. Fibrocystic breast complex may be differentiated from malignancy by the nature of the pain, typical changes in breast and mass size, and the number of lesions. If there is any doubt about the diagnosis, biopsy is indicated. Aspiration often provides symptomatic relief in addition to confirming the diagnosis. If with aspiration clear fluid is obtained, and the mass disappears, follow-up is necessary for at least 3 months to ensure there is no recurrence.[4] If a residual mass or thickening is present, bloody fluid is aspirated, or the mass recurs, excisional biopsy is performed. Milky or clear fluid in a mass that resolves for 3 months represents a cystic lesion. If no fluid is obtained and the mass persists, excisional biopsy is indicated. Mammography and ultrasonography can be diagnostic and should be performed prior to invasive evaluation of any mass. Fine-needle aspiration or excisional biopsy can determine management based on histologic findings. Recurrence of the mass dictates biopsy. Hyperplastic or proliferative lesions with atypical epithelial cells increase the risk for cancer. Fibrocystic breast changes are not otherwise associated with cancer.[5]

Management includes education regarding the benign nature of this condition and symptom relief. Dietary restrictions, such as methylxanthines found in coffee, tea, colas, and chocolate, or limiting dietary fat is controversial. Some women seem to benefit from a reduction of these substances, although there are no consistent randomized controlled studies to support this recommendation. Supplementation with various vitamins such as vitamins B, A, and E, reduction of dietary fat and salt, and an increase in protein, especially soy protein, have been advocated, although there is no evidence of efficacy.[6] The use of low-estrogen, high-progesterone oral contraceptives produces relief in many patients, as does some progestational agents in the luteal phase. Diuretics may provide some relief. The best data support the use of evening primrose oil, a source of γ-linoleic acid (GLA), in doses of up to 3 g per day, which improves symptoms in 44% to 58% of women.[7] Side effects include nausea and bloating. This herbal remedy should not be used during pregnancy.

Danazol, a gonadotropin production inhibitor and weak estrogen antagonist, is the only pharmacologic agent approved by the U.S. Food and Drug Administration (FDA) for pain from fibrocystic breast condition. Although 60% to 90% of women may benefit, danazol is associated with significant side effects including headache, nausea, emotional lability and depression, fluid retention, vaginal dryness, hirsutism, amenorrhea, weight gain, hot flashes, and acne. Its use should be limited to women with severe symptoms. The initial dose of danazol is 200 to 600 mg po qd. Once the desired effect is obtained, 50 to 100 mg/day can be taken as maintenance therapy. More recent studies suggest danazol confined to the luteal phase at a dosage of 200 mg per day can provide a significant reduction in symptoms with a fewer adverse effects than continuous dosing.[8] The medication can be discontinued after 4 to 6 months with a favorable treatment response continuing for months to years.

Tamoxifen, a synthetic nonsteroid antiestrogenic agent, at a dosage 10 mg/day for 3 to 4 months may also be useful; however, adverse effects include menstrual irregularity, menopausal symptoms, endometrial cancer, and deep vein thrombophlebitis.

Bromocriptine has been used based on its role as a prolactin inhibitor and may be effective for women with cyclic breast pain. Side effects (e.g., nausea, vomiting, postural hypotension, constipation, dizziness) are severe enough that this medication is reserved for women with significant symptoms unresponsive to other agents or when associated with hyperprolactinemia.[9]

Fibroadenoma

Fibroadenoma is the most common benign breast tumor. It occurs in young women usually within 20 years of puberty. It is more frequent and occurs at earlier ages in African-American women than in white women. It tends to grow toward the end of a menstrual cycle and during pregnancy. Multiple lesions may occur and grow rapidly. Older women characteristically experience a single, more slowly growing lesion. Fibroadenomas frequently calcify and may involute after menopause. Occasionally they develop in a postmenopausal woman following administration of estrogen. Fibroadenomas contain both fibrous and epithelial elements. They are not cancerous or premalignant. The typical history is that of a painless, smooth, mass generally discovered by the patient. On physical examination, a small, sharply circumscribed, rubbery, movable, nontender 1- to 5-cm mass is palpable generally in the upper quadrant. Ultrasound examination and fine-needle aspiration (FNA) or excisional biopsy are appropriate for the evaluation of women under 40 years of age. The combination of clinical examination, ultrasound assessment and FNA is referred to as the "triple test." In experienced hands the sensitivity and specificity may be 98% to 99%. Unfortunately, mammography is not a useful diagnostic tool for young patients. Excisional biopsy is both diagnostic and curative.[10] A solid mass in a women over 40 years of age necessitates a mammogram for localization and characterization of the mass as well as evaluation of the remaining breast tissue. The absence of a mass on mammography does not exclude cancer (see Chapter 107).

Cystosarcoma phyllodes, a type of rapidly growing fibroepithelial tumor, recurs if not completely excised. There is a 10% malignancy rate, and simple mastectomy may be necessary to achieve complete removal.

Mastitis and Breast Abscess[11]

Mastitis and breast abscesses virtually always occur in lactating women or women with a history of a bite or penetrating trauma; 7% to 11% of breast-feeding women are affected, usually with the first pregnancy. Breast engorgement usually occurs on the second or third postpartum day (see Chapter 15). Mastitis presents 1 week or more after delivery and is ushered in by milk stasis. Usually only one breast is affected by moderate to severe pain. On examination, usually only one quadrant or lobule is tender, reddened, swollen, and warm. True mastitis is accompanied by fever and flu-like symptoms. Axillary adenopathy, purulent drainage, fever, and leukocytosis may be present. Cultures of breast milk are not useful. *Staphylococcus aureus* and streptococci are typically the causative organisms.

Treatment for mild infection includes local compresses and oral antibiotics. Dicloxacillin 500 mg po q6h, a first-generation cephalosporin, or clindamycin for at least 10 days is a reasonable antibiotic option. Warm compresses are soothing and may relieve congestion. The mother should be counseled about proper feeding technique, adequate fluid intake, and the use of acetaminophen for comfort. The clinician should reassess the patient's progress at 48 to 72 hours.

The infant is not at risk for developing infection if there is no abscess present and may continue to breast-feed. An abscess occurs in 10 % of cases. Pitting edema over an area of inflammation and fluctuation suggests abscess development. For patients with infections unresponsive to conservative management, severe infection abscess, or deep infection, the wound should be drained and cultured. Nursing should be discontinued and parenteral antibiotics administered for 2 to 3 days followed by oral antibiotics. If symptoms are suggestive of infection but the clinical setting is atypical, or the patient does not improve as expected with antibiotics, cancer should be excluded by biopsy of indurated areas.

Nipple Discharge[12]

Normal, healthy women commonly have some degree of nipple discharge following pregnancy and lactation. This fluid is typically clear or milky and can occur spontaneously. It can be produced by palpation and breast stimulation as part of sexual activity. This discharge may be more frequently noted just before menses. Galactorrhea may also be associated with medications (Table 106.4). Women who engage in athletic activities may notice galactorrhea as a response to friction between the nipples and clothing or from endorphin release from the hypothalamus, which may stimulate prolactin. Other causes include hypothyroidism, renal disease, and inflammation of the chest wall from thoracotomy, herpes zoster, or severe burns. Pituitary neoplasia is the most significant cause of galactorrhea, though usually the rarest. It must be excluded through appropriate evaluation, which includes a serum prolactin assay to exclude pituitary adenoma, a thyroid-stimulating hormone (TSH) assay to exclude hypothyroidism, and renal function tests. Further endocrine workup is based on the history and the findings of these studies.[13] The history should elicit the nature of the discharge, association with a mass (unilateral or bilateral), single duct or multiple ducts, relation to menses, premenopausal or postmenopausal status, and association with hormonal therapy. The patient should be queried as to whether it occurs spontaneously or only after manipulation. The following characteristics are ominous: spontaneous discharge, unilateral involvement, discharge from a single duct, and presence in a postmenopausal women or women over 50 years of age.

Fluid characteristics of the fluid may assist diagnosis. Green, black, creamy, or mucoid discharge is characteristic of fibrocystic disease. Bloody discharge may indicate malignancy, though discharge associated with malignancy may also be serous. The discharge should be analyzed for the presence of blood (with a guaiac slide). Other diagnostic options include Gram stain (to determine white blood cells to determine infection) or fat stain (to demonstrate fat globules indicative of milk to evaluate for galactorrhea). Cytology is rarely useful.

Occasionally a nontender mass develops in the breast of a lactating woman. The mass should resolve if milk is aspirated. If it does not resolve or recurs, biopsy is considered.

Ductal ectasia (comedomastitis) is a chronic inflammatory reaction that results in permanent distention of the ducts. A typical history is a multiparous woman in her forties, fifties, or older who notes thick, white or discolored, cheesy material draining

from the nipple. Women who smoke cigarettes are more likely to develop this condition. Physical examination reveals induration under the areola; cheesy, thick fluid can be expressed. The major duct systems under the areola can be excised.

Clear, bloody, or brown-green discharge (suggesting old blood) from a single duct opening on one breast must be investigated. It is usually caused by an intraductal papilloma or rarely by an intraductal cancer. A mass may or may not be present. Although a Pap smear may prove positive for papilloma cells, negative fluid analysis does not exclude cancer. A mammogram may or may not reveal a small lesion in a major duct. Papilloma is histologically benign with only a slight potential for malignant degeneration. Management includes surgical exploration of the duct and removal of the papilloma.

The patient's age may be helpful in the aggressiveness of the evaluation. Nipple discharge is an ominous sign in a postmenopausal woman or a woman 50 years of age or older. If the discharge is associated with a mass, evaluation of the mass is the primary focus of the diagnostic workup.

Painful Nipples

Nipple tenderness is common when breast-feeding is begun. Proper positioning and latching on of the baby at the breast and releasing the infant's suction prior to removal from the breast are keys to prevention. The breast-feeding mother should avoid using soap on the breast or nipples. If dried, cracked nipples are present, topical vitamin E ointment and USP modified lanolin are commonly recommended "home remedies" for cracked nipple but may precipitate sensitivity reactions such as lanolin in wool-sensitive individuals. Breast-feeding should be initiated on the uninvolved breast when the infant's suckling effort is stronger.

Breasts that are bleeding, fissured, blistered, or painful throughout the feeding should be examined by the physician. A *Candida* infection requires treatment with topical antifungal cream. Thrush, *Candida* diaper rash, or maternal *Candida* vaginitis should be treated concurrently. Nipple shields are generally avoided. Painful localized irritation and bleeding nipples in the non–breast-feeding woman can occur from friction of clothing and is commonly seen in joggers. Small elastic bandages can be applied before athletic activities. Emollients or low-dose hydrocortisone cream may ameliorate symptoms. Nipple eczema presents with erythema, scaling and weeping crusts, fissures, vesicles, excoriation, or erosions. The typical symptoms are bilateral burning or itching, and a family or personal history of atopic disease is common. Trigger avoidance and topical steroids help manage symptoms in the nonlactating female.[14] A unilateral, weeping, ulcerated, irritated nipple suggests Paget's disease of the breast, especially in middle-aged or older women, and may be associated with an underlying ductal carcinoma. Prompt evaluation is necessary if lesions do not resolve or are accompanied by a mass.

Acutely Painful Breast Lesions

Trauma may produce a hematoma or rupture of a cyst. The patient complains of pain and tenderness. Mild swelling and

Table 106.4. **Medications Associated with Galactorrhea**

Digitalis	Tricyclic antidepressants
Marijuana	Reserpine
Heroin	Methyldopa
Dopamine receptor blockers	Cimetidine
Phenothiazines	Benzodiazepines
Haloperidol	Amphetamines
Metoclopramide	Verapamil
Isoniazid	Cocaine
CNS dopamine depleters	

CNS = central nervous system.

discoloration may be present. Unless a coagulopathy is suspected, no diagnostic tests are indicated. Patients generally respond to mild analgesics. Fat necrosis is suggested by sudden onset of inflammation and pain without a history of trauma, especially with preexisting fibrocystic disease. Physical examination reveals local pain, swelling, and erythema. If symptoms persist longer than a week, a biopsy should be done to exclude malignancy.

Gynecomastia[15]

Most boys develop bilateral gynecomastia during puberty that spontaneously resolves without treatment within 3 years. Up to 40% of men experience gynecomastia with aging, especially if overweight or obese. Men with unilateral gynecomastia, rapid onset or progressive breast enlargement, pain, asymmetry, or associated erectile dysfunction, or boys with rapid progression, onset before puberty, or other signs of precocious puberty must be evaluated further. Drugs and medication that can cause gynecomastia are listed in Table 106.5. Gynecomastia can also be caused by medical conditions (hyperthyroidism, hypogonadism, cirrhosis, renal failure, pulmonary disease, refeeding after starvation); genetic syndromes (Klinefelter syndrome, testicular feminization); and tumors [testicular, liver, bronchial, gastric, pancreatic cancers; human chorionic gonadotropin (hCG)-producing tumors]. Fat deposits may mimic a breast mass in men. Breast cancer, though rare, does occur in men, and biopsy is indicated when a hard mass is palpated. Laboratory evaluation of gynecomastia includes thyroid, renal, and liver function studies. If the results are normal, gonadotropins such as luteinizing hormone (LH), and testosterone should be obtained if there is no feminization; testosterone, LH, estradiol and dehydroepian-drosterone sulfate (DHEAS) if feminization is present. If testosterone is normal to increased and LH is increased, serum hCG should be obtained. If serum hCG is elevated, testicular ultrasonography should be performed as well as searching for other hCG-secreting tumors. If serum estradiol is elevated, an estrogen-secreting tumor should be excluded.

Care of the Lactating Breast

The nipple of the lactating breast should be cleansed before and after nursing using water and a soft cloth. The baby should nurse as soon as possible after delivery and thereafter "on demand." Proper latching on should be ascertained, since this is crucial to ensure adequate nutrition for the infant and prevention of discomfort for the mother. As much of the areola as possible should be in the baby's mouth rather than sucking directly on the nipple. When the baby is removed from the breast, the suction should be broken first by gently inserting a finger into the baby's mouth. Family physicians dealing with breast-feeding mothers should familiarize themselves with lactation consultation resources available in their community. Information concerning local LaLeche affiliates is available at 1-800-LaLeche. The World Wide Web has excellent resources as well.[16–18]

Diagnostic Procedures

Clinical Breast Examination

The clinical breast examination (CBE)[19] has a 45% sensitivity rate for the detection of breast cancer. The U.S. Preventive Services Task Force[20] 2002: noted that "no screening trial has examined the benefits of clinical breast examination alone (without accompanying mammography) compared to no screening . . . the U.S. Preventive Services Task Force could not determine the benefits of clinical breast examination done or the incremental benefit of adding clinical breast examination to mammography . . . [or] . . . whether potential benefits of routine CBE outweigh the potential harms . . . evidence is insufficient to recommend for or against routine CBE alone to screen for breast cancer (I recommendation)."[20] There is no direct evidence of the effectiveness of CBE as a single examination tool in any age group. The American Academy of Family Physicians suggests CBE every 1 to 3 years for women aged 30 to 39 and annually as of the age of 40 but is currently reviewing this recommendation.

Breast Self-Examination[21–24]

Breast self-examination (BSE) has not been demonstrated to decrease mortality, and a large number of false-positive findings are discovered that require further evaluation and often biopsy. Available studies suffer from design limitations. The U.S. Preventive Services Task force "found poor evidence to determine whether breast self examination reduces breast cancer mortality; . . . Fair evidence that BSE is associated with an increased risk of false positive results and biopsies."[20] It judged the evidence as insufficient to recommend for or

Table 106.5. **Medications and Drugs that Can Cause Gynecomastia**

Estrogen (whether taking it himself, or absorbing it from a
   sexual partner who uses vaginal cream or ring)
Anabolic steroids
Corticosteroids
Clomiphene
Marijuana
Heroin
Methadone
Testosterone
Amphetamines
Meprobamate
Spironolactone
Digoxin
Penicillamine
Hydroxyzine
Reserpine
Methyldopa
Metronidazole hydroxyzine
Ketoconazole
Isoniazid
Cimetidine
Phenytoin
Finasteride
Tricyclic antidepressants

Table 106.6. **Breast Self-Examination (BSE)**

1. Perform after the menstrual cycle.
2. Being with inspection of breasts in a mirror looking for evidence of lumps, dimples, retractions, and asymmetry.
3. Then palpate the breasts while lying down. A small pillow or folded towel may be placed under the shoulder of the breast being examined. The arm of the examination side should be extended over the head.
4. Palpate the left breast with the finger pads of the right hand in a systematic fashion. The most common approach is gradually smaller concentric circles. Repeat the process on the opposite breast.
5. Palpation is also recommended in the shower or tub while the hands and breasts are soapy or with the use of mineral oil or talcum to reduce friction and enhance the sensitivity of the fingers.
6. Both axillas should be examined by palpation as well.

Note: The Guide to Clinical Prevention Services Report of the U.S. Preventive Services Task Force published in 1996 found insufficient evidence to recommend for or against teaching BSE during the periodic health examination.

against teaching or performing routine BSE. (I recommendation). The American Academy of Family Physicians is currently reviewing their policy of supporting BSE. The American Cancer Society, the American College of Obstetricians and Gynecologists, and the National Cancer Institute recommend monthly BSE. If BSE is practiced, it must be practiced correctly. The American Cancer Society has developed community health education programs to instruct women in proper BSE (Table 106.6). The woman who chooses to perform SBE should be observed for technique and educated about reporting any unusual finding.

Breast Aspiration

Aspiration is a useful tool in evaluating a breast mass. A negative result does not preclude biopsy of a clinically suspicious lesion (Table 106.7).

Breast Biopsy[25]

Indications for biopsy include any suspicious lesion, blood nipple discharge, or bloody fluid following aspiration of a cyst, a mass that persists following cyst aspiration, persistent dominant mass, suspicious skin changes, inflammatory changes unresponsive to antibiotics, suspicious axillary nodes, or suspicious microcalcifications on mammography. Fine-needle aspiration biopsy determines the cytology of suspicious lesions. Excisional biopsy is indicated when a breast lesion is suspected to be a malignancy and the fine-needle aspiration biopsy and cytologic evaluation are inconclusive or unavailable. Incisional biopsy is performed to confirm the diagnosis of advanced cancer or evaluate a large breast mass that cannot be excised completely and easily by an excisional biopsy.

Mammography[26]

Mammography is discussed in Chapter 107.

References

1. Johnson LA, Hubbard M, Carlton JC. Adolescent medicine. Monograph 187. AAFP Home Study Self-Assessment Program. Kansas City, MO: American Academy of Family Physicians, 1994.
2. Ader D, Browne M. Prevalence and impact of cyclic mastalgia in a United States clinic based sample. Am J Obstet Gynecol 1997;177:126–32.
3. Davies E. The long term course of mastalgia. J R Soc Med 1998;91:424–64.
4. Hindle WH, Arias RD, Florentine B, Whang J. Lack of utility in clinical practice of cytologic examination of non-bloody cyst fluid from palpable breast cysts. Am J Obstet Gynecol 2001; 182:1300–5.
5. Cady B. Steele GD Jr, Morrow M, et al. Evaluation of common breast problems: guidance for primary care providers CA Cancer J Clin 1998;48:49–60.
6. Horner N, Lampe J. Potential mechanisms of diet therapy for fibrocystic breast conditions show inadequate evidence of effectiveness. J Am Diet Assoc 2000;100(111):1368–80.
7. Budeiri D, Li W, Dorman MC. Is evening primrose oil of value in the treatment of premenstrual syndrome? Control Clin Trials 1996;17:60–8.
8. O'Brian P, Shaughn M, Abukhalil IEH. Randomized controlled trial of the management of premenstrual syndrome and premenstrual mastalgia using luteal phase only danazol. Am J Obstet Gynecol 1999;180:18–23.
9. Gateley CA, Miers M, Mansel RE, Hughes LE. Drug treatments for mastalgia: 17 years experience in the Cardiff Mastalgia Clinic. J R Soc Med 1992;85:12–5.
10. Morrow M. The evaluation of common breast problems. Am Fam Physician 2000:61:2371–85.

Table 106.7. **Breast Cyst Aspiration**

1. Grasp lesion between index and second fingers; hold tightly against underlying tissue.
2. Swab region with alcohol.
3. Consider local infiltration with 1% lidocaine (Xylocaine) if near areola.
4. Insert 20- to 22-gauge 1.5-inch needle on a 10- to 20-cc syringe into center of lesion with a single thrust while applying negative pressure on syringe.
5. If no fluid is obtained:
   a. Apply gentle retraction to plunger.
   b. Move needle backward and forward through center of lesion 6–10 times.
   c. Change radial direction of the needle 5–10 degrees with each sweep.
6. Avoid suction of cellular debris from back into barrel of syringe by withdrawing needle and disconnecting it from the syringe.
7. Reattach syringe.
8. Place needle tip against glass slide.
9. Depress plunger of syringe to express specimen onto slide.
10. Press second slide against first slide to smear debris, similar to technique used to make a blood smear.
11. Fix material with cytofixative immediately.
12. Apply pressure to needle site for minutes.
13. Apply a Band-Aid.
14. Send specimen for cytologic evaluation.
15. If no fluid is obtained or the mass persists after aspiration, excisional biopsy is recommended.

11. Kramish Campbell M, Waller L, Andolsek K, Huff P, Bucci K. Infant feeding and nutrition. In: Andolsek KM, ed. Obstetric care: standards of prenatal, intrapartum and postpartum management. Philadelphia: Lea & Febiger, 1990;207–15.

12. Copeland JA. Nipple discharge 11.6. In: Taylor RB, ed. The 10 minute diagnosis manual: symptoms and signs in the time limited encounter. Philadelphia: Lippincott Williams & Wilkins, 2000;236–7.

13. Pena KS, Rosenfeld J. Evaluation and treatment of galactorrhea. Am Fam Physician 2001;63(9):1763–70,1775.

14. Whitaker-Worth D, et al. Dermatologic diseases of the breast and nipple. J Am Acad Dermatol 2000;43:333–51.

15. Neuman JF. Evaluation and treatment of gynecomastia. Am Fam Physician 1997;55(5):1835–44.

16. *http://www.fda.gov/fdac/features/895_brestfeed.html.*

17. *http://www.fda.gov/opacom/lowlit/feedbby.pdf.*

18. *http://www.pareentsplace.com/expert/lactation/.*

19. Barton MB, Harris R, Fletcher SW. Does this patient have breast cancer? The screening clinical breast examination. Should it be done? How? JAMA 1999;282:1270–80.

20. U.S. Preventive Services Task Force. Breast self-exam screening statements, February 9, 2002. Electronically available at: http://www.guideline.gov/FRAMESETS/guideline_fs.asp?guideline=002385&sSearch_string=breast+cancer+screening

21. O'Malley MS, Fletcher SW. Screening for breast cancer with breast self-examination. JAMA 1987;257:2197–203.

22. Coleman EA. Practice and effectiveness of breast self examination: a selective review of the literature. J Cancer Educ 1991;6(2):83–92.

23. Frank JW, Mai V. Breast self examination in young women: more harm than good? Lancet 1985;2:654–7.

24. Hill D, White V, Jolley D, Mapperson F. Self examination of the breast: is it beneficial? Meta-analysis of studies investigating breast self examination and extent of disease in patients with breast cancer. BMJ 1988;297:271–5.

25. Donegan WL. Evaluation of a palpable breast mass. N Engl J Med 1992;327:937–40.

26. Duijm LE, Guit GL, Hendriiks JC, Zaat JO, Mali WP. Value of breast imaging in women with painful breasts: observational follow up study. BMJ 1998;317:1492–5.

107
Breast Cancer

Marla J. Tobin

Incidence

Breast cancer, a fear of most women, is commonly seen by family physicians. It is the second most common female cancer killer, surpassed only by lung cancer in recent years. Except for skin cancer, it is the most commonly seen cancer in women, with approximately 175,000 new cases of invasive breast cancer diagnosed in 1999 and 43,300 deaths.[1] Breast cancer primarily affects women, but 2400 cases a year and 260 deaths annually (fewer than 1% of all breast cancers) occur in men.

Breast cancer incidence rose steadily about 1% per year from 1940 to 1982 and 4% annually between 1982 and 1987. Since 1987 the incidence has stabilized at approximately 110.2 cases per 100,000 women,[2] which gives women a lifetime risk of developing breast cancer of 1 in 8 (12.6%) and a lifetime chance of dying from breast cancer of 1 in 28 (3.6%). The actual risk for a specific woman at any given point in her life is usually much less based on family history, genetics, reproductive factors, external factors, and competing causes of death. Recently, much work with predictive risk models and estimating annual risk of breast cancer has helped to quantitate this for individuals. Models such as the Gail Model are being used to make such predictions.* Breast cancer can be sporadic (70–85% of the time), familial (10–25% of the time), or genetic (5–10% of the time).

Many women do not perceive themselves at risk for breast cancer, perhaps because no one in their family has had it. Realistically, being female is by far the leading risk factor for breast cancer, and increasing age is the next most important factor. Eighty-five percent of women diagnosed with breast cancer have no family history. Every woman is at risk and every family physician must spread the news to women that breast cancer screening is important. When a woman has a mother, sister, or daughters with breast cancer, it increases the relative risk of breast cancer by two- to threefold.

Other risk factors include a history of breast cancer or atypical hyperplasia, first childbirth after age 30, early menarche, late menopause, and possibly hormone use. Family history is especially important for bilateral cancer or premenopausal cancer if it occurs in a mother or sister. Breast cancer clusters in certain genetic pools and ethnic groups. Obesity, diethylstilbestrol (DES) exposure, and childhood upper body irradiation may also be factors. There is controversy over the role of high-fat diet, high alcohol consumption, and hormone use as risk factors for breast cancer.

Detection

One of the most important roles for the family physician is breast screening and early detection of breast cancer to improve survival. Traditionally, women have been taught to do monthly breast self-examinations (BSEs) and have regular examinations by clinicians. The 1996 U.S. Preventative Services Task Force (USPSTF) recommendations cast doubt on the effectiveness of monthly BSEs and clinician-conducted examinations. Its recommendation for breast cancer screening is as follows: "Routine screening for breast cancer every 1–2 years with mammography alone, mammography and annual clinical breast exam is recommended for women aged 50–69."[3] The task force concluded that evidence is not sufficient for or against using screening clinical breast examinations alone or teaching BSEs (see Chapter 7).

There is ongoing debate regarding mammography before age 50 and at age 70 and beyond. The USPSTF thought that the evidence was insufficient to recommend routine mammograms for these age groups. They did suggest that high-risk women ages 40 to 49 and healthy women ages 70 and over may be candidates for mammography.

---

*Gail Model predictor can be obtained from National Cancer Institute, Bldg. 31, Room 10A03, 31 Center Drive. MSC 2580, Bethesda, MD 20892-2508, or *www.nci.nih.org*, or 1-800-4-CANCER.

Many physicians continue to believe that breast cancer awareness and detection can be improved by educating women about the BSE, promoting clinician examinations, and establishing a regular mammogram screening program.

The American Cancer Society (ACS) recommends annual screening mammograms and clinical breast exams on all women ages 40 and older, as well as monthly BSEs. The American Medical Association, the American College of Obstetrics and Gynecology, the American Women's Medical Association, the National Medical Association, and the American Society of Radiology agree with the ACS recommendation to screen women in their forties. However, the American Academy of Family Physicians, the American College of Physicians, and the USPSTF advise annual screening after age 50.

A standard two-view screening mammogram can detect lesions 2 to 4 years before they become palpable. Because of breast density, mammography is not as good a study in women under age 35. Mammography, however, is strongly recommended annually from age 50 to at least age 69. Mammography has been shown to reduce breast cancer deaths by at least 30% in women age 50 and older. Early detection has been credited with the declining breast cancer deaths in recent years. Mammography is of limited value in women on hormonal replacement therapy, younger women, women with dense or fibrotic breasts, and women with breast implants. Mammography, however, is still considered the gold standard diagnostic test for breast cancer even with newer radiology diagnostics.

Any abnormal mammogram requires close follow-up until resolved. Two of the major liability concerns for family physicians in breast cancer is failure to screen and failure to follow up on a breast problem. Table 107.1 lists the current mammography classification.

Careful attention during the breast examination is paid to breast symmetry, lymph nodes, skin changes, discharge, and retraction. Examining the breast in a consistent and overlapping style ensures that each portion of the breast is checked. Because 15% of breast cancers are detected only by BSE or clinician examination, many physicians continue to promote these options to patients.

Ultrasonography can be a helpful modality. Indications for ultrasonography include guidance of fine-needle aspiration, cyst diagnosis, screening of high-risk patients with radiodense breasts, fear of mammography, a palpable mass, young age or pregnancy, nipple discharge, postradiation measurement of tumor size, ambiguous mammographic results, and detection of axillary lymphadenopathy. Some studies have shown ul-

trasonography to be the most accurate single diagnostic test for women with a palpable breast mass, yielding a 99.7% positive predictive value for benign disease.[4] With the advent of high-resolution ultrasound methods, ultrasonography may become the modality of choice for detecting invasive carcinoma, with mammography remaining preferable for localizing intraductal carcinoma. The use of these ultrasound techniques and ultrasound-directed aspirations and biopsies can markedly reduce the number of breast biopsies. It is still crucial to follow breast masses until removed or definitive testing has been done.

Stereotactic breast biopsy is available in some areas to allow three-dimensional computer imaging and needle biopsy of suspicious lesions. It has the advantages of 98% sensitivity, lower cost than biopsy, and a quicker recovery than after biopsy. The standard mammographic needle localization technique for a nonpalpable lesion biopsy has also been helpful. Cytology testing of breast milk duct lavage can be done by an aspiration technique and analyzed much like a Pap smear for tissue evaluation.

Breast Masses

Statistically, breast masses in women under 30 are usually fibroadenomas. Fine-needle aspiration of the breast confirms cystic structures, but any recurring cystic structure needs further evaluation. Breast biopsies are sometimes necessary for definitive diagnosis if masses do not resolve.

Any persistent breast mass in women should be biopsied, but in women over age 50 there is a high degree of concern about malignancy. A mammogram cannot be the final test, as 15% of palpable breast cancers do not visualize. Tracking patients with lumps or abnormal mammograms is key to good follow-up. Many family physicians believe that if breast masses or abnormalities are not resolved in 4 to 6 weeks they should be referred for possible biopsy. Other indications and considerations for referral are listed in Table 107.2.

Table 107.1. **BiRads Classification (Breast Imaging Reporting and Data System)**

0: Additional studies required
I: Negative
II: Benign finding
III: Probably benign
IV: Suspicious
V: Highly suggestive of malignancy.

Table 107.2. **When to Refer**

Possible indications for referral
Aspirated cystic breast lesion with residual or recurrent mass or thickening
Rapidly recurring breast cysts (within 4–6 weeks)
Asymmetric mass or thickening persisting after menstrual cycle in ovulating woman
Asymmetric mass or thickening in nonovulating women
Suspicious nonpalpable mammographic lesion
Discrete palpable abnormality that is not cystic
Cystic lesions with grossly bloody fluid aspirated
Any woman with discrete lesion that cannot be reexamined by primary physician or is at risk for loss of follow-up

Other considerations for referral
Indeterminate nonpalpable mammographic lesion
Bilateral multiple duct nipple discharge
Women with difficult examination
Extremely high-risk women
Worried patient with negative workup
Lack of adequate physician–patient relationship

Nipple Discharge

Bilateral or nonspontaneous breast discharge is unlikely to be breast cancer. Discharge in a postmenopausal woman, especially those over age 60, is most concerning. Spontaneous persistent bloody, pink, multicolored, or watery discharge can be associated with ductal carcinoma. Localizing which duct of the breast discharges and clearly defining its history and cytology, and performing mammography and galactography, may be indicated.

Treatment

The initial diagnosis of breast cancer is done by needle or excisional biopsy. Staging involves dissection of the lymph nodes at the time of tumor removal (Table 107.3). Ductal breast cancer is the most common type. Lobular breast cancer is also seen. Carcinoma in situ of the duct is a precursor to invasive cancer, and lobular carcinoma in situ may be a marker for cancer in either breast. In lieu of excision of all lymph nodes, some centers are offering sentinel node biopsies to certain candidates who may be able to have a less extensive surgery. Paget's disease presents as eczematous nipple changes and is often associated with underlying malignancy.

In addition to the tissue pathology report, the spread of cancer cells to the lymph nodes is an important prognostic sign. Node-negative breast cancer carries an overall 5-year survival of 90%; node-positive disease drops to 60% survival. Testing for estrogen and progesterone receptors in the tumor and evaluation of the tumor dividing rate (ploidy and S-phase) and the nuclear grade (well versus poorly differentiated) are important prognostically. Basic blood tests at the time of diagnosis include liver enzymes and a complete blood count (CBC). If metastatic disease is suspected, CA-15.3 or carcinoembryonic antigen (CEA) markers can be followed, as can the chest radiograph, bone scans, and mammograms. A team that includes the family physician, surgeon, oncologist, radiation oncologist, and other support services offers women the best treatment options. For lesions less than 2.0 to 2.5 cm (stage 1–2), lumpectomy and irradiation offer cure rates as good as those seen with radical mastectomy.[5,6] Involvement of the woman in the surgical planning and informing her about reconstructive options improves the patient's satisfaction. With her meeting new doctors and the urgency of treatment placed on a woman with breast cancer, her family physician can be an excellent resource for assistance with these decisions.[13]

Reconstructive Options

Women with breast cancer face surgery with two major concerns: cure and disfigurement.[20] Family physicians can make a positive impact on the emotional and physical recovery of women with breast cancer by raising the issues of body image and restoring body symmetry early on. Survival and recurrence rates do not differ in patients who undergo reconstruction.[5]

Implants and tissue expanders are commonly used to restore breast symmetry. In large-breasted women reduction of the nonoperative breast is a consideration. Autogenous tissue methods include the latissimus dorsi musculocutaneous flap and the transverse rectus abdominis muscle (TRAM) flap. Outpatient techniques for nipple reconstruction can add finishing touches that help a woman restore her body image.

Chemotherapy and Irradiation

Many chemotherapy protocols and agents are used to treat breast cancer. Commonly used drugs include cyclophosphamide (Cytoxan), doxorubicin HCl (Adriamycin), 5-fluorouracil, and methotrexate. Common side effects include bone marrow depression, oral or gastrointestinal irritation, hair loss, weakness, and weight loss. Adriamycin can be cardiotoxic. Excellent new drugs can significantly decrease the nausea and vomiting. Monitoring and treating chemotherapy side effects and providing emotional support are roles for the family physician. Chemotherapy appears most beneficial in women under age 65 and for node-positive disease.

Preoperative and postoperative radiation therapy is used to treat breast cancer, especially for stage I or II disease with breast-conserving surgery, as well as for recurrent or metastatic disease. Patients can have skin changes as well as the usual radiation side effects of fatigue and tissue irritation.

Adjuvant Therapy

Adjuvant therapy consists of endocrine therapy to decrease tumor potential. The most commonly used agents include tamoxifen and megestrol acetate (Megace). Tamoxifen is a nonsteroidal antiestrogen agent with partial estrogenic agonist properties. Megestrol is a progestational agent. Leuprolide is another antiestrogen agent that is being used. Although 70% of node-negative breast cancers are cured by surgery, there is a 30% recurrence rate. Adjuvant therapy can decrease this recurrence by one third. Adjuvant protocols should begin soon after surgery; some even begin preoperatively.

Tamoxifen has commonly been used for 5-year protocols, although lengths of use vary. Ongoing trials aimed at breast cancer prevention in high-risk women are using tamoxifen. Tamoxifen now has U.S. Food and Drug Administration (FDA) approval for use in women with node-negative breast cancer larger than 1 cm and those with nodal disease. Common tamoxifen side effects include hot flashes, weight gain, fluid retention, vaginal dryness, and menopausal-like symp-

---

Table 107.3. **Stages of Breast Cancer**

Stage 0   Carcinoma in situ (noninvasive cancer cells in lobule or duct)

Stage I   Local lesion 2 cm or less with no lymph node involvement

Stage II   Lesion with minimal local lymph node involvement or local lesion larger than 2 cm without lymph node involvement

Stage III   Locally advanced lesion with positive axillary nodes and skin or chest wall spread

State IV   Metastatic disease (common sites: other breast, liver, lungs, bones, brain)

toms. Taking tamoxifen increases the risk of deep venous thrombosis and endometrial cancer by about threefold over that in the general population. Any vaginal bleeding or swollen, tender legs in women on tamoxifen should be carefully evaluated. Benefits of tamoxifen other than improved cancer survival include decreased bone mineral loss and it may improve cardiovascular risk factors.

Many new adjuvant therapies are currently in protocols for treatment with exciting possibilities. Two new adjuvants, letrozole and anastrozole, have been shown to be at least as effective as tamoxifen, and several others are in clinical trials. Other antiestrogens, aromatase inhibitors, and luteinizing hormone–releasing hormone antagonists are also treatment options.

New chemotherapy agents also continue to be developed. High-dose chemotherapy with bone marrow transplant has not been recommended as often after a report at the 1999 American Society of Oncology meetings showed no improvement over standard therapy. About 25% to 30% of breast cancers have an overexpression of a human epidermal growth factor receptor-2 (HER2) protein that carries a poor prognosis. Trastuzumab is the first immunotherapy agent that targets the HER2 oncogene.

Many natural therapies such as diets high in vegetables, carotenoids, or vitamin E have been suggested to aid breast cancer patients. A low-fat, low-alcohol diet is suggested as one preventative measure.

Chemotherapy seems to be most beneficial and least toxic in young women. Tamoxifen has greater benefits in older, postmenopausal women and those rich in estrogen receptors. Each woman should have an honest assessment of prognostic factors with risks and benefits discussed.

Prognosis

The single most important prognostic factor is the presence or absence of metastatic cancer in axillary lymph nodes. Node-negative disease has an overall survival of 65% to 82% at 10 years; node-positive survival drops to 25% to 40%. Even node-negative women are considered now for chemotherapy or adjuvant therapy (or both) because approximately 30% of these woman have micrometastasis and so benefit from treatment. Increasing numbers of positive nodes and deeper levels of nodal involvement worsen the prognosis.

Prognostically, patients with positive estrogen receptors generally do better. Those with tumors less than 2.5 cm do better as well, but those whose tumors are less than 1 cm have less than a 10% recurrence rate at 10 years. Higher nuclear grade is associated with higher recurrence. Well-differentiated tumors respond more readily to chemotherapy, as they have a lower percentage of tumor cells dividing.[16] A low S-phase and diploid proliferative index are associated with the most favorable prognosis.

The overall prognosis, reflected in relative survival rate, for women diagnosed with breast cancer is approximately 83% at 5 years after diagnosis, 65% after 10 years, and 56% after 15 years.[6] Women under age 45 have a lower 5-year survival (78%) than older women (86% for those diagnosed at age 65 or older).

When breast cancer can be detected at a local stage, the 5-year survival jumps to 96%, and as many as 90% have remained disease-free in some 20-year follow-up studies. Currently only 58% of breast cancers are diagnosed at the local disease stage (stage I or 0). It is hoped that targeting early detection and universal screening would place more women in this group.

Patients with breast cancer in one breast are at higher risk to develop breast cancer in the other breast. Some genetic links have found breast cancer patients also at an increased risk for colon or ovarian cancer. A family history of breast cancer is especially important if it occurred in a mother or sister, was bilateral, or developed before menopause. Of the genetically linked cancers about one third are BRCA linked.[21,22] Genetic testing should be offered to women who

were diagnosed with breast cancer before age 45 and have a relative with ovarian or breast cancer,

have *both* ovarian and breast cancer before age 50,

have a relative with BRCA, or

have a family history of breast/ovarian cancer in several generations, or two or more relatives on either side.

If confirmed to have the BRCA gene, a woman has a 30% to 50% risk of developing breast cancer before age 50 and a 56% to 87% risk of developing breast cancer by age 80. Female Ashkenazi Jews have a rate of mutation of 1 in 40 for BRCA1 and 1 in 100 for BRCA2. Such high-risk women are candidates for prophylactic therapies such as tamoxifen or prophylactic mastectomy.

Racial differences exist for breast cancer survival. The 5-year survival among white women increased from 63% in 1960 to 80% today, whereas for black women the 46% five-year survival of 1960 is now only 63%. Black women are more likely to be diagnosed with regional disease, but even when stage of disease is corrected for, black women have a lower survival rate. Histology types and socioeconomic factors also seem to have contributing roles.

Follow-Up Care

There are more than 2 million breast cancer survivors in the United States. Continuing care of the breast cancer patient is an important role for family physicians. The patient must be examined for local skin recurrence, correlated breast findings, and axillary or supraclavicular node findings. Ask about lung, liver, or central nervous system symptoms. Mammograms are essential, and chest radiographs or bone scans may be indicated if symptomatic. Patients with breast-conserving surgery are advised to have mammograms every 6 months initially.

Office visits occur at least quarterly for the first 2 to 5 years and then stretch to semiannually and annually. Routine use of bone scans, chest radiography, and liver ultrasonography are not indicated. Any time a breast cancer survivor presents to a physician, even with a minor pain or bump, she may be worried about cancer recurrence, and it should be addressed.

Some 400,000 women seek treatment for lymphedema. These women need to take special precautions to avoid infections. Various compression devices and lymphedema ther-

Table 107.4. Breast Cancer Resources

American Cancer Society—*www.cancer.org* or
    1-800-ACS-2345

Breast Cancer Awareness/Solutions—*www.bce.army.mil*

National Alliance of Breast Cancer Organizations—
    www.nabco.org or 1-800-719-9154

National Breast Cancer Coalition—*www.natlbcc.org* or
    1-202-296-7477

National Cancer Institute—*www.nci.nih.org* or
    1-800-4-CANCER

National Coalition of Cancer Survivorship—
    www.cancersearch.org or 1-888-650-9127

Susan C. Komen Breast Cancer Foundation—*www.komen.org*
    or 1-800-IM-AWARE

Y-ME hotline—*www.y-me.org* or 1-800-221-2141

apies are available. In addition to knowing about these resources, family physicians should also be available to assist women needing wigs, prostheses, or other services.

Cancer support groups such as Reach for Recovery are excellent volunteer programs to assist women at all stages of breast cancer; refer patients early. Assistance with prosthesis and postmastectomy wear can be a helpful service to breast cancer patients, but they hesitate to ask for it. Know where such services are available in your area. Educational materials for patients and families about breast cancer are available from a variety of sources. A list of such resources is presented in Table 107.4.

Terminal Care Issues

Every 11 minutes a woman dies of breast cancer.[15] Family physicians are involved in the terminal care of patients with metastatic breast cancer. Advance directives, death with dignity, involvement of the patient when planning her care, treating symptoms, controlling pain, family issues, and hospice care are considerations. Helping families deal with terminal care, grieving, and appraising their own breast cancer risks are key roles for family physicians (see Chapter 62).

Conclusion

Although breast cancer is many women's fear and the second most common female cancer, we are making strides in earlier detection and improved survival. Family physicians have important roles in education, detection, coordinating care, and the continuing care of women with breast cancer.[13]

References

1. Cancer Statistics 1999. American Cancer Society 1999;49:(1): 8–29.
2. Cianfrocca M, Gradishar WJ. Primary care for survivors of breast cancer. Women's Health Prim Care 1998;1(4):371–85.
3. U.S. Preventative Services Task Force. Guide to clinical preventive services, 2nd ed. Baltimore: Williams & Wilkins, 1996; 73–87.
4. Bard R. Multimodality imaging of breast disease. Female Patient 1996;21:17–22.
5. Bell MC, Partridge EE. Early breast carcinoma: risk factors, screening, and treatment. Contemp Obstet Gynecol 1995;Dec: 31–51.
6. Breast cancer special issue. J Am Med Wom Assoc 1992;47: 140–206.
7. Colditz GA, Hankinson SE, Hunter DJ, et al. The use of estrogens and progestins and the risk of breast cancer in postmenopausal women. N Engl J Med 1995;332:1589–93.
8. Eley JW, Hill HA. Chen VW, et al. Racial differences in survival from breast cancer. JAMA 1994;272:947–54.
9. GIVIO Investigators. Impact of follow-up testing on survival and health-related quality of life in breast cancer patients. JAMA 1995;271:1587–97.
10. Jacobson JA, Danforth DN, Cowan KH, et al. Ten-year results of a comparison of conservation with mastectomy in the treatment of stage I and II breast cancer. N Engl J Med 1995; 332:907–11.
11. Kalllove H, Liberati A, Keeler E, Brook RH. Benefits and costs of screening and treatment for early breast cancer. JAMA 1995; 273:142–54.
12. Kopans DB, Marchant DJ, Osborne MP. Breast cancer vigilance, not panic. Patient Care 1993;Nov 15:135–64.
13. Love N. Breast cancer and primary care. Postgrad Med 1995; 98:43–110.
14. Olivotto IA. Adjuvant systemic therapy for women with breast cancer. Female Patient 1996;21:45–52.
15. Parker S, Wingo PA, Heath CW Jr. ACS breast cancer facts and figures. Monograph 95-20M-no. 8610. Atlanta, GA: American Cancer Society, 1996.
16. Phillips DM, Balducci L. Current management of breast cancer. Am Fam Physician 1996;53:657–65.
17. Rimer BK, Trock B, Balshem A, Engstrom PF, Rosan J, Lerman C. Breast screening practices among primary care physicians: reality and potential. J Am Board Fam Pract 1990;3: 26–34.
18. Rosenfeld JA. Evaluation of nonlactational nipple discharge. Female Patient 1995;20:39–49.
19. Utian WH, Wulf H, Ades TB, et al. Overcoming your patients' fear of breast cancer. Menopause Manag 1994;Nov/Dec:18–28.
20. Webb MS. Reconstruction's place in breast cancer management. Contemp Obstet Gynecol 1994;Aug:83–90.
21. Weitzel JN. Genetic counseling for familial cancer risk. Hosp Pract 1996;Feb 15:57–69.
22. Benjamin I, Buzdar AU, Hartmann LC, et al. Safeguarding the health of women at high risk for breast cancer. JCOM 1999;6 (8, suppl):1–48.
23. Rosenthal TC, Puck SM. Screening for genetic risk of breast cancer. Am Fam Physician 1999;59(1):99–104.
24. Love N, Vogel VG, et al. Breast cancer symposium. Postgrad Med 1999;105(5):43–112.
25. Wood AJJ, Hortobagyi GN. Treatment of breast cancer. N Engl J Med 1998;339(14):974–84.
26. Fisher B, Constantino JP, Wicherham DL, et al. Tamoxifen for prevention of breast cancer: report of the National Surgical Adjuvant Breast and Bowel Project P-1 Study. J Natl Cancer Inst 1998;90(18):1371–88.

108
Selected Disorders of the Female Reproductive System

Gary R. Newkirk and Patricia Ann Boken

Pelvic pain is one of the most vexing problems encountered by the family physician. The monetary and psychosocial costs are unknown but are assumed to be high. In the United States about 40% of all laparoscopies are done for the evaluation and treatment of pelvic pain.[1]

Evaluation of Pelvic Pain

Clinical Presentation

Patients with pelvic pain present with a wide variety of complaints and physical findings. To better understand the causes of pelvic pain and assist with the initial evaluation, it is helpful to distinguish acute pelvic pain from chronic pelvic pain. Chronic pelvic pain is present for 6 months or more and acute pelvic pain for less than 6 months. Chronic pelvic pain syndrome is characterized by incomplete response to treatment, impairment at work or home, signs of depression, and pain that is worse than would be expected on the basis of the pathologic process[2] (see Chapter 61).

Diagnosis

Effective evaluation of pelvic pain begins with a search for organic causes that require immediate therapy. An integrative approach that relates psychological, historical, and physical factors from the outset is essential. When taking the history it is helpful to differentiate acute from chronic pelvic pain because this distinction refines the differential diagnoses (Tables 108.1 and 108.2). A detailed history is obtained clarifying the location, severity, and inciting and relieving factors of the pain. Careful menstrual, pregnancy, and sexual histories are sought. Contraceptive use, previous pelvic problems or surgery, and previous diagnostic and therapeutic efforts are clarified. The psychosocial history includes clarification of prior sexual abuse, personal relationships, and exploration of the patient's efforts to cope with, and her fears about, the cause of pain.

Research has shown a high incidence of sexual abuse associated with chronic pain.[3] Furthermore, current psychiatric diagnoses, especially depression, and substance abuse correlate with pelvic pain. Rates of childhood or adult sexual or physical abuse are as high as 48% in patients presenting with chronic pelvic pain.[3]

Formal psychological consultation may be useful for assessing the psychiatric contribution to chronic pelvic pain. In most instances a psychiatric diagnosis modifies the patient's perception and significance of pelvic pain and rarely is the sole cause of symptoms.

Physical Examination

The physical examination includes careful abdominal, musculoskeletal, and pelvic examination. In addition to the routine abdominal examination, the examiner looks for trigger points in the abdominal wall. The abdominal wall has been identified as a common source of pain for both acute and chronic forms of pelvic pain.[4] The abdominal wall is palpated with the patient's abdominal muscles stretched (supine) and relaxed (knees bent), so trigger points typical of the myofascial syndrome can be detected.[2] During the pelvic examination the external genitalia are examined for signs of sexually transmitted diseases or trauma. The bimanual examination evaluates the introitus, levator sling, vaginal walls, cervix, uterus, adnexa, septum, and cul-de-sac. The urethra is palpated from within the vagina, as significant pain in this area implies the urethral syndrome related to chlamydial infection. The patient is requested to contract and relax the vagina around the examining fingers to assist in the detection of vaginismus. An attempt is made to re-create the pain on the bimanual examination including palpation and movement of the cervix. If pressing on the posterior fourchette or bottom

Table 108.1. **Causes of Acute Pelvic Pain and Initial Management**

Pelvic infection—antibiotics

Pregnancy complications
Ectopic pregnancy—laparoscopy or methotrexate
Spontaneous abortion—may need dilation and curettage
Septic abortion—antibiotics, may need dilation and curettage

Adnexal problems
Ovarian torsion—often requires laparoscopy
Ruptured ovarian cyst—may require surgery
Intracapsular or extracapsular ovarian hemorrhage—may require surgery

Endometriosis—specific therapy (see next section)

Acute degeneration or torsion of a leiomyoma—often requires surgery

Nongynecologic causes
Inflammatory bowel disease—specific medical management
Urinary tract stone—may require surgical removal, antibiotics
Acute cystitis—antibiotics

Sexual abuse

Miscellaneous causes—require specific medical treatment
Sickle cell disease, porphyria, diabetes, systemic lupus erythematosus
Hereditary angioneurotic edema

of the vagina reproduces the pain, there is a high likelihood that the pain has a significant psychological or musculoskeletal origin. Pain of pelvic organ origin may be noted ventrally or both dorsally and ventrally but almost never presents as dorsal back pain alone. The cul-de-sac is palpated for abnormalities such as nodules, which can be found with endometriosis. In most instances the cervix is screened or cultured for gonorrhea and *Chlamydia*.

Table 108.2. **Causes of Chronic and Cyclic Pelvic Pain**

Chronic pelvic pain
Endometriosis
Chronic salpingitis
Severe pelvic adhesions
Adenomyosis
Pelvic congestion syndrome
Nongynecologic causes
 Musculoskeletal
 Inflammatory bowel disease
 Irritable bowel syndrome
 Diverticulitis
 Interstitial cystitis
 Referred pain
 Psychological

Cyclic pelvic pain
Mittelschmerz
Primary dysmenorrhea
Secondary dysmenorrhea
 Adenomyosis
 Endometrial polyp
Pedunculated submucous myoma
Premenstrual tension syndrome

Musculoskeletal dysfunction often contributes to the signs and symptoms of chronic pelvic pain and in many cases is the primary factor.[5] King et al[6] found that a typical pattern of faulty posture, termed typical pelvic pain (TPP) posture, was found in 75% of patients studied with chronic pelvic pain. The posture consists of exaggerated lordotic posture of the lumbar spine, anterior tilt of the pelvis, and kyphosis of the thoracic spine. Referred sources of pain must also be considered.[6,7]

Diagnostic Studies

The initial laboratory evaluation for pelvic pain includes a pregnancy test if the patient is of reproductive age, complete blood count (CBC), urinalysis, and erythrocyte sedimentation rate (ESR). Vaginal probe ultrasonography can confirm intrauterine pregnancies as early as 4 to 5 weeks and can assist in the evaluation of women with suspected ectopic pregnancy. The presence of fluid in the posterior cul-de-sac seen on the ultrasound scan suggests a pathologic process, but this finding has poor specificity. Ultrasonography may also be useful for patients who are difficult to examine because of obesity, are unable to relax, or whose pain prevents palpation during the bimanual examination. Unfortunately, abdominal ultrasonography is sometimes overutilized, as the likelihood of positive findings in a patient with completely normal pelvic examination is low and may contribute to further unnecessary imaging and heightened physician and patient anxiety. For example, ovarian cysts are a common finding on ultrasound scans and may be up to 5 cm in diameter; yet they are not the source of pain unless careful bimanual palpation of these cysts duplicates the pain.

Diagnostic laparoscopy remains an important tool for evaluating pelvic pain.[8] Laparoscopy is the gold standard for diagnosing such conditions as pelvic inflammatory disease (PID), ectopic pregnancy, and ovarian torsion. The cause of chronic pelvic pain in patients under age 30 is most often endometriosis or chronic PID. Older patients are most likely to have adenomyosis, leiomyomas, endometriosis, or symptoms due to pelvic relaxation. Pelvic adhesions are the only finding in 10% to 25% of laparoscopies for chronic pelvic pain, but studies are still not clear whether adhesions are incidental findings or are the cause of the pain. Another benefit of diagnostic laparoscopy is to offer the patient reassurance. In one study that followed patients with chronic pelvic pain after laparoscopy had excluded pelvic pathology, 22% were pain-free at their 6 week follow-up appointment, and 40% reported decreased pain.[9]

Other diagnostic studies that may aid in the diagnosis include urine cultures, barium enema, intravenous pyelography, and empiric nerve blocks to help confirm the origin of pain (e.g., symptomatic adenomyosis).

Management

The patient with acute, severe pelvic pain and deteriorating clinical condition often requires abdominal exploration. In most other instances, a careful history and physical examination indicate the most likely nonsurgical causes of acute pelvic pain. Table 108.1 outlines initial management steps for the various causes of acute pelvic pain.

Narcotics can be used with acute pelvic pain on a selective basis, when the diagnosis is assured, and for a short time. Narcotics should not be used for chronic pelvic pain. Nonsteroidal antiinflammatory drugs (NSAIDs) are the best choice for long-term causes of pelvic pain. Antidepressants help with the management of chronic pelvic pain regardless of whether symptoms of classic depression are identified, and they can be tried on an empiric basis. Low-dose amitriptyline (25 mg) was significantly more effective than placebo in reducing such pain.[10]

Hormone treatment with oral contraceptives, Depo-Provera, and gonadotropin-releasing hormone (GnRH) analogues may be helpful in suppressing ovarian function to treat conditions such as endometriosis, adenomyosis, fibroids, dysmenorrhea, and ovarian cysts. Definitive treatment with antibiotics and the occasional need to drain pelvic abscesses surgically are the main strategies for managing PID.

Several studies have reported the importance of a multi-disciplinary management for treatment of chronic pelvic pain (CPP). Sexual and marital counseling, family therapy, and behavior modification therapy are interventions to be considered. Regular office visits should be scheduled to decrease the patient's need to justify visits by experiencing more pain. The frequency of these visits can be gradually tapered as the patient improves. Realistic goals must be established early regarding the management of CPP.[11] Adapting and coping with CPP is considered the therapeutic goal, with complete resolution of symptoms unlikely.

Adjunctive treatment includes nerve blocks and nerve interruption surgery. Paracervical blocks may have a diagnostic and therapeutic value, as a response to this trial of analgesia strongly implies a uterine source for the pelvic pain. Fascial injections were advocated by Ling and Slocumb[4] for myofascial origins of pelvic pain. Laser uterine nerve ablation therapy has had mixed results when used to manage uterine sources of pain. Patients often adamantly demand a hysterectomy, especially when the search for the etiology of CPP becomes nonproductive. Interestingly, in one study looking at the outcome of women undergoing hysterectomy with CPP, 78% showed significant improvement.[12]

Other, less traditional therapies for CPP include physical therapy for musculoskeletal dysfunction, stressing management through lifelong attention to posture, strength, and flexibility; transcutaneous electrical nerve stimulation (TENS) for musculoskeletal abdominal wall or back pain; acupuncture; and relaxation and biofeedback.

Prevention

Early management of the symptoms of acute pelvic pain and identifying the source decreases the possibility of symptoms becoming chronic. In the patient who is sexually active, counseling regarding sexually transmitted diseases (STDs) and their prevention is always prudent. The use of estrogen in postmenopausal women may be helpful for preventing pelvic pain due to vaginismus. The use of NSAIDs for 3 days prior to menstruation and during menses is beneficial in preventing pelvic pain caused by dysmenorrhea. A thorough history

early in the investigation of CPP sufferers, such as clarifying sexual or physical abuse, may avoid extensive medical evaluations and unnecessary surgical procedures (see Chapter 27). Appropriate posture along with good physical conditioning, nutrition, and regular exercise may prevent the musculoskeletal origins of pelvic pain.

Family and Community Issues

The multiple causes of pelvic pain make its treatment and diagnoses challenging. Family physicians are uniquely qualified to care for patients with pelvic pain by virtue of their psychosocial evaluation skills, long-term management potential, and general ability to coordinate care from various consultants. Education of the community about sexual abuse, STDs, PID, endometriosis, depression, and other factors associated with pelvic pain can be offered by the family physician.

Endometriosis: Diagnosis and Therapy

The presence of tissue that is biologically and morphologically similar to normal endometrium in locations beyond the endometrial cavity is termed endometriosis.[13] Endometriosis affects approximately 7% to 10% of premenopausal women.[14] The prevalence in the general population may be underestimated, as not all endometrial lesions exhibit classic morphologic findings at laparoscopy.[15] Endometriosis is found in 30% to 60% of women who present for infertility evaluation.[16] Sixty to seventy percent of women with endometriosis are nulliparous, and most have a family history.[17] The pathophysiology of endometriosis remains incompletely characterized and poorly understood. The most widely accepted explanation for endometriosis focuses on the concept of retrograde flow of menstrual fluid back through the fallopian tubes with implantation of viable endometrial tissue in the free pelvis.[18] This explanation contrasts with the coelomic metaplasia theory, which argues that undifferentiated coelomic epithelial cells remain dormant on the peritoneal surface until the ovaries produce hormones sufficient to stimulate this ectopic tissue.[14] Despite the controversies surrounding pathophysiology, endometriosis remains one of the most common gynecologic diseases in women during their reproductive years.

Clinical Presentation

Endometriosis is rarely life-threatening but frequently becomes life-altering. Patients with endometriosis present a wide range of clinical symptoms, and frequently there is poor correlation between these symptoms and the extent of endometrial implants within the pelvis. Dysmenorrhea (50%), infertility (25–50%), pelvic pain and dyspareunia (20%), and menstrual irregularities (12–14%) are the most common complaints.[19] Pain can be diffuse or localized to the organs involved. Other, less common symptoms include low back pain, dysuria, hematuria, and diarrhea, which classically occur before or during menses. Despite classic descriptions of the disease, endometriosis may present with some, none, or all of these symptoms, which may or may not correlate with the menstrual cycle. Textbooks describe the typical endometriosis patient as in her late twenties or early thirties, Caucasian, and frequently nulliparous. In reality, endometriosis occurs with all races from early adolescence to the perimenopausal period.

Endometriosis should also be considered in women initially presenting for evaluation of infertility.[20] How endometriosis contributes to infertility is not known, and likely more than one mechanism is involved. Explanations include altered anatomy, ovulatory dysfunction, hormonal abnormalities, autoimmunity, toxic pelvic factors, altered sexual functioning, and increased spontaneous abortions.[16,19] Even though it appears that the number of pelvic implants does not correlate well with the severity of dysmenorrhea and dyspareunia, the probability of successful conception appears to be inversely related to the severity of the disease.[21] Recent prospective controlled trials suggest that minimal to mild endometriosis is not associated with reduced fecundity.[22]

Diagnosis

Patients presenting with pelvic pain, dyspareunia, dysmenorrhea, abnormal bleeding, or infertility should prompt the clinician to consider endometriosis as a diagnosis. Physical findings include uterosacral nodularity, retroversion of the uterus, limited pelvic mobility, adnexal masses, and diffuse or focal tenderness. Unfortunately, neither the history nor the physical examination confirms the diagnosis of endometriosis. The diagnosis of endometriosis requires direct visual and histologic confirmation obtained during laparoscopy or laparotomy. A uniform system of classification based on the presence, location, and quality of adhesions, endometriomas, and tubal distortion has been formulated by the American Fertility Society (AFS). The AFS classifies endometriosis as minimal, mild, moderate, and severe (stages I to IV, respectively).[23] During laparoscopy or laparotomy, endometriosis may appear as classic brown lesions that may be focal (e.g., ovarian) or diffuse (e.g., peritoneal). Reddish blue nodules on the peritoneum, uterine ligaments, or pelvic viscera are a common finding as well. Focal scarring or retraction of the peritoneum, diffuse adhesions, and distortion of uterine, ovarian, and tubal anatomy can be seen. Ovarian implants may result in the formation of an endometrioma. These ovarian masses, or "chocolate cysts," can explain the finding of a tender adnexal mass on pelvic examination. The presence of endometriomas is confirmed during laparotomy and may constitute the initial finding for endometriosis. Extrapelvic (e.g., vulva, vagina) or pelvic endometriosis should be considered with any mass or lesion that becomes painful in a cyclic fashion with menses.

Computed tomography (CT) and magnetic resonance imaging (MRI) can provide presumptive evidence of endometriosis but are rarely justified for the initial workup. These expensive imaging studies are not diagnostic, as there is no characteristic appearance or location for endometriosis implants. Pelvic ultrasonography is not diagnostic either but can be helpful in detecting and characterizing pelvic pathology if the pelvic examination is limited owing to tenderness or obesity. Its common availability, lower cost, safety during pregnancy, and nonradiographic nature are general features that prompt many clinicians to include pelvic ultrasonography in the workup of endometriosis.

A cell surface antigen, CA-125, is found on derivatives of coelomic epithelium including endometrial tissue. Despite the correlation of CA-125 levels with both the degree of endometriosis and the response to therapy, the sensitivity of this assay is too low for it to be used as a screening test. The measurement of peritoneal fluid levels appears to be better for detecting minimal and moderate disease.[24] It may be beneficial to utilize this test when evaluating ovarian cysts.[25] Developing a serum endometrial antibody assay continues to be investigated, with its sensitivity and specificity greater than 0.9 in detecting endometriosis.[25]

Management[26,27]

Treatment for endometriosis is preceded by careful confirmation and staging with laparoscopy or laparotomy. Factors to consider prior to treatment include the patient's age and desire for fertility, the severity of symptoms, and the extent, location, and severity of the disease. Even though there is no universally effective cure for this disorder, treatment options do exist that can provide relief of symptoms. The wide variety of treatments for endometriosis betray its poorly defined etiology and pathophysiology. Treatment includes expectant management, conservative surgical therapy, medical therapy, extensive surgery with castration, and superovulation therapies for infertility, such as in vitro fertilization or gamete intrafallopian tube transfer (GIFT). With more advanced endometriosis, there is a greater likelihood that surgical intervention will be required to treat the disease successfully. Surgical removal of both ovaries invariably induces remission of the disease but should be reserved for women with advanced endometriosis who are over 35 years of age and do not intend to become pregnant.

Expectant management, or watchful waiting, may be a reasonable management strategy for the younger woman who desires pregnancy and has mildly symptomatic endometriosis. Efforts can then be spent identifying and correcting any other infertility factors as necessary (see Evaluation of the Infertile Couple, below). This approach has been shown to produce pregnancy rates as high as those achieved with medical therapy or conservative surgery (50%).[28]

Conservative surgery for endometriosis entails either laparoscopy or laparotomy and is indicated (1) for confirmation of diagnosis; (2) if fertility is desired, to determine tubal occlusion or peritubal, pelvic, or ovarian adhesions; (3) for aspiration of chocolate ovarian cysts; and (4) for evaluation of pelvic pain unrelieved by medical therapy.[16] The initial treatment at the time of diagnostic laparoscopy can often be accomplished with electrocoagulation or laser ablation of implants through the laparoscope. Partial ovarian resection for endometriomas and lysis of adhesions are accomplished as necessary. Definitive surgery includes total hysterectomy and bilateral salpingo-oophorectomy and is indicated in women who do not desire pregnancy and for whom all previous medical and conservative surgical efforts have failed.

Medical management of endometriosis includes the use of danazol, progestins, oral contraceptives, and GnRH agonists. The goal of hormonal therapy is to control symptoms or improve fertility, or both. Most medical regimens involve treatment for at least 6 months, allowing for adequate regression of implants.

Endometriotic implants behave like normal endometrial tissue and are supported by ovarian hormones.[29] The effectiveness of hormonal management takes advantage of the biologic response of endometriotic tissue to alterations of the hormonal environment. In either a hypoestrogenic or a hyperandrogenic environment, endometriotic implants become atrophic. Danazol (Danocrine), for instance, induces a hyperandrogenic state, and GnRH agonists produce a hypoestrogenic state. Both agents induce regression of endometriotic implants. Progesterone therapy such as medroxyprogesterone acetate (Cycrin, Provera) induces decidual or atrophic changes in endometriotic implants. Finally, administration of combined estrogen-progestogen contraceptives (pseudopregnancy regimen) produce an acyclic hormonal environment similar to that of pregnancy, which causes endometriotic implants to atrophy.[30] Table 108.3 summarizes various treatment strategies, the common drugs used for therapy, and their potential side effects. Severe endometriosis and infertility often require an organized treatment plan combining surgical and prolonged medical treatment. In a woman whose symptoms are consistent with endometriosis, empiric medical therapy may be tried prior to definitive surgical diagnosis. In a prospective study it was concluded that after failure of initial treatment with oral contraceptives and NSAIDs, empiric therapy with 3 months of a GnRH agonist is appropriate.[31]

Infertility associated with endometriosis has now been treated with advanced reproductive techniques including administration of hyperstimulation gonadotropins, in vitro fertilization, and GIFT techniques.[32–34] The family physician assumes a critical role in managing endometriosis by arranging for appropriate consultation, monitoring medical treatment protocols, and providing long-term emotional support to patients and families troubled by this chronic condition.

Prevention

At present there are no known effective interventions to prevent endometriosis from developing in a given patient. A positive family history and deferring childbearing lead to a higher likelihood for the development of endometriosis. Endometriosis usually recurs despite medical or conservative surgical treatment.[17] Long-term hormonal therapy without surgery can help prevent progression in some patients with severe

Table 108.3. **Major Treatment Modalities for Endometriosis**

Method	Hormonal effect	Drug	Route of administration	Typical daily dose	Problems
Bilateral oophorectomy (often with hysterectomy)	Hypoestrogenic	NA	Laparotomy	NA	Permanent sterility, bone loss, menopausal symptoms
Laser or electro-fulguration ablation of endometrial implants	NA	NA	Laparoscopy or laparotomy	NA	Surgical risks; ? benefit for severe disease, recurrence
GnRH agonist	Hypoestrogenic	Nafarelin (Synarel)	Nasal	0.4–0.8 mg bid × 6 months	Bone loss, hot flashes, decreased libido, vaginal discharge
		Leuprorelin (Lupron)	IM	3.75 mg per month for 6 months	
		Goserelin (Zoladex)	SC	3.6 mg per month for 6 months	
Androgenic agonist	Hyperandrogenic	Danazol (Danocrine)	Oral	400–800 mg	Androgenic side effects, weight gain, oily skin, deep voice
High progesterone	Hyperprogestational (relative low estrogen)	Medroxyprogesterone acetate (Provera), norethindrone acetate (Aygestin)	Oral	30–60 mg	Mood changes, bloating, breakthrough bleeding
Continuous oral contraceptives (pseudo-pregnancy) or cyclic	Combined estrogenic and progestational	Birth control pills (many types)	Oral	e.g., 0.035 mg ethinyl-estradiol/1 mg norethindrone (1–4 per day)	Oral contraceptive side effects: mood changes, weight gain, bloating, hypertension

NA = not available; SC = subcutaneous.

symptoms. Only definitive surgery such as abdominal hysterectomy with bilateral salpingo-oophorectomy, combined with resection of all endometrial implants, yields the highest likelihood for resolution of symptoms. The laparoscopic finding of minimal endometrial disease in a woman not desiring pregnancy can frequently be managed with cyclic birth control pills to lessen further seeding. More advanced disease usually requires 6 months of danazol or medroxyprogesterone acetate followed by cyclic birth control pills.[20]

Family and Community Issues

Education regarding endometriosis ideally begins during early adolescence as part of comprehensive health education. Women should be encouraged to seek medical help for the symptoms of endometriosis. For many women endometriosis becomes a chronic affliction that requires ongoing education, treatment, and compassion. If the patient requests, the physician should meet with other members of the family to offer information and address questions or concerns. Patients and families may benefit from contacting the Endometriosis Association to obtain educational materials and information regarding support groups that deal with the impact of this chronic condition.[35] Women with documented endometriosis who desire pregnancy should be counseled regarding its relation to infertility, so these desires and the timing of childbearing can be discussed. Effectively managing patients with endometriosis challenges the family physician to remain an informed patient advocate, as comprehensive care frequently involves referral and familiarity with long-term treatment modalities not routinely used by family physicians.[36]

Evaluation of the Infertile Couple

Infertility is generally diagnosed when pregnancy has not occurred in a couple trying to conceive after 1 year of unprotected intercourse. It is estimated that nearly 15% of couples in the United States are infertile.[37] The infertility risk doubles for women of ages 35 to 44 compared to women of ages 30 to 34; consequently, about one third of women older than 35 who desire pregnancy experience infertility.[38]

Couples are seeking professional help for infertility on a increasing basis, and family physicians are in an ideal position to begin this evaluation. Their familiarity with partner's family, medical, and physical histories allow the assessment to begin with both partners, which contributes to the cost-effectiveness of the family physician's infertility evaluation. The major goals when evaluating the infertile couple include (1) identifying and correcting causes of infertility, (2) providing accurate information for the couple, (3) providing emotional support during and after the evaluation process, and (4) providing counseling regarding alternatives should pregnancy be unlikely or impossible.[39] This discussion presents the initial workup of the infertile couple, which is sufficient to allow diagnosis in approximately 60% of couples seeking help.[40]

There are various estimates regarding the causes of infertility. Table 108.4 summarizes the experience for infertile couples in the United States.[39–41]

Table 108.4. **Male and Female Infertility Factors**

Male factors (40% of couples)
  Disorders of spermatogenesis
  Obstruction of efferent ducts
  Disorders of sperm motility
  Sexual dysfunction
Female factors (45% of couples)
  Pelvic origin (30–50% of female causes)
    Tubal disorders
    Uterine disorders
    Endometriosis
  Ovulatory origin (40% of female causes)
    Endocrine (adrenal, thyroid, pituitary) disorder
    Ovarian: luteal phase defects
  Cervical origin (10% of female causes)
    Mucous problems
    Infectious problems
Combined factors (15–30% of couples)
Unidentifiable factors (15% of couples)

Initial Fertility Workup

A timely and cost-effective approach to evaluating the infertile couple requires initial evaluation of both the male and female factors for infertility. Table 108.5 summarizes an organized approach to the fertility workup.[39–42] Both partners are scheduled for extended examination times. Ample time is afforded to explain the need and methods for the various initial tests and data collection including (1) semen analysis, (2) documentation of ovulation, (3) postcoital test, and (4) evaluation of tubal patency. The exact sequence in which a physician evaluates a couple's infertility varies based on historical and physical findings ascertained during the initial visit.

A semen sample is analyzed within 2 hours of ejaculation after 48 hours of ejaculatory abstinence. Evaluation should be by persons experienced with fertility semen analysis. If an abnormality is found on this initial assessment, two additional semen analyses are performed 2 weeks apart. If the abnormality persists, urologic consultation is appropriate.[43]

Assessing ovulation can be accomplished by one or more methods: (1) basal body temperature (BBT) assessment; (2) timed serum progesterone levels; (3) urinary luteinizing hormone (LH) screening; and (4) endometrial biopsy. The method of recording BBT data is explained during the initial visit. Serum progesterone levels are measured 7 days after estimated ovulation. Values consistent with ovulation vary with each laboratory, but generally values of more than 15 ng/mL are consistent with normal ovulatory function and levels under 5 ng/mL imply anovulation.

Endometrial biopsy, in addition to histologically detecting ovulation, provides timing of the progestational effect with the day of the cycle and can provide information regarding ovulation and luteal phase defects. Endometrial sampling is easily accomplished using small aspiration catheters (Pipelle, Z-sampler) at as close to 7 days after presumed ovulation as possible (roughly, day 22 of a 28-day cycle).

Postcoital testing requires evaluation of the sperm–mucus interaction. The couple is instructed to have intercourse following 48 hours of abstinence. Pelvic examination is per-

Table 108.5. **Evaluation Plan for the Infertile Couple**

Initial visit (extended visit time for both partners)
   Complete medical, family, drug and sexual history
   Laboratory studies
      Sexually transmitted disease cultures (especially *Chlamydia,*
         Ureaplasma urealyticum, Neisseria gonorrhoeae)
      Assess need for HIV screening
      Consider CBC, FBS, VDRL, urinalysis
      Men: semen analysis
      Women
         Papanicolaou screening
         KOH and wet mount
      Focused studies
         Thyroid history?—thyroid function tests
         Galactorrhea?—prolactin levels
         Abnormal pelvic examination?—ultrasonography,
            laparoscopy
         History PID?—hysterosalpingography
         Endometriosis likely?—laparoscopy
         History sexual dysfunction?—education,, counseling
   Ovulatory monitoring (BBT, urinary LH)
   Education
      Alcohol, drugs, hot tubs, sexual practices/frequency,
         douching, lubricants
      Arrange for postcoital sample analysis with next visit

Second visit (midcycle/ovulatory as predicted by BBT and/or
   urinary LH testing)
   Review laboratory studies, semen analysis, ovulatory
      monitoring data to date
   Analyze postcoital sample
   Consider and discuss need for endometrial biopsy
   Arrange for hysterosalpingography during follicular phase
      (days 7–9); if laparoscopy deemed necessary, HSP often
      accomplished during laparoscopy

Third visit (midluteal phase of cycle, 7–9 days postovulation)
   Review studies to date
   Perform endometrial sampling
   Consider progesterone and prolactin levels if not already done
   Consider HSP or laparotomy; referral often appropriate at
      this time

CBC = complete blood counts; FBS = fasting blood sugar;
LH = luteinizing hormone; HSP = hysterosalpingography;
BBT = basal body temperature; HIV = human immunodeficiency virus; PID = pelvic inflammatory disease.

formed and aspirated cervical mucus is examined within 2 to 8 hours of intercourse. Intercourse should occur within 24 to 48 hours of presumed ovulation as determined by methods outlined above. The postcoital mucus is examined by experienced individuals for quantity, clarity, pH, spinnbarkeit (ability of cervical mucus to stretch), and the number, forms, and motility of sperm. Generally, finding 5 to 10 sperm with linear motility per high-power field in clear, acellular mucus with more than 8 cm spinnbarkeit excludes cervical factors as a major cause of infertility.

During a subsequent office visit, results of the initial laboratory studies, cultures, and semen analysis are discussed. The postcoital sample can be obtained, and an appointment for the endometrial biopsy, luteal progesterone, and prolactin levels scheduled. The results of these studies are carefully reviewed during the third visit, at which time a decision is made to pursue hysterosalpingography, laparoscopy, hysteroscopy,

or laparotomy. The frequency of these visits also facilitates emotional support and encouragement for the couple. RESOLVE (5 Water Street, Arlington, MA 02174), a national nonprofit infertility organization, has chapters throughout the United States and is an excellent resource for support and counseling groups.[42]

Further Evaluation

Hysterosalpingography (HSP) is a safe, high-yield procedure when performed during the early proliferative phase of the cycle. During HSP a special catheter is passed through the vagina into the endocervical canal through which contrast medium is injected and fluoroscopically followed through the endometrial and fallopian tube lumen. An undiagnosed pelvic mass or PID contraindicates this procedure, as does an iodine or radiocontrast dye allergy. HSP can be performed during laparoscopic surgery as well. The appearance of uterine defects on HSP implicates a uterine cause of infertility, which include post-diethylstilbestrol (DES) uterine abnormalities (T-shaped, hypoplastic cavity), intrauterine synechiae (Asherman syndrome), submucous or large intramural myomas, congenital anomalies, and leiomyomas.

Further evaluation of pelvic factors for infertility requires laparoscopy. Laparoscopy is indicated if HSP is contraindicated or abnormal and is also performed if historical (e.g., PID, endometriosis) or physical (e.g., adhesions, tube/ovarian abnormality) findings implicate a pelvic cause. Women with endometriosis are twice as likely to be infertile as women without this condition. Endometriosis is confirmed and staged by laparoscopy. Treatment for endometriosis was discussed earlier in this chapter. Finally, laparoscopy is indicated if no other significant cause of infertility is identified.

Ovulatory causes of infertility include adrenal and thyroid disorders. Fasting blood glucose, thyroid function, follicle-stimulating hormone (FSH), luteinizing hormone (LH), and prolactin levels assist the evaluation of endocrinologic factors for infertility. Drug-related infertility must also be considered, as a number of medications contribute to disruption of thyroid, adrenal, or ovarian functioning in women and thyroid or adrenal functioning in men (e.g., antihypertensive drugs, major tranquilizers, steroids). Therapy for ovulatory factors is directed toward the underlying disorder, including thyroid replacement for hypothyroidism, bromocriptine for hyperprolactinemia (with pituitary macroadenoma ruled out), or clomiphene to induce ovulation.

Cervical factors for infertility are assessed initially by the postcoital test. The finding of leukocytes suggests cervicitis, and cultures for gonorrhea, *Ureaplasma urealyticum,* and *Chlamydia* are useful for directing treatment. Finding nonmotile or nonprogressively motile sperm with a "shaking" pattern suggests sperm antibodies. Miscalculation of ovulation timing is suggested by poor-quality cervical mucus, which is abnormally thick, cloudy, and demonstrates poor spinnbarkeit. A repeat postcoital test is necessary if ovulatory timing is in question.

Despite comprehensive evaluation 5% to 10% of couples have no identifiable cause for their infertility. Often referral to infertility centers for consideration of assisted reproductive technologies (ARTs) is necessary (e.g., in vitro fertilization, GIFT) and appropriate. Attitudes regarding adoption and assisted reproductive technologies should be explored.

Often individual or joint guilt regarding infertility can be underestimated. Family physicians are in an ideal position to utilize established trust and comfort with their patients to explore potential past history and guilt issues that might relate to infertility. Emotional support remains a part of every visit.[44]

Toxic Shock Syndrome

In 1978 an acute, febrile, exanthematous illness associated with multisystem organ failure became known as the toxic shock syndrome (TSS).[45] There are currently no definitive tests or specific serologic markers for diagnosing TSS. The diagnosis requires the presence of the six clinical criteria, outlined in Table 108.6.[46,47] TSS should be suspected in all patients who present with flu-like symptoms, rash, and otherwise unexplained hypotension.

Early reports indicate that more than 90% of the reported TSS cases involved menstruating females.[48] Because of the high correlation of TSS with menstruation and tampon use, the perception of TSS as strictly a "tampon disease" persists. More recent data reveal that only half of the reported cases were female, and many of these cases were not associated with menstruation.[49] Most cases of tampon-related TSS occurred during the teenage years; 97% of reported patients were white, and 42% were adolescents.[50] Physicians must recognize that TSS can occur in nonmenstruating women, men, and children of all ages. Nonmenstrual cases of TSS occur in males and females equally with various sites and types of infection, including surgical wounds, burns, abscesses, sinus infections, bronchopneumonia, influenza A, tracheitis, empyema, septic abortion, intravenous drug injections, pilonidal abscess, nasal packing, insect or human bites, diaphragm use, and even ear piercing. Interestingly, menstruation-related TSS affects Caucasians almost exclusively, whereas non–menstruation-related forms affect the races proportionate to the racial/sexual mix of the population.[51,52]

Pathogenesis

The expression of TSS depends on the interaction of several bacterial and host factors that are incompletely understood.

Table 108.6. **Toxic Shock Syndrome, Criteria for Diagnosis**

Confirmed diagnosis requires that all six criteria be met:
1. Acute fever
2. Scarlatiniform rash
3. Desquamation of palms and soles 1–2 weeks after illness onset
4. Hypotension
5. Clinical or laboratory evidence of involvement of at least three organ systems: hematologic, gastrointestinal, neurologic, cardiovascular, hepatic, renal, muscular
6. Other causes excluded (e.g., sepsis, measles, drug or toxic ingestion)

Source: Data from Todd and Fishaut[45] and Tofte and Williams.[46]

In the original studies, patients with TSS usually had a source of staphylococcal infection. More recent reports have characterized a streptococcal toxic shock–like syndrome caused by toxins elaborated by group A streptococci.[53,54] Both have in common the presence of bacteria-related toxins that appear to initiate the serious multiorgan syndrome characteristic of these disorders. Toxic shock syndrome toxin-1 (TSST-1) has been identified as one of the significant staphylococcal mediators of pathogenicity in TSS,[55] although TSS can occur in the absence of TSST-1. Endotoxin from co-infecting gram-negative or streptococcal bacteria has also been implicated in TSS.[56] Staphylococcal toxins may interact synergistically with these endotoxins. TSST-1 enhances the release of a wide variety of endogenous mediators produced by the host, which partly explains the multiorgan dysfunction characteristic of this syndrome. Finally, the correlation of TSS with vaginal materials such as tampons, barrier sponges, or the diaphragm strongly implies an as yet uncharacterized relation between foreign materials and the induction and maintenance of this condition. TSS apparently results from multiple, cumulative effects of primary and secondary mediators initiated by the continued growth of certain bacteria.

Clinical Presentation

Toxic shock syndrome presents with a broad spectrum of clinical findings ranging from relatively mild symptomatology to a rapidly fatal illness.[56,57] Mortality is about 3%. Patients may progress from onset of symptoms to overt multisystem failure within 48 hours. Hypotension and poor tissue perfusion, with nonhydrostatic leakage of fluid from the intravascular to the interstitial space, accounts for a portion of the multisystem organ failure (renal, hepatic, central nervous system, hematologic). Fatal complications include refractory shock, renal failure, arrhythmias, intravascular coagulopathy, and respiratory distress syndrome. The initial fever, rash, and malaise of TSS may mimic a common viral syndrome early in the disease process. These symptoms typically progress rapidly to include high fever (104°F), pharyngitis, conjunctivitis, diarrhea, vomiting, myalgia, and scarlet fever–like rash. Within a matter of hours orthostatic dizziness, fainting, or overt hypotension may occur; these first symptoms clearly set this syndrome apart from benign infectious processes. The rash of TSS is usually a prominent finding and typically appears as a diffuse scarlatiniform exanthem beginning on the trunk and spreading to the arms and legs with flexural accentuation. Some clinicians have described this rash as having a "sunburn" appearance that blanches with pressure. "Strawberry tongue," as seen with scarlet fever, is a common finding. Erythema of the mucous membranes and intense conjunctival hyperemia without purulence are characteristic. Generalized nonpitting edema accompanies the rash in many cases. Desquamation of the hands and feet is commonly seen within 10 to 21 days after presentation. Reversible patchy alopecia and shedding of fingernails has been described as well.[58]

Toxic shock syndrome is rare in children, but when it does appear the clinical features of the illness do not differ appreciably from those described in adults. There does seem to be a higher likelihood of respiratory involvement in children.[55] The differential diagnosis of TSS in children includes Kawasaki disease, staphylococcal scalded skin syndrome, scarlet fever, Rocky Mountain spotted fever, leptospirosis, erythema multiforme, Stevens-Johnson syndrome, and measles.

Common laboratory findings of TSS reflect widespread organ involvement: sterile pyuria; normocytic anemia; leukocytosis with left shift; prolongation of the prothrombin and partial thromboplastin times; an increase in serum bilirubin, creatinine, and creatine kinase; hyponatremia; hypokalemia; and metabolic acidosis.[59]

Management

Hospitalization is necessary for all patients with presumed TSS, as the illness may progress from mild to life-threatening within a matter of hours. Supportive measures tailored to the patient's symptoms are the mainstay of therapy.[60] A search is made for the potential source of the staphylococcal or streptococcal toxin, and cultures of any suspected source are obtained. Removal of vaginal tampons, pads, sponges, or diaphragms is paramount. Recent surgical wounds are explored even if they appear not to be inflamed or infected. All presumed sources of toxin must be thoroughly drained and irrigated.

Prospective management includes administration of large volumes of colloid and crystalloid fluids with glucose (10–20 mL/kg) over the first hour to reestablish vascular volume. Patients may require 5 to 10 L of fluid during the first 24 hours to maintain tissue perfusion and urinary output. Swan-Ganz catheterization is required for severe cases. After specimens for culture are obtained, antistaphylococcal antibiotics (e.g., methicillin, oxacillin, nafcillin, first-generation cephalosporin, or vancomycin) are given intravenously until oral fluids can be tolerated. Antibiotics are continued for at least 10 days. Steroid therapy (e.g., methylprednisolone 10–30 mg/kg/day) may be given to patients with severe unresponsive shock. Intravenous immune globulin may be also given to patients who are not improving, although the effectiveness of this therapy has not been proved.

Signs of adult respiratory distress syndrome (ARDS) often develop on the second or third day of treatment with severe TSS. Intubation with continuous positive airway pressure may be required; generally, fluids are not restricted. Acute renal failure may require dialysis.

Recurrences of TSS are common but generally milder. Female patients who experience TSS are advised to avoid the use of vaginal devices (tampons, sponges, diaphragms). Prophylactic antistaphylococcal oral antibiotics at the time of menses have been recommended for patients experiencing TSS associated with menses. Oral contraceptives have been shown to decrease the risk of TSS recurrence.[48] These approaches have not yet been conclusively supported by rigorous studies.

References

1. Peterson HB, Hulka JF, Phillips JM. American Association of Gynecologic Laparoscopists' 1988 membership survey on operative laparoscopy. J Reprod Med 1990;35:587–9.
2. Nolan TE, Elkins TE. Chronic pelvic pain: differentiating anatomic from functional causes. Postgrad Med 1993;94:125–8.
3. Toomey TC, Hernandez JT, Gittelman DF, Hulka JF. Relationship of sexual and physical abuse to pain and psychological assessment variables in chronic pelvic pain. Pain 1993;94:125–8.
4. Ling FW, Slocumb JC. Use of trigger point injections in chronic pelvic pain. Obstet Gynecol Clin North Am 1993;20:809–15.
5. King Baker P. Musculoskeletal origins of chronic pelvic pain. Obstet Gynecol Clin North Am 1993;20:719–40.
6. King PM, Myers LA, Ling FW, et al. Musculoskeletal factors in chronic pelvic pain. J Psych Obstet Gynaecol 1991;12:87–98.
7. Basu HK. Major common problems: pelvic pain. Br J Hosp Med 1981;26:150–8.
8. Vercellini P, Fedele L, Arcaini L, et al. Laparoscopy in the diagnoses of chronic pelvic pain in adolescent women. J Reprod Med 1989;34:827–32.
9. Baker PN, Symonds EM. The resolution of chronic pelvic pain. Am J Obstet Gynecol 1992;166:835–9.
10. McQuay HJ, Carroll D, Glynn CJ. Low dose amitriptyline in the treatment of chronic pain. Anesthesia 1992;47:646–52.
11. Parsons L, Stovall T. Surgical management of chronic pelvic pain. Obstet Gynecol Clin North Am 1993;20:765–78.
12. Stovall TG, Ling FW, Crawford DA. Hysterectomy for chronic pelvic pain of presumed uterine etiology. Obstet Gynecol 1990;75:676–81.
13. Sampson JA. Perforating hemorrhagic (chocolate) cysts of the ovary, their importance and especially their relation to pelvic adenomas of the endometrial type. Arch Surg 1921;3:245–323.
14. Saltiel E, Garabedian-Ruffalo SM. Pharmacologic management of endometriosis. Clin Pharm 1991;10:518–30.
15. Rawsn JM. Prevalence of endometriosis in asymptomatic women. J Reprod Med 1991;36:513–5.
16. Dawood MY. Endometriosis. In: Gold JJ, Josimovich JB, eds. Gynecologic endocrinology. New York: Plenum, 1987;387–404.
17. Moghissi KS. Office management of endometriosis. In: Stenchever MA, ed. Office gynecology. St. Louis: Mosby-Year Book, 1992;413–29.
18. National Center for Health Statistics, McCarthey E. Inpatient utilization of short-stay hospitals by diagnosis: United States, 1980. Hyattsville, MD: National Center for Health Statistics, 1982. DHSS Publ. no. (PHS) 83-1735. (Vital and health statistics; series 13: Data from the National Health Survey, no. 74.)
19. Hurst BS, Rock JA. Endometriosis: pathophysiology, diagnosis, and treatment. Obstet Gynecol Surv 1989;44:297–304.
20. Endometriosis and infertility. In: Speroff L, Glass RH, Kase NG, eds. Clinical gynecology, endocrinology, and infertility, 4th ed. Baltimore: Williams & Wilkins, 1989;547–63.
21. Dmowski WP. Endometriosis. In: Glass RH, ed. Office gynecology. Baltimore: Williams & Wilkins; 1987;317–36.
22. Berube S, Marcoux S. Langeuiun M, Maheux R. Fecundity of infertile women with minimal or mild endometriosis and women with unexplained infertility. Canadian Collaborative Group of Endometriosis. Fertil Steril 1998;69:1034–41.
23. American College of Obstetricians and Gynecologists. Management of endometriosis. Technical bulletin no. 85. Washington, DC: ACOG, 1985.
24. Colacurci N, Fortunato N, DeFranciscis P, et al. Serum and peritoneal CA-125 levels as diagnostic test for endometriosis. Eur J Obstet Gynecol Repord Biol 1996;66:41–3.
25. Mathur S. Autoimmunity in endometriosis: relevance to infertility. Am J Reprod Immunol 2000;44:89–95.
26. Koninck PR, Riittinen L, Sepalla M, Cornillie FJ. CA-125 and placental protein 14 concentrations in plasma and peritoneal fluid of women with deeply infiltrating pelvic endometriosis. Fertil Steril 1992;57:523–30.
27. Badawy SZA, Cuenea V, Freliech H, Stefanu C. Endometrial

antibodies in serum and peritoneal fluid of infertile patients with and without endometriosis. Fertil Steril 1990;53:930–2.

28. Seibel MM. Does minimal endometriosis always require treatment? Contemp Obstet Gynecol 1989;34:27–39.

29. DiZerega GS, Barber DL, Hodgen GD. Endometriosis: role of ovarian steroids in initiation, maintenance, and suppression. Fertil Steril 1980;33:649–53.

30. Barbieri RL. Endometriosis 1990: current treatment approaches. Drugs 1990;39:502–10.

31. Ling FW. Randomized controlled trial of depot leuprolide in patients with chronic pelvic pain and clinically suspected endometriosis. Pelvic Pain Study Group. Obstet Gynecol 1999;93: 51–8.

32. Fedele L, Bianchi S, Marchin M, Villa L, Brioschi D, Parazzini F. Superovulation with human menopausal gonadotropins in the treatment of infertility associated with minimal or mild endometriosis: a controlled randomized study. Fertil Steril 1992;58:28–31.

33. Medical Research International Society for Assisted Reproductive Technology, American Fertility Society. In vitro fertilization-embryo transfer (IVF-ET) in the United States: 1989 results from the IVF-ET registry. Fertil Steril 1991;55:14–23.

34. Olive DL, Schwartz BL. Endometriosis. N Engl J Med 1993; 328:1759–69.

35. Overcoming endometriosis: new help from the Endometriosis Association. Milwaukee: Endometriosis Association.

36. American College of Obstetrics and Gynecologists. Important facts about endometriosis. Washington, DC: ACOG.

37. Whitman-Elia GF, Baxley EG. A primary care approach to the infertile couple. J Am Board Fam Pract 2001;14(1):33–45.

38. Mosher WD. Infertility trends among U.S. couples: 1965–1976. Fam Plann Perspect 1982;14:22–7.

39. Speroff L, Glass RH, Kase NG, eds. Female infertility. 6th ed. Baltimore: Williams & Wilkins, 1999;809–39.

40. Zarutskie PW. Evaluation of the infertile couple. In: Stenchever MA, ed. Office gynecology. St. Louis: Mosby Year Book, 1992; 441–70.

41. American College of Obstetricians and Gynecologists. Infertility. Technical bulletin no. 125. Washington, DC: ACOG, 1989.

42. Davajan V. Workup of the infertile couple. In: Mishell DR, Brenner PF, eds. Management of common problems in obstetrics and gynecology. Oradell, NJ: Medical Economics Books, 1984;387–93.

43. Kolettis PN, Sabanegh ES. Significant medical pathology discovered during a male infertility evaluation. J Urol 2001;166(1): 178–80

44. Boivin I, Appleton TC, Baetens P, et al. Guidelines for counseling in infertility: outline version. Hum Reprod 2001;16(6): 1301–4

45. Todd J, Fishaut M. Toxic-shock syndrome associated with phage-group-I staphylococci. Lancet 1978;2:1116–8.

46. Tofte RW, Williams DN. Toxic shock syndrome: evidence of a broad clinical spectrum. JAMA 1981;246:2163–7.

47. Bryner CL Jr. Recurrent toxic shock syndrome. Am Fam Physician 1989;39:157–64.

48. Davis JP, Chesney PJ, Wand PJ, LaVenture M. Toxic shock syndrome: epidemiologic features, recurrence, risk factors, and prevention. N Engl J Med 1980;303:1429–35.

49. Centers for Disease Control. Summary of notifiable disease, United States. MMWR 1988;37:40.

50. Litt IF. Toxic shock syndrome—an adolescent disease. J Adolesc Health Care 1983;4:270–4.

51. Reingold AL, Hargrett NT, Dan BB, Shands KN, Strickland BY, Broome CV. Nonmenstrual toxic shock syndrome: a review of 130 cases. Ann Intern Med 1982;96:871–4.

52. Sion ML, Hatzitolios AI, Toulis EN, Mikoudi KD, Ziakas GN. Toxic shock syndrome complicating influenza A infection: a two-case report with one case of bacteremia and endocarditis. Intensive Care Med 2001;27(2):443–8.

53. Gallo LE, Fontanarosa PB. Toxic streptococcal syndrome. Ann Intern Med 1990;19:1332–4.

54. Wolf J, Rabinowitz L. Streptococcal toxic shock like syndrome. Arch Dermatol 1995;131:73–7.

55. Resnick SD. Toxic shock syndrome: recent developments in pathogenesis. J Pediatr 1990;116:321–8.

56. Parsonnet J. Mediators in the pathogenesis of toxic shock syndrome: overview. Rev Infect Dis 1989;2(suppl 1):s263–9.

57. Herzer CM. Toxic shock syndrome: broadening the differential diagnosis. J Am Board Fam Pract 2001;14(2):131–6.

58. Tofte R, Williams DN. Toxic shock syndrome: clinical and laboratory features in 15 patients. Ann Intern Med 1981;94:149–56.

59. Davis JP, Osterholm MT, Helms CM, et al. Tri-state toxic-shock syndrome study: clinical and laboratory findings. J Infect Dis 1982;145:441–8.

60. Todd JK. Therapy of toxic shock syndrome. Drugs 1990;39: 856–61.

109

Disorders of the Back and Neck

Walter L. Calmbach

Disorders of the Back

Low back pain is a common and costly medical problem. The lifetime prevalence of low back pain is estimated to be 70% to 85%, while the point prevalence is approximately 30%.[1] Each year, 2% of all American workers have a compensable back injury, and 14% lose at least one workday due to low back pain.[2] Among chronic conditions, back problems are the most frequent cause for limitation of activity (work, housekeeping, school) among patients under 45 years of age.[3] Acute low back pain is the fifth most common reason for a visit to the physician, accounting for 2.8% of all physician visits.[4] And nonsurgical low back pain is the fourth most common admission diagnosis for patients over 65.[5] Although difficult to estimate, the direct medical costs due to back pain totaled $33.6 billion in 1994. Indirect costs (i.e., lost productivity and compensation) are estimated to be as high as $43 billion.[6] In most cases, low back pain is treated successfully with a conservative regimen, supplemented by selective use of neuroradiologic imaging, and appropriate surgical intervention for a small minority of patients.[7]

Background

Epidemiology

Low back pain affects men and women equally, with the onset of symptoms between the ages of 30 and 50 years. It is the most common cause of work-related disability in people under 45 years of age, and is the most expensive cause of work-related disability.[8] Risk factors for the development of low back pain include heavy lifting and twisting, bodily vibration, obesity, and poor conditioning; however, low back pain is common even among patients without these risk factors.[1]

In cases of more severe back pain, occupational exposures are much more significant, including repetitive heavy lifting, pulling, or pushing, and exposures to industrial and vehicular vibrations. If even temporary work loss occurs, additional impor-

tant risk factors include job dissatisfaction, supervisor ratings, and job environment (i.e., boring, repetitive tasks).[1] Factors associated with recurrence of low back pain include traumatic origin of first attack, sciatic pain, radiographic changes, alcohol abuse, specific job situations, and psychosocial stigmata.

Of patients with acute low back pain, only 1.5% develop sciatica (i.e., painful paresthesias and/or motor weakness in the distribution of a nerve root). However, the lifetime prevalence of sciatica is 40%, and sciatica afflicts 11% of patients with low back pain that lasts for more than 2 weeks.[9,10] Sciatica is associated with long-distance driving, truck driving, cigarette smoking, and repeated lifting in a twisted posture. It is most common in the fourth and fifth decades of life, and peaks in the fourth decade. Most patients with sciatica, even those with significant neurologic abnormalities, recover without surgery.[11] Only 5% to 10% of patients with persistent sciatica require surgery.[5,12]

Despite the incidence and prevalence of low back pain and sciatica, the major factor responsible for its societal impact is disability.[12] The National Center for Health Statistics estimates that 5.2 million Americans are disabled with low back pain, of whom 2.6 million are permanently disabled.[13] Between 70% and 90% of the total costs due to low back pain are incurred by the 4% to 5% of patients with temporary or permanent disability.[12] Risk factors for disability due to low back pain include poor health habits, job dissatisfaction, less appealing work environments, poor ratings by supervisors, psychologic disturbances, compensable injuries, and history of prior disability.[12] These same factors are associated with high failure rates for treatments of all types.

Natural History

Recovery from nonspecific low back pain is usually rapid. Approximately one third of patients are improved at 1 week, and two thirds at 7 weeks. However, recurrences are common, affecting 40% of patients within 6 months. Thus, "acute low back pain" is increasingly perceived as a chronic medical problem with intermittent exacerbations.[14]

Low back pain may originate from many structures, including paravertebral musculature, ligaments, the annulus fibrosus, the spinal nerve roots, the facet joints, the vertebral periosteum, fascia, or blood vessels. The most common causes of back pain include musculoligamentous injuries, degenerative changes in the intervertebal discs and facet joints, spinal stenosis, and lumbar disc herniation.[14]

The natural history of herniated lumbar disc is usually quite favorable. Only about 10% of patients who present with sciatica have sufficient pain at 6 weeks that surgery is considered. Sequential magnetic resonance imaging (MRI) shows gradual regression of the herniated disc material over time, with partial or complete resolution in two thirds of patients by 6 months.[14] Acute disc herniation has changed little from its description in the classic article of Mixter and Barr: the annulus fibrosus begins to deteriorate by age 30, which leads to partial or complete herniation of the nucleus pulposus, causing irritation and compression of adjacent nerve roots.[5,15,16] Usually this herniation is in the posterolateral position, producing unilateral symptoms. Occasionally, the disc will herniate in the midline, and a large herniation in this location can cause bilateral symptoms. More than 95% of lumbar disc herniations occur at the L4–L5 or L5–S1 levels.[10] Involvement of the L5 nerve root results in weakness of the great toe extensors and dorsiflexors of the foot, and sensory loss at the dorsum of the foot and in the first web space. Involvement of the S1 nerve root results in a diminished ankle reflex, weakness of the plantar flexors, and sensory loss at the posterior calf and lateral foot.

Among patients who present with low back pain, 90% recover within 6 weeks with or without therapy.[17] Even in industrial settings, 75% of patients with symptoms of acute low back pain return to work within 1 month.[17] Only 2% to 3% of patients continue to have symptoms at 6 months, and only 1% at 1 year. However, symptoms of low back pain recur in approximately 60% of cases over the next 2 years.

Demographic characteristics such as age, gender, race, or ethnicity do not appear to influence the natural history of low back pain. Obesity, smoking, and occupation, however, are important influences.[18] Adults in the upper fifth quintile of height and weight are more likely to report low back pain lasting for 2 or more weeks.[9,18] Occupational factors that prolong or delay recovery from acute low back pain include heavier job requirements, job dissatisfaction, repetitious or boring jobs, poor employer evaluations, and noisy or unpleasant working conditions.[16] Psychosocial factors play an important role in the natural history of low back pain, modulating response to pain, and promoting illness behavior. The generally favorable natural history of acute low back pain is significantly influenced by a variety of medical and psychosocial factors that the practicing physician must be familiar with in order to counsel patients regarding prognosis and treatment.

Clinical Presentation

History

Low back pain is a symptom that has many causes. When approaching the patient with low back pain, the physician should consider three important issues: Is a systemic disease causing the pain? Is the patient experiencing social or psychosocial stresses that may amplify or prolong the pain? Does the patient have signs of neurologic compromise that may require surgical evaluation?[14] Useful items on medical history include: age, fever, history of cancer, unexplained weight loss, injection drug use, chronic infection, duration of pain, presence of nighttime pain, response to previous therapy, whether pain is relieved by bed rest or the supine position, persistent adenopathy, steroid use, and previous history of tuberculosis.[14] Factors that aggravate or alleviate low back pain should also be elicited. Nonmechanical back pain is usually continuous, while mechanical back pain is aggravated by motion and relieved by rest. Low back pain that worsens with cough has traditionally been associated with disc herniation, although recent data indicate that mechanical low back pain also worsens with cough. The presence of leg weakness or leg paresthesias in a nerve root distribution is consistent with disc herniation. Bowel or bladder incontinence with or without saddle paresthesias suggests the cauda equina syndrome; this is a surgical emergency and requires immediate referral to a surgeon. Hip pain can mimic low back pain, and is often referred to the groin, the anterior thigh, or the knee, and is worsened with ambulation. Patients with osteoarthritis or degenerative joint disease report morning stiffness, which improves as the day progresses. Patients with spinal stenosis report symptoms suggestive of spinal claudication, that is, neurologic symptoms in the legs that worsen with ambulation. Spinal claudication is differentiated from vascular claudication in that the symptoms of spinal claudication have a slower onset and slower resolution. A history of pain at rest, pain in the recumbent position, or pain at night suggests infection or tumor as a cause for low back pain. Osteoporosis is a consideration among postmenopausal women or women who have undergone oophorectomy. These patients report severe, localized, unrelenting pain after even "minor" trauma. Patients who present writhing in pain suggest the presence of an intraabdominal process or vascular cause for the pain, such as abdominal aortic aneurysm.

Physical Examination

The initial examination is fairly detailed. With the patient standing and appropriately gowned, the examining physician notes the stance and gait, as well as the presence or absence of the normal curvature of the spine (e.g., thoracic kyphosis, lumbar lordosis, splinting to one side, scoliosis). The range of motion of the back is documented, including flexion, lateral bending, and rotation. Intact dorsiflexion and plantar flexion of the foot is determined by observing heel-walk and toe-walk. Intact knee extension is determined by observing the patient squat and rise, while keeping the back straight.

With the patient seated, a distracted straight-leg raising test is applied. With the hip flexed at 90 degrees, the flexed knee is brought to full extension. A positive straight-leg raising test reproduces the patient's paresthesias in the distribution of a nerve root at <60 degrees of knee extension. Sensation to light touch and pinprick are examined and motor strength of hip and knee flexors is tested. The deep tendon reflexes are tested [knee jerk (L4), ankle jerk (S1)] and long tract signs are elicited by applying Babinski's maneuver (Table 109.1).

With the patient in the supine position, the straight-leg rais-

Table 109.1. **Motor, Sensory, and Deep Tendon Reflex Patterns Associated with Commonly Affected Nerve Roots**

Nerve root	Motor reflexes	Sensory reflexes	Deep tendon reflexes
C5	Deltoid	Lateral arm	Biceps jerk (C5,C6)
C6	Biceps, brachioradialis, wrist extensors	Lateral forearm	Brachioradialis
C7	Triceps, wrist flexors, MCP extensors	Middle of hand, middle finger	Triceps jerk
C8	MCP flexors	Medial forearm	—
T1	Abductors and adductors of fingers	Medial arm	—
L4	Quadriceps	Anterior thigh	Knee jerk
L5	Dorsiflex foot and great toe	Dorsum of foot	Hamstring reflex (L5, S1)
S1	Plantarflex foot	Lateral foot, posterior calf	Ankle jerk

MCP = metacarpophalangeal.

ing test is repeated. With the hip and knee extended, the leg is raised (i.e., the hip is flexed). A positive test reproduces the patient's paresthesias in the distribution of a nerve root. Isolated low back pain does not indicate a positive straight-leg raising test. The crossed straight-leg raising test (i.e., reproduction of the patient's symptoms by straight-leg raising of the contralateral leg) is very specific for acute disc herniation, and suggests a large central disc herniation. The examining physician should realize that the straight-leg raising test is sensitive but not specific, while the crossed straight-leg raising test is specific but not sensitive.[14] Hip range of motion is then tested, and pain radiation to the groin, antero-medial thigh, or knee is documented.

A more detailed examination may be necessary in selected patients. If significant pathology is suspected in a male patient, the cremasteric reflex is tested, i.e., application of a sharp stimulus at the proximal medial thigh should normally cause retraction of the ipsilateral scrotum. With the patient in the prone position, the femoral stretch test is applied. While the hip and knee are in extension, the knee is flexed, placing increased stretch on the femoral nerve, which includes elements from the L2, L3, and L4 nerve roots (i.e., the prone knee-bending test). The hamstring reflex is tested by striking the semitendinosus and semimembranosus tendons at the medial aspect of the popliteal fossa. The hamstring reflex involves both the L5 and S1 nerve roots. Thus, an absent or decreased hamstring reflex in the presence of a normal ankle jerk response (S1) implies involvement of the L5 nerve root (Table 109.1). Sensation in the area between the upper buttocks is tested, as well as the anal reflex and anal sphincter tone (S2, S3, S4).

The clinical diagnosis of acute disc herniation requires repeated physical examination demonstrating pain or paresthesias localized to a specific nerve root, with reproduction of pain on straight-leg raising tests, and muscle weakness in the nerve appropriate root distribution.

Diagnosis
Radiology

Plain Radiographs. Plain radiographs are usually not helpful in diagnosing acute low back pain, because they cannot demonstrate soft tissue sprains and strains, or an acute herniated disc. However, plain radiographs are useful in ruling out conditions such as vertebral fracture, spondylolisthesis, spondylolysis, infection, tumor, or inflammatory spondyloarthropathy[5,19] (Fig. 109.1). In the absence of neurologic deficits, plain radiographs

in the evaluation of low back pain should be reserved for patients over 50 years of age, patients with a temperature >38°C, patients with anemia, a history of trauma, previous cancer, pain at rest, or unexplained weight loss, drug or alcohol abuse, steroid use, diabetes mellitus, or any other reason for immunosuppression.[20] For selected patients, initial plain radiographs of the spine in the early evaluation of acute low back pain should include anteroposterior and lateral views of the lumbar spine.[15] Oblique views are used to rule out spondylolysis, particularly when evaluating acute low back pain in young athletic patients active in sports such as football, wrestling, gymnastics, diving, figure skating, or ballet.[21] If the patient's pain fails to improve after 4 to 6 weeks of conservative therapy, radiographs should be obtained; such patients may be at risk for vertebral infection, cancer, or inflammatory disease.[22]

For patients 65 years of age and older, diagnoses such as cancer, compression fracture, spinal stenosis, and aortic aneurysm become more common. Osteoporotic fracture may occur even in the absence of trauma. Because hormone replacement therapy and other medications may prevent further fractures, early radiography is recommended for older patients with back pain.[14]

Radiographic abnormalities are nonspecific and are observed equally in patients with and without symptoms of low back pain.[23] Clinical correlation is essential before symptoms of low back pain can be attributed to radiographic abnormalities.

CT, MRI, and Myelogram. Computed tomography (CT), myelogram, and magnetic resonance imaging (MRI) each has a specific role in evaluating a select subset of patients with low back pain. Physicians must be aware that many asymptomatic patients demonstrate disc bulging, protrusion, and even extrusion.[5,24] For example, 30% to 40% of CT scans and 64% of MRIs demonstrate abnormalities of the intervertebral disc in asymptomatic patients.[7,24]

CT or MRI should be reserved for patients in whom there is strong clinical suggestion of underlying infection or cancer, progressive or persistent neurologic deficit, or cauda equina syndrome therapy.[5,14] CT or MRI should be considered for patients who show no response to a 4- to 6-week course of conservative therapy.[5] CT and MRI are equally effective in detecting disc herniation and spinal stenosis, but MRI is more sensitive in detecting infection, metastatic cancer, and neural tumors.[14] Myelography is useful in differentiating significant disc herniation from incidental disc bulging not responsible for the patient's signs or symptoms, but has largely been replaced

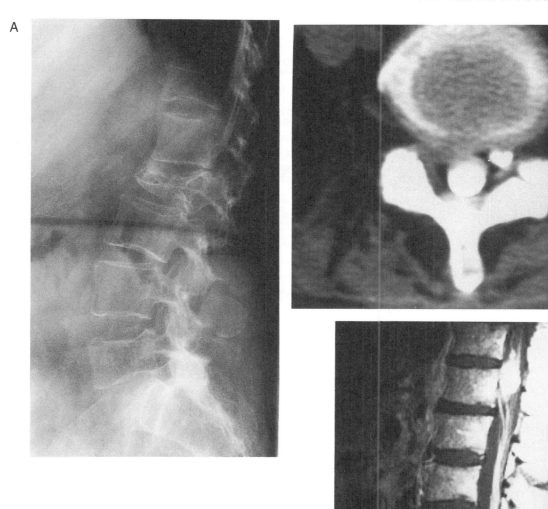

Fig. 109.1. Radiologic studies of the lumbar spine. (A) Plain radiograph demonstrating a compression fracture of the L2 vertebral body due to multiple myeloma. (B) CT scan demonstrating nucleus pulposus herniating posteriorly into the spinal canal. (C) MRI demonstrating an enhancing intramedullary metastatic lesion in the cauda equina at the L1 level.

by noninvasive techniques such as MRI or CT.[15] CT myelography is sometimes used in planning surgery.[14]

Ancillary Tests

Because plain radiographs are not highly sensitive for detection of early cancer or vertebral infection, tests such as erythrocyte sedimentation rate (ESR) and complete blood count (CBC) should be obtained for selected patients.[14,25]

Differential Diagnosis

Osteoarthritis

Osteoarthritis of the vertebral spine is common in later life, and is especially prevalent in the cervical and lumbar spine (also see Chapter 112). Typically, the pain of osteoarthritis of the spine is worse in the morning, increases with motion, but is relieved by rest. It is associated with morning stiffness, and a decreased range of motion of the spine in the absence of systemic symptoms. The severity of symptoms does not correlate well with radiographic findings, and patients with severe degenerative changes on plain radiographs may be asymptomatic, while patients with symptoms suggestive of osteoarthritis of the spine may have minimal radiologic findings. In some patients, extensive osteophytic changes may lead to compression of lumbar nerve roots or may even cause cauda equina syndrome.

Spinal Stenosis

Spinal stenosis is a common cause of back pain among older adults. Symptoms usually begin in the sixth decade, and over time the patient's posture becomes progressively flexed forward. The mean age of patients at the time of surgery for spinal stenosis is 55 years, with an average symptom duration of 4 years.[10] The symptoms of spinal stenosis are often diffuse because the disease is usually bilateral and involves several vertebrae. Pain, numbness, and tingling may occur in one or both legs. Pseudoclaudication is the classic symptom of spinal stenosis. Pseudoclaudication is differentiated from vascular claudication in that pseudoclaudication has a slower onset and a slower resolution of symptoms.[7]

Symptoms are usually relieved with flexion (e.g., sitting, pushing a grocery cart) and exacerbated by back extension. Plain radiographs often show osteophytes at several levels, but as mentioned earlier, caution must be used in ascribing back pain to these degenerative changes. CT or MRI may be used to confirm the diagnosis. Electromyography (EMG) or somatosensory evoked potentials may be used to differentiate the pain of spinal stenosis from peripheral neuropathy. The natural history of spinal stenosis is such that patients tend to remain stable or slowly worsen. Symptoms evolve gradually, but about 15% of patients improve over a period of about 4 years, 70% remain stable, and 15% experience worsening symptoms.[14] Nonoperative therapy for spinal stenosis includes leg strengthening and avoidance of alcohol to reduce the risk of falls, and physical activity such as walking or using an exercise bicycle is also recommended.[27] Decompressive laminectomy may be necessary for selected patients with spinal stenosis who have persistent severe pain. Although treatment for spinal stenosis must be individualized, recent reports suggest that patients treated surgically have better outcomes at 4 years than patients treated nonsurgically, even after adjusting for differences in baseline characteristics.[28] However, at 4-year follow-up, 30% of patients still have severe pain and 10% have undergone reoperation.[28]

Osteoporosis

Osteoporosis is a common problem among seniors, affecting up to 25% of women over 65. Decreased bone mineral density in the vertebral body is associated with an increased risk for spinal compression fractures. In primary care settings, 4% of patients who present with acute low back pain have compression fractures as the cause.[14] Pain symptoms are worse with prolonged sitting or standing, and usually resolve over 3 to 4 months as compression fractures heal.[6] African-American and Mexican-American women have only one fourth as many compression fractures as European-American women.[5] Patients with compression fractures due to osteoporosis usually have no neurologic complaints and do not suffer from neural compression. Plain radiographs document a loss of vertebral body height due to compression fractures. Laboratory tests are normal in primary osteoporosis, and any abnormalities should prompt a search for secondary causes of osteoporosis. The diagnosis of primary osteoporosis is made on clinical grounds, i.e., diffuse osteopenia, compression fractures, and normal laboratory findings[29,30] (also see Chapter 122).

Neoplasia

Multiple myeloma is the most common primary malignancy of the vertebral spine. However, metastatic lesions are the most common cause of cancers of the spine, arising from breast, lung, prostate, thyroid, renal, or gastrointestinal tract primary tumors. Both Hodgkin's and non-Hodgkin's lymphomas frequently involve the vertebral spine. Because the primary site of the tumor is often overlooked, back pain is the presenting complaint for many cancers. In primary care settings, 0.7% of patients who present with low back pain have cancer as the cause.[10,25] Findings significantly associated with cancer as the cause of low back pain include age >50 years, previous history of cancer, pain lasting >1 month, failure to improve with conservative therapy, elevated ESR, and anemia.[25] Patients report a dull constant pain that is worse at night, and not relieved by rest or the recumbent position. Typical radiographic changes may be absent early in the course of vertebral body tumors. A technetium bone scan is usually positive due to increased blood flow and reactive bone formation; however, in multiple myeloma and metastatic thyroid cancer, the bone scan may be negative.[31] Greater diagnostic specificity and improved cost-effectiveness can be achieved by using a higher cut-off point for the ESR (e.g., >50 mm/hr) combined with either a bone scan followed by MRI as indicated, or MRI alone.[32] Symptomatic cancer of the lumbar spine is an ominous sign with a potential for devastating morbidity due to spinal cord injury.[33] Early recognition and treatment are essential if irreversible cord damage is to be avoided.

Posterior Facet Syndrome

The posterior facet syndrome is caused by degenerative changes in the posterior facet joints. These are true diarthrodial joints that sometimes develop degenerative joint changes visible on plain radiographs. Degenerative changes in the posterior facet joints cause a dull achy pain that radiates to the groin, hip, or thigh, and is worsened with twisting or hyperextension of the spine.[34] Steroid injection into the posterior facet joints to relieve presumed posterior facet joint pain is a popular procedure, but the placebo effect of injection in this area is significant and controlled studies have failed to demonstrate benefit from steroid injections.[35,36] The presence of degenerative changes in the facet joints on plain radiographs does not imply that the posterior facets are the cause of the patient's pain. Caution must be used in ascribing the patient's symptoms to these degenerative changes. Historically, the posterior facet syndrome was diagnosed by demonstrating pain relief after injection of local anesthetic into the posterior facet joints, but recent studies cast doubt on the validity of this procedure.[7,34] Several factors have been proposed to identify subjects who might benefit from lidocaine injection into lumbar facet joints: pain relieved in the supine position, age >65, and low back pain not worsened by coughing, hyperextension, forward flexion, rising from flexion, or extension-rotation.[37] However, a recent systematic review concluded that while facet joint injection provided some short-term relief, this benefit was not statistically significant; therefore, convincing evidence is lacking regarding the effects of facet joint injection therapy on low back pain.[38]

Ankylosing Spondylitis

Ankylosing spondylitis is a spondyloarthropathy most commonly affecting men under 40 years of age. Patients present with mild to moderate low back pain that is centered in the back and radiates to the posterior thighs. In its initial presentation, the symptoms are vague and the diagnosis is often over-looked. Pain symptoms are intermittent, but decreased range of motion in the spine remains constant. Early signs of ankylosing spondylitis include limitation of chest expansion, tenderness of the sternum, and decreased range of motion and flexion contractures at the hip. Inflammatory involvement of the knees or hips increases the likelihood of spondylitis.[39] The radiologic hallmarks of ankylosing spondylitis include periarticular destructive changes, obliteration of the sacroiliac joints, development of syndesmophytes on the margins of the vertebral bodies, and bridging of these osteophytes by bone between vertebral bodies, the so-called bamboo spine. Laboratory analysis is negative for rheumatoid factor, but the ESR is elevated early in the course of the disease. Tests for human leukocyte antigen (HLA)-B27 are not recommended because as many as 6% of an unselected population test positive for this antigen.[15]

Visceral Diseases

Several visceral diseases may present with back pain as a chief symptom.[5] These include nephrolithiasis, endometriosis, and abdominal aortic aneurysm. Abdominal aortic aneurysm causes low back pain by compression of surrounding tissues or by extension or rupture of the aneurysm. Patients report dull steady back pain unrelated to activity, which radiates to the hips or thighs. Patients with an acute rupture or extension of the aneurysm report severe tearing pain, diaphoresis, or syncope, and demonstrate signs of circulatory shock.[29]

Cauda Equina Syndrome

The cauda equina syndrome is a rare condition caused by severe compression of the cauda equina, usually by a large midline disc herniation or a tumor.[14] The patient may report urinary retention with overflow incontinence, as well as bilateral sciatica, leg weakness, and sensory loss in a saddle distribution. Patients with these findings represent a true surgical emergency, and should be referred immediately for surgical treatment and decompression.

Psychosocial Factors

Psychological factors are frequently associated with complaints of low back pain, influencing both patient pain symptoms and therapeutic outcome.[40] Features that suggest psychological causes of low back pain include nonorganic signs and symptoms, dissociation between verbal and nonverbal pain behaviors, compensable cause of injury, joblessness, disability-seeking, depression, anxiety, requests for narcotics or other psychoactive drugs, and repeated failure of multiple treatments.[41] Prolonged back pain may be associated with failure of previous treatment, depression, or somatization.[14] Substance abuse, job dissatisfaction, pursuit of disability compensation and involvement in litigation are also associated with persistent unexplained symptoms.[8]

Management

Nonspecific Low Back Pain

For most patients, the best recommendation is rapid return to normal daily activities. However, patients should avoid heavy lifting, twisting, or bodily vibration in the acute phase.[14] A 4- to 6-week trial of conservative therapy is appropriate in the absence of cauda equina syndrome or a rapidly progressive neurologic deficit (Table 109.2).

Bed Rest

Bed rest does not increase the speed of recovery from acute back pain, and sometimes delays recovery.[42,43] Symptomatic relief from back pain may benefit from 1 or 2 days of bed rest, but patients should be told that it is safe to get out of bed even if pain persists.[14]

Medications

Antiinflammatories. Nonsteroidal antiinflammatory drugs (NSAIDs) are effective for short-term symptomatic relief in patients with acute low back pain.[44] There does not seem to be a specific type of NSAID that is clearly more effective than others.[44] Therapy is titrated to provide pain relief at a minimal dose, and is continued for 4 to 6 weeks. NSAIDs should not be continued indefinitely, but rather prescribed for a specific period.[3]

Muscle Relaxants. Although evidence for the effectiveness of muscle relaxants is scant, the main value of muscle relaxants is less for muscle relaxation than for their sedative effect. Diazepam (Valium), cyclobenzaprine (Flexeril), and methocarbamol (Robaxin) are commonly used as muscle relaxants, and carisoprodol (Soma) has documented effectiveness.[3] Muscle relaxants should be prescribed in a time-limited fashion, usually less than 2 weeks. Muscle relaxants and narcotics are not recommended for patients who present with complaints of chronic low back pain (i.e., low back pain of greater than 3 months' duration).[5]

Unproven Treatments

Traction is not recommended for the treatment of acute low back pain.[45] No scientific evidence supports the efficacy of corsets or braces in the treatment of acute low back pain, and these treatments are not recommended.[5] Transcutaneous electrical nerve stimulation (TENS) is not effective in the treatment of low back pain.[46]

Exercise

Back exercises are not useful in the acute phase of low back pain, but are useful later for preventing recurrences.[14] Guidelines from the Agency for Health Care Policy and Research (AHCPR) stress aerobic exercise (e.g., walking, biking, swimming) especially during the first 2 weeks; continuing ordinary activities improves recovery and leads to less disability.[22] However, a recent systematic review concluded that specific back exercises do not improve clinical outcomes.[47] There is moderate evidence that flexion exercises are not effective in the treatment of acute low back pain, and strong evidence that extension exercises are not effective in the treatment of acute low back pain.

Spinal Manipulation

Clinical trials suggest that spinal manipulation has some efficacy.[48,49] Current recommendations are that patients should not be referred for spinal manipulation unless pain persists

Table 109.2. **Nonoperative Treatment Considerations for Low Back Pain and Sciatica**

Treatment	Acute low back pain	Acute sciatica	Subacute low back pain and leg pain	Chronic low back pain and leg pain
Bedrest	Avoid	Avoid	Avoid	Avoid, short-term for flare-ups only
NSAIDs	Symptomatic pain relief, time-limited	Symptomatic pain relief, time-limited	Selected cases if effective	Avoid long-term
Muscle relaxants	Optimal 1 week; maximum 2–4 weeks	Optimal 1 week; maximum 2–4 weeks	Selected cases if effective	Avoid long-term
Opioids	No	Optimal 1–3 days; maximum 2–3 weeks	Selected pre-surgical cases; avoid	Avoid
Antidepressants	No	No	Selected cases	Yes
Local injections	No	No	Selected cases as an adjunct	Flare-ups
Facet injections	No	No	No	Avoid; no long-term effect alone
Epidural corticosteroids	No	Yes	Flare-ups, if effective	Flare-ups only; avoid
Orthoses	Adjunctive	No	Adjunctive	Adjunctive
Cryotherapy (ice)	Adjunctive	Adjunctive	Flare-ups	Flare-ups; self-applied
Thermotherapy	Adjunctive	Adjunctive	Adjunctive	Flare-ups; self-applied
Traction	No	No	No	No
Joint manipulation	Not recommended for first 3–4 weeks	Not with neural signs	If effective; maximum 2–4 months	Flare-ups; time-contingent if effective
Joint mobilization	Yes, if effective	Yes, if effective	If effective; maximum 2–4 months	Flare-ups; time-contingent if effective
Soft tissue techniques (massage, myofascial release, mobilization)	Yes, if effective	Yes, if effective	If effective; maximum 2–4 months	Flare-ups; time-contingent if effective
McKenzie exercises	No	No	Flare-ups, if effective	Flare-ups, if effective
Dynamic lumbar stabilization	No	No	Yes	Yes
Back school	Yes	Yes	Yes	Yes
Functional restoration	No	No	Yes	Optimal 3–4 months; maximum 4–6 months
Pain clinic	No	No	No	Yes

NSAID = nonsteroidal antiinflammatory drug.
Source: Adapted from Wheeler,[41] with permission. Copyright © American Academy of Family Physicians. All rights reserved.

for more than 3 weeks because half of patients spontaneously improve during this time frame.[14]

Back School

A recent systematic review concluded that there is moderate evidence that back schools are not more effective than other treatments for acute low back pain.[50]

Acupuncture (also see Chapter 128)

A recent systematic qualitative review concluded that there is no evidence to show that acupuncture is more effective than no treatment, moderate evidence to show that acupuncture is

not more effective than trigger point injection or TENS, and limited evidence to show that acupuncture is not more effective than placebo or sham procedure for the treatment of chronic low back pain.[51] Therefore, acupuncture is not recommended as a regular treatment for patients with low back pain.

Herniated Intervertebral Disc

Early treatment resembles that for nonspecific low back pain, outlined above. However, for patients with suspected lumbar disc herniation, the role of spinal manipulation is not clear. Narcotic analgesics may be necessary for pain relief for some patients with herniated intervertebral disc, but these medications should be used in a time-limited (i.e., not symptom-limited) manner.[14] Epidural corticosteroid injection may offer temporary symptomatic relief for some patients.[52] However, this invasive procedure offers no significant functional improvement, and does not reduce the need for surgery.[52] If neuropathic pain persists and/or neurologic deficits progress, CT or MRI should be performed, and surgery should be considered.[14]

Surgery

Background. The rate of lumbar surgery in the United States is 40% higher than in most developed nations, and five times higher than in England and Scotland.[53] The lifetime prevalence of lumbar spine surgery ranges between 1% and 3%, and 2% to 3% of patients with low back pain may be surgical candidates on the basis of sciatica alone.[12] Surgery rates vary widely by geographical region in the U.S., and have risen dramatically in the last 10 years.[54] Psychological factors influence postsurgical outcomes more strongly than initial physical examination or surgical findings. Prior to surgery, patients should be evaluated with standard pain indices, activities of daily living scales, and psychometric testing. Surgical results for treating symptomatic lumbar disc herniation unresponsive to conservative therapy are excellent in well-selected patients.[55]

Indications. There is no evidence from clinical trials or cohort studies that surgery is effective for patients who have low back pain unless they have sciatica, pseudoclaudication, or spondylolisthesis.[56] In the absence of cauda equina syndrome or progressive neurologic deficit, patients with suspected lumbar disc herniation should be treated nonsurgically for at least a month.[14] The primary benefit of discectomy is to provide more rapid relief of sciatica in patients who have failed to resolve with conservative management.[56] In well-selected patients, 75% have complete relief of sciatic symptoms after surgery and an additional 15% have partial relief. Patients with clear symptoms of radicular pain have the best surgical outcome, while those with the least evidence of radiculopathy have the poorest surgical outcome.[57] Relief of back pain itself is less consistent. Appropriate patient selection is key to successful surgical outcome.

Options. Standard discectomy is the most common procedure used to relieve symptomatic disc herniation. A posterior longitudinal incision is made over the involved disc space, a variable amount of bone is removed, the ligamentum flavum is incised, and herniated disc material is excised. This procedure allows adequate visualization and yields satisfactory results among 65% to 85% of patients.[11,58] Recent reports suggest that patients who undergo surgical therapy have greater improvement of their symptoms and greater functional recovery at 4 years than patients treated nonoperatively[59]; however, work status and disability status were similar between these two groups. Previous studies have shown that there is no clear benefit to surgery at 10-year follow-up.[11]

Microdiscectomy allows smaller incisions, little or no bony excision, and removal of disc material under magnification. This procedure has fewer complications, fewer unsuccessful outcomes, and permits faster recovery. However, rates of reoperation are significantly higher in patients initially treated with microdiscectomy, presumably due to missed disc fragments or operating at the wrong spinal level.[58] A recent systematic review concluded that the clinical outcomes for patients after microdiscectomy are comparable to those of standard discectomy.[56]

Percutaneous discectomy is an outpatient procedure performed under local anesthesia in which the surgeon uses an automated percutaneous cutting and suction probe to aspirate herniated disc material. This procedure results in lower rates of nerve injury, postoperative instability, infection, fibrosis, and chronic pain syndromes. However, patients undergoing percutaneous discectomy sustain unacceptably high rates of recurrent disc herniation. Only 29% of patients reported satisfactory results after percutaneous discectomy, while 80% of subjects were satisfied after microdiscectomy.[60] A recent systematic review concluded that only 10% to 15% of patients with herniated nucleus pulposus requiring surgery might be suitable candidates for percutaneous discectomy.[56] This procedure is not recommended for patients with previous back surgery, sequestered disc fragments, bony entrapment, or multiple herniated discs.[58,61]

For the time being, automated percutaneous discectomy and laser discectomy should be regarded as research techniques.[56] Arthroscopic discectomy is an emerging technique that shows promising results and effectiveness similar to that of standard discectomy.[62]

Chemonucleolysis is a procedure in which a proteolytic enzyme (chymopapain) is injected into the disc space to dissolve herniated disc material. A recent systematic review concluded that chemonucleolysis is effective for the treatment patients with low back pain due to herniated nucleus pulposus, and is more effective than placebo.[56] However, chemonucleolysis showed consistently poorer results than standard discectomy. Approximately 30% of patients undergoing chemonucleolysis had further disc surgery within 2 years. Proponents of chemonucleolysis have suggested that it may be associated with lower costs, but readmission for a second procedure negates this putative advantage. Chemonucleolysis may be indicated for selected patients as an intermediate stage between conservative and surgical management.[56]

Complications. Complications of surgery on the lumbar spine are largely related to patient age, gender, diagnosis, and type of procedure.[63] Mortality rates increase substantially with age, but are <1% even among patients over 75 years of age. Mortality rates are higher for men, but morbidity rates and likelihood of discharge to a nursing home are significantly higher for women, particularly women over 75. With regard to underlying diagnosis, complications and duration of hospitalization are highest after surgery to correct spinal stenosis, degenerative changes, or instability, and are lowest for procedures to correct herniated disc. With regard to type of procedure, complications and duration of hospitalization are highest for procedures involving arthrodesis with or without laminectomy, followed by laminectomy alone or with discectomy, and are lowest for discectomy alone. Other surgical complications include thromboembolism (1.7%) and infection (2.9%).[5]

Summary

The physician's goal in treating patients with low back pain is to promote activity and early return to work. While it is important to rule out significant pathology as the cause of low back pain, most patients can be reassured that symptoms are due to simple musculoligamentous injury.[14] Patients should be counseled that they will improve with time, usually quite quickly.

Bed rest is not recommended for the treatment of low back pain or sciatica; rather, a rapid return to normal activities is usually the best course.[14] Nonsteroidal antiinflammatory drugs can be used in a time-limited way for symptomatic relief.[44] Back exercises are not useful for acute low back pain, but can help prevent recurrence of back pain and can be used to treat patients with chronic low back pain.[14] Work activities may be modified at first, but avoiding iatrogenic disability is key to successful management of acute low back pain.[5,41] Surgery should be reserved for patients with progressive neurologic deficit or those who have sciatica or pseudoclaudication that persists after nonoperative therapy has failed.[14]

Chronic Low Back Pain

Chronic low back pain (i.e., pain persisting for more than 3 months) is a special problem that warrants careful consideration. Patients presenting with a history of chronic low back pain require an extensive diagnostic workup on at least one occasion, including in-depth history, physical examination, and the appropriate imaging techniques (plain radiographs, CT, or MRI).

Management of patients with chronic back pain should be aimed at restoring normal function.[47] Exercises may be useful in the treatment of chronic low back pain if they aim at improving return to normal daily activities and work.[47] A recent systematic review concluded that exercise therapy is as effective as physiotherapy (e.g., hot packs, massage, mobilization, short-wave diathermy, ultrasound, stretching, flexibility, electrotherapy) for patients with chronic low back pain.[47] And there is strong evidence that exercise is more effective than "usual care." Evidence is lacking about the effectiveness of flexion and extension exercises for patients with chronic low back pain.[47]

Although one literature synthesis cast doubt on the effectiveness of antidepressant therapy for chronic low back pain,[64] it is widely used and recommended.[14] Antidepressant therapy is useful for the one third of patients with chronic low back pain who also have depression. Tricyclic antidepressants may be more effective for treating pain in patients without depression than selective serotonin reuptake inhibitors.[65] However, narcotic analgesics are not recommended for patients with chronic low back pain.[14]

A recent systematic review concluded that there is moderate evidence that back schools have better short-term effects

than other treatments for chronic low back pain, and moderate evidence that back schools in an occupational setting are more effective compared to placebo or "waiting list" controls.[50] Functional restoration programs combine intense physical therapy with cognitive-behavioral interventions and increasing levels of task-oriented rehabilitation and work simulation.[41] Patients with chronic low back pain may require referral to a multidisciplinary pain clinic for optimal management. Such clinics can offer cognitive behavioral therapy, patient education classes, supervised exercise programs, and selective nerve blocks to facilitate return to normal function.[14] Complete relief of symptoms may be an unrealistic goal; instead, patients and physicians should try to optimize daily functioning.

Prevention

Prevention of low back injury and consequent disability is an important challenge in primary care. Pre-employment physical examination screening is not effective in reducing the occurrence of job-related low back pain. However, active aerobically fit individuals have fewer back injuries, miss fewer workdays, and report fewer back pain symptoms.[66] Evidence to support smoking cessation and weight loss as means of reducing the occurrence of low back pain is sparse, but these should be recommended for other health reasons.[66] Exercise programs that combine aerobic conditioning with specific strengthening of the back and legs can reduce the frequency of recurrence of low back pain.[44,66] The use of corsets and education about lifting technique are generally ineffective in preventing low back problems.[67,68] Ergonomic redesign of strenuous tasks may facilitate return to work and reduce chronic pain.[69]

Disorders of the Neck

Cervical Radiculopathy

Cervical radiculopathy is a common cause of neck pain, and can be caused by a herniated cervical disc, osteophytic changes, compressive pathology, or hypermobility of the cervical spine. The lifetime prevalence of neck and arm pain among adults may be as high as 51%. Risk factors associated with neck pain include heavy lifting, smoking, diving, working with vibrating heavy equipment, and possibly riding in cars.[70]

Cervical nerve roots exit the spine above the corresponding vertebral body (e.g., the C5 nerve root exits above C5). Therefore, disc herniation at the C4-C5 interspace causes symptoms in the distribution of C5.[71] Radicular symptoms may be caused by a "soft disc" (i.e., disc herniation) or by a "hard disc" (i.e., osteophyte formation and foraminal encroachment).[71] The most commonly involved interspaces are C5-6, C6-7, C4-5, C3-4, and C7-T1.[70]

The symptoms of cervical radiculopathy may be single or multiple, unilateral or bilateral, symmetrical or asymmetrical.[72] Acute cervical radiculopathy is commonly due to a tear of the annulus fibrosus with prolapse of the nucleus pulposus, and is usually the result of mild to moderate trauma. Subacute symptoms are usually due to long-standing spondylosis accompanied by mild trauma or overuse. The majority of patients with subacute cervical radiculopathy experience resolution of their symptoms within 6 weeks with rest and analgesics. Chronic radiculopathy is more common in middle age or old age, and patients present with complaints of neck or arm pain due to heavy labor or unaccustomed activity.[72–74]

Cervical radiculopathy rarely progresses to myelopathy, but as many as two thirds of patients treated conservatively report persistent symptoms. In severe cases of cervical radiculopathy in which motor function has been compromised, 98% of patients recover full motor function after decompressive laminectomy.[75]

Clinical Presentation

Among patients with cervical radiculopathy, sensory symptoms are much more prominent than motor changes. Typically, patients report proximal pain and distal paresthesias.[71] The fifth, sixth, and seventh nerve roots are most commonly affected. Referred pain caused by cervical disc herniation is usually vague, diffuse, and lacking in the sharp quality of radicular pain. Pain referred from a herniated cervical disc may present as pain in the neck, pain at the top of the shoulder, or pain around the scapula.[72]

On physical examination, radicular pain increases with certain maneuvers such as neck range of motion, Valsalva maneuver, cough, or sneeze. Active and passive neck range of motion is tested, examining flexion, rotation, and lateral bending. Spurling's maneuver is useful in assessing neck pain: the examining physician flexes the patient's neck, then rolls the neck into lateral bending, and finally extends the neck. The examiner then applies a compressive load to the vertex of the skull. This maneuver narrows the cervical foramina posterolaterally, and may reproduce the patient's radicular symptoms.

Diagnosis

The differential diagnosis of cervical nerve root pain includes cervical disc herniation, spinal canal tumor, trauma, degenerative changes, inflammatory disorders, congenital abnormalities, toxic and allergic conditions, hemorrhage, and musculoskeletal syndromes (e.g., thoracic outlet syndrome, shoulder pain).[71,75] In cases of cervical radiculopathy unresponsive to conservative therapy, or in the presence of progressive motor deficit, investigation of other pathologic processes is indicated. Plain radiographs are usually not helpful because abnormal radiographic findings are equally common among symptomatic and asymptomatic patients. CT scan, myelography, and MRI each has a specific role to play in the diagnosis of cervical radiculopathy.[73,74] CT scan is especially useful in delineating bony lesions, CT myelography can effectively demonstrate functional stenoses of the spinal canal, and MRI is an excellent noninvasive modality for demonstrating soft tissue abnormalities (e.g., herniated cervical disc, spinal cord derangement, extradural tumor).

Management

Immobilization. The purpose of neck immobilization is to reduce intervertebral motion which may cause compression,

mechanical irritation, or stretching of the cervical nerve roots.[76] The soft cervical collar or the more rigid Philadelphia collar both hold the neck in slight flexion. The collar is useful in the acute setting, but prolonged use leads to deconditioning of the paracervical musculature. Therefore, the collar should be prescribed in a time-limited manner, and patients should be instructed to begin isometric neck exercises early in the course of therapy.

Bed Rest. Bed rest is another form of immobilization that modifies the patient's activities and eliminates the axial compression forces of gravity.[76] Holding the neck in slight flexion is accomplished by arranging two standard pillows in a V shape with the apex pointed cranially, then placing a third pillow across the apex. This arrangement provides mild cervical flexion, and internally rotates the shoulder girdle, thereby relieving traction on the cervical nerve roots.

Medications. Nonsteroidal antiinflammatory drugs (NSAIDs) are particularly beneficial in relieving acute neck pain. However, side effects are common, and usually two or three medications must be tried before a beneficial result without unacceptable side effects is achieved. Muscle relaxants help relieve muscle spasm in some patients; alternatives include carisoprodol (Soma), methocarbamol (Robaxin), and diazepam (Valium). Narcotics may be useful in the acute setting, but should be prescribed in a strictly time-limited manner.[76] The physician should be alert to the possibility of addiction or abuse.

Physical Therapy. Moist heat (20 minutes, three times daily), ice packs (15 minutes, four times daily or even hourly), ultrasound therapy, and other modalities also help relieve the symptoms of cervical radiculopathy.[76]

Surgery. Surgical intervention is reserved for patients with cervical disc herniation confirmed by neuroradiologic imaging and radicular signs and symptoms that persist despite 4 to 6 weeks of conservative therapy.[71]

Cervical Myelopathy

The cause of pain in cervical myelopathy is not clearly understood but is presumed to be multifactorial, including vascular changes, cord hypoxia, changes in spinal canal diameter, and hypertrophic facets. Therefore, patients with cervical myelopathy present with a variable clinical picture. The usual course is one of increasing disability over several months, usually beginning with dysesthesias in the hands, followed by weakness or clumsiness in the hands, and eventually progressing to weakness in the lower extremities.[72]

Clinical Presentation

In cases of cervical myelopathy secondary to cervical spondylosis, symptoms are usually insidious in onset, often with short periods of worsening followed by long periods of relative stability.[77] Acute onset of symptoms or rapid deterioration may suggest a vascular etiology.[71] Unlike cervical radiculopathy, cervical myelopathy rarely presents with neck pain; instead, patients report an occipital headache that radiates anteriorly to the frontal area, is worse on waking, but improves through the day.[72] Patients also report deep aching pain and burning sensations in the hands, loss of hand dexterity, and vertebrobasilar insufficiency, presumably due to osteophytic changes in the cervical spine.[71,72]

On physical examination, patients demonstrate motor weakness and muscle wasting, particularly of the interosseous muscles of the hand. Lhermitte's sign is present in approximately 25% of patients, i.e., rapid flexion or extension of the neck causes a shock-like sensation in the trunk or limbs.[71] Deep tendon reflexes are variable. Involvement of the anterior horn cell causes hyporeflexia, whereas involvement of the corticospinal tracts causes hyperreflexia. The triceps jerk is the reflex most commonly lost, due to frequent involvement of the sixth nerve root (i.e., the C5-6 interspace). Almost all patients with cervical myelopathy show signs of muscular spasticity.

Diagnosis

Radiologic Diagnosis in Cervical Spondylosis
Intrathecal contrast-enhanced CT scan is a highly specific test that allows evaluation of the intradural contents and the disc margins, and helps differentiate an extradural defect due to disc herniation from that due to osteophytic changes.[73] MRI allows visualization of the cervical spine in both the sagittal and axial planes. Resolution with MRI is sharp enough to identify lesions of the spinal cord and differentiate disc herniation from spinal stenosis.[73] CT scan is preferred in evaluating osteophytes, foraminal encroachment, and other bony changes. CT and MRI complement one another, and their use should be individualized for each patient.[74] Clinical correlation of abnormal neuroradiologic findings is essential because degenerative changes of the cervical spine and cervical disc are common even among asymptomatic patients.[73,74]

Management

Conservative Therapy.
Most patients with cervical myelopathy present with minor symptoms and demonstrate long periods of non-progressive disability. Therefore, these patients should initially be treated conservatively: rest with a soft cervical collar, physical therapy to promote range of motion, and judicious use of NSAIDs. However, only 30% to 50% of patients improve with conservative management. A recent multicenter study comparing the efficacy of surgery versus conservative management demonstrated broadly similar outcomes with regard to activities of daily living, symptom index, function, and patient satisfaction.[77]

Surgery.
Early surgical decompression is appropriate for patients with cervical myelopathy who present with moderate or severe disability, or in the presence of rapid neurologic deterioration.[78] Anterior decompression with fusion, posterior decompression, laminectomy, or laminoplasty is appropriate to particular clinical situations.[79] The best surgical prognosis is achieved by careful patient selection. Accurate diagnosis is essential, and patients with symptoms of relatively short du-

ration have the best prognosis.[71] If surgery is considered, it should be performed early in the course of the disease, before cord damage becomes irreversible.

Surgical decompression is recommended for patients with severe or progressive symptoms; excellent or good outcomes can be expected for approximately 70% of these patients.[77]

Cervical Whiplash

Cervical whiplash is a valid clinical syndrome, with symptoms consistent with anatomic sites of injury, and a potential for significant impairment.[80] Whiplash injuries afflict more than 1 million people in the U.S. each year,[81] with an annual incidence of approximately 4 per 1000 population.[82] Symptoms in cervical whiplash injuries are due to soft tissue trauma, particularly musculoligamentous sprains and strains to the cervical spine. After a rear-end impact in a motor vehicle accident, the patient is accelerated forward and the lower cervical vertebrae are hyperextended, especially at the C5-6 interspace. This is followed by flexion of the upper cervical vertebrae, which is limited by the chin striking the chest. Hyperextension commonly causes an injury to the anterior longitudinal ligament of the cervical spine and other soft tissue injuries of the anterior neck including muscle tears, muscle hemorrhage, esophageal hemorrhage, or disc disruption. Muscles most commonly injured include the sternocleidomastoid, scalenus, and longus colli muscles.

Neck pain and headache are the cardinal features of whiplash injury.[83] Injury to the upper cervical segments may cause pain referred to the neck or the head and presents as neck pain or headache. Injury to the lower cervical segments may cause pain referred to shoulder and or arm. Patients may also develop visual disturbances, possibly due to vertebral, basilar, or other vascular injury, or injury to the cervical sympathetic chain.[81]

After acute injury most patients recover rapidly: 80% are asymptomatic by 12 months, 15% to 20% remain symptomatic after 12 months, and only 5% are severely affected.[83] However this last group of patients generates the greatest health care costs.

Clinical Presentation

On history, patients describe a typical rear-end impact motor vehicle accident with hyperextension of the neck followed by hyperflexion. Pain in the neck may be immediate or may be delayed hours or even days after the accident. Pain is usually felt at the base of the neck and increases over time. Patients report pain and decreased range of motion in the neck, which is worsened by motion or activity, as well as paresthesias or weakness in the upper extremities, dysphagia, or hoarseness.

Physical examination may be negative if the patient is seen within hours of the accident. Over time, however, patients develop tenderness in the cervical spine area, as well as decreased range of motion and muscle spasm. Neurologic examination of the upper extremity should include assessment of motor function and grip strength, sensation, deep tendon reflexes, and range of motion (especially of the neck and shoulder).

Diagnosis

Findings on plain radiographs are usually minimal. Five views of the cervical spine should be obtained: anteroposterior, lateral, right and left obliques, and the odontoid view. Straightening of the cervical spine or loss of the normal cervical lordosis may be due to positioning in radiology, muscle spasm, or derangement of the skeletal alignment of the cervical spine. Radiographs should also be examined for soft tissue swelling anterior to the C3 vertebral body, which may indicate an occult fracture. Signs of preexisting degenerative changes such as osteophytic changes, disc space narrowing, or narrowing of the cervical foramina are also common. Electromyography and nerve conduction velocity tests should be considered if paresthesias or radicular pain are present. Technetium bone scan is very sensitive in detecting occult injuries. However, whiplash injuries usually cause soft tissue injuries that are not demonstrable with most of these studies. For example, MRI of the brain and neck of patients within 2 days of whiplash injury shows no difference between subjects and controls.[84] Therefore, CT or MRI should be reserved for patients with neurologic deficit, intense pain within minutes of injury, suspected spinal cord or disc damage, suspected fracture, or ligamentous injury.[81,82]

Management

Many patients recover within 6 months without any treatment. However, treatment may speed the recovery process and limit the amount of pain the patient experiences during recovery.[82]

Rest. While rest in a soft cervical collar has been the traditional treatment for patients with whiplash injury, recent studies indicate that prolonged rest (i.e., 2 weeks or more) and/or excessive use of the soft cervical collar may be detrimental and actually slow the healing process.[85] Initially, patients should be treated with a brief period of rest and protection of the cervical spine, usually with a soft cervical collar for 3 or 4 days. The collar holds the neck in slight flexion; therefore, the widest part of the cervical collar should be worn posteriorly. The cervical collar is especially useful in alleviating pain if worn at night or when driving. If used during the day, it should be worn 1 or 2 hours and then removed for a similar period in order to preserve paracervical muscle conditioning. The soft cervical collar should not be used for more than a few days; early in the course of treatment, the patient should be encouraged to begin mobilization exercises for the neck.[81]

Medications. NSAIDs are effective in treating the pain and muscle spasm caused by whiplash injuries. Muscle relaxants are a useful adjunct, especially when used nightly, and should be prescribed in a time-limited manner. Narcotics are usually not indicated in the treatment of whiplash injuries.

Physical Therapy. A treatment protocol with proven success involves early active range of motion and strengthening exercises.[86] Patients are instructed to perform gentle rotational exercises 10 times an hour as soon as symptoms allow within 96 hours of injury. Patients who comply with early active treatment protocols report significantly reduced pain and a significantly improved range of motion.

Physical modalities alleviate symptoms of pain and muscle spasm. Early in the course of whiplash injuries, heat modalities for 20 to 25 minutes, every 3 to 4 hours, are useful. However, excessive use of heat modalities can actually delay recovery. Later in the course of whiplash injury, usually 2 to 3 days after injury, cold therapy is indicated to decrease muscle spasm and pain. Range of motion exercises followed by isometric strengthening exercises should be initiated early in the therapy of whiplash injuries, even immediately after injury. Patients should be given specific instructions regarding neck exercises and daily activities. Patient education programs regarding exercises, daily activities, body mechanics, and the use of heat and cold modalities, are also helpful. The patient should be encouraged to remain functional in spite of pain or other symptoms. Any increase in pain following exercise should not be seen as a worsening of the injury. Prolonged physiotherapy should be avoided, because it reinforces the sick role for the patient.[81]

Multimodal treatments maximize success rates after cervical whiplash injury.[82] The goals of therapy are to restore normal function and promote early return to work. Physical therapy is used to reduce inappropriate pain behaviors, strengthen neck musculature, and wean patients off use of a soft cervical collar. Occupational therapy is used to facilitate the patient's return to normal functioning in the workplace. Neuropsychological counseling may be helpful for some patients.

Intraarticular Corticosteroid Injection. Intraarticular injection of corticosteroids is not effective therapy for pain in the cervical spine following whiplash injury.[87]

Prognosis

Most patients with whiplash injuries have negative diagnostic studies but improve, although slowly and irregularly. Patients benefit from a program of rest, immobilization, neck exercises, and return to function. At 2-year follow-up, approximately 82% of patients with whiplash injury can expect to be symptom-free. Patients with persistent symptoms are older, have more signs of spondylosis on cervical radiographs, and probably sustained more severe initial injuries. Patients symptomatic at 2-year follow-up initially reported more pain, a greater variety of pain symptoms, had higher rates of pretraumatic headache, and had more rapid onset of postinjury symptoms. Symptomatic and asymptomatic patients were similar with regard to gender, vocation, and psychological variables.[88] Some patients who sustain a whiplash injury never recover completely, probably due to a combination of the severity of the injury, underlying cervical abnormalities, and psychosocial factors.[81]

References

1. Anderson GBJ. The epidemiology of spinal disorders. In Frymoyer JW, ed. The adult spine: principles and practice, 2nd ed. Philadelphia: Lippincott-Raven, 1997;93–141.
2. Loeser JD, Volinn E. Epidemiology of low back pain. Neurosurg Clin North Am 1991;2:713–18.
3. Deyo RA. Conservative therapy for low back pain. JAMA 1983;250(8):1057–62.

4. Hart LG, Deyo RA, Cherkin DC. Physician office visits for low back pain: frequency, clinical evaluation, and treatment patterns from a U.S. national survey. Spine 1995;20:11–19.

5. Deyo RA, Loeser JD, Bigos SJ. Herniated lumbar inter-vertebral disc. Ann Intern Med 1990;112:598–603.

6. Frymoyer JW, Durett CL. The economics of spinal disorders. In: Frymoyer JW, ed. The adult spine: principles and practice, 2nd ed. Philadelphia: Lippincott-Raven, 1997;143–50.

7. Frymoyer JW. Back pain and sciatica. N Engl J Med 1988; 318(5):291–300.

8. Anderson GBJ. Epidemiologic features of chronic low back pain. Lancet 1999;354:581–5.

9. Deyo RA, Tsui-Wu YJ. Descriptive epidemiology of low back pain and its related medical care in the United States. Spine 1987;12:264–8.

10. Deyo RA, Rainville J, Kent DL. What can the history and physical examination tell us about low back pain? JAMA 1992; 268(6):760–5.

11. Weber H. Lumbar disc herniation: a controlled prospective study with ten years of observation. Spine 1983;8(2):131–40.

12. Frymoyer JW, Cats-Baril WL. An overview of the incidences and costs of low back pain. Orthop Clin North Am 1991;22(2):263–71.

13. National Center for Health Statistics. Prevalence of selected impairments. U.S., 1977, series 10, number 132. Hyattsville, MD. DHHS publication (PHS) 81–1562, 1981.

14. Deyo RA, Weinstein JN. Primary care: low back pain. N Engl J Med 2001;344(5):363–70.

15. Wipf JE, Deyo RA. Low back pain. Med Clin North Am 1995; 79(2):231–46.

16. Mixter WJ, Barr JS. Rupture of inter-vertebral disc with involvement of the spinal canal. N Engl J Med 1934;211(5):210–5.

17. Spitzer WO, LeBlanc FE, Dupuis M, et al. Scientific approach to the assessment and management of activity related spinal disorders. A monograph for clinicians. Report of the Quebec Task Force on Spinal Disorders. Spine 1987;12(suppl 1):S1–59.

18. Frymoyer JW, Nachemson A. Natural history of low back disorders. In: Frymoyer JW, ed. In: The adult spine: principles and practice. New York: Raven Press, 1991;1537–50.

19. Modic MT, Ross JS. Magnetic resonance imaging in the evaluation of low back pain. Orthop Clin North Am 1991;22(2):283–301.

20. Deyo RA, Diehl AK. Lumbar spine films in primary care: current use and effects of selective ordering criteria. J Gen Intern Med 1986;1:20–5.

21. Hensinger RN. Spondylolysis and spondylolisthesis in children and adolescents. J Bone Joint Surg 1989;71A(7):1098–107.

22. Bigos S, Bowyer O, Braen G, et al. Acute low back problems in adults. Clinical practice guideline no. 14. Rockville, MD: Agency for Health Care Policy and Research, December 1994. (AHCPR publication no. 95-0642.)

23. Frymoyer JW, Newberg A, Pope MH, Wilder DG, Clements J, MacPherson B. Spine radiographs in patients with low back pain: an epidemiological study in men. J Bone Joint Surg 1984; 66A(7):1048–55.

24. Jensen MC, Brant-Zawadzki MN, Obuchowski N, Modic MT, Malkasian D, Ross JS. Magnetic resonance imaging in people without back pain. N Engl J Med 1994;331(2):69–73.

25. Deyo RA, Diehl AK. Cancer as a cause of back pain: frequency, clinical presentation, and diagnostic strategies. J Gen Intern Med 1988;3:230–8.

26. Garfin SR, Herkowitz HN, Mirkovic S. Spinal stenosis. Inst Course Lect 2000;49:361–74.

27. Hilibrand AS, Rand N. Degenerative lumbar stenosis: diagnosis and management. J Am Acad Orthop Surg 1999;7:239–49.

28. Atlas SJ, Keller RB, Robson D, Deyo RA, Singer DE. Surgical and nonsurgical management of lumbar spinal stenosis: four-year outcomes from the Maine Lumbar Spine Study. Spine 2000;25(5):556–62.

29. McCowin PR, Borenstein D, Wiesel SW. The current approach to the medical diagnosis of low back pain. Orthop Clin North Am 1991;22(2):315–25.

30. Barth RW, Lane JM. Osteoporosis. Orthop Clin North Am 1988; 19(4):845–58.

31. Bates DW, Reuler JB. Back pain and epidural spinal cord compression. J Gen Intern Med 1988;3:191–7.

32. Joines JD, McNutt RA, Carey TS, Deyo RA, Rouhani R. Finding cancer in primary care outpatients with low back pain: a comparison of diagnostic strategies. J Gen Intern Med 2001; 16(1):14–23.

33. Perrin RG. Symptomatic spinal metastases. Am Fam Physician 1989;39(5):165–72.

34. Jackson RP. The facet syndrome: myth or reality? Clin Orthop 1992;279:110–21.

35. Carette S, Marcoux S, Truchon R, et al. A controlled trial of corticosteroid injections into facet joints for chronic low back pain. N Engl J Med 1991;325(14):1002–7.

36. Lilius G, Laasonen EM, Myllynen P, Harilainen A, Gronlund G. Lumbar facet joint syndrome: a randomized clinical trial. J Bone Joint Surg 1989;71B(4):681–4.

37. Revel M, Poiraudeau S, Auleley GR, et al. Capacity of the clinical picture to characterize low back pain relieved by facet joint anesthesia. Proposed criteria to identify patients with painful facet joints. Spine 1998;23(18):1972–7.

38. Nelemans PJ, deBie RA, deVet HC, Sturmans F. Injection therapy for subacute and chronic benign low back pain. Spine 2001;26(5):501–15.

39. Gran JT. An epidemiological survey of the signs and symptoms of ankylosing spondylitis. Clin Rheumatol 1985;4:161–9.

40. Frymoyer JW, Rosen JC, Clements J, Pope MH. Psychologic factors in low back pain disability. Clin Orthop 1985;195:178–84.

41. Wheeler AH. Diagnosis and management of low back pain and sciatica. Am Fam Physician 1995;52(5):1333–41.

42. Waddell G, Feder G, Lewis M. Systematic reviews of bedrest and advice to stay active for acute low back pain. Br J Gen Pract 1997;47:647–52.

43. Malmivaara A, Hakkinen U, Aro T et al. The treatment of acute low back pain—bedrest, exercises, or ordinary activity? N Engl J Med 1995;332:351–5.

44. van Tulder MW, Scholten RJ, Koes BW, Deyo RA. Nonsteroidal anti-inflammatory drugs for low back pain: a systematic review with the framework of the Cochrane Collaboration Back Review Group. Spine 2000;25(19):2501–13.

45. Beurskens AJ, de Vet HC, Koke AJ, et al. Efficacy of traction for nonspecific low back pain: 12-week and 16-month results of a randomized clinical trial. Spine 1997;22:2756–62.

46. Deyo RA, Walsh NE, Martin DC, Schoenfeld LS, Ramamurthy S. A controlled trial of transcutaneous electrical nerve stimulation (TENS) and exercise for chronic low back pain. N Engl J Med 1990;322(23):1627–34.

47. van Tulder M, Malmivaara A, Esmail R, Koes B. Exercise therapy for low back pain: a systematic review with the framework of the Cochrane Collaboration Back Review Group. Spine 2000;25(21):2784–96.

48. Cherkin DC, Deyo RA, Battie M, Street J, Barlow W. A comparison of physical therapy, chiropractic manipulation, and provision of an educational booklet for the treatment of patients with low back pain. N Engl J Med 1998;339:1021–9.

49. Anderson GBJ, Lucente T, Davis AM, Kappler RE, Lipton JA, Leurgans S. A comparison of osteopathic spinal manipulation with standard care for patients with low back pain. N Engl J Med 1999;341:1426–31.

50. van Tulder MW, Esmail R, Bombardier C, Koes BW. Back

schools for nonspecific low back pain (Cochrane Reivew). In: The Cochrane Library; issue 3. Oxford: Update Software, 1999.

51. van Tulder MW, Cherkin DC, Berman B, Lao L, Koes BW. The effectiveness of acupuncture in the management of acute and chronic low back pain. Spine 1999;24(11):1113–23.

52. Carette S, Leclaire R, Marcoux S. Epidural corticosteroid injections for sciatica due to herniated nucleus pulposus. N Engl J Med 1997;336:1634–40.

53. Cherkin DC, Deyo RA, Loeser JD, Bush T, Waddell G. An international comparison of back surgery rates. Spine 1994; 19(11):1201–6.

54. Taylor VM, Deyo RA, Cherkin DC, Kreuter W. Low back pain hospitalization: recent U.S. trends and regional variations. Spine 1994;19(11):1207–13.

55. Hurme M, Alaranta H. Factors predicting the results of surgery for lumbar inter-vertebral disc herniation. Spine 1987;12(9): 933–8.

56. Gibson JNA, Grant IC, Waddell G. The Cochrane review of surgery for lumbar disc prolapse and degenerative lumbar spondylosis. Spine 1999;24(17):1820–32.

57. Abramovitz JN, Neff SR. Lumbar disc surgery: results of the prospective lumbar discectomy study. Neurosurgery 1991;29(2): 301–8.

58. Hoffman RM, Wheeler KJ, Deyo RA. Surgery for herniated lumbar discs: a literature synthesis. J Gen Intern Med 1993;8: 487–96.

59. Atlas SJ, Chang Y, Kamann E, Keller RB, Deyo RA, Singer DE. Long-term disability and return to work among patients who have a herniated disc: the effect of disability compensation. J Bone Joint Surg 2000;82A(1):4–15.

60. Chatterjee S, Foy PM, Findaly GF. Report of a controlled clinical trial comparing automated percutaneous lumbar discectomy and microdiscectomy in the treatment of contained lumbar disc herniation. Spine 1995;20:734–8.

61. Revel M, Payan C, Vallee C, et al. Automated percutaneous lumbar discectomy vs. chemonucleolysis in the treatment of sciatica. Spine 1993;18(1):1–7.

62. Hermantin FU, Peters T, Quartararo L, Kambin P. A prospective, randomized study comparing the results of open discectomy with those of video-assisted arthroscopic microdiscectomy. J Bone Joint Surg 1999;81A:958–65.

63. Deyo RA, Cherkin DC, Loeser JD, Bigos SJ, Ciol MA. Morbidity and mortality in association with operations on the lumbar spine: the influence of age, diagnosis, and procedure. J Bone Joint Surg 1992;74A(4):536–43.

64. Turner JA, Denny MC. Do antidepressant medications relieve chronic low back pain? J Fam Pract 1993;37(6):545–53.

65. Atkinson JH, Slater MA, Wahlgren DR, et al. Pain 1999;83: 137–45.

66. Lahad A, Malter AD, Berg AO, Deyo RA. The effectiveness of four interventions for the prevention of low back pain. JAMA 1994;272(16):1286–91.

67. Von Poppel MN, Koes BW, van der Ploeg T, Smid T, Bouter LM. Lumbar supports and education for the prevention of low back pain in industry. JAMA 1998;279:1789–94.

68. Daltroy LH, Iversen MD, Larson MG, et al. A controlled trial of an educational program to prevent low back injuries. N Engl J Med 1997;337:322–8.

69. Loisel P, Abenhaim L, Durand P, et al. A population-based, randomized clinical trial on back pain management. Spine 1997;22(24):2911–18.

70. Kelsey JL, Githens PB, Walter SD, et al. An epidemiological study of acute prolapsed cervical intervertebral disc. J Bone Joint Surg 1984;66A:907–14.

71. Clark CR. Degenerative conditions of the spine. In: Frymoyer JW, ed. The adult spine: principles and practice. New York: Raven Press, 1991;1145–64.

72. Lestini WF, Wiesel SW. The pathogenesis of cervical spondylosis. Clin Orthop 1989;239:69–93.

73. Jahnke RW, Hart BL. Cervical stenosis, spondylosis, and herniated disc disease. Radiol Clin North Am 1991;29(4):777–91.

74. Russell EJ. Cervical disc disease. Radiology 1990;177(2): 313–25.

75. Dillin W, Booth R, Cuckler J, Balderston R, Simeone F, Rothman R. Cervical radiculopathy: a review. Spine 1986;11(10): 988–91.

76. Murphy MJ, Lieponis JV. Non-operative treatment of cervical spine pain. In: Sherk HH, ed. The cervical spine. Philadelphia: Lippincott, 1989;670–7.

77. Sampath P, Bendebba M, Davis JD, Ducker TB. Outcome of patients treated for cervical myelopathy. Spine 2000;25(6): 670–6.

78. La Rocca H. Cervical spondylotic myelopathy: natural history. Spine 1988;13(7):854–5.

79. White AA 3rd, Panjabi MM. Biomechanical considerations in the surgical management of cervical spondylotic myelopathy. Spine 1988;13(7):856–69.

80. Hirsch SA, Hirsch PJ, Hiramoto H, Weiss A. Whiplash syndrome: fact or fiction? Orthop Clin North Am 1988;19(4):791–5.

81. Carette S. Whiplash injury and chronic neck pain. N Engl J Med 1994;330(15):1083–4.

82. Eck JC, Hodges SD, Humphreys SC. Whiplash: a review of a commonly misunderstood injury. Am J Med 2001;110(8):651–6.

83. Bogduk N, Teasell R. Whiplash: the evidence for an organic etiology. Arch Neurol 2000;57(4):590–1.

84. Borchgrevink G, Smevik O, Haave I, et al. MRI of cerebrum and spinal column within 2 days after whiplash neck sprain injury. Injury 1997;28:331–5.

85. Borchgrevink GE, Kaasa A, McDonagh D, et al. Acute treatment of whiplash neck sprain injuries. Spine 1998;23:25–31.

86. Rosenfeld M, Gunnarsson R, Borenstein P. Early intervention in whiplash-associated disorders. A comparison of two treatment protocols. Spine 2000;25:1782–7.

87. Barnsley L, Lord SM, Wallis BJ, Bogduk N. Lack of effect of intraarticular corticosteroids for chronic pain in the cervical zygapophyseal joints. N Engl J Med 1994;330(15):1047–50.

88. Radanov BP, Sturzenegger M, DiStefano G. Long-term outcome after whiplash injury: a 2-year follow-up considering features of injury mechanism and somatic, radiologic, and psychosocial findings. Medicine 1995;74(5):281–97.

110
Disorders of the Upper Extremity

Ted C. Schaffer

Because of the functional importance of the upper extremity to human activity, patients with injuries in this region frequently require diagnostic and therapeutic assistance from the family physician. A working knowledge of basic anatomy is helpful for establishing a differential diagnosis for upper extremity complaints. This chapter discusses common disorders in this region, but there are many unusual problems that may also present in an office situation.

Clavicle

The clavicle is the connecting strut that links the arm and shoulder with the axial skeleton. The clavicle is anchored medially by the sternoclavicular and costoclavicular ligaments, while the acromioclavicular and coracoclavicular ligaments anchor it to the scapula. A thorough examination of any shoulder injury should include palpation of the clavicle and evaluation of the acromioclavicular (AC) and the sternoclavicular (SC) joint motion.

Clavicular Fractures

Fractures of the clavicle are often due to a direct blow on the shoulder or occasionally to a fall on an outstretched arm.[1] They account for 5% of all fractures. Eighty percent of clavicular fractures occur in the middle third of the clavicle, especially at the junction of the middle and distal thirds.[2] Even when significant displacement or angulation is present, these fractures heal well with minimal intervention. A figure-of-eight sling or commercial clavicular strap, worn for 3 to 4 weeks by children and 6 weeks by an adult, provides effective immobilization and allows bony union.[1] The patient is advised that a permanent bump may become noticeable at the site of callus formation. Unless there is initial neurovascular injury, operative intervention or reduction is almost never required for fractures in the middle of the clavicle. Fractures of the distal third

(15% of clavicular fractures) sometimes require surgery. Nondisplaced fractures that do not involve the AC joint heal without difficulty using the treatment outlined above. When a displaced or intraarticular fracture causes persistent pain, resection of the distal clavicle may be needed to alleviate discomfort. Fractures of the medial head of the clavicle (5% of fractures) or posterior dislocations at the sternoclavicular joint are fortunately rare. These injuries, caused by a direct blow to that region, may create a medical emergency by compressing the great vessels or compromising the airway. Immediate elevation of the impacted segment and urgent cardiothoracic or orthopedic consultation are recommended.

AC Joint Dislocations

Dislocations of the AC joint result from a direct fall onto the anterior shoulder. Management of this condition is determined by the extent of the dislocation. Specific treatment for this problem is covered in Chapter 52.

AC Joint Arthritis

With advancing age, there is an increased risk of AC joint arthritis, which may be interpreted as shoulder pain. Careful questioning frequently reveals a prior injury such as a grade I or II AC joint dislocation. Another potential source of injury is with extensive weight lifting. Degeneration of the cartilaginous meniscus may contribute to loss of AC joint integrity. On physical examination the patient is point tender over the AC joint. Forward flexion of the arm to 90 degrees followed by adduction of the shoulder, so the hand touches the contralateral shoulder (the crossed arm adduction test) compresses the AC joint and therefore reproduces the pain.

Initial treatment of AC joint arthritis includes rest, ice, and nonsteroidal antiinflammatory drugs (NSAIDs). A corticosteroid injection into the AC joint using an anterior and superior approach may provide some benefit.[3] For cases unresponsive to conservative management, resection of the distal clavicle can alleviate persistent pain.

Scapula

Isolated injuries to the scapula are rare, but occasionally a direct blow over the involved area results in a fracture.[4] Because of the high impact involved, scapular fractures are frequently associated with other thoracic injuries such as rib fractures and pneumothorax. Treatment for fractures of the body of the scapula include immobilization with a sling until subsidence of pain within 2 to 4 weeks, followed by progressive exercises. If the acromion or glenoid is fractured, orthopedic referral is necessary because of potential implications to shoulder mobility and function.[4]

Shoulder

As the pivotal connection between the upper extremity and the axial skeleton, the shoulder is a frequent source of musculoskeletal problems. Its great range of motion is available only at some compromise to bony stability. Most shoulder stability is provided by the periarticular soft tissues. A careful physical examination attempts to identify which components are contributing to a specific problem. Disorders extrinsic to the shoulder may also cause referred pain to this area. An evaluation of the cervical spine should be included for any problem presenting as shoulder pain.

Functionally, the shoulder is composed of four joints: sternoclavicular, acromioclavicular, glenohumeral, and scapulothoracic articulation. The major joint is the glenohumeral joint, in which the humeral head is three times larger than the glenoid socket. A fibrocartilaginous glenoid labrum provides depth to the socket and adds stability. During overhead motion of the arm the humeral head is maintained in the socket by the four muscles of the rotator cuff. Originating from the scapula, these muscles maintain fixation of the humeral head and, based on their humeral insertion, assist in various arm motions. The supraspinatus assists in abduction and forward flexion, the infraspinatus and teres minor create external rotation, and the subscapularis causes internal rotation. Also vital for proper shoulder motion are the scapulothoracic muscles (rhomboid, trapezius, serratus anterior) and the deltoid.[5]

Traumatic Dislocation of the Shoulder

Anterior Dislocation

The major traumatic injury to the shoulder is dislocation of the humerus from the glenohumeral joint. About 95% of such dislocations are anterior,[6] caused by resisted force to the arm when the shoulder is abducted and externally rotated. Examination of this injury reveals a squaring of the shoulder, loss of the roundness of the deltoid muscle, prominence of the acromial edge, and an anterior mass, which is the humeral head. The arm is held in slight external rotation and abduction. Before reduction is attempted, a neurovascular examination assesses function of the anterior axillary nerve, which

can be demonstrated as absent sensation over the deltoid region and loss of deltoid contraction. This injury, present with up to 30% of dislocations, is usually a transient neuropraxia that requires several weeks for neurologic recovery.

If neurologic evaluation of the dislocation reveals no other abnormality, immediate reduction is acceptable. A number of maneuvers have been described to relocate the shoulder.[4] Initial attempts emphasize gentle longitudinal traction on the arm while passive abduction and external rotation is performed. If there has been delay since the dislocation, narcotic analgesia is usually required to overcome muscle spasm. Most important with any maneuver is the caution that excessive torquing of the humerus must be avoided, as it may lead to brachial plexus injury or humeral fracture.

After relocation and repeat neurovascular evaluation, the patient is placed in a sling for a period of immobilization. A rehabilitation program is then instituted to strengthen the supportive musculature, restore motion, and prevent recurrent dislocation. Young patients, especially those under age 20, are at increased risk of recurrence (75–95%)[7] and require 2 to 3 weeks of immobilization before rehabilitation. For adolescents and young adults, failure to undergo and continue a satisfactory rehabilitation program is a frequent cause of recurrent dislocations. A shoulder stabilization procedure is often necessary for recurrent dislocators. In those over age 50, the risk of recurrent dislocation is much less (10%), but the increased risk of adhesive capsulitis and frozen shoulder requires that early shoulder motion be emphasized.[8] In this population an exercise program should be instituted after only 1 week of immobilization. Occasionally, especially in the elderly, there is an associated avulsion fracture of the greater tuberosity.

Subluxation

A more subtle problem is transient subluxation of the humerus, where the humeral head comes partially out of the anterior glenoid rim but then spontaneously reduces. Roentgenographic findings are negative, but the patient describes a transient "dead arm" feeling for several minutes after the initial injury. Later there may be persistent pain in the posterior shoulder due to a tear in the glenoid labrum. On physical examination a positive apprehension sign is noted, with pain when the shoulder is passively placed in abduction and externally rotated. A tear in the glenoid labrum may be a reason for chronic instability of the shoulder.

Those who experience a subluxation should undergo an aggressive rehabilitation program to prevent progression to dislocation. The advent of shoulder arthroscopy has improved the evaluation of patients with this problem.

Posterior Dislocation

Posterior dislocations comprise only 3% of shoulder dislocations but are missed on initial roentgenograms as often as 60% to 80% of the time.[5] They should be particularly suspected if there is a history of seizures, alcohol use, or electrical injury. On physical examination the arm is held in internal rotation, rather than the external rotation of anterior dislocation. Orthopedic consultation should be obtained if this injury is suspected.

Periarticular Shoulder Problems

Most shoulder problems involve the soft tissue periarticular shoulder structures rather than the glenohumeral joint. Because these supporting structures are vital to shoulder stability, a small injury to one component may cause significant problems in the motion and function of the shoulder. Classification is made difficult by the frequent overlap of these problems. At times one of the following specific periarticular shoulder problems is identified.

Rotator Cuff Injuries

Problems associated with the rotator cuff are the most frequent causes of shoulder problems. Impingement occurs chiefly in the supraspinatus as it courses underneath the acromion and coracoacromial ligament. Although this injury is most common in young athletes who engage in throwing or racquet sports, impingement may occur in anyone involved with overhead work or repetitive upper extremity motion. Evaluation of impingement syndromes is discussed in Chapter 52.

As a result of chronic impingement, the rotator cuff may tear. Cuff tears are more common in middle-aged or elderly individuals, often due to a hypovascular supply of the supraspinatus tendon as it inserts on the humerus.[9] One hallmark of cuff tears is continuous pain, especially at night, which may radiate down the lateral humerus. Examination of the patient with a rotator cuff injury reveals painful or limited active abduction (between 60 and 120 degrees), where the cuff comes in greatest contact with the overlying acromial arch.[9] With a significant cuff tear, the patient is frequently unable to hold the arm in 90 degrees of abduction. Atrophy may develop in the supraspinatus or infraspinatus muscles of the scapula. If a cuff tear is suspected, orthopedic referral with arthroscopy or magnetic resonance imaging (MRI) is indicated to delineate potential surgical cases. With any cuff injury an extensive rehabilitation program of 3 to 6 months is needed to gain full motion and strength.

Subacromial Bursitis

The subacromial bursa separates the deltoid muscle from the underlying rotator cuff. Irritation of adjacent structures, most commonly impingement of the rotator cuff, results in inflammatory bursitis. Often there is a history of overuse or trauma followed by pain and limited active motion. Aspiration of excessive bursal fluid followed by corticosteroid injection using a subacromial lateral or posterior approach can provide dramatic relief of this problem.[3] Adequate volume of injection [5 to 10 cc lidocaine (Xylocaine) plus corticosteroid] should be used to optimize injection results.

Calcific tendonitis, usually within the supraspinatus insertion, may cause an acute inflammatory reaction of the overlying subacromial bursa. Roentgenograms demonstrate a calcific deposit superior and lateral to the humerus. The severe pain can be relieved by needle aspiration of the calcific mass along with a lidocaine and corticosteroid injection of the bursa. Occasionally surgical excision of the calcific deposition is required.[10]

Bicipital Tendonitis and Rupture

The long head of the biceps tendon, which is palpable in the bicipital groove, may be irritated as it courses through the glenohumeral joint and below the supraspinatus tendon to its attachment at the superior sulcus of the glenoid. Isolated pain over the long head of the biceps tendon suggests this problem, although usually there is more diffuse tenderness involving the entire subacromial region. The short head of the biceps tendon attaches to the coracoid process and is rarely involved in inflammatory problems of the shoulder. In most cases rupture of the long head of the biceps tendon occurs as a result of advanced impingement in middle-aged or elderly patients. There is a sudden pop associated with a heavy isometric flexion of the arm such as lifting a heavy object with that arm. The patient experiences mild discomfort with ecchymosis in the upper arm and a palpable bulge of the biceps muscle mass. Because the short head remains intact, treatment is symptomatic as little functional loss occurs.[11] Surgical repair is a rare consideration. Rupture of the distal insertion of the biceps tendon can also occur, with pain in the antecubital region. In contrast to proximal long head tear, this injury does warrant surgical repair.[11]

Glenohumeral Disorders

As a non–weight-bearing area, the true glenohumeral joint is subject to less mechanical stress than the lower extremity. When arthritic changes occur, there may have been a prior local injury. Inflammatory arthritis, with erosive changes of the glenohumeral joint and joint effusion, may occur, especially with severe rheumatoid arthritis.[12] Treatment for any degenerative arthritis is primarily aimed at relief of pain and inflammation. Surgical intervention with joint replacement is possible, but functional results are not as satisfactory as with knee and hip joint replacement, and the major goal should be relief of pain.

Adhesive Capsulitis

A poorly understood entity, adhesive capsulitis (also termed frozen shoulder or periarthritis) is characterized by a progressive, painful restriction of shoulder motion. A primary frozen shoulder has no apparent initiating event, is more common in the nondominant shoulder of women ages 40 to 60, and is bilateral in 20% of cases.[13] When there is a secondary cause of shoulder stiffness, such as immobilization, cuff injury, or trauma, the prognosis may not be as good, with permanent loss of shoulder motion. Initial treatment for either kind includes NSAIDs, joint injection, and an aggressive physical therapy program. For refractory cases other management options include manipulation under anesthesia or shoulder arthroscopy to lyse adhesions and enhance shoulder motion.[14]

Osteonecrosis

Although less common than osteonecrosis (avascular necrosis) of the femoral head, osteonecrosis of the humeral head may be caused by a number of illnesses such as alcoholism, sickle cell disease, systemic lupus erythematosus, and long-term steroid use.[15] Bone scan or MRI may be used for early diagnosis, as radiographs do not show subchondral collapse

Fig. 110.1. This impacted humeral fracture in an elderly women is neither displaced nor severely angulated. It was successfully managed with an arm sling for a week followed by range-of-motion exercises and a course of physical therapy.

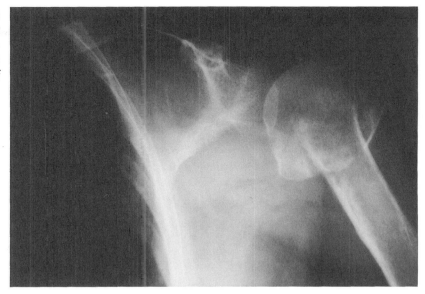

and humeral head flattening until later in the disorder. Treatment includes rest, analgesics, physical therapy for motion, and in severe cases joint replacement.

Humerus

Proximal humeral fractures occur in elderly patients who fall on an outstretched arm, with the fracture line at the surgical neck of the humerus. Although these fractures are frequently impacted, 80% of proximal humeral fractures are nondisplaced.[4] Because brachial plexus injury is possible, neurovascular examination is important with special attention to the axillary nerve. If there is less than 1 cm displacement and less than 45 degrees angulation, treatment is nonoperative (Fig. 110.1). A shoulder immobilizer is provided for 1 to 2 weeks, after which a sling is worn for another 2 weeks.[16] The major complication of these fractures in the elderly is loss of joint mobility, and an early exercise program beginning during the second week is important to maximize shoulder function. Even with rehabilitation some loss of shoulder abduction can be expected.

When a fracture involves the greater or lesser tuberosity or is associated with a humeral head dislocation, there is greater risk of long-term sequelae due to rotator cuff malfunction, and orthopedic consultation should be obtained. With trauma to the humeral shaft, which occurs in young active patients, the integrity of the adjacent radial nerve should be tested.

Elbow

Fractures of the Radial Head

One common uncomplicated elbow injury is a fracture of the proximal radial head. The history of a fall on an outstretched hand accompanies a patient who is reluctant to pronate the hand or to flex the elbow beyond 90 degrees.[17] Radiologic examination of the radial head, especially on the lateral film, is important when the patient is unable to move the elbow

through a complete range of motion. The only roentgenographic evidence for fracture may be a posterior fat pad sign, which occurs when blood that has entered the joint space displaces the fat pad posteriorly (Fig. 110.2).

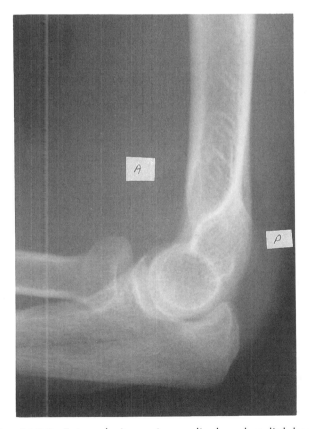

Fig. 110.2. Fat pad signs. A nondisplaced radial head fracture with both a posterior (P) and a prominent anterior (A) fat pad evident on this lateral view. The posterior fat pad is indicative of blood in the joint space from an occult fracture, displacing the fat from the joint space.

Management of a nondisplaced radial head fracture emphasizes pain relief and, in adults, early mobilization. A sling and posterior elbow splint are worn for 1 to 2 weeks, after which range of motion (ROM) exercises are begun while the protective sling is worn for another week.[16] Follow-up of the patient is important for this seemingly trivial problem, as it may take several months for the patient to regain full elbow motion. If displacement of the head or severe angulation has occurred in a child, operative repair may be necessary because the radial head is necessary to provide adequate lengthening of the radius. In adults with radial head displacement or comminution, excision of the radial head is possible to permit adequate pain-free motion at the elbow.

Epicondylitis

Epicondylitis, a frequent elbow complaint, is caused by inflammation of the lateral or medial epicondyle. Although its diagnosis and treatment are covered in Chapter 52, the clinician must understand that epicondylitis is not always related to sports participation. Obtaining an accurate history usually identifies a causative action related to the patient's vocational or recreational activities.

Radial Head Subluxation

The most common elbow complaint in children, known as nursemaid's elbow, occurs when sudden longitudinal traction on the wrist or arm causes the annular ligament to become partially entrapped in the radiohumeral joint. The child younger than 4 years old presents with a painful elbow held in pronation. Gentle rotation of the hand to a supinated position while pressure is applied over the radial head results in a palpable "click" as the radial head is reduced.[18] There is immediate pain relief with full use of the elbow. Radiographs are not necessary; positioning for the radiograph may actually cause reduction of the subluxation. To prevent recurrence, parents and caregivers should be educated about the injury mechanism for this benign entity.

Olecranon Bursitis

Either a single traumatic blow to the elbow or repetitive microtrauma such as leaning on the elbow may result in swelling over the posterior aspect of the elbow. When there is marked inflammation, a septic bursitis is suspected. Treatment for a septic bursitis includes surgical drainage of the bursal fluid and intravenous antibiotics. *Staphylococcus aureus* is the most common infecting organism. For a simple noninfected bursitis, aspiration of clear, straw-colored fluid can be followed by a tight pressure dressing applied to prevent fluid reaccumulation.[19] When recurrent bursitis results in a thickened fibrotic mass, the only recourse may be surgical excision of the entire bursa.

Wrist

Fractures of the Distal Radius

Because of the close proximity to the radiocarpal joint, fractures of the distal radius are considered wrist injuries. In chil-

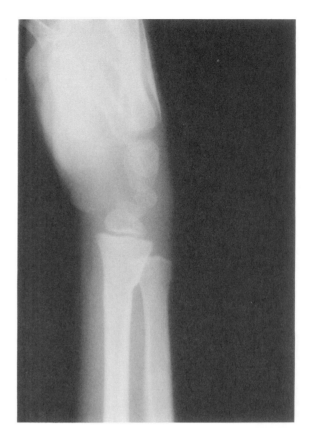

Fig. 110.3. Buckle (torus) fracture. A small cortical disruption is visible in the metaphysis of the distal radius.

dren the most common injury is the buckle, or torus, fracture, which occurs with a fall onto an outstretched hand. Radiographic findings may be subtle, with only a slight cortical disruption of the extraarticular radius seen on the lateral film (Fig. 110.3). Treatment is a short arm cast for 3 weeks; functional return is excellent.[20]

When a child presents with a "sprained wrist," evaluation must be done carefully, as the growth plates are weaker than ligaments during this period of rapid growth. With normal roentgenograms and tenderness over the epiphyseal plate, a Salter I fracture is presumed, and a short arm cast is applied for 2 to 3 weeks.[20]

In adults the most common radial fracture is a Colles' fracture, which occurs when patients over age 50 fall onto an outstretched hand. The "silver fork" deformity is caused by dorsal displacement of the distal fragment. The ulnar styloid may also be fractured. Reduction of a Colles' fracture may be attempted, but the physician must be aware of potential complications of this fracture, including median or ulnar nerve compression, damage to the flexor or extensor tendons, and radioulnar joint arthritis.

Nondisplaced distal radial fractures that are nonarticular can usually be treated with cast immobilization for 6 weeks in adults. Low-impact intraarticular nondisplaced fractures in the elderly may also require only cast immobilization, although the patient is advised that some residual arthritis may occur.[16] For other displaced fractures or intraarticular radial fractures in young patients, treatments such as percutaneous pinning or open reduction internal fixation may be required to minimize long-term problems in the joint.

Carpal Fractures

Sixty percent of carpal bone fractures involve the scaphoid (or carpal navicular) bone. The injury mechanism is a fall on an outstretched hand, usually in an adolescent or young adult. The location of the fracture determines the likelihood of complications. Distal (5%) and middle (waist) scaphoid fractures (80%) carry a good prognosis for healing, whereas proximal (15%) fractures have an incidence of nonunion or avascular necrosis as high as 30% to 50% due to a poor blood supply.

Although a scaphoid fracture is usually identified on a posteroanterior view with the wrist in ulnar deviation, occasionally the fracture is not evident on the initial films. Patients with a "wrist sprain" who have tenderness over the scaphoid tubercle (palmar hand surface) or pain in the anatomic snuffbox, located between the extensor pollicis brevis and extensor pollicis longus tendons, should be immobilized in a short arm cast or splint for 7 to 10 days, at which time repeat films usually demonstrate the fracture. If tenderness continues but plain films remain negative, a bone scan or tomograms may be needed to confirm a suspected fracture. Because of the high risk of nonunion, scaphoid fractures require prolonged immobilization. Clinical opinion varies regarding use of a long arm cast versus a short arm cast, but in general a short arm cast applied for 8 to 12 weeks is acceptable for uncomplicated nondisplaced middle or distal fractures of the scaphoid.[16] The longer time frame is necessary to allow adequate bone healing and to prevent nonunion or avascular necrosis. For patients with a proximal fracture or for those with a treatment delay, orthopedic consultation may be wise because of the high incidence of long-term sequelae.[21] Any scaphoid fracture with displacement more than 1 mm or angulation more than 20 degrees is regarded as unstable and should also be referred for surgical treatment.

Other fractures of the carpal bones are uncommon and frequently require special radiographic views or tomograms for identification. A meticulous examination of the painful area indicates which carpal bones are likely to be involved. Because serious sequelae are common, including ulnar or median neuropathy and chronic wrist stability, orthopedic intervention is usually needed.

Wrist Instability

Although fractures of the carpal bones are unusual, sprains and other minor traumatic wrist injuries are common. A number of serious wrist injuries and carpal instabilities have been described as physicians have gained greater appreciation for the complex interactions of other ligaments and multiple articulations within the carpal complex. Roentgenography may be helpful for delineating certain problems, such as lunate and perilunate dislocations and scapholunate dissociations.[10] More sophisticated procedures, such as arthrography or MRI, may be required to identify other complex problems. Because there may be difficulty distinguishing a serious wrist injury from a minor sprain, the physician should be suspicious of wrist injuries that fail to resolve within a 3- to 4-week period.

In these circumstances an orthopedic consultation is wise to ensure that no significant injury has been overlooked.

TFCC Injuries

The triangulofibrocartilage complex (TFCC) is a small meniscus located distal to the ulna. This tissue serves to absorb impact to forces on the ulnar aspect of the wrist. Injuries can be acute, due to a sudden impact, or chronic, due to repetitive loading such as gymnastics. As with carpal instability, the physician should be suspicious of TFCC injuries when ulnar wrist pain does not respond to 3 to 4 weeks of splinting. Orthopedic consultation, frequently with MRI, may be required to identify the specific problem.[22]

De Quervain's Tenosynovitis

A stenosing tendonitis, de Quervain's tenosynovitis, occurs in the first extensor compartment of the wrist, comprising the abductor pollicis longus and extensor pollicis brevis. As these tendons cross the radial styloid, thickness and swelling may occur. The patient complains of radial wrist pain, and there is often an occupational or vocational history of repetitive hand motion, such as knitting or sewing.

The diagnosis is confirmed by the Finkelstein test, as follows: After passive adduction of the thumb into the palm, ulnar deviation of the wrist elicits a sharp pain that reproduces the patient's symptoms. Initial treatment should include a corticosteroid injection into the tendon sheath. Other treatment options include rest, antiinflammatory medications, and a thumb spica splint. On occasion, surgical release of the tendon sheath is required for symptomatic relief.[23]

Intersection Syndrome

Inflammation can also occur at the crossover of the first and second extensor compartments of the wrist, located 4 to 8 cm proximal to the distal radius.[24] Pain and tenderness are noted in this region, and the problem occurs as an overuse syndrome from repeated wrist extension. This anatomy should be distinguished from the more distal de Quervain's tenosynovitis. Initial treatment should include a thumb spica splint and antiinflammatory medications. Corticosteroid injection is useful for those who do not respond to splinting.[25] This is a contrast to de Quervain's tenosynovitis where injection is the preferred initial treatment.

Carpal Tunnel Syndrome

The most common compression neuropathy of the upper extremity, carpal tunnel syndrome, is discussed in the Chapter 67.

Hand

Metacarpal Fractures

The most common hand fracture is a "boxer's fracture" caused by impaction force and resulting in a fracture of the distal neck of the fifth metacarpal. Because of the mobility of the fourth and fifth metacarpals, volar angulation of the distal fragment of less then 40 degrees is acceptable without the need for bone manipulation.[25]

Whereas angulation is acceptable, a rotation injury around the longitudinal axis of any metacarpal necessitates orthopedic referral for surgical pinning. For a boxer's fracture with mild angulation, an ulnar gutter or volar splint with the metacarpophalangeal (MCP) joint at 90 degrees is applied for 3 to 6 weeks.[25] Midshaft fractures of the fifth metacarpal may be handled in a similar manner if angulation is less than 20 degrees. Nondisplaced fractures of the second and third metacarpals can be treated with a short arm cast, but careful physical examination must be performed to ensure that there is no rotation or angulation present, as these bone problems necessitate surgical correction. The unusual fracture that involves either the articular surface of the metacarpal base or metacarpal head mandates orthopedic consultation because of the potential for later arthritic complications.[16]

Fractures of the thumb metacarpal require surgical correction if they are intraarticular, such as Bennett's fracture (with proximal dislocation of the metacarpal) or Rolando's fracture (a comminuted intraarticular fracture of the metacarpal base). These injuries are less common than the extraarticular metacarpal fracture of the thumb, which if not angulated more than 30 degrees may be treated with a short arm thumb splint cast with the thumb in a flexed position.[26]

Infections

Palmar Hand Infections

Infections of the palmar hand surface are potential disasters. Bacteria can get underneath the dermal layer and then track along the flexor tendon sheaths. In this high glucose medium, the infection can spread rapidly and damage the flexor tendons with subsequent permanent hand impairment. Pain, tenderness, or swelling of the palmar surface suggests a deep hand infection, as does a recent history of minor trauma. Evidence of a palmar space infection mandates tetanus prophylaxis and intravenous antibiotic treatment with early orthopedic consultation for possible drainage.[27] Many physicians believe that animal bites to the palmar region of the hand warrant prophylactic antibiotic treatment to prevent complications (see Chapter 47).

Dorsal Hand Infections

Infections of the dorsal hand may appear worse than palmar infections because of the dramatic swelling within the loose connective tissue, but the prognosis is good. Oral antibiotics and outpatient drainage are usually satisfactory. Before treatment, however, the palmar space is inspected to ensure that the dorsal infection is not originating from a deep palmar infection that has ruptured to the dorsal surface.[27] Lacerations near the MCP joints warrant special precautions, especially those of the fourth or fifth metacarpal. The usual history for this injury is an altercation in which the patient has punched another person in the teeth and sustained a human bite, which may extend into the joint space. The patient frequently denies this history on initial questioning. If unrecognized, the subsequent infection may lead to joint destruction. When this injury is suspected, a hand surgeon should be contacted to consider operative debridement. A good rule to remember is that *all* lacerations over the MCP joints are human bites until proved otherwise.

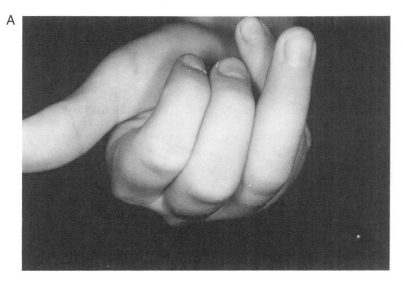
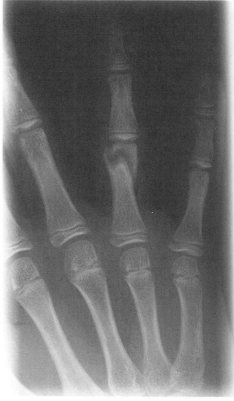

Fig. 110.4. Rotation deformity of the ring finger (A) indicates that surgical fixation is necessary to reduce the fracture. The radiograph (B), with only mild angulation, demonstrates why clinical examination for rotation is necessary for evaluating a finger injury.

Dupuytren's Contracture

Dupuytren's contracture, with thickening of the palmar fascia, results in asymptomatic contractures of the fingers primarily of the MCP joint.[28] The problem often starts with the ring finger and progresses slowly to include other fingers. Although the etiology is unknown, there is a familial tendency with Dupuytren's contracture occurring more frequently in middle-aged men of northern European descent. Pathologically, there is inflammation and subsequent contracture of the palmar aponeurosis, which may progress over years.[28] Although many treatment modalities have been attempted, surgical excision of the contracted region has been the most effective approach. Excision is reserved for those who have some functional hand impairment due to contracture formation.

Finger

Fractures

Distal Tip Fractures

Crush injuries to the tip of the finger cause pain because of the closed space swelling. Even when the fracture is comminuted, the fibrous septa provide stability during bone healing. Protective splinting of the tip for several weeks is usually satisfactory.[29] When fracture fragments are severely displaced, soft tissue interposition may prevent adequate healing unless surgical correction is performed. For any fracture associated with a nail bed injury, the nail bed or matrix must be repaired to minimize aberrant nail growth. Subungual hematomas, with or without an underlying fracture, can be decompressed with an electrocautery device or heated paper clip, creating a hole at the distal tip of the lunula. For any open fracture, such as a nail bed injury or drained subungual hematoma, antibiotic coverage with a cephalosporin is indicated to minimize the risk of osteomyelitis.

Middle and Proximal Phalangeal Fractures

All phalangeal fractures are examined carefully for evidence of angulation (by roentgenography) or rotation (by clinical examination).[26] Angulated or rotated phalangeal fractures are inherently unstable and require orthopedic intervention (Fig. 110.4). Nondisplaced extraarticular fractures of the middle or proximal phalanx can be managed by 1 to 2 weeks of immobilization followed by dynamic splinting with "buddy taping" to an adjacent finger.[16] Large intraarticular fractures involving the middle or proximal phalanx are usually unstable fractures. Small (<25%) avulsion fractures of the volar middle phalangeal base are frequent problems seen in the office that occur with a hyperextension injury (Fig. 110.5). In addition to the fracture is disruption of the distal insertion of the volar plate, a structure that prevents hyperextension of the proximal interphalangeal (PIP) joint. These injuries are managed by 2 to 3 weeks of immobilization with 20 to 30 degrees of flexion at the PIP joint, which allows maximal length of the collateral PIP joint ligaments and permits early finger rehabilitation. A buddy-taping program during activity or sports should continue for an additional 4 to 6 weeks. A gauze pad

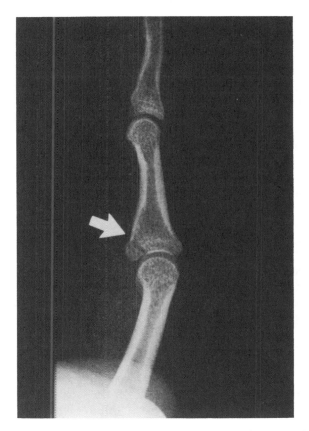

Fig. 110.5. This fracture of the middle phalanx implies that the distal volar plate has been disrupted. A combination of splinting and buddy taping for several weeks is required to allow the volar plate to heal.

should be placed between the fingers in order to prevent skin maceration. Failure of the volar plate to heal properly may result in a swan neck deformity at the PIP joint.

PIP Joint Dislocations

With sudden hyperextension the middle phalanx may dislocate dorsal to the proximal phalanx. This dislocation is easily reduced by gentle traction on the finger followed by flexion of the PIP joint. Because dislocation results in disruption of the distal volar plate, the PIP joint should then be immobilized for 3 to 6 weeks and managed as a volar plate injury as described above.[30] Lateral joint sprains with mild instability (<15 degrees of deviation) can also be managed with flexion splinting and subsequent buddy taping. Treatment of complete lateral dislocations and volar dislocations is more complex and controversial.

Tendon Injuries

Mallet Finger Injuries

Forced flexion of the distal interphalangeal (DIP) joint on an extended finger avulses the extensor tendon as it inserts into the distal phalanx, and the patient cannot extend the distal phalanx. Orthopedic referral is indicated only if there is subluxation of the DIP joint or if there is a large bone fragment involving more than 25% of the articular surface. Usually the roentgenogram demonstrates either no fracture or a small avulsion fragment. This injury is treated by placing the DIP joint in extension for 6 to 8 weeks while the PIP joint is permitted to move freely.[29] A number of commercial or homemade splints are available for application to either the dorsal or volar surface of the DIP joint. Constant prolonged splinting is vital to permit tendon healing. The patient is advised that flexion of the DIP joint even once before adequate repair will result in tendon avulsion and necessitate reinitiation of the entire process. During any splint change, care is exercised to maintain finger extension. Hyperextension of the joint is also avoided, as this position may lead to necrosis of the dorsal skin.

Central Slip Injuries

A laceration or crush of the extensor tendon over the dorsum of the PIP joint or a volar dislocation damages the central portion of the extensor tendon. When this central slip is damaged, subsequent flexion of the PIP joint results in a contracture termed a boutonniere deformity. Tenderness of the central slip region is an injury of this structure until proved otherwise. A dorsal avulsion of the middle phalanx requires orthopedic pinning.[30] A potential central slip injury without fracture is treated by maintaining the PIP joint in extension for 2 to 6 weeks. The stiffness that results from collateral ligament tightening is much easier to treat than is correction of an established boutonniere deformity.

Trigger Fingers

As the flexor tendon courses through the hand, a nodular thickening at the MCP level may prevent free passage of the tendon. The cause is inflammation of the A_1 pulley, the first of five pulleys that guide the flexor tendon into the finger. Although the problem is located at the MCP level, the patient frequently complains of more distal pain at the interphalangeal (IP) joint of the thumb or PIP joint of the finger. During extension of the finger, there is a catching or locking of the PIP joint as the stenosed tendon becomes trapped in the pulley. Initial management is a tendon sheath injection with a small amount of glucocorticoid (e.g., 10 mg triamcinolone) directly into the stenosed area (Fig. 110.6). If the trigger finger persists, surgical release is necessary.[31]

Gamekeeper's Thumb

Damage to the ulnar collateral ligament that occurs with sudden hyperabduction is termed a gamekeeper's or skier's thumb. This ligament is vital for open grasp and pinch action of the hand. Swelling and tenderness of the ulnar side of the MCP joint suggest this injury. A roentgenogram of the thumb is obtained to ensure there is no fracture before the MCP joint is tested. To examine for instability, the MCP joint is stressed with the IP joint of the thumb in both extension and flexion.[16] An unstable joint or a roentgenogram that shows a large avulsion fragment necessitates orthopedic referral for possible surgical exploration. Often the interposition of an adductor aponeurosis between the ends of the torn ligament (termed a Stener lesion) prevents ligament healing unless surgery is performed. Early repair of the ligament, within 1 to 2 weeks, optimizes return of hand function. If there is tenderness but the MCP joint is stable, a thumb spica splint or cast is applied for 2 to 4 weeks and the joint then reassessed for instability.

Infections

Paronychia

A nail bed infection, paronychia is often introduced by minor trauma such as manicuring or nail biting. Redness and swelling occur along the nail folds, and fluctuance is common. Treatment involves a scalpel incision between the nail fold and the nail plate with evacuation of pus; a finger block before incision is optional. The incision is made parallel to the nail plate to avoid damage to the germinal nail matrix. In the unusual event of a subungual abscess, more extensive surgery with partial nail removal is required to drain the abscess. Because an acute paronychia usually involves *Staphylococcus aureus* a short course (5 to 7 days) of an antistaphylococcal antibiotic is often included. Chronic paronychia is often associated with

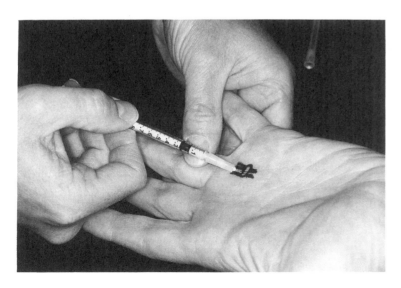

Fig. 110.6. Injection of a trigger finger is performed into the A_1 pulley at the MCP level. The needle can be directed proximally (as shown) or distally.

occupational water exposure, such as by dishwashers or bartenders.[32] The infecting organism is usually *Candida albicans.* Treatment usually includes nail excision.

Felon

Infection of the distal pulp space, or felon, is usually painful because of swelling within a closed space. Minor trauma often provides the nidus for infection. Surgical drainage is required to prevent loss of the entire pulp tissue or to prevent other complications such as osteomyelitis or tenosynovitis. Following a digital block, the felon is drained using one of several surgical techniques.[33] A lateral incision or longitudinal palmar incision is the most common. Incision of the radial side of the index and ulnar side of the thumb and little fingers is avoided to prevent sensory problems in these sensitive areas. Packing material is placed and changed frequently over the next several days, and oral antistaphylococcal antibiotics are administered while the infection resolves.

Tenosynovitis

Infection of a flexor tendon sheath, although an uncommon injury, requires early recognition to prevent serious complications. A position of finger flexion, swelling of the entire finger, and tenderness along the tendon sheath are common findings. The most specific physical finding is severe pain with passive extension of the finger, which leads one strongly to suspect flexor tenosynovitis. In sexually active patients disseminated gonorrhea may also present as tenosynovitis. Emergency orthopedic consultation is suggested for suspected tenosynovitis, as early débridement and aggressive care may allow salvage of the hand, whereas treatment delay of even 24 hours may result in a dramatic loss of finger or hand function.[34]

References

1. Paterson PD, Waters PM. Shoulder injuries in the childhood athlete. Clin Sports Med 2000;19:681–91.
2. Simon RR, Koenigsknecht JJ. Emergency orthopedics: The extremities, 3rd ed. Norwalk, CT: Appleton & Lange, 1995:199–215.
3. Miches WF, Rodriquez RA, Amy E. Joint and soft tissue injections of the upper extremity. Phys Med Rehab Clin North Am 1995;6:823–40.
4. Blake R, Hoffman J. Emergency department evaluation and treatment of the shoulder and humerus. Emerg Med Clin North Am 1999;17:859–786.
5. Woodward TW, Best TM. The painful shoulder: part I. Clinical evaluation. Am Fam Physician 2000;61:3079–88.
6. Greenspan A. Orthopedic radiology: a practical approach, 2nd ed. New York: Gower, 1992;5.1–5.47.
7. Cleeman E, Flatow EL. Shoulder dislocations in the young patient. Orthop Clin North Am 2000;31:217–29.
8. Stayner LR, Cummings J. Should dislocations in patients older than 40 year of age. Orthop Clin North Am 2000;31:231–9.
9. Woodward TW, Best TM. The painful shoulder Part II. Acute and chronic disorders. Am Fam Physician 2000;61:3291–300.
10. Lebrun CM. Common upper extremity injuries. Clin Fam Pract 1999;1 147–84.
11. Carter AM, Erickson SM. Proximal biceps tendon rupture. Phys Sports Med 1999;27:95–101.
12. Klippel JH, ed. Rheumatoid arthritis. In: Primer on the rheumatic diseases, 11th ed. Atlanta: Arthritis Foundation, 1997; 155–61.
13. Harryman DT. Shoulders: frozen and stiff. Instr Course Lect 1993;42:247–57.
14. Sandor R. Adhesive capsulitis: optimal treatment of frozen shoulder. Phys Sports Med 2000;28:23–9.
15. Zuckerman JD, Mirabello SC, Newman D, Gallagher M, Cuomo F. The painful shoulder. Part II. Intrinsic disorders and impingement syndrome. Am Fam Physician 1991;43:497–512.
16. Paras RD. Upper extremity fractures. Clin Fam Pract 2000; 2:637–59.
17. Shapiro MS, Wang JC. Elbow fractures: treating to avoid complications. Physician Sports Med 1995;23:39–50.
18. Thompson GH, Scoles PV. Nursemaid's elbow. In: Behrman RE, Kliegman RM, Jenson HB, eds. Nelson textbook of pediatrics, 16th ed. Philadelphia: WB Saunders, 2000;2092.
19. Simon RR, Koenigskneeht JJ. Soft tissue injuries, dislocations and disorders of the elbow and forearm. In: Emergency orthopedics: The extremities, 4th ed. New York: McGraw-Hill, 2001;253–64.
20. Kocher MS, Waters PM, Michali LJ. Upper extremity injuries in the pediatric athletic. Sports Med 2000;30:117–35.
21. Rettig AC. Management of acute scaphoid fractures. Hand Clinics 2000;16:381–95.
22. Buterbaugh GA, Brown TR, Horn PC. Ulnar-sided wrist pain in athletics. Clin Sports Med 1998;17:567–83.
23. Rettig AC. Elbow, forearm and wrist injuries in the athlete. Sports Med 1998;25:115–30.
24. Hanlon DP, Luellen JR. Intersection syndrome: A case report and review of the literature. J Emerg Med 1999;17:969–71.
25. Petrizzi MJ, Petrizzi MG, Miller A. Making an ulnar gutter splint for a boxer's fracture. Physician Sports Med 1999;27:111–2.
26. Lee S, Jupiter JB. Phalangeal and metacarpal fractures of the hand. Hand Clin 2000;16:323–32.
27. Jebson PL. Deep subfascial space infections. Hand Clin 1998; 14:557–66.
28. Rayan GM. Clinical presentation and types of Dupuytren's disease. Hand Clin 1999;15:87–96.
29. Wang QC, Johnson BA. Fingertip injuries. Am Fam Physician 2001;63:1961–6.
30. Young CC, Raasch WG. Dislocations: diagnosis and treatment. Clin Fam Pract 2000;2:613–35.
31. Moore JS. Flexor tendon entrapment of the digits (trigger finger and trigger thumb). J Occup Enviorn Med 2000;42:526–45.
32. Rockwell PG. Acute and chronic paronychia. Am Fam Physician 2001;63:1113–6.
33. Jebson PJ. Infections of the fingertip. Hand Clin 1998;14: 547–55.
34. Bales SD, Schmidt CC. Pyogenic flexor tenosynovitis. Hand Clin 1998;14:567–78.

111
Disorders of the Lower Extremity

Kenneth M. Bielak and Bradley E. Kocian

The lower extremities facilitate the maintenance of stature and balance, have intimate contact with the ground, and are responsible for movement over that ground. Thus injuries to the lower extremities are more frequent than those to the upper extremities. The bones and muscles of the lower extremity are relatively longer and stronger, and greater forces are required to disrupt the connections between them. This chapter provides basic information on the history, mechanism of injury, and testing procedures necessary to make an accurate diagnosis and formulate a specific management plan for injuries to the lower extremity. The common injuries are described in detail. Reference is made to uncommon and high-impact injuries that should not be missed. Other systemic disorders and sports-related and pediatric injuries are covered in other chapters, though there is some degree of overlap.

Hip and Pelvis

Hip Fractures

Aging is associated with reductions in muscle strength, increased inactivity, and a diminished sense of balance. Moreover, the presence of concomitant medical disorders and their treatments are increased, which are factors that contribute to the increased incidence of falls and fracture of the hip in those 65 years and older (see Chapter 24). Although hip fractures are a common malady of the elderly, anyone subjected to sufficient forces to the hip can be affected. The overall incidence approximates 250,000 hip fractures per year in the United States. In 1996 there were 340,000 hospital admissions for hip fractures in the United States.[1] Hip fractures are associated with more deaths, disability, and medical cost than all other osteoporotic fractures combined. Osteoporosis is the biggest risk factor for hip fracture. Table 111.1 outlines the major risk factors for osteoporotic hip fracture.

The incidence of hip fracture is directly related to the number of risk factors present. In one study women with low bone density and more than five risk factors (Table 111.1)[2] had a hip fracture incidence rate 27 times greater than that of women with fewer than three risk factors and normal bone density. Additionally, geometry (hip axis length) and architecture (Singh grade) further improve determination of hip fracture risk.[3] Simple measurements (reduced thickness of femoral shaft cortex, femoral neck cortex, reduction in an index of tensile trabeculae, and wider trochanteric region) on plain radiographs were as predictive of risk for hip fracture as bone mineral density determinations.[4] Dexa scanning has recently become an important tool in screening for osteoporosis.

The best treatment for osteoporosis is prevention. Preventive measures include hormone replacement therapy, exercise, alendronate, increased calcium intake, and calcitonins (see Chapter 122). Recently, combination therapies of estrogen and alendronate have yielded even greater increases in bone mineral density and are tolerated quite well.[5] Certain facts are important to remember when considering the prescription of preventive measures: Short-term intervention late in the natural course of osteoporosis may have significant effects on the incidence of hip fractures[6]; hip fracture may be associated with reduced muscle strength rather than reduced body mass or fat[7,8]; long-term heavy activity reduces the risk of hip fracture in postmenopausal women[9]; and height appears to be an important independent risk factor for hip fracture among American women and men.[10] Factors that are protective [relative risk (RR) <1] against hip fracture in the elderly are an increase in weight after age 25 and routine walking for exercise.

Fractures of the proximal femur can be classified as femoral neck, intertrochanteric, or subtrochanteric based on anatomic site. Fractures of the femoral neck (cervical or intracapsular) result from an indirect shear force on the angulated femoral neck (Fig. 111.1). They are found more commonly in the elderly and have a high risk for complications, such as avascu-

Table 111.1. Risk Factors for Osteoporotic Hip Fracture

Age >80 years

Family history
Maternal hip fracture

Medical history
Any fracture since age 50
Poor health
Hyperthyroidism
Resting pulse >80 bpm

Current medication use
Anticonvulsants
Benzodiazepines
Caffeine (>2 cups of coffee per day)

Anthropometrics
Current weight less than that at age 25
Height at least 168 cm (5′ 6″) at age 25

Inadequate activity
On feet <4 hours per day
No walking for exercise
Inability to rise from chair without using one's arms

Visual impairment
Lowest quartile of distant depth perception (>2.44 SD)
Lowest quartile of visual contrast perception (<0.7 unit of contrast sensitivity)

lar necrosis. Fractures of the neck of the femur are painful and can be associated with little bruising or swelling. It is important to note that a nondisplaced fracture can be ambulated upon, albeit with some degree of pain. A displaced fracture of the hip causes shortening and external rotation. Extracapsular (intertrochanteric and subtrochanteric) fractures occur with direct trauma to the hip, resulting in immediate pain, inability to ambulate, and generally significant loss of blood. In the elderly, trochanteric fractures have been associated with up to twice the short-term mortality of cervical fractures. In terms of measured bone mineral density (BMD), a relatively low trochanteric BMD or a high femoral neck BMD is asso-ciated with trochanteric hip fracture.[11] Immediate referral for orthopedic surgery is necessary. Treatment options take into account the type and extent of fracture: cervical fractures in the elderly and significant displacements require hip replacement, and extracapsular fractures respond well with repair and internal fixation.

With suspected hip fracture and negative plain radiographs, magnetic resonance imaging (MRI) demonstrated occult femoral and pelvic fractures in 37% and 23% of patients, respectively.[12] Through the use of an immediate MRI in a questionable hip fracture, the prolonged recumbency and inherent costs associated with awaiting a positive bone scan can be avoided.[13] Computed tomography (CT) scan can also be used for the diagnosis of hip fracture that is difficult to see on plain radiographs.

Hip Dislocation

Dislocation of the hip is usually the result of a motor vehicle accident or other severe trauma. Because of the relative strength of the femur in young people, hip dislocations are seen most commonly in young to middle-aged adults. Dislocations occur most commonly in the posterior direction (85–90%) but can also occur in an anterior or central direction.

The type of dislocation is largely determined by the mechanism of injury or the driving force, such as the flexed hip and knee being driven into the dashboard during a motor vehicle accident, forcing the hip to dislocate posteriorly. With a posterior hip dislocation, the physical examination shows a shortened leg that can be internally rotated and adducted. The radiographic examination includes an anteroposterior (AP) view of the pelvis (Fig. 111.2), a cross-table lateral view of the involved hip, and AP and lateral views of the involved femur to the level of the knee. An AP radiograph usually shows the femoral head superior and overlapping the acetabulum with the femur in internal rotation and adduction.[14] Complications of posterior hip dislocations include transient

Fig. 111.1. Femoral neck fracture (intracapsular) with displacement. (Courtesy of A. Allen, M.D., Department of Radiology, University of Tennessee Medical Center.)

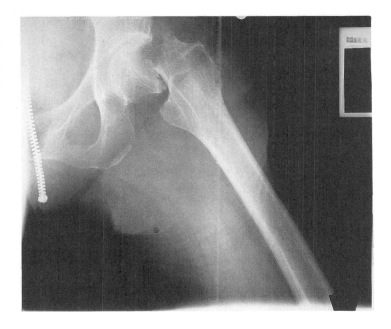

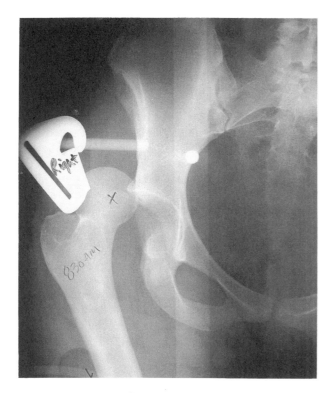

Fig. 111.2. Posterior dislocation of the right hip. Note the internal rotation and adduction of the hip with subsequent loss of the lesser trochanter silhouette. (Courtesy of A. Allen, M.D., Department of Radiology, University of Tennessee Medical Center.)

sciatic neuropathy, avascular necrosis, and periarticular ossification. Orthopedic referral is recommended to decrease the risk of avascular necrosis, which is directly related to the delay in reduction and the patient's age.[15] There may be associated fractures of the pelvis, femur, tibia, patella, and posterior lip of the acetabulum. Because up to 13% of radiographs do not show occult fractures, it is prudent to obtain a CT scan of the hip, if available. However, the CT scan to identify occult fractures is not necessary after reduction of simple posterior hip dislocation because it does not change the treatment plan.[16] In the absence of penetrating trauma, intracapsular gas bubbles on CT are reliable indicators of recent hip dislocation and may be the only objective finding of this injury.[17] MRI can be used for the early detection of osteonecrosis of the femoral head after traumatic hip dislocation or fracture dislocation.[18]

Traumatic anterior dislocation of the hip represents 11% of all hip dislocations and is classified into superior and inferior types. Associated femoral head fractures are common, but acetabular fractures are relatively rare. Whereas inferoanterior hip dislocation is easily recognized on an anteroposterior radiograph of the pelvis, the radiographic appearance of superoanterior hip dislocation is less straightforward. Misinterpretation of a superoanterior hip dislocation can lead to an initial misdiagnosis of posterior hip dislocation, which has implications for the surgical approach and may result in failed closed reduction.[19] The superoanterior dislocation of the femoral head can be distinguished from the posterior dislo-

cation by noting a more lateral orientation to the acetabulum and an externally rotated femur that is not adducted. The lesser trochanter becomes more prominent medially.[20]

Central hip dislocations usually occur with resulting fracture to the iliopubic portion of the acetabulum as a severe lateral blow to the hip drives the femoral head medially. There are usually other skeletal and soft tissue injuries associated with this type of injury.[14]

After closed reduction of a hip dislocation, it is necessary to confirm concentric reduction (the joint space is equidistant on plain radiograph or CT scan). The absence of concentric reduction suggests an interposition of soft tissue in the joint. Early diagnosis and treatment of this serious complication can avoid the poor results of open and deferred treatments.[21]

Pelvic Avulsion Injuries

The bony attachments of the sartorius [anterior superior iliac spine (ASIS)], rectus femoris (anterior inferior iliac spine), and the hamstrings (ischial tuberosity) can be individually avulsed by sudden overloading of the respective muscles (acute muscular contraction against a fixed resistance). The history is typically a sudden onset of extreme pain following sudden, forceful acceleration or deceleration. Localized pain and swelling at the site of injury and increased discomfort with passive stretching and muscle contraction against resistance suggest the diagnosis. Plain radiographs confirm the injury (Fig. 111.3). Subtleties may make the diagnosis obscure, and MRI may be a more sensitive and accurate way to establish the diagnosis. The hamstring avulsion may be espe-

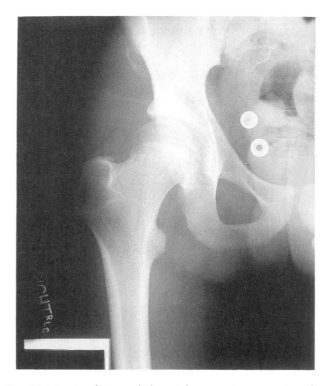

Fig. 111.3. Avulsion of the right anterior superior iliac spine (sartorius muscle origin). (Courtesy of A. Allen, M.D., Department of Radiology, University of Tennessee Medical Center.)

cially common in adolescents, who have apophyses still present. Treatment of avulsion injuries is with ice, rest, and crutches with toe-touch weight-bearing for up to 4 to 6 weeks. Once the pain and swelling subside, stretching and conditioning are best provided by physical therapy before resuming regular activity to prevent formation of bony prominences at the site of injury. If there is significant displacement of the avulsed fragment, consultation with an orthopedic surgeon is recommended.

Muscle Strain, Quadriceps, Hamstring

Common mechanisms of injury to the thigh include excessive tensile forces (strain) or high-velocity compressive forces (contusions, hematoma). There can be significant overload to the quadriceps when there is forceful contraction of the knee extensor muscles against resistance. This situation commonly occurs when landing from a jump, a changing stride misstep, or catching the foot while attempting to kick a ball. The most common injury is to the rectus femoris muscle, which commonly occurs at the distal muscle-tendon unit. The rectus femoris is the most central and superficial of the quadriceps muscles of the anterior thigh, and the distal portion is the leading edge in the flexed knee. Injury to the quadriceps muscles may show a visibly swollen, tender area at the site of the muscle tear. Pain is felt on active contraction and passive stretching. Isolation of this muscle is best done in the prone position with a mild passive stretch to flexion. In the prone position, Ely's test is performed by passive flexion of the knee to 90 degrees while observing the involved hip. Spontaneous hip flexion on the involved side with this maneuver is a positive test, which shows a tight rectus femoris due to spasm or a preexisting flexibility loss due to adaptive soft tissue changes. It is important to rule out avulsed muscles or tendons, especially to the quadriceps and patellar tendons.[22]

Treatment of muscle strain or contusion is geared to preventing further injury by decreasing the amount of bleeding by using the PRICE acronym—protection/pain-free weight bearing, rest, immobilization, ice, compressive wraps, elevation. Aspiration of the hematoma is generally not indicated, as the body resorbs this fluid, and there is increased chance for infection. If there is excessive pressure from the hematoma, which may create a compartment syndrome, elective aspiration may be performed by qualified personnel.

A quadriceps tendon rupture can occur from an off-balance jump that results in an eccentric load on a contracting muscle. Examination may reveal a large hematoma with swelling and tenderness and, possibly, a palpable defect. Incomplete tears can be managed nonoperatively with splints or hinged rehabilitation brace, crutches, and restricted weight-bearing and activity modification. Complete tears are best managed with primary surgical repair within the first 48 to 72 hours to preserve the extensor mechanism of the knee and restore function.

Contusions occur when the thigh is struck directly, resulting in muscle bruising from capillary rupture, edema, inflammation, and infiltrative bleeding. The best outcome occurs with early intervention, such as knee flexion (stretching), pain-free partial weight bearing, applying ice four to five times a day until inflammation stage is completed, restoring

motion with early range of motion exercises, and subsequent aggressive rehabilitation.[23] The most troubling complication of thigh contusions is the development of myositis ossificans, which can occur in 9% to 20% of cases.[24] It can occur fairly quickly following a severe contusion with the development of tenderness, warmth, and loss of range of motion (ROM) to the involved area. If tenderness persists, radiographs obtained at 3 to 4 weeks show flocculent densities similar to a callus. Periosteal reactive changes occur in 60% of cases.[25] Calcifications leading to a mass effect with "zoning" (immature bony rim surrounding an undifferentiated highly cellular central zone)[25] are an early radiographic finding. The risk of heterotopic muscular ossification is directly related to the severity of the trauma. Milder contusions are associated with minimal risk, and severe contusions are associated with increased risk. Acute treatment is with the RICE acronym—rest, ice, compression, and elevation—with an emphasis on compression. Surgical exploration and resection of mature symptomatic heterotopic bone is usually indicated after decreased bone activity is ascertained by bone scan, usually after several months.[26]

The posterior thigh is most commonly injured by strains to the hamstrings, especially to the short head of the biceps. Hamstring strain most commonly occurs with high-velocity movements such as sprinting or hurdling maneuvers. The medial thigh is injured most commonly by strains and less so by contusions, as it is relatively more protected. The lateral thigh is most often injured by contusions because it is more exposed. An inflexible iliotibial band of the lateral thigh can be injured by strain, or chronic overuse, such as in runners on sharply curved tracks or beveled surfaces or increasing their mileage. Commonly the iliotibial band becomes inflamed by excessive friction over the lateral femoral condyle with repetitive knee flexion and extension. It is important to rule out compartment syndromes or traumatic pseudoaneurysms when dealing with injuries to the thigh.

Bursitis

The most common bursal sites that create lower extremity pain are the ischiogluteal, greater trochanter, pes anserine, medial collateral, prepatellar, popliteal, and retrocalcaneal bursae. Typically there is painful swelling that increases in intensity with prolonged weight bearing. The onset may be insidious with overuse or may be acute resulting from trauma. It is essential to rule out other more serious disorders to the underlying structures before commencing a therapeutic program.[27] Treatment consists of the PRICEMM acronym—protection, relative rest, ice, compression, elevation, medication, and modalities (e.g., ultrasonography, high-voltage electrical stimulation, or iontophoresis). Corticosteroid injections can be used effectively if one is mindful of complications such as subcutaneous fat atrophy, skin depigmentation, infection, tendon rupture, hyperglycemia, and steroid flare. It is note-worthy to remember that piriformis bursitis may cause sciatic neuropathy.

Trochanteric bursitis is typically sharply localized over the greater trochanter, and relief of pain after an injection of anesthetic and steroid confirms the diagnosis. Etiologic factors include malalignment of the lower extremity, leg length asymmetry, gluteus medius weakness, and inflexibility of the iliotibial band. Achilles tendonitis is inflammation overlying the Achilles tendon. It can be caused by rubbing the heel against an offending heel counter from new shoes, overtraining, overpronation, or chronically tight heel cords. The examiner finds tenderness, variable swelling, discomfort with movement, and possibly crepitation along the distal tendon. Treatment is to remove the cause by using a temporary $1/4$-inch heel lift, ice, nonsteroidal antiinflammatory drugs (NSAIDs), and iontophoresis or phonophoresis (ultrasonic waves to drive antiinflammatory medication toward the site of injury). Retrocalcaneal bursitis is distinctly different in that the site of inflammation is located anterior to the Achilles tendon at its insertion into the calcaneus. Typically, the shoe is the culprit due to chronic friction, and shoe modification is needed. Additional treatment is similar to that for Achilles tendonitis.

The clinical diagnosis of pes anserine bursitis is based on tenderness over the insertion of the tendons onto the medial tibia (gracilis, sartorius, semitendinosus aponeurosis) along with swelling. Questionable cases ought to have an MRI to rule out other internal derangement of the knee. MRI typically shows fluid underneath the tendons of the pes anserinus at the medial aspect of the tibia near the joint line.[28]

It is important to remember that overuse inflammatory conditions of the lower extremity that occur insidiously secondary to weight-bearing stresses will have an underlying biomechanical cause. Successful treatment evolves around identifying the structural asymmetries, adaptive soft tissue changes, and gait compensations that underlie the overuse injury.

Knee Pain

There are many causes of knee pain, as outlined in Table 111.2. It is helpful to delineate knee pain by determining whether it is anterior, posterior, medial, lateral, intraarticular, or periarticular. Radiographs are usually obtained for acute traumatic knee injuries.

Meniscal Injury

Meniscal injuries are often associated with anterior cruciate ligament (ACL) tears. If a large joint effusion precludes ad-equate examination, prudent management calls for reevaluation in another week or so after a course of PRICE to decrease pain and swelling. Tenderness along the joint line combined with signs of locking, catching, inability to duck walk, pain with passive hyperextension of the knee, or positive McMurray's test is highly suggestive of meniscal damage. McMurray's test is performed with the patient in the supine position and the knee in full flexion. The tibia is internally and externally rotated while placing a mild varus and valgus stress on the knee to induce entrapment of an injured meniscus, resulting in either a snap or pain. Peripheral tears of the lateral meniscus can heal spontaneously, but other meniscal tears require the attention of an orthopedic surgeon. MRI can pick up 90% to 95% of meniscal injuries. For those with contraindications for MRI, CT arthrogram can be used.

Knee Dislocation

Complete knee dislocations are infrequent but serious injuries. Most knee dislocations are associated with posterior cruciate ligament (PCL) and ACL rupture but may occur with neither. Knee dislocation can occur with a low-velocity direct blow to the knee or high-velocity trauma such as in a motor vehicle accident, resulting in obvious distress and deformity. Because of the inherent serious trauma to the surrounding soft tissue, including nerves and blood vessels, it is imperative to act quickly and to provide for immediate transport to a hospital facility. Arteriography in the case of knee dislocation is crucial to rule out disruption of the popliteal artery. Radiography and MRI are necessary to rule out bony fragments or concomitant fracture. Neurovascular examination of the affected limb is important and is compared to the unaffected side. Prompt orthopedic referral is recommended. Treatment options can include surgical repair or immobilization for up to 6 weeks.

Anterior Cruciate Ligament Tear

An ACL tear can result from an external force or intrinsically, from a sudden stop, an abrupt cut, or hyperextension when the knee suddenly "gives out" (Table 111.3). There is typi-

Table 111.2. **Causes of Knee Pain**

Common	Uncommon	Not to be missed
Meniscal tears	Loose body intraarticularly	Stress fracture
Collateral ligament sprains	Tibial spine avulsion	
Contusions	Epiphyseal fracture	
Patellofemoral dysfunction	Popliteal cyst	
Patellar dislocation/subluxation	Tibial plateau fracture	
Anterior cruciate ligament tear	Popliteus tendonitis	
Posterior cruciate ligament tear	Ganglion cyst	
Pes anserine bursitis	Proximal tibiofibular diastasis	
Quadriceps and patellar tendonitis	Chondromalacia patellae	
Patellar bursitis (pre-, infra-)	Neuroma	
Synovitis	Osteochondritis dissecans of the patella	
Arthritis	Bipartite patella	
Plica syndrome	Synovial plica	
Iliotibial band syndrome	Osteochondral injury	
	Discoid meniscus	
	Infrapatellar fat pad syndrome (Hoffa's disease)	

Table 111.3. **Common Causes of Knee Pain and Diagnostic Pearls,**

Injury	History	Examination	Investigation
ACL tear	Audible pop, giving way with twisting, cutting or forced hyperextension	Hemarthrosis (+) Lachman's (+) Pivot shift	Confirm MRI ? Lateral capsule sign ? Tibial eminence fracture
PCL tear	Direct blow to anterior tibia; forced hyperextension	Posterior tibial sag (+) Posterior drawer	? Avulsion fracture Confirm MRI
Patellar subluxation or dislocation	Giving way with knee near extension and externally rotated; direct blow	(+) Apprehension test Hemarthrosis Medial tenderness	?Medial patellar avulsion fracture Malalignment
Collateral ligament tear	Varus or valgus stress to knee	Site tenderness Pain with/without increased laxity on stress test	? Avulsion fragment Confirm MRI
Meniscal tear	Twisting injury with catching, locking, swelling	Joint-line tenderness Mild effusion ±McMurray test	Confirm with arthrogram or MRI

ACL = anterior cruciate ligament; PCL = posterior cruciate ligament.
Source: Adapted from Rothenberg MH. Evaluation of acute knee injuries. Postgrad Med 1993;93:76, with permission.

cally a pop that is felt or heard by the individual with subsequent inability to continue the activity. A tense, bloody effusion within hours of the injury generally occurs. In the hands of an experienced clinician, more than 90% of ACL disruptions can be diagnosed at the time of injury.[29] On examination the Lachman test (an anterior drawer at 30 degrees of flexion) can confirm the diagnosis. A delay in the examination may prevent adequate diagnosis secondary to muscle spasm and severe pain. Anteroposterior, lateral, tunnel, and patellar profile radiographs are recommended to rule out other associated bone injuries. An avulsion of the proximal tibial insertion of the capsule comprises the "lateral capsule sign," or Segond's fracture. It indicates a significant injury to the lateral collateral ligament (LCL) and capsule along with a torn ACL. Occasionally in adolescents there is an avulsion of the ACL off the intercondylar tibial eminence. The degree of joint instability is related to concurrent injury and to stretching of the secondary restraining ligaments of the knee. Some individuals can return to their usual activities within 2 weeks after the effusion resolves. However, further stretching of the secondary ligaments can eventually result in further instability and later to disabling arthritis.

The diagnosis of partial ACL tear on clinical grounds may in reality be a complete rupture of the ACL radiographically.[30] MRI provides unequivocal evidence that ACL tears have associated injuries to the posterolateral femur and soft tissue structures of the knee that may not have been appreciated by arthroscopy alone.[31] In older relatively inactive individuals, nonoperative treatment is a viable option, provided patients are willing to accept a modest amount of instability and an increased risk for meniscal injury and degenerative joint disease.[32] ACL-insufficient knees in active people put them at risk for early degenerative changes. When rehabilitating an ACL tear, emphasis is placed on proper alignment of the lower extremity with a 1:1 strength ratio between quadriceps and hamstrings and on improved balance and proprioception.

Posterior Cruciate Ligament Tear

The PCL can be torn by falling on a flexed knee on a hard surface or when the knee is forced into the dashboard with sudden deceleration of an automobile. There is mild swelling and discomfort with the extremes of flexion and extension of the knee as well as pain posteriorly. The posterior drawer test and the posterior "sag" sign can establish the diagnosis of an isolated tear to the PCL. MRI is an invaluable tool in the diagnosis of PCL disruptions. PCL tears associated with other ligamentous injuries may do better with operative treatment. Isolated PCL tears do reasonably well with symptomatic rest and protection until full, pain-free ROM and equal strength are back to baseline.

Ligamentous Knee Injuries

The ligaments about the knee are the primary stabilizing structures that maintain knee joint stability. The medial collateral ligament (MCL) is the weakest and therefore the most commonly injured of the three major knee stabilizers (ACL, MCL, LCL). Injury most commonly occurs to the MCL with a valgus force on a flexed knee or a direct blow to the lateral knee. MCL tears are graded I to III based on the perceived disruption of the fibers on valgus stress examination (grade I: mild, microscopic disruption; grade II: partial tear; grade III: complete disruption) as well as the degree of tenderness and swelling. Proximal tears occur more frequently than distal tears.[33] The clinical examination is most accurate within minutes of an acutely injured knee. Treatment is conservative with PRICE and return to protected activity with functional improvement.

The mechanism of ski-related ACL injuries is a combination of load forces such that there is an external rotation-valgus force combination such as when the skier catches an inside edge in the snow. Hyperextension and violent quadriceps contraction to recover from an out-of-control sitting-back posture or to gain control after landing a jump may play a role. Isolated rupture of the popliteus is considered in any patient with an acute hemarthrosis, lateral tenderness, and a stable knee, especially after an external rotation injury.[34]

Osteochondritis Dissecans of the Knee

Osteochondritis dissecans (OCD) is a condition in which a segment of bone and the overlying cartilage are separated from underlying vascularized bone. Patients present with poorly localized, aching knee pain and swelling, exacerbated by activity and twisting motions. The physical examination typically shows an intact full ROM, possibly joint effusion, and significant quadriceps atrophy. Plain radiographs with anteroposterior, lateral, axial (sunrise or merchant), and tunnel views are helpful in the diagnosis of this condition. Figure 111.4 shows an articular defect to the medial femoral condyle that is best appreciated on the lateral view. MRI is most helpful for determining the size and viability of defects as well as the stability.[35] OCD of the lateral femoral condyle or patella is referred to an orthopedic surgeon because lateral lesions tend to more weight-bearing, leading to more degenerative changes.

For most young patients brief immobilization followed by activity limitation usually results in gradual healing. "Silent" OCD lesions in the adult are treated surgically to prevent further sloughing of the bony fragment. MRI and bone scans can be reserved for patients who have not improved after 4 to 6 weeks of therapy.[35]

Osteochondral and Chondral Fractures

Osteochondral fractures are a separate entity that are often associated with ligamentous injury and penetrate the articular cartilage to the underlying subchondral bone. These fractures can result from direct trauma or a twisting injury. Patients complain of immediate pain and a snap. Osteochondral fractures can be difficult to diagnose. Multiple radiographic views are often required to isolate the injured area. Acute lesions that are nondisplaced can be treated conservatively with immobilization. Chronic lesions are best left alone unless a loose fragment is identified. It can then be removed surgically.

Chondral fractures involve injuries to the softer cartilaginous layer and are likely to be found at the lateral femoral condyle and the medial surface of the patella. Chondral fractures are found in the skeletally mature, whereas osteochondral fractures tend to be found in the skeletally immature. Diagnosis may be difficult in that the presenting history and symptoms mimic meniscal damage: a traumatic episode with the knee in flexion with subsequent effusion, locking, catching, difficulty ascending stairs, and generalized knee pain. Conservative measures of 4 to 8 weeks of RICEMM is indicated. Those that do not resolve may need arthroscopy for a definitive diagnosis and to develop a plan for further treatment.

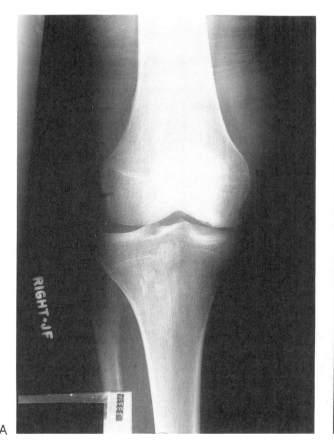

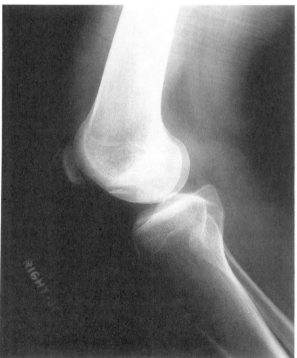

Fig. 111.4. Osteochondritis dissecans of the medial femoral condyle of right knee. Anteroposterior (A) and lateral (B) views. (Courtesy of A. Allen, M.D., Department of Radiology, University of Tennessee Medical Center.)

Patellar Dislocation

When diagnosing patellar dislocation the examiner must rule out other problems, such as ligamentous instability. Radiographic investigation is recommended (skyline and tunnel views). Patellar dislocations respond to immobilization and physical therapy. Patients with concomitant knee problems, such as predisposing patellofemoral malalignment, abnormal patellar configuration, and a history of symptoms of instability are more prone to recurrent dislocation and may benefit from operative intervention.[36] An osteochondral fragment with predisposing signs is managed operatively.[36] Up to 50% of patellar dislocations have an associated osteochondral fracture. Rehabilitation initially includes physical therapy, bracing, taping, and alteration of activities, followed by a maintenance patellar stability program.

Some injuries of the knee may be difficult to detect with simple radiographs alone. Tibial plateau fractures, Segond fractures (avulsion of the LCL from proximal tibial insertion), stress fractures, fibular head fractures, dislocation injuries to the patella and extensor mechanism, and Salter-type fractures are just a few diagnostic possibilities that may require more extensive workup with available MRI.

Lower Leg

Plantaris Tendon/Gastrocnemius Muscle Partial Tear

The tendon of the plantaris muscle can tear with violent contractions due to sudden acceleration and deceleration as is often seen on the tennis court. It is clinically difficult to differentiate between a gastrocnemius muscle tear and a plantaris tendon rupture, as they share the same anatomic location and mechanism of injury. Gastrocnemius muscle tears tend to take longer to heal. These injuries can mimic posterior compartment syndrome and deep venous thrombosis (DVT). DVT may have a palpable cord, and the compartment syndrome may have diminished distal pulses, pallor, and paresthesias. Use of Doppler ultrasonography can rule out DVT,[37] and determining intracompartment pressures can aid in ruling out compartment syndrome. Treatment consists of partial weight-bearing, if pain free, and RICE. Later, increased stretching and ROM exercises are added progressively.

Stress Fractures

Stress fractures are microscopic breaks in the cortex of long bones that have been exposed to mechanical strain due to overuse, such as with prolonged marching during military basic training. Common sites of stress fractures include the tibia, femur, and tarsal navicular and metatarsal bones.[38] Classic symptoms include persistent pain localized to a specific site that is aggravated with activity and relieved by rest and a history of recent increase in level or amount of activity. The examination may be unrevealing or may point to tenderness with compression over the site. The initial radiographs may be negative, although chronic injury may be reflected in periosteal elevation with surrounding edema. A bone scan has been historically the diagnostic procedure of choice. However, MRI has proven to be quite sensitive in diagnosing stress fractures and provides additional information such as marrow edema and actual fracture visualization. MRI is now considered the best choice for diagnosis of stress fractures for the above reasons as well as the fact that it is a noninvasive procedure.[39]

Ankle

Sprains

Ankle sprains are the most common injury to the musculoskeletal system. The lateral ankle with inversion-type mechanism of injury accounts for 85% of ankle sprains. Classification of ankle sprains is made using a grading system: grade I, mild stretch without instability; grade II, moderate stretch of the lateral ligaments resulting in partial disruption of the fibers and mild instability; and grade III, complete tear with gross instability.

Radiographic evaluation is recommended for significant injuries to rule out associated problems such as avulsion fractures, epiphyseal injuries in children, and talar dome injuries from other bony pathology that may occur. Stress radiography may be more beneficial in the chronic instability situation than in the acute setting where edema and inflammation may give a false negative. Proprioception is an important, often overlooked component during rehabilitation of an acute ankle injury and one that may have the most direct bearing on the chronic nature of ankle sprains. When treating the acute ankle sprain it is important to note that patients treated with "dynamic" bracing (protection of lateral motion while allowing full plantar and dorsiflexion) versus those with "static" bracing (i.e., immobilization and casting) have earlier, more comprehensive functional recovery.[40] Early mobilization also allows earlier return to functional capacity and may be more comfortable for the patient.[41] It takes longer to recover from syndesmosis (tibiofibular or "high ankle") sprains than from lateral ankle sprains. Complications can include ossification, which may require surgery to return to full activity.

Achilles Tendon Rupture

Seventy-five percent of Achilles tendon ruptures occur in athletes between the ages of 30 and 40 years, and two thirds are symptomatic prior to rupture. The poorest blood supply to this tendon is 2 to 6 cm proximal to its insertion, and vascularity continues to decrease with age. Risk factors include recent oral or injectable corticosteroid and chronic Achilles tendon injury. This injury usually occurs following a rapid eccentric load, with the patient feeling a "pop," as if struck from behind. There is progressive pain and inability to ambulate. Prior to swelling a palpable defect can be appreciated, and the patient cannot actively plantarflex the foot. By squeezing the relaxed prone calf, there should be movement of the foot into plantarflexion. Absence of this motion describes a positive Thomson test. A plain lateral radiograph may show either collapse of Kager's triangle (triangle formed by the borders of the anterior Achilles tendon, upper part of the calcaneus, and the posterior surface of the deep flexor tendon) or disruption of the shadow of the Achilles tendon.[42] Nonoperative treatment such as casting has recently shown similar results as operative intervention and can be considered a viable option especially in the non-elite athlete. Late ruptures are best treated surgically.[43,44]

Tibial Plafond Fractures

Fractures to the distal tibia that overlie the talus ("tenon") and comprise most of the "mortise" of the ankle joint are termed pilon fractures. The tibial plafond, or pilon fracture, occurs with 7% to 10% of tibial fractures and with only 1% of lower extremity fractures.[45] Typically pilon fractures follow a severe axial load, such as with a fall or a motor vehicle accident, but concomitant rotational forces can result in a wide array of fractures and derangements of the distal tibia and fibula. Clinically there is marked pain, swelling, inability to ambulate, and a history of severe axial loading. Because of the shear forces due to high-energy trauma associated with pilon fractures, the examiner must look for accompanying trauma to the hindfoot, knee, pelvis, and vertebral column. Nondisplaced fractures may respond favorably to casting, but most others require open reduction with internal fixation (ORIF).

Surgical reconstruction should be performed within 8 to 12 hours of injury in a stable patient without significant skin trauma; otherwise, temporizing measures to ensure restoration of length may be implemented for 7 to 10 days prior to ORIF.[46]

Talar Dome Fractures

Fractures to the talus account for 0.14% to 0.90% of all fractures. Because the talus contains seven articulations with adjoining structures, there are a wide variety of injury patterns to the talus: osteochondral defects to the talar dome (Fig. 111.5), posterior tubercle fractures, lateral process fractures, crush fractures, talar neck fractures, and shear fractures to the body of the talus along different planes. Often initial radiographs appear normal, but recurrent pain and instability prompt further investigation to rule out osteochondral injury to the talar dome. The symptoms of pain, recurrent swelling, ankle instability, and "giving way" are highly suggestive of osteochondritis dissecans of the talar dome (Fig. 111.5). Because bony resorption takes time to develop, follow-up radiographs may demonstrate a fracture line, sclerosis, or cyst formation. Bone scans are undertaken if repeat radiographs are unremarkable and the history and physical examination evoke a high index of suspicion.

Staging of OCD of the talar dome is necessary for selecting the appropriate treatment option: stage I, compression of subchondral bone without break in cartilage; stage II, partially detached osteochondral fragment; stage III, totally detached osteochondral fragment remaining in crater; stage IV, displaced osteochondral fragment loose in joint.[47] Stages I, II, and III with a medial talus lesion can be managed with a short leg non–weight-bearing cast for 6 weeks. Referral to an orthopedic surgeon is recommended to deal with the subtleties of operative and nonoperative treatment.

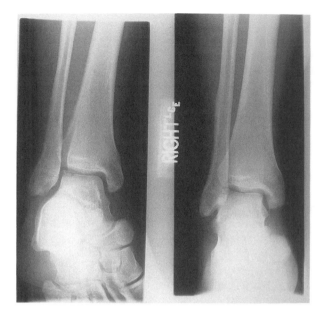

Fig. 111.5. Osteochondral injury (osteochondritis dissecans) of the lateral talar dome. (Courtesy of A. Allen, M.D., Department of Radiology, University of Tennessee Medical Center.)

Foot

Evaluation of foot injuries can be aided by classifying injuries based on the anatomic site on the hindfoot (calcaneus and talus), midfoot (tarsal bones), and forefoot (metatarsals and phalanges) (Table 111.4).

Plantar Fasciitis

Plantar fasciitis refers to disorders involving insertion of the plantar fascia into the medial tubercle of the medial calcaneus. It can present as an inflammation, microtear, or periosteal avulsion. Sharp heel pain is experienced with early morning ambulation and tends to lessen with activity, though a burning sensation or dull ache can occur with activity. Examination shows a specific area of tenderness overlying the medial plantar calcaneus that is aggravated by standing on the tiptoes or dorsiflexing the ankle. Tight heel cords contribute to the chronic nature of this disorder. Lateral radiographs may show heel spurs, but they are rarely the cause of the pain. Treatment options include activity modification, NSAIDs, physical therapy, heel pads, orthotic devices, night splints, and walking casts. Injectable corticosteroids are often used, but long-term efficacy is negligible. Most patients, if not all, find some lessening of symptoms during the first week. Pain relief may last as long as 6 to 7 weeks, but more than half of these patients experience a return to preinjection discomfort.[48]

Haglund's Deformity

Haglund's deformity, or prominence of the posterosuperior os calcis, presents with pain and swelling of the heel made worse by activity. Examination by palpation reveals tenderness, thickening of the overlying skin, and signs of local in-

Table 111.4. **Disorders of the Foot and Ankle**

Common	Uncommon	Not to be missed
Causes of hindfoot pain		
Plantar fasciitis	Calcaneal fracture (traumatic, stress)	Spondyloarthropathies
Fat pad contusion	Compression of the medial branch of the lateral plantar nerve	Osteoid osteoma
	Medial calcaneal nerve entrapment	Reflex sympathetic dystrophy (RSD)
	Tarsal tunnel syndrome	Talar dome fracture
	Talar stress fracture	
	Retrocalcaneal bursitis	
	Haglund's deformity (pump bump)	
	Calcaneal apophysitis (Sever's disease)/(adolescents)	
	Avulsion of Achilles tendon	
	Achilles tendonitis	
Causes of midfoot pain		
Navicular stress fracture	Cuneiform stress fracture	Osteoid osteoma
Midtarsal joint sprain	Cuboid stress fracture	RSD
Extensor tendonitis	Peroneal tendonitis	
Tibialis posterior tendonitis	Abductor hallucis strain	
Plantar fascia strain	Cuboid strain	
	Tarsal coalition (adolescents)	
	Köhler's disease (young children)	
Causes of forefoot pain		
Corns, calluses	Freiberg's osteochondritis	RSD
Onychocryptosis	Joplin's neuritis	Lisfranc fracture/dislocation
Synovitis MTP joints	Stress fracture sesamoids	
First MTP sprain	Toe clawing	
Subungual hematoma	Plantar wart	
Hallux valgus	Subungual exostosis	
Hallux rigidus	Hammer toe	
Morton's neuroma		
Sesamoiditis		
Metatarsal stress fracture		
Jones' fracture (5th MT base)		

MTP = metatarsophalangeal

flammation. There may also be a varus deformity of the heel and a mild degree of cavus of the foot reflected by a high medial arch, making the tuberosity appear more prominent. Conservative treatment includes PRICE, and only those not benefiting from therapy are considered for surgical intervention. Surgical resection of the posterosuperior calcaneus has mixed results with little more than 50% of patients obtaining complete relief of pain.[49]

Tarsal Tunnel Syndrome

Tarsal tunnel syndrome is caused by entrapment of the posterior tibial nerve under the flexor retinaculum or at the site of either of its branches, the medial or lateral plantar nerves. The tunnel is formed by the flexor retinaculum, which is located behind and distal to the medial malleolus. Pain and paresthesias radiate along the plantar aspect of the foot from the medial malleolus and increase with activity. A positive Tinel's sign (paresthesias with percussion over the inflamed nerve) may be found along with increased discomfort from prolonged manual compression of the posterior tibial nerve behind the medial malleolus. There are many causes of this disorder, including posttraumatic deformities, tortuous veins, ganglion, lipoma, edema, the presence of accessory muscles,

and synovial hypertrophy. Careful selection of candidates for resection of a space-occupying lesion has the best chance of success because of the high rate of complications and patient dissatisfaction with results.[50] MRI is helpful when planning the surgery for refractory cases of tarsal tunnel syndrome, as it identifies an inflammatory or mass lesion.[51]

Anterior Tarsal Tunnel Syndrome

Anterior tarsal tunnel syndrome is entrapment of the deep peroneal nerve (or anterior tibial nerve) under the extensor retinaculum at the ankle. The tunnel roof is the inferior extensor retinaculum; the tunnel floor is the fascia overlying the talus and navicular. Within the tunnel are four tendons, an artery, a vein, and the deep peroneal nerve. Most people with this disorder have had recurrent ankle sprains or other trauma, wear tight-fitting shoes or ski boots, carry keys under their shoelace tongue, or do sit-ups with their feet hooked under a bar. Plantar flexion with supination stretches the nerve and contributes to symptomatology. Clinical features include numbness and paresthesias in the first dorsal web space (superficial medial branch of the deep peroneal nerve) and occasionally aching and tightness about the ankle and dorsum of the foot. If the lateral, chiefly motor division of the nerve

Table 111.5. **Nerve Entrapment Conditions of the Foot**

Transient plantar or digital paresthetica (stair-climbing)
Classic tarsal tunnel syndrome
Distal tarsal tunnel syndromes
Medial plantar nerve
First branch of the lateral plantar nerve
Entrapment of the higher tibial nerve
Deep peroneal nerve
Superficial peroneal nerve
Sural nerve
Saphenous nerve

is affected, the syndrome is difficult to recognize, as the characteristic paresthesias are absent. The patient experiences only aching pain over the dorsum of the foot that is worse in some positions or less severe in others. On examination, there may be sensory loss in the first dorsal web space with a positive Tinel's sign over the area of the nerve injury, which is usually at the level of the ankle (the nerve runs a few millimeters medial to the dorsalis pedis artery). Treatment includes such conservative measures as protecting the area, rest, judicious ice, NSAIDs, and possibly surgical release of the nerve if all else fails. Table 111.5 shows other nerve impingement syndromes of the foot.[52]

Midfoot Injuries

Lisfranc Injury

The Lisfranc injury involves the articulation of the forefoot and midfoot, the tarsometatarsal joint (TMT), with or without associated fractures. This injury should be ruled out in any injury to the midfoot. The two major mechanisms of injury are direct (crushing) and the more common indirect (violent abduction or plantarflexion of the forefoot).

The midfoot sprain can be identified by mild to moderate midfoot swelling and an inability to bear weight. The TMT joint can be stressed with passive plantar and dorsiflexion, pronation, and abduction of the first and second metatarsal rays. Positive results of tenderness with these maneuvers identifies potential midfoot pathology. With no radiographic evidence of diastasis (grade III injury), treatment consists of a non–weight-bearing cast until the patient is asymptomatic. Persistent discomfort warrants a weight-bearing radiographic view to evaluate for articulation instability. The radiograph should document a space between the first and second metatarsal base that may be widened 2 to 5 mm. An ankle block may be necessary for the patient not able to tolerate weight-bearing. For more subtle injuries, diagnostic studies can be postponed for 1 to 2 weeks without a compromise in treatment. Nonoperative treatment consists of casting and the use of crutches for 4 to 6 weeks. It may take up to 4 months for a return to full activity.[53] Medial and global tenderness often requires a longer recovery time,[54] in contrast to injuries to the lateral aspect of the midfoot.[55] Any significant diastasis or other local soft tissue injuries require referral to an orthopedic surgeon. A history of a significant foot injury associated with persistent pain and swelling markedly out of proportion to the radiographic findings raises the suspicion of

a dislocation. Comparison views with and without weight-bearing may be helpful for determining the subtle widening between the first and second metatarsal shafts.

Osteoid Osteoma

An osteoid osteoma is a benign bone lesion that can occur on any bone of the foot but is seen most often on the tarsal bones. It causes chronic pain, and one third of patients describe nocturnal pain. Many patients with osteoid osteoma fail to respond to restriction of activity. Radiography may reveal reactive cortical changes and may show a central, round, radiopaque nidus surrounded by a thin, rarefied zone usually less than 1 cm. Bone scan, CT, or MRI may add to further localization of the lesion. Referral to an orthopedic surgeon is indicated, as most of these lesions respond to local excision of the nidus.

Forefoot Injuries

Turf Toe

Hyperextension of the first metatarsophalangeal (MTP) joint or severe hallux valgus stress can result in a painful, swollen joint that becomes more severe with time. Turf toe generally refers to a sprain of the plantar capsular ligament of the big toe. Joint rest is the foremost treatment with immobilization, ice, and compression. Later, ultrasound, contrast baths, or paraffin baths offer some benefit. Taping that restricts extension of the toe may allow return to full activity.

Sesamoids

A fall from a height or forced dorsiflexion may create inflammation of the sesamoids of the foot or possibly even fracture. The pain is localized over the plantar aspect of the first metatarsal head with weight-bearing and palpation. Radiographs may show a bipartite medial sesamoid. A bone scan may be needed to rule out a stress fracture. Treatment consists of unloading the metatarsal head with padding and NSAIDs. Chronic cases may require surgery to débride or repair nonhealing fractures.

Metatarsals

The metatarsals may be injured from direct trauma, severe shear forces, and overuse. Stress fractures are common and result usually from inordinate increases in distance traveled by running or hiking. Tenderness is localized over the specific metatarsal and not within the interspace. Plain radiographs are positive within 3 to 6 weeks, but a bone scan or MRI can establish the diagnosis within days. The treatment is rest and use of a firm, flat-soled shoe. Based on symptoms, a return to activity is usually accomplished within 6 weeks.

Metatarsalgia

Metatarsalgia is pain under the metatarsals that is exacerbated with functional activities. It can present as burning and is more commonly seen in women and in the second metatarsal. The most common cause is increased weight-bearing pressure over the metatarsal head. It is important to rule out stress fracture, neuroma, and avascular necrosis of the metatarsal head.

Treatment lies in correcting any shoe deformity that may be causing the problem; relieving the pressure point by using shoe inserts, metatarsal pads, or orthotics; and trimming any adjacent calluses. Hot soaks and NSAIDs are of proved benefit in the acute setting.

Bunion

A bunion is an excessive bony growth (exostosis) on the head of the first metatarsal with callous formation and bursal inflammation. It is the result of a tight shoe box compressing the toes or faulty foot dynamics with late pronation and push-off from the medial forefoot. Basic treatment is to find shoes with an ample toe box to decrease constriction of the MTP joint. Severe symptoms may require surgical correction. A bunionette is a bony prominence on the lateral aspect of the fifth metatarsal head.

Fracture of the Fifth Metatarsal

Fracture of the fifth metatarsal base can occur either at the base or the tuberosity. It is typically an avulsion fracture of the peroneus tendon resulting from a violent inversion stress to that side of the foot. Symptomatic treatment for 3 to 4 weeks is all that is needed prior to return to full activity. A transverse fracture at the base (Jones fracture) is associated with more complications resulting from nonunion or delayed union (Fig. 111.6). It is managed closely with immobilization. A bone graft is considered if nonunion is suspected.

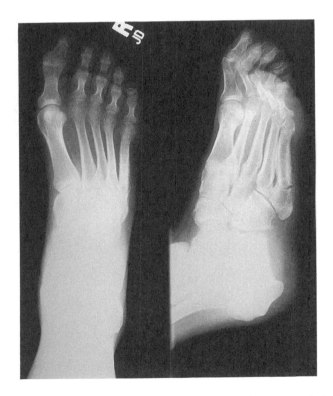

Fig. 111.6. Transverse fracture (Jones' fracture) of the base of the fifth metatarsal. (Courtesy of M. Holt, M.D., Department of Orthopedics, University of Tennessee Medical Center.)

Interdigital Neuritis (Morton's Neuroma)

Interdigital neuritis is compressive neuropathy of the interdigital nerve caused by recurrent impingement underneath the intermetatarsal ligament. It is usually seen in the third to fourth digital web space.[49] Conservative measures include rest from the offending activity, increased use of sole shock-absorbing shoes, a metatarsal pad placed proximal to the lesion, NSAIDs, or injection with anesthetic and steroids. Surgical neurolysis is used as a last resort.

References

1. Graves EJ, Owings MF. 1996 Summary: National Hospital Discharge Survey. Advance data from vital and health statistics; no. 301. Hyattsville, MD: National Center for Health Statistics, 1996.
2. Cummings SR, Browner WS, Stone K, et al. Risk factors for hip fracture in white women. N Engl J Med 1995;332:767–73.
3. Peacock M, Liu G, Manatunga AK, Timmerman L, Johnston CC Jr. Better discrimination of hip fracture using bone density, geometry, and architecture. Osteoporos Int 1995;5:167–73.
4. Gluer CC, Pressman A, Li J, et al. Prediction of hip fractures from pelvic radiographs: the study of osteoporotic fractures: the study of Osteoporotic Fractures Research Group. J Bone Miner Res 1994;9:671–7.
5. Lindsay R, Cosman F, Lobo RA, et al. Addition of alendronate to ongoing hormone replacement therapy in the treatment of osteoporosis: a randomized, controlled clinical trial. J Clin Endocrinol Metab 1999;V84(9):3076.
6. Kanis JA, Gullberg B, Allander E, et al. Evidence for efficacy of drugs affecting bone metabolism in preventing hip fracture. BMJ 1992;305:1124–8.
7. Bean N, Lehman AB. Habitus and hip fracture revisited: skeletal size, strength and cognition rather than thinness? Age Ageing 1995;24:481–4.
8. Robinovitch SN, Hayes WC. Force attenuation in trochanteric soft tissues during impact from a fall. J Orthop Res 1995;13:959–62.
9. Jaglal SB, Darlinton GA. Lifetime occupational physical activity and risk of hip fracture in women. Ann Epidemiol 1995;5:321–4.
10. Hemenway D, Colditz GA. Body height and hip fracture: a cohort study of 90,000 women. Int J Epidemiol 1995;24:783–6.
11. Greenspan SL, Maitland LA, Kido TH, Krasnow MB, Hayes WC. Trochanteric bone mineral density is associated with type of hip fracture in the elderly. J Bone Miner Res 1994;9:1889–94.
12. Bogost GA, Cures JV III. MR imaging in evaluation of suspected hip fracture: frequency of unsuspected bone and soft-tissue injury. Radiology 1995;197:263–7.
13. Guancre CA, Kozin SH, Levy AS, Brody LA. The use of MRI in the diagnosis of occult hip fractures in the elderly: a preliminary review. Orthopedics 1994;17:327–30.
14. Norris MA. Fractures and dislocations of the hip and femur. Semin Roentgenol 1994;29:100–12.
15. Mitchell MJ, Resnick D. Diagnostic imaging of lower extremity trauma. Radiol Clin North Am 1989;27:909–28.
16. Frick SL. Is computed tomography useful after simple posterior hip dislocation? J Orthop Trauma 1995;9:388–91.
17. Fairbairn KJ, Murphey MD, Resnik CS. Gas bubbles in the hip joint on CT: an indication of recent dislocation. AJR 1995;164:931–4.
18. Poggi JJ, Spritzer CE, Roark T, Goldner RD. Changes on magnetic resonance images after traumatic hip dislocation. Clin Orthop Relat Res 1995;319:249–59.

19. Erb RE, Nance EP Jr, Edwards JR. Traumatic anterior dislocation of the hip: spectrum of plain film and CT findings. AJR 1995;165:1215–19.
20. Rogers LF, ed. The hip and femoral shaft. In: Radiology in skeletal trauma, vol. 2. New York: Churchill Livingstone, 1992:653–712.
21. Burgos J, Ocete G. Traumatic hip dislocation with incomplete reduction due to soft-tissue interposition in a 4-year-old boy. J Pediatr Orthop 1995;4:216–8.
22. Zarins B. Acute muscle and tendon injuries in athletes. Clin Sports Med 1983;2:167–82.
23. Young LY, Rock MG. Thigh injuries in athletes. Mayo Clin Proc 1993;68:1099–106.
24. Ryan JB, Hopkinson WJ, Arciero RA, Kolakowski KR. Quadriceps contusions. Am J Sports Med 1991;19:299–304.
25. Lipscomb AB, Johnston RK. Treatment of myositis ossificans traumatica in athletes. Am J Sports Med 1976;4:111–20.
26. Arrington ED. Skeletal muscle injuries. Orthop Clin North Am 1995;26:411–22.
27. Butcher JD, Lillegard WA. Lower extremity bursitis. Am Fam Physician 1996;53:2317–24.
28. Forbes JR, Janzen DL. Acute pes anserine bursitis: MR imaging. Radiology 1995;104:525–7.
29. Johnson DL. Diagnosis for anterior cruciate ligament surgery. Clin Sport Med 1993;12:671–84.
30. Lintner DM, Moseley JB, Noble PC. Partial tears of the anterior cruciate ligament. Am J Sports Med 1995;23:111–6.
31. Speer KP, Bassett FH, Feagin JA, Garrett WE. Osseous injury associated with acute tears of the anterior cruciate ligament. Am J Sports Med 1992;20:382–9.
32. Buss DD, Skyhar M, Galinat B, Warren RF, Wickiewicz TL. Nonoperative treatment of acute anterior cruciate ligament injuries in a selected group of patients. Am J Sports Med 1995;23:160–5.
33. Schwietzer ME, Deely DM, Hume EL. Medial collateral ligament injuries: evaluation of multiple signs, prevalence and location of associated bone bruises, and assessment with MR imaging. Radiology 1995;194:825–9.
34. Geissler WB, Caspari RB. Isolated rupture of the popliteus with posterior tibial nerve palsy. J Bone Joint Surg 1992;74:811–13.
35. Ralston BM, Bach BR, Bush-Joseph CA, Knopp WD. Osteochondritis dissecans of the knee. Physician Sport Med 1996;24:73–84.
36. Hawkins RJ, Anisette G. Acute patellar dislocations: the natural history. Am J Sports Med 1986;14:117–20.
37. Helms CA, Garvin GJ. Plantaris muscle injury: evaluation with MR imaging. Radiology 1995;195:201–3.
38. Johnson AW, Wheeler DL. Stress fractures of the femoral shaft in athletes-more common than expected. Am J Sports Med 1994;22:248–56.
39. Deutsch AL, Coel MN, Mink JH. Imaging of stress injuries to bone. Radiography, scintigraphy, and MR imaging. Clin in Sports Med 1997;16(2)275–91.
40. Regis D, Magnan B, Spagnol S, Bragantini A. Dynamic orthopaedic brace in the treatment of ankle sprains. Foot Ankle Int 1995;16:422–6.
41. Eiff MP, Smith AT, Smith GE. Early mobilization versus immobilization in the treatment of lateral ankle sprains. Am J Sports Med 1994;22:83–8.
42. Cetti R. Roentgenographic diagnoses of ruptured Achilles tendons. Clin Orthop 1993;286:215–21.
43. Soma CA. Repair of acute Achilles tendon injuries. Orthop Clin North Am 1995;26:239–47.
44. Howard CB, Winston I, Bell W, et al. Late repair of calcaneal tendon with carbon fiber. J Bone Joint Surg 1984;66B:206–208.
45. McFerran MA, Boulas HJ. Complications encountered in the treatment of pilon fractures. J Orthop Trauma 1992;6:195–200.
46. Brumback RJ. Fractures of the tibial plafond. Orthop Clin North Am 1995;26:273–85.
47. Berndt AL. Transchondral fractures (osteochondritis dissecans) of the talus. J Bone Joint Surg 1959;41A:988–1020.
48. Miller RA, McGuire M. Efficacy of first time steroid injection for painful heel syndrome. Foot Ankle Int 1995;16:610–2.
49. Nesse E. Poor results after resection of Haglund's heel: analysis of 35 heels in 23 patients after 3 years. Acta Orthop Scand 1994;65:107–9.
50. Pfeiffer WH. Clinical results after tarsal tunnel decompression. J Bone Joint Surg 1994;76A:1222–30.
51. Frey C. Magnetic resonance imaging and the evaluation of tarsal tunnel syndrome. Foot Ankle 1993;14:159–64.
52. Schon LC. Nerve entrapment, neuropathy, and nerve dysfunction in athletes. Orthop Clin North Am 1994;25:47–59.
53. Shapiro MS, Finerman GAM. Rupture of Lisfranc's ligament in athletes. Am J Sports Med 1994;22:687–91.
54. Trevino SG. Controversies in tarsometatarsal injuries. Orthop Clin North Am 1995;26:229–38.
55. Meyer SA, Albright JP, Crowley ET, et al. Midfoot sprains in collegiate football players. Am J Sports Med 1994;22:392–401.

112
Osteoarthritis

Alicia D. Monroe and John B. Murphy

Epidemiology

Arthritis affects an estimated 43 million persons in the United States.[1] Osteoarthritis (OA) is the most common rheumatic disease, and the third most common principal diagnosis recorded by family practitioners for office visits made by older patients.[2,3] Hip and knee OA are a leading cause of activity limitation, disability, and dependence among the elderly.[3,4] Population-based studies of OA demonstrate that the prevalence of radiographic OA is much higher than clinically defined or symptomatic OA, and there is a progressive increase in the prevalence of OA with advancing age.[3,5] The prevalence, pattern of joint involvement, and severity of OA has been observed to vary among populations by ethnicity and race, but some of the data are conflicting. [4,6] Europeans have higher prevalence rates of radiographic hip OA (7–25%), compared to Hong Kong Chinese (1%), and Caribbean and African black populations (1–4%).[4] The National Health and Nutrition Examination Survey (NHANES I) study, showed higher rates of knee OA for U.S. black women, but no racial differences in hip OA. In the Johnson County Arthritis Study, African Americans and whites showed similar high rates of radiographic hip OA (29.9% versus 26.4%) and knee OA (37.4% versus 39.1%).[7]

Pathophysiology

Systemic factors (age, sex, race, genetics, bone density, estrogen replacement therapy, and nutritional factors) may predispose joints to local biomechanical factors (obesity, muscle weakness, joint deformity, injury) and the subsequent development of OA.[4,6] The degenerative changes seen in osteoarthritic cartilage are clearly distinct from those seen with normal aging.[8] The pathologic changes in OA cartilage appear to be mediated by complex interactions between me-chanical and biologic factors including excessive enzymatic degradation, decreased synthesis of cartilage matrix, increased levels of cytokines and other inflammatory molecules, and dysregulation of OA chondrocytes. The net result includes disorganization of the cartilage matrix and fibrillation.[8,9] As the disease advances, disorganization gives way to fissures, erosion, ulceration, and eventually cartilage is irreversibly destroyed. As the cartilage degenerates, joint stresses are increasingly transmitted to the underlying bone, initiating the bony remodeling process, which results in marginal osteophytes, subchondral sclerosis, and cysts.

Clinical Presentation and Diagnosis

Signs and Symptoms

Osteoarthritis, classified as primary (idiopathic) or secondary, represents a "final common pathway" for a number of conditions of diverse etiologies.[6] Primary OA is further classified as localized (e.g., hands, feet, knees, or other single sites) or generalized including three or more local areas. Secondary OA is classified as (1) posttraumatic, (2) congenital or developmental, (3) metabolic, (4) endocrine, (5) other bone and joint diseases, (6) neuropathic, and (7) miscellaneous. Commonly affected joints include the interphalangeal, knee, hip, acromioclavicular, subtalar, first metatarsophalangeal, sacroiliac, temporomandibular, and carpometacarpal joint of the thumb. Joints usually spared include the metacarpophalangeal, wrist, elbow, and shoulder. Early during the symptomatic phase, OA pain is often described as a deep, aching discomfort. It occurs with motion, particularly with weight-bearing, and is relieved by rest. As the disease progresses, pain can occur with minimal motion and at rest. OA pain is typically localized to the joint, although pain associated with hip OA is often localized to the anterior inguinal region, and the medial or lateral thigh, but it may also radiate to the buttock, anterior thigh, or knee. OA pain of the spine may be associated with radicular symptoms including pain, paresthesias, and muscle weakness. Although joint stiffness can occur, it is usually of short duration (<30 minutes).

Physical examination of an affected joint may show decreased range of motion, joint deformity, bony hypertrophy, and occasionally an intraarticular effusion. Crepitance and pain on passive and active movement and mild tenderness may be found. Inflammatory changes including warmth and redness are usually absent. During late stages there may be demonstrable joint instability. Physical findings associated with hand OA include Heberden's nodes of the distal interphalangeal joints, representing cartilaginous and bony enlargement of the dorsolateral and dorsomedial aspects. Bouchard's nodes are similar findings at the proximal interphalangeal joints. Physical findings of knee OA can also include quadriceps muscle atrophy, mediolateral joint instability, limitation of joint motion, initially with extension, and varus angulation resulting from degenerative cartilage in the medial compartment of the knee. The patient with OA of the hip often holds the hip adducted, flexed, and internally rotated, which may result in functional shortening of the leg and the characteristic limp (antalgic gait).

Radiographic Features and Laboratory Findings

During early stages of OA plain radiographs may be normal. As the disease progresses, joint space narrowing becomes evident as articular cartilage is lost. Marginal osteophyte formation is seen as a result of bone proliferation. Subchondral bony sclerosis appears radiographically as increased bone density. Subchondral bone cysts develop and vary in size from several millimeters to several centimeters, appearing as translucent areas in periarticular bone. Bony deformity, joint subluxation, and loose bodies may be seen in advanced cases. Computed tomography, magnetic resonance imaging, and ultrasonography provide powerful tools for the assessment of OA, although the diagnosis of OA rarely requires such expensive modalities. There are no specific laboratory tests for OA. Unlike with the inflammatory arthritides, with OA the erythrocyte sedimentation rate (ESR) and hemogram are normal and autoantibodies are not present. If there is joint effusion, the synovial fluid is noninflammatory, with fewer than 2000 white blood cells (WBCs), a predominance of mononuclear WBCs, and a good mucin clot. The diagnosis of OA is usually based on clinical and radiologic features, with the laboratory assessment being useful for excluding other arthritic conditions or secondary causes of OA.

Management

The goals of OA management are pain control, prevention of joint damage, maximizing function and quality of life, and minimizing therapeutic toxicity.[10] An appropriate treatment plan for OA combines oral medications, exercise, and patient education. Nonpharmacologic management strategies for OA include periods of rest (1–2 hours) when symptoms are at their worst, avoidance of repetitive movements or static body positions that aggravate symptoms, heat (or cold) for the control of pain, weight loss if the patient is overweight, adaptive mobility aids to diminish the mechanical load on joints, adaptive equipment to assist in activities of daily living (ADL), range of motion exercises, strengthening exercises, and endurance

Table 112.1 **Pharmacologic Treatment of Osteoarthritis**

Drug	Dosage range/frequency	Relative cost/30days
Acetaminophen	750–1000 mg qid	$
Aspirin, enteric coated	975 mg qid	$
Extended release aspirin	800 mg qid	$
Salicylsalicylic acid	3–4 g/day 2 or 3 doses	$
Choline magnesium trisalicylate	3 g/day in 1, 2, or 3 doses	$$
Celecoxib (Celebrex)	100–200mg bid	$$$$
Diclofenac (Voltaren)	150–200 mg/day in 2 or 3 doses	$$
Diflunisal (Dolobid)	500–1000 mg/day in 2 doses	$$
Etodolac (Lodine)	300 mg bid–tid	$$
Fenoprofen (Nalfon)	300–600 mg tid–qid	$$
Flurbiprofen (Ansaid)	200–300 mg/day in 2, 3, or 4 doses	$$
Ibuprofen (Motrin)	1200–3200 mg/day in 3 or 4 doses	$
Indomethacin (Indocin)	25–50 mg tid–qid	$
Ketoprofen (Orudis)	50 mg qid or 75 mg tid	$$
Meclofenamate sodium	200–400 mg in 3 or 4 doses	$$$
Meloxicam (Mobic)	7.5–15 mg/day	$$$
Nabumetone (Relafen)	1000 mg once/day to 2000 mg/day	$$$
Naproxen (Naprosyn)	250–500 mg bid–tid	$
Naproxen sodium (Anaprox)	275–550 mg bid	$
Oxaprozin (Daypro)	600 mg once/day to 1800 mg/day	$$
Piroxicam (Feldene)	20 mg once/day	$$
Rofecoxib (Vioxx)	25–50 mg once/day	$$$
Sulindac (Clinoril)	150–200 mg bid	$
Tolmetin (Tolectin)	600–1800 mg/day in 3 or 4 doses	$$

$ = 18–35; $$ = 36–55; $$$ = 56–80; $$$$ = 81–145.

exercises.[11,12] Immobilization should be avoided. The use of adaptive mobility aids (e.g., canes, walkers) is an important strategy, but care must be taken to ensure that the mobility aid is the correct device, properly used, appropriately sized, and in good repair. Medial knee taping to realign the patella in patients with patellofemoral OA, and the use of wedged insoles for patients with medial compartment OA and shock absorbing footwear may help reduce joint symptoms.[10,13]

Pharmacologic approaches to the treatment of OA include acetaminophen, salicylates, nonselective nonsteroidal anti-inflammatory drugs (NSAIDs), cyclooxygenase-2 (COX-2) specific inhibitors, topical analgesics, and intraarticular steroids.[14,15] Acetaminophen is advocated for use as first-line therapy for relief of mild to moderate pain, but it should be used cautiously in patients with liver disease or chronic alcohol abuse. Salicylates and NSAIDs are commonly used as first-line medications for the relief of pain related to OA. Compliance with salicylates can be a major problem given their short duration of action and the need for frequent dosing; thus NSAIDs are preferable to salicylates. There is no justification for choosing one nonselective NSAID over another based on efficacy, but it is clear that a patient who does not respond to an NSAID from one class may well respond to an NSAID from another. The choice of a nonselective NSAID versus a COX-2 specific inhibitor should be made after assessment of risk for GI toxicity (e.g., age 65 or older, history of peptic ulcer disease, previous GI bleeding, use of oral corticosteroids, or anticoagulants). For patients at increased risk for upper GI bleeding, the use of a nonselective NSAID and gastroprotective therapy or a COX-2 specific inhibitor is indicated. NSAIDs should be avoided or used with extreme caution in patients at risk for renal toxicity (e.g., intrinsic renal disease, age 65 or over, hypertension, congestive heart failure, and concomitant use of diuretics or angiotensin-converting enzyme (ACE) inhibitors].[10]

Topical capsaicin may improve hand or knee OA symptoms when added to the usual treatment; however, its use may be limited by cost and the delayed onset of effect requiring multiple applications daily and sustained use for up to 4 weeks. Intraarticular steroids are generally reserved for the occasional instance when there is a single painful joint or a large effusion in a single joint, and the pain is unresponsive to other modalities. For patients who do not respond to NSAIDs or acetaminophen, tramadol can be considered, but seizures have been reported as a rare side effect. Narcotics should be avoided if at all possible, but they may be considered in patients unresponsive to or unable to tolerate other medications. Glucosamine sulfate, chondrotin sulfate, or acupuncture may be effective in reducing pain symptoms from OA, and glucosamine may prevent progression of knee OA.[10,16] Osteotomy, arthroscopy, arthrodesis, and total joint replacement are the primary surgical approaches for OA. Candidates for arthroplasty are individuals with severe pain, impaired joint function, or those who have experienced declines in functional status that do not improve with nonpharmacologic and pharmacologic measures.

The costs of OA can be substantial (Table 112.1). The direct costs for drug therapy (which can easily exceed $60 per month)[17] are added to lost income related to time spent on physician and physical therapy visits, disability-related work absences, and absences related to surgery. The pain and functional disability associated with OA can contribute to social isolation and depression. Potentially modifiable risk factors include obesity, mechanical stress/repetitive joint usage, and joint trauma.[4] Weight reduction, avoidance of traumatic injury, prompt treatment of injury, and work-site programs designed to minimize work-related mechanical joint stress may be effective interventions for preventing OA.

References

1. CDC. Prevalence of arthritis—United States, 1997. MMWR 2001;50(17):334–6.
2. Facts about family practice. Kansas City, MO: AAFP, 1987; 30–7.
3. Lawrence RC, Helmick CG, Arnett FC, et al. Estimates of the prevalence of arthritis and selected musculoskeletal disorders in the United States. Arthritis Rheum 1998;41(5):778–99.
4. Felson DT, Zhang Y. An update on the epidemiology of the knee and hip osteoarthritis with a view to prevention. Arthritis Rheum 1998;41:1343–55.
5. Croft P. Review of UK data on the rheumatic diseases: osteoarthritis. Br J Rheumatol 1990;29:391–5.
6. Felson DT, conference chair. Osteoarthritis: new insights. Part I: The disease and its risk factors. Ann Intern Med. 2000;133: 635–46.
7. Jordan JM, Linder GF, Renner JB, Fryer JG. The impact of arthritis in rural populations. Arthritis Care Res 1995;8:242–50.
8. Hamerman D. The biology of osteoarthritis. N Engl J Med 1989; 320:1322–30.
9. Piperno M, Reboul P, LeGraverand MH, et al. Osteoarthritic cartilage fibrillation is associated with a decrease in chrondrocyte adhesion to fibronectin. Osteoarthritis Cartilage 1998;6: 393–99.
10. Felson DT, conference chair. Osteoarthritis: new insights. Part 2: Treatment approaches. Ann Intern Med 2000;133:726–37.
11. Dunning RD, Materson RS. A rational program of exercise for patients with osteoarthritis. Semin Arthritis Rheum 1991; 21(suppl 2):33–43.
12. Kovar PA, Allegrante JP, MacKenzie CR, Petersan MGE, Gutin B, Charlson ME. Supervised fitness walking in patients with osteoarthritis of the knee: a randomized controlled trial. Ann Intern Med 1992;116:529–34.
13. Brandt KD. Nonsurgical management of osteoarthritis, with an emphasis on nonpharmacologic measures. Arch Fam Med 1995; 4:1057–64.
14. Bradley J, Brandt K, Katz B, Kalasinski L, Ryan S. Comparison of an anti-inflammatory dose of ibuprofen, an analgesic dose of ibuprofen and acetominophen in the treatment of patients with osteoarthritis. N Engl J Med 1991;325:87–91.
15. Griffin MR, Brandt KD, Liang MH, Pincus T, Ray WA. Practical management of osteoarthritis: integration of pharmacologic and nonpharmacolic measures. Arch Fam Med 1995;4:1049–55.
16. Reginster JY, Deroisy R, Rovati LC, et al. Long-term effects of glucosamine sulphate on osteoarthritis progression: a randomized, placebo-controlled clinical trial. Lancet 2001;357:251–56.
17. Med Lett 2000;42:57–64.

113
Rheumatoid Arthritis and Related Disorders

Joseph W. Gravel Jr., Patricia A. Sereno, and Katherine E. Miller

Joint pain is a common presenting complaint to the family physician. The importance of accurate diagnosis of chronic joint pain (>6 weeks) has been even more accentuated in recent years by earlier use of drugs other than nonsteroidal antiinflammatory drugs (NSAIDs) for treatment of rheumatoid arthritis. Continuity in the doctor–patient relationship is also particularly important, as treatment must be continually reassessed and modified over time.

Joint Pain

Differential Diagnosis

The physician's first task for a patient presenting with complaints of chronic joint pain, stiffness, redness, warmth, or swelling (in the absence of trauma) is to precisely localize the pain. Pain in small joints (hands and feet) is usually pinpointed more easily than in large joints such as the shoulder, hip, or spine. If the pain is in fact periarticular, it may be characterized as local (e.g., bursitis, tendonitis, or carpal tunnel) or diffuse (e.g., polymyalgia rheumatica, polymyositis, fibromyalgia).

If the joint pain is truly articular, the differential diagnosis is narrowed by determining whether involvement is monarticular or oligoarticular (osteoarthritis, gout, pseudogout, septic arthritis) or polyarticular. Asymmetric polyarticular arthritides include ankylosing spondylitis, psoriatic arthritis, Reiter syndrome, and spondyloarthropathies. Symmetric polyarticular distribution suggests rheumatoid arthritis, systemic lupus erythematosus (SLE), Sjögren syndrome, polymyositis, and scleroderma. When pain is diffuse, not relatable to specific anatomic structures, or described in vague terms, fibromyalgia or psychological factors must be considered (see Chapter 114).

Correlation of joint pain with activity or at rest can differentiate inflammatory from mechanical conditions. In addition to joint pain, it is important to inquire about other symptoms, including joint stiffness, limitation of motion, swelling, weakness, and fatigue or other systemic symptoms. Stiffness is discomfort associated with joint movement after a period of inactivity. Morning stiffness and its duration (especially if >60 minutes) suggest an inflammatory arthritis such as rheumatoid arthritis, while patients with degenerative joint disease may complain of joint stiffness during the day rather than upon awakening. With neurologic conditions such as Parkinson's disease, this stiffness tends to be relatively constant (see Chapter 66). Finally, constitutional symptoms such as fatigue, malaise, weight loss, and fever are common with rheumatologic diseases. The patient's functional ability can be addressed by asking: "What is hard to do now that you could do before, and how does this affect your daily life?"[1] It is also useful to take an occupational history as well as inquire about hobbies or other activities requiring repetitive joint movements.

Physical Examination

A thorough physical examination is performed on all patients who present with joint pain, including the asymptomatic joints. Joints are examined for swelling, tenderness, deformity, instability, and limitation of motion. Synovial thickening or an articular effusion must be differentiated from periarticular soft tissue swelling. Joint instability can be tested by moving adjacent bones opposite to the direction they normally move; an unstable joint's adjacent bones move more than normally. Arthritic joints often have greater passive ranges of motion (ROMs) than active ROMs. The clinician must be familiar with normal ROMs to identify arthritic joints' limitations. Grip strength can be assessed with a blood pressure (BP) cuff inflated to 20 mm Hg. The maximal grip force (in millimeters of mercury) may be recorded to identify changes over time. It is also recommended to search for signs of systemic disease by looking for liver, spleen, or lymph node enlargement, neurologic abnormalities, oral or nasal ulcerations, rashes, nodules, and pericardial or pulmonary rubs.

Biologic factors contribute to examination variability, such as circadian changes in joint size and grip strength, among patients with rheumatoid arthritis observed over a 24-hour interval.[2] Hence it may be prudent to record the time of the examination in the medical record. Accurately recording the physical examination is important but can be cumbersome, particularly if many joints are involved. One way to address this problem is to use skeleton diagrams or draw stick figures in the medical record to illustrate involved joints.

From the history and physical examination the family physician may arrive at a short differential diagnosis of the patient's presenting joint complaints. Laboratory tests and imaging studies help to further reduce the diagnostic possibilities, but the initial history and physical examination remain the hallmarks of the diagnostic process.

Rheumatoid Arthritis

Rheumatoid arthritis (RA) is a chronic, systemic, inflammatory disease that affects mainly synovial joints in a symmetric distribution. In most patients the disease is chronic and progressive, although recent changes in the treatment of RA may serve to improve long-term outcomes. Rheumatoid arthritis occurs in all racial and ethnic groups. It is seen more commonly in women by a 3:1 ratio, and estimates of its worldwide prevalence generally are around 1%. RA occurs in all age groups but is more common with increasing age, peaking between the fourth and sixth decades of life.

The cause of RA is unknown, but there probably is not a single etiology. There appears to be a genetic predisposition, which is then triggered by unknown stimuli. This leads to proliferation of the synovial-lining cells and subsynovial vessels, forming a "pannus." Mononuclear and polymorphonuclear leukocytes invade, followed by a further inflammatory cascade involving such factors as proteases and cytokines.

Diagnosis

The diagnosis of RA is based primarily on clinical grounds rather than on the results of any gold standard test. The 1987 American College of Rheumatology (ACR) criteria for classification of RA (Table 113.1) may be used to assist the family physician with an early clinical diagnosis of RA. The temperature over RA-involved joints is often elevated, but the joints are usually not red. A pannus (caused by proliferating synovium) can sometimes be felt, as can soft tissue swelling. Early diagnosis and subsequent aggressive treatment of RA may reduce joint destruction and disability. Patients may also demonstrate classic late changes such as swan-neck and boutonniere deformities and ulnar deviation of the metacarpophalangeal (MCP) joints due to ligamentous laxity. The swan-neck deformity is characterized by flexion of the distal interphalangeal (DIP) and MCP joints and hyperextension of the proximal interphalangeal (PIP) joint, probably due to shortening of the interosseous muscles and tendons and shortening of the dorsal tendon sheath. The boutonniere deformity results from avulsion of the extensor hood of the PIP due to chronic inflammation, causing the PIP to pop up in flexion. The DIP stays in hyperextension. Hand flexor tenosynovitis is also common with RA. Atlantoaxial (C1-2) subluxation caused by ligamentous laxity is underrecognized and is a diagnostic consideration when RA patients complain of arm or leg weakness.

Extraarticular Manifestations

Because RA is a systemic inflammatory disease, it is not surprising that there are multiple extraarticular manifestations that help with the diagnosis; systemic symptoms such as fatigue, malaise, anorexia, weight loss, and fever may be prominent. Serious infections and hematologic malignancies such as non-Hodgkin's lymphoma are also more common in patients with RA. Renal disease is usually secondary to drug toxicities or amyloidosis. RA can cause pericardial effusions, pericarditis, myocarditis, and coronary arteritis. Pulmonary

---

Table 113.1. **1987 American College of Rheumatology Revised Criteria for Classification of Rheumatoid Arthritis**

Criterion	Definition
1. Morning stiffness	Morning stiffness in and around the joints lasting at least 1 hour before maximal improvement
2. Arthritis of three or more joint areas	At least three joint areas with simultaneous soft tissue swelling or fluid (not bony overgrowth alone) observed by a physician; the 14 possible joint areas are right or left PIP, MCP, wrist, elbow, knee, ankle, and MTP joints
3. Arthritis of hand joints	At least one joint area swollen as above in a wrist, MCP, or PIP
4. Symmetric arthritis	Simultaneous involvement of the same joint areas on both sides of the body; bilateral involvement of PIP, MCP, or MTP joints is acceptable without absolute symmetry
5. Rheumatoid nodules	Subcutaneous nodules over bony prominences or extensor surfaces or juxtaarticular regions, observed by a physician
6. Serum rheumatoid factor	Demonstration of abnormal amounts of serum rheumatoid factor by any method that has been positive in fewer than 5% of normal control subjects.
7. Radiologic changes	Radiologic changes typical of rheumatoid arthritis on posteroanterior hand and wrist roentgenograms, which must include erosions or unequivocal bony decalcification localized to or most marked adjacent to the involved joints (osteoarthritis changes alone do not qualify)

For classification of rheumatoid arthritis, at least four of these seven criteria must be met. Criteria 1 through 4 must have been present for at least 6 weeks. Patients with two clinical diagnoses are not excluded.
MCP = metacarpophalangeal; MTP = metatarsophalangeal; PIP = proximal interphalangeal.

complications include pleural effusions, pulmonary fibrosis, nodular lung disease, and possibly small airways disease. RA can also cause secondary Sjögren syndrome.

Subcutaneous nodules are present in 25% of patients and tend to occur in areas subject to pressure, such as the elbows and sacrum, although nodules have been found in many other areas, including (rarely) the heart and lungs. Sometimes these nodules need to be biopsied to differentiate from other entities such as gouty tophi and xanthomas.

Clinical Presentations

About 55% to 70% of patients with RA experience an insidious onset over weeks to months, 8% to 15% have an acute onset, and 15% to 20% have an intermediate onset, with symptoms developing over days to weeks.[3] Patients usually first experience small joint involvement in the hands and feet, particularly the PIPs and MCPs. Morning stiffness lasting more than 1 hour in these joints is suggestive of RA. Edema and inflammatory products are absorbed by lymphatics and venules with motion. Patients often have constitutional symptoms as well. Large joints become symptomatic later in the course of the disease. Symmetry of involvement is an important diagnostic feature that helps differentiate RA from other rheumatologic conditions. Muscle atrophy may develop around affected joints, causing weakness out of proportion to the pain. Finally, symptoms must present for more than 6 weeks to establish the diagnosis.

Other less common presentations include acute-onset RA and palindromic attacks. Acute-onset RA has the best long-term prognosis. Palindromic attacks are characterized by sudden, brief episodes of swelling of a large joint such as a knee, wrist, or ankle, thereby mimicking gout. Twenty to forty percent of patients with palindromic attacks progress to the chronic joint pain of RA.[4]

Clinical Course

The course of RA ranges from an intermittent type, marked by partial or complete remissions without need for continuous therapy (approximately 20% of patients), to either rapidly or slowly progressive disease. It is unclear whether treatment alters the final result of disabling arthritis in this progressive subset of patients, although pharmacologic treatment and other factors such as lowering environmental temperatures and humidity may lessen symptoms.

Laboratory Studies

Selected laboratory studies are best undertaken only after a careful history and physical examination are done. Rheumatoid factor (RF), antinuclear antibody (ANA), and erythrocyte sedimentation rate (ESR) are normally the most helpful laboratory tests to aid in the diagnosis of RA. However, positive results are not specific to RA and may be elevated with other connective tissue diseases. Further, the frequency of abnormal results in the absence of disease increases with age. Thus "arthritis panels" often confuse rather than clarify the situation.

Rheumatoid factor, an immunoglobulin M (IgM) antibody, is present in 80% to 90% of patients with RA; it is usually associated with severe, advanced disease. However, between 10% and 25% of patients with RA never have an abnormal RF. ANA titers should only be ordered in patients with systemic symptoms. ANA titers may be elevated in up to 30% of patients with RA; if abnormal, it is important to entertain the diagnoses of SLE, Sjögren syndrome, and scleroderma as well. Hemolytic complements (CH_{50}), C3 and C4 are normal or increased with early RA, whereas these levels are decreased in patients with SLE. The ESR is nonspecific and a rather insensitive marker for disease activity, although it may be helpful to differentiate exacerbations from other noninflammatory etiologies. Levels of C-reactive protein (CRP) reflect RA activity and may change more rapidly than the ESR—within 24 hours rather than days or weeks.

A complete blood count (CBC) can be helpful. Many patients with RA have a chronic, mild, normochromic normocytic anemia. Most have normal white blood cell (WBC) counts. Thrombocytosis may wax and wane along with disease activity.

Finally, synovial fluid analysis in RA shows yellowish white, turbid but sterile fluid without crystals, with more than 2000 WBC/mm^3 (but typically between 10,000 and 20,000) and with more than 75% polymorphonuclear leukocytes. Synovial fluid CH_{50} is lower than that in serum, and the synovial glucose is usually at least 30 mg/dL less than the serum glucose.

Imaging Studies

Plain radiographs are not helpful for most patients early in the course of RA, as they generally show only soft tissue swelling or osteoporosis. Radiographs are indicated only to help rule out infection or fracture, when the patient has a history of malignancy, when the physical examination fails to localize the source of pain, or when pain continues despite conservative treatment. Over time, radiographs of the hands and feet in particular may show joint space narrowing, periarticular osteoporosis, and eventually marginal bony erosions.

Rheumatoid Arthritis and Osteoarthritis

Because early rheumatoid arthritis and OA (see Chapter 112) are both common entities, the family physician must often differentiate between them. With RA a predominant early symptom is morning stiffness, whereas with OA pain increases through the day and with use. Joints are symmetrically involved in RA and are usually, in order of frequency, MCPs, wrists, and PIPs; DIPs are almost never affected. OA is often less symmetric and involves weight-bearing joints (hips, knees) and DIPs. Soft tissue swelling and warmth strongly suggest RA, as do periarticular osteopenia and marginal erosions on plain films. OA patients often have bony osteophytes on physical examination or radiography more commonly than soft tissue swelling. Laboratory findings in OA are normal, whereas RA patients often have elevated ESR, RF, CRP, CH_{50}, C3, and C4, as well as anemia, eosinophilia, and thrombocytosis.

Nonpharmacologic Treatment

There are numerous ways to measure treatment success for RA, including measurement of various laboratory parameters such as RF titer, ESR, and number of bony erosions on radiographs; but ultimately the patient's perception of success matters much more. The American Rheumatism Association Medical Information System (ARAMIS) and several multipurpose arthritis centers employ "the five D's" as dimensions for describing patient outcome: death, disability, discomfort, drug toxicity, and dollar cost. Different patients value each of these outcomes differently, which the family physician must keep in mind when proposing treatment options. Optimal management of RA utilizes community resources as well as a variety of treatment modalities.

Because RA is a chronic disease with no known cure, patients often are vulnerable to quack practitioners and charlatans. With the rising popularity of the Internet, patients have access to hundreds of unregulated Web sites, many of them commercial, which advertise thousands of (often expensive) "miracle cures." Patient education and an open relationship with the family physician help protect patients from misinformation.

Concomitant anxiety and depression are common among RA patients and are important to treat. The patient's psychological status is often more influenced by control of pain, socioeconomic factors, and the patient's support mechanisms (social and family support, sense of control, and coping skills) than by changes in disease status.[5]

Rest and Exercise

Resting affected joints during periods of exacerbation, including the use of splinting, may be helpful. At other times exercise to minimize periarticular muscle atrophy is necessary, often with the help of physical and occupational therapists. Water exercise has been found to help symptoms in some patients.

Dietary Therapy

There have been many proposed diets for RA, with only a few small studies showing positive effects with specific dietary manipulations. Clearly, excessive weight places more strain on inflamed joints, and dietary recommendations can be made to promote weight loss. Diets with supplemental fatty acids to eliminate precursors of arachidonic acid (and therefore diminish leukotrienes and prostaglandins) have been proposed to help, as have fasting and vegetarian diets,[6,7] but large studies have yet to be done.

Psychological Support

The same progression of responses observed with normal grieving (shock, anger, denial, resignation, and acceptance) is seen with chronic illnesses such as RA. Patients commonly fear becoming crippled, an issue that needs to be explicitly addressed by the family physician by providing education about the disease and available treatment options. It is important to consider the diagnosis of depression, and to treat if present. Sexuality may be affected because of pain, constitutional symptoms such as fatigue, and poor self-image secondary to deformities; the patient's partner may be reluctant to engage in sexual intimacy from fear of causing discomfort. So long as it does not prevent obtaining needed treatments, acting as "normal" as possible, rather than thinking of one-

self as a "rheumatoid patient," is often psychologically healthy. Families often need help coping with patients, particularly those with severe disease. If the RA patient becomes overly dependent on family or on the physician, the development of coping mechanisms will be delayed. Group psychotherapy, structured group support, and relaxation therapy, among other psychoeducational approaches, have been shown to strengthen coping strategies and to improve compliance with treatment regimens.[8]

Some particularly useful therapeutic modalities include local support groups and patient education. One specific example is the Arthritis Self-Help Course, organized by the Arthritis Foundation, which provides information on isometric exercise, relaxation techniques, joint protection, nutrition and techniques for coping with chronic illness. The Arthritis Foundation (800-283-7800) and the National Institute of Health's National Arthritis Clearinghouse (301-495-4484) are also good sources of information for patients.

Pharmacotherapy

Pharmacologic treatment of the RA patient has undergone a transformation during the last several years. Observations that radiographically detectable irreversible joint damage progresses most rapidly during the first years of RA have led to growing enthusiasm for early treatment with disease-modifying antirheumatic drugs (DMARDs). These agents may minimize synovitis and ultimately prevent irreversible joint damage.

Initiating early treatment by recognizing early signs of synovitis may be the physician's most important task. Two problems hinder the early use of these potentially valuable drugs. First, selecting the patients who should receive DMARDs and those who would do equally well with less toxic drugs is still problematic. Second, differentiating early RA from other entities is often clinically difficult and can delay treatment until after it could potentially help the most.

Aspirin and NSAIDs

There is no one consistently superior NSAID for treatment of RA. Some patients who do not respond to or tolerate a particular NSAID may respond to or better tolerate another; treatment is empiric (Table 113.2). It is important to keep in mind that aspirin-allergic asthmatic patients may develop severe bronchospasm and anaphylactoid reactions with any NSAID.[9]

An adequate trial with an NSAID requires the patient take a maximal dose for 3 weeks before changing to a different NSAID. It is usually best to switch to an NSAID from a different class. All NSAIDs can cause dyspepsia and gastrointestinal (GI) toxicity, and all except nonacetylated salicylates and selective cyclooxygenase-2 (COX-2) inhibitors can interfere with platelet function and prolong bleeding times. Other common side effects include renal toxicity and central nervous system (CNS) symptoms such as drowsiness, dizziness, and confusion. Misoprostol (Cytotec), a prostaglandin analogue, can prevent gastric ulceration caused by NSAIDs, although this combination has become less common since the introduction of the selective COX-2 inhibitors.[10]

Which NSAID is best to use for RA? Fries and colleagues[11]

Table 113.2. **Common NSAIDs Used for Rheumatoid Arthritis**

Arylcarboxylic acids
- Salicylic acids
  - Acetylated
    - Aspirin, extended release/enteric coated
  - Nonacetylated
    - Diflunisal (Dolobid)
    - Salsalate (Disalcid, Mono-Gesic)

Arylalkanoic acids
- Arylacetic acids
  - Diclofenac (Cataflam/Voltaren)
  - Naproxen (Aleve, Naprosyn)
  - Naproxen sodium (Anaprox)
- Arylpropionic acids
  - Ibuprofen (Advil, Motrin, Nuprin)
  - Ketoprofen (Orudis)
- Oxazolepropionic acids
  - Oxaprozin (Daypro)
- Heteroarylacetic acids
  - Tolmetin (Tolectin)
- Indole and indene acetic acids
  - Sulindac (Clinoril)
- Pyranocarboxylic acids
  - Etodolac (Lodine)

Enolic acids–oxicams
- Piroxicam (Feldene)

Nonacidic agents
- Nabumetone (Relafen)

Selective COX-2 inhibitors
- Celecoxib (Celebrex)
- Rofecoxib (Vioxx)

---

analyzed 2747 patients with RA who were followed up for an average of 3.5 years.[11] Consistently, the least toxic NSAIDs were coated or buffered aspirin, salsalate, and ibuprofen. The most toxic were indomethacin, tolmetin sodium, meclofenamate sodium, and ketoprofen. Drugs identified in this study as having high toxicity were no more clinically effective for RA treatment than those with lower toxicity.

Cyclooxygenase-2 Inhibitors. Traditional NSAIDs inhibit both COX-1 and -2. While COX-2 is a primary enzyme in the synthesis of prostaglandins which cause joint inflammation and pain, COX-1 leads to production of other prostaglandins, including those that are gastric-protective. Patients using selective COX-2 inhibitors experience fewer GI complications, but have similar pain relief, when compared with those using traditional NSAIDS.[12] As such, these medications are particularly useful in patients who are intolerant of the GI effects of older NSAIDs, or who are at high risk of GI complications (elders, patients with a history of GI bleeding, or who are taking corticosteroids).

Glucocorticoids.

Glucocorticoids are used in a variety of ways for treatment of RA. Glucocorticoid articular injections are often used for temporary suppression of RA in a joint, but generally this technique is not recommended more than three times per year. Common drugs for injection include short-acting preparations

such as hydrocortisone acetate; intermediate-acting preparations such as triamcinolone acetonide (Kenalog), triamcinolone diacetate (Aristocort), and methylprednisolone acetate (Depo-Medrol); and long-acting preparations such as dexamethasone acetate (Decadron-LA), and betamethasone sodium phosphate and acetate (Celestone, Soluspan). Lidocaine is usually injected with the steroid to maximize patient comfort.

Systemic glucocorticoids, most commonly prednisone, are often used as "bridge therapy," when initiating therapy with DMARDs, to keep patients comfortable for the 3 to 6 months before the DMARD takes effect. Systemic glucocorticoids may need to be continued for longer periods in patients with mostly constitutional symptoms compared to those with predominantly joint symptoms.

Low-dose prednisone may be especially useful in elderly patients as an alternative to other second-line drugs that carry more risk. Oral prednisone is given in as low a dose as is clinically effective; side effects are minimized if the dose is kept at or below 7.5 mg/day. Prednisone is usually given in a single morning dose as there is no clear advantage to dividing doses. Low-dose alternate-day therapy minimizes hypothalamic-pituitary axis suppression and infection risk, although other long-term side effects such as osteoporosis and cataract formation are unaffected.[13] Increased osteopenia probably occurs even with low-dose therapy, but measures such as vitamin D and calcium supplementation may help avoid it.

DMARDs

Radiographically detectable irreversible joint damage progresses most rapidly during the first years of RA.[14] One challenge is to develop early prognostic indicators to identify the patients who will develop severe RA and those who will not, so as to initiate needed treatment in the former group and avoid overtreatment in the latter. Evidence is growing that until these indicators are refined, in general the earlier that DMARDs are started by the family physician, usually in cooperation with a rheumatologist, the better the outcome (Table 113.3). There are few data available involving direct comparison of various DMARDs' effects on the long-term outcome of disease, and short-term trials often fail to detect significant differences.

Clinical responses to DMARDs vary considerably, ranging from complete remission to no response. Most clinicians give a trial of 4 to 6 months before changing therapy, either by increasing the dose, adding an additional DMARD, or substituting completely with a different DMARD. A relapse in symptoms usually occurs with discontinuation of these drugs, necessitating continuation even when patients are doing well. Patients often have relapses even without medication changes, necessitating frequent modification of treatment. In addition, toxic side effects may develop at any time necessitating changes in therapy.

Two of the newest DMARDs are the tumor necrosis factor (TNF) inhibitors and the pyrimidine synthesis inhibitor leflunomide. TNF is a cytokine which causes inflammation; it is present in the synovium of RA patients. TNF inhibitors have been used with good success in patients with refractory RA. However, they are expensive (a wholesale cost in 1999

Table 113.3. **Commonly Used Disease-Modifying Antirheumatic Drugs**

Type/generic (trade) name	Usual dosage	Toxic effects	Recommended monitoring
Gold compounds/ gold Na thiomalate (Myochrysine) Aurothioglucose (Solganal)	IM: 10 to 50 mg weekly until there is toxicity, major clinical improvement, or cumulative dose of 1 g; if effective, interval between doses is increased	Pruritus, dermatitis (up to 1/3 or patients), stomatitis, nephrotoxicity, blood dyscrasias, "nitroid" reaction: flushing, weakness, nausea, dizziness 30 min after injection	CBC, platelet count and U/A before each to every other dose
Antimalarial/ hydroxychloroquine (Plaquenil)	PO: 400–600 mg qd with meals, when good response obtained (usually 4–12 weeks) decrease to 200–400 mg qd	Retinopathy, dermatitis, muscle weakness, hypoactive DTRs, CNS	Ophthalmologic exam every 3 months (visual acuity, slit-lamp, funduscopic, visual field test), neuromuscular exam
Methotrexate (Rheumatrex)	PO: 7.5–15.0 mg weekly	Pulmonary toxicity, ulcerative stomatitis, leukopenia, thrombocytopenia, GI distress, malaise, fatigue, chills, fever, CNS, elevated LFTs/liver disease, ?lymphoma, infection, teratogenic	CBC with platelets, LFTs weekly for 6 weeks then monthly LFTs, U/A periodically, hCG prn
Azathioprine (Imuran)	PO: 50–100 mg qd, increase at 4-week intervals by 0.5mg/kg/day up to 2.4 mg/kg/day	Leukopenia, thrombocytopenia, GI, ?neoplasia if previous treatment with alkylating agents, teratogenic	CBC with platelets weekly for 1 month, 2×/month for 2 months then monthly, hCG prn
Sulfasalazine (Azulfidine)	PO: 500 mg/day, then increase up to 3 g/day	GI, skin rash, pruritus, blood dyscrasias, oligospermia	CBC, U/A q2 weeks for 3 months, then monthly for 9 months, then every 6 months.
Pyrimidine synthesis inhibitor/leflunomide (Arava)	PO: 20 mg/d	Diarrhea, rash, hepatic toxicity, teratogenic	LFTs regularly
TNF inhibitors/ etanercept (Enbrel)	SC: 25 mg twice weekly	Injection-site reaction, auto-antibody formation, infection	Only as indicated for symptoms of infection
Infliximab (Remicade)	IV: 3–10 mg/kg at 0, 2, and 6 weeks, then every 8 weeks	Headache, infusion reaction. lupus-like syndrome, infection	

CBC = complete blood count; CNS = central nervous system; DTR = deep tendon reflex; GI = gastrointestinal; hCG = human chorionic gonadotropin; LFTs = liver function tests; TNF = tumor necrosis factor; U/A = urinalysis.

of $1000–1300 per month) and have common local and systemic side effects.[9]

Leflunomide has been shown to be superior to methotrexate and sulfasalazine for symptomatic relief of rheumatoid arthritis, with serious adverse effects taking place in 0% to 2% of users.[15] It is teratogenic, and female patients who want to become pregnant after having taken the drug must take cholestyramine to bind the drug. Without the cholestyramine, the medication can be present in the body for up to 2 years.[9]

Surgery

When pharmacologic therapy and all other modalities have been attempted, surgery sometimes provides relief of pain. Ninety percent of elderly patients with severe incapacitating rheumatoid joint disease can expect excellent pain relief and satisfactory motion following total hip or knee replacement.[16]

Experimental Treatment and Therapy of the Future

Because of the chronicity, lack of a cure, and associated disability of RA, patients are vulnerable to many unproved "alternative" therapies. There is definitely a need for better therapies, making RA an intensely active area of current research.

Borrowing an idea from oncology to suppress immune responses maximally, combination therapy with DMARDs is being actively investigated. Other experimental therapies include high-dose intravenous prednisolone, total lymphoid irradiation, interferon-γ, interleukin-1 (IL-1) inhibitors, cyclosporine. monoclonal antibody antagonists against T-cell receptors, and phenytoin. Tetracyclines have been investigated for years based on the theory that infectious agents such as *Mycoplasma* or *Chlamydia* may cause RA.[17] The antibody-absorbing column Prosorba is used with plasmapheresis, and is Food and Drug Administration (FDA) approved for moderate to severe RA in patients refractory to methotrexate. It is expensive, and long-term efficacy is unknown.

Juvenile Rheumatoid Arthritis

Juvenile rheumatoid arthritis (JRA), a heterogeneous group of diseases formerly known as Still's disease, is clinically distinct from RA in adults. The cause is unknown. Hypotheses concerning etiology include infection, hypersensitivity, an autoimmune reaction, or a combination of these factors. Fortunately, at least 75% of children with JRA eventually have long remissions without significant residual deformity or loss of function. About 5% of patients with adult RA have symptoms beginning in childhood.

Clinical manifestations of JRA fall into three major categories: pauciarticular (40–50%), polyarticular (25–40%), and systemic (10–20%). These classifications are helpful for determining diagnosis, treatment, and prognosis in children with chronic arthritis. Consideration of other possibilities for arthritis, including mechanical or degenerative disorders, septic arthritis, reactive arthritis to extraarticular infection, connective tissue diseases, neoplastic disorders, endocrine disorders (type 1 diabetes mellitus, hyperthyroidism, hypothyroidism), and idiopathic pediatric joint pain syndromes is recommended. Diagnosis may be difficult without persistent, objective joint swelling. JRA is largely a diagnosis of exclusion.

In pauciarticular-onset disease, children have four or fewer joints involved during the first 6 months of symptoms. Large joints are primarily affected, often asymmetrically. Pauciarticular type I JRA affects girls 80% of the time, usually before age 4. Pauciarticular type II JRA affects boys 90% of the time, usually at age 8 or older, and many go on to develop spondyloarthropathies such as ankylosing spondylitis. There is a 10% to 30% risk of chronic iridocyclitis with this disease, and many authorities recommend frequent slit-lamp examinations to prevent scarring and loss of vision.

Polyarticular-onset JRA occurs mostly in girls, involving multiple joints including small joints. RF-positive polyarticular JRA tends to be more severe than RF-negative disease, both acutely and with long-term risk of severe arthritis.

Systemic-onset JRA is characterized by high intermittent fevers (>102°F), rash, hepatosplenomegaly, lymphadenopathy, arthralgias, and leukocytosis. Arthritis becomes chronic but the systemic symptoms generally dissipate with time.

The NSAIDs are generally used as first-line treatment for JRA as concerns about Reye's syndrome have discouraged use of salicylates, the drugs of choice in the past. As in adults, low-dose methotrexate is being used more frequently as the second-line drug of choice. Sulfasalazine has also been used with success. Gold compounds and antimalarials are probably less effective in JRA than in adult RA and are used less commonly. Long-term systemic glucocorticoids are effective for symptom relief but do not prevent joint damage and are best avoided in children if possible. Topical steroids are used for associated iridocyclitis. Physical and occupational therapy are important for protecting joint mobility; this is particularly important in JRA as children often do not complain of pain but simply stop using affected joints. The ultimate goal is to utilize these various treatments to encourage children with JRA to live active, normal lives. The family physician coordinates care with other members of the treatment team and offers necessary support to the child and family.

Systemic Lupus Erythematosus

Systemic lupus erythematosus (SLE) is a complicated rheumatologic disorder with a broad range of presentations. The incidence of SLE has more than tripled in the past 30 years, from 1.5/100,000 in 1950–79 to 5.6/100,000 in 1980–92.[18] The incidence among female patients is three times that of male patients, resulting in a prevalence of 1 in 700 for women between the ages of 20 and 64 years.[19,20] The disease incidence in African-American and Hispanic women in the same age group is higher than in their Caucasian counterparts.

The pathogenesis of SLE is not completely understood. Current theories include polyclonal B-cell activation and antigen stimulation resulting in the immune response that characterizes this complex disorder. Studies have pointed to a genetic factor contributing to the development of SLE. Twin studies have revealed a concordance rate among monozygotic twins to be as high as 30% to 50%. An association with human leukocyte antigen (HLA) groups DR2, DR3, DR4, and DR5 has also been found.

Laboratory Findings

Detection of antinuclear antibodies is a highly sensitive screening test for SLE, although it is not specific for SLE. A marginally elevated antinuclear antibodies titer is found in 2% to 5% of normal individuals.[20] About 95% of SLE patients have positive antinuclear antibodies titers that are more than two times higher than the normal limit identified by any given laboratory. Other antibodies identified in SLE patients include anti–double-stranded DNA, anti-DNA–histone complex, anti-Sm (Smith antigen), and anti-Ro (Robert antigen). Antibodies to dsDNA and Sm antigen are specific for SLE and have been associated with more severe cases. Anti-Ro antibodies are associated with various dermatologic manifestations of SLE. Anti–single-stranded DNA is not specific for SLE and therefore plays no role in diagnosis.

Up to 30% of SLE patients also have circulating antiphospholipid antibodies. These antibodies, known as the "lupus anticoagulant" may result in prolonged partial thromboplastin (PTT) and prothrombin (PT) times yet paradoxically result in an increased risk of thrombotic events. When counseling female patients who have circulating antiphospholipid antibodies, it is important to discuss the increased risk of spontaneous abortions. In fact, a history of recurrent spontaneous midtrimester abortions should trigger testing for antiphospholipid antibodies.

Systemic lupus erythematosus is characterized by a wide variety of presentations. The SLE classification system, revised in 1982 and updated in 1997, identifies 11 symptoms of the disease or systems affected in SLE patients. To con-

Table 113.4. **1982 American College of Rheumatology Revised Criteria for Classification of Systemic Lupus Erythematosus (updated 1997)**

Criterion	Definition
1. Malar rash	Fixed erythema, flat or raised, over the malar eminences, tending to spare the nasolabial folds
2. Discoid rash	Erythematous raised patches with adherent keratotic scaling and follicular plugging; atrophic scarring may occur in older lesions
3. Photosensitivity	Skin rash as a result of unusual reaction to sunlight, by patient history or physician observation
4. Oral ulcers	Oral or nasopharyngeal ulceration, usually painless, observed by physician
5. Arthritis	Nonerosive arthritis involving two or more peripheral joints, characterized by tenderness, swelling or effusion
6. Serositis	Pleuritis—convincing history of pleuritic pain or rub heard by a physician or evidence of pleural effusion
	OR
	Pericarditis—documented by electrocardiogram or rub or evidence of pericardial effusion
7. Renal disorder	Persistent proteinuria greater than 500 mg/24 hours or greater than 3+ on dipstick
	OR
	Cellular casts—may be red cell, hemoglobin, granular, tubular or mixed—on urine sediment
8. Neurologic disorder	Seizures or psychosis in the absence of offending drugs or known metabolic derangements
9. Hematologic disorder	Hemolytic anemia with reticulocytosis
	OR
	Leukopenia—less than 4,000/mm³ on 2 or more occasions
	OR
	Lymphopenia—less than 1,500/mm³ on 2 or more occasions
	OR
	Thrombocytopenia—less than 100,000/mm³ in the absence of offending drugs
10. Immunologic disorder	Anti-DNA in abnormal titer
	OR
	Anti-Smith antibody
	OR
	Positive finding of antiphospholipid antibodies based on:
	1. An abnormal serum level of IgG or IgM anticardiolipin antibodies
	2. A positive test result for lupus anticoagulant using a standard method
	3. A confirmed false-positive serologic test for syphilis known to be positive for at least 6 months
11. Positive ANA test	An abnormal titer of ANA by immunofluorescence or an equivalent assay at any point in time and in the absence of drugs known to be associated with drug-induced lupus syndrome.

For classification of SLE at least four of these 11 criteria must be met, either serially or simultaneously, during any interval of observation.

ANA = antinuclear antibody.

firm a diagnosis of SLE, patients must have at least four of the 11 criteria present either serially or simultaneously (Table 113.4).

Mucocutaneous Manifestations

The classic malar butterfly rash is present in only one third of patients. It usually presents abruptly after exposure to sunlight and lasts for several days or weeks. More commonly, patients have a patchy maculopapular rash on sun-exposed areas. Subacute cutaneous lupus erythematosus presents with a unique rash characterized by photosensitivity and superficial, nonindurated, nonscarring lesions.

One third to two thirds of SLE patients are markedly photosensitive, and sun exposure not only results in rash but also may induce a flare of systemic manifestations. Seventy percent of patients with photosensitivity have anti-Ro antibodies.[21]

Discoid lesions are raised plaques that may result in scarring. Other skin manifestations include alopecia, hyperpigmentation, and hives. Biopsy shows immunoglobulin deposition at the dermoepidermal junction. This finding is known as the lupus band test.[22]

Arthritis

Arthralgias are the most common complaint of SLE patients and are often present at the time of initial diagnosis. Up to 76% of patients develop arthritis associated with disease activity. It is difficult to differentiate the joint complaints of SLE patients from those of RA patients, but SLE patients usually present with pain out of proportion to the degree of synovitis. Also, in contrast to RA patients, SLE patients have soft tissue involvement that can result in joint deformity without evidence of cartilage involvement (Jaccoud arthropathy). Tendon rupture can also occur.

Serositis

SLE patients can have inflammation of the pleural, pericardial, and peritoneal membranes. Exudative pleural effusions are common but are usually small and therefore of little clinical importance.[22] Up to 29% of SLE patients have symptoms of pericarditis including pain, friction rub, and electrocardiographic changes.

Renal Disease

Renal involvement occurs in as many as 75% of patients, and the resulting glomerulonephritis is a major determinant of morbidity and mortality[23] (see Chapter 97). Immune complex deposition along the glomerular basement membrane results in an inflammatory response resulting in the characteristic glomerular findings. SLE patients should have an annual urinalysis to look for early evidence of proteinuria. Because of renal compensatory mechanisms, even urinalysis and measurement of serum creatinine or creatinine clearance may underestimate actual parenchymal damage. Renal biopsy obviously can document the type of lesion present in symptomatic patients, but biopsy results have not been useful for predicting disease progression. A persistently elevated serum creatinine level (>2 mg/dL) is the best predictor of future renal morbidity.[19]

Neurologic Disorder

Neurologic complaints among SLE patients vary from headache to seizures. Neuropsychiatric findings in SLE patients can be the result of direct injury from immune complexes and thrombotic events or of other organ dysfunction. Cognitive dysfunction has been documented in 20% to 70% of patients. Progressive decline in cognitive function leading to dementia has been reported but is rare. Laboratory studies in symptomatic patients are significant for antineuronal antibodies. Most patients have normal cerebrospinal fluid (CSF) findings, but CSF studies are important to exclude infectious causes of neurologic manifestations. Immunologic CSF studies (i.e., oligoclonal bands) are not specific in SLE patients. Studies comparing magnetic resonance imaging (MRI) to computed tomographic (CT) in symptomatic SLE patients have met with conflicting results. CT is more than adequate for diagnosing mass lesions or intracranial hemorrhage. MRI is more sensitive for picking up the signs of chronic vascular injury but may also identify incidental or clinically insignificant lesions.[23]

Hematologic Disorder

It is not surprising that most SLE patients have anemia of chronic disease. Up to 25% of SLE patients may also have an autoimmune thrombocytopenia; and 5% of these patients have severe thrombocytopenia with a platelet count as low as 20,000 cells/mm.[3,23] Further, SLE patients have higher incidences of both arterial and venous thromboembolic events. Some studies have shown up to a 50-fold increase in risk of myocardial infarction among reproductive-aged women with SLE, compared to age-matched controls.[18] Some investigators have recommended prophylactic aspirin or other anticoagulation treatment for all SLE patients, regardless of antiphospholipid status,[24] and aggressive anticoagulation with warfarin [with a goal international normalized ratio (INR) of 2.5–3.5] for patients with known antiphospholipid antibodies.[18]

Treatment

Treatment of SLE is best tailored to individual patients and their specific symptoms. Current treatment regimens have in general been successful in decreasing the morbidity and mortality associated with SLE. Current data indicate that more than 90% of patients survive at least 15 years.

All SLE patients are encouraged to minimize sun exposure and to use sunscreen. The most common complaint, arthralgias, can often be adequately treated with NSAIDs. Patients being treated long term with NSAIDs should be monitored periodically for renal and hepatic side effects. Glucocorticoids have also been used to treat severe symptoms, but they increase the risk of side effects. Cutaneous manifestations of SLE generally respond well to treatment with antimalarials (i.e., hydroxychloroquine or quinacrine). For treatment of skin disease resistant to either of these agents, small studies have used dapsone, azathioprine, gold, intralesional interferon, and retinoids. Methotrexate is more effective that placebo for moderate SLE without renal involvement.[18]

The foundation of treatment of SLE patients with renal disease has long been glucocorticoid therapy; however, this practice is being challenged. Patients with mild disease can often be managed with low-dose prednisone; patients with diffuse proliferative or severe focal proliferative glomerulonephritis may require a 2-month course of high-dose prednisone (1 mg/kg) followed by a prolonged taper. However, studies using cyclophosphamide have shown this drug to be effective as either a single agent or in combination with glucocorticoids, and more effective than glucocorticoids alone.[18,23]

Like treatment of renal disease, the mainstay for treating thrombocytopenia has long been glucocorticoids. Patients with disease resistant to glucocorticoid treatment may respond to splenectomy, but prior to consideration of splenectomy providers must weigh the benefits against the risks posed by decreased immune function. Cyclophosphamide and chemotherapeutic agents such as vincristine and procarbazine have also been used in patients with severe disease.[23]

Reiter Syndrome

Reiter syndrome, a form of reactive arthritis, is defined as "an acute, sterile synovitis associated with a localized infection elsewhere in the body"—generally a venereal infection.[25] The hallmark of Reiter syndrome is the triad of arthritis, conjunctivitis, and urethritis. Other symptoms found in patients with Reiter syndrome include sacroiliitis, enthesopathic symptoms with the most common sites being the Achilles' tendon and planter fascia, dactylitis, mucocutaneous lesions including stomatitis, circinate balanitis, and nail lesions.

The exact prevalence and incidence of Reiter syndrome is unknown. It has a five- to ninefold higher incidence in men and the prevalence is increased in patients positive for HLA-B27.[26] Laboratory findings in Reiter syndrome patients are usually nonspecific and do not confirm the diagnosis. There is no cure for Reiter syndrome, but the underlying illness should be treated.

Raynaud's Disease

During the late nineteenth century Maurice Raynaud described digital vasospasm that seemed to be cold-induced. He believed that this phenomenon, now known as Raynaud's disease, was due to changes in the CNS control over vascular innervation. Raynaud's phenomenon is classically described in patients who develop extremity blanching and numbness with cold exposure, followed by cyanosis and then erythema on rewarming. The fingers are affected most commonly, but the toes and ears may also be involved.

Raynaud's disease has been divided into primary and secondary forms. Primary Raynaud's is more common than the secondary form, occurring in 3% to 16% of the general population.[27] Secondary Raynaud's disease is far less common, developing in only 3% to 9% of patients; it is defined as Raynaud's phenomenon associated with the development of a connective tissue disease (most commonly scleroderma).

Evaluation of a patient in whom Raynaud's disease is suspected includes a thorough history and physical examination. Changes consistent with the disease can be reproduced in the office by immersing the patient's affected extremity in ice water. Antinuclear antibodies are positive in 17% to 26% of patients but do not predict disease progression.[28]

Investigations into the pathophysiology of Raynaud's disease have led to identification of a number of abnormalities, but the complete mechanism has not been fully established. Studies have shown that patients with this disorder have an abnormal adrenergic response. Neuropeptide release (possibly due to sensory nerve system damage) and endothelial factors have also been identified.[27–29]

It is important to discuss with patients the role of behavior modification. Conservative approaches to treatment include warm socks or mittens and cold avoidance. Patients are encouraged to stop smoking and to avoid vasoconstrictive drugs, such as amphetamines, cocaine, and over-the-counter decongestants. Caffeine may also exacerbate symptoms by causing a rebound vasoconstriction after an initial vasodilatation. In patients with vasospasm associated with emotional stress, relaxation and stress management strategies have also been helpful.

When conservative strategies fail, patients may respond to calcium channel blockers. Nifedipine has been the most widely studied at doses of 10 mg sublingually for immediate treatment of acute vasospasm or 30 to 60 mg of nifedipine taken on a chronic basis, although care must be taken to avoid symptomatic hypotension.

Scleroderma

Scleroderma, or systemic sclerosis, is a connective tissue disorder whose hallmark is tissue fibrosis. Systemic scleroderma is characterized by progressive fibrosis of the skin, lungs, heart, gastrointestinal tract, and kidneys. An association of limited skin involvement and late visceral involvement is known as CREST syndrome (*c*alcinosis, *R*aynaud's phenomenon, *e*sophageal dysmotility, *s*clerodactyly, and *t*elangiectasias). A localized form of scleroderma, known as linear scleroderma or morphea, exists when fibrotic changes are localized to the skin; it does not involve the GI tract.[30]

As with many other connective tissue diseases, scleroderma affects women three times as often as men, and the incidence in the United States is estimated to be 1/100,000 persons per year. The incidence peaks in women between the fifth and sixth decades of life.[31] Clinically, patients with systemic involvement present earlier in the disease course with mostly skin complaints.

The histopathologic features found in patients with scleroderma include diffuse small artery and arteriolar vasculitis with fibrinoid necrosis, intimal thickening, and mucopolysaccharide deposition. The exact mechanism responsible for excess deposition is unknown.

Because there is no cure for scleroderma, treatment goals are to optimize function of involved organ systems. The skin is involved in most patients, so it is important that patients use moisturizers to help maintain skin integrity. For patients with Raynaud's phenomenon, refer to the treatment guidelines discussed above. Patients may require antihypertensive drugs and treatment for gastroesophageal reflux. Immunosuppressive agents may slow disease progression.

Sjögren Syndrome

Sjögren syndrome is a rare, chronic inflammatory autoimmune disorder characterized by the combination of keratoconjunctivitis sicca (dry eyes), xerostomia (dry mouth), and rheumatoid arthritis or connective tissue disease. Vaginal dryness is also common, and restrictive lung disease is also associated.[32] Sjögren syndrome affects women 10 times more often than men. Other causes of xerostomia (i.e., drug-related) must be excluded prior to diagnosis. Unfortunately, treatment options are limited. The mainstay of treatment has long been the use of lubricants for the affected areas, as well as combined care provided by a rheumatologist, ophthalmologist, and family physician.

Ankylosing Spondylitis

Ankylosing spondylitis is an inflammatory disease of the spine that can also involve other joints and extraarticular organs. Ankylosing spondylitis is considered a seronegative spondyloarthropathy because patients with this disorder do not usually have a positive rheumatoid factor. The disease most commonly affects men (male/female ratio 5:1) and usually presents during adulthood (in the thirties). Onset after age 40 is unusual. More than 90% of Caucasian patients with ankylosing spondylitis have HLA-B27; however, it is important to remember that most patients with back pain who are positive for HLA-B27 do not have ankylosing spondylitis.

The key to diagnosis of ankylosing spondylitis is having a high clinical suspicion. More than half of the patients with ankylosing spondylitis initially present complaining of low back pain. Features that distinguish the low back pain associated with ankylosing spondylitis are morning stiffness, pain unrelieved with rest (rather, patients may try to "work the pain out"), and awakening from sleep with pain. Patients may also complain of pain in the buttocks or hips but usually do not complain of pain radiating below the knees. Many patients also have peripheral joint involvement. Large joints are more commonly involved than the small joints of the hands and feet. Enthesopathy is also common and can be demonstrated radiographically. Uveitis is a common extraarticular manifestation and often precedes joint disease.

The diagnosis can be confirmed radiographically if there is evidence of sacroiliitis. If the disease has progressed, patients have the "bamboo spine" seen on radiographs. The ESR is elevated. It is easy to measure the flexibility of the spine, which is decreased in most patients. The two most commonly used tests to assess spinal flexion are Schober's flexion test and Moll's lateral flexion test. Schober's test is performed by identifying, with the patient standing, the top of the sacrum and marking on the spine points 10 cm above this point and 5 cm below. In normal individuals, with forward flexion this distance increases by at least 5 cm. The Moll's lateral flexion test is performed by marking the point in the midaxillary line of the iliac crest and the point 20 cm above this site. When the normal patient bends to the opposite side, this distance increases by at least 3 cm.[33]

The goals of treatment of ankylosing spondylitis are to decrease pain and maintain functional status. NSAIDs are the drugs of choice to control inflammation and decrease pain. Oral prednisone has not been shown to be helpful. It is also important in the preservation of functional status to encourage the patient to strengthen back extensor muscles. At the present time, spinal ossification cannot be prevented, but function is better preserved if the patient's spine is ossified in an erect position in contrast to stooped over.

Psoriatic Arthritis

Psoriatic arthritis is a form of inflammatory arthritis seen in approximately 20% of psoriasis patients (see Chapter 115). Like ankylosing spondylitis, patients with psoriatic arthritis have serum negative for rheumatoid factor. Psoriatic arthritis is usually a mild form of arthritis that is sometimes difficult to distinguish from rheumatoid arthritis. Points for differentiating psoriatic arthritis from rheumatoid arthritis are as follows. Psoriatic arthritis is found in patients with psoriasis, distal joint involvement, tenosynovitis, and enthesopathy. Psoriatic arthritis is generally treated with NSAIDs or antimalarials. In up to one third of patients a flare in the skin disease may precede a flare of joint symptoms.[34]

Polymyalgia Rheumatica

Patients with polymyalgia rheumatica are usually over age 50 and present with complaints of myalgias and arthralgias referable to the hips and shoulders. The pain usually has been present for several months, and patients may suffer from constitutional symptoms including fatigue, weight loss, and low-grade fever. Patients complain that these muscles or joints are achy, and that they have morning stiffness.

Polymyalgia rheumatica has a prevalence of approximately 1 in 150 persons over age 50.[35] On clinical examination, patients are tender to palpation, but their strength is intact and creatine phosphokinase levels are normal, ruling out muscle destruction. The most characteristic finding in polymyalgia rheumatica is an elevated ESR. In fact, many patients have ESRs in excess of 100 mm/hr. It is estimated that one fourth to one half of patients with polymyalgia rheumatica also have temporal arteritis.

Some patients with polymyalgia rheumatica respond to NSAIDs, but the key to treatment has traditionally been a prolonged course of a corticosteroid. Patients generally respond quickly to prednisone at a dose of 10 to 20 mg/day. If a patient does not respond quickly to corticosteroids, consider other diagnoses. Patients often require daily steroids for a minimum of 2 years. When attempts are made to wean a patient off prednisone, the dose is decreased by only 1 mg/month.

Temporal Arteritis

Temporal, or giant cell, arteritis, like polymyalgia rheumatica, presents in persons over 50 years of age with an annual incidence 18/100,000 people over age 50. It is more common among the Caucasian population but has been reported in nonwhite patients; it occurs more commonly in women with a female/male ratio of 3:1. Most patients present with headache and may have tenderness to palpation over the temporal artery (see Chapter 63). Patients may also have visual symptoms including diplopia, hemianopia, or amaurosis fugax (visual changes usually described as a window shade being pulled down over one eye).

As with polymyalgia rheumatica, patients with temporal arteritis usually have an elevated ESR to levels higher than 100 mm/hr; confirmation of this diagnosis requires biopsy of the temporal artery. Biopsy results are more likely to be positive if specimens are obtained less than 24 hours after beginning treatment. It is recommended not to withhold treatment pending biopsy results in patients with a high clinical suspicion because of the risk of blindness. Patients are started on prednisone 1 mg/kg/day, and the dosage is decreased based on symptoms and the ESR.[36]

References

1. American College of Rheumatology Ad Hoc Committee on Clinical Guidelines. Guidelines for the initial evaluation of the adult patient with acute musculoskeletal symptoms. Arthritis Rheum 1996;39:1–8.
2. Boardman PL, Hart FD. Clinical measurement of the antiinflammatory effects of salicylates in rheumatoid arthritis. BMJ 1967;4:264–7.
3. Smith CA, Arnett FC. Diagnosing rheumatoid arthritis: current criteria. Am Fam Physician 1991;44:863–70.
4. Harris ED Jr. Clinical features of rheumatoid arthritis. In: Kel-

ley WN, Harris ED Jr, Ruddy S, Sledge CB, eds. Textbook of rheumatology, 5th ed. Philadelphia: Saunders, 1997;898–932.

5. Yelin E, Callahan LF. The economic cost and social and psychological impact of musculoskeletal conditions. Arthritis Rheum 1995;38:1351–62.

6. Volker D, Fitzgerald P, Major G, et al. Efficacy of fish oil concentrate in the treatment of rheumatoid arthritis. J Rheumatol 2000;27:2343–6.

7. Muller H, de Toledo FW, Fesch KL. Fasting followed by vegetarian diet in patients with rheumatoid arthritis: a systematic review. Scand J Rheumatol 2001;30:1–10.

8. Smedstand LM, Liang, MH. Psychosocial management of rheumatic diseases. In: Kelley WN, Harris ED Jr, Ruddy S, Sledge CB, eds. Textbook of rheumatology, 5th ed. Philadelphia: Saunders, 1997;534–9.

9. Abramowicz M, ed. Drugs for rheumatoid arthritis. Med Lett 2000;42:57–64.

10. Graham DY, White RH, Moreland LW, et al. Duodenal and gastric ulcer prevention with misoprostol in arthritis patients taking NSAIDs. Ann Intern Med 1993;119:257–61.

11. Fries JF, Williams CA, Bloch DA. The relative toxicity of nonsteroidal antiinflammatory drugs. Arthritis Rheumatol 1991;34: 1353–60.

12. Simon LS, Weaver AL, et al. Anti-inflammatory and upper gastrointestinal effects of celecoxib in rheumatoid arthritis: a randomized controlled trial. JAMA 1999;282;1921–8.

13. Bello CS, Garrett, SD. Therapeutic and adverse effects of glucocorticoids. U.S. Pharmacist Continuing Education Program no. 430-000-99-028-H01, August 1999.

14. Van der Heijde DM, van Leeuwen MA, van Riel PL, et al. Biannual radiographic assessments of hands and feet in a three-year prospective follow-up of patients with early rheumatoid arthritis. Arthritis Rheum 1992;35:26–34.

15. Shadic N. New developments in rheumatoid arthritis therapy. American College of Rheumatology anual scientific meeting, 1999.

16. Harris WH, Sledge CB. Total hip and total knee replacement. N Engl J Med 1990;323:725–31,801–7.

17. Langevitz, P, Livneh A, Bank I, Pras M. Benefits of minocycline in rheumatoid arthritis. Drug Saf 2000;22:405–14.

18. Ruiz-Irastorza G, Khamashta MA, Castellino G, et al. Systemic lupus erythematosus. Lancet 2001;357:1027–31.

19. Mills J. Systemic lupus erythematosus. N Engl J Med 1994;330: 1871–9.

20. Condemi J. The autoimmune diseases. JAMA 1992;268:2882–92.

21. Boumpas D, Fessier B, Austin H, et al. Systemic lupus erythematosus. Part 2. Dermatologic and joint disease, the antiphospholipid antibody syndrome, pregnancy and hormonal therapy, morbidity and mortality, and pathogenesis. Ann Intern Med 1995;123:42–53.

22. Osial T, Cash J, Eisenbeis C. Arthritis associated syndromes. Prim Care 1993;20:857–82.

23. Boumpas D, Austin H, Fessler B, et al. Systemic lupus erythematosus: emerging concepts. Part 1. Renal, neuropsychiatric, cardiovascular, pulmonary, and hematologic disease. Ann Intern Med 1995;122:940–50.

24. Wahl DG, Bounameaux H, et al. Prophylactic antithrombotic therapy for patients with systemic lupus erythematosus with or without antiphospholipid antibodies: Do the benefits outweigh the risks? A decision analysis. Arch Intern Med 2000;160(13): 2042–8.

25. Hughes R, Keat A. Reiter's syndrome and reactive arthritis: a current view. Semin Arthritis Rheum 1994;24(3):190–210.

26. Kirchner J. Reiter's syndrome. Postgrad Med 1995;97:111–21.

27. Kahaleh B, Matucci-Cerinic M. Raynaud's phenomenon and scleroderma. Arthritis Rheum 1995;38:1–4.

28. Adee A. Managing Raynaud's phenomenon: a practical approach. Am Fam Phys 1993;47(4):823–9.

29. Dowd P. Raynaud's phenomenon. Lancet 1995;346:283–90.

30. Sjögren R. Gastrointestinal motility disorders in scleroderma. Arthritis Rheum 1994;37:1265–82.

31. Edwards J, Porter J. Raynaud's syndrome and small vessel arteriopathy. Semin Vasc Surg 1993;6:56–65.

32. Lehrer S, Bogursky E, Yemmini M, et al. Gynecologic manifestations of Sjögren's syndrome. Am J Obstet Gynecol 1994; 170:835–7.

33. Merritt J, McLean T, Erickson R, et al. Measurement of trunk flexibility in normal subjects: reproducibility of three clinical methods. Mayo Clin Proc 1986;61:192–7.

34. Gladman D. Toward unraveling the mystery of psoriatic arthritis. Arthritis Rheum 1993;36:881–3.

35. Salvarini C, Gabriel S, O'Fallon M, Hunder G. Epidemiology of polymyalgia rheumatica in Olmstead County, Minnesota, 1970–1991. Arthritis Rheum 1995;38:369–73.

36. Pountain G, Hazleman B. Polymyalgia rheumatica and giant cell arteritis. BMJ 1995;310:1057–9.

114

Selected Disorders of the Musculoskeletal System

Jeffrey G. Jones and Doug Poplin

Problems of the Soft Tissues

Fibromyalgia

Fibromyalgia (FM) is a common musculoskeletal syndrome characterized by generalized pain, fatigue, and a number of associated symptoms. The condition has formerly been called fibrositis and psychogenic rheumatism. The condition is confusing in that there is considerable overlap between FM symptoms and those of other conditions such as myofascial pain syndrome, temporomandibular joint syndrome, and chronic fatigue syndrome.

Diagnostic Criteria

The diagnosis of FM has been standardized through the use of specific accepted diagnostic criteria (Table 114.1, Fig. 114.1).

Epidemiology

At any given time, approximately 3% to 6% of the general population meet the criteria for diagnosis of FM.[1] Studies also show that women more commonly meet the diagnostic criteria.[2] The condition most commonly begins during the thirties or forties, although it may occur at any age. There is a familial aggregation of fibromyalgia, suggesting that there is a genetic predisposition to the condition.[3]

Clinical Features

Widespread pain and tenderness are the cardinal features of FM. Stiffness after being in one position for a prolonged period, including morning stiffness, is common. Frequently weather changes, emotional stress, unaccustomed physical activity, and menses worsen the symptoms. Although patients often report a sensation of swelling, there is usually no objective evidence of this on examination. People with FM may be more sensitive to pain throughout the body, not just in the areas of tender points. For example, it is common to see increased visceral pain in patients with FM, so associated syndromes and symptoms, such as irritable bowel syndrome, dysmenorrhea, mitral valve pro-

lapse, interstitial cystitis, and migraine headaches are more common.[1] One must also be aware that tender points are common sites for pain even in the general population, who have an average of 3.7 positive tender points.[4] Pain perception is also influenced by a number of other factors including aerobic fitness, quality of sleep, and depression.[5] Thus a condition based on pain sensation may encompass a number of other conditions.

Most patients with FM complain of fatigue (see Chapter 55), and many have poor-quality sleep (see Chapter 56). The relation between FM and sleep disturbance is not as clear as once thought.[1] Improvement in FM symptoms with pharmacologic treatment does not necessarily correlate with an improvement in sleep.[6] FM patients also have a higher incidence of migraine and tension headaches than the general population[1] (see Chapter 63). Approximately 84% of people with FM complain of numbness or tingling somewhere in the body.[7] Echocardiographic evidence of mitral valve prolapse is seen in up to 75% of FM patients.[8] Patients with FM have a higher incidence of depression, and controversy remains as to whether FM symptoms are a manifestation of a psychosomatic syndrome, or, conversely, depression results from chronic pain (see Chapters 32 and 61).

Differential Diagnosis

Early rheumatoid arthritis (and other rheumatic conditions), polymyalgia rheumatica, and hypothyroidism are included in the differential diagnosis and can generally be excluded with an appropriate history and laboratory analysis. Infections, especially human immunodeficiency virus (HIV), hepatitis, and subacute bacterial endocarditis, can also present similarly to FM. Neoplastic conditions and endocrine problems may cause similar clinical presentations.

Diagnosis

Fibromyalgia can usually be reliably diagnosed by a typical history, physical examination consistent with the appropriate number of tender points, and appropriate laboratory studies.

Table 114.1. **1990 American College of Rheumatology Diagnostic Criteria for Fibromyalgia**

1. History of widespread pain of at least 3 months' duration. This pain must be present in the axial skeleton as well as all four quadrants of the body.
2. Pain must be present in at least 11 of 18 of the following paired tender points on digital palpation.
   a. Occiput: at the suboccipital muscle insertions
   b. Cervical: at the anterior aspects of the intertransverse spaces at C5–C7
   c. Trapezius: at the midpoint of the upper border
   d. Supraspinatus: at the origins above the scapular spine near the medial border
   e. Second rib: at the second costochondral junctions
   f. Lateral epicondyle: 2 cm distal to the epicondyles
   g. Gluteal: in upper outer quadrants of buttocks in anterior fold of muscle
   h. Greater trochanter: posterior to trochanteric prominences
   i. Knees: at the medial fat pad proximal to the joint line

These points should be palpated with approximately 4 kg of pressure. For the tender point to be considered painful, the patient must state that it is painful and not merely tender.

Source: Wolfe F, Smythe HA, Yunus MB, et al. The American College of Rheumatology 1990 Criteria for the Classification of Fibromyalgia. 1990;33:160–72, with permission.

The laboratory evaluation, which should include a thyroid-stimulating hormone (TSH) assay, erythrocyte sedimentation rate (ESR), and an antinuclear antibody (ANA) test, helps to rule out other conditions but does not rule in FM.

Management

Patient Education. Important to the management of this condition is a thorough explanation of the condition. Patients have often seen many physicians while trying to "find a cure." It is often therapeutic for patients to find a physician who can provide them with a diagnosis. The Arthritis Foundation (1314 Spring Street NW, Atlanta, GA 30309) can provide additional information.

Behavior Modification. Modifying behavior often involves emphasis on activities that help to lessen symptoms. Patients often must be reminded that caffeine, especially near bedtime, may worsen an already poor sleep pattern. Helping patients to reframe their situation into one with less victimization, along with other cognitive therapy interventions, can also be useful. Directing the patient toward self-management of symptoms through relaxation training, meditation, or electromyographic (EMG) biofeedback can help control symptoms while shifting the locus of control back to the patient.

Medication. Amitriptyline (Elavil and others) and cyclobenzaprine (Flexeril) have been studied and found to be helpful for FM. They are both tricyclic compounds, although cyclobenzaprine does not have antidepressant activities. Although it is generally acknowledged that these medicines are helpful, the mechanism of action is not clear. Low doses are recommended to start, and the doses can be slowly increased. The goal of therapy is to improve sleep and lessen symptoms but not cause a "hangover." The drugs are sometimes not well tolerated, usually due to anticholinergic side effects or vivid dreams. Zolpi-

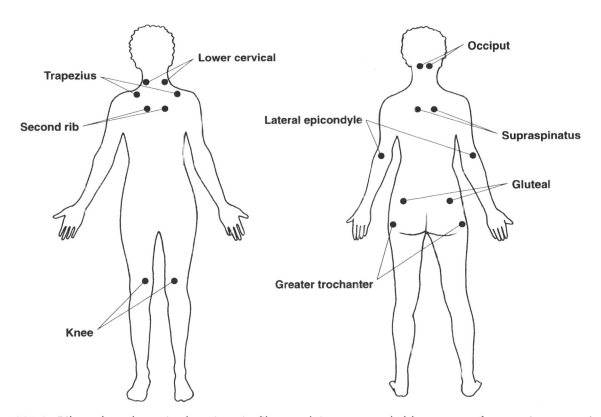

Fig. 114.1. Bilateral tender point locations in fibromyalgia are remarkably constant from patient to patient.

dem (Ambien) may be a reasonable alternative.[1] If one is not able to control symptoms with the above medicines, the selective serotonin reuptake inhibitors offer another potential option. The nonsteroidal antiinflammatory drugs (NSAIDs) are not usually highly effective in treating this condition.

Exercise. Because it is rare for patients to have lasting improvements without exercise,[1] this modality should be emphasized in all cases. Often these patients are deconditioned, and one must start at a low work load to avoid flaring symptoms. Water exercise classes, especially in heated pools, tend to be effective. Other exercises to consider include walking, riding stationary bicycles, and engaging in low-impact aerobics. Exercise programs that incorporate elements of muscle stretching, muscular endurance, and aerobic fitness tend to be most effective. Regardless of the specific exercise program, it must be approached slowly and consistently to produce optimal results.

Prognosis

Generally, FM patients have chronic symptoms, but their resulting disability is a function of their willingness to accept responsibility for managing these symptoms. A sense of helplessness is a strong negative predictor of outcome in FM patients.[9] Only about 5% of FM patients have a complete remission.[10] Patients may need to be guided away from costly and untested treatments. Patients should be counseled vocationally into returning to nonphysically demanding work. As with many other chronic conditions, the empathetic, optimistic physician's guidance and support can be therapeutic and help to empower FM patients to cope effectively with their conditions.

Myofascial Pain Syndrome

Definition

Myofascial pain syndrome (MPS) is the name given to the common clinical syndrome of persistent regional or local pain in muscle(s) accompanied by "trigger points" on palpation of the involved muscles. The trigger point has local tenderness, the presence of a "taut band," and a twitch response. Palpation of the trigger point characteristically produces pain referred beyond it.[11] The syndrome may be acute and is often seen after strain or trauma to a muscle. Nonmusculoskeletal symptoms, such as fatigue, are unusual. The pathophysiology is not well understood.

The terminology used to describe this and related problems is not standardized, adding to the confusion. Many authors see MPS as an entity distinct from FM, although there is some thought that MPS and FM represent two extremes of a single disorder.[12] It is not unusual for a patient to have symptoms characteristic of both syndromes.

Clinical Features

Patients generally present to the physician with complaints of localized pain and stiffness. The pain may be related to specific muscle activity and may be progressive. It may eventually become chronic and result in a sleep disorder or chronic pain syndrome. Physical examination of the patient generally reveals local muscle pain. Trigger points may not be noted unless specifically sought. Knowledge of typical pain radiation patterns and trigger point locations is useful to the physician (Fig. 114.2). In our experience, MPS involving the shoulder and neck is most common, although it may involve any muscle.[13]

Management

Patients with MPS generally enjoy a good prognosis. The most critical elements of treatment include patient education and stretching of the involved muscle. Physical therapy may be useful for patient education, stretching instruction, and perhaps "spray and stretch," a procedure where a local vapocoolant spray is used over the involved area immediately before stretching. In resistant cases, injection of the trigger point with local anesthetic, followed immediately by stretching, can

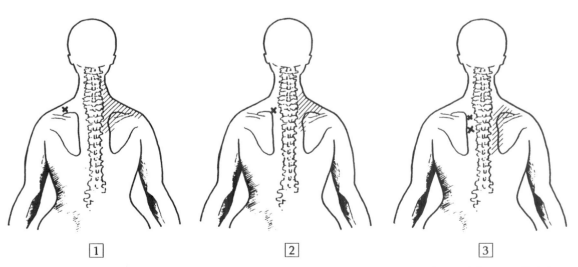

|1| |2| |3|

Fig. 114.2. Myofascial pain syndromes involving the neck and shoulder girdle. The involved muscles are (1) trapezius, (2) levator scapula, and (3) rhomboids. The distribution of pain is indicated by parallel lines, and the common trigger points are indicated by an X.

produce dramatic, prolonged relief. Multiple injections may be required. For some muscle groups, physical strengthening may help resolve the condition and help to prevent recurrence. MPS is less often associated with other medical conditions, including psychological conditions, than is FM. In MPS patients the use of biofeedback and relaxation therapy may help to teach them to discriminate between unnecessarily tense muscles and relaxed ones. Improved skills in dealing with life's stresses may be useful for treatment and prevention in these patients.

Complex Regional Pain Syndrome

Complex regional pain syndrome (CRPS) has replaced reflex sympathetic dystrophy (RSD) as the designation for a syndrome characterized by pain that is out of proportion to the inciting event, loss of function, and evidence of autonomic dysfunction. CRPS is subdivided into types I and II based on the nature of the initial injury. Cases of CRPS type I develop after nonspecific and often minor trauma to the affected area. Cases of CRPS type II evolve from definite injuries to peripheral nerves.[14]

Diagnosis

The clinical criteria[14] for diagnosis include the following: (1) diffuse pain, which is often nonanatomic and is frequently out of proportion to the initial injury; the pain may develop at any time relative to the injury; (2) loss of function, which can include any activity or motion impairment associated with the pain; and (3) sympathetic dysfunction, which includes some objective evidence of an autonomic dysfunction as represented by skin, soft tissue, or blood flow changes. It might also include atrophy of the skin or subcutaneous tissue, edema, Sudeck's osteoporosis, or a characteristic bone scan.

Complex regional pain syndrome usually has three phases: acute, dystrophic, and atrophic.[14] The *acute phase* is generally thought to be associated with signs of sympathetic denervation or underactivity, resulting in increased skin temperature, increased hair and nail growth, and edema. The acute phase usually lasts up to 3 months after the injury. The *dystrophic phase* is associated with hyperactivity of the sympathetic nervous system, which commonly translates into a burning pain, cold intolerance, cool skin, decreased hair and nail growth, hyperhidrosis, decreased range of motion, and atrophy. Behavioral and emotional changes are often seen during this phase and are often related to protecting the painful body part. The *atrophic phase* may be associated with decreased pain but is generally associated with irreversible changes in skin, subcutaneous tissue, and muscle. Fibrosis and contractures may develop. Testing helpful in documenting CRPS includes objective measurement of skin temperature (e.g., with thermography); measurement of blood flow (e.g., plethysmography or Doppler assessment); roentgenographic changes (e.g., with a three-phase bone scan or on plain radiographs); and response to neural blockade. Referral to an anesthesiologist for a trial of blockade, when accompanied by objective verification of a successful block and associated decrease in signs and symptoms, can be helpful from both diagnostic and treatment points of view.[15]

Management

Treatment of CRPS often requires multiple modalities and should not be associated with a further increase in pain or use of narcotics. For optimal effects, any treatment requires active participation of the patient. Effective treatment generally involves the following.

Physical Therapy. The early use of physical therapy is a mainstay of the successful treatment of patients with CRPS. Pain control can be enhanced through desensitization exercises and transcutaneous electrical nerve stimulator (TENS) units. Functional loss and atrophy can be minimized through exercises to mobilize and strengthen the affected area.[14]

Invasive Treatments. Chemical blockade, such as a stellate ganglion blockade or a regional Bier block, is often helpful early in the course of CRPS.[15] Multiple blocks may be required. Persistent cases have been treated with surgical sympathectomies and with implanted spinal cord electrical stimulators.[16]

Noninvasive Medications. A variety of medications have been used for CRPS,[17] but none is consistently effective, making treatment choices a largely empiric process. This inconsistency may represent varied pathophysiologic mechanisms in CRPS. The most commonly used oral medications include NSAIDs for nonnarcotic pain relief, low-dose tricyclic antidepressants, and membrane-stabilizing anticonvulsants such as gabapentin.[14] Other medications that have resulted in some success include short-term use of corticosteroids, calcium channel blockers, α- and β-adrenergic antagonists, and intramuscular calcitonin. Useful topical regimens include lidocaine patches and capsaicin cream 0.025% applied four times daily to the affected area.[17]

Psychotherapy. It is important for the patient to maintain a positive emotional outlook, and psychotherapy directed to this goal may be useful. Additionally, therapy directed against some of the associated emotional consequences of CRPS may be useful, as anxiety, depression, and even suicide attempts are not uncommon in this group of patients.[17] Biofeedback is sometimes useful for dealing with CRPS.

Prevention

Although primary prevention is not possible for CRPS, secondary prevention is helpful. The earlier CRPS is diagnosed and treatment started, the better is the prognosis. Because psychological issues become more predominant the longer CRPS continues, addressing these issues early may also help minimize suffering and prevent suicide.

Family Issues

Family members may need help understanding why inconsequential trauma may cause such major problems. Including the family members in explanations may help ensure understanding and facilitate rapport, which is essential for treatment of this condition. Occasionally, the family, along with many health care professionals, views the symptoms of CRPS as somatization. Explanations to the family that CRPS is not primarily a psychological problem (but that it may have marked psychological implications) may help preserve family function.

Neuroma

A neuroma is a benign mass composed of disorganized axons and scar tissue. In any location it may cause pain but is especially sensitive when at a location that receives trauma or pressure. Neuromas commonly occur after trauma to a nerve or in the proximal portion of the nerve if it has been transected. The neuroma may form long after the initial nerve trauma. In the upper extremity, the most common locations for a neuroma are in the thumb (bowler's thumb) and the sensory branches of the radial nerve in the distal forearm. Treatment depends on the degree of symptoms, but it is not unusual for symptomatic neuromas of the upper extremities to require surgical excision. In the lower extremities, Morton's neuroma (MN) is the most common type. It represents an entrapment neuropathy of the interdigital nerve and is a common cause of forefoot pain, especially in women. The nerve is normally about 2 mm in diameter and generally does not cause symptoms until it reaches a size of 5 mm.[18]

Diagnosis

Morton's neuroma can usually be diagnosed clinically because of its characteristic sharp or burning pain on the plantar aspect of the foot, radiating to the tip of one or two toes. It most commonly involves the nerve in the third–fourth intermetatarsal space. The pain is usually made worse by walking, standing, or postures with the toes extended (e.g., standing on tiptoes). The physical findings include tenderness or reproduction of the pain when the interspace is compressed in a dorsoplantar or lateral direction. Numbness or tingling of the involved toes is common.

Management

This condition can often be managed through conservative means. Initially, a broad, soft shoe without elevated heels is used. A metatarsal bar support that removes pressure from the metatarsal head is also helpful. NSAIDs may also be useful. An orthotic device that stabilizes the foot in a neutral position is often helpful. Local injections of steroids may also be effective.[19] In cases that do not respond to conservative treatment, surgical resection of the neuroma (interdigital neurectomy), which leaves a residual numbness of the innervated toes, or release of the metatarsal ligament may be used. Approximately 80% of patients respond favorably to surgery.[20]

Prevention

The factor most conducive to prevention of MN is shoe selection. People should be encouraged to use a shoe wide enough to accommodate the foot comfortably and to avoid high-heeled shoes.

Dupuytren's Contracture

Dupuytren's contracture (DC) is a disease of the palmar and digital fascia characterized by a progressive fibrosis of the palmar aponeurosis, resulting in a flexion deformity of the fingers. The condition is most common in white-skinned races, especially those of Celtic origin.[21] It is two to seven times more common in men than women. It is seen most commonly between the ages of 50 and 70 years. DC is commonly seen in association with alcoholism, hyperlipidemia, epilepsy, and diabetes. One researcher found a 40% co-occurrence between Dupuytren's and epilepsy.[22] This connection is thought to be due to the genetic transmission common to the two conditions. In another study, DC was noted in 42% of 150 diabetics, compared to 18% of a control group.[23] This association is strong enough that physicians need to be vigilant about diagnosing diabetes when treating patients with DC (see Chapter 120). The pathognomonic sign of DC is a nodule in the palm, usually located at the base of the ring finger. The other fingers or thumb may also be involved but less commonly than the ring finger. This nodule may be painful or pruritic. The right hand is more commonly affected (regardless of hand dominance), but the condition is bilateral about half of the time. The diagnosis is usually easy and is made by palpating a characteristic nodule or cord in the typical palmar location (Fig. 114.3). If left untreated, the flexion contracture progresses. There are no proved nonsurgical methods for treating DC.[21] No one surgical technique has been found that is universally effective, but some type of fasciotomy is generally required. The optimal timing of surgical therapy is also not clear, but most authors recommend surgery when the metacarpophalangeal (MCP) joint contracture reaches 30 degrees or more. After surgery, the recurrence rate is about 50% if the patients are followed up for at least 5 years.[24]

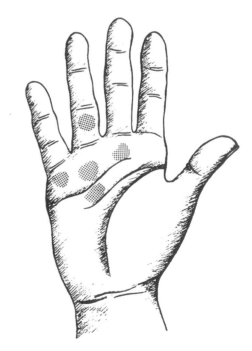

Fig. 114.3. Characteristic sites of palmar nodules (stippled areas) of Dupuytren's contracture. The right hand is more commonly involved, regardless of hand dominance.

Ganglion Cysts

Ganglion cysts, which are common benign tumors, may arise from a joint capsule or the synovial sheath of a tendon. They may maintain their connection to the synovial sheath or joint, in which case they may vary in size. The dorsal or volar wrist is the region where most ganglia occur. Ganglia may occur at any age but are most commonly seen between the ages of 20 and 40 and in women.[25] Ganglia may be obvious or occult. With occult cysts, patients may complain of a dull ache and tenderness, but no mass is palpable.[26] They may become evident by causing a compression neuropathy or compartment syndrome. This condition should be kept in mind when wrist pain of unknown etiology is encountered. Magnetic resonance imaging (MRI) or ultrasound techniques may be helpful in assessing the anatomy of the wrist when an occult cyst is suspected.

With obvious cysts the onset is usually insidious, although some patients report a history of acute onset associated with heavy use or trauma. Patients may report weakness or altered range of motion of the wrists or fingers. Radiation of pain into the forearm is not unusual. The examination reveals a firm, usually nontender cyst that feels like a small marble under the skin. A characteristic history and physical examination is usually sufficient to make the diagnosis, but aspiration of jelly-like fluid confirms the diagnosis. A large-bore needle is usually required because of the viscous nature of the fluid. Instillation of steroids into the cyst may be helpful. If patients are symptomatic or if the appearance is unacceptable to the patient, surgical removal is the treatment of choice. When counseling patients or assessing the effectiveness of treatment, one must remember that approximately half of these cysts disappear without therapy[26] and that regardless of therapy recurrence is common.

Abnormalities of Bone

Benign Tumors

The primary care physician refers most of the patients found to have tumors involving bone, but it is helpful to have some understanding of these conditions in order to have a better idea of what to expect for the patient. No one system of classification is entirely satisfactory for all tumors, and a comprehensive inclusion of all types of tumors is beyond the scope of this chapter. Thus only the most common representatives of bone-related problems are discussed: benign tumors, neoplastic tumors, and miscellaneous problems.

Osteochondroma

Osteochondroma, also called exostosis, may be thought of as a developmental aberration of epiphyseal bone growth.[27] Bony projections, covered with cartilage caps, are found. Males are affected three times more commonly than females. The lesions are often single but can be part of a hereditary condition called osteochondromatosis. The lesions occur most commonly in the long bones of the extremities. They occasionally result in derangement of epiphyseal growth, causing bowing or shortening of the bones.

Growth of the osteochondroma usually stops at the time of epiphyseal closure.

Osteoma

Osteomas are benign projections of densely sclerotic bone from cortical surfaces, usually the facial bones or skull.[27] They may arise at any age and are usually of little clinical significance unless they obstruct a sinus, impinge on the brain, or cause some cosmetic concern. They do not tend to transform into other types of lesions and do not usually require treatment unless they cause symptoms.

Osteoid Osteoma

Osteoid osteomas are usually found in young adults. They are twice as common in males as females. They are usually painful, which prompts the patient to seek medical help. The pain is usually nocturnal and dramatically responsive to aspirin. They are usually located at the ends of the tibia and femur. They appear as small radiolucent foci surrounded by densely sclerotic bone (Fig. 114.4). They can usually be managed by local excision.[28] When the lesions are larger than 2 cm in greatest dimension, they are, by definition, osteoblastomas.

Chondroma

Chondromas are composed of mature hyaline cartilage. They frequently arise within the interior of a bone and so are called enchondromas. They occur singly in either sex and most commonly between the ages of 20 and 50. There are genetic conditions where these tumors occur multiply, the most common of which is Ollier's disease. With the single chondroma, transformation into a sarcoma is rare. Most of the single lesions occur in the small bones of the hands or feet. Most of the lesions are asymptomatic and may be noticed incidentally or by some bone deformation. They rarely result in pain through pathologic fracture. Excision of the lesions may be required to exclude the possibility of chondrosarcoma,[27] a rare transformation except in individuals with Ollier's disease, where multiple enchondromas are seen.

Giant Cell Tumor

A relatively rare lesion, the giant cell tumor is most commonly seen in individuals between the ages of 20 and 50. Patients usually present with local pain or functional dysfunction related to the location of the tumor. About half of these tumors occur in the knee. Radiographs reveal the typical, large lytic "soap-bubble" lesions. The cell of origin of these tumors is not clear, and the biologic behavior is somewhat erratic. Although most of these tumors are benign, they may be aggressive, eroding into the joint space and surrounding tissues. Treatment is usually conservative, with curettage or conservative resection. However, after treatment, the tumors commonly recur, although it may be years later. Up to 4% of these tumors metastasize to the lungs, usually after surgical resection.[27]

Malignant Bone Tumors

Malignant tumors of bone may originate in the bone or metastasize to the bone. There are definite patterns in tumor type based on the age of the patient.

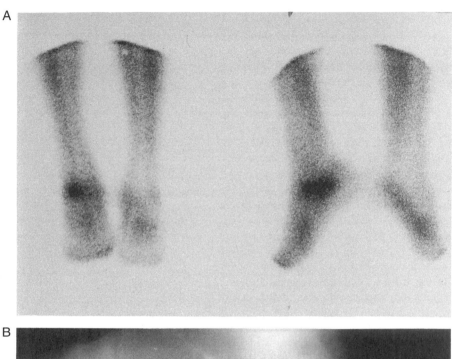

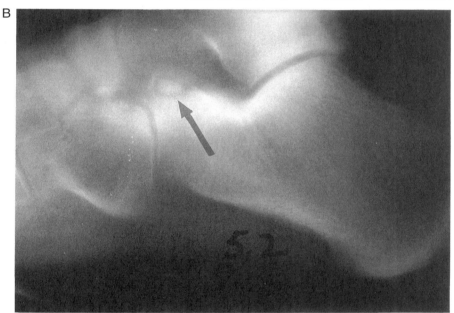

Fig. 114.4. Young woman with persistent foot pain and normal plain films of the foot. (A) Bone scan revealed a focus of uptake. (B) Tomography confirmed the presence of an osteoid osteoma (arrow).

Ewing's Sarcoma

Ewing's sarcoma is a tumor of uncertain origin. It is most common in children and young adults. It is more common in whites than blacks. The tumor may occur in any bone but has some predilection for long tubular bones and the pelvis. The presenting complaints include pain, swelling, tenderness, and erythema, which makes it resemble osteomyelitis. Early there may be no radiographic abnormalities, but later a typical lytic lesion with an "onion-skin" appearance of the periosteum is seen. The prognosis is improving with the use of surgery, chemotherapy, and in some cases radiotherapy. Long-term cures are now seen in about 50% of 5-year survivors.[27]

Primary Chondrosarcoma

A cartilage-producing bone tumor, primary chondrosarcoma occurs most commonly during middle to late life. It occurs most commonly in the central skeleton. The tumors are slow-growing and late in metastasizing, resulting in a relatively favorable prognosis. They are graded on the basis of anaplasia, and most of the tumors fall into the low anaplastic categories.[27] Because they are slow-growing, patients may present with a bony mass that has been present for years. Radiographs demonstrate radiolucent lesions with increased uptake on bone scintigraphy.[29] Successful treatment requires total removal of the tumor. The specimen's pathologic analysis has prognostic value, with the lower grades of anaplasia being associated with a higher 5-year survival.

Osteosarcoma

Osteosarcoma is an aggressive tumor of mesenchymal cell origin characterized by formation of bone by the tumor. Except for myeloma, it is the most common primary bone cancer. These tumors can generally be split into primary and secondary types. Primary osteosarcomas occur most commonly in children and young adults and are most common in males. There appears to be a genetic predisposition. The secondary osteosarcomas generally develop in adults in areas of abnormal bone (e.g., Paget's disease) or in response to some sort of carcinogen exposure (most commonly irradiation). The most common presenting complaints of patients with osteosarcoma are local pain, tenderness, and swelling. It most often occurs in the medullary cavity of the metaphyseal end of the long bones of the extremities. Radiographs, computed tomography (CT) scans, or MRI scans often provide a characteristic picture of subperiosteal or soft tissue penetration of the tumor with extraosseous bone density. To confirm the diagnosis, however, biopsy is required. Great advances have been made in treatment recently, with a combination of surgery, radiotherapy, and chemotherapy (depending on the specific type of lesion) providing the best chances for survival.[27]

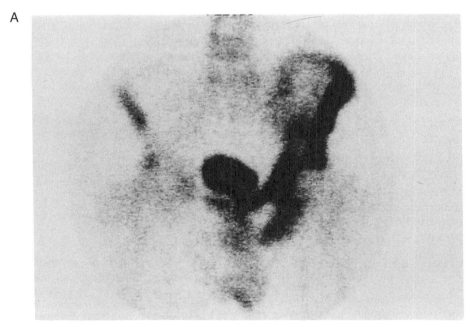

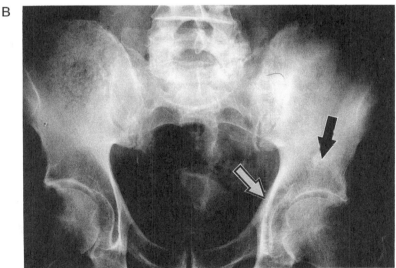

Fig. 114.5. (A) Bone scan shows extensive uptake in half of the pelvis in this patient with nocturnal pelvic pain. (B) Plain film shows coarse trabeculae over the acetabulum (black arrow) and a thickening of the iliopectineal line (white arrow), findings seen with Paget's disease.

Chordoma

Chordoma is a malignant bone tumor seen most commonly in the sacrum and spine. It is thought to arise from remnants of the notochord. These tumors are usually seen in middle-aged and elderly adults. Radiographs, CT scans, or MRI scans usually show the mixed lytic and sclerotic lesions of the chordoma.[30]

Metastatic Malignant Tumors

Tumors that commonly metastasize to bone include thyroid, breast, prostate, bronchus, kidney, bladder, uterus, ovary, testicle, and adrenal tumors. Lymphomas most commonly spread to bone from primary involvement of lymph nodes but also are seen rarely primarily in the skeleton. Bone scans are thought to be the best screening test for patients suspected of having skeletal metastasis.[31] Patients with metastatic bone disease most often present with pathologic fracture or pain. The radiographic appearance of these lesions tends to be sclerotic in prostate and breast metastasis and lytic in lung, bowel, kidney, and thyroid. Biopsy of the bony lesion is helpful for determining whether the lesion is metastatic.

Miscellaneous Bone Conditions

Nonossifying Fibroma

A common condition, nonossifying fibroma is also called a fibrous cortical defect. It is considered a developmental aberration rather than a neoplasm. It is seen primarily in children and occurs most commonly in the femur, tibia, and fibula. The diagnosis can usually be made by the radiographic picture, and a large number of these lesions are found while obtaining a radiograph for another purpose. The lesions are sharply demarcated, lobular, radiolucent defects in the metaphyseal cortex. There is often an intact, thin layer of subperiosteal cortical bone. The lesions may range in size from a few millimeters to 5 cm. They are usually asymptomatic and are seen in approximately one third of children.[27] The larger lesions may cause pain and predispose the child to fracture. These lesions do not tend to transform into neoplasms and often disappear spontaneously.

Paget's Disease of Bone

Osteitis deformans (Paget's disease of bone) is characterized by excessive bone destruction and disorganized repair, resulting in mottled increased density and bony deformity.[27] There is a genetic component to this lesion, although many people develop clinically insignificant lesions. The condition is thought to be related to a canine distemper (paramyxovirus) infection.[32]

Diagnosis. Paget's disease is often asymptomatic and discovered incidentally by radiography. When symptomatic, nighttime bone pain is usually the first symptom. Because of bone softening, bowing of the tibias, pathologic fractures, and increased kyphosis are commonly seen. An increasing head circumference, deafness, and a waddling gait are other relatively common symptoms. A markedly elevated serum alkaline phosphatase level and normal calcium and phosphorus are the usual laboratory pattern. An elevated 24-hour urinary hydroxyproline level, indicative of rapid bone turnover, is also seen. Radiographic findings include expanded bone with increased density. Early on, radiolucent lesions are common, especially in the skull and pelvis (Fig. 114.5). Later mixed, then sclerotic lesions are seen.[27] A bone scan can detect lesions before they become apparent on plain radiographs.

Complications. The complications of Paget's disease include fractures, spinal cord compression, malignant degeneration, and hypercalcemia-related problems such as renal stones. The latter complication is seen primarily if there is excessive calcium intake along with immobilization.

Treatment. Treatment is warranted only if significant symptoms are present. NSAIDs can be of value in suppressing bone activity and controlling mild symptoms. Calcitonins and diphosphonates suppress bone resorption mediated by osteoclasts and are effective in Paget's disease. These treatments have significant potential side effects and complications. The alkaline phosphatase level can be used to monitor disease activity.

Prognosis. The later in life that Paget's disease begins, the better is the prognosis. The progression is usually slow, over years. Renal complications and malignant degeneration of lesions are associated with a poor prognosis.

References

1. Clauw DJ. Fibromyalgia: more than just a musculoskeletal disease. Am Fam Physician 1995;52:843–51.
2. Goldenberg DL. Fibromyalgia syndrome: an emerging but controversial condition. JAMA 1987;257:2782–7.
3. Stormorken H, Brosstad F. Fibromyalgia: family clustering and sensory urgency with early onset indicate genetic predisposition and thus a "true" disease [letter]. Scand J Rheumatol 1992;21:207–11.
4. Silman A, Schollum J, Croft P. The epidemiology of tender point counts in the general population [abstract]. Arthritis Rheum 1993;36(suppl):48.
5. Granges G, Littlejohn GO. A comparative study of clinical signs in fibromyalgia/fibrositis syndrome, healthy and exercising subjects. J Rheumatol 1993;20:344–51.
6. Reynolds WJ, Moldofsky H, Saskin P, et al. The effects of cyclobenzaprine on sleep physiology and symptoms in patients with fibromyalgia. J Rheumatol 1991;18:452–4.
7. Simms RW, Goldenberg DL. Symptoms mimicking neurologic disorders in fibromyalgia syndrome. J Rheumatol 1988;15:1271–3.
8. Pellegrino MJ, Van Fossen D, Gordon C, et al. Prevalence of mitral valve prolapse in primary fibromyalgia: a pilot investigation. Arch Phys Med Rehabil 1989;70:541–3.
9. Goldenberg DL. Management of fibromyalgia syndrome. Rheum Dis Clin North Am 1989;15:499–512.
10. Felson DT, Goldenberg DL. The natural history of fibromyalgia. Arthritis Rheum 1986;29:1522–6.
11. Yunus MB, Kalyan-Raman UP, Kalyan-Raman K. Primary fibromyalgia syndrome and myofascial pain syndrome: clinical features and muscle pathology. Arch Phys Med Rehabil 1988;69:451–4.

12. Thompson JM. Tension myalgia as a diagnosis at the Mayo Clinic and its relationship to fibrositis, fibromyalgia, and myofascial pain syndrome. Mayo Clin Proc 1990;65:1237–48.

13. Harden RN, Bruehl SP, Gass S, Niemiec C, Barbick B. Signs and symptoms of the myofascial pain syndrome: a national survey of pain management providers. Clin J Pain 2000;16(1):64–72.

14. Lederhaas G. Complex regional pain syndrome: new emphasis. Emerg Med 2000;32:18–22.

15. Warfield CA. The sympathetic dystrophies. Hosp Pract 1984;May:52c–j.

16. Kemler MA, Barendse GAM, Kleef M, et al. Spinal cord stimulation with chronic reflex sympathetic dystrophy. N Engl J Med 2000;343(9):618–24.

17. Haddox JD, Van Alstine D. Pharmacologic therapy for reflex sympathetic dystrophy. Phys Med Rehabil 1996;10:297–309.

18. Redd RA, Peters VJ, Emery SF, et al. Morton neuroma: sonographic evaluation. Radiology 1989;171:415–17.

19. Strong G, Thomas PS. Conservative treatment of Morton's neuroma. Orthop Rev 1987;16:343–5.

20. Mann RA. Pain in the foot. 2. Causes of pain in the hindfoot, midfoot, and forefoot. Postgrad Med 1987;82:167–74.

21. Riolo J, Young VL, Ueda K, et al. Dupuytren's contracture. South Med J 1991;84:983–96.

22. James JIP. The relationship of Dupuytren's contracture and epilepsy. Hand 1969;1:47–9.

23. Noble J, Heathcote JG, Cohen H. Diabetes mellitus in the aetiology of Dupuytren's disease. J Bone Joint Surg 1984;66B:322–5.

24. McFarlane RM. The current status of Dupuytren's disease. J Hand Surg 1983;8:703–8.

25. Smith CL, Wernick R. Common nonarticular syndromes in the elbow, wrist, and hand. Postgrad Med 1994;95:173–91.

26. Jennings CD. Deciding whether and how to treat painful ganglia. J Musculoskel Med 1986;3:39–46.

27. Rosenberg AE. Skeletal system and soft tissue tumors. In: Cotran RS, Kumar V, Robbins SL, eds. Robbins' pathologic basis of disease. Philadelphia: Saunders, 1994;1213–46.

28. Healey JH, Ghelan B. Osteoid osteoma and osteoblastoma. Clin Orthop 1986;204:76–85.

29. Vande Streek PR, Carretta RF, Weiland FL. Nuclear medicine approaches to musculoskeletal disease. Radiol Clin North Am 1994;32:227–53.

30. Tumors and infiltrative lesions of the lumbosacral spine. In: Borenstein DG, Wiesel SW, Boden SD, eds. Low back pain. Philadelphia: Saunders, 1995;390–5.

31. Ell PJ. Bones and joints. In: Maisey MN, Britton KE, Gilday DL, eds. Clinical nuclear medicine. Philadelphia: Saunders, 1983;135–65.

32. Cartwright EJ, Gordon MT, Freemont AJ, et al. Paramyxoviruses and Paget's disease. J Med Virol 1993;40:133–41.

115
Common Dermatoses

Daniel J. Van Durme

Acne Vulgaris

Acne is the most common dermatologic condition presenting to the family physician's office. There are an estimated 40 to 50 million people in the United States affected with acne, including about 85% of all adolescents between the ages of 12 and 25.[1] It can present with a wide range of severity and may be the source of significant emotional and psychological, as well as physical, scarring. As adolescents pass through puberty, and develop their self-image, the physical appearance of the skin can be critically important (see Chapter 22). Despite many effective treatments for this disorder, patients (and their parents) often view acne as a normal part of development and do not seek treatment. The importance of early treatment to prevent the physical and emotional scars cannot be overemphasized.

The multifactorial pathogenesis of acne is important to understand, as most treatments are not curative but rather are directed at disrupting selected aspects of development. Acne begins with abnormalities in the pilosebaceous unit. There are four key elements involved in acne development: (1) keratinization abnormalities, (2) increased sebum production, (3) bacterial proliferation, and (4) inflammation. Each may play a greater or lesser role and manifests as a different type or presentation of acne. Initially, there is an abnormality of keratinization and increased sebum. Cohesive hyperkeratosis of the cells lining the pilosebaceous unit combines with increased sebum to block the follicular canal with "sticky" cells and thus a microcomedo develops. This blocked canal leads to further buildup of sebum behind the plug. This sebum production can be increased by androgens and other factors as well. The plugged pilosebaceous unit is seen as a closed comedone ("whitehead"), or as an open comedone ("blackhead") when the pore dilates and the fatty acids in the sebaceous plug become oxidized. The normal bacterial flora of the skin, especially *Proprionybacterium acnes*, proliferates in this plug and releases chemotactic factors drawing in leukocytes. The plug may also lead to rupture of the pilosebaceous unit under the skin, which in turn causes an influx of leukocytes. The resulting inflammation leads to the development of papular or pustular acne. This process can be marked and accompanied by hypertrophy of the entire pilosebaceous unit, leading to the formation of nodules and cysts. There are also factors that can aggravate or trigger acne, such as an increase in androgens during puberty, cosmetics, mechanical trauma, or medications.[2,3]

Diagnosis

Diagnosis is straightforward and is based on the finding of comedones, papules, pustules, nodules, or cysts primarily on the face, back, shoulders, or chest, particularly in an adolescent patient. The presence of comedones is considered a necessity for the proper diagnosis of acne vulgaris. Without comedones, one must consider rosacea, steroid acne, or other acneiform dermatoses. It is important for choice of therapy and for long-term follow-up to describe and classify the patient's acne appropriately. Both the quantity and the type of lesions are noted. The number of lesions indicates whether the acne is mild, moderate, severe, or very severe (sometimes referred to as grades I–IV). The predominant type of lesion should also be noted (i.e., comedonal, papular, pustular, nodular, or cystic).[3] Thus a patient with hundreds of comedones on the face may have "very severe comedonal acne," whereas another patient may have only a few nodules and cysts and have "mild nodulocystic acne."

Management

Prior to pharmacologic management it is important to review and dispel some of the misperceptions that many patients (and parents) have about acne. This condition is not due to poor hygiene, nor are blackheads a result of "dirty pores." Aggressive and frequent scrubbing of the skin may actually aggravate the condition. Mild soaps should be used regularly, and the face should be washed gently and dried well prior to the application of topical medication. Several studies have failed to implicate diet as a significant contributor to acne,[4] and fatty foods and chocolate have not been found to be significant causative agents. Nevertheless, if patients are aware of something in their diet that triggers a flare-up, they should avoid it.

All patients should be taught that acne can be suppressed or controlled when medicines are used regularly, but that the initial therapy usually takes several weeks to show significant benefit. As the current lesions heal, the medications work to prevent the eruption of additional lesions. Typically, a noticeable response to medication is seen in about 6 weeks, and patients must be informed of this time lapse so they do not give up too soon. Some patients may have some initial worsening in the appearance of the skin when they first start treatment.

The treatment options for acne are based on several factors, including the predominant lesion and skin type, the distribution of lesions, individual patient preferences, and some trial and error. Benzoyl peroxide has both antibacterial and mild comedolytic activity and serves as the foundation of most acne therapy. This agent is available as cleansing liquids and bars and as gels or creams, with strengths ranging from 2.5% to 10%. The increase in strength increases the drying (and often the irritation) of the skin. It does not provide additional antibacterial activity. This agent can be used once or twice daily as basic therapy in most patients, although 1% to 2% of patients may have a contact allergy to it.[2]

Because all acne starts with some degree of keratinization abnormality and microcomedone formation, it is prudent to start with a comedolytic agent. Currently, the most effective agents are the topical retinoids—tretinoin (Retin-A, Avita), adapalene (Differin), and tazarotene (Tazorac). They are generally started at the lowest dose possible and thinly applied every night. Mild erythema and irritation are common at first. If they are severe, the frequency can be decreased to three times per week or less, and then slowly increased to every night. The strength of the preparation can also be gradually increased as needed and as tolerated over several weeks to months. Patients should be warned about some degree of photosensitivity with tretinoin and should use sun blocks as needed. Tazarotene is in pregnancy category X and must be avoided in pregnant women due to potential teratogenic effects. If benzoyl peroxide is also used, it is crucial to separate the application of these compounds by several hours. When applied close together, these preparations cause more irritation to the skin while inactivating each other, rendering treatment ineffective.

Antibiotics are recommended for papular or pustular (papulopustular) acne. They act by decreasing the proliferation of *P. acnes* and by inactivating the neutrophil chemotactic factors released during the inflammatory process. Topical agents include erythromycin (A/T/S 2%, Erycette solution), clindamycin (Cleocin T), tetracycline (Topicycline), and sodium sulfacetamide with sulfur (Novacet, Sulfacet-R). These agents are available in a variety of delivery vehicles and are applied once (sometimes twice) a day in conjunction with benzoyl peroxide. With both topical and oral antibiotics, some degree of trial and error is necessary. Some patients respond well to clindamycin, whereas another patient may respond only to erythromycin. Azelaic acid (Azelex) topical cream has been Food and Drug Administration (FDA) approved since 1996 for inflammatory acne and has some antibacterial and comedolytic activity. It should be used with caution in patients with a dark complexion, due to potential hypopigmentation. Additionally, benzoyl peroxide is available as a combination gel with erythromycin (Benzamycin) or with clindamycin (BenzaClin) and can be convenient and effective, but somewhat expensive.

Oral antibiotics are indicated for patients with severe or widespread papulopustular acne or patients with difficulty reaching the affected areas on their body (i.e., on the back). The most commonly used oral antibiotics are tetracycline and erythromycin, which are started at 1 g/day in divided doses. Tetracycline patients are warned of the photosensitivity side effect and advised to take the medicine on an empty stomach, without dairy products. Erythromycin patients should be warned of potential gastrointestinal (GI) upset. Other options for oral medications are doxycycline (50–100 mg twice a day), minocycline (50–100 mg twice a day), and occasionally trimethoprim-sulfamethoxazole (Bactrim DS or Septra DS 1 tablet once daily) for the refractory cases. As the acne improves, the dose of the oral medications can often be gradually decreased to about one-half the original dose for long-term maintenance therapy.[5,6]

Oral contraceptives have also been shown to have substantial benefits in many young women with acne. The nonandrogenic progestins, norgestimate (Ortho-Cyclen, Ortho-TriCyclen) or desogestrel (Ortho-Cept, Desogen) should be used, and may take 2 to 4 months to show benefit.[6,7]

Nodulocystic acne requires initial therapy with benzoyl peroxide, tretinoin, and antibiotics. If these agents fail to control the acne adequately, oral isotretinoin (Accutane) may be used. This agent has been extremely effective in decreasing the production of sebum and shrinking the hypertrophied sebaceous glands of nodulocystic acne. In most patients it induces a remission for many months or cures the condition. If lesions remain, they are usually more susceptible to conventional therapy as described above. Accutane treatment consists of a 16- to 20-week course at 0.5 to 2.0 mg/kg/day. Although this medicine can be profoundly effective, it has "black box" warnings about its teratogenicity and its association with pseudotumor cerebri. There are also numerous less severe side effects, including xerosis, cheilitis, epistaxis, myalgias, arthralgias elevated liver enzymes, and others. Liver function tests, triglyceride levels, and complete blood counts should be frequently monitored. The highly teratogenic potential must be made clear to all female patients, and this medication must be used with extreme caution in all women with childbearing potential. Patient selection guidelines for women include (negative) serum pregnancy tests before starting, maintenance of two highly effective methods of contraception throughout therapy and for 1 to 2 months after therapy, and signed informed consent by the patient.[7,8]

Atopic Dermatitis

Atopic dermatitis (AD) is a common, chronic, relapsing skin condition with an estimated incidence of 10% in the United States. It usually arises during childhood, with about 85% of patients developing it during the first 5 years of life.[9] The disease presents with severe pruritus, followed by various morphologic features. It has been described as "the itch that rashes." Although AD can be found as an isolated illness in some individuals, it is often a manifestation of the multisystemic process of atopy, which includes asthma, allergic rhinitis, and atopic dermatitis (see Chapters 36 and 83). A family or personal history of atopy can be a key element in making the diagnosis.

While there are questions as to the specifics of the role of the immune system and allergies in AD, there is some type of abnormality in the cell-mediated immune system (a T-cell defect) in these patients. They have an increased susceptibility to cutaneous viral (and fungal) infections, especially herpes simplex, molluscum contagiosum, and papillomavirus.[10,11] However, even though about 80% of patients with AD have an elevated immunoglobulin E (IgE) level, there is not enough evidence to conclude what specific role allergies play in the development of this disease.[12,13] Thus even though many people are under the misperception that their skin is allergic to just about everything, they should be taught that the process is not a true allergy but rather a reaction of genetically abnormal skin to environmental stressors.

The eruption is eczematous and usually symmetric. It is erythematous, may have papules and plaques, and often has secondary changes of excoriations and lichenification. The persistent excoriations can lead to secondary bacterial infection, which may be noted by more exudative and crusting lesions. In infants and children, AD is commonly seen on the face and the extensor areas, whereas in older children and adults it is more commonly seen in flexural areas of the popliteal and antecubital fossae and the neck and wrists (Fig. 115.1). Patients with AD may also have numerous other features including generalized xerosis, cheilitis, hand dermatitis, palmar hyperlinearity, and sensitivity to wool and lipid solvents (e.g., lanolin).[9,10]

Treatment of atopic dermatitis begins with attempts at moisturizing the skin. Bathing is done only when necessary and then with cool or tepid water and a mild soap (e.g., Dove or Purpose) or a soap substitute (e.g., Cetaphil). Immediately after bathing and gently patting the skin dry, an emollient is applied to the skin to help seal in the moisture. This emollient should have no fragrances, no alcohol, and no lanolin (e.g., Aquaphor, Keri lotion, Lubriderm) and should be used daily to maintain well-lubricated skin. If the affected areas are particularly severe in an acute outbreak, wet dressings with aluminum acetate solution (Burow's solution) can be applied two or three times daily. If the affected area has dry, noninflamed skin, a moisturizer with lactic acid (e.g., Lac-Hydrin) can be of such help that steroids can be avoided.

Controlling the intense pruritus is important. Keeping the nails trimmed short, and the use of mittens at night can decrease the excoriations in children. Topical steroids can control the inflammatory process. Generally the lowest possible potency should be used, but often high-potency creams may be needed on lichenified areas. In infants and children, one can often maintain good control with 0.25% to 2.5% hydrocortisone cream or ointment, applied two or three times a day. For more severe cases and in adults, 0.1% triamcinolone cream or ointment (or an equivalent-strength steroid) may be needed. Only rarely should fluorinated steroid preparations be used. While the underlying pathogenesis and the pruritus of AD are not primarily histamine mediated, many authors recommend the use of antihistamines that can be adjusted and titrated to balance the antipruritic effect with any potential sedating effects.[9–11] The more traditionally sedating antihistamines such as diphenhydramine (Benadryl) or hydroxyzine (Atarax, Vistaril) can be used at night and loratadine (Claritin) or cetirizine (Zyrtec) can be used during the day. Doxepin hydrochloride 5% cream (Zonalon) has both H_1 and H_2 blocking effects and may help to control pruritus without the

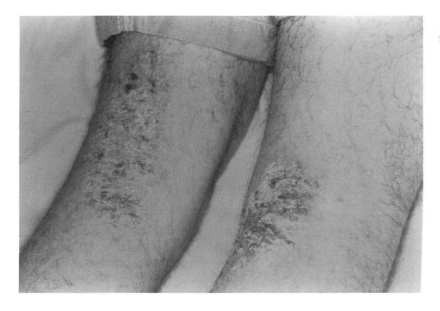

Fig. 115.1. Atopic dermatitis in the popliteal fossae.

problems of long-term topical steroid use; however, absorption of this agent leads to drowsiness in some patients, particularly if a large amount of the skin is treated. Tacrolimus ointment (Protopic) is an immunomodulating agent that was FDA approved for AD in 2001. It works similarly to cyclosporine and has been shown to be safe and effective for both long- and short-term use in AD.[14]

If the AD suddenly becomes much worse, development of a secondary infection or a possible contact dermatitis must be considered. If there is secondary infection, antibiotics directed at *Staphylococcus aureus* are used. Dicloxacillin, erythromycin, cephalexin, and topical mupirocin (Bactroban) are good choices. For patients prone to recurrent impetigo, it is reasonable to have a usual supply of mupirocin at home for any outbreaks. If these measures fail to provide adequate control, it is reasonable to pursue possible specific provocative factors such as foods, contact allergens or irritants, dust mites, molds, or possible psychological stressors.[9]

This condition can produce a great deal of anxiety and frustration in both patients and parents, and the stress can further aggravate the condition. Although psychological factors aggravate the condition, it is important to emphasize that the condition is not caused by "nerves." It is an inherited condition that can be aggravated by emotional stress. This supportive counseling for the patient and the family can be crucial. Furthermore, although affected children may appear "fragile," they are not, and they may desperately need some affectionate handling to help ease their own anxieties about their condition.[15]

Miliaria

Miliaria (heat rash) is a common condition resulting from the blockage of eccrine sweat glands. There is an inflammatory response to the sweat that leaks through the ruptured duct into the skin, and papular or vesicular lesions result. It usually occurs after repeated exposure to a hot and humid environment. Miliaria can occur at any age but is especially common in infants and children.[16]

One of the most common forms of miliaria is miliaria crystallina, in which the blockage occurs near the skin surface and the sweat collects below the stratum corneum. A thin-walled vesicle then develops, but there is little to no erythema. This situation is often seen in infants or bedridden patients and can be treated with cool compresses and good ventilation to control perspiration.

Miliaria rubra (prickly heat or heat rash) is more commonly seen in susceptible patients of any age group when exposed to sufficient heat. In this case the occlusion is at the intraepidermal section of the sweat duct. As a result there is more erythema, sometimes a red halo, or just diffuse erythema with papules and vesicles. Occasionally, the eruptions become pustular, resulting in miliaria pustulosa. There is usually more of a mild stinging or "prickly" sensation than real pruritus. The condition is self-limited but can be alleviated by cool wet to dry soaks. A low-strength steroid lotion (e.g., 0.025% or 0.1% triamcinolone lotion) is often helpful for alleviating the symptoms in these patients.[10]

Pityriasis Rosea

Pityriasis rosea (PR) is a benign, self-limited condition primarily found in patients between the ages of 10 and 35. The cause is unknown, but a viral etiology is suspected as some patients have a prodrome of a viral-like illness with malaise, low-grade fever, cough, and arthralgias; there is an increased incidence in the fall, winter, and spring.[17]

This disorder typically starts with a single, 2- to 10-cm, oval, papulosquamous, salmon-pink patch (or plaque) on the trunk or proximal upper extremity. This "herald patch" is followed by a generalized eruption of discrete, small, oval plaques on the trunk and proximal extremities, sparing the palms and soles and oral cavity. These plaques align their long axis with the skin lines, thus giving the rash a characteristic "Christmas tree" appearance (Fig. 115.2). The plaques often have a fine, tissue-like "collarette" scale at the edges.

The differential diagnosis includes tinea corporis, as the initial herald patch can be confused with ringworm. The diffuse eruption of PR may resemble secondary syphilis but can often be distinguished by the sparing of the palms and soles in PR. It may also give the appearance of psoriasis (especially guttate psoriasis) but has much finer plaques that are not clustered on the extensor areas. Finally, the eruption may be confused with tinea versicolor. Skin scrapings for a potassium chloride (KOH) preparation should be strongly considered in any patient with

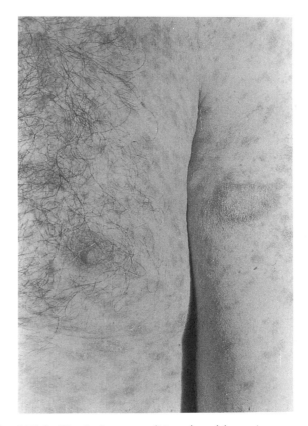

Fig. 115.2. Pityriasis rosea. (Note herald patch on arm.)

apparent PR, as well as serologic testing for syphilis in any sexually active patient (see Chapters 41 and 116).

The management of PR is fairly easy. Pruritus is generally mild and can be controlled with oral antihistamines or topical low-potency steroid preparations. Patients can be reassured that the lesions will fade within about 6 weeks, but may last up to 10 weeks. They should be warned, however, that postinflammatory hypo- or hyperpigmentation (especially in those with more darkly pigmented skin) is possible.[17]

Psoriasis

Psoriasis is a chronic, recurrent disorder characterized by an inflammatory, scaling, hyperproliferative papulosquamous eruption. Lesions are well-defined plaques with a thick, adherent, silvery white scale. If the scale is removed, pinpoint bleeding can be seen (Auspitz's sign). Psoriasis occurs in about 1% to 3% of the worldwide population.[18] The etiology is unknown, although some genetic link is suspected, as one third of patients have a positive family history for the disease. It may start at any age, with the mean age of onset during the late twenties.[19]

Lesions most commonly occur on the extensor surfaces of the knees and elbows but are also typically seen on the scalp and the sacrum and can affect the palms and soles as well. The nails may show pitting, onycholysis, or brownish macules ("oil spots") under the nail plate. Finally, up to 20% of these patients may develop psoriatic arthritis, which can be severe, even crippling.[20]

Although psoriasis is usually not physically disabling and longevity is not affected, the patient's physical appearance can be profoundly affected and may cause significant psychological stress as the patient withdraws from social activities. Attention to the psychosocial implications of this chronic disease is crucial for every family physician.

The classic presentation, chronic plaque psoriasis or psoriasis vulgaris, demonstrates erythematous plaques and silvery adherent scales on elbows, knees (Fig. 115.3), scalp, or buttocks. It is usually easy to diagnose when in the classic form, but there are numerous morphologic variants. Discoid, guttate, erythrodermic, pustular, flexural (intertriginous), light-induced, and palmar-plantar psoriasis are among the many clinical presentations of this condition. The plaques may be confused with seborrheic or atopic dermatitis, and the guttate variant may resemble pityriasis rosea or secondary syphilis. If the diagnosis is unclear, referral to a dermatologist or a biopsy (read by a dermatopathologist, if possible) is in order.

The lesions often appear on areas subjected to trauma (Koebner phenomenon). Other precipitating factors include infections, particularly upper respiratory infections, and stress. Several drugs, particularly lithium, beta-blockers, angiotensin-converting enzyme (ACE) inhibitors, and antimalarial agents are well known to trigger an outbreak or exacerbate existing psoriasis in some patients.[18,19] The nonsteroidal antiinflammatory drugs (NSAIDs) used for psoriatic arthritis may worsen the skin manifestations. Systemic corticosteroids can initially clear the psoriasis, but a "rebound phe-

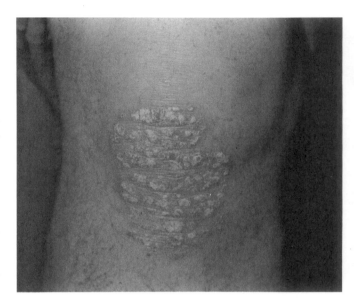

Fig. 115.3. Typical psoriatic plaque.

nomenon," or worsening of the lesions, even after slowly tapering the dose is common.

Management

Patients must understand that there is no cure for psoriasis. All treatments are suppressive (i.e., designed to control the manifestations, improve the cosmetic appearance for the patient, and, it is hoped, induce a remission). Therapy should start with liberal use of emollients and mild soaps. Moderate exposure to sunlight, while avoiding sunburn, can also improve the condition. After this start, treatment modalities are divided into topical agents and systemic therapies. The decision to use systemic agents is usually based on the percent of body surface area involved, with 20% often being used as the cutoff for changing to systemic treatment. In practice, however, the decision to use systemic therapy is based on the severity of the disease, the resistance to topical treatments, the availability of other agents, and a complex of social and psychological factors.[18–22] This decision is usually best made by an experienced dermatologist in consultation with the patient and the family physician.

Keratolytic preparations such as those with salicylic acid (Keralyt gel) or urea-based (Lac-Hydrin) can soften plaques and increase the efficacy of other topical agents. With the exception of emollients, the topical treatments for chronic plaque psoriasis should be applied to the lesions only and not the surrounding skin. It should be carefully explained to the patient that the medications that stop the overgrowth of the psoriatic skin have side effects on the normal surrounding skin and application should be done carefully.

Topical steroid preparations are a typical starting point for psoriasis, and while they can provide prompt relief, it is often temporary. Tolerance to these agents is common (tachyphylaxis), and one must remain vigilant for the long-term side effects of thinning of the skin, hypopigmentation, striae, and telangiectasia. The lowest effective strength is used, always using caution with higher strengths on the face, groin, and intertriginous areas. Increased efficacy is seen when ointments are used under occlusion, but this practice can also lead to enough systemic absorption to suppress the pituitary-adrenal system.[20]

The topical agent calcipotriene 0.005% (Dovonex) has shown good results with mild to moderate plaque psoriasis. It is a derivative of vitamin D and works by inhibiting keratinocyte and fibroblast proliferation. It is available as a cream, ointment, or scalp solution and is applied as a thin layer twice a day with most improvement noted within 1 month. Side effects include itching or burning in 10% to 20% of patients and rare cases of hypercalcemia (<1%), particularly when large amounts are used (>100 g/week).[21]

Tazarotene (Tazorac) is a topical retinoid gel that inhibits epidermal proliferation and inflammation in psoriasis (and is also FDA approved for acne vulgaris). Tazarotene alone has shown only modest benefit and can often cause irritation. Optimal benefit from this agent is obtained by combining it with a medium-potency steroid, such that tazarotene is applied each night and the steroid is applied each morning. This drug must be avoided in pregnant women due to potential teratogenic effects.[21]

Chronic plaques can often be managed by using the antimitotic agents of anthralin or coal tar. Anthralin preparations (e.g., Anthra-Derm, Drithocreme, Dritho-Scalp) can be applied to thick plaques in the lowest dose possible for about 15 minutes a day and then showered off. Care must be taken to avoid the face, genitalia, and flexural areas. The duration and strength of the preparation is gradually increased as tolerated until irritation occurs. This preparation is messy and can stain normal skin, clothing, and bathroom fixtures. Coal tar preparations can be used alone or, more successfully, in combination with ultraviolet B (UVB) light therapy (Goeckerman regimen).[19] Coal tar may be found in both crude and refined preparations, such as bath preparations, gels, ointments, lotions, creams, solutions, soaps, and shampoos. In general, the treatment is similar to that with anthralin; progressively higher concentrations are used as needed until irritation or improvement results. The preparations are left on overnight, and staining can be a problem.

When systemic therapy is needed, treatment with ultraviolet (UV) light can be extremely effective. There are two basic regimens: One uses UVB (alone or with coal tar or anthralins) and the other uses UVA light therapy with oral psoralens (PUVA) therapy. The psoralen acts as a photosensitizer, and the UVA is administered in carefully measured amounts via a specially designed unit. Phototherapy and photochemotherapy can be expensive and carcinogenic. Thus they are administered only by an experienced dermatologist. Other systemic agents include the retinoid acitretin (Soriatane), methotrexate, etretinate (Tegison), and cyclosporine.[18–21] Due to the numerous side effects of these medicines, their use is generally best left to an experienced dermatologist and is beyond the scope of this text.

The lesions of psoriasis may disappear with treatment, but residual erythema, hypopigmentation, or hyperpigmentation is common. Patients must be instructed to continue treatment until there is near or complete resolution of the induration and not to always expect complete disappearance of the lesions.

Family and Community Issues

Proper patient and family education is crucial for managing the physical and psychosocial manifestations of this disease. The patient should be allowed to participate in the decision of which treatment modalities will be used and must be carefully instructed on the proper use of the one(s) chosen. The ongoing emotional support the family physician provides can help prevent the emotional scars that psoriasis may leave behind. The National Psoriasis Foundation (6600 SW 92nd, Suite 300, Portland, OR 97223; phone 800-723-9166, *www.psoriasis.org*) is a nonprofit organization dedicated to supporting research and education in this field. It provides newsletters and other educational material for patients and their families. A written prescription with the address and Web site can be one of the most effective long-term "treatments" for these patients.

Poison Ivy, Poison Oak, and Sumac (Rhus Dermatitis)

Plant-related contact dermatitis can be triggered by numerous plant compounds, but the most common allergen is the urishiol resin found in the genus *Toxicodendron* (formerly *Rhus*) containing the plants poison ivy, poison oak, and poison sumac. These three plants cause more allergic contact dermatitis than all other contact materials combined.[10] The oleoresin urishiol, which serves as the allergen (and rarely as a primary irritant), is located within all parts of the plant.[23]

The clinical presentation varies with the amount of the allergen and the patient's own degree of sensitivity. About 70% to 80% of Americans are mildly to moderately sensitive to the allergen, with about 10% to 15% at each end of the spectrum—either very sensitive or completely tolerant.[24] The eruption is erythematous with papules, wheals, and often vesicles. In severe cases, large bullae or diffuse urticarial hives are seen. The distribution is often linear or streak-like on exposed skin from either direct contact with the plant or by inadvertent spreading of the resin by the patient.

A history of exposure to the plant or to any significant activities outdoors helps in the diagnosis. It must be remembered, however, that the resin adheres to animal hair, clothing, and other objects and can then cling to the patient's skin after this indirect contact. Thus the patient may not be aware of any direct exposure. The thick, calloused skin on the hands often prevents eruption on the palms while the resin is transferred to another part of the body, where an eruption does occur. Outbreaks typically occur within 8 to 48 hours of the exposure. Alternatively, the initial exposure may sensitize the patient so the rash occurs a couple of weeks after exposure in response to the resin remaining on or in the skin.[23] The ability of the resin to remain on the skin (even after washing) and cause a later eruption has led to the mistaken belief that the fluid of the vesicles can cause spreading of the lesions.

Treatment begins with removal of any remaining allergen by thorough skin cleansing with soap and water as soon after exposure as possible. Rubbing (isopropyl) alcohol can be even more effective in dispersing the oily resin. Any clothing that may have come in contact with the plant should also be washed. If the affected area is small, and there is no significant vesicular formation, topical steroids (medium to high potency, such as triamcinolone 0.1–0.5%) are sufficient. The blisters can be relieved by frequent use of cool compresses with water or with Burow's solution (one packet or tablet of Domeboro in 1 pint of water). Oral antihistamines (e.g., diphenhydramine 25–50 mg or hydroxyzine 10–25 mg, four times a day) can help relieve the pruritus. If the outbreak is severe or widespread, or it involves the face and eyes, oral steroids may be needed. A tapering dose of prednisone (starting at 0.5–1.0 mg/kg/day) can be used over 5 to 7 days if the outbreak started a week or more after exposure. A longer, tapering course should be used (10–14 days) if treating an outbreak that started within 1 to 2 days of exposure. This regimen treats the lesions that are present and should suppress further development of lesions as the skin is sensitized.[24]

Prevention is best done by avoidance of the plants altogether or using clothing (that is then carefully removed to avoid rubbing the resin on the skin) as a barrier. The FDA has approved the first medication proved to prevent outbreak, bentoquatam (IvyBlock). This nonprescription lotion is applied before potential exposure and dries on the skin to form a protective barrier. This lotion does not irritate or sensitize the skin and provides 4 to 8 hours of protection. Desensitization attempts have not been successful and are not recommended.

Seborrheic Dermatitis

Seborrheic dermatitis, a chronic, recurrent scaling eruption, is common (incidence 3–5%) and typically occurs on the face, scalp, and the areas of the trunk where sebaceous glands are more prominent. It is usually seen in two age groups: infants during the first few months of life (may present as "cradle cap") and adults ages 30 to 60 (dandruff). It causes mild pruritus, is generally gradual in onset, and is fairly mild in its presentation. An increased incidence (up to 80%) has been described in patients with acquired immunodeficiency syndrome (AIDS), and these patients often present with a severe, persistent eruption[25] (see Chapter 42). The etiology is unknown, but there appears to be some link to the proliferation of the yeast *Pityrosporum ovale*, in the *Malassezia* genus. While this organism is present as normal flora for all people, the response of seborrheic dermatitis to antifungals agents strongly suggests a role for *P. ovale*.[26]

The lesions are scaling macules, papules, and plaques. They may be yellowish, thick and greasy, or sometimes white, dry, and flaky. Thick, more chronic lesions occasionally crust and then fissure and weep. Secondary bacterial infection leading to impetigo is not uncommon. The differential diagnosis includes atopic dermatitis, candidiasis, or a dermatophytosis. When the scalp is involved, the plaques are often confused with psoriasis, and the two conditions may overlap, referred to as seboriasis or sebopsoriasis. When the trunk is involved, the lesions may appear similar to those of pityriasis rosea.

Periodic use of shampoos containing selenium sulfide (Selsun, Selsun Blue), pyrithione zinc (Sebulon, Head and Shoulders), salicylic acid and sulfur combinations (Sebulex), or coal tar (Denorex, Neutrogena T-Gel) can be effective, not just on the scalp, but also on the trunk. The antifungal agent ketoconazole (Nizoral) is also available as a shampoo and can be highly effective. These shampoos are used two or three times a week and must be left on the skin (scalp) for about 5 to 10 minutes prior to rinsing. They are used alternating with regular soaps/shampoos as needed. This regimen may prevent the tachyphylaxis that can occur with daily use. After about 1 month the frequency of use can be decreased as tolerated to maintain control. Low-potency topical steroid creams or lotions such as 2.5% hydrocortisone or 0.01% fluocinolone (also available as a shampoo) can be used once or twice a day in the scalp or in other areas such as the face, groin, and chest. Topical ketoconazole cream (Nizoral) or terbinafine cream or spray (Lamisil) twice daily can also be helpful. Thick scales, such as may be found on the scalps of infants, can be gently scrubbed off with a soft toothbrush after soaking the area for 5 minutes with warm mineral oil or a salicylic acid shampoo. In severe and unresponsive cases, isotretinoin (Accutane) has been shown to be very effective in seborrheic dermatitis by markedly shrinking the size of the sebaceous glands and demonstrating some antiinflammatory effect. As compared to treatment for acne vulgaris, these patients often respond to lower doses (0.1 to 0.3 mg/kg/day) and shorter courses (4 weeks).[26] The same precautions, especially regarding pregnancy, that are described above must be observed.

Rosacea (Acne Rosacea)

A chronic facial dermatosis, acne rosacea typically appears in patients between the ages of 30 and 60. It is characterized by acneiform lesions such as papules, pustules, and occasionally nodules (Fig. 115.4). It is more common in those of Celtic, Scandinavian, or Northern European descent—those with fair skin who tend to flush easily. In addition to the facial flushing, generalized erythema, and telangiectasias, they may have moderate to severe sebaceous gland hyperplasia. Ocular manifestations such as conjunctivitis, blepharitis, and episcleritis can be found in more than half of the patients. Severe involvement of the nose can lead to soft tissue hypertrophy and rhinophyma. Otherwise, most lesions are on the forehead, cheeks, and nose. The pathogenesis is unknown, but increasing evidence suggests that it is primarily a cutaneous vascular disorder that leads to lymphatic damage followed by edema, erythema, and finally papules and pustules.[27] Despite popular conception, alcohol is not known to play a causative role, but the vasodilatory effects of alcohol may make the condition appear worse. There is also some vasomotor instability in response to stress, sun exposure, hot liquids, and spicy foods, and these should be avoided.[28]

Treatment with oral erythromycin or tetracycline 1 g/day in divided doses or with minocycline or doxycycline at 50 to

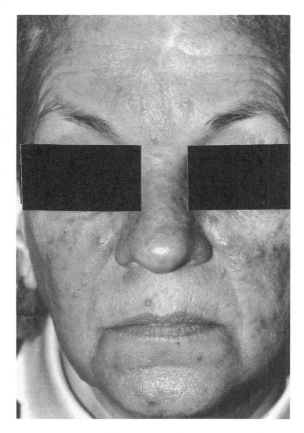

Fig. 115.4. Acne rosacea.

100 mg twice a day can help alleviate both the facial and ocular manifestations of the disease. Response is variable, with some patients showing a prompt response followed by weeks or months of remission and others requiring long-term suppression with antibiotics. If long-term treatment is needed, the dose is titrated down to the minimal effective amount. Topical agents include clindamycin and erythromycin, but some of the better responses are seen with metronidazole 0.75% gel, lotion or cream (MetroGel, MetroLotion, Metrocream), or 1% cream (Noritate) in mild to moderate cases.[29] Topical sodium sulfacetamide and sulfur lotion is available in a unique preparation (Sulfacet-R) that includes a color blender for patients to add tint to the lotion to match their own skin coloration. This agent is popular with women in particular who may wish to hide the erythema and lesions. Oral metronidazole (Flagyl) may be used with caution in resistant cases. Topical tretinoin (Retin-A) and oral isotretinoin (Accutane) have shown promising results in patients with severe, refractory rosacea.[29–31]

Dyshidrotic Eczema (Pompholyx)

Dyshidrotic eczema, a recurrent eczematous dermatosis of the fingers, palms, and soles, is more common in the young population (under age 40) and typically presents with pruritic, often tiny, deep-seated vesicles. The etiology is unknown, but despite the name and the fact that many patients may have associated hyperhidrosis, it is not a disorder of sweat retention. Many of these patients have a history of atopic dermatitis, and it is considered a type of hand/foot eczema. Emotional stress plays a role in some cases, as does ingestion of certain allergens (e.g., nickel and chromate).[10]

The onset is typically abrupt and lasts a few weeks, but the disorder can become chronic and lead to fissuring and lichenification. Secondary bacterial infection can also occur. The vesicles are usually small but can be bullous and may give the appearance of tapioca. The most common site is the sides of the fingers in a cluster distribution (Fig. 115.5). The nails can also show involvement with dystrophic changes such as ridging, pitting, or thickening.

Controlling this disorder can be difficult and frustrating for the physician and patient alike. Attempts should be made to remove the inciting stressor whenever possible. Further treatment is similar to that for atopic dermatitis: Cool compresses may provide relief, and topical steroids can alleviate the inflammation and pruritus. It is one of the dermatoses in which high-potency fluorinated or halogenated steroids (in the ointment or gel formulation) are often needed to penetrate the thick stratum corneum of the hands. If secondary infection is present, erythromycin or cephalexin can be helpful. Rarely, oral steroids may be needed, but these drugs are reserved for the more severe, recalcitrant cases.

Drug Eruptions

Rashes of various types are common reactions to medications. The dermatologic manifestations can be highly variable: maculopapular (or morbilliform) eruptions; urticaria; fixed, hyperpigmented lesions; photosensitivity reactions; vesicles and bullae; acneiform lesions; and generalized pruritus, among others. Serious and even life-threatening dermatologic reactions can occur as well, such as Stevens-Johnson syndrome, toxic epidermal necrolysis, hypersensitivity syndrome, and serum sickness.[31,32]

Definitively assigning a diagnosis of a particular eruption to a single agent can be difficult, as patients may take multiple medications, they may have coexistent illnesses, and the drug eruption may not manifest until the patient has been taking it for several days (sometimes weeks). Only when the eruption follows the administration a particular agent, resolves with removal of the agent, recurs with readministration, and other causes have been excluded can one say that the eruption is definitely due to a specific drug. Caution must be used prior to any rechallenge with an agent, and so readministration is often not recommended. Subsequently, many patients mistakenly believe they have dermatologic reactions or allergies to certain medications when their rash may have had nothing to do with their medication.

Table 115.1 lists several of the typical drug reactions to some of the more common drugs in clinical practice.[10,15,24,32–34] Treatment consists of stopping the offending (or suspected) medication. Topical low- to mid-potency steroids and oral antihistamines can relieve the pruritus that accompanies many eruptions.

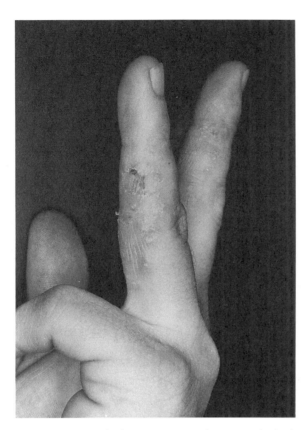

Fig. 115.5. Dyshidrotic eczema (or pompholyx).

Contact Dermatitis

Contact dermatitis is the clinical response of the skin to an external stimulant. It is an extremely common condition. Chemically caused dermatitis is responsible for an estimated 30% of all occupational illness.[35] The condition is such a problem with a wide variety of mechanisms of pathogenesis and potential products involved that an international journal, *Contact Dermatitis*, is devoted specifically to this topic. By suspecting virtually everything and anything and taking a thorough history, the family physician nevertheless should be able to diagnose and manage most of these patients.

While some authors describe several different subtypes of contact dermatitis, the two most common types are irritant contact dermatitis and allergic contact dermatitis. Morphologically and histologically, they can appear identical, and the difference to the clinician is more conceptual.[36] Irritant contact dermatitis accounts for the majority of cases of contact dermatitis, and results from a break in the skin's integrity and subsequent local absorption of an irritant. There is no true demonstrable allergen present. A single exposure can induce an inflammatory response if the agent is caustic enough or if there is a marked degree of exposure. Often the response is the result of prolonged exposure with repeated minor damage to the skin, such as in those who must wash their hands frequently. Common offending agents include soaps, industrial solvents, and topical medications (e.g., benzoyl peroxide, tretinoin, lindane, benzyl benzoate, anthralin).[37,38]

The second most common type is allergic contact dermatitis. It is a delayed hypersensitivity reaction that occurs

Table 115.1. **Common Reactions to Common Drugs**

Anaphylaxis	Maculopapular (morbilliform)	Serum sickness
Aspirin	Barbiturates	Aspirin
Sulfonamides	Isoniazid	Penicillin
NSAIDs	Phenothiazines	Sulfonamide
Serum (animal derived)	Sulfonamides and sulfonylureas	Urticaria
Penicillins	Lithium	Antibiotics
Fixed drug eruptions	NSAIDs	Opiates
Antibiotics—penicillins, sulfonamides,	Phenytoin	Blood products
tetracyclines	Thiazides	Radiocontrast agents
Phenolphthalein	Gentamicin	NSAIDs
Barbiturates	Penicillin compounds	Vesicular eruption
Dextromethorphan	Quinidine	Barbiturates
NSAIDs	Photosensitivity	Clonidine
Allopurinol	Carbamazepine	Naproxen
Lupus-like eruptions	Methotrexate	Sulfonamides
Hydralazine	Coal tar compounds	Captopril
Methyldopa	Oral contraceptives	Furosemide
Hydrochlorothiazide	Furosemide	Penicillin
Procainamide	NSAIDs	Cephalosporins
Isoniazid	Quinidine	Nalidixic acid
Quinidine	Tetracyclines	Piroxicam
	Griseofulvin	
	Phenothiazines	
	Sulfonamides and sulfonylureas	
	Thiazides	

NSAID = nonsteroidal antiinflammatory drug.

after the body is sensitized to the offending agent. The reaction is thus often delayed somewhat from the time of exposure. The response varies depending on the individual's sensitivity, the amount and concentration of the allergen, and the degree of penetration. Poison ivy dermatitis is perhaps the most common form of allergic contact dermatitis (discussed earlier in the chapter). Other common offenders are nickel, fragrances, rubber chemicals, neomycin, thimerosal, parabens (found in sunscreens and lotions), and benzocaine (topical anesthetic).[36–38] Even topical steroid preparations have been reported to cause allergic contact dermatitis in some patients.[39]

Physical findings may be identical or may vary somewhat with different forms of contact dermatitis. The irritant type often causes an erythematous scaling eruption with a typically indistinct margin (Fig. 115.6), whereas the allergic type may cause more erythema, edema, vesicular formation, and weeping. The offending agent is often identified more by the shape of the eruption than the appearance of the skin (e.g., a watchband or the elastic band of some article of clothing).

Treatment is symptomatic after removal of the irritant or allergen. Cool compresses can provide relief from the pruritus, particularly if there is any weeping. Oral antihistamines may be needed along with topical steroids. Ointment compounds are recommended, as they are less irritating and sensitizing than most creams or lotions. The patient should avoid any topical preparations with benzocaine or other -caines, as

they may aggravate the condition. In severe cases a tapering course of oral steroids over 1 to 2 weeks is necessary. Subacute and chronic cases may also be colonized with *Staphylococcus aureus*, and an oral antibiotic (e.g., dicloxacillin, erythromycin, or cephalexin) may speed resolution.

Avoidance of the irritant or allergen is sometimes difficult for patients. Their job may require some exposure, or it may be difficult to verify the specific agent. Testing with a commercially available patch test kit (T.R.U.E. Test Allergen Patch Test Panel) is the most reliable method of identifying a true allergic contact dermatitis and its causative agent.[39] This is particularly useful in developing a long-term plan of avoidance.

Urticaria

Urticaria, a common skin condition affecting about 20% of the population, is characterized by transient wheals or hives.[40] It is typically a type I immunologic reaction (mediated by IgE) but may be from physical or environmental exposure (pressure- or cold-induced). Urticaria can be acute (lasting less than 6 weeks) or chronic. Perhaps the most frustrating issue for the patient and physician faced with urticaria is that the underlying cause is often difficult to ascertain. In only about 20% of cases of chronic urticaria can the specific etiology be determined.[41,42]

A generalized eruption of pruritic wheals with erythema and localized edema and lesions lasting less than 24 hours establishes the diagnosis. Angioedema is a closely related process in which deeper tissues may be involved, particularly mucous membranes. Severe generalized urticaria can be a systemic illness leading to cardiac problems and even death.

One should search carefully to find the underlying etiology by doing a thorough comprehensive history and physical examination. Common causes include medications (antibiotics, NSAIDs, narcotics, radiocontrast dyes), illnesses (viral hepatitis, streptococcal, parasitic), connective tissue disorders (lupus, juvenile rheumatoid arthritis), endocrine disorders (hyper- or hypothyroidism), neoplastic disorders (lymphoma, leukemia, carcinoma), physical agents (pressure, cold, heat, exercise, menstruation), skin contacts (chemicals, fragrances, dyes, soaps, lotions, feathers, animal dander), insect bites and bee stings, foods (chocolate, shellfish, strawberries, nuts), and psychological stress.[10,15,40,41,43] The amount of laboratory work and other testing recommended can be highly variable and depends in part on the clinical utility of finding the underlying trigger(s). In general, an extensive workup is not advised during the first 6 weeks. Once the condition has persisted into chronic urticaria, a thorough history is as effective as an extensive and costly laboratory workup in finding the underlying cause.[40,44]

Treatment consists of avoidance of any known or suspected precipitant and the use of medications as needed for comfort. The H_1-blockers such as cetirizine (Zyrtec), loratadine (Claritin), diphenhydramine, or hydroxyzine can be used alone or in combination with an H_2-blocker such as cimetidine (Taga-

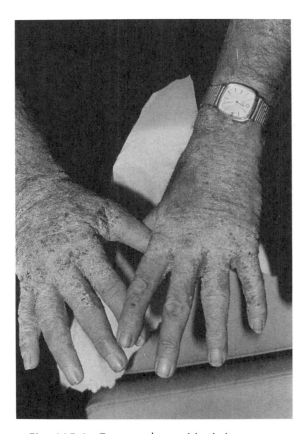

Fig. 115.6. Contact dermatitis, irritant type.

met). Doxepin, a tricyclic antidepressant, can also be helpful at 25 mg once or twice a day. For severe, acute urticaria, a tapering dose of prednisone over 2 weeks can be helpful. Chronic urticaria may require a great deal of maintenance emotional support, as the condition can make normal activities difficult. Patients must be reassured, and medications may be needed on a long-term daily basis.

References

1. White GM Recent findings in the epidemiologic evidence, classification, and subtypes of acne vulgaris. J Am Acad Dermatol 1998;39:S34–7.
2. Russell JJ. Topical therapy for acne. Am Fam Physician 2000; 61:357–66.
3. Leyden JJ. New understandings of the pathogenesis of acne. J Am Acad Dermatol 1995;32:S15–25.
4. Rosenberg EW. Acne diet reconsidered. Arch Dermatol 1981;117:193–5.
5. Johnson BA, Nunley JR. Use of systemic agents in the treatment of acne vulgaris. Am Fam Physician 2000;62:1823–30, 1835–6.
6. Leyden JJ. Therapy for acne vulgaris. N Engl J Med 1997; 336(16):1156–62.
7. Thiboutot D. New treatments and therapeutic strategies for acne. Arch Fam Med 2000;9:179–83.
8. Van Durme DJ. Family physicians and Accutane. Am Fam Physician 2000;62:1772–7.
9. Kristal L, Klein PA. Atopic dermatitis in infants and children. An update. Pediatr Clin North Am 2000;47:877–95.
10. Habif TP. Clinical dermatology: a color guide to diagnosis and therapy, 3rd ed. St. Louis: Mosby-Year Book, 1996.
11. Fleischer AB. Atopic dermatitis. Perspectives on a manageable disease. Postgrad Med 1999;106:49–55.
12. Borirchanyavat K, Kurban AK. Atopic dermatitis. Clin Dermatol 2000;18:649–55.
13. Halbert AR, Weston WL, Morelli JG. Atopic dermatitis: is it an allergic disease? J Am Acad Dermatol 1995;33:1008–18.
14. Leicht S, Hanggi M. Atopic dermatitis. Postgrad Med 2001;109(6):119–27.
15. Goldstein BG, Goldstein AO. Practical dermatology, 2nd ed. St. Louis: Mosby-Year Book, 1997.
16. Feng E, Janniger CK. Miliaria. Cutis 1995;55:213–6.
17. Bjornberg A, Tenger E. Pityriasis rosea. In: Freedberg IM, Eisen AZ, Wolff K, et al, eds. Dermatology in general medicine, 5th ed. New York: McGraw-Hill, 1999;541–6.
18. Greaves MW, Weinstein GD. Treatment of psoriasis. N Engl J Med 1995;332:581–8.
19. Christophers E, Moreweitz U. Psoriasis. In: Freedberg IM, Eisen AZ, Wolff K, et al, eds. Dermatology in general medicine. 5th ed. New York: McGraw-Hill, 1999;495–522.
20. Linden KG. Weinstein GD. Psoriasis: current perspectives with an emphasis on treatment. Am J Med 1999;107:595–605.
21. Pardasani AG, Feldman SR, Clark AR. Treatment of psoriasis: an algorithm-based approach for primary care physicians. Am Fam Physician 2000;61:725–33,736.
22. American Academy of Dermatology. Committee on Guidelines of Care, Task Force on Psoriasis. Guidelines of care for psoriasis. J Am Acad Dermatol 1993;28:632–7.
23. Tanner TL. Rhus (Toxicodendron) dermatitis. Prim Care 2000; 27:493–502.
24. Pariser RJ. Allergic and reactive dermatoses. Postgrad Med 1991;89:75–85.
25. Janniger CK, Schwartz RA. Seborrheic dermatitis. Am Fam Physician 1995;52:149–59.
26. Johnson BA, Nunley JR. Treatment of seborrheic dermatitis. Am Fam Physician 2000;61:2703–10, 2713–14.
27. Wilkin JK. Rosacea: pathophysiology and treatment. Arch Dermatol 1994;130:359–62.
28. Zuber TJ. Rosacea. Prim Care 2000;27:309–18.
29. Thiboutot DM. Acne and rosacea. New and emerging therapies. Dermatol Clin 2000;18:63–71.
30. Ertl GA, Levine N, Kligman AM. A comparison of the efficacy of topical tretinoin and low dose oral isotretinoin in rosacea. Arch Dermatol 1994;130:319–24.
31. Hirsch RJ, Weinberg JM. Rosacea 2000. Cutis 2000;66:125–8.
32. Roujeau JC, Stern RS. Severe adverse cutaneous reactions to drugs. N Engl J Med 1994;33:1272–85.
33. Manders SM. Serious and life-threatening drug eruptions. Am Fam Physician 1995;51:1865–72.
34. Crowson AN. Recent advances in the pathology of cutaneous drug eruptions. Dermatol Clin 1999;17:537–60.
35. Anonymous. Contact dermatitis and urticaria from environmental exposures: Agency for Toxic Substances and Diseases Registry. Am Fam Physician 1993;48:773–80.
36. Rietschel RL Comparison of allergic and irritant contact dermatitis. Immunol Allergy Clin North Am 1997;17:359–64.
37. Oxholm A, Maibach MI. Causes, diagnosis, and management of contact dermatitis. Compr Ther 1990;16:18–24.
38. Adams RM. Recent advances in contact dermatitis. Ann Allergy 1991;67:552–66.
39. Belsito DV. The diagnostic evaluation, treatment, and prevention of allergic contact dermatitis in the new millennium. J Allergy Clin Immunol 2000;105:409–20.
40. Greaves MW. Chronic urticaria. N Engl J Med 1995;332: 1767–72.
41. Beltrani VS. Allergic dermatoses. Med Clin North Am 1998;82:1105–33.
42. Huston DP, Bressler RB. Urticaria and angioedema. Med Clin North Am 1992;76:805–40.
43. Mahmood T. Urticaria. Am Fam Physician 1995;51:811–6.
44. Kozel MM, Mekkes JR, Bossuyt PM, Bos JD. The effectiveness of a history-based diagnostic approach in chronic urticaria and angioedema. Arch Dermatol 1998;134:1575–80.

116
Skin Infections and Infestations

Michael L. O'Dell

The skin is the body's largest and most visible organ. It is possibly the most assailed organ as well, as it is in constant contact with the outside environment. This constant exposure leaves skin subject to innumerable challenges. Nevertheless, the skin is remarkably impervious, and it reliably protects against infection and infestation in most normal individuals. The skin's ability to prevent infection is a result of its structure. The skin's continuity and integrity on the body's surface are largely unbroken unless trauma intervenes. The skin surface is dry under normal conditions, and this dry state is combined with a low surface pH. The acidity and dryness of the skin militate against colonization by most pathogens. Secretions exuded by the pilosebaceous apparatus are also inhibitors of bacterial growth. The normal skin flora is of low virulence and contributes to the suppression of more virulent organisms.

Skin infection or infestation is nevertheless a common complaint in most family physicians' offices. Physicians must remain mindful that such illnesses are often related to a break in the skin through trauma. Environmental conditions, such as hygiene, also contribute to contracting skin infections or infestation. Additionally, in patients who lack adequate immune defenses, organisms that are not generally considered pathogens may gain access.

Many infectious illnesses and infestations potentially cause skin eruption. This chapter addresses only those conditions where the primary illness is one localized to the skin. Many other illnesses with skin manifestations, such as gonorrhea, are covered throughout the text (see Chapter 41).

Pyodermas and Bacterial Skin Infection

Purulent skin infections (pyoderma) and other bacterial skin infections represent some of the most common or serious skin infections seen by family physicians. These skin infections include erythrasma, impetigo, ecthyma, folliculitis, erysipelas, cellulitis, and necrotizing fasciitis.[1-5]

Erythrasma and Other Bacterial Diseases Due to *Corynebacterium* and *Propionibacterium*

Erythrasma is a superficial, often asymptomatic skin infection that causes reddish brown macular skin discoloration, generally in the genital area (Fig. 116.1). The infection, easily confused with tinea cruris, may also affect the axillae and intertriginous skinfolds, particularly in obese individuals. Erythrasma is more common in males. Individuals affected notice skin color changes and present with this complaint. Wood's light examination is helpful, as the infected area glows a coral-pink color. The causative agent of infection is *Corynebacterium minutissimum*, a porphyrin-producing bacterium, and this porphyrin production accounts for the fluorescence under Wood's light illumination. Effective treatment can generally be accomplished with topical erythromycin. Erythrasma will generally also respond to imidazole cream, which lessens the significance of confusing this bacterial infection with tinea cruris. A study has found that single-dose treatment with 1 g of clarithromycin orally is effective.[1] Treatment with erythromycin for 7 days is also effective but is not necessarily more effective than topical treatment.

Trichomycosis axillaris affects the axillary area in persons with hyperhydrosis or poor hygiene. The infection results in a disagreeable rancid smell. The affected individual may also notice thickening of the axillary hair. Examination of axillary hair reveals coating of the hair shaft with black, yellow-white, or red deposits that are firmly adherent to the hair shaft. These deposits are the result of heavy colonization with *Corynebacterium tenuis*. Measures that improve body hygiene along with antiseptic soaps quickly ameliorate the condition and prevent its return. Occasionally the use of a topical imidazole cream or erythromycin is warranted.

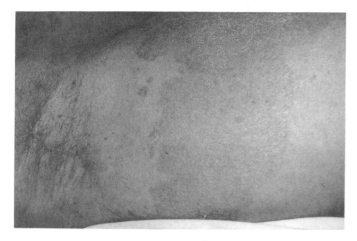

Fig. 116.1. Erythrasma.

Pitted keratolysis, a disorder causing painful burning sensation of weight-bearing surfaces, often affects the feet of individuals exposed to warm and damp climates while wearing occlusive foot wear. It is most common in soldiers and workers wearing boots. Long-distance runners and other athletes are also affected. Patients often complain of malodor and "sliminess" in affected areas.[2] Examination of the symptomatic patient reveals tenderness to minimal pressure over affected areas of the soles, and these affected areas are on the weight-bearing aspect of the foot. Pitted lesions of the keratinized layer of callused areas are present, and the overall appearance of the infected areas is whitish and macerated. Hyperhydrosis and malodor are present. *Corynebacterium* and *Dermatophilus congolensis* are among the agents responsible for this illness. Topical therapy with antimicrobial agents such as erythromycin is generally effective, provided it is supplemented with at least daily washing of the feet with soap or acidic detergents.

Impetigo

Impetigo is a common superficial skin infection subclassified according to whether large bullae are present. This subclassification is not as useful as once believed because *Staphylococcus aureus* has been found with either pattern. The illness is most common in children but is occasionally seen in adults. Individuals affected by the disease are usually not systemically ill, although lymph node swelling is occasionally present.

Small-vesicle impetigo contagiosa begins with small, reddened macules that progress to water-filled vesicles. The vesicles, which are surrounded by a thin band of erythema, soon rupture, leaving a honey-colored crusted area. With bullous impetigo the initial lesion tends to be a large, flaccid blister, which quickly becomes cloudy and purulent.

Systemic antibiotics are often not required for impetigo, and topical therapy with agents such as mupirocin (Bactroban) is sufficient. Where cases of streptococcal postinfectious nephritis have been noted in the community, treatment with oral or parenteral antibiotics may be more urgent. Systemic treatment is given to patients with eczema, as the recurrence rate with topical treatment in one series was 38% with topical treatment and 17.8% with systemic treatment. The illness is contagious among children, and so it represents a significant problem for schools, day-care centers, and nurseries. The risk of spread may also warrant more aggressive oral treatment. Trimming nails and frequent changing of clothing and bed linens may also prevent further spread.

Certain strains of *Staphylococcus* produce an exotoxin that causes exfoliation. Staphylococcal scalded skin syndrome may result, and exfoliation of large areas of skin may occur. This illness occurs more commonly in infants and immunosuppressed patients. With such a group of patients, early systemic therapy of impetigo with an antistaphylococcal agent is warranted along with other supportive measures.[6]

If systemic therapy is warranted, antistaphylococcal agents are used. Recommended systemic agents include penicillinase-resistant synthetic penicillins (i.e., dicloxacillin), erythromycin, oral first-generation cephalosporins (e.g., cephalexin), or clindamycin. Laboratory evidence of resistance to erythromycin is now common among *S. aureus* cultures, but treatment failure remains rare (Fig. 116.2).[7,8] Upon healing, residual discoloration or erythema may persist for several weeks at the site.

Ecthyma

Ecthyma usually occurs on the legs as small bullae followed by an adherent crust. Ecthyma is more common in debilitated individuals. It is likely initiated by minor areas of trauma, allowing entry of streptococci or staphylococci. The adherent crust gives way to a purulent ulcerated lesion that heals slowly. Resolution is aided by use of antistaphylococcal antibiotics and attention to improvement of nutritional status.

Folliculitis, Furuncles, Carbuncles

Folliculitis describes yellowish pustules that form around hair follicles, especially in intertriginous areas. The illness affects males most commonly, particularly those living in humid and warm climates. Diabetics are particularly prone to such lesions. The pustules are surrounded by a thin band of erythema.

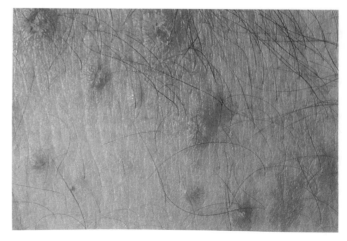

Fig. 116.2. Impetigo that has responded poorly to erythromycin.

Adequate treatment generally consists of improved hygiene measures and application of antiseptics or topical antimicrobials such as mupirocin or bacitracin. If the illness affects the area of the beard, frequent changing of the razor is indicated. With extensive involvement, systemic antistaphylococcal antibiotics are of value.

Hot-tub folliculitis, a special type of folliculitis, may occur following exposure to a poorly maintained hot-tub or Jacuzzi. Pool maintenance, including limiting the use of cyanuric acid, is key to preventing this illness.[3] The causative agent for the folliculitis is *Pseudomonas aeruginosa*. The illness is self-limited in most patients, and resulting serious illness is rare. Cases of sepsis have occurred with this illness, although sepsis usually occurs only in immunosuppressed patients.

Furuncles (boils) may be considered an extension of folliculitis—a more aggressive form of this process. Furuncles are areas of inflammation and infection that may extend through the dermis to the subcuticular tissue. Furuncles may occur on any non–weight-bearing surface, and they are particularly common on areas of friction, the nasal area, and the external ear. Furuncles are more common in adolescent patients and patients with poor hygiene, seborrhea, diabetes, or immunodeficiency. Occasionally, widespread and numerous boils may occur among groups that share common bathing facilities, such as athletes and others.[4] On examination a painful, fluctuant lesion is noted that exhibits central necrosis and liquefaction. Surrounding erythema may be present, and lymphadenopathy is often seen. The preferred treatment of a furuncle is drainage; antibiotic therapy is generally not needed following drainage. Certain facial lesions have the potential to result in cavernous sinus thrombosis as a result of venous drainage through the vena angularis. Thus furuncles located above an imaginary line from the corner of the mouth to the ear lobe are treated aggressively with antistaphylococcal antibiotics in addition to drainage. Recommended systemic agents include penicillinase-resistant synthetic penicillins (e.g., dicloxacillin), erythromycin, oral first-generation cephalosporins (e.g., cephalexin), or clindamycin. Occasionally admission and intravenous antibiotics are required, and such measures should be considered for patients who appear systemically ill.

Carbuncles are localized collections of furuncles, with the lesions having multiple connecting sinuses. Carbuncles are most common on the back of the neck in men over age 40. The size of many carbuncles and the multiple sinuses make surgical treatment complicated. Antistaphylococcal antibiotics and local measures are used in addition to drainage. Large lesions may require extensive débridement, and surgical consultation is useful.

Hidradenitis suppurativa is pathologically related to furuncles. The disease generally does not involve the sweat glands themselves and tends to be limited to the pilosebaceous structures. The disease is more common in males and in individuals afflicted with acne conglobata. Examination reveals furunculoid lesions that are often multiple in the axillae, inguinal area, scrotum, labia, or mons pubis. Drainage is necessary, and topical clindamycin or systemic antistaphylococcal antibiotics are warranted.[5] Treatment with retinoic acid is useful, particularly in milder cases.[6] The moistness of the area

of occurrence often supports gram-negative secondary infections, cultures of drainage may help direct antibiotic treatment. Surgical consultation and excision of the infected area is often necessary, particularly when multiple recurrences of the infection have led to scarring and multiple sinus tracts.

Erysipelas

Erysipelas is a common acute illness marked by a red, painful, swollen, spreading, irregular lesion with a sharply defined border in the infected area (Fig. 116.3). The illness affects all age groups, although it is somewhat more common during childhood. Fever is generally present, as is prominent lymphatic involvement. Elevation of the white blood cell count (WBC) is common. Sepsis is unusual but is more likely in children, the elderly, diabetics, or immunosuppressed patients. Cultures of the lesion are rarely positive. The process is nearly always caused by group A streptococci, although group G streptococci and *S. aureus* may rarely cause a similar picture. As such, treatment is generally with oral penicillin or erythromycin. Extra precautions must be taken when erysipelas involves the face, as cavernous sinus thrombosis may result [9]

Cellulitis

Cellulitis refers to a group of acute bacterial illnesses involving a spreading infection of the epidermis and subcutaneous tissue. Cellulitis generally begins with a break in the skin, and the source of this break may be important when determining the empiric therapy. Common breaks in the skin of the lower leg include intertrigo from tinea pedis, leg ulcers or wounds, and dermatitis involving the leg. Other factors that are associated with leg cellulites include lymphedema, venous insufficiency, and being overweight.[7] The patient complains of pain, redness, and warmth in the affected area. Systemic complaints, such as fever, are also common. Examination reveals cutaneous erythema that lacks the sharply demarcated border so characteristic of erysipelas. The infected area is warm, edematous, and painful. Culture is generally not beneficial in normal patients. However, in patients with under-

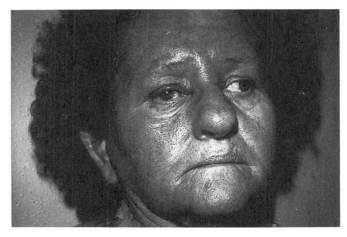

Fig. 116.3. Erysipelas.

lying illness, such as diabetes or human immunodeficiency virus (HIV) infection, aspiration of the lesion for culture is useful and more likely to be positive. Cellulitis is characteristically caused by group A streptococci or *S. aureus*. Inoculation with many other pathogens, including *Haemophilus influenzae* or marine vibrios, may also lead to cellulitis.

Treatment of cellulitis generally involves elevation of the affected body area as well as antibiotic treatment. In otherwise normal patients, treatment with antistaphylococcal antibiotics is warranted. If the patient is immunocompromised or otherwise at risk, other pathogens should be considered. A history of injury in brackish water followed by findings of cellulitis should prompt institution of coverage for various halophilic vibrios. Tetracyclines, augmented by antistaphylococcal agents, are instituted when vibrio infection is suspected. Irrespective of the causative agent, after an initial episode of cellulitis the patient remains at risk for recurrence in the same area due to damage to lymphatics.

Cellulitis involving the tissues near the eye may result in serious sequelae. If possible, a distinction should be made between periorbital (preseptal) and orbital (postseptal) cellulitis. Distinguishing between postseptal and preseptal cellulitis is not always an easy task. Hallmarks of late postseptal cellulitis include proptosis, pain on motion of the eye, marked chemosis, and fever. Postseptal cellulitis generally results from spread of an underlying sinusitis, whereas preseptal cellulitis usually follows trauma to the periorbital area. *S. aureus*, *Streptococcus*, and *H. influenzae* are common pathogens involved in either pre- or postseptal cellulitis. Infection involving the postseptal spaces may quickly spread and result in cavernous sinus thrombosis and other central nervous system (CNS) involvement. Thus postseptal cellulitis is an emergent condition and warrants inpatient treatment. Treatment involves intravenous administration of a penicillinase-resistant synthetic penicillin and an aminoglycoside for at least 7 days. Drainage may also be required. Treatment of preseptal cellulitis may also require drainage. However, antibiotic coverage for preseptal cellulitis is generally limited to a penicillinase-resistant synthetic penicillin or a cephalosporin such as cefuroxime. Hospitalization may not be required for preseptal cellulitis.

Cellulitis involving the face or neck also raises special concerns. Such infections may be the result of trauma, although many of the infections involving the face and neck are secondary to poor dental hygiene. Infections related to an odontogenic source may quickly spread to the submental spaces and the lateral and retropharyngeal spaces. With involvement of the spaces surrounding the pharynx collapse of the airway may occur. Severe systemic symptoms may also appear. Aggressive antibiotic therapy is warranted, as is surgical drainage.[8] Antibiotic therapy generally consists of penicillin to provide coverage for *Bacteroides melaninogenicus*, and additional anaerobic coverage with metronidazole or clindamycin is wise.

Abscess

Abscesses are commonly seen in busy family medicine practices. Often patients present with a localized area of redness and induration well before central fluctuance appears. The process of abscess formation results from localized pyogenic infection and may occur on any aspect of the skin. Although abscesses may involve many body organs and pathogens, the skin abscess generally results from a staphylococcal infection. Culture almost invariably reveals mixed flora, despite staphylococci being the suspected initiating organism.

Infection generally begins as a cellulitis with diffuse erythema and inflammation but little central necrosis or fluctuance. Lymphangitis and other cardinal signs of cellulitis may be present. If treated as for cellulitis with antibiotics, small areas of abscess may resolve without drainage.

The clinician must remain mindful of the site of the abscess. Chest wall abscess may represent empyema in an acutely ill patient. In such cases drainage of the empyema is required. Abscess and drainage over the parotid gland may represent suppurative parotitis. Penicillinase-resistant penicillins and milking of the parotid gland assist in recovery. Cervical and facial abscesses are particularly worrisome and may herald airway compromise. Sublingual and submandibular abscess represents an emergent situation, as airway compromise often ensues. Abscess of the palmar aspect of the hand may signify underlying flexor tendon sheath involvement. Involvement of the palmar flexor tendon sheath requires surgical drainage, and disability may result. Perineal abscesses can be deceiving and involve extensive tissue. Perirectal and perineal abscesses are notoriously difficult to drain and treat, and it is wise to consider hospitalization and surgical consultation in such cases.

Treatment of abscess requires drainage, which is often curative; antibiotic treatment may not be required after drainage. However, drainage prior to central loculation and "pointing" may paradoxically spread infection. Antibiotic treatment, application of moist heat, and watchful waiting are often required for an uncomplicated abscess prior to drainage. With infections involving critical areas, such as lung, neck, and hand, any such watchful waiting should be done in a hospitalized setting. Perineal or perianal abscesses should be carefully assessed as to their size and the extent of spread, and hospitalization should be considered.

Necrotizing Fasciitis

Necrotizing fasciitis is a relatively rare disease but is significant and life-threatening when it occurs. Most commonly the infection involves the perineum or abdominal wall. The illness usually follows an episode of trauma, although patients with diabetes or alcoholism may contract the illness with no preceding trauma. Distinguishing between simple abscess, cellulites, and necrotizing fasciitis is not always clear. An elevated white blood count ($>14,000/mm^3$), low sodium (<135 mmol/l), and an elevated blood urea nitrogen (BUN) (>15 mg/dL) are often found in patients with necrotizing fasciitis.[9] Group A β-hemolytic *Streptococcus* (GABHS) has received much notoriety and has been labeled the "flesh-eating bacteria." GABHS infection often accompanies varicella infection and is characterized by violaceous bullae surrounded by edema and erythema. GABHS is particularly dangerous as multisystem failure occurs due to toxin production. In most cases of necrotizing fasciitis, however, several bacteria usually are present, including streptococci groups A, C, and G. Anaerobic bacteria exist in combination with aerobic or gram-negative bacteria on culture. Clostridial organisms are occasionally found, and when they are found, subcutaneous gas production is usually present (gas gangrene). Necrosis of infected tissue occurs rapidly and includes affected muscle, particularly if clostridial organisms are present. Surgical removal of devitalized tissue is required, as is high-dose parenteral antibiotic therapy.[6] Antibiotic therapy consists of clindamycin and penicillin. Hyperbaric oxygen therapy may be a useful therapy in addition to antibiotics and debridement.

Viral Skin Diseases

Skin diseases caused by viruses are common, especially in children (see Chapter 18). Many of the "six diseases" of childhood (measles, scarlet fever, rubella, scarlatina, erythema infectiosum, exanthema subitum) are caused by viruses. Other common viral pathogens include herpes simplex virus 1 and 2 and varicella. Warts, caused by papillomaviruses, are common, and a busy family physician usually sees several patients with warts in a week's practice. Importantly, there is increasing evidence that certain subtypes of papillomavirus cause malignant transformation in infected cells.[10]

Rubella

The incidence of rubella has decreased due to effective vaccination and recent outbreaks have largely been in communities of immigrants from countries with ineffective vaccination programs.[11] Rubella is in many instances similar to measles, and it is common for lay persons to call rubella "German measles" and refer to measles as "hard measles" (also see Chapter 18). Rubella is a less significant illness than measles, but it can be profoundly detrimental to a fetus exposed during the first trimester. The illness of rubella generally begins as a rash 16 to 18 days after exposure, and, unlike measles, there is virtually no prodrome. The rash is similar to that of measles; it begins on the face and exhibits a butterfly pattern. The rash of rubella often affects the perioral area, and this distinction is useful if a concern about scarlet fever also exists. Lymphadenopathy may become prominent during the illness, particularly postauricular adenopathy. In adults arthralgia of the wrist, finger, and knee joints is commonly seen during the infection. Treatment is symptomatic, although special considerations are necessary for the affected pregnant woman. Pregnant women exposed to rubella should be advised to receive rubella immunoglobulin. Pregnant women who experience the illness should be carefully studied for evidence of fetal damage and appropriately counseled regarding potential fetal outcomes. Reimmunization or testing for immunity should be considered for adolescents. Testing for immunity is a routine aspect of preconception and prenatal screening.

Erythema Infectiosum

Erythema infectiosum, or fifth disease, occurs sporadically and in clustered groups. Years may elapse between cases seen by a busy family physician only to have several cases appear within a short time. The illness is caused by B19 parvovirus. The illness generally appears suddenly and without a prodrome. The onset of the illness follows exposure by 6 to 14 days. The exanthem begins on the face with a characteristic "slapped-face" distribution and appearance. Bright red discoloration of both cheeks is seen at the onset of the illness. No adenopathy is present. The facial rash disappears within hours to 2 days, followed by lace-like, ring-shaped macular lesions that are approximately 1 to 2 cm in diameter and intertwined with adjacent lesions. This second phase of the illness lasts up to 1 week, after which the rash fades without sequelae. Blood counts obtained during the illness often show leukopenia, lymphopenia, and decreased reticulocytes and platelets. No treatment is generally warranted. The infection may pose significant risk during pregnancy, where the fetus may be spontaneously aborted or experience hydrops fetalis. Approximately 35% of pregnant women are susceptible to human parvovirus infection during pregnancy, and their greatest risk of exposure comes from their other children during epidemics of fifth disease.[12] The infected pregnant woman should be carefully evaluated and appropriately counseled regarding potential outcomes for the fetus. Of concern is increasing evidence that implicates human parvovirus in onset of rheumatoid arthritis.[13]

Other Morbilliform Rashes

A variety of other viral illnesses are capable of producing measles-like (morbilliform) rashes. Morbilliform rashes may be related to infection with various enterocytopathogenic human orphan (ECHO) viruses, as well as several Coxsackieviruses. In an adequately immunized child measles and rubella should be considered less likely than other causes of morbilliform rashes.

Human Herpesvirus Infections

Two forms of infection are caused by varicella-zoster virus (VZV): chickenpox and shingles. Chickenpox is the primary infection, whereas zoster is thought to be a recrudescence of latent virus in dorsal nerve root ganglia. Infection with VZV may be especially serious in patients who are immunocompromised. Vaccination appears to be effective and is now widespread in practice.[14]

The primary infection, chickenpox, is generally acquired by droplet spread (see Chapter 18). After an incubation period of approximately 14 days, children begin to experience the exanthem. Adults may experience a prodrome of headache, vomiting, and high temperature. A prodrome is rare in children but may appear in a child who is likely to progress to varicella pneumonia. Scattered red spots occur all over the body particularly on the head and trunk. Over the course of a few hours, the spots become small papules and then thin-walled vesicles. Surrounding each vesicle is a thin ring of erythema. As the infection continues, successive crops of vesicles occur as the older vesicles rupture and then crust over. New lesions continue to appear for up to 5 days in immunocompetent patients. Over a period of 2 weeks the last of the skin lesions crusts over with a brownish crust that falls off at the end of 2 to 3 more weeks without scarring.

Healthy children generally recover well from varicella infection and antiviral treatment is of marginal benefit. Adolescents and adults, however, tend to have a more difficult and severe course of illness and should be started on antiviral therapy promptly.[15] Significant intrauterine limb deformities can occur with varicella in early pregnancy. Acyclovir is considered a category B drug during pregnancy and has been used for treatment of varicella during pregnancy.[12] Transmission of vaccine modified varicella to a pregnant woman has been reported following vaccination of her 12-month-old child, and a delay in immunization may be warranted when a pregnant woman resides in the household of the child to be immunized.[16]

Most patients with chickenpox recover without difficulty, although several complications can occur. Secondary bacterial infection of the skin lesions with *Streptococcus* or *S. aureus* may occur, and such secondary infections may require antibiotic treatment. CNS involvement may also occur, including transverse myelitis, ataxia with meningeal irritation, aseptic meningitis, and Reye's syndrome. Varicella pneumonia, a serious complication, is more common in adults. The complications of myocarditis, corneal lesions, nephritis, arthritis, bleeding diatheses, acute glomerulonephritis, and hepatitis are more common in adults.

Immunization is now available and recommended for chickenpox.[14] Immunization programs for the illness appear effective. Immunization may dramatically decrease the incidence of chickenpox and its complications in future years.

Zoster is thought to be the result of reactivation of VZV residing in the dorsal nerve root ganglia. In immunocompetent patients, lesions of the illness follow a segmental pattern as defined by the distribution of sensory nerves emanating from the dorsal nerve root ganglia. A prodrome may occur that consists of malaise and slight temperature elevation. Pain, which follows the dermatome of the affected nerve root, may also occur as a prodromal symptom or at any time during the illness. A rash, similar to that of chickenpox, occurs along the affected dermatome (Fig. 116.4). The rash typically is uni-

lateral and does not cross the midline. The duration of the rash and the presence of subsequent crusts are of shorter duration than seen with chickenpox, with the entire illness lasting no more than 10 days. Valacyclovir is more effective than acyclovir in preventing postherpetic neuralgia and is the current agent of choice, and some advocate use of concurrent steroids for patients over 50 years of age.[15,17] Immunocompromised patients are generally treated with parenteral acyclovir, famciclovir, or valacyclovir. An unfortunate and feared complication is postherpetic neuralgia, where long-term pain is noted on the area of the eruption. Topical capsaicin is useful for treating postherpetic neuralgia.[10]

Various patterns are common or of note with zoster, including zoster ophthalmicus, zoster of the second and third trigeminal nerve branch, and zoster oticus. With zoster ophthalmicus the first branch of the trigeminal nerve is involved. Thus the forehead, periorbital area, and nose may be affected. A zoster lesion on the tip of the nose indicates that the patient is at increased risk for corneal and conjunctival involvement as well. Such patients should be promptly seen by an ophthalmologist. Zoster of the second and third trigeminal nerve branch is common and frequently involves the oral mucous membranes as well. Finally zoster oticus involves the outer ear and occasionally the inner ear. Acoustic and facial nerve paralysis may occur, producing Ramsay Hunt syndrome. More than two thirds of patients with Ramsay Hunt syndrome experience hearing loss.

The characteristic appearance of lesions induced by VZV is usually sufficient evidence to conclude that VZV is the cause. Culture is available for difficult cases, as are various immunologic tests.

Immunization for varicella has been introduced, and reports of its efficacy have been encouraging. The incidence of zoster, even in patients at risk because of cancer, appears significantly lessened through immunization.

Two types of herpes simplex virus (HSV) commonly cause infection: HSV-1 and HSV-2. HSV-1 is more commonly associated with oral lesions and HSV-2 more commonly with genital lesions, but either type may be found in either location. The infectious agents are neurotropic. Partly as a result of this neurotropism, the rash tends to be confined to defined areas. As with varicella, another member of the human herpesvirus family, a primary and secondary disease state occurs. The virus remains forever in the host after the primary infection. The immune status of the infected individual is important in determining the severity of recrudescent infections.

The primary infection of genital herpes is generally symptomatic and is usually caused by HSV-2 (see Chapter 41). Systemic signs of fever, headache, and myalgias occur in 40% of men and 70% of women. Local genital symptoms of severe pain, itching, dysuria, vaginal or urethral discharge, distal penile lesions, and tender, bilateral, inguinal adenopathy occurs. When an individual engages in anal intercourse, the primary lesions may begin in the rectum. Sequential stages of rash are noted with papules, vesicles, wet ulcers, and finally healing ulcers (Fig. 116.5). Healing occurs over 2 to 3 weeks, although viral shedding persists for approximately 12 days from the onset of symptoms. Diagnosis of genital her-

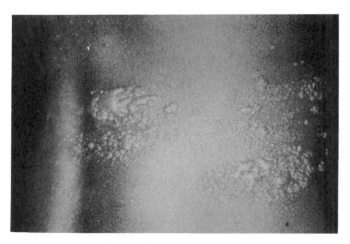

Fig. 116.4. Herpes zoster.

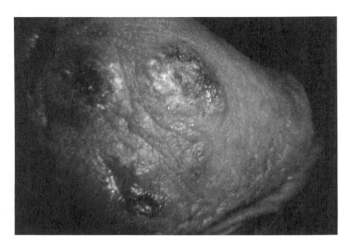

Fig. 116.5. Herpes progenitalis.

pes is preferably made by viral culture or polymerase chain reaction, although Papanicolaou or Tzanck smears, immunofluorescent staining of cells, or immunologic testing is useful in selected circumstances. Patients should be counseled that they are likely to be contagious periodically, even without symptoms, and that sexual contact may spread the illness to a previously uninfected partner. The use of condoms diminishes but does not negate the chance for spread of the infection. Given the obvious implications for the patient and sexual partners, clear, preferably culture-based evidence that a patient is indeed infected should be sought (see Chapter 41). Initial infections may be treated efficaciously with acyclovir, famciclovir, or valacyclovir, with all being equally efficacious. The choice between these three agents can be largely based on patient preferences as to cost and frequency of administration. Reactivation of genital herpes is common, and on any given day approximately 1% of infected individuals are actively shedding virus. Virus may be shed during asymptomatic periods, and most recurrences are asymptomatic. Recurrences may be treated and, if the recurrences are frequent, suppressed with acyclovir, famciclovir, or valacyclovir.[18] Women with genital HSV infection are at higher risk for cervical carcinoma, although the relation between infection and cervical cancer is not known to be causal.[10]

Of particular importance to family physicians is the chance that a mother with genital HSV infection will transmit the virus to her infant during the delivery process. Such maternal-to-neonate transmission may result in the neonate developing serious illness, such as herpetic encephalitis. Initial infection late in pregnancy confers the highest risk of neonatal infection. Large series studying the use of cervical cultures near the time of delivery have shown the practice of obtaining weekly cultures to be futile.[18] Thus prevention of transmission is problematic, and the clinician is left to rely on heightened suspicion of infection when managing the newborn. If active lesions are present at the onset of labor, many would opt for cesarean section to reduce the risk of neonatal infection.[19]

The primary infection of oral herpes (herpes labialis) is an episode of gingivostomatitis accompanied by systemic symptoms of headache, fever, and upper respiratory symptoms.

Early onset of infection is somewhat more common in lower socioeconomic classes, with 90% having evidence of infection by young adulthood, whereas fewer than 50% of young adults in higher socioeconomic classes have evidence of infection. Treatment of the initial episode is often desirable and is usually with oral acyclovir. Approximately 20% of adults have recurrent outbreaks and these may be provoked by stress, fever, illness, or excessive exposure to sun. Occasionally the infection involves the eye, and in this circumstance urgent ophthalmologic consultation is needed (see Chapter 71). Penciclovir is a topical cream that, if applied at the prodromal or early erythema stage, can shorten the duration of symptoms and viral shedding.[20]

HSV infections are major causes of morbidity and mortality among immunosuppressed patients. Frequent or severe recurrences of HSV infections should prompt consideration of HIV infection, Hodgkin's disease, or other immunosuppressive illness. Up to 10% of patients with HIV and recurrent HSV infections have HSV strains that are resistant to acyclovir. Such strains are usually sensitive to foscarnet.[18]

Exanthema subitum, which is also known as sixth disease or roseola infantum, is caused by human herpesvirus 6. Human herpesvirus 6 infections, and its alarming accompanying fever, are now thought to account for up to 10% to 40% of all pediatric emergency room visits.[21] Up to 70% of infants infected in North America do not experience the characteristic rash during the illness.[22] The illness occurs within 3 to 7 days following exposure, with the onset marked by elevation of the temperature up to 40°C. This elevated temperature may last up to 3 days and is accompanied by malaise. The rash occurs as the temperature falls. The rash, which begins on the trunk and then spreads to the extremities, is noted after the prodrome. The face is often spared, but otherwise the rash may be difficult to distinguish from that of measles. It persists less than 2 days before fading without sequelae.[2]

Human herpesvirus 7 may also cause exanthema subitum, and is now suspected as a causative agent for pityriasis rosea.[22] Pityriasis rosea often begins with the so-called herald patch on the trunk (see Chapter 115). Within 4 to 10 days after the truncal lesion occurs, a fine, scaly, often salmon colored rash appears on the trunk and limbs. Infection is also associated with chronic fatigue syndrome and childhood recurrent fever. HSV-7 infection is ubiquitous and 85% of U.S. citizens have antibody evidence of prior infection.

Hand, Foot, and Mouth Disease

Hand, foot, and mouth disease is a curious illness affecting the body parts noted in its name. The incubation period for the illness is not known, although it is known to be caused by the enterovirus, coxsackie A16 virus, and, recently, enterovirus 71. The illness does not have a true prodrome, and the systemic symptoms of fever, headache, and malaise accompany the rash if they occur at all. The rash affects the palms of the hands, soles of the feet, and oral mucosa. A polyhedral grayish yellow vesicle with a surrounding rim of erythema occurs on the soles and palms. The vesicles may be more rounded in the oral mucosa. Coxsackievirus may be recovered from the lesions and is also found in the stool. In children the rash may become more generalized. The rash generally lasts 3 to 5 days, after which it quickly fades, although ulceration of the vesicles may occur. Enterovirus 71 associated infections may be severe and fatal. Cases with complications of pulmonary edema and significant neurologic involvement have been reported.[23]

Warts

Warts are virus-induced areas of epithelial hyperplasia and are generally benign. Human papillomavirus, the causative agent of warts, occurs as many different types. Selected types of the papillomavirus may be capable of inducing malignant transformation, and cervical cancer associated with condyloma is the most well-documented example of malignancy associated with papillomavirus.[10] Common types of warts are common warts (verrucae vulgaris), plantar or mosaic warts (verrucae plantares), juvenile warts (verrucae plana juveniles), genital or condyloma warts, and mucosal papillomas. In general, the appearance of warts is distinctive. Shaving a section of the wart with a scalpel reveals a characteristic thrombosed capillary network. Biopsy is warranted if confusion exists as to whether a lesion is a wart or a cancerous lesion.

Common warts are the most frequently seen wart. Common warts are generally flesh colored and hyperkeratotic with a papillomatous surface that is often peppered with central black dots. Although diagnostic criteria have been developed, the experienced practitioner intuitively has a higher sensitivity and specificity in making the diagnosis of warts than one who applies strict guidelines.[24] There is a tendency for these warts to be located on the extremities, as these areas may be more susceptible to inoculation and mount a poorer immune response than the trunk or face. Nonetheless, such warts occur on any skin surface. In fact, the shape of the wart is somewhat dependent on the area in which it is located. Lesions on the face tend to be filiform, whereas warts on the extremity areas subject to friction tend to be more mosaic in appearance. The mosaic appearance of the extremity warts is a function of closely proximate multiple warts that are also abraded to reveal the capillary network supporting the warty growth. Common warts spontaneously resolve, although the resolution may occur years after the onset. The lesions resolve spontaneously without scarring.

Plantar warts occur on the soles and are distinguished from mosaic warts by being solitary lesions surrounded by hyperkeratotic, callus-like skin. The wart tends to occur on the ball of the foot, and so the patient experiences pain while walking. Occasionally the warts become large, and large warts are more common when the warts involve the area of the heel.

Juvenile or plane warts are flat papules, usually 1 to 4 mm across that are relatively inconspicuous in color. They usually appear suddenly and propagate quickly, often into hundreds of lesions. They are, as their name suggests, most commonly seen in adolescents and children. These warts have a predilection for the facial area and distal upper extremities.

Condylomas are warts in the intertriginous areas of mucous membranes. The most common form of condyloma is condyloma acuminata. The infection is fostered by moist conditions, maceration, and epithelial defects. Sexual transmission is common. The lesion begins as a small papule that, when macerated, is generally whitish. The lesion becomes multiple and grows, eventually forming a cauliflower-like structure that may be large. Vegetations develop, and when moist the "leaves" of the vegetation may be separated and distinguished. The labia minora and majora, as well as the vaginal introitus are often involved in women. Cervical lesions are now recognized as common, and certain types of papillomavirus are associated with the development of cervical cancer. Infection of the cervix by human papillomavirus is often not discernible without a colposcope. The coronal sulcus, frenulum, and urethral orifice are common sites for condylomas in males. Rectal lesions are also common. Occasionally the condyloma becomes large and destroys surrounding tissues.

A rare syndrome involving warts has also been described. Epidermodysplasia verruciformis is an autosomal-recessive disorder that affects individuals unable to terminate a human papillomavirus infection. The skin lesions resemble juvenile warts and appear during early childhood. The wart lesions continue to spread and become confluent, particularly on light-exposed skin surfaces. Infection with HPV-5 or -8 often results in malignant transformation of the lesions and the development of Bowen's disease and squamous cell carcinoma.

Treatment of warts should involve therapies that do not induce scarring, as the lesions resolve spontaneously without scarring. Imiquod is a new therapy based on immune modulation that has shown excellent effectiveness in resolving genital condyloma.[25] Imiquimod treatment is well accepted by patients and has a low rate of recurrence of genital warts. Imiquimod will likely become the treatment of choice for condyloma, given that other treatments of genital warts are often painful, prolonged, and have a high rate of recurrence. Early studies have shown it to be effective in common warts as well.[26] Various treatments for condyloma and for common warts are at least partially effective, including freezing with liquid nitrogen, use of keratolytic agents such as salicylic acids, use of 5-fluorouracil alone or in combination with salicylic acid, use of podophyllin, sharp curetting of the lesion, laser ablation, desquamative agents such as retinoic acid, photochemotherapy with methoxypsoralen and UV light, psychotherapy or hypnosis, and hot water.[27] Given the presence of such an extensive list, the experienced clinician can recognize that no single therapy always works well, and so several trials involving differing therapies may be required in a difficult case. Freezing with liquid nitrogen is a particularly attractive option in that it may be quickly performed in the office, generally does not require local anesthetic agents, and the extended use of potentially toxic agents, such as podophyllin, is not required. Retreatment is frequently necessary for bulky warts, but there is little chance of scarring, such as with sharp curet or electrocoagulation. Ideally a 2-mm rim of normal tissue around the wart shows evidence of freeze during the procedure, thus ensuring that potentially infected surrounding tissue is also removed. However, use of liquid nitrogen is only 80% to 90% effective, and other therapies are necessary for many patients.

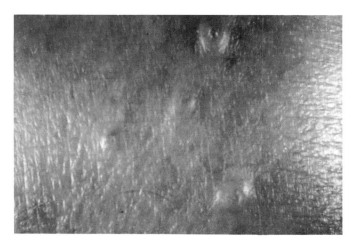

Fig. 116.6. Molluscum contagiosum.

Molluscum Contagiosum

Although the lesions of molluscum contagiosum resemble those of warts, the causative agent here is a poxvirus, related to smallpox. The lesions are communicable from person to person and may be sexually transmitted. An incubation period of weeks to months is noted. The infection is more common among children and adolescents but may be seen in any age group. Those who are immunocompromised, particularly those infected with HIV, are at particular risk for acquiring molluscum contagiosum.[28] Patients with HIV often have quite large and multiple lesions when infected. Molluscum contagiosum lesions are hard, pearl-like nodules with a characteristic dimple on top (Fig. 116.6). Treatment of the lesions involves removing the nodules, which can generally be accomplished by squeezing them with a curved forceps. Use of a sharp curet or freezing the lesion with liquid nitrogen is also an effective means of removing nodules.[10] Imiquimod has also been shown to be effective in the treatment of molluscum lesions.[26,29]

Fungal and Yeast Infections

Various fungi are capable of infecting skin structures and the resulting infections are generically termed dermatomycoses. The most important and frequently found fungi are *Candida albicans, Trichophyton, Epidermophyton*, and *Microsporum* genera. A few molds are also capable of inducing disease.

The diagnosis of many dermatomycoses can generally be made visually and requires little if any further testing. Diagnosis of dermatomycoses also relies heavily on the use of potassium hydroxide (KOH) preparations and on culture. The KOH preparation, in particular, is a useful diagnostic test. Skin scrapings are placed on a microscopic slide and covered with a coverslip; a few drops of 15% KOH are allowed to seep under the cover glass. The sample is allowed to stand for approximately 1 hour and then is gently heated. This preparation allows dissolution of the keratin in the cells, leaving a clearer view of the fungal elements. Some examiners prefer to add blue-black ink to the preparation as it enhances identification of the fungal elements.

Dermatophytoses

The dermatophytoses are the most commonly encountered fungal illnesses in a family physician's office. The site of the illness specifies the name of the illness as follows: tinea capitis (hair-bearing portions of head), tinea barbae (scalp), tinea faciei (face), tinea corporis (body), tinea cruris (groin), tinea manus (hands), tinea pedis (feet), and tinea unguium (nails). Fungal infections generally itch, and this symptom often brings the patient to seek attention. The most common pathogens causing these illnesses are the *Trichophyton* species, especially *Trichophyton mentagrophytes*. Many of the *Trichophyton* species are noted in domestic animals, and their spread by these sources may be more common in children.

Tinea capitis is most commonly seen in infants and young children. The disease has reached epidemic proportions in Northern California, England, and Wales recently.[30–32] The infection can be transmitted to others in school, day-care, and household settings. Circular lesions with a distinct border and the impression of central clearing are noted. Where the fungi have penetrated especially deeply around hair follicles, a nodular-inflammatory lesion may occur, known as a kerion. Microsporosis is noninflamed-appearing variant of tinea capitis caused by *Microsporum audouinii*. Microsporosis is more common among school-aged boys and is contagious in this population. Whitish dusted patches of hair loss that become confluent are noted with microsporosis, with hairs broken just above the scalp. The lesions of microsporosis fluoresce greenish white under the Wood's light, and this distinction is helpful for distinguishing the illness from other forms of alopecia. Fungal cultures are obtained to aid in directing therapy and confirming the diagnosis of tinea capitis. Tinea capitis generally requires systemic therapy, and severely inflamed lesions are treated with systemic or intralesional steroids. For small, noninflammatory lesions in children, a potent topical imidazole may be tried while cultures are pending. Terbinafine should now be considered the agent of choice for tinea capitis, and is administered to adults in a 250 mg per day dose for 2 weeks for *Trichosporum tonsurans* infection and 4 to 8 weeks for *Microsporum* infections. For children who weigh less than 20 kg (but who are older than 2 years of age) the dose is 62.5 mg daily, for those 20 to 40 kg the dose is 125 mg daily for durations similar to those of the adult dosing. Ketoconazole, itraconazole, or griseofulvin are also useful.

Tinea barbae appears first as a pustular folliculitis involving the beard. The illness spreads across much of the beard area, leaving the hairs looking dusty and appearing as wicks sticking out from a pustular base. The illness may last more than 6 weeks and is occasionally accompanied by mild systemic signs. Gradually, and likely secondary to an immune response, the illness resolves without scarring. This illness has become rarer and is most often associated with animal handlers, but it should be considered in the differential diagnosis of pustular facial lesions.[33] Although the disease is self-limited, treatment as for tinea capitis should be considered.

Tinea corporis and tinea faciei are most commonly seen in children. Lesions with reddish, scaling, raised borders surround a central zone that is faded but often scaling (Fig. 116.7). This classic "ringworm" appearance is characteristic,

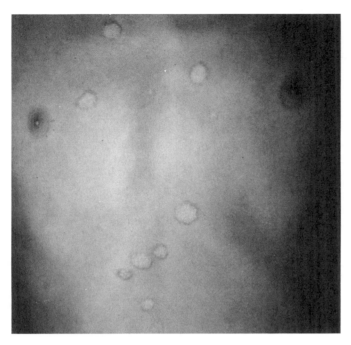

Fig. 116.7. Tinea corporis.

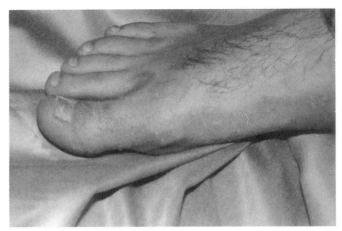

Fig. 116.9. Tinea pedis.

although confirmation with KOH scraping is wise. Topical treatment with imidazole creams is all that is generally required for this illness. If a refractory illness occurs, the use of terbinafine 250 mg daily for 2 weeks is effective. Fluconazole and ketoconazole are also useful agents.

Tinea cruris, also known as "jock itch," usually affects the groin area, perianal area, and upper inner thighs while sparing the scrotum and penis (Fig. 116.8). Other intertriginous areas may also be affected, such as the axillae. It is more common in overweight individuals or those with excessive sweating. It is commonly confused with erythrasma, a distinction that may have treatment implications. For resistant cases, confirmation of the infection with fungal culture is wise. Additionally, erythrasma fluoresces a characteristic coral-pink under the Wood's light, and so use of such a light may be helpful. Tinea cruris generally responds well to imidazole creams, par-

ticularly when the patient is advised to wear loose cotton undergarments. Talc powder may also be useful, but inhalation of the powder is to be avoided. If a refractory illness occurs, terbinafine at 250 mg per day for 2 weeks should be prescribed. Ketoconazole or fluconazole are also useful agents.

Tinea pedis may be the most common skin lesion in North America and Europe, with an estimate of 15% to 30% of the adult population being affected (Fig. 116.9). Although much less common than tinea pedis, tinea manus is a similar disease, so the two are discussed together. The illnesses manifest in three ways, which are sometimes all seen in selected patients. One is the intertriginous variety, where the interdigital spaces are primarily affected. Maceration and cracking of the interdigital spaces is noted with this variety. A second variety, with squamous hyperkeratosis, is also noted. Here irregular but sharply defined areas of hyperkeratosis appear on the sole, heels, or tips of the toes with tinea pedis and on the palms and volar and lateral surfaces of the fingers with tinea manus. In the third variety, itchy, dyshidrotic vesicles may form. This dyshydrotiform variety generally affects the same surfaces as seen with the hyperkeratotic form. Treatment includes use of imidazole creams, reduction of perspiration, and avoidance of occlusive clothing items such as rubberized boots or gloves. If a refractory illness occurs, terbinafine at 250 mg per day for 2 weeks should be prescribed. Ketoconazole and fluconazole are also useful agents.

Tinea unguium is also referred to as onychomycosis. This disease involves invasion of the nail plate and results in thickened, hyperkeratotic, brittle nails. The toenails are more commonly involved than the fingernails. The changes in the nail first appear distally and then move back to the nail bed. This retrograde progression of the process aids in distinguishing it from psoriasis, which otherwise may have a similar appearance. Generally, little functional disability is involved, and patients seek medical attention for cosmetic purposes. The illness is persistent and notoriously difficult to treat. Systemic treatment is necessary when cure is desirable, but recurrences are common. For fingernail infections, terbinafine at 250 mg daily for 6 weeks is generally effective.[34] For toenail infections, the duration of treatment is doubled to 12 weeks. Some physicians

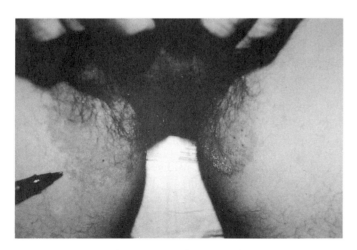

Fig. 116.8. Tinea cruris.

prefer a regime involving 1 week of treatment monthly with fluconazole 150 to 300 mg per day during the week of treatment. Using this 1 week per month regimen, treatment of fingernails requires 3 to 6 months and toenails 6 to 12 months. Itraconazole is also an effective agent.

Diseases Caused by Yeasts

Various yeasts are capable of causing skin disease in humans, the most common of which is *Candida albicans*. Candidosis occurs worldwide and has acquired special significance with increasing numbers of immunosuppressed patients for whom infection can be lethal. Another yeast commonly seen as causing disease is *Pityrosporum (Malassezia) furfur*, the causative agent of tinea versicolor, more properly known as pityriasis versicolor.

Oral thrush is a common finding during infancy, and it commonly affects immunosuppressed individuals. Angular cheilitis is caused by oral *C. albicans* as well. With thrush, a whitish, curd-like coating is noted primarily on the tongue. In severe cases, usually in individuals with immunosuppression, the coating may spread throughout the oropharynx and be associated with painful swallowing. With angular cheilitis, cracking and fissuring occur at the corners of the mouth. Nearly pure cultures of *C. albicans* are often obtained from these areas. Angular cheilitis is more common in older individuals with poor-fitting teeth. Oral thrush and angular cheilitis can generally be treated a single 200-mg dose of fluconazole. Nystatin pastilles or clotrimazole troches are also useful. Immunosuppressed patients often require prolonged systemic therapy with fluconazole, 200 mg on day 1 followed by 100 mg daily for 14 days.

Candidal vulvovaginosis is commonly noted in women. The affected woman seeks attention for relief of vaginal itching and burning, dysuria, and discharge (see Chapter 102). The illness is more common among women who are diabetic or who use douches. The external genitalia may be reddened, and candidal intertrigo or folliculitis may be present in the groin. The vaginal mucous membrane is often reddened. A whitish, creamy to cheesy consistency vaginal discharge is noted. A single oral dose of fluconazole 150 mg or itraconazole 200 mg is quite effective. Alternatively, treatment with imidazole (topical vaginal preparation) is effective in 80% of cases. Chronic candidal vulvovaginitis occurs in less than 5% of healthy women, but may require long-term suppressive therapy with fluconazole, ketoconazole, itraconazole, or intravaginal clotrimazole.[35] Occasionally the male sexual partner requires treatment to prevent recurrent infection.

Candidal balanitis primarily occurs in uncircumcised men who are obese, elderly, diabetic, or have phimosis. Inadequate hygiene or a sexual partner with candidal vulvovaginosis increases the risk for this illness. The prepuce and glans are affected, and reddened patches with grayish white deposits are noted. Secondary bacterial infections and phimosis related to inflammation may also occur. Thorough cleansing followed by antifungal creams (not ointments!) usually is sufficient to clear the disease. Circumcision should be considered upon resolution of the inflammation.

Candidal intertrigo may occur where skinfolds are moist and macerated. Obesity, diabetes mellitus, and immunosuppression are important predisposing conditions. An area of redness and maceration is usually surrounded by a scaly area, often with small satellite lesions. Keeping the affected area dry and clean and applying topical antifungal agents generally clear the rash promptly.

Candidal diaper rash is common among infants, especially when close-fitting, poorly absorbent diapers are used (see Chapter 17). Scattered small lesions with a surrounding scaly "collarette" are noted with this illness, and occasionally a larger central area of macerated lesions is present as well. Various antifungal creams are effective, particularly if paired with frequent diaper changes and exposure to air. Rubber pants are avoided. The use of combined steroid and antifungal cream remains controversial given that long-term use may theoretically result in sufficient absorption of steroid to suppress the adrenal axis.

Chronic paronychia may occur when *C. albicans* infects the nail bed. Such infections are more common among individuals whose hands are frequently moistened (e.g., bartenders and dentists). The nail fold is reddened and inflamed. Without culture or examination of the pathogen microscopically, it is difficult to differentiate between paronychia caused by dermatophytes and those caused by *C. albicans*. Drainage, sometimes involving removal of the nail, is necessary. Drainage and adequate drying of the hands generally is sufficient to effect cure.

Tinea versicolor is a common infection that is more properly referred to as pityriasis versicolor. "Tinea" is incorrectly used, as the rash is not one caused by a dermatophyte. Rather, it is due to infection by the yeast *Pityrosporum (Malassezia) furfur*. The illness is rare before puberty. It is more common in humid, warm environments, and the causative organism requires an environment rich in lipids. Thus the rash of the illness is found on the chest and back and may spread to the lateral buttocks. The skin lesions are generally coffee-colored and are up to 1 cm in size. As the rash spreads, the lesions become confluent and slightly scaly (Fig. 116.10). The skin lesions themselves show little change in color seasonally, al-

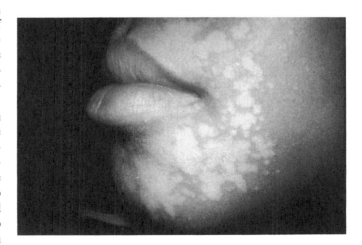

Fig. 116.10. Pityriasis versicolor.

though the pigmentation of surrounding skin makes the lesions appear lighter during months where skin becomes tan and darker during nontanning months. The lesions are chronic without treatment but are also asymptomatic. The organism is mildly contagious. Treatment with selenium-based shampoos, imidazole creams, or a single 400-mg dose of ketoconazole is often effective.

Dermal Mycoses

Various mycoses are capable of causing deep infection. Examples of such infections include chromomycosis, mycetoma, protothecosis, and sporotrichosis. Sporotrichosis, though unusual in North America and Europe, is the most common of these illnesses.

Sporotrichosis is a chronic, deep infection with *Sporothrix schenckii*, a fungus found throughout the world on rotting wood products and baled hay. The infection occurs sporadically in North America and Europe but is the most common deep mycotic infection in Mexico. The illness results from traumatic inoculation, usually on the hands or feet. Five variations of the infection have been described. Lymphocutaneous sporotrichosis is the most common, and with this illness multiple bluish red swellings occur along the lymph node chain draining the primary inoculation site.[36] Fixed cutaneous sporotrichosis may occur when prior immunity to the organism contains the lesion to a cluster of wart-like growths at the inoculation site. Disseminated sporotrichosis may occur in patients who are immunodeficient, and multiple inflamed papulonodules occur over the body following hematogenous spread. Mucocutaneous sporotrichosis occurs when both skin and mucous membrane involvement are noted. Finally, extracutaneous systemic sporotrichosis may involve bone, large joint, eyes, muscle, and kidney. This last illness is particularly dangerous but rare. Itraconazole is now the agent of choice for sporotrichosis. Potassium iodide orally is often sufficient in forms of the disease limited to skin.

Infestations

A variety of insects cause or spread illness and rash in humans. Although far more common in temperate climates, infestations may be found globally. Good hygiene tends to prevent such infestations, but even well-groomed individuals may be affected. Many insects are capable of producing rash in humans, including fleas, *Cimex lectularius* (bed bug), and *Hymenoptera* (bees and wasps). These insect-related rashes are not related to true infestation. The insects that cause infestation or skin manifestations of significant duration include *Sarcoptes scabiei* (scabies), lice (*Pediculosis capitis, P. corporis, Phthirus pubis*), *Demodex folliculorum*, and chigger mites. Various helminths also cause skin rashes, but they are rarely seen in the United States. *Ancylostoma* sp. and other hookworms cause cutaneous larva migrans. *Wuchereria bancrofti* infestation results in filariasis, a common cause of elephantiasis in certain countries. *Onchocerca volvulus* is the cause of onchocerciasis, a debilitating multiorgan illness with significant skin manifestations. Most family physicians are unlikely to see these last three infestations in their practices, and so they are not discussed further.

Scabies

The most common infestation is that of scabies, caused by the mite *S. scabiei*. The female mite burrows under the skin to lay her eggs, which are fertilized by the male mite. The eggs hatch within a few days. By 2 weeks after infestation, extensive colonization has occurred accompanied by intense itching. The mite is transmissible skin to skin through close contact, such as sexual intercourse. The finger webs, wrists, genitalia, nipples, abdomen, buttocks, and ankles are commonly affected, although spread to nearly any region other than the head and neck may be seen (Fig. 116.11). The mite almost never affects the head and neck region in adults. A burrow 5 to 10 mm long is almost pathognomonic for the illness, although burrows may be difficult to find as a result of excoriation. Skin scrapings or aspiration of a vesicle may reveal the female mite or parts under the microscope. In fair-skinned individuals the mite may be seen as a dark dot at the end of the burrow. Permethrin or lindane are preferred treatments for the infestation. Lindane is used cautiously in young children and should not be used on infants or pregnant women. Ivermectin is also an effective agent, and has extensively been given orally outside of the United States.[37] Ivermectin, while generally safe, can have serious toxicity and should be reserved for resistant or otherwise unusual cases.[38] Careful cleansing of bedclothes and treatment of frequent household contacts is also recommended.

Pediculosis

Three species of lice are parasitic in humans: the head louse (*P. capitis*), body louse (*P. humanus corporis*), and pubic louse (*Phthirus pubis*). Lice attach themselves to hair by means of three pairs of strong, grasping legs. The female lays her eggs embedded in a water-insoluble glue that adheres the eggs to the hair shaft. Eggs hatch after a period of 1 week. The lice ingest blood every few hours.

Head lice are commonly seen in children and individuals

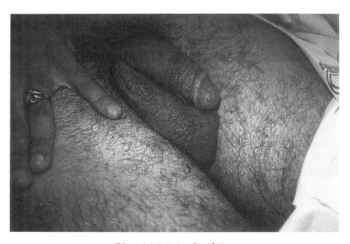

Fig. 116.11. Scabies.

with long hair. Small epidemics are common in schools, and these epidemics are aided by poor hygiene. Symptomatic individuals generally complain of itching behind the ears, a favorite site for the louse's blood meal. Small, intensely red papules may be noted in this area, which is a reaction to the saliva of the louse. Nits, which are small, white-to-clear, oval concretions on the hair shaft, are common.

Body lice are most common among the homeless. These lice do not actually attach to the body but to clothing, particularly the seams. Intense pruritus from exposure to the louse saliva during blood meals results in widespread excoriations arranged in a linear fashion. Pediculosis humanus corporis is capable of transmitting various rickettsial diseases, including spotted fever, typhus, and trench fever.[38]

Pubic lice are most commonly spread during sexual intercourse but may be spread by other means as well. The lice favor the apocrine regions and therefore are found in the pubic and anogenital area, axillary region, and uncommonly in the scalp, eyebrows, and eyelashes. Itching is less intense than with other louse diseases, but nits are easily apparent. A distinctive slate-gray lesion may also occur at the area of bites. This lesion probably represents digested blood breakdown products.

The treatment of lice infestation is generally with permethrin, lindane, or pyrethrins. Permethrin (Nix) is the most effective of the three agents.[39] Lindane is used cautiously in young children and should not be used at all on infants or pregnant women. A 5% malathion lotion preparation (Ovide Topical) has recently been reintroduced as a prescription agent in the U.S. Malathion is an organophosphate and must be used with caution. Instituting adequate hygiene is important. Ivermectin may be used as well, but is considered less safe than permethrin.[38] Treatment of clothes and bed sheets, especially for body lice, is also important. Control of school-based infestation is aided by discussing the case with school health officials.

Demodex

Demodex folliculorum is a small mite that lives as a saprophyte in sebaceous glands. It may be associated with the pathogenesis of rosacea, and it has also been implicated in blepharitis and pustular eruptions around the mouth. Treatments that anecdotally are successful include 5% sulfurated zinc, lindane, and crotamiton. Such treatment is generally reserved for refractory forms of rosacea (see Chapter 115).

Chiggers

Chiggers is a common and extraordinarily pruritic rash, occurring most commonly among those who are active in outdoor activities. The illness is caused by infestation with the larval form of the chigger mite, the most common of which is *Trombicula alfreddugesi*. The mite is most commonly found in low-lying bottom lands. The larval form attaches to the skin, where it feeds on digested epidermal cells. During this feeding stage the mite may appear as a bright red dot on the skin. Although the chigger mite is not a blood feeder, it is capable of transmitting rickettsial diseases, such as rick-

ettsialpox. Although scratching generally removes the mite, if any mites are present they should be removed with a needle. Lindane and crotamiton also are effective in killing the mite, the latter agent also providing some relief from itching. The use of clothes that fit tight at the neck, wrist, and ankle helps prevent the infestation, as the mite cannot cross such constricted areas. DEET and other insect repellents are also useful for prevention.[40]

References

1. Wharton JR, Wilson PL, Kincannon JM. Erythrasma treated with single-dose clarithromycin. Arch Dermatol 1998;134(6): 671–2.
2. Takama H. Pitted keratolysis: clinical manifestations in 53 cases. Br J Dermatol 1997;137(2):282–5.
3. Pseudomonas dermatitis/folliculitis associated with pools and hot tubs—Colorado and Maine, 1999–2000. MMWR 2000;49(48): 1087–91.
4. Landen MG. Outbreak of boils in an Alaskan village: a case-control study [see comments]. West J Med 2000;172(4):235–9.
5. Jemec GB, Wendelboe P. Topical clindamycin versus systemic tetracycline in the treatment of hidradenitis suppurativa. J Am Acad Dermatol 1998;39(6):971–4.
6. Boer J, van Gemert MJ. Long-term results of isotretinoin in the treatment of 68 patients with hidradenitis suppurativa [see comments]. J Am Acad Dermatol 1999;40(1):73–6.
7. Dupuy A. Risk factors for erysipelas of the leg (cellulitis): case-control study. BMJ 1999;318(7198):1591–4.
8. Chow AW, Roser SM, Brady FA. Orofacial odontogenic infections. Ann Intern Med 1978;88(3)392–402.
9. Wall DB. Objective criteria may assist in distinguishing necrotizing fasciitis from nonnecrotizing soft tissue infection. Am J Surg 2000;179(1):17–21.
10. zur Hausen H. Papillomaviruses causing cancer: evasion from host-cell control in early events in carcinogenesis. J Natl Cancer Inst 2000;92(9):690–8.
11. Centers for Disease Control and Prevention. Rubella among Hispanic adults—Kansas, 1998, and Nebraska, 1999. JAMA 2000; 283(14):1819–20.
12. Ely JW, Yankowitz J, Bowdler NC. Evaluation of pregnant women exposed to respiratory viruses. Am Fam Physician 2000; 61(10) 3065–74.
13. Takahashi Y. Human parvovirus B19 as a causative agent for rheumatoid arthritis. Proc Natl Acad Sci USA 1998;95(14): 8227–32.
14. Prevention of varicella. Update recommendations of the Advisory Committee on Immunization Practices (ACIP). MMWR 1999;48(RR-6):1–5.
15. Cohen JI. Recent advances in varicella-zoster virus infection. Ann Intern Med 1999;130(11):922–32.
16. Salzman MB. Transmission of varicella-vaccine virus from a healthy 12-month-old child to his pregnant mother [see comments]. J Pediatr 1997;131(1 pt 1):151–4.
17. Alper BS, Lewis PR. Does treatment of acute herpes zoster prevent or shorten postherpetic neuralgia? [see comments]. J Fam Pract 2000;49(3):255–64.
18. Drake S. Improving the care of patients with genital herpes. BMJ 2000;321(7261):619–23.
19. Brown ZA. The acquisition of herpes simplex virus during pregnancy N Engl J Med 1997;337(8):509–15.
20. Spruance SL. Penciclovir cream for the treatment of herpes simplex labialis. A randomized, multicenter, double-blind, placebo-controlled trial. Topical Penciclovir Collaborative Study Group. JAMA 1997;277(17):1374–9.

21. Berger M, Global infectious disease epidemiology network. San Francisco: C. Y. Informatics, 2001.
22. Drago F, Rebora A. The new herpesviruses: emerging pathogens of dermatological interest. Arch Dermatol 1999;135(1):71–5.
23. Huang CC. Neurologic complications in children with enterovirus 71 infection [see comments]. N Engl J Med 1999;341(13):936–42.
24. Young R, Jolley D, Marks R. Comparison of the use of standardized diagnostic criteria and intuitive clinical diagnosis in the diagnosis of common viral warts (verrucae vulgaris). Arch Dermatol 1998;134(12):1586–9.
25. Edwards L. Self-administered topical 5% imiquimod cream for external anogenital warts. HPV Study Group. Human Papillomavirus. Arch Dermatol 1998;134(1):25–30.
26. Hengge UR, Goos M, Arndt R. Topical treatment of warts and mollusca with imiquimod [letter; comment]. Ann Intern Med 2000;132(1):95.
27. Beutner KR, Ferenczy A. Therapeutic approaches to genital warts. Am J Med 1997;102(5A):28–37.
28. Cotell SL, Roholt NS. Images in clinical medicine. Molluscum contagiosum in a patient with the acquired immunodeficiency syndrome. N Engl J Med 1998;338(13):888.
29. Buckley R, Smith K. Topical imiquimod therapy for chronic giant molluscum contagiosum in a patient with advanced human immunodeficiency virus 1 disease. Arch Dermatol 1999;135(10):1167–9.
30. Lamagni T, Evans B, Campbell C. Tinea capitis should be on the public health agenda [letter]. BMJ 2000;321(7258):451.
31. Gibbon KL. Unnecessary surgical treatment of fungal kerions in children. BMJ 2000;320(7236):696–7.
32. Lobato MN, Vugia DJ, Frieden IJ. Tinea capitis in California children: a population-based study of a growing epidemic. Pediatrics 1997;99(4):551–4.
33. Glaser DA, Riordan AT. Images in clinical medicine. Tinea barbae: man and beast [see comments]. N Engl J Med 1998;338(11):735.
34. Ellis MR, Kane KY. Oral treatment of onychomycosis. J Fam Pract 1999;48(4):252.
35. Sobel JD. Vaginitis [see comments]. N Engl J Med 1997;337(26):1896–903.
36. Saxena M, Rest EB. An ulcerating nodule on the arm. Lymphocutaneous sporotrichosis. Arch Dermatol 1998;134(10):1281, 1284.
37. Chouela EN. Equivalent therapeutic efficacy and safety of ivermectin and lindane in the treatment of human scabies [see comments]. Arch Dermatol 1999;135(6):651–5.
38. Chosidow O. Scabies and pediculosis [see comments]. Lancet 2000;355(9206):819–26.
39. Dawes M. Evidence based case report: treatment for head lice [see comments]. BMJ 1999;318(7180):385–6.
40. Jones JG. Chiggers. Am Fam Physician 1987;36(2):149–52.

117
Skin Tumors

Michael Herbst, Denise K.C. Sur, and Allen S. Yang

Skin tumors are very common, often dangerous, and sometimes disfiguring. Family physicians are particularly well equipped to prevent, diagnose, treat, and follow skin tumors. For example, advising patients to limit their recreational and occupational sun exposure can prevent skin cancers. Knowledge of patients' risk factors for skin tumors and performing screening skin examinations permits early diagnosis. The procedural skills of family physicians are effective for treatment of most skin tumors. Continuity of care provides the ideal setting for follow-up of these tumors and prevention of their sequelae.

Benign Skin Tumors

Acrochordons (Skin Tags)

Acrochordons are extremely common. They are small, benign, flesh-colored to hyperpigmented, pedunculated skin tags, characteristically attached by short, thin stalks. They are most common on the neck, in the axilla, and in skinfolds. Acrochordons are more frequent in women and the obese. They are uncommon before 30 years of age. Acrochordons can be treated by simple excision with scissors, by electrodesiccation, or using cryotherapy.

Dermatofibroma

Dermatofibromas are common skin lesions that are often found on the anterior surface of the leg. They are more frequent in women than in men. They present as pink- to brown-colored, firm nodules 3 to 10 mm in diameter. Their surface is usually smooth but may be scaly. They are a localized, nodular, fibrous response to what may be an insignificant skin injury or inflammation. They usually develop over several months and rarely resolve spontaneously. The Fitzpatrick's or "dimple" sign (dimpling of the lesion with lateral compres-

sion between the thumb and forefinger) is typical but not pathognomonic of dermatofibroma. The treatment of choice is elliptical excision. It is reserved for instances where irritation, erosion, or a rapid increase in size arouses concern about the possibility of skin cancer. Intralesional corticosteroids should not be used because the results are unpredictable and often unsatisfactory.

Hemangioma

Hemangiomas are localized vascular lesions resulting from hyperplasia of cutaneous blood vessels. The different types are distinguished clinically by their depth and color. Hemangiomas occur in approximately 10% of newborns with a 3:1 preponderance in females.[1] Salmon patches are superficial midline capillary hemangiomas that appear commonly at the nape of the neck or on the glabella or forehead of newborns. Approximately 50% resolve spontaneously and many of the rest become quite faint; treatment is not usually indicated. Strawberry hemangiomas are collections of dilated vessels in the dermis that appear as raised, bright red lesions. They are often present at birth but may also appear within the first few months of life. Complete involution occurs in more than 90% of these lesions, usually commencing before age 3 years.[2] Observation and reassurance are the usual management. Cavernous hemangiomas are collections of dilated vessels deep in the dermis and the subcutaneous tissue; they are easily confused with dermal and subcutaneous venous malformations, which can appear very similar but have a different natural history.[3] Compared to strawberry hemangiomas, venous hemangiomas present later in infancy and grow more slowly. Most cavernous hemangiomas spontaneously involute, although involution can be delayed and incomplete.

Treatment of both strawberry and cavernous hemangiomas is reserved for large lesions or lesions involving vital organs. Strawberry hemangiomas and some cavernous hemangiomas respond well to intralesional steroids. A 2- to 4-week course of oral corticosteroids is also often effective; the high doses used previously do not appear to be necessary.[4] Large or cosmetically unacceptable lesions may be treated with pulsed-dye laser therapy.

Nevus flammeus (port wine stains) are congenital hemangiomas, usually unilateral, that consist of capillaries near the skin surface. They are present at birth and persist lifelong. Port wine stain lesions are most commonly associated with branches of the trigeminal nerve and may be associated with Sturge-Weber syndrome. Nevus flammeus appears as flat, red to red-blue, initially smooth patches that may eventually assume a cobblestone surface. Pulsed-dye laser therapy is often successful in ablating port wine stains with minimal scarring; this treatment is suitable for children as well as adults.

Cherry angiomas, which appear as small, smooth, firm, deep red papules, are the most common of all the vascular lesions of skin. Their frequency increases with age. If they are cosmetically unacceptable, they can be easily ablated by electrodesiccation.

Keloid

Keloids are smooth, raised, red, firm overgrowths of fibroblastic tissue that arise in traumatized areas of a predisposed person. Unlike hypertrophic scars, keloids proliferate into the surrounding normal skin, extending beyond the area of injury. They commonly occur on the anterior chest, shoulders, neck, and earlobes. They are more common in African Americans and those with a family history of keloids. The initial treatment of choice is intralesional corticosteroids every 2 to 4 weeks for a total of three to five injections. This can be accomplished with a 27- or 30-gauge needle using triamcinolone acetonide 10 mg/mL. This treatment works best for early, small, or narrow lesions and usually stops keloid growth and leads to significant flattening. For larger lesions, consider referral to a dermatologist or plastic surgeon.

Lipomas

Lipomas are common, soft, encapsulated, subcutaneous fatty tumors that occur in all sizes. Malignant degeneration, with large, rapidly growing tumors, is very rare. Simple excision, which is facilitated by the presence of the capsule, is the treatment of choice. It is usually reserved for cosmetically troubling lesions or to establish the diagnosis in symptomatic or rapidly growing lesions.

Melanocytic Nevocellular Nevus (Mole)

Moles are small, circumscribed collections of melanocytes that may appear as macules, papules, or nodules. The average white adult has approximately 20 moles, but they may be present in large numbers. They are classified according to the location of the melanocytes. In junctional nevi, which predominate during early childhood, the melanocytes cluster in the epidermis. In dermal nevi, which predominate in adult life, the melanocytes cluster in the dermis. In compound nevi the melanocytes have a mixed epidermal and dermal location.

Because malignant melanoma cannot be excluded by inspection, histologic evaluation is required for all nevi with atypical features or which itch, burn, or bleed. Moles should never be treated with cryotherapy or electrodesiccation because these techniques do not permit pathologic evaluation of the lesion. Punch biopsy(s) may be sufficient to establish the diagnosis if total excision is cosmetically unacceptable.

Seborrheic Keratosis

Seborrheic keratosis (SK) is one of the most common skin tumors. The etiology is unknown, although there is often a familial tendency. They become common in middle age and are frequent in older patients. Histologically, they are confined to the epidermis and have no malignant potential.

SKs may be a few millimeters to 3 cm in size. The surface may vary from a smooth, finely cobblestoned pattern to a rough, velvety surface, which may be dry, fissured, and irregularly pigmented. They have sharp borders and appear to be "stuck on" to the skin surface, which helps to distinguish them from other pigmented lesions. The thickness of an SK and the degree of trauma from contact with skin or clothing can alter their surface appearance and cause inflammation in surrounding tissue.

Treatment with cryosurgery or electrocautery is usually highly effective, and if care is taken to avoid injury to the deeper layers of the skin, scarring is minimal. Occasionally biopsy is required to rule out melanoma.

Premalignant Lesions

Actinic Keratosis

Actinic keratosis (AK), also known as solar keratosis, is the most common premalignant skin lesion.[5,6] The prevalence of AKs increases with ultraviolet light exposure and with age. Fair-skinned individuals have a higher incidence of AKs. AKs are most frequent on sun-exposed areas of the body, including the scalp of men with male-pattern baldness, the face, the ears, and the dorsum of the hands. AKs are also common on the upper chest, extensor surface of the forearms, and the legs.

Clinically, AKs appear as single or multiple erythematous macules with adherent scale or as keratotic papules with a roughened surface that may be more easily felt than seen. They are usually asymptomatic. Although the risk of malignant transformation is uncertain, it is estimated that 10% of people with AKs eventually develop cutaneous squamous cell carcinoma (SCC).[7] AKs are not the only precursors to SCC. Studies have shown that 40% may arise de novo in normal skin.[5,8] Infiltration, elevation, or tenderness of an AK suggests malignant change. The presence of AKs should prompt the physician to examine the patient closely for other skin cancers.

Minimizing ultraviolet exposure and the use of sunscreens and protective clothing are essential for prevention. The goal of therapy is to completely eradicate the lesions while minimizing scarring. Cryosurgery and electrodesiccation and curettage are both effective. If multiple or poorly defined lesions are present, topical application of 2% solution or 5% 5-fluorouracil (5-FU) cream, applied twice daily for 2 to 3 weeks may be effective. Erythematous reactions, which may be uncomfortable and unsightly, develop after several days. 5-FU therapy is continued until the keratoses crust; a low potency, nonfluorinated topical steroid such as 1% hydrocortisone ointment is then applied twice daily for 2 to 3 weeks. The latter speeds healing and minimizes discomfort. This protocol is especially effective for AKs on the face, ears, and scalp. AKs on the forearms and dorsum of the hands respond less well to 5-FU therapy, although a 5% preparation of 5-FU cream may be used. Pretreatment with topical 0.05% to 0.10% tretinoin cream twice daily for a few months enhances the therapeutic effect of subsequently applied 5-FU cream.[5] All patients in with a history of AKs should undergo periodic skin examinations to detect new lesions.

Keratoacanthoma

Keratoacanthomas are common, rapidly growing, round, flesh-colored lesions with a characteristic central crater covered by a keratotic plug. They occur most commonly in Caucasian men with fair complexions and sun-damaged skin. Clinically and histologically, keratoacanthomas are low-grade or abortive SCCs. In contrast to SCCs, keratoacanthomas do not usually exceed 3 cm in size. Keratoacanthomas may regress within 2 to 6 months or progress to SCC. Excisional or shave biopsy is advisable; they are difficult to distinguish from SCCs, and spontaneous resolution may leave a disfiguring pitted scar. All tissue should be submitted for histologic evaluation. Immunosuppressed patients are at increased risk of developing keratoacanthomas and invasive SCCs.

Leukoplakia

Leukoplakia is a nonspecific term that describes any hyperkeratotic, fixed, white patch on a mucosal surface that cannot be characterized as another disease. The usual lesion is a white patch that ranges from a flat, slightly translucent area to palpable lesions that are indurated and fissured. Some lesions are papillomatous or wrinkled and have a rough quality on palpation. Although the color is generally white, leukoplakia may appear gray, yellow, or even brown in heavy cigarette smokers. Leukoplakia must be differentiated from candidiasis, which appears similar but wipes easily from the mucosal surface with a gauze sponge, and lichen planus, which cannot be wiped away. Biopsy is essential to the diagnosis.

The term *leukoplakia* implies cellular atypia and therefore carcinoma in situ for most dermatopathologists. Many clinicians, however, use the term to describe lesions that range from benign hyperkeratotic conditions to carcinoma.

The incidence of leukoplakia is highest in males and in persons over 40. Approximately 50% of leukoplakic lesions are found on the buccal mucosa, mandibular alveolar ridge, or tongue. The lower lip, maxillary alveolar ridge, and palate are also common sites of involvement. Leukoplakia is associated with the use of tobacco (smoked or chewed) and alcohol, oral infection, chronic irritation of the oral mucosa from mal-

occlusion or poorly fitting dentures, and ultraviolet exposure to the mucosa of the lower lip.[9]

Approximately 10% of leukoplakic lesions show invasive carcinoma on initial biopsy or subsequently undergo malignant transformation.[9] Preventive therapy should be directed toward removal of causative factors such as ultraviolet light exposure, malocclusion, tobacco, and alcohol. Once dysplasia or atypia is identified in a lesion, therapeutic options include cryotherapy and surgical excision.

Hairy Leukoplakia

Oral hairy leukoplakia (OHL) is an important lesion strongly associated with HIV/AIDS. It also is a clinical marker for advanced HIV disease. OHL resembles other leukoplakias clinically, most often presenting as an asymptomatic, whitish, wrinkled lesion on the lateral aspects of the tongue. It may also involve the buccal mucosa, floor of the mouth, or palate. The differential diagnosis includes candidiasis, other leukoplakias, lichen planus, and traumatic hyperplasia. The diagnosis is made by biopsy. The word *hairy* refers to the histologic finding of hair-like projections of keratinized epithelium.

Epstein-Barr virus (EBV) is strongly associated with OHL. EBV is typically present and actively replicating in these lesions; HIV has not been recovered.[10] *Candida* infections often coexist and hyphal elements are common on histologic examination. Treatment is directed at the underlying HIV infection.

Squamous Intraepidermal Neoplasia

The histologic finding of full-thickness epidermal cellular atypia without dermal invasion is characteristic of a group of lesions broadly categorized as squamous intraepidermal neoplasia (SIN), SCC in situ, and intraepidermal SCC. Bowen's disease, erythroplasia of Queyrat, and bowenoid papulosis are examples of these cutaneous SIN lesions.

Bowen's Disease

Bowen's disease typically appears as erythematous, scaling or crusting macules, patches, or plaques that are sharply demarcated and vary in size from a few millimeters to several centimeters in diameter.[11] Bowen's disease may appear on any part of the body, including mucous membranes, nail beds, and anogenital areas. While cutaneous bowenoid lesions are generally unpigmented, mucosal lesions appear as velvety red plaques or hyperpigmented papules resting on a velvety base.

Ultraviolet light exposure is presumed to be a major etiologic factor in the development of Bowen's disease. It typically arises during the sixth decade of life, predominantly among fair-skinned persons. Although 75% of the lesions of Bowen's disease occur on sun-exposed surfaces (50% on the head) they also can arise from chemical or human papillomavirus (HPV) exposure.[11] Because HPV-16 has been isolated from some Bowen's lesions, a role as an etiologic agent or cofactor is suspected.

The differential diagnosis of Bowen's disease includes psoriasis, nummular eczema, multicentric superficial basal cell carcinoma (BCC), lichen simplex chronicus, Paget's disease, and actinic keratosis. Pigmented lesions can resemble lentigo maligna melanoma and pigmented BCC. Histologically, bowenoid lesions resemble SCC in situ. Invasive SCC arising from lesions of Bowen's disease is reported in 5% to 20% of cases.[11] Nodularity in a Bowen's lesion suggests that invasive changes may have occurred. Bowen's disease has long been considered a harbinger of a primary internal malignancy. Controversy continues regarding the association of Bowen's disease and primary internal malignancy; more recent studies have failed to confirm the association.[11]

The treatment of choice for small Bowen's lesions is excision with a margin of 5 mm clear of disease on pathologic examination. Electrodesiccation followed by curettage and cryotherapy is also used, but because Bowen's lesions can extend down the outer sheaths of hair follicles, these treatments may incompletely eradicate some lesions. Topical application of either 2% solution or 5% 5-FU cream twice daily for 4 to 12 weeks has also been successful in treating some Bowen's lesions. Regardless of the therapy, close follow-up and regular skin examination is indicated.

Erythroplasia of Queyrat

Erythroplasia, meaning "red patch," is a nonspecific term analogous to leukoplakia. As with leukoplakia, erythroplasia occurs on mucosal surfaces. The glans penis is a modified mucosal surface. When Bowen's disease affects the glans penis it is referred to as erythroplasia of Queyrat. These lesions typically present as bright, erythematous, velvety, nonscaly plaques in elderly men. Erythroplasia of Queyrat has a greater tendency than Bowen's disease to invade and metastasize, with rates up to 30%. Treatment options vary according to the size of the lesion but are the same as for Bowen's disease presenting elsewhere on the body. Because the lesions always contain atypia, they should be treated to ensure complete eradication of the epidermal abnormality.

Bowenoid Papulosis

Bowenoid papulosis represents another unique form of intraepidermal SCC. It appears on the genitalia of both men and women as multiple flat-topped or dome-shaped papules, often pigmented, with a roughened surface ranging up to a few millimeters in diameter. HPV types 16 and 18 have been isolated in 80% of Bowenoid papules and may be a factor or cofactor in their development. Treatment options are the same as for Bowen's disease.

Lentigo Maligna

Lentigo maligna presents during middle to late life as a single macule on an exposed area of skin, characteristically with irregularly irregular borders and colors that vary within the lesion from tan to black. The sizes of the macules vary from one to several centimeters. Histologically, lentigo maligna shows a profuse proliferation of melanocytes in the basal layer of the epidermis. The differential diagnosis includes early seborrheic keratosis, café-au-lait spots, and nevi.

As the term implies, lentigo maligna may develop into malignant melanoma. If simple excisional biopsy of the entire lesion is not possible because of size or location, one or more small punch biopsies may be utilized to establish the diagnosis. Referral to an experienced dermatologist or plastic surgeon is warranted in some instances for treatment of large lesions.

Congenital Nevomelanocytic Nevi

Congenital nevomelanocyclic nevi (CNN) are nevi present at birth. They are categorized as either small or large, with large lesions defined as those >1.5 cm in diameter.[12] The lifetime risk of developing malignant melanoma in small CNNs is much less than 5%. Very large CNNs are also known as giant congenital nevi, bathing trunk nevi, or garment nevi. The lifetime risk of developing melanoma in a giant nevus is 6.3% to 10%.[12] If possible, large CNNs should be completely excised during childhood to eliminate the potential of melanoma.

Malignant Lesions

The most common malignant neoplasms of the skin are basal cell carcinoma, squamous cell carcinoma, and malignant melanoma. The annual incidence of nonmelanoma skin cancers in the United States is approximately one million, and it is believed that this is an underestimate due to underreporting. Nonmelanoma skin cancers are largely basal cell carcinomas, but deaths are predominantly due to SCC. Nonmelanoma skin cancers cause approximately 2300 deaths per year in the United States.[13] Malignant melanoma is a much less common but more lethal skin cancer. The incidence of melanoma in the United States in 1998 was 41,600 cases, but it caused 7300 deaths. Melanoma, representing only about 3% of all skin cancers, accounts for two thirds of all skin cancer deaths.[14] The most important etiologic agent for skin cancer is ultraviolet radiation from sun exposure. The cumulative total skin exposure to UV radiation seems to be the most important environmental risk factor for nonmelanoma skin cancer, though some recent data suggest that severe blistering sunburns in childhood may be more important for basal cell cancer. Although sun exposure is believed to play a role in causing melanoma, some evidence suggests that ultraviolet radiation exposure is not as important as it is for nonmelanoma skin cancer.[15] Other risk factors for malignant skin cancer include psoralen-ultraviolet light treatment (PUVA), tobacco use, living near the equator, and ionizing radiation exposure.[16] Host factors are as important as environmental risk factors. Fair-skinned patients are at increased risk for skin cancer. Other risk factors include blue eyes, red hair, freckles, the presence of pigmented nevi, family history of skin cancer, male gender, and xeroderma pigmentosa.[16]

Basal Cell Carcinoma

Basal cell carcinoma (BCC) accounts for nearly 75% of all skin cancers.[12] Ninety percent of lesions occur on sun-exposed areas of the head and neck and one third occur on the nose.[17]

The typical BCC lesion appears during the fourth decade of life in persons with fair skin and poor ability to tan. Patients who had severe, intermittent sunburns as children or young adults are at particularly high risk for BCC, but it can occur in anyone. The nodular form of the disease presents as a "pearly" or translucent, slightly pink papule or nodule with a telangiectatic surface. The nodular form may evolve into a rodent ulcer, which appears as an ulcer with a "rolled" border that may be crusted and bleed. Both the nodular and the rodent ulcer types are amenable to elliptical excision or a shave procedure followed by curettage and fulguration. It is important to recognize that over a 5-year period there is a 44% incidence of recurrent BCC.[18] Lesions that recur at the original site are often more aggressive than the primary lesions.

Though metastasis is rare, local spread of BCC can be both destructive and disfiguring. The Mohs technique of in vivo fixation, excision, and simultaneous histologic evaluation may be helpful for management of recurrent BCC and for lesions in precarious places such as the nasolabial folds, the medial and lateral canthi, and the external auditory canal.

Three true variants of BCC exist, though their incidence is much lower than the nodular and rodent ulcer types. The first, morpheaform or sclerosing BCC, presents as a plaque-like lesion with ill-defined margins, often giving the appearance of a scar. Because of the extensive, dense fibrous stroma that extends into the surrounding tissue, simple excision of sclerosing BCC is frequently inadequate and a wide excision or Mohs procedure is necessary. The second variant, superficial BCC, may be confused with eczema or psoriasis because of its papulosquamous appearance. Also known as the superficial multicentric type, this variant often occurs as multiple lesions on the trunk in non–sun-exposed areas. It is the least common form of BCC. Because there is no true dermal involvement, this lesion may respond well to topical 5% 5-FU cream applied twice daily for 3 to 6 weeks; application may be required for as long as 12 weeks to eradicate the lesion. The third variant, pigmented BCC, may be difficult to differentiate from melanoma. These highly pigmented lesions occur in individuals with both dark and light complexions. The diagnosis is established by biopsy. They are managed the same way as other basal cell lesions.

Squamous Cell Carcinoma

Squamous cell carcinoma (SCC) is defined as a malignant tumor of epithelial keratinocytes. The incidence of squamous cell carcinoma is highest among fair-skinned Caucasians exposed to intense sunlight. SCCs may arise de novo in areas of previous actinic damage, such as actinic keratoses, leukoplakia, cutaneous horns, and old scars, particularly burn scars. Although the distribution of SCC is similar to that of BCC, it also occurs frequently in non-sun-exposed areas and in darker-pigmented individuals. The incidence of SCC is highest in males and in persons over the age of 55. Unlike BCC, SCC lesions grow rapidly and may metastasize widely. They appear initially as a simple macule or papule that evolves into lesions with a thick, keratinized scale, which may ulcerate, crust, or erode. Because of their more aggressive nature, the treatment of choice for SCCs is careful excision and complete eradication.

Malignant Melanoma

Malignant melanoma (MM) is the most serious of all skin malignancies. It metastasizes frequently and has a high mortality rate. MM tends to occur in those at risk for the other cutaneous malignancies: those with high sun exposure, who burn rather than tan, and who have a family history of melanoma. The incidence of MM has climbed exponentially since the early 1980s, though its mortality has risen only linearly. The overall survival rate for MM is 80%, but the 5-year survival rate is <5% for disseminated disease.[19]

The keys to prevention of MM are avoidance of ultraviolet light exposure and excision of lentigo maligna lesions and dysplastic nevi.[20] Most melanomas occur on sun-exposed areas, although it may occur on any body surface and 5% of all genital cutaneous malignancies are melanomas. Children at risk for MM are those with congenital nevi, particularly giant congenital nevi, and those with familial dysplastic nevi syndrome.[21]

When evaluating a pigmented lesion for melanoma, certain features are especially important. These features are often summarized as the ABCDE rule: *a*symmetric lesions, lesions with irregular *b*orders, lesions with variegated *c*olor, lesions with a *d*iameter greater than 6 mm, and lesions showing an *e*levated surface with irregularities are potential melanomas.[20] All new pigmented lesions are suspect. A mole is worrisome if it itches, burns, or hurts, has a change in contour, or is scaling, crusting, or bleeding. Any significant combination of these factors should lead one to perform a biopsy or wide excision, or both. All pigmented genital lesions warrant biopsy. After the diagnosis is established, referral for staging and definitive treatment should be instituted immediately.

There are four subtypes of MM. Superficial spreading melanomas account for 70% of all MMs. These lesions typically have asymmetry, irregular borders, variable color and contour, and size greater than 6 mm. They commonly occur on the trunk in both sexes and on the lower extremities in women. Superficial spreading melanomas evolve over several years. Initially they spread horizontally but may develop deep invasion or "vertical" spread. Acral lentiginous melanomas account for 5% to 10% of all MMs. They occur as flat, pigmented lesions on the soles, palms, nail beds, and mucous membranes. Acral lentiginous melanoma is the most common type of melanoma in nonwhites. It has a poor prognosis, possibly secondary to delayed diagnosis. Nodular melanoma is the fastest growing of the MMs. It is unique because it has no horizontal growth stage. It occurs as a nodule that simultaneously extends both superficially and deep into the tissues. Nodular melanoma accounts for 10% to 15% of all melanomas. It has a higher metastatic rate and worse prognosis than other types. Lentigo maligna melanoma (LMM) occurs in older persons on sun-exposed areas and accounts for 5% of all MMs. This variant arises from lentigo maligna, which is considered by many to be MM in situ. A slow-growing macular lesion may be present for years prior to diagnosis. In contrast to BCC and SCC, which are found in areas that have had high-dose, intermittent sun exposure, LMM occurs in sun-exposed areas that have been heavily sun-damaged with evidence of thickened skin, telangiectasias, and keratosis.

Prevention of Skin Cancer

The single most important method for prevention of skin cancer is to avoid exposure to ultraviolet radiation from sunlight. All patients, and especially those at risk for skin cancer, should be given the following recommendations:

- Avoid sun exposure, especially from 10 A.M. to 4 P.M., when solar UV intensity is at its maximum.
- Use a sunscreen with an SPF (solar protection factor) of at least 15.
- Wear protective clothing, including large-brim hats, sunglasses, long-sleeved shirts, and long pants.
- Avoid sun tanning outdoors and in tanning booths.

The role of the primary care physician in skin cancer screening is not entirely clear. The American Academy of Dermatology and the Skin Cancer Foundation recommend complete skin examinations for all patients annually. The U.S. Preventative Services Task Force states there is insufficient evidence to recommend for or against routine complete skin exams. The American Cancer Society seems to compromise by recommending complete exams every 3 years between the ages of 20 to 40, and then annually after the age of 40.[17]

Patient education is probably more important than is screening by physicians. The delay in diagnosis patients with melanoma is more likely to be late presentation of patients rather than physician misdiagnosis.[15] Patients often present late in the course of skin cancer when pain or bleeding develops. The ABCDE rule is helpful for both patients and physicians in screening for skin cancer. Additional information for patients is available through the following Internet sites:

- American Academy of Family Physicians: *http://familydoctor.org/*
- American Cancer Society: *http://www.cancer.org*
- The Skin Cancer Foundation: *http://www.skincancer.org*
- American Academy of Dermatology: *http://www.aad.org/*

Kaposi's Sarcoma

Kaposi's sarcoma (KS), which was previously found primarily in those of African and southern European ethnicity, has become one of the diseases most commonly associated with AIDS. At the beginning of the AIDS epidemic, 35% to 40% of all AIDS patients also had KS. More recently the incidence of KS in AIDS patients has fallen to about 15%. Kaposi's sarcoma occurs in nearly half of homosexual men with HIV infection, but less than 5% of other persons infected with HIV infection.[22] A tumor of the vascular endothelium, KS can occur on any body surface including the palms, soles, and mucous membranes. The etiology of Kaposi's sarcoma is likely related to the human herpesvirus-8, which is found in most cases of KS.[23] KS has also been reported in all organs of the body except the brain. The lesions typically appear as violaceous or erythematous macules with associated cutaneous edema. They can be easily confused with other pigmented skin lesions. Biopsy is essential during the initial evaluation of such lesions.

KS cannot now be cured, so it is a lifelong problem. Its primary treatment is antiviral therapy of the HIV infection itself. Localized KS requires no treatment, but lesions that are painful or interfere with ambulation can be managed with local excision, irradiation, or intralesional chemotherapy. Newer therapeutic agents include retinoic acids, human chorionic gonadotropin, and antiangiogenic factors. Rapidly progressive KS (more than 10 new lesions per month), lymphedema, pulmonary KS, or disseminated KS may be treated with systemic chemotherapy, but pancytopenia and immunosuppression are common in these immunocompromised patients.[24]

Biopsy Techniques

Excisional Biopsy

Larger and deeper lesions are best removed by sharp excision within a full-thickness ellipse of skin that is approximately two to three times as long as it is wide. Obtaining cosmetically favorable scars requires placement of the incision so that it is parallel to lines of skin stress (Langer's lines) (Fig. 117.1). It is important to handle the tissue gently and use noncrushing instruments. Good cosmesis is also dependent on skin closure that minimizes tissue tension. For larger lesions it may be necessary to carefully undermine the skin to achieve this. Deep structures should be closed in layers using absorbable suture material, as potential spaces within the wound may become hematomas or seromas. These can become infected or produce scars with surface defects. Deep sutures should also approximate the skin margins as much as possible to minimize the tension on superficial sutures and to limit later widening of the scar. The skin margins themselves should be closed using the finest size of monofilament, nonabsorbable suture material that is practical. Eversion of skin margins is essential to avoid dehiscence and "trapdoor" scars, in which one side of the wound is higher than the other. Subcuticular suture techniques are particularly useful for avoiding suture-induced crosshatch scars, and they may permit the sutures to be removed after a somewhat longer period of wound healing. Skin closure with staples or clips is less precise and more traumatic and should be avoided. Steri-Strips or similar dressings, applied at right angles to the incision, will support wounds after closure. Many experts advise the application of ointments to the wound.[25,26] Ointments can speed wound healing and minimize scar formation by occluding the wound and keeping it moist. There is a risk of contact dermatitis from antibacterial ointments,[27] however, particularly for neomycin-containing ointments.

Shave Biopsy

Shave biopsy is best adapted to lesions known to be nonmalignant. If a lesion is found to be malignant on pathologic examination, a shave biopsy specimen may not be adequate to assess the depth and extent of the malignancy. Postsurgical changes may also confound the pathologist examining tissue from a reexcision.

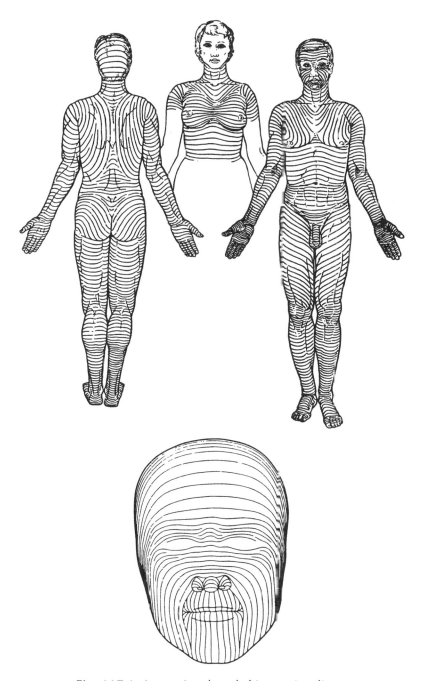

Fig. 117.1. Langer's relaxed skin tension lines.

Local anesthesia is produced by skin infiltration underneath the lesion and into the dermis. The lesion is then shaved off with a scalpel or a loop tip of an electrosurgical generator in cutting mode. Hemostasis may be obtained with the electrosurgical unit in fulguration mode using a ball tip.

Punch Biopsy

Punch biopsy is used to obtain diagnostic tissue from lesions that are either too large to excise primarily or to minimize cosmetic damage. Small lesions may be completely removed by this technique. The area is first infiltrated with a local anesthetic. If a small (2–3 mm) specimen is removed, there is lit-

tle need for sutures. For larger punch biopsies, the skin may be stretched perpendicular to Langer's lines before obtaining the specimen. After releasing the skin tension the defect is elliptical and may be closed with one or more sutures. For large or heterogeneous lesions, or when melanoma is suspected, complete excision of the lesion is preferred because it permits full pathologic evaluation. Alternatively, one may obtain several punch biopsy specimens from the lesion.

Electrosurgery

Electrosurgical generators produce a variety of current types. "Cutting" settings produce low lateral heat and spare surrounding tissue. "Blend" settings produce moderate lateral heat and both cut and coagulate. "Coagulation" settings produce the highest lateral heat and allow effective cautery and fulguration (electrosurgical tissue destruction). Various tip designs are available to perform special tasks. Needles concentrate electrosurgical energy and are used to cut, as are the fine square or circular loops. Tips with larger surface areas are used for coagulation.

Cryosurgery

Freezing is especially useful for ablating common benign skin lesions such as warts, seborrheic keratoses, and acrochordons. Generally, skin lesions are destroyed when one can see a 2- to 3-mm rim of frozen tissue extending beyond the lesion itself, although deeper lesions or thicker skin may require larger margins. There are several methods of cryosurgery, including direct application of liquid nitrogen and contact with nitrous oxide cryoprobes. Insulated flasks of liquid nitrogen with spray nozzles may be used to destroy superficial, flat lesions, but care must be taken to aim them accurately. The cotton tip of a large stick applicator, such as those used in office gynecology, can be pulled into a fine point, dipped into liquid nitrogen, and used to freeze tissue with a high degree of speed and accuracy. It is important to hold the applicator vertically so that the liquid nitrogen flows readily onto the tissue. This technique makes it unnecessary to press the cotton tip against the skin, and permits the physician to closely observe the skin being treated. Nitrous oxide cryoprobes come with a variety of probe tips so one can adequately cover the lesion. Special cold-conducting jellies must be used with the probe to provide good skin contact. Infiltration with local anesthesia before cryosurgery is contraindicated as it distorts tissue fluids and the pattern of the freeze. Topical anesthesia may be used but is rarely needed.

References

1. Esterly NB. Cutaneous hemangiomas, vascular stains, malformations, and associated syndromes. Curr Probl Dermatol 1995;3:69–107.
2. Bowers RE, Graham EA, Tomlinson KM. The natural history of the strawberry nevus. Arch Dermatol 1960;62:667–80.
3. Dohil MA. Vascular and pigmented birthmarks. Pediatr Clin North Am 2000;47(4):783–812, v–vi.
4. Akyuz C, Yaris N, Kutluk MT, Buyukpamukcu M. Management of cutaneous hemangiomas: a retrospective analysis of 1109 cases and comparison of conventional dose prednisolone with high-dose methylprednisolone therapy. Pediatr Hematol Oncol 2001;18(1):47–55.
5. Beacham BE. Solar-induced epidermal tumors in the elderly. Am Fam Physician 1990;42:153–60.
6. Thomas JM. Premalignant and malignant epithelial tumors. In: Sams WM Jr, Lynch PJ, eds. Principles and practice of dermatology. New York: Churchill Livingstone, 1990;199–213.
7. Glogau RG. The risk of progression to invasive disease. J Am Acad Dermatol 2000;42(1 pt 2):23–4.
8. Marks R. The role of treatment of actinic keratoses in the prevention of morbidity and mortality due to squamous cell carcinoma. Arch Dermatol 1991;127:1031–3.
9. Yeatts D, Burns JC. Common oral mucosal lesions in adults. Am Fam Physician 1991;44:2043–50.
10. Triantos D, Porter SR, Scully C, Teo CG. Oral hairy leukoplakia: clinicopathologic features, pathogenesis, diagnosis, and clinical significance. Clin Infect Dis 1997;25(6):1392–6.
11. Lee M, Wick MM. Bowen's disease. CA Cancer J Clin 1990;40:237–42.
12. Fitzpatrick TB, Johnson RA, Wolff K, Suurmond D. Color atlas and synopsis of clinical dermatology. New York: McGraw-Hill, 2000.
13. Rhodes AR. Public education and cancer of the skin: what do people need to know about melanoma and non-melanoma skin cancer? Cancer 1995;75(suppl):613–36.
14. Borenza SJ, Waterman G, Fenske NA. Malignant melanoma: management guidelines. Geriatrics 1990;45:55–62.
15. Goldstein AM, Tucker MA. Etiology, epidemiology, risk factors, and public health issues of melanoma. Curr Opin Oncol 1993;5:358–63.
16. Bruce AJ, Brodland DG. Overview of skin cancer detection and prevention for the primary care physician. Mayo Clin Proc 2000;75:491–500.
17. Mora R. Non-melanoma skin cancer. Prim Care 1989;16:665–84.
18. Marcil I, Stern RS. Risk of developing a subsequent non-melanoma skin cancer in patients with a history of non-melanoma skin cancer: a critical review of the literature and meta-analysis. Arch Dermatol 2000;136(12):1524–30.
19. Friedman RJ, Rigel DS, Silverman MK, Kopf AW, Vossaert KA. Malignant melanoma in the 1990's: the continued importance of early detection and the role of physician examination and self-examination of the skin. CA Cancer J Clin 1991;41:201–26.
20. Jerant AF, Johnson JT, Sheridan CD, Cafrey TJ. Early detection and treatment of skin cancer. Am Fam Physician 2000;357–68.
21. Roth ME, Grant-Kels JM. Important melanocytic lesions in childhood and adolescence. Pediatr Clin North Am 1991;38:791–809.
22. Safai B, Diaz B, Schwartz J. Malignant neoplasms associated with the human immunodeficiency virus infection. CA Cancer J Clin 1992;42:74–95.
23. Prieto VG, Shea CR. Update on dermatopathology: selected cutaneous vascular neoplasms. Dermatol Clin 1999;17:507–20.
24. Gascon P, Schwartz RA. Kaposi's sarcoma: new treatment modalities. Dermatol Clin 2000;18:169–75.
25. Thakur N. Topical ointments and wound healing. J Fam Pract 1997;44(1):26–7.
26. Cho CY, Lo JS. Dressing the part. Dermatol Clin 1998;16(1):25–47.
27. Smack DP, et al. Infection and allergy incidence in ambulatory surgery patients using white petrolatum vs. bacitracin ointment. JAMA 1996;276(12):972–7.

118
Selected Disorders of the Skin

Aubrey L. Knight

Disorders of Hypopigmentation

Vitiligo

Vitiligo is an acquired loss of pigmentation and the most common cause of hypopigmentation. Histologically, the disorder is characterized by a lack of melanocytes in the epidermis. The pigment loss can be diffuse or localized. The incidence peaks between the ages of 10 and 30. The course of the disease is extremely variable.

The etiology of vitiligo is unknown, but it may be an autoimmune disorder with antibodies to melanocytes. There is a positive family history in 30% of cases. Vitiligo is thought to be more prevalent in dark-skinned individuals, but this may be due to easier recognition of the skin manifestations in dark-skinned persons. Vitiligo is associated with thyroid disorders in up to 30% of cases, and there are reported associations with alopecia areata, pernicious anemia, other autoimmune disorders, diabetes mellitus, Addison's disease, premature graying, and melanoma. Potential precipitating events include emotional stress, physical illness, sunburn, or other forms of cutaneous trauma occurring 2 to 3 months prior to the onset of pigment loss. On physical examination hypopigmented lesions often are seen initially on the hands, forearms, feet, and lips. Acquired depigmented hairs are seen within vitiliginous patches. Rarely, there is an associated uveitis.

The laboratory examination is aimed at uncovering associated systemic disorders such as adrenal insufficiency, diabetes mellitus, pernicious anemia, and thyroid disorders. The diagnosis is made by careful examination and can be confirmed with use of a Wood's light, which accentuates the hypopigmented areas. Skin biopsy reveals normal skin except for the absence of melanocytes.

Management

Treatment is important to restore as much as possible the normal appearance, morphology, and function of the skin, as vitiligo is of cosmetic and social concern. Sunscreens are recommended for all patients, as the hypopigmentation becomes more accentuated with tanning of the normal skin. There are three treatment choices. The first involves the use of cosmetics to mask the hypopigmented areas. Repigmentation with topical steroids for isolated lesions or topical or oral psoralen plus ultraviolet A radiation (PUVA) photochemotherapy for more extensive disease is a second option.[1] Since melanocytes are indolent and slow to respond to such therapy, treatment must continue for 6 to 12 months. Finally, those individuals with extensive disease may obtain better cosmetic results from depigmentation. This involves destruction of the remaining melanocytes with monobenzone. With this therapy there is irreversible depigmentation resulting in photosensitivity.

Pityriasis Alba

Pityriasis alba is common skin disorder in prepubertal children with a history of atopic dermatitis (see Chapter 115). The lesions begin with erythema and progress to hypopigmentation and are located primarily on the cheeks and lateral arms. It is more common in dark-skinned individuals in sunny climates. The condition is transient and nonscarring, gradually fading after puberty. Treatment is not mandatory, but when inflammation appears topical steroids are helpful.

Tuberous Sclerosis

The presence of hypopigmented macules is one of the earliest signs of tuberous sclerosis. Tuberous sclerosis is an autosomal-dominant disease characterized by involvement of the skin, central nervous system, kidneys, heart, and retina. The disease affects 1 in 10,000 people. The classic triad of mental retardation, epilepsy, and angiofibromas occurs in 25% of affected individuals. The hypopigmented lesions tend to be oval or ash-leaf shaped; they are present in 40% to 90% of individuals and are often present at birth. Skin biopsy shows melanocytes, thereby excluding vitiligo. The prognosis is variable, but the survival curves are decreased when compared to the general population. There is no treatment for the skin manifestations, but anticonvulsants can be used to control seizures.

Tinea Versicolor

Tinea versicolor is a common fungal infection of the skin with a characteristic pattern and distribution. The lesions can be white, pink, or brown and occur on the sternal skin, back, and lateral neck. The lesions are often scaly and sometimes pruritic. Treatment can be topical or oral; oral therapy provides better cure and lower recurrence rates. Topical treatment includes selenium sulfide 2.5% suspension applied 10 minutes every day for 10 days, antifungals for 2 to 4 weeks, or sulfur-salicylic shampoo applied at bedtime and washed off in the morning for 1 week. Oral medications include ketoconazole or itraconazole, both at doses of 200 mg/day for 5 days. These regimens result in better than 90% cure rates.

Photosensitivity Dermatitis

Medications, both topical and systemic, can cause a photosensitivity reaction. The eruption is confined to the sun-exposed areas and results in severe erythema within 24 hours of sun exposure. Some of the more common medications that cause a photosensitivity reaction are furosemide, nonsteroidal antiinflammatory drugs (NSAIDs), sulfonamides, tetracyclines, and thiazides. The reaction gradually fades with discontinuation of the medication, but steroids may be necessary in particularly severe cases with a significant inflammatory reaction.

Lichen Planus

Lichen planus is an inflammatory disorder of the skin and mucous membranes. It is characterized by 1- to 10-mm shiny, flat, oval, pruritic papules. The lesions tend to be located on the ventral surface of the wrists and forearms, dorsal feet, groin, sacrum, shins, and scalp. Mucous membrane involvement occurs in 40% to 60% of individuals. Lichen planus occurs most commonly in the 40- to 60-year-old age group. The etiology is unknown, but approximately 10% have a positive family history. Many consider it to be an autoimmune disorder. The attacks may be preceded by stress, and the disorder is associated with lupus erythematous and hepatitis C. Certain drug eruptions, chemical exposures, and skin effects after bone marrow transplantation have a similar appearance and are referred to as lichenoid.

Clinical Presentation

There are several clinically distinct patterns of lichen planus. *Localized* lichen planus is the most commonly encountered cutaneous pattern. This disorder is characterized by papules on the flexor surfaces of the wrists and forearms and immediately above the ankles. The course is unpredictable with

some patients experiencing spontaneous remission. *Hypertrophic* lichen planus is most typically found on the pretibial areas of the legs but can occur in any location. Pruritus is more prevalent with this form of the disorder, and a hypertrophic plaque appears. Lichen planus of the palms and soles generally occurs as an isolated condition. Pruritus is a prominent feature and is often intractable. This pattern of lichen planus is particularly resistant to treatment. *Mucosal* lichen planus can occur with or without the cutaneous manifestations. Lesions may be located on the buccal mucosa, tongue, lips, glans penis, vulvovaginal region, and anus. The lesions can be nonerosive or erosive. Nonerosive mucosal lichen planus is generally asymptomatic but can progress to the more extensive and painful erosive form. Candidal superinfection is found in around 20% of erosive mucosal lichen planus, and malignant transformation occurs in 1.2%.[2] *Generalized* lichen planus is a form of the disorder that can occur abruptly with diffuse involvement including the nails. A highly characteristic, dark brown pigmentation remains as the disease clears.

Treatment

One of the goals of management is symptomatic relief with oral or topical antipruritics. More specific therapies for cutaneous and mucosal lichen planus includes topical steroids, intralesional steroids, PUVA, and systemic steroids. Cyclosporine may be used for severe cases of cutaneous lichen planus, with dapsone, hydroxychloroquine (Plaquenil), or azathioprine reserved for severe mucosal lichen planus.

Cutaneous Lupus Erythematosus

Lupus erythematosus (LE) is a heterogeneous autoimmune disease marked with autoantibody production that can affect one or more organs (systemic LE) as well as the skin. The skin is the second most commonly affected organ and skin manifestations are the second most common presenting complaint. Two distinct cutaneous forms of lupus erythematosus exist. Chronic cutaneous LE (discoid LE) carries a low incidence of systemic disease (see Chapter 113). It is more common in females and has a peak incidence during the fourth decade of life. The incidence of chronic cutaneous LE is 3/100,000 in Caucasian females and 8/100,000 in black females. The antinuclear antibody (ANA), anti–double-stranded (ds) DNA, and erythrocyte sedimentation rate (ESR) are all usually within normal limits.

Subacute cutaneous LE is a less well defined disorder that can encompass the full spectrum of manifestations associated with LE. ANA, dsDNA, LE preparation, and ESR are more likely to be positive in this subgroup. Additionally, there are cutaneous manifestations of systemic lupus erythematosus.

Clinical Presentation

The face is the most commonly affected area with chronic cutaneous LE, but lesions can occur on any body surface. Lesions usually begin as well-demarcated, red, flat-topped plaques with a firmly adherent scale. The scale penetrates the hair follicles, resulting in follicular plugs. Epidermal and dermal atrophy occurs, resulting in smooth white or hypopigmented depressed scars with telangiectasia and scarring alopecia. When the plaques become thick, it is referred to as hypertrophic discoid LE and can resemble keratoacanthoma.

Subacute cutaneous LE can occur in a papulosquamous pattern or an annular-polycyclic pattern. Both forms tend to occur on the trunk, with lesions rarely below the waist. Additionally, the lesions are likely to occur on the sun-exposed areas of the arms, legs, and face. Follicular plugging, atrophy, and scarring are much less likely to occur with subacute cutaneous LE than with chronic cutaneous LE. Annular-polycyclic subacute cutaneous LE is occasionally confused with erythema multiforme. The hypopigmentation that occurs with this disorder is also likely to fade. Subacute cutaneous LE, however, tends to be more likely to recur. Other manifestations include photosensitivity, telangiectasias, arthritis, and vasculitis.

In addition to the autoimmune serology mentioned earlier, a skin biopsy may be helpful in determining the etiology of lesions typical of cutaneous LE. The skin can be examined for specific lesional histopathology and immunopathology.

Treatment

Patients with all forms of LE should avoid direct exposure to sunlight and should routinely use sunscreens that provide at least 15 UVB protection. Topical corticosteroids are the agents of choice for cutaneous LE. The steroid is applied to the active lesions alone. Antimalarials and dapsone can be considered when topical corticosteroids fail. Hydroxychloroquine (Plaquenil) is considered safe, but patients should have periodic eye examinations.[3] Second- and third-line therapies include oral corticosteroids, gold, azathioprine, methotrexate, and isotretinoin.

Corns and Calluses

Corns and calluses develop from foot abnormalities, overuse, and poorly fitting footwear as a result of pressure, shearing forces, and friction. Such foot abnormalities as bunion deformities, hammer toes, claw toes, elevated metatarsals, pes cavovarus (high arch with inverted hindfoot), planovalgus (flat arch with everted hindfoot), and varus or valgus ankle positions render an individual at risk for developing corns and calluses.[4] Both corns and calluses consist of an abnormal proliferation of keratin at the stratum corneum layer of the epidermis. Corns are caused by abnormal pressure and are usually located over the non–weight-bearing surfaces. In contrast, calluses are a thickening of the epidermis over the weight-bearing areas.

Clinical Presentation

The evaluation of corns and calluses begins with a thorough examination of the affected foot and ankle, looking for evidence of structural abnormalities of the foot. This phase is followed by a closer examination of the corn or callus. Corns located over the condyles in the web spaces are referred to as "soft corns." They are most frequently caused by wearing a shoe that is too tight across the toe. "Hard corns," most often occurring dorsolateral on the fifth toe, have sharp borders and a loss of the normal dermal ridges. They are most often overlying bony prominences or due to shoes that impinge on the tips of the toes. Corns are painful when direct pressure is applied. Calluses usually occur on the heel and over the metatarsal heads or sesamoid bones of the great toe. As with corns, calluses can cause pain and interfere with an individual's activities.

In the diabetic patient or the individual with peripheral arterial disease, corns and calluses can cause serious morbidity. This is primarily due to the decreased perception of pain and the increased risk of tissue breakdown and infection.

Management

Removal of pressure is the first step in the conservative management of these lesions. If there is a foot abnormality such as excessive pronation, the use of orthotic devices can decrease the pressure with regression of the lesion. For persons with soft corns, wearing shoes with a wider toe box or using lamb's wool between the toes can decrease the pain. If the problem is primarily on the sole of the foot over the metatarsal heads, low-heeled shoes with pads or metatarsal bars are helpful.

Methods for removing the excessive keratin include the use of keratinolytic medications (e.g., salicylic acid) and trimming the lesion with a sharp blade. Patients, excluding diabetics, can be taught to pare their own lesions with an emery board or pumice stone.

When conservative management does not control the symptoms, surgery may be necessary. The surgical procedure should correct the cause rather than simply excise the hyperkeratotic area. A number of procedures exist that serve to realign the metatarsal heads, reduce hammer toes, remove osteophytes or metatarsal condyles, and correct claw toes.

Nail Problems

A number of medical conditions have manifestations in the nails. Examination of the nails, however, is frequently overlooked by physicians. The three most common conditions of the nails the family physician encounters are onychomycosis, ingrown toenails, and subungual hematomas.

Onychomycosis

Fungal infections can occur in the fingernails or toenails but are much more common in the latter. Toenail infections occur in 15% to 20% of the population aged 40 to 60 years. Onychomycosis can occur in association with trauma, systemic disease, or immunocompromised states. The etiologic agents responsible for these infections are usually *Candida albicans, Trichophyton mentagrophytes,* or *Trichophyton rubrum.* There are four distinct clinical patterns of nail infections.[5] The most common is distal subungual onychomycosis, the earliest signs of which are white patches along one edge of the nail plate. Gradually, there is lifting of the nail plate, striations in the nail, and hyperkeratosis under the nail. Finally, the nail becomes yellowish, mottled, and powdery; and the patient complains of pain and an inability to wear shoes. White superficial onychomycosis is caused by *T. mentagrophytes*. The nail plate is not thickened. Proximal subungual onychomycosis is most commonly caused by *T. rubrum* and is seen in patients with acquired immunodeficiency syndrome (AIDS). Infection occurs within the substance of the nail plate, and the surface remains intact. Candidal onychomycosis is seen in association with chronic mucocutaneous candidiasis and typically involves all of the fingernails.

Because fungal infections of the nails require long-term treatment with expensive medications, one should confirm the presence of fungi prior to initiating antifungal therapy. The cornified cells of the nail bed contain the greatest concentration of fungi, so the sample is taken from the nail bed after trimming the distal nail.[6] The diagnosis can then be established by potassium hydroxide (KOH) examination and culture.

Management

Treatment of fungal infections of the nails is difficult. Topical medications have proved ineffective in eradicating the infection. Oral therapy with griseofulvin (Fulvicin P/G, Grifulvin V, Grisactin, Gris-PEG) for 6 to 18 months is often necessary to eradicate the infection. The recommended dosage of the ultramicrosize form is 10 to 15 mg/kg/day. As a result of the length of therapy required, periodic monitoring of liver enzymes and blood counts is recommended. The newer antifungals are likely as effective as griseofulvin with shorter durations of treatment. Itraconazole (Sporanox) at 200 mg/day for 3 months (fingernail) or 6 months (toenail) or "pulse dosing" at 400 mg/day for 7 days each month for 4 months has produced good response rates.[7] Similar results are seen with terbinafine (Lamisil) at 250 mg/day for 12 weeks[8,9] and fluconazole (Diflucan) 150 mg/week for 12 weeks.[10] After a clinical response with an oral agent, long-term topical antifungal agents may prevent reinfection.[11]

Another option in the treatment of onychomycosis is removal of the entire nail. This alternative is reserved for patients with extremely painful or distorted nails. After removal of the nail, 60% phenol can be applied, destroying the matrix and inhibiting further nail growth. Topical antifungals are used after removal.

Ingrown Toenails

The nail of the great toe is the most common site of an ingrown nail. The condition is usually caused by trauma, tight shoes, or improper nail trimming, allowing the soft tissue to overgrow and obliterating the nail sulcus. As the nail continues to grow, a spicule irritates the soft tissue, causing pain, soft tissue proliferation, and infection (paronychia).

If treatment is begun early, conservative management with soaks, loosely fitting shoes, and elevation of the offending edge of the nail with a wisp of cotton can be curative.[12] This treatment should continue until the nail grows beyond the soft tissue reaction. Patients are then instructed on proper trimming techniques to avoid a recurrence.

When there is a great deal of granulation tissue, making conservative management painful and difficult, removal of a portion of the nail becomes necessary. If there is a significant paronychial infection, pretreatment with systemic antimicrobials for several days helps to decrease the soft tissue reaction. The use of antibiotics to control infection without removing a portion of the offending nail, however, is not curative.[13]

The procedure is performed under digital block anesthesia with a rubber-band tourniquet at the base of the toe for hemostasis. With a hemostat the nail is separated from the nail bed and then divided with nail-splitting scissors. The offending portion of the nail is then removed together with the matrix, and the hypertrophic granulation tissue is excised. The toe is dressed with Vaseline gauze and a bulky dressing that is removed in 2 to 3 days. At that time, a protective dressing can be used until the wound has healed. In patients with recurrent ingrown toenail, the matrix may be destroyed with 60% phenol to prevent further nail growth.

Subungual Hematoma

Subungual hematoma is caused by trauma to the nail plate. The resultant bleeding causes immediate pain due to separation of the nail plate. When faced with a patient with a subungual hematoma, a radiograph to rule out fracture to the distal phalanx is obtained if the history suggests a fracture. Treatment consists of draining the trapped blood, which can be accomplished using the tip of a red-hot paper clip or fine-tip surgical cautery. The patient is informed that the blood stain will persist until the nail has completely grown out.

Alopecia

Alopecia, defined as the absence of hair from areas where it is normally present, is a multifactorial problem that can affect all age groups. Hair has a distinct growth cycle, and knowledge of this cycle can aid the primary care physician in determining the etiology of alopecia in the individual patient. Growing hairs are called anagen hairs and are securely anchored. Approximately 85% of hairs are in the anagen phase, which lasts about 3 years. The resting or telogen phase lasts about 100 days, and approximately 15% of hairs are in this phase at any one time. The human scalp is a mosaic of hairs in these phases and the transition (catagen) phase.

Scalp hair is the fastest-growing organ system in the body, with a growth rate of 0.3 mm/day. Normal shedding occurs at a rate of 100 hairs lost per day. When hair is shed, new hair growth occurs in the same follicle. Abnormal hair loss can be pathologic or physiologic.

Pathologic Hair Loss

There are three major categories of pathologic hair loss that are related to the degree of involvement and the presence or absence of scarring. The individual patient can usually be placed in the proper category based on the physical examination. Early recognition of the type of hair loss may lead to more timely treatment and serve to prevent further hair loss.

Telogen Effluvium

Telogen effluvium is the most common form of pathologic hair loss. It is a process that leads to decreased hair density but not usually to complete baldness. With this condition there is anagen arrest, resulting in a larger percentage of hairs entering the telogen phase. Consequently, more hairs than normal are lost on a daily basis. The telogen phase lasts approximately 100 days, so the onset of hair loss is about 100 days after the inciting event. Conversely, when the precipitating event is no longer present, the hair thinning corrects itself after about 100 days.

The most common cause of telogen effluvium is stress, either physical or psychological. Drugs such as oral contraceptives, anticoagulants, beta-blockers, and retinoids can also lead to this condition. Other causes of telogen effluvium include pregnancy and the postpartum state, fever, dieting, infection, malnutrition, and hypo- or hyperthyroidism.

When telogen effluvium is suspected, biopsy is usually not necessary; instead, a search for the underlying cause is undertaken. The patient is reassured that this form of alopecia is not permanent. Treatment involves identification and elimination of the cause. The hair regenerates within 3 to 4 months. Patients are reassured that, unless the cause cannot be eliminated, the hair will grow back.

Anagen Defluvium

Anagen defluvium manifests as patchy or diffuse hair loss. The hair loss tends to be sudden and in large amounts. The most common cause of this form of hair loss is medications, primarily antimitotic chemotherapeutic agents. Other causes include drugs such as allopurinol, bromocriptine, and levodopa; radiation therapy; and certain endocrine disorders. In contrast to telogen effluvium, the hair loss occurs soon after the inciting event. This condition is usually reversible after removal of the underlying cause.

Alopecia areata, a common form of anagen defluvium, can occur at any age but is more common in individuals under the age of 25. There are patches of complete hair loss, and the affected scalp appears normal. Hairs at the borders of the patch are easily plucked and have a thin base, which has led to the descriptive term *exclamation-point hairs*, considered characteristic of this disorder.

The cause of alopecia areata is unknown; it is currently thought, however, to be an autoimmune phenomenon. There is an association between alopecia areata and such conditions as diabetes mellitus, Hashimoto's thyroiditis, pernicious anemia, and inflammatory bowel disease.

The course of alopecia areata is unpredictable. The disease usually resolves within 5 years without treatment; recurrences, however, are common.[14] A number of therapeutic interventions have been studied in this condition with no single best treatment available. Systemic, intralesional, and topical corticosteroids have been used with varying success. Long-term use of these agents is discouraged because of their local and systemic side effects. Topical and oral cyclosporine and oral incsiplex, a synthetic immunomodulator, have been used with some success in the treatment of alopecia areata. Topical miroxidil has been evaluated and found to stimulate hair growth within 12 weeks with a maximal response in 1 year.[15] Other treatments include anthralin, dinitrochlorobenzene, and tars, which induce an irritant or allergic contact dermatitis that promotes hair growth during healing.[16]

Cicatricial (Scarring) Alopecia

There is a diverse group of conditions that can lead to hair loss with scarring. Primary dermatologic conditions such as lichen planus, lupus erythematosus, dermatomyositis, dermatologic neoplasms, and pemphigoid are among the most common causes of scarring alopecia. Trauma due to chemicals or burns, certain developmental defects, and infections can also cause scarring. These conditions have in common follicular destruction that leads to dermal scarring. The scarring is irreversible, and in most instances the only effective treatment is surgical. Further permanent hair loss can frequently be prevented if prompt action is taken. When scarring alopecia is present, biopsy is necessary to determine the etiology.

Traumatic Alopecia

Traumatic alopecia is due to compulsive hair pulling (trichotillomania) or the use of braids or curlers that place undue stress on the hair (traction alopecia). Trichotillomania is common in normal children but can be a sign of serious psychological disorders in adults. Clinically affected areas demonstrate broken, twisted hairs sometimes with an associated folliculitis. Trichotillomania is treated by patient education and, at times, psychiatric intervention. Traction alopecia can be reversed with discontinuation of the practice that led to the hair trauma.

Fungal Infection

Fungal infections can lead to scarring or nonscarring alopecia. The diagnosis is confirmed by 10% KOH examination, Wood's lamp fluorescence, or fungal culture. Treatment usually involves a 4- to 12-week course of oral griseofulvin. Alternatives include oral ketoconazole or itraconazole (see Chapter 116).

Physiologic Hair Loss

Androgenic alopecia, or male pattern baldness, is exceedingly common and manifests as bitemporal thinning of the hair followed by loss of hair over the crown. This type of thinning can occur in women as well as men, although the hair loss is generally less severe in women. Male pattern baldness can begin as early as the adolescent years with more than 50% of Caucasian men having noticeable hair loss by age 50. The condition follows an autosomal-dominant pattern of inheritance with incomplete penetrance.[17] Certain ethnic groups, including Japanese, Chinese, and American Indians, are relatively immune to the condition.

The treatment of androgenic alopecia can be surgical or

medical. Surgical approaches, such as hair transplantation, scalp reduction, transposition flap, and soft tissue expansion, are used to camouflage the hair loss.[16] These procedures are usually done in individuals with well-developed, stable baldness. Although androgenic alopecia is the most frequent indication for surgical treatment, these methods have also been employed for the treatment of traumatic hair loss.

Topical minoxidil (Rogaine) received the first U.S. Food and Drug Administration (FDA) approval for the medical management of androgenic alopecia. Several large-scale clinical trials have demonstrated statistically significant increases in hair growth in men and women with androgenic alopecia using topical minoxidil versus placebo.[18–21] Ideal candidates for the use of topical minoxidil are under the age of 30 with less than 5 years of hair loss. Minoxidil is available in 2% and 5% topical solutions. Two studies have compared the two strengths and found the higher strength to lead to greater hair mass.[22,23]

Side effects of minoxidil are minimal and due primarily to local irritation. Topical absorption of minoxidil is only 1.4%.[24] It is recommended, however, that topical minoxidil not be used in persons with unstable hypertension or other unstable cardiovascular problems.

More recently, oral finasteride (Proscar) has been approved for use in androgenic alopecia. Several studies have demonstrated mild to moderate increases in hair count, especially in the frontal area.[25] Finasteride has been well tolerated, with sexual side effects being the most common; 3.8% experience at least one sexual side effect. Finasteride should not be used in women or children.

With either medication, 6 months of therapy may be necessary before the desired effects are evident. Discontinuation of either medication leads to resumption of the balding process.[26] Further study is needed to determine the long-term benefit of these medications as well as the safety and effectiveness of their use in combination.

References

1. Drake LA, Ceiley RI, Dorner W, et al. Guidelines of care for phototherapy and photochemotherapy. J Am Acad Dermatol 1994;31:643–8.
2. Habif TP. Clinical dermatology: a color guide to diagnosis and therapy, 3rd ed. St. Louis: Mosby, 1996;211–27.
3. Potter B. Hydroxychloroquine. Cutis 1993;52:229–31.
4. Brainard BJ. Managing corns and plantar calluses. Phys Sportsmed 1991;19:61–7.
5. Habif TP. Clinical dermatology: a color guide to diagnosis and therapy. 3rd ed. St. Louis: Mosby, 1996;765–9.
6. Zaias N. Onychomycosis. Arch Dermatol 1972;105:263–74.
7. Korting HC, Schafer-Korting M, Zienicke H, Georgii A, Ollert MW. Treatment of tinea unguium with medium and high doses of ultramicrosize griseofulvin compared with that with itraconazole. Antimicrob Agents Chemother 1993;37:2064–8.
8. Goodfield MJD, Andrew L, Evans EGV. Short term treatment of dermatophyte onychomycosis with terbinafine. BMJ 1992; 304:1151–4.
9. Van Der Schroeff JG, Cirkel PKS, Van Dijk TJA, et al. A randomized treatment duration-finding study of terbinafine in onychomycosis. Br J Dermatol 1992;126:36–9.
10. Nahass GT, Sisto M. Onychomycosis: successful treatment with once-weekly fluconazole. Dermatology 1993;186:59–61.
11. Zaias N, Drachman D. A method for the determination of drug effectiveness in onychomycosis: trials with ketoconazole and griseofulvin ultramicrosize. J Am Acad Dermatol 1983;9: 912–19.
12. Ruoff AC. Foot and ankle. In: Wolcott MW, ed. Ambulatory surgery. Philadelphia: Lippincott, 1988.
13. Hefland AE. Nail and hyperkeratotic problems in the elderly foot. Am Fam Physician 1989;39:101–10.
14. Atton AV, Tunnessen WW. Alopecia in children: the most common causes. Pediatr Rev 1990;12:25–30.
15. Price VH. Treatment of hair loss. N Engl J Med 1999;341: 964–71.
16. Burke KE. Hair loss: what causes it and what can be done about it? Postgrad Med 1989;85:52–77.
17. Caserio RJ, Hordinsky MK. Disorders of hair. J Am Acad Dermatol 1988;19:895–903.
18. DeVillez RL. Topical minoxidil therapy in hereditary androgenic alopecia. Arch Dermatol 1985;121:197–202.
19. Olsen EA, Weiner MS, DeLong ER, Pinnell S. Topical minoxidil in early male pattern baldness. J Am Acad Dermatol 1985;13:185–92.
20. Olsen EA, DeLong ER, Weiner MS: Dose-response study of topical minoxidil in male pattern baldness. J Am Acad Dermatol 1986;15:30–7.
21. Price VH, Menefee E. Quantitative estimation of hair growth. I. Androgenic alopecia in women: effect of minoxidil. J Invest Dermatol 1990;95:683–7.
22. Price VH, Menefee E. Quantitative estimation of hair growth: comparative changes in weight and hair count with 5 percent and 2 percent minoxidil, placebo and no treatment. In: Van Neste D, Randall VA, eds. Hair research for the next millenium. New York: Elsevier, 1996;67–71.
23. Trancik RJ. Update on topical minoxidil in hair loss. Proceedings of the annual meeting of the American Academy of Dermatology, February 27–March 4, 1998, Orlando, FL.
24. Franz TJ. Percutaneous absorption of minoxidil in man. Arch Dermatol 1985;121:203–6.
25. Scow DT, Nolte RS, Shaughnessy AF. Medical treatments for balding in men. Am Fam Physician 1999;58:2189–94.
26. Olsen EA, Weiner MS. Topical minoxidil in male pattern baldness: effects of discontinuation of treatment. J Am Acad Dermatol 1987;17:97–101.

119
Dyslipidemias

Patrick E. McBride, Gail Underbakke, and James H. Stein

Dyslipidemias, which include lipoprotein overproduction or deficiencies, are primary disorders of lipoprotein metabolism or secondary disorders induced by behavioral or other metabolic causes. These disorders are a common clinical problem, with 25% to 30% of adults in the United States having total cholesterol (TChol) levels of 240 mg/dL or higher and over half having TChol levels exceeding 200 mg/dL.[1] The four major classes of lipoproteins include the triglyceride-rich particles—chylomicrons and very low density lipoprotein (VLDL)—and the cholesterol-rich particles—low-density lipoprotein (LDL) and high-density lipoprotein (HDL). Evidence from epidemiologic, pathologic, animal, genetic, and metabolic studies strongly support a causal relation between serum lipoprotein concentrations and atherosclerosis.[2]

Optimum and at-risk lipoprotein levels are shown in Table 119.1. These levels are based on population percentiles and a vast research base, but are still arbitrary because the associated risk is linear. Lipoproteins act synergistically with environmental and metabolic factors, e.g., smoking, diabetes mellitus (DM), obesity, and high blood pressure, to promote atherosclerosis and thrombosis.[1,3]

Treatment of dyslipidemias has been proven to reduce coronary heart disease (CHD) morbidity and mortality, and total mortality, in many primary and secondary prevention trials.[3–8] These studies and others have demonstrated that treatment of lipoprotein disorders leads to plaque stabilization, improved endothelial function, prevention of atherosclerotic lesion formation, and regression of existing plaques, reducing CHD symptoms and adverse clinical events.[5,7–10] The patients who benefit most from lipid treatment are those who have CHD or noncoronary atherosclerosis, genetic dyslipidemias, diabetes mellitus, or multiple risk factors, including multiple lipoprotein abnormalities.[3] The benefits of lipid therapy have been demonstrated in men and women, and in older patients.[4,5,11]

The National Cholesterol Education Program Adult Treatment Panel III (NCEP ATP III) guidelines recommend evaluation for underlying atherosclerosis and comprehensive risk assessment for all patients prior to determining lipoprotein goals.[3] LDL cholesterol (LDL-C) treatment goals are risk-stratified, using 10-year risk estimates derived from Framingham Heart Study data. CHD risk can be estimated using downloadable risk calculators (for desktop or handheld computers) and paper handouts available at *http://www.nhlbi.nih.gov/guidelines/cholesterol/index.htm*. A 10-year CHD risk >20% is termed a "CHD-risk equivalent," as this is the same CHD event risk as a person with known CHD. High-risk primary prevention patients, including those with diabetes mellitus or noncoronary atherosclerosis, and individuals with a 10-year CHD risk >20%, have the same lipoprotein goals as a person with CHD. Patients with a 10-year risk of 10% to 20% or <10% have higher LDL-C goals and are therefore not treated as aggressively (Table 119.2).

The presence of multiple risk factors exponentially increases overall atherosclerotic risk. A clinical evaluation, including a personal and family history, nutritional evaluation, focused physical examination, assessment of potential secondary causes of the dyslipidemia, and confirmation of lipoprotein abnormalities, is essential to characterize overall risk, identify genetic and environmental influences on dyslipidemias, and to determine treatment.

Screening

Current recommendations are that all adults age 20 years and older and children from high-risk families have a fasting lipoprotein profile every 5 years.[3] If a patient presents to the clinic in nonfasting state, an acceptable alternative is to measure TChol and HDL cholesterol (HDL-C) levels, since these measures are reliable in non-fasting individuals and provide important information for an initial risk assessment. A fasting lipoprotein profile should be obtained if the patient has a

Table 119.1. **National Cholesterol Education Program Adult Treatment Panel III (ATP III) Classification of LDL, Total, and HDL Cholesterol, and Triglycerides (mg/dL)**

LDL-cholesterol—primary target of therapy
<100	Optimal
100–129	Near optimal/above optimal
130–159	Borderline high
160–189	High
≥190	Very high

Total cholesterol
<200	Desirable
200–239	Borderline high
≥240	High

HDL cholesterol
<40	Low
≥60	High

Triglycerides
<150	Normal
150–199	Borderline high
200–499	High
>499	Very high

HDL = high-density lipoprotein; LDL = low-density lipoprotein.

TChol >200 or HDL-C <40 mg/dL, or a family history of premature CHD or dyslipidemia. Because people who have TChol less than 200 mg/dL may develop atherosclerosis due to low HDL-C, abnormalities of other lipoproteins, or multiple risk factors, a lipoprotein profile is necessary for a thorough risk evaluation for patients with atherosclerosis or risk factors.[1,3] Lipoprotein profile evaluation is especially important for individuals with a personal history of atherosclerosis, two or more CHD risk factors, a family history of dyslipidemia, or premature CHD in a first-degree relative (grandparent, parent, sibling, or child), or a TChol averaging greater than 200 mg/dL on two occasions. It is important to note that approximately 50% of CHD events occur in individuals with no family history of CHD,[12] so the entire risk factor history and laboratory profile should guide assessment and treatment.

Evidence indicates that HDL-C and LDL-C remain important risk factors past age 65, particularly in the presence of atherosclerosis.[11,13] Evaluation of older adults for dyslipidemia treatment is based on the individual's motivation, prognosis, comorbidities, and potential improvement in quality and quantity of life.[11,13]

Dyslipidemias include a variety of common primarily autosomal-dominant genetic disorders that are influenced by both genetic and environmental factors (e.g., lifestyle) and may affect multiple members of high-risk families.[12,14] The presence of a family history of premature atherosclerosis (prior to age 55–65 years old) requires a thorough screening evaluation of the patient and first-degree relatives due to the high incidence of dyslipidemias and other risk factors in these families. Children or adolescents in families with premature atherosclerosis or with dyslipidemias in parents, grandparents, and siblings should be screened in childhood for lipid disorders and other risk factors. Detailed guidelines are available for screening and treatment in children and adolescents.[15] Routine screening of all children remains controversial, but measurement and treatment is recommended for children from families with premature atherosclerosis or genetic cholesterol disorders.

Office cholesterol testing is practical and reliable owing to the availability of advanced testing equipment and national standardization programs. Patients who are acutely or chronically ill, including a recent myocardial infarction, surgery, a mild viral illness, and even those who are pregnant or have had significant weight loss, will have fluctuating lipoprotein levels and should not be tested until they are stabilized.[3] It takes approximately 3 months for cholesterol levels to return to baseline levels after a major illness. Proper phlebotomy technique, such as avoiding prolonged tourniquet time (>1 min), or "milk-

Table 119.2. **LDL-Cholesterol Goals Plus Cutpoints for Initiating Lifestyle Changes or Medical Therapy**

Patient risk group	LDL-C goal (mg/dL)	LDL-C level at which to start lifestyle changes (mg/dL)	LDL-C level at which to consider starting medical therapy (mg/dL)
CHD or CHD risk equivalent[a] (10-year risk >20%)	<100	≥100	≥130 (100–129; medical therapy optional)[b]
2+ risk factors (10-year risk ≤20%)	<130	≥130	≥130 (if 10-yr risk = 10–20%) ≥160 (if 10-yr risk = <10%)
0–1 risk factors[c]	<160	≥160	≥190 (160–189: medical therapy optional)

[a]A CHD risk equivalent is a condition that carries an absolute risk for developing new CHD equal to the risk for having recurrent CHD events in persons with established CHD.

[b]Some authorities recommend the use of LDL-lowering medications in this category if levels of <100 mg/dL cannot be achieved by lifestyle changes alone. Others prefer use of medications that primarily modify TGs and HDL, e.g., nicotinic acid or fibrate. Clinical judgment also may call for deferring medications for some patients in this subcategory.

[c]Almost all people with 0–1 risk factor have a 10-year risk <10%; thus, 10-year risk assessment in people with 0–1 risk factor is not necessary.

Note: Risk calculators can be downloaded for the office at *www.nhlbi.nih.gov/guidelines/cholesterol/profmats.htm.*

CHD = coronary heart disease; LDL-C = low-density lipoprotein cholesterol; TG = triglyceride.

ing" the finger for a fingerstick, may also influence cholesterol measures. Biologic variation and standard measurement errors produce a 6% to 9% daily variance for TChol, making it important to average at least two cholesterol measures from different days prior to management decisions.

A TChol higher than 240 mg/dL, if LDL-C is higher than 160 mg/dL, is associated with a marked increase in atherosclerotic risk and is called "high blood cholesterol" for adults[1,3] (Table 119.1). A TChol of 200 to 239 mg/dL, with LDL-C 130 to 159 mg/dL, is considered "borderline" due to increasing risk in this range, particularly in the presence of other risk factors. A TChol of 200 mg/dL or more (with LDL-C >130 mg/dL) in children and adolescents (ages 2–19 years) is higher than the 90th percentile and is considered "high blood cholesterol," whereas a TChol of 170 to 199 mg/dL is considered a borderline elevation for children.[15]

Lipoprotein profiles must be done after a 12- to 14-hour fast because triglyceride (TG) measurements are variable in the nonfasting state. When TChol, TG, and HDL-C are measured, LDL-C can be estimated using the formula:

$$LDL\text{-}C = TChol - HDL\text{-}C - TG/5$$

Dividing clinical TG levels by 5 provides an estimate of VLDL-C cholesterol. These LDL-C calculations are not accurate if the TG exceeds 400 mg/dL.

A lipoprotein profile usually is sufficient to develop a clinical classification and treatment approach for dyslipidemias. Lipoprotein phenotyping to determine the specific biochemical abnormality, using the Fredrickson-Levy classification, may be useful to direct treatment when the TG level is more than 400 mg/dL. It is important to recognize that when TG is >400 mg/dL, the TChol, HDL-C, and LDL-C are much less accurate in most clinical laboratories, and should not be relied on for clinical decisions.

Secondary Causes of Abnormal Cholesterol Levels

The following secondary causes of dyslipidemias should be considered prior to extensive testing or treatment:

Uncontrolled diabetes mellitus
Obesity and the metabolic syndrome
Medications (steroids including estrogen, progesterone, prednisone, anabolic steroids, and others; beta-blockers, or *cis*-retinoic acid)
Obstructive liver disease
Nephrotic syndrome
Multiple myeloma
Hypothyroidism
Excess dietary alcohol, fat, or caloric intake

A directed medical history, nutrition history, thyroid-stimulating hormone (TSH) assay, and fasting chemistry survey (including glucose, liver enzymes, and creatinine) can rule out most of the common secondary causes of dyslipidemias. Hypothyroidism should be considered especially in an older patient or a patient with previously normal lipid levels who develops a sudden elevation of LDL-C or TG. Treatment of secondary causes usually results in a marked improvement, or normalization, of abnormal lipoprotein levels.

Dyslipidemia Classification

A practical system of dyslipidemia classification yields four categories based on clinical, genetic, and biochemical parameters, as listed in Table 119.3 and discussed below. This approach uses screening lipoprotein results and is compatible with the more complex Fredrickson-Levy system. Each of the four dyslipidemia categories has a specific therapeutic approach.

Table 119.3. **Classifications of Dyslipidemias**

Lipoprotein levels (mg/dL)	Fredrickson-Levy class	Genetic disorder
LDL-C elevated		
LDL-C >130	IIA	Familial hypercholesterolemia (LDL >200)
TG <150		Primary hypercholesterolemia (LDL 130–199)
HDL-C >40		
Triglycerides elevated		
TG >500[a]	I, V	LPL deficiency
LDL-C NA		Apo C-III deficiency
HDL-C NA		Familial hypertriglyceridemia
HDL-C decreased		
HDL-C <40	—	Hypo-α-lipoproteinemia
TG <150		
LDL-C <130		
Combined dyslipidemias		
LDL-C >130	IIB, IV, III	Familial combined hyperlipidemia
TG >150		Familial dysbetalipoproteinemia
HDL-C <40		

[a]LDL-C, HDL-C and Total cholesterol levels are not accurate when TG >500 mg/dL.

NA = not applicable.

Elevated LDL-C Cholesterol (LDL-C >130 mg/dL, TG <150 mg/dL)

Elevation of LDL-C, without an elevation of TG, is considered either primary or familial hypercholesterolemia. Familial hypercholesterolemia (FH) is a relatively common disorder caused by defects in the LDL receptor gene, with the heterozygous form affecting approximately 1 in 500 Americans and 1 in 200 French Canadians. FH is expressed during childhood and is autosomal dominant, with selective elevation of LDL-C (usually >220 mg/dL), and often extensor tendon thickening (primarily the Achilles tenderness) or xanthomas. Most individuals with isolated LDL-C elevations <200 mg/dL do not have FH and are considered to have primary hypercholesterolemia, likely due to multiple factors, including nutrition, obesity, and genetic factors.

Very High Triglyceride (TG >500 mg/dL)

Hypertriglyceridemias are elevations of either chylomicrons, intermediate-density lipoproteins (IDL), or VLDL. Because all of these forms of dyslipidemia result in elevated TG, lipoprotein electrophoresis (phenotyping) may be useful for distinguishing among these disorders (Table 119.3). Fasting TG levels over 1000 mg/dL can be due to genetic influences, or a combination of genetic predisposition and secondary causes, such as alcohol abuse, poorly controlled diabetes, obesity, renal disease, or corticosteroids in patients with an underlying moderate hypertriglyceridemia.[14,16]

Patients with TG levels over 1000 mg/dL have a relatively low risk of CHD, but have a high risk of associated pancreatitis (10–15% annually), most likely due to lipemia and subsequent hyperviscosity, which results in obstruction of the microvasculature in the pancreas.[17] The priority of medical therapy in these patients is the prevention of pancreatitis. It is important to note that TG levels drop precipitously during acute attacks, which may mask the etiology of this life-threatening condition (see Chapter 89). A careful family history, family lipid screening, and remeasurement of TG levels after recovery can identify hypertriglyceridemia as the cause of pancreatitis.

Combined Dyslipidemias (LDL-C >130 mg/dL, TG >150 mg/dL, HDL-C <40 mg/dL)

Combined dyslipidemia, a very common and important disorder, is found in a high percentage of patients who survive myocardial infarction or have coronary revascularization.[18] Combined dyslipidemias include abnormalities of several lipoproteins, usually elevated LDL-C and TG with low HDL-C. Family history will often include the presence of multiple first-degree family members with CHD. As these disorders may be polygenic, affected patients and family members often present with a variety of dyslipidemias, including approximately one third with elevated TG, one third with elevated LDL-C alone, and the rest with a combined dyslipidemia.[14] This disorder is not usually expressed until adulthood, although it is now identified in children due to the recent increase in childhood obesity in the U.S.

Although TG is not metabolically independent of other lipoproteins, research documenting increased atherosclerosis risk while accounting for the interaction of TG, LDL-C, HDL-C, and other risk factors has led to the designation of TG as an independent CHD risk factor.[3,10] Moderate-range hypertriglyceridemia (TG 200–499 mg/dL) is usually associated with alteration of LDL and VLDL into highly atherogenic forms (small, dense particles), low HDL-C due to reduced HDL production, and altered HDL effectiveness in reverse cholesterol transport.[3,10]

Non-HDL cholesterol, equal to TChol − (HDL-C), can be used to monitor treatment of patients who have had an initial TG measurement of 200 to 499 mg/dL. The non–HDL-C estimate includes all of the atherogenic lipoproteins, and should be <30 points higher than the LDL-C goals. Therefore, for a patient with CHD or DM or for a patient with a 10-year risk greater than 20%, the non–HDL-C cholesterol goal is <130 mg/dL, and for a patient with a 10-year CHD risk of 10% to 20%, the non–HDL-C cholesterol goal is <160 mg/dL. Because only TChol and HDL-C are necessary, the non–HDL-C calculation does not require a fasting blood test, and the non–HDL-C value more accurately assesses risk in patients with TG of 200 to 499 mg/dL.[3]

The metabolic syndrome is a high-risk, common syndrome that resembles familial combined hyperlipidemia and frequently results in premature clinical manifestations. Previously called syndrome X or the insulin-resistance syndrome, this syndrome includes a combined dyslipidemia and metabolic abnormalities associated with central obesity and insulin resistance (glucose intolerance or type II DM, hypertension, and hyperuricemia). Specific measures that identify this syndrome are listed in Table 119.4. Patients with metabolic syndrome can be effectively detected in the office by measuring the waist circumference at the iliac crest (on exhalation). The lipoprotein profile common to the metabolic syndrome includes small, dense LDL particles, which are more easily oxidized and recognized by scavenger macrophages, rather than

Table 119.4. **Clinical Identification of the Metabolic Syndrome—Any Three of the Following:**

Risk factor	Defining level
Abdominal obesity[a]	Waist circumference
Men	>102 cm (>40 in)
Women	>88 cm (>35 in)
Triglycerides	≥150 mg/dL
HDL cholesterol	
Men	<40 mg/dL
Women	<50 mg/dL
Blood pressure	≥130/≥85 mm Hg
Fasting glucose	≥110 mg/dL

[a]Overweight and obesity are associated with insulin resistance and the metabolic syndrome. However, the presence of abdominal obesity is more highly correlated with the metabolic risk factors than is an elevated body mass index (BMI). Therefore, the simple measure of waist circumference is recommended to identify the body weight component of the metabolic syndrome.

the usual lipoprotein receptors, and therefore are more likely to cause atherosclerosis.[18]

In addition to the metabolic syndrome, other causes of combined dyslipidemias are a lack of physical activity, hypothyroidism, DM, alcohol abuse, nephrotic syndrome, and use of glucocorticoids. A rare subtype of the combined dyslipidemias, associated with premature CHD and peripheral arterial disease, is familial dysbetalipoproteinemia (type III). The type III disorder is characterized by elevations of both fasting TChol and TG levels (exceeding 300 mg/dL) and the presence of xanthomas. Lipoprotein electrophoresis is recommended when levels of both LDL-C and TG are very high because treatment recommendations differ from those for other combined dyslipidemias (see below).

Low HDL Cholesterol (HDL-C <40 mg/dL, TG <150 mg/dL)

HDL-C is an independent risk factor and is the most powerful predictor of premature CHD.[19] Low HDL-C is associated with genetic factors, male sex, hypertriglyceridemias, smoking, obesity, and a sedentary lifestyle. Familial hypoalphalipoproteinemia (low HDL-C) is a syndrome found in 7% to 10% of CHD patients less than age 60. This disorder is characterized by an HDL-C level of less than 40 mg/dL, a TG level less than 200 mg/dL, and an autosomal-dominant inheritance.[18] Many other genetic forms of HDL-C deficiency exist but are far less common. Medications, including beta-blockers (nonsympathomimetic), retinoids, progestins, and anabolic steroids can significantly lower HDL-C.

Nonpharmacologic Management of Dyslipidemias

Nutrition and Weight Management

Lifestyle changes are the cornerstone of any treatment program to modify serum lipids. The U.S. Dietary Guidelines and the Food Pyramid recommend food choices that will reduce the risk of heart disease in the general population, and form the foundation for diet guidelines to treat dyslipidemias.[20] Patients with dyslipidemias or a diagnosis of CHD should use the Food Pyramid as a guide, but further limit saturated fat to <7% of calories, and dietary cholesterol to <200 mg/day. See Table 119.5 for a summary of diet recommendations. Trans fat, created during hydrogenation of vegetable oils, raises LDL-C and may reduce HDL-C, so it should be limited by considering it part of the daily saturated fat intake. The major sources of trans fats in the American diet are commercial baked goods, fried foods, and stick margarines.[21] Weight management through caloric reduction and increased activity is encouraged if needed to achieve a body mass index (BMI) of <25. The addition of water-soluble (viscous) fibers and plant stanols/sterols (usually found in margarines) is encouraged if lipids are not normalized by a reduction of saturated fat and cholesterol. Because omega-3 fat found in fish lowers TG levels and is associated with a lower risk for CHD, consumption of two to three fish meals per week is recommended. Inclusion of soy protein is encouraged because it helps reduce LDL-C levels and has other health benefits.[22]

There is debate about the optimal fat content of the diet for the treatment of dyslipidemia. A diet very low in fat (<10% of calories) can reduce LDL-C, but may also reduce HDL-C and increase TG due to a higher carbohydrate content.[23] A Mediterranean-type diet (30–40% of calories as total fat, an emphasis on monounsaturated fat, and saturated fat limited to <7% of calories) can reduce LDL-C without decreasing HDL-C and increasing TG, but the higher fat intake may make calorie control and weight loss more difficult. Medical nutrition therapy in consultation with a registered dietitian is recommended to tailor guidelines and maximize the lipid response to diet.

Serum cholesterol reduction from diet modification varies significantly between individuals, but averages 10% to 15%.[3] Triglycerides are very responsive to diet change, weight loss, and exercise, while the main dietary influences on HDL-C are weight loss and the balance of fat and carbohydrate in the diet. Diet recommendations for dyslipidemia should be individualized based on the patient's lipid pattern, body weight, food preferences, and level of motivation.

Elevated LDL-C

Patients with familial hypercholesterolemia are less responsive to diet changes than those with other forms of hypercholesterolemia, but all patients with elevated TChol should reduce their intake of saturated fat, trans fat, and cholesterol, as they are the primary dietary elements that raise LDL-C.

Increased consumption of foods high in soluble (viscous)

Table 119.5. **Nutritional Recommendations**

	AHA/NCEP general population[a]	AHA/NCEP dyslipidemia or CHD[b]	Very low fat diet	Mediterranean dietary pattern
Total fat (% of calories)	<30%	<30%	10%	30–40%
Saturated fat	<10%	<7%	—	7–10%
Monounsaturated fat	10–15%	10–15%	—	15–30%
Polyunsaturated fat	≤10%	≤10%	—	<10%
Carbohydrate	50–60%	50–60%	70–75%	40–55%
Protein	10–20%	10–20%	15–20%	15–20%
Cholesterol	<300 mg/day	<200 mg/day	5 mg/day	<200 mg/day

[a]American Heart Association/National Cholesterol Education Program guidelines for the general, healthy American population.
[b]AHA/NCEP guidelines for anyone with CHD, CHD risk equivalent, or dyslipidemia.

fiber may be beneficial for some patients with LDL-C elevations. The primary sources of water-soluble fiber are oats, barley, legumes (dried beans and peas), fruits, and some vegetables. Including 20 to 30 g of dietary fiber per day, of which 10 to 25 g is soluble, could result in an additional 5% to 15% reduction in TChol and LDL-C.[24] Fiber supplements (psyllium) may be recommended for patients who are not able to consume adequate fiber through their diet, but it is preferable to obtain fiber from food because of the additional nutrients provided by high-fiber foods. Plant stanols and sterols reduce the absorption of dietary cholesterol, and can reduce LDL-C by up to 15% when used in a dose of 2 to 3 g/day.[21] Stanols and sterols are currently marketed in margarines. To prevent weight gain, patients should take care to compensate for the extra calories that these products contain. Soy protein can reduce LDL-C levels in some people, especially when soy is substituted for foods higher in saturated fat and cholesterol. Studies indicate that 25 g of soy protein per day can reduce LDL-C by 5%.[24]

Very High Triglycerides

TG levels are influenced by the total amount of fat and carbohydrate consumed, but not by the type of fat. For patients with triglycerides between 150 and 500 mg/dL, emphasis is on weight reduction. Very low fat (and consequently higher carbohydrate) diets can lead to significant increases in serum triglycerides in some patients, usually those with the metabolic syndrome. For these patients, nutritional plans of no more than 30% fat with an emphasis on monounsaturated fat are recommended. Patients who do not experience increased TG with higher carbohydrate intakes achieve the best results on a diet containing 20% of calories as fat. Optimal therapy is determined on an individual basis and requires follow-up to allow adjustment. Limitation or avoidance of alcohol is recommended for patients with high TG, and limitation of concentrated sweets is recommended for patients with glucose intolerance and high TG.

A strict control of total fat to 10% of calories is recommended for the patient with very high TG (TG >500 mg/dL) to prevent pancreatitis. Because medium-chain triglycerides (MCTs) are directly absorbed into the portal vein and do not increase chylomicron production, MCT oil (obtained from a pharmacy) can be used by patients who are not overweight to make food more palatable and to provide adequate calories. Consultation with a registered dietitian is recommended to ensure that the very low fat diet is nutritionally adequate.

Combined Dyslipidemias

Patients with combined dyslipidemia and the metabolic syndrome should make weight control and regular exercise a priority, since these changes will have a favorable impact on all serum lipoproteins and the other risks often noted with this pattern (abdominal obesity, glucose intolerance, and hypertension). Patients do not have to reach goal weight to see benefits, since a 10% reduction in body weight is associated with up to a 30% reduction in abdominal obesity. Patients should

attempt to reduce body weight by limiting total fat intake to 25% to 30% of calories and saturated fat to <7% of calories. Total carbohydrate intake should not exceed 60% of calories, with an emphasis on complex carbohydrates (whole grains, vegetables, legumes) rather than simple carbohydrates (sugars, sweetened drinks, desserts). Serving sizes of starchy foods (pasta, bread, rice, potatoes, etc.) should be monitored, since they can often be a source of excess calories and may raise TG due to their refined carbohydrate content. Alcohol restriction or avoidance is recommended for reduction of caloric intake and TG.

Low HDL-C

No specific foods or nutrients increase HDL-C levels, with the exception of ethanol. However, ethanol is addictive, myotoxic, raises blood pressure and TG levels, and has variable effects on subspecies of HDL-C.[25] Alcohol should not be recommended as a treatment for low HDL-C. Because HDL-C levels are reduced in patients who are overweight or who have the metabolic syndrome, the normalization of body weight through calorie restriction and increased exercise is the primary goal for patients with low HDL-C. HDL-C levels may also increase in response to a diet higher in monounsaturated fats (nuts, avocado, canola, or olive oil) or the omega-3 polyunsaturated fats found in fish. If fat intake is increased, the quantity of carbohydrate foods will need to be decreased in order to maintain a consistent calorie intake and prevent weight gain.

Other Nutritional CVD Benefits

Plant foods (fruits, vegetables, whole grains, legumes, nuts) contain nutrients and other chemicals that help reduce the risk of heart disease, stroke, and high blood pressure. Antioxidant nutrients can reduce lipoprotein atherogenicity by protecting LDL-C from oxidation but are best obtained by consuming foods containing these vitamins rather than by taking supplements.[26–28] Flavonoids and fish oils reduce platelet aggregation and may reduce inflammation and CHD events.[29] Adequate intake of folic acid (400 μg/day) can help prevent elevations of serum homocysteine, which increases the risk of CHD and stroke.[30] The identity, function, and safe doses of protective nutrients are not completely understood, so it is not possible to establish appropriate guidelines for supplement use. Until more information is available, reasonable amounts of these and other potentially beneficial nutrients can be obtained by consuming at least five servings of fruits and vegetables per day, at least six servings of grain products (with at least half being whole grain), soy or legumes several times per week, fish two to three times per week, and a handful of nuts several times per week.

The practical application of nutritional guidelines by patients and health care providers requires counseling for behavior change and translation of recommendations based on percentage of calories to actual food choices. Table 119.6 lists the daily total fat and saturated fat gram allowances at different calorie levels and fat recommendations. The five food categories listed in Table 119.7 account for more than

Table 119.6. **Percentage of Calories as Fat Translated to Fat Grams**

Calorie intake	30% of calories (g)	10% of calories (g)	7% of calories (g)
1500	50	17	12
1800	60	20	14
2000	67	22	16
2400	80	27	19

90% of the fat, saturated fat, and cholesterol consumed in the typical American diet.[31] Counseling for low-fat and low-cholesterol eating should focus on substitution in these five food categories because of their significant contribution to dietary fat, and on recommendations to increase the consumption of plant-based foods.

Exercise

Physical activity is associated with improvement in the lipoprotein profile, but results depend on baseline lifestyle habits, presence of obesity or diabetes, type of dyslipidemia, and the specific exercise program. Both endurance and resistance exercise are helpful in achieving weight reduction and in reducing triglycerides and raising HDL-C, but have little influence on LDL-C unless there is significant weight loss.[14] Daily physical activity increases the clearance of TG-rich lipoproteins and glucose, and is often moderately effective in treating hypertriglyceridemia and combined dyslipidemia. Exercise of moderate intensity, longer duration,

Table 119.7. **Major Food Group Sources of Saturated Fat and Cholesterol**

Food group	Suggestions
Meats	Smaller portions (6–8 oz/day) Use lean meats, trim fat Broil, bake, or grill Include fish several times per week Plan some meatless meals using soy, dried beans, or peas
Dairy products	Use skim or low-fat products Use part-skim or low-fat cheeses as a meat substitute Substitute low-fat frozen desserts for ice cream
Eggs	Limit yolks to four per week Use egg whites or egg substitute when baking
Fats/oils	Use smaller amounts of all fats Substitute unsaturated fats like olive oil, canola oil, or soft margarine for butter, stick margarine, or shortening Use reduced-fat mayonnaise/salad dressings
Snacks/desserts	Substitute low-fat snack foods (pretzels, popcorn, fruit) for deep fried snacks Use smaller servings of desserts Substitute fruit for other desserts Eat small amounts of nuts or seeds several times per week

and increased frequency appears to have more benefit for dyslipidemia and weight loss than higher intensity, less frequent activity.[14] However, both resistance and endurance activity will improve dyslipidemias, and any regular activity that the patient enjoys should be encouraged. A clear physician message about the importance of physical activity has a significant impact in increasing patient's physical activity.[32]

Smoking Cessation

Cigarette smoking is associated with a number of metabolic processes that affect lipoproteins, including increasing plasma free fatty acids, glucose, and VLDL-C, and lowering HDL-C. Smoking cessation is associated with an average increase in HDL-C of 6 to 8 mg/dL.[33]

Pharmacologic Management

Indications

The use of medications for cholesterol treatment should follow careful consideration and implementation of the nonpharmacologic methods discussed above. The following guidelines are general recommendations and cannot specifically address every clinical situation. Treatment recommendations do not replace the physician's clinical judgment in dealing with an individual patient. Treatment is individualized based on overall risk, pattern of dyslipidemia, and associated medical conditions. Other important factors include cost, prognosis, and patient motivation. Medication use is recommended for those at highest risk who fail to reach goal cholesterol levels after an adequate trial of lifestyle change (usually 3 to 6 months). Any recommendation for early pharmacologic treatment (with lifestyle changes) is focused on the highest risk individuals: those with prior CHD events or "CHD-risk equivalents" (patients with DM or multiple risk factors and a 10-year risk of CHD events >20%), and those with genetic lipid disorders (LDL-C >220, TG >1000, or HDL-C <30 mg/dL).[3]

The new NCEP ATP III guidelines use 10-year CHD risk estimates to stratify risk for primary prevention patients with two or more CHD risk factors into LDL-C treatment goal categories to guide treatment decisions (Table 119.2).[3] The risk estimate tools are simple and risk can be calculated using these tools in a minimal amount of time. Patients with one risk factor, or none, usually have a 10-year CHD risk of <10%, so they usually do not require risk calculations. Patients with a 10-year CHD risk of less than 10% have a recommended goal LDL-C of <160 mg/dL, while those with a 10-year risk of 10% to 20% have a goal LDL-C of <130 mg/dL. For patients with a 10-year CHD risk of greater than 20% ("CHD-risk equivalents") the LDL-C goal is <100 mg/dL, the same as for patients with known CHD, as the risk for future CHD is similar (Table 119.2).

Medications

The cholesterol-lowering medications are listed in Table 119.8. Given the limited choice of medications and their

Table 119.8. **Cholesterol-Lowering Medications**

Medication	Dose range	LDL reduction (%)	Cost	Side effects and special considerations
HMG-CoA reductase inhibitors (statins)[a]				
Atorvastatin (Lipitor)	10 mg qd min 80 mg qd max	35–38 50–60	$$$–$$$$	*Note:* this list is for all statins: Increased hepatic transaminases and other minor GI effects (2–3%) May continue if liver function tests (LFTs) are elevated but <2–3 times normal—remonitor Myalgias/arthralgias (2–3%)[b,c]
Fluvastatin (Lescol)	20 mg qhs min 40 mg bid or 80 mg XL max	20–25 35–38	$$+	[b,c]
Lovastatin (Mevacor)	10 mg qhs min 80 mg qhs or 40 mg bid max	25–30 35–40	$$–$$$$	[b,c]Lovastatin is now available as a generic medication
Pravastatin (Pravachol)	10 mg qhs min 40 mg qhs max	25–32 30–35	$$$–$$$$	[b]*Note:* Only statin without CYP450 metabolism; less interaction with other meds
Simvastatin (Zocor)	10 mg qhs min 80 mg qhs max	35–40% 45–50%	$$$–$$$$	[b,c]
Bile acid sequestrants				Second line for LDL-C disorders Potent combination with statins
Colestipol (Colestid)	4–8 g bid–tid	10–25%	$$$–$$$$	May increase TG Bloating, constipation
Cholestyramine (Questran)	5–10 g bid–tid (start at a low dose)	TG may increase moderately	$$–$$$	Interferes with some medication and fat-soluble vitamin absorption
Colesevelam (Welchol)	6 capsules (3 capsules bid or 6 qd with meal)		$$$$	Colesevelam has less GI toxicity and may interference less with absorption of other medications
Psyllium	5–15 g bid–tid	0–10%	$	Bloating, diarrhea/constipation
Plant stanols or sterols (dietary supplement Benecol Take Control	3 tablespoons of margarine tid or used as salad dressing bid	8–15%	$–$$	Minimal to no side effects Weight gain may occur due to increased calorie intake
Niacin				
Niacin plain	500–1500 bid–tid (starting dose: 100 mg)	20–25%	$	Flushing, dry skin, rash Glucose intolerance Elevated uric acid
Extended release (Niaspan only SR-formulation recommended)	Extended release, 500–2000 mg qhs	Also: 50% TG decrease, 25% HDL-C increase	$$–$$$	Dyspepsia or ulcer Caution with diabetes, gout, history of gastritis or peptic ulcer
Fibrates		TG 50% decrease; HDL-C 5–20% increase; LDL-C 10% increase to 20% decrease	$$–$$$	Nausea
Gemfibrozil (Lopid)	600 mg bid			Myositis (2–6%) with statins and cyclosporine
Fenofibrate (Tricor)	67–201 mg qd			

[a]All statins have moderate TG lowering (15–40+%) and HDL raising (5–12%) effects.

[b]Increased myositis with gemfibrozil, and possibly fenofibrate and niacin.

[c]Cytochrome CYP450 metabolism with interaction with other medications that are metabolized there; may result in higher statin levels and possible myositis and/or rhabdomyolysis.

specificity, family physicians must be familiar with all these medication classes to effectively treat dyslipidemias. More detailed prescribing information and management principles are available through many current resources.[3,14,16] Some of the medications are expensive, but cost-effective therapy is possible with good working knowledge of the medications.[34]

Medications within each class listed in Table 119.8 have similar intraclass effects and side effects. However, if side effects occur, medications may be substituted within a class with caution, since pharmacokinetics vary. The statins primarily reduce LDL-C, but also moderately reduce TG and raise HDL. The bile acid resins primarily lower LDL-C, but may exacerbate TG elevations. Plant sterols and psyllium are food derivatives that lower LDL-C modestly, but this effect can be enhanced in combination with other medications. Niacin is effective for elevated TG and low HDL-C, but lowers LDL-C only at higher doses, and is somewhat limited by side effects. Gemfibrozil primarily reduces TG (and subse-

quently raises HDL-C), but may also raise LDL-C as TG is lowered. Fenofibrate (Tricor) is effective for TG, HDL-C, and LDL-C, but may also elevate LDL-C if the baseline TG is high (>300 mg/dL). Due to safety concerns raised in clinical trials, clofibrate (Atromid-S), also a fibrate, is limited to use for high-risk patients with hypertriglyceridemias who cannot take other fibrates or niacin.[14] Medications such as the statins and niacin have recently been shown to have effects beyond lipid-lowering, including antiinflammatory effects, that appear to contribute to their effectiveness in reducing CHD events.[35]

Medication Use for Specific Dyslipidemia Classification

The pattern of dyslipidemia dictates the appropriate choice of medication as discussed below and presented in Table 119.3 and Fig. 119.1.

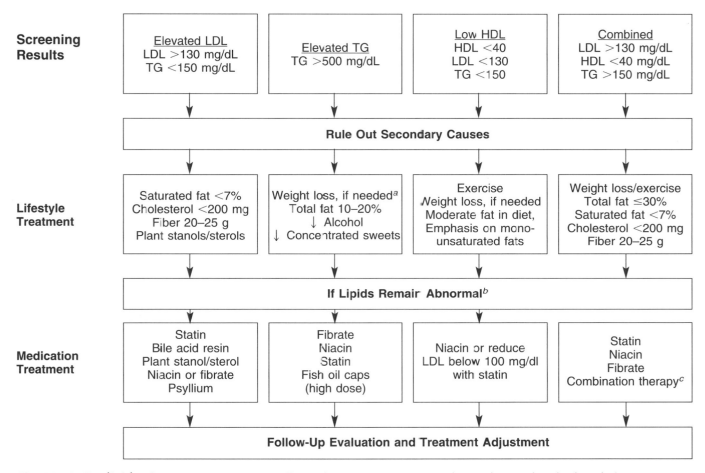

Fig. 119.1. Dyslipidemia treatment summary. [a]Exception: immediate medication (gemfibrozil or niacin) for patients with TG >1000 mg/dL due to high risk of pancreatitis, or LDL-C >220 mg/dL due to genetic basis, and resistance to nonpharmacologic treatment after ruling out secondary causes. [b]Notes: (1) Goal LDL-C <100 with CHD/noncoronary atherosclerosis; diabetes mellitus, 10-yr CHD-risk >20%; (2) goal LDL-C <130 if no known CHD or noncoronary atherosclerosis but high risk (LDL-C >160 mg/dL with two or more risk factors or LDL-C >190 mg/dL in isolation). [c]See text; statins and fibrates and/or niacin may be used in combination with close monitoring for hepatitis or myositis (risk of interaction 2–6%; cerivastatin should not be used in combination with a fibrate).

Elevated LDL-C

For isolated LDL-C elevations, or elevated LDL-C after TG is controlled with combined dyslipidemias, medications that primarily lower LDL-C are recommended. Statins are the most effective treatment. The bile acid resins, plant sterols, and psyllium are modest in efficacy (5–20% mean LDL-C reductions), but side effects are limited to the gastrointestinal tract. Niacin is a potent and inexpensive agent, especially in low-dose combination with bile acid resins, but high doses are generally required to lower LDL-C significantly. Estrogen may effectively reduce LDL-C in postmenopausal women but may also significantly exacerbate TG elevations. Hormone replacement therapy currently is contraindicated in women with CHD due to clinical trial evidence of increased thrombotic events, including CHD events, in three clinical trials.[3,36] Elevated LDL-C in combination with elevated HDL-C in older women is associated with only a modestly increased risk, and nutritional assessment and counseling may be adequate.

Hypertriglyceridemias

After secondary causes are evaluated and treated, niacin and gemfibrozil are the treatments of choice for TG >400 to 500 mg/dL. It is important to realize that when TG is greater than 400 mg/dL, TG usually must be controlled before TChol and LDL-C lowering can be successful. Fibrates are the treatment of choice for hypertriglyceridemia associated with diabetes, gout, gastritis, or ulcer disease due to the potential for niacin to exacerbate these conditions. However, patients with well-controlled diabetes may tolerate niacin without significant worsening of hyperglycemia. Caution and careful monitoring is still advised, however. Note that if TGs are reduced with gemfibrozil, often the LDL-C level rises and may require additional treatment. Fenofibrate will also be effective in these patients, but is more expensive. Omega-3 fish oil capsules (minimum 5.4 g DHA or EPA daily) also can lower TG safely and effectively (though not as effectively as niacin or the fibrates), but may cause abdominal bloating, belching, flatulence, or loose stools. Bile acid resins or estrogens may exacerbate TG elevations, and estrogens, progestins, and other steroids are contraindicated for patients with hypertriglyceridemia (TG >300–400 mg/dL) because they may significantly elevate TG and the high TG may lead to pancreatitis.

Combined Dyslipidemia

This pattern is commonly associated with the metabolic syndrome and premature CHD. The treatments of choice for this disorder are statins, niacin, gemfibrozil, and fenofibrate. Combined dyslipidemias are frequently associated with glucose intolerance and gout, which are relative contraindications to niacin use. Fibrates may be effective but are often limited by a variable response of LDL-C, so treatment may require fibrates in combination with psyllium, a bile acid resin, or a low-dose statin to reduce LDL-C effectively. Statins may be useful if TG levels are moderately elevated but may not be effective if the TG level is over 300 to 400 mg/dL. Patients put on oral contraceptives or hormone replacement therapy should have baseline lipoprotein screening and follow-up testing to ensure that triglycerides are not significantly elevated

Low HDL-C

The only medication that effectively raises isolated low HDL-C (<40 mg/dL) is niacin.[37] Isolated HDL-C deficiencies are slow to respond to treatment, if they respond at all. Patients with documented atherosclerosis or a high-risk family profile with low HDL-C may be candidates for a prolonged trial of low- to moderate-dose niacin (250–500 mg bid) to determine if HDL-C can be increased without significant side effects. Many studies demonstrate CHD event reduction by lowering LDL-C below target levels with statins when HDL-C cannot be raised.[4,5,7]

Combination Therapy

Combining medications to treat cholesterol may be effective when a single agent is insufficient, or to reduce the dosage and side effects of a single medication. Combinations of a statin or other medication that reduces lipoprotein production (i.e., niacin or fibrate) with a medication that reduces bile acid reabsorption (bile acid resin, a plant stanol or sterol, or psyllium) are synergistic in reducing LDL-C levels. Other statins can be combined with niacin or fibrates, but careful education of the patient about identifying and reporting myalgia symptoms is needed, as are more frequent follow-up visits (every 3 to 4 months) to monitor blood chemistry. Combinations of either gemfibrozil or niacin with fluvastatin, pravastatin, or simvastatin increases the risk of myositis to 1% to 2% and combinations with lovastatin increase myositis risk to 5% to 6%.

Monitoring Medications

Patients on medications should be monitored every 4 to 6 weeks to adjust medication doses and evaluate side effects until lipid goals are reached. Evaluations of liver function and the lipoprotein profile are appropriate monitoring tests. Levels of liver function tests such as alanine aminotransferase (ALT) or aspartate aminotransferase (AST) that are less than two to three times normal and that are not progressive can be tolerated with the use of cholesterol medications, especially the statins. More frequent monitoring is recommended for those with severe underlying clinical disease, with liver enzyme elevations or underlying liver disease, on combination cholesterol therapy, or taking other medications that could interact to cause drug-induced hepatitis. Most of the cholesterol medications are metabolized in the liver, with the exception of those that are not absorbed (e.g., resins, stanols, or sterols), and fibrates, which have mixed hepatic and renal metabolism. Due to frequent benign elevations of creatinine kinase (CK) that occur from physical activity, CK levels are only recommended if patients complain of generalized myalgias. When the lipoprotein levels reach treatment goals, monitoring every 4 to 6 months is appropriate to assess side effects and laboratory studies, and to verify diet and medication adherence. Since dyslipidemias are an asymptomatic condition, an initial visit 4 to 6 weeks after initiation of therapy provides an opportunity for valuable patient feedback on medication effectiveness. If patients do not get feedback within that time frame, there is a significant drop in medication adherence.[3]

References

1. American Heart Association. 2001 Heart and Stroke Statistical Update. Dallas, Texas: American Heart Association.
2. LaRosa JC, Hunninghake D, Bush D, et al. The cholesterol facts. A summary of the evidence relating dietary fats, serum cholesterol, and coronary heart disease. A joint statement by the American Heart Association and the National Heart, Lung, and Blood Institute. The Task Force on Cholesterol Issues, American Heart Association. Circulation 1990;81:1721–33.
3. National Cholesterol Education Program (NCEP) Expert Panel (ATP III). Executive summary of the third report of the National Cholesterol Education Program (NCEP) expert panel on detection, evaluation and treatment of high blood cholesterol in adults (Adult Treatment Panel III). JAMA 2001;285:2486–97.
4. Downs JR, Clearfield M, Weis S. Primary prevention of acute coronary events with lovastatin in men and women with average cholesterol levels: results of AFCAPS/TexCAPS. JAMA 1998;279:1615–22.
5. Scandanavian Simvastatin Survival Study Group. Randomised trial of cholesterol lowering in 4444 patients with coronary heart disease. Lancet 1994;344:1383–9.
6. Shepherd J, Cobbe S, Ford I. Prevention of coronary heart disease with pravastatin in men with hypercholesterolemia. West of Scotland Coronary Prevention Study Group. N Engl J Med 1995;333:1301–7.
7. Sacks FM, Pfeffer MA, Moye LA, et al. The effect of pravastatin on coronary events after myocardial infarction in patients with average cholesterol levels. Cholesterol and Recurrent Events (CARE) Trial investigators. N Engl J Med 1996;335:1001–9.
8. Lipid Research Clinics Coronary Primary Prevention Trial Results I. Reduction in incidence of coronary heart disease. JAMA 1984;251:351–64.
9. Superko HR, Krauss RM. Coronary artery disease regression. Convincing evidence for the benefit of aggressive lipoprotein management. Circulation 1994;90:1056–69.
10. Ferguson EE. Preventing, stopping, or reversing coronary artery disease—triglyceride-rich lipoproteins and associated lipoprotein and metabolic abnormalities: the need for recognition and treatment. Dis Mon 2000;46:421–503.
11. Carlsson CM, Carnes M, McBride PE, Stein JH. Managing dyslipidemia in older adults. J Am Geriatr Soc 1999;47:1458–65.
12. Williams RR, Hunt SC, Heiss G, et al. Usefulness of cardiovascular family history data for population-based preventive medicine and medical research (the Health Family Tree Study and the NHLBI Family Study). Am J Cardiol 2001;87:129–35.
13. Pacala JT. The relation of serum cholesterol to risk of coronary heart disease: implications for the elderly. J Am Board Fam Pract 1990;3:271–82.
14. Oberman A, Kreisberg RA, Henkin Y. Principles and management of lipid disorders: a primary care approach. Baltimore: Williams & Wilkins, 1992.
15. National Cholesterol Education Program (NCEP) Expert Panel (ATP II). Highlights of the report of the expert panel on blood cholesterol levels in children and adolescents. Am Fam Physician 1992;45:2127–36.
16. Knopp RH. Drug treatment of lipid disorders. N Engl J Med 1999;341:498–511.
17. Brown WV, Ginsburg H. Classification and diagnosis of the hyperlipidemias. In Steinberg D, Olefsky JM, eds. Hypercholesteremia and atherosclerosis: pathogenesis and prevention. New York: Churchill Livingstone, 1987;143–68.
18. Genest J, Martin-Munley S, McNamara JR, Salem DN, Schaefer EJ. Frequency of genetic dyslipidemias in patients with premature coronary artery disease. Arteriosclerosis 1989;9:701A.
19. Boden WE. High-density lipoprotein cholesterol as an independent risk factor in cardiovascular disease: assessing the data from Framingham to the Veterans Affairs High-Density Lipoprotein Intervention Trial. Am J Cardiol 2000;86:19L–22L.
20. USDA and US Department of Health and Human Services. Dietary guidelines for Americans, 5th ed. Home and Garden bulletin no. 232. Washington, DC: DHHS, 2000.
21. Lichtenstein AH, Deckelbaum RJ. AHA Science Advisory. Stanol/sterol ester-containing foods and blood cholesterol levels. A statement for healthcare professionals from the Nutrition Committee of the Council on Nutrition, Physical Activity, and Metabolism of the American Heart Association. Circulation 2001;103:1177–9.
22. Krauss RM, Ecked RH, Howard B, et al. AHA Dietary Guidelines: revision 2000: a statement for healthcare professionals from the Nutrition Committee of the American Heart Association. Circulation 2000;102:2284–99.
23. Grundy SM. The optimal ratio of fat-to-carbohydrate in the diet. Annu Rev Nutr 1999;19:325–41.
24. Jenkins DJ, Kendall CW, Vidgen E, et al. The effect on serum lipids and oxidized low-density lipoprotein of supplementing self-selected low-fat diets with soluble-fiber, soy, and vegetable protein foods. Metab Clin Exp 2000;49:67–72.
25. Pearson TA. Alcohol and heart disease. Circulation 1996;94:3023–5.
26. Tribble DL. Antioxidant consumption and risk of coronary heart disease: emphasis on vitamin C, vitamin E, and β-carotene. Circulation 1999;99:591–5.
27. Adams AK, Wermuth EO, McBride PE. Antioxidant vitamins and the prevention of coronary heart disease. Am Fam Physician 1999;60:895–904.
28. Jialal I, Abate N. Therapy and clinical trials. Curr Opin Lipidol 2000;11:93–7.
29. Stone NJ. The Gruppo Italiano per lo Studio della Sopravvivenza nell'Infarto Miocardio (GISSI)-Prevenzione Trial on fish oil and vitamin E supplementation in myocardial infarction survivors. Curr Cardiol Rep 2001;2:445–51.
30. Stein JH, McBride PE. Hyperhomocysteinemia and atherosclerotic vascular disease: pathophysiology, screening and treatment. Arch Intern Med 1998;158:1301–6.
31. Subar AF, Krebs-Smith SM, Cook A, Kahle LL. Dietary sources of nutrients among US adults, 1989 to 1991. J Am Diet Assoc 1998;93:537–47.
32. Ockene IS, Hebert JR, Ockene JK, Merriam PA, Hurley TG, Saperia GM. Effect of training and a structured office practice on physician-delivered nutrition counseling: the Worcester-Area Trial for Counseling in Hyperlipidemia (WATCH). Am J Prev Med 1996;12:252–8.
33. McBride PE. The health consequences of smoking. Cardiovascular diseases. Med Clin North Am 1992;76:333–53.
34. Jacobsen TA, Schein JR, Williamson A, Ballantyne CM. Maximizing the cost-effectiveness of lipid-lowering therapy. Arch Intern Med 1998;158:1977–89.
35. Ridker PM, Rifai N, Clearfield M. Measurement of C-reactive protein for the targeting of statin therapy in the primary prevention of acute coronary events. N Engl J Med 2001;344:1959–65.
36. Hulley S, Grady D, Bush T, et al. Randomized trial of estrogen plus progestin for secondary prevention of coronary heart disease in postmenopausal women. Heart and Estrogen/progestin Replacement Study (HERS) Research Group. JAMA 1998;280:605–13.
37. Martin-Jadraque R, Tato F, Mostaza JM, Vega GL, Grundy SM. Effectiveness of low-dose crystalline nicotinic acid in men with low high-density lipoprotein cholesterol levels. Arch Intern Med 1996;156:1081–8.

120
Diabetes Mellitus

Charles Kent Smith, John P. Sheehan, and Margaret M. Ulchaker

Diabetes mellitus (DM) affects 12 million to 15 million individuals in the United States, incurring an immense cost in terms of morbidity and premature death. The most prevalent form, type 2 DM, previously called adult-onset DM, has racial preponderances, female predilection, and strong associations with obesity. During the 1980s there was a revolution in DM management with the advent of home blood glucose monitoring devices, human insulin, and reliable laboratory markers of long-term glycemic control. Additionally, published national and international standards of care have been disseminated directly to patients and physicians, heightening the importance of adequate care and glycemic control to minimize devastating long-term complications.[1,2] Table 120.1 describes diagnostic criteria for diabetes mellitus, impaired glucose tolerance, and gestational diabetes.

Heightened clinical awareness of the genetics and predisposing factors should foster early diagnosis and adequate metabolic control of the type 2 patient. In contrast, the type 1 DM patient generally presents with a more precipitous clinical picture of ketoacidosis. Declining islet cell secretory function is more gradual, however, and can evolve over a 10-year period. Understanding the autoimmune nature of islet destruction has led to experimental protocols attempting to interrupt this process. Occasionally, there is diagnostic confusion owing to a lack of a family history, the absence of significant ketosis, and the absence of significant obesity and other diagnostic hallmarks. The measurement of C-peptide levels, islet cell antibodies, and glutamic acid decarboxylase (GAD) antibodies provides useful diagnostic clarification.[3] C-peptide is the fragment produced when proinsulin, produced by the islets of Langerhans, is cleaved to produce insulin. For every molecule of insulin produced, a molecule of C-peptide has to exist; therefore, C-peptide is a marker of endogenous insulin production. Measurement of a C-peptide level is very useful in documenting insulin secretory capacity in the insulin-treated individual, in whom an insulin level would measure both endogenous and exogenous insulin. Careful clinical follow-up can clarify evolving absolute insulin deficiency even in the absence of these laboratory markers.

Pathophysiology

Previously, type 1 DM was considered to be an acute event. Viral associations were invoked with regard to the seasonal trends in its incidence. However, patients can have markers of islet destruction in the form of islet cell antibodies for up to 10 years prior to the development of overt DM. Islet cell, insulin, and GAD autoantibodies, along with the loss of first-phase insulin secretion in response to an intravenous glucose tolerance test, are highly predictive of evolving type 1 DM.[4] Attempts to interrupt this autoimmune process with immunosuppressive agents have been tried with some encouraging results, but toxicity remains a concern. Insulin has been given to experimental animals that have autoimmune islet destruction without overt DM in an attempt to suppress the autoimmune process. A pilot study of 12 patients demonstrated exciting promise for clinical applicability of this approach in humans.[5] However a nationwide clinical trial of prophylactic insulin in individuals at high risk to develop type 1 DM disappointingly showed no effect on the rate of progression to type 1 DM. A group of investigators in Edmonton, Alberta, Canada have treated seven patients with type 1 DM with islet cell transplantation. These patients who are initially on triple immunosuppression therapy have normal ambient glucose levels. However, on intravenous glucose tolerance testing, they have impaired glucose tolerance. The key to islet cell transplantation is developing safe immunosuppressives or modifying the process to eliminate the need for immunosuppressives.[6]

In contrast, type 2 DM is associated with genetic predispositions, advancing age, obesity, and lack of physical exercise. The importance of caloric intake and energy expendi-

Table 120.1. **Diagnostic Criteria for Diabetes Mellitus, Impaired Glucose Tolerance, and Gestational Diabetes**

Nonpregnant adults

Criteria for diabetes mellitus: Diagnosis of diabetes mellitus in nonpregnant adults should be restricted to those who have one of the following:

Fasting plasma glucose ≥126 mg/dL. Fasting is defined as no caloric intake for at least 8 hours.

Symptoms of diabetes mellitus (such as polyuria, polydipsia, unexplained weight loss) coupled with a casual plasma glucose level of ≥200 mg/dL. Casual is defined as any time of day without regard to time interval since the last meal.

2-hour postprandial plasma glucose ≥200 mg/dL during an oral glucose tolerance test. The test should be performed by World Health Organization criteria using a glucose load containing the equivalent of 75 g anhydrous glucose dissolved in water.

Note: In the absence of unequivocal hyperglycemia with acute metabolic decompensation, these criteria should be confirmed by repeat testing on a second occasion. The oral glucose tolerance test is not recommended for routine clinical use.

Criterion for impaired glucose tolerance: 2-hour postprandial plasma glucose ≥140 mg/dL and ≤199 mg/dL during an oral glucose tolerance test. The test should be performed by World Health Organization criteria using a glucose load containing the equivalent of 75 g anhydrous glucose dissolved in water.

Pregnant Women

Criteria for gestational diabetes: After an oral glucose load of 100 g, gestational diabetes is diagnosed if two plasma glucose values equal or exceed:

Fasting: 105 mg/dL
1 Hour: 190 mg/dL
2 Hour: 165 mg/dL
3 Hour: 145 mg/dL

Source: Clinical practice recommendations: 2001.[1]

ture has been clearly established.[7] Although type 2 DM is a syndrome of insulin resistance and islet secretory defects, in any given individual it is not possible to define the degree of insulin resistance versus secretory defects with any precision. The earliest metabolic defect found in first-degree relatives of individuals with type 2 DM is defective skeletal muscle glucose uptake with later increased insulin resistance at the level of the liver and resultant uncontrolled hepatic glucose output. The ensuing hyperglycemia can have a toxic effect called glucotoxicity on the islets, resulting in secondary secretory defects with declining insulin secretion and self-perpetuating hyperglycemia. Hyperglycemia may also down-regulate glucose transporters. To become hyperglycemic, insulin secretion must be insufficient to overcome the insulin resistance; it has been estimated that insulin secretory capacity is reduced by 50% at the time of diagnosis with type 2 DM.[8] It is unclear whether secretory defects or insulin resistance is the primary defect even for type 2 DM. Patients may exhibit many abnormalities, including loss of first-phase insulin secretion and loss of the pulsatility of insulin secretion.[9–12] Additionally, both men and women tend to have abdominal obesity, which is associated with hyperinsulinemia and insulin resistance.[13] Type 2 DM is a syndrome not only of disordered glucose metabolism but also of lipid metabolism; many patients have a concurrent dyslipidemia manifesting elevations in serum triglycerides, depressions in high-density lipoprotein (HDL) cholesterol, and marginal increases in total cholesterol. This dyslipidemia results from uncontrolled hepatic very low density lipoprotein (VLDL) secretion and defective clearance of lipoprotein molecules. The associations of hyperinsulinemia and insulin resistance with essential hypertension have been documented[14] along with the marked tendency for patients with essential hypertension to develop DM and the converse—patients with type 2 DM developing essential hypertension. A central unifying hypothesis focuses on hyper-

insulinemia and insulin resistance being primary metabolic aberrations that result not only in hyperglycemia but also hypertension and dyslipidemia. Thus our current understanding of type 2 DM and the cardiodysmetabolic syndrome, formerly known as syndrome X[15] (hyperinsulinemia, dyslipidemia, hypertension, and hyperglycemia) highlights the important issue not only of primary prevention of type 2 DM but also secondary prevention.

Importance of Glycemic Control

The relation between microvascular complications of DM and glycemic control has been debated for decades. Many studies suggested an association between poor long-term glycemic control and retinopathy, neuropathy, and nephropathy. Unfortunately, many of these studies were not randomized, and the role of genetic factors was unclear. However, positive trends with glycemic control had been described. Small human studies and several animal studies link sustained metabolic control to the prevention of complications. One study showed, however, that early poor control despite later good control results in diabetic complications.[16] The Diabetes Control and Complications Trial (DCCT) in individuals with type 1 DM proved the profound impact of intensive therapy on reducing the risk of microvascular complications.[17] Decades of questions about the glucose hypothesis are therefore finally answered, with the obvious recommendation that most individuals with type 1 DM be treated with intensive therapy. A potential negative aspect of attempts to achieve optimum glycemic control by intensive insulin therapy is the potential for severe hypoglycemia. An educated and motivated patient working with a multidisciplinary health care team can significantly reduce the risk of this. Glycemic goals may need to be modified in the individual with poor hypoglycemia awareness. The United Kingdom Prospective Diabetes Study (UKPDS), a 20-year prospective study in type 2 DM, demonstrated that both intensive glycemic control and intensive blood pressure control reduced the risk of microvascular and macrovascular complications of DM.[18–20] Excellent metabolic control as defined by normal hemoglobin A_{1c} (HbA_{1c}) levels without significant hypoglycemia is an achievable goal.

Defining Control

The definition of DM control has varied. During the bygone era of urine testing, predominantly negative urine tests were indicative of good glycemic control. However, because blood glucose can be twice normal in the absence of glycosuria, urine glucose monitoring is now outmoded. Home blood glucose monitoring (HBGM) provides positive feedback of daily glycemic control to patients and physicians. Patients engaged in intensive insulin therapy can monitor themselves four to ten times per day and make adjustments in their regimen to optimize blood glucose control. The precision and accuracy of the home units has improved considerably, as has the simplicity and duration of the test. Some systems enable users to obtain the blood sample from the forearm. Each system has its inherent weaknesses and limitations in such areas as blood volume, timing, hematocrit, temperature, and humidity. It is important that patients adhere strictly to the manufacturers' guidelines because attention to proper calibrations, strip handling, and ongoing maintenance are critical. Minimally invasive HBGM is the wave of the future, with the Glucowatch Biographer being the first to reach market. The HbA_{1c}, the marker of long-term glycemic control, measures the degree of glycosylation of the A_{1c} subfraction of hemoglobin and reflects the average blood glucose over the preceding 60 to 90 days. It also allows for identification of possible falsification of or errors in HBGM results. It is a useful motivating tool for patients; it often becomes a perceived challenge to reduce the result within the constraints of hypoglycemia. The National Glycosylated Hemoglobin Standardization Program is responsible for standardizing and correlating various assays to the DCCT methodology.[21]

Hemoglobinopathies can skew HbA_{1c} results, and can be detected via inspection of the chromatograms in the laboratory. The American Diabetes Association recommends that the HbA_{1c} be performed at least two to four times per year in all patients. Given that the DCCT demonstrated a linear relation between the HbA_{1c} (all the way into the normal, nondiabetic range) and microvascular complication risk, the ideal is therefore normalization of the HbA_{a1c} within the constraints of hypoglycemia. In addition to markers of glycemic control, it is critical to monitor other clinical parameters. Annual lipid profiles are an integral part of overall DM care in view of the high prevalence of dyslipidemia especially in the patient with type 2 DM. In type 1 DM patients, lipid disturbances are uncommon unless patients are in poor glycemic control, have a familial dyslipidemia, or have renal insufficiency. Markers of nephropathy are also important to measure. The earliest marker, microalbuminuria, is not only a forerunner of overt clinical nephropathy but also a marker for greatly increased cardiovascular risk in both type 1 and type 2 patients.[22,23] Microalbuminuria can be conveniently measured in spot urine specimens or by overnight albumin excretion rates,[24] rather than the more cumbersome 24-hour urine collection.

Patient Education

Patient attention to management principles decidedly affects short-term metabolic control and ultimately has an impact on long-term complications. The interactions of patients with registered nurses and dietitians (preferably certified diabetes educators) are critical. The presence of family members and significant others during the educational sessions is vital to a successful outcome. Education must encompass a comprehensive understanding of the pathophysiology of DM and its complications and the importance of attaining and sustaining metabolic control. Accurate HBGM is critical; after initial instruction, periodic reassessment of performance technique helps to ensure continued accuracy. The results stored in the memory of most meters can be downloaded to a computer, via a meter-specific computer program. However, the traditional written glucose log actually provides more information when an educated, motivated patient records glucose results, times of day, medication administered, and notes regarding activity and other variables. Education must also focus on dietary principles. For individuals with diabetes, the current dietary recommendations are a diet containing at least 50% of the calories from carbohydrate, less than 30% fat, and 20% or less protein. Caloric requirements are based on ideal body weight (IBW)—not actual body weight. We calculate IBW by the Hamwi formula.[25]

Women
  100 pounds for 5 feet
  5 pounds for every additional inch
  Example: Woman 5'3" = 115 pounds IBW

Men
  106 pounds for 5 feet
  6 pounds for every additional inch
  Example: Man 5'8" = 154 pounds IBW

Based on anthropometric measures, 10% may be subtracted or added based on small body frame or large body frame, respectively.

Basal caloric requirements then are as follows.

Woman 5'3": IBW = 115 pounds
115 × 10 kcal = 1150 kcal/day

Add 300 to 400 kcal/day for moderate to strenuous activity. Subtract 500 kcal/day for 1 pound per week weight loss.

Because individuals with DM type 2 are generally hyperinsulinemic, diet prescriptions for weight loss and maintenance require a lower caloric level than previously mentioned. The activity factor in kilocalories (300–400 kcal/day) can be modified in these individuals. For the type 2 DM patient, caloric restriction is of major importance. In contrast, diet for the type 1 DM patient should involve careful consistency of carbohydrate intake. Achieving this degree of dietary education generally requires several sessions with a dietitian/nutrition specialist. Dietary principles are an ongoing exercise, and eradication of myths and misconceptions is a major task. Unfortunately, many patients still perceive that "sugar-free" implies carbohydrate-free and that "sugar-free" foods cannot affect blood glucose control. This belief fails to recognize the monomer/polymer concept and the fact that most carbohydrates are ultimately digested into glucose. In addition to maintaining carbohydrate consistency, patients must learn carbohydrate augmentation for physical activity in the absence of insulin reduction. Patients also need instruction on carbohydrate strategies for dealing with intercurrent illness when the usual complex carbohydrate may be substituted with simple carbohydrate. Although it has long been said that diet is the cornerstone of DM management,[26] effective DM dietary education is still problematic owing to time constraints and reimbursement problems.

Insulin-treated patients must be aware of the many facets of insulin therapy. Accurate drawing-up and mixing of insulin is an assumption that is often not founded in reality. Site selection, consistency, and rotation are crucial. Insulin absorption is most rapid from the upper abdomen; the arms, legs, and buttocks, respectively, are next. We find that administering the premeal insulin in the abdomen optimizes postmeal control (assuming the use of lispro, insulin aspart, or regular insulin). In contrast, the buttocks, as the slowest absorption site, is not a good choice for premeal injections. However, the lower buttocks is an ideal site for bedtime injections of intermediate-acting insulin [neutral protamine Hagedorn (NPH)/lente] to minimize nocturnal hypoglycemia. Haphazard site selection and rotation can lead to erratic glycemic control. Because of the variability in absorption among sites, we suggest site consistency—using the same anatomic site at the same time of day (all breakfast injections in the abdomen, all dinner injections in the arms, all bedtime injections in the lower buttocks). Broad rotation within the sites is important to eliminate local lipohypertrophy.[27] The fast-acting insulin analogues, lispro with its peak action 1 hour postinjection and the new insulin aspart with its peak action 30 to 90 minutes postinjection, significantly improve postprandial glycemic control. This facilitates insulin injection timing as it is injected 0 to 10 minutes premeal. In contrast, regular insulin requires premeal timing of insulin injections (generally 30 minutes) to optimize postprandial glycemic control, as its peak effect is 3 to 4 hours after injection. Patients need a comprehensive perspective on insulin adjustments[28] for hyperglycemia, altered physical activity, illness management, travel, and alcohol consumption.

Patients need education on the pathophysiology, prevention, and treatment of microvascular complications. Education on macrovascular risk factors and their modification for prevention of cardiovascular, cerebrovascular, and peripheral vascular disease is also critical. Patients can have a considerable impact on decreasing foot problems and amputations

with simple attention to hygiene (avoidance of foot soaks), daily foot inspection, and the use of appropriate footwear. These measures can greatly reduce the incidence of trauma, sepsis, and ultimately amputations.[29]

Diabetic Complications

Complications of DM include those that are specific to DM and those that are nonspecific but are accelerated by the presence of DM. The microvascular complications of DM are diabetes specific—the triad of retinopathy, neuropathy, and nephropathy. Macrovascular disease—atherosclerosis—a common complication in patients with DM, is not specific to DM but is greatly accelerated by its presence. A major misconception among patients and even physicians is that the complications of DM tend to be less severe in patients with type 2 DM. Patients with type 2 DM or impaired glucose tolerance have greatly accelerated macrovascular disease and also suffer significant morbidity from microvascular complications.

Retinopathy

Retinopathy, the commonest cause of new-onset blindness during middle life, is broadly classified as nonproliferative (background) and proliferative. In addition, macular edema may be present in either category. Macular edema is characterized by a collection of intraretinal fluid in the macula, with or without lipid exudates (hard exudates). In nonproliferative retinopathy, ophthalmoscopic findings may include microaneurysms, intraretinal hemorrhages, and macular edema. In more advanced nonproliferative retinopathy, cotton wool spots reflecting retinal ischemia can be noted. In proliferative retinopathy, worsening retinal ischemia results in neovascularization, preretinal or vitreous hemorrhage and fibrous tissue proliferation. Macular edema can also occur in proliferative retinopathy. Early diagnosis and treatment with laser therapy has been shown to be vision sparing in patients with macular edema and/or proliferative retinopathy. Several studies clearly document the importance of annual examinations by an ophthalmologist for all patients.[30] Good visual acuity does not exclude significant retinal pathology; unfortunately, many patients, and health care providers alike, believe good visual acuity implies an absence of significant retinal disease.

Neuropathy

Diabetic neuropathy is discussed in Chapter 67. The clinical spectrum of diabetic neuropathy is outlined in Table 120.2.

Nephropathy/Hypertension

Diabetic nephropathy may first manifest as microalbuminuria, detected on a spot urine determination or by the timed overnight albumin excretion rate. The presence of microalbuminuria should alert the patient and physician to the need for stringent glycemic control; such control has been shown to decrease the progression from microalbuminuria to clinical proteinuria and attendant evolution of hypertension. Hypertension increases the rate of deterioration of renal function

Table 120.2. **Classification of Diabetic Neuropathy**

Type	Signs and symptoms
Sensory peripheral polyneuropathy	Pain and dysesthesia Glove and stocking sensory loss Loss of reflexes Muscle weakness/wasting
Autonomic	Orthostatic hypotension Gastroparesis, diarrhea, atonic bladder, impotence, anhidrosis, gustatory sweating, cardiac denervation on ECG
Mononeuropathy	Cranial nerve palsy Carpal tunnel syndrome Ulnar nerve palsy
Amyotrophy	Acute anterior thigh pain Weakness of hip flexion Muscle wasting
Radiculopathy	Pain and sensory loss in a dermatomal distribution

in patients with DM, and aggressive treatment is mandatory. The Captopril Diabetic Nephropathy Study demonstrated that treatment with the angiotensin-converting enzyme inhibitor (ACEI) captopril was associated with a 50% reduction in the risk of the combined end points of death, dialysis, and transplantation in macroproteinuric (>500 mg/24 hr) type 1 DM patients. Overall, the risk of doubling the serum creatinine was reduced by 48% in captopril-treated patients. The beneficial effects were seen in both normotensive and hypertensive patients such that captopril at a dose of 25 mg po tid is approved for use in normotensive proteinuric (>500 mg/24 hr) type 1 DM patients.[31] In light of this and other studies in both type 1 and type 2 DM patients, the use of ACEI for prevention of progression of microalbuminuria and macroalbuminuria is recommended, unless there is a contraindication. For antihypertensive therapy ACEI is the antihypertensive of choice, unless contraindicated, given the data not only in nephropathy but also in retinopathy. The recent Heart Outcomes Prevention Evaluation (HOPE) study demonstrated a reduced risk of microvascular and macrovascular events in individuals with DM treated with the ACEI ramipril.[32,33]

Given the macrovascular benefits alone, we should probably be looking for reasons not to prescribe ACEIs, rather than reasons to prescribe them. In patients intolerant of ACEIs due to cough, angiotensin receptor blockers and calcium channel blockers are good alternatives in light of data that show decreasing proteinuria with many of these agents over and above that achievable with conventional antihypertensive therapy. Additionally, beta-blockers have a favorable metabolic and side-effect profile. Avoidance of excessive dietary protein intake is also important, as excessive dietary protein may be involved in renal hypertrophy and glomerular hyperfiltration. Strict glycemic control even over a 3-week period can decrease renal size (as seen on ultrasonography) and decrease the hyperfiltration associated with amino acid infusions to levels comparable to those of normal, non-DM individuals.[34] Nationwide clinical trials with pimagedine (an inhibitor of protein glycosylation and cross-linking) in diabetic nephropathy

were discontinued due to adverse events and efficacy issues. Newer generation inhibitors of glycosylation and cross-linking are under clinical development.

Patients with DM in general are salt-sensitive, having diminished ability to excrete a sodium load with an attendant rise in blood pressure; therefore, avoidance of excessive dietary sodium intake is important. Hyperinsulinemia and insulin resistance are also important in the genesis of hypertension, with insulin-resistant patients having higher circulating insulin levels to maintain normal glucose levels. Associated with this insulin resistance and hyperinsulinemia is the occurrence of elevated blood pressures even in nondiabetic individuals. Insulin is antinatriuretic and stimulates the sympathetic nervous system; both mechanisms may be important in the genesis of hypertension. Hypertension exacerbates retinopathy, nephropathy, and macrovascular disease and must be diagnosed early and managed aggressively. When lifestyle modifications fail to control blood pressure, the pharmacologic agent chosen should be not only efficacious but kind to the metabolic milieu. Diuretics are very useful in edematous states. Beta-blockers have an important role in the post–myocardial infarction/anginal patient and in the heart failure patient. The benefits of beta-blockade in these patients outweigh the theoretical problems of masking of hypoglycemia, delay in recovery of hypoglycemia, and the worsening of insulin resistance. ACEIs inhibitors are a good choice in the proteinuric patient; calcium channel blockers are a good choice for the angina patient. Alpha-blockers are a good choice in the patient with benign prostatic hyperplasia, however, they are generally not used as monotherapy given the data suggesting increased risk of congestive heart failure.[35] Monotherapy of hypertension is frequently unsuccessful, especially in the setting of nephropathy, such that combination therapy is frequently needed with special attention to underlying concomitant medical problems (see Chapter 75).

Macrovascular Disease

Macrovascular disease is the major cause of premature death and considerable morbidity in individuals with DM, especially those with type 2 DM. Conventional risk factors for macrovascular disease warrant special attention in DM; they include smoking, lack of physical activity, dietary fat intake, obesity, hypertension, and hyperlipidemia. Correction and control of hyperlipidemia through improved metabolic control and the use of diet or pharmacotherapy are mandatory for the DM patient. The National Cholesterol Education Program guidelines[36] are of special importance to the diabetic, as are the American Diabetes Association guidelines[1] for the treatment of hypertriglyceridemia, with pharmacotherapy now being indicated for patients with persistent elevation in triglycerides above 200 mg/dL. LDL cholesterol lowering has been demonstrated to confer greater coronary event risk reduction and mortality reduction in diabetic patients than in nondiabetic patients. DM is one of the few diseases in which women have greater morbidity and mortality than men, especially in terms of macrovascular disease, with black women bearing the greatest load.

Foot Problems

Foot problems in the diabetic are a major cause of hospitalization and amputations. They generally constitute a combination of sepsis, ischemia, and neuropathy. The presence of significant neuropathy facilitates repetitive trauma without appropriate pain and ultimately nonhealing. Additionally, neuropathy may mask manifestations of peripheral vascular disease (PVD) (e.g., claudication and rest pain) such that patients may have critical ischemia with minimal symptoms. Therefore, PVD may be difficult to diagnose on the usual clinical grounds alone. Not only may neuropathy mask clinical symptoms, the clinical signs may be somewhat confusing. Patients with less severe neuropathy may exhibit cold feet related to arteriovenous shunting, and patients with more severe neuropathy may exhibit cutaneous hyperemia related to autosympathectomy. Noninvasive vascular testing along with clinical evaluation is helpful for the diagnosis and management of PVD. Calcific medial arterial disease is common and can cause erroneously high blood pressure recordings in the extremities, confusing the assessment of the severity of PVD. Severe ischemia with symptoms and nonhealing wounds generally requires surgical intervention. Milder symptoms and disease may respond favorably to enhanced physical activity and the use of one of the hemorheologic agents—pentoxifylline or cilostazol. Appropriate podiatric footwear and management are important to both ulcer healing and prevention of repetitive trauma.[29,37] Early PVD can readily be detected by ankle-brachial indices using a hand-held Doppler. A reduced ankle-brachial index at the posterior tibial artery in isolation has been demonstrated to be an important marker, conferring a 3.8-fold increased risk of cardiovascular death.

Achieving Glycemic Control

A recent consensus conference of the American College of Endocrinology issued revised goals for glycemic control focusing on an HbA_{1c} <6.5% and a fasting blood glucose <110 mg/dL. These new goals are in line with the International Diabetes Federation standards, which in turn are in accord with the clinical trials data.

Type 1 DM

Optimal management of type 1 DM requires an educated, motivated patient and a physiologic insulin regimen. The major challenge is physiologic insulin replacement matched to dietary carbohydrate with appropriate compensation for variables such as exercise. Physiologic insulin replacement involves intensive insulin therapy with multiple injections (three or more per day) or the use of continuous subcutaneous insulin infusion (CSII) pumps. Several regimens have been utilized to achieve glycemic control (Table 120.3). The conventional split-mix regimen combining lispro/regular and an intermediate-acting insulin in the morning before breakfast and in the evening before supper is antiquated. Its major limitation is nocturnal hypoglycemia from the pre-supper intermediate-acting insulin when stringent control of the fasting blood glucose is sought. This regimen was one of those used in the conventional group in the DCCT and was inferior at reducing the risk of complications.

Taking the split-mix regimen and then dividing the evening insulin dose—delivering lispro/regular insulin before supper and the intermediate-acting insulin at bedtime—can afford a significant reduction in the risk of nighttime hypoglycemia.[38] Most patients require 0.5 to 0.8 units/kg body weight to achieve acceptable glycemic control. There are numerous options for dosing insulin in an intensive therapy regimen. One option is to distribute two thirds of the insulin in the morning and one third of the insulin in the evening, with (1) one third of the morning dose being lispro/regular and two thirds being intermediate-acting insulin; (2) 50% of the evening insulin as lispro/regular insulin before supper; and (3) the remaining 50% as intermediate-acting insulin at bedtime (10 P.M. to 1 A.M.). These doses are modified according to individual dietary preferences and carbohydrate distribution. See Table 120.3 for other options.

Additionally, patients need algorithms to adjust their insulin for hyperglycemia, varying physical activity, and intercurrent illnesses. These individualized algorithms are based on the unit/kg insulin dose. Many episodes of severe hypoglycemia occur in the context of unplanned physical activity and dietary errors; likewise, many episodes of ketoacidosis occur during episodes of minor intercurrent illness. For physical activity, a reduction in insulin dosage of 1 to 2 units per

Table 120.3. **Commonly Used Physiologic Insulin Programs**

Insulin program	Breakfast	Lunch	Dinner	Bed (10 P.M.–1 A.M.)
Basal-bolus humalog/regular and bid ultralente	H/R + U	H/R	H/R + U	0
Basal-bolus humalog and insulin glargine	H/R	H/R	H/R	G[a]
Tid: Humalog and NPH/lente	H/R + N/L	—	H/R	N/L[b]
Qid: Humalog/regular, ultralente and NPH/lente	H/R + U	H/R	H/R	N/L[b]
Qid: regular and NPH/lente	R	R	R	N/L[b]

[a]Do not mix insulin glargine with any other insulin in a syringe.

[b]Give injection in lower buttocks.

H = humalog; G = glargine; L = lente; N = NPH; R = regular; U = ultralente.

20 to 30 minutes of activity generally suffices pending the intensity of the activity. The other option is to augment carbohydrate intake (i.e., 15 g carbohydrate prior to every 20–30 minutes of activity). During illness it is important that patients appreciate the fact that illness is a situation of insulin resistance and that all of the routine insulin should be administered. Carbohydrate from meals and snacks may be substituted as simple carbohydrate in the form of liquids such as juices and regular ginger ale. It is important that the treatment regimen is individualized and that therapeutic options for insulin administration are discussed with each patient. In this way, patients' lifestyles can be accommodated and appropriate insulin regimens tailored.[28] For example, using a basal-bolus regimen with ultralente or insulin glargine, it is possible to delay the lunchtime injection pending the patient's time constraints; furthermore, the insulin dose can be adjusted depending on carbohydrate intake and physical activity. Inhaled quick-acting insulin is under clinical investigation. Concerns exist, however, about the vasodilatory properties of insulin and the theoretical potential for pulmonary hypotension and pulmonary edema, especially in patients with cardiac dysfunction.[39] In some individuals, a lunchtime injection is not feasible. A schoolchild or a person engaged in construction work might find it difficult to accommodate a prelunch insulin injection and might be better off with a morning intermediate-acting insulin to cover the lunchtime carbohydrate intake, with lispro/regular insulin being taken to cover the breakfast carbohydrate intake as a combined prebreakfast dose.

Severe hypoglycemia in the well-educated, adherent, motivated patient on a physiologic insulin regimen is uncommon. Most severe hypoglycemic episodes are explained on the basis of diet or exercise and insulin-adjustment errors.[40] The individual who is attempting to achieve true euglycemia, however, is at risk for periodic easily self-treated hypoglycemia. See Table 120.4 for management strategies. For the individual with type 1 DM who has been educated thoroughly, is on a physiologic insulin regimen with an agreed diet plan, and has algorithms for illness and physical activity, failure to attain the desired degree of glycemic control is largely related to psychosocial variables or, occasionally, altered and unpredictable insulin kinetics.

Type 2 DM

In most instances, type 2 DM is a syndrome of insulin resistance coupled with variable secretory defects, both of which can be compounded by glucotoxicity. As insulin resistance is related to genetic factors, obesity, and sedentary lifestyle, the mainstay of treatment for the type 2 DM patient is correction of insulin resistance through diet and exercise and reversal of glucotoxicity acutely through reestablishment of euglycemia. Many patients still perceive themselves to be more absolutely insulin-deficient than insulin-resistant and are willing to accept insulin therapy as a compromise in the context of failed weight loss efforts. Additionally, many patients perceive pharmacotherapy to be equivalent to a diet and exercise regimen alone, assuming the desired degree of glycemic control is achieved. Chronic nonadherence to a diet regimen with resultant failure of weight loss or progressive obesity frequently leads to mislabeling the patient as a "brittle diabetic." It is important to avoid premature and unnecessary insulin therapy in these individuals and to stress to them the importance of diet and exercise as the most physiologic approach to controlling their metabolic disorder.

Pharmacotherapy for Type 2 DM

Pharmacotherapy for type 2 DM can be directed at (1) decreasing insulin resistance and increasing insulin sensitization (metformin hydrochloride and the thiazolidinediones), (2) interference with the digestion and absorption of dietary carbohydrate (α-glucosidase inhibitors), (3) augmentation of insulin secretion and action (sulfonylureas, repaglinide, and nateglinide), and (4) insulin therapy (Table 120.5).

Decreasing Insulin Resistance/Increasing Insulin Sensitivity

Metformin hydrochloride and the thiazolidinediones work via different mechanisms. Metformin mainly inhibits the uncontrolled hepatic glucose production, while the thiazolidinediones mainly enhance skeletal muscle glucose uptake—the earliest defect in evolving type 2 DM.

Metformin (Glucophage), a true insulin sensitizer, decreases hepatic glucose production and enhances peripheral glucose

---

Table 120.4. **Hypoglycemia Management Strategies**

Causes	Signs and symptoms	Treatment
Insulin/OHA overdose	Sympathomimetic	Conscious—15 g
Carbohydrate omission	Coldness	Simple carbohydrate
Missed/late meal	Clamminess	Juice 4 oz
Missed/late snack	Shaking	Regular soda 6 oz
	Diaphoresis	3 B-D glucose tablets
	Headaches	7 Lifesavers
Uncompensated	Neuroglycopenic	Unconscious
activity/exercise	Confusion	Glucagon SC[a]
	Disorientation	D_{50} 50 cc IV
	Loss of consciousness	

[a]We do not recommend the use of gel products (e.g., Monojel) for treatment of unconscious hypoglycemia, as aspiration is a potential hazard.

OHA = oral hypoglycemic agent.

utilization. It is an antihyperglycemic agent and does not stimulate insulin secretion; hence, when used as monotherapy it cannot induce hypoglycemia. Ideal candidates for treatment are overweight or obese type 2 DM patients. The potentially fatal side effect of lactic acidosis generally occurs only when metformin is used in contraindicated patients: those with renal insufficiency, liver disease, alcohol excess, or underlying hypoxic states (congestive heart failure, chronic obstructive pulmonary disease, significant asthma, acute myocardial infarction). Metformin should be discontinued the morning of (1) elective surgery that may require general anesthesia and (2) elective procedures using contrast materials (e.g., intravenous pyelogram, cardiac catheterization), and should not be restarted for 48 to 72 hours after the surgery/procedure, pending documentation of a normal serum creatinine. Adjustments in the individual's diabetes regimen will have to be made for this time period to maintain glycemic control. In the UKPDS, despite similar levels of glycemic control, the subset of obese type 2 DM patients treated with metformin had a statistically significantly lower cardiovascular event and death rate than the other groups.[41] Thus, metformin must be modulating other aspects of the cardiodysmetabolic syndrome.

Thiazolidinediones [pioglitazone (ACTOS) and rosiglitazone (Avandia)] are antihyperglycemic insulin-sensitizing agents that bind to the peroxisome proliferator-activated receptor (PPAR) and amplify the insulin signal. In addition to glucose lowering properties, they have purported beneficial effects on the other components of the cardiodysmetabolic syndrome. These agents may also assist in preservation of β-cell function via reduction in lipid deposition within the islets of Langerhans—a concept called lipotoxicity, a finding documented in animals. These agents can be safely used in patients with renal insufficiency without the need for dosage adjustment. A contraindication to their use is liver disease or elevations in hepatic transaminases. Edema is the commonest clinical adverse effect. Although the risk of transaminase elevation is rare, monitoring should be done every 2 months for the first year, and periodically thereafter. These agents are contraindicated in patients with New York grade III or grade IV congestive heart failure. Clinically, glucose lowering is very gradual with these agents, such that individualized downward titration in insulin dosage in insulin-treated type 2 DM patients may not be needed for at least 2 weeks, and the maximum effect may not be seen for up to 12 weeks.

α-Glucosidase Inhibition

α-Glucosidase inhibition by acarbose (Precose) and miglitol (Glyset) has a primary mode of action of decreasing postprandial blood glucoses via direct interference with the digestion and absorption of dietary carbohydrate. These agents are most commonly used as adjunctive therapy rather than monotherapy. Both of these agents need to be dosed with the first bite of the meal. Increased intestinal gas formation, the most common side effect, is minimized with slow dose titration and does improve with continued administration.

Augmentation of Insulin Secretion

Sulfonylureas enhance insulin secretion and action. First-generation sulfonylureas (chlorpropamide, tolazamide, tolbu-

tamide), although efficacious, have a higher risk of side effects, such as sustained hypoglycemia, the chlorpropamide flush (an Antabuse-like reaction), protein binding interference with certain medications, and syndrome of inappropriate diuretic hormone (SIADH) secretion. The second- and third-generation sulfonylureas are preferred owing to their increased milligram potency, shorter duration of action, and better side-effect profile.

Prior concerns about possible cardiotoxicity of sulfonylureas related to the University Group Diabetes Program (UGDP) Study have generally disappeared, given the emergence of data to support the safety of these agents from the cardiovascular prospective in the UKPDS. Glimepiride, a third-generation sulfonylurea, has theoretical benefits in terms of reduced risk of hypoglycemia, potentially lower risk of adverse cardiovascular effects, and perhaps reduced potential for secondary failure.

The insulin secretagogue in the meglitinide class, repaglinide (Prandin), is dosed prior to meals, producing an abrupt spurt of insulin secretion, designed to assist in the control of postprandial glucose levels. There is a potential, although unproven, for a reduction in weight gain so frequently seen with sulfonylureas. Theoretical potential to reduce secondary failure rates is also a purported benefit.

Nateglinide (Starlix), a phenylalanine derivative, is an insulin secretagogue, the effects of which are glucose-dependent. Nateglinide dosed prior to meals produces an abrupt spurt of insulin. However, in contrast to repaglinide, nateglinide restores early insulin secretion that is lost as β-cell function is declining prior to the development of type 2 DM. Early insulin secretion is important, shutting off hepatic glucose production in preparation for the prandial glucose rise. Weight gain is attenuated and hypoglycemia is very rare. Switching from a sulfonylurea to nateglinide can result in a slight rise in fasting glucoses; however, as postprandial glucoses are significantly improved, the HbA$_{1c}$ may be maintained or lowered. This is due to the fact that postprandial glucose contributes more to the HbA$_{1c}$ than fasting or preprandial glucoses do.

Insulin Therapy

To achieve the American Diabetes Association (ADA) goal HbA$_{1c}$, the vast majority of type 2 DM patients will require combination therapy. The concept of initiating pharmacotherapy with an insulin-sensitizing agent appears physiologically logical and, it is hoped, will assist in delaying or preventing sulfonylurea failure, frequently seen after 5 to 6 years of sulfonylurea monotherapy. Additionally, insulin sensitization will ameliorate many of the other components of the cardiodysmetabolic syndrome, thus, it is hoped, translating to reduced macrovascular disease. This hypothesis is currently being tested in several clinical trials.

Can type 2 DM be prevented? The Diabetes Prevention Program in type 2 DM is ongoing with metformin being used in the treatment group. In the HOPE trial, that nondiabetic patients at high risk to develop cardiovascular disease who were treated with ramipril 10 mg daily had a 34% risk reduction in the development of type 2 DM.[33] In the West of Scotland trial, the use of pravastatin reduced the risk of developing type 2 DM

Table 120.5. **Oral Medications Commonly Used to Treat Type 2 DM**

Parameter	Metformin	Pioglitazone	Rosiglitazone	Sulfonylurea
Mode of action	↓ Hepatic glucose ↑ Skeletal muscle glucose utilization	↑ Skeletal muscle glucose utilization ↓ Hepatic glucose	↑ Skeletal muscle glucose utilization ↓ Hepatic glucose	↑ Insulin secretion ↓ Hepatic glucose production
Glucose effects	Fasting and postprandial	Fasting and postprandial	Fasting and postprandial	Fasting and postprandial
Hypoglycemia as monotherapy	No	No	No	Yes
Weight gain	No	Possible	Possible	Possible
Insulin levels	↓	↓	↓	↑
Side effects	GI (self-limiting symptoms of nausea, diarrhea, anorexia)	? Elevation in hepatic transaminases	? Elevation in hepatic transaminases	Potential allergic reaction if sulfa allergy Potential drug interactions (first-generation agents) SIADH
Lipid effects	↓	↑ HDL, ↓ Trigs LDL concentration unaltered	Increase in total cholesterol, LDL and HDL concentration ? Change in particle composition	↑ or ↓
Usual starting dose for a 70-kg man	500 mg bid with meals or XR 500 mg with the evening meal	15 mg qd	4 mg daily either single or divided dose Better results with divided dose	Varies with each agent Glyburide 2.5 mg qd Glucotrol XL 5 mg qd Glynase 3 mg qd Amaryl 2 mg qd
Maximum dose	850 mg tid with meals or XR 2000 mg with the evening meal	45 mg qd	8 mg daily as either single or divided dose Better results with divided dose	Varies with each agent Glyburide 10 mg bid Glucotrol XL 20 mg qd Glynase 6 mg bid Amaryl 8 mg qd
Contraindications	Type 1 diabetes Renal dysfunction Hepatic dysfunction History of EtOH abuse Chronic conditions associated with hypoxia (asthma, COPD, CHF) Acute conditions associated with potential for hypoxia (CHF, acute MI, surgery) Situations associated with potential renal failure	Type 1 diabetes Liver disease Class III and IV CHF	Type 1 diabetes Liver disease Class III and IV CHF	Type 1 diabetes Hepatic dysfunction

by 30%.[42] A recent Finnish lifestyle modification study demonstrated a 58% risk reduction in developing type 2 DM in patients with impaired glucose tolerance who were randomized to a program of intensive diet and exercise.[43]

Insulin therapy in type 2 DM patients is indicated in situations where patients are acutely decompensated and are more insulin-resistant due to intercurrent illnesses. Clearly, short-term insulin therapy can reestablish glycemic control acutely in many individuals. However, reevaluation of endogenous insulin production with C-peptide determinations is impor-

Parameter	Repaglinide	Nateglinide	Acarbose	Miglitol
Mode of action	↑ Insulin secretion	↑ Insulin secretion	α-Glucosidase inhibition ↓ carbohydrate digestion and absorption from GI tract	α-glucosidase inhibition ↓ carbohydrate digestion and absorption from GI tract
Glucose effects	Postprandial and fasting	Postprandial	Postprandial	Postprandial
Hypoglycemia as monotherapy	Yes; less than that seen with sulfonylureas	No	No	No
Weight gain	No		No	No
Insulin levels	↑	↑	↓ or ▽®	↓ or ▽®
Side effects	Rare hypoglycemia	Very rare hypoglyemia, as effects are glucose-dependent	GI (flatulence, abdominal distention, diarrhea)	GI (flatulence, abdominal distention, diarrhea)
Lipid effects	No change	No change	↓ or ▽®	↓ or ▽®
Starting dose for a 70-kg man	0.5 mg prior to meals	120 mg tid prior to meals	25 mg tid with first bite of each meal	25 mg tid with first bite of each meal
Maximum dose	16 mg daily in divided doses at meals/snacks	120 mg tid prior to meals	100 mg tid with first bite of each meal	100 mg tid with first bite of each meal
Contraindications	Type 1 diabetes	Type 1 diabetes	Type 1 diabetes Inflammatory bowel disease Bowel obstruction Cirrhosis Chronic conditions with maldigestion or malabsorption	Type 1 diabetes Inflammatory bowel disease Bowel obstruction Cirrhosis Chronic conditions with maldigestion and malabsorption

tant. Most obese patients with type 2 DM have normal or fairly elevated C-peptide levels, assuming they are not glucotoxic from antecedent chronic hyperglycemia. The initiation of insulin therapy in a type 2 DM patient remains controversial in terms of indications and optimum insulin reg-imen. The dilemma revolves around the obese C-peptide–positive patient who was achieving good glycemic control in the short term with insulin. This individual often suffers pro-gressive obesity and worsening glycemic control owing to worsening insulin resistance. thereby increasing requirements for exogenous insulin. Thus frequently insulin therapy in an obese C-peptide–positive patient fails to achieve its primary goal of sustained improved glycemic control. Additionally, perpetuation of the obese state, or indeed worsening thereof, in conjunction with progressive hyperinsulinemia raises concerns about the impact of this worsened metabolic milieu on hypertension, dyslipidemia, and the atherosclerotic process. Initiation of insulin therapy should therefore be undertaken cautiously in most patients and progress carefully monitored in terms not only of glycemic control but also of hypertension, dyslipidemia, and obesity.

Many insulin regimens have been used to treat type 2 DM, most being similar to those used in the type 1 setting. Trends have focused on the use of bedtime insulin therapy in these individuals on the grounds that it can maximally affect the dawn hepatic glucose output/disposal and peak insulin resistance, thereby achieving the best possible fasting blood glucose and minimizing glucotoxicity. Minimizing glucotoxicity facilitates daytime islet secretory function and minimizes the need for daytime insulin therapy.[44] Combination therapy with insulin-sensitizing agents and insulin seems theoretically sound, reducing the need for exogenous insulin. The data, however, support modest improvements in glycemic control and modest reduction in insulin requirements. It is the exceptional patient who is able to discontinue insulin therapy. One such regimen has been the use of a bedtime dose of intermediate-acting insulin at a dose of 0.2 units/kg of body weight coupled with daytime oral agents. An alternative to the bedtime intermediate-acting insulin is the use of insulin glargine starting at a dose of 10 units and titrating accordingly. Although hypoglycemia is relatively uncommon in type 2 DM patients owing to their fundamental insulin resistance, it can occur in those on insulin or sulfonylureas. Sulfonylureas should be used with caution in patients with hepatic or renal impairment and the elderly.

Gestational Diabetes Mellitus

Gestational DM (GDM) is an important entity in terms of maternal morbidity, fetal macrosomia, associated obstetric complications, and neonatal hypoglycemia. GDM should be sought in all patients using current screening and diagnostic guidelines (Table 120.1). Early, aggressive management can significantly improve outcome. The initial strategy for the patient with GDM is dietary control; when the goals of pregnancy are not being achieved (i.e., premeal and bedtime glucose <90 mg/dL and 1 hour postprandial glucose <120 mg/dL), insulin therapy is initiated. Given the data linking postprandial blood glucose levels to macrosomia, it is important that postprandial glucose levels are controlled adequately and that target glucose levels are achieved.[45,46] In our center the postprandial goal is most readily and predictably reached with premeal lispro insulin. To cover basal requirements we use a small dose of prebreakfast ultralente insulin and an overnight intermediate-acting insulin. As an alternative, premeal regular insulin and overnight intermediate-acting insulin can be used. Most women with GDM have reestablishment of euglycemia immediately postpartum. These individuals, however, should be counseled on the long-

term risks of prior GDM for developing overt type 2 DM, which may occur in as many as 70% of these individuals.[47] Additionally, the hazards of persistent obesity, associated insulin resistance, dyslipidemia, hypertension, and potential for premature cardiovascular death must be addressed[48] (see Chapter 10).

Individuals with type 1 DM who are contemplating pregnancy should be in optimal glycemic control prior to conception to decrease the risk of congenital malformations and the incidence of maternal-fetal complications. The achievement of two consecutive HbA$_{1c}$ levels in the nondiabetic range is recommended before conception. Alternatively, CSII may be used to readily achieve these goals. Careful follow-up by a skilled management team is essential to an optimum outcome.[46] Insulin glargine has a category C rating for pregnancy and should not be used. The team approach to the care of the pregnant individual with diabetes is also discussed in Chapter 10.

Contraception and DM

The use of oral contraceptives (OCs) in women with type 1 or type 2 DM has been an area of controversy,[46] with many believing that significant elevations occur in blood glucose along with an increased risk of vascular complications. In our experience the incidence of such problems is minimal given a woman who is normotensive and has an absence of vascular disease; therefore, we believe OCs can be safely used. Even for a woman in poor glycemic control, OCs are still the most effective form of contraception (also see Chapter 101).

Diabetic Ketoacidosis

Diabetic ketoacidosis (DKA) is the ultimate expression of absolute insulin deficiency resulting in uncontrolled lipolysis, free fatty acid delivery to the liver, and ultimately accelerated ketone body production. Insulin deficiency at the level of the liver results in uncontrolled hepatic glucose output via gluconeogenesis and glycogenolysis. With insulin-mediated skeletal muscle glucose uptake being inhibited, hyperglycemia rapidly ensues. The attendant osmotic diuresis due to hyperglycemia results in progressive dehydration and a decreasing glomerular filtration rate. Dehydration may be compounded by gastrointestinal fluid losses (e.g., emesis from ketones or a primary gastrointestinal illness with concurrent diarrhea). Insensible fluid losses from febrile illness may further compound the dehydration.

Diagnosis of DKA is fairly characteristic in the newly presenting or established type 1 DM patient. The history of polydipsia, polyuria, weight loss, and Kussmaul's respirations are virtually pathognomonic. Physical examination is directed at assessing the level of hydration (e.g., orthostasis) and the underlying precipitating illness. Measurement of urine ketone, urine glucose, and blood glucose levels can rapidly confirm the clinical suspicion, with arterial pH, serum bicarbonate, and ketones validating the diagnosis. A thorough search for an underlying precipitating illness remains axiomatic (e.g., urosepsis, respiratory tract infection, or silent myocardial infarction). Treatment is directed at correcting (1) dehydration/hypotension; (2) ketonemia/acidosis; (3) uncontrolled hepatic glucose output/hyperglycemia; and (4) insulin resistance of the DKA/underlying illness. Of course specific treatment is directed to any defined underlying illnesses.

Dehydration and hypotension require urgent treatment with a 5- to 6-L deficit to be anticipated in most individuals. Initial treatment is 0.9% NaCl, with 1 to 2 L/hr being given for the first 2 hours and flow rates thereafter being titrated to the individual's clinical status. Use of a Swan-Ganz catheter is prudent in the individual with cardiac compromise. Potassium replacement at a concentration of 10 to 40 mEq/L is critical to replace the usual deficits of more than 5 mEq/kg once the patient's initial serum potassium level is known and urine output is documented. Giving 50% of the potassium as KCl and 50% as KPO_4 appears theoretically sound, but routine phosphate replacement has not been shown to alter the clinical outcome. Bicarbonate therapy is generally reserved for patients with a pH of less than 7.0, plasma bicarbonate less than 5.0 mEq/L, severe hyperkalemia, or a deep coma. Bicarbonate is administered by slow infusion 50 to 100 mEq over 1 to 2 hours with the therapeutic end point being a pH higher than 7.1 rather than normalization of the pH. Overzealous use of bicarbonate can result in severe hypokalemia with attendant cardiac arrhythmogenicity, paradoxical central nervous system acidosis, and possible lactic acidosis due to tissue hypoxia. Intravenous insulin therapy is initiated at a dose of 0.1 U/kg/hr with rapid titration every 1 to 2 hours should a 75 to 100 mg/dL/hr decrease in glucose not be achieved. Insulin therapy at this relatively high dose is needed to combat the insulin resistance of the hormonal milieu of DKA (i.e., high levels of glucagon, cortisol, growth hormone, and catecholamines). Given that hepatic glucose output is more rapidly controlled than ketogenesis, the insulin infusion rate can be maintained by switching the intravenous infusion to dextrose 5% to 10% when blood glucose is less than 250 mg/dL. The insulin infusion is continued until the patient is ketone-free, clinically well, and able to resume oral feeding. It is of paramount importance that subcutaneous insulin be instituted promptly at the time of refeeding.

Flow sheets should be generated documenting the following:

1. Patient admission weight relative to previous weights with serial weights every 6 to 12 hours, urine ketones, and fluid balance
2. Vital signs and mental status every 1 to 2 hours
3. Bedside glucose monitoring every 1 to 2 hours
4. Urine ketones every 1 to 2 hours
5. Fluid balance
6. Blood gases and arterial pH on admission, repeating until pH is over 7.1
7. Serum potassium on admission and then every 2 to 4 hours
8. Serum ketones on admission and then every 2 to 4 hours
9. Complete blood count, serum chemistries, chest roentgenogram, electrocardiogram, and appropriate cultures on admission
10. Abnormal chemistries other than potassium repeated every 4 hours until normal.[49,50]

References

1. Clinical practice recommendations: 2001. Diabetes Care 2001; 24(suppl 1):S1–S133.
2. The European patient's charter. Diabetic Med 1991;8:782–3.
3. Landin-Olsson M, Nilsson KO, Lernmark A, Sunkvist G. Islet cell antibodies and fasting C-peptide predict insulin requirement at diagnosis of diabetes mellitus. Diabetalogia 1990;33:561–8.
4. Zeigler AG, Herskowitz RD, Jackson RA, Soeldner JS, Eisenbarth GS. Predicting type I diabetes. Diabetes Care 1990;13: 762–75.
5. Keller RJ, Eisenbarth GS, Jackson RA. Insulin prophylaxis in individuals at high risk of type I diabetes. N Engl J Med 1993; 341:927–8.
6. Shapiro AMJ, Lakey BS, Ryan EA, et al. Islet transplantation in seven patients with type 1 diabetes mellitus using a glucocorticoid-free immunosuppressive regimen. N Engl J Med 2000; 343:230–8.
7. Helmrich SP, Ragland DR, Leung RW, Paffenbarger RS. Physical activity and reduced occurrence of non-insulin-dependent diabetes mellitus. N Engl J Med 1991;325:147–52.
8. UKPDS Group. UK prospective diabetes study XI: biochemical risk factors in type 2 diabetic patients at diagnosis compared with age-matched normal subjects. Diabetic Med 1994;11:533–44.
9. DeFronzo RA. The triumvirate: B-cell, muscle, and liver: a collusion responsible for NIDDM. Diabetes 1988;37:667–87.
10. Eriksson J, Franssila-Kallunki A, Ekstrand A. Early metabolic defects in persons at increased risk for non-insulin-dependent diabetes mellitus. N Engl J Med 1989;321:337–43.
11. DeFronzo RA, Bonadonna RC, Ferrannini E. Pathogenesis of NIDDM. Diabetes Care 1992;15:318–68.
12. Clark PM, Hales CN. Measurement of insulin secretion in type 2 diabetes: problems and pitfalls. Diabetic Med 1992;9:503–12.
13. Bjornstorp P. Metabolic implications of body fat distribution. Diabetes Care 1991;14:1132–43.
14. Ferrannini E, Buzzigoli G, Bonadonna B, et al. Insulin resistance in essential hypertension. N Engl J Med 1987;317:350–7.
15. Zavaroni I, Bonora E, Pagliara M, et al. Risk factors for coronary artery disease in healthy persons with hyperinsulinemia and normal glucose tolerance. N Engl J Med 1989;320:703–6.
16. Kern TS, Engerman RL. Arrest of glomerulonephropathy in diabetic dogs by improved glycemic control. Diabetologia 1990; 33:522–5.
17. Diabetes Control and Complications Trial Research Group. The effect of intensive treatment of diabetes on the development and progression of long-term complications in insulin-dependent diabetes mellitus. N Engl J Med 1993;329:977–86.
18. UKPDS Group. Intensive blood-glucose control with sulfonylureas or insulin compared with conventional treatment and risk of complications in patients with type 2 diabetes (UKPDS 33). Lancet 1998;352:837–53.
19. UKPDS Group. Association of glycaemia with macrovascular and microvascular complications of type 2 diabetes (UKPDS 35): prospective observational study. BMJ 2000;321:405–11.
20. UKPDS Group. Association of systolic blood pressure with macrovascular and microvascular complications of type 2 diabetes (UKPDS 36): prospective observational study. BMJ 2000;321:412–9.
21. National committee for clinical laboratory standards. Development of designated comparison methods for analytes in the clinical laboratory, 2nd ed., proposed guideline. NCCLS publication NRSCL6-P2 Villanova, PA: NCCLS, 1993.

22. Viberti GC. Etiology and prognostic significance of albuminuria in diabetes. Diabetes Care 1988;11:840–8.
23. Deckert T, Feldt-Rasmussen B, Borch-Johnson K, Jensen T, Kofoed-Gnevoldsen A. Albuminuria reflects widespread vascular damage: the Steno hypothesis. Diabetologia 1989;32:219–26.
24. Marshall SM. Screening for microalbuminuria: which measurement? Diabetic Med 1991;8:706–11.
25. Hamwi GL. Changing dietary concepts in therapy. In: Danowski TS, ed. Diabetes mellitus: diagnosis and treatment. New York: American Diabetes Association, 1964;73–8.
26. Wood FC, Bierman EL. Is diet the cornerstone in management of diabetes? N Engl J Med 1986;1244–7.
27. Zehrer C, Hansen R, Bantl J. Reducing blood glucose variability by use of abdominal injection sites. Diabetes Educator 1990;16:474–7.
28. Skyler JS, Skyler DL, Seigler DE, O'Sullivan M. Algorithms for adjustment of insulin dosage by patients who monitor blood glucose. Diabetes Care 1981;4:311–8.
29. Frykberg RG. Management of diabetic foot problems (Joslin Clinic). Philadelphia: Saunders, 1984.
30. Singerman LJ. Early-treatment diabetic retinopathy study: good news for diabetic patients and health care professionals [editorial]. Diabetes Care 1986;9:426–9.
31. Lewis EJ, Hunsicker LG, Bain RE, Rohde RD. The effect of angiotensin-converting enzyme inhibition on diabetic nephropathy. N Engl J Med 1993;329:1456–62.
32. The Heart Outcomes Prevention Evaluation (HOPE) Study Investigators. Effects of an angiotensin-converting enzyme inhibitor, ramipril, on cardiovascular events in high risk patients. Lancet 2000;342:145–53.
33. The Heart Outcomes Prevention Evaluation (HOPE) Study Investigators. Effects of ramipril on cardiovascular and microvascular outcomes in people with diabetes mellitus: results of the HOPE study and MICRO-HOPE sub-study. Lancet 2000;345:253–9.
34. Tuttle KR, Bruton JL, Perusek MC, Lancaster JL, Kopp DT, DeFronzo RA. Effect of strict glycemic control on renal enlargement in insulin-dependent diabetes mellitus. N Engl J Med 1991;324:1626–32.
35. ALLHAT Collaborative Research Group. Major cardiovascular events in hypertensive patients randomized to doxazosin vs. chlorthalidone: the antihypertensive and lipid-lowering treatment to prevent heart attack trial (ALLHAT). JAMA 2000;283:1967–75.
36. Expert panel on detection, evaluation, and treatment of high blood cholesterol in adults. Executive summary of the third report of the national cholesterol education program (NCEP) expert panel on detection, evaluation, and treatment of high blood cholesterol in adults. JAMA 2001;285:2486–97.
37. Flynn MD, Tooke JE. Aetiology of diabetic foot ulceration: a role for the microcirculation? Diabetic Med 1992;9:320–9.
38. Skyler JS. Insulin treatment: therapy for diabetes mellitus and related disorders. Alexandria, VA: American Diabetes Association, 1991;127–37.
39. Chan NH, Baldeweg S, Tan TMM, Hurel SI. Inhaled insulin in type 1 diabetes. Lancet 2001;357:1979.
40. Bhatia V, Wolfsdorf JI. Severe hypoglycemia in youth with insulin-dependent diabetes mellitus: frequency and causative factors. Pediatrics 1991;88:1187–93.
41. UKPDS Group. Effect of intensive blood-glucose control with metformin on complications in overweight patients with type 2 diabetes (UKPDS 34). Lancet 1998;352(9131):854–65.
42. Freeman DJ, Norrie J, Sattar N, et al. Pravastatin and the development of diabetes mellitus: evidence for a protective treatment effect in the West of Scotland Coronary Prevention Study. Circulation 2001;103:346–7.
43. Tuomilehto J, Lindstorm J, Eirksson JG, et al. Prevention of type 2 diabetes mellitus by changes in lifestyle among subjects with impaired glucose tolerance. N Engl J Med 2001;344:1343–50.
44. Groop LC, Widèn E, Ekstrand A, et al. Morning or bedtime NPH insulin combined with sulfonylureas in treatment of NIDDM. Diabetes Care 1992;15:831–4.
45. Proceedings of the Third International Workshop-Conference on Gestational Diabetes Mellitus. Diabetes 1991;40(suppl 2):1–201.
46. Jovanovic-Peterson L, Peterson CM. Pregnancy in the diabetic woman: guidelines for a successful outcome. Endocrinol Metab Clin North Am 1992;33:433–56.
47. Kaufmann RC, Amankwah KS, Woodrum J. Development of diabetes in previous gestational diabetic [abstract]. Diabetes 1991;40:137A.
48. Kaufmann RC, Amankwah KS, Woodrum J. Serum lipids in former gestational diabetics [abstract]. Diabetes 1991;40:192A.
49. Kozak GP, Rolla AR. Diabetic comas. In: Kozak GP, ed. Clinical diabetes mellitus. Philadelphia: Saunders, 1982;109–45.
50. Siperstein MD. Diabetic ketoacidosis and hyperosmolar coma. Endocrinol Metab Clin North Am 1992;33:415–32.

121
Thyroid Disease

Michael B. Harper and E. J. Mayeaux Jr.

Thyroid diseases are among the most common endocrine disorders.[1] They may seriously affect patients' health and often require lifelong treatment and monitoring. This chapter reviews the most common thyroid problems, with emphasis on clinical presentation, diagnosis, treatment, and follow-up.

Screening for Thyroid Disease

In 2000, the American Thyroid Association released consensus recommendations on screening asymptomatic adults for thyroid disease.[2] Even though they note a serious lack of efficacy data, especially in men and younger women, they recommend measuring a thyroid-stimulating hormone (TSH) level in all patients at age 35 and every 5 years thereafter. These recommendations have not been generally accepted to date. The American Academy of Family Physicians, American College of Physicians, U.S. Preventative Services Task Force, and the Royal College of Physicians conclude there is not enough evidence to recommend screening in the general population.[3] Screening patients who are at higher risk for thyroid disease is recommended. Patients with atrial fibrillation or hyperlipidemia should be screened at least once. Annual screening is recommended for patients with diabetes or Down syndrome. Those taking amiodarone or lithium require periodic monitoring.[4]

Hyperthyroidism

Thyrotoxicosis results from excess thyroid hormone. The prevalence of this condition in the United States among adults over 55 years of age is 2%. Two thirds of these patients were taking thyroid hormone preparation.[1] Excluding excess hormone ingestion, approximately 90% of hyperthyroidism is caused by Graves' disease, and thyrotoxic nodules and thyroiditis account for almost all other cases.[5] Women are more commonly affected by hyperthyroidism than men, with reported ratios varying from 4:1 to 10:1.[5,6]

Health Risks

Hyperthyroidism causes or exacerbates several other health problems, with cardiovascular complications being most important. Atrial fibrillation is the most common complication, occurring in 8% to 22% of thyrotoxic patients, and these patients are at increased risk of stroke from atrial thromboembolism.[7] Cardiac failure, angina, myocardial infarction, and sudden death have been associated with thyrotoxicosis.[8] Thyroid storm causes multisystem involvement and carries a high risk of mortality (10–75%).[5] Calcium and bone metabolism are affected by thyrotoxicosis, leading to osteoporosis and an increased risk of bone fracture. Atrial fibrillation and osteoporosis may occur with even subclinical hyperthyroidism.[9] Periodic paralysis is a rare complication of thyrotoxicosis, occurring mostly in Orientals.[10]

Family Impact

As with any chronic disease, hyperthyroidism places stress on the family system. Among other symptoms, the affected family member may experience emotional lability, heat intolerance, and fatigue, all of which strain relationships within the family. Hyperthyroidism may be especially stressful prior to diagnosis, when the patient and family do not know an illness is responsible for these changes. Additional stress may result from reduced job performance or loss of income.

Clinical Presentation

Symptoms of thyrotoxicosis, arranged in order of frequency, are listed in Table 121.1, and the chief complaint can be any one of these symptoms. A directed history usually reveals up to eight symptoms, although some patients, especially in the geriatric age group, may report only a few.[5,11]

Table 121.1. **Signs and Symptoms of Thyrotoxicosis (in Order of Frequency)**

Symptoms/signs	Percent of patients
Symptoms	
Nervousness	88
Weight loss	83
Heat intolerance	75
Dyspnea	70
Palpitation	69
Increased sweating	62
Fatigue	58
Tachycardia	51
Eye complaints	49
Weakness	47
Increased appetite	45
Vomiting	44
Swelling of legs	38
Chest pain	36
History of fever	36
Nausea	28
Diarrhea	26
Frequent bowel movements	21
Abdominal pain	20
Swelling in neck	16
Anorexia	13
Constipation	12
Dysphagia	12
Hair loss	4
Signs	
Goiter	96
Skin changes (smooth, moist)	85
Tremor	79
Tachycardia (>100 bpm) (heart rate ≥80 bpm)	76 (HR >100)
Systolic murmur	76
Ocular signs (e.g., lid lag)	60
Brisk deep tendon reflexes	56
Pulse pressure ≥70 mm Hg	52
Bruit over thyroid	47
Atrial fibrillation	8
Gynecomastia	7
Splenomegaly	7

Source: Harper MB. Vomiting, nausea and abdominal pain: unrecognized symptoms of thyrotoxicosis. J Fam Pract 1989;29: 382–6.

Patients often report weight loss, even with a history of increased appetite. Heat intolerance is usually described as preferring room temperatures cooler than do other family members or preferring winter to summer. Fatigue and weakness of proximal muscles can be reported as difficulty climbing stairs.

It is of note that abdominal symptoms of vomiting, nausea, and abdominal pain, although previously thought to be rare or present only preceding thyroid storm, may be relatively common.[11] Patients who present with these abdominal symptoms as their chief complaint may be at higher risk of missed diagnosis. Vomiting can occur without nausea and tends to be postprandial. Abdominal pain is usually epigastric or left upper quadrant in location, unrelated to meals, and described as sharp or cramping.[11]

Physical findings of thyrotoxicosis are listed in Table 121.1, and five or more are typically present. Goiter is the most frequent sign, but the enlargement may be only mild or difficult to appreciate, especially when it occupies a substernal location. The skin tends to be warm, moist, and velvety smooth. A fine tremor of outstretched hands is usually present, and deep tendon reflexes are often brisk with a rapid relaxation phase. Lid lag may be present with any cause of thyrotoxicosis; exophthalmos is specific to Graves' disease. Onycholysis may be present, typically of the ring fingers, causing separation of the nail from the distal nailbed and difficulty cleaning the nails (Plummer's nails).[5,10,11]

Laboratory Evaluation

Confirmation of clinical thyrotoxicosis is accomplished by measuring thyrotropin (TSH) by a highly sensitive assay and is further substantiated with measurement or estimate of free thyroxine (T_4) and sometimes free triiodothyronine (T_3). These hormones are clinically active only when they are not protein bound. A diagnostic approach to the patient with thyrotoxicosis is shown in Fig. 121.1. Along with the TSH, initial tests are usually free T_4 and free T_3. Although the reliability of some methods has been questioned in the past, newer assays of free T_4 and free T_3 are more dependable.[5,12] Alternately, free T_4 can be estimated with the free thyroxine index (FTI). This value is obtained by measuring total T_4 and thyroid hormone–binding ratio (THBR, also known as T_3 resin uptake), which is an indirect measure of thyroid-binding protein. The FTI is calculated from the first two measurements. When THBR is normal, an elevated T_4 level confirms thyrotoxicosis. However, euthyroid patients may have an elevated total T_4 due to excess thyroid-binding proteins, such as during pregnancy, with use of estrogens, or with some inherited disorders.

Through pituitary feedback mechanisms, TSH levels inversely follow free T_4 levels. Measurement of TSH by a highly sensitive assay in patients with hyperthyroidism yields a value far below the normal range and helps confirm the diagnosis. The sensitive TSH is especially useful in patients with concomitant illnesses or on medications that can alter T_4 and THBR values.[12] Because TSH is a more sensitive measure of thyroid status, patients may have an abnormally low TSH with a normal FTI. They are considered to have subclinical hyperthyroidism.[5,9] TSH can also be moderately low as a result of nonthyroidal illness or medications (glucocorticoids and dopamine) and is occasionally low in healthy people, particularly the elderly.[13] The TSH level in these settings is usually not less than 0.1 μU/mL. When the TSH level is less than the lower limit of a sensitive assay (undetectable), thyrotoxicosis is usually present.[5] Rarely, a TSH-secreting adenoma causes hyperthyroidism with an elevated TSH.

When TSH is low but free T_4 (or FTI) is normal, measurement of free T_3 should be obtained and, if elevated, confirms clinical thyrotoxicosis. This condition, known as T_3 toxicosis, occurs occasionally in patients with early Graves' disease or a thyrotoxic nodule.[5,10]

Nuclear medicine scans of the thyroid are useful for assessing thyroid size to determine if thyroid nodules are function-

Fig. 121.1. Diagnostic approach to the patient with thyrotoxicosis.

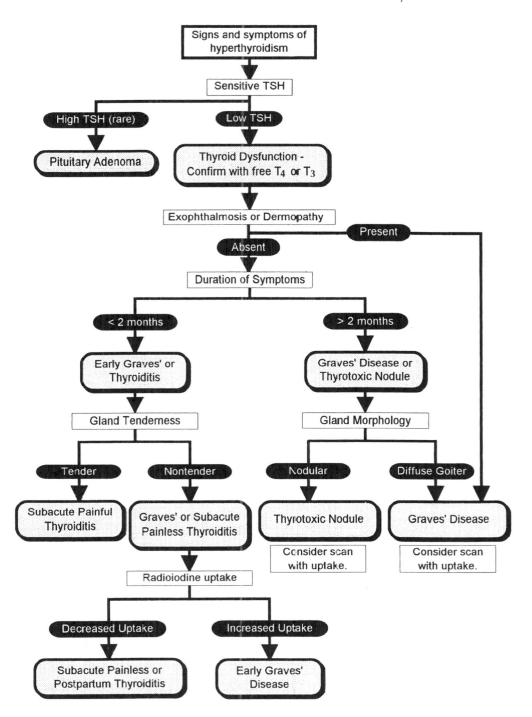

ing (hot) or nonfunctioning (cold) and to measure the level of thyroid function (thyroid uptake). Of the radionuclides available for thyroid scans, iodine 123 (^{123}I) is probably optimal. Technetium may also be used for thyroid imaging, but measurement of function is less reliable, as a nonfunctioning nodule by the ^{123}I scan may demonstrate function with technetium.[5]

Graves' Disease

The disease described by Robert Graves in 1835 is the most common cause of hyperthyroidism.[10] Its etiology is an autoimmune process, closely related to chronic lymphocytic (Hashimoto's) thyroiditis. The onset of Graves' disease may follow some physical or psychological stress, and a family history of thyroid disease is often present.[5,10]

Signs and Symptoms

All the clinical manifestations of thyrotoxicosis may be present in Graves' disease, with additional specific findings of ophthalmopathy and dermopathy. A diffuse goiter occurs in most patients and may cause neck swelling or dysphagia. On palpation, the thyroid is nontender and somewhat soft. Eye problems occur in more than 50% of patients and include pressure sensation, irritation, gritty feeling, lacrimation, a change in appearance, and occasional blurred vision or diplopia (see Chapter 71). The exophthalmos occasionally causes marked eye irritation or even blindness. Dermopathy occurs in 1% to 2% of patients and causes raised, firm, nontender, intradermal nodules on the anterior surfaces of the lower legs. Clubbing of the nails (acropachy) is a rare manifestation of Graves' disease.[5,10]

Diagnosis

Graves' disease is diagnosed by confirming hyperthyroidism with thyroid function tests (FTI or free T_4), along with one or more physical findings specific to the disease. If a goiter is present without exophthalmos or dermopathy, Graves' disease may be difficult to distinguish from subacute painless thyroiditis or postpartum thyroiditis. A reliable history of chronic hyperthyroid symptoms strongly suggests Graves' disease, and an elevated thyroid uptake confirms this diagnosis when it remains in doubt.[5,10] Thyrotropin receptor (TSH-R) antibodies are present in most patients with Graves' disease but they are of limited diagnostic value. High titers of these antibodies may identify those patients who are unlikely to go into remission. Measurement of TSH-R antibodies in pregnant patients with thyrotoxicosis may be useful.[5]

Treatment

Therapy of Graves' disease is directed toward controlling the effects of excess thyroid hormone and reducing the production of additional hormone.[13] Beta-blockers are especially effective in controlling the tachycardia, tremor, and other symptoms related to excess hormone. Propranolol is begun at 20 to 40 mg two to four times daily and increased every few days until the heart rate is within the normal range.[10] When beta-blockers are contraindicated, diltiazem or clonidine may be effective.[14,15] Controlling hormone production may be accomplished with antithyroid medications, radioiodine ablation, or surgery. Choice of treatment is influenced by the clinical presentation, the age of the patient, and the patient's ability and willingness to comply with a treatment regimen.[5,10]

Antithyroid medications available in the United States to control thyroid hormone production are methimazole or propylthiouracil. In addition to blocking production of thyroid hormone, these medications may alter the course of the disease via their immunosuppressive effects.[16] Reported remission rates vary widely and are probably higher in patients with less severe hyperthyroidism, short duration of illness, and small goiter. The duration of treatment is usually 6 months to 2 years. The remission rate can be as high as 60% if treatment is continued for 2 years. Failure to achieve remission after 2 years of treatment is an indication for alternate therapy.[5,10,16]

Initial adult dosage of methimazole is 20 to 30 mg/day divided into two doses. In patients with severe hyperthyroidism and a large goiter, the higher dose is warranted. Euthyroid status, determined clinically and with thyroid function tests (T_4 and T_3), is usually achieved within 4 to 6 weeks, and the dosage is reduced incrementally every 4 to 6 weeks to a maintenance dose of 2.5 to 10 mg/day given in a single dose. TSH is not useful for following the response to treatment, as it may remain suppressed for months after T_4 and T_3 normalize. The initial dose of propylthiouracil is usually 300 mg/day, and maintenance is 50 to 100 mg/day. Both must be divided into

three doses.[5,10] Either of these drugs may cause rash, leukopenia, and (rarely) agranulocytosis. Patients should be cautioned about these side effects. Methimazole has the advantages of lower risk of agranulocytosis, a longer half-life allowing usage on a once-a-day schedule, and more rapid return to euthyroid status. Propylthiouracil may be preferable during pregnancy, lactation or thyroid storm.[5,10]

Concomitant administration of thyroxine 100 to 200 μg/day has been proposed to avoid frequent adjustments in antithyroid dosage and possibly reduce recurrence of hyperthyroidism, but data demonstrating the effectiveness of this treatment regimen are limited and have not been reproduced.[5,13,17]

Iodine 131 ablation can be used to permanently destroy thyroid tissue sufficiently to reduce hormone production to normal levels. This method has become the most commonly used initial therapy for Graves' disease in the United States.[3,10] The amount of radiation used can be calculated based on the patient's weight, gland size, and thyroid uptake. In practice, this method is not strictly used because results are not as precise as desirable.[10] A major disadvantage of this treatment is the high prevalence of hypothyroidism (>90%), which continues to increase with the passage of time.[5] Therefore, a patient's ability to comply with lifelong replacement therapy should be considered when choosing this treatment.

Controversy exists regarding the use of ^{131}I ablation in children and young adults, owing to the fear of increased risk of thyroid cancer later in life. Studies to date have not confirmed this increased risk, and use of radioiodine ablation in patients under the age of 20 is common.[5,12] Pregnancy is a contraindication to [131]I. Patients who are elderly or markedly hyperthyroid should be initially treated with antithyroid drugs because ^{131}I ablation can induce a temporary exacerbation of thyrotoxicosis or thyroid storm.[10]

Subtotal thyroidectomy is an alternate method of permanently controlling thyroid hormone production. This treatment is indicated when the goiter is large, particularly if obstructive symptoms are present. Surgery is also indicated in children who fail a trial of antithyroid medication. The disadvantages of surgery include the cost and risk of surgical complications. Following surgery for Graves' disease, hypothyroidism has been reported in 53% of patients and recurrence of hyperthyroidism in 3.4%.[10]

Follow-up

Regardless of the treatment used, Graves' disease requires lifelong monitoring. Patients treated with antithyroid medications who go into remission must be followed for possible relapses and are at a small risk of late hypothyroidism. After treatment with ^{131}I ablation or surgery, patients require chronic periodic monitoring for development of hypothyroidism. Once hypothyroidism occurs, lifelong hormone replacement is necessary.[5,10]

Thyrotoxic Nodule

An autonomously functioning thyroid nodule may cause thyrotoxicosis with typical hyperthyroid symptoms. Physical examination reveals a thyroid nodule, and findings specific to Graves' disease are absent. The diagnosis is confirmed with elevated FTI (or free T_4), low TSH, and a hot nodule on

Fig. 121.2. Diagnostic approach to the euthyroid patient with a thyroid nodule.

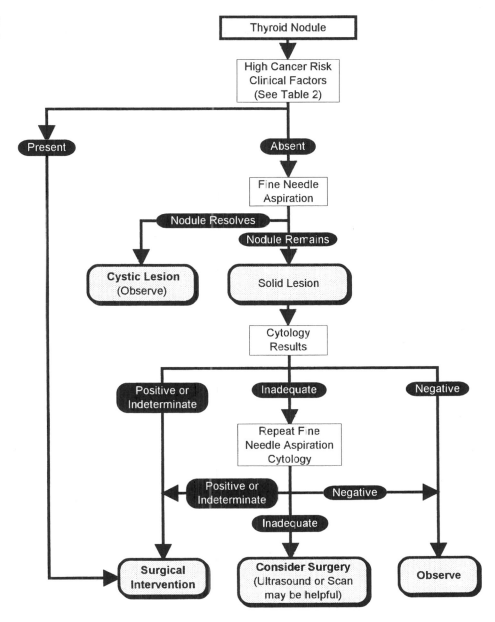

radioiodine scan. Fine-needle aspiration is indicated if the nodule is not hot on nuclear medicine scan, as with other non-toxic nodules (Fig. 121.2).

Treatment is with ^{131}I ablation or occasionally surgery. Antithyroid medications are not usually indicated for thyrotoxic nodules. Hypothyroidism following ^{131}I ablation is less common than with Graves' disease, although a 40% long-term prevalence of hypothyroidism has been reported.[18] Indications for surgery include a thyrotoxic nodule that is very large or progressively enlarging or other signs suggestive of thyroid cancer.[5]

The nodule may persist after ablation treatment, and ongoing monitoring by physical examination is needed to identify any increase in size. Should the nodule or adjacent tissue enlarge, further evaluation for possible thyroid cancer is required. Periodic monitoring for possible hypothyroidism also is necessary.

Thyroiditis

Thyroiditis is defined as an inflammatory process involving the thyroid gland. This inflammation may cause thyrotoxicosis due to unregulated release of thyroid hormone from an injured gland. There are several types of thyroiditis, each with a different clinical picture; three are discussed below. Hashimoto's thyroiditis is discussed in the next section, and postpartum thyroiditis is discussed in the section on pregnancy. Measurement of ^{123}I thyroid uptake is useful in any patient with thyrotoxicosis and suspected thyroiditis. Elevated FTI (or free T_4) with diminished thyroid uptake confirms thyrotoxicosis due to thyroiditis.

Subacute painful (granulomatous) thyroiditis is probably caused by a viral infection and is the thyroiditis that most commonly results in thyrotoxicosis. Patients present with an exquisitely tender, firm, asymmetric nodular thyroid gland.

They have symptoms of neck pain, a flu-like syndrome, and symptoms of thyrotoxicosis. The erythrocyte sedimentation rate is elevated, and antithyroid antibodies are absent. These patients usually go through four phases: (1) hyperthyroidism lasting 3 to 6 weeks; (2) euthyroid status for a few weeks; (3) hypothyroidism lasting weeks to months; and (4) euthyroid state again. The clinical diagnosis is usually made during the hyperthyroid phase and is confirmed with an elevated FTI and decreased uptake on ^{123}I scans. Treatment of inflammation is accomplished with aspirin, other nonsteroidal antiinflammatory agents, or corticosteroids (prednisone 20 mg twice daily for 1 week then tapered over 2–4 weeks). Patients may require β-blocker therapy to control symptoms and tachycardia initially, but there are usually no long-term sequelae requiring treatment or monitoring.[5,19]

Subacute painless (lymphocytic) thyroiditis is an autoimmune process that may cause thyrotoxicosis. Physical examination usually reveals a mildly enlarged thyroid gland that is somewhat firm and nontender, although nearly 50% of patients have no goiter. Antibodies to thyroid peroxidase are present in about 50% of patients. These patients may go through the same four phases as subacute painful thyroiditis, but the euthyroid phase preceding hypothyroidism may be brief or absent. Some patients do not return to euthyroid status after hypothyroidism occurs and require chronic thyroid hormone replacement.[5,19]

Acute thyroiditis, caused by a bacterial infection, is a rare condition in developed countries because of the availability of antibiotic therapy. Patients present with acute thyrotoxicosis, fever, and a tender, enlarged thyroid gland. Treatment is directed toward controlling effects of excess thyroid hormone with beta-blockers and treating the infection with broad-spectrum antibiotics. Needle aspiration for culture is indicated, and abscess drainage may be necessary.[5,19]

Hypothyroidism

A deficiency of thyroid hormone can be caused by several conditions, all of which can produce the same clinical picture of hypothyroidism. The most common causes of hypothyroidism are autoimmune thyroid diseases, including Hashimoto's thyroiditis, and previous treatment for Graves' disease. Other thyroiditis, congenital hypothyroidism, and central hypothyroidism are uncommon causes.

Approximately 1% to 2% of the general population have spontaneous hypothyroidism: 1.9% of the female population, and 0.1% of the male population.[6] Hypothyroidism is more common with advancing age, affecting 6.9% to 7.3% of patients age 55 or over.[1,6] Women are affected 10 times more frequently than men. Congenital hypothyroidism occurs in 1/3000 to 1/4000 live births in the United States.[20]

Health Risks

Severe hypothyroidism may lead to coma and death if untreated. Hypothyroidism can cause bradycardia, hearing impairment, carpal tunnel syndrome, and hypercholesterolemia with increased risk of atherosclerotic heart disease. Demen-

tia, depression, and suicide can be a sequela of hypothyroidism. Hashimoto's thyroiditis may be associated with primary thyroid lymphoma.[19] Elderly patients are at increased risk because concomitant illnesses are common and because the symptoms of hypothyroidism may remain unrecognized.[1]

Family Issues

The depression often associated with hypothyroidism has a devastating effect on the family. Withdrawal, vegetative disturbances, apathy, and loss of motivation can affect the entire family unit. This situation is especially a problem when the diagnosis is delayed.

Clinical Presentation

Symptoms of hypothyroidism include generalized weakness, fatigue, memory loss or slowed thinking, intolerance to cold, dry skin, hair loss, hoarseness, dyspnea, anorexia, deafness, chest pain, and facial or peripheral edema. A modest weight gain of approximately 10 pounds is typical, but patients may actually lose weight early in the disease process due to anorexia.[2] Constipation is a common complaint. Depression is often the presenting symptom, so hypothyroidism must be considered during any depression workup[21,22](see Chapter 32). Women may have heavy, prolonged menstrual periods that can lead to severe anemia.[5]

Periorbital edema, peripheral edema, and pale, thick, dry skin are often the first physical signs noted. Hyperkeratosis of the knees and elbows is also common. Diastolic hypertension may be present. Delayed relaxation phase of deep tendon reflexes is common but may be subtle. When hypothyroidism is severe, mucopolysaccharides deposit in subcutaneous tissue, causing the nonpitting edema known as myxedema. Pleural and pericardial effusions, cardiomegaly, bradycardia, and prolonged QT interval are possible cardiac manifestations.[5]

Laboratory Evaluation

Hypothyroidism is diagnosed by finding an elevated TSH and a low free T_4 or low serum FTI.[12]

Treatment

Oral synthetic L-thyroxine is the treatment of choice for hypothyroidism.[3,12,19,20,23] The usual starting dosage is approximately 75 μg/day, but elderly patients and patients with heart disease are started at a much lower dose (25 μg/day). The TSH is measured every 6 weeks and the dosage of thyroxin is adjusted upward by 25 μg/day until the TSH is within the normal range, indicating the patient has returned to a euthyroid state. The target dose for most patients is approximately 1.6 to 1.7 μg/kg/day. Most forms of hypothyroidism are lifelong problems and continued replacement is necessary. Once the patient is on a stable dose, the TSH level should be assayed annually to monitor appropriateness of replacement therapy.[12]

There is preliminary evidence that treatment with a combination of thyroxine and triiodothyronine (12.5 μg/day) may improve mood and neuropsychological functioning in patients on replacement therapy.[24] These effects must be reproduced in larger trials before specific recommendations can be made. Addition of triiodothyronine may prove useful for patients with depression or those patients currently on desiccated thyroid preparations who are resistant to switching to thyroxine alone.

Subclinical Hypothyroidism

Subclinical hypothyroidism is defined as the presence of a high TSH with a free T_4 (or FTI) in the normal range. Some authors feel these patients are functionally hypothyroid relative to their own bodily requirements.[12,22,25] There is still some debate about whether to treat subclinical hypothyroidism. Patients often feel better with therapy, and treatment is usually indicated, especially if antithyroid antibodies are present.[3,4] Asymptomatic patients who have mild TSH elevation (<10 μU/mL), negative antithyroid antibodies, and no goiter may be followed without replacement.[3,5,19] Since subclinical hypothyroidism may be associated with reversible hypercholesterolemia,[26] depression,[21] and atherosclerosis,[27] treatment is warranted for patients with these conditions.

Hashimoto's Thyroiditis

Hashimoto's thyroiditis was first described in 1912 in four patients with lymphocyte infiltration, fibrosis, and follicular cell degeneration. It causes most cases of adult-onset hypothyroidism.[6,19] The etiology of the disease is autoimmune, with antibodies to thyroid peroxidase (antimicrosomal antibodies) and thyroglobulin usually present.[19,23] Like most autoimmune diseases, there is a genetic predisposition. It is most common in women (8:1) and is usually diagnosed between the ages of 30 and 50. Its incidence is increasing in developing countries.[19]

Signs and Symptoms

Patients usually present with a painless, diffuse, firm goiter. Patients may complain of tenderness or fullness of the anterior neck. Dysphagia and hoarseness are occasionally present. Although hyperthyroidism is found in up to 5% of patients during the acute stages of the disease, hypothyroidism with its various signs and symptoms is more common.[19] The presence of pain suggests the development of a primary B-cell lymphoma, a cancer associated with chronic autoimmune thyroiditis.[5]

Diagnosis

The diagnosis is suspected in patients with a characteristic goiter and is confirmed in 90% of cases by finding antibodies to thyroid peroxidase. Antithyroglobulin antibodies are also present in up to 70% of patients, but they are rarely present alone. Therefore, this latter assay is not usually necessary for diagnosis.[25] FTI (or free T_4) and the TSH level should be obtained to determine thyroid function.[19,23] If the goiter is very large, lobulated, or painful, fine-needle aspiration or biopsy may be indicated.[5]

Treatment

Treatment of hypothyroidism is described above and requires lifelong replacement. Thyrotoxicosis usually does not occur with this type of thyroiditis, and if present is of short duration requiring only symptomatic treatment. Graves' disease may precede or follow this illness and require additional treatment.

Congenital Hypothyroidism

Thyroid dysgenesis is the cause of congenital hypothyroidism in 80% of patients, and various problems with thyroid hormone production and regulation account for the rest. Severe growth and mental retardation (cretinism) can occur, but these sequelae are avoided if replacement therapy is started within the first 3 months of life. Undiagnosed congenital hypothyroidism has become rare in industrialized countries owing to neonatal screening. Transient perinatal hypothyroidism may result when mothers are given iodine or iodine-containing contrast agents.[20]

Euthyroid Sick Syndrome

Many severely ill patients have a low T_3 level or T_3 and T_4 levels below normal range. Free T_4 is usually normal if measured by a reliable, sensitive assay, and TSH is also usually normal. This so-called euthyroid sick syndrome is not indicative of true tissue hypothyroidism, and replacement is unnecessary unless the TSH level becomes markedly elevated (>20 μU/mL).[28]

Thyroid Nodules and Thyroid Cancer

Benign thyroid nodules are frequently encountered in primary care. They are estimated to occur in 4% to 8% of the adult population. In contrast, clinically significant thyroid cancer is infrequent, comprising only 1% of all malignancies and ranking 35th among causes of cancer death. Clinically insignificant thyroid cancers are more common, with American autopsy studies revealing a prevalence of 6% to 13%.[29]

Health Risks and Family Issues

Providing cost-effective yet thorough management for patients with thyroid nodules represents a distinct challenge to family physicians. Although thyroid nodules carry a low risk of mortality due to thyroid cancer, patients and their families must struggle with the knowledge that a potentially malignant growth is present. The anxiety produced by this fear not only causes stress in the patient but also has major implications for the family. Therefore, the evaluation should reveal adequate information not only to satisfy the physician but to alleviate the fears of patients and their family members.

Evaluation

Table 121.2 lists the findings that indicate high and moderate risks of cancer. When two or more of these factors are found, the probability of thyroid cancer is high. Laryngoscopy to evaluate vocal cord function is indicated, especially if any hoarseness or voice change has occurred. A history of neck irradiation increases the risk of both benign and malignant thyroid nodules. Multiple thyroid nodules suggest a benign process.

Table 121.2. **Clinical Factors Suggesting Malignancy in Thyroid Nodules**

High probability
  Rapid growth of nodule
  Vocal cord paralysis
  Fixation to adjacent tissue
  Enlarged regional lymph node(s)
  Very firm nodule
  Family history of multiple endocrine neoplasia type II
    (MEN-II) or medullary carcinoma
  Distant metastases (lungs or bones)
Moderate probability
  Age <15 years
  Age >70 years
  History of neck irradiation
  Diameter of nodule >4 cm
  Male sex and solitary nodule

Laboratory Studies

Thyroid function tests and the TSH assay are useful for confirming the clinical impression of thyroid status. Thyrotoxic nodules are only rarely malignant,[5,30] although Graves' disease has been associated with an increased incidence of thyroid cancer. Measurement of antibodies to thyroid peroxidase is useful for identifying autoimmune thyroiditis when there is also diffuse enlargement of the gland. A calcitonin assay is important in patients with a family history of multiple endocrine neoplasia type II (MEN-II) or medullary carcinoma, as calcitonin is usually elevated under these conditions. Genetic testing and calcitonin elevation may identify family members with this type of thyroid cancer before clinical manifestations appear.[5,29]

Workup

The workup of a solitary nontoxic thyroid nodule is outlined in Fig. 121.2. It may include nuclear medicine scans, ultrasonography, surgery, or fine-needle aspiration cytology (FNAC). The latter method has become the initial procedure of choice because it is the most accurate and most cost-effective. The FNAC technique is relatively simple and low risk,[5,29] and its sensitivity is reported to be more than 90%.[31,32] The most worrisome limitation is that a false-negative result may cause a malignancy to be missed, although the false-negative rate has been less than 10% in most studies and in one study as low as 0.7%. There is particular difficulty differentiating follicular adenoma from follicular carcinoma with FNAC, as finding evidence of invasion is required to diagnose the latter. A skilled and experienced cytopathologist is required for reliable results.

Results of FNAC are classified as positive when malignant cells are identified, negative when adequate benign glandular tissue is present, indeterminate when tissue is present and criteria for positive or negative reports are not met, and inadequate when insufficient tissue is present.[32]

Nuclear medicine scans have traditionally been part of the routine workup of thyroid nodules because a cold nodule was thought to indicate malignancy. In practice, however, scans have not proved to be as useful as expected. Because 84% of all thyroid nodules are cold on scan, most cold nodules are benign. Some thyroid cancers (1–4%) are hot on scan. Therefore nuclear medicine scans do not reliably distinguish benign from malignant nodules and so are not indicated for the routine initial workup of euthyroid patients.[5,30]

Ultrasonography can be used to determine if a thyroid nodule is solid or cystic, but this finding does not differentiate benign from malignant nodules. Studies have demonstrated that 9% to 14% of cystic nodules contain cancer compared to 10% to 20% of solid nodules being cancerous.[30] Cystic degeneration occurs in 25% of papillary carcinomas. Therefore, ultrasonography is not indicated for the routine initial workup. Ultrasonography may be used to seek the presence of other nodules, guide needle biopsy, document and follow the size of a nodule, and evaluate for metastasis.

Management

The decision regarding when to remove a thyroid nodule surgically should take into account several factors, including clinical findings, availability of FNAC with cytopathologic support, degree of anxiety of the patient and family, and ability to have reliable long-term follow-up. Reasonable guidelines are as follows: (1) Surgery is recommended for patients with one or more high-risk clinical factors or FNAC yielding positive or indeterminate results. (2) Observation is recommended for benign FNAC. Should the nodule increase in size, repeat FNAC or surgery is indicated. (3) Repeat the FNAC if the initial results are inadequate. Consider surgery if repeat FNAC is inadequate. (4) Consider surgery or repeat the FNAC for a persistent nodule after aspiration of a cyst.

Ultrasonography and nuclear medicine scans may be useful for the latter two situations when FNAC does not provide clear guidance (Fig. 121.2). Suppression of benign thyroid nodules with thyroid hormone replacement is often recommended, but the effectiveness of this treatment is questionable. If suppression is initiated, treatment for more than 12 months may be necessary to determine whether any benefit is achieved.[33] Thyroid nodules associated with Hashimoto's thyroiditis have been shown to respond to suppression.[5]

Thyroid Cancer

Four cell types of thyroid cancer are possible, each with a considerably different natural course and prognosis:

1. Papillary carcinoma accounts for 60% to 80% of all thyroid cancer. The tumor is slow-growing, and there is good long-term survival if surgical removal is performed while the cancer is still confined to the thyroid gland. Papillary carcinoma spreads by lymphatic means.
2. Follicular carcinoma accounts for 10% to 15% of all thyroid cancers. It is slightly more aggressive than the papillary variety and spreads by the hematogenous route. A subcategory of follicular carcinoma is the Hürthle cell type, which is more aggressive and more common in iodine-deficient countries.
3. Medullary carcinoma accounts for only 2% to 5% of thy-

roid cancers. Most of these lesions are sporadic, but some are familial; 20% are part of the MEN-II syndrome, which has an autosomal-dominant inheritance pattern. The latter can be identified early with elevated calcitonin levels and genetic testing. Screening with these tests should be performed on all family members if MEN-II or familial medullary carcinoma is diagnosed. If medullary carcinoma is not diagnosed prior to a palpable mass being present, the cure rate is less than 50%.[29,33,34]

4. Anaplastic thyroid carcinoma is the most aggressive type but accounts for only 2% to 7% of cases. It has the worst prognosis of any thyroid cancer, with a median survival time of 4 to 7 months and a 5-year survival rate of only 4%.

Surgery is the treatment of choice for all thyroid carcinoma when excision is possible. Controversy remains as to whether total or partial thyroidectomy is preferable. Near-total resection is probably the procedure of choice.[34] Radioiodine ablation is recommended for patients with known residual tumor and probably also for those at high risk of recurrence. Some patients with anaplastic thyroid cancer will respond to combined radiation and chemotherapy after thyroidecotmy.[5,24]

Thyroid Disease During Pregnancy

Both hypothyroidism and hyperthyroidism can complicate pregnancy (see Chapter 12). Thyroid-binding globulin increases during pregnancy, and so total T_3 and T_4 increase as well; hence, tests for these substances are not sufficient to diagnose or follow pregnant patients with thyroid disease.[35,36] Any use of radioactive iodine is contraindicated during pregnancy.

Hypothyroidism causes anovulation and rarely coincides with pregnancy. When hypothyroidism occurs, it is associated with gestational hypertension, premature labor, and low birth weight. Treatment consists of replacement with L-thyroxine to maintain the TSH level in the normal range on a sensitive assay.[35,36]

Hyperthyroidism during pregnancy is caused by the same etiologies as in nonpregnant patients, with Graves' disease being the most common cause. Thyrotoxicosis may lead to spontaneous abortion, stillbirth, neonatal death, and low birth weight.[35,36] Antithyroid drugs (usually propylthiouracil), propranolol, and occasionally thyroid resection may be used for treatment.[36]

Postpartum thyroiditis is a transient autoimmune thyroid dysfunction that occurs within the first postpartum year (see Chapter 15). It is probably an exacerbation of a preexisting subclinical autoimmune thyroiditis.[5,35] The true incidence is probably 5% to 10%, although it is frequently underdiagnosed.[32] The most common complaints are depression, poor memory, and impaired concentration. The clinical course consists of a hyperthyroid phase (which may be absent), followed by a hypothyroid phase and eventually a return to euthyroid status. The diagnosis is usually made with a sensitive TSH measurement. Patients with antibodies to thyroid peroxidase and thyroglobulin are at increased risk of developing this syndrome.[36] Patients who have one episode of postpartum thyroiditis are at increased risk for recurrence with future pregnancies and may develop permanent hypothyroidism.[35]

References

1. Bagchi N, Brown TR, Parish RF. Thyroid dysfunction in adults over age 55 years. Arch Intern Med 1990;150:785–7.
2. Ladenson PW, Singer PA, Ain KB, et al. American Thyroid Association guidelines for detection of thyroid dysfunction. Arch Intern Med 2000;160:1573–5.
3. Arbelle JE, Porath A. Practice guideline for the detection and management of thyroid dysfunction. A comparative review of the recommendations. Clin Endocrinol 1999;51:11–18.
4. Tunbridge WM, Vanderpump PJ. Population screening for autoimmune thyroid disease. Endocrinol Metab Clin North Am 2000;29:239–53.
5. Braverman LE, Utiger RD, eds. The thyroid: a fundamental and clinical text. 8th ed. New York: Lippincott, 2000.
6. Tunbridge WM, Evered DC, Hall R, et al. The spectrum of thyroid disease in a community: the Whickham survey. Clin Endocrinol (Oxf) 1977;7:481–93.
7. Bar-Sela S, Ehrenfeld M, Eliakim M. Arterial embolism in thyrotoxicosis with atrial fibrillation. Arch Intern Med 1981;141:1191–2.
8. Terndrup TE, Heisig DG, Garceau JP. Sudden death associated with undiagnosed Graves' disease. J Emerg Med 1990;8:553–5.
9. Sawin CT, Geller A, Wolf PA, Belanger AJ, Baker E, Bacharach P. Low serum thyrotropin concentrations as a risk factor for atrial fibrillation in older persons. N Engl J Med 1994;331:1249–52.
10. McDougall IR. Graves' disease: current concepts. Med Clin North Am 1991;75:79–95.
11. Harper MB. Vomiting, nausea and abdominal pain: unrecognized symptoms of thyrotoxicosis. J Fam Pract 1989;29:382–6.
12. Surks MI, Chopre IJ, Mariash CN, Nicoloff JT, Solomon DH. American Thyroid Association guidelines for use of laboratory tests in thyroid disorders. JAMA 1990;263:1529–32.
13. Franklyn JA. Management of hyperthyroidism. N Engl J Med 1994;330:1731–8.
14. Milner MR, Gelman KM, Phillips RA, Fuster V, Davies TF, Goldman ME. Double blind crossover trial of diltiazem versus propranolol in the management of thyrotoxic syndromes. Pharmacotherapy 1990;10:100–6.
15. Hermar VS, Joffee BI, Kalk WJ, Panz V, Wing J, Seftel HC. Clinical and biochemical responses to nadolol and clonidine in hyperthyroidism. J Clin Pharmacol 1989;29:1117–20.
16. Allanic H, Fauchet J, Orgiazzi J, et al. Antithyroid drugs and Graves' disease: a prospective randomized evaluation of the efficacy of treatment duration. J Clin Endocrinol Metab 1990;8:553–5.
17. Hashizume K, Ichikawa K, Sakurai A, et al. Administration of thyroxine in treated Graves' disease. N Engl J Med 1991;324:947–53.
18. Berglund J, Christensen SB, Dymling JF, Hallengren B. The incidence of recurrence and hypothyroidism following treatment with antithyroid drugs, surgery or radioiodine in all patients with thyrotoxicosis in Malmo during the period 1970–1974. J Intern Med 1991;229:435–42.
19. Singer PA. Thyroiditis: acute, subacute, and chronic. Med Clin North Am 1991;75:61–77.
20. Gruters A. Congenital hypothyroidism. Pediatr Ann 1992;21:15–28.
21. Whybrow PC, Prange AJ, Tredway CR. Mental changes accompanying thyroid gland dysfunction. Arch Gen Psychiatry 1969;20:48–63.

22. Gold MS, Pottash AL, Extein I. Hypothyroidism and depression: evidence from complete thyroid function evaluation. JAMA 1981;245:1919–22.

23. Rapoport B. Pathophysiology of Hashimoto's thyroiditis and hypothyroidism. Annu Rev Med 1991;42:91–6.

24. Bunevicius R, Kazanavicius G, Zalinkevicius R, Prange AJ. Effects of thyroxine as compared with thyroxine and triiodothyroxine in patients with hypothyroidism. N Engl J Med 1999;340: 424–9.

25. Ladenson PW. Optimal laboratory testing for diagnosis and monitoring of thyroid nodules, goiter, and thyroid cancer. Clin Chem 1996;42:183–7.

26. Tanis BC, Westindorp GJ, Smelt HM. Effect of thyroid substitution on hypercholesterolemia in patients with subclinical hypothyroidism: effect of levothyroxine therapy. Arch Intern Med 1990;150:2097–100.

27. Hak AE, Pols HAP, Visser TJ, Drexhage HA, Hofman A, Witteman CM. Subclinical hypothyroidism is an independent risk factor for atherosclerosis and myocardial infarction in elderly women: the Rotterdam study. Ann Intern Med 2000;132:270–8.

28. Cavalieri RR. The effects of nonthyroid disease and drugs on thyroid function tests. Med Clin North Am 1991;75:28–39.

29. Harvey HK. Diagnosis and management of the thyroid nodule. Otolaryngol Clin North Am 1990;23:303–37.

30. Cox MR, Marshal SG, Spence RA. Solitary thyroid nodule: a prospective evaluation of nuclear scanning and ultrasonography. Br J Surg 1991;78:90–3.

31. Hamming JF, Goslings BM, Steenis GJ, Claasen H, Hermans J, Velde CJ. The value of fine needle aspiration biopsy in patients with nodular thyroid disease divided into groups of suspicion of malignant neoplasms on clinical grounds. Arch Intern Med 1990;150:113–6.

32. Grant CS, Hay ID, Cough IR, McCarthy PM, Goellner JR. Long term follow-up of patients with benign fine-needle aspiration cytologic diagnoses. Surgery 1989;106:980–6.

33. Cheung PS, Lee JM, Boey JH. Thyroxine suppressive therapy of benign solitary thyroid nodules: a prospective randomized study. World J Surg 1989;13:818–22.

34. Kaplan MM. Progress in thyroid cancer. Endocrinol Metab Clin North Am 1990;19:469–77.

35. Lowe TW, Cunningham FG. Pregnancy and thyroid disease. Clin Obstet Gynecol 1991;34:72–81.

36. Bishnoi A, Sachmechi I. Thyroid disease in pregnancy. Am Fam Physician 1996;53:215–20.

122
Osteoporosis

Paula Cifuentes Henderson and Richard P. Usatine

Osteoporosis is a major health concern affecting approximately 20 million people in the United States. It is responsible for more than 1.3 million fractures annually,[1] with $15 billion in direct financial expenditures to treat these fractures.[2] The clinical consequences of an osteoporotic fracture include increased mortality, disability, and the need for long-term nursing care. After a hip fracture the mortality rate of patients 65 to 79 years old at 1 year is between 20% and 30%, and these rates worsen with increased age.[3] Among those who survive, 50% won't be able to work without some type of assistance. After a collapsed osteoporotic vertebra, 30% of patients will experience chronic disabling back pain and spinal deformity.[4,5] Osteoporotic fractures have a profound impact on quality of life, decreasing the physical, functional, and psychological performance secondary to pain, deformities, and inability to perform the activities of daily living (ADL)[6] (see Chapter 23, Table 23.1).

Osteoporosis is a disease characterized by low bone mass and michroarchitectural deterioration of bone tissue leading to enhanced bone fragility and a consequent increase in fracture risk.[7] It can be a silent disease because it is often asymptomatic until a fracture occurs. The lifetime risk of a 50-year-old white woman of having an osteoporotic fracture is 40%. Fractures secondary to osteoporosis are more common in women than in men and in Caucasians and Asians than in African Americans and Latinos.[8] These fractures most commonly occur at the hip, vertebrae, and wrists.

Primary osteoporosis is related to aging and not associated with chronic illness. Secondary osteoporosis is related to chronic conditions that contribute to accelerated bone loss such as with hyperparathyroidism, malignancy, renal failure, and hyperthyroidism.[9]

Assessment and Diagnosis

Risk Factor Assessment

Start with the medical history and ask questions about:

Menopause (surgical and natural)
Family history of osteoporosis (especially mother)
Exercise
Diet
Smoking
Alcohol intake

Other risk factors such as age, gender, ethnicity, and slender body habitus can usually be observed without asking specific questions. The physical exam includes the measurement of height and weight, and the examination of the spine looking for any signs of deformity such as kyphosis, scoliosis, and limited range of motion. Screening for secondary forms of osteoporosis may be helpful. Assess the patient's risk of falling by asking about a history of falls and a decrease in visual acuity.[10,11]

Genetic Issues

The prevalence of osteoporosis varies by sex, ethnicity, and race.[12] Decreased bone density is more common in women of Northern European or Asian descent. Women and men experience age-related decrease in bone mass density starting at midlife, but women experience more rapid bone loss after the menopause.[13] Genetic syndromes like Turner's (45,X0) syndrome patients have streak ovaries and decreased estrogen production leading to the early development of osteoporosis.[14]

Endocrine Factors

Risk factors associated with decreased bone density include early estrogen deficiency secondary to surgery or to early menopause, hyperthyroidism, hyperparathyroidism, hypercortisolism, Addison's disease, and Cushing's syndrome.[14]

Medications

Chronic use of certain medications that affect the bone metabolism, such as corticosteroids, exogenous thyroid hormone, gonadotropin-releasing hormone (GnRH) analogues, anticoagulants, and anticonvulsants, increase the risk of osteoporosis and subsequent fractures.[15]

Lifestyle

Excessive use of alcohol depresses osteoblastic function and increases the risk of osteoporosis. Physical activity early in life contributes to higher peak bone mass and reduces the risk of falls by approximately 25%.[16] Good nutrition with a balanced diet is necessary for the development of healthy bones. Calcium and vitamin D are required for the prevention and treatment of osteoporosis. There are data to support recommendations (found later in the chapter) for specific dietary calcium intakes at various stages in life.[17,18] Patients at high risk also include those who pursue thinness excessively, have a history of an eating disorder,[19] restrict their intake of dairy products, don't consume enough vegetables and fruits, and have a high intake of low-calcium/high-phosphorus beverages like sodas. These beverages have a negative effect on calcium balance.

Laboratory Assessment

If the history and physical exam suggests secondary causes of osteoporosis, the physician should consider tests such as thyroid-stimulating hormone (TSH), parathyroid hormone (PTH), calcium, vitamin D, urine N-teloptide, complete blood count (CBC), chem panel, cortisol, erythrocyte sedimentation rate (ESR) or serum protein electrophoresis, based on the differential diagnosis.[20,21]

Bone Densitometry Assessment

To prevent osteoporosis, the physician should attempt to establish early detection of low bone mineral density (BMD). Currently there is no accurate measure of bone strength, but BMD is the accepted method to establish a diagnosis of osteoporosis and predict future fracture risk.[22,23] The World Health Organization (WHO) defines osteoporosis as a BMD 2.5 standard deviations (SDs) below the mean for young white adult women. This definition does not apply to other ethnic groups, men, or children.[7,24] The U.S. Preventive Services Task Force suggests that the primary reason to screen postmenopausal women is to check for a low BMD so that early intervention may be initiated to slow the further decrease of the bone density.[25] The ultimate goal is to prevent vertebral and hip fractures.

The most thoroughly studied and most widely used technique to measure BMD is the dual-energy x-ray absortiometry (DEXA) scan. This is considered to be the gold standard screening test to measure the BMD of the hip and spine. It is less expensive and involves less radiation exposure than the quantitative computed tomography (CT). Since some patients don't respond to therapy for osteoporosis, the BMD results can also

Table 122.1. World Health Organization (WHO) Diagnostic Criteria for Osteoporosis

Diagnosis	Bone Mineral Density (BMD) T score[a]
Normal	≤1
Osteopenia	1–2.5
Osteoporosis	≥2.5
Severe osteoporosis	≥2.5 and history of fracture

[a]Standard deviation (SD) below the mean in healthy young adults.

Source: WHO Study Group.[7]

be used to follow them and evaluate their response to treatment. Bone mass should be measured in postmenopausal women 1 to 2 years following the initiation of therapy.

The report of the DEXA provides a T score and a Z score. The T score is defined as the number of SDs above or below the mean BMD for sex- and race-matched young controls (not age matched). This should be distinguished from a Z score, which is defined as the number of SDs above or below the average BMD comparing the patient with the population adjusted for age, sex, and race. These results can be used to classify patients into three categories: normal, osteopenic, and osteoporotic (Table 122.1). Osteoporosis is diagnosed using the patient's T score, because the T score is a measure of current fracture risk. A T score of 1 SD below the age-predicted mean is associated with a two- to threefold increased risk of fracture. Patients with T scores more than 2 SDs below the mean have an exponential increase in their risk of fracture. Z scores have little significant value for clinical practice.

Table 122.2. Indications for Bone Mineral Density (BMD) Screening

National Osteoporosis Foundation guidelines[a]
  Women >65 willing to start therapy if BMD low
  Women <65 postmenopausal with at least one additional risk factor
  All postmenopausal women with fractures
  Women considering therapy for osteoporosis, and BMD would affect decision
  Women who have received HRT for a prolonged period
  No formal guideline developed in premenopausal women

American Association of Clinical Endocrinologists clinical practice guidelines[b]
  Perimenopausal women willing to start therapy if BMD low
  X-ray evidence of bone loss
  Asymptomatic hyperparathyroidism
  Monitoring therapeutic response and BMD would affect decision
  Long-term use of glucocorticoid

BMD = bone mineral density; HRT = hormone replacement therapy.

[a]National Osteoporosis Foundation (NOF). Physician's guide to prevention and treatment of osteoporosis. Washington, DC: NOF, 1998, 2000

[b]American Association of Clinical Endocrinologists (AACE). Clinical practice guidelines for the prevention and treatment of postmenopausal osteoporosis. Endocrinol Pract 1996;2(2):157–71.

Newer measures of bone strength, such as the ultrasound, are being introduced as an alternative screening method to the DEXA scan. This measurement of bone mass is being done through peripheral bone mass assessment. In 1998, the Food and Drug Administration (FDA) approved the use of a portable ultrasound to assess bone mass through the measurement of the calcaneous. If a patient has a low T score in the ultrasound of a peripheral bone, the current recommendation is to obtain a DEXA of the hip and spine for further evaluation and treatment.[11]

The diagnosis and treatment of osteoporosis should be individualized based on each patient's risk factors rather than the assessment of a T score alone.

Indications for bone mineral density assessment include:

Women ≥65 years old who are willing to start drug therapy if BMD is found to be low
Women <65 who have at least one additional risk factor for osteoporosis
Postmenopausal women with a fracture
Radiographic evidence of bone loss
Long-term steroid use
Hyperparathyroidism
Monitoring therapeutic response if the results would affect the clinical decision.

Although there is no evidence to support this, some clinicians screen premenopausal women with BMD for the following conditions:

Prolonged oligo/amenorrhea
A long-standing history of eating disorders
Stress fractures
Chronic use of medications that promote bone resorption.

There is a lack of evidence to support the cost-effectiveness of universal routine bone density screenings or to support the efficacy of early preventive medications to prevent fractures. Therefore, an individualized approach is recommended[25] (Table 122.2).

Bone Remodeling Assessment

Another way to assess bone strength is to measure markers of bone remodeling (turnover) in the blood or urine. There is some evidence that bone turnover rate predicts the risk of osteoporotic fractures in postmenopausal women.[26] These markers include indices of bone resorption such as serum and urine levels of C- and N-telopeptide, and indices of bone formation such as osteocalcin and bone-specific alkaline phosphatase. These markers of bone turnover may be particularly useful if obtained prior to starting treatment and then repeated in 3 to 6 months to measure the response. Despite the fact that these markers may identify changes in bone remodeling, they do not predict fracture risk.

These tests are very expensive and are not recommended for screening or as the first-line studies to follow treatment response. However, if the BMD does not increase with treatment, one might order the turnover markers for further assessment.

Prevention and Treatment

Nonpharmacologic

Nonpharmacologic therapy for prevention and treatment of osteoporosis includes adequate dietary intake of calcium and vitamin D, weight-bearing exercise, fall precautions, no smoking, and avoidance of excessive alcohol intake. These steps should be started early in life and continued through menopause because BMD peaks at about age 35 and then begins to decline with accelerated bone loss after menopause.

Calcium

According to the National Institutes of Health (NIH) Consensus Development Conference, the optimal recommended dose of elemental calcium is the amount that each person needs to maintain adult bone mass and minimizes bone loss later in life (Table 122.3). The recommended dose for postmenopausal women <65 years old who are on hormone replacement therapy (HRT) is 1000 mg/day and 1500 mg/day for all other postmenopausal women.[27] Calcium supplements are advisable if diet cannot supply the recommended amount necessary. Calcium citrate should be taken between meals while calcium carbonate should be taken with meals because it is best absorbed with gastric acid. Calcium should not be taken with iron because the iron decreases the absorption. Several studies show that calcium supplements can reduce bone loss in postmenopausal women and will reduce the risk of fractures.[27] The effect is not strong enough to recommend calcium alone for osteoporosis prevention.

Table 122.3. **Optimal Calcium Intake**[a]

Population		NIH	RDA
Infants, children, and young adults			
0–6 Months		400	400
6–12 Months		600	600
1–10 years		800–1200	800
11–24 years		1200–1500	1200
Adult women			
Pregnant and lactating			
<24 years		1200–1500	1200
>24 years		1200	800
Premenopausal			
25–49 years		1000	800
Postmenopausal			
50–64 years	On Estrogen	1000	800
	Not on estrogen	1500	800
≥65 years		1500	
Adult men			
25–64 years		1000	800
≥65 years		1500	800

[a]Calcium recommendations in mg/day.

NIH = National Institutes of Health; RDA = Recommended Daily Allowance.

Adapted from the NIH Consensus Conference, 1994.[18]

Vitamin D

The recommended daily intake of vitamin D needed for adequate calcium absorption is 400 to 800 IU. Vitamin D deficiency can occur in patients with inadequate sunlight exposure. Sunlight exposure is shown to be useful in preventing hip fractures, especially in elderly institutionalized women.[28]

Physical Activity

Adequate physical activity may exert a positive influence on bone mass and is necessary for bone acquisition and maintenance. The extent of this influence and the most effective type of program are not fully understood. Most trials of exercise intervention show that a reduction of falls is likely to be secondary to improved muscular strength and balance. Low-impact exercise like walking has minimal effect on BMD; high-impact exercise like weight training stimulates the increase of BMD. Women who exercise regularly are at a lower risk of hip fractures.[29] However, excessive exercise by competitive athletes can also be a risk factor for bone loss, particularly if they have hypoestrogenic oligo/amenorrhea.

Fall Prevention

Most osteoporotic fractures result from a fall. Risk factors for falling include visual or hearing problems, gait disturbances, underlying conditions that predispose the patient to syncope, cognitive impairment, and the use of certain medications like diuretics, antihypertensive, benzodiazepines, and antidepressants. Home safety precautions may help to prevent falls. External hip protectors have been shown to provide protection against hip fractures in frail elderly adults (see Chapter 24).

Pharmacologic Treatment

Pharmacologic treatment should be initiated in women with:

No risk factors and who have T scores below 2 SDs
Risk factors and T scores below 1.5 SD
A history of vertebral or hip fractures
Multiple risk factors over 70 years of age without BMD measurement.

The pharmacologic agents for treatment and prophylaxis of osteoporosis include HRT, calcium and vitamin D supplements, bisphosphonates, selective estrogen receptor modulators (SERMs), intranasal calcitonin, and parathyroid hormone (PTH). While the most widely prescribed regimen is HRT with calcium and vitamin D, there are many reasons to consider using the other medications.

Inhibitors of Bone Resorption

Hormonal

Hormone Replacement Therapy (HRT)

In the PEPI trial, HRT increased BMD at the hip by 1.7 % and at the spine by 3.5% to 5.0% over a 3-year period compared to placebo. HRT inhibits bone loss for the duration of the therapy, which recurs once therapy is discontinued. In premenopausal women with osteoporosis secondary to hypoestro-

genic stages, early intervention with estrogen to achieve return of menses, is critical since bone loss may be irreversible.

Observational studies consistently suggest that postmenopausal HRT reduces the risk of hip and other types of fractures.[30] Evidence from randomized controlled trials (RCTs), especially for vertebral fracture prevention, is less available. In a Danish RCT, HRT reduced forearm fracture incidence in recent postmenopausal women.[31] In another randomized trial, HRT and vitamin D prevented nonvertebral fractures in postmenopausal women.[32] A meta-analysis published in 2001 suggests that estrogen reduces risk of nonvertebral fractures by 27%. Estrogen seemed to reduce the risk of fractures by 33% in younger women, but had no significant effect in women aged 60 years or older.[33]

Before starting a patient on HRT the physician and the patient need to consider all the risks and benefits. Common adverse effects like breakthrough bleeding and breast tenderness or enlargement should be discussed. The risk of breast cancer and heart disease are very important issues. The relationship of HRT to breast cancer and heart disease is still controversial. HRT should be used with caution in patients who have a personal or family history of breast or endometrial cancer, or a history of a hypercoagulable state or thromboembolic episodes. Informed consent should be given to all patients (see Chapter 104).

In postmenopausal women without contraindications to HRT, any of the three recommended regimens could be used: estrogen alone in women without a uterus, estrogen with progestin daily, and estrogen with progestin in a cyclic manner (estrogen every day and progestin only for 10 to 14 days of the month). The most common regimen is conjugated estrogen at a daily dose of 0.625 mg or its equivalent. This dose can be used if the therapy begins at the onset of menopause in order to prevent the rapid bone loss that occurs early. If the postmenopausal woman is older at the time of starting the HRT, she might be more sensitive to the standard dose. One might consider starting at half the dose (0.3 mg) to avoid discontinuation secondary to adverse effects. Estrogen alone is avoided in women with a uterus in order to prevent endometrial cancer. Estrogen given with progesterone may actually decrease the risk of endometrial cancer.

Selective Estrogen Receptor Modulators (SERMs)

SERMs are an important alternative for women with contraindications or intolerance to estrogen therapy. Tamoxifen and raloxifene were FDA approved in 2000 for treatment of postmenopausal osteoporosis. The main goal is to maximize the beneficial estrogenic effect in bone and minimize the effect on the breast and endometrium.

One study showed that raloxifene may decrease the risk of vertebral fracture by 36%, but there has been no published evidence for hip fracture reduction.[34] Both SERMs are contraindicated in women at risk for deep venous thrombosis.

Bisphosphonates

Alendronate (Fosamax)

Alendronate was approved by the FDA in 1995 for treatment of postmenopausal osteoporosis. It reduces the risk of vertebral fractures by 30% to 50% and increases the BMD at the spine and hip.[35] Alendronate also reduces the risk of fractures in men and women with osteoporosis secondary to the chronic use of steroids.[36]

One study evaluated the addition of alendronate to HRT in the treatment of postmenopausal women with low BMD despite ongoing treatment with estrogen.[37] Compared with HRT alone, at 12 months alendronate plus HRT produced significantly greater increases in BMD of the lumbar spine (3.6% vs. 1.0%, $p < .001$) and hip trochanter (2.7% vs. 0.5%, $p < .001$). This study suggests that alendronate may be beneficial when added to HRT in postmenopausal women with low BMD despite ongoing treatment with HRT. However, it should be noted that the outcome measured was BMD and not fractures.

The recommended starting dose for postmenopausal osteoporosis prevention is 5 mg/day with a maintenance dose of 10 mg/day. The most common side effect is esophageal irritation secondary to reflux. Therefore, the patient should take alendronate with a full glass of water without food and remain upright for at least 30 minutes to avoid reflux. Another available regimen is 70 mg once a week. This weekly dose was demonstrated to be as effective with fewer gastrointestinal side effects.[38] At this time, the use of alendronate has not been approved for premenopausal women.

Risedronate (Actonel)

Risedronate is a newer biphosphonate approved in 2000 by the FDA for treatment of postmenopausal osteoporosis. While the indications are the same as alendronate, it has fewer gastrointestinal side effects. Both agents cost over $50 a month. In a randomized, double-blind, placebo-controlled trial of 2458 ambulatory postmenopausal women younger than 85 years with at least 1 vertebral fracture at baseline, risedronate decreased the relative incidence of new vertebral fractures by 41% over 3 years. The absolute risk reduction was from 16.3% to 11.3%. The cumulative incidence of nonvertebral fractures over 3 years was reduced by 39% (5.2 % vs 8.4%). The overall safety profile of risedronate, including gastrointestinal safety, was similar to that of placebo. The most effective dose was 5 mg/day.[39]

Calcitonin

Calcitonin is helpful when treating painful osteoporosis due to its significant analgesic effect. This hormone inhibits bone resorption by acting directly on the osteoclasts. The PROOF study is controversial; it demonstrates a reduction of vertebral fractures with calcitonin.[40] It is available in nasal spray at a recommended dose of 200 IU/day that corresponds to one squirt through one nostril every day alternating nostrils; or in the injectable form (200 units/mL) to be used three to five times/week at a dose of 50 to 100 IU/dose.

Stimulators of Bone Formation

Parathyroid Hormone (PTH)

PTH is the most promising anabolic agent that stimulates bone formation. It is still undergoing clinical trials. Even though it

increases the BMD of the lumbar spine,[41] there are no data on fracture risk. One disadvantage is that it must be administered by subcutaneous injection. It is not yet approved by the FDA.

Fluoride

Fluoride stimulates bone formation but does not decrease the risk of a fracture. A meta-analysis showed that fluoride increases bone mineral density at the lumbar spine and does not reduce the number of vertebral fractures. Increasing the dose of fluoride actually increased the risk of nonvertebral fractures and gastrointestinal side effects.[42] It is not approved by the FDA for osteoporosis prevention and treatment.

Conclusion

Fractures of the hip, vertebrae, and wrists from osteoporosis cause significant decreases in the quality of life for many older individuals. The complications of hip fractures can also lead to death. Better methods for prevention, early detection, and treatment now exist. Healthy lifestyles, including no smoking, exercise, good diet, and calcium intake, can help to prevent osteoporosis. By assessing family history, ethnicity, body type, and other risk factors, physicians can target prevention and screening efforts to patients at highest risk for osteoporosis. Patients at higher risk should probably be screened using a DEXA scan. Pharmacologic therapies such as hormone replacement, calcium, vitamin D, bisphosphonates, SERMs, and calcitonin can help prevent BMD loss and may reduce the risk of fractures. Currently, the data for fracture prevention are stronger for the bisphosponates than for hormonal therapy. Every family physician should feel comfortable screening for, preventing, and treating osteoporosis.

Suggested Web Sites

The National Institutes of Health Osteoporosis and Related Bone Diseases: National Resource Center *www.osteo.org*

The National Osteoporosis Foundation. *www.nof.org*

References

1. Riggs BL, Melton LJ III. The worldwide problem of osteoporosis: insights afforded by epidemiology. Bone 1995;17:505S–11S.
2. Chrischilles E, Shireman T, Wallace R. Costs and health effects of osteoporotic fractures. Bone 1994;15:377–87.
3. Lu Yao GL, Baron JA, Barrett JA. Treatment and survival among elderly Americans with hip fractures: a population-based study. Am J Public Health 1994;84:1287–91.
4. Watts NB. Hip fracture prevention in nursing homes: clinical importance and management strategies. Consult Pharm 1996;11:944–5.
5. Cummings SR, Kelsey JL, Nevitt MC. Epidemiology of osteoporosis and osteoporotic fractures. Epidemiol Rev 1985;7178–208.

6. Gold DT. The clinical impact of vertebral fractures. Bone 1996; 18:185–90.

7. World Health Organization (WHO) Study Group. Assessment of fracture risk and its application to screening for post-menopausal osteoporosis. Geneva, Switzerland: WHO Technical Report Series, 1994;843.

8. National Osteoporotic Foundation, 2025 osteoporosis prevalence figures: state by state report. January 1997. Women's Health Matters 1998;2(30):1.

9. Harper KD, Weber TJ. Secondary osteoporosis. Diagnostic considerations. Endocrinol Metab Clin North Am 1998;27(2):325–48.

10. World Health Organization (WHO). Assessment of fracture risk and its application to screening for postmenopausal osteoporosis. WHO technical report series 843. Geneva: WHO, 1994.

11. Heinemann DF. Osteoporosis. An overview of the National Osteoporosis Foundation clinical practice guide. Geriatrics 2000; 55(5):31–6.

12. Pocock NA, Eisman JA, Hopper JL. Genetic determinants of bone mass in adults. J Clin Invest 1987;80:706–10.

13. Seeman E. Growth in bone mass and size: Are racial and gender differences in bone density more apparent than real? J Clin Endocrinol Metab 1998;83:1414–18.

14. Harper KD, Weber TJ. Secondary osteoporosis. Diagnostic considerations. Endocrinol Metab Clin North Am 1998;27(2):325–48.

15. Saag KG, Emkey R, Schinitzer A. For the glucocorticoid-induced osteoporosis intervention study group. Alendronate for the prevention and treatment of glucocorticoid-induced osteoporosis. N Engl J Med 1998;339:292–9.

16. Bassey EJ, Rothwell MC, Littlewood JJ. Pre- and post-menopausal women have different bone mineral density responses to the same high impact exercise. J Bone Miner Res 1998;13:1805–13.

17. Dawson B, Harris SS, Krall EA. Effect of calcium and vitamin D supplementation on bone density in men and women 65 years of age or older. N Engl J Med 1997;337:670–6.

18. NIH Consensus Development Panel on Optimal Calcium Intake. NIH Consensus Conference: optimal calcium intake. JAMA 1994;272:1942–8.

19. Hotta M, Shibasaki T, Sato K. The importance of body weight history in the occurrence and recovery of osteoporosis in patients with anorexia nervosa: evaluation by dual x-ray absorptiometry and bone metabolic markers. Eur J Endocrinol 1998; 139:276–83.

20. Consensus Development Conference. Diagnosis, prophylaxis and treatment of osteoporosis. Am J Med 1993;94:646–50.

21. Nattiv A. Osteoporosis: its prevention, recognition, and management. Family Pract Recert 1998;20(2):17–41.

22. Black DM, Cummings SR, Genant HK. Axial and appendicular bone density predict fractures in older women. J Bone Miner Res 1996;11:707–30.

23. AACE Clinical Practice guidelines for the prevention and treatment of postmenopausal osteoporosis. Endocrinol Pract 1996; 2(2):157–71.

24. National Osteoporosis Foundation. Physicians guide to prevention and treatment of osteoporosis. Bele Mead, NJ: Experta Medica, 1998.

25. NIH Consensus Conference. Osteoporosis prevention, diagnosis and therapy. JAMA 2001;285(6):785–94.

26. Garnero P, Hauserr E,Chapui MC. Markers of bone resorption predict hip fracture in elderly women: the EPIDOS prospective study. J Bone Miner Res 1996;11:1531–8.

27. Reid R, Ames RW, Evans MC. Effect of calcium supplementation on bone loss in postmenopausal women. N Engl J Med 1993;328:460–4.

28. Chapuy MC, Arlot ME, Duboeuf F. Vitamin D3 and calcium to prevent hip fractures in the elderly women. N Engl J Med 1992; 327:1637–42.

29. Paganini-Hill A, Chao A, Ross RK. Exercise and other factors in the prevention of hip fracture: the Leisure World study. Epidemiology 1991;2:16–25.

30. Grady D, Cummings SR. Postmenopausal hormone therapy for prevention of fractures: how good is the evidence? JAMA 2001;285(22):2909–10.

31. Mosekilde L, Beck-Nielsen H, Sorensen OH, et al. Hormonal replacement therapy reduces forearm fracture incidence in recent postmenopausal women—results of the Danish Osteoporosis Prevention Study. Maturitas 2000;36(3):181–93.

32. Komulainen MH, Kroger H, Tuppurainen MT, et al. HRT and Vit D in prevention of non-vertebral fractures in postmenopausal women; a 5 year randomized trial. Maturitas. 1998;31(1):45–54.

33. Torgerson DJ, Bell-Syer SEM. Hormone replacement therapy and prevention of nonvertebral fractures: a meta-analysis of randomized trials. JAMA 2001;285:2891–7.

34. Ettinger B, Black DM, Mitlak BH. Reduction of vertebral fracture risk in postmenopausal women with osteoporosis treated with raloxifene: results from a 3-year randomized clinical trial. JAMA 1999;282:637–45.

35. Karpf DB, Shapiro DR, Seeman E. Prevention of nonvertebral fractures by alendronate: a meta-analysis. JAMA 1997;277:1159–64.

36. Saag KG, Emkey R, Schnitzer TJ, et al. Alendronate for the prevention and treatment of glucocorticoid-induced osteoporosis. Glucocorticoid-Induced Osteoporosis Intervention Study Group. N Engl J Med 1998;339(5):292–9.

37. Lindsay R, Cosman F, Lobo RA, et al. Addition of alendronate to ongoing hormone replacement therapy in the treatment of osteoporosis: a randomized, controlled clinical trial. J Clin Endocrinol Metab 1999;84(9):3076–81.

38. Baran D. Osteoporosis. Efficacy and safety of a bisphosphonate dosed once weekly. Geriatrics 2001;56(3):28–32.

39. Harris ST, Watts NB, Genant HK. Effects of risedronate treatment on vertebral and nonvertebral fractures in women with postmenopausal osteoporosis. JAMA 1999;282:1344–52.

40. Chestnut CH, Silverman SL, Andriano K. Salmon calcitonin nasal spray reduces the rate of new vertebral fractures independently of known major pre-treatment risk factors: accrued 5 year analysis of the PROOF study. Bone 1998;23(5):S290.

41. Lindsay R, Cosman F, Nieves J. Does treatment with parathyroid hormone increases vertebral size? Osteoporosis International 2000. World Congress on Osteoporosis 2000;11(2):556, S206.

42. Haguenauer D, Welch V, Shea B, Tugwell P, Adachi JD, Wells G. Fluoride for the treatment of postmenopausal osteoporotic fractures: a meta-analysis. Osteoporos Int 2000;11(9):727–38.

123
Gout

James F. Calvert, Jr.

Gout encompasses a spectrum of diseases caused by precipitation of uric acid crystals in tissue. The gouty disorders include (1) acute monarticular arthritis caused by uric acid crystals in joints, (2) nephrolithiasis, (3) soft tissue deposits of urate crystals known as tophi, and (4) uric acid renal disease. Gout occurs in about 1.3% of men over 40, making it the most common form of inflammatory arthritis in men. The prevalence in women is about half that in men,[1] although there is evidence that the relative prevalence of gout in women has increased.[2] The prevalence of gout increases with age, and it is more common in persons of African or Polynesian ancestry.

Hyperuricemia

Hyperuricemia is caused by either increased production of uric acid or decreased ability to excrete it; some of the more common disorders characterized by hyperuricemia are listed in Table 123.1. Hyperuricemia is defined as the presence of a serum uric acid over 7.0 mg/dL (420 μmol/L). Uric acid is less likely to form crystals at concentrations below this level. The risk of having all the gouty disorders increases proportionately to the serum uric acid level.[3] Prophylactic treatment to lower the uric acid level incurs no benefit to patients with asymptomatic hyperuricemia and is more risky and expensive than no treatment,[4] although the discovery that a patient has hyperuricemia should lead to an attempt to determine its etiology and significance. An exception to this rule is that patients with lymphoproliferative disorders or those about to undergo chemotherapy for other malignancies should be treated prophylactically with allopurinol.[5,6] Uric acid levels are often elevated prior to the development of heart disease, stroke, hyperlipidemia, diabetes, and hyperinsulinism, but whether the hyperuricemia is an innocent bystander in these disorders or part of their cause is a matter of controversy.[7–9]

Acute Gout

Acute gout is characterized by severe pain in a single joint that develops over a period of a few hours. Uric acid is more likely to crystalize at lower temperatures, so the metatarsophalangeal joint of the great toe, the coolest part of the body, is the most common site of gouty attacks, but other joints, typically a knee, shoulder, hand, or another part of the foot or ankle, are the site of presentation in 30% to 50% of cases.[10] Gout can present in any joint, and the inflammation can be extremely subtle in some cases; hence a search for crystals should be undertaken for all arthritis of unknown etiology. More than half of women with gout have polyarticular disease,[11] a presentation that is also common in the elderly. Chronic gout is uncommon but does occur, most often in postmenopausal women. Attacks of acute gout commonly follow trauma or surgery, especially in patients with hyperuricemia.

Diagnosis of Acute Gout

With acute oligoarticular gout the skin over the affected joint is usually red and warm; peeling of the skin is common, and pain is typically so severe the patient does not allow anything to touch the affected joint. Low-grade fever, elevated peripheral white blood cell (WBC) count, and elevated erythrocyte sedimentation rate (ESR) are commonly seen in patients with acute gout. Because of these characteristics the appearance of acute oligoarticular gout is distinctive, and the most important item in the differential diagnosis is joint infection. This distinction can be particularly troublesome in the hand.[12]

Diagnostic Studies

The serum uric acid level is not helpful for excluding or confirming a diagnosis of gout. Although clinical diagnostic criteria have been developed for acute gout, examination of syn-

Table 123.1. **Some Possible Causes of Hyperuricemia**

Endogenous causes
    Family history
    Overproduction or underexcretion of urate
    Large body build
    Rapid cell turnover (malignancy)
    Renal failure
    Hypertension
Exogenous causes
    Dietary purine: organ meats, kale, spinach, shellfish, beans
    Alcohol, especially beer
    Medications: especially diuretics and antimetabolites (e.g.,
        cyclosporine)
    Poisons: lead, others

ovial fluid under polarized light provides the only definitive diagnosis.[13] Acute synovitis due to deposition of pyrophosphate crystals (pseudogout) becomes more common after age 65, so joint aspiration is particularly important for this age group.

Synovial fluid can easily be obtained by passing an 18-gauge or smaller needle into the joint and aspirating it. Many clinicians prefer to numb the surrounding soft tissue with lidocaine before attempting joint entry. Joint fluid is then sent for crystal examination, cell count, Gram stain, and culture. The cell count is over 20,000/cu mL in those with gout or infection, and counts as high as 100,000/cu mL may be seen with either; the presence of crystals is the only reliable indicator that gout rather than infection is present. The needle-shaped crystals of gout have a unique appearance under polarized light; they are about the size of a neutrophil and are commonly seen inside them. In patients with acute gout the joint radiographs may be normal, but the erosions seen with chronic gout are fairly specific and can be helpful in making that diagnosis (Fig. 123.1). Radiographs can help identify unsuspected fractures or osteomyelitis in patients with acute arthritis.[14]

Treatment of Gout and Hyperuricemia

Treatment of gout specifically addresses one of three clinical entities: (1) acute gout, (2) the intercritical period that occurs for 2 to 3 months after an acute attack, or (3) long-term management of chronic hyperuricemia.

Treatment of Acute Gout

Attacks of acute gout are most commonly managed by nonsteroidal antiinflammatory drugs (NSAIDs) (see Chapter 112). High doses are needed. Although all NSAIDs are probably effective for acute gout, indomethacin (Indocin) is commonly used. One regimen involves giving indomethacin 50 mg four times a day for the first 2 days, then 50 mg three times a day for a week, then 50 mg twice a day for a week, then 25 mg two or three times a day for 2 to 3 weeks (or more). Acute gout can also be treated with colchicine in a dose of 0.6 mg/hr by mouth up to a total of 5 or 6 mg until relief or severe gastrointestinal side effects occur. At one time it was thought that colchicine was effective only for acute

gouty arthritis, and so its use had utility in the differential diagnosis; it is now known that colchicine is at times successful for any form of acute arthritis.[15] Colchicine can be given intravenously, a method that reduces side effects; but the drug is potentially toxic in this form, and it is recommended that physicians considering the use of intravenous colchicine carefully review the instructions for its use.[16] For patients who are unlikely to tolerate treatment with NSAIDs or colchicine (e.g., those with gastrointestinal disease or renal failure), intraarticular or even systemic steroids can be used. Another option is the use of a single dose of 60 mg of depo-triamcinolone (Kenalog) intramuscularly.[17] Adrenocorticotropic hormone (ACTH) is also effective in a dose of 0.4 mg (40 units) IM, which may have to be repeated every 12 hours for 2 to 3 days.[13,18]

Management of Intercritical Gout

Patients who have had resolution of an acute gouty attack are susceptible to a recurrence in the same joint for the next 2 to 3 months, a period known as the intercritical period. Hence, preventive therapy is indicated for several months after an acute attack. Oral colchicine at 0.6 mg one or two times a day is effective for this purpose and is unlikely to have any side effects. Low-dose colchicine can be started along with NSAIDs at the time of an acute attack. Another alternative is low-dose NSAID therapy, such as indomethacin 25 mg twice a day, though this alternative is more likely to cause side effects.

Hypouricemic agents (e.g., allopurinol or probenecid) worsen an acute gouty attack and are never used during one. After some weeks of intercritical treatment the possibility of starting chronic drug therapy to lower the serum uric acid level can be considered. In patients who have only an occa-

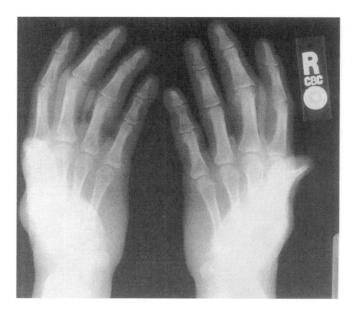

Fig. 123.1. Radiograph of the hand of a patient with gout. There are typical margin erosions and areas of radiolucency at the proximal interphalangeal joints of the index and long fingers bilaterally.

sional gouty attack and have no complication of gout such as tophi or gouty renal disease (see section below), treatment of hyperuricemia is optional; some patients prefer the risk of an occasional attack to taking medicine on a long-term basis. Patients who believe their attacks are frequent enough to justify treatment or in whom treatment is indicated because of tophi or gouty renal disease should undergo treatment directed at hyperuricemia. Most experts believe that dietary therapy is of marginal benefit in lowering uric acid levels,[19] although patients should be advised to lose weight and reduce consumption of alcohol, meats, fat, and cholesterol. Hydration is important. Avoidance of medications that elevate the serum uric acid level is also helpful. Low-dose aspirin, niacin, and diuretics are the most common of these agents, and cyclosporine is another offender.

Hyperuricemia

Medical treatment of hyperuricemia involves use of either uricosuric agents or allopurinol (Zyloprim), an agent that interferes with uric acid metabolism. The choice of agent depends on patient characteristics. Allopurinol is indicated in patients with nephrolithiasis, tophi, or renal disease. It is also indicated in patients with congenital overproduction of uric acid. These patients can be identified by collecting a 24-hour urine specimen for uric acid assay; the uric acid content is more than 1 g in overproducers (some clinicians use 600 or 800 mg as the cutoff).

Patients with hyperuricemia who excrete less than 1 g/24 hr are considered to be underexcreters and can be treated with a uricosuric agent instead of allopurinol unless they have nephrolithiasis, tophi, or renal failure. Probenecid (Benemid), the most commonly used uricosuric agent, is started at 250 mg twice a day for a few days, then increased to 500 mg twice a day, and gradually increased up to a total of 3 g/day if needed. The goal of therapy is to get the serum uric acid below 6.0 mg/dL (360 μmol/L), although a level of 5 mg/dL (300 μmol/L) or less more effectively dissolves uric acid crystals. Gastric intolerance to probenecid is fairly common, and many drug interactions occur; for example, aspirin eliminates the uricosuric effect of probenecid. The cost of probenecid is also slightly higher than that of allopurinol. For this reason, many clinicians prefer to use allopurinol even in underexcreters. It is effective against any form of hyperuricemia.

Allopurinol should be started at a dose of 100 mg/day and increased gradually up to 300 mg/day if needed to keep the serum uric acid under 6.0 mg/dL (360 μmol/L). If the serum uric acid remains elevated in a patient on allopurinol 300 mg/day, noncompliance should be suspected,[20] although doses up to 800 mg/day are occasionally needed. The most common side effect of allopurinol is a rash; a vasculitic syndrome affecting the skin and kidneys accompanied by fever, leukocytosis, eosinophilia, and hepatitis may be seen. This syndrome is more common among the elderly and in patients with renal failure or on diuretic therapy; in these patients use of the lowest possible dose of allopurinol and a goal of 7 mg/dL (420 μmol/L) rather than 6 mg/dL (360 μmol/L) can be considered. When this syndrome occurs, it is treated with high-dose steroids.

Acute attacks of gout are common when either uricosuric agents or allopurinol are started, even if several months have elapsed since the patient's last attack. It is important to warn patients of this possibility. Continuing prophylactic therapy with colchicine at 0.6 mg once or twice a day for the first year of hypouricemic therapy is advised. Starting with low doses of hypouricemic agents, as noted above, is also helpful. Urate-lowering drugs should not be started until a month has passed since the last acute attack of gout, and, if possible, colchicine should be started first and continued for the first few months of treatment with urate-lowering therapy, although the risk of possible toxicity to colchicine needs to be considered.[13]

Finally, patient education is an important component in the management of gout. Patients need to understand the difference between the agents used to control acute gout, the intercritical period, and chronic therapy with urate-lowering agents, or there will be substantial confusion and worsening of their condition.[20] Patients need to be followed regularly by the same provider with frequent monitoring of their uric acid levels for those on urate-lowering therapy; patient education can occur during these visits.

Uric Acid Nephropathy

Uric acid nephropathy is caused by precipitation of uric acid crystals in the renal tubules (see Chapter 97). It is usually due to a sudden overproduction of uric acid in a dehydrated patient (e.g., following vigorous exercise).[21] Uric acid nephropathy can also be seen in patients with aggressive leukemia or during chemotherapy leading to rapid cell turnover. Uric acid nephropathy can be treated with vigorous hydration, diuretics, and alkalinization of urine; prevention is often possible if patients at risk are kept well hydrated.

Tophi

Tophi are aggregates of uric acid crystals surrounded by a giant cell foreign-body reaction. They gradually enlarge with time and eventually become first radiopaque and then obvious on physical examination. They appear around joints and in the subcutaneous tissues. Their presence is an indication for allopurinol therapy, which gradually leads to their dissolution. Tophi are much less common now than previously, probably because hyperuricemia is treated more aggressively.[13]

Pseudogout

Arthritis due to deposition of calcium pyrophosphate dihydrate, or calcium pyrophosphate deposition disease (CPDD), is often called pseudogout. The knee is the most commonly affected joint; the disease is much more common in the elderly. Radiographs show chondrocalcinosis. The diagnosis is made by synovial fluid analysis; the joint fluid is similar to that seen in gout except that the crystals are characteristic. Treatment of an acute attack is the same as that for acute gout, and colchicine prophylaxis can prevent recurrence.

References

1. Peacock DJ, Cooper C. Epidemiology of the rheumatic diseases. Curr Opin Rheumatol 1995;7(2):82–6.
2. Gabriel SE. Update on the epidemiology of the rheumatic diseases. Curr Opin Rheumatol 1996;8(2):96–100.
3. Harris MD, Siegel LB, Alloway JA. Gout and hyperuricemia. Am Fam Physician 1999;59(4):925–34.
4. Campion EW, Glynn RJ, DeLarby DO. Asymptomatic hyperuricemia: risks and consequences in the Normative Aging Study. Am J Med 1987;82:421–6.
5. Van Doomum S, Ryan PFJ. Clinical manifestations of gout and their management. Med J Aust 2000;172:493–7.
6. Davis JC. A practical approach to gout. Postgrad Med 1999; 106(4):115–23.
7. Berkowitz D. Gout, hyperlipidemia, and diabetes interrelationships. JAMA 1966;197:41:227–42.
8. Johnson RJ, Kivlighn SD, Kim Y, et al. Reappraisal of the pathogenesis and consequences of hyperuricemia in hypertension, cardiovascular disease, and renal disease. Am J Kidney Dis 1999;33(2):225–34.
9. Pittman JR, Bross MH. Diagnosis and management of gout. Am Fam Physician 1999;59(7):1799–806.
10. Snaith ML. Gout, hyperuricemia, and crystal arthritis. BMJ 1995;310:521–4.
11. Joseph J, McGrath H. Gout or 'pseudogout': how to differentiate crystal-induced arthropathies. Geriatrics 1995;50(4):13–39.
12. Louis DS, Jebson DL. Mimickers of hand infections. Hand Clin 1998;14(4):519–29.
13. Fam AG. Managing problem gout. Ann Acad Med Singapore 1998;27:93–9.
14. Beutler A, Schumacher HR. Gout and 'pseudogout': when are arthritic symptoms caused by crystal deposition? Postgrad Med 1994;2:103–20.
15. Ben-Chetrit E, Micha L. Colchicine: 1998 update. Semin Arthritis Rheum 1998;28(1):48–59.
16. Milne ST, Meek PD. Fatal colchicine overdose: report of a case and review of the literature. Am J Emerg Med 1998;16(6): 603–8.
17. Alloway JA, Moriarty MJ, Hoogland YT, et al. Comparison of triamcinolone acetonide with indomethacin in the treatment of acute gouty arthritis. J Rheumatol 1993;20:1383–5.
18. Axelrod D, Preston D. A comparison of parenteral adrenocorticotrophic hormone with indomethacin in the treatment of acute gout. Arthritis Rheum 1988;31:803–5.
19. Emmerson BT. The management of gout. N Engl J Med 1996; 334(7):445–51.
20. Corkill MM. Gout. NZ Med J 1994;107:337–9.
21. Wortmann RL. Effective management of gout: an analogy. Am J Med 1998;105:513–14.

124
Selected Disorders of the Endocrine and Metabolic System

Richard D. Blondell

The endocrine system governs the metabolic activities of the body, affects tissue growth, regulates the functioning of many organ systems, and influences behavior and cognition. Because the endocrine system is involved in an extraordinary range of physiologic processes, it is important to consider an endocrine disorder in many clinical situations, especially when a patient presents with vague multisystem complaints.

Pituitary

The pituitary (hypophysis) has two distinct parts—an anterior lobe (adenohypophysis) and a posterior lobe (neurohypophysis)—that have different embryologic origins. There is also a vestigial intermediate lobe. The neurohypophysis is not a true gland. Instead, macroneurons of the hypothalamus project to the posterior pituitary and release either vasopressin (also called antidiuretic hormone, ADH) or oxytocin, two similar 9-amino-acid peptides, into capillary beds. Neurons of the hypothalamus secrete hormones (e.g., gonadotropin-releasing hormone, GnRH) that are carried to the adenohypophysis via a tiny portal vein system and regulate the production and pulsatile release of hormones (Table 124.1) by the different cell types of the adenohypophysis. Excess secretion of anterior pituitary hormones may be due to hypothalamic stimulation, loss of hypothalamic inhibition, or a hormone-secreting adenoma. If an adenoma is secretory, usually only one hormone is produced, which is typically prolactin, growth hormone (GH), or adrenocorticotropin (ACTH).

Hyperprolactinemia and Galactorrhea

Prolactin is a 198-amino-acid hormone that is required for lactation but not breast development. Hyperprolactinemia may be noted during the evaluation of breast discharge (see Chapter 106), menstrual disorders, infertility, or impotence. Because the hypothalamus inhibits pituitary prolactin release, any condition that affects the hypothalamus or the pituitary stalk causing hypopituitarism (e.g., neurosarcoidosis) may

lead to hyperprolactinemia. Also the pituitary may be prompted to secrete prolactin when the sensory nerves of the breast are stimulated by trauma, scars, breast implants, neoplasms, or herpes zoster or with nipple stimulation from loose-fitting clothes or during sexual foreplay. Physiologic causes of prolactin release include pregnancy, hypoglycemia, stress, food ingestion, and sleep. Pituitary prolactin release can be induced pharmacologically by drugs commonly used in clinical practice: narcotics, estrogens, verapamil, α-methyldopa, reserpine, tricyclic antidepressants, and dopamine receptor antagonists, such as phenothiazines, butyrophenones (haloperidol), and thioxanthenes. Hyperprolactinemia is also associated with certain chronic diseases: renal failure, cirrhosis, and hypothyroidism (see Chapters 90, 97, and 121). Prolactin may be secreted by pituitary adenomas and, on rare occasions, by nonpituitary neoplasms.

Clinical Presentation

The principal clinical features of hyperprolactinemia are stimulation of milk production and suppression of gonadal function through processes that are not well understood. Women present with galactorrhea, amenorrhea or oligomenorrhea, infertility, vaginal dryness, and dyspareunia. Men present with infertility loss of libido, impotence, and occasionally galactorrhea. If hyperprolactinemia is due to a pituitary adenoma, women usually present early because of menstrual abnormalities, whereas men may not present until there are symptoms or signs of the pituitary mass (e.g., headaches or visual difficulties).

Diagnosis

Serum prolactin levels can vary with age, gender, and reproductive status, but normal values are typically <20 ng/mL. To distinguish between nonpregnant patients who may have spuriously elevated serum prolactin levels (usually <50 ng/mL) from those with pathologically elevated levels, baseline values several hours after awakening, before a meal, and under minimal distress are obtained. Serum prolactin values

Table 124.1. **Hormones of the Adenohypophysis**

Cell type (staining characteristics)	Hormone(s) secreted	Target site	Clinical consequence of excess	Clinical consequence of deficiency
Somatotrophs (eosinophilic)	GH	Bones Glucose metabolism	Gigantism, acromegaly Glucose intolerance	Dwarfism Fasting hypoglycemia
Lactotrophs (eosinophilic)	Prolactin	Breasts	Galactorrhea	Inability to lactate
Corticotrophs (basophilic)	ACTH β-Lipoprotein	Adrenal cortex Skin	Cushing syndrome Hyperpigmentation	Adrenal insufficiency Hypopigmentation
Thyrotrophs (chromophobic)	TSH	Thyroid	Hyperthyroidism[a]	Hypothyroidism
Gonadotrophs (chromophobic)	FSH, LH	Females: ovaries Male: testes	Precocious puberty	Delayed puberty, infertility, loss of secondary sexual characteristics

GH = growth hormone; ACTH = adrenocorticotropin hormone; TSH = thyroid-stimulating hormone; FSH = follicle-stimulating hormone; LH = luteinizing hormone.

[a]Secondary hyperthyroidism is a rare condition. Chromophobe adenomas are usually nonsecretory.

greater than 200 ng/mL are usually due to pituitary adenomas, which are best visualized by magnetic resonance imaging (MRI).[1] A detailed clinical history and physical examination often provide clues of the cause of hyperprolactinemia when values are between 20 and 200 ng/mL. The patient is asked about drug use, visual problems, and sexual practices or clothing that might cause nipple stimulation. The chest is inspected for lesions and scars. Thyroid function tests, a mammogram, or MRI of the sella and hypothalamus may be required.

Management

Explanation, reassurance, advice, or medication change may be sufficient treatment for patients who have hyperprolactinemia due to local stimulation or medication. An underlying condition should be treated if possible. Dopamine-agonist drugs suppress prolactin secretion and restore gonadal function. For more than 20 years, bromocriptine has been the standard treatment for hyperprolactinemia-associated dysfunctions and minimally symptomatic prolactin-secreting microadenomas (i.e., <1 cm). The usual dose is 2.5 to 15.0 mg/day. Side effects (nausea, dizziness, and orthostatic hypotension) are limiting factors in 5% to 10% of patients.[2] Pergolide and cabergoline are dopamine agonists that may be better tolerated than bromocriptine. Quinagolide is a well-tolerated, long-acting selective dopamine D2 receptor agonist that has been used in Europe for several years.[3] Transsphenoidal surgery remains the mainstay of treatment for the majority of pituitary adenomas; however, up to 10% of adenomas may recur following surgery.[4]

Acromegaly and Gigantism

Excessive secretion of GH (hypersomatotropism) typically presents between the third and fifth decade of life, and is nearly always caused by a pituitary adenoma and can result in acromegaly. Hypersomatotropism is rare among children, but if it occurs in a child before the closure of the epiphyses,

it causes exaggerated skeletal growth known as pituitary gigantism.

Clinical Presentation

Acromegaly typically presents with the insidious onset of excessive bone growth of the hands, feet, face, and skull. Patients may note the need for larger hats, gloves, rings, and shoes. Overgrowth of the mandible leads to dental malocclusion and a protrusion of the jaw known as prognathism. Family members may note a change in the patient's appearance, which may be obvious from old photographs. The skin becomes thickened with an increase in coarse body hair and an increase in sweat and sebaceous gland function, which can lead to an offensive body odor. There is stimulation of cartilage growth; articular cartilage can undergo necrosis and erosion, causing joint pain; nasopharyngeal overgrowth can cause hoarseness and sleep apnea; and enlargement of the larynx leads to a deep voice. The tongue is enlarged and furrowed. Hypersomatotropism also causes the enlargement of the soft tissues and most viscera.

Diagnosis

The diagnosis can be made through recognition of the constellation of clinical symptoms and signs and is confirmed by the laboratory. Serum levels of GH and insulin-like growth factor I (IGF-I) will be elevated. A morning fasting level of serum GH should be obtained and compared to one obtained 90 minutes after the oral administration of 75 g of glucose, which will normally suppress GH production. The cause is usually due to a macroadenoma (i.e., an adenoma greater than 1 cm in diameter) and is best demonstrated by MRI.

Management

Transsphenoidal surgical resection is generally the preferred treatment, and it usually produces a substantial reduction of GH and IGF-I secretion and an improvement in symptoms.[2] However, some patients will have persistent or recurrent hypersecretion after surgery. Ablative radiotherapy is also used, but hormone levels may take years to decrease. The medications that have been used to reduce GH hypersecretion include dopamine agonists (e.g., bromocriptine, cabergoline) and the somatostatin analogues (e.g., octreotide, lanreotide). Pegvisomant, a genetically engineered GH-receptor antagonist, has been developed for the treatment of acromegaly, which is given by daily subcutaneous injections.[5]

Hypopituitarism

Hypofunction of the pituitary is a rare disorder that may be either partial or complete (panhypopituitarism). It is caused by a number of disorders that disturb the gland directly (primary hypopituitarism) or the hypothalamus (secondary hypopituitarism) (Table 124.2).

Clinical Presentation

Children may present with growth failure and delayed puberty. Adults typically present with a confusing array of psychological problems, family or social difficulties, and multisystem somatic complaints that are due to hormonal deficiencies and the underlying disease that causes the hypopituitarism. Common complaints include fatigue, weight loss, dry skin, menstrual abnormalities, and sexual dysfunction. Symptoms may develop abruptly (as in the Sheehan syndrome) or

Table 124.2. **Selected Causes of Hypopituitarism**

Neoplastic causes
Adenoma
Craniopharyngioma
Metastases

Ischemic causes
Sheehan syndrome (postpartum pituitary necrosis)
Diabetic microvascular disease
Temporal arteritis

Granulomatous causes
Sarcoidosis
Wegener's granulomatosis
Hand-Schüller-Christian syndrome

Developmental causes
Congenital malformation
Developmental cyst
Hydrocephalus

Infectious causes
Tuberculosis
Syphilis
Fungal disease
Meningitis, abscess

Physical causes
Trauma, especially basal skull fractures
Radiation therapy
Surgery, hypophysectomy
Toxic atmosphere (vincristine)

Miscellaneous causes
Pituitary apoplexy
Cavernous sinus thrombosis
Primary empty sella syndrome
Immunologic (lymphocytic hypophysitis)
Idiopathic (occasionally familial)

slowly (as with a slow-growing nonsecretory adenoma). Partial loss of pituitary function might mimic primary failure of the target site. Panhypopituitarism is ultimately fatal. Patients appear pale and chronically ill with a loss of secondary sexual characteristics. Galactorrhea can occur in secondary hypopituitarism (e.g., hypothalamic sarcoidosis) because the hypothalamus inhibits pituitary prolactin. Lack of ADH produces polydipsia and polyuria.

Diagnosis

If the patient is viewed as a whole, the diagnosis is suggested by the clinical history and examination and can be confirmed by simultaneously measuring serum pituitary and target gland hormone levels.[6] MRI is the preferred method for evaluating hypothalamic and pituitary anatomy.

Management

Treatment is aimed at the underlying condition and replacement of target gland hormones (Table 124.3). A deficiency of glucocorticoids is corrected before thyroid hormone replacement to prevent precipitating an adrenal crisis. Because aldosterone secretion is unaffected, mineralocorticoids are not necessary. Sex hormones can be started once the patient is euthyroid, but gonadotropins are required to restore fertility. In children, GH is required. In adults, replacement of GH reduces body fat, increases muscle mass and bone density, and improves exercise tolerance in the short term; the long-term benefits have not been evaluated. These patients should wear a medical identification bracelet or necklace.

Empty Sella Syndrome

With empty sella syndrome the pituitary is flattened against the unyielding bone by the arachnoid space, which, for unknown reasons, herniates into the sella. Because the gland is not destroyed, there may be little if any pituitary dysfunction. The condition is noted occasionally as an incidental radiologic finding. Pituitary function can be monitored clinically or by periodically measuring pituitary hormone levels if indicated.

Water Balance and the Neuroendocrine System

The neuroendocrine system plays a role in regulating water balance by three interrelated mechanisms: vasopressin, renal function, and thirst. Abnormalities of this regulation may present clinically as hyponatremia, hypernatremia, or polyuria and polydipsia (see Chapter 96). Hyponatremia may be due to excessive sodium excretion (e.g., Addison's disease) or to reduced water excretion as with the syndrome of inappropriate secretion of ADH (SIADH).

Polyuria

Polyuria may be due to central diabetes insipidus (DI), nephrogenic DI, an osmotic diuresis, or primary polydipsia.[7]

1066 Richard D. Blondell

Table 124.3. **Hormone Replacement Therapy**

Class of medication	Usual adult dose[a]
Glucocorticoids[b]	
Hydrocortisone[c]	10–20 q A.M.; 5–10 mg q P.M.[e]
Cortisone[d]	25 mg q A.M.; 12.5 mg q P.M.[e]
Prednisone[d]	5 mg q A.M.; 2.5 mg q P.M.[e]
Therapeutic end point: elimination of clinical signs and symptoms	
Overtreatment: development of Cushing syndrome	
Mineralocorticoids[f]	
Fludrocortisone (Florinef)	0.1 mg qd–qod
Therapeutic end point: normalization of blood pressure without postural hypotension, and normalization of serum sodium and potassium	
Overtreatment: edema, hypertension, hypokalemia	
Thyroid hormone	
Levothyroxine (Levoxyl, Synthroid)	1.6 μg/kg/day
Therapeutic end point: minimum dose required to normalize serum TSH[g] in primary hypothyroidism, normal serum T_4 levels in secondary hypothyroidism	
Overtreatment: symptoms of hyperthyroidism, suppressed serum TSH[g] or elevated serum T_4	
Estrogens[h]	
Conjugated estrogens (Premarin)	0.625–1.25 mg qd
Estradiol	0.5–2 mg qd
Estropipate (Ortho-Est, Ogen)	1.5–9 mg qd
Estradiol (Climara, Vivelle) (transdermal)	0.05–0.1 mg/day patch (twice weekly)
Therapeutic end point: restoration of secondary sexual characteristics, elimination of vasomotor symptoms, production of menstruation (if uterus present)	
Overtreatment: edema, nausea, vomiting, dysfunctional bleeding	
Progestogens[h]	
Medroxyprogesterone (Provera, Cycrin)	2.5–10 mg qd
Norethindrone (Micronor, Nor-QD)	0.35 mg qd
Therapeutic end point: production of withdrawal bleeding without breakthrough	
Overtreatment: breast tenderness, nonspecific gastrointestinal symptoms	
Testosterones[i]	
Testosterone cypionate or enanthate (IM)	200–400 mg q2–4 weeks
Testosterone (transdermal)	One 5 mg patch qd
Therapeutic end point: restoration of secondary sexual characteristics	
Overtreatment: excessive acne and aggressive behavior	
Antidiuretics	
Desmopressin[j] (DDAVP) (intranasal)	10–40 μg/day (divided BID–TID)
Therapeutic end point: lowest possible dose needed to control symptoms	
Overtreatment: Water intoxication	

[a]All doses are oral unless otherwise noted.

[b]Acute treatment: hydrocortisone 100 mg IV.

[c]Has some mineralocorticoid effect.

[d]Has little mineralocorticoid effect; can be given as single daily dose.

[e]Double dose during moderate illnesses (fevers, gastroenteritis).

[f]Not required for secondary hypoadrenalism (i.e., hypopituitarism).

[g]As measured by a highly sensitive TSH assay.

[h]When given clinically to produce menses: estrogens are given qd on days 1 to 25 each month; progestogens are given qd during the final 7–14 days (e.g., days 16 to 25). Estrogen/progestogen combination products or birth control pills can be used as an alternative.

[i]Because of potential liver toxicity, oral androgens are not considered to be first-line treatment.

[j]Injectable also available.

Nephrogenic DI may be congenital or acquired. Common causes of the acquired form are chronic renal disease, systemic diseases causing nephropathy (e.g., myeloma, hypercalcemia, sickle cell disease), nephrotoxins (e.g., aminoglycosides, meclocycline, lithium), and postobstructive nephropathy. Polyuria is also seen with the osmotic diuresis of diabetes mellitus (see Chapter 120) and with poorly resorbed solutes (e.g., mannitol, sorbitol).

Polydipsia

Secondary polydipsia is protective for patients with polyuria from any cause. When access to water is limited, dehydration, hypernatremia, and death can result. Primary polydipsia is common among psychiatric patients, but the pathophysiology is not completely understood.[8] The disorder is voluntary in some patients, but in others it may be related to psychotic delusions (psychogenic polydipsia) or to some unknown abnormality in the thirst mechanism (dipsogenic polydipsia). The anticholinergic effects of the medications used in psychiatric patients may cause or exacerbate polydipsia. The clinician must not automatically assume that psychogenic polydipsia is the cause of polyuria or hyponatremia in a given psychiatric patient and should search for some other underlying disease. Although a water deprivation test could be helpful for diagnosis, it may be difficult or impossible to perform in psychiatric patients. In such situations the clinician could evaluate the patient for hypopituitarism biochemically and radiographically. The function of the thyroid, adrenals, and kidneys may also need to be evaluated.

Central Diabetes Insipidus

There are several types of familial DI, but all are rare. Over 95% of the cases of central DI are due to an acquired deficiency of ADH by the disorders causing hypopituitarism (Table 124.1). This deficiency can occur through the loss of the large hypothalamic neurons that synthesize ADH or via the destruction of the posterior pituitary capillary beds.[9] Central DI may be partial or complete, transient or permanent, associated with other pituitary deficiencies or the sole abnormality. A transient form is associated with pregnancy.[10] There are two types of ADH receptors. V_1 receptors mediate the pressor effects of ADH and V_2 receptors are responsible for the antidiuretic and hemostatic effects (i.e., release of factor VIII and von Willebrand's factor).

Clinical Presentation

Depending on the underlying etiology, the onset of central DI may be gradual or abrupt. Polyuria and polydipsia are the only findings in the idiopathic form, but acquired central DI may also present with the symptoms and signs of the associated pituitary lesion. Large volumes (>30 mL/kg) of dilute urine (specific gravity <1.010, osmolality <300 mOsm/L) are excreted over a 24-hour period. Nocturia is usually present.

Diagnosis

A water deprivation test is used to distinguish DI from other causes of polyuria. In a controlled setting water intake is restricted, and the weight and the sodium and osmolarity of the plasma and urine are measured hourly. The patient should not be allowed to lose more than 5% of body weight. Dilute urine in the face of concentrated serum suggests DI. Then vasopressin (5 units SC) is administered to differentiate central DI from nephrogenic DI.

Management

The treatment of central DI is directed at the underlying cause if possible. Synthetic analogs of ADH (Table 124.3) that can be given intranasally are used to treat central DI. Absorption may be erratic with a common cold or allergic rhinitis. Partial central DI may be treated successfully with diuretics (thiazides) or ADH-releasing drugs (e.g., chlorpropamide, carbamazepine). Patients with DI should wear medical identification.

Disorders of Secondary Sexual Characteristics

Puberty is the process leading to physical and sexual maturation that involves the development not only of secondary sexual characteristics but also skeletal growth, alterations in lean body mass, and psychological changes (see Chapter 22). Normal puberty consists of two main endocrinologic events: adrenarche and gonadarche. Adrenarche is the increased secretion of adrenal androgens that normally occurs in both genders between 6 and 8 years of age, usually preceding gonadarche. It is associated with bone growth and changes in pilosebaceous units. Although the adrenals account for some pubic hair growth, the biologic role of adrenarche is not completely understood.[11] Gonadarche is initiated by the hypothalamus. Episodic secretion of GnRH by the hypothalamus results in the pulsatile secretion of the gonadotropins follicle-stimulating hormone (FSH) and luteinizing hormone (LH) by the anterior pituitary. In boys LH stimulates testosterone secretion by the Leydig cells, and after spermarche FSH supports the maturation of spermatozoa. In girls FSH stimulates follicle formation and estrogen secretion. After the onset of ovulation, LH stimulates the development of the corpus within a ruptured graafian follicle. Normal puberty begins between the ages of 8 and 13 in girls and 9 and 14 in boys. Puberty that begins before the lower end of these ranges is deemed precocious, and puberty that does not start before the upper end of these ranges is considered delayed. In girls puberty is heralded by breast development and skeletal growth, followed by the appearance of pubic and axillary hair and then menarche. In boys it is announced by testicular enlargement and is followed by the appearance of pubic hair and enlargement of the penis. Skeletal growth is a late event of male puberty (see Chapter 22). The etiology of a pubertal disorder can often be determined by a focused medical history, a directed physical examination, and appropriate diagnostic tests.[12] Disorders of puberty cause much apprehension. Treatment is determined by the underlying cause.

Precocious Puberty

Precocious puberty could be caused by either a central process [central nervous system (CNS), pituitary] or a peripheral process (Table 124.4). Central precocious puberty is due to the premature production of gonadotropins, which is often physiologic except in young children, when pathologic processes are more likely. Peripheral precocious puberty, always a pathologic condition, is caused by the early appearance of sex hormones. To distinguish between central and peripheral precocious puberty, the order of appearance of the various sexual characteristics are noted as well as the ages of the onset of puberty in family members. The height, weight,

Table 124.4. **Causes of Precocious Puberty**

Central precocious puberty
  True precocious puberty
  Central nervous system lesions
  Gonadotropin-secreting tumor
  Profound hypothyroidism
  Chronic adrenal insufficiency

Peripheral (pseudo) precocious puberty
  Girls
    Ovarian tumor
    Follicular cysts
    Exogenous estrogens
  Boys
    Testicular tumor
    Autonomous Leydig cell function
    Exogenous androgens
  Either
    Polyostotic fibrous dysplasia
    Adrenal tumor
    Adrenal hyperplasia

Tanner stages of breast development, axillary and pubic hair growth, and the genitalia are documented (see Tables 22.1 and 22.2). Radiographs of the left wrist for bone age may be useful, and a difference of more than 2 standard deviations is considered abnormal.

Girls with breast development and pubic hair are likely to have true precocious puberty that is either constitutional (often familial) or idiopathic (i.e., without other pathologic findings). The latter accounts for about 75% of the cases. In either situation, normal pubertal serum levels of FSH, LH, and estradiol are noted. Pathologic causes are not likely to produce both feminization and sexual hair growth. Hyperandrogenism is considered if acne or virilization occurs in the absence of feminization. A pathologic cause is sought if puberty occurs in girls aged ≤6 years.

Boys with precocious puberty have a benign central cause about half of the time, characterized by symmetrically enlarging testicles, virilization, and pubertal levels of FSH, LH, and testosterone. Headaches may be an important diagnostic clue for a CNS abnormality. Participation in sports may lead to abuse of androgens in an effort to "bulk up."[13] Androgens of exogenous or adrenal origin cause physical and sexual development without testicular enlargement. Unilateral testicular enlargement suggests neoplasia. If a pathologic cause for central precocious puberty is suspected, diagnostic images of the head and tests of pituitary function are essential. If a peripheral cause is suspected, biochemical and radiographic evaluation of the adrenals may be worthwhile.

Delayed Puberty

Boys who have not demonstrated testicular enlargement by the age of 14 or for whom 5 years or more have passed between the initial and complete growth of the genitalia have delayed puberty. Girls who have not developed breast buds by the age of 13 or who exhibit primary amenorrhea (passage of 5 years or more between the appearance of breast buds and menarche) have delayed puberty. An appropriate initial as-

sessment consists of a medical history, a complete physical examination with particular attention to the timing of pubertal milestones, and a graph of height and weight. A radiograph of the left wrist for bone age should be obtained. Children with delayed puberty may then be grouped according to the initial assessment: those who appear normal, those who appear to have chromosomal abnormalities (e.g., Turner syndrome in girls, Klinefelter syndrome in boys), and those who appear to have a chronic disease (e.g., hypopituitarism, malignancies, chronic infections, malnutrition, anorexia nervosa). Those who seem normal except for pubertal delay may have a constitutional pubertal delay, primary hypogonadism (e.g., congenital defects, tumors, injuries, infections), or secondary hypogonadism (i.e., gonadotropin deficiency). Appropriate diagnostic tests include serum FSH, LH, estradiol (in girls), or testosterone (in boys); a GnRH stimulation test; and MRI if a CNS lesion is suspected.

Hypogonadism in Adults

Adults may present to their physicians with infertility and loss of secondary sexual characteristics. In men, primary hypogonadism is most often caused by exposure to physical agents (cytotoxic drugs, radiation, or alcohol), infections (mumps), or trauma requiring castration.[13] Women lose gonadal function following oophorectomy and during menopause, but ovarian failure before the age of 40 is considered premature. The serum pituitary gonadotropins (i.e., FSH and LH) are elevated with gonadal failure. Hormone replacement therapy (Table 124.3) can restore secondary sexual characteristics but not fertility. Unexplained loss of secondary sexual characteristics should prompt an evaluation for secondary hypogonadism (i.e., hypopituitarism) consisting of hormonal studies of the hypothalamic-pituitary axis and possibly MRI of the sella.

Hirsutism and Virilization

Traditionally physicians were taught to distinguish between familial or idiopathic hypertrichosis (a generalized increase in terminal hair density), and androgen-induced hirsutism or drug-induced hirsutism. Although certain drugs can cause excessive hair growth, it now appears that most women who have this problem have excess circulating or peripheral androgens.[14] Excessive hair growth can occur with anticonvulsants (e.g., phenytoin), androgenic progestins [medroxyprogesterone (Provera and others), norethindrone], antihypertensives (e.g., minoxidil), phenothiazine derivatives, danazol, and drugs that have androgenic activity (e.g., testosterone, anabolic steroids). An increased sensitivity of pilosebaceous units to androgens causes some forms of hirsutism.[15] Androgen-dependent hair growth is influenced by the ratio of estrogens and androgens and thus may be physiologic (e.g., as in menopause or obesity).

Clinical Presentation

Unwanted hair growth causes many women great concern. Hirsutism is the excessive growth of androgen-dependent hair (face, axilla, chest, suprapubic region) and may be associated with acne. Virilization refers to the androgen-dependent masculinization of a woman. It is characterized by clitoromegaly, voice deepening, increased muscle mass, increased libido, temporal balding, and hirsutism. When accompanied by defeminization (decrease in breast size and vaginal atrophy), it is always pathologic.

Diagnosis

Women with hirsutism and virilization are evaluated for hyperandrogenism. The source of androgens may be exogenous (anabolic steroids) or endogenous from the adrenals (adrenal tumor, adrenogenital syndrome) or ovaries (polycystic ovarian disease). Neoplasms of the adrenals, ovaries, and other locations may secrete androgens or gonadotropins (see Chapter 105). Appropriate initial tests include ultrasound images of the pelvis and selected serum assays: early morning cortisol (to screen for Cushing syndrome), testosterone, androstenedione, and dehydroepiandrosterone sulfate (DHEAS). If the patient with hirsutism has normal basal serum concentrations of testosterone, DHEAS, and androstenedione, an adrenal tumor is unlikely.[16] In women in whom these concentrations are elevated, a tumor is unlikely if the DHEAS and urinary 17-ketosteroid excretion are in the normal basal range and the serum cortisol concentration is less than 3.3 μg/dL after dexamethasone administration (0.5 mg q6h for 48 hours). Mildly elevated serum androgens that are promptly suppressed to the normal range after dexamethasone are most consistent with idiopathic hirsutism or polycystic ovaries, whereas moderately elevated serum 17-hydroxyprogesterone and testosterone values that are only partially suppressed are diagnostic of congenital adrenal hyperplasia. A tumor is likely if dexamethasone does not suppress hormone levels and the cortisol level remains $\geq$3.3 μg/dL.

Management

Treatment is directed at the underlying abnormality. Idiopathic hirsutism, a cosmetic problem, can be managed with shaving, plucking, or epilating wax. Skin irritation and odor tend to limit the use of chemical depilatories. Electrolysis offers a permanent, though expensive, low-risk solution. Hormone replacement can be offered to menopausal women. Selected patients are given spironolactone, a GnRH agonist, or an antiandrogen (e.g., finasteride).

Parathyroids and Calcium Metabolism

The parathyroids are four tiny glands located in the neck close to the thyroid that secrete parathyroid hormone (PTH), an 84-amino-acid peptide also called parathormone. PTH and vitamin D (a prohormone) are the principal regulators of calcium and phosphate. The actions of PTH include (1) osteoclast activation with liberation of calcium from bones; (2) enhancement of reabsorption of calcium from renal tubules; (3) stimulation of intestinal absorption of calcium directly and by promoting the production of renal calcitriol [1,25-dihydroxycholecalciferol (1,25-DHCC)]; and (4) inhibition of renal reabsorption of phosphates. Calcitonin, which inhibits bone resorption by a direct action on osteoclasts, is produced in response to hypercalcemia by perifollicular cells of the thy-roid. Excessive secretion of calcitonin does not usually cause hypocalcemia. It is rare with thyroid medullary carcinoma, which typically secretes large amounts of calcitonin.

Hyperparathyroidism and Hypercalcemia

The hypercalcemia of primary hyperparathyroidism is due to an autonomously functioning benign sporadic adenoma 85% of the time. Idiopathic or familial parathyroid hyperplasia account for most of the rest.[17] Rarely there may be multiple adenomas (as in multiple endocrine neoplasia type 1), a carcinoma of the parathyroid, or ectopic production of PTH by a malignancy. Other causes of hypercalcemia due to increased bone resorption include metastatic cancer, Paget's disease, hyperthyroidism, and immobilization. Hypercalcemia may also occur because of decreased renal excretion of calcium (thiazide diuretics, lithium) or with increased absorption of calcium from the gut (sarcoidosis, vitamin D intoxication). Prolonged tourniquet use can cause measured serum calcium levels to appear elevated.

Clinical Presentation

Hyperparathyroidism often becomes apparent on the basis of hypercalcemia discovered via "routine" multichemistry testing (see Chapter 7). A careful history may reveal the subtle psychological symptoms of hypercalcemia: anxiety, indecision, malaise, excessive worry, and irritability. Hypercalcemia may present as an acute or chronic illness with lethargy, nausea, vomiting, polydipsia, polyuria, impaired renal function, nephrocalcinosis, muscle atrophy, bradycardia, and electrocardiographic (ECG) changes (i.e., short QT).

Diagnosis

Elevated serum calcium levels are more than 10.5 mg/dL in most laboratories. Because almost half of the total serum calcium is protein-bound, an adjustment may be required if a variation in the serum protein level also exists. An increase of protein by 1 g/dL raises the measured total serum calcium by about 0.8 mg/dL. Since the ionized fraction of serum calcium is the biologically active form, it is the preferred diagnostic test of hypercalcemia and should be obtained at the same time as a serum PTH level. If cancer is a diagnostic possibility, a chest radiograph, a bone scan, and, in men, serum prostate-specific antigen (PSA) and alkaline phosphatase levels are useful tests. Patients with Paget's disease have characteristic radiographs of bones, and patients with sarcoidosis or tuberculosis may have abnormal chest radiographs. If hyperparathyroidism is suspected, measuring the serum PTH level is essential.

Management

The cornerstone of the management of hypercalcemia is treatment of the underlying disease. The options for the medical management of patients with minimal or no symptoms include maintenance of hydration, avoidance of immobilization, a modest dietary calcium intake, loop diuretics (thiazide diuretics are contraindicated because they enhance renal reabsorption of calcium), oral phosphates, estrogen replacement (for postmenopausal women), and calcitonin (for Paget's disease). Oral glucocorticoids in the lowest effective dose can be used for patients with malignancies or sarcoidosis. Acutely symptomatic patients usually require treatment in a hospital setting.[18] Bisphosphonates (e.g., pamidronate), gallium nitrate, plicamycin, etidronate, or acute dialysis may have a therapeutic role in some of these patients. Intravenous phosphates are used with caution as a last resort for patients with severe hypercalcemia.

The surgical treatment of hyperparathyroidism is controversial.[19] Patients who are asymptomatic or mildly symptomatic may be treated medically. Surgical treatment is usually indicated for symptomatic patients with parathyroid adenomas or hyperplasia. Minimally invasive procedures are becoming an alternative to conventional neck exploration.[20]

Hypoparathyroidism and Hypocalcemia

Hypoparathyroidism (usually following surgical removal of the parathyroids) results in hypocalcemia and, at times, hypomagnesemia. Hypoparathyroidism may also be inherited (DiGeorge syndrome) or it may be idiopathic, which occurs sporadically. Target organ unresponsiveness to PTH can be inherited. Because maintenance of appropriate serum calcium levels requires intestinal absorption of calcium, vitamin D deficiency, intestinal diseases, or poor dietary intake may also lead to hypocalcemia. Hypocalcemia can occur with renal tubular acidosis, renal failure, hypomagnesemia, and pancreatitis.

Clinical Presentation

The symptoms and signs of hypoparathyroidism are related to the degree of hypocalcemia and are primarily neurologic: paresthesias, Chvostek's sign, carpopedal spasms, tetany, delirium, seizures. Patients with mild symptoms might mimic patients with dementia, depression, or psychosis. A prolonged QT interval may be noted on ECG.

Diagnosis

Hypoalbuminemia is a common cause of an abnormally low serum calcium value. For every 1 g/dL decrease in total serum protein, the measured total serum calcium decreases by 0.8 mg/dL. An ionized serum calcium can be helpful. If it is abnormally low and hypoparathyroidism is suspected, a serum PTH assay is obtained at the same time as another ionized calcium level. Appropriately elevated PTH values are found with hypocalcemia associated with pancreatitis, hyperphosphatemia, and vitamin D deficiency (secondary hyperparathyroidism).

Management

Treatment is aimed at the underlying disease. One gram of calcium carbonate can be given with each meal and increased to 9 to 12 g/day (constipation can be a problem). Modest dietary restriction of protein decreases phosphorus absorption. Intravenous calcium is required for acutely ill patients.

Adrenal Dysfunction

The adrenals are complex glands and play a role in many endocrine and metabolic activities of the body. Although adrenal disease is uncommon, adrenal dysfunction may be the cause of a wide range of clinical problems. The adrenals are composed of an outer layer (the cortex) and an inner core (the medulla). The adrenal cortex secretes three main groups of steroid hormones: glucocorticoids, mineralocorticoids, and sex hormones. Glucocorticoid secretion is under pituitary control. The mineralocorticoids are part of the renin-angiotensin system. Control of sex hormone production is not well understood. The adrenal medulla secretes catecholamines (epinephrine, norepinephrine) and is controlled by the autonomic nervous system.

Adrenocortical Insufficiency

Adrenal hypofunction may be due to primary adrenal insufficiency (Addison's disease), or secondary adrenal insufficiency either from hypopituitarism or from suppression by long-term exogenous glucocorticoids. Addison's disease is uncommon in Western countries; most cases are idiopathic, but others are due to pathologic causes: tuberculosis, amyloidosis, neoplasia. Adrenal insufficiency may also be congenital or familial.

Clinical Presentation

Addison's disease typically has an insidious onset. Early symptoms and signs include malaise, fatigue, weakness, and orthostatic hypotension. Hyperpigmentation is also common with early disease; pale skin is typical of hypopituitarism. Late findings include anorexia, nausea, vomiting, diarrhea, hyponatremia, hyperkalemia, and fasting hypoglycemia. Because early disease may go unrecognized, patients may come to medical attention only during an adrenal crisis following some physical stress (e.g., surgery). An adrenal crisis is characterized by muscle weakness, severe abdominal pain, and hypotension followed by shock, renal shutdown, and death.

Diagnosis

Addison's disease is diagnosed by demonstrating the inability of the adrenal cortex to increase cortisol production during an ACTH stimulation test. Synthetic ACTH 0.25 mg is administered intramuscularly or intravenously before 10 A.M., and serum cortisol levels are determined at baseline and after 30, or preferably 60, minutes. There is some disagreement over the definition of a normal response, but adrenal function is considered to be normal if the basal or the post-ACTH plasma cortisol concentration is at least 18 to 20 μg/dL or greater.[21] If this test is abnormal, simultaneous 8:00 A.M. cortisol and ACTH levels can help to distinguish primary from secondary adrenal insufficiency. Low serum cortisol levels alone are not diagnostic of Addison's disease unless accompanied by persistently elevated levels of ACTH.

Management

Addison's disease is treated with glucocorticoid and mineralocorticoid hormone replacement therapy (Table 124.3). Glucocorticoids are administered if there is a suspicion of an adrenal crisis, which may also require fluid and electrolyte therapy and vasopressors. Patients who will be away from medical care should carry glucocorticoids for self-administration (injection or per rectum), and they should always wear medical identification.

Cushing Syndrome

Cushing syndrome commonly results from the long-term use of exogenous glucocorticoids. On rare occasions it may be caused by a glucocorticoid-producing adrenal adenoma or carcinoma, an ACTH-secreting pituitary adenoma (Cushing disease), or another ACTH-producing neoplasm (usually lung).

Clinical Presentation

Characteristically, affected patients demonstrate rounded "moon" facies, truncal obesity with a prominent dorsal cervical fat pad ("buffalo hump"), hypertension, hirsutism, osteoporosis, glucose intolerance, hypokalemia, and psychiatric disturbances. Patients may complain of proximal muscle weakness, menstrual abnormalities, and sexual dysfunction.

Diagnosis

Confirmation of the clinical diagnosis of adrenocorticoid excess and determining the cause may require the performance of a variety of tests.[22] If there is a clinical suspicion of Cushing syndrome, a 24-hour urine specimen for free cortisol assay or a rapid low-dose dexamethasone suppression test may be obtained. For the latter, the patient is instructed to take 1 mg of dexamethasone between 11:00 P.M. and midnight, and a serum cortisol level is obtained at 8:00 A.M. the next morning. A value ≤5 µg/dL is normal. Values ≥5 µg/dL require further evaluation with a 2-day dexamethasone suppression test.[23]

Management

Therapy is directed at eliminating the source of the excessive glucocorticoids through medication change or surgery for a neoplasia, if indicated.

Hyperaldosteronism

The prevalence of primary hyperaldosteronism is about 1% to 2% in unselected patients with hypertension and is caused by an aldosterone-secreting neoplasia (Conn syndrome) or hyperplasia of the adrenal gland.[24] Secondary hyperaldosteronism is associated with renin hypersecretion (e.g., renal artery stenosis). Some patients may have minimal symptoms, but spontaneous or profound diuretic-induced hypokalemia in a patient with diastolic hypertension is suggestive of hyperaldosteronism. Other patients may exhibit muscle weakness and transient paralysis, paresthesia, tetany, diastolic hypertension, hypernatremia, and hypokalemia. The diagnosis is complicated and involves measuring plasma aldosterone and renin concentrations, conducting imaging studies, and sometimes selective adrenal vein catheterization. Idiopathic aldosteronism is treated medically with spironolactone, but Conn syndrome is treated surgically.

Pheochromocytoma

Pheochromocytomas are rare chromaffin cell tumors that secrete catecholamines. Most pheochromocytomas are found in the adrenal medulla, but approximately 20% originate from extraadrenal neural crest tissue.[25] These tumors can be found in association with neurofibromatosis (von Recklinghausen's disease). Patients are typically middle-aged. Hypertension is the hallmark sign of these tumors and is persistent in about half of the patients. The other half may exhibit paroxysmal hypertension associated with the classic features of catecholamine excess: flushing of the skin, diaphoresis, headache, palpitations, nausea, vomiting, dyspnea, and a sense of impending doom. Urinary metanephrines, urinary vanillylmandelic acid, or plasma catecholamines are elevated in this disorder, but results can be difficult to interpret. Dietary vanilla, exogenous catecholamines, α-methyldopa, rauwolfia alkaloids, and other drugs may also cause elevations, and false-negative results can also occur.[26] Provocative tests are considered to be too hazardous for routine clinical use. Diagnostic imaging is often used to localize the tumor before laparoscopic surgery, the standard treatment.[27] Catecholamine blockage with phenoxybenzamine and metyrosine generally ameliorates symptoms and is necessary to prevent hypertensive crisis during surgery.

Hypoglycemia

Hypoglycemic disorders are not associated with the treatment of diabetes mellitus and are characterized by "Whipple's triad": (1) a low plasma glucose level; (2) symptoms of neuroglycopenia; and (3) relief of these symptoms by carbohydrate intake.[28] Causes in otherwise healthy-appearing patients include insulinoma, factitious factors (health care personnel), and intense exercise. Causes in ill-appearing patients include hypopituitarism, isolated GH deficiency, Addison's disease, sepsis, renal failure, starvation, anorexia nervosa, glycogen storage disease, and many others. Medications (salicylates, quinine, haloperidol, pentamidine, sulfonamides via intentional overdose, accidental overdose, or dispensing error) may mediate hypoglycemia in anybody, whether they appear healthy or ill.[29] Most authorities do not consider "functional hypoglycemia," "early-diabetes hypoglycemia," and "alimentary hypoglycemia" to be actual clinical entities.

Clinical Presentation

The symptoms of hypoglycemia are due to two main processes: an adrenergic response (which usually occurs first when serum glucose levels begin to fall) and CNS dysfunction (which usually occurs later at lower glucose levels). Adrenergic symptoms and signs include anxiety, hunger, a feeling of warmth, nausea, palpitations, tremulousness, pallor, and diaphoresis. Neuroglycopenic symptoms and signs include dizziness, diplopia, blurred vision, inability to concentrate, amnesia, confusion, behavior changes, seizures, and coma. The patient's history about symptoms in relation to meals and recovery after carbohydrate ingestion can be confusing.

Diagnosis

Because many patients present with vague symptoms or with a self-diagnosis of hypoglycemia, an important first step is to determine if there is a relation between symptoms and plasma glucose levels.[30] Although what constitutes a low plasma glucose is debated, values less than 50 mg/dL for men, less than 45 mg/dL for women, and less than 40 mg/dL for children can be considered abnormal for clinical purposes. Ideally, a plasma blood glucose value is obtained at the time the patient has symptoms, but many times it is not practical. Some patients can be taught how to measure blood glucose levels at home and are asked to keep a diary of symptoms, blood glucose levels, and responses to carbohydrate ingestion. A hypoglycemic disorder is suspected if the patient exhibits Whipple's triad. Patients who have vague symptoms after meals not associated with hypoglycemia are said to have "idiopathic postprandial syndrome." The supervised 72-hour fast is the classic diagnostic test for a hypoglycemic disorder, but the 5-hour glucose tolerance test is not considered to have diagnostic value.[28] During the 72-hour fast the patient is allowed only calorie-free and caffeine-free beverages. All medications are stopped. Levels of plasma glucose, insulin, C peptide, and proinsulin are determined every 6 hours until the plasma glucose is 60 mg/dL or lower and then every 1 to 2 hours. The test is ended when hypoglycemic plasma values are noted and the patient has symptoms of hypoglycemia. The absence of typical signs or symptoms precludes the diagnosis of a hypoglycemic disorder. A low plasma glucose level alone is not a sufficient finding for this diagnosis.

Management

Treatment is directed at the underlying cause. Sometimes an explanation of the cause and advice to have frequent meals are all that is required. Individuals who exercise intensely may need to "carbohydrate-load" the day before and ingest carbohydrates during exercise. Medications may need to be discontinued or be given in a lower dose. Patients who have an alcohol use disorder may require specific treatment. Those with factitious hypoglycemia require psychiatric help. Patients with insulinomas are rare (about 4 per million person-years) and require surgery.

References

1. Weinstein J, Issacs S, Shore D, Blevins LS Jr. Diagnosis and management of pituitary tumors. Compr Ther 1997;23:594–604.
2. Colao A, Lombardi G. Growth-hormone and prolactin excess. Lancet 1998;352:1455–61.
3. Webster J. Cabergoline and quinagolide therapy for prolactinomas. Clin Endocrinol 2000;53:549–50.
4. Ciric I, Rosenblatt S, Kerr W Jr, Lamarca F, Pierce D, Baumgartner C. Perspective in pituitary adenomas: an end of the century review of tumorigenesis, diagnosis, and treatment. Clin Neurosurg 2000;47:99–111.
5. Trainer PJ, Drake WM, Katznelson L, et al. Treatment of acromegaly with the growth hormone-receptor antagonist pegvisomant. N Engl J Med 2000;342:1171–7.
6. Vance ML. Hypopituitarism. N Engl J Med 1994;330:1651–62 [published erratum in N Engl J Med 1994;331:487].
7. Robertson GL. Diabetes insipidus. Endocrinol Metab Clin North Am 1995;24:549–72.
8. Illowsky BP, Kirch DG. Polydipsia and hyponatremia in psychiatric patients. Am J Psychiatry 1988;145:675–83.
9. Baylis PH, Cheetham T. Diabetes insipidus. Arch Dis Child 1998;79:84–9.
10. Krege J, Katz VL, Bowes WA Jr. Transient diabetes insipidus of pregnancy. Obstet Gynecol Surv 1989;44:789–95.
11. Parker LN. Adrenarche. Endocrinol Metab Clin North Am 1991;20:71–83.
12. Blondell RD, Foster MD, Dave KC. Disorders of puberty. Am Fam Physician 1999;60:209–18, 223–4.
13. Bagatell CJ, Bremner WJ. Androgens in men—uses and abuses. N Engl J Med 1996;334:707–14.
14. Bergfeld WF. Hirsutism in women. Postgrad Med 2000;107:93–4, 99–104.
15. Toscano V. Hirsutism: pilosebaceous unit dysregulation. Role of peripheral and glandular factors. J Endocrinol Invest 1991;14:153–70.
16. Derksen J, Nagesser SK, Meinders AE, Haak HR, van de Velde CJ. Identification of virilizing adrenal tumors in hirsute women. N Engl J Med 1994;331:968–73.
17. Marx SJ. Hyperparathyroid and hypoparathyroid disorders. N Engl J Med 2000;343:1863–75.
18. Bilezikian JP. Management of acute hypercalcemia. N Engl J Med 1992;326:1196–203.
19. Irvin GL 3rd, Carneiro DM. Management changes in primary hyperparathyroidism. JAMA 2000;284:934–6.
20. Smit PC, Rinkes IH, van Dalen A, van Vroonhoven JM. Direct, minimally invasive adenomectomy for primary hyperparathyroidism: an alternative to conventional neck exploration? Ann Surg 2000;231:559–65.
21. Oelkers W. Adrenal insufficiency. N Engl J Med 1996;335:1206–12.
22. Kirk LF Jr, Hash RB, Katner HP. Cushing's disease: clinical manifestations and diagnostic evaluation. Am Fam Physician 2000;62:1119–27, 1133–4.
23. Boscaro M, Barzon L, Fallo F, Sonino N. Cushing's syndrome. Lancet 2001;357:783–91.
24. Ganguly A. Primary aldosteronism. N Engl J Med 1998;339:1828–34.
25. Whalen RK, Althausen AF, Daniels GH. Extra-renal pheochromocytoma. J Urol 1992;147:1–10.
26. Young WF Jr. Pheochromocytoma and primary aldosteronism: diagnostic approaches. Endocrinol Metab Clin North Am 1997;26:801–27.
27. Walther MM, Keiser HR, Linehan WM. Pheochromocytoma: evaluation, diagnosis, and treatment. World J Urol 1999;17:35–9.
28. Service FJ. Hypoglycemic disorders. N Engl J Med 1995;332:1144–52.
29. Service FJ. Classification of hypoglycemic disorders. Endocrinol Metab Clin North Am 1999;28:501–17.
30. Service FJ. Diagnostic approach to adults with hypoglycemic disorders. Endocrinol Metab Clin North Am 1999;28:519–32.

125
Anemia

Daniel T. Lee and Angela W. Tang

Anemia is a reduction in blood hemoglobin (Hgb) concentration or hematocrit (Hct). Hgb values less than 14 g/dL for men and 12 g/dL for women are widely accepted to indicate anemia. However, data from large samples selected to represent the population of the United States suggests that a lower limit of 13.2 g/dL in men and 11.7 g/dL in women may be more appropriate. The lower limit of normal for children ages 1 to 2 years is 10.7 g/dL, with the cutoff rising to adult values by age 15 to 18 years. African-American references are 0.5 to 0.6 g/dL lower than for whites. There is a small decline in normal values for men but not women after age 65.[1] However, when evaluating the elderly it is advisable to use usual adult reference ranges to avoid missing important underlying disorders. In addition, it is important to evaluate results in the context of previous data. A low-normal Hgb may be significant if the value 1 week earlier was higher.

On occasion, the Hgb and Hct may not accurately reflect red cell mass. For example, patients with expanded plasma volume, as in pregnancy or congestive heart failure, may have falsely low values. Conversely, patients with plasma contraction, as in burns or dehydration, may have falsely elevated values. Finally, in the setting of acute blood loss, both red blood cells (RBCs) and plasma are lost equally, and the true degree of anemia may not be appreciated until plasma volume has time to expand.

Anemia may be categorized by cause: acute blood loss, hemolysis, or marrow underproduction. Central to this task are measurements of cell size (mean corpuscular volume, MCV) and reticulocyte count (an indicator of marrow RBC production).

Clinical Presentation

Symptoms

The degree of symptoms in anemia is highly variable, depending on the degree of anemia and the rapidity of its development. Patients may experience fatigue, weakness, and a decrease in exercise tolerance. Dizziness, headache, tinnitus, palpitations, syncope, and impaired concentration may occur. Some patients experience abdominal discomfort, nausea, and bowel irregularity as blood is shunted from the splanchnic bed. Decreased blood flow to the skin may result in cold intolerance. Patients with preexisting vascular disease are prone to exacerbations of angina, claudication, or cerebral ischemia. Those with mild or gradually developing anemias may be completely or nearly asymptomatic.

History

Historical clues assist in determining the cause of anemia. A family history of anemia or onset of anemia in childhood suggests an inherited etiology. Chronic medical conditions such as hepatic, renal, endocrine, or inflammatory disorders can lead to anemia. Malignancies and infections may cause anemia. A history of gallstones or jaundice points to hemolysis. Exposure to some medications, alcohol, and toxins (e.g., lead) can lead to anemia. Dietary intake of iron, folate, and vitamin B_{12} (cobalamin) should be obtained. Pica, especially of ice, suggests iron deficiency. Blood loss through menstruation or the gastrointestinal (GI) tract must be ascertained. Chronic diarrhea or a history of GI conditions associated with malabsorption suggests a nutritional deficiency anemia. Paresthesias of the extremities or alteration in mental status may point to vitamin B_{12} deficiency. Frequent blood donations may contribute to anemia.

Physical Examination

Tachycardia and wide pulse pressure may be present in the anemic patient. The skin and conjunctiva may demonstrate pallor. In very severe anemias, retinal hemorrhages may be seen. A systolic ejection murmur and venous hum may be heard. Jaundice may suggest hemolysis or liver disease. Glossitis can be present in vitamin B_{12} and iron deficiency. Lymphadenopathy may occur in the presence of hematologic malignancies and infections such as HIV and tuberculosis. Signs of liver disease and splenomegaly should be sought. The stool should be examined for blood. Proprioception and balance deficits may occur in vitamin B_{12} deficiency.

Laboratory Data

Complete Blood Count

Once a patient is determined to be anemic by Hgb and Hct, the MCV should be checked. Normal MCV for adults is 82 to 98 fL. MCV in children is lower, starting at 70 fL at 1 year of age and increasing 1 fL/year, until adult values are reached at puberty. Table 125.1 divides common causes of anemia into microcytic (<82 fL), normocytic (82–98 fL), and macrocytic (>98 fL).

The red cell distribution width (RDW) quantifies the variation in size of the RBCs. Normal RDW is less than 14.5%. An elevation of the RDW may make the MCV by itself less reliable. An example is a patient who has both iron and B_{12} deficiencies. In this case, the MCV may be normocytic, but the RDW will be elevated.[2]

Platelet and white blood cell (WBC) counts should be noted. Platelet and WBC deficiencies point to a global marrow disorder affecting all cell lines, for example aplastic anemia. Elevations suggest infection. Elevated platelet counts are often seen in iron deficiency.

Reticulocyte Count

Reticulocytes, which are newly formed RBCs, normally account for about 1% of circulating RBCs. Reticulocyte formation is increased in a normal individual who loses blood, with the degree of reticulocytosis increasing as anemia becomes more severe. Therefore, a patient's reported reticulocyte percentage should be adjusted for the degree of anemia to determine if the bone marrow response is appropriate:

Corrected Reticulocyte %
$$= \text{Reticulocyte \%} \times \text{Patient's Hct/Normal Hct.}$$

A corrected reticulocyte percentage (also known as reticulocyte index) greater than 1% indicates appropriate bone marrow response to anemia. If the value is less than 1%, causes of hypoproliferative bone marrow should be sought. Increased reticulocyte counts are present in hemolysis, acute hemorrhage, and response to treatment in anemias from other causes. An alternative to corrected reticulocyte percentage is the absolute reticulocyte count, which equals the reported reticulocyte percentage multiplied by the RBC count. The absolute reticulocyte count is normally 50,000 to 75,000/mm^3.

Table 125.1. **Classification of Anemia Based on Mean Corpuscular Volume (MCV)**

Microcytic	Macrocytic
Iron deficiency	Nonmegaloblastic
Thalassemia	Alcoholism
Anemia of chronic disease*	Chronic liver disease
Hemoglobin E*	Bone marrow disorders
Sideroblastic anemia*	Hypothyroidism*
Lead poisoning*	Sideroblastic anemias*
Hereditary*	Marked reticulocytosis
Myelodysplastic syndrome*	Spurious*
Severe alcoholism*	Normal variant*
Medications*	Neonatal period
Normocytic	Megaloblastic
Elevated reticulocyte count	Folate deficiency
Acute blood loss	Poor intake
Hemolysis	Malabsorption
Decreased reticulocyte count	Ethanol
Anemia of chronic disease	Medications
Chronic renal failure	Pregnancy
Chronic liver failure	Infancy
Endocrine disease	High folate requirement
Iron deficiency	B_{12} (cobalamin) deficiency
Myelodysplastic syndromes	Pernicious anemia
Aplastic anemia*	Gastric or ileal surgery*
Pure red cell aplasia*	Ileal disease*
Myelophthisic anemia*	Strict veganism*
Sideroblastic anemia*	Fish tapeworm infection*
	Bacterial overgrowth*
	Pancreatic insufficiency*
	Medications*
	Congenital disorders*
	Medications (anticonvulsants chemotherapy, zidovudine)

*Less common.

Peripheral Smear

Abnormalities in the peripheral smear can assist in determining the etiology of anemia (Fig. 125.1).

Other Laboratory Tests

Further laboratory testing may be warranted, depending on the MCV and reticulocyte count. Bone marrow biopsy is reserved for situations in which anemia remains unexplained or is suspected to arise from marrow dysfunction. Algorithms for evaluation of microcytic, normocytic, and macrocytic anemias are provided in Figs. 125.2, 125.3, and 125.4.

Microcytic Anemias (Fig. 125.2)

Iron Deficiency Anemia

Iron deficiency anemia (IDA) is probably the most common cause of anemia in the U.S. The recommended dietary allowance (RDA) for iron is 10 mg daily for men and 15 mg daily for women.[3] Daily requirements increase during pregnancy, lactation, and adolescence. Meats, eggs, vegetables, legumes, and cereals are principal sources of iron in the American diet, with iron from meats being much more available for absorption.

IDA is always a symptom of an underlying process that should be identified. In the U.S., IDA may be seen in infants fed primarily cow's milk because the iron content is low and the milk causes GI irritation with blood loss and malabsorption. IDA can be seen in children and adolescents whose iron needs are increased due to their rapidly growing bodies. Females lose iron in menstrual blood. Pregnancy places additional demands on a woman's iron stores as the placenta and fetus require iron and blood is lost during childbirth. In men and postmenopausal women, GI blood loss is the most likely cause of IDA. In these patients, a diligent search for occult GI bleeding is imperative when another source of bleeding is not readily appreciated. This should include upper and lower endoscopy with small bowel biopsy. Radiologic tests may substitute if endoscopy is not practical. In over one third of patients with IDA, no source of blood loss will be found despite this evaluation.[4] In these patients, prognosis is good, with anemia resolving in more than two thirds without recurrence.[5] Further search for the source of GI blood loss is required only for persistent bleeding or transfusion dependency. IDA is also seen in decreased absorption states such as celiac disease and gastrectomy. IDA can develop in long-distance runners, probably due to blood loss from the GI tract.[6]

Physician examination may reveal glossitis and angular stomatitis. Esophageal webs, splenomegaly, and koilonychias (spoon-shaped nails) may occur rarely. The most sensitive and specific laboratory test for IDA is serum ferritin, which reflects iron stores. Ferritin below 15 µg/L is diagnostic. Since ferritin is an acute-phase reactant, however, falsely normal levels may occur with coexisting inflammatory conditions. Nonetheless, a ferritin level above 100 µg/L practically rules out IDA.[7] A decreased serum iron and increased total iron binding capacity (TIBC) are helpful but less reliable indicators of IDA. The transferrin saturation (iron/TIBC) should be less than 0.15, but this ratio may be reduced in anemia of chronic disease as well. The MCV is usually normal in early iron deficiency and typically decreases after the Hct drops. The MCV then changes in proportion to the severity of anemia. The RDW is often increased.

Occasionally, ferritin values fall in the indeterminate range of 15 to 100 µg/L and the diagnosis remains uncertain. Bone marrow biopsy is the gold standard to determine iron stores but is rarely necessary. An alternative is a several-week trial of iron replacement. Reticulocytosis should peak after 1 week, and the Hct should normalize in about a month. If no response to therapy occurs, iron should be discontinued to prevent potential iron overload. Soluble serum transferrin receptor (TfR) rises in IDA and is a promising but not widely available test that may assist diagnosis in difficult cases.[8]

Oral iron replacement is available in ferrous and ferric forms. Ferrous forms are preferred due to superior absorption and include ferrous sulfate, gluconate, and fumarate. Ferrous sulfate 325 mg tid is the cheapest and provides the needed 150 to 200 mg of elemental iron per day. However, recent studies suggest that as little as 60 mg elemental iron once or twice a week may suffice.[9] Although Hct should normalize in a few weeks, iron replacement should continue until ferritin reaches 50 µg/L or at least 4 to 6 months. Many patients experience nausea, constipation, diarrhea, or abdominal pain. To minimize these effects, iron may be started once a day and titrated up. In addition, iron may be taken with food, although this can decrease absorption by 40% to 66%.[10] Taking iron with vitamin C may help increase absorption.[11] Liquid iron preparations may be tried. Despite these measures, 10% to 20% of patients do not tolerate oral iron replacement.[12] Enteric-coated iron preparations are not well absorbed and should be avoided. Bran, eggs, milk, tea, caffeine, calcium-rich antacids, H_2-blockers, proton pump inhibitors, and tetracyclines can interfere with iron absorption and should not be taken at the same time. Also, iron supplementation can interfere with the absorption of other medications, including quinolones, tetracycline, thyroid hormone, levodopa, methyldopa, and penicillamine.

Most patients respond well to oral replacement of iron. Treatment failures may result from poor adherence, continued blood loss, interfering substances listed above, or gastrointestinal disturbances limiting absorption. In the rare case where poor absorption or severe intolerance to iron cannot be overcome, parenteral replacement may be needed. Iron dextran may be given IV or as a painful IM injection. The total dose (ml) required to replenish stores equals

$$0.0442 \times (\text{Desired Hgb} - \text{Measured Hgb}) \times \text{Weight} + (0.26 \times \text{Weight})$$

where 1 mL contains 50 mg elemental iron, and weight is lean body weight in kilograms. Adverse reactions include headache; flushing; dyspnea; nausea; vomiting; fever; hypotension; seizures; and chest, back, and abdominal pain. Urticaria and anaphylaxis can occur. A test dose (0.5 mL =

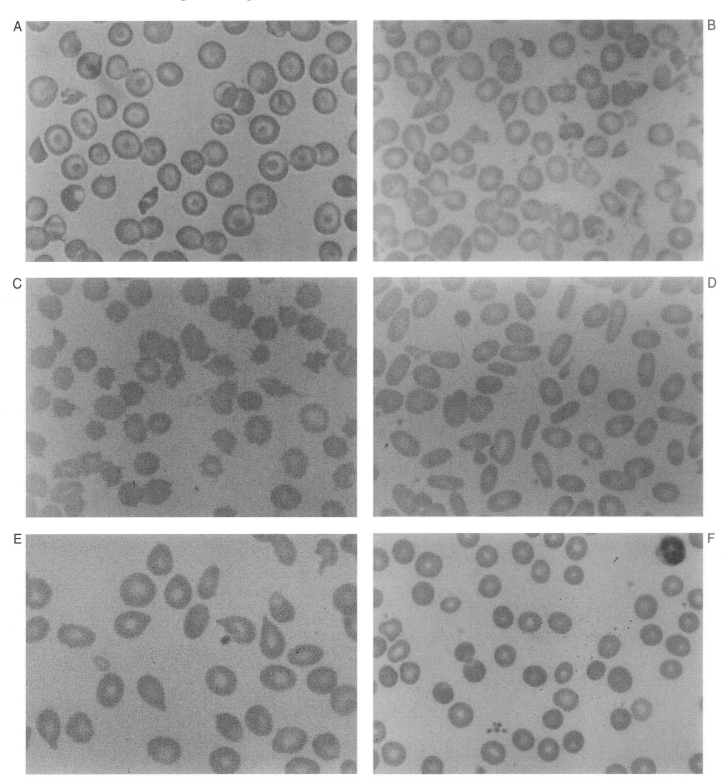

25 mg) should be given to determine whether anaphylaxis will occur. If tolerated, the remainder of the dose may be given, up to a maximum daily dose of 100 mg over 2 minutes or more. If possible, intravenous iron is preferred over intramuscular due to a lower incidence of local reactions and more consistent absorption.

Thalassemia

The thalassemias are inherited disorders of hemoglobin synthesis that are more common in people of Mediterranean, Asian, and African descent. The rare thalassemia majors cause severe anemia and are discovered early in life. Family physicians are more likely to encounter thalassemia trait (tha-

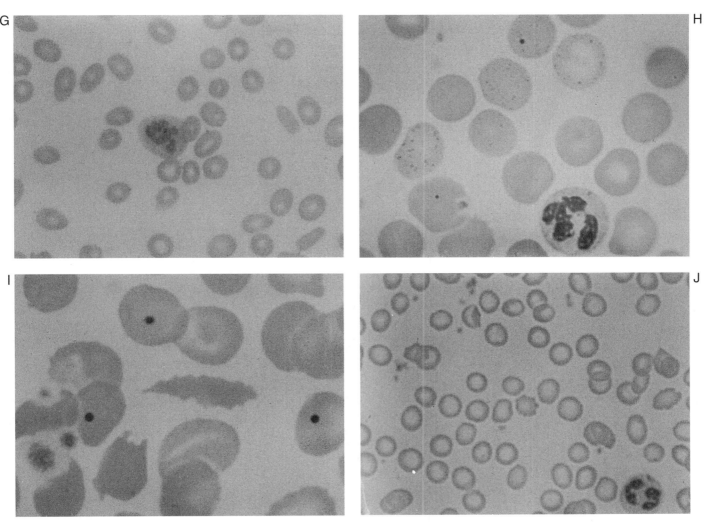

Fig. 125.1. Peripheral smear abnormalities in anemia. (A) Target cells in Hgb C, SC, E, thalassemias, and liver disease. (B) Schistocytes in microangiopathic (DIC, TTP, HUS) or traumatic hemolysis (cardiac valves). (C) Spur cells in end-stage liver disease, abetalipoproteinemia, anorexia nervosa, hypothyroidism, and splenectomy. (D) Elliptocytes in hereditary elliptocytosis. (E) Teardrop cells in myelofibrosis. (F) Spherocytes in hereditary spherocytosis and autoimmune hemolytic anemia. (G) Macroovalocytes and hypersegmented neutrophils in vitamin B_{12} and folate deficiencies. (H) Basophilic stippling in lead poisoning, thalassemia, and sideroblastic anemia. (I) Howell-Jolly bodies in asplenia and megaloblastic anemia. (J) Hypochromia and microcytosis in iron deficiency. (DIC = disseminated intravascular coagulation; TTP = thrombotic thrombocytopenia purpura; HUS = hemolytic uremic syndrome. (Photographs courtesy of Kouichi Tanaka, MD; Harbor-UCLA Medical Center, Torrance, CA.)

lassemia minor) occurring in individuals heterozygous for α- or β-globin chain mutations.

Thalassemia trait should be suspected in an asymptomatic patient with mild anemia and a disproportionately low MCV (56–74 fL). The RDW is usually normal, and the RBC count is normal or increased by 10% to 20%. Iron studies are normal. Blood smear may show target cells, ovalocytes, and basophilic stippling. If a precise diagnosis is required (for prenatal counseling, for example), hemoglobin electrophoresis may be performed. In β-thalassemia trait, elevated levels of Hgb A2 and occasionally Hgb F will be seen. In α-thalassemia trait, the hemoglobin electrophoresis will be normal, and the diagnosis is made by exclusion. Treatment such as potentially harmful iron therapy is not necessary for patients with thalassemia trait.

Hemoglobin E

Hgb E has a prevalence of 5% to 30% in certain groups from Southeast Asia. The heterozygote has mild microcytosis and normal Hct. Homozygotes have marked microcytosis (MCV 60–70 Fl) and mild anemia. Target cells may be present on peripheral smear. Hgb electrophoresis reveals the presence of Hgb E, establishing the diagnosis. Hgb E is important pri-

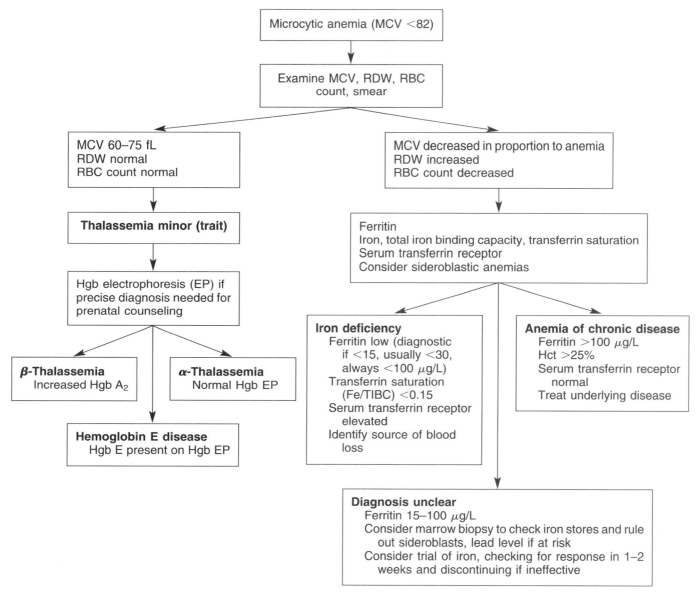

Fig. 125.2. Evaluation of microcytic anemia. MCV = mean corpuscular volume; RBC = red blood cell; RDW = red cell distribution width; TIBC = total iron-binding capacity.

marily in combination with β-thalassemia; in these double heterozygotes, a severe transfusion-dependent anemia occurs.

Sideroblastic Anemia

Sideroblastic anemias are a heterogeneous group of disorders in which ringed sideroblasts are found on bone marrow staining. Sideroblastic anemia may be X linked or due to toxins or medications (lead, alcohol, isoniazid, chloramphenicol, chemotherapy). It may be related to neoplastic, endocrine, or inflammatory diseases or a part of myelodysplastic syndrome. The MCV is usually low but may range from low to high. Iron saturation and ferritin are normal to high. Marrow examination is diagnostic, and treatment is aimed at the underlying cause. In the case of lead poisoning, anemia is microcytic and basophilic stippling may be seen on peripheral

smear. This diagnosis should be suspected and serum lead levels sent in high-risk groups such as children ingesting paint, soil, and dust, and adults with occupational exposure.

Normocytic Anemias (Fig. 125.3)

The absolute reticulocyte count or corrected reticulocyte percentage is important in determining the cause of a normocytic anemia.

Normocytic Anemia with Elevated Reticulocytes

Acute Blood Loss

Acute blood loss is usually obvious but can be missed in cases such as hip fractures and retroperitoneal or pulmonary hemorrhages. The true degree of anemia may not be revealed in the Hct at first, since RBCs and plasma are lost equally. It may take several days for equilibration of blood volume and Hct to reflect fully the degree of bleeding.

Hemolysis

There are many causes of hemolytic anemia (Table 125.2). Laboratory values consistent with hemolysis include elevated serum lactate dehydrogenase (LDH) and indirect bilirubin. Haptoglobin, a plasma protein that binds and clears Hgb, drops precipitously in the presence of hemolysis. If hemolysis is suspected, the peripheral smear should be examined for schistocytes (mechanical hemolysis) and spherocytes (autoimmune hemolysis or hereditary spherocytosis), as in Fig. 125.1. A direct Coombs' test will reveal an autoimmune basis for hemolysis. Further confirmatory testing may be performed as appropriate (Fig. 125.3), usually with the guidance of a hematologist. Treatment of hemolytic anemias is directed at the underlying cause and providing supportive care. Corticosteroids and splenectomy may be indicated for specific causes.

Normocytic Anemias with Decreased Reticulocytes

Anemia of Chronic Disease

Anemia of chronic disease (ACD), which results from chronic inflammatory disorders, infections, and malignancies, is the second most common cause of anemia after iron deficiency. It is probably the most common form of anemia in the elderly.[13] The pathogenesis of ACD is multifactorial and not fully understood. Proposed mechanisms include reduction in RBC life span, impaired utilization of iron stores, and a relative erythropoietin deficiency. Although the anemia is customarily normocytic, it can be microcytic in 30% to 50% of cases.[14] The degree of anemia is usually mild, with Hgb between 7 and 11 g/dL. The serum iron, total iron binding capacity, and transferrin saturation are usually low and not helpful in distinguishing ACD from IDA. More useful is the ferritin level, which is normal or high in ACD. Ferritin greater than 100 μg/L essentially rules out IDA, whereas levels less than 15 μg/L are diagnostic of IDA. In cases of uncertain fer-

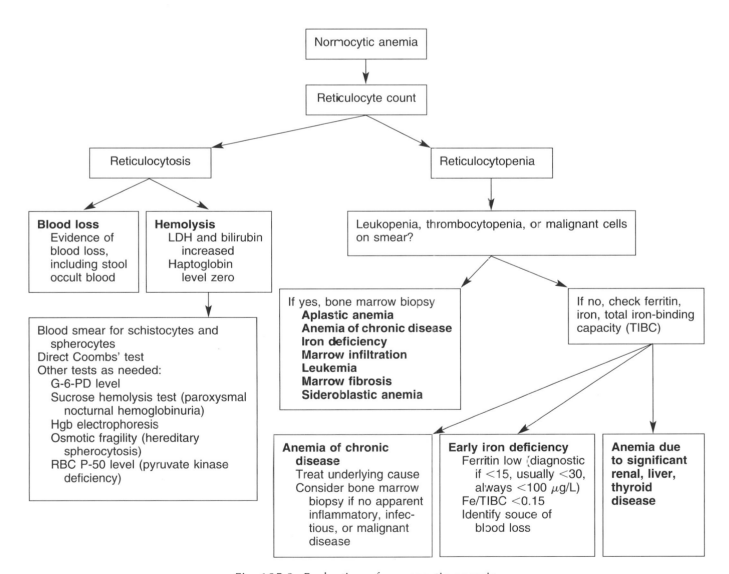

Fig. 125.3. Evaluation of normocytic anemia.

Table 125.2. **Causes of Hemolysis**

Intrinsic (defect in RBCs)	Extrinsic (defect external to RBCs)

Hemoglobinopathies
    Sickle syndromes
    Unstable hemoglobins
    Methemoglobinemia
Membrane disorders
    Paroxysmal nocturnal hemoglobinuria
    Hereditary spherocytosis
    Elliptocytosis
    Pyropoikilocytosis
    Stomatocytosis
Enzyme deficiencies
    Glucose-6-phosphate dehydrogenase (G-6-PD)
    Pyruvate kinase
    Glucose phosphate isomerase
    Congenital erythropoietic porphyria
	Immune
	    Autoimmune
	    Lymphoproliferative
	    Malignancy
	    Collagen vascular disorders
	    Drug induced (methyldopa, procainamide, quinidine, levodopa, sulfas,
	        penicillin, NSAIDs)
	Mechanical
	    Disseminated intravascular coagulation (DIC)
	    Thrombotic thrombocytopenia purpura (TTP)
	    Hemolytic uremic syndrome (HUS)
	    Prosthetic heart valves
	    Disseminated neoplasms
	    Burns
	    Malignant hypertension
	    Vasculitis
	    Severe hypophosphatemia
	    Physical activity ("march" hemoglobinuria)
	Hypersplenism
	Infections
	    Clostridium, Plasmodium, Borrelia,
	        Mycoplasma, Babesia, Haemophilus, Bartonella
	Bites
	    Snakes
	    Spiders

RBCs = red blood cells.

ritin levels (15–100 μg/L), a brief therapeutic trial of iron or a bone marrow biopsy may help with the diagnosis.

Treatment of ACD is directed toward management of the underlying disorder. Erythropoietin is effective in raising Hct in certain cases. Iron treatment will not improve the anemia, since iron stores are adequate. If the anemia is more severe than expected, one should search for a coexisting cause. For example, a patient with rheumatoid arthritis may develop concomitant IDA from GI blood loss due to chronic nonsteroidal antiinflammatory drug (NSAID) use.

Chronic Renal Failure

Anemia occurs frequently in chronic renal failure, due primarily to the kidney's inability to secrete erythropoietin (also see Chapter 97). Generally, the creatinine is above 3 mg/dL. The peripheral smear is usually normal, but burr cells can be seen. The ferritin is typically increased. If a low to low-normal ferritin is noted, concomitant IDA should be entertained.

Therapy consists of ameliorating the renal failure and replacing erythropoietin. Hemodialysis may improve RBC production, but erythropoietin is the mainstay of treatment, even before dialysis is required. Complications of erythropoietin include increased blood pressure. It is important to remember that renal failure patients often have coexisting iron deficiency, and ferritin should be monitored during therapy.

Chronic Liver Disease

Chronic liver disease causes a normocytic or occasionally macrocytic anemia (also see Chapter 90). Target cells can be seen on peripheral smear. Spur cells are seen in severe liver failure (Fig. 125.1). Treatment is directed at improving liver function. Alcoholics with liver disease have additional causes

for anemia that are discussed under nonmegaloblastic macrocytic anemias.

Endocrine Disease

Various endocrine diseases such as hypothyroidism, hyperthyroidism, hypogonadism, hypopituitarism, hyperparathyroidism, and Addison's disease are associated with anemia. The anemia is readily corrected with treatment of the underlying endocrine problem.

Aplastic Anemia

Aplastic anemia is due to an injury or destruction of a common pluripotential stem cell resulting in pancytopenia. Bone marrow biopsy reveals severe hypoplasia and fatty infiltration. In the U.S., approximately half the cases are idiopathic. Other causes include viral infections [e.g., HIV, hepatitis, Epstein-Barr virus (EBV)], drugs and chemicals (e.g., chemotherapy, benzene, chloramphenicol), radiation, pregnancy, immune diseases (e.g., eosinophilic fasciitis, hypoimmunoglobulinemia, thymoma, thymic carcinoma, graft-versus-host disease), paroxysmal nocturnal hemoglobinuria, systemic lupus erythematosus, and inherited disorders.

Treatment includes managing the underlying cause and supportive care, in conjunction with a hematologist. Judicious use of transfusions may be needed if the anemia is severe. Immunosuppressive therapy and bone marrow transplantation are indicated in certain cases.

Myelophthisic Anemia

Myelophthisic anemias result from bone marrow infiltration by invading tumor cells (hematologic malignancies or solid tumor metastases), infectious agents (tuberculosis, fungal infections), or granulomas (sarcoidosis). Less common causes include lipid storage diseases, osteopetrosis, and myelofibrosis. Treatment is directed at the underlying cause.

Red Cell Dysplasia

Pure red cell dysplasias involve a selective failure of erythropoiesis. The granulocyte and platelet counts are normal. Red cell dysplasias share many causes with aplastic and myelophthisic anemia, including malignancies, connective tissue disorders, infections, and drugs. There is an idiopathic form and a congenital form. One infection that specifically targets red cell production specifically is parvovirus B19. This virus also causes erythema infectiosum (fifth disease), an acute polyarthropathy syndrome, and hydrops fetalis. Anemia results from parvovirus B19 infection primarily in those with chronic hemolysis (e.g., sickle cell disease), by suppressing erythropoiesis and disrupting a tenuous balance needed to keep up with RBC destruction. In this situation, anemia can be profound but is usually self-limited. Parvovirus B19 infections may become chronic in immunosuppressed individuals who cannot form antibodies to the virus. Treatment concepts for red cell aplasia are similar to aplastic anemia.

Myelodysplastic Syndromes

The myelodysplastic syndromes (MDS) are a group of clonal hematologic diseases of unknown etiology that result in the inability of bone marrow to produce adequate erythrocytes, leukocytes, platelets, or some combination of these. Patients are usually over 60 years of age and have an increased risk for leukemia. Bone marrow biopsy is diagnostic, revealing characteristic dysplastic blood precursor cells. Treatment is largely supportive.

Macrocytic Anemias (Fig. 125.4)

Macrocytic anemias may be separated into megaloblastic and nonmegaloblastic types, based on peripheral smear findings (Table 125.1). A sensitive and specific sign of megaloblastic anemia is hypersegmented neutrophils, in which neutrophils contain nuclei with more than 5 lobes. A marked elevation of MCV (>120 fL) is also highly suggestive of megaloblastosis. RBCs of megaloblastic anemias, in addition to being increased in size, are often oval in shape (macroovalocytes). Most macrocytosis, however, results from nonmegaloblastic causes. In a recent survey, drug therapy and alcoholism accounted for >50% of macrocytosis, whereas vitamin B_{12} and folate deficiencies accounted for only 6% of cases.[15]

Megaloblastic Anemias

Vitamin B_{12} Deficiency

Vitamin B_{12} (cobalamin) is ingested from primarily animal sources, including meats, eggs, and dairy products. U.S. RDA is 2 μg of vitamin B_{12} daily. A typical Western diet provides 5 to 30 μg/day. After ingestion, B_{12} is bound by intrinsic factor, which is produced by gastric parietal cells. Bound vitamin is absorbed in the terminal ileum. Body stores of vitamin B_{12} total 2000 to 5000 μg. Thus, B_{12} deficiency takes years to develop and rarely occurs from dietary insufficiency except in strict vegans. The majority of B_{12} deficiency is due to

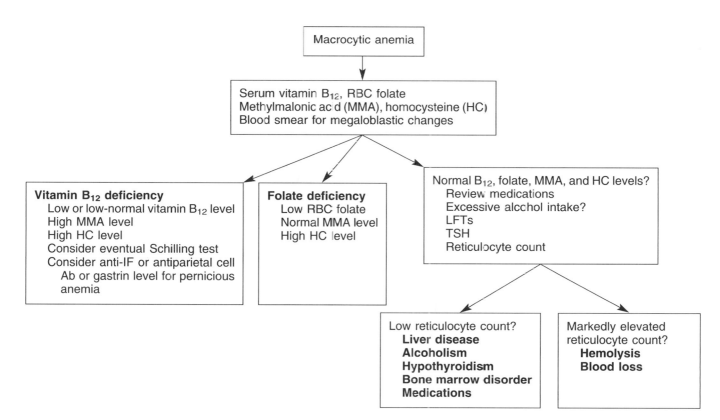

Fig. 125.4. Evaluation of macrocytic anemia. LFT = liver function test; TSH = thyroid-stimulating hormone.

pernicious anemia, which occurs primarily in the elderly and is due to atrophy of the gastric mucosa and intrinsic factor deficiency. Other causes of B_{12} deficiency include gastric and ileal surgeries, ileal absorption problems such as Crohn's disease, sprue, and tapeworm infection.

Signs and symptoms of B_{12} deficiency include glossitis, sore mouth, and GI disturbances such as constipation, diarrhea, and indigestion. Neurologic symptoms such as paresthesias of the extremities and subacute combined degeneration (loss of lower extremity vibration and position sense) may occur. Dementia and subtle neuropsychiatric changes may be present. Importantly, anemia or macrocytosis are absent in 28% of patients with neurologic abnormalities due to B_{12} deficiency.[16]

In addition to peripheral smear changes of hypersegmented neutrophils and macroovalocytes, laboratory findings include a low B_{12} level ($<$200 pg/mL) and reticulocyte count. However, low-normal B_{12} levels ($<$350 pg/mL) are present in many patients with neurologic disease or anemia, so further workup may be indicated if the diagnosis is still suspected. Falsely low B_{12} levels may be found in folate deficiency, pregnancy, and myeloma. Elevated serum methylmalonic acid (MMA) levels are highly sensitive and essentially rule out B_{12} deficiency if normal. In one study, elevated MMA levels occurred in 98% of cases of clinically defined B_{12} deficiency. Falsely elevated levels occur in renal failure and hypovolemia, and spot urine MMA levels may be superior in this setting. Homocysteine level rises with B_{12} deficiency (96% of cases in one study) but are less specific, occurring in folate deficiency and renal disease as well.[17–19] Occasionally, a mild thrombocytopenia and leukopenia, along with an elevated LDH and indirect bilirubin from ineffective erythropoiesis, are present.

Traditionally, the Schilling test is performed to determine the etiology of B_{12} efficiency. However, B_{12} replacement effectively treats deficiencies from all causes. This test, which measures 24-hour urinary excretion of radiolabeled B_{12} given orally, distinguishes pernicious anemia from bacterial overgrowth and other absorption problems. Although the test is expensive, difficult to perform properly, and no longer available in some centers, many experts feel that it should be performed at some point during a patient's course. Alternatively, antibodies to intrinsic factor may be measured. These antibodies are highly specific for pernicious anemia but present in only about 50% of cases. Antibodies to gastric parietal cells are found in about 85% of cases of pernicious anemia but also in 3% to 10% of healthy persons.[19] Extremely elevated serum gastrin levels and low pepsinogen-1 levels also suggest pernicious anemia.

B_{12} replacement regimens vary. One common method is 1000 μg vitamin B_{12} IM daily for 1 week, then weekly for 1 month, then every 1 to 3 months for life. Hematocrit should return to normal in 2 months. Failure to normalize should trigger a search for coexisting iron deficiency, which occurs in up to one third of patients. Six months or more may be needed for neurologic improvement, and up to 80% of patients will have at least partial resolution of neurologic manifestations. An alternative to parenteral B_{12} is high-dose oral therapy. Pa-

tients with pernicious anemia can absorb 1% to 2% of oral B_{12} without the addition of intrinsic factor, so treatment with daily oral B_{12} 1000 to 2000 μg can be considered in adherent patients.[20] B_{12} maintenance can also be accomplished with an intranasal gel preparation 500 μg once weekly, although this form is more costly than parenteral and oral forms.

Folate Deficiency

Folate is found in a wide variety of unprocessed foods. Especially rich sources include green leafy vegetables, citrus fruits, liver, and certain beans and nuts. The RDA for folate is about 200 μg daily and is increased to 400 μg in pregnancy. In contrast to vitamin B_{12}, folate stores remain adequate for only 2 to 4 months, so folate deficiency anemia is often the result of inadequate dietary intake. The typical Western diet provides only 200 to 300 μg of folate daily. Persons at risk for folate deficiency include malnourished alcoholics, neglected elderly, and the homeless. Patients who are pregnant or have certain malabsorption disorders are also at risk. Impaired absorption may occur in patients taking oral contraceptives or anticonvulsants, such as phenobarbital and phenytoin. Cirrhosis can lead to deficiency through decreased storage and metabolism capabilities of the liver. Dialysis can cause loss of folate and deficiency.

The clinical findings of folate deficiency are similar to B_{12} deficiency except neurologic symptoms are generally absent. The laboratory findings are similar except that the homocysteine level is elevated (methylmalonic acid remains normal). The serum folate can rise to normal after a recent folate-rich meal, vitamin ingestion, or hemolysis, so serum folate should not be used for diagnosis. RBC folate level is felt to be more accurate, but confirmation with homocysteine levels should be obtained if the diagnosis is suspected.

Treatment is aimed at the underlying problem. Replacement is usually 1 mg orally daily. Concurrent vitamin B_{12} deficiency must be treated as well, because folate replacement can resolve hematologic abnormalities while permitting neurologic damage from cobalamin deficiency to progress.

Drugs

Certain drugs cause megaloblastic anemia. Most common causes are chemotherapy agents. Infrequent causes are phenytoin, sulfasalazine, zidovudine, trimethoprim, pyrimethamine, methotrexate, triamterine, sulfa compounds, and oral contraceptives.

Nonmegaloblastic Anemias
Alcoholism

The most common cause of nonmegaloblastic macrocytic anemia is alcoholism (also see Chapter 59). Anemia in alcoholics arises from several causes. Alcohol suppresses erythropoiesis and decreases folate absorption in patients whose diets are often poor. Alcoholics often lose blood from varices and ulcers. Anemia is worsened if liver failure occurs. Moreover, alcoholics are prone to develop sideroblastic or hemolytic anemia. They are also at increased risk for developing infections that can lead to anemia of chronic disease. Comprehensive therapy includes reduction of alcohol intake, folate supplementation, and treatment of complications.

Miscellaneous

The anemia of hypothyroidism, chronic liver disease, post-splenectomy, and primary bone marrow disorders may be macrocytic instead of normocytic. Hemolytic anemia or hemorrhage can result in macrocytosis when reticulocytes, which are larger than normal RBCs, are markedly increased. Certain drugs occasionally cause nonmegaloblastic macrocytic anemia.

Summary

Discovery of anemia should lead the physician to investigate the underlying cause of anemia. Conversely, it may be reasonable to check for anemia in patients who develop certain acute or chronic medical conditions. The history and physical examination combined with the CBC, peripheral smear, and reticulocyte count reveal the etiology in most cases. It is not uncommon to find multifactorial causes for a patient's anemia. If the type of anemia remains unclear or there is additional evidence of marrow dysfunction (pancytopenia), a bone marrow biopsy or hematology consultation may be indicated.

References

1. Dallman PR, Yip R, Johnson C. Prevalence and causes of anemia in the United States, 1976 to 1980. Am J Clin Nutr 1984;39:437–45.
2. Bessman JD, Gilmer PR, Gardner FH. Improved classification of anemias by MCV and RDW. Am J Clin Pathol 1983;80:322–6.
3. Lee GR, Herbert V. Nutritional factors in the production and function of erythrocytes. In: Lee GR, Foerster J, Lukens J, Paraskevas F, Greer JP, Rodgers GM, eds. Wintrobe's clinical hematology. Philadelphia: Lippincott Williams & Wilkins, 1999;232t.
4. Rockey DC, Cello JP. Evaluation of the gastrointestinal tract in patients with iron-deficiency anemia. N Engl J Med 1993;329: 1691–5.
5. Fireman Z, Kopelman Y, Sternberg A. Editorial: endoscopic evaluation of iron deficiency anemia and follow-up in patients older than 50. J Clin Gastroenterol 1998;26(1):7–10.
6. Stewart JG, Ahlquist DA, McGill DB, Ilstrup DM, Schwartz S, Owen RA. Gastrointestinal blood loss and anemia in runners. Ann Intern Med 1984;100:843–5.
7. Guyatt GH, Oxman AD, Ali M, Willan A, McIlroy W, Patterson C. Laboratory diagnosis of iron-deficiency anemia: an overview. J Gen Intern Med 1992;7:145–53.
8. Punnonen K, Irjala K, Rajamaki A. Serum transferrin receptor and its ratio to serum ferritin in the diagnosis of iron deficiency. Blood 1997;89(3):1052–7.
9. Gross R, Schultink W, Juliawati. Treatment of anemia with weekly iron supplementation [letter]. Lancet 1994;344:821.
10. Iron-containing products. In: drug facts and comparisons staff, eds. Drug facts and comparisons. St. Louis: Facts and comparisons, 2000;31–41.
11. Hallberg L, Brune M, Rossander-Hulthen L. Is there a physiological role of vitamin C in iron absorption? Ann NY Acad Sci 1987;493:324–32.
12. Little DR. Ambulatory management of common forms of anemia. Am Fam Physician 1999;59(6):1598–604.
13. Joosten E, Pelemans W, Hiele M, Noyen J, Verghaeghe R, Boogaerts MA. Prevalence and causes of anaemia in a geriatric hospitalized population. Gerontology 1992;38:111–17.
14. Krantz SB. Pathogenesis and treatment of the anemia of chronic disease. Am J Med Sci 1994;307:353–9.
15. Savage DG, Ogundipe A, Allen R, Stabler S, Lindenbaum J. Etiology and diagnostic evaluation of macrocytosis. Am J Med Sci 2000;319(6):343–52.
16. Lindenbaum J, Healton EB, Savage DG, et al. Neuropsychiatric disorders caused by cobalamin deficiency in the absence of anemia or macrocytosis. N Engl J Med 1988;318(26):1720–8.
17. Savage DJ, Lindenbaum J, Stabler SP, Allen RH. Sensitivity of serum methylmalonic acid and total homocysteine determinations for diagnosing cobalamin and folate deficiencies. Am J Med 1994;96:239–46.
18. Klee GG. Cobalamin and folate evaluation: Measurement of methylmalonic acid and homocysteine vs. vitamin B_{12} and folate. Clin Chem 2000;46(8B):1277–83.
19. Snow CF. Laboratory diagnosis of vitamin B_{12} and folate deficiency. Arch Intern Med 1999;159:1289–98.
20. Elia M. Oral or parenteral therapy for B_{12} deficiency. Lancet 1998;352:1721–2.

Selected Disorders of the Blood and Hematopoietic System

Paul M. Paulman, Layne A. Prest, and Cheryl A. Abboud

Bleeding Disorders: Congenital

Disorders of Coagulation

Hemophilia A

Hemophilia A is an autosomal X-linked recessive deficiency of factor VIII. Because of the mode of transmission and gene expression, males have hemophilia A, and females are usually asymptomatic carriers of the hemophilia A gene. All daughters of a hemophiliac father are carriers of the hemophilia A gene; all his sons are normal. The children of a female hemophilia A carrier have a 50% chance of being affected by the gene. Hemophilia A affects approximately 1 in 10,000 to 1 in 20,000 males in the United States.[1]

Hemophilia A usually presents with hemorrhage into a joint or a muscle. Excessive bleeding following minor cuts or abrasions is rare because of normally functioning platelets and normal vessel walls. Common first presentations are either a hemarthrosis or large bruise following a fall during the first 2 years of life or prolonged bleeding following neonatal circumcision. The most common bleeding sites are joints (knees, elbows, ankles, shoulder, hips, wrists), muscles, renal tract, nervous system, gastrointestinal tract, and the oral cavity following tooth extraction.

Screening coagulation tests reveal a normal platelet count, normal bleeding time, normal prothrombin time (PT), and a prolonged activated partial thromboplastin time (APTT) (Table 126.1). The diagnosis is confirmed by obtaining a serum factor VIII assay (normal 1.0 U/mL). The disease is classified as mild, moderate, or severe depending on the serum level of factor VIII activity.[2]

Hemorrhage in hemophilia is prevented by intravenous infusion of recombinant factor VIII or human-derived factor VIII concentrates treated to inactivate or remove viruses. The plasma factor VIII level is maintained at 0.3 U/mL if the patient experiences minor hemorrhage, 0.5 U/mL with severe hemorrhage, and 0.8 to 1.0 U/mL with life-threatening hemorrhage. Intravenous deamino-γ-D-arginine vasopressin (DDAVP) (desmopressin acetate 0.3 μg/kg) is the treatment of choice for the patient with mild hemophilia; the mechanism of action is unclear.[3] Complications of bleeding are managed conservatively or by drainage depending on the site and severity. Surgical and dental procedures can be performed for the patient with hemophilia A. The following factors should be considered.

1. The procedure should be done in a facility with an adequate blood bank and surgeons and dentists experienced in treating patients with hemophilia A.
2. No intramuscular medications are prescribed, and no salicylate is given.
3. The factor VIII level should be maintained at 80% to 100% of normal (0.8–1.0 U/mL).
4. ϵ-Aminocaproic acid (4 g PO q4–6h for 2–8 days) can be used as single or adjunctive postoperative therapy for dental procedures.[4] ϵ-Aminocaproic acid is a potent inhibitor of fibrinolysis (inhibits plasminogen activation) and enhances hemostasis in hemophiliacs.

Hemophilia A is preventable only via genetic counseling (see Chapter 16). A family genogram is invaluable for tracking the illness across generations. Women who are at risk for being carriers for hemophilia A can be identified as normal or carriers through factor VIII antibody studies and DNA analysis, with a detection rate of 70% to 100%.[4] Hemophilia A can usually be detected in a male fetus using chromosome studies when there is a family history of hemophilia A (i.e., the mother is at risk of being a carrier). Detection of de novo cases, with no family history, is difficult. In addition to the many severe somatic problems patients with hemophilia A face, there are severe psychosocial problems associated with this disease that affect the functioning of the patient and family unit. These problems include the following[5]:

1. Responses of the patient and family to a chronic illness, including overprotection

Table 126.1. **Laboratory Abnormalities Seen with Bleeding Disorders**

Disease	Platelet count	Bleeding time	PT	APTT
Hemophilia A and B	Normal	Normal	Normal	Prolonged
von Willebrand's disease	Normal	Prolonged	Normal	Normal
Thrombocytopenia	Low	Prolonged	Normal	Normal
Vitamin K deficiency	Normal	Normal	Prolonged	Normal or prolonged

PT = prothrombin time; APTT = activated partial thromboplastin time.
Normal values: platelet count 250,000 to 500,000/mm³; bleeding time: Ivy 2 to 7 minutes, Duke 1 to 4 minutes; APTT 34 to 54 seconds; PT 10 to 14 seconds.

2. "Daredevil syndrome"—patient taking risks above those expected for the developmental stage
3. School and vocational problems
4. Financial burdens (treatment cost $10,000–$50,000/year)
5. Concern about infections from blood products [human immunodeficiency virus (HIV) infection prior to 1985, hepatitis B and C]
6. Peer and sibling relationship problems

Referral to a hemophilia support group or a family counselor may improve the patient's and family's level of functioning and compliance. Gene transfer therapy may offer a hope for a cure for the hemophilias in the future.[1]

von Willebrand's Disease

von Willebrand's disease (vWD) is an inherited hemorrhagic disorder characterized by deficiency of von Willebrand factor (vWF). vWF is necessary for normal interaction of platelets with vessel walls. vWD is inherited in an autosomal-dominant pattern, with males and females equally affected. The prevalence of vWD may be as high as 1.5% of the population; the most severe form has a prevalence rate of 1 in 1 million. There are four types and multiple subtypes of vWD. Many patients with vWD also have low levels of factor VIII.[6]

Hemorrhage with vWD is highly variable. Epistaxis, gastrointestinal bleeding, easy bruising, and menorrhagia are characteristic of vWD. Hemarthroses are rare. Bleeding following trauma, dental extractions, or operations may be severe. Patients with vWD types I and II platelet type usually have mild or no bleeding problems. Patients with type III disease have severe bleeding problems.

The diagnosis of vWD is confirmed by laboratory findings of prolonged bleeding time, decreased factor VIII levels, decreased vWF activity, and decreased vWF antigen. The PT, APTT, and platelet count are usually normal (Table 126.1).

The goals of therapy for vWD are to correct coagulation abnormalities, prevent hemorrhage, and return the levels of vWF and factor VIII to normal. For patients with mild vWD, DDAVP administered intranasally or intravenously at a dose of 0.2 to 0.3 µg/kg body weight can be effective.[7] Oral contraceptives can increase plasma levels of factor VIII and vWF and are useful for women with vWD whose primary problem is menstrual bleeding. Intravenous factor VIII is used to treat patients with more severe bleeding problems. Treatment is titrated to the clinical status of the patient. Surgical and dental procedures can be safely performed in most patients with vWD. Treatment is started (DDAVP or factor VIII) 1 hour prior to the procedure and is continued for 2 to 3 days after the procedure. The goal of perioperative therapy is to keep the bleeding time within the normal range. vWD is preventable only through genetic counseling. It is passed via an autosomal-dominant pattern, with 50% of the children of a parent with vWD at risk to inherit the disease. vWD can be detected in utero via chromosomal analysis. The family and community issues are similar to concerns faced by patients with hemophilia A.

Hemophilia B

Hemophilia B is an X-linked recessive factor IX deficiency. It has an incidence of approximately 1 in 30,000 males and is diagnosed by factor IX assay. Hemophilia B is clinically indistinguishable from hemophilia A. Treatment of hemophilia B is intravenous recombinant or human-derived factor IX concentrate. DDAVP has no value in hemophilia B.[3]

Acquired Disorders of Coagulation Factors: Vitamin K Deficiency

Vitamin K is a fat-soluble compound essential to the synthesis of factors II, VII, IX, and X. The sources of vitamin K are dietary (especially green, leafy vegetables) and synthesis of vitamin K by intestinal bacteria. The daily adult requirement of vitamin K is 100 to 200 µg/day. Deficiency states of vitamin K can be seen in the newborn (hemorrhagic disease), the elderly, patients with liver disease, after ingestion of vitamin K antagonists (i.e., warfarin), or with long-term antibiotic use (elimination of gastrointestinal flora).

Vitamin K deficiency presents with bleeding in the skin or from mucosal surfaces. Internal bleeding and hemarthroses are rare. The PT is prolonged; the bleeding time and platelet count are usually normal; and the APTT may be prolonged (Table 126.1).

Vitamin K deficiency is diagnosed by correcting clinical and laboratory abnormalities with vitamin K replacement. A direct laboratory assay for vitamin K is also available.[8]

In the case of life-threatening hemorrhage, fresh frozen plasma is given intravenously to return the PT to normal and stop the bleeding. In less urgent situations, vitamin K can be given by the intramuscular, intravenous, or oral route (AquaMEPHYTON 10–15 mg). The goal of therapy is to prevent further bleeding and to return the PT to normal. Treatment with vitamin K usually corrects the PT within 24 to 48 hours.

A diet with adequate amounts of vitamin K–containing foods (especially green, leafy vegetables), avoidance of hepatotoxic agents, and judicious use of long-term antibiotics can prevent vitamin K deficiency. Vitamin K 0.5 to 1 mg IM should be given to all newborns to prevent hemorrhagic disease of the newborn.[9] Vitamin K supplementation is also recommended during pregnancy for women on anticonvulsant therapy or prolonged treatment with certain antibiotics.[10]

Vitamin K deficiency may be a sign of neglect in the elderly patient, whose diet may be deficient.

Disorders of Platelets

Platelets play a crucial role in hemostasis through adhesion, "platelet plug" formation, and release of substances that promote platelet aggregation. Bleeding due to platelet disorders is usually in the skin or from mucosal surfaces. Thrombocytopenia is defined as a platelet count below 100,000/mm³. The causes of thrombocytopenia are listed in Table 126.2. Platelet colony-stimulating factors may become an option for the treatment of thrombocytopenia in the future. Aspirin, clopidogrel, and ticlopidine can cause clinically significant platelet dysfunction.

Idiopathic Thrombocytopenic Purpura

Idiopathic thrombocytopenic purpura (ITP) is caused by interaction of immunoglobulin G (IgG) and other antibodies with megakaryocytes or platelets, resulting in increased platelet destruction. ITP can present as a primary problem or be associated with such condition as malignancies, collagen vascular disease, or viral illnesses. Acute ITP is most common in children, and chronic ITP is more common in adults, with a male/female ratio of 1:3.[11] Acute ITP occurs most commonly between the ages of 2 and 9 years; chronic ITP occurs chiefly between the ages of 20 and 50 years.

Patients with ITP may be asymptomatic, or they may present with persistent skin bleeding (especially in areas exposed to trauma) or mucosal surface bleeding (i.e., epistaxis, menorrhagia, ecchymoses). Internal hemorrhage and hemarthroses

Table 126.2. **Causes of Thrombocytopenia**

Acquired amegakaryocytic thrombocytopenic purpura
Aplastic anemia
Leukemia
Marrow infiltration/replacement
Hypersplenism
Idiopathic thrombocytopenic purpura
Collagen-vascular diseases
Lymphomas and solid tumors
Infection (HIV and others)
Disseminated intravascular coagulation (DIC)
Thrombotic thrombocytopenic purpura
Chemical agents
Congenital
Cavernous hemangioma
Cardiopulmonary bypass
Hemolytic-uremic syndrome

are rare. Intracranial hemorrhage, though rare, can be a serious complication of ITP.

Diagnosis

The diagnosis is established through the history, physical examination findings, and platelet count. Atraumatic bleeding usually is not a problem with a platelet count above 20,000/mm³. Traumatic bleeding can occur with platelet counts of 40,000 to 60,000/mm³. Other routine clotting studies are usually normal except for a prolonged bleeding time.

Treatment

Treatment is unnecessary in patients with mild thrombocytopenia and is reserved for the patient who is bleeding because of thrombocytopenia or whose platelet count is below 20,000/mm³. The goal of therapy is to stop the bleeding and return the platelet count to more than 20,000/mm³.

Corticosteroids. Prednisone in a dose of 1 to 2 mg/kg/day (up to 100 mg/day) can be used for up to 6 weeks and has a success rate of up to 80%.

Splenectomy. Splenectomy is reserved for patients who fail conservative therapy or who have hypersplenism. It has a success rate of 60% to 80% if all accessory splenic tissue is identified and removed.[12] Patients should receive pneumococcal and *Haemophilus influenzae* B vaccine at least 2 weeks prior to splenectomy.

Danazol. Danazol has a mechanism of action probably similar to that of corticosteroids. It can be used concomitantly with corticosteroids and allows a lower dose of corticosteroid to be used. The dosage is 400 to 800 mg/day for up to 3 months, with tapering to 50 to 200 mg/day if a response is seen.[13]

Immunosuppressive Agents. Immunosuppressive agents are used if thrombocytopenia persists despite treatment with steroids, danazol, or splenectomy. Vincristine and vinblastine are the most commonly used agents.

γ-Globulin. Intravenous γ-globulin in doses of 400 to 1000 mg/kg/day has been used successfully in cases of recalcitrant ITP.

Other Therapeutic Options. Plasmapheresis and colchicine have been used with limited success in patients with ITP.[14] Monoclonal antibody therapy for ITP is in the experimental stages.[15] ITP is not preventable. If ITP becomes a chronic condition, patients and their families face psychosocial issues that are virtually identical to those faced by patients with hemophilia A and other bleeding disorders.

Thrombotic Thrombocytopenic Purpura

Thrombotic thrombocytopenic purpura (TTP) is primarily a disease of adults of largely unknown etiology. The hallmark of TTP is widespread platelet thrombi occurring throughout the microcirculation. Although rare, TTP can be fatal in up to 90% of untreated patients.

The clinical manifestations of TTP may include hemorrhage, hemolytic anemia, neurologic problems (headache, mental status changes, seizures, coma, and focal neurologic changes), hematuria, renal failure, and fever.

The diagnosis of TTP is made based on the clinical findings and laboratory findings including severe thrombocytopenia, red cell fragmentation, reticulocytosis, elevated indirect serum bilirubin, decreased haptoglobin, and proteinuria. Disseminated intravascular coagulation is usually not associated with TTP. Severe TTP is treated with prednisone (1 to 2 mg/kg/day) and plasmapheresis.

The hemolytic-uremic syndrome (HUS) is clinically similar to TTP. HUS is usually seen in children following infections by viruses, *Escherichia coli*, or *Shigella* species. The clinical picture of HUS includes thrombocytopenia and hemolytic anemia. Neurologic symptoms are less common in HUS than in TTP. The treatment for patients with HUS is plasma exchange. Syndromes resembling TTP/HUS have been seen in patients receiving certain chemotherapeutic agents.[15]

Disorders of the Vascular Wall

The integrity of the vascular wall is essential for maintenance of normal coagulation. Some causes of vascular wall disruption are listed in Table 126.3. Vascular causes of bleeding (purpura) tend to manifest most often on the lower extremities. Purpura of the head and neck is usually caused by fat emboli, amyloidosis, or mechanical stresses. Bleeding from vascular causes (with some exceptions) is usually confined to the skin.

Congenital Disorders

Hereditary hemorrhagic telangiectasia (Osler-Weber-Rendu disease) is a congenital disorder. Bleeding in patients with hereditary hemorrhagic telangiectasia (HHT) occurs because of malformations of small veins in the skin and mucosa (telangiectases). Transmission of HHT is autosomal dominant, with males and females affected equally (incidence 1/50,000).[16] Epistaxis and gastrointestinal (GI) tract bleeding are the most common presentations. The lesions of HHT usually become clinically significant during the second or third decade of life. Examination may reveal lesions in the mouth, face, hands, and feet. The lesions are 1 to 3 mm in diameter, nonpulsatile, red to purplish and flat, round, or spider-like. HHT lesions are also found in the lungs of 15% to 20% of patients and can occur in virtually any organ.

The diagnosis of HHT is established via the history and clinical examination. The family history is often positive. Screening coagulation studies are usually normal. Therapy for HHT is symptomatic. Whenever possible, pressure is applied to bleeding sites. Cautery or surgical therapy of nasal mucosal lesions yields mixed results. GI bleeding can be treated by resection or embolectomy. HHT is not preventable.

The family and community issues are similar to those faced by patients with other bleeding disorders.

Table 126.3. **Bleeding from Vascular Abnormalities**

Congenital causes
  Hereditary hemorrhagic telangiectasia
  Angiokeratoma corporis diffusum
  Ataxia telangiectasia
  Cavernous hemangioma
  Ehlers-Danlos syndrome
  Pseudoxanthoma elasticum
  Osteogenesis imperfecta
  Marfan syndrome

Acquired causes
  Mechanical
    Trauma
    Increased venous pressure
  Decreased supporting tissue
    Senile purpura
    Scurvy
    Corticosteroids
    Amyloidosis
  Chemical agents
    Warfarin (Coumadin)
    Snake venoms
  Infections: meningococcus, rickettsiae, streptococci, shigellae, gram-negative bacteria, measles, rubella, diphtheria
  Vasculitis: Henoch-Schönlein purpura
  Vascular obstruction
    DIC
    Fat emboli
    Leukostasis
    Paraproteinemia
    Proliferative retinopathy
  Idiopathic causes

Acquired Disorders

Senile purpura is a characteristic lesion of the elderly.[17] The lesion is caused by progressive loss of collagen in vessels and skin, possibly hastened by ultraviolet (sun) exposure. The lesions of senile purpura usually occur on the upper extremities, especially the back of the hands, wrists, and forearms. The lesions are large, dark, and well demarcated. The diagnosis is made clinically. Screening coagulation studies are usually normal. There is no specific treatment. Most lesions of senile purpura resolve slowly. Counseling the patient regarding the benign nature of the illness is recommended. Minimizing sun exposure may slow some of the skin changes of aging.

Vasculitis

Vasculitis (vascular inflammation) can be caused by many disease processes, including immune causes, infections, drugs, neoplasms, connective tissue diseases, and cold exposure. Henoch-Schönlein purpura (HSP) (allergic purpura) is considered the model for the study of vasculitis. It primarily affects the kidneys, GI tract, and joints. The etiology is unknown. HSP has been seen after viral and streptococcal infections. Drugs (sulfonamides and penicillin) have been implicated as causative agents, and there are data to support an immune mechanism as a cause.[18] HSP is most often seen in children aged 2 to 10 years (male/female ratio 2:1) but can occur at any age. There is an increased incidence during early spring and early autumn.

Henoch-Schönlein presents with fever followed by a macular or urticarial rash on the buttocks, legs, and arms that becomes purpuric. Lesions can occur in crops. Other findings include edema (legs, hands, scalp, eyes), abdominal pain, vomiting, diarrhea, intussusception, arthritis, and hypertension. Kidney involvement is manifested by proteinuria, hematuria, renal failure, or nephrotic syndrome. Iritis, pericarditis, pleurisy, and neurologic disorders are seen less frequently.

Most patients recover spontaneously within 1 month, although relapses are frequent. Treatment is symptomatic. Penicillin is often used because of the association of HSP with streptococcal infections. Glucocorticoids and immunosuppressive agents can be used for the 5% to 10% of patients who develop progressive renal failure. Dapsone is being studied as a possible treatment for HSP.[19]

Other Bleeding Disorders

Simple, Easy Bruising (Devil's Pinches)

Simple, easy bruising is an ill-defined condition that presents with bruises on the lower extremities and trunk.[20] It is most common in women during their reproductive years. The suspected etiology is platelet dysfunction owing to aspirin ingestion. If no abnormality is found on routine coagulation studies, patients can be counseled to avoid aspirin and can be reassured that the disease has only cosmetic complications.

Disseminated Intravascular Coagulation

Disseminated intravascular coagulation (DIC) is a syndrome of accelerated fibrin deposition in blood vessels and lysis of red blood cells. Disorderly production of fibrin monomers and polymer leads to diffuse and damaging fibrin deposits and plugs in the microvasculature. Bleeding in DIC is caused by the consumption of fibrin and its procoagulants. It is a hemorrhagic

Table 126.4. **Causes of Disseminated Intravascular Coagulation**

Tissue injury	Immunologic phenomena
Obstetric problems	**Drugs**
Amniotic fluid embolism	Fibrinolytic agents
Abruptio placentae	Ancrod
Uterine rupture	Warfarin (Coumadin)
Eclampsia	Heparin
Retained dead fetus	Lipid emulsion
Septic abortion	Clotting factor concentrate
Midtrimester abortion	**Other causes**
Malignancies	Liver disease
Infections	Pancreatic disease
Bacterial	Pulmonary disease
Fungal	Neurologic disease
Viral	Envenomation
Protozoal	Transfusions
Cardiovascular disease or injury	

complication of many serious illnesses (Table 126.4). Hemorrhage may occur in the skin, central nervous system (CNS), GI system, genitourinary system, or elsewhere. DIC may be associated with a high mortality rate depending on the nature and severity of the cause. The diagnosis is suspected clinically and confirmed by laboratory findings of elevated fibrin degradation products, prolonged prothrombin and partial thromboplastin times, decreased fibrin levels, and thrombocytopenia.

Treatment of DIC consists of maintaining the vital functions of the patient and treating the underlying disease process. Heparin is used if there is evidence of thrombosis (gangrene of the extremities or digits).[21] Because DIC depletes coagulation factors, replacement with cryoprecipitate may be considered if there is no evidence of thrombosis and indications of coagulation factor depletion.[22] Platelets are replaced for any patient with a count less than 20,000/mm^3 or any patient with a count less than 50,000/mm^3 with bleeding.[22]

Neutropenia

Neutropenia is defined as an absolute neutrophil count (ANC) of less than 1500/mm^3:

White Blood Cell Count
$$\times \ (\% \ \text{Bands} + \% \ \text{Mature Neutrophils}) \times 0.01$$

An ANC of 1500/mm^3 or more is the standard for all ages and all races, with some exceptions: newborns have elevated neutrophil counts during the first days of life, and certain populations of blacks and Yemenite Jews may have low neutrophil counts. An ANC of 500 to 1000/mm^3 puts patients at increased risk for bacterial infection, whereas an ANC of 500/mm^3 or less may put patients at significant risk for bacterial infection that requires inpatient management.[23] Neutropenia can be either acquired or intrinsic and can result from decreased production, margination, or shift from blood to tissue, increased destruction, or a combination of causes.

Acquired Neutropenia

Postinfectious Neutropenia

Neutropenia is commonly seen with viral infections including varicella, measles, rubella, hepatitis A and B, mononucleosis, influenza, and Kawasaki disease. Neutrophil counts usually return to normal after resolution of the viremia. More than 70% of patients with acquired immunodeficiency syndrome (AIDS) have neutropenia.[24] Bacterial infections (especially those due to *Staphylococcus aureus* and *Mycobacterium tuberculosis* plus brucellosis, tularemia, and rickettsia) can cause neutropenia. Sepsis is a cause of marked neutropenia, particularly in debilitated patients and newborns.

Drug-Induced Neutropenia

Table 126.5 lists agents associated with neutropenia.

Chronic Benign Neutropenia of Childhood

Chronic benign neutropenia of childhood is probably an autoimmune disease with mature neutrophil depletion and in-

Table 126.5. **Drugs that Cause Neutropenia**

Nonsteroidal antiinflammatory drugs	Bacampicillin
Ibuprofen	Capreomycin
Indomethacin	Carbenicillin
Meclofenamate	Cefaclor
Mefenamic acid	Cefadroxil
Oxyphenbutazone	Cefamandole
Phenylbutazone	Cefazolin
Anticonvulsants	Cefotaxime
Carbamazepine	Cephalexin
Mephenytoin	Cephaloglycin
Paramethadione	Cephaloridine
Phenobarbital	Cephalothin
Phenytoin	Cephradine
Valproate	Chloramphenicol
Antipsychotics	Clindamycin
Acetophenazine	Cyclacillin
Carphenazine	Dapsone
Chlorprothixene	Demeclocycline
Fluphenazine	Doxycycline
Haloperidol	Flucytosine
Loxapine	Furazolidone
Mesoridazine	Griseofulvin
Molindone	Hetacillin
Perphenazine	Lincomycin
Piperacetazine	Methacycline
Thiethylperazine	Metronidazole
Thioridazine	Mezlocillin
Thiothixene	Moxalactam
Trimeprazine	Nafcillin
Trifluoperazine	Novobiocin
Triflupromazine	Oxacillin
Antidepressants	Oxytetracycline
Amitriptyline	Paraaminosalicylic acid
Amoxapine	Penicillin G
Desipramine	Penicillin V
Doxepin	Pyrimethamine
Imipramine	Quinine
Nortriptyline	Quinacrine
Protriptyline	Rifampin
Maprotiline	Tetracycline
Trimipramine	Ticarcillin
Antiarrhythmics	Trimethoprim
Procainamide	Vidarabine
Quinidine	Zidovudine
Tocainide	**Antineoplastic agents**
Anxiolytics	**Other drugs**
Diazepam	Allopurinol
Tybamate	Clofibrate
Diuretics	Dantrolene
Diazoxide	Ethanol
Ethacrynate	Levamisole
Mercaptomerin	Levodopa
Antimicrobials	Methyldopa
Amoxicillin	Methysergide
Ampicillin	Nifedipine
	Penicillamine
	Podophyllin
	Sulfonamides

creased immature granulocytes in the bone marrow.[25] The disease can present during the first 3 years of life; 90% of patients are diagnosed before the age 14 months. There is a slight female predominance (3:2). ANCs as low as 500/mm³ are rel-

atively common, although they are usually normal at birth. Children with chronic benign neutropenia of childhood may present with fever, infections (skin infection, oral ulcers, otitis, sinusitis), or hepatosplenomegaly. Treatment of this disorder centers around appropriate management of infections. In patients with severe infections, raising the neutrophil count with glucocorticoids, γ-globulin, or granulocyte colony-stimulating factor may be necessary.[23] Some experts believe this disorder is identical to chronic idiopathic neutropenia.

Autoimmune Neutropenia

Autoimmune neutropenia can occur with medication ingestion, other autoimmune diseases, infection, or as a separate entity.[26] Hepatosplenomegaly is seen in about half the patients. The time of presentation varies from early childhood to old age. The propensity for infection is related to the degree to neutropenia. Therapy centers around appropriate treatment of the related condition(s). If patients have severe neutropenia and severe recurrent infections, treatment with glucocorticoids or γ-globulins (or both) may be warranted.[27,28]

Alloimmune (Isoimmune) Neutropenia

This neutropenia is secondary to transplacental IgG antibody transfer. Newborns with alloimmune neutropenia may experience moderate to severe recurrent infections; treatment with glucocorticoids or γ-globulins (or both) may be warranted.[27,28] This process is similar to the hemolysis in the newborn caused by Rh isoimmunization. The condition affects 1 in 2000 infants and usually resolves by age 15 weeks.

Treatment includes antibiotics if there is any concern about sepsis. Exchange transfusion to decrease antibody titers or transfusions of maternal neutrophils may be helpful.

Nutritional Neutropenia

Neutropenia has been associated with deficiencies of vitamin B_{12}, folate, copper, and thiamine. Neutrophil counts usually return to normal following correction of these deficiencies. Mild neutropenia has also been associated with anorexia nervosa.

Intrinsic Defects

Cyclic neutropenia is an autosomal-dominant inherited disorder characterized by neutropenia that recurs every 15 to 35 days. The disease is usually benign, but patients may have recurrent fever, pharyngitis, stomatitis, gingivitis, and other bacterial infections.[29] The severity of infection usually parallels the severity of the neutropenia, and there have been several deaths due to infections in patients with cyclic neutropenia. Therapy is supportive and includes antibacterial mouthwash to decrease gingivitis. Patients with severe neutropenia and severe infection may be considered for bone marrow transplantation or therapy with colony-stimulating factors.[30,31]

Other Hematologic Disorders

Hemochromatosis

Hemochromatosis is the most common iron storage disease in the United States. In patients of European origin, hemochromatosis is an autosomal-recessive inherited disorder linked to the human leukocyte antigen (HLA) locus and is known as primary or hereditary hemochromatosis. Secondary hemochromatosis is seen with a variety of anemias, particularly with β-thalassemia, associated with increased iron absorption and inefficient erythropoiesis. The signs and symptoms of hemochromatosis result from organ damage due to excessive iron deposition. Hemochromatosis affects approximately 1 in 5000 people in the United States, with symptoms manifesting usually between the ages of 40 and 60 years. Men are affected more frequently than women; menstruation delays the onset of symptoms in affected women.

The clinical manifestations of hemochromatosis include brown or gray skin discoloration, hepatosplenomegaly, carcinoma of the liver, hepatic cirrhosis, abdominal pain, congestive cardiomyopathy, insulin-dependent diabetes mellitus, arthralgias, loss of libido, and hypogonadism. The diagnosis of hemochromatosis is supported by laboratory findings of increased serum iron and increased serum ferritin, along with the history and physical examination findings. The definitive diagnosis requires a liver biopsy.[32]

Treatment of hereditary hemochromatosis is usually weekly phlebotomy to return iron stores to normal. With secondary hemochromatosis, phlebotomy may not be indicated owing to the anemia that often accompanies the disease. Chelation with desferrioxamine is the recommended treatment for most cases of secondary hemochromatosis. Because hereditary hemochromatosis is an inherited disorder and the prognosis for the disease improves dramatically with early treatment, all family members of a patient with hereditary hemochromatosis should be screened for the disease with a serum iron and a serum ferritin. Patients at risk for developing the complication of hemochromatosis can be followed via appropriate monitoring and treatment protocols.

Polycythemia

Polycythemia is defined as an increased red blood cell (RBC) mass 36 mL/kg or more (hematocrit >51%) for men and 32 mL/kg or more (hematocrit >48%) for women.[33] The causes of polycythemia include polycythemia vera (a hematologic malignancy) and secondary causes (lung disease, heart disease, kidney disease, and other malignancies). Patients living at high altitudes exhibit high hematocrits owing to decreased oxygen tension with increasing elevation. Polycythemia vera is a rare disorder with a prevalence of 5 to 17 cases per 1 million population.[34] Secondary polycythemia is seen most commonly after age 60 years and in the newborn. Apparent polycythemia describes increased hemoglobin and packed cell volume with normal red cell mass. This condition is caused by decreased plasma volume and may be associated with alcohol and tobacco use and therapy with diuretics.

Clinical problems for patients with polycythemia are caused by vascular thrombosis due to the increased RBC mass. The risk of thrombosis increases with age and increasing hematocrit. Thrombotic events occur in the CNS and peripheral vascular systems, leading to strokes and pulmonary emboli. Thrombosis can occur in the vena cava and the splenic, hepatic, portal, mesenteric, and coronary vessels. Patients with polycythemia may present with a variety of symptoms, including headache, weakness, pruritus, dizziness, excessive sweating, visual disturbances, paresthesias, joint symptoms, epigastric distress, and weight loss. Physical examination may reveal ruddy cyanosis, conjunctival plethora, hepatomegaly, splenomegaly, and hypertension. Laboratory findings reveal a hematocrit of more than 48% to 51% and thrombocytosis. Patients with polycythemia vera may also be prone to hemorrhagic complications due to platelet dysfunction.[35] Patients with polycythemia may develop hyperuricemia due to increased RBC destruction after treatment.[36]

The treatment of polycythemia is aimed at correcting the secondary cause. Phlebotomy is indicated for patients who are symptomatic to maintain the hematocrit at 42% to 45%. Patients who suffer from hypoxia due to chronic lung or heart disease may see improvement of their polycythemia after oxygen therapy. Therapy for patients with polycythemia vera may include radioactive phosphorus or alkylating agents in addition to phlebotomy.[37] The prognosis usually depends on the severity of the secondary cause. Median survival of patients with polycythemia vera varies from 10 to 14 years. There is no effective strategy for preventing polycythemia vera. Prevention of secondary polycythemia centers around preventing the causes of lung and heart disease, especially tobacco smoking.

Sickle Cell Anemia

Sickle cell anemia is an autosomal-dominant inherited disease caused by a substitution of one amino acid in the hemoglobin molecule.[38] The RBCs of patients with sickle cell anemia assume a sickle shape and become dysfunctional when deoxygenated. Patients who are homozygous for the sickle cell gene have sickle cell anemia, and those who are heterozygous have sickle cell trait. Sickle cell trait, which appears to offer patients protection against malaria, is found in 2.5 million people in the United States (8% of African Americans).[39] Because the distribution of sickle cell trait appears to be related to protection from malaria and not race, sickle cell trait is found in nonblacks.[40] β-Thalassemia may be inherited with sickle cell anemia.

The clinical characteristics of sickle cell anemia are due to the malformation of RBCs when they are deoxygenated and include bone pain, anemia, infections, cardiomegaly, CNS infarctions, gallstones, renal infarction, retinopathy, and avascular necrosis of the hip. The sickled cells lead to vascular occlusion or hemolytic anemia (or both). Almost every organ system can be affected in sickle cell anemia. Patients with sickle cell anemia are at increased risk of pneumococcal infections due to splenic infarctions. The mortality for untreated sickle cell anemia is 10% to 15% during the first decade of life.[41] Patients with sickle cell trait usually have few clinical problems. Microinfarctions of the kidney, spleen, and CNS have been reported with decreased oxygen tension, as has an association with an increased incidence of sudden death in some patients with sickle cell trait during intense physical activity.[42]

Table 126.6. **Treatment for Patients with Sickle Cell Disease**

General treatment
Caloric supplements
Folic acid (5 mg/day)
Prophylactic penicillin, daily (children)
Pneumococcal vaccine
Haemophilus influenzae B vaccine
Hepatitis B vaccine
Transfusions to maintain hemoglobin between 10 and 12 g/dL
Chelation therapy as needed for iron overload
Antidepressants for chronic pain
Psychological support
Crisis treatment
Hydration
Oxygen if hypoxic
Antibiotics if fever or infection is present
Analgesia: consider patient-controlled analgesia with narcotics
Crisis prevention
Hydroxyurea

The treatment of patients with sickle cell anemia is outlined in Table 126.6. Curative therapy may be offered to patients with sickle cell anemia in the future through gene therapy, bone marrow transplantation, cord blood stem cell infusion, or nonablative marrow infusion.[43] Hydroxyurea has been found to be effective in decreasing the number of sickle cell crises.[44] Other agents, such as erythropoietin, vanillin, arginine butypyrate, poloxamer 188, and nitric oxide are being investigated for prevention or treatment of sickle cell crises. Vitamin E and vasodilators have not been effective in sickle cell anemia.

Sickle cell anemia cannot be prevented, but it can be detected in utero.[45] Genetic counseling should be offered to the parents of a child with sickle cell anemia.

As with management of all chronic diseases, physicians should expect both the patient and family to go through significant adjustments to the diagnosis. Many aspects of this adjustment correspond to those typically seen in a grief-loss process. Physicians and families must encourage the patient to be as active as possible, promoting independence and confidence in his or her abilities as well as decreasing withdrawal, regression, and the potential for depression. This independence also minimizes the tendency for anger and resentment to build up if the patient–family relationship becomes overly dependent. Other attempts to help that can become problematic occur when family members consistently try to protect the patient by putting his or her needs first. Family members may also become vigilant and attentive to every need. The decision to take on these functions is often made without an overt discussion within the family. Power struggles can ensue and can manifest in various behavioral-emotional symptoms (i.e., school problems, family dysfunction, caregiver burnout. The pain that results from chronic, relapsing conditions like sickle cell can be one of the most troubling symptoms patients and their families confront.[46–50] It can also be difficult for physicians to assess and manage. This is because chronic pain is a subjective perceptual experience involving the interactions among physiologic, psychological, and sociocultural factors. Aside from a purely organic etiology, chronic pain can have its origins in the patient's psychological distress (e.g., anxiety, depression, substance abuse), caregiver burnout, and/or secondary gain (e.g., malingering). The diagnostic question that emerges is, How much of this pain is real and how much is psychological? The physician can sort out the issues and answer this question by taking a careful history, paying attention to the patient's affect and caregivers' verbal and nonverbal signals, assessing the patient for psychosocial problems, and maintaining continuity of care.[51]

It is crucial that all family members be given adequate and clear information regarding the nature of the disease. Major decisions about caregiving, symptom management, and range of activities should be negotiated, with physician assistance if necessary. Ultimately, families are helped by the physician assisting them to adjust to, but not be consumed by, this chronic illness.[46,47]

Table 126.7. **Leukemias**

Disease	Incidence	Treatment	Prognosis
Acute			
Acute myeloid leukemia (AML)	Common in elderly; 10–15% of childhood leukemia	Systemic chemotherapy Bone marrow transplantation (selected patients)	5–30% long-term survival (age-dependent)
Acute lymphocytic leukemia (ALL)	Common in children	Systemic chemotherapy, Bone marrow transplantation (selected patients)	20–80% long-term survival (dependent on gender, extent of disease, and other factors)
Chronic			
Chronic myeloid leukemia (CML)	More common in middle age	Systemic chemotherapy Bone marrow transplantation (selected patients) Splenic irradiation (selected patients),	20% long-term survival (dependent on stage of disease)
Chronic lymphocytic leukemia (CLL)	Common in elderly; 25% of all leukemias	Systemic chemotherapy Radiation therapy (selected patients)	3–12 years survival (dependent on stage of disease)

Hematologic Malignancies

Multiple Myeloma

Multiple myeloma is a plasma cell (β-lymphoid) malignancy. Expansion of the plasma cell mass and the secreted products of the cells cause the symptoms associated with multiple myeloma.

Presenting problems in multiple myeloma include bone pain, anemia, recurrent infection, hypercalcemia, azotemia, bleeding disorders, or paralysis secondary to spinal cord fractures. Multiple myeloma occurs most often in middle-aged or older patients. It is slightly more common in men than women. The annual incidence is approximately 3 in 100,000.

The definitive diagnosis of multiple myeloma requires demonstration of plasmacytosis in the bone marrow or a soft tissue lesion with positive urine or serum M protein and an indication of invasive tumor (i.e., lytic bone lesion). Supporting diagnostic studies for multiple myeloma include serum and 24-hour urine protein electrophoresis (demonstrating M protein) and complete skeletal radiographs (demonstrating lytic lesions). Other laboratory abnormalities may include an elevated erythrocyte sedimentation rate (ESR), low hemoglobin, elevated serum calcium, and elevated serum creatinine. Most patients with multiple myeloma present with advanced disease and require systemic chemotherapy. The median survival varies from 3 to 5 years depending on the clinical stage and response to chemotherapy. Autologous stem cell transplantation is the treatment of choice for younger patients with multiple myeloma.[52]

Myelodysplastic Syndromes

Myelodysplastic syndromes (MDS) is the term applied to a large group of acquired neoplastic disorders of red blood cell, white blood cell, and platelet cell lines.[53] MDS is characterized by ineffective hemopoiesis in the presence of normal or increased cellularity of the bone marrow. Some patients progress to acute myeloid leukemia. Most cases arise de novo, but there is an association of myelodysplastic syndrome with previous treatment for malignancy.

There are five subgroups of MDS determined by the portion of blasts in the blood and marrow and other parameters. Most patients with MDS are men over age 70. The patient with MDS may present with refractory anemia, recurrent infection due to neutropenia, or easy bruising due to thrombocytopenia.

Treatment has been disappointing. Several agents, including erythropoietin, granulocyte colony-stimulating factor, low-dose chemotherapy, and bone marrow transplantation have been tried with variable responses. A referral to a hematologist familiar with the current treatment protocols may be beneficial for the patient with MDS.

Leukemias

The leukemias are neoplasms characterized by large numbers of abnormal white blood cells (WBCs) in the bone marrow and other organs. Common features include an elevated WBC count, abnormal WBCs in the peripheral blood, evidence of bone marrow failure, and involvement of other organs (liver, spleen, lymph tissue, meninges, brain, skin, testes). The leukemias are classified as acute or chronic. Their features are listed in Table 126.7.

Signs and symptoms of acute leukemia may include pallor, lethargy, fever, malaise, bleeding or bruising, bone pain, lymphadenopathy, hepatosplenomegaly, and hypertrophy of the gums. Chronic leukemia may present with weight loss, anorexia, splenomegaly, pallor, bruising, hyperuricemia, bacterial or fungal infection, excessive reaction to vaccination or insect bites, tonsillar enlargement, herpes zoster, or no symptoms.[54]

The role of the family physician in managing leukemia is to refer patients, as appropriate, to a hematologist or oncologist for initial treatment, provide ongoing treatment and monitoring in the patient's home community, provide ongoing care for the patient's other medical problems, and provide information and other support for the patient and the patient's family.

References

1. Mannucci PM, Tuddenham, Eg. The hemophilias: progress and problems. Semin Hematol 1999;36(4)(suppl 7):104–17.
2. Williams WJ, Beutler E, Erslev AJ, Lichtman MA. Hematology. New York: McGraw-Hill, 1990.
3. Association of Hemophilia Clinic Directors of Canada. Hemophilia and von Willebrand's disease. 2. Management. Can Med Assoc J 1995;153:147–57.
4. Brocker-Briende AJHT, Briët E, Quadt R. Genotype assignment of hemophilia A by use of intragenic and extragenic restriction fragment length polymorphisms. Thromb Haemost 1987;57:131–6.
5. Leahey M, Wright LM. Intervening with families with chronic illness. Fam Syst Med 1985;3:60–9.
6. Bowie EJW, Didishem P, Thompson JH, Owen CA. von Willebrand's disease: a critical review. Hematol Rev 1968;1:1–50.
7. Batlle J, Fernanda M, Lopez-Fernandez F, et al. Proteolytic degradation of von Willebrand factor after DDAVP administration in normal individuals. Blood 1987;70:173–6.
8. Bertina RM, Van Der Marel-Van Nieuwkoop W, Dubbeldam J, Boekhout-Musser J, Verltkamp JJ. New method for the rapid detection of vitamin K deficiency. Clin Chim Acta 1980;105:93–8.
9. Zipursky A. Review: prevention of vitamin K deficiency bleeding in newborns. Br J Haematol 1999;104:430–7.
10. Thorp JA, Gaston L, Caspers DR, Pal ML. Current concepts and controversies in the use of vitamin K. Drugs 1995;49:376–87.
11. George JN, Raskob GE. Idiopathic thrombocytopenic purpura: diagnosis and management. Am J Med Sci 1998;3(2):87–93.
12. Akwari OE, Itani KMF, Coleman RE, Rosse WF. Splenectomy for primary and recurrent immune thrombocytopenic purpura (ITP): current criteria for patient selection and results. Ann Surg 1987;206:529–39.
13. Nalli G, Sajeva R, Carnevale MG, Ascari E. Danazol therapy for idiopathic thrombocytopenic purpura (ITP). Haematologica 1988;73:55–7.
14. Blanchette VS, Hogan VA, McCombie NE, et al. Intensive plasma exchange therapy in ten patients with idiopathic thrombocytopenic purpura. Transfusion 1984;24:388–94.
15. Tieney LM, McPhee SJ, Papadalic MA. Current medical diagnosis and treatment, 38th ed. Stamford, CT: Lange, 1999;522–4.
16. Bird RM, Hammarsten JF, Marshall RA, Robinson RR. A study of hereditary hemorrhagic telangiectasia. N Engl J Med 1957;275:105–9.
17. Tattersall RN, Seville R. Senile purpura. Q J Med 1950;19:151–9.
18. Levinsky RJ, Barratt TM. IgA immune complexes in Henoch-Schönlein purpura. Lancet 1979;2:1100–3.

19. Saulsbury FT. Henoch-Schönlein purpura in children. Medicine 1999;78:395–409.
20. Lackner H, Karpatkin S. On the "easy bruising" syndrome with normal platelet count: a study of 75 patients. Ann Intern Med 1975;83:190–6.
21. Coleman RW, Robboy SJ, Minna JD. Disseminated intravascular coagulation (DIC): an approach. Am J Med 1972;52:679–89.
22. deJonge E, Levi M, Stoutenbeck CP, von Devester SJH. Current drug treatment strategies for disseminated intravascular coagulation. Drugs 1998;55(6):767–77.
23. Dale DC, Guerry D, Wewerka JR, Bull JM, Cusid MJ. Chronic neutropenia. Medicine (Baltimore) 1979;58:128–44.
24. Murphy MF, Metcalfe P, Waters AH, et al. Incidence and mechanism of neutropenia and thrombocytopenia in patients with human and immunodeficiency virus infection. Br J Haematol 1987;66:337–40.
25. Pincus SH, Boxer LA, Stossel TP. Chronic neutropenia in childhood. Am J Med 1976;61:849–61.
26. Conway LT, Clay ME, Kline WE, Ramsay NKC, Krivit W. McCullough J. Natural history of primary autoimmune neutropenia in infancy. Pediatrics 1987;79:728–33.
27. Bussel J, Lalezari P, Fikrig S. Intravenous treatment with gamma globulin of autoimmune neutropenia of infancy. J Pediatr 1988;112:298–301.
28. Lalevari P, Murphy GB, Allen FH. NBI, a new neutrophil-specific antigen involved in the pathogenesis of neonatal neutropenia. J Clin Invest 1971;50:1108–15.
29. Minchinton RM, McGrath KM. Alloimmune neonatal neutropenia—a neglected diagnosis. Med J Aust 1987;147:139–41.
30. Dale DC, Hammond WP. Cyclic neutropenia: a clinical review. Blood Rev 1988;2:178–85.
31. Williams WJ, Beutler E, Erslev AV, Lichtner MA. Hematology. New York: McGraw-Hill, 1990.
32. Motulsky AG. Hemochromatosis. In: Wyngaarden JB, Smith LH, eds. Cecil textbook of medicine, 18th ed. Philadelphia: Saunders, 1988;1189–92.
33. Williams WJ, Beutler E, Erslev AV, Lichtner MA. Hematology. New York: McGraw-Hill, 1990.
34. Modan B. An epidemiological study of polycythemia vera. Blood 1965;26:657–67.
35. Schafer AI. Bleeding and thrombosis in the myeloproliferative disorders. Blood 1984;64:1–12.
36. Yu TF. Secondary gout associated with myeloproliferative diseases. Arthritis Rheum 1965;8:765–71.
37. Provan D, Weatherall D. Red cells 11: acquired anaemia and polycythaemia. Lancet 2000;355:1260–8.
38. Dean J, Schecter AN. Sickle-cell anemia: molecular and cellular bases of therapeutic approaches. N Engl J Med 1978;299:752–63.
39. Heller P, Best WR, Nelson RB, Becktel J. Clinical implications of sickle-cell trait and glucose-6-phosphate dehydrogenase deficiency in hospitalized black male patients. N Engl J Med 1979;18:1001–5.
40. Dunston T, Rowland R, Huntsman RG, Yawson G. Sickle-cell haemoglobin C disease and sickle-cell beta thalassemia in white South Africans. S Afr Med J 1972;46:1423–6.
41. Powars DR. Natural history of sickle cell disease—the first ten years. Semin Hematol 1975;12:267–85.
42. Kark JA, Posey DM, Schumacher HR, Ruchle CJ. Sickle-cell trait as a risk factor for sudden death in physical training. N Engl J Med 1987;317:781–7.
43. Wethers DL. Sickle cell disease in childhood: part II. Diagnosis and treatment of major complications and recent advances in treatment. AAFP 2000;62(6):1309–14.
44. Charache S, Tevin MC, Moore RD, et al. Effect of hydroxyurea on the frequency of painful crisis in sickle cell anemia. N Engl J Med 1995;332:1318–22.
45. Levitan M. Textbook of human genetics, 3rd ed. New York: Oxford University Press, 1988.
46. Penn P. Coalitions and binding interactions in families with chronic illness. Fam Syst Med 1983;1:16–25.
47. Leahey M, Wright LM. Interviewing with families with chronic disease. Fam Syst Med 1985;3:60–9.
48. Ballas SK. Management of sickle pain. Curr Opin Hematol 1997;4(2):104–11.
49. Sickle cell center provides model for management of chronic disease. Clin Rescur Manag 2001;2(1):13–6, 1.
50. Day, SW, Wynn LW. Sickle cell pain and hydroxyurea. Am J Nurs 2000;100(11):34–8.
51. Walco GA, Dampier CD. Chronic pain in adolescent patients. J Pediatr Psychol 1987;12(2):215–25.
52. Tricot G. Unique role of cytogenics in the prognosis of patients with myeloma receiving high dose therapy and autotransplants. J Clin Oncol 1997;15:26–59.
53. Koettler HP, ed. Myelodysplastic syndrome. Hematol Oncol Clin North Am 1992;6:485–728.
54. Hoffebrand AV, Pettit JE, eds. The acute leukemias and chronic leukemias. In: Essential haematology. Oxford: Blackwell, 1993;209–50.

Part III

Family Medicine Applications

127
Medical Informatics, the Internet, and Telemedicine

Joseph E. Scherger

Jeremy's right ear began to hurt in the middle of a school day. Rather than call a parent to leave work and try to get a quick appointment with Jeremy's family physician, the school nurse obtained a faxed permission from the mother. She then set up a video link with the family physician's office and called up Jeremy's medical record on a computer. With the school nurse's help and hands, the family physician was able to examine Jeremy. She checked his ears with an electronic otoscope, looked at his throat, and listened to his heart and lungs with an electronic stethoscope. The right tympanic membrane was red and bulging. She talked with Jeremy to assess his level of pain. The electronic medical record contained a history of multiple ear infections and an allergy to penicillin. The family physician diagnosed a recurrent ear infection and determined that Jeremy's classmates were not at risk. The latest clinical guideline on acute otitis media, available to the family physician over her consultant Web site, informed her that Jeremy could be observed and did not need an antibiotic. However, because of Jeremy's history of repeated infections, including one recently, the family physician chose to treat the infection. When Jeremy took the school bus home, he had printed instructions and a slip for a follow-up appointment with the family physician. An antibiotic prescription, based on the current clinical guideline, was transmitted electronically to the pharmacy. Jeremy's father picked up the medication on his way home.

Medical informatics, the Internet, and telemedicine offer the potential to make health care more convenient, safer, and of higher quality. Electronic tools are changing the way information is shared and used throughout society, and health care is no exception. Just like the automobile and telephone radically changed how health care was delivered in the 20th century, computers and the Internet will radically change health care in the 21st century. The medical informatics story has been building for decades. The development of the Internet in the 1990s and the reduction in size and cost of computers and video equipment have accelerated change, and leave no doubt that electronic health care is for real.

Definitions

Medical informatics is the use of computers to share, retrieve, and use medical information. **Telemedicine**, or more broadly, **telehealth**, is the provision of health care services,

clinical information, and education over a distance using telecommunication technology.[1] Telemedicine existed long before the Internet, but has been greatly accelerated by digital technology using the Internet. **eHealth** has emerged as a popular term and refers to the use of electronics in health care, especially Internet-based health care delivery. The **Internet** is a collection of interconnected networks that speak the same computer language. The **World Wide Web** is a global extension of the Internet.[1]

Telehealth and Telemedicine

Robert Brooks is director of the health department for the state of Florida. When he wants to meet with all the nurses in the public health clinics throughout the state, he arranges for a video conference. The nurses use a satellite feed to connect from rural and urban clinics. New immunization policies are discussed and procedural questions are answered.

The only labor and delivery unit in Colusa County, California, shut down due to lack of a provider. Faculty at the University of California–Davis recruited two family physicians to reopen the unit. To avoid isolation and elevate the quality of care, a telemedicine unit was installed linking Colusa Community Hospital to the university medical center. Fetal monitor strips and other patient data are routinely shared with online consultation, which is always available.

Telemedicine can be traced to the early 1900s when radio communications were used for providing medical services in Antarctica. In 1924, researchers were describing a remote "radio doctor" who could both see and be seen by the patient. In 1950, x-ray images were transmitted for the first time in Pennsylvania.[1]

The National Aeronautics and Space Administration (NASA) pioneered modern telemedicine technologies to monitor astronauts in space. These technologies were applied to remote Indian reservations and earthquake victims in Mexico City in 1985.[1]

Telemedicine was further advanced in 1991 when the governor of Georgia asked Dr. Jay Sanders to develop a statewide telemedicine program. By 1993, there were 10 telemedicine programs using interactive video conferencing technology. The rise has been exponential since then. Telemedicine offers the ability to open access to care and bring high-quality care to remote or any distant area.[1]

Most telemedicine applications are contained within a health care system through an intranet, or a private network of interlinked computers. Family physician offices can be linked now that technology is getting smaller and less expensive.[2,3] As telemedicine moves to the Internet, and digital images become commonplace on computers, many applications, such as treating Jeremy's earache, will become routine in a family physician's office.

eHealth and the Internet

The concerns about Y2K at the turn of the millennium made society realize its dependence on computers. Health care is no exception, and while health care has lagged behind other service industries in computer usage, the movement to new information and communication technologies is now rapid and offers real benefits. Three applications of particular importance to the family physician are electronic communication, information retrieval, and clinical decision support.

Electronic Communication (E-Mail)

Within a few years, electronic communication (e-mail) has exceeded paper mail in volume. This explosion, coupled with access to seemingly unlimited information on the Internet, is rapidly changing human civilization globally. This chapter was written at the World Organization of Family Doctors (WONCA) conference in Durban, South Africa. From there, the author communicated daily by e-mail with patients and with colleagues around the world.

E-mail brings the power of asynchronous communication to health care, done in a few minutes and at little expense. The current methods of health care delivery, visits, and telephone require synchronous presence, often just for the sharing of information. E-mail allows the family physician to shift work to asynchronous communication, enabling a transformation of the work schedule to a more selective use of visits and telephone. This new communication tool is likely to radically transform how doctors work, and has the potential to enhance patient relationships and allow for fewer, more time-intensive visits.[4,5] Reimbursement models for medicine are being developed to support e-mail.[6]

E-mail is an imperfect form of communication in that sight and sound are not yet readily available. E-mail does not substitute for necessary face-to-face visits. Rather, it extends the communication options. The American Academy of Family Physicians (AAFP) has developed guidelines for the proper use of e-mail with patients, available in the quality module of the AAFP Web site.[7] The key elements of these guidelines, developed by the American Medical Informatics Association (AMIA),[8] are:

Do not use e-mail for emergencies or urgent matters.
Establish a turnaround time for responses.

Inform patients of privacy considerations, including e-mail as part of the medical record, and who besides the addressee may see the e-mail.
Establish acceptable and unacceptable types of e-mail transactions.
Print all e-mails as part of the medical record.
Avoid anger, sarcasm, harsh criticism, or libelous references to third parties.

For risk management and medical legal considerations:

Obtain a patient's informed consent for use of e-mail.
Use password-protected screen savers on all desktop workstations in the office, hospital, and home.
Never forward patient identifiable information to a third party without the patient's expressed permission [key Health Insurance Portability and Accountability Act (HIPAA) regulation].
Use encryption for all messages as it becomes available. Any practice can now have an interactive Web site for secure messaging. Another option is to use a secure messaging service such as *healinx.com*.

Physician use of e-mail with patients has been increasing rapidly, and patients generally appreciate the convenience and added service.[9] E-mail expands patient's access to information and care. Imagine a future family physician's office with a limited number of time-intensive appointments that start on time, relatively quiet telephones, and staff processing most information and communication over computers.[5]

Information Retrieval

The Internet provides an instantaneous global connection to information, for patients and physicians alike. Awash in information, a quotation from T.S. Eliot has become prophetic: "Where is the wisdom we've lost in information? Where is the knowledge we've lost in information?"[10] Physicians are becoming less a source of information, and more a patient advisor as to what information is worthwhile. While there is lots of misinformation on the Internet, many Web sites contain useful patient education and discovery information for a patient to obtain a diagnosis and the latest treatments.[11,12] Indeed, almost all patient education is moving to the Internet in order to be current. The family physician has a new duty to direct patients to useful Internet sites, and the modern office should provide a "library" of Internet-based information.[13,14]

Clinical Decision Support

The complexity of modern medicine exceeds the inherent limitations of an unaided human mind.

David Eddy[15]

Prior to the 21st century, most physicians practiced medicine "off the top of their heads." References books were available, but were generally not convenient to use at the time of service. Often, reference books did not answer the specific clinical question at hand, such as the latest guideline for treating a disease like asthma, or the potential interactions of adding a new drug to a patient taking three others. The growing list of medications that interact with each other or prolong the QT interval is impossible to remember. Quality medical search engines can provide a scientific answer to almost any clinical question in a few minutes. Such applications can be accessed almost anywhere, making the entire medical library, continually updated, readily accessible to even a remote rural physician. Computerized clinical decision support is rapidly becoming a new standard of care that could revolutionize the consistency and quality of care delivered by family physicians.

Privacy, Confidentiality, and Security

Computers offer the potential for great privacy and security, but also the risk that confidential patient information could be sent to the wrong people. The Health Insurance Portability and Accountability Act of 1996 (HIPAA) called for protections of the privacy of medical information. HIPAA privacy guidelines have been developed by the US. Department of Health and Human Services (DHHS) and were implemented in 2001. These guidelines applied to all sources of medical information, including paper, and will have a great impact on physician offices. No longer will the fax machine sit out in the open with a patient's lab results in a tray for all to see. Patient consent will be required for sharing patient information with anyone, even consultants brought in to evaluate the patient. E-mail communication with patients will require consent and guidelines to ensure confidentiality and security. The modern family physician's office will have a Web site that offers secure messaging, using measures such as encryption, authentication, firewalls, and electronic signatures.[1] All such measures are becoming more available at lower cost, and will make computerization the most secure means of storing and transmitting patient information.

Quality of Care

The Institute of Medicine (IOM) of the National Academy of Sciences has released two reports calling for radical measures to improve the quality of health care in the United States.[16,17]

Information technology will play a major role in these changes, and provide a means to developing quality systems. Quality in any industry can be divided into these dimensions: safety, effectiveness, and service.

Safety

Patient safety is critically important in health care, and the IOM reports that between 44,000 and 98,000 patients die each year in hospitals due to errors.[16,17] This makes hospital errors among the top 10 causes of death. The reasons for the high error rate, which are mostly avoidable, are the lack of safety systems to override an expected rate of human error. Health care operates 24 hours a day, 7 days a week, doing repeated critical tasks. Despite an understanding of safety systems and

available technologies such as bar coding and computerized order entry, most hospitals and physician offices still use handwriting and person-to-person handoffs without double-checking for accuracy. Family physicians should begin investing in the technologies to make their practice safer, such as electronic medical records with built-in reminders and drug interaction knowledge tools, and electronic prescribing. All office staff should be trained and empowered to action in making a safer office.

Effectiveness

Effectiveness means that a patient receives the latest evidence-based care every time in any clinical setting. Customization of care comes from patient preferences rather than variation in physician knowledge.[17] Computerized clinical decision support gives family physicians the tools to provide the latest and best care at all times. A 21st century standard of care is likely to require this.[17,18]

Service

Receiving health care has become increasingly inconvenient. Patients often wait on the telephone for a long time before negotiating their care needs with a person who does not know them. Then they take 2 to 3 hours out of their day just to receive 10 minutes of time with a physician. Just as shopping and service industries have gone online providing access to service 24 hours a day, so will health care. Electronic communication and a fully interactive Web site allow a family physician to provide service any time, while the physician can work at his or her convenience. While face-to-face visits remain a fundamental means of care, and the telephone is still necessary for urgent matters, much routine care can be shifted to the Internet, making the service of health care far more convenient for the patient and physician alike.[15,19]

Summary

Bill Gates has said, "The Internet changes everything."[20] While we may not appreciate the significance of a dramatic change in history while living through it, the Internet's impact on human civilization may be as great as the invention of movable type. Andrew Grove, Intel chairman, has called the Internet the "New World," making its discovery comparable to Columbus discovering America.[20]

A family physician's office is likely to become outdated within a decade without making changes using medical informatics and the Internet. Electronic medical records are an important, but not the most important, initial step. E-mail and using the Internet for patient education and clinical decision support are the top priorities to improving quality and service. Electronic prescribing will reduce medical errors. As electronic communication becomes visual, telemedicine, the first innovation in telecommunications in health care, will become part of every family physician's office. Patients will not need to come to the office. This future for family physicians is exciting and promises to allow for an unprecedented quality of care in a more satisfying manner. Medical informatics, the Internet, and telemedicine are a new frontier for family practice and may help bring about a renaissance in the specialty.

References

1. Maheu MM, Whitter P, Allen A. E-health, telehealth, and telemedicine: a guide to start-up and success. San Francisco: Jossey-Bass, 2001.
2. Nesbitt TS, Hilty DM, Kuenneth CA, Siefkin A. Development of a telemedicine program. West J Med 2000;173:169–74.
3. Strode SW, Gustke S, Allen A. Technical and clinical progress in telemedicine. JAMA 1999;281:1066–8.
4. Scherger JE. E-mail enhanced relationships: getting back to basics. Hippocrates 1999;13(9):7–8. Available at *www.hippocrates. com.*
5. Scherger JE. Primary care in 2010. Hippocrates 2000;14(3):26–32. Available at *www.hippocrates.com.*
6. Baldwin FD. Will pay for e-mail: preferred provider organization offers cash incentives for e-mail consultations. eMD 2000; Fall:21–5. Available at *www.edotmd.com.*
7. American Academy of Family Physicians. E-mail communicaton module. Available at *www.aafp.org/quality/module/mod6/,* September 16, 2000.
8. Kane B, Sands DZ. Guidelines for the clinical use of electronic mail with patients. J Am Med Inform Assoc 1998;5:104–11.
9. Morasch LJ. Making the most of physician-patient e-mail. Hippocrates 2000;14(11):33–9. Available at *www.hippocrates.com.*
10. Rules-happy cabinet: Rumsfeld, Powell, and O'Neill weigh in. Wall Street Journal March 2, 2001; 237(43):1.
11. Media Matrix. Top health care information sites in January (2001). Internet Health Care Magazine 2001;April:8. Available at *www.internethealthcare.mag.com.*
12. Brunk D. Internet databases can answer most clinical questions. Family Practice News 2000;November 1:3.
13. McKenna MK. Worth While Web: 50 useful sites for family physicians. Family Practice Management 2001;April:23–38. Available at *www.aafp.org/fpm/.*
14. Ferguson T. Online patient helpers and physicians working together: a new partnership for high quality health care. BMJ 2000;321:1129–32.
15. Millenson ML. Demanding medical excellence: doctors and accountability in the information age. Chicago: University of Chicago Press, 1997.
16. Kohn LT, Corrigan JM, Donaldson, MS, eds. To err is human: building a safer health system. Institute of Medicine. Washington, DC: National Academy Press, 2000.
17. Corrigan JM, Donaldson MS, eds. Crossing the quality chasm: a new health system for the 21st century. Institute of Medicine. Washington, DC: National Academy Press, 2001.
18. Hunt DL, Jaeschke R, McKibbon KA. User's guide to the medical literature: XXI. Using electronic health informatics resources in evidence-based practice. JAMA 2000;283:1875–9.
19. Lowes R. Putting your practice online is easier than ever. Med Econ 2000; December 4:45–63. Available at *www.memag.com.*
20. Gates B. Business at the speed of thought: using a digital nervous system. New York: Warner Books, 1999.

128

Complementary and Alternative Medicine

Lisa Grill Dodson and Meg Hayes

Alternative medicine is a diverse collection of more than 100 practices that are used as a form of healing. These techniques and practices are not generally taught in allopathic medical schools or used by Western medical doctors. Table 128.1 lists some of the more common practices of alternative medicine. The preferred term, *complementary and alternative medicine* (CAM), is in keeping with the actual use of these therapies since CAM is frequently used as a complement to, rather than as a replacement for, allopathic medicine. An estimated 40% the United States population utilizes some form of alternative therapy each year spending more than $27 billion (1998).[1]

The Cochrane Collaboration has adopted the following definition: "Complementary and alternative medicine (CAM) is a broad domain of healing resources that encompasses all health systems, modalities, and practices and their accompanying theories and beliefs, other than those intrinsic to the politically dominant health system of a particular society or culture in a given historical period. CAM includes all such practices and ideas self-defined by their users as preventing or treating illness or promoting health and well-being. Boundaries within CAM and between the CAM domain and that of the dominant system are not always sharp or fixed."[2] What may be considered as alternative by one person may be another's primary source of health care, and practices that are mainstream for one condition may be alternative for another.

This chapter outlines current use of CAM and provides a brief description of more commonly used methods of CAM. A full discussion of each of the methods is beyond the scope of this chapter. Table 128.2 lists additional information resources. In addition, we will present some guidelines for selection of alternative providers as colleagues. CAM is an area of rapidly growing interest and widespread use among patients,[3] and physicians are well advised to become knowledgeable in these areas.

Herbal Medicine

Herbs and plants have been used medicinally by humans for centuries. Herbal products account for billions of dollars in sales each year and are widely used for many conditions. The popularity of herbal medications relates to increasing availability and acceptability of CAM by the general population, concerns regarding use of allopathic medications, increasing desire for preventative medicine, and self-advocacy by patients seeking alternatives to allopathic medications that have failed to treat conditions or have caused side effects. Herbal products may be viewed as "natural" and therefore healthier and safer than allopathic medications. Patients may not notify their physicians of their use of herbal medications for fear of nonacceptance of this practice. Herb–drug interactions are well documented, and it is important for patients to be explicitly queried about all substances and treatments taken, whether prescribed or over the counter.

Standardization of herbal medication is complicated by the natural properties of plants, which contain numerous chemical compounds. The conditions under which the plant is grown, harvested, and processed can affect the chemical composition, and the various components of the plant, leaves, roots, and flowers may have different effects or uses. In addition, it is frequently not known which of the components is responsible for the desired effect. Standardized extracts are available and should be used preferentially, but many herbal preparations are not labeled to include the precise composition.[4] In the United States, the Food and Drug Administration (FDA) does not regulate herbal medications. The 1994 Dietary Supplement Health and Education Act (DSHEA) placed herbal products into a new class identified as "dietary supplements," and limited the authority of the FDA to regulate herbs as medications. Dietary supplements, including herbals and botanicals, vitamins, minerals, and amino acids, are exempt from FDA approval or monitoring, provided that they do not claim to treat or prevent disease. Dietary supplements must carry the following disclaimer: "This statement has not been evaluated by the Food and Drug Administration. This product is not intended to diagnose, treat, cure, or prevent any disease." Supplement labels can claim to maintain health or function, such as "maintains normal cardiovascular function," but cannot claim to "reduce blood pressure" without FDA-approved proof.

Table 128.1. **Common Complementary and Alternative Therapies**

Acupressure	Environmental	Nutritional therapy
Acupuncture	medicine	Reflexology
Aromatherapy	Herbal medicine	Reiki
Ayurveda	Homeopathy	Relaxation therapy
Biofeedback	Massage	Shiatsu
Chiropractic	Mind–body	Therapeutic touch
Cranial osteopathy	Naturopathy	Yoga

The most definitive source of information on herbal medicine is the German Commission E. This commission has examined the evidence for use of more than 350 herbs. Evidence considered included clinical studies, chemical data, experimental pharmacologic studies, traditional use, case reports, and other data available to assess the safety and efficacy of herbal medications. While criticism has been leveled that many of these sources lack scientific rigor, the Commission E monographs remain the most authoritative source of information on these widely used compounds. The monographs are available in paper and electronic formats.[5]

Table 128.3 lists documented uses for some commonly used herbal medication, as well as contraindications and side effects.

Naturopathy

Naturopathy is not a single discipline, but represents a wide variety of practices and techniques that are combined into a philosophy of healing.[6] Naturopaths may utilize herbal medications, homeopathy, diet and exercise, stress management, hydrotherapy, massage, and many other modalities in an individualized approach for each patient. The principles of naturopathy are as follows:

Table 128.2. **Sources of Information on Complementary and Alternative Practitioners**

American Chiropractic Association
www.amerchiro.org

American Association of Naturopathic Physicians
www.naturopathic.org

American Massage Therapy Association
www.amtamassage.org

American Academy of Medical Acupuncture (MD and DO
    acupuncturists)
www.medicalacupuncture.org

National Acupuncture and Oriental Medicine Alliance
www.acupuncturealliance.org

National Center for Homeopathy
www.homeopathic.org

American Academy of Family Physicians Alternative Medicine
    Database
www.familydoctor.org

National Institute of Health, National Center for
    Complementary and Alternative Medicine
www.nccam.nih.gov

Holistic approach to patient care
Identification of underlying causes rather than symptomatic
    treatment
Use of therapy to promote the body's self-restorative powers
Emphasis on self-care and prevention
Interdisciplinary cooperation with other medical providers

Five schools in the U.S. and Canada grant doctor of naturopathy (ND) degrees after a prescribed 4-year course of study. There are a number of correspondence and home study courses that also offer an ND degree, but with no Council on Naturopathic Medical Education (CNME) accreditation or standardization, and the quality of these programs must be highly suspect. The American Association of Naturopathic Physicians does not recognize these degrees, which do not make one eligible for board examination or licensure in states that license naturopaths. Therefore, it is incumbent on the patient and/or referring physician to determine the source of the degree and whether it represents a valid level of training. Twelve states currently license naturopathic physicians.

Homeopathy

First developed in the 18th century, homeopathy has been rising in popularity again since the latter part of the 20th century due largely to a general increase in the popularity and acceptability of CAM. The basic tenets of homeopathy include curing illness with highly dilute substances that at full strength cause similar illness, creating a "healing crisis" in which symptoms may worsen before improving, and avoidance of substances and conditions that counteract homeopathic medicines (called antidotes). Many allopathic medications and treatments may function as antidotes and may make patients taking homeopathic remedies reluctant to take other medications.

Classical homeopathy is highly individualized and relies on the skill of the practitioner to determine the remedy for a particular person. Similar patients might require different approaches. This has complicated attempts to standardize treatments for scientifically controlled trials, and there is little evidence that compares homeopathy to allopathic medications.[7,8] Homeopathic medications are available over the counter for specific conditions, but because classical homeopathy is highly individualized, consultation with an experienced practitioner is recommended.

Numerous training courses and programs provide instruction in homeopathy, but no diploma or certification is currently recognized in the U.S. as a license to practice homeopathy. There are no national standards or licensing requirements, but both allopathic and naturopathic physicians may use homeopathy as a part of their practice.

Traditional Chinese Medicine

Traditional Chinese medicine (TCM) includes the practice of acupuncture, moxibustion (the burning of the herb mugwort to tonify acupuncture needles, or used alone to warm acupunc-

Table 128.3. **Uses of Common Herbal Medications**

System and herb	Uses/effects	Contraindications	Side effects
Cardiovascular			
Garlic	Lower lipids Increase vascular resistance Mild hypertension	None	Avoid before surgery Potentiates warfarin
Gastrointestinal			
Ginger root	Treatment and prophylaxis of nausea and vomiting	Caution in gallstones	None known
Milk thistle	Dyspepsia, chronic inflammatory liver disease	None known	Mild laxative effect
Mental health			
Ginkgo biloba	Organic brain disorders (dementia), vascular occlusive disease, vertigo, tinnitus, Raynaud disease	Known hypersensitivity to ginkgo; caution in depression	Stomach upset, headache, skin reaction
Ginseng	Fatigue, weakness, convalescence	Hypertension, excessive caffeine use	Possible interaction with MAOI
St. John's Wort	Mild to moderate depressive mood, anxiety	None known, not recommended in combination with other antidepressants	None known
Valerian	Restlessness, sleep disorders	None known	None known
Immune			
Echinacea	Promote natural resistance to infection	Systemic illness such as HIV, TB, MS	Chills, fever, nausea, allergic reaction
Endocrine			
Black cohosh	Premenstrual discomfort, menopausal symptoms	None known	Gastric upset
Saw palmetto	Symptoms of benign prostatic hypertrophy	None known	None known

HIV = human immunodeficiency virus; MAOI = monoamine oxidase inhibitor; MS = multiple sclerosis; TB = tuberculosis.

ture points), massage, herbal therapy, and qi gong, a meditative physical exercise. All of these modalities are employed to improve the flow of qi (pronounced "chee") through 12 primary and eight accessory channels known as meridians. Qi is thought to be the vital force that circulates throughout the meridians to protect, nourish, and animate living beings. Although TCM treatments are used to mend disease states, the central purpose, or higher wisdom, is to maintain the body's order and balance by preserving the conditions within which life thrives. Disease states are thought to result from internal and external causes that disturb balance, such as that between yin and yang. Treatment is aimed at correcting the imbalance through disbursement or replenishment of the disrupted element within the body.

TCM practice is based on thousands of years of practice and recorded case histories, or "wisdom that has stood the test of time." Due to historic religious, cultural and philosophical constraints in China, TCM practices have historically not been experimental based.

For the treatment of pain, acupuncture analgesia has been shown to be more effective than placebo, indicating that there is a physiologic mechanism present.[9] It is postulated that the penetration of the acupuncture needle stimulates small-diameter nerves in muscles, which then send impulses to the spinal cord. These impulses activate three centers—the spinal cord, midbrain, and pituitary—to release endorphins and the monoamines serotonin and norepinephrine, which act to suppress pain transmission to the cortex at multiple synaptic levels.[10] Further, at the level of the pituitary gland, adrenocorticotropic hormone (ACTH) is released in eqimolar amounts to endorphin thus stimulating cortisol production by the adrenal cortex.[11] This may explain why acupuncture has been found to be helpful in the relief of bronchospasm in asthma and inflammation of arthritis.

The World Health Organization recognizes more than 40 conditions for which acupuncture may be useful (Table 128.4). Areas of active research regarding acupuncture treatment efficacy include addiction, stroke rehabilitation, hypertension, attention-deficit/hyperactivity disorder, and major depressive disorder. Americans most commonly seek acupuncture treatment for the relief of chronic pain, particularly for arthritis and low back pain.[12] Clinical studies have demonstrated efficacy in chemotherapy- and anesthesia-induced nausea, and for postsurgical dental pain. In some cases it has been found that the combination of acupuncture and standard pharmaceutical treatment is superior to either modality used singly. Prelimi-

Table 128.4. **The World Health Organization Recognizes Traditional Chinese Medicine (TCM) Treatment of Over 43 Common Disorders**

Gastrointestinal disorders
Food allergies, peptic ulcer, chronic diarrhea, constipation, indigestion, gastrointestinal weakness, anorexia, gastritis
Urogenital disorders
Stress incontinence, urinary tract infection, sexual dysfunction
Gynecological disorders
Dysfunctional uterine bleeding, infertility in women and men, premenstrual syndrome
Respiratory disorders
Emphysema, sinusitis, allergies, asthma, bronchitis
Musculoskeletal and neurologic disorders
Arthritis, migraine headaches, neuralgia, insomnia, dizziness, low back pain, neck pain, shoulder pain
Cardiovascular disorders
Hypertension, angina pectoris, arteriosclerosis, anemia
Emotional and psychological disorders
Depression and anxiety, attention-deficit/hyperactivity disorder
Addictions
Alcohol, nicotine, and drugs
Eye, ear, nose, and throat disorders
Ear infection, serous otitis, sinusitis, tinnitus

nary research suggests effectiveness in acupuncture treatment of fibromyalgia,[13] the correction of breech presentation in primigravidas,[14] and painful rheumatologic conditions including osteoarthritis and rheumatoid arthritis.[15]

In 1996 the FDA reclassified acupuncture needles from the investigational class III status to a class II device, and required the use of sterile, nontoxic needles that bear a labeling statement restricting their use to qualified practitioners. In the year 2000 there were an estimated 20,000 nationally certified acupuncturists in the U.S., and approximately one third of those are medical doctors.[16] Complications associated with acupuncture are relatively rare. The reported occurrence of adverse events is only about 50 cases over a 20-year period in the United States.[17] Reported complications have included pneumothorax and other organ puncture, transmission of infectious disease, syncope, bleeding, dyspnea, chest pain, dermatitis, and migration of broken needle fragments.[15] Contraindications to acupuncture include bleeding disorders, skin infections, and valvular heart disease (insertion of semipermanent needles only). Electro-acupuncture should not be used for patients with pacemakers, cardiac arrhythmias, or epilepsy. Caution also must be exercised in pregnant women, as stimulation of some acupuncture points may stimulate uterine contractions.

Manipulation

Massage therapy and osteopathic and chiropractic manipulation are widely used for musculoskeletal complaints such as headache, neck, and low back pain. Manipulation has also been found to be of value in repetitive strain injury, chronic fatigue syndrome, fibromyalgia, rheumatoid, and osteoarthritis. The benefit of manipulation is likely due to both the local effects on muscles and ligaments as well as psychological relaxation, both of which can reduce pain and increase function.[18] Studies also demonstrate patient preference for manual treatment for acute low back pain, both chiropractic and massage. Satisfaction is thought to be linked to the amount of time spent by the practitioner, the laying on of hands, and the frequency of visits as well as the end result in pain and disability reduction.

Massage Therapy

Massage therapy is the manipulation of soft tissue and connective tissue with the intention of maintaining or improving health by affecting changes in relaxation, circulation, lymph flow, and increased range of motion. Empirical support exists for the efficacy of massage therapy in reducing pain, increasing alertness, diminishing depression and anxiety, enhancing immune function, and improving sleep patterns. Specifically, massage therapy has been found to be valuable in reducing both psychological and physiologic anxiety levels in patients undergoing surgery under local anesthesia,[17] facilitating mother–infant interaction for mothers with postpartum depression,[18] and decreasing pain and anxiety and improving sleep in patients with low back pain.[19]

Massage therapy can be considered for a number of conditions, including troubled neonates, for parent–infant bonding, recovery from trauma and abuse, relaxation effect, treatment of injuries, end-of-life palliative care, and to aid independence in the elderly.[20,21] Contraindications to massage include bleeding disorders, contagious or irritated skin disorders, edema due to heart or kidney failure, fever, infections spread by blood or lymph circulation, and leukemia or lymphoma.

Chiropractic

Chiropractic treatments focus on the relationship between the structure of the spine and healthy body function. Chiropractic treatment may include spinal manipulation, applications of heat or cold, dietary recommendations, and prescription of nutritional supplements. Chiropractors are licensed in every state since 1975 and have accredited education standards. The profession enjoys a high level of recognition and public utilization, with an estimated 1 in 15 Americans seeing a chiropractor annually. There are more than 50,000 chiropractors in practice in the United States, and the World Federation of Chiropractic has representation from 70 countries. Medicare, workers' compensation programs, and many private insurers pay for chiropractic services.

Chiropractic treatment has integrated into the health care system as the result of a professional emphasis on research that has defined the benefits and risks of spinal manipulation using accepted outcome measures. Studies have demonstrated beneficial effect of spinal manipulation on the duration and severity of acute low back pain and short-term positive results in chronic low back pain,[22] although studies have not demonstrated substantial long-term effects on pain.[23]

Consider referral to a chiropractor for treatment of acute,

uncomplicated back and neck pain, or for a short course of treatment for chronic pain and nonprogressive sciatica. Other conditions that may be improved include acute and chronic neck pain, headaches that originate from the cervical spine, and symptoms of otitis media.[24]

Chiropractic treatment of nonmusculoskeletal conditions is controversial and to date there are not adequate data on effectiveness. Reports of anecdotal improvement for menstrual cramps, asthma, and functional gastrointestinal symptoms exist, but it will be some time before data concerning any definitive effect in these disorders are available. Contraindications to chiropractic manipulation include conditions where bony structures are susceptible to trauma such as acute fractures, bone tumors, severe rheumatoid arthritis, and osteoporosis. Manipulation should also be avoided in patients with a progressive neurologic deficit and in those who have a deteriorating condition without a clear diagnosis.

Mind-Body Medicine

The field of mind-body medicine includes a number of techniques and interventions that affect the physiology of the autonomic nervous system (ANS). Divided into the sympathetic and parasympathetic nervous systems, the ANS was long thought to relate to bodily functions that operated below the level of one's conscious awareness or control. In 1974 it was demonstrated that experienced meditators could produce remarkable changes in their physiology including decreased pulse and respiratory rates, decreased oxygen consumption and blood lactate levels, as well as a change in electroencephalographic (EEG) patterns[25] with a decrease in anxiety and hostility accompanying these physiologic changes. This "relaxation response" can provide benefit in a variety of conditions such as heart disease, prematurity, surgical patients, functional bowel disease, chronic fatigue syndrome, headache, depression and anxiety, chronic pain, and dysmenorrhea. The response can be elicited through progressive muscle relaxation, meditation, guided imagery, breathing exercises, cognitive behavioral therapy, and hypnosis. The following techniques are easily learned and can be incorporated into daily life for cost-effective health benefit[26]:

- Progressive muscle relaxation and body scan are used to reduce muscle tone. In progressive relaxation the patient first holds tension in a muscle group for several seconds and then consciously relaxes it before moving on to repeat this exercise throughout the body. In body scan the patient starts at the head or feet and consciously relaxes a portion of the body one segment at a time. These techniques can be aided by the use of a scripted audiotape to guide the patient through the complete exercise.
- Guided imagery cues the imagination to stimulate physiologic changes. Just as one may experience sympathetic arousal with images such as a frightening scene in a movie, the opposite can be achieved with appropriate images. For example, learning to warm the hands by imagery suggesting the holding of a warm mug of cocoa or the ambient heat of a campfire can result in a significant temperature change

in the fingertips due to increased blood flow. This technique is helpful to migraine headache patients in ablating an early headache without medication, or as an adjunct to medication, and in the treatment of Raynaud disease.[27]
- Breathing exercises are useful in focusing a patient's attention on the process of inhalation and exhalation. For patients who suffer panic disorder and anxiety, this exercise gives a focus to the thought process that can replace any troubling thought or images that may have preceded an episode of hyperventilation, while slowing the breath, prolonging the expiratory phase, and resolving an associated alkalosis
- Cognitive behavioral therapy (CBT) addresses thoughts and beliefs that may impair recovery while encouraging action that may be beneficial to recovery. CBT that includes a cognitive restructuring with graded increase in activity has been shown to be beneficial in treating chronic fatigue syndrome[28] (also see Chapter 55).
- Hypnosis is a method of helping patients to move beyond conscious and subconscious blocks that may thwart their healing process. Under hypnosis, patients are active problem solvers who incorporate their moral and cultural ideas into their behavior while exhibiting a heightened responsiveness to the expectations expressed by the therapist.[29] This technique may be useful in such diverse situations as tobacco cessation, chronic pain, and irritable bowel syndrome.

Mind-body interventions pose little risk or contraindication. The interventions can offer significant symptom relief from pain and chronic illness while providing patients with a powerful sense of control, thus engaging them in active participation in their health care. These techniques are frequently useful alone, and may also be employed as adjunctive treatment to standard care. Mind-body interventions can be taught in brief office visits and have the potential to improve the quality and decrease the cost of health care.[30]

Conclusion

CAM is a diverse collection of practices, procedures, and philosophies of healing. There is widespread use of CAM, although there is not yet a large body of scientific study to confirm that these practices are safe and effective. Physicians should be aware of the CAM practices used by their patients and work to become knowledgeable in the legitimate uses of alternative medicine. Physicians should remain open to discussion of CAM with patients and assist them in selecting CAM practices and practitioners that have demonstrated effectiveness and safety.

References

1. Eisenberg DM, Davis RB, Ettner SL, Appel S, Wilkey S, Van Rompay M, Kessler RC. Trends in alternative medicine use in the United States. JAMA 1998;280(18):1569–75.
2. Zollman C, Vickers A. ABC of complementary medicine. BMJ 1999;319(7211):693–96.

3. Elder N, Gillcrist A, Minz R. Use of alternative health care by family practice patients. Arch Fam Med 1997;6:181–4.

4. Talalay P. The importance of using scientific principles in the development of medicinal agents from plants. Acad Med 2001;76(3):238–47.

5. Blumenthal M, Goldberg A, Brinckmann J, eds. Herbal medicine: expanded Commission E monographs. Newton, MA: Integrative Medicine Communications, 2000. *www.onemedicine.com.*

6. American Association of Naturopathic Physicians. *History of Naturopathic Medicine,* 2001 Available at *www.naturopathic.org.*

7. Linde K, Melchart D. Randomized controlled trials of individualized homeopathy: a state-of-the-art review. J Alternative Complement Med 1998;4(4):371–88.

8. Linde K, Clausius N, Ramirez G, et al. Are the clinical effects of homeopathy placebo effects? A meta-analysis of placebo-controlled trials. Lancet 1997;350(9081):834–43.

9. Birch S, Hammerschlag R, Berman BM. Acupuncture in the treatment of pain. J Alternative Complement Med 1996;2(1):101–24.

10. Stux G, Pomeranz B. *Basics of acupuncture, 4th ed.* New York: Springer, 1998;7–15.

11. Rossier J, French ED, Rivier C, Ling N, Guillemin R, Bloom FE. Foot-shock induced stress increases beta-endorphin levels in blood but not brain. Nature 1977;270(5638):618–20.

12. Diehl DL, Kaplan G, Coulter I, Glik D, Hurwitz EL. Use of acupuncture by American physicians. J Alternative Complement Med 1997;3(2):119–26.

13. Berman BM, Ezzo J, Hadhazy V, Swyers JP. Is acupuncture effective in the treatment of fibromyalgia? J Fam Pract 1999;48(3):213–8.

14. Cardini F, Weixin H. Moxibustion for correction of breech presentation: a randomized controlled trial. JAMA 1998;280(18):1580–4.

15. Berman BM, Swyer JP, Ezzo J. The evidence for acupuncture as a treatment for rheumatologic conditions. Rheumatol Dis Clin North Am 2000;26(1):103–15.

16. Culliton PD. Current utilization of acupuncture by United States patients. *National Institutes of Health Consensus Development Conference on Acupuncture, program and abstracts,* Bethesda, MD, November 3–5, 1997.

17. Lytle CD. An overview of acupuncture. Washington, DC: U.S. Government Printing Office, Department of Health and Human Services, Public Health Service, Food and Drug Administration, 1993.

18. Fiechtner JJ, Brodeur RR. Manual and manipulation techniques for rheumatic disease. Rheum Dis Clin North Am 2000;26(1):83–96.

19. Kim MS, Cho KS. Effects of hand massage on anxiety in cataract surgery using local anesthesia. J Cataract Refract Surg 2001;27(6):884–90.

20. Onozawa K, Glover V, Adams D, Modi N, Kumar RC. Infant massage improves mother-infant interaction for mothers with postnatal depression. J Affect Disord 2001;63(1–3):201–7.

21. Hernandez-Reif M, Field T, Krasnegor J, Theakston H. Lower back pain is reduced and range of motion increased after massage therapy. Int J Neurosci 2001;106(3–4):131–45.

22. Koes BW, Assendelft WJ, van der Heijden GJ, Bouter LM. Spinal manipulation for low back pain. An updated systematic review of randomized clinical trials. Spine 1996;21(24):2860–71.

23. Bronfort G. Spinal manipulation: current state of research and its indications. Neurol Clin 1999;17(1):91–111.

24. Froehle RM. Ear infection: a retrospective study examining improvement from chiropractic care and analyzing for influencing factors. J Manipulative Physiol Ther 1996;19(3):169–77.

25. Benson J, Beary JF, Carol MP. The relaxation response. Psychiatry 1974;37(1):37–46.

26. Friedman R, Sobel D, Myers P, Caudill M, Benson H. Behavioral medicine, clinical health psychology, and cost offset. Health Psychol 1995;14(6):509–18.

27. Bilkis MR, Mark KA Mind-body medicine. Practical applications in dermatology. Arch Dermatol 1998;134(11):1437–41.

28. Price JR, Couper J. Cognitive behaviour therapy for adults with chronic fatigue syndrome. Cochrane Database Syst 2000; issue 2.

29. Nash MR. The truth and the hype of hypnosis. Sci Am 2000;285(1):47–55.

30. Chiaramonte DR. Mind-body therapies for primary care physicians. Prim Care 1997;24(4):787–807.

129
The Family Physician's Role in Responding to Biologic and Chemical Terrorism

Alan L. Melnick

In April 2000, the Centers for Disease Control and Prevention (CDC) warned physicians and public health officials against ignoring the possibility of chemical and biologic terrorism.[1] The CDC based its warning on terrorist activities over the previous 10 years, including the sarin gas attack in the Tokyo subway and the discovery of military bio-weapons programs in Iraq and the former Soviet Union. While noting these events, the report stated that the public health system must be prepared to detect covert biologic and chemical attacks and prevent the accompanying illness and injury. In addition, the CDC reminded primary health care providers throughout the United States to be "vigilant because they will probably be the first to observe and report unusual illnesses or injuries."

In spite of this and other warnings, most family physicians have spent little time planning for terrorism. One reason may be the rarity of these events, especially on U.S. soil. Until recently, the only reported case of bioterrorism in the United States occurred in 1985, when members of the Rajneesh cult infected hundreds of people with salmonella in rural Oregon in an attempt to influence a local election.[2] It is unlikely that authors of family medicine textbooks written before September 2001 considered devoting significant space for discussions about how family physicians should respond to terrorist attacks.

The September 11, 2001 events in New York City and Washington, D.C., abruptly changed our perspectives about the likelihood that terrorists could direct weapons of mass destruction against civilian communities in the United States. The public, including physicians, suddenly began to recognize the consequences of being unprepared for such terrorist attacks, especially those associated with chemical and biologic weapons. Shortly after the September attacks, the CDC recommended heightened surveillance for any unusual disease occurrence or increased numbers of illnesses that might be associated with terrorist attacks.

On October 4, 2001, the CDC and its state and local partners reported a case of inhalational anthrax in Florida.[3] Over the following several weeks, public health authorities reported additional cases from Florida and New York City. Investigations revealed that the intentional release of *Bacillus anthracis* was responsible for these cases.[4] By November 9, a total of 22 cases (17 confirmed and five suspected) of bioterrorism-related anthrax were reported from Washington, D.C., Florida, New Jersey, and New York City.[5] Ten of these cases were the inhalational form, resulting in four deaths; the other 12 cases were cutaneous anthrax. Of the 10 inhalation cases, most were people who had processed, handled, or received letters containing *B. anthracis* spores.

The association of anthrax with mail increased the level of public alarm. State and territorial public health officials responding to a CDC survey from September 11 through October 17 estimated their health departments had received 7000 reports of potential bioterrorist threats. Potential threats included suspicious packages, letters containing powder, and potential dispersal devices. Nearly 5000 of these reports required telephone follow-up and about 1000 of the reports led to testing of suspicious materials at a public health laboratory.[6] Public health officials were not alone. Patients deluged physicians' offices with concerns about suspicious envelopes and packages and concerns about anthrax symptoms. Although only four areas of the United States had identified bioterrorism-associated anthrax infections, physicians and public health officials across the nation were obliged to respond to bioterrorist hoaxes and threats, as well as anxious patients.

These events illustrate how family physicians and other primary care physicians have been and will be on the front line in detecting and responding to terrorist threats and events. We can summarize their roles:

- Addressing patients' concerns about their risk of terrorist-caused illness
- Reporting credible risks to law enforcement and public health authorities
- Detecting terrorist-caused illness

- Providing effective prophylactic therapy to exposed patients
- Providing effective treatment for patients with terrorist-caused illness
- Recommending actions families can take to protect themselves from future risks
- Providing counseling to families traumatized by terrorist threats and activities

This chapter provides information useful for family physicians in performing these roles, including:

- The features of terrorist attacks distinguishing them from other forms of disasters
- The type of biologic or chemical agent terrorists are likely to use
- The clinical manifestations of these agents, including the routes of exposure
- How to provide effective preventive treatment for those exposed
- How to treat terrorist-caused illness
- How to identify patients at risk of exposure
- Resources available for families traumatized by terrorism

Features of Terrorist Attacks

Historically, most planning for an emergency response to terrorism has focused on overt attacks such as bombings and attacks using chemicals. Chemical events are also likely to be overt because inhalation or skin/mucous membrane absorption of chemicals produces effects that are usually immediate and obvious. For obvious reasons, explosive and chemical attacks elicit an immediate response by law enforcement, fire, and emergency medical services personnel. In comparison to chemicals and explosives, the impact of biologic agents is more likely to be covert and delayed. As the recent anthrax events demonstrated, biologic agents do not have an immediate impact due to the interval between exposure and the onset of illness (the incubation period).[1] Consequently, the most likely responders to future biologic attacks will be family physicians and other health care providers. For example, after an intentional, covert release of variola virus, some infected patients would arrive at their doctors' offices and local emergency rooms 1 to 2 weeks later. Other infected people may have traveled, and they would probably show up at emergency rooms distant from their homes. Their symptoms would appear at first to be an ordinary viral infection, including fever, back pain, headache and nausea. As the disease progressed, many physicians would not recognize the characteristic early-stage papular rash of smallpox. After the rash became pustular and patients began dying, the terrorists could be continents away, and patients would be disseminating the disease further through person-to-person contact. Soon after, secondary cases would begin to occur, resulting in dissemination throughout the world.

Table 129.1 summarizes the distinguishing features of explosive, chemical, and biologic attacks, pointing out why early detection and response to biologic terrorism are critical. With-

Table 129.1. **Features Distinguishing Biologic Attacks from Chemical and Explosive Attacks**

Chemical/explosive agents	Biological agents
Overt	Covert
Immediate	Delayed (incubation period)
Police/fire/EMS detection and response	Medical/public health detection and response
Injuries occur at once	Continuing new cases due to transmission
Cases at location of event	Cases at multiple locations

EMS = emergency medical service.

out adequate preparation, a large-scale attack could overwhelm the public health and health care system. Large numbers of infected patients would seek medical care, resulting in a corresponding need for medical supplies, equipment, diagnostic tests, and hospital beds. The October 2001 anthrax events revealed that the "worried well" would also seek medical attention, causing additional strain on physician and public health resources. First responders and medical personnel could also be at risk of exposure, and widespread panic and fear of contagion would disrupt everyday life.[1]

Besides an aerosol release, terrorists could deliver some chemical agents covertly by contaminating food or water. The accidental contamination of chicken feed with dioxin-contaminated fat in Europe shows how this could occur. Because dioxin does not cause immediate symptoms, authorities did not discover the contamination for months in 1999, and Europeans probably consumed the dioxin in chicken meat and eggs sold that year. One lesson learned from this event is that physicians and public health officials need to recognize and report unusual or suspicious health problems in animals as well as humans.[1] The 1999 West Nile virus epidemic in birds and humans in New York City reinforced this lesson. Fortunately, chemical contamination of public water supplies will pose little risk due to dilution by the large volume of water.

Family physicians must be vigilant for indications that terrorists have released a biologic agent. These indications include[7]:

1. An unusual temporal or geographic cluster of illness. For example, the occurrence of similar symptoms in people who attended the same public event or gathering or patients presenting with clinical signs and symptoms suggestive of an infectious disease outbreak should raise suspicion. One indication may be two or more patients presenting with an unexplained febrile illness associated with sepsis, pneumonia, respiratory failure, rash, or a botulism-like syndrome with flaccid muscle paralysis. Suspicion should be heightened if these symptoms occurred in previously healthy persons.
2. An unusual age distribution for common diseases. For example, an increase in what looks like chickenpox in adult patients, but may be smallpox.
3. A large number of cases of acute flaccid paralysis with prominent bulbar palsies, suggestive of a release of botulinum toxin.

Biologic or Chemical Agent Terrorists Are Likely to Use

Terrorists can choose from countless biologic and chemical agents, and the list can seem overwhelming. However, to best protect our patients and their families, family physicians should focus their attention on the agents that terrorist are most likely to use and that have the greatest potential for mass casualties. The CDC has defined three categories of agents, A, B, and C, with potential as weapons, based on several criteria[1]:

- Ease of dissemination or transmission
- Potential for major public health impact such as high mortality
- Potential for public panic and social disruption
- Requirements for public health preparedness

Based on these criteria, category A contains seven agents of highest concern for the CDC:

- *Bacillus anthracis* (anthrax)
- *Yersinia pestis* (plague)
- *Variola major* (smallpox)
- *Clostridium botulinum* toxin (botulism)
- *Francisella tularensis* (tularemia)
- Filoviruses (Ebola hemorrhagic fever, Marburg hemorrhagic fever)
- Arenaviruses [Lassa (Lassa fever), Junin (Argentine hemorrhagic fever), and related viruses]

This chapter focuses on these biologic agents. Those interested in additional information on agents not covered in this chapter, including those in categories B and C, should visit the CDC Web site at *http://www.bt.cdc.gov*.

Anthrax

Exposure Evaluation

After the October 2001 terrorist release of anthrax, thousands of patients called physicians' offices with concerns about possible anthrax. Some were asymptomatic, while others were experiencing upper respiratory or other symptoms suggestive of a viral infection. Concern about recent exposure to suspicious mail was a theme common to many of these cells. Given the number of actual anthrax cases, the "worried well" generated the vast majority of these calls, taxing the resources of physicians and other health care providers.

Figures 129.1 and 129.2 summarize the recommended clinical evaluation for patients with possible inhalational anthrax and cutaneous anthrax, respectively.[6] Clearly, taking a history is the most essential step in the clinical evaluation. When taking a history, family physicians should ask questions regarding the patient's concern about exposure with two goals in mind:

1. Assess the probability of exposure. By doing so, physicians can determine whether the patient is at risk for anthrax disease, whether to notify public health officials and

law enforcement agencies, and whether to begin preventive or curative treatment. Given the volume of patient telephone calls, physicians should consider training their nursing staff to triage the calls to reduce the number of patients requiring evaluation that is more extensive.
2. Review with patients their level of risk. If patients come to the office for further evaluation, the visit provides opportunities to educate them and the public on how to evaluate their risk and how to take reasonable measures to protect themselves and their families.

In a telephone call or during an office visit, physicians and their staff should ask their patients the following questions:

- Have you been exposed to a situation where anthrax transmission has been confirmed or under investigation?
- Have you had any contact with a substance believed to be contaminated with anthrax?
- When, where, and under what circumstances did the contact occur?
- What was the nature of the contact (skin, inhalation, ingestion)?
- Was any powder suspended in the air?
- Did other people come into contact with the substance?
- Were you exposed to a suspicious package/mail item? If so, why was it suspicious?
- Were you exposed to something else? Why do you believe it was contaminated?
- Where is the substance/package? Is it contained safely (e.g., in a plastic zip-lock bag)?

To assist physicians and other responders in evaluating exposure, local, state, and federal law enforcement authorities have released guidelines on identification of packages/envelopes potentially contaminated with anthrax. Characteristics of suspicious packages include:

- Inappropriate or unusual labeling
- Excessive postage
- Handwritten or poorly typed addresses
- Misspellings of common words
- Strange return address or no return address
- Incorrect titles or title without a name
- Not addressed to a specific person
- Marked with restrictions, such as "Personal," "Confidential," or "Do not x-ray"
- Marked with any threatening language
- Postmarked from a city or state that does not match the return address
- Powdery substance felt through or appearing on the package or envelope
- Oily stains, discoloration, or odor
- Lopsided or uneven envelope
- Excessive packaging material such as masking tape, string, etc.
- Other suspicious signs
- Excessive weight
- Ticking sound
- Protruding wires or aluminum foil

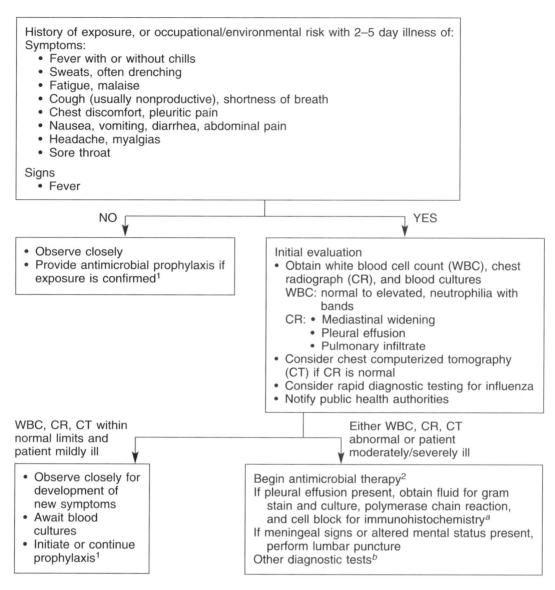

History of exposure, or occupational/environmental risk with 2–5 day illness of:
Symptoms:
- Fever with or without chills
- Sweats, often drenching
- Fatigue, malaise
- Cough (usually nonproductive), shortness of breath
- Chest discomfort, pleuritic pain
- Nausea, vomiting, diarrhea, abdominal pain
- Headache, myalgias
- Sore throat

Signs
- Fever

NO

- Observe closely
- Provide antimicrobial prophylaxis if exposure is confirmed[1]

YES

Initial evaluation
- Obtain white blood cell count (WBC), chest radiograph (CR), and blood cultures
  WBC: normal to elevated, neutrophilia with bands
  CR: • Mediastinal widening
      • Pleural effusion
      • Pulmonary infiltrate
- Consider chest computerized tomography (CT) if CR is normal
- Consider rapid diagnostic testing for influenza
- Notify public health authorities

WBC, CR, CT within normal limits and patient mildly ill

- Observe closely for development of new symptoms
- Await blood cultures
- Initiate or continue prophylaxis[1]

Either WBC, CR, CT abnormal or patient moderately/severely ill

Begin antimicrobial therapy[2]
If pleural effusion present, obtain fluid for gram stain and culture, polymerase chain reaction, and cell block for immunohistochemistry[a]
If meningeal signs or altered mental status present, perform lumbar puncture
Other diagnostic tests[b]

[a]Available through CDC or LRN. Cell block obtained by centrifugation of pleural fluid.
[b]Serologic testing available at CDC may be an additional diagnostic technique.

Fig. 129.1. Clinical evaluation of persons with possible inhalational anthrax.[6]

Clinical Presentation

Anthrax can present as one of three types of infection in humans: inhalational, cutaneous, and gastrointestinal. Cutaneous anthrax is the most common naturally occurring form, with about 224 cases reported between 1944 and 1994 in the United States. Until the recent terrorist attacks, inhalational anthrax had not been reported since 1978. Gastrointestinal anthrax, which follows ingestion of insufficiently cooked contaminated meat, is relatively uncommon, with outbreaks reported in Africa and Asia.

Inhalational Anthrax

Inhalational anthrax results from the deposition of spores into the alveolar spaces. The estimated LD_{50} (lethal dose sufficient to kill 50% of exposed persons) is 2500 to 55,000 inhaled spores.[8] Inhalational anthrax does not cause a typical bronchopneumonia, so the term *anthrax pneumonia* is misleading. Postmortem study of those who died following the 1979 accidental release of anthrax spores in Sverdlovsk (in the former Soviet Union) revealed hemorrhagic thoracic lymphadenitis and hemorrhagic mediastinitis in all patients. About half of the patients had hemorrhagic meningitis as well. Early diagnosis is difficult and requires a high index of suspicion. The clinical presentation of inhalational anthrax is in two stages. Patients first develop nonspecific symptoms, including fever, dyspnea, cough, headache, vomiting, chills, weakness, abdominal pain, and chest pain. Signs of illness and laboratory studies are nonspecific during the first stage, which could last from hours to a few days. The second stage develops abruptly, with sudden fever, dyspnea, diaphoresis, and

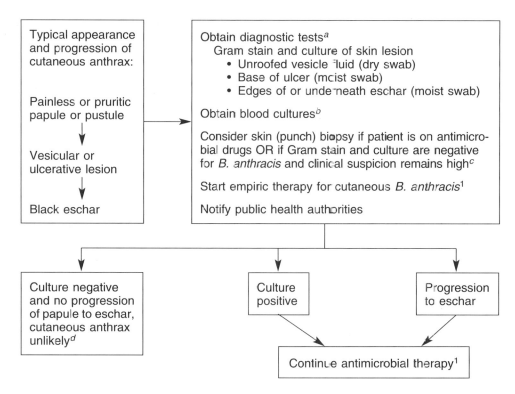

^aSerologic testing available at CDC may be an additional diagnostic technique for confirmation of cases of cutaneous anthrax.
^bIf blood cultures are positive for *B. anthracis*, treat with antimicrobials as for inhalational anthrax.[1]
^cPunch biopsy should be submitted in formalin to CDC. Polymerase chain reaction can also be done on formalin-fixed specimen. Gram stain and culture are frequently negative for *B. anthracis* after initiation of antimicrobials.
^dContinued antimicrobial prophylaxis for inhalational anthrax for 60 days if aerosol exposure to *B. anthracis* is known or suspected.[2]

Fig. 129.2. Clinical evaluation of persons with possible cutaneous anthrax.[6]

shock. Stridor may result from massive lymphadenopathy and expansion of the mediastinum. A chest radiograph most often shows a widened mediastinum consistent with lymphadenopathy.[8]

The mortality rate of occupationally acquired inhalational anthrax cases in the United States is 89%, but most of these cases occurred before the development of critical care units, and in some cases, before the advent of antibiotics. During the October 2001 terrorist-caused outbreak, six out of 10 of the early inhalational anthrax cases survived, signifying that early diagnosis and treatment is critical to improving survival.

Many patients with a low risk of exposure but concerned about anthrax will have symptoms of an influenza-like illness. Physicians evaluating these patients must consider epidemiologic, clinical, and, if indicated, laboratory and radiographic findings to differentiate between influenza-like illness and inhalational anthrax.[9] Influenza-like illness (ILI) is a nonspecific respiratory illness characterized by fever, fatigue, cough, and other symptoms.[9] Besides influenza, ILI has many other causes including other viruses, such as rhinoviruses, respiratory syncytial virus (RSV), adenoviruses, and parainfluenza virus. Other, less common causes of ILI are bacterial, such as *Legionella* spp., *Chlamydia pneumoniae*, *Mycoplasma pneumoniae*, and *Streptococcus pneumoniae*. Each year, adults can average three and children can average six episodes of ILI. Some causes of ILI, specifically influenza, RSV, and some

bacterial infections, can lead to serious complications requiring hospitalization, making them particularly difficult to differentiate from inhalational anthrax.

The 10 cases of inhalational anthrax following the October 2001 terrorist event provide epidemiologic clues helping physicians differentiate inhalational anthrax from ILI. Nine of the 10 cases occurred among postal workers, persons exposed to letters or areas known to be contaminated with anthrax spores, and media employees. Inhalational anthrax is not transmissible from person to person. Consequently, nine of the 10 cases were located in only a few communities. In comparison, viral causes of ILI are spread person to person, causing millions of cases each year across all communities. In addition, nonanthrax causes of ILI have a typical seasonal pattern. Pneumococcal disease, influenza, and RSV infection generally peak in the winter, mycoplasma and legionellosis are more common in the summer and fall, rhinoviruses and parainfluenza virus infections usually peak during the fall and spring, and adenoviruses circulate throughout the year.

Table 129.2 shows how clinical signs and symptoms identified in the October 2001 cases can help physicians distinguish other causes of ILI from inhalational anthrax. Most cases of nonanthrax ILI are associated with nasal congestion and rhinorrhea. In comparison, only one of the 10 patients in the October 2001 outbreak complained of rhinorrhea.

A history of influenza vaccination does not help differen-

Table 129.2. **Clinical Findings of Inhalational Anthrax, Laboratory Confirmed Influenza, and Other Causes of Influenza-Like Illness (ILI)[9]**

Symptom/sign	Inhalational anthrax (n = 10)	Laboratory-confirmed influenza	ILI from other causes
Elevated temperature	70%	68%–77%	40%–73%
Fever or chills	100%	83%–90%	75%–89%
Fatigue/malaise	100%	75%–94%	62%–94%
Cough (minimal or nonproductive)	90%	84%–93%	72%–80%
Shortness of breath	80%	6%	6%
Chest discomfort or pleuritic chest pain	60%	35%	23%
Headache	50%	84%–91%	74%–89%
Myalgias	50%	67%–94%	73%–94%
Sore throat	20%	64%–84%	64%–84%
Rhinorrhea	10%	79%	68%
Nausea or vomiting	80%	12%	12%
Abdominal pain	30%	22%	22%

tiate inhalational anthrax from other causes of ILI. The vaccine does not prevent ILI caused by infectious agents other than influenza, and many persons vaccinated against influenza will still get ILI. Therefore, receipt of vaccine does not increase the probability of inhalational anthrax as a cause of ILI, especially among persons who have no probable exposure to anthrax.

Chest radiographic findings can help differentiate nonanthrax ILI from inhalational anthrax. In the October 2001 outbreak, all 10 inhalational anthrax patients presented with abnormal chest radiographs, seven with mediastinal widening, seven with infiltrates, and eight with pleural effusion. The radiographic findings were easier to discern with posteroanterior and lateral views, compared to portable anteroposterior views. In comparison, most cases of ILI are not associated with radiographic findings of pneumonia, which occurs most often among the very young, the elderly, or those with chronic pulmonary disease.[9]

The most useful microbiologic test for anthrax is a standard blood culture, which should show growth within 6 to 24 hours. Physicians should order blood cultures only for patients in situations where they suspect bacteremia and not routinely on all patients with ILI symptoms who have no probable exposure to anthrax. When ordering blood cultures, physicians must alert the laboratory to the possibility of anthrax, so that the lab performs appropriate biochemical testing and species identifi-

cation. Rapid diagnostic tests for anthrax are not available, so physicians need to be vigilant about recognizing unusual radiologic findings. A chest radiograph showing a widened mediastinum in a previously healthy person with evidence of severe flu-like symptoms is essentially pathognomonic of advanced inhalational anthrax. Although the patient's prognosis may be poor even with treatment, immediate reporting may lead to earlier diagnosis in others.

Table 129.3 summarizes the epidemiology and clinical presentation of inhalational anthrax.[8,10]

Cutaneous Anthrax[8]

Cutaneous anthrax follows the deposition of the organism into the skin, especially areas with previous cuts or abrasions. Exposed areas, such as the arms, hands, face, and neck, are the most frequently affected. There are no data suggesting a prolonged latency period, and in Sverdlovsk, no cutaneous cases occurred more than 12 days after the aerosol release. After the spore begins germinating in the skin, toxin production causes local edema. The initial pruritic macule or papule enlarges into an ulcer by day two. Next, 1- to 3-mm vesicles may appear, discharging clear or serosanguineous fluid containing numerous organisms on Gram stain. A painless, depressed, black eschar follows, frequently associated with extensive local edema. Over the next 1 to 2 weeks, the eschar dries, loosens, and falls off, most often leaving no permanent

Table 129.3. **Epidemiology and Presentation of Inhalational Anthrax[8,10]**

Epidemiology	Incubation period	Clinical syndrome	Diagnostic studies	Microbiology	Pathology
Sudden appearance of multiple cases of severe flu-like illness with fulminant course and high mortality	Average: 1–7 days Range: 2–60 days	Nonspecific "viral" syndrome followed in 2–5 days by severe respiratory distress, mediastinitis, shock and death	CXR: widened mediastinum; peripheral blood smear; gram + bacili on unspun smear	Blood culture growth of large gram + baccili with preliminary identification of *Bacillus* species	Hemorrhagic mediastinitis, hemorrhagic thoracic lymphadenitis, hemorrhagic meningitis

CXR = chest x-ray.

scar. Lymphangitis and painful lymphadenopathy can occur with associated systemic symptoms. Antibiotic therapy does not change the course of the skin manifestations, but it does reduce the likelihood of systemic disease, reducing the mortality rate from 20% to near zero. Figure 129.2 summarizes the clinical evaluation of persons with possible cutaneous anthrax.[6]

Gastrointestinal Anthrax

Gastrointestinal anthrax results from the deposition and germination of spores in the upper or lower gastrointestinal tract. Infection in the upper tract causes the oral-pharyngeal form, with development of an oral or esophageal ulcer and accompanying regional lymphadenopathy, edema, and sepsis. Lower tract infections cause intestinal lesions predominantly in the terminal ileum or cecum. These infections present initially with malaise, nausea, and vomiting, progressing rapidly to hematochezia, acute abdomen, or sepsis. Some patients develop massive ascites. The mortality rate is high, given the difficulty of early diagnosis.[8]

Treatment

A high index of suspicion, prompt diagnosis, and immediate initiation of effective antimicrobial treatment are critical for treating inhalational anthrax. Physicians must report suspected or confirmed cases of anthrax to local and state public health authorities immediately to prompt an epidemiologic investigation. Because of the rarity of the disease, neither adequate clinical experience nor controlled trials are available to validate current recommendations for treatment. Because of the high associated mortality, the CDC recommends two or more known effective antibiotics. Table 129.4 summarizes the recommendations for the October 2001 anthrax outbreak. The recommendations could change as we gather more experience with treating anthrax. Ciprofloxacin or doxycycline is recommended for initial intravenous therapy until susceptibility results are available. Other antibiotics suggested for use in combination with ciprofloxacin or doxycycline include rifampin, vancomycin, imipenem, chloramphenicol, penicillin and ampicillin, clindamycin, and clarithromycin. Cephalosporins and trimethoprim-sulfamethoxazole are not recommended as therapy.[11] Although penicillin is labeled for use to treat inhalational anthrax, data from the October 2001 outbreak revealed the presence of β-lactamases in B. anthracis isolates from Florida, New York City, and Washington, D.C. Therefore, penicillin alone is not recommended for treatment of systemic anthrax infection.[11] The recommendations for gastrointestinal anthrax, including oropharyngeal anthrax, are the same as those for inhalational anthrax.

The toxin produced by B. anthracis is a major cause of the morbidity associated with the disease. One study suggested corticosteroids as adjunct therapy for inhalational anthrax associated with extensive edema, respiratory failure, and meningitis.[11,12]

Ciprofloxacin and doxycycline are also the drugs of choice for cutaneous anthrax (Table 129.5). For patients with signs of systemic involvement, such as extensive edema or head and neck lesions, the CDC recommends intravenous therapy

with multiple antibiotics. Although treatment causes skin lesions to become culture negative within 24 hours, the lesions still develop into eschars. Corticosteroids may be helpful for toxin-mediated morbidity associated with extensive edema or swelling of the head and neck areas. A 7- to 10-day course of antibiotics is typically effective for cutaneous anthrax. However, the CDC recommends 60 days of treatment for patients with bioterrorist-induced cutaneous anthrax, because many of these patients are also at risk for aerosol exposure.[11]

Preventive Therapy

To protect the public, the highest priority is to identify people at risk of exposure and respond appropriately to protect them. The circumstances of any potential exposure rather than laboratory test results should be the main factor in decisions regarding antibiotic prophylaxis. After taking a history, physicians should offer antibiotic prophylaxis to patients with an exposure or contact with an item or environment known or suspected to be contaminated with B. anthracis, regardless of laboratory tests.[11] Although nasal swabs for anthrax culture can detect anthrax spores, negative cultures do not rule out exposure. Therefore, nasal cultures are useful for epidemiologic purposes, but not for determining whether individual patients should receive antibiotic prophylaxis.

The latest recommendation from the CDC[13] is to initiate antimicrobial prophylaxis pending additional information when:

- A patient is exposed to an air space where a suspicious material may have been aerosolized (e.g., near a suspicious powder-containing letter during opening)
- A patient has shared the air space likely to be the source of an inhalational anthrax case

After initial prophylaxis, physicians should continue antimicrobial prophylaxis for 60 days for:

- Patients exposed to an air space known to be contaminated with aerosolized B. anthracis
- Patients exposed to an air space known to be the source of an inhalational anthrax case
- Patients along the transit path of an envelope or other vehicle containing B. anthracis that may have been aerosolized (e.g., a postal sorting facility in which an envelope containing B. anthracis was processed)
- Unvaccinated laboratory workers exposed to confirmed B. anthracis cultures

Physicians should not provide antimicrobial prophylaxis:

- For prevention of cutaneous anthrax
- For autopsy personnel examining bodies infected with anthrax when appropriate isolation precautions and procedures are followed
- For hospital personnel caring for patients with anthrax
- For persons who routinely open or handle mail in the absence of a suspicious letter or credible threat

Table 129.4. **Inhalational Treatment Protocol for Cases Associated with the October 2001 Bioterrorism Attack[11]**

Category	Initial therapy (intravenous)*[1]	Duration

Adults	Ciprofloxacin 400 mg every 12 hr†
	 or
	 Doxycycline 100 mg every 12 hr††
	 and
	 One or two additional antimicrobials¶
		IV treatment initially**. Switch to oral antimicrobial therapy when clinically appropriate:
		     Ciprofloxacin 500 mg po bid
		     or
		     Doxycycline 100 mg po bid
		 Continue for 60 days (IV and po combined)‡‡

Children	Ciprofloxacin 10–15 mg/kg every 12 hr¶¶,***
	 or
	 Doxycycline:†††,††
	     >8 yr and >45 kg: 100 mg every 12 hr
	     >8 yr and ≤45 kg: 2.2 mg/kg every 12 hr
	     ≤8 yr: 2.2 mg/kg every 12 hr
	     and
	 One or two additional antimicrobials¶
		IV treatment initially**. Switch to oral antimicrobial therapy when clinically appropriate:
		     Ciprofloxacin 10–15 mg/kg po every 12 hrs***
		     or
		     Doxycycline:†††
		       >8 yr and >45 kg: 100 mg po bid
		       >8 yr and ≤45 kg: 2.2 mg/kg po bid
		       ≤8 yr: 2.2 mg/kg po bid
		 Continue for 60 days (IV and po combined)¶¶

Pregnant women†††	Same for nonpregnant adults (the high death rate from the infection outweighs the risk posed by the antimicrobial agent)	IV treatment initially. Switch to oral antimicrobial therapy when clinically appropriate.† Oral therapy regimens same for nonpregnant adults
Immunocompromised persons	Same for nonimmunocompromised persons and children	Same for nonimmunocompromised persons and children

*For gastrointestinal and or oropharyngeal anthrax, use regimens recommended for inhalational anthrax.

†Ciprofloxacin or doxycycline should be considered an essential part of first-line therapy for inhalational anthrax.

‡Steroids may be considered as an adjunct therapy for patients with severe edema and for meningitis based on experience with bacterial meningitis of other etiologies.

¶Other agents with in vitro activity include rifampin, vancomycin, penicillin, ampicillin, chloramphenicol, imipenem, clindamycin, and clarithromycin. Because of concerns of constitutive and inducible β-lactamases in *Bacillus anthracis*, penicillin and ampicillin should not be used alone. Consultation with an infectious disease specialist is advised.

**Initial therapy may be altered based on clinical course of the patient: one or two antimicrobial agents (e.g., ciprofloxacin or doxycycline) may be adequate as the patient improves.

††If meningitis is suspected, doxycycline may be less optimal because of poor central nervous system penetration.

‡‡Because of the potential persistence of spores after an aerosol exposure, antimicrobial therapy should be continued for 60 days.

¶¶If intravenous ciprofloxacin is not available, oral ciprofloxacin may be acceptable because it is rapidly and well absorbed from the gastrointestinal tract with no substantial loss by first-pass metabolism. Maximum serum concentrations are attained 1–2 hours after oral dosing but may not be achieved if vomiting or ileus are present.

***In children, ciprofloxacin dosage should not exceed 1 g/day.

†††The American Academy of Pediatrics recommends treatment of young children with tetracyclines for serious infections (e.g., Rocky Mountain spotted fever).

‡‡‡Although tetracyclines are not recommended during pregnancy, their use may be indicated for life-threatening illness. Adverse effects on developing teeth and bones are dose related; therefore, doxycycline might be used for a short time (7–14 days) before 6 months of gestation.

Table 129.6 summarizes the CDC recommendations for initial and continued postexposure prophylaxis.

The antibiotic of choice for preventing inhalational anthrax in exposed pregnant women is ciprofloxacin 500 mg twice a day for 60 days. Physicians may consider prophylactic therapy with amoxicillin 500 mg three times daily for 60 days for instances in which the specific *B. anthracis* strain has been proven penicillin sensitive (*MMWR* 11/2/01, notice to readers).

Physicians must be careful in prescribing prophylactic antibiotics because they have been associated with adverse health effects among patients taking them for short-term treatment of bacterial infections. However, few data exist regarding the use of these antimicrobials for longer periods, such as the 60 days recommended for anthrax prophylaxis. Because of the large number of patients that may receive anthrax prophylaxis, the CDC is recommending enhanced surveillance programs to detect and monitor adverse events associated with the medications. In addition, the CDC hopes to gain information on how to design programs to promote completion of the recommended prophylactic regimens.

Table 129.5. **Cutaneous Anthrax Treatment Protocol[a] for Cases Associated with the October 2001 Bioterrorism Attack[11]**

Category	Initial therapy (oral)[b]	Duration
Adults[c]	Ciprofloxacin 500 mg bid or Doxycycline 100 mg bid	60 days[c]
Children[c]	Ciprofloxacin 10–15 mg/kg every 12 hr (not to exceed 1 g/day)[b] or Doxycycline:[d] >8 yr and >45 kg: 100 mg every 12 hr >8 yr and ≤45 kg: 2.2 mg/kg every 12 hr ≤8 yr: 2.2 mg/kg every 12 hr	60 days[c]
Pregnant women[c,e]	Ciprofloxacin 500 mg bid or Doxycycline 100 mg bid	60 days[c]
Immunocompromised persons[c]	Same for nonimmunocompromised persons and children	60 days[c]

[a]Cutaneous anthrax with signs of systemic involvement, extensive edema, or lesions on the head or neck require intravenous therapy, and a multidrug approach is recommended (see Table 129.1).

[b]Ciprofloxacin or doxycycline should be considered first-line therapy. Amoxicillin 500 mg po tid for adults or 80 mg/kg/day divided every 8 hours for children is an option for completion of therapy after clinical improvement. Oral amoxicillin dose is based on the need to achieve appropriate minimum inhibitory concentration levels.

[c]Previous guidelines have suggested treating cutaneous anthrax for 7–10 days, but 60 days is recommended in the setting of this attack, given the likelihood of exposure to aerosolized *B. anthracis*.[6]

[d]The American Academy of Pediatrics recommends treatment of young children with tetracyclines for serious infections (e.g., Rocky Mountain spotted fever).

[e]Although tetracyclines or ciprofloxacin are not recommended during pregnancy, their use may be indicated for life-threatening illness. Adverse effects on developing teeth and bones are dose related; therefore, doxycycline might be used for a short time (7–14 days) before 6 months of gestation.

Anthrax vaccination requires an initial six-dose series and an annual booster. Current supplies are limited and the production capacity is modest. Given the costs and logistics of a large-scale vaccination program, the low likelihood of an attack in any given community, and the effectiveness of prophylactic antibiotics for those exposed, the CDC does not recommend vaccination of the population. Consequently, the vaccine is available only to the military.

Plague

Table 129.7 summarizes the clinical presentation and diagnosis of pneumonic plague, the most likely clinical presentation of *Yersinia pestis* infection associated with a terrorist attack. This clinical presentation is different from that of naturally occurring plague, which is associated with the presence of painful infected lymph nodes, or buboes. Another difference from the naturally acquired infection is that pneumonic plague is transmissible from person to person through respiratory droplets. A pneumonic plague outbreak would result with symptoms initially resembling those of other serious respiratory illnesses.[14] After an incubation period of 1 to 6 days, patients present with an acute and often fulminant course of malaise, fever, headache, myalgia, and cough with mucopurulent sputum, hemoptysis, chest pain, and clinical sepsis. Prominent gastrointestinal symptoms, including nausea, vomiting, abdominal pain, and diarrhea might be present. The pneumonia rapidly progresses to dyspnea, stridor, and cyanosis. Gram-negative rods may be seen on Gram stain of the sputum, and the chest radiograph will show evidence

Table 129.6. **CDC Recommendations for Postexposure Prophylaxis for Prevention of Inhalational Anthrax After Intentional Exposure to *Bacillus Anthracis*[4]**

Category	Initial therapy	Duration
Adults (including immunocompromised persons)	Ciprofloxacin 500 mg po bid Or Doxycycline 100 mg po bid	60 days
Pregnant women	Ciprofloxacin 500 mg po bid	60 days
Children	Ciprofloxacin 10–15 mg/kg po q12h (maximum 1 g per day) Or Doxycycline: >8 yr and 45 kg: 100 mg po bid >8 yr and ≤45 kg: 2.2 mg/kg po bid ≤8 yr: 2.2 mg/kg po bid	60 days

Table 129.7. **Clinical Presentation and Diagnosis of Pneumonic Plague[10,14]**

Epidemiology	Incubation period	Clinical signs	Diagnostic studies	Pathology
Sudden appearance of many persons with fever, cough, dyspnea, hemoptysis and chest pain Gastrointestinal symptoms are common (nausea, vomiting, abdominal pain and diarrhea) Patients have fulminant course with high mortality	1–7 days, usually 2–4 days	Acute onset of cough with hemoptysis, tachypnea, dyspnea and cyanosis Sepsis, shock and organ failure Infrequent presence of a cervical bubo (purpuric skin lesions and necrotic digits only in advanced disease)	Pulmonary infiltrates or consolidation on chest radiograph Sputum, blood or lymph node aspirate for culture and Gram stain Gram-negative bacilli with bipolar (safety pin) staining on Wright, Giemsa, or Wayson stain Rapid diagnostic tests available only at some health departments, the CDC and military labs	Lobular exudation, bacillary aggregation and areas of necrosis in pulmonary parenchyma

of bronchopneumonia.[14] Patients rapidly progress to respiratory failure, shock, and a bleeding diathesis.[10] Without appropriate therapy, the mortality rate is 100%.

As with anthrax, early diagnosis is critical and requires a high index of suspicion. The sudden appearance of previously healthy patients with fever, cough, chest pain, and a fulminant course should suggest the possibility of inhalational anthrax or pneumonic plague. There are no readily available rapid diagnostic tests for plague, and microbiologic studies are important in the diagnosis. Cultures of sputum, blood, or lymph node aspirates should demonstrate growth within 24 to 48 hours after inoculation.

Although the plague vaccine was effective in preventing or ameliorating bubonic disease, it was not effective in preventing pneumonic plague or reducing its morbidity. Production of the vaccine ceased in 1999. Table 129.8 summarizes the recommendations for postexposure prophylaxis and therapy for patients with pnemonic plague.

During a pneumonic plague epidemic, all persons developing a fever of 38.5°C (101.3°F) or above or a new cough should begin parenteral antibiotics. In mass epidemics, if parenteral antibiotics are unavailable, physicians may prescribe oral antibiotics according to the mass casualty recommendations in Table 129.8. Infants with tachypnea should also receive treatment.

Asymptomatic persons having household, hospital, or other close contact (within 2 m) with untreated patients should receive prophylactic therapy for 7 days. Physicians should watch case contacts closely, and begin treating for disease at the first sign of a fever or cough within 7 days of exposure. Contacts refusing antibiotic prophylaxis do not require isolation but should also receive treatment at the first sign of infection. Doxycycline is the drug of choice for postexposure prophylaxis. Table 129.8 lists the alternatives. Doxycycline is also the drug of choice as prophylaxis for exposed children and pregnant women. Pregnant women unable to take doxycycline should receive ciprofloxacin or another fluoroquinolone.[14]

The Working Group on Civilian Biodefense bases its recommendations for treatment of pneumonic plague on reports in the literature of human disease, reports of studies in animal models, reports on in vitro susceptibility testing, and antibiotic safety. Aminoglycosides are the most efficacious treatment for pneumonic plague. In a limited, contained outbreak, parenteral streptomycin or gentamicin are the drugs of choice. In a mass outbreak, in which parenteral therapy may not be available, the Working Group recommends oral therapy with doxycycline (or tetracycline) or ciprofloxacin (Table 129.8). In addition, patients with pneumonic plague require supportive care to treat complications of gram-negative sepsis, including adult respiratory distress syndrome, disseminated intravascular coagulation, shock, and multiorgan failure.[14] Because the potential benefits outweigh the risks, in limited or contained situations, streptomycin or gentamicin are the drugs of choice for children; in mass outbreaks, children should receive doxycycline (Table 129.8). Due to its association with irreversible deafness in children following fetal exposure, physicians should avoid using streptomycin in pregnant women and instead give gentamicin. If gentamicin is not available, doxycycline is the drug of choice for pregnant women, because the benefits outweigh the risk of fetal toxicity.

Wearing masks was effective in preventing person-to-person transmission of pneumonic plague in outbreaks early in the 20th century. Therefore, current guidelines recommend the use of surgical masks to prevent transmission in future outbreaks. Close contacts of confirmed cases who have received less than 48 hours of antibiotic therapy should wear masks and follow droplet precautions (gowns, gloves, and eye protection). In addition, people should avoid unnecessary close contact until cases receive at least 48 hours of antibiotic therapy and exhibit some clinical improvement. In the event of large outbreaks, public health officials will work with private physicians to cohort cases while they receive antibiotic therapy.

Table 129.8. **The Working Group on Civilian Biodefense Recommendations**[a] **for Treatment of Patients with Pneumonic Plague in the Contained and Mass Casualty Settings and for Postexposure Prophylaxis**[14]

Patient category	Recommended therapy
	Contained casualty setting
Adults	Preferred choices
	Streptomycin, 1 g IM twice daily
	Gentamicin, 5 mg/kg IM or IV once daily or 2 mg/kg loading dose followed by 1.7 mg/kg IM or IV 3 times daily[b]
	Alternative choices
	Doxycycline, 100 mg IV twice daily or 200 mg IV once daily
	Ciprofloxacin, 400 mg IV twice daily[c]
	Chloramphenicol, 25 mg/kg IV 4 times daily[d]
Children[e]	Preferred choices
	Streptomycin, 15 mg/kg IM twice daily (maximum daily dose, 2 g)
	Gentamicin, 2.5 mg/kg IM or IV 3 times daily[b]
	Alternative choices
	Doxycycline,
	If ≥45 kg, give adult dosage
	If <45 kg, give 2.2 mg/kg IV twice daily (maximum, 200 mg/d)
	Ciprofloxacin, 15 mg/kg IV twice daily[c]
	Chloramphenicol, 25 mg/kg IV 4 times daily[d]
Pregnant women[f]	Preferred choice
	Gentamicin, 5 mg/kg IM or IV once daily, or 2 mg/kg loading dose followed by 1.7 mg/kg IM or IV 3 times daily[b]
	Alternative choices
	Doxycycline, 100 mg IV twice daily or 200 mg IV once daily
	Ciprofloxacin, 400 mg IV twice daily[c]
	Mass casualty setting and postexposure prophylaxis[g]
Adults	Preferred choices
	Doxycycline, 100 mg orally twice daily[i]
	Ciprofloxacin, 500 mg orally twice daily[c]
	Alternative choice
	Chloramphenicol, 25 mg/kg orally 4 times daily[d,h]
Children	Preferred choice
	Doxycycline[i]
	If ≥45 kg, give adult dosage
	If <45 kg, then give 2.2 mg/kg orally twice daily
	Ciprofloxacin, 20 mg/kg orally twice daily
	Alternative choices
	Chloramphenicol, 25 mg/kg orally 4 times daily[d,h]
Pregnant women	Preferred choices
	Doxycycline, 100 mg orally twice daily[i]
	Ciprofloxacin, 500 mg orally twice daily
	Alternative choices
	Chloramphenicol, 25 mg/kg orally 4 times daily[d,h]

[a]These are consensus recommendations of the Working Group on Civilian Biodefense and are not necessarily approved by the Food and Drug Administration. See "Therapy" section for explanations. One antimicrobial agent should be selected. Therapy should be continued for 10 days. Oral therapy should be substituted when patient's condition improves. IM indicates intramuscularly; IV, intravenously.

[b]Aminoglycosides must be adjusted according to renal function. Evidence suggests that gentamicin, 5 mg/kg IM or IV once daily, would be efficacious in children, although this is not yet widely accepted in clinical practice. Neonates up to 1 week of age and premature infants should receive gentamicin, 2.5 mg/kg IV twice daily.

[c]Other fluoroquinolones can be substituted at doses appropriate for age. Ciprofloxacin dosage should not exceed 1 g/d in children.

[d]Concentration should be maintained between 5 and 20 μg/mL. Concentrations greater than 25 μg/mL can cause reversible bone marrow suppression.

[e]Refer to "Management of Special Groups" for details. In children, ciprofloxacin dose should not exceed 1 g/d, chloramphenicol should not exceed 4 g/d. Children younger than 2 years should not receive chloramphenicol.

[f]Refer to "Management of Special Groups" for details and for discussion of breastfeeding women. In neonates, gentamicin loading dose of 4 mg/kg should be given initially.

[g]Duration of treatment of plague in mass casualty settings is 10 days. Duration of postexposure prophylaxis to prevent plague infection is 7 days.

[h]Children younger than 2 years should not receive chloramphenicol. Oral formulation available only outside the United States.

[i]Tetracycline could be substituted for doxycycline.

Smallpox (Variola)

Acute smallpox symptoms resemble those of other acute viral infections such as influenza. After an incubation period of 12 to 14 days (range 7 to 17 days), smallpox begins with a 2- to 4-day nonspecific prodrome of fever, myalgias, headache, and backache before rash onset. Severe abdominal pain and delirium may be present. Physicians who have never seen the characteristic smallpox rash might confuse smallpox with chickenpox, but the rashes do have distinct features. The typical varicella rash has a centripetal distribution, with lesions most prominent on the trunk and rarely seen on the palms and soles. The varicella rash develops in successive groups of lesions over several days, resulting in lesions of various stages of development and resolution. Varicella lesions are superficial. In contrast, the vesicular/pustular variola rash has a centrifugal distribution, most prominent on the face and extremities. Variola lesions develop at one time, and the pustules are characteristically round, tense, and deeply embedded in the dermis. Secondary bacterial infection is uncommon. Death usually results from the toxemia associated with circulating immune complexes and soluble variola antigens. The case fatality rate in the unvaccinated population is 30%.[15]

Smallpox spreads from person to person by droplet nuclei or aerosols from the oropharynx of infected people and by direct contact. Contaminated clothing or bed linens can spread the virus. Patients are most infectious from rash onset through the first 7 to 10 days of rash.

The United States discontinued routine smallpox vaccinations in 1972. Five years later, in 1977, international efforts eradicated smallpox from the world. The susceptibility of people who received the vaccine 29 or more years ago is uncertain, because clinical studies have never measured the duration of immunity following vaccination. Therefore, we must assume that the U.S. population is highly susceptible to infection. Given the high case-fatality rate, physicians suspecting a single case must treat it as an international health emergency and immediately contact local and state public health authorities.

Public health authorities do not recommend mass vaccination for smallpox at this time for several reasons:

- Current supplies are inadequate to vaccinate the entire population.
- The risks of vaccine complications outweigh the likelihood of a smallpox attack. Potential complications include, but are not limited to, postvaccinial encephalitis, progressive vaccinia infection, eczema vaccinatum, generalized vaccinia, and inadvertent inoculation (transmission of vaccinia infection to close contacts or autoinoculation from the vaccine site to other areas, including the eyes). Certain populations are at greater risk of complications, including patients with eczema, immune deficiency, and pregnant women.
- Vaccinia immune globulin (VIG) is useful in treating some of the vaccine complications. However, like the vaccine itself, VIG is in short supply, and not enough is available to treat all the complications that could occur.

Currently, the only available treatments for patients with smallpox infection are supportive therapy and antibiotics for occasional superimposed bacterial infections. A smallpox attack would pose difficult problems for public health officials due to the ability of the virus to continue to spread unless stopped by isolation of patients and vaccination/isolation of their close contacts.

Given the incubation period and the lag time before physicians recognized the rash as smallpox, 2 weeks or more could pass between the release of the virus and the diagnosis of the first cases. With each generation of transmission, the number of cases could expand by a factor of 10 to 20.[15] The best way to interrupt disease transmission is to identify, vaccinate, and observe those at greatest risk of infection. Clearly, as soon as physicians make the first diagnosis, they should isolate their patients and vaccinate their household and other face-to-face contacts. Whenever possible, physicians should isolate patients in their home or other nonhospital facility to avoid further disseminating of the disease. In addition, hospitals and health care facilities treating patients with smallpox should take special precautions to ensure that all bedding and clothing of smallpox patients is autoclaved or laundered in hot water with bleach. Standard disinfectants, such as hypochlorite or quaternary ammonia, are effective for cleaning viral-contaminated surfaces.

After an aerosol release of smallpox, public health authorities will make vaccine supplies available to affected communities. Postexposure vaccination is effective in preventing infection or lowering mortality up to 4 days after exposure. Physicians should give the vaccine to suspected cases to ensure that a mistaken diagnosis does not place patients at risk for smallpox. An emergency vaccination program should also include:

- Health care workers at clinics or hospitals that could receive patients
- Other essential disaster response personnel, such as police, firefighters, transit workers, public health staff, emergency management staff, and mortuary staff that may have to handle bodies
- Because of the risk of dissemination, in an outbreak situation all hospital employees and patients should receive vaccination. Immunocompromised patients or patients with other contraindications for vaccination should receive VIG.

Botulism

Patients with botulism classically present with difficulty seeing, speaking, and swallowing.[16] Clinical features of botulism include:

- Symmetrical cranial neuropathies, such as ptosis, weakened jaw clench, dysarthria, dysphonia and dysphagia, and often enlarged or sluggishly reactive pupils
- Blurred vision or diplopia
- Symmetric descending weakness in a proximal to distal pattern

- Respiratory dysfunction from respiratory muscle paralysis or upper airway obstruction
- Dry mouth and injected pharynx resulting from peripheral parasympathetic cholinergic blockade
- No sensory deficit[7] except for rare circumoral and peripheral paresthesias secondary to hyperventilation as patients become anxious from paralysis
- No fever (botulism is an intoxication)

As the paralysis extends, patients lose head control, become hypotonic, and develop generalized weakness. Dysphagia and loss of the gag reflect may necessitate intubation and usually mechanical ventilation. Deep tendon reflexes present initially and gradually diminish, and patients may develop constipation. The case fatality rate is 60% without respiratory support. Death results from upper airway obstruction (due to pharyngeal and upper airway muscle paralysis) and inadequate tidal volume (diaphragmatic and accessory respiratory muscle paralysis).[16] Botulinum toxin does not penetrate the brain, so severely ill patients are not confused or obtunded. However, the associated bulbar palsies create communication difficulties and can make patients appear lethargic. Physicians can recognize botulism by its classic triad[16]:

- Symmetric, descending flaccid paralysis with prominent bulbar palsies (the four D's—diplopia, dysarthria, dysphonia, and dysphagia)
- Afebrile patient
- Clear sensorium

Inhalational botulism, resulting from an aerosol release of botulinum toxin, would have a similar clinical presentation as foodborne botulism, but perhaps without accompanying gastrointestinal symptoms. A waterborne release of botulinum toxin, in spite of its potency, would unlikely cause illness for a couple of reasons. First, standard water treatments, such as chlorination and aeration, would rapidly inactivate the toxin. Second, the large volume of water would require a very large, expensive inoculum, so it would not be an efficient way for terrorists to distribute the toxin.

Early recognition of an intentional airborne release of botulinum toxin requires heightened clinical suspicion. Certain features are particularly suggestive[16]:

- Outbreak of a large number of cases of acute flaccid paralysis with prominent bulbar palsies
- Outbreak with an unusual botulinum toxin type
- Outbreak with a common geographic factor among cases (for example, airport or work location) but without a common dietary exposure
- Multiple simultaneous outbreaks with no common source

Physicians seeing patients with findings suggestive of botulism should take a careful travel history, activity history, and a dietary history. They should ask patients if they know of anyone with similar symptoms. A single case of suspected botulism is a potential public health emergency because it reflects the possibility of contaminated food, available to others, or a release of aerosolized toxin. Therefore, physicians must immediately report suspect cases to their hospital epidemiologist and to their local and state public health departments, who can coordinate shipping of antitoxin, laboratory testing, and epidemiologic investigation. Laboratory testing is only available at the CDC and some state public health laboratories.

Treatment includes supportive care and passive immunization with equine antitoxin. Patients must receive antitoxin at the first suspicion of botulism to minimize neurologic damage. The antitoxin will not reverse already existing paralysis. Physicians can obtain antitoxin from the CDC through their state and local health departments. Because the recommended dosage has changed over time, physicians should review the package insert with public health authorities before administering the antitoxin. Potential side effects include anaphylaxis, serum sickness, urticaria, and other reactions suggestive of hypersensitivity, necessitating a small challenge dose before giving the full dose. Supportive care may include enteral tube or parenteral nutrition, intensive care, mechanical ventilation, treatment of secondary infections, and monitoring for impending respiratory failure. Pregnant patients and children should receive the standard treatment, including antitoxin. The potential adverse effects of antitoxin and its limited availability outweigh its use as a prophylaxis for exposed patients without symptoms. In an outbreak situation, physicians should closely observe potentially exposed asymptomatic patients.

Tularemia

After inhalation of contaminated aerosol, *F. tularensis* causes an abrupt onset of an acute, nonspecific febrile illness beginning 3 to 5 days after exposure. Nearly half the patients have a dissociation of pulse and temperature. Symptoms include headaches, chills, and rigors; generalized body aches (often prominent in the low back); coryza; and sore throat. Patients frequently develop a dry or slightly productive cough, with or without objective signs of pneumonia, such as purulent sputum, dyspnea, tachypnea, pleuritic pain, or hemoptysis. Gastrointestinal symptoms, including nausea, vomiting, and diarrhea, may occur. Symptoms of untreated, continuing illness include sweats, fever, chills, progressive weakness, malaise, anorexia, and weight loss. Many cases develop pleuropneumonitis over the ensuing days and weeks. The earliest chest radiograph findings may be peribronchial infiltrates, typically advancing to bronchopneumonia in one or more lobes, often accompanied by pleural effusions and hilar adenopathy.[17]

However, clinical signs may be minimal or absent, and some patients will show only one or several small, discrete infiltrates or scattered granulomatous lesions of the lung parenchyma or pleura. In previous studies, only 25% to 50% of patients had radiographic evidence of pneumonia in the early stages of the disease. In some patients, however, the pneumonia can progress rapidly to respiratory failure and death. The case fatality rate with treatment is about 2%. Person-to-person transmission has not been documented.

Inhalation can occasionally cause the oropharyngeal form of tularemia, associated with stomatitis and exudative pharyngitis, sometimes with ulceration. Patients may develop pronounced cervical or retropharyngeal lymphadenopathy.

Because of the nonspecific symptoms, physicians and public health authorities would have difficulty distinguishing between a terrorist attack and a natural outbreak of community acquired infection, especially influenza and some atypical pneumonia. Several clues that would indicate an intentional cause would include:

- Abrupt onset in large numbers of acutely ill people
- Rapid progression of many cases from upper respiratory symptoms and bronchitis to life-threatening pleuropneumonitis and systemic infection
- An unusual number of cases with findings of atypical pneumonia, pleuritis, and hilar adenopathy
- Cases among young, previously healthy adults and children

Physicians who suspect inhalational tularemia should do the following:

- Promptly collect specimens of respiratory secretions and blood and alert the laboratory of the need for special diagnostic and safety procedures
- Immediately notify the hospital epidemiologist or infection control practitioner
- Immediately notify their state and local health departments

Table 129.9 summarizes the Working Group for Civil Biodefense recommendations for antibiotic treatment in a contained casualty situation, where resources are adequate for individual case management. Streptomycin is the drug of choice, with gentamicin as an alternative in children and adults. Gentamicin is the drug of choice for pregnant women.[17]

Table 129.10 summarizes the Working Group recommendations for treatment in a mass casualty situation. Oral doxycycline or ciprofloxacin is the treatment of choice for adults and children. In mass situations, oral ciprofloxacin is the best choice for pregnant women.

Due to the short incubation period and incomplete protection by available vaccines, the Working Group on Civilian Biodefense does not recommend tularemia vaccination for postexposure prophylaxis. Treatment begun with streptomycin, gentamicin, doxycycline, or ciprofloxacin during the incubation period is protective against symptomatic infection. Once public health officials become aware that terrorists have released a *F. tularensis* aerosol, they will attempt to identify people at risk of exposure. Those exposed patients who are still asymptomatic should receive prophylactic treatment with 14 days of doxycycline or ciprofloxacin. If health officials fail to detect the release until people start becoming ill, physicians should instruct their patients to begin a fever watch. Those who develop an unexplained fever or flu-like illness within 14 days of exposure should begin treatment as outlined in Tables 129.9 and 129.10. Close contacts of cases do not require prophylaxis because person-to-person transmission does not occur.[17]

Table 129.9. Recommendations for Tularemia Treatment[a] in Contained Casualty Situations[17]

Contained casualty recommended therapy
Adults
Preferred choices
Streptomycin, 1 g IM twice daily
Gentamicin, 5 mg/kg IM or IV once daily[b]
Alternative choices
Doxycycline, 100 mg IV twice daily
Chloramphenicol, 15 mg/kg IV 4 times daily[b]
Ciprofloxacin, 400 mg IV twice daily[b]
Children
Preferred choices
Streptomycin, 15 mg/kg IM twice daily (should not exceed 2 g/d)
Gentamicin 2.5 mg/kg IM or IV 3 times daily[b]
Alternative choices
Doxycycline: if weight ≥45 kg, 100 mg IV twice daily; if weight <45 kg, give 2.2 mg/kg IV twice daily
Chloramphenicol, 15 mg/kg IV 4 times daily[b]
Ciprofloxacin, 15 mg/kg IV twice daily[b,c]
Pregnant women
Preferred choices
Gentamicin, 5 mg/kg IM or IV once daily[b]
Streptomycin, 1 g IM twice daily
Alternative choices
Doxycycline, 100 mg IV twice daily
Ciprofloxacin, 400 mg IV twice daily[b]

[a]Treatment with streptomycin, gentamicin, or ciprofloxacin should be continued for 10 days; treatment with doxycycline or chloramphenicol should be continued for 14–21 days. Persons beginning treatment with intramuscular (IM) or intravenous (IV) doxycycline, ciprofloxacin, or chloramphenicol can switch to oral antibiotic administration when clinically indicated.

[b]Not a U.S. Food and Drug Administration–approved use.

[c]Ciprofloxacin dosage should not exceed 1 g/d in children.

Table 129.10. Recommendations for Tularemia Treatment[a] in Mass Casualty Situations and for Postexposure Prophylaxis[17]

Mass Casualty Recommended Therapy
Adults
Preferred choices
Doxycycline, 100 mg orally twice daily
Ciprofloxacin, 500 mg orally twice daily[b]
Children
Preferred choices
Doxycycline; if ≥45 kg, give 100 mg orally twice daily; if <45 kg, give 2.2 mg/kg orally twice daily
Ciprofloxacin, 15 mg/kg orally twice daily[b,c]
Pregnant women
Preferred choices
Ciprofloxacin, 500 mg orally twice daily[b]
Doxycycline, 100 mg orally twice daily

[a]One antibiotic, appropriate for patient age, should be chosen from among alternatives. The duration of all recommended therapies in Table 129.3 is 14 days.

[b]Not a U.S. Food and Drug Administration–approved use.

[c]Ciprofloxacin dosage should not exceed 1 g/d in children.

Hemorrhagic Viruses

Viral hemorrhagic fevers (VHFs) are illnesses that can cause severe, fatal disease in humans. The CDC has focused its efforts on four pathogens that are potential bioterrorist agents: Ebola, Marburg, Lassa, and South American VHF viruses. Ebola and Marburg viruses are in the filovirus family, while Lassa and the South American VHF viruses are in the arenavirus family. None of these is native to the United States, so an outbreak that epidemiologists cannot link to travel must raise suspicion of bioterrorism. Although person-to-person spread is not common through the inhalational route in a typical outbreak situation, a bioterrorist-released aerosol could cause an outbreak through inhalational exposure.

After an incubation period of usually 5 to 10 days (range 2 to 19 days), the infection causes the abrupt onset of fever, myalgias, and headache.

The filoviruses (Ebola and Marburg) are probably zoonotic illnesses (acquired from animals) that can be transmitted person to person through contact with blood or body secretions of infected persons. The incubation period for Ebola and Marburg viruses ranges from several days to 3 weeks following exposure. Clinical signs of Ebola and Marburg VHFs include the abrupt onset of fever, fatigue, stomach pain, headache, and myalgias. Other signs and symptoms include nausea, vomiting, abdominal pain, diarrhea, chest pain, cough, and pharyngitis. Most patients develop a maculopapular rash, prominent on the trunk, approximately 5 days after onset of illness. As the disease progresses, bleeding manifestations, such as petechiae, ecchymoses, and hemorrhages, appear.[7] Severe cases may have chest pain and show signs of bleeding under the skin, in internal organs, and from body openings. The case-fatality rate for Ebola hemorrhagic fever is 36% to 88% and may be strain dependent. Marburg hemorrhagic fever has a reported case-fatality rate around 25%.

In nature, direct contact with infected rodents or their urine and droppings causes infection with arenaviruses (Lassa and South American VHFs). Infection can also result from inhalation of particles contaminated with rodent excretions. Direct contact with blood or body secretions from infected patients can also cause person-to-person transmission. The incubation period for the Lassa and Junin viruses is typically 1 to 3 weeks. In addition to the symptoms typical of Ebola and Marburg VHFs (see above), Lassa fever frequently causes neurologic symptoms, including hearing loss, tremors, and encephalitis, as well as signs of respiratory distress. South American VHFs can cause severe hemorrhagic fever, and a spotted rash may be a prominent feature. Lassa virus infections cause mild or undetectable illness in most infected people, but about 20% of people develop severe disease. Overall case-fatality rates are about 1%, but 15% to 20% of persons requiring hospitalization for Lassa fever may die. Pregnant women are more at risk for severe Lassa infection. The South American VHFs such as Junin (the cause of Argentine hemorrhagic fever) have case-fatality rates of 15% to 30%.

Immediate notification of a suspected case of VHF to local or state health departments and the CDC is essential for rapid diagnosis, investigation, and control activities. Other than supportive therapy, there is no effective treatment for Ebola or Marburg infections. Specifically, patients will require appropriate maintenance of fluids and electrolytes and careful monitoring of blood pressure. Physicians and other health care staff must avoid contact with body fluids from infected patients, including blood, saliva, urine, and feces. Strict barrier procedures are required for suspected VHF patients. Health care staff should wear gowns and gloves when attending patients, and they should consider using face masks to prevent small-droplet exposure. Hospitals must separate VHF patients from other patients. Close personal contacts or medical personnel exposed to blood or body secretions from VHF patients require monitoring for fever or other symptoms during the established incubation period.

According to the World Health Organization, ribavirin may be effective for treating some patients with Lassa fever. Patients must receive ribavirin within the first 6 days of illness and they must continue the treatment intravenously for 10 days. Treatment with convalescent-phase plasma may be effective for some patients with Junin virus infections. A vaccine has been developed for Junin virus, but it is not licensed for use in the United States. Additional information about viral hemorrhagic fever viruses is available online at *http://www.bt.cdc.gov/Agent/VHF/VHF.asp*.[18]

Chemical Agents

Chemical agents that terrorists might use range from warfare agents to toxic chemicals commonly used in industry.[1] The CDC Strategic Planning Workgroup criteria for determining priority chemical agents include the following:

- Chemical agents already known to be used as weaponry
- Availability of chemical agents to potential terrorists
- Chemical agents likely to cause major morbidity or mortality
- Potential of agents for causing public panic and social disruption
- Agents that require special action for public health preparedness

Categories of chemical agents include the following:

- Nerve agents: tabun (ethyl N,N-dimethylphosphoramidocyanidate), sarin (isopropyl methylphosphorofluoridate), soman (pinacolyl methylphosphorofluoridate), GF (cyclohexylmethylphosphorofluoridate), VX (o-ethyl-[S]-[2-diisopropylaminoethyl]-methylphosphorothiolate)
- Blood agents: hydrogen cyanide, cyanogen chloride
- Blister agents: Lewisite (an aliphatic arsenic compound, 2-chlorovinyldichloroarsine), nitrogen and sulfur mustards, phosgene oxime
- Heavy metals: arsenic, lead, mercury
- Volatile toxins: benzene, chloroform, trihalomethanes
- Pulmonary agents: phosgene, chlorine, vinyl chloride
- Incapacitating agents: BZ (3-quinuclidinyl benzilate)
- Pesticides: persistent and nonpersistent
- Dioxins, furans, and polychlorinated biphenyls (PCBs)

- Explosive nitro compounds and oxidizers: ammonium nitrate combined with fuel oil
- Flammable industrial gases and liquids: gasoline, propane
- Poison industrial gases, liquids, and solids: cyanides, nitriles
- Corrosive industrial acids and bases: nitric acid, sulfuric acid

Industry introduces hundreds of new chemicals internationally each month, making it impossible for family physicians to prepare for each of them. Instead, physicians should concentrate on treating exposed persons by clinical syndrome (e.g., burns and trauma, cardiorespiratory failure, neurologic damage, and shock) rather than by specific agent. As with biologic attacks, physicians must be vigilant in recognizing an unusual temporal or geographic cluster of chemically induced illness. For example, the occurrence of similar symptoms in people who attended the same public event or gathering or patients presenting with clinical signs and symptoms suggestive of clinical syndrome related to chemical exposure should raise suspicion. Because of the public health risk, physicians must notify their local and state health departments if they suspect a nerve agent release. In addition, when evaluating and treating potentially exposed patients, physicians should coordinate their activities with authorities responsible for sampling and decontaminating the environment.

This chapter discusses several of the chemical agents that terrorists might use, such as nerve agents and blister agents. Further information is available on the CDC Web site at *http://www.bt.cdc.gov/Agent/Agentlist.asp*.

Nerve Agents

Regardless of the route of exposure, nerve agents cause symptoms due to potent inhibition of anticholinesterase.[19] Symptoms and signs include:

- Rhinorrhea
- Chest tightness
- Pinpoint pupils
- Shortness of breath
- Excessive salivation and sweating
- Nausea, vomiting, and abdominal cramps
- Involuntary defecation and urination
- Muscle twitching
- Confusion
- Seizures
- Flaccid paralysis
- Coma
- Respiratory failure and death

The initial effects of nerve agents depend on the dose and route of exposure. For example, inhalation causes respiratory effects within seconds to minutes, including rhinorrhea, chest tightness, and shortness of breath. Therefore, asymptomatic patients arriving at the hospital do not require admission or treatment if the only possible exposure was through inhalation. In addition, patients with inhalation exposure exhibiting only miosis or mild rhinorrhea do not require admission. On

the other hand, a large exposure due to absorption through skin exposure may first present an hour later with abdominal pain, nausea, and vomiting.[9]

Exposed patients with contaminated skin or clothing can contaminate rescuers and health care providers through direct contact or through off-gassing vapor. Therefore, all patients should undergo contamination of eyes, clothing, and skin before entering the hospital or emergency room treatment area. Health care providers, especially first responders at risk of exposure should wear the appropriate personal protective equipment. In addition, atropine administered repeatedly as necessary and pralidoxime (2-PAM Cl) are antidotes for nerve agent toxicity. Pralidoxime is effective only if patients receive it within minutes to a few hours following exposure. Additional treatment consists of supportive measures, including airway support and mechanical ventilation. Some patients will exhibit resistance to ventilation due to bronchial constriction and spasm. This resistance lessons after atropine administration. Table 129.11 summarizes the emergency department management of nerve agent toxicity. Additional information in decontamination, first aid, personal protective equipment, and treatment is available from the Agency for Toxic Substances and Disease Registry (ATSDR) Web site at *http://www.bt.cdc.gov/agent/nerve/Nervesfnl.pdf*.

Blister Agents: Nitrogen and Sulfur Mustards

Nitrogen and sulfur mustards are vesicants that injure the skin, eye, and respiratory tract. Within several minutes after exposure, they can cause cellular changes, although the clinical effects occur 1 to 24 hours later. Table 129.12 summarizes the clinical effects of nitrogen and sulfur mustards.[20]

Medical Management of Nitrogen and Sulfur Mustard Exposures

Because of the delayed effects, most patients with severe exposures to nitrogen or sulfur mustards will go home or elsewhere after their exposure and may present only later at emergency rooms or physicians' offices when they begin developing symptoms. Like other chemical agents, patients with nitrogen or sulfur mustard-contaminated skin or clothing can contaminate rescuers and health care providers by direct contact or through off-gassing vapor. Therefore, once health care providers are aware of an exposure, they should require all patients to undergo decontamination of eyes, clothing, and skin before allowing them to enter the treatment area. Decontamination can also reduce tissue damage. Health care providers, especially first responders at risk of exposure, should wear the appropriate personal protective equipment.

There are no antidotes for nitrogen mustard or sulfur mustard toxicity. The medical management is only supportive for skin, ocular, and respiratory exposure. One guideline physicians can follow is to keep skin, eye, and airway lesions free from infection. Severe skin burns may require care in a burn unit. Patients with airway damage below the pharynx require oxygen and assisted ventilation as necessary with positive

Table 129.11. **Recommendations for Nerve Agent Therapy in the Emergency Rom[19]**

| Patient age | Antidotes | | Other treatment |
	Mild/moderate symptoms[a]	Severe symptoms[b]	
Infant (0–2 yr)	Atropine: 0.05 mg/kg IM or 0.02 mg/kg IV 2-PAM Cl: 15 mg/kg IV slowly	Atropine: 0.1 mg/kg IM or 0.02 mg/kg IV 2-PAM Cl: 15 mg/kg IV slowly	Assisted ventilation as needed
Child (2–10 yr)	Atropine: 1 mg IM 2-PAM Cl: 15 mg/kg IV slowly	Atropine: 2 mg IM 2-PAM Cl: 15 mg/kg IV slowly	Repeat atropine (2 mg IM or 1 mg IM for infants) at 5–10 minute intervals until secretions have diminished and breathing is comfortable or airway resistance has returned to near normal
Adolescent (>10 yr)	Atropine: 2 mg IM 2-PAM Cl: 15 mg/kg IV slowly	Atropine: 4 mg IM 2-PAM Cl: 15 mg/kg IV slowly	
Adult	Atropine: 2 to 4 mg IM 2-PAM Cl: 15 mg/kg (1 g) IV slowly	Atropine: 6 mg IM 2-PAM Cl: 15 mg/kg (1 g) IV slowly	Phentolamine for 2-PAM Cl induced hypertension: 5 mg IV for adults 1 mg IV for children
Elderly, frail	Atropine: 1 mg IM 2-PAM Cl: 5 to 10 mg/kg IV slowly	Atropine: 2 mg IM 2-PAM Cl: 5 to 10 mg/kg IV slowly	Diazepam for convulsions: 0.2 to 0.5 mg IV for children ≤5 yr 1 mg IV for children >5 yr 5 mg IV for adults

[a]Mild/moderate symptoms include localized sweating, muscle fasciculations, nausea, vomiting, weakness, dyspnea.

[b]Severe symptoms include unconsciousness, convulsions, apnea, flaccid paralysis.

Source: Agency for Toxic Substances and Disease Registry (ATSDR) *http://www.bt.cdc.gov/agent/nerve/Nervesfnl.pdf.*

2-PAM Cl = pralidoxime chloride; also called pyridine aldoxine methyl chloride.

end-expiratory pressure (PEEP). At the first sign of damage at or below the larynx, patients will require intubation and transfer to the critical care unit. Bronchodilators may be helpful for bronchoconstriction. Steroids are not of proven value, but they can be used if bronchodilators are ineffective. Due to the risk of bleeding and perforation, emesis induction is contraindicated. Further information regarding decontamination, first aid, personal protective equipment, and treatment is available from the ATSDR at *http://www.bt.cdc.gov/Agent/Blister/NMUSTARDfnl.pdf* for nitrogen mustard, and *http://www.bt.cdc.gov/Agent/Blister/SMUSTARDfnl.pdf* for sulfur mustard.

Blister Agents: Lewisite and Mustard-Lewisite Mixture

Unlike the other blister agents, sulfur and nitrogen mustards, lewisite and the mustard-lewisite mixture cause symptoms immediately. Lewisite, a systemic poison, and mustard-lewisite mixture are irritating to the skin, eyes, and airways. Contact with the liquid or vapor forms can cause skin erythema and blistering, corneal damage and iritis, damage to the airway mucosa, pulmonary edema, diarrhea, capillary leakage, and

subsequent hypotension.[21] Table 129.13 summarizes the health effects of the mixture.

Management

Patients with lewisite or mustard-lewisite–contaminated skin or clothing can contaminate rescuers and health care providers by direct contact or through off-gassing vapor. Therefore, as with other blister agents, once health care providers are aware of an exposure, they should require all patients to undergo decontamination of eyes, clothing, and skin before allowing them to enter the treatment area. Decontamination can also help reduce tissue damage. Health care providers, especially first responders at risk of exposure, should wear the appropriate personal protective equipment.

Management of lewisite or mustard-lewisite exposure is similar to that of nitrogen and sulfur mustard exposures with two exceptions. First, patients exposed to lewisite or the mixture will have an abrupt onset of symptoms and will likely present to emergency rooms immediately after exposure. As with the other blister agents, patients will require supportive care for eye, skin, ingestion, and airway exposures. The second exception is that an antidote is available for lewisite exposure. British anti-

Table 129.12. **Health Effects of Exposure to Nitrogen and Sulfur Mustards[20]**

	Nitrogen mustard	Sulfur mustard
Dermal	Erythema and blistering. Rash develops in several hours, followed by blistering in 6–12 hr. Severe exposure can cause second- and third-degree burns.	Erythema and blistering. Pruritic rash develops in 4–8 hours, followed by blistering in 2–18 hours. Severe exposure can cause second- and third-degree burns.
Ocular	Intense conjunctival and scleral inflammation, pain, swelling, lacrimation, photophobia, and corneal damage.	Most sensitive tissue to sulfur. Intense conjunctival and scleral pain, swelling, lacrimation, blepharospasm, and photophobia. Miosis may occur. Severe exposure can cause corneal edema, perforation, scarring, and blindness.
Respiratory	Mucosal damage within hours that may progress over days. Nasal and sinus pain or discomfort, pharyngitis, laryngitis, cough, and dyspnea. Pulmonary edema is uncommon.	Upper and lower airway inflammation within hours of exposure and progressing over several days. Burning nasal pain, epistaxis, sinus pain, laryngitis, loss of taste and smell, cough, wheezing, and dyspnea. Pseudomembrane formation and local airway obstruction.
Gastrointestinal (GI)	Ingestion can cause chemical burns and hemorrhagic diarrhea. Nausea and vomiting may occur after ingestion, dermal or inhalation exposure.	Ingestion can cause chemical burns and cholinergic stimulation. Nausea and vomiting may occur after ingestion or inhalation. Early nausea and vomiting is usually transient and not severe. Nausea, vomiting, and diarrhea occurring several days after exposure indicates GI tract damage and is a poor prognostic sign.
Central nervous system (CNS)	High doses have caused tremors, seizures, incoordination, ataxia, and coma in laboratory animals.	High doses can cause hyperexcitability, convulsions, and insomnia.
Hematopoietic	Bone marrow suppression and increased risk for infection, hemorrhage, and anemia.	Bone marrow suppression and increased risk for infection, hemorrhage, and anemia.
Delayed effects	Potential menstrual irregularities, alopecia, hearing loss, tinnitus, jaundice, impaired spermatogenesis, generalized swelling, and hyperpigmentation.	Years after apparent healing of severe eye lesions, relapsing keratitis or keratopathy may develop.
Potential sequelae	Chronic respiratory and eye conditions following large exposures.	Persistent eye conditions, loss of taste and smell, and chronic respiratory illness, including asthmatic bronchitis, recurring respiratory infections, and pulmonary fibrosis.

lewisite (BAL), also known as dimercaprol, is a chelating agent than can reduce systemic effects from lewisite. However, because of toxic side effects, only patients who have signs of shock or significant pulmonary injury should receive BAL. Only trained personnel, in consultation with a regional poison control center, should provide chelation therapy. Additional information regarding decontamination, first aid, personal protective equipment, and treatment is available from the ATSDR at *http://www.bt.cdc.gov/Agent/Blister/Lewisitefnl.pdf.*

How to Take Care of the "Worried-Well" Patient

The deluge of patient calls following the bioterrorist events in October 2001, mostly from the worried well, illustrate how family physicians have continued to work on the front lines of responding to terrorism, real and imagined. By answering questions and addressing concerns, physicians can easily reassure patients and reduce the trauma that many families have already experienced. Table 129.14 contains a list of suggested answers for questions patients are likely to ask. Physicians should consider consulting with their local public health officials for updates and additional information useful for addressing patient concerns.

In addition to addressing patient concerns, family physicians play an essential role in addressing symptoms related to trauma from real or imagined events. Patients can suffer from posttraumatic stress disorder (PTSD), even if their families and friends are not immediate victims of violent events. According to the *Diagnostic and Statistical Manual of Mental Disorders*, 4th edition (DSM-IV), the first six criteria for the diagnosis of PTSD requires patient exposure to a traumatic event in which both of the following were present:

Table 129.13. Health Effects of Exposure to Lewisite and Mustard-Lewisite Mixture[21]

	Lewisite and Mustard-Lewisite Mixture
Dermal	Pain and skin irritation within seconds to minutes. After exposure to the liquid form, erythema within 15–30 minutes and blisters within several hours, developing fully by 12–18 hours. Slightly longer response times for the vapor. The blister begins as a small blister in the center of the erythematous area and expands to include the entire area.
Ocular	Immediate pain and blepharospasm. Edema of conjunctiva of eyelids follows, and the eyes may be swollen shut within an hour. High doses can cause corneal damage and iritis. Lacrimation, photophobia, and inflammation of the conjunctiva and cornea may occur.
Respiratory	Burning nasal pain, epistaxis, sinus pain, laryngitis, cough, and dyspnea may occur. Necrosis can lead to pseudomembrane formation and local airway obstruction. High levels of exposure can result in pulmonary edema.
GI	Ingestion or inhalation of lewisite can cause nausea and vomiting. Ingestion of the mixture causes severe abdominal pain, vomiting, and hematochezia after 15–20 minutes.
Cardiovascular	Lewisite shock due to increased capillary permeability and subsequent intravascular volume loss, hypovolemia, and organ congestion.
Hepatic	Necrosis due to shock and hypoperfusion.
Renal	Decreased renal function secondary to hypotension.
Hematopoietic	Bone marrow suppression.
Potential sequelae	Chronic respiratory and eye conditions.

- The person experienced, witnessed, or was confronted with an event or events that involved actual or threatened death or serious injury, or a threat to the physical integrity of self or others.
- The person's response involved intense fear, helplessness, or horror. In children, this may be expressed instead by disorganized or agitated behavior.

Certainly, these features characterized the public's experience with recent terrorist events, including the September 2001 World Trade Center attack and the October 2001 anthrax attacks. Following such events, family physicians are likely to see increasing numbers of patients with symptoms related to PTSD. Because the diagnosis of PTSD may be challenging, family physicians will need to have a good understanding of its diagnostic features so they can provide the appropriate care or preventive interventions for people at risk. Fortunately, information is available from the American Academy of Family Physicians, including an excellent article on the primary care treatment of PTSD,[22] and a patient handout available at *http://www.aafp.org/afp/20000901/1035.html*. The Web site also includes additional resources for families traumatized by terrorism.

Summary

This chapter has discussed some of the common causes and presentations of terrorist caused illness. Clearly, family physicians are on the front lines of detecting and responding to biologic and chemical attacks. Their roles include:

- Addressing patient concerns about their risks of terrorist-caused illness
- Participation in surveillance to detect an attack. This includes reporting potential exposures and any unusual cases or clusters of cases to local and state public health officials and law enforcement as necessary.
- Working with public health officials to identify patients at risk of exposure and provide preventive treatment.
- Working with public health officials to identify patients with terrorist-caused disease and providing effective treatment.
- Educating patients and the community on the risks of biologic and chemical terrorism, and how to protect themselves and their families
- Detecting symptoms of psychological trauma following terrorist events, and providing compassionate counseling and treatment to address these symptoms

In several ways, family physicians are particularly well suited to respond to terrorism. First, family physicians are widely dispersed, in rural and urban areas, making them accessible for patients wherever terrorist events might occur. Second, family physicians provide continuity care, essential for the appropriate care of patients and families with ongoing physical and emotional outcomes from violent events. Third, family physicians provide comprehensive care, and can take care of most of the health problems, including emotional issues, facing victims of terrorism. Fourth, family physicians understand how to coordinate care for patients, and can refer victims of terrorist attacks to other appropriate services as necessary. Most importantly, family physicians understand how to provide care in the context of family and community.[23] As the events of September/October 2001 demonstrated, terrorism affects entire communities, whether or not individuals directly experience physical outcomes from the attacks. Family physicians, who understand how their patients and families interact with their community, can help identify and treat problems at the community level. Although horrible, past terrorist events illustrate the pivotal role that family

Table 129.14. **Common Patient Questions and Suggested Answers**

Question	Answer
What is my risk of getting anthrax from the mail?	The current risk of anthrax from exposure to an envelope or other object containing anthrax is low, because transmission from secondary aerosolization of anthrax spores is unlikely. Primary aerosolization results from the initial release of anthrax, whereas secondary aerosolization is due to the agitation (from wind or human activities) of particles that have settled after the primary release. The particles that have settled tend to be large and require large amounts of energy to be resuspended in air. Therefore, residue on mail or packages is unlikely to cause any additional infections.
How do I know if an item of mail is suspicious?	Share the FBI criteria with patients (see page 1109).
How should I handle a suspicious envelope or package?	Do not shake or empty the contents of a suspicious package or envelope. Do not carry the package or envelope, show it to others, or allow others to examine it. Put the package or envelop on a stable surface; do not sniff, touch, taste, or look closely at it or any contents that may have spilled. Alert others in the area about the suspicious package or envelope. Leave the area, close any doors, and take actions to prevent others from entering the area. If possible, shut off the ventilation system. Wash hands with soap and water to prevent spreading potentially infectious material to face or skin. Seek additional instructions for exposed or potentially exposed persons. If at work, notify a supervisor, a security officer, or a law enforcement official. If at home, contact your local law enforcement agency. If possible, create a list of persons who were in the room or area when this suspicious letter or package was recognized and a list of persons who also may have handled this package or letter. Give the list to both the local public health authorities and law enforcement officials.
Should my family purchase gas masks?	Gas masks are generally ineffective against communicable disease. In addition, they provide protection against chemicals only when properly fitted and tested. For complete protection, people would have to wear them 24 hours per day, 7 days per week, because we cannot predict the time and location of a terrorist attack. Therefore, we do not recommend purchasing gas masks.
Should my family be vaccinated for bioterrorist-used germs?	At this time, the risk of vaccine complications and the cost of vaccinating the entire population outweigh the benefits of vaccinating everyone in the United States. In addition, only the CDC and the military have the vaccines—they are not available in physicians' offices or at local health departments. In the case of a terrorist attack, public health authorities and physicians will quickly identify people at risk of exposure, and make vaccines and preventive antibiotics available to them.
Should my family stockpile antibiotics just in case?	There are several reasons why public health authorities and most physicians recommend against stockpiling antibiotics. Specific antibiotics are effective only against specific infections, and we cannot predict which agents terrorists will use. People must take the antibiotics at the proper time after exposure for them to be effective, which means that they must know when they have been exposed. Antibiotics taken inappropriately can lead to resistant bacteria, which can put the entire community at risk. The CDC has stockpiled large amounts of antibiotics, and we will make these available immediately to exposed people within 12 hours of the recognition of an attack.
Should I get a laboratory test for anthrax?	No, and here is why: Nasal swabs and blood tests are inaccurate. • You can be exposed and still have a negative test. • On the other hand, a positive test *does not* mean you have inhaled enough germs to get sick. Therefore, decisions on whether to give preventive antibiotics must be based upon risk assessment rather than testing results. Testing is done only as part of the public health investigation into a confirmed or highly probable exposure. • The decision to test is a public health and law enforcement decision. • The public health lab will do the testing only in case of a credible threat.
Is our water supply safe from terrorism?	Yes. In general, routine water treatment (chlorine, filtering) in our public water systems would take care of biologic agents terrorists might place in the system, just as they handle natural germs. If terrorists were to add chemical agents, the water would so dilute the chemicals that they would pose little threat.
What can my family do to protect itself?	The best thing for families to do: develop a disaster plan just as they would for natural disasters. The disaster plan should include an emergency communications plan, a meeting place, and a disaster supplies kit. Parents should check with their children's school to get a copy of the emergency plan of the school. More information is obtainable at the local Red Cross chapter or at the Red Cross Web site: *http://www.redcross.org/services/disaster/keepsafe/unexpected.html.*

physicians play, working in partnership with public health officials to protect and promote the health of families and communities.

References

1. Centers for Disease Control and Prevention. Biological and chemical terrorism: strategic plan for preparedness and response. Recommendations of the CDC Strategic Planning Workgroup. MMWR 2000;49(RR-04):1–14.
2. Oregon Department of Human Services. Bioterrorism: could it happen here? Communicable Disease Summary 50(1), January 2, 2001. Available at *http://www.ohd.hr.state.or.us/cdsum/2001/ohd5001.pdf*.
3. Centers for Disease Control and Prevention. Ongoing investigation of anthrax—Florida, October 2001. MMWR 2001;40: 877.
4. Centers for Disease Control and Prevention. Update: investigation of anthrax associated with intentional exposure and interim public health guidelines. MMWR 2001;41:889–93.
5. Centers for Disease Control and Prevention. Update: investigation of bioterrorism-related anthrax and adverse events from antimicrobial prophylaxis. MMWR 2001;44:973–6.
6. Centers for Disease Control and Prevention. Update: investigation of bioterrorism-related anthrax and interim guidelines for clinical evaluation of persons with possible anthrax. MMWR 2001;43:941–8.
7. Centers for Disease Control and Prevention. Recognition of illness associated with the intentional release of a biologic agent. MMWR 2001;41:893–7.
8. Inglesby TV, Henderson DA, Bartlett JG, et al. Anthrax as a biological weapon. Medical and public health management. JAMA 1999;281(18):1735–45. Also available at *http://www.bt.cdc.gov*.
9. Centers for Disease Control and Prevention. Notice to readers: considerations for distinguishing influenza-like illness from inhalational anthrax. MMWR 2001;44:984–6.
10. Henning KJ, Layton M. Bioterrorism. In: APIC text of infection control and epidemiology. Washington, DC: Association of Professionals in Infection Control and Epidemiology, 2001: 1–11.
11. Centers for Disease Control and Prevention. Update: investigation of bioterrorism-related anthrax and interim guidelines for exposure management and antimicrobial therapy, October 2001. MMWR 2001;42:909–19.
12. Dixon TC, Meselson M, Guillemin J, Hanna PC. Anthrax. N Engl J Med 1999;341:815–26.
13. Centers for Disease Control and Prevention. Notice to readers: interim guidelines for investigation of and response to Bacillus anthracis exposures. MMWR 2001;44:987–90.
14. Inglesby TV, Dennis DT, Henderson DA, et al. Plague as a biological weapon: medical and public health management. JAMA 2000;283:2281–90. Also available at *http://www.bt.cdc.gov*.
15. Henderson DA, Inglesby TV, Bartlett JG, et al. Smallpox as a biological weapon: medical and public health management. JAMA 1999;281:2127–37. Also available at *http://www.bt.cdc.gov*.
16. Arnon SS, Schechter R, Inglesby TV, et al. Botulinum toxin as a biological weapon: medical and public health management. JAMA 2001;285:1059–70. Also available at *http://www.bt.cdc.gov*.
17. Dennis DT, Inglesby TV, Henderson DA, et al. Tularemia as a biological weapon: medical and public health management. JAMA 2001;285:2763–73. Also available at *http://www.bt.cdc.gov*.
18. Centers for Disease Control and Prevention. Viral hemorrhagic fevers: fact sheets. *http://www.cdc.gov/ncidod/dvrd/spb/mnpages/factmeru.htm*
19. Nerve Agents. Agency for Toxic Substances and Disease Registry. *http://www.bt.cdc.gov/agent/nerve/Nervesfnl.pdf*.
20. Blister Agents. Agency for Toxic Substances and Disease Registry. Nitrogen mustard (HN-1) (C6H13Cl2N) CAS 538-07-8, UN 2810; nitrogen mustard (HN-2) (C5H11Cl2N) CAS 51-75-2, UN 2927; and nitrogen mustard (HN-3) (C6Hl2C13N) CAS 555-77-1, UN 2810. *http://www.bt.cdc.gov/Agent/Blister/NMUSTARDfnl.pdf*.
21. Blister Agents. Lewisite (L) (C2H2AsCl3) CAS 541-25-3, UN 1556; and mustard-lewisite mixture (HL) CAS number not available, UN 2810 Agency for Toxic Substances and Disease Registry. *http://www.bt.cdc.gov:80/Agent/Blister/Lewisitefnl.pdf*.
22. Lange JT, Lange CL, Cabaltica RBG. Primary care treatment of post-traumatic stress disorder. Am Fam Physician 2000;62(5): 1035–40.
23. Saultz JW, ed. Textook of Family Medicine. New York: McGraw-Hill, 2000.

130
Profile of Family Physicians in the United States

Daniel J. Ostergaard, Gordon T. Schmittling, and Darrell L. Henderson

The production of fully trained family physicians in the United States began in 1969 with 15 pilot family practice residency programs.[1] There were 1754 residents in training in 164 approved programs by 1973,[2] and these numbers passed 7000 in 386 programs only eight years later in 1981. The number of residents in family practice residency programs surpassed 10,000 in 1996 with a total of 10,102 in 452 programs.[3] By 1996 each state, the District of Columbia, and the Commonwealth of Puerto Rico had at least one family practice residency.[4] The number of family practice residencies and residents peaked in 1998 at 475 programs of 10,687 residents.[3] By July 2001, 63,930 physicians had completed family practice residency programs since 1970.[5]

Family practice residency programs numbered 469 in July 2001, and residents in those programs numbered 10,262. The first-year fill rate in 2001 was 96.3%, 3399 positions filled of a total of 3528 approved first-year positions (Table 130.1).[5]

Family practice residency programs in the United States differ from those of many other specialties in their utilization of community hospitals for a major portion of residency training. Approximately 84% of family practice residency programs are based in community hospitals, most of which have varying levels of medical school affiliation,[3] and 43% of residencies are in institutions in which family practice is the only residency.[6]

The demographic composition of family practice residency classes with regard to sex and minority status has shifted dramatically since 1981. Fewer than 10% of residents in training during each year prior to 1976 were women.[2] More than 30% of residents in training each year were women after 1987 and more than 40% after 1993.[3] By 2001, 47.5% of residents in family practice residency programs were women.[7]

Since 1973 the American Academy of Family Physicians (AAFP) has collected information about the minority status of family practice residents in training. Residency program directors tell the AAFP how many residents in their programs are minorities, i.e., black, Asian/Pacific Islander, American Indian/Eskimo/Aleut, or Hispanic. (The directors provide only the number of minorities.) Before 1977, fewer than 10% of the residents in training during any particular year belonged to minority groups.[2] By 2001, 32.0% of family practice residents in training were minorities.[7]

The changing demographic composition of residents in family practice training programs is a reflection of the changing composition of students in medical schools. In the 1975–76 academic year, 20.5% of medical students were women and this percentage had increased to 42.6% by the 1997–98 academic year. Unfortunately, the growth in the number of minority students (with the exception of Asian and Pacific Islanders) in each class was modest during the same time.[8] Although minorities and women constitute higher proportions of the medical student population and residents in training during each succeeding year, the overall effect of this change is not yet apparent in the composition of family physicians in practice. In 1970, for example, women constituted only 4.2% of all physicians in family practice, increasing to 12.7% in 1980 and 27.3% in 1999.[9]

During the 1980s, 11% to 13% of graduates from U.S. medical schools each year entered a family practice residency program.[10] The percentage peaked at 16.6% when 2634 of 15,894 medical school graduates between June 1996 and June 1997 were residents in family practice in October 1997, but declined to 12.8% in October 2000.[3] The percentage varied from school to school, but was generally higher for medical schools that had a department or division of family medicine than medical schools with no organized structure for family medicine. The number of medical schools with academic departments or divisions of family medicine increased rapidly from 1990 to 2000. Approximately 81% of medical schools had either a department or a division of family medicine in 1990 and the percentage increased to approximately 92% in 2000.[11]

Table 130.1. Results of the Annual Survey of Family Practice Residency Programs: 2001, American Academy of Family Physicians

Survey item	No.
Programs	
Total accredited programs	469
Newly accredited programs not yet accepting residents	0
Program structure types	
Community hospital-based	24
Community-based/medical school affiliated	274
Community-based/medical school-administered	98
Medical school–based	59
Military programs	14
Residents	
Total residents	10,262
First-year residents	3,399
Second-year residents	3,410
Third-year residents	3,453
Total approved first-year positions	3,528
First-year fill rate	96.3%

Increase/decrease class size by year

	1999–2000	2000–2001	2001–2002
2002 Class	3,538	3,513	3,453
2003 Class		3,475	3,410
2004 Class			3,399
Residency graduates as of July 2001			3,513

Total graduates from family practice residency programs since January 1, 1970	63,930

Source: Report on survey of 2001 graduating family practice residents. Leawood, KS: American Academy of Family Physicians, reprint 150. Reprinted with permission.

Practice Patterns of Residency Graduates

One of the signature characteristics of family practice residency graduates is an apparent commitment to remain in family practice. Of all graduates of Accreditation Council on Graduates Medical Education (ACGME) accredited family practice residencies between 1969 and 1993, 91% identified themselves as practicing family practice in January 1994.[12] These data provide excellent evidence that family practice residencies produce doctors who continue to provide primary care services and therefore contribute to access to primary health services in the United States.

Graduates of family practice residency programs practice in a variety of practice arrangements and choose communities of varying populations. More than 10% of graduating family practice residents during each year prior to 1988 entered solo practice. For each year after 1988 fewer than 10% of graduating family practice residents chose to practice alone, and fewer than 6% between 1995 and 2001. The percentage of graduates choosing a family practice group increased from 20% in 1984 to 39% in 2001 (Table 130.2).[13] Without question, the major trend among graduates is to enter group practice rather than solo practice, unlike the general practitioners of previous years. Of all family physicians practicing in 2000,

those who did not complete a family practice residency program were more than twice as likely to have a solo practice as graduates of family practice residency programs: 41% to 16%, respectively.[3] It is worthy of note that all American family practice residents have their ambulatory training in a group practice environment.

Family physicians settle in communities that represent the spectrum of size and location of communities in the United States. Approximately 37% of graduates in 2001 located in towns of less than 25,000 in population and 17% settled in large metropolitan areas of more than 500,000 population (Table 130.3).[13]

Ambulatory Practice of Family Physicians Compared to Other Generalist Physicians

The United States Department of Health and Human Services, National Center for Health Statistics compiles data comparing the ambulatory practice patterns of various specialties. The data are collected in the annual (since 1989) National Ambulatory Medical Care Survey (NAMCS). The survey measures characteristics of visits to the offices of nonfederally employed physicians classified by the American Medical Association (AMA) or the American Osteopathic Association

Table 130.2. Practice Arrangements of 2001 Graduating Residents[a]

Practice arrangements	No. of reporting graduates	Percent of total reporting graduates
Family practice group	906	38.9
Multispecialty group	294	12.6
Two-person family practice group (partnership)	213	9.1
Solo	139	6.0
Practice arrangement not specified	187	8.0
Military	128	5.6
Teaching	42	1.8
U.S. Public Health Service	29	1.3
Emergency room	68	2.9
Hospital staff	82	3.5
Research	4	0.2
Administrative	2	0.1
Further training or fellowship in family practice	105	4.5
Further training or fellowship in another specialty	49	2.1
None of the above	80	3.4
Total	2,328	100.0

[a]The number of "practice arrangements" responses exceeds the number of reporting graduates (2045) because of multiple responses.

Source: Report on survey of 2001 graduating family practice residents. Leawood, KS: American Academy of Family Physicians, reprint 155aa. Reprinted with permission.

Table 130.3. **Distribution of 2001 Graduating Residents by Community Size**

Character and population of community	Reporting graduates		
	No.	%	Cumulative %
Rural area or town (<2,500)			
Not within 25 miles of large city	79	4.0	4.0
Within 25 miles of large city	36	1.8	5.8
Small town (2,500–10,000)			
Not within 25 miles of large city	194	9.8	15.6
Within 25 miles of large city	130	6.6	22.2
Small city (10,000–25,000)			
Not within 25 miles of large city	138	7.0	29.2
Within 25 miles of large city	151	7.6	36.8
Medium city (25,000–100,000)	306	15.5	52.3
Suburb of small metropolitan area	87	4.4	56.7
Small metropolitan area (100,000–500,000)	239	12.1	68.8
Suburb of large metropolitan area	273	13.8	82.6
Large metropolitan area (500,000 or more)	208	10.6	93.2
Inner city/low income area (500,000 or more)	135	6.8	100.0
Total	1,976	100.0	

Source: Report on survey of 2001 graduating family practice residents. Leawood, KS: American Academy of Family Physicians, reprint 155aa. Reprinted with permission.

(AOA) as being in office-based patient care. Internists who do not indicate a subspecialty are considered in this discussion to be general internists. All pediatricians are included in this discussion regardless of whether they have a subspecialty within pediatrics.[14]

During the 12-month period from December 29, 1998 through December 27, 1999, patients made an estimated 756.7 million ambulatory visits to nonfederally employed office-based physicians (Table 130.4). Visits to family physicians accounted for 22.5% of ambulatory visits (170.6 million), of which 17.9% (30.6 million) were to doctors of osteopathy.[15] The members of the osteopathic medical profession are designated as "physicians and surgeons, DO." They are qualified to render complete health care. Osteopathic medicine is a complete system of medical care with a philosophy that combines the needs of the patient with the current practice of medicine, surgery, and obstetrics. Osteopathic philosophy also emphasizes the interrelationship of structure and function, as well as the body's ability to heal it-

Table 130.4. **Distribution of Office Visits by Physician Specialty and Professional Identity, United States, 1999**

	Office visits: no. (in thousands)			
	Doctor of medicine	Doctor of osteopathy	Total	Percent of total
All visits	709,071	47,663	756,734	100.0
Physician specialty				
General and family practice (GFP)	140,003	30,568	170,571	22.5
Internal medicine (IM)[a]	133,624	1,983	135,607	17.9
Pediatrics (PD)	71,187	2,858	74,045	9.8
Obstetrics and gynecology (OBG)	57,998	1,520	59,518	7.9
Ophthalmology (OPH)	51,165	—[b]	51,165	6.8
Orthopedic surgery (ORS)	38,925	1,591	40,516	5.4
Dermatology (D)	30,797	1,907	32,704	4.3
Psychiatry (P)	21,791	555	22,346	3.0
General surgery (GS)	20,127	1,047	21,174	2.8
Urology (U)	17,415	—[b]	17,415	2.3
Cardiovascular diseases (CD)	16,547	—[b]	16,566	2.2
Otolaryngology (OTO)	16,254	—[b]	16,369	2.2
Neurology (N)	8,298	—[b]	8,298	1.1
All other specialties	84,941	5,499	90,440	12.0
Professional identity				
Doctor of medicine (M.D.)			709,071	93.7
Doctor of osteopathy (D.O.)			47,663	6.3

[a]General internal medicine.

[b]The estimated number was greater than 30% of the relative standard error or based on fewer than 30 cases in a survey sample.

Source: U.S. Department of Health and Human Services, Public Health Service, Centers for Disease Control and Prevention, National Center for Health Statistics, 1999 data.

Table 130.5. **Office Visits by Sex and Age of Patients to All Physicians and Selected Specialties: United States, 1999**

Patient age (years)	Office visits (no. in thousands)				
	All physicians	GFP	PD	IM[a]	OB
Total	756,734	170,571	74,045	135,607	59,518
Under 3 years	44,506	6,589	31,290	1,973	—[b]
3–17 years	91,121	21,034	40,141	3,356	1,351
18–24 years	40,983	10,906	—[b]	4,054	10,566
25–44 years	186,022	48,932	—[b]	29,415	32,172
45–64 years	201,911	47,793	—[b]	44,008	11,342
65–74 years	92,642	17,629	—[b]	24,725	2,013
75 years and over	99,548	17,687	—[b]	28,076	1,909
Male, total	311,168	73,039	38,803	56,785	—[b]
Under 3 years	23,279	2,949	16,904	—[b]	—[b]
3–17 years	46,532	10,456	20,935	1,446	—[b]
18–24 years	13,031	4,159	—[b]	2,290	—[b]
25–44 years	66,938	20,169	—[b]	13,327	—[b]
45–64 years	82,487	20,589	—[b]	19,125	—[b]
65–74 years	40,973	8,123	—[b]	10,289	—[b]
75 years and over	37,926	6,593	—[b]	9,450	—[b]
Female, Total	445,566	97,532	35,242	78,822	59,518
Under 3 years	21,227	3,641	14,386	1,115	—[b]
3–17 years	44,589	10,577	19,206	1,910	1,351
18–24 years	27,952	6,747	—[b]	1,765	10,566
25–44 years	119,084	28,763	—[b]	16,087	32,172
45–64 years	119,424	27,204	—[b]	24,883	11,342
65–74 years	51,669	9,506	—[b]	14,436	2,013
75 years and over	61,621	11,094	—[b]	18,626	1,909

See Table 130.4 for abbreviations.

[a]General internal medicine.

[b]The estimated number was greater than 30% of the relative standard error or based on fewer than 30 cases in a survey sample.

Source: U.S. Department of Health and Human Services, Public Health Service, Centers for Disease Control and Prevention, National Center for Health Statistics, 1999 data, unpublished.

self.[16] The AOA and the American College of Osteopathic Family Physicians (ACOFP) are the two professional organizations of osteopathic physicians that are relevant to this discussion. Currently, there are 19 AOA-accredited colleges of osteopathic medicine in the United States.[16,17]

Family physicians had more ambulatory visits than general internists among adults 18 to 64 years, 107.6 million (25.1%) compared to 77.5 million (18.1%). Family physicians and general practitioners had more ambulatory visits than obstetrician/gynecologists among women age 45 and older, 47.8 million (20.5%) compared to 15.3 million (6.6%). Family physicians had 20.3% (27.6 million) of visits by children and adolescents from birth to age 17, compared to 52.7% of visits (71.4 million) to pediatricians (Table 130.5). When the teenage years of 13 to 19 are examined, 28.5% of ambulatory visits were to family physicians, 18.7% to pediatricians, and 52.8% to all other physicians.[15]

Reason for Office Visit

When categorizing the principal reason for patient visits to offices of primary care physicians, one sees that many of the most common reasons and symptoms are presented more often in the offices of family physicians than other generalist specialties (Table 130.6). The same can be said for the most common diagnoses (Table 130.7).[15]

Tests and Procedures

One or more diagnostic or screening service was ordered or performed during approximately 81.8% of office visits to family physicians. Blood pressure tests were given in 67.8% of all office visits, urinalysis in 9.8%, skin examinations in 8.0%, and x-rays in 6.1% (Table 130.8).[15]

Approximately one in four visits (25.7%) to family physicians resulted in one or more pharmacologic agents ordered or provided.[15]

Preventive and Therapeutic Services

Nearly one in three, 31.2%, of visits to family physicians included some form of preventive or therapeutic service ordered or provided. Diet and nutrition counseling was included in 14.9% of visits to family physicians, exercise counseling in 11.2%, and tobacco use/exposure counseling in 4.0%. Physiotherapy was ordered or provided in 3.3% of visits (Table 130.9).[15]

Disposition, Follow-Up, and Duration of Visit

The patient was scheduled to return at a specified time in 45.0% of visits to family physicians, and 38.2% to return if needed. The family physician referred the patient to another

Table 130.6. Office Visits by 20 Most Frequent Principal Reasons for Visit to Family Physicians: United States, 1999

Principal reason for visit of patient	No. of visits (in thousands)						
	To all specialties	To M.D. GFP	To D.O. GFP	To all GFP	To all PD	To all IM[a]	To all OBG
Total	756,734	140,003	30,568	170,571	74,045	135,607	59,518
General medical examination	46,039	9,972	1,912	11,884	6,651	13,091	6,997
Cough	20,654	6,133	1,471	7,604	6,387	4,346	—[b]
Symptoms referable to throat	15,315	4,796	1,243	6,039	4,134	2,888	—[b]
Progress visit	33,975	3,669	667	4,336	—[b]	9,859	—[b]
Hypertension	11,130	3,440	—[b]	4,026	—[b]	5,615	—[b]
Back symptoms	10,482	2,732	1,244	3,976	—[b]	2,322	—[b]
Stomach and abdominal pain, cramps, and spasms	10,077	2,857	—[b]	3,466	—[b]	2,603	—[b]
Headache (excludes migraine and sinus)	8,599	2,600	845	3,445	—[b]	1,333	—[b]
Medications (excludes allergy and injections)	9,284	2,460	962	3,422	—[b]	1,987	—[b]
Sinus problems	7,506	2,793	—[b]	3,262	—[b]	2,083	—[b]
Blood pressure test	6,789	2,425	—[b]	3,022	—[b]	2,497	—[b]
Head cold, upper respiratory infection (coryza)	6,767	2,090	845	2,935	1,517	1,557	—[b]
Skin rash	10,446	2,395	—[b]	2,888	2,128	1,401	—[b]
Earache, or ear infection	11,047	2,060	732	2,792	4,865	1,543	—[b]
Diabetes mellitus	8,400	2,408	—[b]	2,408	—[b]	2,712	—[b]
Low back symptoms	9,186	1,747	—[b]	2,384	—[b]	1,543	—[b]
Fever	9,963	1,738	—[b]	2,346	6,005	—[b]	—[b]
Knee symptoms	11,778	2,055	—[b]	2,055	—[b]	1,658	—[b]
Nasal congestion	9,067	1,434	—[b]	2,051	2,675	1,602	—[b]
Physical exam required for school or employment	3,634	1,600	—[b]	2,040	—[b]	—[b]	—[b]

See Table 130.4 for abbreviations.

[a]General internal medicine.

[b]The estimated number was greater than 30% of the relative standard error or based on fewer than 30 cases in a survey sample.

Source: U.S. Department of Health and Human Services, Public Health Service, Centers for Disease Control and Prevention, National Center for Health Statistics, 1999 data.

Table 130.7. Office Visits by 20 Most Frequent Principal Diagnoses by Family Physicians: United States, 1999

Principal diagnosis	To all specialties	No. of visits (in thousands)					
		To M.D. GFP	To D.O. GFP	To all GFP	To PD	To IM[a]	To OBG
Total	756,734	140,003	30,568	170,571	74,045	135,607	59,518
Essential hypertension	31,962	10,164	2,434	12,598	—[b]	14,075	—[b]
Acute URIs of multiple or unspecified sites	17,691	6,708	1,397	8,105	6,764	1,999	—[b]
General medical examination	13,405	4,740	755	5,495	—[b]	2,460	3,382
Diabetes mellitus	19,585	3,980	1,081	5,061	—[b]	8,537	—[b]
Chronic sinusitis	10,797	4,306	—[b]	4,924	1,498	2,538	—[b]
Health supervision of infant or child	22,626	2,905	902	3,807	18,000	—[b]	—[b]
Bronchitis, not specified as acute or chronic	8,083	2,487	692	3,179	1,295	2,861	—[b]
General symptoms	9,008	2,717	—[b]	3,178	—[b]	2,421	—[b]
Disorders of lipoid metabolism	7,788	2,495	—[b]	2,851	—[b]	4,015	—[b]
Special investigations and examinations	14,609	2,569	—[b]	2,777	—[b]	1,215	6,539
Acute pharyngitis	7,835	1,609	1,131	2,740	2,303	1,776	—[b]
Contact dermatitis and other eczema	7,590	2,254	—[b]	2,651	—[b]	—[b]	—[b]
Suppurative unspecified otitis media	11,843	1,688	912	2,600	7,427	—[b]	—[b]
Sprains and strains of other and unspecified parts of back	5,624	1,555	901	2,456	—[b]	—[b]	—[b]
Other and unspecified disorders of back	8,627	1,978	—[b]	2,419	—[b]	2,349	—[b]
Other disorders of urethra and urinary tract	7,111	1,941	—[b]	2,350	—[b]	1,615	—[b]
Influenza	4,027	2,074	—[b]	2,322	—[b]	—[b]	—[b]
Allergic rhinitis	16,662	1,476	—[b]	1,866	—[b]	2,923	—[b]
Depressive disorder, not elsewhere classified	6,461	1,552	—[b]	1,844	—[b]	1,552	—[b]
Normal pregnancy	16,402	1,453	—[b]	1,838	—[b]	—[b]	14,508

See Table 130.4 for abbreviations.

[a]General internal medicine.

[b]The estimated number was greater than 30% of the relative standard error or based on fewer than 30 cases in a survey sample.

Source: U.S. Department of Health and Human Services, Public Health Service, Centers for Disease Control and Prevention, National Center for Health Statistics, 1999 data.

Table 130.8. **Office Visits by Screening/Diagnostic Service(s),[a] Tests and Procedures Performed or Ordered: United States, 1999**

Diagnostic/screening services	No. of visits (in thousands)						
	All specialties	M.D. GFP	D.O. GFP	All GFP	PD	IM[b]	OBG
Total visits	756,734	140,003	30,568	170,571	74,045	135,607	59,518
Visits with a service	556,636	114,075	25,503	139,578	31,597	113,289	53,389
Visits without a service	200,097	25,928	5,065	30,993	42,448	22,318	6,129
Examinations reported							
Breast	48,835	7,538	1,039	8,577	1,566	7,327	23,277
Pelvic	49,720	6,043	1,016	7,059	1,225	5,216	33,347
Rectal	30,575	5,588	1,065	6,653	—[c]	6,333	9,420
Skin	75,557	12,545	1,143	13,688	5,286	11,230	5,944
Visual acuity	59,267	3,484	798	4,282	3,696	2,541	1,960
Glaucoma	29,055	—[c]	—[c]	—[c]	—[c]	—[c]	—[c]
Hearing	12,395	1,723	313	2,036	3,229	2,418	—[c]
Tests and measurements reported							
Blood pressure	339,342	94,967	20,743	115,710	9,909	98,853	39,243
Strep	10,908	2,946	—[c]	3,577	5,180	—[c]	—[c]
Pap	26,771	4,288	990	5,278	—[c]	1,874	19,264
Urinalysis	62,240	14,478	2,239	16,717	4,244	11,462	14,166
Pregnancy	3,061	—[c]	—[c]	—[c]	—[c]	—[c]	2,021
PSA test	9,640	2,437	—[c]	2,752	—[c]	3,015	—[c]
Blood lead level	1,631	—[c]	—[c]	—[c]	—[c]	—[c]	—[c]
Cholesterol	27,035	6,578	356	7,434	—[c]	13,799	—[c]
HIV serology	2,307	—[c]	—[c]	—[c]	—[c]	—[c]	1,167
Other STD test	3,322	—[c]	—[c]	—[c]	—[c]	—[c]	2,536
Hematocrit/hemoglobin	43,452	8,970	1,022	9,992	6,230	13,895	2,953
Other blood test	103,033	22,172	4,422	26,594	2,947	39,095	7,291
EKG test	22,593	3,559	—[c]	4,116	—[c]	9,429	—[c]
Imaging							
X-ray	51,918	8,688	1,755	10,443	1,939	9,551	—[c]
CT scan/MRI	12,778	1,720	—[c]	1,959	—[c]	1,749	—[c]
Mammography	12,733	2,530	—[c]	3,101	—[c]	2,497	5,758
Ultrasound	16,609	1,682	—[c]	2,298	—[c]	2,390	5,674
Other diagnostic/screening services	102,860	12,224	4,008	16,232	7,377	15,715	7,082

See Table 130.4 for abbreviations.

[a]The sum of the diagnostic/screening services exceeds the total number of visits because more than one service could be performed or ordered per visit.

[b]General internal medicine.

[c]The estimated number was greater than 30% of the relative standard error or based on fewer than 30 cases in a survey sample.

Source: U.S. Department of Health and Human Services, Centers for Disease Control and Prevention, National Center for Health Statistics, 1999 data.

physician in 6.3% of visits. Visits to family physicians resulted in hospitalization in less than 1% of visits.[15]

The average duration of an office visit in which the physician had direct contact with the patient was 19.3 minutes for all specialties, 17.7 minutes for family physicians, 15.4 minutes for pediatricians, 20.7 minutes for general internists, and 17.9 minutes for obstetricians/gynecologists.[15]

In the late 1990s significant investigation was done by Kurt Stange and colleagues[18] in which the actual physician patient encounter was directly observed by a trained observer. Among the findings from the Direct Observation of Primary Care (DOPC) work was the determination that prevision of care to a second family member is relatively common in family practice even when that family member was not present during office visit. Care was provided to a nonpresent patient during 18% of observed outpatient visits.

The nature of care provided for patients has changed over the past 40 years by virtue of new technology and other med-

ical advances. However, there was little change between 1961 and 2001 regarding the proportion of patients who visited a physician's office relative to those who are admitted to an academic medical-center hospital. In both 1961 and 2001 almost 25% of the American population visited a physician's office but less than one person in 1000 is admitted to the hospital of an academic medical center.[19]

Method of Payment

Physicians in the United States can expect payment from several sources. In 1999 family physicians were the attending physician in 18.8% of all office visits in which one source of payment was Medicare, 25.5% of all office visits in which one source of payment was Medicaid, and 23.2% of all office visits in which one source of payment was private insurance (Table 130.10).[15]

Table 130.9. **Office Visits by Preventive/Therapeutic Service(s)[a] Performed or Ordered: United States 1999**

Preventive/Therapeutic Services	No. of visits (in thousands)						
	All specialties	M.D. GFP	D.O. GFP	GFP	PD	IM[b]	OBG
Total visits	756,734	140,003	30,568	170,571	74,045	135,607	59,518
Visits with a service	242,946	43,555	9,702	53,257	20,342	50,414	
Visits without a service	513,788	96,448	20,866	117,314	53,703	85,193	36,430
Counseling/education							
Diet and nutrition counseling	103,885	21,312	4,142	25,454	13,801	33,861	11,006
Exercise counseling	74,005	16,683	2,425	19,108	3,510	24,208	5,880
HIV/STD transmission counseling	5,034	1,803	—[c]	1,875	—[c]	1,241	—[c]
Family planning/contraception counseling	8,428	1,993	—[c]	2,211	—[c]	—[c]	4,595
Prenatal counseling	8,399	1,180	—[c]	1,298	—[c]	—[c]	7,044
Breast self examination counseling	10,089	2,357	—[c]	2,718	—[c]	1,872	3,879
Tobacco use/exposure counseling	21,717	6,114	780	6,894	1,614	9,121	—[c]
Growth and development counseling	16,034	1,869	—[c]	2,260	11,052	1,304	—[c]
Mental health counseling	16,631	2,560	—[c]	2,748	—[c]	4,741	—[c]
Stress management counseling	17,320	2,978	—[c]	3,266	—[c]	6,972	—[c]
Skin cancer prevention counseling	14,611	1,404	—[c]	1,506	—[c]	1,630	—[c]
Injury prevention counseling	22,842	3,656	—[c]	4,086	6,929	2,246	—[c]
Other therapy							
Psychotherapy	20,711	—[c]	—[c]	—[c]	—[c]	3,371	—[c]
Psychopharmacotherapy	18,279	—[c]	—[c]	—[c]	—[c]	1,656	—[c]
Physiotherapy	26,343	3,658	1,929	5,587	—[c]	3,085	—[c]
Complementary	2,922	—[c]	—[c]	1,025	—[c]	—[c]	—[c]
Other therapeutic and preventive therapy	24,878	3,356	682	4,038	1,688	3,526	1,682

See Table 130.4 for abbreviations.

[a]Number of individual visits exceeds the number of all services because more than one service could be provided at each visit.

[b]General internal medicine.

[c]The estimated number was greater than 30% of the relative standard error or based on fewer than 30 cases in a survey sample.

Source: U.S. Department of Health and Human Services, Public Health Service, Centers for Disease Control and Prevention, National Center for Health Statistics, 1999 data.

Hospital Admission Privileges

Most family physicians in the United States spend most of their professional time working in their ambulatory setting, whether that be a group practice or as solo physician in a medical office. However, most family physicians in the United States also have part of their practice in the hospital and ad-

mit selected patients from the ambulatory setting to the hospital setting and provide care for those patients in the hospital. In recent years there is an emerging trend in the United States toward "hospitalists," physicians who spend most of their time in the hospital taking care of patients admitted by other physicians. Hospitalists may be family physicians, internists, or other physicians. There is mixed opinion as to

Table 130.10. **Office Visits to All Physicians and Selected Specialties by Expected Source of Payment: United States 1999**

Expected source of payments[a]	No. of visits (in thousands)				
	All specialties	GFP	PD	IM[b]	OBG
Total visits	756,734	170,571	74,045	135,607	59,518
Private insurance	417,620	96,915	53,750	64,956	42,749
Medicare	156,720	29,396	—[c]	41,176	3,670
Medicaid	56,809	14,496	12,232	8,236	6,322
Worker's compensation	15,639	2,597	—[c]	—[c]	—[c]
Self-pay	40,658	12,108	3,272	3,151	2,131
No charge	7,194	—[c]	—[c]	—[c]	—[c]
Other source of pay	35,616	6,856	1,923	10,384	2,514
Unknown source of pay	14,627	4,447	—[c]	4,344	—[c]
Not reported	11,851	3,386	2,032	2,589	—[c]

See Table 130.4 for abbreviations.

[a]More than one source of payment can be reported; the sum of the sources exceeds the number of visits.

[b]General internal medicine.

[c]The estimated number was greater than 30% of the relative standard error or based on fewer than 30 cases in a survey sample.

Source: U.S. Department of Health and Human Services, Public Health Service, Centers for Control and Prevention, National Center for Health Statistics, 1999 data.

Table 130.11. **Types of Patient Care in Family Physicians'**[a] **Hospital Practices, by Urban/Rural Area, May 2000**

Privilege	Percentage		
	Total	Urban	Rural
Obstetrics			
Routine delivery	23.3	22.5	25.5
Forceps delivery	9.9	9.3	11.7
High risk	8.2	7.7	9.5
C-sections	5.1	4.9	5.7
VBAC	16.3	15.5	‾8.6
Augmentation	19.8	15.0	22.3
Induction	19.0	18.0	21.9
Dilatation and curettage	12.0	11.3	14.2
Tubal ligation	5.6	5.3	6.5
Vacuum extraction	18.0	16.9	21.5
Surgery			
Assisting	26.2	26.1	26.5
Minor	36.8	36.3	38.5
Major	3.6	3.3	4.7
Coronary care unit	48.0	49.1	44.5
Intensive care unit	51.9	53.2	48.0
Emergency room	59.3	59.8	58.1
Psychiatry	37.3	38.4	34.2
Newborn care	62.3	63.4	58.9
Attend at C-section	30.7	30.1	32.4
Neonatal ICU	5.7	5.6	5.9
Interpret ECGs	35.3	35.7	34.0
Gastroenterologic			
Flexible sigmoidoscopy	28.8	29.1	27.9
Colonoscopy	3.3	3.3	3.4
EGD	3.5	3.1	4.7
Colposcopy	17.2	17.6	16.0

[a]Includes only active member respondents of the American Academy of Family Physicians.

Source: American Academy of Family Physicians Practice Profile Survey I, May 2000. Reprinted with permission.

whether patient care is best served by family physicians providing their own care to their patients when hospitalized versus turning the care of their patients over to hospitalists when hospitalization is necessary. All physicians in all specialties must apply to officials of each hospital to gain privileges to care for patients in the hospital setting.

The AAFP surveys its members each year to ascertain the extent of their hospital practices and their satisfaction with their hospital privileges. Although family physicians practice primarily in office settings, approximately 86% of active members of the AAFP had hospital admission privileges in May 2000. Approximately 85% of those physicians indicated that they considered their privileges to be "generally about right."[3] The types of privileges held by family physicians varied by census division, and by urban-rural settings (Table 130.11). In May 2000 the percentage of family physicians in each census division with hospital admission privileges ranged from a high of 92.3% in the West North Central Division (Iowa, Kansas, Minnesota, Missouri, Nebraska, and the Dakotas) to a low of 79.2% in the East South Central Division (Alabama, Kentucky, Mississippi, and Tennessee).[3]

A higher proportion of family physicians in the West North Central Division had privileges in routine obstetric care and most of the more complicated obstetric care than family physicians in other census divisions. The majority of family physicians who did not have obstetrical privileges of any kind indicated that they did not want the privileges.[3]

Family physicians in the nonmetropolitan areas of each census division were more likely to have hospital privileges with more procedures than their urban counterparts.[3]

Conclusion

From late in the 1980s through the late 1990s the specialties of family practice, general internal medicine, and general pediatrics experienced a resurgence of interest from several quarters. The United States government's Council on Graduate Medical Education called for more generalist physicians.[20] Major medical organizations such as the AMA and Association of American Medical Colleges analyzed the need for increased access to medical care in the United States and made similar pronouncements about the need for more generalist physicians.[21,22] Major national health-oriented foundations increased their efforts toward this end in both philanthropy and analysis of the nation's health care needs. The AAFP, after a detailed study and periodic reviews of population and work-force trends, set forth recommendations in 1998 to achieve a family physician supply of 35.1 M.D. family physicians per 100,000 population by the year 2015. To reach that goal it is necessary to produce 3332 to 3682 M.D. family physicians per year by ACGME-accredited family practice residencies. The academy recommends that 50% of physicians completing their training in the United States practice as generalists and that 50% of those generalists be family physicians.[23]

Partly in response to these stimuli, and partly in response to the importance of gatekeeper generalists in managed care payers, family practice was attractive to medical students, residency programs multiplied, and the number of family practice residents increased through the mid-1990s.

Although the number of family practice residencies and family practice residents increased through the mid-1990s, during 1999 through 2001 the number of residency positions and the number of family practice residents declined. The number of first-year family practice positions filled in 1998 was 3575 compared to 3399 in 2001. Reasons for the decline over the past 4 years are under analysis and multifactorial, among them being a series of changes in the managed care environment in the United States during the past few years. It should be noted, however, that there remain more family practice residency positions available and filled in 2001 than in most previous years and family practice remains the most prominent specialty choice among medical students seeking a career in primary care.[24]

References

1. Ostergaard DJ, Schmittling GT. Profile of family physicians in the United States. In: Taylor RB, ed. Family medicine: principles and practice, 5th ed. New York: Springer-Verlag, 1998; 1144–52.

2. American Academy of Family Physicians. Facts about family practice: 1998. Kansas City, MO. AAFP, 1998.

3. American Academy of Family Physicians. Facts about family practice. Leawood, KS: AAFP, 2001. Available at *URL:http://www.aafp.org/facts.*

4. American Academy of Family Physicians. 1996 directory of family practice residency programs. Leawood, KS: AAFP, 1996.

5. American Academy of Family Physicians. Family practice residency programs, reprint 150. Kansas City, MO: AAFP, 2001.

6. American Academy of Family Physicians. 2001 directory of family practice residency programs. Leawood, KS: AAFP, 2001.

7. American Academy of Family Physicians. Cumulative results of annual surveys of family practice residency programs, reprint 151. Leawood, KS: AAFP, 2001.

8. Association of American Medical Colleges. Statistical information related to medical education. Washington, DC: AAMC, 1998.

9. American Medical Association. Physician characteristics and distribution in the US, 2001–2002 ed. Chicago: AMA, 2001.

10. American Academy of Family Physicians. Facts about family practice. Kansas City, MO: AAFP, 1990.

11. Pugno PA, Schmittling GT, Graham R, McPherson DS, Kahn NB Jr. Entry of US medical school graduates into family practice residencies: 2000–2001 and three-year summary. Family Med 2001;33:585–93.

12. Kahn NB Jr, Schmittling GT, Ostergaard DJ, Graham R. Specialty practice of family practice residency graduates, 1969 through 1993: a national study. JAMA 1996;275:713–15.

13. American Academy of Family Physicians. Reports on surveys of graduating family practice residents, reprints 155a–155aa. Leawood, KS: AAFP, 1975–2001.

14. National Center for Health Statistics, Centers for Disease Control and Prevention, Public Health Service, U.S. Department of Health and Human Services. National ambulatory medical care survey. 1999 NAMCS micro-data file documentation. Available at *http://www.cdc.gov/nchs/datawh/ftpdata/ftpdata.htm.*

15. National Center for Health Statistics, Centers for Disease Control and Prevention, Public Health Service, U.S. Department of Health and Human Services. National ambulatory medical care survey, 1999. Available at *http://www.cdc.gov/nchs/datawh/ftpdata/ftpdata.htm.*

16. American Osteopathic Association. AOA fact sheet. The DO. January 2001. Chicago: AOA, 2001. Available at *http://www.aoa-net.org/AOA, General/general.htm.*

17. American College of Osteopathic Family Physicians. ACFP osteopathic. Arlington Heights, IL: AOA, 2001.

18. Stange K, Zyzanski S, Jaen C, et al. Illuminating the "black box": a description of 4,454 patient visits to 138 family physicians. J Family Pract 1998;46:377–89.

19. Green LA, Fryer GE, Yawn BP, Lanier D, Dovey SM. The ecology of medical care revisited. N Engl J Med 2001;344:2021–5.

20. Council on Graduate Medical Education, U.S. Department of Health and Human Services. Recommendations to improve access to health care through physician workforce reform. Washington, DC: COGME, 1994.

21. Primary Care Task Force. Report of the medical schools section. JAMA 1992;268:1092–4.

22. Generalist Physician Task Force. AAMC policy of the generalist physician: as adopted October 8, 1992. Acad Med 1993;68:1–6.

23. American Academy of Family Physicians. Family Physician Workforce Reform: Recommendations of the American Academy of Family Physicians. Kansas City, MO: AAFP, September 1998.

24. Pugno PA, McPherson DS, Schmittling GT, Kahn NB Jr. Results of the 2001 National Resident Matching Program: family practice. Family Med 2001;33:594–601.

131
Chronology of the Evolution of Family Practice as a Specialty in the United States

Robert B. Taylor

Year	Event	Significance
1900	At least 80% of American physicians were general practitioners: one general practitioner for every 600 people.	General practice was the predominant model of medical care.
1910	Publication of the *Flexner Report* by the Carnegie Foundation, with cooperation of the American Medical Association (AMA)	Prompted changes in methods and quality of medical education: premedical education, biomedical research, and postgraduate training.
1940	Generalists comprised 76% of private medical practitioners:	Decline of generalism paralleled the rise of specialty practice.
	1950—62% of practitioners were generalists 1960—45% of practitioners were generalists 1970—21% of practitioners were generalists	
	AMA petitioned to approve a general practice specialty board.	Request refused.
1941	General Practice Certifying Board proposed in American Medical Association (AMA) House of Delegates.	First call for a certifying board for generalists.
1946	Section on General Practice of the AMA organized.	An early organization of generalists with nationwide representation.
1947	American Academy of General Practice (AAGP) founded by a small group (no more than 150) of family physicians meeting in Atlantic City, New Jersey.	First major medical organization to require continuing medical education as a condition of membership.
1950	First residency training programs in general practice established.	Signified need for post-graduate generalist training beyond the internship year.
	Publication of journal *GP*.	First scientific journal for generalists.
1958	Family Health Foundation of America incorporated.	Early funding for conferences on family medicine education.

Year	Event	Significance
1960	American Board of General Practice formed.	First effort to obtain general practice board status.
1964	19% of U.S. medical graduates entered general practice.	Continued decline in numbers of general practitioners.
	American Board of Family Practice Advisory Group formed.	Developed objectives for the American Board of Family Practice (see 1969).
1965	National Family Health Conference sponsored by Family Health Foundation of America.	Studied unmet needs of American family for comprehensive health care, what practitioner can meet this need, and how he or she can best be trained.
1966	Report of Citizens' Commission on Graduate Medical Education: *The Graduate Education of Physicians* (Millis Commission Report).	Identified fragmentation in health care and proposed concept of a "primary physician."
	Report of the Ad Hoc Committee on Education for Family Practice of the Council on Medical Education: *Meeting the Challenge of Family Practice* (Willard Commission Report).	Recommended training of a "family physician."
1967	Formation of Society of Teachers of Family Medicine (STFM).	First organization of family medicine educators.
1969	STFM published *Family Medicine Times* (*FMT*).	First publication (newsletter) for family medicine educators.
	American Board of Family Practice (ABFP) founded.	Organized as official certifying board for the new specialty.
	Recognition of family practice as a specialty February 6, 1969, based upon approval of the Liaison Committee for Specialty Boards.	The 20th American medical specialty.
	Fifteen approved family practice residencies in the U.S.	Model graduate training programs established.
1970	First examination by ABFP.	Successful candidates sitting for 1970 and 1971 examinations became charter diplomates.
1971	American Academy of General Practice changed its name to American Academy of Family Physicians (AAFP).	The Academy recognized shift in emphasis to family practice.
1972	AAFP fellowships first awarded.	Recognized "interest and participation in special educational programs designed to enhance professional competence and the quality of health care provided to the people of America."
	First meeting of North American Primary Care Research Group (NAPCRG).	Forum for presentation of family practice research results.
	WONCA (World Organization of Family Doctors) formed.	Worldwide organization begins with 18 members.
1973	Publication of *Family Practice* (Conn, Rakel, Johnson, editors).	First major family practice textbook.
	First National Conference of Family Practice Residents and Student Members.	First national meeting of family practice trainees.
1974	*Journal of Family Practice* began publication.	First family practice peer-reviewed journal.

Year	Event	Significance
	Medical students and residents gain seats in AAFP Congress of Delegates.	First major specialty to reorganize medical student and resident delegates.
1975	Residency Assistance Program (RAP) initiated.	Family medicine educators develop guidelines and offer consultation to family practice residency training programs.
	STFM Foundation formed.	The charitable arm of STFM.
1976	First recertification examination by ABFP.	First recertification examination by any medical specialty.
	Publication of the Virginia Study in the Journal of Family Practice.	First major report of doctor-patient contacts in family practice.
1977	Doctors Ought to Care (DOC) founded.	Championed positive health strategies for the clinic, classroom, and community.
1978	Publication of *Family Medicine: Principles and Practice*, 1st edition (Taylor, editor; Buckingham, Donatelle, Jacott, Rosen, associate editors).	Second major family practice textbook.
	Practice eligible route to ABFP certification expired.	Candidates for the ABFP certification examination subsequently must have satisfactorily completed a 3-year approved family practice residency.
	Association of Departments of Family Medicine established.	First organization of family medicine academic units.
1979	End of first decade as a specialty: Residency training programs: 364 FP residents in training: 6531 Members of AAFP: 43,956 Diplomates of ABFP: 22,246	Continuing growth of the specialty.
	Family Medicine Teacher established.	Official journal of STFM.
1980	26% of active allopathic practitioners were generalists.	Beginning upward trend in number of generalists.
	Graduate Medical Education National Advisory Committee (GMENAC) report published.	"Near balance" of general practitioners/family physicians vs. need was predicted for 1990; no change recommended for family practice residencies.
1981	*Family Medicine Teacher* became *Family Medicine*.	Society's publication becomes an academic journal.
	Family Practice Research Journal began publication.	Third academic journal in family practice.
1982	Report of the Study Group on Family Medicine Research: *Meeting the Challenge of Research in Family Medicine*.	Documented past achievements and current status; indicated future directions in family medicine research.
1983	Publication of *Family Medicine: Principles and Practice*, 2nd edition (Taylor, editor; Buckingham, Donatelle, Jacott, Rosen, associate editors).	Principles and practice of discipline integrated as "Family Medicine Content"

Year	Event	Significance
1984	Conjoint meeting of STFM and NAPCRG.	First joint assembly of family medicine educators and researchers.
	Keystone I Conference held at Keystone, Colorado.	A time for FP leaders to meditate and reflect.
1985	Liaison Committee on Medical Education (LCME) report *Functions and Structure of a Medical School* called for predoctoral training "necessary to enter graduate medical education programs in family medicine . . . "	Official recognition of need for medical schools to present family medicine knowledge, skills, attitudes, and behaviors.
	FM student interest groups established at U.S. medical schools.	Emphasis on recruitment of medical students to careers in family practice.
1986	Family Practice redefined by AAFP and ABFP.	New definition affirms independence from other specialties.
	More than 20,000 physicians were graduates of 3-year family practice residencies.	Record number of residency trained family physicians.
	"Michigan lawsuit" won in United States Supreme Court after 10-year battle.	Successful challenge of a Medicare statute that discriminated against family physicians on basis of different fees for the same procedure.
1987	First Leadership Skills Development Conference held by the AAFP.	Emphasis on enhancing the skills of family physician leaders.
1988	*Journal of the American Board of Family Practice* began publication.	Fourth U.S. academic journal in the specialty.
	More than half of all AAFP members were certified by ABFP (26,500 ABFP diplomates).	Predominant practitioner had become board-certified family physician.
	Keystone II Conference held in Keystone, Colorado.	FP leaders meet to reflect and inspire.
	First examination for Certificate of Added Qualifications (CAQ) in Geriatric Medicine.	Joint venture of American Board of Family Practice and American Board of Internal Medicine.
	Publication of *Family Medicine: Principles and Practice*, 3rd edition. (Taylor, editor; Buckingham, Donatelle, Johnson, Scherger, associate editors).	Core problems and procedures in family medicine identified.
1989	Anniversary of 20 years as a specialty: 384 residency training programs 7,392 FP residents in training.	Family medicine entered third decade as residency trained physicians began to assume leadership roles.
	New active members of AAFP required to be residency trained family physicians.	Affirmed the distinction between family physicians vs general practitioners and others.
	Association of Family Practice Residency Directors (AFPRD) formed.	First organization of directors of family practice residency programs.
1990	President George Bush signed into law Medicare Physician Payment Reform based on Resource Based Relative Value Scale (RBRVS).	Projected Medicare payment to be based on resource costs integral to providing a service.
	AMA adopted policy that every U.S. medical school should have a family practice department.	Recognition of need for medical student exposure to family medicine content and family physician role models.
	33% of active allopathic physicians were generalists.	Increasing trend toward generalist practice.

Year	Event	Significance
1991	AMA resolved "to develop recommendations for adequate reimbursement of primary care physicians, improved recruitment of medical school graduates, and training a sufficient number of primary care physicians to meet projected national needs."	Evidence of AMA support of family practice and primary care.
1992	Medicare physician payment reform began.	Beginning phase-in Medicare fee schedule, eliminating specialty differentials.
	Council on Graduate Medical Education (COGME) recommended that half of all medical school graduates enter primary care careers.	Recognition that medical schools must meet health care needs of the nation.
	Archives of Family Practice began publication.	American Medical Association affirmed value of family medicine research through support of a new specialty journal.
1993	First examination for CAQ in Sports Medicine for primary care physicians.	Joint venture of the American Boards of Family Practice, Emergency Medicine, Internal Medicine, and Pediatrics.
	Liaison Committee on Medical Education document *Functions and Structure of a Medical School* changed to read: "Clinical education programs involving patients should include disciplines such as family medicine, internal medicine, obstetrics and gynecology, pediatrics, psychiatry, and surgery."	Family medicine achieved parity with other specialties in requirements for the medical school curriculum.
	Number of family practice residencies exceeded 400.	New residencies included inner city, rural, and health maintenance organization.
1994	Publication of *Family Medicine: Principles and Practice*, 4th edition (Taylor, editor; David, Johnson, Phillips, Scherger, associate editors).	Emphasis on core problems in clinical family medicine.
	End of practice pathway to CAQ in Geriatric Medicine.	Candidates must complete formal accredited geriatric fellowship program.
1995	American Boards of Family Practice and Internal Medicine called for educational resource sharing and collaborative training.	Indicated trend for family physicians to teach our knowledge and skills to other specialists.
1996	Publication of *Fundamentals of Family Medicine* (Taylor, editor; David, Johnson, Phillips, Scherger, associate editors).	First predoctoral clerkship textbook based on health problems of a single extended family.
	Alaska's first graduate medical education program was a family practice residency.	Family practice became the first specialty to have residency programs established in all 50 states.
1997	Fiftieth anniversary of the AAGP/AAFP.	Fifty years since 1947 founding of AAGP in Kansas City, Missouri.
	Revised Program Requirements for Residency Education in Family Practice.	Changes reflect the evolution of the discipline by no longer defining training elements as derivatives of other specialties and emphasizing the use of family physicians as teachers.
	Graduates of U.S. family practice residency programs top 50,000.	AAFP annual survey confirms that 50,002 physicians have graduated from FP residencies since the 1960s.

Year	Event	Significance
1998	Publication of *Family Medicine: Principles and Practice*, 5th edition (Taylor, editor; David, Johnson, Phillips, Scherger, associate editors).	Expanded emphasis on clinical problems in generalist health care.
	AAFP Research Initiative begun.	AAFP commits $7.7 million to support family practice research.
	Center for Policy Studies in Family Practice and Primary Care begun in Washington, D.C.	AAFP initiative intended to bring a family practice and primary care perspective to national health policy deliberations.
1999	Anniversary of 30 years as a specialty: Residency training programs: 474 FP residents in training: 10,632 Graduates of FP residency programs: 56,859.	Family medicine continues to prosper as it enters the new millennium.
	AAFP begins national practice-based network for primary care research.	The network's mission will be "conduct, support, promote and advocate primary care research in practice-based settings that (1) addresses questions of importance to the discipline of family medicine and (2) improves the health care delivery to and health status of patients, their families and communities."
	Practice pathway to CAQ in Sports Medicine ends.	One-year sports medicine fellowship required for eligibility.
2000	112 Departments of family medicine in U.S. medical schools. 476 U.S. family practice residency programs. 61,000 Board-certified family physicians.	Continued success of family practice at the beginning of the new millennium.
	Keystone III Conference held in Colorado Springs, Colorado.	A forum for family physicians to share ideas and strengthen the specialty.
2001	Certificate of Added Qualifications in Adolescent Medicine begun.	Collaborative effort of ABFP, the American Board of Pediatrics and the American Board of Internal Medicine.
2002	Thirtieth anniversary of the founding of WONCA, which comprises 58 member organizations in 53 countries.	World organization of family doctors has total membership exceeding 150,000 general practitioners/family physicians.
2003	*Annals of Family Medicine* began publication.	New research journal co-sponsored by the AAFP, ABFP, AFPRD, NAPCRG, ADFM, and STFM.
	Publication of *Family Medicine: Principles and Practice*, 6th edition (Taylor, editor; David, Fields, Phillips, Scherger, associate editors).	Emphasis on evidence-based health care and patient/community centered practice in the new millennium.
2004	AAFP-WONCA combined meeting in Orlando, Florida, USA.	Largest meeting in the history of family and general physicians worldwide.

Index

ISBN 0-387-95400-7

ICD-9 Codes for Family Practice 2001-2002: The *FPM* Short List

FAMILY PRACTICE
MANAGEMENT®

I. Infectious and Parasitic Diseases

052.9	Chickenpox, NOS
111.9	Dermatomycosis, unspec.
009.1	Gastroenteritis, infectious
007.1	Giardiasis
098.0	Gonorrhea, acute, lower genitourinary tract
054.9	Herpes simplex, any site
053.9	Herpes zoster, NOS
042	HIV disease
V08	HIV positive, asymptomatic
075	Infectious mononucleosis
136.9	Infectious/parasitic diseases, unspec.
487.1	Influenza w/ upper respiratory symptoms
007.9	Intestinal protozoa, NOS
132.0	Lice, head
088.81	Lyme disease
055.9	Measles, NOS
112.0	Moniliasis, oral
112.3	Moniliasis, skin/nails
112.1	Moniliasis, vulva/vagina
072.9	Mumps, NOS
132.9	Pediculosis, unspec.
127.4	Pinworms
138	Polio, late effects
795.5	Positive PPD
082.0	Rocky mountain spotted fever
056.9	Rubella, NOS
003.0	Salmonella gastroenteritis
135	Sarcoidosis
133.0	Scabies
038.9	Septicemia, NOS
005.0	Staphylococcal food poisoning
034.0	Strep throat
097.9	Syphilis, unspec.
111.0	Tinea versicolor
131.9	Trichomoniasis, unspec.
011.90	Tuberculosis, pulmonary, NOS
099.9	Venereal disease, unspec.
077.99	Viral conjunctivitis
057.9	Viral exanthems, other, NOS
070.9	Viral hepatitis, NOS
079.99	Viral infection, unspec.
078.10	Warts, all sites
078.11	Warts, condyloma

II. Neoplasms
Malignant Neoplasms

188.9	Bladder, unspec.
174.9	Breast, female, unspec.
153.9	Colon, unspec.
184.9	Female genital, unspec., CIS excluded
159.0	Gastrointestinal tract, unspec.
201.90	Hodgkin's, NOS
208.90	Leukemia, w/o remission, NOS
162.9	Lung, unspec.
187.9	Male genital, unspec.
185	Prostate
165.9	Respiratory tract, NOS
173.9	Skin, unspec.
199.1	Unspec.
189.9	Urinary, unspec.

Benign Neoplasms

211.3	Colon
214.9	Lipoma, any site
239.9	Neoplasm, unspec.
216.9	Skin, unspec.
239.2	Skin, soft tissue neoplasm, unspec.
229.9	Unspec.
218.9	Uterus (leiomyoma, unspec.)

III. Endocrine, Nutritional & Metabolic Disorders

266.2	B12 deficiency w/o anemia
276.5	Dehydration
250.91	Diabetes mellitus, I, complications
250.01	Diabetes mellitus, I, uncomplicated
250.90	Diabetes mellitus, II, complications
250.00	Diabetes mellitus, II, uncomplicated
250.13	Diabetic ketoacidosis
271.9	Glucose intolerance
240.9	Goiter, unspec.
274.9	Gout, unspec.
275.42	Hypercalcemia
272.0	Hypercholesterolemia, pure
276.7	Hyperkalemia
272.4	Hyperlipidemia, NOS
276.0	Hypernatremia
252.0	Hyperparathyroidism
242.90	Hyperthyroidism, NOS
272.1	Hypertriglyceridemia, pure
275.41	Hypocalcemia
250.80	Hypoglycemia, diabetic, unspec.
251.2	Hypoglycemia, nondiabetic, unspec.
276.8	Hypokalemia
276.1	Hyponatremia
244.9	Hypothyroidism, unspec.
269.9	Nutritional deficiencies, unspec.
278.00	Obesity, NOS
790.6	Other abnormal blood chemistry
241.0	Thyroid nodule

IV. Blood Diseases

288.9	Abnormal white blood cells, unspec.
285.1	Anemia, acute blood loss
285.29	Anemia, chronic illness
280.9	Anemia, iron deficiency, unspec.
285.9	Anemia, other, unspec.
281.0	Anemia, pernicious
289.9	Blood disease, unspec.
287.9	Hemorrhagic conditions, unspec.
289.1	Lymphadenitis, chronic
238.4	Polycythemia vera
282.60	Sickle-cell anemia, unspec.
282.5	Sickle-cell trait

V. Mental Disorders

309.9	Adjustment reaction, unspec.
305.00	Alcohol abuse, unspec.
303.90	Alcoholism, unspec.
331.0	Alzheimer's
307.1	Anorexia nervosa
300.00	Anxiety state, unspec.
314.01	Attention deficit, w/ hyperactivity
314.00	Attention deficit, w/o hyperactivity
307.51	Bulimia
312.9	Conduct disorder, unspec.
311	Depressive disorder, NOS
290.0	Dementia, senile, uncomplicated
290.40	Dementia, multi-infarct, uncomplicated
305.90	Drug abuse, unspec.
307.40	Insomnia/nonorganic sleep disorder, unspec.
315.9	Learning disability/developmental delay, NOS
319	Mental retardation, unspec.
300.9	Neurosis, NOS
300.01	Panic disorder
301.9	Personality disorder, unspec.
298.9	Psychosis, unspec.
295.90	Schizophrenia, unspec.
302.70	Sexual dysfunction, unspec.
308.3	Situational disturbance, acute
780.53	Sleep apnea w/ hypersomnia
307.81	Tension headache
305.1	Tobacco abuse

VI. Nervous System & Sense Organ Disorders
Nervous System Diseases

351.0	Bell's palsy
354.0	Carpal tunnel
438.9	CVA, late effect, unspec.
345.90	Epilepsy, unspec., not intractable
310.1	Memory/cognitive change
322.9	Meningitis, unspec.
346.90	Migraine, unspec., w/o intractable migraine
333.90	Movement disorder, unspec.
340	Multiple sclerosis
359.9	Myopathy, unspec.
349.9	Nervous system, NOS
357.9	Neuropathy, unspec.
332.0	Parkinsonism, primary
333.99	Restless legs
333.1	Tremor, essential/familial
781.0	Tremor/spasms, NOS
350.1	Trigeminal neuralgia

Eye Diseases

373.00	Blepharitis, unspec.
366.9	Cataract, unspec.
373.2	Chalazion
372.30	Conjunctivitis, unspec.
918.1	Corneal abrasion
370.00	Corneal ulcer, unspec.
379.90	Eye disorder, unspec.
930.9	Eye foreign body, external, unspec.
378.9	Eye movement disorder, unspec.
365.9	Glaucoma, unspec.
373.11	Hordeolum (stye)
367.9	Refractive errors, unspec.
362.9	Retinal disorder, unspec.
368.10	Visual disturbance, unspec.
369.9	Visual loss, unspec.

Ear Diseases

388.9	Ear disorder, unspec.
381.50	Eustachian salpingitis, unspec.
389.9	Hearing loss, unspec.
380.10	Otitis externa, unspec.
382.00	Otitis media, acute
382.01	Otitis media, acute w/ rupture of ear drum
381.10	Otitis media, chronic serous
386.2	Vertigo, central
386.10	Vertigo, peripheral, unspec.
380.4	Wax in ear

VII. Circulatory System

794.31	Abnormal electrocardiogram
410.10	Acute myocardial infarction, anterior, NOS (to 8 weeks)
410.40	Acute myocardial infarction, inferior, NOS (to 8 weeks)
410.70	Acute myocardial infarction, subendocardial (to 8 weeks)
410.60	Acute myocardial infarction, true posterior (to 8 weeks)
410.90	Acute myocardial infarction, unspec. (to 8 weeks)
428.1	Acute pulmonary edema
413.9	Angina pectoris, NOS
411.1	Angina, unstable
441.9	Aortic aneurysm, unspec.
447.9	Arterial disorder, other, unspec.
440.9	Atherosclerosis, NOS (excludes heart/brain)
427.31	Atrial fibrillation
861.01	Cardiac contusion
434.91	Cerebral artery occlusion, w/ infarction, unspec.
414.9	Chronic ischemic heart disease, unspec.
459.9	Circulatory disorder, unspec.
426.9	Conduction disorder, unspec.
428.0	Congestive heart failure
424.1	Disease of heart valve, aortic, not rheumatic
424.0	Disease of heart valve, mitral, not rheumatic
424.3	Disease of heart valve, pulmonary, not rheumatic
424.2	Disease of heart valve, tricuspid, not rheumatic
796.2	Elevated BP w/o hypertension
429.9	Heart disease, other, unspec.
401.1	Hypertension, benign
401.0	Hypertension, malignant
403.91	Hypertension, renal disease, unspec., w/ renal failure
402.91	Hypertensive cardiac w/ congestive heart failure
432.9	Intracranial hemorrhage, NOS
412	Myocardial infarction, old
458.0	Orthostatic hypotension
427.0	Paroxysmal supraventricular tachycardia
420.91	Pericarditis, acute, nonspecific
443.9	Peripheral vascular disease, unspec.
427.60	Premature beats, unspec.
415.19	Pulmonary embolism, not iatrogenic
416.9	Pulmonary heart disease, chronic, unspec.
398.90	Rheumatic heart disease, unspec.
427.81	Sick sinus syndrome
451.9	Thrombophlebitis, unspec.
435.9	Transient ischemic attack, unspec.
454.9	Varicose veins w/o ulcer/inflammation
459.81	Venous insufficiency, unspec.

VIII. Respiratory System

478.1	Abscess/ulcer of nose
493.90	Asthma, unspec.
493.02	Asthma, extrinsic, acute exacerbation
493.12	Asthma, intrinsic, acute exacerbation
466.11	Bronchiolitis, acute, due to RSV
466.0	Bronchitis, acute
491.9	Bronchitis, chronic, unspec.
496	Chronic obstructive pulmonary disease, NOS
464.4	Croup
492.8	Emphysema
464.00	Laryngitis, acute, no obstruction
475	Peritonsillar abscess
462	Pharyngitis, acute
511.9	Pleural effusion, NOS
511.0	Pleurisy, NOS
486	Pneumonia, unspec.
512.8	Pneumothorax, spontaneous
519.9	Respiratory disease, other, NOS
477.9	Rhinitis, allergic, cause unspec.
472.0	Rhinitis, chronic
461.1	Sinusitis, acute, frontal
461.0	Sinusitis, acute, maxillary
461.9	Sinusitis, acute, NOS
473.1	Sinusitis, chronic, frontal
473.0	Sinusitis, chronic, maxillary
473.9	Sinusitis, chronic, NOS
474.9	Tonsil/adenoid disease, chronic, unspec.
463	Tonsillitis, acute
465.9	Upper respiratory infection, acute, NOS

IX. Digestive System

565.0	Anal fissure, nontraumatic
540.9	Appendicitis, unspec.
575.0	Cholecystitis, acute
574.20	Cholelithiasis, NOS
571.9	Chronic liver disease, unspec.
571.5	Cirrhosis, NOS
564.00	Constipation, unspec.
555.9	Crohn's disease, NOS
521.00	Dental caries, unspec.
522.5	Dental abscess
525.9	Dental, unspec.
562.11	Diverticulitis of colon, NOS
562.10	Diverticulosis of colon
536.8	Dyspepsia
530.9	Esophageal disease, unspec.
530.10	Esophagitis, unspec.
564.9	Functional disorder intestine, unspec.
575.9	Gallbladder disease, unspec.
535.50	Gastritis, unspec., w/o hemorrhage
558.9	Gastroenteritis, noninfectious, unspec.
530.81	Gastroesophageal reflux, no esophagitis
455.6	Hemorrhoids, NOS
553.3	Hernia, hiatal, noncongenital
550.90	Hernia, inguinal, NOS
553.9	Hernias, other, NOS
560.1	Ileus
560.9	Intestinal obstruction, unspec.
564.1	Irritable bowel syndrome
528.9	Oral, soft tissue diseases, unspec.
529.9	Oral, tongue diseases, unspec.
577.0	Pancreatitis, acute
533.90	Peptic ulcer disease, unspec., w/o obstruction
569.1	Rectal prolapse
524.60	Temporomandibular joint disorder, unspec.
556.9	Ulcerative colitis, unspec.

X. Genitourinary System
Urinary System Diseases

595.0	Cystitis, acute
595.1	Cystitis, interstitial, chronic
580.9	Glomerulonephritis, acute, unspec.
582.9	Glomerulonephritis, chronic, unspec.
791.0	Proteinuria, nonpostural, nonobstetric
590.10	Pyelonephritis, acute, no necrosis
593.9	Renal disease, NOS
584.9	Renal failure, acute, unspec.
585	Renal failure, chronic
597.81	Urethral syndrome, nonvenereal disease, NOS
592.9	Urinary calculus, unspec.
599.6	Urinary obstruction, unspec.

Male Genital Organ Diseases

607.1	Balanitis
603.9	Hydrocele, unspec.
302.72	Impotence, psychosexual dysfunction
607.84	Impotence, organic
608.82	Hematospermia
608.9	Male genital disease, other, unspec.
604.90	Orchitis/epididymitis, unspec.
605	Phimosis
600.0	Prostatic hypertrophy, benign
601.9	Prostatitis, NOS
099.40	Urethritis, nongonococcal, unspec.
456.4	Varicocele

Source: Daugird A, Spencer D, Whitecar PS. ICD-9 Codes for Family Practice, The FPM Short List. Family Practice Management 2001: 8(9); 20-22. Used with permission.